A REFERENCE GUIDE TO FETAL AND NEONATAL RISK

Briggs

Drugs in **Pregnancy** and **Lactation** Thirteenth Edition

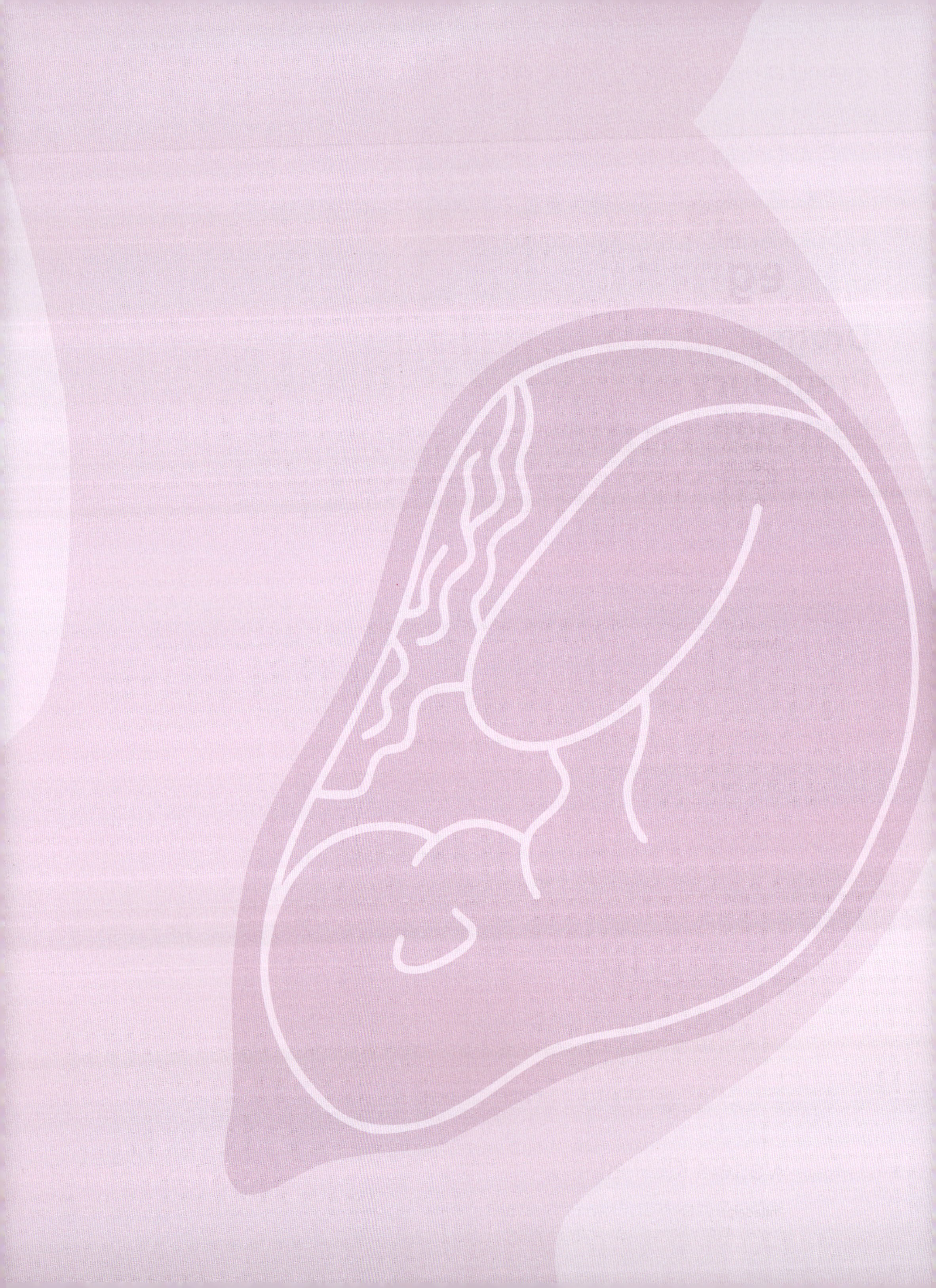

A REFERENCE GUIDE TO FETAL AND NEONATAL RISK

Briggs Drugs in Pregnancy and Lactation

Thirteenth Edition

Craig V. Towers, MD, FACOG
Retired Fellow of the American College of Obstetrics and Gynecology
Emeritus of the Society for Maternal-Fetal
Medicine Specialists
Retired Professor of Obstetrics and Gynecology
Knoxville, Tennessee

Alicia B. Forinash, PharmD, FCCP, BCPS, BCACP
Professor of Pharmacy Practice
St. Louis College of Pharmacy at the University of Health Sciences and Pharmacy
Clinical Pharmacy Specialist
Maternal Fetal Care Center and WISH Center at SSM Health St. Mary's
St. Louis, Missouri

Carrie A. Brusseau, PharmD
Assistant Professor, College of Pharmacy
The University of Tennessee Health Science Center
Pharmacist Specialist, Women and Infants
University of Tennessee Medical Center
Knoxville, Tennessee

Wolters Kluwer

Philadelphia • Baltimore • New York • London
Buenos Aires • Hong Kong • Sydney • Tokyo

Acquisitions Editor: Nicole Dernoski, Tulie McKay
Development Editor: Cindy Yoo
Editorial Coordinator: Yamini Balabaskar
Senior Production Project Manager: Alicia Jackson
Manager, Graphic Arts & Design: Stephen Druding
Manufacturing Coordinator: Lisa Bowling
Prepress Vendor: S4Carlisle Publishing Services

Thirteenth edition

9 8 7 6 5 4 3 2 1

Printed in Mexico

Library of Congress Cataloging-in-Publication Data

ISBN-13: 978-1-975207-03-8

Cataloging in Publication data available on request from publisher.

shop.lww.com

QUADM0526

Dedication

It is with a heavy heart that we inform the readers and patrons of Briggs Drugs in Pregnancy and Lactation *that we lost Gerald "Jerry" G. Briggs to cancer in the late summer of 2023 during the early planning stages of the 13th edition. He was a giant in the field of Maternal-Child Health, and we, especially I, will truly miss him.*

Thank you, Jerry, for all the years of tireless work in improving the outcomes
for millions of pregnant women and their newborns worldwide!

Craig V. Towers, MD

Foreword

We lost Jerry as we were in the planning stages of this edition. I am grateful for having the opportunity to work with him for 10 years on this book and other professional endeavors. He will be missed and will be remembered as a legacy for perinatal pharmacists. Thank you, Jerry, for everything you have done to help improve maternal-infant care.

I am excited to contribute to the 13th edition of this book. We have updated every drug and added several new medications to this edition. Several of the drug monographs include contact information for enrolling patients into studies or registries. Please encourage your pregnant and lactating patients to enroll in these studies/registries, as this will continue aiding our understanding of the safety and/or efficacy of these medications. I would like to thank my husband, Brian, and my children, Riley and Cole, for all their support while I have been working on this edition. Also, I would like to thank all the exceptional health care professionals and staff that I collaborate with every day at the Maternal Fetal Care Center and Women and Infant Substance Help (WISH) Center at SSM Health St. Mary's, as well as my colleagues at the St. Louis College of Pharmacy. Finally, thank you to all the wonderful pharmacy and premed students who assisted with research, and I look forward to seeing the amazing things you accomplish in your careers. Finally, thank you to my wonderful coauthors, Craig and Carrie, for all of the hard work and collaboration to complete this edition.

Alicia B. Forinash, PharmD, FCCP, BCPS, BCACP
Professor of Pharmacy Practice
St. Louis College of Pharmacy
Clinical Pharmacy Specialist
Maternal Fetal Care Center and WISH Center at SSM Health St. Mary's
St. Louis, Missouri

It is with immense gratitude that I write this foreword for the 13th edition of *Briggs Drugs in Pregnancy and Lactation*. As a new author contributing to this long-standing and respected reference, it is an honor and privilege to continue the important work of Gerald G. Briggs, whose decades-long commitment to supporting safe medication use in pregnancy and lactation has served as the foundation for this edition.

I have also been incredibly fortunate to collaborate with Dr Towers and Dr Forinash, whose depth of knowledge, dedication to scientific accuracy, and remarkable patience have been both a guide and an inspiration throughout this process. I am sincerely thankful for their mentorship and support.

Together, we have performed an extensive and updated review of the current literature, with the goal of ensuring that this new edition remains a trusted and up-to-date resource. We have worked diligently to provide a comprehensive summary of the available evidence for each drug included, offering valuable, clinically relevant information to assist health care professionals in making informed decisions when caring for patients during pregnancy and lactation.

To all who have contributed, directly or indirectly, thank you. This book stands as a collective effort—grounded in science, enriched by experience, and driven by our shared commitment to maternal and infant health.

Carrie A. Brusseau, PharmD
Assistant Professor, College of Pharmacy
The University of Tennessee Health Science Center
Pharmacist Specialist, Women and Infants
University of Tennessee Medical Center
Knoxville, Tennessee

Preface

I was blessed to receive my maternal-fetal medicine training at one of the field's pioneering programs—Long Beach Memorial Women's Hospital in Long Beach, California, and the University of California, Irvine. I was also fortunate to be mentored by several leaders in the field, including Roger K. Freeman, MD (a former author of this reference guide), Thomas J. Garite, MD, Michael P. Nageotte, MD, and Gerald G. "Jerry" Briggs. Jerry was the one who first inspired me to study the effects of drugs used during pregnancy, which led to numerous peer-reviewed publications on this topic. The first edition of this book was published in the middle of my residency, and it became the first comprehensive reference guide on drugs used during pregnancy and/or lactation. I was honored when he asked me to join the authorship team in late 2013 for the 10th edition, which was published in 2015.

This 13th edition represents more than 10,000 hours of work over a 2-year 6-month period. After removing drugs from the 12th edition that have been withdrawn from the US market or are not prescribed, we added 362 new drugs, bringing the total for the 13th edition to 1,606. In this new edition, readers will see that every drug is presented. Another important update involves how contraindications are addressed. While numerous drugs are labeled "contraindicated" by manufacturers, this designation is not always absolute in clinical practice. For example, certain antineoplastic agents may be used under specific circumstances despite such labeling. The potential risks and benefits of such agents should be discussed with the pregnant mother so that an informed decision can be made.

To me, it is beyond amazing what pregnant women can endure and how many of these women are often ready to do it all over again, soon after giving birth. As I have stated in numerous lectures over my 37-year career as a maternal-fetal medicine specialist, "if the role of childbirth was relegated to men, the human race would have gone extinct eons ago!" As detailed in other editions, there will always be drugs, and there will always be pregnant and lactating women. It is our hope that all prescribed medications will improve outcomes for both the mother and newborn—in short, "produce more good than harm."

This subject matter is complicated by the lack of drug studies during pregnancy and lactation for fear of harming the mother, fetus, or newborn. It is not ethically possible to create a new drug, pair it with a placebo, and blindly randomize patients during the early stages of gestation or while breastfeeding (essentially a randomized placebo-controlled trial), to determine whether the drug increases the risk of fetal anomalies or neonatal complications. Thus, most available data on pregnant or lactating women comes from case reports or series or studies that analyze the use of drugs in patients with a specific medical condition, often making the control group different in many clinical scenarios.

The expected "normal" major birth defect rate in the United States ranges from about 2% to 4%. However, some disease states (poorly controlled diabetes or autoimmune disorders, etc) have increased rates for anomalies or newborn complications, which need to be considered. Numerous studies have compared outcomes between pregnant or lactating women who used a particular drug with those who did not. In some instances, a significantly higher rate of fetal anomalies or neonatal complications was found in the drug-exposed group. However, when looking closer, the anomaly rate in the nonexposed group may be 1%, while the rate in the exposed group is 3%. Although this difference may reach significance, it does not necessarily indicate that the drug is a true teratogen. For a drug to be strongly suspected as being teratogenic in the overall pregnancy population, the anomaly rate should exceed 4%. Furthermore, a consistent pattern of defects should emerge. Many control groups are assembled differently, and birth anomaly surveillance postdelivery in these control groups may not be as thorough or systematic as the drug-exposed population. This can potentially lead to biased comparisons.

Additionally, for a drug to have the potential for being a teratogen, it must be present in the maternal circulation at the time when a specific organ system is forming. For example, if a medication is first taken at 10 weeks' gestation and the newborn is found to have a major cardiac defect postdelivery, the drug was not the cause because fetal heart formation was complete prior to drug exposure. When evaluating potential risks, the primary concern for the neonate is major malformations that can affect life and quality of life. Minor defects, in some cases, may be variations of anatomy with little or no clinical significance. True teratogens will usually produce much higher rates of specific types of birth abnormalities, such as severe limb anomalies with thalidomide or central nervous system defects with isotretinoin.

Briggs Drugs in Pregnancy and Lactation remains the only reference guide that includes information on the use of medications during both pregnancy and breastfeeding. It has been an honor to work alongside Dr Alicia Forinash, who (like me) has been with the book since the 10th edition. We were pleased to add the experience and knowledge of Dr Carrie Brusseau from the Pharmacy Department at the University of Tennessee Medical Center, Knoxville. Both Alicia and Carrie have specialized expertise in maternal-infant pharmacy. I can honestly say that this edition would not have occurred without their tremendous wisdom, proficiency, and relentless work. I sincerely thank both of you. I would also like to personally thank Kelsey Grabeel, Laura Wolfe, Riley Forinash, and Nathan Brusseau.

Without their support with literature searches, obtaining needed articles, collecting information from prior editions and other sources, and photocopying, this book would also be incomplete. Lastly, I must genuinely thank my wife, children, and extended family for tolerating me and enduring these past two-and-a-half years. To close, we will truly miss the passion, experience, intelligence, and mentorship of Jerry. The world lost a great clinician with his passing.

Craig V. Towers, MD, FACOG
Retired Fellow of the American College of Obstetrics and Gynecology
Emeritus of the Society for Maternal-Fetal Medicine Specialists
Retired Professor of Obstetrics and Gynecology

Contents

Instructions for Use of the Reference Guide

This Reference Guide is arranged so that the user can quickly locate a monograph. The American generic name needs to be known, and the medications are listed in alphabetical order. Trade names are no longer used because they often change, and many drugs have numerous labels. If a specific drug is not listed, the user should refer to the manufacturer's product information for the specific ingredients and pregnancy/lactation information. Nowhere in this reference guide do we, the authors, "recommend" that certain drugs be administered during pregnancy and/or lactation. There are medications that improve pregnancy outcome, such as insulin in a person with diabetes who is insulin-dependent. However, ALL decisions regarding the use of a drug during pregnancy or while breastfeeding are those made by the patient in conjunction with the health care providers. The material presented in this book is also static, and in many cases, new research is published that could affect overall conclusions. The authors have done their best to provide information that was found through literature searches at the time of monograph development and present that material here.

Each monograph contains seven parts:

- **Generic Name (United States)**
- **Pharmacologic Class**
- **Pregnancy Recommendation**
- **Breastfeeding Recommendation**
- **Pregnancy Summary**
- **Breastfeeding Summary**
- **References**

PREGNANCY AND BREASTFEEDING RECOMMENDATIONS

The pregnancy and breastfeeding recommendations are not really "recommendations" in that they do not tell women or health care providers that a specific drug should be used during gestation or postdelivery. Rather, they are intended to assist the reader in determining the level of risk for a specific drug. Also, they only apply to the usual therapeutic dose of the drug in a typical patient. Because genetic makeup, medical condition, ability to metabolize a drug, and other factors may significantly alter the risk, the recommendations may not apply to the entire population. In addition to the animal reproduction data and known human pregnancy outcomes, the assessment of risk includes, when relevant, other major factors such as route of administration, metabolism to active metabolites, species differences, type of defects, pharmacokinetics, effects of other agents in the drug class, and the embryofetal effects of untreated or undertreated maternal disease. Moreover, drug exposures represent different levels of risk depending on the gestational age of the pregnancy, and thus, the timing of the exposure is critical in determining risk. Because short statements of risk may not always adequately assess the risk throughout the pregnancy, readers are encouraged to review the entire monograph before estimating the risk for a specific patient. Furthermore, not all drugs fit into the provided recommendations listed below.

PREGNANCY SUMMARY

The Pregnancy Summary is meant to support the Pregnancy Recommendation. The Pregnancy Summary provides a brief overview of available human data (if any), a sentence or two on placental transfer, a summary of animal reproduction studies, and information on use during pregnancy. We tried to add any information on statements provided by the American College of Obstetrics and Gynecology, Society for Maternal-Fetal Medicine specialists, American Academy of Pediatrics, Food and Drug Administration (FDA), Centers for Disease Control and Prevention (CDC), and other medical agencies and organizations. If a pregnancy exposure registry exists, we tried to supply this contact information because the more data we collect, the better health care we can provide. For animal data, the FDA has stated that animal drug exposure doses above 10 times the recommended human dose are not clinically meaningful. Furthermore, because animal data only relate to human pregnancy outcome about 20% of the time, we have noted whether or not embryofetal toxicity was observed in animal studies rather than the specifics since it may not correlate. Therefore, we tried to report animal reproduction data based on this parameter. Regardless, from a clinical standpoint, drug exposure at doses greater than the maximum recommended human dose is not likely to be healthy for any human pregnancy. Because few absolutes are possible in human teratology, the reader must carefully weigh the evidence, or lack thereof, before utilizing any drug in a pregnant woman. Readers who require more details than are presented should refer to the specific references listed at the end of the monograph.

BREASTFEEDING SUMMARY

The Breastfeeding Summary is meant to support the Breastfeeding Recommendation. The Breastfeeding Summary provides a brief overview of available human data (if any), a sentence or two on whether the medication is or might be found in human breast milk, and a statement on possible side effects that could be seen in an exposed breastfeeding infant. Animal studies on breastfeeding have not been found to be clinically helpful. Readers who require more details than are presented should refer to the specific references listed at the end of the monograph.

The risks for a specific drug used during breastfeeding may be different than what is listed for use during pregnancy. The recommendations for breastfeeding are based on the known toxicity of the drug or similar drugs in adults or children (when known) and the amount of drug excreted into breast milk (if known). Although most drugs taken by the mother are probably found in human breast milk, the concentrations are usually unknown. Fortunately, the amounts in many instances are usually too low to cause toxicity. However, the therapeutic dose for infants of most drugs is rarely known. Therefore, we used a proposal from the literature (Ito S. *N Engl J Med* 2000;343:118-128) to classify exposures as clinically insignificant if, in the absence of data suggesting otherwise, the estimated dose ingested by a nursing infant was no more than 10% of the mother's weight-adjusted dose. However, in some cases, this infant dosage amount may not be relevant.

DEFINITIONS OF PREGNANCY RECOMMENDATIONS

HUMAN DATA SUGGEST COMPATIBLE OR COMPATIBLE

The human pregnancy experience, either for the drug itself or drugs in the same class or with similar mechanisms of action, is adequate to demonstrate that the embryofetal risk is very low or nonexistent. Animal reproduction data are not relevant.

HUMAN DATA SUGGEST LOW RISK

There is some human pregnancy experience, either for the drug itself or drugs in the same class or with similar mechanisms of action, including the first trimester, suggesting that the drug does not represent a significant risk of developmental toxicity (structural anomalies, growth restriction, functional and/or behavioral defects, or death) at any time in pregnancy. The available human pregnancy data outweigh any animal reproduction data.

HUMAN DATA SUGGEST RISK (FIRST, SECOND, OR THIRD TRIMESTER)

Evidence (for the drug or similar drugs) suggests that there may be an embryofetal risk for developmental toxicity (structural anomalies, growth restriction, functional and/or behavioral deficits, or death) throughout pregnancy or in the noted trimester(s). The human pregnancy data outweigh any animal reproduction data. Usually, pregnancy exposure should be avoided, but the risk may be acceptable if the maternal condition requires the drug.

NO/LIMITED HUMAN DATA—ANIMAL DATA SUGGEST LOW RISK

There is no or limited human pregnancy experience, and the few pregnancy exposures have not been associated with developmental toxicity (structural anomalies, growth restriction, functional and/or behavioral deficits, or death). The drug does not cause developmental toxicity (at doses that did not cause maternal toxicity) in all animal species studied at doses less than 10 times the recommended human dose.

NO/LIMITED HUMAN DATA—ANIMAL DATA SUGGEST POTENTIAL RISK

There is no or limited human pregnancy experience, and the few pregnancy exposures have not been associated with developmental toxicity (structural anomalies, growth restriction, functional and/or behavioral deficits, or death). The drug causes developmental toxicity (at doses that did not cause maternal toxicity) in one animal species at doses less than 10 times the recommended human dose.

NO/LIMITED HUMAN DATA—ANIMAL DATA SUGGEST RISK

There is no or limited human pregnancy experience, and the few pregnancy exposures have not been associated with developmental toxicity (structural anomalies, growth restriction, functional and/or behavioral deficits, or death). The drug causes developmental toxicity (at doses that did not cause maternal toxicity) in two or more animal species at doses less than 10 times the recommended human dose.

NO HUMAN DATA AND NO RELEVANT ANIMAL DATA

There are no human pregnancy data or relevant data in animals (no animal studies performed; or the animal doses exceeded 10 times the recommended human dose; or the doses administered to animals caused maternal toxicity). The risk in pregnancy cannot be assessed.

CONTRAINDICATED (FIRST, SECOND, OR THIRD TRIMESTER)

Human exposures at any time in pregnancy or in the noted trimester(s), either to the drug itself or to drugs in the same class or with similar mechanisms of action, have been associated with developmental toxicity (structural anomalies, growth restriction, functional and/or behavioral deficits, or death). Animal reproduction data, if available, confirm the risk. The drug should not be used in pregnancy or in the specified trimester.

(MATERNAL BENEFIT MAY OUTWEIGH EMBRYOFETAL RISK)

There may or may not be human pregnancy experience with the drug, but the potential maternal benefit outweighs the known or unknown embryofetal risk.

DEFINITIONS OF BREASTFEEDING RECOMMENDATIONS

COMPATIBLE

Either the drug is not excreted in clinically significant amounts into human breast milk or its use during lactation does not, or is not expected to, cause toxicity in a nursing infant.

PROBABLY COMPATIBLE

Either there are no human data or the human data are limited. The available data suggest that the drug does not represent a significant risk to a nursing infant.

POTENTIAL TOXICITY

Either human data suggest a risk to a nursing infant or human data are limited, but characteristics of the drug suggest that it could represent a clinically significant risk to a nursing infant or mother. The drug is best avoided during breastfeeding due to its effect on the infant or potential risk to the mother, such as further loss of essential vitamins or nutrients. However, depending on the drug and the clinical circumstances, short-term use by the mother may be possible, but the infant should be closely monitored for potential adverse side effects.

CONTRAINDICATED

There may or may not be human experience, but the combined data suggest that the drug may cause severe toxicity in a nursing infant, or breastfeeding is contraindicated because of the maternal condition for which the drug is indicated. Women should not breastfeed if they are taking the drug or have the condition.

(HOLD BREASTFEEDING)

The drug may or may not be excreted into human breast milk, but the maternal benefit of therapy outweighs the benefits of breast milk to an infant. Breastfeeding can be held until maternal therapy is completed and the drug has been eliminated (or reaches a low concentration) from her system. The star symbol (*) is occasionally used under some Recommendations to clarify a point that is discussed in the Summary below. When mentioning that an infant should be monitored for potential side effects, if the side effects list nausea, headache, abdominal pain, and others, we notate these and then, in parentheses, state "leading to irritability." For the side effect of decreased appetite, we list this and, in parentheses, state "monitor infant growth," and for fatigue, we state "lethargy" in parentheses.

ABBREVIATIONS USED IN THIS REFERENCE BOOK

AAP	American Academy of Pediatrics
ACIP	Advisory Committee on Immunization Practices
ACOG	American College of Obstetrics and Gynecology
AIDS	Acquired immune deficiency syndrome
BSA	Body surface area
CDC	Centers for Disease Control and Prevention
FDA	Food and Drug Administration
FHR	Fetal heart rate
HDL	High-density lipoprotein
HIV	Human immunodeficiency virus
ICU	Intensive care unit
IM	Intramuscular
IUGR	Intrauterine growth restriction
IV	Intravenous
LDL	Low-density lipoprotein
LLQ	Lower limit of quantification
LMP	Last menstrual period
LMWH	Low-molecular-weight heparin
MRHD	Maximum recommended human dose
MRHID	Maximum recommended human inhalation dose
MRHOD	Maximum recommended human ophthalmic dose
MW	Molecular weight
NICU	Neonatal intensive care unit
NSAID	Nonsteroidal anti-inflammatory drug
PEG	Polyethylene glycol
RBC	Red blood cell
REMS	Risk evaluation and mitigation strategy
RHD	Recommended human dose
RID	Relative infant dose
SC	Subcutaneous
SMFM	Society for Maternal-Fetal Medicine
SSRI	Selective serotonin reuptake inhibitor

APPENDIX

The Appendix arranges the drugs by their pharmacologic category. This allows a reader to identify all the drugs that have been reviewed within a specific medication classification, such that comparisons can occur, if desired.

In conclusion, this reference guide is no substitute for individual patient assessment based upon health care professionals' examination of each patient and consideration of current or prior medical conditions, medication history, laboratory data, and other factors unique to the patient. This book is merely a reference tool. Health care professionals, and not the authors, are solely responsible for the use of this work, including all medical judgments and for any resulting diagnoses and treatments.

Acknowledgments

We would like to thank the following student research assistants and other individuals associated with this 13th edition:

For Alicia B. Forinash, PharmD, FCCP, BCPS, BCACP:
Caitlin Brewster, PharmD
Abigail Herman, PharmD
Sarah Schiewer, PharmD
Emilee Thurman, PharmD
Mackenzie Wagner, PharmD

For Carrie A. Brusseau, PharmD:
Olivia Bray, PharmD
Tori Hashimura, PharmD
Katie Medley, PharmD
Katherine Pleines, PharmD
Allison Smith, PharmD
Kayla Tolbert, PharmD
Jordan Whaley, PharmD

For Craig V. Towers, MD, FACOG (*Retired*):
Nathan Brusseau
Riley Forinash

Kelsey Grabeel, Professor
Preston Medical Library/Health Information Center, University of Tennessee Health Science Center College of Medicine, Knoxville/University of Tennessee Medical Center

Laura Wolfe, Senior Library Associate
Preston Medical Library/Health Information Center, University of Tennessee Health Science Center College of Medicine, Knoxville/University of Tennessee Medical Center

A

ABACAVIR

Antiretroviral (Nucleoside Reverse Transcriptase Inhibitor)

PREGNANCY RECOMMENDATION: Human Data Suggest Low Risk (Maternal Benefit May Outweigh Any Potential Embryofetal Risk)

BREASTFEEDING RECOMMENDATION: *Contraindicated

PREGNANCY SUMMARY

Data from the Antiretroviral Pregnancy Registry (APR) show that there have been more than 2,000 exposures to abacavir in human pregnancy. Of these, over 1,000 were in the first trimester with an overall congenital birth anomaly rate of about 2.7%, which falls within the expected range in the United States. Several other smaller studies have also not shown an increased rate. No pattern to the defects has been identified. The drug crosses the placenta, so some fetal exposure will occur. Animal studies did not show any embryofetal toxicity in two species at doses of less than 10 times the recommended human dose (RHD). In order to decrease the risk of perinatal transmission of HIV-1 to the neonate, this drug should not be withheld if a pregnant woman is infected with HIV-1 with a positive viral load, or is failing her current treatment regimen, and is a candidate for this drug's usage. There is a pregnancy exposure registry that monitors pregnancy outcomes in patients using antiretroviral medicines during pregnancy. Health care providers are encouraged to call the APR at 1-800-258-4263.

BREASTFEEDING SUMMARY

Two studies have been located that described the use of abacavir during human lactation. A total of 26 women have been tested, and the drug has been found in breast milk, but at low levels. Median breast milk levels ranged from about 57 to 91 ng/mL. All of the calculated relative infant doses (RIDs) were less than 1%. *However, the current Centers for Disease Control and Prevention (CDC) recommendation is that mothers infected with HIV should not breastfeed their infants in order to reduce the risk of postnatal transmission of the virus to the neonate. In a clinical setting where a mother is not infected with HIV (or in cases where the HIV viral load is negative), the drug by itself is probably compatible. If the clinical decision is to use this drug while breastfeeding, the infant should be monitored for the most common reported adult side effects of nausea and headache (both leading to irritability), fatigue (lethargy), vomiting, poor sleep, and rash.

References

1. Prescribing Information. Abacavir sulfate. Aurobindo Pharma USA, Inc; 2020.
2. Chappuy H, Treluyer JM, Jullien V, et al. Maternal-fetal transfer and amniotic fluid accumulation of nucleoside analogue reverse transcriptase inhibitors in human immunodeficiency virus-infected pregnant women. *Antimicrob Agents Chemother*. 2004;48:4332-4336.
3. Bawdon RE. The *ex vivo* human placental transfer of the anti-HIV nucleoside inhibitor abacavir and the protease inhibitor amprenavir. *Infect Dis Obstet Gynecol*. 1998;6:244-246.
4. Antiretroviral Pregnancy Registry Steering Committee. Antiretroviral Pregnancy Registry international interim report for 1 January 1989 through 31 July 2009. Registry Coordinating Center. Published 2009. Accessed May 29, 2010. http://www.apregistry.com
5. Carpenter CCJ, Fischi MA, Hammer SM, et al. Antiretroviral therapy for HIV infection in 1996. *JAMA*. 1996;276;146-154.
6. Minkoff H, Augenbraun M. Antiretroviral therapy for pregnant women. *Am J Obstet Gynecol*. 1997;176:478-489.
7. Minkoff H. Human immunodeficiency virus infection in pregnancy. *Obstet Gynecol*. 2003;101:797-810.
8. Panel on Treatment of HIV During Pregnancy and Prevention of Perinatal Transmission. Recommendations for the use of antiretroviral drugs during pregnancy and interventions to reduce perinatal HIV transmission in the United States. *Department of Health and Human Services*. Accessed July 25, 2023. https://clinicalinfo.hiv.gov/en/guidelines/perinatal.
9. Sibiude J, Mandelbrot L, Blanche S, et al. Association between prenatal exposure to antiretroviral therapy and birth defects: an analysis of the French perinatal cohort study (ANRS C01/C011). *PLoS Med*. 2014;11:e1001635.
10. Shapiro RL, Rossi S, Ogwu Moss M, et al. Therapeutic levels of lopinavir in late pregnancy and abacavir passage into breast milk in the Mma Bana Study, Botswana. *Antiviral Ther*. 2013;18:585-590.
11. Brown ZA, Watts DH. Antiviral therapy in pregnancy. *Clin Obstet Gynecol*. 1990;33:276-289.
12. De Martino M, Tovo P-A, Pezzotti P, et al. HIV-1 transmission through breast-milk: appraisal of risk according to duration of feeding. *AIDS*. 1992; 6:991-997.
13. Van de Perre P. Postnatal transmission of human immunodeficiency virus type 1: the breast feeding dilemma. *Am J Obstet Gynecol*. 1995;173:483-487.

ABALOPARATIDE

Bone Health (Osteoporosis)

PREGNANCY RECOMMENDATION: Contraindicated

BREASTFEEDING RECOMMENDATION: Contraindicated

PREGNANCY SUMMARY

No reports describing the use of abaloparatide in human pregnancy have been located. The drug will probably not cross the placenta. However, the absence of human pregnancy experience prevents a complete assessment of any embryofetal risk. Animal reproduction studies have not been performed. Nevertheless, the drug is not indicated for use in women with reproductive potential.

BREASTFEEDING SUMMARY

No reports describing the use of abaloparatide during human lactation have been located. The drug will probably not enter breast milk. In addition, because it is a peptide, if the drug were to be ingested through breastfeeding, it probably would be digested in the infant's gastrointestinal tract and not be absorbed. Nevertheless, the drug is not indicated for use in women with reproductive potential.

Reference

1. Prescribing Information. Tymlos. Radius Health, Inc; 2017.

ABAMETAPIR

Dermatologic/Anti-Infective (Topical—Pediculicide)

PREGNANCY RECOMMENDATION: No Human Data—Animal Data Suggest Low Risk

BREASTFEEDING RECOMMENDATION: Probably Compatible

PREGNANCY SUMMARY

No reports describing the use of abametapir in human pregnancy have been located. The drug will probably cross the placenta; however, based on the topical use of the drug and low plasma levels seen following systemic absorption, fetal exposure is probably negligible. Animal data did not show fetotoxic effects, even when administered orally. However, the absence of human pregnancy experience prevents a complete assessment of the embryofetal risk.

BREASTFEEDING SUMMARY

Abametapir probably enters breast milk. However, the total drug amount found in breast milk is likely to be negligible because the drug is for topical use, with low plasma levels found following systemic absorption. The topical lotion contains benzyl alcohol, which has been associated with serious and possibly fatal reactions in neonates, including "gasping syndrome" when consumed orally. Benzyl alcohol was found to be systemically absorbed following topical usage, but plasma levels were low (<4 mcg/mL). In addition, benzyl alcohol would be rapidly metabolized to benzoic acid in the maternal liver, and therefore, exposure to a breastfeeding newborn is not likely. Breastfeeding while using abametapir should be based on the mother's clinical need for treatment.

References

1. Prescribing Information. Xeglyze. Groupe Parima, Inc, for Dr. Reddy's Laboratories, S.A.; 2020.
2. Nair B. Final report on the safety assessment of benzyl alcohol, benzoic acid, and sodium benzoate. *Int J Toxicol*. 2001;20(suppl 3):23-50.

ABATACEPT

Immunologic (Fusion Protein)

PREGNANCY RECOMMENDATION: Limited Human Data—Animal Data Suggest Low Risk

BREASTFEEDING RECOMMENDATION: Potential Toxicity

PREGNANCY SUMMARY

A few studies have been located that describe the use of abatacept during human pregnancy. The largest involved patients reported to the manufacturer, which may produce a bias toward the reporting of poor outcomes. In 132 exposed pregnancies (excluding elective terminations), there were 44 (33%) spontaneous losses and 2 pregnancies lost to follow-up. Of the 86 live births, there were 6 (7%) major anomalies, and all were different (no pattern). The spontaneous loss rate is high, but many of these pregnancies were on numerous other drugs, including methotrexate. Abatacept has been shown to cross the placenta. This is consistent with the drug having the Fc fragment of an immunoglobulin G (IgG)1 antibody. Therefore, some fetal exposure will occur. However, this limited human pregnancy experience prevents a complete assessment of the embryofetal risk. Animal data did not show any embryofetal toxicity or malformations in three species at doses of less than 10 times the RHD in one species and more than 10 times the RHD in the other two. Using this drug during pregnancy should be based on the pros and cons of the mother's clinical need for treatment versus any potential fetal risk that might occur from exposure. It is contraindicated if abatacept is combined with methotrexate or leflunomide. There is a pregnancy exposure registry that monitors pregnancy outcomes in women using this drug. Health care providers are encouraged to call the Orencia Pregnancy Exposure Registry at 1-877-311-8972.

BREASTFEEDING SUMMARY

Two studies have been located that described the use of abatacept during human lactation. A total of three women using the drug had breast milk samples tested. The peak levels ranged from 100 to 256 ng/mL, and the trough levels ranged from 50 to 170 ng/mL. The calculated RIDs were all below 3%. In addition, no adverse effects on the neonates were reported. It is known that the Fc fragment of IgG antibodies facilitates transport, so some of the drug may be found in human breast milk. Regardless, if any of this fusion protein were to be ingested through breastfeeding, it would probably be digested in the infant's gastrointestinal tract and not be absorbed. Despite this, due to a concern for potential serious adverse effects that might be seen in a breastfed infant, the manufacturer recommends that women not breastfeed while being treated with this drug. However, breastfeeding while using this drug should be based on the mother's clinical need for treatment versus any potential infant risks that might occur. If used, the infant should be monitored for the most common reported adult side effects of nausea (leading to irritability) and upper respiratory tract infection.

References

1. Ostensen M, Lockshin M, Doria A, et al. Update on safety during pregnancy of biological agents and some immunosuppressive anti-rheumatic drugs. *Rheumatology*. 2008;47(suppl 3):iii28-iii31.
2. Ostensen M, Förger F. Management of RA medications in pregnant patients. *Nat Rev Rheumatol*. 2009;5:382-390.
3. Makol A, Wright K, Amin S. Rheumatoid arthritis and pregnancy—safety considerations in pharmacological management. *Drugs*. 2011;71:1973-1987.
4. Pham T, Bachelez H, Barthelot JM, et al. Abatacept therapy and safety management. *Joint Bone Spine*. 2012;72(suppl 1):3-84.
5. Furst DE, Keystone EC, So AK, et al. Updated consensus statement on biological agents in the treatment of rheumatic disease, 2012. *Ann Rheum Dis*. 2013;72(suppl 2):ii2-ii34.
6. Product Information. Orencia. E.R. Squibb & Sons; 2018.
7. Ojeda-Uribe M, Afif N, Dahan E, et al. Exposure to abatacept or rituximab in the first trimester of pregnancy of three women with autoimmune diseases. *Clin Rheumatol*. 2013;32:695-700.
8. Kumar M, Ray L, Vemuri S, Simon TA. Pregnancy outcomes following exposure to abatacept during pregnancy. *Semin Arthritis Rheum*. 2015;45:351-356.
9. Prescribing Information. Orencia. Bristol-Myers Squibb; 2018.

ABEMACICLIB

Antineoplastic (Kinase Inhibitor)

PREGNANCY RECOMMENDATION: No Human Data—Animal Data Suggest Potential Risk

BREASTFEEDING RECOMMENDATION: Potential Toxicity

PREGNANCY SUMMARY

No reports describing the use of abemaciclib in human pregnancy have been located. Some amount of the drug will probably cross the placenta, so fetal exposure will likely occur. However, the absence of human pregnancy experience prevents a complete assessment of the embryofetal risk. Animal studies showed embryofetal toxicity and teratogenicity. Based on these animal studies and the drug's mechanism of action, the manufacturer recommends that women with reproductive potential use effective contraception during treatment and for 3 weeks after the last dose. However, using this drug during pregnancy should be based on the pros and cons of the mother's clinical need for treatment versus any potential fetal risk that might occur from exposure.

BREASTFEEDING SUMMARY

No reports describing the use of abemaciclib during human lactation have been located. Some amount of the drug probably enters breast milk, so infant exposure will likely occur. However, due to the concern for potential serious adverse effects in a breastfed infant, the manufacturer recommends that women not breastfeed while being treated with abemaciclib and for at least 3 weeks after the last dose. Nevertheless, breastfeeding while using this drug should be based on the mother's clinical need for treatment. If used, the infant should be monitored for the most common reported adult side effects of nausea, headache, and abdominal pain (all leading to irritability), decreased appetite, diarrhea, vomiting, alopecia, lethargy, and infections.

Reference

1. Prescribing Information. Verzenio. Eli Lilly and Company; 2021.

ABIRATERONE ACETATE

Antineoplastic (Androgen Biosynthesis Inhibitor)

PREGNANCY RECOMMENDATION: *Contraindicated

BREASTFEEDING RECOMMENDATION: *Contraindicated

PREGNANCY SUMMARY

No reports describing the use of abiraterone acetate in human pregnancy have been located. The drug will probably cross the placenta, so some fetal exposure will likely occur. Therefore, the absence of human pregnancy experience prevents a complete assessment of the embryofetal risk. The drug was found to cause embryofetal toxicity in one animal species at doses less than 10 times the RHD. *However, based on the drug's approved indication, use during pregnancy is contraindicated. Based on animal studies and the drug's mechanism of action, the manufacturer recommends that males with female partners of reproductive potential use effective contraception during treatment and for 3 weeks after the last dose.

BREASTFEEDING SUMMARY

No reports describing the use of abiraterone acetate during human lactation have been located. The drug would probably be found in breast milk, so some infant exposure could occur. *However, because of the drug's approved indication, breastfeeding is contraindicated with this drug.

Reference

1. Prescribing Information. Abiraterone acetate. Janssen Biotech; 2020.

ABROCITINIB

Dermatologic (Janus Kinase Inhibitor)

PREGNANCY RECOMMENDATION: No Human Data—Animal Data Suggest Low Risk

BREASTFEEDING RECOMMENDATION: Potential Toxicity

PREGNANCY SUMMARY

No reports describing the use of abrocitinib in human pregnancy have been located. Some amount of the drug will probably cross the placenta, so fetal exposure will likely occur. However, the absence of human pregnancy experience prevents a complete assessment of the embryofetal risk. Animal studies did not show any embryofetal toxicity. Using this drug during pregnancy should be based on the pros and cons of the mother's clinical need for treatment versus any potential fetal risk that might occur from exposure. There is a pregnancy exposure registry that monitors pregnancy outcomes in women using this drug. Health care providers are encouraged to call 1-877-311-3770.

BREASTFEEDING SUMMARY

No reports describing the use of abrocitinib during human lactation have been located. Some of the drug probably enters breast milk, so infant exposure will likely occur. However, due to the concern for potential serious adverse effects seen in adults, the manufacturer recommends that women not breastfeed while being treated with abrocitinib and for 1 day after the last dose. Nevertheless, breastfeeding while using this drug should be based on the mother's clinical need for treatment. If used, the infant should be monitored for the most common reported adult side effects of nausea, headache, and abdominal pain (all leading to irritability), vomiting, lethargy, urinary tract infection, and various laboratory abnormalities (see Prescribing Information [PI]).

Reference

1. Prescribing Information. Cibinqo. Pfizer Labs; 2022.

ACALABRUTINIB

Antineoplastic (Bruton Tyrosine Kinase Inhibitor)

PREGNANCY RECOMMENDATION: No Human Data—Animal Data Suggest Low Risk

BREASTFEEDING RECOMMENDATION: Potential Toxicity

PREGNANCY SUMMARY

No reports describing the use of acalabrutinib in human pregnancy have been located. Some amount of the drug will probably cross the placenta, so fetal exposure will likely occur. However, the absence of human pregnancy experience prevents a complete assessment of the embryofetal risk. Animal studies did not show any embryofetal toxicity at doses that did not produce maternal toxicity. However, based on the animal studies and the drug's mechanism of action, the manufacturer recommends that women with reproductive potential use effective contraception during treatment and for 1 week after the last dose. Nevertheless, using this drug during pregnancy should be based on the pros and cons of the mother's clinical need for treatment versus any potential fetal risk that might occur from exposure.

BREASTFEEDING SUMMARY

No reports describing the use of acalabrutinib during human lactation have been located. Some amount of the drug probably enters breast milk, so infant exposure will likely occur. However, due to the concern for potential adverse effects in a breastfed infant, the manufacturer recommends that women not breastfeed while being treated with acalabrutinib and for at least 2 weeks after the last dose. Nevertheless, breastfeeding while using this drug should be based on the mother's clinical need for treatment. If used, the infant should be monitored for the most common reported adult side effects of nausea, musculoskeletal pain, abdominal pain, and headache (all leading to irritability), diarrhea, vomiting, constipation, lethargy, rash, and upper respiratory tract infection.

Reference

1. Prescribing Information. Calquence. AstraZeneca Pharmaceuticals LP; 2019.

ACAMPROSATE

Miscellaneous (Anti-Alcohol)

PREGNANCY RECOMMENDATION: Limited Human Data—Animal Data Suggest Risk (Maternal Benefit May Outweigh Embryo–Fetal Risk)

BREASTFEEDING RECOMMENDATION: Probably Compatible

PREGNANCY SUMMARY

One study of patients from Australia reported on 54 exposures to acamprosate during pregnancy that were compared with pregnancies with alcohol use and a nonusing control group. Overall, the major malformation rate was no different between the groups. In addition, there was no difference in neonatal birth weight or preterm delivery. Small amounts of the drug will likely cross the placenta, so some fetal exposure may occur. However, this limited human pregnancy experience prevents a complete assessment of the embryofetal risk. Animal data showed embryofetal toxicity with malformations in three species at doses less than 10 times the RHD, but this was not seen in a fourth species with higher doses. Ethanol (alcohol) use during pregnancy is well known to cause dose-related developmental toxicity (fetal alcohol syndrome). Even in the absence of obvious structural defects, alcohol use during gestation is associated with marked neurotoxicity in the offspring. Therefore, in pregnant women with alcohol dependency, the benefit of using this drug to maintain sobriety may outweigh the embryofetal risk in some cases.

BREASTFEEDING SUMMARY

No reports describing the use of acamprosate during human lactation have been located. The drug will probably be excreted into breast milk, so some infant exposure will likely occur. However, since the oral bioavailability is only 11%, the total amount may be small. The effect on a nursing infant from exposure in breast milk is unknown. However, alcohol is excreted into breast milk and has the potential to cause neonatal harm. Thus, if a lactating woman requires acamprosate to refrain from drinking, the benefit to the nursing infant may outweigh the unknown risk from the drug. If the clinical decision is to use this drug while breastfeeding, the infant should be monitored for the most common reported adult side effects of anxiety (leading to irritability), decreased appetite (monitor infant growth), vomiting, and insomnia.

References

1. Prescribing Information. Acamprosate. Teva Pharmaceuticals USA; 2018.
2. Kelty E, Tran D, Lavin T, et al. Prevalence and safety of acamprosate use in pregnant alcohol-dependent women in New South Wales, Australia. *Addiction*. 2019;114:206-215.

ACARBOSE

Antidiabetic (α-Glucosidase Inhibitor)

PREGNANCY RECOMMENDATION: Limited Human Data—Animal Data Suggest Low Risk

BREASTFEEDING RECOMMENDATION: Probably Compatible

PREGNANCY SUMMARY

A few reports describing the use of acarbose during human pregnancy have been located. In four first-trimester exposures, no birth anomalies or pregnancy complications were described. A few other reports have described the use of the drug in the second and third trimesters without any adverse effects related to the drug being identified. A small amount of the drug may cross the placenta, but the levels are likely to be clinically insignificant (oral bioavailability less than 2%). However, this limited human pregnancy experience prevents a complete assessment of the embryofetal risk. Animal studies did not show any embryofetal toxicity in one species at doses of less than 10 times the RHD. The American College of Obstetricians and Gynecologists (ACOG) recommends that insulin be used for type 1 and type 2 diabetes occurring during pregnancy and, if diet therapy alone is not successful, for gestational diabetes.

BREASTFEEDING SUMMARY

No reports describing the use of acarbose during human lactation have been located. The amount of drug excreted into human breast milk is likely to be clinically insignificant. However, due to a concern for potential serious adverse effects that might be seen in a breastfed infant, the manufacturer recommends that women not breastfeed while being treated with this drug. Nevertheless, breastfeeding while using this drug should be based on the mother's clinical need for treatment versus any potential infant risks that might occur. If used, the infant should be monitored for the most common reported adult side effects of abdominal pain (leading to irritability), diarrhea, and flatulence.

References

1. American College of Obstetricians and Gynecologists. ACOG practice bulletin No. 60: pregestational diabetes mellitus. *Obstet Gynecol*. 2005;105:675-685.
2. American College of Obstetricians and Gynecologists. ACOG practice bulletin No. 30: gestational diabetes. *Obstet Gynecol*. 2001;98:525-538.
3. Prescribing Information. Acarbose. Actavis Pharma; 2017.
4. Bertini AM, Silva JC, Taborda W, et al. Perinatal outcomes and the use of oral hypoglycemic agents. *J Perinat Med*. 2005;33:519-523.
5. Nicholson W, Bolen S, Witkop CT, et al. Benefits and risks of oral diabetes agents compared with insulin in women with gestational diabetes: a systematic review. *Obstet Gynecol*. 2009;113:193-205.
6. Brown J, Martis R, Hughes B, Rowan J, Crowther CA. Oral anti-diabetic pharmacological therapies for the treatment of women with gestational diabetes. *Cochrane Database Syst Rev*. 2017;1(1):CD011967.
7. Liang HL, Ma SJ, Xiao YN, Tan HZ. Comparative efficacy and safety of oral antidiabetic drugs and insulin in treating gestational diabetes mellitus: an update PRISMA-compliant network meta-analysis. *Medicine (Baltimore)*. 2017;96:e7939.
8. Wilton LV, Pearce GL, Martin RM, et al. The outcomes of pregnancy in women exposed to newly marketed drugs in general practice in England. *Br J Obstet Gynaecol*. 1998;105:882-889.
9. De Veciana M, Trail PA, Evans AT, Dulaney K. A comparison of oral acarbose and insulin in women with gestational diabetes mellitus (abstract). *Obstet Gynecol*. 2002;99(suppl):5S.
10. Yaris F, Yaris E, Kadioglu M, et al. Normal pregnancy outcome following inadvertent exposure to rosiglitazone, gliclazide, and atorvastatin in a diabetic and hypertensive woman. *Reprod Toxicol*. 2004;18:619-621.

ACEBUTOLOL

Antihypertensive/Cardiovascular (Cardioselective β-Blocker)

PREGNANCY RECOMMENDATION: Limited Human Data—Animal Data Suggest Low Risk

BREASTFEEDING RECOMMENDATION: Potential Toxicity

PREGNANCY SUMMARY

Several studies have been located that describe the use of acebutolol during human pregnancy. One case report described the use of the drug at the time of conception and through to delivery. No birth anomalies were identified, and no adverse effects related to the drug were described. Nearly all the other reports describe the use of the drug in the second and third trimesters. Some β-blockers may cause intrauterine growth restriction (IUGR), which was reported in a few studies, but not in others. A few publications described a few adverse neonatal effects shortly after delivery, including hypotension, bradycardia, and respiratory issues. The elimination half-lives of the drug and active metabolite (diacetolol) are also longer in newborns when compared with adults at 13 hours (versus 3.5 hours for acebutolol) and 20 hours (versus 10 hours for diacetolol). The drug crosses the placenta, so some fetal exposure will occur. However, this limited human pregnancy experience prevents a complete assessment of the embryofetal risk. Animal studies did not show any embryofetal toxicity in one species at doses of more than 10 times the RHD. Embryofetal toxicity was seen in a second species at doses less than 10 times the RHD, but maternal toxicity also occurred. Using this drug during pregnancy should be based on the pros and cons of the mother's clinical need for treatment versus any potential fetal risk that might occur from exposure. The ACOG recommends labetalol and nifedipine as first-line treatments for hypertension in pregnancy. If the drug is being used for ventricular arrhythmia and the patient is in good control, maintaining the drug may be the best treatment approach, but close fetal observation is recommended.

BREASTFEEDING SUMMARY

A few case reports describing the use of acebutolol during human lactation were located. In four lactating women, the drug and active metabolite (diacetolol) were found in all breast milk samples. The diacetolol levels were usually higher than the acebutolol levels. The breast milk levels for acebutolol ranged from about 40 ng/mL to 4 mcg/mL, whereas the levels for diacetolol ranged from about 60 ng/mL to nearly 7 mcg/mL. Using the highest combined values for a sampling, the level for both drugs was about 11 mcg/mL, which would suggest a calculated RID of about 9.5%. Due to a concern for potential serious adverse effects that might be seen in a breastfed infant, the manufacturer recommends that women not breastfeed while being treated with this drug. Nevertheless, breastfeeding while using this drug should be based on the mother's clinical need for treatment versus any potential infant risks that might occur. If used, the infant should be monitored for the most common reported adult side effects of nausea, headache, and dizziness (all leading to irritability), fatigue (lethargy), constipation, and insomnia.

References

1. Dubois D, Petitcolas J, Temperville B, Klepper A. Beta blockers and high-risk pregnancies. *Int J Biol Res Pregnancy*. 1980;1:141-145.
2. Dubois D, Petitcolas J, Temperville B, et al. Treatment of hypertension in pregnancy with beta-adrenoceptor antagonists. *Br J Clin Pharmacol*. 1982; 13(suppl 2):375S-378S.
3. Bianchetti G, Dubruc C, Vert P, et al. Placental transfer and pharmacokinetics of acebutolol in newborn infants (abstract). *Clin Pharmacol Ther*. 1981; 29:233-234.
4. Boutroy MJ. Fetal and neonatal effects of the beta-adrenoceptor blocking agents. *Dev Pharmacol Ther*. 1987;10:224-231.
5. Williams ER, Morrissey JR. A comparison of acebutolol with methyldopa in hypertensive pregnancy. *Pharmatherapeutica*. 1983;3:487-491.
6. Prescribing Information. Acebutolol. Marlex Pharmaceuticals; 2017.
7. Dumez Y, Tchobroutsky C, Hornych H, Amiel-Tison C. Neonatal effects of maternal administration of acebutolol. *Br Med J*. 1981;283:1077-1079.
8. Yassen H, Boutroy MJ, Monin P, Vert P. Hemodynamic and renal adaptation of newborn infants of hypertensive mothers treated with acebutolol. *Arch Fr Pediatr*. 1992;49:351-355.
9. Lee LC, Bathgate SL, Macri CJ. Arrhythmogenic right ventricular dysplasia in pregnancy: a case report. *J Reprod Med*. 2006;51:725-728.
10. Boutroy MJ, Bianchetti G, Dubruc C, et al. To nurse when receiving acebutolol: is it dangerous for the neonate? *Eur J Clin Pharmacol*. 1986;30:737-739.
11. American Academy of Pediatrics Committee on Drugs. The transfer of drugs and other chemicals into human milk. *Pediatrics*. 2001;108:776-789.

ACETAMINOPHEN

Pain (Analgesic/Antipyretic)

PREGNANCY RECOMMENDATION: Human Data Suggest Low Risk (Short-Term Use)

BREASTFEEDING RECOMMENDATION: Probably Compatible

PREGNANCY SUMMARY

Acetaminophen is commonly used in all stages of pregnancy. Combined data from 7 large studies reported a rate of congenital birth anomalies of about 4% in more than 48,000 first-trimester exposures. No pattern to the defects was seen in any of the studies. There have been questions about the use of acetaminophen during pregnancy, increasing the risk for cryptorchidism, childhood asthma, childhood intelligence quotient, and attention deficit hyperactivity disorder (ADHD), but no consistent findings for these have been found. The drug crosses the placenta, so fetal exposure will occur. Animal studies have shown some embryofetal toxicity in two species at doses of less than 10 times the RHD. Using this drug during pregnancy should be based on the pros and cons of the mother's clinical need for treatment versus any potential fetal risk that might occur from exposure. Many of the exposures in the reported studies involved short-term usage, consistent with the need for fever reduction and in treating mild to moderate pain. Long-term usage has not been fully analyzed and could lead to liver injury if not closely monitored.

BREASTFEEDING SUMMARY

Several studies have been located that describe the use of acetaminophen during human lactation. A total of about 37 women had breast milk samples analyzed, and the drug was found in all cases shortly after use. If the drug is stopped, breast milk levels are usually negative by 12 to 15 hours. The concentrations in breast milk vary from a low of about 2 ng/mL to 15 mcg/mL. The calculated RIDs were under 3% in most instances. However, in these studies, the lactating women received single doses that ranged from 500 to 1,000 mg. Breast milk levels are likely to be higher if the mother is using 3,000 mg/d, which might produce RIDs that could exceed 10%. The maximum daily dose in adults for acetaminophen is 4,000 mg. There have been 18 infants tested for the drug following exposure through breastfeeding. Blood levels have not been analyzed. The drug was not detected in the urine in 12 infants following a dose of 650 mg. It was detected in the urine of six infants following maternal doses of 1,000 to 2,000 mg. Breastfeeding while using this drug should be based on the mother's clinical need for treatment versus any potential infant risks that might occur. If used, the infant should be monitored for the most common reported adult side effects of nausea, headache, and pruritus (all leading to irritability), vomiting, insomnia, and constipation.

References

1. Prescribing Information. Tylenol. Johnson & Johnson Consumer, Inc, McNeil Consumer Healthcare Division; 2017.
2. Saad A, Hegde S, Kechichian T, et al. Is there a causal relation between maternal acetaminophen administration and ADHD? *PLoS One*. 2016;11: e0157380.
3. Hay-Schmidt A, Finkielman O, Jensen B, et al. Paracetamol/acetaminophen impairs brain masculinisation. *Reproduction*. 2017;154:145-152. doi:10.1530/REP-17-0165
4. Wu K, Guo C, Lu X, et al. Impact of perinatal exposure to acetaminophen on hepatocellular metabolic function in offspring. *Am J Transl Res*. 2016; 8:5646-5652.
5. Levy G, Garretson LK, Soda DM. Evidence of placental transfer of acetaminophen. *Pediatrics*. 1975;55:895.
6. Nitsche JF, Patil AS, Langman LJ, et al. Transplacental passage of acetaminophen in term pregnancy. *Am J Perinatol*. 2017;34:541-543.
7. Char VC, Chandra R, Fletcher AB, Avery GB. Polyhydramnios and neonatal renal failure-a possible association with maternal acetaminophen ingestion. *J Pediatr*. 1975;86:638-639.
8. Rollins DE, Von Bahr C, Glaumann H, et al. Acetaminophen: potentially toxic metabolite formed by human fetal and adult liver microsomes and isolated fetal liver cells. *Science*. 1979;205:1414-1416.
9. Haibach H, Akhter JE, Muscato MS, et al. Acetaminophen overdose with fetal demise. *Am J Clin Pathol*. 1984;82:240-242.
10. Wang P-H, Yang M-J, Lee W-L, et al. Acetaminophen poisoning in late pregnancy. A case report. *J Reprod Med*. 1997;42:367-371.
11. Byer AJ, Taylor TR, Semmer JR. Acetaminophen overdose in the third trimester of pregnancy. *JAMA*. 1982;247:3114–5.
12. Stokes IM. Paracetamol overdose in the second trimester of pregnancy. Case report. *Br J Obstet Gynaecol*. 1984;91:286-288.
13. Ludmir J, Main DM, Landon MB, Gabbe SG. Maternal acetaminophen overdose at 15 weeks of gestation. *Obstet Gynecol*. 1986;67:750-751.
14. Rosevear SK, Hope PL. Favourable neonatal outcome following maternal paracetamol overdose and severe fetal distress: case report. *Br J Obstet Gynaecol*. 1989;96:491-493.
15. Friedman S, Gatti M, Baker T. Cesarean section after maternal acetaminophen overdose. *Anesth Analg*. 1993;77:632-634.
16. Riggs BS, Bronstein AC, Kulig K, et al. Acute acetaminophen overdose during pregnancy. *Obstet Gynecol*. 1989;74:247-253.
17. McElhatton PR, Sullivan FM, Volans GN. Paracetamol overdose in pregnancy analysis of the outcomes of 300 cases referred to the teratology information service. *Reprod Toxicol*. 1997;11:85-94.
18. Wilkes JM, Clark LE, Herrera JL. Acetaminophen overdose in pregnancy. *South Med J*. 2005;98:1118-1122.
19. Taney J, Anastasio H, Paternostro A, et al. Placental abruption with delayed fetal compromise in maternal acetaminophen toxicity. *Obstet Gynecol*. 2017; 130:159-162.
20. Kang EM, Lundsberg LS, Illuzzi JL, Bracken MB. Prenatal exposure to acetaminophen and asthma in children. *Obstet Gynecol*. 2009;114:1295-1306.
21. Scialli AR, Ang R, Breitmeyer J, Royal MA. Childhood asthma and use during pregnancy of acetaminophen. A critical review. *Reprod Toxicol*. 2010; 30:508-519.
22. Lourido-Cebreiro T, Salgado FJ, Valdes L, Gonzalez-Barcala FJ. The association between paracetamol and asthma is still under debate. *J Asthma*. 2017;54:32-38.
23. Heinonen OP, Slone D, Shapiro S. *Birth Defects and Drugs in Pregnancy*. Publishing Sciences Group; 1977.
24. Golden NL, King KC, Sokol RJ. Propoxyphene and acetaminophen: possible effects on the fetus. *Clin Pediatr*. 1982;21:752-754.
25. Aselton P, Jick H, Milunsky A, Hunter JR, Stergachis A. First-trimester drug use and congenital disorders. *Obstet Gynecol*. 1985;65:451-455.
26. Thulstrup AM, Sorensen HT, Nielsen GL, et al; EuroMap Study Group. Fetal growth and adverse birth outcomes in women receiving prescriptions for acetaminophen during pregnancy. *Am J Perinatol*. 1999;16:321-326.
27. Cleves MA, Savell VH Jr, Raj S, et al; National Birth Defects Prevention Study. Maternal use of acetaminophen and nonsteroidal anti-inflammatory drugs (NSAIDs), and muscular ventricular septal defects. *Birth Defects Res A Clin Mol Teratol*. 2004;70:107-113.
28. Rebordosa C, Kogevinas M, Horvath-Puho E, et al. Acetaminophen use during pregnancy: effects on risk for congenital abnormalities. *Am J Obstet Gynecol*. 2008;198:178.E1–178.E7.
29. Feldkamp ML, Meyer RE, Krikov S, Botto LD. Acetaminophen use in pregnancy and risk of birth defects. Findings from the National Birth Defects Prevention Study. *Obstet Gynecol*. 2010;115:109-115.
30. Adjei AA, Gaedigk A, Simon SD, et al. Interindividual variability in acetaminophen sulfation by human fetal liver: implications for pharmacogenetic investigations of drug-induced birth defects. *Birth Defects Res A Clin Mol Teratol*. 2008;82:155-165.
31. Lind DV, Main KM, Kyhl HB, et al. Maternal use of mild analgesics during pregnancy associated with reduced anogenital distance in sons: a cohort study of 1027 mother-child pairs. *Hum Reprod*. 2017;32:223-231.
32. Dreier JW, Andersen AM, Berg-Beckhoff G. Systematic review and meta-analysis: fever in pregnancy and health impacts in the offspring. *Pediatrics*. 2014;133:e674-e688.
33. Jensen MS, Rebordosa C, Thulstrup AM, et al. Maternal use of acetaminophen, ibuprofen, and acetylsalicylic acid during pregnancy and risk of cryptorchidism. *Epidemiology*. 2010;21:779-785.
34. Kristensen DM, Hass U, Lesne L, et al. Intrauterine exposure to mild analgesics is a risk factor for development of male reproductive disorders in human and rat. *Hum Reprod*. 2011;26:235-244.
35. Gurney J, Richiardi L, McGlynn KA, et al. Analgesia use during pregnancy and risk of cryptorchidism: a systematic review and meta-analysis. *Hum Reprod*. 2017;32:1118-1129.
36. Streissguth AP, Treder RP, Barr HM, et al. Aspirin and acetaminophen use by pregnant women and subsequent child IQ and attention decrements. *Teratology*. 1987;35:211-219.
37. Liew Z, Ritz B, Virk J, Arah OA, Olsen J. Prenatal use of acetaminophen and child IQ: a Danish cohort study. *Epidemiology*. 2016;27:912-918.
38. Brandlistuen RE, Ystrom E, Nulman I, et al. Prenatal paracetamol exposure and child neurodevelopment: a sibling-controlled cohort study. *Int J Epidemiol*. 2013;42:1702-1713. doi:10.1093/ije/dyt183
39. Liew Z, Ritz B, Rebordosa C, et al. Acetaminophen use during pregnancy, behavioral problems, and hyperkinetic disorders. *JAMA Pediatr*. 2014;168:313-320.
40. Avella-Garcia CB, Julvez J, Fortuny J, et al. Acetaminophen use in pregnancy and neurodevelopment: attention function and autism spectrum symptoms. *Int J Epidemol*. 2016;45:1987-1996.
41. Ystrom E, Gustavson K, Brandlistuen RE, et al. Prenatal exposure to acetaminophen and risk of ADHD. *Pediatrics*. 2017;140:e20163840.
42. Good P. Did acetaminophen provoke the autism epidemic? *Altern Med Rev*. 2009;14:364-372.
43. Andrade C. Use of acetaminophen (paracetamol) during pregnancy and the risk of autism spectrum disorder in the offspring. *J Clin Psychiatry*. 2016; 77:e152-e154.
44. Stergiakouli E, Thapar A, Smith GD. Association of acetaminophen use during pregnancy with behavioral problems in childhood: evidence against confounding. *JAMA Pediatr*. 2016;170:964-970.

45. Beale DJ. Acetaminophen in pregnancy and adverse childhood neurodevelopment. *JAMA Pediatr*. 2017;171:394-395.
46. Saunders NR, Habgood MD. Acetaminophen in pregnancy and adverse childhood neurodevelopment. *JAMA Pediatr*. 2017;171:395.
47. Little MO, Wickremsinhe MN, Lyerly AD. Acetaminophen in pregnancy and adverse childhood neurodevelopment. *JAMA Pediatr*. 2017;171:395-396.
48. Damkier P, Scialli AR, Lusskin SI. Acetaminophen in pregnancy and adverse childhood neurodevelopment. *JAMA Pediatr*. 2017;171:396.
49. Stergiakouli E, Thapar A, Smith GD. Acetaminophen in pregnancy and adverse childhood neurodevelopment. *JAMA Pediatr*. 2017;171:396-397.
50. Liew Z, Ritz B, Virk J, Olsen J. Maternal use of acetaminophen during pregnancy and risk of autism spectrum disorders in childhood: a Danish National Birth Cohort study. *Autism Res*. 2016;9:951-958.
51. Hornig M, Bresnahan MA, Che X, et al. Prenatal fever and autism risk. *Mol Psychiatry*. 2018;23:759-766.
52. Vienterie R, Wood ME, Brandlistuen RE, et al. Neurodevelopmental problems at 18 months among children exposed to paracetamol *in utero*: a propensity score matched cohort study. *Int J Epidemol*. 2016;45:1998-2008. doi:10.1093/ije/dyw192
53. Pearson H. Comparative effects of aspirin and acetaminophen on hemostasis. *Pediatrics*. 1978;62(suppl):926-929.
54. Rudolph AM. Effects of aspirin and acetaminophen in pregnancy and in the newborn. *Arch Intern Med*. 1981;141:358-363.
55. Rumack CM, Guggenheim MA, Rumack BH, et al. Neonatal intracranial hemorrhage and maternal use of aspirin. *Obstet Gynecol*. 1981;58(suppl):52S-56S.
56. Kirshon B, Moise KJ Jr, Wasserstrum N. Effect of acetaminophen on fetal acid-base balance in chorioamnionitis. *J Reprod Med*. 1989;34:955-959.
57. Matheson I, Lunde PKM, Notarianni L. Infant rash caused by paracetamol in breast milk? *Pediatrics*. 1985;76:651-652.
58. Berlin CM Jr, Yaffe SJ, Ragni M. Disposition of acetaminophen in milk, saliva, and plasma of lactating women. *Pediatr Pharmacol*. 1980;1:135-141.
59. Findlay JWA, DeAngelis RL, Kearney MF, et al. Analgesic drugs in breast milk and plasma. *Clin Pharmacol Ther*. 1981;29:625-633.
60. Bitzen PO, Gustafsson B, Jostell KG, et al. Excretion of paracetamol in human breast milk. *Eur J Clin Pharmacol*. 1981;20:123-125.
61. Notarianni LJ, Oldham HG, Bennett PN. Passage of paracetamol into breast milk and its subsequent metabolism by the neonate. *Br J Clin Pharmacol*. 1987;24:63-67.
62. American Academy of Pediatrics Committee on Drugs. The transfer of drugs and other chemicals into human milk. *Pediatrics*. 2001;108:776-789.

ACETAZOLAMIDE

Cardiovascular/Central Nervous System/Ophthalmic (Carbonic Anhydrase Inhibitor/Antiseizure/Glaucoma)

PREGNANCY RECOMMENDATION: Limited Human Data—Animal Data Suggest Potential Risk

BREASTFEEDING RECOMMENDATION: Probably Compatible

PREGNANCY SUMMARY

The Collaborative Perinatal Project (CPP) reported no major anomalies in 12 first-trimester exposures to acetazolamide. Two retrospective surveys on the use of acetazolamide during gestation have not demonstrated any increased fetal risks. There are cases reports that have shown no adverse effects and some with abnormal fetal effects. However, these are not likely related to the drug except for one possible case with ectrodactyly and syndactyly. The drug will probably cross the placenta, so some fetal exposure will likely occur. Therefore, this limited first-trimester human pregnancy experience prevents a complete assessment of the embryofetal risk. Animal data have shown some embryofetal toxicity in three species but some of these do not report a human exposure comparison or state that it was less than 10 times the RHD. Using this drug during pregnancy should be based on the pros and cons of the mother's clinical need for treatment versus any potential fetal risk that might occur from exposure. The drug has been widely used for years during pregnancy.

BREASTFEEDING SUMMARY

Three case reports were located that describe the use of acetazolamide during human lactation. The drug was found to be excreted into breast milk in all three women. Breast milk levels ranged from about 0.2 mcg/mL to a little more than 4 mcg/mL. The calculated RIDs were all less than 3%. However, due to a concern for potential serious adverse effects that might be seen in a breastfed infant, the manufacturer recommends that women not breastfeed while being treated with this drug. Nevertheless, breastfeeding while using this drug should be based on the mother's clinical need for treatment versus any potential infant risks that might occur. If used, the infant should be monitored for the most common reported adult side effects of nausea, headache, and dizziness (all leading to irritability), diarrhea, fatigue (lethargy), vomiting, decreased appetite (monitor infant growth), fever, drowsiness, and various laboratory abnormalities (see PI).

References

1. Prescribing Information. Acetazolamide. Alembic Pharmaceuticals; 2019.
2. Prescribing Information. Acetazolamide. Sagent Pharmaceuticals; 2018.
3. Lee AG, Pless M, Falardeau J, Capozzoli T, Wall M, Kardon RH. The use of acetazolamide in idiopathic intracranial hypertension during pregnancy. *Am J Ophthalmol*. 2005;139:855-859.
4. Falardeau J, Lobb BM, Golden S, Maxfield SD, Tanne E. The use of acetazolamide during pregnancy in intracranial hypertension patients. *J Neuroophthalmol*. 2013;33:9-12.
5. Kesler A, Kupferminc M. Idiopathic intracranial hypertension and pregnancy. *Clin Obstet Gynecol*. 2013;56:389-396.
6. Golan S, Maslovitz S, Kupferminc MJ, Kesler A. Management and outcome of consecutive pregnancies complicated by idiopathic intracranial hypertension. *Isr Med Assoc J*. 2013;15:160-163.
7. Jacopin-Bruneau L, Gommier B, Pierre F, Boog G. Idiopathic intracranial hypertension and pregnancy. A report of two cases. *J Gynecol Obstet Reprod (Paris)*. 2010;39:246-250.
8. Shepard TH. *Catalog of Teratogenic Agents*. 6th ed. Johns Hopkins University Press; 1989:5-6.
9. Nakatsuka T, Komatsu T, Fujii T. Axial skeletal malformations induced by acetazolamide in rabbits. *Teratology*. 1992;45:629–636.
10. Miller TA, Scott WJ Jr. Abnormalities in ureter and kidney development in mice give acetazolamide-amiloride or dimethadione (DMO) during embryogenesis. *Teratology*. 1992;46:541-550.
11. Worsham GF, Beckman EN, Mitchell EH. Sacrococcygeal teratoma in a neonate. Association with maternal use of acetazolamide. *JAMA*. 1978;240: 251-252.

12. Favre-Tissot M, Broussole P, Robert JM, Dumont L. An original clinical study of the pharmacologic-teratogenic relationship. *Ann Med Psychol.* 1964;1:389. As cited in Nishimura H, Tanimura T, eds. *Clinical Aspects of the Teratogenicity of Drugs.* Excerpta Medica; 1976:210.
13. McBride WG. The teratogenic action of drugs. *Med J Aust.* 1963;2:689-693.
14. Heinonen OP, Slone D, Shapiro S. *Birth Defects and Drugs in Pregnancy.* Publishing Sciences Group; 1977.
15. Merlob P, Litwin A, Mor N. Possible association between acetazolamide administration during pregnancy and metabolic disorders in the newborn. *Eur J Obstet Gynecol Reprod Biol.* 1990;35:85-88.
16. Al-Saleem AI, Al-Jobar AM. Possible association between acetazolamide administration during pregnancy and multiple congenital malformations. *Drug Des Devel Ther.* 2016;10:1471-1476.
17. Soderman P, Hartvig P, Fagerlund C. Acetazolamide excretion into human breast milk. *Br J Clin Pharmacol.* 1984;17:599-560.

ACETYLCYSTEINE

Antidote (Acetaminophen)/ Respiratory (Mucolytic)

PREGNANCY RECOMMENDATION: Limited Human Data—Animal Data Suggest Low Risk (Maternal Benefit Probably Outweighs Any Embryofetal Risk With Overdose)

BREASTFEEDING RECOMMENDATION: Probably Compatible

PREGNANCY SUMMARY

No reports describing the use of acetylcysteine with inhalation use during human pregnancy have been located. A few publications on its use in treating acetaminophen overdose were found. Over 60 pregnancy exposures have been described, but only a few were in the first trimester and no outcome data specific for these were provided. Overall, no major adverse effects related to the drug were found. Most of the poor outcomes were due to adverse effects caused by the drug overdose. The drug will probably cross the placenta, so some fetal exposure will likely occur. Therefore, this limited human pregnancy experience prevents a complete assessment of the embryofetal risk. Animal data did not show any embryofetal toxicity in two species at doses of less than 10 times the RHD. However, due to the severe consequences related to acetaminophen overdose, the drug should be used in the same manner as it is used in nonpregnant patients.

BREASTFEEDING SUMMARY

No reports describing the use of acetylcysteine during human lactation have been located. The drug will likely be found in breast milk, so some infant exposure will likely occur. The amount of the drug in breast milk is likely to be much lower with inhalation use than with levels following intravenous (IV) use. In addition, IV use is for treating an acetaminophen overdose, which is not likely to occur often in a breastfeeding woman. Moreover, acetylcysteine has been administered to preterm neonates for therapeutic indications, without causing any toxicity, at doses far above those that would be obtained from breast milk following inhalation use. Breastfeeding while using this drug should be based on the mother's clinical need for treatment versus any potential infant risks that might occur. If used, the infant should be monitored for the most common reported adult side effects of nausea (leading to irritability), cough, vomiting, fever, rhinorrhea, and sweating.

References

1. Zed PJ, Krenzelok EP. Treatment of acetaminophen overdose. *Am J Health Syst Pharm.* 1999;56:1081–1091.
2. Product Information. Acetylcysteine solution. Hospira; 2017.
3. Product Information. Acetylcysteine injection. Paddock Laboratories; 2016.
4. Acetylcysteine (N-acetylcysteine). In: *Drug Facts and Comparisons.* Facts and Comparisons; 2000.
5. Domingo JL. Developmental toxicity of metal chelating agents. *Reprod Toxicol.* 1998;12:499-510.
6. Horowitz RS, Dart RC, Jarvie DR, et al. Placental transfer of *N*-acetylcysteine following human maternal acetaminophen toxicity. *Clin Toxicol.* 1997;35:447-451.
7. Byer AJ, Traylor TR, Semmer JR. Acetaminophen overdose in the third trimester of pregnancy. *JAMA.* 1982;247:3114-3115.
8. Ludmir J, Main DM, Landon MB, Gabbe SG. Maternal acetaminophen overdose at 15 weeks of gestation. *Obstet Gynecol.* 1986;67:750-751.
9. Rosevear SK, Hope PL. Favourable neonatal outcome following maternal paracetamol overdose and severe fetal distress. Case report. *Br J Obstet Gynaecol.* 1989;96:491-493.
10. Riggs BS, Bronstein AC, Kulig K, et al. Acute acetaminophen overdose during pregnancy. *Obstet Gynecol.* 1989;74:247-253.
11. McElhatton PR, Sullivan FM, Volans GN. Paracetamol overdose in pregnancy: analysis of the outcomes of 300 cases referred to the teratology information service. *Reprod Toxicol.* 1997;11:85-94.
12. Crowell C, Lyew RV, Givens M, Deering SH. Caring for the mother, concentrating on the fetus: intravenous *N*-acetylcysteine in pregnancy. *Am J Emerg Med.* 2008;26:735.e1-735.e2.
13. Forrester MB, Stanley SK. Exposures and treatments among women of childbearing age and pregnant women reported to Texas poison centers. *Vet Hum Toxicol.* 2004;46:210-212.
14. Rumiris D, Purwosunu Y, Wibowo N, et al. Lower rate of preeclampsia after antioxidant supplementation in pregnant women with low antioxidant status. *Hypertens Pregnancy.* 2006;25:241-253.
15. Amin AF, Shaaban OM, Bediawy MA. *N*-acetyl cysteine for treatment of recurrent unexplained pregnancy loss. *Reprod Biomed Online.* 2008;17:722-726.
16. Shahin AY, Hassanin IMA, Ismail AM, et al. Effect of oral N-acetyl cysteine on recurrent preterm labor following treatment for bacterial vaginosis. *Int J Gynaecol Obstet.* 2009;104:44-48.
17. Ahola TM, Fellman V, Laaksonen R, et al. Pharmacokinetics of intravenous N-acetylcysteine in preterm neonates (abstract). *Pediatr Res.* 1998;43(suppl 2):163.
18. Isbister GK, Bucens IK, Whyte IM. Paracetamol overdose in a preterm neonate. *Arch Dis Child Fetal Neonat Ed.* 2001;85:F70-F72.

ACITRETIN

Dermatologic (Retinoid)

PREGNANCY RECOMMENDATION: Contraindicated (Human Data)

BREASTFEEDING RECOMMENDATION: Potential Toxicity

PREGNANCY SUMMARY

Several case reports and small series have been published regarding the use of acitretin during human pregnancy. Acitretin is a known teratogen, primarily involving the fetal central nervous system, face, limbs, cardiac, and bone development, with a rate of 25% or higher with first-trimester exposure. Case reports have described these defects when the drug was used in the first trimester. In one review, there were 238 pregnancy exposures to etretinate and acitretin that occurred after the last dose. Pregnancies were included if the drug was stopped within 3 years prior to conception. Excluding lost to follow-up, early spontaneous abortions, and elective terminations, there were 15 (12.7%) major anomalies (several consistent with retinoid embryopathy) in 118 cases. For acitretin exposure only, there were 3 (7%) major anomalies in 43 cases where the drug was stopped more than a year prior to conception but less than 2 years. No anomalies were seen in the four cases where the drug was stopped more than 2 years from conception. The drug and active metabolite cross the placenta, so some fetal exposure will occur. Acitretin was not found to cause any embryofetal toxicity or teratogenicity in one species at doses of less than 10 times the RHD. Of critical importance is the fact that a high percentage of the recipients of this drug are women with childbearing potential. Due to the high risk of life-threatening birth defects, the manufacturer recommends that women with reproductive potential who are taking acitretin be advised to use two effective forms of contraception at least 1 month prior to treatment, during treatment, and for at least 3 years after the last dose. The drug carries an extensive boxed warning for a contraindication for use in pregnancy. There is a program called "Do Your P.A.R.T"—Pregnancy Prevention Actively Required during and after Treatment that should be followed prior to use. It explains the number of required negative pregnancy tests, the types of pregnancy tests used, that two forms of contraception are required, and that a patient agreement/informed consent for females is signed. See PI for more details or call 888-784-3335 (888-STIEFEL). It also carries a boxed warning for an increased risk of hepatotoxicity; thus, liver function tests should be monitored.

BREASTFEEDING SUMMARY

One case regarding the use of acitretin during human lactation was located. The mother stopped breastfeeding to start the drug, and had breast milk levels obtained. Her daily dose was 40 mg, and the mean breast milk level at steady state was about 35 ng/mL. The calculated RID was less than 1%. Because some amount of the drug may be stored in subcutaneous fat, the actual elimination of these compounds may take much longer. The manufacturer recommends a contraception period of 3 years after acitretin therapy is stopped, but a similar recommendation for breastfeeding has not been made. Using an alternative drug to treat the various dermatologic conditions is an option for some patients. Nevertheless, breastfeeding while using this drug should be based on the mother's clinical need for treatment versus any potential infant risks that might occur.

References

1. Prescribing Information. Soriatane. Stiefel Laboratories; 2019.
2. Geiger JM, Walker M. Is there a reproductive safety risk in male patients treated with acitretin (Neotigason®/Soriatane®)? *Dermatology*. 2002;205:105-107.
3. Sturkenboom MC, DeJong-Van Den Berg LT, Van Voorst-Vader PC, et al. Inability to detect plasma etretinate and acitretin is a poor predictor of the absence of these teratogens in tissue after stopping acitretin treatment. *Br J Clin Pharmacol*. 1994;38:229-235.
4. De Die-Smulders CEM, Sturkenboom MC, Veraart J, et al. Severe limb defects and craniofacial anomalies in a fetus conceived during acitretin therapy. *Teratology*. 1995;52:215-219.
5. Geiger JM, Baudin M, Saurat JH. Teratogenic risk with etretinate and acitretin treatment. *Dermatology*. 1994;189:109-116.
6. Maradit H, Geiger JM. Potential risk of birth defects after acitretin discontinuation. *Dermatology*. 1999;198:3-4.
7. Barbero P, Lotersztein V, Bronberg R, et al. Acitretin embryopathy: a case report. *Birth Defects Res A Clin Mol Teratol*. 2004;70:831-833.
8. Berbis P, Bun H, Geiger JM, et al. Acitretin (RO10-1670) and oral contraceptives: interaction study. *Arch Dermatol Res*. 1988;280:388-389.
9. Rollman O, Pihl-Lundin I. Acitretin excretion into human breast milk. *Acta Derm Venereol*. 1990;70:487-490.

ACLIDINIUM BROMIDE

Respiratory (Anticholinergic—Inhalation)

PREGNANCY RECOMMENDATION: No Human Data—Animal Data Suggest Low Risk

BREASTFEEDING RECOMMENDATION: Probably Compatible

PREGNANCY SUMMARY

No reports describing the use of aclidinium bromide in human pregnancy have been located. The drug will probably cross the placenta, but the overall amount is likely to be clinically insignificant. Therefore, the absence of human pregnancy experience prevents a complete assessment of the embryofetal risk. Animal studies did not show any embryofetal toxicity in two species at doses of more than 10 times the RHD. Using this drug during pregnancy should be based on the pros and cons of the mother's clinical need for treatment versus any potential fetal risk that might occur from exposure.

BREASTFEEDING SUMMARY

No reports describing the use of aclidinium during human lactation have been located. The drug may be found in breast milk, but the overall amount is likely to be clinically insignificant. Breastfeeding while using this drug should be based on the mother's clinical need for treatment. If used, the infant should be monitored for the most common reported adult side effects of headache (leading to irritability) and cough.

Reference

1. Prescribing Information. Tudorza Pressair. AstraZeneca; 2020.

ACYCLOVIR

Antiviral (Herpes/Varicella-Zoster)

PREGNANCY RECOMMENDATION: Human Data Suggest Low Risk

BREASTFEEDING RECOMMENDATION: Probably Compatible

PREGNANCY SUMMARY

Numerous studies have been located that describe the use of acyclovir during human pregnancy. From two large databases (Michigan Medicaid Surveillance study [MMSS] and the Acyclovir Pregnancy Registry), a total of 36 (3.7%) major anomalies were described in 1,074 first-trimester drug exposures. Several other smaller studies have not shown an increased risk for birth defects. In addition, no pattern to the anomalies has been identified. The drug crosses the placenta, so fetal exposure will occur. Animal studies did not show any embryofetal toxicity or teratogenicity in three species at doses of more than 10 times the RHD. Using this drug during pregnancy should be based on the pros and cons of the mother's clinical need for treatment versus any potential fetal risk that might occur from exposure. Systemic IV treatment is indicated for life-threatening disseminated herpes simplex virus infections, as well as varicella pneumonia, both of which can be fatal in some cases.

BREASTFEEDING SUMMARY

A few reports describing the use of acyclovir during human lactation were located. In a total of five women, the drug was found in all samples, with a range of about 400 ng/mL to a high of 7.3 mcg/mL. All of the calculated RIDs were less than 3%. Infant serum levels have not been located, but the drug was found to be excreted in the urine of one infant whose only exposure was through breast milk. No adverse infant effects related to the drug were described. Breastfeeding while using this drug should be based on the mother's clinical need for treatment versus any potential infant risks that might occur. If used, the infant should be monitored for the most common reported adult side effects of nausea (leading to irritability), vomiting, diarrhea, and fatigue (lethargy).

References

1. Prescribing Information. Zovirax. Prestium Pharma; 2019.
2. Moore HL, Szczech GM, Rodwell DE, et al. Preclinical toxicology studies with acyclovir: teratologic, reproductive, and neonatal tests. *Fund Appl Toxicol*. 1983;3:560-568.
3. Stahlmann R, Klug S, Lewandowski C, et al. Prenatal toxicity of acyclovir in rats. *Arch Toxicol*. 1988;61:468-479.
4. Chahoud I, Stahlmann R, Bochert G, et al. Gross-structural defects in rats after acyclovir application on day 10 of gestation. *Arch Toxicol*. 1988;62:8-14.
5. Stahlmann R, Korte M, Van Loveren H, et al. Abnormal thymus development and impaired function of the immune system in rats after prenatal exposure to acyclovir. *Arch Toxicol*. 1992;66:551-559.
6. Clive D, Turner NT, Hozier J, et al. Preclinical toxicology studies with acyclovir: genetic toxicity tests. *Fund Appl Toxicol*. 1983;3:587-602.
7. Stahlmann R, Chahoud I, Thiel R, et al. The developmental toxicity of three antimicrobial agents observed only in nonroutine animal studies. *Reprod Toxicol*. 1997;11:1-7.
8. Henderson GI, Hu Z-Q, Johnson RF, et al. Acyclovir transport by the human placenta. *J Lab Clin Med*. 1992;120:885-926.
9. Landsberger EJ, Hager WD, Grossman JH III. Successful management of varicella pneumonia complicating pregnancy: a report of three cases. *J Reprod Med*. 1986;31:311-314.
10. Utley K, Bromberger P, Wagner L, Schneider H. Management of primary herpes in pregnancy complicated by ruptured membranes and extreme prematurity: case report. *Obstet Gynecol*. 1987;69:471-473.
11. Greffe BS, Dooley SL, Deddish RB, Krasny HC. Transplacental passage of acyclovir. *J Pediatr*. 1986;108:1020-1021.
12. Haddad J, Simeoni U, Messer J, Willard D. Transplacental passage of acyclovir. *J Pediatr*. 1987;110:164.
13. Kingsley S. Fetal and neonatal exposure to acyclovir (abstract). Paper presented at: Second World Congress on Sexually Transmitted Diseases; June 1986; Paris. As cited in Haddad J, Simeoni U, Messer J, Willard D. Transplacental passage of acyclovir. *J Pediatr*. 1987;110:164.
14. Frenkel LM, Brown ZA, Bryson YJ, et al. Pharmacokinetics of acyclovir in the term human pregnancy and neonate. *Am J Obstet Gynecol*. 1991;164:569-576.
15. Fletcher CV. The placental transport and use of acyclovir in pregnancy. *J Lab Clin Med*. 1992;120:821-822.

16. Stone KM, Reiff-Eldridge R, White AD, et al. Pregnancy outcomes following systemic prenatal acyclovir exposure: conclusions from the International Acyclovir Pregnancy Registry, 1984-1999. *Birth Defects Res A Clin Mol Teratol*. 2004;70:201-207.
17. Brown ZA, Baker DA. Acyclovir therapy during pregnancy. *Obstet Gynecol*. 1989;73:526-531.
18. Brown ZA, Watts DH. Antiviral therapy in pregnancy. *Clin Obstet Gynecol*. 1990;33:276-289.
19. Arvin AM, Hensleigh PA, Prober CG, et al. Failure of antepartum maternal cultures to predict the infant's risk of exposure to herpes simplex virus at delivery. *N Engl J Med*. 1986;315:796-800.
20. Carney O, Mindel A. Screening pregnant women for genital herpes. *BMJ*. 1988;296:1643.
21. Canadian Task Force on the Periodic Health Examination. Periodic health examination, 1989 update: 4. Intrapartum electronic fetal monitoring and prevention of neonatal herpes simplex. *Can Med Assoc J*. 1989;141:1233-1240.
22. Brocklehurst P, Kinghorn G, Carney O, et al. A randomised placebo controlled trial of suppressive acyclovir in late pregnancy in women with recurrent genital herpes infection. *Br J Obstet Gynaecol*. 1998;105:275-280.
23. Workowski KA, Bolan GA; Centers for Disease Control and Prevention. Sexually transmitted diseases treatment guidelines, 2015. *MMWR Recomm Rep*. 2015;64:1-137.
24. Lagrew DC Jr, Furlow TG, Hager WD, Yarrish RL. Disseminated herpes simplex virus infection in pregnancy. *JAMA*. 1984;252:2058-2059.
25. Grover L, Kane J, Kravitz J, Cruz A. Systemic acyclovir in pregnancy: a case report. *Obstet Gynecol*. 1985;65:284-287.
26. Berger SA, Weinberg M, Treves T, et al. Herpes encephalitis during pregnancy: failure of acyclovir and adenine arabinoside to prevent neonatal herpes. *Isr J Med Sci*. 1986;22:41-44.
27. Anderson H, Sutton RNP, Scarffe JH. Cytotoxic chemotherapy and viral infections: the role of acyclovir. *J R Coll Physicians Lond*. 1984;18:51-55.
28. Hockberger RS, Rothstein RJ. Varicella pneumonia in adults: a spectrum of disease. *Ann Emerg Med*. 1986;15:931-934.
29. Glaser JB, Loftus J, Ferragamo V, et al. Varicella-zoster infection in pregnancy. *N Engl J Med*. 1986;315:1416.
30. Tschen EH, Baack B. Treatment of herpetic whitlow in pregnancy with acyclovir. *J Am Acad Dermatol*. 1987;17:1059-1060.
31. Kundsin RB, Falk L, Hertig AT, Horne HW Jr. Acyclovir treatment of twelve unexplained infertile couples. *Int J Fertil*. 1987;32:200-204.
32. Chazotte C, Andersen HF, Cohen WR. Disseminated herpes simplex infection in an immunocompromised pregnancy: treatment with intravenous acyclovir. *Am J Perinatol*. 1987;4:363-364.
33. Cox SM, Phillips LE, DePaolo HD, Faro S. Treatment of disseminated herpes simplex virus in pregnancy with parenteral acyclovir: a case report. *J Reprod Med*. 1986;31:1005-1007.
34. Bernuau J, Caujolle B, Rouzioux C, et al. Severe acute hepatitis due to herpes-simplex in the third trimester of pregnancy: combating with acyclovir (abstract). *Gastroenterol Clin Biol*. 1987;11:79.
35. Hankins GDV, Gilstrap LC III, Patterson AR. Acyclovir treatment of varicella pneumonia in pregnancy. *Crit Care Med*. 1987;15:336-337.
36. Hankey GR, Bucens MR, Chambers JSW. Herpes simplex encephalitis in third trimester of pregnancy: successful outcome for mother and child. *Neurology*. 1987;37:1534-1537.
37. Frieden FJ, Ordorica SA, Goodgold AL, et al. Successful pregnancy with isolated herpes simplex virus encephalitis: case report and review of the literature. *Obstet Gynecol*. 1990;75:511-513.
38. Glorioso DV, Molloy PJ, Van Thiel DH, Kania RJ. Successful empiric treatment of HSV hepatitis in pregnancy. Case report and review of the literature. *Dig Dis Sci*. 1996;41:1273-1275.
39. Leen CLS, Mandal BK, Ellis ME. Acyclovir and pregnancy. *Br Med J*. 1987;294:308.
40. Eder SE, Apuzzio JJ, Weiss G. Varicella pneumonia during pregnancy: treatment of two cases with acyclovir. *Am J Perinatol*. 1988;5:16-18.
41. Boyd K, Walker E. Use of acyclovir to treat chickenpox in pregnancy. *BMJ*. 1988;296:393-394.
42. Key TC, Resnik R, Dittrich HC, Reisner LS. Successful pregnancy after cardiac transplantation. *Am J Obstet Gynecol*. 1989;160:367-371.
43. Stray-Pedersen B. Acyclovir in late pregnancy to prevent neonatal herpes simplex. *Lancet*. 1990;336:756.
44. Brocklehurst P, Carney O, Helson K, et al. Acyclovir, herpes, and pregnancy. *Lancet*. 1990;336:1594-1595.
45. Stray-Pedersen B. Acyclovir, herpes, and pregnancy. *Lancet*. 1990;336:1595.
46. Greenspoon JS, Wilcox JG, McHutchison LB. Does acyclovir improve the outcome of disseminated herpes simplex virus during pregnancy (abstract)? *Am J Obstet Gynecol*. 1991;164:400.
47. Broussard RG, Payne DK, George RB. Treatment with acyclovir of varicella pneumonia in pregnancy. *Chest*. 1991;99:1045-1047.
48. Smego RA Jr, Asperilla MO. Use of acyclovir for varicella pneumonia during pregnancy. *Obstet Gynecol*. 1991;78:1112-1116.
49. Ciraru-Vigneron N, Nguyen Tan Lung R, et al. Interest in the prescription acyclovir in the end of pregnancy in the case of genital herpes: a new protocol of the prevention of risks of herpes neonatal. *Presse Med*. 1987;16:128.
50. Haddad J, Langer B, Astruc D, et al. Oral acyclovir and recurrent genital herpes during late pregnancy. *Obstet Gynecol*. 1993;82:102-104.
51. Esmonde TF, Herdman G, Anderson G. Chickenpox pneumonia: an association with pregnancy. *Thorax*. 1989;44:812-815.
52. Horowitz GM, Hankins GDV. Early-second-trimester use of acyclovir in treating herpes zoster in a bone marrow transplant patient. A case report. *J Reprod Med*. 1992;37:280-282.
53. Gilbert GL. Chickenpox during pregnancy. *BMJ*. 1993;306:1079-1080.
54. Moling O, Mayr O, Gottardi H, et al. Severe pneumonia in pregnancy three months after resolution of cutaneous zoster. *Infection*. 1994;22:216-218.
55. Greenspoon JS, Wilcox JG, McHutchison LB, Rosen DJD. Acyclovir for disseminated herpes simplex virus in pregnancy. A case report. *J Reprod Med*. 1994;39:311-317.
56. Randolph AG, Hartshorn RM, Washington AE. Acyclovir prophylaxis in late pregnancy to prevent neonatal herpes: a cost-effectiveness analysis. *Obstet Gynecol*. 1996;88:603-610.
57. Scott LL, Sanchez PJ, Jackson GL, et al. Acyclovir suppression to prevent cesarean delivery after first-episode genital herpes. *Obstet Gynecol*. 1996;87:69-73.
58. Whitty JE, Renfroe YR, Bottoms SF, et al. Varicella pneumonia in pregnancy: clinical experience (abstract). *Am J Obstet Gynecol*. 1993;168:427.
59. Chandra PC, Patel H, Schiavello HJ, Briggs SL. Successful pregnancy outcome after complicated varicella pneumonia. *Obstet Gynecol*. 1998;92:680-682.
60. Wilton LV, Pearce GL, Martin RM, et al. The outcomes of pregnancy in women exposed to newly marketed drugs in general practice in England. *Br J Obstet Gynaecol*. 1998;105:882-889.
61. Anderson R, Lundqvist A, Bergstrom T. Successful treatment of generalized primary herpes simplex type 2 infection during pregnancy. *Scand J Infect Dis*. 1999;31:210-212.
62. Balfour HH Jr. Antiviral drugs. *N Engl J Med*. 1999;340:1255-1268.
63. Smith JR, Cowan FM, Munday P. The management of herpes simplex virus infection in pregnancy. *Br J Obstet Gynaecol*. 1998;105:255-260.
64. American College of Obstetricians and Gynecologists. ACOG practice bulletin No. 82: management of herpes in pregnancy. *Obstet Gynecol*. 2007;109:1489-1498.
65. Bork K, Kaiser T, Benes P. Transfer of aciclovir from plasma to human breast milk. *Drug Res*. 2000;50:656-658.
66. Lau RJ, Emery MG, Galinsky RE. Unexpected accumulation of acyclovir in breast milk with estimation of infant exposure. *Obstet Gynecol*. 1987;69:468-471.
67. Meyer LJ, de Miranda P, Sheth N, Spruance S. Acyclovir in human breast milk. *Am J Obstet Gynecol*. 1988;158:586-588.
68. Bork K, Benes P. Concentration and kinetic studies of intravenous acyclovir in serum and breast milk of a patient with eczema herpeticum. *J Am Acad Dermatol*. 1995;32:1053-1055.
69. Taddio A, Klein J, Koren G. Acyclovir excretion in human breast milk. *Ann Pharmacother*. 1994;28:585-587.
70. American Academy of Pediatrics Committee on Drugs. The transfer of drugs and other chemicals into human milk. *Pediatrics*. 2001;108:776-789.

ADAGRASIB

Antineoplastic (KRAS G12C Inhibitor)

PREGNANCY RECOMMENDATION: No Human Data—Animal Data Suggest Potential Risk

BREASTFEEDING RECOMMENDATION: Potential Toxicity

PREGNANCY SUMMARY

No reports describing the use of adagrasib in human pregnancy have been located. Some amount of the drug will probably cross the placenta, so fetal exposure will likely occur. However, the absence of human pregnancy experience prevents a complete assessment of the embryofetal risk. Animal studies did show embryofetal toxicity, but maternal toxicity also occurred. Using this drug during pregnancy should be based on the pros and cons of the mother's clinical need for treatment versus any potential fetal risk that might occur from exposure. The drug may also prolong the cardiac QT interval.

BREASTFEEDING SUMMARY

No reports describing the use of adagrasib during human lactation have been located. Some amount of the drug probably enters breast milk, so infant exposure will likely occur. However, due to the concern for potential serious adverse effects in a breastfed infant, the manufacturer recommends that women not breastfeed while being treated with this drug and for at least 1 week after the last dose. Nevertheless, breastfeeding while using this drug should be based on the mother's clinical need for treatment. If used, the infant should be monitored for the most common reported adult side effects of musculoskeletal pain and nausea (both leading to irritability), vomiting, decreased appetite (monitor growth), diarrhea, lethargy, edema, dyspnea, and several laboratory abnormalities (see PI).

Reference

1. Prescribing Information. Krazati. Mirati Therapeutics, Inc; 2022.

ADALIMUMAB

Immunologic (TNF-α Inhibitor—Monoclonal Antibody)

PREGNANCY RECOMMENDATION: Limited Human Data—Animal Data Suggest Low Risk (Maternal Benefit May Outweigh Any Embryofetal Risks)

BREASTFEEDING RECOMMENDATION: Probably Compatible

PREGNANCY SUMMARY

Numerous case reports and series have been located that describe the use of adalimumab during human pregnancy. The rate of major congenital malformations was about 4.4% in more than 270 pregnancies with first-trimester exposure. No pattern to the defects was identified. The drug has been shown to cross the placenta at delivery, with cord blood levels usually a little higher than the maternal serum concentrations. In addition, the drug may be detectable in the serum of infants for several weeks postdelivery. Therefore, this limited human pregnancy experience prevents a complete assessment of the embryofetal risk. Animal data did not show any embryofetal or teratogenicity in one species at doses of more than 10 times the RHD. In many circumstances, the maternal benefits from treatment with adalimumab, a tumor necrosis factor alpha (TNF-α) antagonist, appear to outweigh the unknown embryofetal risks. The World Congress of Gastroenterology and European League Against Rheumatism (EULAR) state that the use of biologic TNF inhibitors (including adalimumab) is overall compatible for use in pregnancy for many immunologic disorders. Because of the long elimination half-life, use before conception may result in inadvertent exposure to an unplanned pregnancy. If adalimumab is used in pregnancy for the treatment of rheumatoid arthritis, health care professionals are encouraged to call the toll-free number (877-311-8972) for information about patient enrollment in the Organization of Teratology Information Specialists (OTIS) Rheumatoid Arthritis study and pregnancy registry.

BREASTFEEDING SUMMARY

A few studies have been located that describe the use of adalimumab during human lactation. From three studies, the breast milk of 24 mothers was evaluated. The drug was not detected in the breast milk in 19 women (lower limit of quantification [LLQ] of 10 ng/mL). In the remaining five cases, the peak level for the drug was about 700 ng/mL. The calculated RIDs were all less than 1%. In two cases, the breast milk concentration was less than 0.1% of the maternal serum concentration. Therefore, exposure is negligible. Additionally, if any IgG antibodies were to be ingested through breastfeeding, they would probably be digested in the infant's gastrointestinal tract and not be absorbed. This is consistent with the drug not being detected in the blood (LLQ of 65 ng/mL) in two breastfeeding infants whose mothers were receiving treatment with adalimumab. Breastfeeding while using this drug should be based on the mother's clinical need for treatment versus any potential infant risks that might occur. If used, the infant should be monitored for the most common reported adult side effects of headache (leading to irritability), infections, and rash.

References

1. Gisbert JP. Safety of immunomodulators and biologics for the treatment of inflammatory bowel disease during pregnancy and breast-feeding. *Inflamm Bowel Dis*. 2010;16:881-895.

2. El Mourabet M, El-Hachem S, Harrison JR, Binion DG. Anti-TNF antibody therapy for inflammatory bowel disease during pregnancy: a clinical review. *Curr Drug Targets*. 2010;234-241.
3. Mahadevan U, Cucchiara S, Hyams JS, et al. The London position statement of the World Congress of Gastroenterology on biological therapy for IBD with the European Crohn's and Colitis Organization: pregnancy and pediatrics. *Am J Gastroenterol*. 2011;106:214-223.
4. Gotestam Skorpen C, Hoeltzenbein M, Tincani A, et al. The EULAR points to consider for use of antirheumatic drugs before pregnancy, and during pregnancy and lactation. *Ann Rheum Dis*. 2016;75:795-810.
5. Khanna D, McMahon M, Furst DE. Safety of tumour necrosis factor-α antagonists. *Drug Saf*. 2004;27:307-324.
6. Prescribing Information. Humira. AbbVie; 2019.
7. Mahadevan U, Wolf DC, Dubinsky M, et al. Placental transfer of anti-tumor necrosis factor agents in pregnant patients with inflammatory bowel disease. *Clin Gastroenterol Hepatol*. 2013;11:286-292.
8. Vesga L, Terdiman JP, Mahadevan U. Adalimumab use in pregnancy. *Gut*. 2005;54:890.
9. Mishkin D, Van Deinse W, Becker J, Farraye FA. Successful use of adalimumab (Humira) for Crohn's disease in pregnancy. *Inflamm Bowel Dis*. 2006;12:827-828.
10. Coburn LA, Wise PE, Schwartz DA. The successful use of adalimumab to treat active Crohn's disease of an ileoanal pouch during pregnancy. *Dig Dis Sci*. 2006;51:2045-2047.
11. Hyrich KL, Symmons DPM, Watson KD, Silman AJ. Pregnancy outcome in women who were exposed to anti-tumor necrosis factor agents: results from a national population register. *Arthritis Rheum*. 2006;54:2701-2702.
12. Roux CH, Brocq O, Breuil V, et al. Pregnancy in rheumatology patients exposed to anti-tumour necrosis factor (TNF)-α therapy. *Rheumatology*. 2007; 46:695-698.
13. Kraemer B, Abele H, Hahn M, et al. A successful pregnancy in a patient with Takayasu's arteritis. *Hypertens Pregnancy*. 2008;27:247-252.
14. Velinov M, Zellers N. The fetal mycophenolate mofetil syndrome. *Clin Dysmorphol*. 2008;17:77-78.
15. Berthelot JM, De Bandt M, Goupille P, et al; On behalf of CRI (Club Rhumatismes et Inflammation). Exposition to anti-TNF drugs during pregnancy: outcome of 15 cases and review of the literature. *Joint Bone Spine*. 2009;76:28-34.
16. Jurgens M, Brand S, Filik L, et al. Safety of adalimumab in Crohn's disease during pregnancy: case report and review of the literature. *Inflamm Bowel Dis*. 2010;16:1634-1636.
17. Carter JD, Ladhani A, Ricca LR, et al. A safety assessment of tumor necrosis factor antagonists during pregnancy: a review of the Food and Drug Administration database. *J Rheumatol*. 2009;36:635-641.
18. Dessinioti C, Stefanaki I, Stratigos AJ, et al. Pregnancy during adalimumab use for psoriasis. *J Eur Acad Dermatol Venereol*. 2011;25:738-739.
19. Ben-Horin S, Yavzori M, Katz L, et al. Adalimumab level in breast milk of a nursing mother. *Clin Gastroenterol Hepatol*. 2010;8:475-476.
20. Winger EE, Reed JL, Ashoush S, et al. Treatment with adalimumab (Humira) and intravenous immunoglobulin improves pregnancy rates in women undergoing IVF. *Am J Reprod Immunol*. 2009;61:113-120.
21. Bortlik M, Machkova N, Duricova D, et al. Pregnancy and newborn outcome of mothers with inflammatory bowel diseases exposed to anti-TNF-α therapy during pregnancy: three-center study. *Scand J Gastroenterol*. 2013;48:951-958.
22. Casanova MJ, Chaparro M, Domenech E, et al. Safety of thiopurines and anti-TNF-α drugs during pregnancy in patients with inflammatory bowel disease. *Am J Gastroenterol*. 2013;108:433-440.
23. Zelinkova Z, van der Ent C, Bruin KF, et al; Dutch Delta IBD Group. Effects of discontinuing anti-tumor necrosis factor therapy during pregnancy on the course of inflammatory bowel disease and neonatal exposure. *Clin Gastroenterol Hepatol*. 2013;11:318-321.
24. Chambers C, Johnson D, Luo Y, Xu R, Jones K. Pregnancy outcome in women treated with adalimumab for the treatment of rheumatoid arthritis: an update on the OTIS autoimmune diseases in pregnancy project. *Am J Gastroenterol*. 2014;109(suppl):S638.
25. Giacuzzo S, Padovan M, Capucci R, et al. Pregnancy outcome of mothers with rheumatic diseases exposed to biological agent during pregnancy: a single-centre study. *Ann Rheum Dis*. 2014;73(suppl 2):414.
26. Kelly O, Hartery K, Boland K, et al. TNF alpha inhibitor use in pregnancy: experience in a European cohort. *J Crohn's Colitis*. 2014;8:S204-S205.
27. Seirafi M, de Vroey B, Amiot A, et al. Factors associated with pregnancy outcome in anti-TNF treated women with inflammatory bowel disease. *Aliment Pharmacol Ther*. 2014;40:363-373.
28. Diav-Citrin O, Otcheretianski-Volodarsky A, Schechtman S, Ornoy A. Pregnancy outcome following gestational exposure to TNF-α–inhibitors: a prospective, comparative, observational study. *Reprod Toxicol*. 2014;43:78-84.
29. Weber-Schoendorfer C, Oppermann M, Wacker E, et al. Pregnancy outcome after TNF-α inhibitor therapy during the first trimester: a prospective multicenter cohort study. *Br J Clin Pharmacol*. 2015;80:727-729.
30. Bazzani C, Scrivo R, Andreoli L, et al. Prospectively-followed pregnancies in patients with inflammatory arthritis taking biological drugs: an Italian multicenter study. *Clin Exp Rheumatol*. 2015;33:688-693.

ADAPALENE

Dermatologic (Retinoid—Topical)

PREGNANCY RECOMMENDATION: Limited Human Data—Animal Data Suggest Low Risk

BREASTFEEDING RECOMMENDATION: Probably Compatible

PREGNANCY SUMMARY

Three reports were located that describe the use of adapalene during human pregnancy. The manufacturer reported on four unintended pregnancies with first-trimester exposure that delivered healthy newborns with no major malformations identified. In a second study, of 119 pregnancies (excluding elective terminations), there were 7 (6%) spontaneous abortions and 2 (1.8%) congenital anomalies in the 112 that delivered live newborns. However, the gestational ages of the exposures were not provided. The third was a case report of an anomalous fetus that was exposed in the first trimester, but the defects did not fit what is usually seen with retinoid-induced malformations. The amount of drug that might cross the placenta is likely to be negligible due to the minimal systemic absorption seen with topical use. Therefore, this limited human pregnancy experience prevents a complete assessment of the embryofetal risk. Animal data did not show any embryofetal toxicity in two species with topical use at doses of less than 10 times the RHD in one and more than 10 times the RHD in the second. Using this drug during pregnancy should be based on the pros and cons of the mother's clinical need for treatment versus any potential fetal risk that might occur from exposure. Some experts question the treatment of acne during pregnancy.

BREASTFEEDING SUMMARY

No reports describing the use of adapalene during human lactation have been located. Any amount of drug that may be found in breast milk will likely be clinically insignificant due to low systemic absorption with topical use. Breastfeeding while using this drug should be based on the mother's clinical need for treatment versus any potential infant risks that might occur. Due to the topical use, systemic side effects were not evaluated.

References

1. Prescribing Information. Differin. Galderma Laboratories; 2020.
2. Weiss JS, Mallavalli S, Meckfessel MH, et al. Safe use of adapalene 0.1% gel in a non-prescription environment. *J Drus Dermatol*. 2021;20:1330-1335.
3. Autret E, Berjot M, Jonville-Bera AP, et al. Anophthalmia and agenesis of optic chiasma associated with adapalene gel in early pregnancy. *Lancet*. 1997; 350:339.

ADEFOVIR

Antiviral (Hepatitis B/HIV)

PREGNANCY RECOMMENDATION: Limited Human Data—Animal Data Suggest Low Risk (Maternal Benefit Probably Outweighs Any Embryofetal Risk)

BREASTFEEDING RECOMMENDATION: Probably Compatible (Hepatitis B)/*Contraindicated (HIV)

PREGNANCY SUMMARY

The APR reported, for the period January 1989 through January 2024, prospective data (before the outcomes were known) involving 12,314 live births that had been exposed during the first trimester to one or more antiretroviral agents. No congenital defects were noted in 82 cases with the use of adefovir. The overall birth anomaly rate for the entire registry is about 2.96% in 12,314 pregnancies. No pattern to the anomalies has ever been identified. In a second study evaluating the use of adefovir in treating hepatitis B virus (HBV) infections, no anomalies were seen in 11 pregnancies with early exposure to adefovir. Lastly, from data submitted to the US Food and Drug Administration (FDA) Adverse Event Reporting System, no increased signal for congenital birth defects was seen in 242 cases with adefovir use in treating HBV infections. The drug will likely cross the placenta, so some fetal exposure will probably occur. However, this limited human pregnancy experience prevents a complete assessment of the embryofetal risk. For HIV, in order to decrease the perinatal transmission of HIV-1 to the neonate, this drug should not be withheld if a pregnant woman is infected with HIV-1, especially if she has a positive viral load, or is failing her current treatment regimen, and is a candidate for this drug's usage. There is a pregnancy exposure registry that monitors pregnancy outcomes in patients using antiretroviral medicines, including adefovir during pregnancy. Health care providers are encouraged to call the APR at 1-800-258-4263.

BREASTFEEDING SUMMARY

No reports describing the use of adefovir during human lactation have been located. The drug will likely be excreted into breast milk, so some infant exposure will probably occur. Women infected with hepatitis B can breastfeed without additional risk for the transmission of hepatitis B to the infant as long as the newborn receives the hepatitis B immunoglobulin and the hepatitis B vaccine. However, due to a concern for potential serious adverse effects that might be seen in a breastfed infant, the manufacturer recommends that women not breastfeed while being treated with this drug. Nevertheless, breastfeeding while using this drug should be based on the mother's clinical need for treatment versus any potential infant risks that might occur. If used, the infant should be monitored for the most common reported adult side effects of nausea and asthenia (both leading to irritability), and vomiting. *Regarding HIV, the current CDC recommendation is that mothers infected with HIV should not breastfeed their infants in order to reduce the risk of postnatal transmission of the virus to the neonate. In a clinical setting where a mother is not infected with HIV (or in cases where the HIV viral load is negative), the drug by itself is probably compatible.

References

1. Prescribing Information. Hepsera. Gilead Sciences; 2019.
2. Horowitz HW, Telzak EE, Sepkowitz KA, Wormser GP. Human immunodeficiency virus infection, part II. *Dis Mon*. 1998;44:677-716.
3. Lee JS, Mullaney S, Bronson R, et al. Transplacental antiretroviral therapy with 9-(2-phosphonylmethoxyethyl)adenine is embryotoxic in transgenic mice. *J Acquir Immune Defic Syndr*. 1991;4:833-838.
4. Antiretroviral Pregnancy Registry Steering Committee. Antiretroviral Pregnancy Registry international interim report for 1 January 1989 through 31 January 2024. Registry Coordinating Center. Published 2009. Accessed January 23, 2025. www.apregistry.com
5. Carpenter CCJ, Fischi MA, Hammer SM, et al. Antiretroviral therapy for HIV infection in 1996. *JAMA*. 1996;276;146-154.
6. Minkoff H, Augenbraun M. Antiretroviral therapy for pregnant women. *Am J Obstet Gynecol*. 1997;176:478-489.
7. Minkoff H. Human immunodeficiency virus infection in pregnancy. *Obstet Gynecol*. 2003;101:797-810.
8. Panel on Treatment of HIV During Pregnancy and Prevention of Perinatal Transmission. Recommendations for the use of antiretroviral drugs during pregnancy and interventions to reduce perinatal HIV transmission in the United States. *Department of Health and Human Services*. Accessed July 25, 2023. https://clinicalinfo.hiv.gov/en/guidelines/perinatal

9. Brown ZA, Watts DH. Antiviral therapy in pregnancy. *Clin Obstet Gynecol.* 1990;33:276-289.
10. De Martino M, Tovo P-A, Pezzotti P, et al. HIV-1 transmission through breast-milk: appraisal of risk according to duration of feeding. *AIDS.* 1992; 6:991-997.
11. Van de Perre P. Postnatal transmission of human immunodeficiency virus type 1: the breast feeding dilemma. *Am J Obstet Gynecol.* 1995;173:483-487.
12. Gao X, Duan X, Cai H, et al. Pregnancy outcomes for pregnant women with hepatitis B exposing to entecavir or adefovir dipivoxil therapy or in early pregnancy. *J Matern Fetal Neonatal Med.* 2022;35:476-480.
13. Yang R, Yin N, Zhao Y, et al. Adverse events during pregnancy associated with entecavir and adefovir: new insights from a real-world analysis of cases reported to FDA adverse event reporting system. *Front Pharmacol.* 2022;12:772768.

ADENOSINE

Cardiovascular (Antiarrhythmic/Diagnostic)

PREGNANCY RECOMMENDATION: Limited Human Data and No Relevant Animal Data (Maternal Benefit May Outweigh Any Embryofetal Risk)

BREASTFEEDING RECOMMENDATION: Probably Compatible

PREGNANCY SUMMARY

Numerous case reports and series have been located that describe the use of adenosine during human pregnancy in all trimesters. Most exposures were in the second and third trimesters to convert supraventricular tachycardia (SVT) in the mother with good outcomes. A few first-trimester exposures have occurred with no reported anomalies found in the newborns at delivery. The drug has also been used in treating malignant fetal tachycardias by direct injection with some success. Endogenous adenosine has been found in cord blood, and the drug should cross if it reaches the placental interface. However, with an elimination half-life of less than 10 seconds, the amounts are likely to be clinically insignificant. Therefore, this limited first-trimester human pregnancy experience prevents a complete assessment of the embryofetal risk. Animal reproduction and fertility studies have not been conducted. Using this drug during pregnancy should be based on the pros and cons of the mother's clinical need for treatment versus any potential fetal risk that might occur from exposure. However, the risks for poor pregnancy outcomes with significant maternal SVT are likely to be high if left untreated.

BREASTFEEDING SUMMARY

No reports describing the use of adenosine during human lactation have been located. Because adenosine is only used by IV injection in acute care situations, it is doubtful that any reports will be located. In addition, with an elimination half-life of less than 10 seconds, the drug will be out of the maternal blood system in 1 to 2 minutes. Therefore, this would not likely affect any ability to breastfeed, if desired, and she is capable of breastfeeding.

References

1. Page RL, Joglar RL, Al-Khatib SM, et al. 2015 ACC/AHA/HRS guideline for the management of adult patients with supraventricular tachycardia: a report of the American College of Cardiology/American Heart Association Task Force on Clinical Practice Guidelines and the Heart Rhythm Society. *Circulation.* 2015;132:1-131.
2. Prescribing Information. Adenosine. Sagent Pharmaceuticals; 2019.
3. Shepard TH. *Catalog of Teratogenic Agents.* 6th ed. Johns Hopkins University Press; 1989:194.
4. Bissonnette JM, Hohimer AR, Knopp SJ. The effect of centrally administered adenosine on fetal breath movements. *Respir Physiol.* 1991;84:273-285.
5. Mason B, Ogunyemi D, Punla O, Koos B. Maternal and fetal cardiovascular effects of intravenous adenosine (abstract). *Am J Obstet Gynecol.* 1993;168:439.
6. Mason BA, Ogunyemi D, Punla O, Koos BJ. Maternal and fetal cardiorespiratory responses to adenosine in sheep. *Am J Obstet Gynecol.* 1993;168: 1558-1561.
7. Landauer M, Phernetton TM, Rankin JHG. Maternal ovine placental vascular responses to adenosine. *Am J Obstet Gynecol.* 1986;154:1152-1155.
8. Ross Russell RI, Greenough A, Lagercrantz H, et al. Fetal anaemia and its relation with increased concentrations of adenosine. *Arch Dis Child Fetal Neonatal.* 1993;68:35-36.
9. Podolsky SM, Varon J. Adenosine use during pregnancy. *Ann Emerg Med.* 1991;20:1027-1028.
10. Harrison JK, Greenfield RA, Wharton JM. Acute termination of supraventricular tachycardia by adenosine during pregnancy. *Am Heart J.* 1992;123: 1386-1388.
11. Mason BA, Ricci-Goodman J, Koos BJ. Adenosine in the treatment of maternal paroxysmal supraventricular tachycardia. *Obstet Gynecol.* 1992;80: 478-480.
12. Afridi I, Moise KJ Jr, Rokey R. Termination of supraventricular tachycardia with intravenous adenosine in a pregnant woman with Wolff-Parkinson-White syndrome. *Obstet Gynecol.* 1992;80:481-483.
13. Leffler S, Johnson DR. Adenosine use in pregnancy. Lack of effect on fetal heart rate. *Am J Emerg Med.* 1992;10:548-549.
14. Propp DA, Broderick K, Pesch D. Adenosine during pregnancy. *Ann Emerg Med.* 1992;21:453-454.
15. Adair RF. Fetal monitoring with adenosine administration. *Ann Emerg Med.* 1993;22:1925.
16. Matfin G, Baylis P, Adams P. Maternal paroxysmal supraventricular tachycardia treated with adenosine. *Postgrad Med J.* 1993;69:661-662.
17. Hagley MT, Cole PL. Adenosine use in pregnant women with supraventricular tachycardia. *Ann Pharmacother.* 1994;28:1241-1242.
18. Elkayam U, Goodwin TM Jr. Adenosine therapy for supraventricular tachycardia during pregnancy. *Am J Cardiol.* 1995;75:521-523.
19. Hagley MT, Haraden B, Cole PL. Adenosine use in a pregnant patient with supraventricular tachycardia. *Ann Pharmacother.* 1995;29:938.
20. Kohl T, Tercanli S, Kececioglu D, Holzgreve W. Direct fetal administration of adenosine for the termination of incessant supraventricular tachycardia. *Obstet Gynecol.* 1995;85:873-874.
21. Hubinont C, Debauche C, Bernard P, Sluysmans T. Resolution of fetal tachycardia and hydrops by a single adenosine administration. *Obstet Gynecol.* 1998;92(part 2):718.
22. Dangel JH, Roszkowski T, Bieganowska K, et al. Adenosine triphosphate for cardioversion of supraventricular tachycardia in two hydropic fetuses. *Fetal Diagn Ther.* 2000;15:326-330.

ADO-TRASTUZUMAB EMTANSINE

Antineoplastic (HER2 Targeted Antibody-Drug Conjugate—Monoclonal Antibody)

PREGNANCY RECOMMENDATION: Limited Human Data Suggest Risk—Animal Data Suggest Risk

BREASTFEEDING RECOMMENDATION: Potential Toxicity

PREGNANCY SUMMARY

Postmarketing studies and case reports have described findings of fetal renal failure producing severe oligohydramnios leading to pulmonary hypoplasia and poor pregnancy outcome with trastuzumab, pertuzumab, and ado-trastuzumab emtansine. It is not known if this is related to first-trimester use or if it occurs later in pregnancy, as seen with angiotensin-converting enzyme (ACE) and angiotensin II receptor blocker (ARB) inhibitors. Human IgG antibodies are known to cross the placenta, especially during the second and third trimesters, which suggests that some transfer will occur. It is also not known how much emtansine disassociates from the antibody prior to entering the cancer cell, but some levels are found systemically. This drug component will also likely cross by itself, and because it is a microtubule disruptor, it could produce some fetal harm. Based on animal studies and the drug's mechanism of action, the manufacturer recommends that women with reproductive potential use effective contraception during treatment and for 6 months after the last dose. The drug carries a boxed warning for an increased risk of hepatotoxicity, cardiac toxicity, and embryofetal toxicity. Using this drug during pregnancy should be based on the pros and cons of the mother's clinical need for treatment versus any potential fetal risk that might occur from exposure. If pregnancy occurs when taking this drug, the manufacturer requests that this be reported to the adverse event line at 888-835-2555. In addition, if pregnancy exposure to ado-trastuzumab emtansine occurs, health care providers are encouraged to enroll patients in the MotHER Pregnancy Registry by calling 800-690-6720.

BREASTFEEDING SUMMARY

No reports describing the use of ado-trastuzumab emtansine during human lactation have been located. It is known that IgG antibodies can be found in human breast milk, but are not found in the neonatal or infant circulation. Additionally, if any IgG antibodies were to be ingested through breastfeeding, they would probably be digested in the infant's gastrointestinal tract and not be absorbed. Nevertheless, the concern with this drug is DM1 mertansine, which is a microtubule disrupter with a MW of only 738. This drug, if found separate from the antibody, could cross and theoretically be harmful to the newborn. Due to a concern for potential serious adverse effects that might be seen in a breastfed infant, the manufacturer recommends that women not breastfeed while being treated with this drug and for at least 7 months after the last dose. Breastfeeding while using this drug should be based on the mother's clinical need for treatment versus any potential infant risks that might occur. If used, the infant should be monitored for the most common reported adult side effects of nausea, headache, and musculoskeletal pain (all leading to irritability), fatigue (lethargy), constipation, and various laboratory abnormalities (see PI).

References

1. Prescribing Information. Kadcyla. Genentech Incorporation; 2018.
2. Gougis P, Grandal B, Jochum F, et al. Treatments during pregnancy targeting ERBB2 and outcomes of pregnant individuals and newborns. *JAM Netw Open*. 2023;6:e2339934.

ADUCANUMAB

Central Nervous System (Monoclonal Antibody—Alzheimer)

PREGNANCY RECOMMENDATION: No Human Data and No Relevant Animal Data

BREASTFEEDING RECOMMENDATION: Probably Compatible

PREGNANCY SUMMARY

No reports describing the use of aducanumab in human pregnancy have been located. As an IgG, it likely crosses the placenta, so some fetal exposure will probably occur. Therefore, the absence of human pregnancy experience prevents a complete assessment of the embryofetal risk. Animal data did not show any embryofetal toxicity, but the relevance to humans is limited as the pharmacologic target (aggregated amyloid β) is not present in rats. Using this drug during pregnancy should be based on the pros and cons of the mother's clinical need for treatment versus any potential fetal risk that might occur from exposure.

BREASTFEEDING SUMMARY

No reports describing the use of aducanumab during human lactation have been located. It is known that IgG antibodies can be found in human breast milk, but are not found in the neonatal or infant circulation. Additionally, if any IgG antibodies were to be ingested through breastfeeding, they would probably be digested in the infant's gastrointestinal tract and not be absorbed. Breastfeeding while using this drug should be based on the mother's clinical need for treatment. If used, the infant should be monitored for the most common reported adult side effects of headache (leading to irritability) and edema.

Reference

1. Prescribing Information. Aduhelm. Biogen, Inc; 2022.

AFAMELANOTIDE

Dermatologic (Implant)

PREGNANCY RECOMMENDATION: No Human Data—Animal Data Suggest Low Risk

BREASTFEEDING RECOMMENDATION: Probably Compatible

PREGNANCY SUMMARY

No reports describing the use of afamelanotide during human pregnancy were located. The drug will not likely cross the placenta, especially in the first trimester. However, because it is a peptide, some fetal exposure might occur in the third trimester. Therefore, this limited human pregnancy experience prevents a complete assessment of the embryofetal risk. Animal studies did not show any embryofetal toxicity in one species at doses of more than 10 times the RHD. Using this drug during pregnancy should be based on the pros and cons of the mother's clinical need for treatment versus any potential fetal risk that might occur from exposure.

BREASTFEEDING SUMMARY

No reports describing the use of afamelanotide during human lactation have been located. The drug will not likely be found in breast milk. Additionally, because it is a peptide consisting of 13 amino acids, if the drug were to be ingested through breastfeeding, it would probably be digested in the infant's gastrointestinal tract and not be absorbed. Breastfeeding while using this drug should be based on the mother's clinical need for treatment versus any potential infant risks. If used, the infant should be monitored for the most common reported adult side effects of nausea and oropharyngeal pain (both leading to irritability), somnolence, fatigue (lethargy), cough, and skin irritation.

References

1. Prescribing Information. Scenesse. Clinuvel; 2020.
2. Bioclati G, Marchesini E, Sorge F, et al. Long-term observational study of afamelanotide in 115 patients with erythropoietic protoporphyria. *Br J Dermatol*. 2015;172:1601-1612.

AFATINIB

Antineoplastic (Tyrosine Kinase Inhibitor)

PREGNANCY RECOMMENDATION: Limited Human Data—Animal Data Suggest Risk

BREASTFEEDING RECOMMENDATION: Potential Toxicity

PREGNANCY SUMMARY

One case report of first-trimester exposure to afatinib was located. She ultimately delivered at term, a healthy newborn with no identified anomalies or complications. The child was progressing well at 16 months of age. The drug will likely cross the placenta, so some fetal exposure will probably occur. However, this limited human pregnancy experience prevents a complete assessment of the embryofetal risk. Animal studies did show embryofetal toxicity in two species at doses less than 10 times the RHD. Based on animal studies and the drug's mechanism of action, the manufacturer recommends that women with reproductive potential use effective contraception during treatment and for 2 weeks after the last dose. Nevertheless, using this drug during pregnancy should be based on the pros and cons of the mother's clinical need for treatment versus any potential fetal risk that might occur from exposure. There is a registry for women who are pregnant and have cancer. For more information, women and health care providers are encouraged to contact the Cancer and Pregnancy Registry at 1-877-635-4499.

BREASTFEEDING SUMMARY

No reports describing the use of afatinib during human lactation have been located. The drug will likely be found in breast milk, so some infant exposure will probably occur. Due to the concern for potential serious adverse effects that might be seen in a breastfed infant, the manufacturer recommends that women not breastfeed while being treated with this drug and for at least 2 weeks after the last dose. Nevertheless, breastfeeding while using this drug should be based on the mother's clinical need for treatment. If used, the infant should be monitored for the most common reported adult side effects of nausea and pruritus (both leading to irritability), diarrhea, vomiting, rash, and decreased appetite.

References

1. Prescribing Information. Gilotrif. Boehringer Ingelheim Pharmaceuticals; 2020.
2. Pina PS, Lara-Mejis L, Matias-Cruz V, et al. Case report: osimertinib administration during pregnancy in a woman with advanced EGFR-mutant non-small cell lung cancer. *Front Oncol*. 2023;13:1108124.

AFLIBERCEPT OPHTHALMIC

Ophthalmic (Intravitreal—VEGF Receptor Inhibitor)

PREGNANCY RECOMMENDATION: Limited Human Data—Animal Data Suggest Low Risk

BREASTFEEDING RECOMMENDATION: Probably Compatible

PREGNANCY SUMMARY

Two reports were located that described the use of aflibercept during human pregnancy. In one publication, two patients used the drug, one in the first trimester and the second at 13 weeks' gestation. Both delivered at term with no newborn malformations noted. The second study was a disproportionality analysis of the FDA Adverse Event Reporting System that found an increased signal for pregnancy loss with the use of vascular endothelial growth factor (VEGF) inhibitors, bevacizumab, ranibizumab, and aflibercept, which requires further study. The drug will likely cross the placenta in the second half of gestation, so some fetal exposure will probably occur. Therefore, this limited human pregnancy experience prevents a complete assessment of the embryofetal risk. Animal data did not show any embryofetal toxicity in one species at doses of more than 10 times the recommended human intraocular dose. Using this drug during pregnancy should be based on the pros and cons of the mother's clinical need for treatment versus any potential fetal risk that might occur from exposure.

BREASTFEEDING SUMMARY

One report describing the use of aflibercept ophthalmic during human lactation was located. The drug was not detected until day 4 at a concentration of about 11 ng/mL. This level is consistent with the levels found following systemic absorption with intravitreal use. However, because it is primarily a protein, if ingested through breastfeeding, it would probably be digested in the infant's gastrointestinal tract and not be absorbed. Regardless, due to a concern for potential serious adverse effects that might be seen in a breastfed infant, the manufacturer recommends that women not breastfeed while being treated with this drug. Nevertheless, breastfeeding while using this drug should be based on the mother's clinical need for treatment versus any potential infant risks that might occur. Because of the ophthalmic use of the drug, systemic side effects were not evaluated.

References

1. Prescribing Information. Eylea. Regeneron Pharmaceuticals; 2017.
2. Ong AY, Kilre CA, Frise C, et al. Intravitreal anti-vascular endothelial growth factor injections in pregnancy and breastfeeding: a case series and systematic review of the literature. *Eye (Lond)*. 2024;38:951-963.
3. Sakai T, Mori C, Ohtsu F. Potential safety signal of pregnancy loss with vascular endothelial growth factor inhibitor intraocular injections: a disproportionality analysis using the Food and Drug Administration Adverse Event Reporting System. *Front Pharmacol*. 2022;13:1063625.
4. SakaiJuncal VR, Paracha Q, Bamakrid M, et al. Ranibizumab and aflibercept levels in breast milk after intravitreal injection. *Ophthalmology*. 2020: 127:278-280.

AGALSIDASE BETA

Genetic/Metabolic (Fabry Disease—Enzyme)

PREGNANCY RECOMMENDATION: Limited Human Data—Animal Data Suggest Low Risk (Maternal Benefit May Outweigh Any Embryofetal Risk)

BREASTFEEDING RECOMMENDATION: Probably Compatible

PREGNANCY SUMMARY

The successful use of agalsidase beta during human pregnancy has been described in a few reports. Four infants were exposed throughout most of the pregnancy, and no major anomalies were identified at delivery. In addition, there have been a few studies published on pregnancy exposure to agalsidase alfa. A total of 10 pregnancies had exposure again throughout most of the pregnancy, and no major malformations were described at birth. Because it is a protein, it is not known whether some placental transfer might occur in the second half of pregnancy, so fetal exposure may occur. However, this limited human pregnancy experience prevents a complete assessment of the embryofetal risk. Animal data did not show any embryofetal toxicity in one species at doses of less than 10 times the RHD. Fabry disease is a debilitating condition that can be markedly improved by the use of enzyme replacement therapy. If a woman requires enzyme replacement therapy and gives informed consent, the enzyme should not be withheld because of pregnancy.

BREASTFEEDING SUMMARY

No reports describing the use of agalsidase beta during human lactation have been located. One study did describe the use of agalsidase alfa in six lactating women who had Fabry disease. No breast milk drug levels were analyzed, but overall, none of the six infants had any major side effects from exposure. Overall, excretion into breast milk should be negligible. However, if any of this protein were to be ingested through breastfeeding, it would probably be digested in the infant's gastrointestinal tract and not be absorbed. Even if not fully digested, there is poor oral absorption of this enzyme. The endogenous enzyme, α-galactosidase A, is present in the maternal bloodstream and also found in newborns. Breastfeeding while using this drug should be based on the mother's clinical need for treatment versus any potential infant risks that might occur. If used, the infant should be monitored for the most common reported adult side effects of headache, dizziness, myalgia, and musculoskeletal pain (all leading to irritability), fatigue (lethargy), cough, peripheral edema, and rash. Moreover, the indication for enzyme replacement therapy implies that the mother may be dependent on this treatment and received it during pregnancy. The overall risk to a nursing infant from maternal use is likely to be negligible.

References

1. Prescribing Information. Fabrazyme. Genzyme; 2012.
2. Lee K, Jin X, Zhang K, Copertino L, et al. A biochemical and pharmacological comparison of enzyme replacement therapies for the glycolipid storage disorder Fabry disease. *Glycobiology*. 2003;13:305-313.
3. Wendt S, Whybra C, Kampmann C, et al. Successful pregnancy outcome in a patient with Fabry disease receiving enzyme replacement therapy with agalsidase alfa. *J Inherit Metab Dis*. 2005;28:787-788.
4. Kalkum G, Macchiella D, Reinke J, et al. Enzyme replacement therapy with agalsidase alfa in pregnant women with Fabry disease. *Eur J Obstet Gynecol Reprod Biol*. 2009;144:92-93.
5. Germain DP, Bruneval P, Tran TC, et al. Uneventful pregnancy outcome after enzyme replacement therapy agalsidase beta in a heterozygous female with Fabry disease: a case report. *Eur J Med Genet*. 2010;53:111-112.
6. Politei JM. Treatment with agalsidase beta during pregnancy in Fabry disease. *J Obstet Gynaecol Res*. 2010;36:428-429.
7. Thurberg BL, Politei JM. Histologic abnormalities of placental tissues in Fabry disease: a case report and review of the literature. *Hum Pathol*. 2012;43:610-614.
8. Tasci ES, Bicik Z. Safe and successful treatment with agalsidase beta during pregnancy in Fabry disease. *Iran J Kidney Dis*. 2015;9:406-408.
9. Iwafuchi Y, Maruyama H, Morioka T, et al. Enzyme replacement therapy in a patient of heterozygous Fabry disease: clinical and pathological evaluations by repeat kidney biopsy and a successful pregnancy. *CEN Case Rep*. 2017;6:210-214.
10. Fernandez P, Fernandez SO, Gonzalez JGM, Enzyme replacement therapy in pregnant women with Fabry disease: a case series. *JIMD Rep*. 2019;45:77-81.

AIR POLYMER-TYPE A

Diagnostic (Ultrasound Contrast Agent)

PREGNANCY RECOMMENDATION: Contraindicated

BREASTFEEDING RECOMMENDATION: Probably Compatible

PREGNANCY SUMMARY

No reports describing the use of air polymer-type A in human pregnancy have been located. Because cellulose is not systemically absorbed, this substance would not be expected to cross the human placenta. Glycerol exists naturally in the bloodstream, and because plasma levels would not change following absorption, this would also not affect placental transfer. Nevertheless, because the preparation is used to determine fallopian tube patency, use of this agent is contraindicated during pregnancy. When used, the patient needs to be in the preovulatory phase of her menstrual cycle and have a negative pregnancy test.

BREASTFEEDING SUMMARY

Because cellulose is not systemically absorbed and glycerol exists naturally in the bloodstream, if the clinical decision were to use this product in a lactating woman, continued breastfeeding could probably occur.

Reference

1. Prescribing Information. ExEm Foam. ExEm Foam, Inc; 2019.

ALBENDAZOLE

Anti-Infective (Anthelmintic)

PREGNANCY RECOMMENDATION: Limited Human Data—Animal Data Suggest Potential Risk

BREASTFEEDING RECOMMENDATION: Probably Compatible

PREGNANCY SUMMARY

Several studies have been located that describe the use of albendazole during human pregnancy. Three (3.7%) major congenital anomalies were found in more than 80 first-trimester exposures. Several reports exist that describe use in the second and third trimesters with no reported major complications seen related to the drug. Albendazole is rapidly metabolized before it reaches the systemic circulation. However, the active metabolite, albendazole sulfoxide, does reach the circulation and is the primary therapeutic agent. This metabolite will probably cross the placenta, so some fetal exposure will likely occur. Therefore, this limited human pregnancy experience prevents a complete assessment of the embryofetal risk. Animal data did show some embryofetal toxicity in one species at doses of less than the RHD. The same was seen in a second species, but significant maternal toxicity also occurred. No embryofetal toxicity was seen in a third species at doses of less than the RHD. Because parenchymal neurocysticercosis and cystic hydatid disease can lead to long-term medical consequences, using this drug, especially in the second and third trimesters, should be considered.

BREASTFEEDING SUMMARY

One study was located that evaluated breast milk levels for albendazole sulfoxide in 33 women. The mean peak concentration for the drug was about 352 ng/mL. The average level at about 36 hours after a dose was 57 ng/mL. The calculated RID was less than 1%. Infant blood levels have not been analyzed. Breastfeeding while using this drug should be based on the mother's clinical need for treatment versus any potential infant risks that might occur. If used, the infant should be monitored for the most common reported adult side effects of nausea, headache, dizziness, and abdominal pain (all leading to irritability), vomiting, and elevated liver function tests.

References

1. Mantovani A, Ricciardi C, Stazi AV, Macri C. Effects observed on gestational day 13 in rat embryos exposed to albendazole. *Reprod Toxicol*. 1995;9:265-273.
2. de Silva N, Guyatt H, Bundy D. Anthelmintics. A comparative review of their clinical pharmacology. *Drugs*. 1997;53:769-788.
3. Prescribing Information. Albenza. Ameda Pharmaceuticals; 2018.
4. Mantovani A, Macri C, Stazi AV, Ricciardi C. Effects of albendazole on the early phases of rat organogenesis in vivo: preliminary results (abstract). *Teratology*. 1992;46:25A.
5. Horton J. The use of antiprotozoan and anthelmintic drugs during pregnancy and contraindications. *J Infect*. 1993;26:104-105.
6. Torlesse H, Hodges M. Anthelmintic treatment and haemoglobin concentrations during pregnancy. *Lancet*. 2000;356:1083.
7. Auer H, Kollaritsch H, Juptner J, Aspock H. Albendazole and pregnancy. *Appl Parasitol*. 1994;35:146-147.
8. Cowden J, Hotez P. Mebendazole and albendazole treatment of geohelminth infections in children and pregnant women. *Pediatr Infect Dis J*. 2000;19:659-660.
9. Torlesse H, Hodges M. Albendazole therapy and reduced decline in haemoglobin concentration during pregnancy (Sierra Leone). *Trans R Soc Trop Med Hyg*. 2001;95:195-201.
10. Montes H, Soetkino R, Carr-Locke DL. Hydatid disease in pregnancy. *Am J Gastroenterol*. 2002;97:1553-1555.
11. Can D, Oztekin O, Oztekin O, et al. Hepatic and splenic hydatid cyst during pregnancy: a case report. *Acta Gynecol Obstet*. 2003;268:239-240.
12. Gyapong JO, Chinbuah MA, Gyapong M. Inadvertent exposure of pregnant women to ivermectin and albendazole during mass drug administration for lymphatic filariasis. *Trop Med Int Health*. 2003;8:1093-1101.
13. Elliott AM, Quigley MA, Nampijja M, et al. Helminth infection during pregnancy and development of infantile eczema. *JAMA*. 2005;294:2032-2034.
14. Yilmaz N, Kiymaz N, Etlik O, Yazici T. Primary hydatid cyst of the brain during pregnancy—case report. *Neurol Med Chir (Tokyo)*. 2006;46:415-417.
15. Choe JS, Han JY, Ahn HK, et al. Foetal outcomes after exposure to albendazole in early pregnancy. *J Obstet Gynaecol*. 2017;17:1108-1111.
16. Abdel-Tawab AM, Bradley M, Ghazaly EA, et al. Albendazole and its metabolites in the breast milk of lactating women following a single oral dose of albendazole. *Br Clin Pharmacol*. 2009;68:737-742.
17. Allen HE, Crompton DWT, de Silva N, et al. New policies for using anthelmintics in high risk groups. *Trends Parasitol*. 2002;18:381-382.

ALBIGLUTIDE

Antidiabetic (GLP-1 Receptor Agonist)

PREGNANCY RECOMMENDATION: No Human Data and No Relevant Animal Data

BREASTFEEDING RECOMMENDATION: Probably Compatible

PREGNANCY SUMMARY

No reports describing the use of albiglutide in human pregnancy have been located. The drug is not likely to cross the placenta; however, because it consists of a protein, it is not known whether some fetal exposure could occur in the third trimester. Therefore, the absence of human pregnancy experience prevents a complete assessment of the embryofetal risk. Animal studies did show some embryofetal toxicity, but at doses greater than 10 times the RHD. Using this drug during pregnancy should be based on the pros and cons of the mother's clinical need for treatment versus any potential fetal risk that might occur from exposure. ACOG recommends that insulin be used for types 1 and 2 diabetes during pregnancy and, if diet therapy alone is not successful, for gestational diabetes.

BREASTFEEDING SUMMARY

No reports describing the use of albiglutide during human lactation have been located. The drug will likely not be found in breast milk. Additionally, if any drug were to be ingested through breastfeeding, because it is a protein, it would probably be digested in the infant's gastrointestinal tract and not be absorbed. However, due to the theoretical concern for adverse effects that might be seen in a breastfed infant exposed to this drug, the manufacturer recommends that women not breastfeed while using this drug or discontinue the drug. Nevertheless, breastfeeding while using this drug should be based on the mother's clinical need for treatment. If used, the infant should be monitored for the most common reported adult side effects of nausea, back pain, and arthralgia (all leading to irritability), diarrhea, upper respiratory tract infection, and cough.

References

1. Prescribing Information. Tanzeum. GlaxoSmithKline; 2019.
2. Gestational Diabetes Mellitus. ACOG practice bulletin no. 190. American College of Obstetricians and Gynecologists. *Obstet Gynecol*. 2018;131:e49-e64.
3. Pregestational Diabetes Mellitus. ACOG practice bulletin no. 201. American College of Obstetricians and Gynecologists. *Obstet Gynecol*. 2018;132:e228-e248.

ALBUTEROL

Respiratory (β_2-Adrenergic Agonist)

PREGNANCY RECOMMENDATION: Human Data Suggest Low Risk

BREASTFEEDING RECOMMENDATION: Probably Compatible

PREGNANCY SUMMARY

Numerous studies were located that describe the use of albuterol during human pregnancy. From the Michigan Medicaid Surveillance Study (MMSS), there were 48 (4.4%) anomalies identified in 1,090 first-trimester exposures. No real pattern to the defects was seen. Most other publications describe the use of albuterol in treating asthma later in pregnancy. It has also been used in treating preterm labor. Similar to other betamimetics, the drug can cause maternal and fetal tachycardia and hyperglycemia. Nevertheless, the amount of drug that may cross the placenta with inhalation use is likely to be clinically insignificant due to low bioavailability. Animal data did not show any embryofetal toxicity or teratogenicity in one species administered inhalation doses of more than 10 times the recommended human inhaled dose (RHID). Using this drug during pregnancy should be based on the pros and cons of the mother's clinical need for treatment versus any potential fetal risk that might occur from exposure. The drug should not be withheld because of pregnancy, in the case of acute bronchospasm related to asthma and other reversible obstructive airway disease. There is a pregnancy exposure registry that monitors pregnancy outcomes in women using this drug. Health care providers are encouraged to call the Mothers-to-Baby Pregnancy study at 1-877-311-8972.

BREASTFEEDING SUMMARY

No reports describing the use of albuterol during human lactation have been located. Some amount of the drug may be found in breast milk, but the amount that might be present based on blood levels following inhalation use is likely to be clinically insignificant. Breastfeeding while using this drug should be based on the mother's clinical need for treatment versus any potential infant risks that might occur. If used, the infant should be monitored for the most common reported adult side effects of headache and dizziness (both leading to irritability), elevated heart rate, and tremors. Other drugs in the class (see Terbutaline) are considered compatible with breastfeeding.

References

1. Liggins GC, Vaughan GS. Intravenous infusion of salbutamol in the management of premature labor. *J Obstet Gynaecol Br Commonw*. 1973;80:29-33.
2. Korda AR, Lynerum RC, Jones WR. The treatment of premature labor with intravenous administered salbutamol. *Med J Aust*. 1974;1:744-746.
3. Hastwell G. Salbutamol aerosol in premature labour. *Lancet*. 1975;2:1212-1213.
4. Hastwell GB, Halloway CP, Taylor TLO. A study of 208 patients in premature labor treated with orally administered salbutamol. *Med J Aust*. 1978;1:465-469.
5. Hastwell G, Lambert BE. A comparison of salbutamol and ritodrine when used to inhibit premature labour complicated by ante-partum haemorrhage. *Curr Med Res Opin*. 1979;5:785-789.
6. Ng KH, Sen DK. Hypotension with intravenous salbutamol in premature labour. *Br Med J*. 1974;3:257.
7. Pincus R. Salbutamol infusion for premature labour—the Australian trials experience. *Aust NZ Obstet Gynaecol*. 1981;21:1-4.
8. Gummerus M. The management of premature labor with salbutamol. *Acta Obstet Gynecol Scand*. 1981;60:375-377.
9. Crowhurst JA. Salbutamol, obstetrics and anaesthesia: a review and case discussion. *Anaesth Intensive Care*. 1980;8:39-43.
10. Lind T, Godfrey KA, Gerrard J, Bryson MR. Continuous salbutamol infusion over 17 weeks to pre-empt premature labour. *Lancet*. 1980;2:1165-1166.

11. Kuhn RJP, Speirs AL, Pepperell RJ, et al. Betamethasone, albuterol, and threatened premature delivery: benefits and risks. Study of 469 pregnancies. *Obstet Gynecol*. 1982;60:403-408.
12. Eggers TR, Doyle LW, Pepperell RJ. Premature labour. *Med J Aust*. 1979; 1:213-216.
13. Prescribing Information. Proventil HFA. Merck Sharpe & Dohme: 2018.
14. Prescribing Information. Albuterol. Mylan Pharmaceuticals; 2010.
15. Sodha RJ, Schneider H. Transplacental transfer of β-adrenergic drugs studied by an in vitro perfusion method of an isolated human placental lobule. *Am J Obstet Gynecol*. 1983;147:303-310.
16. Haukkamaa M, Gummerus M, Kleimola T. Serum salbutamol concentrations during oral and intravenous treatment in pregnant women. *Br J Obstet Gynaecol*. 1985;92:1230-1233.
17. Felicity Ashworth M, Spooner SF, Verkuyl DAA, et al. Failure to prevent preterm labour and delivery in twin pregnancy using prophylactic oral salbutamol. *Br J Obstet Gynaecol*. 1990;97:878-882.
18. Boylan P, O'Discoll K. Long-term salbutamol or successful Shirodkar suture? *Lancet*. 1980;2:1374.
19. Addis GJ. Long-term salbutamol infusion to prevent premature labor. *Lancet*. 1981;1:42-43.
20. Edmonds DK, Letchworth AT. Prophylactic oral salbutamol to prevent premature labour. *Lancet*. 1982;1:1310-1311.
21. Wager J, Fredholm B, Lunell NO, Persson B. Metabolic and circulatory effects of intravenous and oral salbutamol in late pregnancy in diabetic and non-diabetic women. *Acta Obstet Gynecol Scand Suppl*. 1982;108:41-46.
22. Whitehead MI, Mander AM, Hertogs K, et al. Acute congestive cardiac failure in a hypertensive woman receiving salbutamol for premature labour. *Br Med J*. 1980;280:1221-1222.
23. Poole-Wilson PA. Cardiac failure in a hypertensive woman receiving salbutamol for premature labour. *Br Med J*. 1980;281:226.
24. Fogarty AJ. Cardiac failure in a hypertensive woman receiving salbutamol for premature labour. *Br Med J*. 1980;281:226.
25. Davies PDO. Cardiac failure in a hypertensive woman receiving salbutamol for premature labour. *Br Med J*. 1980;281:226-227.
26. Robertson M, Davies AE. Cardiac failure in a hypertensive woman receiving salbutamol for premature labour. *Br Med J*. 1980;281:227.
27. Crowley P. Cardiac failure in a hypertensive woman receiving salbutamol for premature labour. *Br Med J*. 1980;281:227.
28. Whitehead MI, Mander AM, Pettingale KW. Cardiac failure in a hypertensive woman receiving salbutamol for premature labour (reply). *Br Med J*. 1980; 281:227.
29. Davies AE, Robertson MJS. Pulmonary oedema after the administration of intravenous salbutamol and ergometrine—case report. *Br J Obstet Gynaecol*. 1980;87:539-541.
30. Milliez J, Blot Ph, Sureau C. A case report of maternal death associated with betamimetics and betamethasone administration in premature labor. *Eur J Obstet Gynaecol Reprod Biol*. 1980;11:95-100.
31. Thomas DJ, Dove AF, Alberti KG. Metabolic effects of salbutamol infusion during premature labour. *Br J Obstet Gynaecol*. 1977;84:497-499.
32. Wager J, Lunell NO, Nadal M, Ostman J. Glucose tolerance following oral salbutamol treatment in late pregnancy. *Acta Obstet Gynecol Scand*. 1981;60:291-294.
33. Lunell NO, Joelsson I, Larsson A, Persson B. The immediate effect of a beta-adrenergic agonist (salbutamol) on carbohydrate and lipid metabolism during the third trimester of pregnancy. *Acta Obstet Gynecol Scand*. 1977;56:475-478.
34. Procianoy RS, Pinheiro CE. Neonatal hyperinsulinism after short-term maternal beta sympathomimetic therapy. *J Pediatr*. 1982;101:612-614.
35. Barnett AH, Stubbs SM, Mander AM. Management of premature labour in diabetic pregnancy. *Diabetologia*. 1980;188:365-368.
36. Wager J, Fredholm BB, Lunell NO, Persson B. Metabolic and circulatory effects of oral salbutamol in the third trimester of pregnancy in diabetic and non-diabetic women. *Br J Obstet Gynaecol*. 1981;88:352-361.
37. Desgranges M-F, Moutquin J-M, Peloquin A. Effects of maternal oral salbutamol therapy on neonatal endocrine status at birth. *Obstet Gynecol*. 1987;69:582-584.
38. Hastwell GB. Apgar scores, respiratory distress syndrome and salbutamol. *Med J Aust*. 1980;1:174-175.
39. Hastwell G. Salbutamol and respiratory distress syndrome. *Lancet*. 1977; 2:354.
40. Wallace RL, Caldwell DL, Ansbacher R, Otterson WN. Inhibition of premature labor by terbutaline. *Obstet Gynecol*. 1978;51:387-392.
41. Freysz H, Willard D, Lehr A, et al. A long term evaluation of infants who received a beta-mimetic drug while in utero. *J Perinat Med*. 1977;5:94-99.
42. Michie CA, Braithwaite S, Schulenberg E, Harvey D. Do maternal β-sympathomimetics influence the development of retinopathy in the premature infant? *Arch Dis Child*. 1994;71:F149.
43. Rayburn WF, Atkinson BD, Gilbert KA, Turnbull GL. Acute effects of inhaled albuterol (Proventil) on fetal hemodynamics (abstract). *Teratology*. 1994; 49:370.
44. Rayburn WF, Atkinson BD, Gilbert K, Turnbull GL. Short-term effects of inhaled albuterol on maternal and fetal circulations. *Am J Obstet Gynecol*. 1994;171:770-773.
45. Baker ER, Flanagan MF. Fetal atrial flutter associated with maternal beta-sympathomimetic drug exposure. *Obstet Gynecol*. 1997;89:861.
46. Witter FR, Zimmerman AW, Reichmann JP, Connors SL. In utero beta 2 adrenergic agonist exposure and adverse neurophysiologic and behavioral outcomes. *Am J Obstet Gynecol*. 2009;210:553-559.

ALCAFTADINE OPHTHALMIC

Antihistamine/Ophthalmic (Topical)

PREGNANCY RECOMMENDATION: No Human Data—Animal Data Suggest Low Risk

BREASTFEEDING RECOMMENDATION: Probably Compatible

PREGNANCY SUMMARY

No reports describing the use of alcaftadine ophthalmic in human pregnancy have been located. The drug will probably cross the placenta, so some fetal exposure will likely occur. However, the amount is probably clinically insignificant. However, the absence of human pregnancy experience prevents a complete assessment of the embryofetal risk. Animal studies did not show any embryofetal toxicity in two species at doses well above the recommended human oral dose (RHOD). Using this drug during pregnancy should be based on the pros and cons of the mother's clinical need for treatment versus any potential fetal risk that might occur from exposure. If used during pregnancy, consider placing pressure over the tear duct in the corner of the eye for at least 1 minute, and then remove any excess solution with absorbent tissue to decrease the amount of drug reaching the systemic circulation even further.

BREASTFEEDING SUMMARY

No reports describing the use of alcaftadine ophthalmic during human lactation have been located. The drug may be found in breast milk. However, the amount of the parent drug and active metabolite is likely to be negligible. Antihistamines, in general, are considered compatible with breastfeeding. Breastfeeding while using this drug should be based on the mother's clinical need for treatment. If used, the infant should be monitored for the most common reported adult systemic side effect of nausea (leading to irritability). A method to decrease some systemic absorption with ophthalmic use is described above in the Pregnancy Summary.

Reference

1. Prescribing Information. Lastacaft. Allergan; 2018.

ALDESLEUKIN

Antineoplastic (Interleukin-2 Peptide)

PREGNANCY RECOMMENDATION: No Human Data—Animal Data Suggest Low Risk

BREASTFEEDING RECOMMENDATION: Probably Compatible (Hold Breastfeeding)

PREGNANCY SUMMARY

No reports describing the use of aldesleukin in human pregnancy have been located. The drug is not likely to cross the placenta; however, because it consists of a peptide, it is not known whether some fetal exposure could occur in the third trimester. Therefore, the absence of human pregnancy experience prevents a complete assessment of the embryofetal risk. Animal studies did not show any embryofetal toxicity in one species at doses of greater than 10 times the RHD. However, maternal toxicity in animals was seen at doses of less than 10 times the RHD. Using this drug during pregnancy should be based on the pros and cons of the mother's clinical need for treatment versus any potential fetal risk that might occur from exposure. There is a registry for women who are pregnant and have cancer. For more information, women and health care providers are encouraged to contact the Cancer and Pregnancy Registry at 1-877-635-4499.

BREASTFEEDING SUMMARY

No reports describing the use of aldesleukin during human lactation have been located. The drug will not likely be found in breast milk. Additionally, if any drug were to be ingested through breastfeeding, because it is a peptide, it would probably be digested in the infant's gastrointestinal tract and not be absorbed. However, due to the theoretical concern for adverse effects that might be seen in a breastfed infant exposed to this drug, the manufacturer recommends that women not breastfeed while using this drug or discontinue the drug. Nevertheless, breastfeeding while using this drug should be based on the mother's clinical need for treatment. If used, the infant should be monitored for the most common reported adult side effects of nausea, abdominal pain, and pruritus (all leading to irritability), diarrhea, vomiting, fever, rash, lethargy, tachycardia, and various laboratory abnormalities (see PI)

Reference

1. Prescribing Information. Proleukin. Prometheus Laboratories; 2020.

ALECTINIB

Antineoplastic (Tyrosine Kinase Inhibitor)

PREGNANCY RECOMMENDATION: Limited Human Data—Animal Data Suggest Potential Risk

BREASTFEEDING RECOMMENDATION: Potential Toxicity

PREGNANCY SUMMARY

A total of eight case reports were located that describe the use of alectinib during nine human pregnancies. Of these, seven had first-trimester exposure, and no major birth anomalies were identified at delivery. The drug was started in the second trimester in the other two cases, and both newborns did well. The drug has been shown to cross the placenta at term, but fetal levels were less than 25% of the maternal concentrations. However, this limited human pregnancy experience prevents a complete assessment of the embryofetal risk. Animal studies did show some embryofetal toxicity in two species at doses of less than 10 times the RHD, but maternal toxicity also occurred. Based on the animal studies and the drug's mechanism of action, the manufacturer recommends that women with reproductive potential use effective contraception during treatment and for 1 week after the last dose. They also recommend that males with female partners of reproductive potential use effective contraception during treatment and for 3 months after the last dose. Nevertheless, using this drug during pregnancy

(*continued*)

should be based on the pros and cons of the mother's clinical need for treatment versus any potential fetal risk that might occur from exposure. Hyperglycemia was seen in about 36% of patients in the clinical trials. Therefore, if used, glucose levels need to be monitored.

BREASTFEEDING SUMMARY

Two studies have been located that found alectinib in colostrum after delivery. The breast milk levels were 152 ng/mL (maternal serum level of 259 ng/mL) and about 12 ng/mL (maternal serum level of 155 ng/mL). This shows that the drug can be found in breast milk if it is present in the maternal circulation. Therefore, infant exposure would occur. Due to a concern for potential serious adverse effects that might be seen in a breastfed infant, the manufacturer recommends that women not breastfeed while being treated with this drug and for at least 1 week after the last dose. Nevertheless, breastfeeding while using this drug should be based on the mother's clinical need for treatment versus any potential infant risks that might occur. If used, the infant should be monitored for the most common reported adult side effects of myalgia (leading to irritability), fatigue (lethargy), constipation, and various laboratory abnormalities (see PI).

References

1. Prescribing Information. Alecensa. Genentech; 2021.
2. Scarfone G, Fumagalli M, Imbimbo M, et al. First case report of pregnancy on alectinib in a woman with metastatic ALK-rearranged lung cancer: a case report. *J Thorac Oncol*. 2021;16:873-877.
3. Shang M, Luo X, Wu J, et al. The safety and efficacy for the treatment of alectinib in a woman with ALK-positive lung cancer delivered a healthy male neonate throughout pregnancy: a case report. *Lung Cancer*. 2023;180:107188.
4. Kato M, Yamaura T, Mine H, et al. Anaplastic lymphoma kinase-tyrosine kinase inhibitor treatment for metastatic non-small cell lung cancer throughout the entire gestation. *Cureus*. 2024;16:e63592.
5. Carlier S, Carestia L, Marot JC, Wieers G. Unplanned pregnancy in an HIV positive woman undergoing alectinib treatment for metastatic non-small-cell Lung cancer. *BMJ Case Rep*. 2022;15:e247530.
6. Weidenbaum C, Cann CG, Osmundson S, et al. Two uncomplicated pregnancies on alectinib in a woman with metastatic ALK-rearranged NSCLC: a case report. *JTO Clin Res Rep*. 2022;3(8):100361.
7. De Smedt F, Dessy F, Carestia L, et al. A pregnant patient with ALK-positive non-small cell lung cancer treated with alectinib: a case report and review of the literature. *Oncol Lett*. 2022;25(2):54.
8. Wu F, Rittberg R, Lim K, Ho C. Treating anaplastic lymphoma kinase (ALK) fusion-driven metastatic non-small cell lung cancer (NSCLC) with alectinib through pregnancy. *BMJ Case Rep*. 2024;17:e255575.
9. Gonzalez-Mosquera LF, Rous FA, Rogers A, et al. ALK rearrangement positive lung adenocarcinoma in pregnancy treated with alectinib: a case report. *Clin Lung Cancer*. 2024;25:e77-e80.

ALEMTUZUMAB

Antineoplastic (CD52 Receptor Inhibitor—Monoclonal Antibody)

PREGNANCY RECOMMENDATION: Limited Human Data—Animal Data Suggest Potential Risk

BREASTFEEDING RECOMMENDATION: Probably Compatible

PREGNANCY SUMMARY

One study was located that described the use of alemtuzumab during 12 pregnancies at various stages of gestation. No major birth anomalies were identified. As an IgG antibody, it likely crosses the placenta, especially during the second half of gestation, so some fetal exposure will probably occur. Therefore, this limited human pregnancy experience prevents a complete assessment of the embryofetal risk. Animal studies did show some embryofetal toxicity, but no teratogenicity, in one species at doses of less than 10 times the RHD. However, dosing was daily in mice for about 6 days, whereas normal dosing in humans is about every other day. It is not possible to determine any effect of this dosing frequency difference. Based on animal studies and the drug's mechanism of action, the manufacturer recommends that women with reproductive potential use effective contraception during treatment and for 3 months after the last dose. Nevertheless, using this drug during pregnancy should be based on the pros and cons of the mother's clinical need for treatment versus any potential fetal risk that might occur from exposure. A potential fetal consequence of exposure to alemtuzumab is depletion of B and T lymphocytes, which should be evaluated if used near delivery.

BREASTFEEDING SUMMARY

No reports describing the use of alemtuzumab during lactation have been located. It is known that IgG antibodies can be found in human breast milk, but are not found in the neonatal or infant circulation. Additionally, if any IgG antibodies were to be ingested through breastfeeding, they would probably be digested in the infant's gastrointestinal tract and not be absorbed. However, due to a concern for potential serious adverse effects that might be seen in a breastfed infant, the manufacturer recommends that women not breastfeed while being treated with this drug and for at least 3 months after the last dose. Nevertheless, breastfeeding while using this drug should be based on the mother's clinical need for treatment versus any potential infant risks that might occur. If used, the infant should be monitored for the most common reported adult side effects of nausea (leading to irritability), diarrhea, vomiting, insomnia, infections, and rash.

References

1. Prescribing Information. Campath. Genzyme; 2017.
2. Tuohy O, Costelloe L, Hill-Cawthome G, et al. Alemtuzumab treatment of multiple sclerosis: long-term safety and efficacy. *J Neurol Neurosurg Psychiatry*. 2015;86:208-215.

ALENDRONATE

Bone Health (Bisphosphonate)

PREGNANCY RECOMMENDATION: Limited Human Data—Animal Data Suggest Potential Risk

BREASTFEEDING RECOMMENDATION: Probably Compatible

PREGNANCY SUMMARY

A few studies that describe the use of alendronate during human pregnancy were located. In about 50 exposures to the drug, many involved alendronate use prior to conception. However, with the long elimination half-life, the drug was likely to be present. No major birth defects were described, and in many cases, all of the bone analyses and tests were also normal. If the drug is in the maternal circulation, then some of it will likely cross the placenta. However, this limited human pregnancy experience prevents a complete assessment of the embryofetal risk. Animal studies did show some embryofetal toxicity in one species at doses of less than 10 times the RHD, but not in a second species at doses of more than 10 times the RHD. In most cases, a low-level, continuous exposure throughout gestation will probably occur. Using this drug during pregnancy for Paget disease of the bone and for glucocorticoid-induced osteoporosis should be based on the pros and cons of the mother's clinical need for treatment versus any potential fetal risk that might occur from exposure.

BREASTFEEDING SUMMARY

No reports describing the use of alendronate during human lactation have been located. The drug may be found in breast milk. However, oral bioavailability is low at less than 1% and the amount of maternal drug released from bone is only 25% of the amount systemically absorbed with oral use. Therefore, the overall concentrations are very limited. Based on the drugs approved use, it would only occur in Paget disease of the bone and for glucocorticoid-induced osteoporosis, which are uncommon disorders. Breastfeeding while using this drug should be based on the mother's clinical need for treatment versus any potential infant risks that might occur. If used, the infant should be monitored for the most common reported adult side effects of nausea, musculoskeletal pain, and abdominal pain all leading to irritability), and constipation.

References

1. Ornoy A, Wajnberg R, Diav-Citrin O. The outcome of pregnancy following pre-pregnancy or early pregnancy alendronate treatment. *Reprod Toxicol*. 2006;22:578-579.
2. Product information. Fosamax. Merck Sharp & Dohme; 2016.
3. Green SB, Pappas AL. Effects of maternal bisphosphonate use on fetal and neonatal outcomes. *Am J Health Syst Pharm*. 2014;71:2029-2036.
4. Minsker DH, Manson JM, Peter CP. Effects of the bisphosphonate, alendronate, on parturition in the rat. *Toxicol Appl Pharmacol* 1993;121:217-223.
5. Patlas N, Golomb G, Yaffe P, Pinto T, Breuer E, Ornoy A. Transplacental effects of bisphosphonates on fetal skeletal ossification and mineralization in rats. *Teratology*. 1999;60:68-73.
6. Rutgers-Verhage AR, deVries TW, Torringa MJL. No effects of bisphosphonates on the human fetus. *Birth Defects Res A Clin Mol Teratol*. 2003;67:203-204.
7. Djokanovic N, Klieger-Grossmann C, Koren G. Does treatment with bisphosphonates endanger the human pregnancy? *J Obstet Gynaecol Can*. 2008;30:1146-1148.
8. Hassen-Zrour S, Korbaa W, Bejia I, Saidani Z, Bergaoui N. Maternal and fetal outcome after long-term bisphosphonate exposure before conception. *Osteoporos Int*. 2010;21:709-710.
9. Gerin M, Jambon G, Fouque-Aubert A, et al. Neonatal transient hypophosphatemic hypercalciuric rickets in dizygous twins: a role for maternal alendronate therapy before pregnancy or antireflux medications? *Arch Pediatr*. 2016;23:957-962.

ALGLUCOSIDASE ALFA

Genetic/Metabolic (Enzyme—Pompe Disease)

PREGNANCY RECOMMENDATION: Limited Human Data—Animal Data Suggest Low Risk (Maternal Benefit May Outweigh Any Potential Embryofetal Risk)

BREASTFEEDING RECOMMENDATION: Probably Compatible

PREGNANCY SUMMARY

One case report was located that described the use of alglucosidase alfa in human pregnancy. The patient had Pompe disease and was treated throughout gestation with the drug. A healthy infant with no identified birth anomalies was delivered at term. Because it is a protein, it is not known whether some placental transfer might occur in the second half of gestation. However, this limited human pregnancy experience prevents a complete assessment of the embryofetal risk. Animal studies did not show any embryofetal toxicity or teratogenicity in two species at doses of less than 10 times the RHD. Using this drug during pregnancy should be based on the pros and cons of the mother's clinical need for treatment versus any potential fetal risk that might occur from exposure. If a woman requires continued administration of alglucosidase alfa for the treatment of Pompe disease, it should probably not be withheld because of pregnancy.

BREASTFEEDING SUMMARY

Alglucosidase alfa is an endogenous enzyme, and some levels would normally be expected in human breast milk. One report describing the use of alglucosidase alfa during human lactation was located. A mother with Pompe disease was being treated with alglucosidase alfa. The enzyme activity in the breast milk prior to treatment was about 10% of the activity seen in the breast milk of an unaffected woman. Following drug administration, the activity increased by about 82-fold. Therefore, the enzyme appears to have entered the breast milk. Because it is a large polypeptide, if the drug were to be ingested through breastfeeding, it would probably be digested in the infant's gastrointestinal tract and not be absorbed. Breastfeeding while using this drug should be based on the mother's clinical need for treatment versus any potential infant risks that might occur. If used, the infant should be monitored for the most common reported adult side effects of pruritus, neck pain, and extremity pain (all leading to irritability), diarrhea, lethargy, flushing, and rash. If a woman requires continued administration of alglucosidase alfa for the treatment of Pompe disease, it should not be withheld because of breastfeeding.

References

1. Prescribing Information. Myozyme. Genzyme; 2018.
2. de Vries JM, Brugma JDC, Ozkan L, et al. First experience with enzyme replacement therapy during pregnancy and lactation in Pompe disease. *Mol Genet Metab*. 2011;104:552-555.

ALIROCUMAB

Antilipemic (Monoclonal Antibody)

PREGNANCY RECOMMENDATION: Limited Human Data—Animal Data Suggest Low Risk

BREASTFEEDING RECOMMENDATION: Probably Compatible

PREGNANCY SUMMARY

One case report with first-trimester exposure to alirocumab (along with rosuvastatin and ezetimibe) was located. An unplanned pregnancy occurred, and the drugs were stopped at about 6 weeks' gestation. The infant was delivered at term with agenesis of the corpus callosum, though the child was developing normally at the last follow-up of 9 months of age. It is not possible in this case to determine if any of the drugs or a combination led to the anomaly. However, monoclonal antibodies of the IgG class do not cross the placenta in the first trimester. Antibodies do cross the placenta, especially during the second half of gestation. Therefore, fetal exposure can occur then. Therefore, this limited human pregnancy experience prevents a complete assessment of the embryofetal risk. Animal studies did not show any embryofetal toxicity in one animal species. Using this drug during pregnancy should be based on the pros and cons of the mother's clinical need for treatment versus any potential fetal risk that might occur from exposure.

BREASTFEEDING SUMMARY

No reports describing the use of alirocumab during human lactation have been located. It is known that IgG antibodies can be found in human breast milk, but are not found in the neonatal or infant circulation. Additionally, if any IgG antibodies were to be ingested through breastfeeding, they would probably be digested in the infant's gastrointestinal tract and not be absorbed. Breastfeeding while using this drug should be based on the mother's clinical need for treatment versus any potential infant risks. If used, the infant should be monitored for the most common reported adult side effects of nasopharyngitis and influenza-like symptoms.

References

1. Prescribing Information. Praluent. Sanofi-Aventis U.S.; 2020.
2. Vuignier Y, Beaud F, Kosinski C, et al. Exposure to alirocumab during the first trimester of pregnancy: a case report. *Birth Defects Res*. 2021;113:1156-1160.

ALISKIREN

Antihypertensive (Renin Inhibitor)

PREGNANCY RECOMMENDATION: No Human Data (*Potential Risk Second and Third Trimesters)

BREASTFEEDING RECOMMENDATION: Probably Compatible

PREGNANCY SUMMARY

Although there is no published human pregnancy experience with aliskiren, the drug will probably cross the placenta, so some fetal exposure will likely occur. Therefore, the absence of human pregnancy experience prevents a complete assessment of the embryofetal risk. *Because aliskiren acts directly on the renin-angiotensin system, exposure in the second and third trimesters should be avoided except in those rare incidences in which the mother requires therapy with this agent. Two other classes of agents that act on this system, ACE inhibitors and ARBs, are known to cause marked fetal renal insufficiency in the second and third trimesters. Therefore, the use of aliskiren during the second and third trimesters may theoretically cause fetal and neonatal toxicity identical to that seen with ACE inhibitors and ARB drugs. These effects include fetal renal toxicity leading to oligohydramnios, pulmonary hypoplasia, limb contracture deformities, and facial deformations. The drug carries a boxed warning for these risks. These findings are not always permanent, and some cases have shown reversal, even when the drug was not discontinued until well past 20 weeks of gestation. However, if possible, the drug should not be used after 20 weeks of gestation.

BREASTFEEDING SUMMARY

No reports describing the use of aliskiren during human lactation have been located. The drug will probably be found in human breast milk, so some infant exposure will likely occur. Due to a concern for potential serious adverse effects that might be seen in a breastfed infant, the manufacturer recommends that women not breastfeed while being treated with this drug. Nevertheless, breastfeeding while using this drug should be based on the mother's clinical need for treatment versus any potential infant risks that might occur. If used, the infant should be monitored for the most common reported adult side effect of diarrhea.

References

1. Product information. Tekturna. Novartis Pharmaceuticals; 2017.
2. Azizi M, Webb R, Nussberger J, Hollenberg NK. Renin inhibition with aliskiren: where are we now, and where are we going? *J Hypertens*. 2006;24:243-256.

ALLOPURINOL

Antineoplastic/Antigout (Xanthine Oxidase Inhibitor)

PREGNANCY RECOMMENDATION: Limited Human Data—Animal Data Suggest Low Risk

BREASTFEEDING RECOMMENDATION: Potential Toxicity

PREGNANCY SUMMARY

A few case reports and one series have been located that describe the use of allopurinol during human lactation. From about 39 first-trimester exposures, 2 (5.3%) cases of multiple fetal anomalies were described. A few other studies have described use in the second and third trimesters with no serious adverse fetal effects seen. Allopurinol and the active metabolite, oxipurinol, both cross the placenta, so some fetal exposure will occur. However, this limited human pregnancy experience prevents a complete assessment of the embryofetal risk. Animal studies did not show any embryofetal toxicity or teratogenicity in two species at doses of less than 10 times the RHD. Using this drug during pregnancy should be based on the pros and cons of the mother's clinical need for treatment versus any potential fetal risk that might occur from exposure.

BREASTFEEDING SUMMARY

One case report was located that described the use of allopurinol during human lactation. The peak allopurinol and oxipurinol concentrations were 0.9 and 53.7 mcg/mL, respectively. In infants, the normal dosing of allopurinol is about 10 mg/kg/d, and from these breast milk values, the overall exposure is about 8.19 mg/kg/d. In this case, the infant's blood was analyzed. Allopurinol was not detected (LLQ of 0.5 mcg/mL), but the oxipurinol level was about 6.6 mcg/mL (about 40% of the maternal blood level). Due to a concern for potential serious adverse effects that might be seen in a breastfed infant, the manufacturer recommends that women not breastfeed while being treated with this drug and for 1 week after the last dose. However, some mothers may need treatment with this drug. Therefore, if the clinical decision is to use this drug while breastfeeding, the infant should be monitored for the most common reported adult side effects of nausea (leading to irritability), diarrhea, and elevated liver function tests.

References

1. Prescribing Information. Zyloprim. Prometheus Laboratories; 2009.
2. Fujii T, Nishimura H. Comparison of teratogenic action of substances related to purine metabolism in mouse embryos. *Jpn J Pharmacol*. 1972;22:201-206.
3. Chaube S, Murphy ML. The teratogenic effects of the recent drugs active in cancer chemotherapy. In: Woollam DHM, ed. *Advances in Teratology*. Academic Press; 1968;3:181-237. As cited in Shepard TH. *Catalog of Teratogenic Agents*. 6th ed. Johns Hopkins University Press; 1989:58.
4. Torrance HL, Benders MJ, Derks JB, et al. Maternal allopurinol during fetal hypoxia lowers cord blood levels of the brain injury marker S-100B. *Pediatrics*. 2009;124:350-357.
5. Awidi AS, Tarawneh MS, Shubair KS, et al. Acute leukemia in pregnancy: report of five cases treated with a combination which included a low dose of adriamycin. *Eur J Cancer Clin Oncol*. 1983;19:881-884.
6. Ali R, Kimya Y, Koksal N, et al. Pregnancy in chronic lymphocytic leukemia: experience with fetal exposure to chlorambucil. *Leuk Res*. 2009;33:567-569.
7. AlKindi S, Dennison D, Pathare A. et al. Two cases of acute leukaemia in pregnancy. *Acta Haematol*. 1979;61:298-300.
8. Boros SJ, Reynolds JW. Intrauterine growth retardation following third-trimester exposure to busulfan. *Am J Obstet Gynecol*. 1977;129:111-112.
9. Farber M, Knuppel RA, Binkiewicz A, Kennison RD. Pregnancy and von Gierke's disease. *Obstet Gynecol*. 1976;47:226-228.
10. Coddington CC, Albrecht RC, Cefalo RC. Gouty nephropathy and pregnancy. *Am J Obstet Gynecol*. 1979;133:107-108.
11. Gülmezoğlu AM, Hofmeyr GJ, Oosthuisen MMJ. Antioxidants in the treatment of severe pre-eclampsia: an explanatory randomized controlled trial. *Br J Obstet Gynaecol*. 1997;104:689-696.
12. Kaandorp JJ, Benders MJNL, Rademaker CMA, et al. Antenatal allopurinol for reduction birth asphyxia induced brain damage (ALLO-Trial); a randomized double blind placebo controlled multicenter study. *BMC Pregnancy Childbirth*. 2010;10:8.
13. Boda D. Results of and further prevention of hypoxic fetal brain damage by inhibition of xanthine oxidase enzyme with allopurinol. *J Perinat Med*. 2011;39:441-444.
14. Kozenko M, Grynspan D, Oluyomi-Obi, et al. Potential teratogenic effects of allopurinol: a case report. *Am J Med Genet*. 2011;155:2247-2252.
15. Hoeltzenbein M, Stieler K, Panse M, et al. Allopurinol use during pregnancy—outcome of 31 prospectively ascertained cases and a phenotype possible indicative for teratogenicity. *PLoS One*. 2013;8:e66637.
16. Seinen ML, de Boer NKH, van Hoorn ME, et al. Safe use of allopurinol and low-dose mercaptopurine therapy during pregnancy in an ulcerative colitis patient. *Inflamm Bowel Dis*. 2013;19(3):E37. doi:10.1002/ibd. 22945
17. Fazal MW, Dooque MP, Leong RW, et al. Allopurinol use in pregnancy in three women with inflammatory bowel disease: safety and outcomes: a case series. *BMC Gastroenterol*. 2013;13:172.
18. Kamilli I, Gresser U, Schaefer C, Zollner N. Allopurinol in breast milk. *Adv Exp Med Biol*. 1991;309A:143-145.
19. Kamilli I, Gresser U. Allopurinol and oxypurinol in human breast milk. *Clin Investig*. 1993;71:161-164.

ALMOTRIPTAN

Central Nervous System (Antimigraine—Triptan)

PREGNANCY RECOMMENDATION: No Human Data—Animal Data Suggest Low Risk

BREASTFEEDING RECOMMENDATION: Probably Compatible

PREGNANCY SUMMARY

No reports describing the use of almotriptan in human pregnancy have been located. The drug will probably cross the placenta, so some fetal exposure will likely occur. Therefore, the absence of human pregnancy experience prevents a complete assessment of the embryofetal risk. Animal studies did not show any embryofetal toxicity or teratogenicity in two species at doses of more than 10 times the RHD. Using this drug during pregnancy should be based on the pros and cons of the mother's clinical need for treatment versus any potential fetal risk that might occur from exposure.

BREASTFEEDING SUMMARY

One report was located that described the use of almotriptan during human lactation. The drug was found in the breast milk of a single patient with a peak level of about 106 ng/mL and a mean breast milk level of about 30 ng/mL. The calculated RID was about 1.8%. Breastfeeding while using this drug should be based on the mother's clinical need for treatment versus any potential infant risks that might occur. If used, the infant should be monitored for the most common reported adult side effects of nausea, headache, dizziness, and dry mouth (all leading to irritability), somnolence, and vomiting.

References

1. Prescribing Information. Axert. Janssen Pharmaceutical; 2018.
2. Soldin OP, Dahlin J, O'Mara DM. Triptans in pregnancy. *Ther Drug Monit*. 2008;30:5-9.
3. Amundsen S, Nordeng H, Fuskevag OM, et al Transfer of triptans into human breast milk and estimation of infant drug exposure through breastfeeding. *Basic Clin Pharmacol Toxicol*. 2021;128:795-804.

ALOGLIPTIN

Antidiabetic (DPP4 Inhibitor)

PREGNANCY RECOMMENDATION: No Human Data—Animal Data Suggest Low Risk

BREASTFEEDING RECOMMENDATION: Probably Compatible

PREGNANCY SUMMARY

No reports describing the use of alogliptin in human pregnancy have been located. The drug will probably cross the placenta, so some fetal exposure will likely occur. Therefore, the absence of human pregnancy experience prevents a complete assessment of the embryofetal risk. Animal studies did not show any embryofetal toxicity in two species at doses greater than 10 times the RHD. Using this drug during pregnancy should be based on the pros and cons of the mother's clinical need for treatment versus any potential fetal risk that might occur from exposure. ACOG recommends that insulin be used for types 1 and 2 diabetes during pregnancy and, if diet therapy alone is not successful, for gestational diabetes.

BREASTFEEDING SUMMARY

No reports describing the use of alogliptin during human lactation have been located. The drug will probably be excreted into breast milk, so some infant exposure will likely occur. Breastfeeding while using this drug should be based on the mother's clinical need for treatment. If used, the infant should be monitored for the most common reported adult side effects of headache and arthralgia (both leading to irritability), hypoglycemia, elevated liver function tests, and upper respiratory tract infections.

References

1. Product information. Nesina. Takeda Pharmaceuticals; 2019.
2. Gestational Diabetes Mellitus. ACOG practice bulletin no. 190. American College of Obstetricians and Gynecologists. *Obstet Gynecol*. 2018;131: e49-e64.
3. Pregestational Diabetes Mellitus. ACOG practice bulletin no. 201. American College of Obstetricians and Gynecologists. *Obstet Gynecol*. 2018;132: e228-e248.

ALOSETRON

Gastrointestinal (Serotonin 5-HT_3 Receptor Antagonist)

PREGNANCY RECOMMENDATION: No Human Data—Animal Data Suggest Low Risk

BREASTFEEDING RECOMMENDATION: Potential Toxicity

PREGNANCY SUMMARY

No reports describing the use of alosetron in human pregnancy have been located. Because the drug is restricted by the manufacturer to severe diarrhea-predominant irritable bowel syndrome, pregnancy exposures are probably infrequent. The drug will probably cross the placenta, so some fetal exposure will likely occur. Therefore, the absence of human pregnancy experience prevents a complete assessment of the embryofetal risk. Animal studies did not show any embryofetal toxicity in two species at doses of much greater than 10 times the RHD. Using this drug during pregnancy should be based on the pros and cons of the mother's clinical need for treatment versus any potential fetal risk that might occur from exposure.

BREASTFEEDING SUMMARY

No reports describing the use of alosetron during human lactation have been located. The drug will probably be found in breast milk, so some infant exposure will likely occur. Breastfeeding while using this drug should be based on the mother's clinical need for treatment versus any potential infant risks. If used, the infant should be monitored for the most common reported adult side effects of nausea and abdominal pain (both leading to irritability) and constipation. However, because of the boxed warning risks, if the clinical decision is to use alosetron during lactation, close infant monitoring should occur.

Reference

1. Prescribing Information. Lotronex. Prometheus Laboratories; 2018.

ALPELISIB

Antineoplastic (Phosphatidylinositol 3-Kinase Inhibitor)

PREGNANCY RECOMMENDATION: No Human Data—Animal Data Suggest Risk

BREASTFEEDING RECOMMENDATION: Potential Toxicity

PREGNANCY SUMMARY

No reports describing the use of alpelisib in human pregnancy have been located. The drug will probably cross the placenta, so some fetal exposure will likely occur. Therefore, the absence of human pregnancy experience prevents a complete assessment of the embryofetal risk. Animal studies did show embryofetal toxicity in two species at doses less than 10 times the RHD. Based on animal studies and the drug's mechanism of action, the manufacturer recommends that women with reproductive potential use effective contraception during treatment and for 1 week after the last dose. They also recommend that males with female partners of reproductive potential use effective contraception during treatment and for 1 week after the last dose. Nevertheless, using this drug during pregnancy should be based on the pros and cons of the mother's clinical need for treatment versus any potential fetal risk that might occur from exposure. The drug can also produce hyperglycemia, so close observation of glucose levels should occur.

BREASTFEEDING SUMMARY

No reports describing the use of alpelisib during human lactation have been located. The drug will probably be found in breast milk, so some infant exposure will likely occur. Due to the concern for potential serious adverse effects that might be seen in a breastfed infant, the manufacturer recommends that women not breastfeed while being treated with this drug and for at least 1 week after the last dose. However, breastfeeding while using this drug should be based on the mother's clinical need for treatment versus any potential infant risks. If used, the infant should be monitored for the most common reported adult side effects of stomatitis (leading to irritability), diarrhea, and elevated glucose levels.

Reference

1. Prescribing Information. Piqray. Novartis Pharmaceuticals; 2022.

ALPHA-GALACTOSIDASE (ORAL)

Gastrointestinal (Dietary Supplement—Antiflatulence)

PREGNANCY RECOMMENDATION: No Human Data and No Relevant Animal Data

BREASTFEEDING RECOMMENDATION: Probably Compatible

PREGNANCY SUMMARY

No reports describing the use of oral α-galactosidase in human pregnancy have been located. This supplement will not likely cross the placenta in any clinically significant amounts. However, the absence of human pregnancy experience prevents a complete assessment of the embryofetal risk. No animal reproduction or fertility studies have been conducted with this supplement. Using this supplement during pregnancy should be based on the pros and cons of the mother's clinical need for treatment versus any potential fetal risk that might occur from exposure.

BREASTFEEDING SUMMARY

No reports describing the use of oral α-galactosidase during human lactation have been located. Any amount of this supplement that might be found in breast milk is likely to be clinically insignificant. In addition, if any of this protein were to be ingested through breastfeeding, it would probably be digested in the infant's gastrointestinal tract and not be absorbed. Breastfeeding while using this supplement should be based on the mother's clinical need for treatment versus any potential infant risks that might occur. If used, the infant should be monitored for the most common reported adult side effect of diarrhea. The overall risk to a nursing infant from maternal use of this supplement is likely to be negligible.

Reference

1. Supplement Information. Beano. Prestige Consumer Healthcare, Inc; 2023.

ALPRAZOLAM

Central Nervous System (Benzodiazepine)

PREGNANCY RECOMMENDATION: Human Data Suggest Potential Risk (Third Trimester)

BREASTFEEDING RECOMMENDATION: Potential Toxicity

PREGNANCY SUMMARY

A few studies and case reports have been located that describe the use of alprazolam during human pregnancy. In one large study of data collected prospectively by the manufacturer from worldwide surveillance, a total of 542 exposures to the drug occurred in the first trimester. After excluding patients lost to follow-up and elective terminations, there were 47 (14.6%) spontaneous losses, which falls within the expected range. Of the remaining 276 live births, there were 13 (4.7%) with congenital birth defects described, but not all of these were major malformations. In addition, no pattern to the defects was seen. The drug will probably cross the placenta, so some fetal exposure will likely occur. However, this limited human pregnancy experience prevents a complete assessment of the embryofetal risk. Animal studies did not show any embryofetal toxicity or teratogenicity in one species at doses of more than 10 times the RHD. When alprazolam is used close to delivery, neonatal withdrawal has been reported postbirth that includes lethargy, decreased respirations, irritability, poor eating, and tremors. The drug does have a risk for dependence and withdrawal when it is discontinued (usually seen after 3 months of use). It is classified as a Schedule IV controlled substance. Acute withdrawal can lead to seizures; therefore, a tapered drop in drug dosage is indicated (if possible). Lastly, the elimination half-life of other benzodiazepines (see Diazepam) can be long in the fetus, and this can lead to a decrease in fetal heart rate (FHR) variability that can last for many hours, in some cases.

BREASTFEEDING SUMMARY

Four studies were located that describe the use of alprazolam during human lactation. In a total of 11 women, the drug was found in breast milk in all cases, with maximum breast milk levels ranging from 1 to about 25 ng/mL. However, maternal doses were less than 1 mg/d in all cases except for one. Therefore, the calculated RIDs ranged from about 2% to about 10%. The elimination half-life of the drug in breast milk was about 15 hours. Due to a concern for potential serious adverse effects that might be seen in a breastfed infant, the manufacturer recommends that women not breastfeed while being treated with this drug. If the clinical decision is to use this drug while breastfeeding, the infant should be monitored for the most common reported adult side effects of drowsiness, lethargy, and decreased heart rate. If possible, if a benzodiazepine drug is needed, using one with a shorter elimination half-life might be considered.

References

1. Prescribing Information. Alprazolam. Apotex; 2017.
2. Esaki K, Oshio K, Yanagita J. Effects of oral administration of alprazolam (TUS-1) on the rat fetus: experiment on drug administration during the organogenesis period. *Preclin Rep Cent Inst Exp Anim*. 1981;7:65-77. As cited in Shepard TH. *Catalog of Teratogenic Agents*. 6th ed. Johns Hopkins University Press; 1989:32.
3. Gonzalez C, Smith R, Christensen HD, Rayburn WF. Prenatal alprazolam induces subtle impairment in hind limb balance and dexterity in C57BL/6 mice (abstract). *Teratology*. 1994;49:390.
4. Christensen HD, Pearce K, Gonzalez C, Rayburn WF. Does prenatal alprazolam exposure increase anxiety in adult mice offspring (abstract)? *Teratology*. 1994;49:390.
5. Rayburn W, Gonzalez C, Christensen D. Social interactions of C57BL/6 mice offspring exposed prenatally to alprazolam (Xanax) (abstract). *Am J Obstet Gynecol*. 1995;172:389.
6. Christensen HD, Gonzalez CL, Rayburn WF. Effects from prenatal exposure to alprazolam on the social behavior of mice offspring. *Am J Obstet Gynecol*. 2003;189:1452-1457.
7. Rayburn WF, Christensen HD, Gold KM, Gonzalez CL. Neurobehavior effects in four strains of mice offspring exposed prenatally to alprazolam. *Am J Obstet Gynecol*. 2002;187:968-972.
8. Barry WS, St Clair SM. Exposure to benzodiazepines in utero. *Lancet*. 1987;1:1436-1437.
9. Ayd FJ Jr, ed. Exposure to benzodiazepines in utero. *Int Drug Ther Newslett*. 1987;22:37-38.
10. St. Clair SM, Schirmer RG. First-trimester exposure to alprazolam. *Obstet Gynecol*. 1992;80:843-846.
11. Bergman U, Rosa FW, Baum C, et al. Effects of exposure to benzodiazepine during fetal life. *Lancet*. 1992;340:694-696.
12. Oo CY, Kuhn RJ, Desai N, et al. Pharmacokinetics in lactating women: prediction of alprazolam transfer into milk. *Br J Clin Pharmacol*. 1995;40:231-236.
13. Anderson PO, McGuire GG. Neonatal alprazolam withdrawal—possible effects of breast feeding. *DICP Ann Pharmacother*. 1989;23:614.
14. American Academy of Pediatrics Committee on Drugs. The transfer of drugs and other chemicals into human milk. *Pediatrics*. 2001;108:776-789.

ALTEPLASE

Hematologic (Thrombolytic—Tissue Plasminogen Activator)

PREGNANCY RECOMMENDATION: Limited Human Data—Animal Data Suggest Potential Risk (Maternal Benefit May Outweigh Any Embryofetal Risk)

BREASTFEEDING RECOMMENDATION: Probably Compatible

PREGNANCY SUMMARY

Several case reports and small series have been located that describe the use of alteplase during human pregnancy. In about 30 pregnancy exposures, most of the uses occurred in the second and third trimesters. Of those that had exposure in the first trimester, nearly all occurred in the last 4 weeks of that trimester. No major malformations have been reported, and no major complications related specifically to the drug were described. Some complications have occurred in these cases, but it

(continued)

is difficult to determine if these were related to the disease, other drugs used in the treatment, or the use of alteplase (or all three). Transplacental passage of the drug is not expected. However, because it is a protein, it is not known whether some placental transfer might occur in the second half of gestation. Therefore, this limited human pregnancy experience prevents a complete assessment of the embryofetal risk. Animal studies did show some embryofetal toxicity in one species at doses of less than 10 times the RHD. Due to the indication for use of the drug, pregnancy would not be a contraindication for use in treating acute ischemic stroke, acute myocardial infarction (MI), or pulmonary embolism.

BREASTFEEDING SUMMARY

No reports describing the use of alteplase during human lactation have been located. The drug is essentially the same as endogenous tissue plasminogen activator, which is normally found in colostrum. Regardless, because it is a protein, if the drug were to be ingested through breastfeeding, it would probably be digested in the infant's gastrointestinal tract and not be absorbed. Due to the indication for use of the drug, breastfeeding would not be a contraindication for use in treating acute ischemic stroke, acute MI, or pulmonary embolism. If the clinical decision is to use this drug while breastfeeding, the infant should be monitored for the most common reported adult side effect of bleeding (bruising).

References

1. Prescribing Information. Activase. Genentech, 2018.
2. Shepard TH. *Catalog of Teratogenic Agents*. 8th ed. Johns Hopkins University Press; 1995:416.
3. Flossdorf T, Breulmann M, Hopf H-B. Successful treatment of massive pulmonary embolism with recombinant tissue type plasminogen activator (rt-PA) in a pregnant woman with intact gravidity and preterm labour. *Intensive Care Med*. 1990;16:454-456.
4. Barclay GR, Allen K, Pennington CR. Tissue plasminogen activator in the treatment of superior vena caval thrombosis associated with parenteral nutrition. *Postgrad Med J*. 1990;66:398-400.
5. Baudo F, Caimi TM, Redaelli R, et al. Emergency treatment with recombinant tissue plasminogen activator of pulmonary embolism in a pregnant woman with antithrombin III deficiency. *Am J Obstet Gynecol*. 1990;163:1274-1275.
6. Seifried E, Gabelmann A, Ellbrück D, et al. Thrombolytische Therapie einer Lungenarterienembolie in der Frühschwangerschaft mit rekombinantem Gewebe-Plasminogen-Aktivator. *Geburtshilfe Frauenheilkd*. 1991;51:655. As cited in Turrentine MA, Braems G, Ramirez MM. Use of thrombolytics for the treatment of thromboembolic disease during pregnancy. *Obstet Gynecol Surv*. 1995;50:534-541.
7. Schumacher B, Belfort MA, Card RJ. Successful treatment of acute myocardial infarction during pregnancy with tissue plasminogen activator. *Am J Obstet Gynecol*. 1997;176:716-719.
8. Fleyfel M, Bourzoufi K, Huin G, et al. Recombinant tissue type plasminogen activator treatment of thrombosed mitral valve prosthesis during pregnancy. *Can J Anaesth*. 1997;44:735-738.
9. Huang WH, Kirz DS, Gallee RC, Gordey K. First trimester use of recombinant tissue plasminogen activator in pulmonary embolism. *Obstet Gynecol*. 2000;96:838.
10. Elford K, Leader A, Wee R, Stya PK. Stroke in ovarian hyperstimulation syndrome in early pregnancy treated with intra-arterial rt-PA. *Neurology*. 2002;59:1270-1272.
11. Song JY, Valentino L. A pregnant patient with renal vein thrombosis successfully treated with low-dose thrombolytic therapy: a case report. *Am J Obstet Gynecol*. 2005;192:2073-2075.
12. Weilbach C, Rahe-Meyer N, Raymondos K, Piepenbrock S. Delivery of a healthy child 30 weeks after resuscitation for thromboembolism and treatment with danaparoid: 5-year follow up. *J Perinat Med*. 2006;34:505-506.
13. Turrentine MA, Braems G, Ramirez MM. Use of thrombolytics for the treatment of thromboembolic disease during pregnancy. *Obstet Gynecol Surv*. 1995;50:534-541.

ALVIMOPAN

Gastrointestinal (μ-Opioid Receptor Antagonist)

PREGNANCY RECOMMENDATION: No Human Data—Animal Data Suggest Low Risk

BREASTFEEDING RECOMMENDATION: Probably Compatible

PREGNANCY SUMMARY

No reports describing the use of alvimopan in human pregnancy have been located. The drug will probably cross the placenta, so some fetal exposure will likely occur. Therefore, the absence of human pregnancy experience prevents a complete assessment of the embryofetal risk. Animal data did not show any embryofetal toxicity in two species at doses of less than and greater than 10 times the RHD. Using this drug during pregnancy should be based on the pros and cons of the mother's clinical need for treatment versus any potential fetal risk that might occur from exposure.

BREASTFEEDING SUMMARY

No reports describing the use of alvimopan during human lactation have been located. The drug will probably be found in breast milk, so some infant exposure will likely occur. Breastfeeding while using this drug should be based on the mother's clinical need for treatment versus any potential infant risks. If used, the infant should be monitored for the most common reported adult side effects of back pain and abdominal discomfort (both leading to irritability), urinary retention, and hypokalemia.

Reference

1. Prescribing Information. Entereg. Cubist Pharmaceuticals; 2019.

AMANTADINE

Antiviral/Central Nervous System (Influenza A/Anti-Parkinson)

PREGNANCY RECOMMENDATION: Limited Human Data—Animal Data Suggest Potential Risk

BREASTFEEDING RECOMMENDATION: Potential Toxicity

PREGNANCY SUMMARY

A few studies were located that describe the use of amantadine during human pregnancy. From these, there were 5 (7.1%) major anomalies in about 70 pregnancies with first-trimester exposure. Of seven case reports, two involved infants with multiple congenital defects. No pattern to these defects has been identified. The drug will probably cross the placenta, so some fetal exposure will likely occur. Therefore, this limited human pregnancy experience prevents a complete assessment of the embryofetal risk. Animal data did show some embryofetal toxicity with malformations in one species at doses of less than the RHD. ACOG and CDC no longer recommend amantadine for treating influenza A in pregnancy because of the high levels of resistance.

BREASTFEEDING SUMMARY

According to the manufacturer, amantadine is excreted into human breast milk in low concentrations. No reports of adverse effects in nursing infants have been located. The manufacturer recommends that amantadine should not be used during breastfeeding. However, if the clinical decision is to use this drug while breastfeeding, the infant should be monitored for the most common reported adult side effects of nausea and dizziness (both leading to irritability), and insomnia. The drug is a dopamine agonist and could cause adverse effects with breastfeeding initiation and maintenance.

References

1. Prescribing Information. Amantadine. Alembic Pharmaceuticals; 2018.
2. Nora JJ, Nora AH, Way GL. Cardiovascular maldevelopment associated with maternal exposure to amantadine. *Lancet*. 1975;2:607.
3. Golbe LI. Parkinson's disease and pregnancy. *Neurology*. 1987;37:1245-1249.
4. Levy M, Pastuszak A, Koren G. Fetal outcome following intrauterine amantadine exposure. *Reprod Toxicol*. 1991;5:79-81.
5. Pandit PB, Chitayat D, Jefferies AL, et al. Tibial hemimelia and tetralogy of Fallot associated with first trimester exposure to amantadine. *Reprod Toxicol*. 1994;8:89-92.
6. Rosa F. Amantadine pregnancy experience. *Reprod Toxicol*. 1994;8:531.
7. Greer LG, Sheffield JS, Rogers VL, et al. Maternal and neonatal outcomes after antepartum treatment of influenza with antiviral medications. *Obstet Gynecol*. 2010;115:711-716.

AMBRISENTAN

Cardiovascular (Pulmonary Arterial Hypertension)

PREGNANCY RECOMMENDATION: *No Human Data and No Relevant Animal Data

BREASTFEEDING RECOMMENDATION: Potential Toxicity

PREGNANCY SUMMARY

No reports describing the use of ambrisentan in human pregnancy have been located. The drug will probably cross the placenta, so some fetal exposure will likely occur. Therefore, the absence of human pregnancy experience prevents a complete assessment of the embryofetal risk. Animal studies did show teratogenicity in two species at doses of more than 10 times the maximum recommended human dose (MRHD) based on weight. *However, the drug carries a boxed warning for a contraindication for use in pregnancy. Based on these animal studies, the manufacturer states that pregnancy must be excluded prior to use and recommends that women with reproductive potential use two forms of effective contraception during treatment and for 1 month after the last dose. Regardless, pregnant women with pulmonary hypertension are extremely high-risk with an increased risk for mortality and poor pregnancy outcomes. Therefore, using this drug during pregnancy should be based on the pros and cons of the mother's clinical need for treatment versus any potential fetal risk that might occur from exposure.

BREASTFEEDING SUMMARY

No reports describing the use of ambrisentan during human lactation have been located. The drug will likely be found in human breast milk, so some infant exposure will probably occur. However, due to a concern for potential serious adverse effects that might be seen in a breastfed infant, the manufacturer recommends that women not breastfeed while being treated with this drug. Nevertheless, postpartum women with pulmonary hypertension are extremely high-risk patients, and breastfeeding while using this drug should be based on the mother's clinical need for treatment versus any potential infant risks that might occur. If used, the infant should be monitored for the most common reported adult side effects of abdominal pain (leading to irritability), constipation, peripheral edema, and flushing.

Reference

1. Prescribing Information. Letairis. Gilead Sciences; 2018.

AMIFAMPRIDINE

Miscellaneous (Potassium Channel Blocker)

PREGNANCY RECOMMENDATION: Limited Human Data—Animal Data Suggest Potential Risk

BREASTFEEDING RECOMMENDATION: Potential Toxicity

PREGNANCY SUMMARY

One case of human pregnancy exposure to amifampridine was located. A mother used the drug at the time of conception and throughout the pregnancy until delivery. A healthy term newborn was delivered with no identified anomalies, and the infant was progressing normally at 5 months. The drug will probably cross the placenta, so some fetal exposure will likely occur. Therefore, this limited human pregnancy experience prevents a complete assessment of the embryofetal risk. Animal data did show an increase in stillbirth and some neonatal toxicity with use throughout pregnancy and into lactation in one species at doses less than 10 times the RHD. However, no embryofetal toxicity or malformations were seen in two animal species using the drug at conception and through organogenesis at doses less than 10 times the RHD. Using this drug during pregnancy should be based on the pros and cons of the mother's clinical need for treatment versus any potential fetal risk that might occur from exposure. There is a pregnancy exposure registry that monitors pregnancy outcomes in patients using this drug during gestation. Health care providers are encouraged to call the Pregnancy Registry at 1-855-212-5856.

BREASTFEEDING SUMMARY

No reports describing the use of amifampridine during human lactation have been located. The drug will probably be found in breast milk, so some infant exposure will likely occur. Breastfeeding while using this drug should be based on the mother's clinical need for treatment versus any potential infant risks. If used, the infant should be monitored for the most common reported adult side effects of nausea, abdominal pain, back pain, paresthesia, and headache (all leading to irritability), diarrhea, and elevated liver function tests.

References

1. Prescribing Information. Firdapse. Catalyst Pharmaceuticals; 2022.
2. Pelufo-Pellicer A, Monte-Boquet E, Roma-Sanchez, et al. Fetal exposure to 3,4-diaminopyridine in a pregnant woman with congenital myasthenia syndrome. *Ann Pharmacother*. 2006;40:762-766.

AMIFOSTINE

Antidote (Cytoprotectant)

PREGNANCY RECOMMENDATION: No Human Data—Animal Data Suggest Potential Risk

BREASTFEEDING RECOMMENDATION: Potential Toxicity

PREGNANCY SUMMARY

No reports describing the use of amifostine in human pregnancy have been located. The drug will probably cross the placenta, so some fetal exposure will likely occur. Therefore, the absence of human pregnancy experience prevents a complete assessment of the embryofetal risk. Animal studies did show embryofetal toxicity in one species at doses less than 10 times the RHD. Using this drug during pregnancy should be based on the pros and cons of the mother's clinical need for treatment versus any potential fetal risk that might occur from exposure.

BREASTFEEDING SUMMARY

No reports describing the use of amifostine during human lactation have been located. The drug will probably be found in breast milk, so some infant exposure could occur. Breastfeeding while using this drug should be based on the mother's clinical need for treatment versus any potential infant risks. If used, the infant should be monitored for the most common reported adult side effects of nausea (leading to irritability), diarrhea, lethargy, somnolence, vomiting, hypotension, hypocalcemia, fever, and rash. However, due to the very short elimination half-life and because the drug is given as a short IV infusion immediately before chemotherapy or radiation (when breastfeeding would be unlikely to occur), the risk of exposing an infant to amifostine when nursing is later resumed is likely to be negligible.

Reference

1. Prescribing Information. Ethyol. Cumberland Pharmaceuticals; 2019.

AMIKACIN

Antibacterial (Aminoglycoside—Mycoplasma Avium Complex)

PREGNANCY RECOMMENDATION: Limited Human Data—Animal Data Suggest Low Risk

BREASTFEEDING RECOMMENDATION: Potential Toxicity

PREGNANCY SUMMARY

No reports linking the use of amikacin to congenital defects have been located. Ototoxicity and nephrotoxicity, which are known to occur with aminoglycoside therapy in humans, have not been reported as an effect of in utero exposure to amikacin. The drug crosses the placenta, so some fetal exposure will occur. However, this limited human pregnancy experience prevents a complete assessment of the embryofetal risk. Animal studies did not show any embryofetal toxicity in two species at doses of more than 10 times the RHD. Serum levels following oral inhalation use are less than 10% of the serum concentrations seen with intramuscular (IM) use. Using this drug during pregnancy should be based on the pros and cons of the mother's clinical need for treatment versus any potential fetal risk that might occur from exposure.

BREASTFEEDING SUMMARY

Three studies were located that describe the use of amikacin during human lactation. A total of five women had breast milk analyzed following either a 100 or 200 mg IM dose. The drug was detected in every patient, but in trace amounts in four (detectable but less than 1 mcg/mL). In the fifth case, the concentration was 1.5 mcg/mL. However, blood levels with inhalation use are less than 10% of those seen with IM administration. Therefore, the overall amount that may be found in breast milk is likely to be minimal. Regardless, the amount of drug that is needed to cause ototoxicity or nephrotoxicity is not fully known. Breastfeeding while using this drug should be based on the mother's clinical need for treatment versus any potential infant risks that might occur. If used, the infant should be monitored for the most common reported adult side effects of nausea, headache, and musculoskeletal pain (all leading to irritability), cough, fatigue (lethargy), and diarrhea.

References

1. Prescribing Information. Amikacin. West-Ward Pharmaceuticals; 2016.
2. Mallie JP, Coulon G, Billerey C, et al. In utero aminoglycosides-induced nephrotoxicity in rat neonates. *Kidney Inter*. 1988;33:36-44.
3. Bernard B, Abate M, Ballard C, Wehrle P. Maternal-fetal pharmacology of BB-K8. Presented at: Antimicrobial Agents and Chemotherapy 14th Annual Conference; 1974, Abstract 71; Montreal, Quebec Canada.
4. Matsuda C, Mori C, Maruno M, Shiwakura T. A study of amikacin in the obstetrics field. *Jpn J Antibiot*. 1974;27:633-636.
5. Bernard B, Abate M, Thielen P, et al. Maternal-fetal pharmacological activity of amikacin. *J Infect Dis*. 1977;135:925-931.
6. Flores-Mercado F, Garcia-Mercado J, Estopier-Jauregin C, et al. Clinical pharmacology of amikacin sulphate: blood, urinary and tissue concentrations in the terminal stage of pregnancy. *J Int Med Res*. 1977;5;292-294.
7. Pacifici GM. Placental transfer of antibiotics administered to the mother: a review. *Int J Clin Pharmacol Ther*. 2006;44:57-63.
8. Yuasa M. A study of amikacin in obstetrics and gynecology. *Jpn J Antibiot*. 1974;27;377-381.
9. Matsuda S. Transfer of antibiotics into maternal milk. *Biol Res Pregnancy Perinatol*. 1984;5:57-69.

AMILORIDE

Cardiovascular (Diuretic)

PREGNANCY RECOMMENDATION: Limited Human Data—Animal Data Suggest Low Risk

BREASTFEEDING RECOMMENDATION: Probably Compatible

PREGNANCY SUMMARY

Several case reports and data from the Michigan Medicaid Surveillance Study (MMSS) described a total of 36 pregnancies with first-trimester exposure to amiloride. Of these, there were two major congenital birth defects, both different. The others all delivered healthy appearing infants with no identified anomalies. The drug probably crosses the placenta, so some fetal exposure will likely occur. However, this limited human pregnancy experience prevents a complete assessment of the

(continued)

embryofetal risk. Animal studies did not show any embryofetal toxicity or teratogenicity in two species at doses of more than 10 times the RHD. Using this drug during pregnancy should be based on the pros and cons of the mother's clinical need for treatment versus any potential fetal risk that might occur from exposure. In general, diuretics are not recommended in the treatment of gestational hypertension because of the maternal hypovolemia characteristic of this disease.

BREASTFEEDING SUMMARY

No reports describing breast milk drug levels with the use of amiloride during human lactation have been located. One study did evaluate serum potassium levels in an infant exposed to the drug through breastfeeding, and the potassium level was slightly elevated when she was on the drug, with a return to normal levels when she stopped. This is suggestive that some of the drug was in the breast milk. If the clinical decision is to use this drug while breastfeeding, the infant should be monitored for the most common reported adult side effects of nausea, headache, and abdominal pain (all leading to irritability), vomiting, diarrhea, and elevated potassium serum levels.

References

1. Prescribing Information. Amiloride hydrochloride. Par Pharmaceutical; 2018.
2. Miller TA, Scott WJ Jr. Abnormalities in ureter and kidney development in mice given acetazolamide-amiloride or dimethadione (DMO) during embryogenesis. *Teratology*. 1992;46:541-550.
3. Duminy PC, Burger PT. Fetal abnormality associated with the use of captopril during pregnancy. *S Afr Med J*. 1981;60:805.
4. Almeida OD Jr, Spinnato JA. Maternal Bartter's syndrome and pregnancy. *Am J Obstet Gynecol*. 1989;160:1225-1226.
5. Robson DJ, Jeeva Raj MV, Storey GCA, Holt DW. Use of amiodarone during pregnancy. *Postgrad Med J*. 1985;61:75-77.
6. Deruelle P, Dufour P, Magnenant E, et al. Maternal Bartter's syndrome in pregnancy treated with amiloride. *Eur J Obstet Gynecol Reprod Biol*. 2004;115:106-107.
7. Mascetti L, Bettinelli A, Simonetti GD, et al. Pregnancy in inherited hypokalemic salt-losing renal tubular disorder. *Obstet Gynecol*. 2011;117:512-516.
8. Mathen S, Venning M, Gillham J. Outpatient management of Gitelman's syndrome in pregnancy. *BMJ Case Rep*. 2013;2013:bcr2012007927. doi:10.1136/bcr-2012-007927
9. Krysiak R, Samborek M, Stojko R. Primary aldosteronism in pregnancy. *Acta Clin Belg*. 2012;67:130-134.
10. Ibrahim A, Rodan AR, Westenfelder C, Al-Rabadi L. Gitelman syndrome patient managed with amiloride during pregnancy and lactation. *BMC Nephrol*. 2024;25:403.

AMINOCAPROIC ACID

Hematologic (Fibrinolysis Inhibitor)

PREGNANCY RECOMMENDATION: Limited Human Data—No Relevant Animal Data (Maternal Benefit May Outweigh Any Embryofetal Risk)

BREASTFEEDING RECOMMENDATION: Potential Toxicity (Hold Breastfeeding)

PREGNANCY SUMMARY

A few case reports have described the use of aminocaproic acid during human pregnancy in the second and third trimesters. No fetal toxicity was reported. The drug will probably cross the placenta, so some fetal exposure will likely occur. Therefore, this limited human pregnancy experience prevents a complete assessment of the embryofetal risk. No animal reproduction studies have been conducted. Use of the drug is uncommon but is indicated in conditions that can be life-threatening. Therefore, pregnancy should probably not be a reason for preventing use.

BREASTFEEDING SUMMARY

No reports describing the use of aminocaproic acid during human lactation have been located. The drug will probably be found in human breast milk, so some infant exposure will likely occur. Aminocaproic acid is usually needed in life-threatening situations and should probably not be withheld due to breastfeeding. If the clinical decision is to use this drug while breastfeeding, the infant should be monitored for the most common reported adult side effects of headache, nausea, and abdominal pain (all leading to irritability), peripheral edema, vomiting, diarrhea, decreased heart rate, and hypotension.

References

1. Prescribing Information. Aminocaproic acid. VersaPharm; 2013.
2. Willoughby JS. Sodium nitroprusside, pregnancy and multiple intracranial aneurysms. *Anaesth Intensive Care*. 1984;12:358-360.

AMINOPHYLLINE

Respiratory

SEE THEOPHYLLINE

(PARA)-AMINOSALICYCLIC ACID

Antibacterial (Antituberculosis)

PREGNANCY RECOMMENDATION: Limited Human Data—Animal Data Suggest Risk (Maternal Benefit May Outweigh Any Potential Embryofetal Risk)

BREASTFEEDING RECOMMENDATION: Probably Compatible

PREGNANCY SUMMARY

Several studies have been located that describe the use of *para*-aminosalicylic acid during human pregnancy. With combined data from a few larger series, the congenital birth anomaly rate is slightly higher than the expected rate, but no pattern to the defects has been described. This finding may be related to the maternal disease state. The drug will probably cross the placenta, so some fetal exposure will likely occur. Therefore, this limited human pregnancy experience prevents a complete assessment of the embryofetal risk. Animal studies did show some embryofetal toxicity with malformations in two species at doses of about equal to the RHD. However, because tuberculosis (TB), especially multidrug-resistant TB, is a serious infection, withholding the drug because of pregnancy could have adverse consequences.

BREASTFEEDING SUMMARY

Para-aminosalicylic acid was found to be excreted into human breast milk. The breast milk level was about 1.1 mcg/mL, resulting in a calculated RID that was less than 1%. Due to a concern for potential serious adverse effects that might be seen in a breastfed infant, the manufacturer recommends that women not breastfeed while being treated with this drug. Nevertheless, breastfeeding while using this drug should be based on the mother's clinical need for treatment versus any potential infant risks that might occur. If used, the infant should be monitored for the most common reported adult side effects of nausea (leading to irritability), diarrhea, vomiting, rash, and fever.

References

1. Prescribing Information. Paser. Jacobus Pharmaceutical; 2010.
2. Heinonen OP, Slone D, Shapiro S. *Birth Defects and Drugs in Pregnancy*. Publishing Sciences Group; 1977:299.
3. Varpela E. On the effect exerted by first line tuberculosis medicines on the foetus. *Acta Tuberc Pneumol Scand*. 1964;35:53-69.
4. Lowe CR. Congenital defects among children born to women under supervision or treatment for pulmonary tuberculosis. *Br J Prev Soc Med*. 1964;18:14-16.
5. Wilson EA, Thelin TJ, Ditts PV. Tuberculosis complicated by pregnancy. *Am J Obstet Gynecol*. 1973;115:526-529.
6. Scheinhorn DJ, Angelillo VA. Antituberculosis therapy in pregnancy. Risk to the fetus. *West J Med*. 1977;127:195-198.
7. Drobac PC, del Castillo H, Sweetland A, et al. Treatment of multi-drug resistant tuberculosis during pregnancy: long-term follow-up of 6 children with intrauterine exposure to second-line agents. *Clin Infect Dis*. 2005;40:1689-1692.
8. Cassina M, Fabris L, Okolicsanyl L, et al. Therapy of inflammatory bowel diseases in pregnancy and lactation. *Expert Opin Drug Saf*. 2009;8:695-707.
9. Nielsen OH, Maxwell C, Hendel J. IBD medications during pregnancy and lactation. *Nat Rev Gastroenterol Hepatol*. 2014;11:116-127.
10. Cury DB, Moss AC. Treatment of Crohn's disease in pregnant women: drug and multidisciplinary approaches. *World J Gastroenterol*. 2014;20:8790-8795.
11. Holdiness MR. Antituberculosis drugs and breast-feeding. *Arch Intern Med*. 1984;144:1888.

AMIODARONE

Cardiovascular (Antiarrhythmic)

PREGNANCY RECOMMENDATION: Limited Human Data—Animal Data Suggest Risk

BREASTFEEDING RECOMMENDATION: Potential Toxicity

PREGNANCY SUMMARY

Numerous case reports and small series have been published that describe the use of amiodarone during human pregnancy. Regarding use in treating maternal arrhythmias, over 25 cases have been identified, with about 17 having exposure at the time of conception and through the first trimester. One spontaneous abortion occurred, and one major malformation was described (a muscular ventricular septal defect [VSD]). The remaining infants did well. The remainder of uses occurred in the second and third trimesters. Overall, most infants did well. Many had thyroid function tests performed postdelivery, and again, most were in the normal range; however, in several cases where iodine levels were analyzed, most values were markedly elevated. Many infants were also delivered preterm or were growth restricted, but this could also have been related to maternal disease. The drug and its active metabolite, desethylamiodarone (DEA), cross the placenta, so some fetal exposure

(continued)

will occur. However, this limited human pregnancy experience still prevents a complete assessment of the embryofetal risk. Animal studies did show some embryofetal toxicity in three species at doses of less than 10 times the RHD. This drug is often used in life-threatening situations in many instances. Therefore, using this drug during pregnancy should be based on the pros and cons of the mother's clinical need for treatment versus any potential fetal risk that might occur from exposure. Depending on the maternal dose, a significant amount of free iodine can be released in some cases, so newborn thyroid function should be evaluated postdelivery. Long-term use can be more complicated, especially with an elimination half-life that might be up to 2 months in some cases. In the clinical trials, the drug was also found to prolong the QT interval.

BREASTFEEDING SUMMARY

Numerous studies have been located that describe the use of amiodarone during human lactation in 13 women. The drug and active metabolite, DEA, were found in nearly every breast milk sample tested. Concentrations for amiodarone ranged from about 0.15 mcg/mL to a high of about 25 mcg/mL, but most were in the 1 to 3.5 mcg/mL range. Concentrations for DEA ranged from about 0.01 mcg/mL up to a high of about 5.7 mcg/mL, but most were in the 0.5 to 1.8 mcg/mL range. The calculated RIDs ranged from about 3% up to 45%, with a median of about 11%. Infant serum levels were also analyzed in four cases with a range for amiodarone of about 10 to 400 ng/mL versus 10 to 300 ng/mL for DEA. Due to a concern for potential serious adverse effects that might be seen in a breastfed infant, the manufacturer recommends that women not breastfeed while being treated with this drug. Nevertheless, this drug is often used in life-threatening situations in many instances. Breastfeeding while using this drug should be based on the mother's clinical need for treatment versus any potential infant risks that might occur. If used, the infant should be monitored for the most common reported adult side effects of dizziness and blurred vision (both leading to irritability), cough, vomiting, tachycardia, and elevated liver function tests. Also, depending on the maternal dose, a significant amount of free iodine can be released in some cases, so infant thyroid function should be monitored. It is thought that a single dose during breastfeeding will likely be tolerated. Long-term use may be more complicated, especially with an elimination half-life that might be up to 2 months in some cases.

References

1. Prescribing Information. Amiodarone. Cameron Pharmaceuticals; 2018.
2. Candelpergher G, Buchberger R, Suzzi GL, Padrini R. Trans-placental passage of amiodarone: electrocardiographic and pharmacologic evidence in a newborn. *G Ital Cardiol*. 1982;12:79-82.
3. McKenna WJ, Harris L, Rowland E, et al. Amiodarone therapy during pregnancy. *Am J Cardiol*. 1983;51:1231-1233.
4. Pitcher D, Leather HM, Storey GAC, Holt DW. Amiodarone in pregnancy. *Lancet*. 1983;1:597-598.
5. Robson DJ, Jeeva Raj MV, Storey GAC, Holt DW. Use of amiodarone during pregnancy. *Postgrad Med J*. 1985;61:75-77.
6. Arnoux P, Seyral P, Llurens M, et al. Amiodarone and digoxin for refractory fetal tachycardia. *Am J Cardiol*. 1987;59:166-167.
7. Penn IM, Barrett PA, Pannikote V, et al. Amiodarone in pregnancy. *Am J Cardiol*. 1985;56:196-197.
8. Strunge P, Frandsen J, Andreasen F. Amiodarone during pregnancy. *Eur Heart J*. 1988;9:106-109.
9. Plomp TA, Vulsma T, de Vijlder JJM. Use of amiodarone during pregnancy. *Eur J Obstet Gynecol Reprod Biol*. 1992;43:201-207.
10. Gembruch U, Manz M, Bald R, et al. Repeated intravascular treatment with amiodarone in a fetus with refractory supraventricular tachycardia and hydrops fetalis. *Am Heart J*. 1989;118:1335-1338.
11. Rey E, Bachrach LK, Burrow GN. Effects of amiodarone during pregnancy. *Can Med Assoc J*. 1987;136:959-960.
12. Widerhorn J, Bhandari AK, Bughi S, et al. Fetal and neonatal adverse effects profile of amiodarone treatment during pregnancy. *Am Heart J*. 1991;122:1162-1166.
13. Wladimiroff JW, Steward PA. Treatment of fetal cardiac arrhythmias. *Br J Hosp Med*. 1985;34:134-140. As cited by Widerhorn J, Bhandari AK, Bughi S, et al. Fetal and neonatal adverse effects profile of amiodarone treatment during pregnancy. *Am Heart J*. 1991;122:1162-1166.
14. Foster CJ, Love HG. Amiodarone in pregnancy: case report and review of literature. *Int J Cardiol*. 1988;20:307-316.
15. De Wolf D, De Schepper J, Verhaaren H, et al. Congenital hypothyroid goiter and amiodarone. *Acta Paediatr Scand*. 1988;77:616-618.
16. Ovadia M, Brito M, Hoyer GL, Marcus FI. Human experience with amiodarone in the embryonic period. *Am J Cardiol*. 1994;73:316-317.
17. Rey E, Duperron L, Gauthier R, et al. Transplacental treatment of tachycardia-induced fetal heart failure with verapamil and amiodarone: a case report. *Am J Obstet Gynecol*. 1985;153:311-312.
18. Laurent M, Betremieux P, Biron Y, LeHelloco A. Neonatal hypothyroidism after treatment by amiodarone during pregnancy. *Am J Cardiol*. 1987;60:942.
19. Flack NJ, Zosmer N, Bennett PR, et al. Amiodarone given by three routes to terminate fetal atrial flutter associated with severe hydrops. *Obstet Gynecol*. 1993;82:714-716.
20. Fulgencio JP, Hamza J. Anaesthesia for caesarean section in a patient receiving high dose amiodarone for fetal supraventricular tachycardia. *Anaesthesia*. 1994;49:406-408.
21. Magee LA, Taddio A, Downar E, et al. Pregnancy outcome following gestational exposure to amiodarone (abstract). *Teratology*. 1994;49:398.
22. Magee LA, Downar E, Sermer M, et al. Pregnancy outcome after gestational exposure to amiodarone in Canada. *Am J Obstet Gynecol*. 1995;172:1307-1311.
23. Ito S, Magee L, Smallhorn J. Drug therapy for fetal arrhythmias. *Clin Perinatol*. 1994;21:543-572.
24. Sloskey GE. Amiodarone: a unique antiarrhythmic agent. *Clin Pharm*. 1983;2:330-340.
25. Rotmensch HH, Rotmensch S, Elkayam U. Management of cardiac arrhythmias during pregnancy: current concepts. *Drugs*. 1987;33:623-633.
26. Ward RM. Maternal drug therapy for fetal disorders. *Semin Perinatol*. 1992;16:12-20.
27. American Academy of Pediatrics Committee on Drugs. The transfer of drugs and other chemicals into human milk. *Pediatrics*. 2001;108:776-789.

AMITRIPTYLINE

Mental Health (Antidepressant/Tricyclic)

PREGNANCY RECOMMENDATION: Limited Human Data—Animal Data Suggest Risk

BREASTFEEDING RECOMMENDATION: Potential Toxicity

A

PREGNANCY SUMMARY

Several studies have been identified regarding the use of amitriptyline during human pregnancy. From 3 large databases (CPP, MMSS, and the European Network of Teratology Information Services [ENTIS]), there were 577 first-trimester exposures to the drug, with 26 (4.5%) major anomalies identified. No pattern to the defects was seen. The drug crosses the placenta, so some fetal exposure will occur. Therefore, based on the slightly increased risk for major anomalies overall, further human pregnancy experience needs to be collected for a more complete assessment of the embryofetal risk. Animal studies did show some embryofetal toxicity in two species at doses of less than 10 times the RHD, but this was not seen in two different species at doses of more than 10 times the RHD. Using this drug during pregnancy should be based on the pros and cons of the mother's clinical need for treatment versus any potential fetal risk that might occur from exposure. Neonatal withdrawal after in utero exposure in the third trimester to other antidepressants (see Imipramine) has been reported, but not with amitriptyline as of yet. However, the potential for this complication exists because of the close similarity among these agents.

BREASTFEEDING SUMMARY

Several case reports were located that have described the use of amitriptyline during human breastfeeding. In six lactating women, the drug and its active metabolite, nortriptyline, were found in nearly every breast milk sample analyzed. Breast milk levels ranged from about 13 to 197 ng/mL for amitriptyline and for nortriptyline ranged from undetectable to 72 ng/mL. All of the calculated RIDs were less than 2%. Breastfeeding while using this drug should be based on the mother's clinical need for treatment versus any potential infant risks that might occur. If used, the infant should be monitored for the most common reported adult side effects of nausea (leading to irritability), diarrhea, vomiting, and rash. The drug can increase prolactin levels in some patients, but this should not have any adverse effect on breastfeeding.

References

1. Prescribing Information. Amitriptyline. Accord Healthcare; 2017.
2. Elia J, Katz IR, Simpson GM. Teratogenicity of psychotherapeutic medications. *Psychopharmacol Bull*. 1987;23:531-586.
3. Shepard TH. *Catalog of Teratogenic Agents*. 6th ed. Johns Hopkins University Press; 1989:44-45.
4. McBride WG. Limb deformities associated with iminodibenzyl hydrochloride. *Med J Aust*. 1972;1:492.
5. Freeman R. Limb deformities: possible association with drugs. *Med J Aust*. 1972;1:606.
6. Australian Drug Evaluation Committee. Tricyclic antidepressants and limb reduction deformities. *Med J Aust*. 1973;1:768-769.
7. Heinonen OP, Slone D, Shapiro S. *Birth Defects and Drugs in Pregnancy*. Publishing Sciences Group; 1977:336-337.
8. Idanpaan-Heikkila J, Saxen L. Possible teratogenicity of imipramine/chloropyramine. *Lancet*. 1973;2:282-283.
9. Rachelefsky GS, Glynt JW, Ebbin AJ, Wilson MG. Possible teratogenicity of tricyclic antidepressants. *Lancet*. 1972;1:838.
10. Banister P, Dafoe C, Smith ESO, Miller J. Possible teratogenicity of tricyclic antidepressants. *Lancet*. 1972;1:838-839.
11. Scanlon FJ. Use of antidepressant drugs during the first trimester. *Med J Aust*. 1969;2:1077.
12. Crombie DL, Pinsent R, Fleming D. Imipramine in pregnancy. *Br Med J*. 1972;1:745.
13. Kuenssberg EV, Knox JDE. Imipramine in pregnancy. *Br Med J*. 1972;2:292.
14. Golden SM, Perman KI. Bilateral clinical anophthalmia: drugs as potential factors. *South Med J*. 1980;73:1404-1407.
15. Wertelecki W, Purvis-Smith SG, Blackburn WR. Amitriptyline/perphenazine maternal overdose and birth defects (abstract). *Teratology*. 1980;21:74A.
16. Rafla NM, Meehan FP. Thanatophoric dwarfism: drugs and antenatal diagnosis. A case report. *Eur J Obstet Gynecol Reprod Biol*. 1990;38:161-165.
17. McElhatton PR, Garbis HM, Elefant E, et al. The outcome of pregnancy in 689 women exposed to therapeutic doses of antidepressants. A collaborative study of the European Network of Teratology Information Services (ENTIS). *Reprod Toxicol*. 1996;10:285-294.
18. Shearer WT, Schreiner RL, Marshall RE. Urinary retention in a neonate secondary to maternal ingestion of nortriptyline. *J Pediatr*. 1972;81:570-572.
19. Nulman I, Rovet J, Stewart DE, et al. Child development following exposure to tricyclic antidepressants or fluoxetine throughout fetal life: a prospective, controlled study. *Am J Psychiatry*. 2002;159:1889-1895.
20. Bader TF, Newman K. Amitriptyline in human breast milk and the nursing infant's serum. *Am J Psychiatry*. 1980;137:855-856.
21. Wilson JT, Brown D, Cherek DR, et al. Drug excretion in human breast milk. Principles, pharmacokinetics and projected consequences. *Clin Pharmacokinet*. 1980;5:1-66.
22. Brixen-Rasmussen L, Halgrener J, Jorgensen A. Amitriptyline and nortriptyline excretion in human breast milk. *Psychopharmacology (Berlin)*. 1982;76:94-95.
23. Breyer-Pfaff U, Nill K, Entenmann A, Gaertner HJ. Secretion of amitriptyline and metabolites into breast milk. *Am J Psychiatry*. 1995;152:812-813.
24. Yoshida K, Smith B, Craggs M, Kumar RC. Investigation of pharmacokinetics and of possible adverse effects in infants exposed to tricyclic antidepressants in breast-milk. *J Affect Disord*. 1997;43:225-237.
25. Wisner KL, Perel JM, Findling RL. Antidepressant treatment during breast-feeding. *Am J Psychiatry*. 1996;153:1132-1137.
26. Erickson SH, Smith GH, Heidrich F. Tricyclics and breast feeding. *Am J Psychiatry*. 1979;136:1483.
27. American Academy of Pediatrics Committee on Drugs. The transfer of drugs and other chemicals into human milk. *Pediatrics*. 2001;108:776-789.

AMIVANTAMAB

Antineoplastic (Monoclonal Antibody)

PREGNANCY RECOMMENDATION: No Human Data—Animal Data Suggest Potential Risk

BREASTFEEDING RECOMMENDATION: Probably Compatible

PREGNANCY SUMMARY

No reports describing the use of amivantamab in human pregnancy have been located. As an IgG antibody, the drug is likely to cross the placenta, so some fetal exposure will probably occur. However, the absence of human pregnancy experience prevents a complete assessment of the embryofetal risk. Animal reproduction studies have not been conducted. However, in animals, epidermal growth factor is critically important for blastocyst implantation, placental development, and embryofetal/postnatal survival. Therefore, embryofetal toxicity could occur. Because of this, the manufacturer recommends that women with reproductive potential who are taking amivantamab use effective contraception during treatment and for at least 3 months after the last dose. Nevertheless, using this drug during pregnancy should be based on the pros and cons of the mother's clinical need for treatment versus any potential fetal risk that might occur from exposure. Elevated glucose levels have been reported in patients treated with this drug. Therefore, if used during pregnancy, glucose levels should be monitored.

BREASTFEEDING SUMMARY

No reports describing the use of amivantamab during human lactation have been located. It is known that IgG antibodies can be found in human breast milk, but are not found in the neonatal or infant circulation. Additionally, if any IgG antibodies were to be ingested through breastfeeding, they would probably be digested in the infant's gastrointestinal tract and not be absorbed. However, due to the potential for adverse effects that might be seen in a breastfed infant, the manufacturer recommends that women should not breastfeed while being treated with amivantamab and for at least 3 months after the last dose. Nevertheless, breastfeeding while using this drug should be based on the mother's clinical need for treatment. If used, the infant should be monitored for the most common reported adult side effects of musculoskeletal pain and nausea (both leading to irritability), dyspnea, edema, lethargy, cough, constipation, vomiting, rash, and various laboratory abnormalities (see PI).

Reference

1. Prescribing Information. Rybrevant. Janssen Biotech; 2022.

AMISULPRIDE

Gastrointestinal (Antiemetic)

PREGNANCY RECOMMENDATION: Limited Human Data—Animal Data Suggest Low Risk

BREASTFEEDING RECOMMENDATION: Probably Compatible

PREGNANCY SUMMARY

No studies have been found regarding the IV use of amisulpride in human pregnancy. Amisulpride is available orally as an atypical antipsychotic in Europe. The drug crosses the placenta; thus, fetal exposure occurs. Animal data did not show fetotoxic effects. However, the absence of human pregnancy experience prevents a complete assessment of the embryofetal risk. Amisulpride can cause prolongation of the QT interval. Its use should be avoided in patients with congenital long QT syndrome.

BREASTFEEDING SUMMARY

No reports of IV amisulpride use in human lactation have been reported. Amisulpride is excreted into human breast milk, producing a high breast milk to plasma ratio of 11:20. Three case reports of nursing mothers taking oral amisulpride found the RID to be low, with a range between 4.7% and 10.7% of the maternal weight-adjusted dose. However, due to the high breast milk to plasma ratio, the manufacturer recommends that breastfeeding women consider interrupting breastfeeding, pumping, and discarding breast milk for 48 hours after receiving amisulpride to minimize exposure to the infant.

References

1. Prescribing Information. Barhemsys. Acacia Pharma, Inc; 2021.
2. Nandakumaran M, Challier JC, Rey E, et al. In vitro transfer of six benzamides in the human placenta. *Dev Pharmacol Ther*. 1984;7(suppl 1):60-66.
3. Damkier P, Videbech P. The safety of second-generation antipsychotics during pregnancy: a clinically focused review. *CNS Drugs*. 2018;32(4):351-366.
4. Ilett KF, Watt F, Hackett LP, et al. Assessment of infant dose through milk in a lactating woman taking amisulpride and desvenlafaxine for treatment-resistant depression. *Ther Drug Monit*. 2010;32(6):704-707.
5. Teoh S, Ilett KF, Hackett LP, Kohan R. Estimation of race-amisulpride transfer into milk and of infant dose via milk during its use in a lactating woman with bipolar disorder and schizophrenia. *Breastfeed Med*. 2011;6(2):85-88.
6. O'Halloran SJ, Wong A, Joyce DA. A liquid chromatography-tandem mass spectrometry method for quantifying amisulpride in human plasma and breast milk, applied to measuring drug transfer to a fully breast-fed neonate. *Ther Drug Monit*. 2016;38(4):493-498.
7. Uguz F. Breastfed infants exposed to combined antipsychotics: two case reports. *Am J Ther*. 2016;23(6):e1962-e1964.

AMLODIPINE

Cardiovascular (Calcium Channel Blocker)

PREGNANCY RECOMMENDATION: Limited Human Data—Animal Data Suggest Potential Risk (Maternal Benefit May Outweigh Any Potential Embryofetal Risk)

BREASTFEEDING RECOMMENDATION: Probably Compatible

PREGNANCY SUMMARY

A few case reports and studies have been located that described the use of amlodipine during human pregnancy. No major birth anomalies were identified in four first-trimester exposures. In a multicenter cohort prospective observational study from ENTIS, 299 pregnant women were exposed to calcium channel blockers during the first trimester. The four most common agents were nifedipine 76, verapamil 62, diltiazem 41, and amlodipine 38. The rate of major birth defects (3.5%) was not elevated, and no pattern to the anomalies was seen. However, specific information on the individual drugs was not provided. The drug will probably cross the placenta, so some fetal exposure will likely occur. Therefore, this limited human pregnancy experience prevents a complete assessment of the embryofetal risk. Animal studies did show some embryofetal toxicity in one species at doses of less than 10 times the RHD when administered prior to conception and throughout the entire gestation. Uncontrolled hypertension and serious coronary artery disease can lead to a high rate of poor pregnancy outcomes. Therefore, the use of this drug in many cases may outweigh any potential fetal risks.

BREASTFEEDING SUMMARY

A few studies describing the use of amlodipine during human lactation were found. The breast milk of 45 lactating women was analyzed, and the drug was not detected in six cases (LLQ of 100 pg/mL). In the remaining 39 women, amlodipine concentrations ranged from about 2 to 20 ng/mL. These levels seem low, but the normal human dose in a 70 kg person ranges from about 70 to 140 mcg/kg. Thus, the calculated RIDs range from about 1% up to 15%. Regardless, a total of 18 infants had serum levels checked following exposure to amlodipine through breastfeeding. In every case, the drug was not detected (LLQ ranging from 100 to 400 pg/mL). However, due to a concern for potential serious adverse effects that might be seen in a breastfed infant, the manufacturer recommends that women not breastfeed while being treated with this drug. Nevertheless, breastfeeding while using this drug should be based on the mother's clinical need for treatment versus any potential infant risks that might occur. If used, the infant should be monitored for the most common reported adult side effects of nausea, headache, and abdominal pain (all leading to irritability), peripheral edema, fatigue (lethargy), and somnolence.

References

1. Prescribing Information. Amlodipine besylate. Amneal Pharmaceuticals; 2019.
2. Rosbotham JL, Johnson A, Haque KN, Holden CA. Painful subcutaneous fat necrosis of the newborn associated with intra-partum use of a calcium channel blocker. *Clin Exp Dermatol*. 1998;23:19-21.
3. Ahn HK, Nava-Ocampo AA, Han JY, et al. Exposure to amlodipine in the first trimester of pregnancy and during breastfeeding. *Hypertens Pregnancy*. 2007;26:179-187.
4. Nahapetian A, Oudiz RJ. Serial hemodynamics and complications of pregnancy in severe pulmonary arterial hypertension. *Cardiology*. 2008; 109:237-240.
5. Weber-Schoendorfer C, Hannemann D, Meister R, et al. The safety of calcium channel blockers during pregnancy: a prospective, multicenter, observational study. *Reprod Toxicol*. 2008;26:24-30.
6. Vigil-De Gracia P, Dominguez L, Solis A. Management of chronic hypertension during pregnancy with furosemide, amlodipine or aspirin: a pilot clinical trial. *J Matern Fetal Neonatal Med*. 2014;27:1291-1294.
7. Yu P, Diao W, Tang Q, Jiang X. A successful pregnancy and parturition in a patient with anuria undergoing maintenance hemodialysis for 6 years: a case report of a 3-year-follow-up. *BMC Pregnancy Childbirth*. 2015;15:218.
8. Jiang N, Liu Q, Lin L, et al. The effect of calcium channel blockers on prevention of preeclampsia in pregnant women with chronic hypertension. *Clin Exp Obstet Gynecol*. 2015;42:79-81.
9. Szucs KA, Axline SE, Rosenman MB. Maternal membranous glomerulonephritis and successful exclusive breastfeeding. *Breastfeed Med*. 2010;5: 123-126.
10. Vasa R, Ramirez M. Amlodipine exposure through breastfeeding in a 32 week preterm newborn. *Breastfeed Med*. 2013;8(suppl 1):S15.
11. Naito T, Kubono N, Deguchi S, et al. Amlodipine passage into breast milk in lactating women with pregnancy-induced hypertension and its estimation of infant risk for breastfeeding. *J Hum Lact*. 2015;31:301-306.
12. Morgan JL, Kogutt BK, Meek C, et al. Pharmacokinetics of amlodipine besylate at delivery and during lactation. *Pregnancy Hypertens*. 2018;11:77-80.
13. American Academy of Pediatrics Committee on Drugs. The transfer of drugs and other chemicals into human milk. *Pediatrics*. 2001;108:776-789.

AMMONIUM CHLORIDE

Metabolic (Electrolyte Supplement)

PREGNANCY RECOMMENDATION: Limited Human Data and No Relevant Animal Data

BREASTFEEDING RECOMMENDATION: Probably Compatible

PREGNANCY SUMMARY

The CPP reported 11 (3.0%) major congenital malformations in 365 first-trimester exposures to ammonium chloride. No pattern to the defects was seen. No reports describing the use of the IV infusion were located. Ammonium chloride will probably cross the placenta, so some fetal exposure will likely occur. Therefore, this limited human pregnancy experience prevents a complete assessment of the embryofetal risk. No animal reproduction studies have been conducted. Using this drug during pregnancy should be based on the pros and cons of the mother's clinical need for treatment versus any potential fetal risk that might occur from exposure. The drug is contraindicated in patients with impaired renal function and in patients whose alkalosis came from vomiting. During infusion, patients should also be watched for signs of ammonia toxicity (sweating, pallor, bradycardia, irregular breathing, tremor, arrhythmias, and coma).

BREASTFEEDING SUMMARY

No reports describing the use of ammonium chloride IV infusion during human lactation have been located. The drug will probably be found in breast milk, so some infant exposure will likely occur. The drug is also absorbed well from the gastrointestinal tract (97% oral bioavailability). Breastfeeding while using this drug should be based on the mother's clinical need for treatment versus any potential infant risks that might occur. If used, the infant should be monitored for the most common reported adult side effects of nausea (leading to irritability), vomiting, and diarrhea.

References

1. Prescribing Information. Ammonium chloride. Hospira, Inc; 2019.
2. Heinonen OP, Slone D, Shapiro S. *Birth Defects and Drugs in Pregnancy*. Publishing Sciences Group; 1977.
3. Goodlin RC, Kaiser IH. The effect of ammonium chloride induced maternal acidosis on the human fetus at term. I. pH, hemoglobin, blood gases. *Am J Med Sci*. 1957;233:666-674.
4. Kaiser IH, Goodlin RC. The effect of ammonium chloride induced maternal acidosis on the human fetus at term. II Electrolytes. *Am J Med Sci*. 1958; 235:549-554.

AMOXAPINE

Mental Health (Tricyclic Antidepressant)

PREGNANCY RECOMMENDATION: Limited Human Data—Animal Data Suggest Risk

BREASTFEEDING RECOMMENDATION: Potential Toxicity

PREGNANCY SUMMARY

In a surveillance study of Michigan Medicaid recipients, 19 newborns had been exposed to amoxapine during the first trimester. Three (16%) major birth defects were observed (one expected). However, no pattern to the anomalies was seen, and though the total incidence of anomalies is high, the number of exposures is too small to draw any conclusion. The drug will likely cross the placenta, so some fetal exposure will probably occur. Therefore, this limited human pregnancy experience prevents a complete assessment of the embryofetal risk. Animal studies did not show any teratogenicity, but embryofetal toxicity was seen in three species at doses less than 10 times the RHD. Using this drug during pregnancy should be based on the pros and cons of the mother's clinical need for treatment versus any potential fetal risk that might occur from exposure. There is a pregnancy exposure registry that monitors pregnancy outcomes in women using antidepressant drugs during pregnancy. Health care providers are encouraged to call the National Pregnancy Registry for Antidepressants at 1-844-405-6185.

BREASTFEEDING SUMMARY

No reports describing the use of amoxapine during human lactation have been located. The drug has been found to cause hyperprolactinemia, leading to galactorrhea, and in one case, amoxapine and its metabolite were found to be excreted into the milk of a woman with galactorrhea. Therefore, the drug will likely be found in the breast milk of a breastfeeding mother. Breastfeeding should be based on the mother's clinical need for treatment versus any potential infant risks. If used, the infant should be monitored for the most common reported adult side effects of nausea and headache (both leading to irritability), lethargy, constipation, somnolence, dry mouth, and elevated prolactin levels.

References

1. Prescribing Information. Amoxapine. Actavis Pharma; 2019.
2. Jaffe K, Zisook S. Galactorrhea in a patient treated with amoxapine. *J Clin Psychiatry*. 1978;39:821.
3. Gelenberg AJ, Cooper DS, Doller JC, et al. Galactorrhea and hyperprolactinemia associated with amoxapine therapy: report of a case. *JAMA*. 1979;242:1900-1901.
4. Gelenberg AJ. Amoxapine, a new antidepressant, appears in human milk. *J Nerv Ment Dis*. 1979;167:635-636.

AMOXICILLIN

Antibacterial (Penicillin)

PREGNANCY RECOMMENDATION: Human Data Suggest Compatible

BREASTFEEDING RECOMMENDATION: Compatible

PREGNANCY SUMMARY

Numerous large studies have been located describing the use of amoxicillin during human pregnancy. From more than 16,000 first-trimester exposures, the rate of congenital anomalies was 3.5% and not all of these were major defects. No pattern to the anomalies was found. Amoxicillin has been used in treating infections during pregnancy for several decades. Amoxicillin crosses the placenta, so fetal exposure will occur. Animal studies did not show any increased risk for embryofetal toxicity or teratogenicity in two species at doses of less than 10 times the RHD. Using this drug during pregnancy should be based on the pros and cons of the mother's clinical need for treatment versus any potential fetal risk that might occur from exposure.

BREASTFEEDING SUMMARY

Amoxicillin was found in human breast milk in one patient following a single 1-g dose. The levels ranged from a low of about 0.4 mcg/mL up to a peak of 1.3 mcg/mL. Using the peak concentration, the total amount of amoxicillin received in a day would be less than 1 mg/kg/d. Amoxicillin can be used in treating newborns with a normal infant dose of about 30 mg/kg/d. Therefore, infant exposure through breastfeeding is minimal. Breastfeeding while using this drug should be based on the mother's clinical need for treatment versus any potential infant risks that might occur. If used, the infant should be monitored for the most common reported adult side effects of nausea (leading to irritability), vomiting, diarrhea, and rash.

References

1. Prescribing Information. Amoxicillin. Ranbaxy Pharmaceutical; 2008.
2. Heinonen OP, Slone D, Shapiro S. *Birth Defects and Drugs in Pregnancy*. Publishing Sciences Group; 1977.
3. Masterton RG, Evans DC, Strike PW. Single-dose amoxycillin in the treatment of bacteriuria in pregnancy and the puerperium-a controlled clinical trial. *Br J Obstet Gynaecol*. 1985;92:498-505.
4. Jakobi P, Neiger R, Merzbach D, Paldi E. Single-dose antimicrobial therapy in the treatment of asymptomatic bacteriuria in pregnancy. *Am J Obstet Gynecol*. 1987;156:1148-1152.
5. Almeida L, Schmauch A, Bergstrom S. A randomised study on the impact of peroral amoxicillin in women with prelabour rupture of membranes preterm. *Gynecol Obstet Invest*. 1996;41:82-84.
6. Magwali TL, Chipato T, Majoko F, et al. Prophylactic augmentin in prelabor preterm rupture of the membranes. *Int J Gynecol Obstet*. 1999;65:261-265
7. Magat AH, Alger LS, Nagey DA, et al. Double-blind randomized study comparing amoxicillin and erythromycin for the treatment of *Chlamydia trachomatis* in pregnancy. *Obstet Gynecol*. 1993:81:745-749.
8. Alary M, Joly J-M, Mondor M, et al. Randomised comparison of amoxycillin and erythromycin in treatment of genital chlamydia infection in pregnancy. *Lancet*. 1994;344:1461-1465.
9. Turrentin MA, Newton ER. Amoxicillin or erythromycin for the treatment of antenatal chlamydial infection: a meta-analysis. *Obstet Gynecol*. 1995;86:1021-1025.
10. Kenyon SL, Taylor DJ, Tarnow-Mordi W; for the ORACLE Collaborative Group. Broad-spectrum antibiotics for preterm, prelabour rupture of fetal membranes: the ORACLE I randomised trial. *Lancet*. 2001;357:979-988.
11. Jepsen P, Skriver MV, Floyd A, et al. A population-based study of maternal use of amoxicillin and pregnancy outcome in Denmark. *Br J Clin Pharmacol*. 2003;55:216-221.
12. Berkovitch M, Diav-Citrin O, Greenberg R, et al. First-trimester exposure to amoxycillin/clavulanic acid: a prospective, controlled study. *Br J Clin Pharmacol*. 2004;58:298-302.
13. Cooper WO, Hernandez-Diaz S, Arbogast PG, et al. Antibiotics potentially used in response to bioterrorism and the risk of major congenital malformations. *Paediatr Perinat Epidemiol*. 2009;23:18-28.
14. Lin KJ, Mitchell AA, Yau W-P, et al. Maternal exposure to amoxicillin and the risk of oral clefts. *Epidemiology*. 2012;23:699-705.
15. Whatling R, Fearne JM. Molar incisor hypomineralization: a study of aetiological factors in a group of UK children. *Int J Paediatr Dent*. 2008;18:155-162.
16. Kafetzis D, Siafas C, Georgakopoulos P, Papadatos C. Passage of cephalosporins and amoxicillin into the breast milk. *Acta Paediatr Scand*. 1981;70:285-288.
17. Ito S, Blajchman A, Stephenson M, et al. Prospective follow-up of adverse reactions in breast-fed infants exposed to maternal medication. *Am J Obstet Gynecol*. 1993;168:1393–1399.

AMOXICILLIN/CLAVULANIC ACID

Antibacterial (Penicillin—β-Lactamase Inhibitor)

PREGNANCY RECOMMENDATION: Human Data Suggest Low Risk

BREASTFEEDING RECOMMENDATION: Probably Compatible

PREGNANCY SUMMARY

Numerous large studies have been published describing the use of amoxicillin during human pregnancy. From more than 16,000 first-trimester exposures, the rate of congenital anomalies was 3.5% and not all of these were major defects.

(*continued*)

No pattern to the anomalies was found. Clavulanic acid has not been specifically studied for any adverse effects during human pregnancy, including birth anomalies. However, based on its mechanism of action and long-term use over 40 years, it is not thought to be a teratogen. Amoxicillin/clavulanic acid has been used in treating infections during pregnancy for several decades. Amoxicillin crosses the placenta, so fetal exposure will occur. Clavulanic acid will also likely cross the placenta, so some fetal exposure to this drug will also probably occur. Animal studies did not show any increased risk for embryofetal toxicity or teratogenicity in two species at doses of less than 10 times the RHD. Using this drug during pregnancy should be based on the pros and cons of the mother's clinical need for treatment versus any potential fetal risk that might occur from exposure.

BREASTFEEDING SUMMARY

Amoxicillin was found in human breast milk in one patient following a single 1-g dose. The levels ranged from a low of about 0.4 mcg/mL to a peak of 1.3 mcg/mL. Using the peak concentration, the total amount of amoxicillin received in a day would be less than 1 mg/kg/d. Amoxicillin can be used in treating newborns with a normal infant dose of about 30 mg/kg/d. Therefore, infant exposure is minimal. Though it has not been fully evaluated, clavulanic acid will also probably be found in breast milk. This antibacterial drug combination can also be used in newborns. Breastfeeding while using this drug should be based on the mother's clinical need for treatment versus any potential infant risks that might occur. If used, the infant should be monitored for the most common reported adult side effects of nausea (leading to irritability), vomiting, diarrhea, and rash.

References

1. Prescribing Information. Augmentin. USAntibiotics, LLC; 2024.
2. Heinonen OP, Slone D, Shapiro S. *Birth Defects and Drugs in Pregnancy*. Publishing Sciences Group; 1977.
3. Masterton RG, Evans DC, Strike PW. Single-dose amoxycillin in the treatment of bacteriuria in pregnancy and the puerperium-a controlled clinical trial. *Br J Obstet Gynaecol*. 1985;92:498-505.
4. Jakobi P, Neiger R, Merzbach D, Paldi E. Single-dose antimicrobial therapy in the treatment of asymptomatic bacteriuria in pregnancy. *Am J Obstet Gynecol*. 1987;156:1148-1152.
5. Almeida L, Schmauch A, Bergstrom S. A randomised study on the impact of peroral amoxicillin in women with prelabour rupture of membranes preterm. *Gynecol Obstet Invest*. 1996;41:82-84.
6. Magwali TL, Chipato T, Majoko F, et al. Prophylactic augmentin in prelabor preterm rupture of the membranes. *Int J Gynecol Obstet*. 1999;65:261-265.
7. Magat AH, Alger LS, Nagey DA, et al. Double-blind randomized study comparing amoxicillin and erythromycin for the treatment of *Chlamydia trachomatis* in pregnancy. *Obstet Gynecol*. 1993:81:745-749.
8. Alary M, Joly J-M, Mondor M, et al. Randomised comparison of amoxycillin and erythromycin in treatment of genital chlamydia infection in pregnancy. *Lancet*. 1994;344:1461-1465.
9. Turrentin MA, Newton ER. Amoxicillin or erythromycin for the treatment of antenatal chlamydial infection: a meta-analysis. *Obstet Gynecol*. 1995; 86:1021-1025.
10. Kenyon SL, Taylor DJ, Tarnow-Mordi W; for the ORACLE Collaborative Group. Broad- spectrum antibiotics for preterm, prelabour rupture of fetal membranes: the ORACLE I randomised trial. *Lancet*. 2001;357:979-988.
11. Jepsen P, Skriver MV, Floyd A, et al. A population-based study of maternal use of amoxicillin and pregnancy outcome in Denmark. *Br J Clin Pharmacol*. 2003;55:216-221.
12. Berkovitch M, Diav-Citrin O, Greenberg R, et al. First-trimester exposure to amoxycillin/clavulanic acid: a prospective, controlled study. *Br J Clin Pharmacol*. 2004;58:298-302.
13. Cooper WO, Hernandez-Diaz S, Arbogast PG, et al. Antibiotics potentially used in response to bioterrorism and the risk of major congenital malformations. *Paediatr Perinat Epidemiol*. 2009;23:18-28.
14. Lin KJ, Mitchell AA, Yau W-P, et al. Maternal exposure to amoxicillin and the risk of oral clefts. *Epidemiology*. 2012;23:699-705.
15. Whatling R, Fearne JM. Molar incisor hypomineralization: a study of aetiological factors in a group of UK children. *Int J Paediatr Dent*. 2008;18:155-162.
16. Kafetzis D, Siafas C, Georgakopoulos P, Papadatos C. Passage of cephalosporins and amoxicillin into the breast milk. *Acta Paediatr Scand*. 1981; 70:285-288.
17. Ito S, Blajchman A, Stephenson M, et al. Prospective follow-up of adverse reactions in breast-fed infants exposed to maternal medication. *Am J Obstet Gynecol*. 1993;168:1393-1399.

AMPHETAMINE

Central Nervous System (Stimulant)

PREGNANCY RECOMMENDATION: Human Data Suggest Potential Risk (Medicinal Use)/Contraindicated (Nonmedical Use)

BREASTFEEDING RECOMMENDATION: Potential Toxicity (Medicinal Use)/Contraindicated (Nonmedical Use)

PREGNANCY SUMMARY

From the CPP, there were 26 (3.9%) major malformations seen with first-trimester exposure in 671 pregnancies. No specific pattern was identified. Numerous other series and case reports have described an array of various birth defects in mothers who misused amphetamines along with other drugs and alcohol. No specific study that has analyzed a large number of patients using medicinal amphetamine doses for narcolepsy and attention-deficit/hyperactivity disorder (ADHD) was located. The drug class is vasoconstricting, and this could lead to birth anomalies where this might be a factor, but drug dosages, purity, lifestyle, co-use of other drugs, and many other factors may play a role. Amphetamines should not be used in patients with underlying hypertension or who have gestational hypertension. The drug crosses the placenta, so fetal exposure will occur. Therefore, this limited human pregnancy experience (with medicinal use) prevents a complete assessment of the embryofetal risk. Animal studies using medicinal amphetamine dosages did show some embryofetal toxicity in two species, one with doses of less than 10 times the RHD and the other at 10 times the RHD, but maternal toxicity occurred in both of these evaluations. No embryofetal toxicity was seen in a third species using medicinal dosages of more than 10 times the RHD. Amphetamines can lead to dependence and misuse and are classified as Schedule II controlled substances. The drug carries a boxed warning for the potential risk of misuse. Using amphetamines for nonmedical purposes is contraindicated.

BREASTFEEDING SUMMARY

Two case reports were located that described the use of medicinal amphetamine during human lactation. In one mother using 20 mg/d for narcolepsy, the maximum drug level in breast milk was about 138 ng/mL, producing an RID of about 7%. In the second patient using 35 mg/d for narcolepsy, the peak breast milk concentration was about 82 ng/mL, with a calculated RID of about 2%. Breastfeeding with amphetamines is generally discouraged. Therefore, breastfeeding while using this drug for medicinal purposes should be based on the mother's clinical need for treatment versus any potential infant risks that might occur. If used, the infant should be monitored for the most common reported adult side effects of nausea, dizziness, headache, and abdominal pain (all leading to irritability), vomiting, diarrhea, sweating, fever, and decreased appetite (monitor infant growth). Nonmedical use and misuse of amphetamines can be harmful for a breastfed infant.

References

1. Burchfield DJ, Lucas VW, Abrams RM, et al. Disposition and pharmacodynamics of methamphetamine in pregnant sheep. *JAMA*. 1991;265:1968-1973.
2. Stek A, Fisher B, Clark KE. Maternal and fetal cardiovascular responses to methamphetamine (abstract). *Am J Obstet Gynecol*. 1993;168:333.
3. Nora JJ, Trasler DG, Fraser FC. Malformations in mice induced by dexamphetamine sulphate. *Lancet*. 1965;2:1021-1022.
4. Nora JJ, McNamara DG, Fraser FC. Dextroamphetamine sulphate and human malformations. *Lancet*. 1967;1:570-571.
5. Nora JJ, Vargo T, Nora A, et al. Dextroamphetamine: a possible environmental trigger in cardiovascular malformations. *Lancet*. 1970;1:1290-1291.
6. Nora JJ, Nora AH, Sommerville RJ, et al. Maternal exposure to potential teratogens. *JAMA*. 1967;202:1065-1069.
7. Matera RF, Zabala H, Jimenez AP. Bifid exencephalia: teratogen action of amphetamine. *Int Surg*. 1968;50:79-85.
8. Gilbert EF, Khoury GH. Dextroamphetamine and congenital cardiac malformations. *J Pediatr*. 1970;76:638.
9. Levin JN. Amphetamine ingestion with biliary atresia. *J Pediatr*. 1971;79:130-131.
10. McIntire MS. Possible adverse drug reaction. *JAMA*. 1966;197:62-63.
11. Bogdanoff B, Rorke LB, Yanoff M, Warren WS. Brain and eye abnormalities: possible sequelae to prenatal use of multiple drugs including LSD. *Am J Dis Child*. 1972;123:145-148.
12. Nelson MM, Forfar JO. Associations between drugs administered during pregnancy and congenital abnormalities of the fetus. *Br Med J*. 1971;1:523-527.
13. Milkovich L, van den Berg BJ. Effects of antenatal exposure to anorectic drugs. *Am J Obstet Gynecol*. 1977;129:637-642.
14. Eriksson M, Larsson G, Winbladh B, Zetterstrom R. The influence of amphetamine addiction on pregnancy and the newborn infant. *Acta Paediatr Scand*. 1978;67:95-99.
15. Larsson G, Eriksson M, Zetterstrom R. Amphetamine addiction and pregnancy: psycho-social and medical aspects. *Acta Psychiatr Scand*. 1979;60:334-345.
16. Billing L, Eriksson M, Larsson G, Zetterstrom R. Amphetamine addiction and pregnancy. III. One year follow-up of the children: psychosocial and pediatric aspects. *Acta Paediatr Scand*. 1980;69:675-680.
17. Eriksson M, Larsson G, Zetterstrom R. Amphetamine addiction and pregnancy. II. Pregnancy, delivery and the neonatal period: socio-medical aspects. *Acta Obstet Gynecol Scand*. 1981;60:253-259.
18. Larsson G. The amphetamine addicted mother and her child. *Acta Paediatr Scand Suppl*. 1980;278:7-24.
19. Heinonen OP, Slone D, Shapiro S. *Birth Defects and Drugs in Pregnancy*. Publishing Sciences Group; 1977.
20. Briggs GG, Samson JH, Crawford DJ. Lack of abnormalities in a newborn exposed to amphetamine during gestation. *Am J Dis Child*. 1975;129:249-250.
21. Steiner E, Villen T, Hallberg M, Rane A. Amphetamine secretion in breast milk. *Eur J Clin Pharmacol*. 1984;27:123-124.
22. Tenorio GM, Nazvi M, Bickers GH, Hubbird RH. Intrauterine stroke and maternal polydrug abuse: case report. *Clin Pediatr*. 1988;27:565-567.
23. Ghidini A, Sicherer S, Willner J. Congenital abnormalities (VATER) in baby born to mother using lovastatin. *Lancet*. 1992;339:1416-1417.
24. Little BB, Snell LM, Gilstrap LC III. Methamphetamine abuse during pregnancy: outcome and fetal effects. *Obstet Gynecol*. 1988;72:541-544.
25. Ramin SM, Little BB, Trimmer KJ, et al. Methamphetamine use during pregnancy in a large urban population (abstract). *Am J Obstet Gynecol*. 1992;166:353.
26. Dearlove JC, Betteridge T. Stillbirth due to intravenous amphetamine. *BMJ*. 1992;304:548.
27. Sussman S. Narcotic and methamphetamine use during pregnancy: effect on newborn infants. *Am J Dis Child*. 1963;106:325-330.
28. Neuberg R. Drug dependence and pregnancy: a review of the problems and their management. *J Obstet Gynaecol Br Commonw*. 1970;66:1117-1122.
29. Ramer CM. The case history of an infant born to an amphetamine-addicted mother. *Clin Pediatr*. 1974;13:596-597.
30. Oro AS, Dixon SD. Perinatal cocaine and methamphetamine exposure: maternal and neonatal correlates. *J Pediatr*. 1987;111:571-578.
31. Dixon SD, Bejar R. Echoencephalographic findings in neonates associated with maternal cocaine and methamphetamine use: incidence and clinical correlates. *J Pediatr*. 1989;115:770-778.
32. Chernoff GF, Jones KL. Fetal preventive medicine: teratogens and the unborn baby. *Pediatr Ann*. 1981;10:210-217.
33. Kalter H, Warkany J. Congenital malformations (second of two parts). *N Engl J Med*. 1983;308:491-497.
34. Zierler S. Maternal drugs and congenital heart disease. *Obstet Gynecol*. 1985;65:155-165.
35. Ayd FJ Jr. Excretion of psychotropic drugs in human breast milk. *Int Drug Ther News Bull*. 1973;8:33-40.

AMPHOTERICIN B

Anti-Infective (Antifungal)

PREGNANCY RECOMMENDATION: Limited Human Data—Animal Data Suggest Potential Risk

BREASTFEEDING RECOMMENDATION: Probably Compatible

A

PREGNANCY SUMMARY

Numerous case reports and series have been located that describe the use of amphotericin B during human pregnancy. Overall, in more than 30 pregnancies, no adverse effects on the pregnancy related to the drug were reported. No major malformations were described in the few cases with first-trimester exposure. The drug crosses the placenta, so some fetal exposure will occur. However, this limited human pregnancy experience prevents a complete assessment of the embryofetal risk. Animal studies did show some embryofetal toxicity in one species at doses of less than 10 times the RHD. Using this drug during pregnancy should be based on the pros and cons of the mother's clinical need for treatment versus any potential fetal risk that might occur from exposure.

BREASTFEEDING SUMMARY

No reports describing the use of amphotericin B during human lactation have been located. The drug will probably be found in human breast milk, so some infant exposure may occur. Regardless, because the drug is not absorbed systemically through oral use, effects on a breastfeeding infant are likely to be negligible. However, due to a concern for potential serious adverse effects that might be seen in a breastfed infant, the manufacturer recommends that women not breastfeed while being treated with this drug. Nevertheless, breastfeeding while using this drug should be based on the mother's clinical need for treatment versus any potential infant risks that might occur. If used, the infant should be monitored for the most common reported adult side effects of nausea, pruritus, and abdominal pain (all leading to irritability), diarrhea, vomiting, decreased appetite (monitor infant growth), and rash.

References

1. Prescribing Information. Ambisome. Astellas Pharma US; 2019.
2. Prescribing Information. Abelcet. Leadiant Biosciences; 2018.
3. McCoy MJ, Ellenberg JF, Killam AP. Coccidioidomycosis complicating pregnancy. *Am J Obstet Gynecol*. 1980;137:739-740.
4. Ismail MA, Lerner SA. Disseminated blastomycosis in a pregnant woman. Review of amphotericin B usage during pregnancy. *Am Rev Respir Dis*. 1982;126:350-353.
5. Hager H, Welt SI, Cardasis JP, Alvarez S. Disseminated blastomycosis in a pregnant woman successfully treated with amphotericin-B: a case report. *J Reprod Med*. 1988;33:485-488.
6. Heinonen OP, Slone D, Shapiro S. *Birth Defects and Drugs in Pregnancy*. Publishing Sciences Group; 1977:297.
7. Neiberg AD, Maruomatis F, Dyke J, Fayyad A. Blastomyces dermatitidis treated during pregnancy. *Am J Obstet Gynecol*. 1977;128:911-912.
8. Philpot CR, Lo D. Cryptococcal meningitis in pregnancy. *Med J Aust*. 1972;2:1005-1007.
9. Aitken GWE, Symonds EM. Cryptococcal meningitis in pregnancy treated with amphotericin. A case report. *Br J Obstet Gynaecol*. 1962;69:677-679.
10. Feldman R. Cryptococcosis (torulosis) of the central nervous system treated with amphotericin B during pregnancy. *South Med J*. 1959;52:1415-1417.
11. Kuo D. A case of torulosis of the central nervous system during pregnancy. *Med J Aust*. 1962;1:558-560.
12. Crotty JM. Systemic mycotic infections in Northern Territory aborigines. *Med J Aust*. 1965;1:184.
13. Littman ML. Cryptococcosis (torulosis). Current concepts and therapy. *Am J Med*. 1959;27:976-978.
14. Mick R, Muller-Tyl E, Neufeld T. Comparison of the effectiveness of nystatin and amphotericin B in the therapy of female genital mycoses. *Wien Med Wochenschr*. 1975;125:131-135.
15. Silberfarb PM, Sarois GA, Tosh FE. Cryptococcosis and pregnancy. *Am J Obstet Gynecol*. 1972;112:714-720.
16. Curole DN. Cryptococcal meningitis in pregnancy. *J Reprod Med*. 1981;26:317-319.
17. Sanford WG, Rasch JR, Stonehill RB. A therapeutic dilemma: the treatment of disseminated coccidioidomycosis with amphotericin B. *Ann Intern Med*. 1962;56:553-563.
18. Harris RE. Coccidioidomycosis complicating pregnancy. Report of 3 cases and review of the literature. *Obstet Gynecol*. 1966;28:401-405.
19. Smale LE, Waechter KG. Dissemination of coccidioidomycosis in pregnancy. *Am J Obstet Gynecol*. 1970;107:356-359.
20. Hadsall FJ, Acquarelli MJ. Disseminated coccidioidomycosis presenting as facial granulomas in pregnancy: a report of two cases and a review of the literature. *Laryngoscope*. 1973;83:51-58.
21. Daniel L, Salit IE. Blastomycosis during pregnancy. *Can Med Assoc J*. 1984;131:759-761.
22. Peterson CW, Johnson SL, Kelly JV, Kelly PC. Coccidioidal meningitis and pregnancy: a case report. *Obstet Gynecol*. 1989;73:835-836.

AMPICILLIN

Antibacterial (Penicillin)

PREGNANCY RECOMMENDATION: Human Data Suggest Compatible

BREASTFEEDING RECOMMENDATION: Compatible

PREGNANCY SUMMARY

Numerous large studies have been published describing the use of ampicillin during human pregnancy. From more than 14,000 first-trimester exposures, the rate of congenital anomalies was 3.8% and not all of these were major defects. No pattern to the anomalies was found. Ampicillin has been used in treating infections during pregnancy for several decades. The drug crosses the placenta, so fetal exposure will occur. Animal studies did not show any increased risk for embryofetal toxicity or teratogenicity in three species at doses up to 10 times the RHD. Using this drug during pregnancy should be based on the pros and cons of the mother's clinical need for treatment versus any potential fetal risk that might occur from exposure.

BREASTFEEDING SUMMARY

Several studies have been located that describe the use of ampicillin during human lactation. More than 50 women have been evaluated, and the drug was found in nearly every breast milk sample tested. Breast milk concentrations ranged from about 30 ng/mL to 3 mcg/mL. Nearly every calculated RID was less than 1%. Using the highest recorded breast milk concentration, the RID was only 1.6%. In addition, ampicillin can be administered to neonates with doses up to 100 mg/kg/d. Therefore, infant exposure through breastfeeding is minimal. Breastfeeding while using this drug should be based on the mother's clinical need for treatment versus any potential infant risks that might occur. If used, the infant should be monitored for the most common reported adult side effects of nausea (leading to irritability), vomiting, diarrhea, and rash.

References

1. Bray R, Boc R, Johnson W. Transfer of ampicillin into fetus and amniotic fluid from maternal plasma in late pregnancy. *Am J Obstet Gynecol.* 1966;96:938-942.
2. MacAulay M, Abou-Sabe M, Charles D. Placental transfer of ampicillin. *Am J Obstet Gynecol.* 1966;96:943-950.
3. Biro L, Ivan E, Elek E, Arr M. Data on the tissue concentration of antibiotics in man. Tissue concentrations of semi-synthetic penicillins in the fetus. *Int Z Klin Pharmakol Ther Toxikol.* 1970;4:321-324.
4. Elek E, Ivan E, Arr M. Passage of penicillins from mother to foetus in humans. *Int J Clin Pharmacol Ther Toxicol.* 1972;6:223-228.
5. Kraybill EN, Chaney NE, McCarthy LR. Transplacental ampicillin: inhibitory concentrations in neonatal serum. *Am J Obstet Gynecol.* 1980;138:793-796.
6. Jordheim O, Hagen AG. Study of ampicillin levels in maternal serum, umbilical cord serum and amniotic fluid following administration of pivampicillin. *Acta Obstet Gynecol Scand.* 1980;59:315-317.
7. Philipson A. Pharmacokinetics of ampicillin during pregnancy. *J Infect Dis.* 1977;136:370-376.
8. Noschel VH, Peiker G, Schroder S, et al. Untersuchungen zur pharmakokinetik von antibiotika und sulfanilamiden in der schwangerschaft und unter der geburt. *Zentralbl Gynakol.* 1982;104:1514-1518.
9. Willman K, Pulkkinen M. Reduced maternal plasma and urinary estriol during ampicillin treatment. *Am J Obstet Gynecol.* 1971;109:893-896.
10. Boehn F, DiPietro D, Goss D. The effect of ampicillin administration on urinary estriol and serum estradiol in the normal pregnant patient. *Am J Obstet Gynecol.* 1974;119:98-101.
11. Sybulski S, Maughan G. Effect of ampicillin administration on estradiol, estriol and cortisol levels in maternal plasma and on estriol levels in urine. *Am J Obstet Gynecol.* 1976;124:379-381.
12. Aldercreutz H, Martin F, Lehtinen T, et al. Effect of ampicillin administration on plasma conjugated and unconjugated estrogen and progesterone levels in pregnancy. *Am J Obstet Gynecol.* 1977;128:266-271.
13. Van Look PFA, Top-Huisman M, Gnodde HP. Effect of ampicillin or amoxycillin administration on plasma and urinary estrogen levels during normal pregnancy. *Eur J Obstet Gynecol Reprod Biol.* 1981;12:225-233.
14. Dossetor J. Drug interactions with oral contraceptives. *Br Med J.* 1975; 4:467-468.
15. DeSano EA Jr, Hurley SC. Possible interactions of antihistamines and antibiotics with oral contraceptive effectiveness. *Fertil Steril.* 1982;37:853-854.
16. Friedman CI, Huneke AL, Kim MH, Powell J. The effect of ampicillin on oral contraceptive effectiveness. *Obstet Gynecol.* 1980;55:33-37.
17. Back DJ, Breckenridge AM, MacIver M, et al. The effects of ampicillin on oral contraceptive steroids in women. *Br J Clin Pharmacol.* 1982;14:43-48.
18. Rothman KJ, Fyler DC, Goldblatt A, Kreidberg MB. Exogenous hormones and other drug exposures of children with congenital heart disease. *Am J Epidemiol.* 1979;109:433-439.
19. Zierler S. Maternal drugs and congenital heart disease. *Obstet Gynecol.* 1985;65:155-165.
20. Heinonen OP, Slone D, Shapiro S. *Birth Defects and Drugs in Pregnancy.* Publishing Sciences Group; 1977.
21. Boyer KM, Gotoff SP. Prevention of early-onset neonatal group B streptococcal disease with selective intrapartum chemoprophylaxis. *N Engl J Med.* 1986;314:1665-1669.
22. Amon E, Lewis SV, Sibai BM, et al. Ampicillin prophylaxis in preterm premature rupture of the membranes: a prospective randomized study. *Am J Obstet Gynecol.* 1988;159:539-543.
23. Morales WJ, Angel JL, O'Brien WF, Knuppel RA. Use of ampicillin and corticosteroids in premature rupture of membranes: a randomized study. *Obstet Gynecol.* 1989;73:721-726.
24. Heim K, Alge A, Marth C. Anaphylactic reaction to ampicillin and severe complication in the fetus. *Lancet.* 1991;337:859.
25. Czeizel AE, Rockenbauer M, Sorensen HT, Olsen J. A population-based case-control teratologic study of ampicillin treatment during pregnancy. *Am J Obstet Gynecol.* 2001;185:140-147.
26. Wilson J, Brown R, Cherek D, et al. Drug excretion in human breast milk: principles, pharmacokinetics and projected consequences. *Clin Pharmacokinet.* 1980;5:1-66.
27. Knowles J. Excretion of drugs in milk-a review. *J Pediatr.* 1965;66:1068-1082.
28. Williams M. Excretion of drugs in milk. *Pharm J.* 1976;217:219.
29. Ito S, Blajchman A, Stephenson M, et al. Prospective follow-up of adverse reactions in breast-fed infants exposed to maternal medication. *Am J Obstet Gynecol.* 1993;168:1393-1399.

AMPICILLIN/SULBACTAM

Antibacterial (Penicillin—β-Lactamase Inhibitor)

PREGNANCY RECOMMENDATION: Human Data Suggest Low Risk

BREASTFEEDING RECOMMENDATION: Probably Compatible

PREGNANCY SUMMARY

Numerous large studies have been located describing the use of ampicillin during human pregnancy. From more than 14,000 first-trimester exposures, the rate of congenital anomalies was 3.8% and not all of these were major defects. No pattern to the anomalies was found. Sulbactam has not been specifically studied for any adverse effects during human pregnancy, including birth defects. However, based on its mechanism of action and long-term use over 35 years, it is not thought to be a teratogen. Ampicillin/sulbactam has been used in treating infections during pregnancy for over three decades. Ampicillin crosses the placenta, so fetal exposure will occur. Sulbactam will also likely cross the placenta, so some fetal exposure to this drug will also probably occur. Animal studies did not show any increased risk for embryofetal toxicity or teratogenicity in three species at doses up to 10 times the RHD. Using this drug during pregnancy should be based on the pros and cons of the mother's clinical need for treatment versus any potential fetal risk that might occur from exposure.

BREASTFEEDING SUMMARY

Several studies have been located that describe the use of ampicillin during human lactation. More than 50 women have been evaluated, and the drug was found in nearly every breast milk sample tested. Breast milk concentrations ranged from about 30 ng/mL to 3 mcg/mL. Nearly every calculated RID was less than 1%. Using the highest recorded breast milk concentration, the RID was only 1.6%. Sulbactam has also been evaluated in a few lactating women. Breast milk levels ranged from about 10 ng/mL up to 2.8 mcg/mL. Using the highest recorded breast milk concentration, the RID was only 2.9%. In addition, ampicillin/sulbactam can be administered to neonates with doses up to 100 mg/kg/d (for ampicillin) and 50 mg/kg/d (for sulbactam). Therefore, infant exposure through breastfeeding is minimal. Breastfeeding while using this drug should be based on the mother's clinical need for treatment versus any potential infant risks that might occur. If used, the infant should be monitored for the most common reported adult side effects of nausea (leading to irritability), vomiting, diarrhea, and rash.

References

1. Bray R, Boc R, Johnson W. Transfer of ampicillin into fetus and amniotic fluid from maternal plasma in late pregnancy. *Am J Obstet Gynecol.* 1966;96:938-942.
2. MacAulay M, Abou-Sabe M, Charles D. Placental transfer of ampicillin. *Am J Obstet Gynecol.* 1966;96:943-950.
3. Biro L, Ivan E, Elek E, Arr M. Data on the tissue concentration of antibiotics in man. Tissue concentrations of semi-synthetic penicillins in the fetus. *Int Z Klin Pharmakol Ther Toxikol.* 1970;4:321-324.
4. Elek E, Ivan E, Arr M. Passage of penicillins from mother to foetus in humans. *Int J Clin Pharmacol Ther Toxicol.* 1972;6:223-228.
5. Kraybill EN, Chaney NE, McCarthy LR. Transplacental ampicillin: inhibitory concentrations in neonatal serum. *Am J Obstet Gynecol.* 1980;138:793-796.
6. Jordheim O, Hagen AG. Study of ampicillin levels in maternal serum, umbilical cord serum and amniotic fluid following administration of pivampicillin. *Acta Obstet Gynecol Scand.* 1980;59:315-317.
7. Philipson A. Pharmacokinetics of ampicillin during pregnancy. *J Infect Dis.* 1977;136:370-376.
8. Noschel VH, Peiker G, Schroder S, et al. Untersuchungen zur pharmakokinetik von antibiotika und sulfanilamiden in der schwangerschaft und unter der geburt. *Zentralbl Gynakol.* 1982;104:1514-1518.
9. Willman K, Pulkkinen M. Reduced maternal plasma and urinary estriol during ampicillin treatment. *Am J Obstet Gynecol.* 1971;109:893-896.
10. Boehm F, DiPietro D, Goss D. The effect of ampicillin administration on urinary estriol and serum estradiol in the normal pregnant patient. *Am J Obstet Gynecol.* 1974;119:98-11
11. Sybulski S, Maughan G. Effect of ampicillin administration on estradiol, estriol and cortisol levels in maternal plasma and on estriol levels in urine. *Am J Obstet Gynecol.* 1976;124:379-381.
12. Aldercreutz H, Martin F, Lehtinen T, et al. Effect of ampicillin administration on plasma conjugated and unconjugated estrogen and progesterone levels in pregnancy. *Am J Obstet Gynecol.* 1977;128:266-271.
13. Van Look PFA, Top-Huisman M, Gnodde HP. Effect of ampicillin or amoxicillin administration on plasma and urinary estrogen levels during normal pregnancy. *Eur J Obstet Gynecol Reprod Biol.* 1981;12:225-233.
14. Dossetor J. Drug interactions with oral contraceptives. *Br Med J.* 1975;4:467-468.
15. DeSano EA Jr, Hurley SC. Possible interactions of antihistamines and antibiotics with oral contraceptive effectiveness. *Fertil Steril.* 1982;37:853-854.
16. Friedman CI, Huneke AL, Kim MH, Powell J. The effect of ampicillin on oral contraceptive effectiveness. *Obstet Gynecol.* 1980;55:33-37.
17. Back DJ, Breckenridge AM, MacIver M, et al. The effects of ampicillin on oral contraceptive steroids in women. *Br J Clin Pharmacol.* 1982;14:43-48.
18. Rothman KJ, Fyler DC, Goldblatt A, Kreidberg MB. Exogenous hormones and other drug exposures of children with congenital heart disease. *Am J Epidemiol.* 1979;109:433-439.
19. Zierler S. Maternal drugs and congenital heart disease. *Obstet Gynecol.* 1985;65:155-165.
20. Heinonen OP, Slone D, Shapiro S. *Birth Defects and Drugs in Pregnancy.* Publishing Sciences Group; 1977.
21. Boyer KM, Gotoff SP. Prevention of early-onset neonatal group B streptococcal disease with selective intrapartum chemoprophylaxis. *N Engl J Med.* 1986;314:1665-1669.
22. Amon E, Lewis SV, Sibai BM, et al. Ampicillin prophylaxis in preterm premature rupture of the membranes: a prospective randomized study. *Am J Obstet Gynecol.* 1988;159:539-543.
23. Morales WJ, Angel JL, O'Brien WF, Knuppel RA. Use of ampicillin and corticosteroids in premature rupture of membranes: a randomized study. *Obstet Gynecol.* 1989;73:721-726.
24. Heim K, Alge A, Marth C. Anaphylactic reaction to ampicillin and severe complication in the fetus. *Lancet.* 1991;337:859.
25. Czeizel AE, Rockenbauer M, Sorensen HT, Olsen J. A population-based case-control teratologic study of ampicillin treatment during pregnancy. *Am J Obstet Gynecol.* 2001;185:140-147.
26. Wilson J, Brown R, Cherek D, et al. Drug excretion in human breast milk: principles, pharmacokinetics and projected consequences. *Clin Pharmacokinet.* 1980;5:1-66.
27. Knowles J. Excretion of drugs in milk-a review. *J Pediatr.* 1965;66:1068-1082.
28. Williams M. Excretion of drugs in milk. *Pharm J.* 1976;217:219.
29. Ito S, Blajchman A, Stephenson M, et al. Prospective follow-up of adverse reactions in breast-fed infants exposed to maternal medication. *Am J Obstet Gynecol.* 1993;168:1393-1399.

AMYL NITRITE

Cardiovascular (Vasodilator—Angina Pectoris)

PREGNANCY RECOMMENDATION: Limited Human Data—No Relevant Animal Data (Maternal Benefit May Outweigh Embryofetal Risk)

BREASTFEEDING RECOMMENDATION: Probably Compatible

PREGNANCY SUMMARY

The CPP reported 15 first-trimester exposures to 6 cardiac vasodilators (one of which was amyl nitrite), and 2 (13%) newborns were identified who had malformations. However, no specific pattern was noted, and coexposures to other drugs were not described. In addition, it was not stated whether amyl nitrite was taken by the two mothers of the affected infants. The number of cases is too small to assess the risk of amyl nitrite in pregnancy. Some amount of the drug will likely cross the placenta, so a limited amount of fetal exposure may occur. Therefore, this limited human pregnancy experience prevents a complete assessment of the embryofetal risk. Because the drug produces smooth muscle vasodilation, there has been a report that its use during difficult preterm cesarean section may be beneficial and poses no threat to the mother or fetus. Animal reproduction studies have not been conducted with amyl nitrite. Using this drug during pregnancy should be based on the pros and cons of the mother's clinical need for treatment versus any potential fetal risk that might occur from exposure.

BREASTFEEDING SUMMARY

No reports describing the use of amyl nitrite during human lactation have been located. Some amount of the drug will likely be found in breast milk, so a limited amount of infant exposure may occur. Breastfeeding while using this drug should be based on the mother's clinical need for treatment versus any potential infant risks. If used, the infant should be monitored for the most common reported adult side effects of nausea, headache, and dizziness (all leading to irritability), hypotension, tachycardia, flushing, vomiting, and weakness (lethargy). However, it is doubtful if maternal use would represent any risk to a nursing infant, whereas the maternal benefit could be substantial.

References

1. Prescribing Information. Amyl nitrate inhalation. James Alexander Corporation; 2023.
2. Heinonen OP, Slone D, Shapiro S. *Birth Defects and Drugs in Pregnancy*. Wright PSB; 1983:371-373.
3. Kumar D, Zourlas PA, Barnes AC. In vivo effect of amyl nitrite on human pregnant uterine contractility; an objective evaluation. *Am J Obstet Gynecol*. 1965;91:1066-1068.
4. Hendricks SK, Ross B, Colvard MA, et al. Amyl nitrite: use as a smooth muscle relaxant in difficult preterm cesarean section. *Am J Perinatol*. 1992; 9:289-292.

ANACAULASE

Dermatologic (Topical—Enzyme)

PREGNANCY RECOMMENDATION: **No Human Data—Animal Data Suggest Low Risk**

BREASTFEEDING RECOMMENDATION: **Probably Compatible**

PREGNANCY SUMMARY

No reports describing the use of anacaulase in human pregnancy have been located. Most of the drug components are not likely to cross the placenta; therefore, fetal exposure is probably nonexistent or extremely limited. However, bromelain (the primary protein) is absorbed systemically with topical use and will probably cross the placenta in limited amounts. Therefore, the absence of human pregnancy experience prevents a complete assessment of the embryofetal risk. Animal studies did not show embryofetal toxicity with IV administration. Using this topical drug during pregnancy should be based on the pros and cons of the mother's clinical need for treatment versus any potential fetal risk that might occur from exposure.

BREASTFEEDING SUMMARY

No reports describing the use of anacaulase during human lactation have been located. Most of the components of the drug will likely not appear in breast milk. However, bromelain, the primary protein, will probably be found in breast milk in limited amounts. Nevertheless, because they are proteins, if any were to be ingested through breastfeeding, they would most likely be digested in the infant's gastrointestinal tract and not be absorbed. Breastfeeding while using this topical drug should be based on the mother's clinical need for treatment. If used, the infant should be monitored for the most common reported adult side effects of pruritus (leading to irritability) and pyrexia.

Reference

1. Prescribing Information. Nexobrid. Vericel Corporation; 2022.

ANAGRELIDE

Hematologic (Antiplatelet)

PREGNANCY RECOMMENDATION: **Limited Human Data—Animal Data Suggest Low Risk**

BREASTFEEDING RECOMMENDATION: **Potential Toxicity**

PREGNANCY SUMMARY

A total of about 12 first-trimester exposures to anagrelide were located in seven publications. Of these, there were 2 first-trimester spontaneous abortions, and the remaining 10 delivered healthy newborns with no reported birth anomalies. The drug will probably cross the placenta, so some fetal exposure will likely occur. Therefore, this limited human pregnancy experience prevents a complete assessment of the embryofetal risk. Animal studies did not show any embryofetal toxicity in one species at doses of more than 10 times the RHD. Some embryofetal toxicity was seen in a second species, but again at doses of more than 10 times the RHD. Based on the drug's mechanism of action, the manufacturer recommends that women with reproductive potential use effective contraception during treatment. Nevertheless, using this drug during pregnancy should be based on the pros and cons of the mother's clinical need for treatment versus any potential fetal risk that might occur from exposure.

BREASTFEEDING SUMMARY

No reports describing the use of anagrelide during human lactation have been located. The drug will probably be found in breast milk, so some infant exposure will likely occur. However, due to a concern for potential serious adverse effects that might be seen in a breastfed infant, the manufacturer recommends that women not breastfeed while being treated with this drug. Nevertheless, breastfeeding while using this drug should be based on the mother's clinical need for treatment versus any potential infant risks that might occur. If used, the infant should be monitored for the most common reported adult side effects of nausea, headache, dizziness, and abdominal pain (all leading to irritability), diarrhea, vomiting, fever, peripheral edema, and rash.

References

1. Prescribing Information. Agrylin. Shire US Manufacturing; 2018.
2. Wright CA, Tefferi A. A single institutional experience with 43 pregnancies in essential thrombocythemia. *Eur J Hematol*. 2001;66:152-159.
3. Doubek M, Brychtova Y, Doubek R, et al. Anagrelide therapy in pregnancy: report of a case of essential thrombocythemia. *Ann Hematol*. 2004;83:726-727.
4. Alkindi S, Dennison D, Pathare A. Successful outcome with anagrelide in pregnancy. *Ann Hematol*. 2005;84:758-759.
5. Sobas MA, Perez Encinas MM, Rabunal Martinez MJ, et al. Anagrelide treatment in early pregnancy in a patient with JAK2V617F-positive essential thrombocythemia: case report and literature review. *Acta Haematol*. 2009;122:221-222.
6. Cornet N, Vialard F, Mir O, Berveiller P. Is anagrelide safe during pregnancy? *J Gynecol Obstet Hum Reprod*. 2017;45:697-699.
7. Bohiltea RE, Cirstoiu MM, Ionescu CA, et al. Primary myelofibrosis and pregnancy outcomes after low molecular-weight heparin administration: a case report and literature review. *Medicine (Baltimore)*. 2017;96:e8735.

ANAKINRA

Immunologic (Human Interleukin-1 Receptor Antagonist)

PREGNANCY RECOMMENDATION: Limited Human Data—Animal Data Suggest Low Risk

BREASTFEEDING RECOMMENDATION: Probably Compatible

PREGNANCY SUMMARY

A few case reports and series were located that describe the use of anakinra during human gestation. Of about 39 first-trimester pregnancies (one set of twins—40 newborns), there were 2 spontaneous abortions and 36 infants born with no anomalies described. A few were growth restricted or preterm, but overall, they did well. There was one intrauterine fetal death (IUFD) of one of the twins that had bilateral renal agenesis, and one of live birth with unilateral renal agenesis. Therefore, fetal renal issues may need further evaluation. Based on ex vivo placental perfusion, a minimal amount of interleukin-1 receptor antagonist (IL-1RA) may cross to the fetus at term. Therefore, this limited human pregnancy experience prevents a complete assessment of the embryofetal risk. Animal studies did not show any embryofetal toxicity or teratogenicity in two species at doses of more than 10 times the RHD. Using this drug during pregnancy should be based on the pros and cons of the mother's clinical need for treatment versus any potential fetal risk that might occur from exposure.

BREASTFEEDING SUMMARY

A few studies have been located that describe the use of anakinra during human lactation. None of the infants were reported to have any drug-related adverse effects. Endogenous IL-1RA is normally found in human breast milk. In one study of 88 normal lactating mothers, IL-1RA was found in colostrum with a mean level of about 670 ng/mL. The concentration was lower in mature breast milk. Because endogenous IL-1RA is normally found in human breast milk, there appears to be no risk to a nursing infant from maternal administration of anakinra. Furthermore, because it is a protein, if the drug were to be ingested through breastfeeding, it would probably be digested in the infant's gastrointestinal tract and not be absorbed. If the clinical decision is to use this drug while breastfeeding, the infant should be monitored for the most common reported adult side effects of nausea, headache, arthralgia, and abdominal pain (all leading to irritability), diarrhea, fever, upper respiratory tract infection, and rash.

References

1. Prescribing Information. Kineret. Swedish Orphan Biovitrum; 2016.
2. Romero R, Gomez R, Galasso M, et al. The natural interleukin-1 receptor antagonist in the fetal, maternal, and amniotic fluid compartments: the effect of gestational age, fetal gender, and intrauterine infection. *Am J Obstet Gynecol*. 1994;171:912-921.
3. Bry K, Lappalainen U, Waffarn F, et al. Influence of fetal gender on the concentration of interleukin-1 receptor antagonist in amniotic fluid and in newborn urine. *Pediatr Res*. 1994;35:130-134.
4. Brown NL, Alvi SA, Elder MG, et al. Regulation of prostaglandin production in intact fetal membranes by interleukin-1 and its receptor antagonist. *J Endocrinol*. 1998;159:519-526.
5. Simon C, Frances A, Piquette GN, et al. Embryonic implantation in mice is blocked by interleukin-1 receptor antagonist. *Endocrinology*. 1994;134:521-528.
6. Simon C, Valbuena D, Krussel J, et al. Interleukin-1 receptor antagonist prevents embryonic implantation by a direct effect on the endometrial epithelium. *Fertil Steril*. 1998;70:896-906.
7. Romero R, Tartakovsky B. The natural interleukin-1 receptor antagonist prevents interleukin-1-induced preterm delivery in mice. *Am J Obstet Gynecol*. 1992;167:1041-1045.
8. Fidel PL Jr, Romero R, Cutright J, et al. Treatment with interleukin-1 receptor antagonist and soluble tumor necrosis factor receptor Fc fusion protein does not prevent endotoxin-induced preterm parturition in mice. *J Soc Gynecol Invest*. 1997;4:22-26.
9. McDuffie RS Jr, Davies JK, Leslie KK, et al. A randomized controlled trial of interleukin-1 receptor antagonist in a rabbit model of ascending infection in pregnancy. *Infect Dis Obstet Gynecol*. 2001;9:233-237.
10. Zaretsky MV, Alexander JM, Byrd W, Bawdon RE. Transfer of inflammatory cytokines across the placenta. *Obstet Gynecol*. 2004;103:546-550.
11. Unfried G, Tempfer C, Schneeberger C, et al. Interleukin 1 receptor antagonist polymorphism in women with idiopathic recurrent miscarriage. *Fertil Steril*. 2001;75:683-687.
12. Karhukorpi J, Laitinen T, Kivela H, et al. IL-1 receptor antagonist gene polymorphism in recurrent spontaneous abortion. *J Reprod Immunol*. 2003;58:61-67.
13. Berger CT, Recher M, Steiner U, Hauser TM. A patient's wish: anakinra in pregnancy. *Ann Rheum Dis*. 2009;68:1794-1795.
14. Chang Z, Spong C, Jesus AA, et al. Anakinra use during pregnancy in patients with Cryopyrin-associated periodic syndromes (CAPS). *Arthritis Rheumatol*. 2014;66:3227-3232.
15. Gotestam-Skorpen C, Hoeltzenbein M, Tincani A, et al. The EULAR points to consider for use of antirheumatic drugs before pregnancy, and during pregnancy and lactation. *Ann Rheum Dis*. 2016;75:795-810.
16. Ligen U, Kucuksahin O. Anakinra use during pregnancy: report of a case with Familial Mediterranean Fever and infertility. *Eur J Rheumatol* 2017;4:66–67.
17. Youngstein T, Hoffmann P, Gul A, et al. International multi-centre study of pregnancy outcomes with interleukin-1 inhibitors. Rheumatology (Oxford) 2017;56:2102–8.
18. Smith CJF, Chambers CD. Five successful pregnancies with antenatal anakinra exposure. *Rheumatology (Oxford)*. 2018;57:1271-1275. doi:10.1093/rheumatology/key093
19. Buescher ES, Malinowska I. Soluble receptors and cytokine antagonists in human milk. *Pediatr Res*. 1996;40:839-844.
20. Srivastave MD, Srivastava A, Brouhard B, et al. Cytokines in human milk. *Res Commun Mol Pathol Pharmacol*. 1996;93:263-287.
21. Buescher ES, Hair PS. Human milk anti-inflammatory component contents during acute mastitis. *Cell Immunol*. 2001;210:87-95.

ANGIOTENSIN II

Cardiovascular (Vasoconstrictor)

PREGNANCY RECOMMENDATION: No Human Data and No Relevant Animal Data

BREASTFEEDING RECOMMENDATION: Probably Compatible

PREGNANCY SUMMARY

No reports describing the use of angiotensin II in human pregnancy have been located. A limited amount of the drug will probably cross the placenta, so some fetal exposure may occur. However, the absence of human pregnancy experience prevents a complete assessment of any embryofetal risk. Animal reproduction studies have not been performed. Because septic and other distributive shock have high rates of mortality, this drug should not be withheld if clinically needed by the mother.

BREASTFEEDING SUMMARY

No reports describing the use of angiotensin II during human lactation have been located. A limited amount of the drug will probably enter breast milk. However, because it is an octapeptide, if the drug were to be ingested through breastfeeding, it would probably be digested in the infant's gastrointestinal tract and not be absorbed. Nevertheless, septic and other distributive shock have high rates of mortality. Therefore, this drug should not be withheld if clinically needed by the mother.

Reference

1. Prescribing Information. Giapreza. La Jolla Pharmaceutical Company; 2017.

ANIDULAFUNGIN

Anti-Infective (Antifungal)

PREGNANCY RECOMMENDATION: No Human Data—Animal Data Suggest Potential Risk

BREASTFEEDING RECOMMENDATION: Potential Toxicity

PREGNANCY SUMMARY

No reports describing the use of anidulafungin in human pregnancy have been located. A limited amount of the drug will probably cross the placenta, so some fetal exposure may occur. Therefore, the absence of human pregnancy experience prevents a complete assessment of the embryofetal risk. Animal studies did show some embryofetal toxicity in one species at doses of less than 10 times the RHD, but maternal toxicity also occurred. No embryofetal toxicity was seen in a second species at doses less than 10 times the RHD (and no maternal toxicity). Using this drug during pregnancy should be based on the pros and cons of the mother's clinical need for treatment versus any potential fetal risk that might occur from exposure.

BREASTFEEDING SUMMARY

One case report was located that evaluated the use of anidulafungin during breastfeeding. The highest drug level obtained in the breast milk after the drug was discontinued was 240 ng/mL. The levels then decreased and were undetectable at 38 hours. The infant displayed no adverse effects. In addition, the drug is a lipopeptide of six amino acids and may undergo some degradation in the infant's gastrointestinal tract. Breastfeeding while using this drug should be based on the mother's clinical need for treatment versus any potential infant risks. If used, the infant should be monitored for the most common reported adult side effects of nausea, headache, and abdominal pain (all leading to irritability), diarrhea, vomiting, fever, insomnia, hypokalemia, and anemia.

References

1. Prescribing Information. Eraxis. Roerig Pfizer, Inc; 2020.
2. Eijsink JFH, Wieringa A, Vries-Koenjer MTLM, Ter Horst PGJ. Anidulafungin levels in breast milk after cessation of treatment: a case report. *Breastfeed Med*. 2024;19:134-136.

ANIFROLUMAB

Immunologic (Interferon Receptor Antagonist, Type I—Monoclonal Antibody)

PREGNANCY RECOMMENDATION: No Human Data—Animal Data Suggest Low Risk

BREASTFEEDING RECOMMENDATION: Probably Compatible

PREGNANCY SUMMARY

No reports describing the use of anifrolumab in human pregnancy have been located. As an IgG, anifrolumab is likely to cross the placenta, so some fetal exposure will probably occur. Therefore, the absence of human pregnancy experience prevents a complete assessment of the embryofetal risk. Animal data did not show any embryofetal toxicity. Using this drug during pregnancy should be based on the pros and cons of the mother's clinical need for treatment versus any potential fetal risk that might occur from exposure. Systemic lupus erythematosus during pregnancy is associated with a worsening of the underlying disease, spontaneous abortion, preeclampsia, premature birth, IUGR, and stillbirth. There is a pregnancy exposure registry that monitors pregnancy outcomes in women using this drug. Health care providers and women who are pregnant and have taken anifrolumab at any time during pregnancy are encouraged to contact the Saphnelo registry at 1-877-693-9268.

BREASTFEEDING SUMMARY

No reports describing the use of anifrolumab during human lactation have been located. It is known that IgG antibodies can be found in human breast milk, but are not found in the neonatal or infant circulation. Additionally, if any IgG antibodies were to be ingested through breastfeeding, they would probably be digested in the infant's gastrointestinal tract and not be absorbed. Breastfeeding while using this drug should be based on the mother's clinical need for treatment. If used, the infant should be monitored for the most common reported adult side effects of various infections and cough.

Reference

1. Prescribing Information. Saphnelo. AstraZeneca Pharmaceuticals; 2022.

ANSUVIMAB

Antiviral (Monoclonal Antibody—Ebola)

PREGNANCY RECOMMENDATION: No Human Data and No Relevant Animal Data (Maternal Benefit May Outweigh Embryo–Fetal Risk)

BREASTFEEDING RECOMMENDATION: *Contraindicated

PREGNANCY SUMMARY

Two studies that total 424 adult and pediatric patients infected with Zaire ebolavirus and administered ansuvimab have been reported. Pregnant women were included in both studies. However, specific information for the pregnancy population subset regarding birth anomalies, pregnancy loss, and adverse maternal/fetal outcomes was not supplied because of the high mortality rate associated with this infection. Because it is an antibody of the IgG class, it probably crosses the placenta. Animal reproduction studies have not been performed. If a pregnant woman were to be infected with the Zaire ebolavirus, treatment should not be withheld.

BREASTFEEDING SUMMARY

Ansuvimab probably enters breast milk. However, it is known that IgG antibodies can be found in human breast milk, but are not found in neonatal or infant circulation. Additionally, if any IgG antibodies were to be ingested through breastfeeding, they would probably be digested in the infant's gastrointestinal tract and not be absorbed. *However, the current CDC recommendation is that mothers should NOT breastfeed their infants (with a confirmed infection of Zaire ebolavirus) in order to reduce the risk of postnatal transmission of the virus. The drug itself, outside of an Ebola virus infection, is probably compatible.

References

1. Prescribing Information. Ebanga. Ridgeback Biotherapeutics, LP; 2020.
2. Mulangu S, Dodd LE, Davey RT Jr, et al. A randomized, controlled trial of Ebola virus disease therapeutics. *N Engl J Med*. 2019;381(24):2293-2303.

ANTHRALIN

Dermatologic (Topical—Antipsoriatic)

PREGNANCY RECOMMENDATION: No Human Data and No Relevant Animal Data

BREASTFEEDING RECOMMENDATION: Potential Toxicity

PREGNANCY SUMMARY

No reports describing the use of anthralin in the first trimester of human pregnancy have been located. A case of contact dermatitis from inadvertent exposure to anthralin was reported. However, no information on the pregnancy outcome was provided. If systemic absorption occurs (which it probably does when applied to psoriatic-affected skin), then the drug will likely cross the placenta, and fetal exposure will probably occur. Therefore, the absence of human pregnancy experience prevents a complete assessment of the embryofetal risk. Animal reproduction studies have not been conducted. Using this drug during pregnancy should be based on the pros and cons of the mother's clinical need for treatment versus any potential fetal risk that might occur from exposure.

BREASTFEEDING SUMMARY

No reports describing the use of anthralin during human lactation have been located. The drug will likely be found in breast milk, but levels would depend on the amount of systemic absorption. Breastfeeding while using this drug should be based on the mother's clinical need for treatment versus any potential infant risks. Because it has not been determined how much anthralin is absorbed after topical use, systemic side effects have not been reported.

References

1. Prescribing Information. Zithranol-RR cream. Elorac Inc; 2020.
2. Strauss RM, Bate J, Pring D. Connubial contact dermatitis: an unusual pregnancy dermatosis. *Acta Derm Venereol*. 2003;83:316.

ANTIHEMOPHILIC FACTOR (HUMAN)

Hematologic (Recombinant Factor VIII)

PREGNANCY RECOMMENDATION: No Human Data and No Relevant Animal Data

BREASTFEEDING RECOMMENDATION: Probably Compatible

PREGNANCY SUMMARY

No reports describing the use of antihemophilic factor (human) in human pregnancy have been located. The drug will probably not cross the placenta in any clinically significant amounts. However, the absence of human pregnancy experience prevents a complete assessment of the embryofetal risk. Animal reproduction studies have not been conducted. Using this drug during pregnancy should be based on the pros and cons of the mother's clinical need for treatment versus any potential fetal risk that might occur from exposure.

BREASTFEEDING SUMMARY

No reports describing the use of antihemophilic factor (human) during human lactation have been located. Excretion into breast milk will likely be minimal, if it occurs at all. However, even if small amounts were excreted into breast milk, they should be digested in the infant's gastrointestinal tract and have no effect on a nursing infant. Thus, if a mother with this condition chooses to breastfeed her infant, the drug should not be withheld. If the clinical decision is to use this drug while breastfeeding, the infant should be monitored for the most common reported adult side effects of dizziness (leading to irritability), flushing, and rash.

Reference

1. Prescribing Information. Afstyla. CSL Behring; 2023.

ANTITHROMBIN (HUMAN/RECOMBINANT)

Hematologic (Factor in Blood Clotting)

PREGNANCY RECOMMENDATION: **Limited Human Data—Animal Data Suggest Low Risk (Maternal Benefit May Outweigh Any Embryofetal Risk)**

BREASTFEEDING RECOMMENDATION: **Probably Compatible**

PREGNANCY SUMMARY

A few reports describing the use of antithrombin during human pregnancy were located. In two, the drug was used in about 80 pregnant women as a potential treatment for preeclampsia. No adverse newborn effects related to the drug were described. The manufacturer reported data from the clinical trials that about 22 women received antithrombin at delivery. No adverse maternal or neonatal effects related to the drug were identified. The drug should not cross the placenta in the first half of gestation in any clinically significant amounts. However, because it is a protein, it is not known whether some placental transfer might occur in the second half of gestation. However, the absence of the first-trimester human pregnancy experience prevents a complete assessment of the embryofetal risk. Animal studies did not show any embryofetal toxicity or teratogenicity in two species at doses of less than 10 times the RHD. Using this drug during pregnancy should be based on the pros and cons of the mother's clinical need for treatment versus any potential fetal risk that might occur from exposure.

BREASTFEEDING SUMMMARY

No reports describing the use of antithrombin during human lactation have been located. The drug is not likely to be found in human breast milk in clinically significant amounts. The manufacturer states that the concentration of antithrombin in breast milk will only be about one-fiftieth to one-hundredth the maternal blood concentration. However, even if small amounts did enter breast milk, they would likely be digested in the infant's gastrointestinal tract and not be absorbed. Therefore, the risk to a nursing infant from this agent appears to be negligible. If the clinical decision is to use this drug while breastfeeding, the infant should be monitored for the most common reported adult side effects of pruritus (leading to irritability), flushing, peripheral edema, and rash.

References

1. Prescribing Information. Thrombate III. Grifols USA; 2017.
2. Prescribing Information. ATryn. GTC Biotherapeutics, Inc; 2018.
3. Nakabayashi M, Asami M, Nakatani A. Efficacy of antithrombin replacement therapy in severe early-onset preeclampsia. *Semin Thromb Hemost.* 1999;25:463-466.
4. Maki M, Kobayashi T, Terao T, et al. Antithrombin therapy for severe preeclampsia. Results of a double-blind, randomized, placebo-controlled trial. *Thromb Haemost.* 2000;84:583-590.

APALUTAMIDE

Antineoplastic (Androgen Receptor Inhibitor)

PREGNANCY RECOMMENDATION: ***Contraindicated**

BREASTFEEDING RECOMMENDATION: ***Contraindicated**

PREGNANCY SUMMARY

No reports describing the use of apalutamide in human pregnancy have been located, and based on the approved use for the drug, studies will not likely ever occur. The drug will probably cross the placenta, so some fetal exposure would likely occur. *However, the drug is contraindicated for use in women. Animal studies did show some embryofetal toxicity in one species at doses less than 10 times the RHD. Based on animal studies and the drug's mechanism of action, the manufacturer recommends that males with female partners of reproductive potential use effective contraception during treatment and for 3 months after the last dose.

BREASTFEEDING SUMMARY

No reports describing the use of apalutamide during human lactation have been located. *Although the the drug would likely be found in breast milk, the drug is contraindicated for use in women.

Reference

1. Prescribing Information. Erleada. Janssen Products; 2023.

APIXABAN

Hematologic (Anticoagulant)

PREGNANCY RECOMMENDATION: No Human Data—Animal Data Suggest Low Risk

BREASTFEEDING RECOMMENDATION: Potential Toxicity

PREGNANCY SUMMARY

No reports describing the use of apixaban in human pregnancy have been located. The drug appears to cross the placenta, so fetal exposure will occur. Therefore, the absence of human pregnancy experience prevents a complete assessment of the embryofetal risk. In most cases. oral anticoagulants are not recommended for use in pregnancy because they can cross the placenta, which could theoretically be a risk for in utero fetal bleeding. Animal studies did not show any embryofetal toxicity or teratogenicity in three species at doses of less than 10 times the RHD in two, and more than 10 times the RHD in one. However, some maternal bleeding did occur in these animals. In humans, maternal bleeding during pregnancy and at delivery, as well as fetal and newborn bleeding, is a risk because there is no established way to reverse the anticoagulant effect that may persist for up to 24 hours. Low-molecular-weight heparin (LMWH) and heparin are usually the treatments of choice in pregnancy.

BREASTFEEDING SUMMARY

Two reports were located that describe the use of apixaban during human lactation. In four breastfeeding women, all using about 10 mg/d, peak breast milk levels ranged from 200 to 250 ng/mL. The calculated RIDs ranged from 14% to 21%. Due to a concern for potential serious adverse effects that might be seen in a breastfed infant, the manufacturer recommends that women not breastfeed while being treated with this drug. Because the drug is found in breast milk and because other anticoagulant options are available, alternative medications should be considered. If the clinical decision is to use this drug while breastfeeding, the infant should be monitored for the most common reported adult side effect of bleeding.

References

1. Greer IA. Thrombosis in pregnancy: updates in diagnosis and management. *Hematology Am Soc Hematol Educ Program*. 2012;2012:203-207. doi:10.1182/asheducation-2012.1.203
2. Prescribing Information. Eliquis. E.R. Squibb & Sons; 2019.
3. Wang L, He K, Maxwell B, et al. Tissue distribution and elimination of [^{14}C] apixaban in rats. *Drug Metab Dispos*. 2011;39:256-264.
4. Bapat P, Pinto LSR, Lubetsky A, et al. Examining the transplacental passage of apixaban using the dually perfused human placenta. *J Thromb Haemost*. 2016;14:1436-1441.

APOMORPHINE

Central Nervous System (Anti-Parkinson)

PREGNANCY RECOMMENDATION: Limited Human Data—Animal Data Suggest Potential Risk

BREASTFEEDING RECOMMENDATION: Potential Toxicity

PREGNANCY SUMMARY

No reports describing the use of apomorphine in early human pregnancy have been located. The drug has been used during labor (with scopolamine) and has not been associated with any adverse events, maternal or fetal/neonatal effects. The drug will probably cross the placenta, so some fetal exposure will likely occur. Therefore, this limited first-trimester human pregnancy experience prevents a complete assessment of the embryofetal risk. Animal studies did show embryofetal toxicity and malformations in one species at doses of less than the RHD. Using this drug during pregnancy should be based on the pros and cons of the mother's clinical need for treatment versus any potential fetal risk that might occur from exposure. Apomorphine has been shown to prolong the QT interval.

BREASTFEEDING SUMMARY

No reports describing the use of apomorphine during human lactation have been located. The drug will probably be found in breast milk. Apomorphine is a dopamine agonist and may increase serum prolactin levels, but this should not adversely affect lactation. Breastfeeding while using this drug should be based on the mother's clinical need for treatment versus any potential infant risks that might occur. If used, the infant should be monitored for the most common reported adult side effects of nausea and dizziness (both leading to irritability), peripheral edema, vomiting, decreased blood pressure, somnolence, and rhinorrhea.

References

1. Prescribing Information. Apokyn. US WorldMeds; 2017.
2. Holdsworth JD, Furness RM, Roulston RG. A comparison of apomorphine and stomach tubes for emptying the stomach before general anaesthesia in obstetrics. *Br J Anaesth*. 1974;46:526-529.
3. Sharpley HF. Scopolamine in obstetrics. *J S C Med Assoc (Columbia)*. 1951; 47:393-401.
4. White R. The use of apomorphine with scopolamine in labor. *Am J Obstet Gynecol*. 1952;64:91-100.

APRACLONIDINE OPHTHALMIC

Ophthalmic/Autonomic (α_2-Adrenergic Agonist—Topical)

PREGNANCY RECOMMENDATION: No Human Data and No Relevant Animal Data

BREASTFEEDING RECOMMENDATION: Probably Compatible

PREGNANCY SUMMARY

No reports describing the use of apraclonidine in human pregnancy have been located. The drug will probably cross the placenta, so some fetal exposure may occur. However, due to the low plasma levels seen with systemic absorption following ophthalmic use, fetal exposure is probably clinically insignificant. However, the absence of human pregnancy experience prevents a complete assessment of the embryofetal risk. No relevant animal studies have been conducted. Using this drug during pregnancy should be based on the pros and cons of the mother's clinical need for treatment versus any potential fetal risk that might occur from exposure. If used during pregnancy, consider placing pressure over the tear duct in the corner of the eye for at least 1 minute, and then remove any excess solution with absorbent tissue to decrease the amount of drug reaching the systemic circulation even further.

BREASTFEEDING SUMMARY

No reports describing the use of apraclonidine ophthalmic during human lactation have been located. The drug may be found in breast milk, but the low levels of systemic absorption following ophthalmic use suggest that the overall amount is likely to be clinically insignificant. Breastfeeding while using this drug should be based on the mother's clinical need for treatment versus any potential infant risks. If used, the infant should be monitored for the most common reported adult systemic side effects of nausea, headache, chest pain, and myalgia (all leading to irritability), constipation, dry mouth, and insomnia. A method to decrease some systemic absorption with ophthalmic use is described above in the Pregnancy Summary.

Reference

1. Prescribing Information. Apraclonidine. Alcon Laboratories, Inc; 2020.

APREMILAST

Immunologic (Phosphodiesterase-4 Enzyme Inhibitor—Antipsoriatic)

PREGNANCY RECOMMENDATION: No Human Data—Animal Data Suggest Risk

BREASTFEEDING RECOMMENDATION: Potential Toxicity

PREGNANCY SUMMARY

No reports describing the use of apremilast in human pregnancy have been located. The drug will probably cross the placenta, so some fetal exposure will likely occur. Therefore, the absence of human pregnancy experience prevents a complete assessment of the embryofetal risk. Animal studies did show some embryofetal toxicity with malformations in two species at doses of less than 10 times the RHD. Using this drug during pregnancy should be based on the pros and cons of the mother's clinical need for treatment versus any potential fetal risk that might occur from exposure. There is a pregnancy exposure registry that monitors pregnancy outcomes in women using this drug. Health care providers are encouraged to call the Otezla Pregnancy Exposure Registry at 1-877-311-8972.

BREASTFEEDING SUMMARY

No reports describing the use of apremilast during human lactation have been located. The drug will probably be found in breast milk, so some infant exposure will likely occur. Breastfeeding while using this drug should be based on the mother's clinical need for treatment versus any potential infant risks that might occur. If used, the infant should be monitored for the most common reported adult side effects of nausea and headache (both leading to irritability), diarrhea, and upper respiratory tract infection.

Reference

1. Prescribing Information. Otezla. Celgene; 2019.

APREPITANT

Gastrointestinal (Antiemetic)

PREGNANCY RECOMMENDATION: No Human Data—Animal Data Suggest Low Risk

BREASTFEEDING RECOMMENDATION: Probably Compatible

PREGNANCY SUMMARY

No reports describing the use of aprepitant in human pregnancy have been located. The drug will probably cross the placenta, so some fetal exposure will likely occur. Therefore, the absence of human pregnancy experience prevents a complete assessment of the embryofetal risk. Animal studies did not show any embryofetal toxicity in two species at doses less than 10 times the RHD. Using this drug during pregnancy should be based on the pros and cons of the mother's clinical need for treatment versus any potential fetal risk that might occur from exposure.

BREASTFEEDING SUMMARY

No reports describing the use of aprepitant during human lactation have been located. The drug will probably be found in breast milk, so some infant exposure will likely occur. Due to a potential for tumorigenicity seen in rodent carcinogenic studies, the manufacturer recommends that women not breastfeed while using this drug. Nevertheless, breastfeeding while using this drug should be based on the mother's clinical need for treatment versus any potential infant risks. If used, the infant should be monitored for the most common reported adult side effects of headache and pruritus (both leading to irritability), constipation, and fever.

Reference

1. Prescribing Information. Emend. Merck Sharp & Dohme Corp; 2020.

APROCITENTAN

Antihypertensive (Vasodilator)

PREGNANCY RECOMMENDATION: *No Human Data—Animal Data Suggest Potential Risk

BREASTFEEDING RECOMMENDATION: Potential Toxicity

PREGNANCY SUMMARY

No reports describing the use of aprocitentan during human pregnancy have been located. In five studies reporting on a total of eight first-trimester exposures to other endothelin receptor agonist (ERA) drugs (five bosentan and three ambrisentan

(continued)

cases) treated for pulmonary hypertension, all delivered healthy infants with no fetal anomalies identified (six preterm and two term). The drug will probably cross the placenta, so some fetal exposure will likely occur. However, the absence of human pregnancy experience prevents a complete assessment of the embryofetal risk. Animal studies did show embryofetal toxicity in one species at doses of less than 10 times the RHD. *Based on the drug's mechanism of action, the manufacturer states that the drug is contraindicated for use in pregnancy. They recommend that women with reproductive potential use effective contraception during treatment and for 1 month after the last dose. A negative pregnancy test is needed prior to drug initiation, and it is only available through a REMS program (TRYVIO REMS). The drug carries a boxed warning for this increased risk of embryofetal toxicity. However, there is increasing evidence that suggests a role of the endothelin system in preeclampsia, and blockage of the endothelin receptor may result in physiologic improvement. Therefore, using this drug during pregnancy should be based on the pros and cons of the mother's clinical need for treatment versus any potential fetal risk that might occur from exposure.

BREASTFEEDING SUMMARY

No reports describing the use of aprocitentan during human lactation were located. The drug will probably be excreted into breast milk, so some infant exposure will likely occur. However, due to the concern for potential serious adverse effects that might be seen in a breastfed infant, the manufacturer recommends that women not breastfeed while being treated with this drug. Nevertheless, breastfeeding while using this drug should be based on the mother's clinical need for treatment. If used, the infant should be monitored for the most common reported adult side effects of anemia and peripheral edema.

References

1. Prescribing Information. Tryvio. Indorsia Pharmaceuticals, Ltd; 2024.
2. Hitzerd E, Neuman RI, Broekhuizen M, et al. Transfer and vascular effect of endothelin receptor agonists in the human placenta. *Hypertension*. 2020;75:877-884.
3. Molelekwa V, Akhter P, McKenna P, et al. Eisenmenger's syndrome in a 27 week pregnancy—management with bosentan and sildenafil. *Ir Med J*. 2005;98:87-88.
4. Elliot CA, Stewart P, Webster VJ, et al. The use of iloprost in early pregnancy in patients with pulmonary hypertension. *Eur Respir J*. 2005;26:168-173.
5. Streit M, Speich R, Fischler M, Ulrich S. Successful pregnancy in pulmonary arterial hypertension associated with systemic lupus erythematosus: a case report. *J Med Case Rep*. 2009;3:7255.
6. Tokgoz HC, Kaymaz C, Poci N, et al. A successful cesarean delivery without fetal or maternal morbidity in an Eisenmenger patient with cor triatriatum sinistrum, double-orifice mitral valve, large ventricular septal defect, and single ventricle who was under long-term bosentan treatment. *Turk Kardiyol Dem Ars*. 2017;45:184-188.
7. Amann U, Wentzell N, Kollhorst B, Haug U. Prescribing of endothelin receptor antagonists and riociguat in women of childbearing age in a large German claims database study. *Reprod Toxicol*. 2023;119:108415.

ARFORMOTEROL

Respiratory (Inhalation—COPD)

PREGNANCY RECOMMENDATION: No Human Data—Animal Data Suggest Low Risk

BREASTFEEDING RECOMMENDATION: Probably Compatible

PREGNANCY SUMMARY

No reports describing the use of arformoterol during human pregnancy have been located. Some amount of the drug may cross the placenta; however, the total amount is likely to be clinically insignificant due to the minimal levels absorbed systemically with inhalation use. Therefore, the absence of human pregnancy experience prevents a complete assessment of the embryofetal risk. Animal data did not show any embryofetal toxicity or teratogenicity in one species at doses well above 10 times the maximum recommended human daily inhaled dose (MRHDID). There was some teratogenicity in a second species, but again, the doses were more than 300 times the MRHDID. Using this drug during pregnancy should be based on the pros and cons of the mother's clinical need for treatment versus any potential fetal risk that might occur from exposure.

BREASTFEEDING SUMMARY

No reports describing the use of arformoterol during human lactation have been located. The drug might be found in breast milk. However, the total amount is likely to be clinically insignificant due to the minimal levels absorbed systemically with inhalation use. If the clinical decision is to use this drug while breastfeeding, the infant should be monitored for the most common reported adult side effects of back pain, dyspepsia, and leg cramps (all leading to irritability), diarrhea, rash, and peripheral edema.

Reference

1. Prescribing Information. Brovana. Sunovion Pharmaceuticals; 2019.

ARGATROBAN

Hematologic (Anticoagulant)

PREGNANCY RECOMMENDATION: Limited Human Data—No Relevant Animal Data (Maternal Benefit May Outweigh Any Embryofetal Risk)

BREASTFEEDING RECOMMENDATION: Probably Compatible

PREGNANCY SUMMARY

A few case reports and a small series were located that described the use of argatroban in about seven human pregnancies. One exposure occurred at around 9 weeks' gestation, and no birth anomalies were identified at delivery. The other cases all occurred in the second and third trimesters. No adverse effects related to the drug were described. The drug will probably cross the placenta, so some fetal exposure will likely occur. Therefore, this limited human pregnancy experience prevents a complete assessment of the embryofetal risk. Animal studies did not show any embryofetal toxicity or teratogenicity in two species, but at doses of only about 20% to 30% of the RHD dose. No studies have been performed to see what might occur with doses equal to the RHD. Using this drug during pregnancy should be based on the pros and cons of the mother's clinical need for treatment versus any potential fetal risk that might occur from exposure. If a pregnant woman requires argatroban therapy, the benefits to her in many clinical cases may outweigh the theoretical risks to the embryo or fetus.

BREASTFEEDING SUMMARY

No studies describing the use argatroban during human lactation have been located. The drug will probably be found in breast milk, so some infant exposure will likely occur. However, oral bioavailability is less than 1%, so any drug absorbed through breastfeeding is likely to be clinically insignificant. Regardless, due to a concern for potential serious adverse effects that might be seen in a breastfed infant, the manufacturer recommends that women not breastfeed while being treated with this drug. Nevertheless, breastfeeding while using this drug should be based on the mother's clinical need for treatment versus any potential infant risks that might occur. If used, the infant should be monitored for the most common reported adult side effects of nausea, headache, and back pain (all leading to irritability), diarrhea, vomiting, fever, and decreased blood pressure.

References

1. Prescribing Information. Argatroban. Sandoz; 2018.
2. Taniguchi S, Fukuda I, Minakawa M, et al. Emergency pulmonary embolectomy during the second trimester of pregnancy: report of a case. *Surg Today*. 2008;38:59-61.
3. Young SK, Al-Mondhiry HA, Vaida SJ, et al. Successful use of argatroban during the third trimester of pregnancy: case report and review of the literature. *Pharmacotherapy*. 2008;28:1531-1536.
4. Ekbatani A, Asaro LR, Malinow AM. Anticoagulation with argatroban in a parturient with heparin-induced thrombocytopenia. *Int J Obstet Anesth*. 2010;19:82-117.
5. Darki A, Kodali PP, McPheters JP, et al. Hypereosinophilic syndrome with cardiac involvement. *Tex Heart Inst J*. 2011;38:163-165.
6. Tanimura K, Ebina Y, Sonoyama A, et al. Argatroban therapy for heparin-induced thrombocytopenia during pregnancy in a woman with hereditary antithrombin deficiency. *J Obstet Gynaecol Res*. 2012;38:749-752.
7. Chaudhary RK, Nepal C, Khanal N, et al. Management and outcome of heparin-induced thrombocytopenia in pregnancy: a systematic review. *Cardiovasc Hematol Agents Med Chem*. 2015;13:92-97.

ARIMOCLOMOL

Genetic/Central Nervous System (Heat Shock Protein Coinducer—Pharmacologic Chaperone)

PREGNANCY RECOMMENDATION: No Human Data—Animal Data Suggest Potential Risk (Maternal Benefit May Outweigh Any Embryofetal Risk)

BREASTFEEDING RECOMMENDATION: Probably Compatible

PREGNANCY SUMMARY

No reports describing the use of arimoclomol in human pregnancy have been located. The drug will likely cross the placenta, so fetal exposure will probably occur. However, the absence of human pregnancy experience prevents a complete assessment of the embryofetal risk. Animal reproduction studies did show some embryofetal toxicity in one species at doses of less than 10 times the RHD, in the absence of maternal toxicity. Using this drug during pregnancy should be based on the pros and cons of the mother's clinical need for treatment versus any potential fetal risk that might occur from exposure.

BREASTFEEDING SUMMARY

No reports describing the use of arimoclomol during human lactation have been located. The drug will probably be excreted into breast milk, so some infant exposure will likely occur. Breastfeeding while using this drug should be based on the mother's clinical need for treatment versus any potential infant risks that might occur. If used, the infant should be monitored for the most common reported adult side effects of decreased appetite (monitor infant growth), diarrhea, and urinary tract infection.

Reference

1. Prescribing Information. Miplyffa. Geron Corp; 2024.

ARIPIPRAZOLE

Mental Health (Atypical Antipsychotic)

PREGNANCY RECOMMENDATION: Limited Human Data—Animal Data Suggest Potential Risk/Human Data Suggest Potential Risk (Third Trimester)

BREASTFEEDING RECOMMENDATION: Potential Toxicity

PREGNANCY SUMMARY

Several case reports and series were located that describe the use of aripiprazole during human pregnancy. The rate of major birth anomalies was about 3.7% in more than 140 first-trimester exposures. No pattern to the defects was identified. The drug will cross the placenta, so fetal exposure will occur. However, this limited human pregnancy experience prevents a complete assessment of the embryofetal risk. Animal data were confusing in that some embryofetal toxicity with malformations was found in two species at doses of less than 10 times the RHD based on body surface area (BSA) in two evaluations. However, this was not found at the same dosages in the same species in two other evaluations. There is a risk of extrapyramidal signs and/or withdrawal symptoms (agitation, hypertonia, hypotonia, tremor, somnolence, decreased respirations, and feeding difficulties) in the newborn if the drug is used in the third trimester near delivery. Using this drug during pregnancy should be based on the pros and cons of the mother's clinical need for treatment versus any potential fetal risk that might occur from exposure. If the mother's condition requires treatment with aripiprazole, using the lowest effective dose is recommended. There is a pregnancy exposure registry that monitors pregnancy outcomes in women using atypical antipsychotic drugs. Health care providers are encouraged to contact the National Pregnancy Registry for Atypical Antipsychotics at 1-866-961-2388.

BREASTFEEDING SUMMARY

A total of six women from five studies were located where aripiprazole was used during human lactation. Breast milk levels for aripiprazole ranged from undetectable (LLQ 10 ng/mL) to about 54 ng/mL. In one analysis, the active metabolite was also analyzed with reported concentrations of 9 and 6 ng/mL. Using the combined levels of the drug and metabolite, the calculated RID would be about 65%. All other calculated RIDs were less than 10%. In one study, the infant's blood level was evaluated, showing a concentration of 7.6 ng/mL. However, this was obtained on day 6 postpartum of a mother using 18 mg daily through the pregnancy and postpartum, so some of this may still have been from transplacental transfer (due to an elimination half-life of about 3 days).

References

1. Prescribing Information. Abilify. Otsuka America Pharmaceutical; 2019.
2. Windhager E, Kim SW, Saria A, et al. Perinatal use of aripiprazole. *J Clin Psychopharmacol*. 2014;34:637-641.
3. Mendhekar DN, Sharma JB, Srilakshmi P. Use of aripiprazole during late pregnancy in a woman with psychotic illness. *Ann Pharmacother*. 2006;40:575.
4. Mendhekar DN, Sunder K, Andrade C. Aripiprazole use in a pregnant schizoaffective woman. *Bipolar Disord*. 2006;8:299-300.
5. Mervak B, Collins J, Valenstein M. Case report of aripiprazole usage during pregnancy. *Arch Womens Ment Health*. 2008;11:249-250.
6. Lutz UC, Hiemke C, Wiatr G, et al. Aripiprazole in pregnancy and lactation. A case report. *J Clin Psychopharmacol*. 2010;30:204-205.
7. Watanabe N, Kasahara M, Sugibayashi R, et al. Perinatal use of aripiprazole. A case report. *J Clin Psychopharmacol*. 2011;31:377-379.
8. Gentile S, Tofani S, Bellantuono C. Aripiprazole and pregnancy. A case report and literature review. *J Clin Psychopharmacol*. 2011;31:531-532.
9. Nguyen T, Teoh S, Hackett P, Ilett K. Placental transfer of aripiprazole. *Aust N Z J Psychiatry*. 2011;45:500-501.
10. Widschwendter CG, Hofer A. Aripiprazole use in early pregnancy: a case report. *Pharmacopsychiatry*. 2012;45:299-300.
11. Bellet F, Beyens MN, Bernard N, et al. Exposure to aripiprazole during embryogenesis: a prospective multicenter cohort study. *Pharmacoepidemiol Drug Safety*. 2015;24:368-380.
12. Ennis ZN, Damkler P. Pregnancy exposure to olanzapine, quetiapine, risperidone, aripiprazole and risk of congenital malformations. A systematic review. *Basic Clin Pharmacol Toxicol*. 2015;116:315-320.
13. Uguz F. Second-generation antipsychotics during the lactation period. A comparative systematic review on infant safety. *J Clin Psychopharmacol*. 2016;36:244-252.
14. Frew JR. Psychopharmacology of bipolar I disorder during lactation: a case report of the use of lithium and aripiprazole in a nursing mother. *Arch Womens Ment Health*. 2015;18:135-136.
15. Klinger G, Stahl B, Fusar-Poli P, Merlob P. Antipsychotic drugs and breastfeeding. *Pediatr Endocrinol Rev*. 2013;10:308-317.

ARMODAFINIL

Central Nervous System (Stimulant)

PREGNANCY RECOMMENDATION: Limited Human Data—Animal Data Suggest Potential Risk

BREASTFEEDING RECOMMENDATION: Potential Toxicity

PREGNANCY SUMMARY

No reports describing the use of armodafinil in human pregnancy have been located. The manufacturer described three cases where the drug was used, resulting in a spontaneous abortion in one case and two others that were growth restricted but with no reported anomalies. The drug will probably cross the placenta, so some fetal exposure will likely occur. Therefore, this limited human pregnancy experience prevents a complete assessment of the embryofetal risk. Animal studies did not find any embryofetal toxicity or teratogenicity in two species at doses of more than 10 times the RHD based on weight, but these doses were less than the MRHD. Some maternal toxicity was also seen in both species at these doses. Using this drug during pregnancy should be based on the pros and cons of the mother's clinical need for treatment versus any potential fetal risk that might occur from exposure. Avoiding armodafinil during pregnancy, if possible, may be the best clinical course.

BREASTFEEDING SUMMARY

No reports describing the use of armodafinil during human lactation have been located. However, two studies analyzing the use of modafinil were located. In two lactating women, modafinil was used at daily doses of 250 and 400 mg. Because modafinil is a 1:1 mixture of the R-enantiomer (which is armodafinil), this would be a daily dose of about 125 and 200 mg of armodafinil. Breast milk levels for armodafinil ranged from about 0.4 mcg/mL to about 4.1 mcg/mL (this peak was in the higher dose patient). The calculated RIDs for armodafinil using mean concentrations were both about 10% (but were both about 20% using peak values). In one infant exposed through breastfeeding, a serum concentration of about 190 ng/mL was reported. Breastfeeding while using this drug should be based on the mother's clinical need for treatment versus any potential infant risks that might occur. If used, the infant should be monitored for the most common reported adult side effects of headache (leading to irritability), diarrhea, vomiting, and insomnia.

Reference

1. Prescribing Information. Nuvigil. Cephalon; 2017.

ARTESUNATE

Anti-Infective (Antimalarial—Artemisinin Derivative)

PREGNANCY RECOMMENDATION: Human Data Suggest Low Risk (Maternal Benefit May Outweigh Any Embryofetal Risk)

BREASTFEEDING RECOMMENDATION: Probably Compatible

PREGNANCY SUMMARY

Per the manufacturer, there are reports describing the use of IV artesunate in the first trimester along with published trials and studies of 1,300 women with first-trimester exposure and over 6,500 women exposed in the second and third trimesters to oral artesunate, and other artemisinin class drugs (via various routes of administration). They state that no increased risk for major birth defects, miscarriage, or adverse pregnancy outcomes was identified. In addition, a recent meta-analysis of 7 studies concluded that artemisinin-based treatment (ABT) in 737 pregnancies in the first trimester had a lower rate (though not significant) of adverse pregnancy outcomes and major congenital anomalies when compared with the non-ABT group (n = 1,076) or quinine (n = 917). However, due to animal embryofetal toxicity data, first-trimester use has been limited to the treatment of severe malaria. The drug will probably cross the placenta, so some fetal exposure will likely occur. The CDC considers IV artesunate low risk for use in pregnant women in the second and third trimester. The CDC and World Health Organization (WHO) also currently recommend its use for the treatment of severe malaria in all trimesters of pregnancy. There is a pregnancy safety study for artesunate. Health care providers should report artesunate exposure by contacting Amivas LLC at 1-855-526-4827 (1-855-5AMIVAS).

BREASTFEEDING SUMMARY

One abstract was located that reported an analysis of artesunate use during lactation. The drug itself was not detected, whereas dihydroartemisinin (DHA) was found at low levels producing an RID of less than 1%. Another study stated that infants exposed to the drug though breastfeeding may experience increased vomiting. Breastfeeding while using this drug should be based on the mother's clinical need for treatment versus any potential infant risks that might occur. The CDC considers IV artesunate safe for use during lactation.

References

1. Product information. Artesunate. Amivas LLC; 2022.
2. Centers for Disease Control and Prevention. Malaria treatment (United States). Accessed May 7, 2023. https://www.cdc.gov/malaria/diagnosis_treatment/treatment.html
3. WHO guidelines for malaria, 13 August 2025. Geneva: World Health Organization; 2025. https://doi.org/10.2471/ B09514. *WHO guidelines for malaria*, August 13, 2025. Geneva: World Health Organization; 2025. https://doi.org/10.2471/ B09514.
4. Saito M, McGready R, Tinto H, et al. Pregnancy outcomes after first-trimester treatment with artemisinin derivatives versus non-artemisinin antimalarials: a systematic review and individual patient data meta-analysis. *Lancet*. 2023;401:118-130.
5. Saito M, Carrara VI, Gilder ME, et al. A randomized controlled trial of dihydroartemisinin-piperaquine, artesunate-mefloquine and extended artemether-lumefantrine treatments for malaria in pregnancy on the Thailand-Myanmar border. *BMC Med*. 2021;19:132.
6. Rouamba T, Valea I, Bognini JD, et al. Safety profile of drug use during pregnancy at peripheral health centres in Burkina Faso: a prospective observational cohort study. *Drugs Real World Outcomes*. 2018;5:193-206.
7. Moore KA, Simpson JA, Paw MK, et al. Safety of artemisinins in first trimester of prospectively followed pregnancies: an observational study. *Lancet Infect Dis*. 2016;16(5):576-583.
8. Tinto H, Sevene E, Dellicour S, et al. Assessment of the safety of antimalarial drug use during early pregnancy: protocol for a multicenter prospective cohort study in Burkina Faso, Kenya and Mozambique. *Reprod Health*. 2015;12:112.
9. Rulisa S, Kaligirwa N, Agaba S, et al. Pharmacovigilance of artemether-lumefantrine in pregnant women followed until delivery in Rwanda. *Malar J*. 2012;11:225.
10. McGready R, Lee SJ, Wiladphaingern J, et al. Adverse effects of falciparum and vivax malaria and the safety of antimalarial treatment in early pregnancy: a population-based study. *Lancet Infect Dis*. 2011;12:388-396.
11. Mosha D, Mazuguni F, Mrema S, et al. Safety of artemether-lumefantrine exposure in first trimester of pregnancy: an observational cohort. *Malar J*. 2014;13:197.
12. Manyando C, Mkandawire R, Puma L, et al. Safety of artemether-lumefantrine in pregnant women with malaria: results of a prospective cohort study in Zambia. *Malar J*. 2010;9:249.
13. Jansen FH, Jansen-Luts A, Ameye C, et al. Is artesunate or its active metabolite dihydroartemisinin being excreted in the milk of lactating mothers? *Am J Trop Med Hyg*. 2006;75:158.
14. Creek D, Bigira V, Arinaitwe E, et al. Increased risk of early vomiting among infants and young children treated with dihydroartemisinin-piperaquine compared with artemether-lumefantrine for uncomplicated malaria. *Am J Trop Med Hyg*. 2010;83:873-875.

ASCIMINIB

Antineoplastic (Tyrosine Kinase Inhibitor)

PREGNANCY RECOMMENDATION: No Human Data—Animal Data Suggest Risk

BREASTFEEDING RECOMMENDATION: Potential Toxicity

PREGNANCY SUMMARY

No reports describing the use of asciminib in human pregnancy have been located. The drug will likely cross the placenta, so some fetal exposure will probably occur. Therefore, the absence of human pregnancy experience prevents a complete assessment of the embryofetal risk. Animal data did show embryofetal toxicity. Based on animal studies and the drug's mechanism of action, the manufacturer recommends that women with reproductive potential use effective contraception during treatment and for 1 week after the last dose. Nevertheless, using this drug during pregnancy should be based on the pros and cons of the mother's clinical need for treatment versus any potential fetal risk that might occur from exposure. Hypertension and cardiac arrhythmias were seen in 19% and 7% of patients, respectively, in the clinical trials.

BREASTFEEDING SUMMARY

No reports describing the use of asciminib during human lactation have been located. Asciminib will probably be found in breast milk, so some infant exposure will likely occur. The manufacturer recommends that women not breastfeed while being treated with this drug and for at least 1 week after the last dose. Nevertheless, breastfeeding while using this drug should be based on the mother's clinical need for treatment. If used, the infant should be monitored for the most common reported adult side effects of nausea and musculoskeletal pain (both leading to irritability), upper respiratory tract infections, lethargy, rash, diarrhea, and several laboratory abnormalities (see PI).

Reference

1. Prescribing Information. Scemblix. Novartis Pharmaceuticals; 2022.

ASENAPINE

Mental Health (Atypical Antipsychotic)

PREGNANCY RECOMMENDATION: No Human Data—Animal Data Suggest Potential Risk

BREASTFEEDING RECOMMENDATION: Potential Toxicity

PREGNANCY SUMMARY

No reports describing the use of asenapine during human pregnancy have been located. The drug will probably cross the placenta, so some fetal exposure will likely occur. Therefore, the absence of human pregnancy experience prevents a complete assessment of the embryofetal risk. Use of antipsychotic drugs during the third trimester has been associated with extrapyramidal and/or withdrawal symptoms in some neonates after delivery. Animal studies did show some embryofetal toxicity in one species at doses of less than 10 times the RHD. Using this drug during pregnancy should be based on the pros and cons of the mother's clinical need for treatment versus any potential fetal risk that might occur from exposure. There is a pregnancy exposure registry that monitors pregnancy outcomes in women using atypical antipsychotic drugs. Health care providers are encouraged to contact the National Pregnancy Registry for Atypical Antipsychotics at 1-866-961-2388. Use of this drug has been associated with prolongation of the QT interval.

BREASTFEEDING SUMMARY

No reports describing the use of asenapine during human lactation have been located. The drug will probably be found in breast milk, so some infant exposure will likely occur. In a systematic review of 37 reports involving 206 infants with exposure to second-generation antipsychotic drugs during lactation (none involved asenapine), the overall findings suggested that they were relatively safe. Olanzapine comprised 170 (83%) of the cases. In another study of data from the National Pregnancy Registry for Atypical Antipsychotics, 576 women using second-generation antipsychotic drugs during lactation were compared with 818 women using other mental health drugs while breastfeeding. No adverse effects were noted in the infants of both groups. The number exposed to asenapine was not provided. Other studies have evaluated the literature on the use of antipsychotic drugs during breastfeeding and have stated that there are no data on asenapine. Therefore, they recommend using atypical antipsychotic drugs where safety data exist. Nevertheless, breastfeeding while using this drug should be based on the mother's clinical need for treatment versus any potential infant risks. If used, the infant should be monitored for the most common reported adult side effects of nausea and paresthesia (both leading to irritability), somnolence, fatigue (lethargy), extrapyramidal signs, and various laboratory abnormalities (see PI).

References

1. Prescribing Information. Saphris. Allergan USA; 2019.
2. Uguz F. Second-generation antipsychotics during the lactation period: a comparative systematic review on infant safety. *J Clin Psychopharmacol.* 2016;36:244-252.
3. Viguera AC, Vanderkruik R, Gaccione P, et al. Breastfeeding practices among women taking second-generation antipsychotics: findings from the National Pregnancy Registry for Atypical Antipsychotics. *Arch Womens Ment Health*. 2022;25:511-516.
4. Parikh T, Goyal D, Scarff JR, Lippmann S. Antipsychotic drugs and safety concerns for breast-feeding infants. *South Med J.* 2014;107:696-698.
5. Klinger G, Stahl B, Fusar-Poli P, Merlob P. Antipsychotic drugs and breastfeeding. *Pediatr Endocrinol Rev.* 2013;10:308-317.

ASFOTASE ALFA

Endocrine/Metabolic (Enzyme)

PREGNANCY RECOMMENDATION: No Human Data—Animal Data Suggest Low Risk

BREASTFEEDING RECOMMENDATION: Probably Compatible

PREGNANCY SUMMARY

No reports describing the use of asfotase alfa during human pregnancy have been located. The drug will probably not cross the placenta, especially in the first half of gestation. However, the absence of human pregnancy experience prevents a complete assessment of the embryofetal risk. Animal studies did not show any embryofetal toxicity in two species at doses of greater than 10 times the RHD. Using this drug during pregnancy should be based on the pros and cons of the mother's clinical need for treatment versus any potential fetal risk that might occur from exposure.

BREASTFEEDING SUMMARY

No reports describing the use asfotase alfa during human lactation have been located. The drug will likely not be found in breast milk. However, because it is an enzyme consisting of over 1,400 amino acids, if the drug were to be ingested through breastfeeding, it would probably be digested in the infant's gastrointestinal tract and not be absorbed. Nevertheless, breastfeeding while using this drug should be based on the mother's clinical need for treatment versus any potential infant risks. If used, the infant should be monitored for the most common reported adult side effects of hypersensitivity reactions.

Reference

1. Prescribing Information. Strensiq. Alexion Pharmaceuticals; 2020.

ASPARAGINASE

Antineoplastic (Enzyme)

PREGNANCY RECOMMENDATION: Limited Human Data—Animal Data Suggest Risk

BREASTFEEDING RECOMMENDATION: Probably Compatible

PREGNANCY SUMMARY

The reported use of asparaginase during human pregnancy is limited to six pregnancies, all in the second trimester, resulting in the birth of seven infants (one set of twins). In each case, multiple other chemotherapeutic agents were used with asparaginase for the treatment of acute leukemias. Therapy with asparaginase was initiated between 16 and 22 weeks' gestation. The drug will not likely cross the placenta in clinically significant amounts. However, this limited human pregnancy experience prevents a complete assessment of the embryofetal risk. Animal data did show some embryofetal toxicity with malformations in two species at doses of less than 10 times the RHD. Using this drug during pregnancy should be based on the pros and cons of the mother's clinical need for treatment versus any potential fetal risk that might occur from exposure. The drug is also associated with glucose intolerance, and this should be monitored if used in pregnancy.

BREASTFEEDING SUMMARY

No reports describing the use of asparaginase during human lactation have been located. The drug will not likely be excreted into breast milk. However, if any of this enzyme were to be ingested through breastfeeding, it would probably be digested in the infant's gastrointestinal tract and not be absorbed. However, due to a concern for potential serious adverse effects that might be seen in a breastfed infant, the manufacturer recommends that women not breastfeed while being treated with this drug. Nevertheless, breastfeeding while using this drug should be based on the mother's clinical need for treatment versus any potential infant risks that might occur. If used, the infant should be monitored for the most common reported adult side effects of hyperglycemia and other laboratory abnormalities, rash, flushing, and shortness of breath.

References

1. Prescribing Information. Erwinaze. Jazz Pharmaceuticals: 2016.
2. Adamson RH, Fabro S, Hahn MA, et al. Evaluation of the embryotoxic activity of L-asparaginase. *Arch Int Pharmacodyn Ther*. 1970;186:310-320. As cited in Shepard TH. *Catalog of Teratogenic Agents*. 6th ed. Johns Hopkins University Press; 1989:58-59.
3. Ohguro Y, Imamura S, Koyama K, et al. Toxicological studies on L-asparaginase. *Yamaguchi Igaku*. 1969;18:271-292. As cited in Shepard TH. *Catalog of Teratogenic Agents*. 6th ed. Johns Hopkins University Press; 1989:58-59.
4. Okun DB, Groncy PK, Sieger L, Tanaka KR. Acute leukemia in pregnancy: transient neonatal myelosuppression after combination chemotherapy in the mother. *Med Pediatr Oncol*. 1979;7:315-319.
5. Khurshid M, Saleem M. Acute leukaemia in pregnancy. *Lancet*. 1978; 2:534-535.
6. Karp GI, Von Oeyen P, Valone F, et al. Doxorubicin in pregnancy: possible transplacental passage. *Cancer Treat Rep*. 1983;67:773-777.
7. Awidi AS, Tarawneh MS, Shubair KS, et al. Acute leukemia in pregnancy: report of five cases treated with a combination which included a low dose of adriamycin. *Eur J Cancer Clin Oncol*. 1983;19:881-884.
8. Turchi JJ, Villasis C. Anthracyclines in the treatment of malignancy in pregnancy. *Cancer*. 1988;61:435-440.
9. Schleuning M, Clemm C. Chromosomal aberrations in a newborn whose mother received cytotoxic treatment during pregnancy. *N Engl J Med*. 1987; 317:1666-1667.
10. Blatt J, Mulvihill JJ, Ziegler JL, et al. Pregnancy outcome following cancer chemotherapy. *Am J Med*. 1980;69:828-832.
11. Evenson DP, Arlin Z, Welt S, et al. Male reproductive capacity may recover following drug treatment with the L-10 protocol for acute lymphocytic leukemia. *Cancer*. 1984;53:30-36.
12. Green DM, Hall B, Zevon MA. Pregnancy outcome after treatment for acute lymphoblastic leukemia during childhood or adolescence. *Cancer*. 1989;64:2335-2339.
13. Green DM, Zevon MA, Lowrie G, et al. Congenital anomalies in children of patients who received chemotherapy for cancer in childhood and adolescence. *N Engl J Med*. 1991;325:141-146.
14. Mulvihill JJ, McKeen EA, Rosner F, Zarrabi MH. Pregnancy outcome in cancer patients: experience in a large cooperative group. *Cancer*. 1987;60: 1143-1150.
15. Pajor A, Zimonyi I, Koos R, et al. Pregnancies and offspring in survivors of acute lymphoid leukemia and lymphoma. *Eur J Obstet Gynecol Reprod Biol*. 1991;40:1-5.

ASPARAGINASE ERWINIA CHRYSANTHEMI (RECOMBINANT)

Antineoplastic (Enzyme)

PREGNANCY RECOMMENDATION: No Human Data—Animal Data Suggest Potential Risk

BREASTFEEDING RECOMMENDATION: Probably Compatible

PREGNANCY SUMMARY

No reports describing the use of asparaginase *Erwinia chrysanthemi* (recombinant) in human pregnancy have been located. The drug is not likely to cross the placenta; however, because it consists of a protein, it is not known whether some fetal exposure could occur. Therefore, the absence of human pregnancy experience prevents a complete assessment of the embryofetal risk. Embryofetal toxicity with malformations was observed in animal studies. Because of the animal studies, the manufacturer recommends that women with reproductive potential use effective nonhormonal contraception during treatment with this drug and for at least 3 months after the last dose. Nevertheless, using this drug during pregnancy should be based on the pros and cons of the mother's clinical need for treatment versus any potential fetal risk that might occur from exposure. In addition, elevated glucose levels were seen in 21% of patients treated with this drug in clinical trials. Therefore, if used during pregnancy, glucose levels should be monitored.

BREASTFEEDING SUMMARY

No reports describing the use of asparaginase *Erwinia chrysanthemi* (recombinant) during human lactation have been located. The drug is not likely to be excreted into breast milk. However, if any of this enzyme were found in breast milk, it would probably be digested in the infant's gastrointestinal tract and not be absorbed. Regardless, due to the concern for potential serious adverse effects that might be seen in a breastfed infant, the manufacturer recommends that women not breastfeed during treatment with this drug and for 1 week after the last dose. Nevertheless, breastfeeding while using this drug should be based on the mother's clinical need for treatment. If used, the infant should be monitored for the most common reported adult side effects of nausea, musculoskeletal pain, and headache (all leading to irritability), infection, lethargy, decreased appetite (monitor growth), pyrexia, and various laboratory abnormalities (see PI).

Reference

1. Prescribing Information. Rylaze. Jazz Pharmaceuticals; 2022.

ASPIRIN

Pain (Nonsteroidal Anti-Inflammatory)

PREGNANCY RECOMMENDATION: **Human Data Suggest Compatible (Low Dose)/Human Data Suggest Risk (Second and Third Trimesters) (Full Dose)**

BREASTFEEDING RECOMMENDATION: **Probably Compatible (Low Dose)/Potential Toxicity (Full Dose)**

PREGNANCY SUMMARY

Numerous publications have been located that describe the use of aspirin during human pregnancy. Regarding first-trimester exposure, more than 16,500 exposures were reported by the CPP and the MMSS. The major congenital malformation rate was 2.9% and no pattern to the defects was seen. Several studies have analyzed the use of aspirin and risk for cardiac defects. Though results have varied widely, the overall analysis (including the data from the CPP and MMSS) does not support this finding. A large number of studies have also evaluated the use of low-dose aspirin (40-150 mg/d) for the prevention or delay of preeclampsia. If used, especially if started prior to 16 weeks' gestation, the benefit from this daily consumption has been documented. On the other hand, like other NSAIDs, use of full-dose aspirin after 20 weeks' gestation can lead to fetal renal dysfunction, producing oligohydramnios with numerous poor outcomes related to this condition. It can also cause premature closure of the fetal ductus arteriosus, producing persistent pulmonary hypertension and possible fetal or newborn death. Lastly, the use of aspirin in the last 10 days prior to birth can increase the risk for bleeding at the time of delivery. The drug crosses the placenta, so fetal exposure will occur, and in some cases, fetal blood concentrations can be higher than maternal levels. Animal studies did show some embryofetal toxicity with teratogenicity in one species at doses of less than 10 times the RHD, but not in a second species. Using low-dose aspirin during pregnancy is probably compatible, but use of full-dose aspirin after 20 weeks' gestation is not recommended, if at all possible. If an analgesic or antipyretic is needed during pregnancy, acetaminophen should be considered.

BREASTFEEDING SUMMARY

Several studies have been located that describe the use of aspirin during human lactation. The drug has been studied in patients using full doses as well as low-dose aspirin. The drug has been found in breast milk in nearly every sample tested with sensitive assays. Because of the rapid conversion of aspirin to salicylic acid, most breast milk samples have been evaluated for salicylic acid levels. The breast milk of about 25 women has been analyzed. In cases of larger full-dose aspirin use, breast milk levels for salicylic acid ranged from about 1 mcg/mL up to about 39 mcg/mL. Calculated RIDs were on average about 10%. In addition, in a few cases, aspirin was analyzed but was not detected (LLQ of 600 pg/mL). With low-dose aspirin (single 325 mg dose or 81 mg dosages), breast milk levels for salicylic acid ranged from about 0.024 mcg/mL up to about 0.745 mcg/mL. The calculated RIDs were 1% or less. One infant has been analyzed in a case of a mother using 2.4 g/d. The infant serum level was about 65 mcg/mL (or $<$25% of the maternal level). Reye syndrome is associated with the use of aspirin in infants who have viral infections. It is not known if this can occur with aspirin exposure through breastfeeding.

Due to a concern for potential serious adverse effects that might be seen in a breastfed infant, the manufacturer recommends that women not breastfeed while being treated with this drug. However, the use of low-dose aspirin (81 mg) in certain clinical conditions is probably acceptable. If the clinical decision is to use this drug while breastfeeding, the infant should be monitored for the most common reported adult side effects of dyspepsia, abdominal pain (leading to irritability), and bruising (bleeding).

References

1. Corby DG. Aspirin in pregnancy: maternal and fetal effects. *Pediatrics.* 1978;62(suppl):930-937.
2. Palmisano PA, Cassady G. Salicylate exposure in the perinate. *JAMA.* 1969;209:556-558.
3. Forfar JO, Nelson MM. Epidemiology of drugs taken by pregnant women: drugs that may affect the fetus adversely. *Clin Pharmacol Ther.* 1973;14:632-642.
4. Finnigan D, Burry AF, Smith IDB. Analgesic consumption in an antenatal clinic survey. *Med J Aust.* 1974;1:761-762.
5. Collins E, Turner G. Maternal effects of regular salicylate ingestion in pregnancy. *Lancet.* 1975;2:335-337.
6. Slone D, Heinonen OP, Kaufman DW, et al. Aspirin and congenital malformations. *Lancet.* 1976;1:1373-1375.
7. Hill RM, Craig JP, Chaney MD, et al. Utilization of over-the-counter drugs during pregnancy. *Clin Obstet Gynecol.* 1977;20:381-394.
8. Harrison K, Thomas I, Smith I. Analgesic use during pregnancy. *Med J Aust.* 1978;2:161.
9. Bodendorfer TW, Briggs GG, Gunning JE. Obtaining drug exposure histories during pregnancy. *Am J Obstet Gynecol.* 1979;135:490-494.
10. Jackson AV. Toxic effects of salicylate on the foetus and mother. *J Pathol Bacteriol.* 1948;60:587-593.
11. Lewis RN, Schulman JD. Influence of acetylsalicylic acid, an inhibitor of prostaglandin synthesis, on the duration of human gestation and labour. *Lancet.* 1973;2:1159-1161.
12. Rudolph AM. Effects of aspirin and acetaminophen in pregnancy and in the newborn. *Arch Intern Med.* 1981;141:358-363.
13. Stuart MJ, Gross SJ, Elrad H, Graeber JE. Effects of acetylsalicylic-acid ingestion on maternal and neonatal hemostasis. *N Engl J Med.* 1982;307:909-912.
14. Stuart MJ. Aspirin and maternal or neonatal hemostasis. *N Engl J Med.* 1983;308:281.
15. Niebyl JR, Blake DA, Burnett LS, King TM. The influence of aspirin on the course of induced midtrimester abortion. *Am J Obstet Gynecol.* 1976;124:607-610.
16. Castellanos JM, Aranda M, Cararach J, Cararach V. Effect of aspirin on oestriol excretion in pregnancy. *Lancet.* 1975;1:859.
17. Babenerd VJ, Kyriakidis K. Acetylsalicylic acid in the prevention of premature delivery. *Fortschr Med.* 1979;97:463-466.
18. Wolff F, Bolte A, Berg R. Does an additional administration of acetylsalicylic acid reduce the requirement of betamimetics in tocolytic treatment? *Geburtshilfe Frauenheilkd.* 1981;41:293-296.
19. Wolff F, Berg R, Bolte A. Clinical study of the labour inhibiting effects and side effects of acetylsalicylic acid (ASA). *Geburtshilfe Frauenheilkd.* 1981;41:96-100.
20. Buhler M, Papiernik E. Successive pregnancies in women fitted with intrauterine devices who take antiinflammatory drugs. *Lancet.* 1983;1:483.
21. Goodlin RC. Correction of pregnancy-related thrombocytopenia with aspirin without improvement in fetal outcome. *Am J Obstet Gynecol.* 1983;146:862-864.
22. Gant NF. Lupus erythematosus, the lupus anticoagulant, and the anticardiolipin antibody. Supplement No. 6, May/June 1986, to Pritchard JA, MacDonald PC, Gant NF. *Williams Obstetrics.* 17th ed. Appleton-Century-Crofts; 1985.
23. Branch DW, Scott JR, Kochenour NK, Hershgold E. Obstetric complications associated with the lupus anticoagulant. *N Engl J Med.* 1985;313:1322-1326.
24. Elder MG, DeSwiet M, Robertson A, et al. Low-dose aspirin in pregnancy. *Lancet.* 1988;1:410.
25. Lockshin MD, Druzin ML, Qamar T. Prednisone does not prevent recurrent fetal death in women with antiphospholipid antibody. *Am J Obstet Gynecol.* 1989;160:439-443.
26. Beaufils M, Uzan S, Donsimoni R, Colau JC. Prevention of pre-eclampsia by early antiplatelet therapy. *Lancet.* 1985;1:840-842.
27. Beaufils M, Uzan S, Donsimoni R, Colau JC. Prospective controlled study of early antiplatelet therapy in prevention of preeclampsia. *Adv Nephrol.* 1986;15:87-94.
28. Ylikorkala O, Makila U-M, Kaapa P, Viinikka L. Maternal ingestion of acetylsalicylic acid inhibits fetal and neonatal prostacyclin and thromboxane in humans. *Am J Obstet Gynecol.* 1986;155:345-349.
29. Spitz B, Magness RR, Cox SM, et al. Low-dose aspirin. I. Effect on angiotensin II pressor responses and blood prostaglandin concentrations in pregnant women sensitive to angiotensin II. *Am J Obstet Gynecol.* 1988;159:1035-1043.
30. Wallenburg HCS, Rotmans N. Prevention of recurrent idiopathic fetal growth retardation by low-dose aspirin and dipyridamole. *Am J Obstet Gynecol.* 1987;157:1230-1235.
31. Wallenburg HCS, Rotmans N. Prophylactic low-dose aspirin and dipyridamole in pregnancy. *Lancet.* 1988;1:939.
32. Uzan S, Beaufils M, Bazin B, Danays T. Idiopathic recurrent fetal growth retardation and aspirin-dipyridamole therapy. *Am J Obstet Gynecol.* 1989;160:763.
33. Wallenburg HCS, Rotmans N. Idiopathic recurrent fetal growth retardation and aspirin-dipyridamole therapy. Reply. *Am J Obstet Gynecol.* 1989;160:763-764.
34. Sibai BM, Mirro R, Chesney CM, Leffler C. Low-dose aspirin in pregnancy. *Obstet Gynecol.* 1989;74:551-557.
35. Trudinger B, Cook CM, Thompson R, et al. Low-dose aspirin improves fetal weight in umbilical placental insufficiency. *Lancet.* 1988;2:214-215.
36. Romero R, Lockwood C, Oyarzun E, Hobbins JC. Toxemia: new concepts in an old disease. *Semin Perinatol.* 1988;12:302-323.
37. Lubbe WF. Low-dose aspirin in prevention of toxaemia of pregnancy. Does it have a place? *Drugs.* 1987;34:515-518.
38. Wallenburg HCS, Dekker GA, Makovitz JW, Rotmans P. Low-dose aspirin prevents pregnancy-induced hypertension and pre-eclampsia in angiotensin-sensitive primigravidae. *Lancet.* 1986;1:1-3.
39. Benigni A, Gregorini G, Frusca T, et al. Effect of low-dose aspirin on fetal and maternal generation of thromboxane by platelets in women at risk for pregnancy-induced hypertension. *N Engl J Med.* 1989;321:357-362.
40. Schiff E, Peleg E, Goldenberg M, et al. The use of aspirin to prevent pregnancy-induced hypertension and lower the ratio of thromboxane A_2 to prostacyclin in relatively high risk pregnancies. *N Engl J Med.* 1989;321:351-356.
41. Turner G, Collins E. Fetal effects of regular salicylate ingestion in pregnancy. *Lancet.* 1975;2:338-339.
42. Earle R Jr. Congenital salicylate intoxication-report of a case. *N Engl J Med.* 1961;265:1003-1004.
43. Lynd PA, Andreasen AC, Wyatt RJ. Intrauterine salicylate intoxication in a newborn. A case report. *Clin Pediatr (Phila).* 1976;15:912-913.
44. Shapiro S, Monson RR, Kaufman DW, et al. Perinatal mortality and birthweight in relation to aspirin taken during pregnancy. *Lancet.* 1976;1:1375-1376.
45. Arcilla RA, Thilenius OG, Ranniger K. Congestive heart failure from suspected ductal closure in utero. *J Pediatr.* 1969;75:74-78.
46. Collins E. Maternal and fetal effects of acetaminophen and salicylates in pregnancy. *Obstet Gynecol.* 1981;58(suppl):57S-62S.
47. Aterman K, Holzbecker M, Ellenberger HA. Salicylate levels in a stillborn infant born to a drug-addicted mother, with comments on pathology and analytical methodology. *Clin Toxicol.* 1980;16:263-268.
48. Van Marter LJ, Leviton A, Allred EN, et al. Persistent pulmonary hypertension of the newborn and smoking and aspirin and nonsteroidal antiinflammatory drug consumption during pregnancy. *Pediatrics.* 1996;97:658-663.
49. Alano MA, Ngougmna E, Ostrea EM Jr, Konduri GG. Analysis of nonsteroidal antiinflammatory drugs in meconium and its relation to persistent pulmonary hypertension of the newborn. *Pediatrics.* 2001;107:519-523.
50. Bleyer WA, Breckenridge RJ. Studies on the detection of adverse drug reactions in the newborn. II. The effects of prenatal aspirin on newborn hemostasis. *JAMA.* 1970;213:2049-2053.
51. Corby DG, Schulman I. The effects of antenatal drug administration on aggregation of platelets of newborn infants. *J Pediatr.* 1971;79:307-313.
52. Casteels-Van Daele M, Eggermont E, de Gaetano G, Vermijlen J. More on the effects of antenatally administered aspirin on aggregation of platelets of neonates. *J Pediatr.* 1972;80:685-686.
53. Haslam RR, Ekert H, Gillam GL. Hemorrhage in a neonate possible due to maternal ingestion of salicylate. *J Pediatr.* 1974;84:556-557.
54. Ekert H, Haslam RR. Maternal ingested salicylate as a cause of neonatal hemorrhage. Reply. *J Pediatr.* 1974;85:738.
55. Pearson H. Comparative effects of aspirin and acetaminophen on hemostasis. *Pediatrics.* 1978;62(suppl):926-929.

56. Haslam RR. Neonatal purpura secondary to maternal salicylism. *J Pediatr.* 1975;86:653.
57. O'Brien JR. Effects of salicylates on human platelets. *Lancet.* 1968;1:779-783.
58. Weiss HJ, Aledort ML, Shaul I. The effect of salicylates on the haemostatic properties of platelets in man. *J Clin Invest.* 1968;47:2169-2180.
59. Bleyer WA. Maternal ingested salicylates as a cause of neonatal hemorrhage. *J Pediatr.* 1974;85:736-737.
60. Rumack CM, Guggenheim MA, Rumack BH, et al. Neonatal intracranial hemorrhage and maternal use of aspirin. *Obstet Gynecol.* 1981;58(suppl):52S-56S.
61. Soller RW, Stander H. Maternal drug exposure and perinatal intracranial hemorrhage. *Obstet Gynecol.* 1981;58:735-737.
62. Corby DG. Editorial comment. *Obstet Gynecol.* 1981;58:737-740.
63. Levy G, Procknal JA, Garrettson LK. Distribution of salicylate between neonatal and maternal serum at diffusion equilibrium. *Clin Pharmacol Ther.* 1975;18:210-214.
64. Levy G, Garrettson LK. Kinetics of salicylate elimination by newborn infants of mothers who ingested aspirin before delivery. *Pediatrics.* 1974;53:201-210.
65. Garrettson LK, Procknal JA, Levy G. Fetal acquisition and neonatal elimination of a large amount of salicylate. Study of a neonate whose mother regularly took therapeutic doses of aspirin during pregnancy. *Clin Pharmacol Ther.* 1975;17:98-103.
66. Li DK, Liu L, Odouli R. Exposure to non-steroidal anti-inflammatory drugs during pregnancy and risk of miscarriage: population based cohort study. *BMJ.* 2003;327:368-371.
67. Richards ID. Congenital malformations and environmental influences in pregnancy. *Br J Prev Soc Med.* 1969;23:218-225.
68. Nelson MM, Forfar JO. Associations between drugs administered during pregnancy and congenital abnormalities of the fetus. *Br Med J.* 1971;1:523-527.
69. Saxen I. Associations between oral clefts and drugs during pregnancy. *Int J Epidemiol.* 1975;4:37-44.
70. Benawra R, Mangurten HH, Duffell DR. Cyclopia and other anomalies following maternal ingestion of salicylates. *J Pediatr.* 1980;96:1069-1071.
71. McNiel JR. The possible effect of salicylates on the developing fetus. Brief summaries of eight suggestive cases. *Clin Pediatr (Phila).* 1973;12:347-350.
72. Sayli BS, Asmaz A, Yemisci B. Consanguinity, aspirin, and phocomelia. *Lancet.* 1966;1:876.
73. Zierler S, Rothman KJ. Congenital heart disease in relation to maternal use of Bendectin and other drugs in early pregnancy. *N Engl J Med.* 1985;313:347-352.
74. Rothman KJ, Fyler DC, Goldblatt A, Kreidberg MB. Exogenous hormones and other drug exposures of children with congenital heart disease. *Am J Epidemiol.* 1979;109:433-439.
75. Zierler S. Maternal drugs and congenital heart disease. *Obstet Gynecol.* 1985;65:155-165.
76. Werler MM, Mitchell AA, Shapiro S. The relation of aspirin use during the first trimester of pregnancy to congenital cardiac defects. *N Engl J Med.* 1989;321:1639-1642.
77. Kallen BAJ, Olausson PO. Maternal drug use in early pregnancy and infant cardiovascular defect. *Reprod Toxicol.* 2003;17:255-261.
78. Torfs CP, Katz EA, Bateson TF, et al. Maternal medications and environmental exposures as risk factors for gastroschisis. *Teratology.* 1996;54:84-92.
79. Streissguth AP, Treder RP, Barr HM, et al. Aspirin and acetaminophen use by pregnant women and subsequent child IQ and attention decrements. *Teratology.* 1987;35:211-219.
80. Klebanoff MA, Berendes HW. Aspirin exposure during the first 20 weeks of gestation and IQ at four years of age. *Teratology.* 1988;37:249-255.
81. Matt DW, Borzelleca JF. Toxic effects on the female reproductive system during pregnancy, parturition, and lactation. In: Witorsch RJ, ed. *Reproductive Toxicology.* 2nd ed. Raven Press, 1995:175-193.
82. Daewood MY. Nonsteroidal antiinflammatory drugs and reproduction. *Am J Obstet Gynecol.* 1993;169:1255-1265.
83. Hernandez RK, Werler MM, Romitti P, et al; National Birth Defects Prevention Study. Nonsteroidal antiinflammatory drug use among women and the risk of birth defects. *Am J Obstet Gynecol.* 2012;206:228.e1-228.e8.
84. Kwit NT, Hatcher RA. Excretion of drugs in milk. *Am J Dis Child.* 1935;49:900-904.
85. Erickson SH, Oppenheim GL. Aspirin in breast milk. *J Fam Pract.* 1979;8:189-190.
86. Weibert RT, Bailey DN. Salicylate excretion in human breast milk (abstract no. 7). Presented at: The 1979 Seminar of the California Society of Hospital Pharmacists; October 13, 1979; Los Angeles, CA.
87. Findlay JWA, DeAngelis RL, Kearney MF, et al. Analgesic drugs in breast milk and plasma. *Clin Pharmacol Ther.* 1981;29:625-633.
88. Anderson PO. Drugs and breast feeding-a review. *Drug Intell Clin Pharm.* 1977;11:208-223.
89. Clark JH, Wilson WG. A 16-day-old breast-fed infant with metabolic acidosis caused by salicylate. *Clin Pediatr (Phila).* 1981;20:53-54.

ATAZANAVIR

Antiretroviral (Protease Inhibitor—HIV-1)

PREGNANCY RECOMMENDATION: Human Data Suggest Low Risk (Maternal Benefit May Outweigh Any Embryofetal Risk)

BREASTFEEDING RECOMMENDATION: *Contraindicated

PREGNANCY SUMMARY

Interim data from the APR (through January 31, 2024) showed that there were 37 (2.5%) major birth anomalies in 1,485 first-trimester pregnancy exposures. In a second, smaller study, there were 2 (2.2%) major malformations in 89 exposures that occurred at the time of conception. The drug crosses the placenta, so fetal exposure will occur. Animal data did show some embryofetal toxicity in one species at doses of less than 10 times the RHD based on AUC. No embryofetal toxicity was seen in a second species at doses of less than 10 times the RHD. In order to decrease the perinatal transmission of HIV-1 to the neonate, this drug should not be withheld if a pregnant woman is infected with HIV-1 with a positive viral load who is failing her current treatment regimen and is a candidate for this drug's usage. The drug has been associated with prolonging the cardiac PR interval. There is a pregnancy exposure registry that monitors pregnancy outcomes in patients using antiretroviral medicines during pregnancy. Health care providers are encouraged to call the APR at 1-800-258-4263.

BREASTFEEDING SUMMARY

Atazanavir was evaluated in three lactating women. The drug was found in breast milk at a median peak level of about 0.42 mcg/mL. The calculated RID would be about 1.5%. *However, the current CDC recommendation is that mothers infected with HIV should not breastfeed their infants in order to reduce the risk of postnatal transmission of the virus to the neonate.

In a clinical setting where a mother is not infected with HIV (or in cases where the HIV viral load is negative), the drug by itself is probably compatible.

References

1. Prescribing Information. Atazanavir sulfate. Teva Pharmaceuticals; 2017.
2. Antiretroviral Pregnancy Registry Steering Committee. Antiretroviral Pregnancy Registry international interim report for 1 January 1989 through 31 July 2009. Registry Coordinating Center. Published 2009. Accessed May 29, 2010. www.apregistry.com
3. Centers for Disease Control. Public Health Service Task Force recommendations for the use of antiretroviral drugs in pregnant women infected with HIV-1 for maternal health and for reducing perinatal HIV-1 transmission in the United States. *MMWR Recomm Rep*. 1998;47(RR-2):1-30.
4. Fassett M, Kramer F, Stek A. Treatment with protease inhibitors in pregnancy is not associated with an increased incidence of gestational diabetes (abstract). *Am J Obstet Gynecol*. 2000;182:S97.
5. Carpenter CCJ, Fischi MA, Hammer SM, et al. Antiretroviral therapy for HIV infection in 1996. *JAMA*. 1996;276:146-154.
6. Minkoff H, Augenbraun M. Antiretroviral therapy for pregnant women. *Am J Obstet Gynecol*. 1997;176:478-489.
7. Minkoff H. Human immunodeficiency virus infection in pregnancy. *Obstet Gynecol*. 2003;101:797-810.
8. Panel on Treatment of HIV During Pregnancy and Prevention of Perinatal Transmission. Recommendations for the use of antiretroviral drugs during pregnancy and interventions to reduce perinatal HIV transmission in the United States. *Department of Health and Human Services*. Accessed July 25, 2023. https://clinicalinfo.hiv.gov/en/guidelines/perinatal.
9. Williams PL, Crain MJ, Yildirim C, et al. Congenital anomalies and in utero antiretroviral exposure in human immunodeficiency virus-exposed uninfected infants. *JAMA Pediatr*. 2015;169:48-55.
10. Rice ML, Zeldow B, Siberry GK, et al; Pediatric HIV/AIDS cohort study (PHACS). Evaluation of risk for late language emergence after in utero antiretroviral drug exposure in HIV-exposed uninfected infants. *Pediatr Infect Dis J*. 2013;32:e406-e413.
11. Sirois PA, Huo Y, Williams PL, et al. Safety of perinatal exposure to antiretroviral medications: developmental outcomes in infants. *Pediatr Infect Dis J*. 2013;32:648-655.
12. Himes SK, Huo Y, Siberry GK, et al. Meconium atazanavir concentrations and early language outcomes in HIV-exposed uninfected infants with prenatal atazanavir exposure. *J Acquir Immune Defic Syndr*. 2015;69:178-186.
13. Samuel M, Bradshaw D, Perry M, et al. Antenatal atazanavir: a retrospective analysis of pregnancies exposed to atazanavir. *Infect Dis Obstet Gynecol*. 2014;2014:1-7.
14. Eley T, Bertz R, Hardy H, Burger D. Atazanavir pharmacokinetics, efficacy and safety in pregnancy: a systematic review. *Antiviral Ther*. 2013;18:361-375.
15. Else LJ, Jackson V, Brennan M, et al. Therapeutic drug monitoring of atazanavir/ritonavir in pregnancy. *HIV Med*. 2014;15:604-610.
16. Brown ZA, Watts DH. Antiviral therapy in pregnancy. *Clin Obstet Gynecol*. 1990;33:276-289.
17. De Martino M, Tovo P-A, Pezzotti P, et al. HIV-1 transmission through breast-milk: appraisal of risk according to duration of feeding. *AIDS*. 1992;6:991-997.
18. Van de Perre P. Postnatal transmission of human immunodeficiency virus type 1: the breast feeding dilemma. *Am J Obstet Gynecol*. 1995;173:483-487.

ATENOLOL

Autonomic (β_1-Adrenergic Blocker)

PREGNANCY RECOMMENDATION: Human Data Suggest Potential Risk (Second and Third Trimesters)

BREASTFEEDING RECOMMENDATION: Potential Toxicity

PREGNANCY SUMMARY

Numerous studies have been located that describe the use of atenolol during human pregnancy. Nearly all of them report the use of the drug in relation to pregnancy outcome, especially fetal growth and placental weight. From the MMSS, a total of 9 (8.6%) major anomalies were described in 105 first-trimester exposures. All of the defects varied except for a possible elevated risk for hypospadias. In many studies, birth weights at delivery were smaller when compared to other antihypertensive drugs used in treating hypertension during pregnancy, including other β-blockers. In several publications, smaller placental sizes were also seen when compared with other antihypertensive drug exposures for treating hypertension. Again, this was also true when compared with other β-blockers. An interesting concept that has not been fully studied is the use of atenolol in patients with hypertension primarily caused by vasoconstriction versus increased cardiac output. These outcomes may be different if only used in patients with increased cardiac output and not in vasoconstriction related hypertension. The drug crosses the placenta, so fetal exposure will occur. Therefore, this limited first-trimester human pregnancy experience prevents a complete assessment of the embryofetal risk. Animal data did not show any embryofetal toxicity in one species at doses of less than 10 times the RHD. Using this drug during pregnancy should be based on the pros and cons of the mother's clinical need for treatment versus any potential fetal risk that might occur from exposure.

BREASTFEEDING SUMMARY

Several studies have been located that describe the use of atenolol during human lactation. From these reports, a total of more than 60 women had their breast milk analyzed. The drug was found in nearly every sample ranging from 25 ng/mL to 2.1 mcg/mL. The calculated RIDs ranged from about 3% up to a high of about 35%. Atenolol was also analyzed in an infant's blood in 17 cases. In 13 infants, the drug was not detected (LLQ of about 10 ng/mL). In the remaining four infants, drug levels ranged from about 116 ng/mL up to 2 mcg/mL (seen 48 hours after the last nursing). In one case, the drug level in the infant was about 19% of the maternal level. Infants exposed to β-blockers can have an increased risk of decreased heart rate and hypoglycemia. Breastfeeding while using this drug should be based on the mother's clinical need for treatment versus any potential infant risks that might occur. If used, the infant should be monitored for the most common reported adult side effects of nausea, dizziness, headache, and blurred vision (all leading to irritability), diarrhea, fatigue (lethargy), and rash. Because of the wide variation in the amount of drug found in breast milk along with infant blood levels, other β_1 selective blockers might be indicated.

References

1. Prescribing Information. Tenormin. AstraZeneca Pharmaceuticals; 2017.
2. Speiser Z, Gordon I, Rehavi M, Gitter S. Behavioral and biochemical studies in rats following prenatal treatment with β-adrenoceptor antagonists. *Eur J Pharmacol.* 1991;195:75-83.
3. Tabacova SA, Kimmel CA, Wall K, McCloskey CA. Animal-human concordance in the developmental toxicity of two antihypertensive agents (abstract). *Teratology.* 2002;65:304.
4. Melander A, Niklasson B, Ingemarsson I, et al. Transplacental passage of atenolol in man. *Eur J Clin Pharmacol.* 1978;14:93-94.
5. Woods DL, Morrell DF. Atenolol: side effects in a newborn infant. *Br Med J.* 1982;285:691-692.
6. Liedholm H. Transplacental passage and breast milk accumulation of atenolol in humans. *Drugs.* 1983;25(suppl 2):217-218.
7. Lardoux H, Gerard J, Blazquez G, et al. Hypertension in pregnancy: evaluation of two beta blockers atenolol and labetalol. *Eur Heart J.* 1983;4(suppl G):35-40.
8. Thorley KJ. Pharmacokinetics of atenolol in pregnancy and lactation. *Drugs.* 1983;25(suppl 2):216-217.
9. Boutroy MJ. Fetal and neonatal effects of the beta-adrenoceptor blocking agents. *Dev Pharmacol Ther.* 1987;10:224-231.
10. Fowler MB, Brudenell M, Jackson G, Holt DW. Essential hypertension and pregnancy: successful outcome with atenolol. *Br J Clin Pract.* 1984;38:73-74.
11. Hurst AK, Shotan A, Hoffman K, et al. Pharmacokinetic and pharmacodynamic evaluation of atenolol during and after pregnancy. *Pharmacotherapy.* 1998;18:840-846.
12. Schneider H, Proegler M. Placental transfer of B-adrenergic antagonists studied in an in vitro perfusion system of human placental tissue. *Am J Obstet Gynecol.* 1988;159:42-47.
13. Satge D, Sasco AJ, Col JY, et al. Antenatal exposure to atenolol and retroperitoneal fibromatosis (abstract). *Teratology.* 1997;55:103.
14. Satge D, Sasco AJ, Col J-Y, et al. Antenatal exposure to atenolol and retroperitoneal fibromatosis. *Reprod Toxicol.* 1997;11:539-541.
15. Thorley KJ, McAinsh J, Cruickshank JM. Atenolol in the treatment of pregnancy-induced hypertension. *Br J Clin Pharmacol.* 1981;12:725-730.
16. Rubin PC, Butters L, Low RA, Reid JL. Atenolol in the treatment of essential hypertension during pregnancy. *Br J Clin Pharmacol.* 1982;14:279-281.
17. Liedholm H. Atenolol in the treatment of hypertension of pregnancy. *Drugs.* 1983;25(suppl 2):206-211.
18. Rubin PC, Butters L, Clark DM, et al. Placebo-controlled trial of atenolol in treatment of pregnancy-associated hypertension. *Lancet.* 1983;1:431-434.
19. Rubin PC, Butters L, Low RA, et al. Atenolol in the management of hypertension during pregnancy. *Drugs.* 1983;25(suppl 2):212-214.
20. Fabregues G, Alvarez L, Varas Juri P, et al. Effectiveness of atenolol in the treatment of hypertension during pregnancy. *Hypertension.* 1992;19(suppl II):II129-II131.
21. Frishman WH, Chesner M. Beta-adrenergic blockers in pregnancy. *Am Heart J.* 1988;115:147-152.
22. Dubois D, Petitcolas J, Temperville B, Klepper A. Beta blockers and high-risk pregnancies. *Int J Biol Res Pregnancy.* 1980;1:141-145.
23. Dubois D, Petitcolas J, Temperville B, et al. Treatment of hypertension in pregnancy with β-adrenoceptor antagonists. *Br J Clin Pharmacol.* 1982; 13(suppl):375S-378S.
24. Dubois D, Peticolas J, Temperville B, Klepper A. Treatment with atenolol of hypertension in pregnancy. *Drugs.* 1983;25(suppl 2):215-218.
25. Butters L, Kennedy S, Rubin PC. Atenolol in essential hypertension during pregnancy. *BMJ.* 1990;301:587-589.
26. Montan S, Ingemarsson I, Marsal K, Sjoberg N-O. Randomized controlled trial of atenolol and pindolol in human pregnancy: effects on fetal haemodynamics. *BMJ.* 1992;304:946-949.
27. Lip GYH, Beevers M, Churchill D, et al. Effect of atenolol on birth weight. *Am J Cardiol.* 1997;79:1436-1438.
28. Lydakis C, Lip GYH, Beevers M, Beevers DG. Atenolol and fetal growth in pregnancies complicated by hypertension. *Am J Hypertens.* 1999;12: 541-547.
29. Tuimala R, Hartikainen-Sorri A-L. Randomized comparison of atenolol and pindolol for treatment of hypertension in pregnancy. *Curr Ther Res.* 1988;44:579-584.
30. Montan S, Liedholm H, Lingman G, et al. Fetal and uteroplacental haemodynamics during short-term atenolol treatment of hypertension in pregnancy. *Br J Obstet Gynaecol.* 1987;94:312-317.
31. Rubin PC. Beta blockers in pregnancy. *Br J Obstet Gynaecol.* 1987;94: 292-293.
32. Rasanen J, Jouppila P. Uterine and fetal hemodynamics and fetal cardiac function after atenolol and pindolol infusion. A randomized study. *Eur J Obstet Gynecol Reprod Biol.* 1995;62:195-201.
33. Jouppila P, Rasanen J, Alahuhta S, Jouppila R. Vasoactive drugs in obstetrics: a review of data obtained by Doppler and color Doppler methods. *Hyperten Pregnancy.* 1995;14:261-275.
34. Easterling TR, Brateng D, Schmucker B, et al. Prevention of preeclampsia: a randomized trial of atenolol in hyperdynamic patients before onset of hypertension. *Obstet Gynecol.* 1999;93:725-733.
35. Easterling TR, Carr DB, Brateng D, et al. Treatment of hypertension in pregnancy: effect of atenolol on maternal disease, preterm delivery, and fetal growth. *Obstet Gynecol.* 2001;98:427-433.
36. Al Kasab SM, Sabag T, Al Zaibag M, et al. β-Adrenergic receptor blockade in the management of pregnant women with mitral stenosis. *Am J Obstet Gynecol.* 1990;163:37-40.
37. Soderlin MK, Purhonen S, Haring P, et al. Myocardial infarction in a parturient. *Anaesthesia.* 1994;49:870-872.
38. Lubbe WF. More on beta-blockers in pregnancy. *N Engl J Med.* 1982;307:753.
39. Knott PD, Thorpe SS, Lamont CA. Congenital renal dysgenesis possibly due to captopril. *Lancet.* 1989;1:451.
40. Mehta N, Modi N. ACE inhibitors in pregnancy. *Lancet.* 1989;2:96.
41. Smith AM. Are ACE inhibitors safe in pregnancy? *Lancet.* 1989;2:750-751.
42. Briggs GG, Nageotte MP. Fatal fetal outcome with the combined use of valsartan and atenolol. *Ann Pharmacother.* 2001;35:859-861.
43. Ingemarsson I, Liedholm H, Montan S, et al. Fetal heart rate during treatment of maternal hypertension with beta-adrenergic antagonists. *Acta Obstet Gynecol Scand.* 1984;118(suppl):95-97.
44. Rubin PC, Butters L, Clark D, et al. Obstetric aspects of the use in pregnancy-associated hypertension of the B-adrenoceptor antagonist atenolol. *Am J Obstet Gynecol.* 1984;150:389-392.
45. Bakri YN, Ingemansson SE, Ali A, Parikh S. Pheochromocytoma and pregnancy: report of three cases. *Acta Obstet Gynecol Scand.* 1992;71:301-304.
46. Pickrell MD, Sawers R, Michael J. Pregnancy after renal transplantation: severe intrauterine growth retardation during treatment with cyclosporin A. *BMJ.* 1988;296:825.
47. Tabacova SA, Kimmel CA. Atenolol: pharmacokinetic/dynamic aspects of comparative developmental toxicity. *Reprod Toxicol.* 2002;16:1-7.
48. Sibai BM. Chronic hypertension in pregnancy. In reply. *Obstet Gynecol.* 2002;100:1358-1359.
49. Reynolds B, Butters L, Evans J, et al. First year of life after the use of atenolol in pregnancy associated hypertension. *Arch Dis Child.* 1984;59:1061-1063.
50. Liedholm H, Melander A, Bitzen PO, et al. Accumulation of atenolol and metoprolol in human breast milk. *Eur J Clin Pharmacol.* 1981;20:229-231.
51. Kulas J, Lunell NO, Rosing U, et al. Atenolol and metoprolol. A comparison of their excretion into human breast milk. *Acta Obstet Gynecol Scand.* 1984;118(suppl):65-69.
52. White WB, Andreoli JW, Wong SH, Cohn RD. Atenolol in human plasma and breast milk. *Obstet Gynecol.* 1984;63:42S-44S.
53. White WB. Management of hypertension during lactation. *Hypertension.* 1984;6:297-300.
54. Eyal S, Kim JD, Anderson GD, et al. Atenolol pharmacokinetics and excretion in breast milk during the first 6 to 8 months postpartum. *J Clin Pharmacol.* 2010;50:1301-1309.
55. Schmimmel MS, Eidelman AJ, Wilschanski MA, et al. Toxic effects of atenolol consumed during breast feeding. *J Pediatr.* 1989;114:476-478.
56. Diamond JM. Toxic effects of atenolol consumed during breast feeding. *J Pediatr.* 1989;115:336.
57. Koren G. Toxic effects of atenolol consumed during breast feeding. *J Pediatr.* 1989;115:336-337.
58. Anderson PO. Drugs and breast milk. *Pediatrics.* 1995;95:957.
59. American Academy of Pediatrics Committee on Drugs. The transfer of drugs and other chemicals into human milk. *Pediatrics.* 2001;108:776-789.

ATEZOLIZUMAB

Antineoplastic (Programmed Cell Death Ligand 1 Blocking Monoclonal Antibody)

PREGNANCY RECOMMENDATION: No Human Data and No Relevant Animal Data

BREASTFEEDING RECOMMENDATION: Probably Compatible

PREGNANCY SUMMARY

No reports describing the use of atezolizumab during human pregnancy have been located. As an IgG antibody, it likely crosses the placenta, especially during the second half of pregnancy, so some fetal exposure will probably occur. However, the absence of human pregnancy experience prevents a complete assessment of the embryofetal risk. No animal reproduction studies have been conducted. Regarding reproduction, the main function of the programmed cell death ligand 1 (PD-L1)/programmed cell death receptor 1 (PD-1) pathway is to preserve pregnancy by maintaining maternal immune tolerance to a fetus. In the mouse model, blocking this signal during pregnancy resulted in an increase in fetal loss. Based on the drug's mechanism of action, the manufacturer recommends that women with reproductive potential use effective contraception during treatment and for 5 months after the last dose. Nevertheless, using this drug during pregnancy should be based on the pros and cons of the mother's clinical need for treatment versus any potential fetal risk that might occur from exposure. There is a registry for women who are pregnant and have cancer. For more information, women and health care providers are encouraged to contact the Cancer and Pregnancy Registry at 1-877-635-4499.

BREASTFEEDING SUMMARY

No reports describing the use of atezolizumab during human lactation have been located. It is known that IgG antibodies can be found in human breast milk, but are not found in the neonatal or infant circulation. Additionally, if any IgG antibodies were to be ingested through breastfeeding, they would probably be digested in the infant's gastrointestinal tract and not be absorbed. Regardless, based on the drug's mechanism of action and the concern for potential serious adverse effects that might be seen in a breastfed infant, the manufacturer recommends that women not breastfeed while being treated with this drug and for at least 5 months after the last dose. Nevertheless, breastfeeding while using this drug should be based on the mother's clinical need for treatment versus any potential infant risks that might occur. If used, the infant should be monitored for the most common reported adult side effects of nausea (leading to irritability), diarrhea, lethargy, alopecia, constipation, decreased appetite, cough, and various laboratory abnormalities (see PI).

Reference

1. Prescribing Information. Tecentriq. Genentech; 2021.

ATOGEPANT

Central Nervous System (Calcitonin Gene-Related Peptide Receptor Antagonist)

PREGNANCY RECOMMENDATION: No Human Data—Animal Data Suggest Potential Risk

BREASTFEEDING RECOMMENDATION: Potential Toxicity

PREGNANCY SUMMARY

No reports describing the use of atogepant in human pregnancy have been located. Atogepant is likely to cross the placenta, so some fetal exposure will probably occur. Therefore, the absence of human pregnancy experience prevents a complete assessment of embryofetal risk. Animal data did show some embryofetal toxicity. Using this drug during pregnancy should be based on the pros and cons of the mother's clinical need for treatment versus any potential fetal risk that might occur from exposure. In pregnant rats, calcitonin gene-related peptide (CGRP), a potent vasodilator, leads to dilation of the uterine artery. Therefore, the impact of administering a CGRP antagonist on uterine blood flow is unknown. If the drug is used in the latter half of pregnancy, fetal activity and growth can be monitored.

BREASTFEEDING SUMMARY

No reports describing the use of atogepant during human lactation have been located. The drug probably enters breast milk, so some infant exposure will probably occur. The manufacturer recommends that the developmental and health benefits of breastfeeding be considered along with the mother's clinical need for treatment with atogepant. If used while breastfeeding, the infant should be monitored for the most common reported adult side effects of nausea (leading to irritability), constipation, and lethargy.

References

1. Prescribing Information. Qulipta. AbbVie; 2021.
2. Gangula PRR, Thota C, Wimalawansa SJ, et al. Mechanisms involved in calcitonin gene-related peptide-induced relaxation in pregnant rat uterine artery. *Biol Reprod*. 2003;69:1635-1641.

ATOLTIVIMAB/MAFTIVIMAB/ODESIVIMAB

Antiviral (Monoclonal Antibodies—Ebola)

PREGNANCY RECOMMENDATION: No Human Data and No Relevant Animal Data

BREASTFEEDING RECOMMENDATION: *Contraindicated

PREGNANCY SUMMARY

Two studies that total 382 adult and pediatric patients infected with Zaire ebolavirus and administered atoltivimab, maftivimab, and odesivimab have been reported. A few pregnant women were included in both studies. However, specific information for the pregnancy population subset regarding birth anomalies, pregnancy loss, and adverse maternal/fetal outcomes was not supplied because of the high mortality rate associated with this infection. Because these are antibodies of the IgG class, they probably cross the placenta. Animal studies have not been performed. If a pregnant woman were to be infected with the Zaire ebolavirus, treatment should not be withheld.

BREASTFEEDING SUMMARY

Atoltivimab, maftivimab, and odesivimab probably enter breast milk. However, it is known that IgG antibodies can be found in human breast milk, but are not found in neonatal or infant circulation. Additionally, if any IgG antibodies were to be ingested through breastfeeding, they would probably be digested in the infant's gastrointestinal tract and not be absorbed. *Nevertheless, the current CDC recommendation is that mothers should not breastfeed their infants (with a confirmed infection of Zaire ebolavirus) in order to reduce the risk of postnatal transmission of the virus. The drug itself, outside of an Ebola virus infection, is probably compatible.

References

1. Prescribing Information. Inmazeb. Regeneron Pharmaceuticals Inc; 2020.
2. Mulangu S, Dodd LE, Davey RT Jr, et al. A randomized, controlled trial of Ebola virus disease therapeutics. *N Engl J Med*. 2019;381(24):2293-2303.

ATOMOXETINE

Mental Health (Selective Norepinephrine Reuptake Inhibitor)

PREGNANCY RECOMMENDATION: Limited Human Data—Animal Data Suggest Potential Risk

BREASTFEEDING RECOMMENDATION: Potential Toxicity

PREGNANCY SUMMARY

A few studies have evaluated drugs used in treating ADHD during pregnancy. In one study, 480 cases were compared with a population control and a higher rate of spontaneous abortion was seen, but the anomaly rate was no higher. However, specifics for atomoxetine were not provided. In a second study, 453 pregnant patients using atomoxetine did not have a higher rate for preeclampsia, placental abruption, growth restriction, and preterm birth when compared with a population control. The drug will likely cross the placenta, so some fetal exposure will probably occur. Therefore, the absence of first-trimester human pregnancy experience prevents a complete assessment of the embryofetal risk. Animal studies did show some embryofetal toxicity in one species at doses of less than 10 times the RHD, but this was not seen in a second species at doses of less than 10 times the RHD. Using this drug during pregnancy should be based on the pros and cons of the mother's clinical need for treatment versus any potential fetal risk that might occur from exposure.

BREASTFEEDING SUMMARY

No reports describing the use of atomoxetine during human lactation have been located. The manufacturer reported on two exposed infants who, by report, slept longer, but no other adverse effects were noted. Evaluation of breast milk levels for the drug was not performed. The drug will likely be found in human breast milk, so some infant exposure will likely occur. Breastfeeding while using this drug should be based on the mother's clinical need for treatment versus any potential infant risks that might occur. If used, the infant should be monitored for the most common reported adult side effects of nausea, dry mouth, and abdominal pain (all leading to irritability), fatigue (lethargy), vomiting, flushing, somnolence, and decreased appetite (monitor infant growth).

References

1. Prescribing Information. Strattera. Eli Lilly; 2019.
2. Heiligenstein J, Michelson D, Wernicke J, et al. Atomoxetine and pregnancy. *J Am Acad Child Adolesc Psychiatry*. 2003;42:884-885.
3. Haervig KB, Mortensen LH, Hansen AV, Strandberg-Larsen K. Use of ADHD medication during pregnancy from 1999 to 2010: a Danish register-based study. *Pharmacoepidem Drug Saf*. 2014;23:526-533.
4. Cohen JM, Hernandez-Diaz S, Bateman BT, et al. Placental complications associated with psychostimulant use in pregnancy. *Obstet Gynecol*. 2017;130:1192-1201.
5. Ornoy A. Pharmacological treatment of attention deficit hyperactivity disorder during pregnancy and lactation. *Pharm Res*. 2018;35:46. doi:10.1007/s11095-017-2323-z

ATORVASTATIN

Antilipemic (Statin)

PREGNANCY RECOMMENDATION: *Limited Human Data—Animal Data Suggest Potential Risk

BREASTFEEDING RECOMMENDATION: Potential Toxicity

PREGNANCY SUMMARY

Two studies that analyzed statin drug use in general described more than 1,200 first-trimester exposures. After adjusting for confounders, neither teratogenic effects nor organ-specific malformations were observed with statin use. However, the number of cases that used atorvastatin was small. Numerous case reports exist that describe newborns with first-trimester exposure resulting in some with normal outcomes and some with birth anomalies. However, no pattern has been seen, and these reports are often biased toward the reporting of poor outcomes. The drug will likely cross the placenta, so some fetal exposure will probably occur. Therefore, this limited human pregnancy experience prevents a complete assessment of embryofetal risk. Embryofetal toxicity was observed in one animal species at doses of less than 10 times the RHD. Cholesterol and other products of cholesterol biosynthesis are essential components for fetal development. Moreover, maternal cholesterol levels increase during pregnancy. Hyperlipidemia treatment is not generally necessary during pregnancy. Atherosclerosis is a chronic process, and stopping lipid-lowering therapy during pregnancy should have little impact on the outcome of long-term therapy of primary hyperlipidemia for most patients. *Based on the drug's mechanism of action, the manufacturer states that the use of atorvastatin is contraindicated during pregnancy. Nevertheless, using this drug during pregnancy (especially with cardiovascular disorders) should be based on the pros and cons of the mother's clinical need for treatment versus any potential fetal risk that might occur from exposure.

BREASTFEEDING SUMMARY

One study was located that describe the use of atorvastatin during human lactation. Three lactating women were administered 20, 40, and 80 mg doses of atorvastatin and the absolute infant levels were about 0.07, 0.19, and 0.27 mcg/kg/d. The calculated RIDs were all well below 1%. Due to a concern for potential serious adverse effects that might be seen in a breastfed infant, the manufacturer recommends that women not breastfeed while being treated with this drug. However, breastfeeding while using this drug should be based on the mother's clinical need for treatment versus any potential infant risks that might occur. If used, the infant should be monitored for the most common reported adult side effects of arthralgia, myalgia, and extremity pain (all leading to irritability), and diarrhea.

References

1. Prescribing Information. Lipitor. Parke-Davis Div of Pfizer; 2019.
2. Henck JW, Craft WR, Black A, et al. Pre- and postnatal toxicity of the HMG-CoA reductase inhibitor atorvastatin in rats. *Toxicol Sci*. 1998;41:88-99.
3. Dostal LA, Schardein JL, Anderson JA. Developmental toxicity of the HMG-CoA reductase inhibitor, atorvastatin, in rats and rabbits. *Teratology*. 1994;50:387-394.
4. Yaris F, Yaris E, Kadioglu M, et al. Normal pregnancy outcome following inadvertent exposure to rosiglitazone, gliclazide, and atorvastatin in a diabetic and hypertensive woman. *Reprod Toxicol*. 2004;18:619-621.
5. Edison RJ, Muenke M. Mechanistic and epidemiologic considerations in the evaluation of adverse birth outcomes following gestational exposure to statins. *Am J Med Genet A*. 2004;131:287-298.
6. Edison RJ, Muenke M. Gestational exposure to lovastatin followed by cardiac malformation misclassified as holoprosencephaly. *N Engl J Med*. 2005;352:2759.
7. McElhatton P. Preliminary data on exposure to statins during pregnancy (abstract). *Reprod Toxicol*. 2005;20:471-472.
8. Taguchi N, Rubin ET, Hosokawa A, et al. Prenatal exposure to HMG-CoA reductase inhibitors: effects on fetal and neonatal outcomes. *Reprod Toxicol*. 2008;26:175-177.
9. Bartels A, Egan N, Khashan A, et al. Maternal cholesterol levels are elevated throughout normal pregnancy (abstract). *Am J Obstet Gynecol*. 2011;240:S98-S99; Poster Session. S98.
10. Lecarpentier E, Morel O, Foumier T, et al. Statins and pregnancy: between supposed risks and theoretical benefits. *Drugs*. 2012;72:773-788.
11. Godfrey LM, Erramouspe J, Cleveland KW. Teratogenic risk of statins in pregnancy. *Ann Pharmacother*. 2012;46:1419-1424.

ATOVAQUONE

Anti-Infective (Antiprotozoal)

PREGNANCY RECOMMENDATION: Limited Human Data—Animal Data Suggest Potential Risk (Maternal Benefit May Outweigh Any Potential Embryofetal Risk)

BREASTFEEDING RECOMMENDATION: Potential Toxicity

PREGNANCY SUMMARY

Most of the studies reporting on the use of atovaquone during human pregnancy have been related to its use combined with proguanil (see atovaquone Proguanil). Use in the first trimester is limited. In addition, studies on the use of atovaquone in treating *Pneumocystis carinii* pneumonia during pregnancy were also not located. Use in treating malaria in the second and third trimesters has not shown an increased risk for adverse fetal effects. The drug will probably cross the placenta, so some fetal exposure will likely occur. Therefore, the absence of human pregnancy experience prevents a complete assessment of the embryofetal risk. Animal studies did not show any embryofetal toxicity or teratogenicity in one species at doses of less than 10 times the RHD. However, in a second species, embryofetal toxicity was seen at doses less than the RHD, but maternal toxicity was also present. Using this drug during pregnancy should be based on the pros and cons of the mother's clinical need for treatment versus any potential fetal risk that might occur from exposure. Because the maternal benefit appears to exceed any unknown embryofetal risk, atovaquone should probably not be withheld because of pregnancy.

BREASTFEEDING SUMMARY

No reports describing the use of atovaquone during human lactation have been located. Some amount of the drug will probably be found in human breast milk, so some infant exposure will likely occur. The severity of the mother's illness, such as infection with HIV, may preclude breastfeeding. Breastfeeding while using this drug should be based on the mother's clinical need for treatment versus any potential infant risks that might occur. If used, the infant should be monitored for the most common reported adult side effects of nausea, headache, pruritus, and abdominal pain (all leading to irritability), diarrhea, cough, and vomiting.

References

1. Rosenblatt JE. Antiparasitic agents. *Mayo Clin Proc*. 1999;74:1161-1175.
2. Irvine MH, Einarson A, Bozzo P. Prophylactic use of antimalarials during pregnancy. *Can Fam Physician*. 2011;57:1279-1281.
3. Proscribing Information. Mepron. GlaxoSmithKline; 2019.
4. McGready R, Stepniewska K, Edstein MD, et al. The pharmacokinetics of atovaquone and proguanil in pregnant women with acute falciparum malaria. *Eur J Clin Pharmacol*. 2003;59:545-552.
5. McGready R, Keo NK, Villegas L, White NJ, Looareesuwan S, Nosten F. Artesunate-atovaquone-proguanil rescue treatment of multidrug-resistant *Plasmodium falciparum* malaria in pregnancy: a preliminary report. *Trans R Soc Trop Med Hyg*. 2003;97:592-594.
6. McGready R, Ashley EA, Moo E, et al. A randomized comparison of artesunate-atovaquone-proguanil versus quinine in treatment of uncomplicated falciparum malaria during pregnancy. *J Infect Dis*. 2005;192:846-853.
7. Na-Bangchang K, Manyando C, Ruengweerayut R, et al. The pharmacokinetics and pharmacodynamics of atovaquone and proguanil for the treatment of uncomplicated falciparum malaria in third-trimester pregnant women. *Eur J Clin Pharmacol*. 2005;61:573-582.
8. Pasternak B, Hviid A. Atovaquone-proguanil use in early pregnancy and the risk of birth defects. *Arch Intern Med*. 2011;171:259-260.

ATOVAQUONE/PROGUANIL

Anti-Infective (Antiprotozoal)

PREGNANCY RECOMMENDATION: Limited Human Data—Animal Data Suggest Potential Risk (Maternal Benefit May Outweigh Any Potential Embryofetal Risk)

BREASTFEEDING RECOMMENDATION: Potential Toxicity

PREGNANCY SUMMARY

Several studies regarding the use of atovaquone/proguanil during human pregnancy have been located. Use in the first trimester is limited. Use in treating malaria in the second and third trimesters has not shown an increased risk for adverse fetal effects. Both drugs will probably cross the placenta, so some fetal exposure will likely occur. Therefore, the absence of human pregnancy experience prevents a complete assessment of the embryofetal risk. Animal studies did not show any embryofetal toxicity or teratogenicity in one species at doses of less than 10 times the RHD. However, in a second species, embryofetal toxicity was seen at doses less than the RHD, but maternal toxicity was also present. Using this drug during pregnancy should be based on the pros and cons of the mother's clinical need for treatment versus any potential fetal risk that might occur from exposure. Because the maternal benefit appears to exceed any unknown embryofetal risk, atovaquone/proguanil should probably not be withheld because of pregnancy.

BREASTFEEDING SUMMARY

No reports describing the use of atovaquone/proguanil during human lactation have been located. Some amount of both drugs will probably be found in human breast milk, so infant exposure will likely occur. The severity of the mother's illness, such as infection with HIV, may preclude breastfeeding. Breastfeeding while using this drug should be based on the mother's clinical need for treatment versus any potential infant risks that might occur. If used, the infant should be monitored for the most common reported adult side effects of nausea, headache, pruritus, and abdominal pain (all leading to irritability), diarrhea, cough, and vomiting.

References

1. Rosenblatt JE. Antiparasitic agents. *Mayo Clin Proc*. 1999;74:1161-1175.
2. Irvine MH, Einarson A, Bozzo P. Prophylactic use of antimalarials during pregnancy. *Can Fam Physician*. 2011;57:1279-1281.
3. Prescribing Information. Malarone. GlaxoSmithKline; 2019.
4. McGready R, Stepniewska K, Edstein MD, et al. The pharmacokinetics of atovaquone and proguanil in pregnant women with acute falciparum malaria. *Eur J Clin Pharmacol*. 2003;59:545-552.
5. McGready R, Keo NK, Villegas L, White NJ, Looareesuwan S, Nosten F. Artesunate- atovaquone-proguanil rescue treatment of multidrug-resistant *Plasmodium falciparum* malaria in pregnancy: a preliminary report. *Trans R Soc Trop Med Hyg*. 2003;97:592-594.
6. McGready R, Ashley EA, Moo E, et al. A randomized comparison of artesunate-atovaquone-proguanil versus quinine in treatment of uncomplicated falciparum malaria during pregnancy. *J Infect Dis*. 2005;192:846-853.
7. Na-Bangchang K, Manyando C, Ruengweerayut R, et al. The pharmacokinetics and pharmacodynamics of atovaquone and proguanil for the treatment of uncomplicated falciparum malaria in third-trimester pregnant women. *Eur J Clin Pharmacol*. 2005;61:573-582.
8. Pasternak B, Hviid A. Atovaquone-proguanil use in early pregnancy and the risk of birth defects. *Arch Intern Med*. 2011;171:259-260.

ATRACURIUM

Musculoskeletal (Muscle Relaxant)

PREGNANCY RECOMMENDATION: Limited Human Data—Animal Data Suggest Potential Risk

BREASTFEEDING RECOMMENDATION: Probably Compatible

PREGNANCY SUMMARY

No reports describing the use of atracurium during the first trimester of human pregnancy were located. Numerous case reports and series have described use during surgical procedures in the second and third trimesters, with no adverse effects related to the drug being described. Atracurium has also been used for minimizing fetal movements during intrauterine procedures with good success. The drug has been shown to cross the placenta at delivery with drug levels from 3% to 33% maternal concentrations, so some fetal exposure will occur. Therefore, this limited human pregnancy experience prevents a complete assessment of the embryofetal risk. Animal studies did show embryofetal toxicity and teratogenicity at doses less than the RHD. However, these dosages were administered daily for 13 days, whereas in humans, it would only occur once with a given surgery. It is not possible to determine if this increased dosing frequency affects the overall animal response. Using this drug during pregnancy should be based on the pros and cons of the mother's clinical need for treatment versus any potential fetal risk that might occur from exposure. Based on the available data, use of atracurium during the latter portion of human pregnancy appears to represent little, if any, risk.

BREASTFEEDING SUMMARY

No reports describing the use of atracurium during human lactation have been located. The drug may be found in breast milk, but the overall amount is likely to be minimal. Although usage in a lactating woman is possible, the drug should be out of the maternal system in less than 2 hours after the drug is stopped (five plus elimination half-lives). Therefore, breastfeeding should be able to resume fairly soon after the patient recovers from anesthesia. If the clinical decision is to use this drug while breastfeeding, the infant should be monitored for the most common reported adult side effects of pruritus (leading to irritability), rash, flushing, and cough.

References

1. Prescribing Information. Atracurium besylate. Meitheal Pharmaceuticals; 2018.
2. Drenck NE, Viby-Mogensen J, Ostergaard D, Seraj M. Atracurium (tracrium). *Middle East J Anesthesiol*. 1988;9:457-465.
3. Anonymous. Atracurium. *Lancet*. 1983;1:394-395.
4. Skarpa M, Dayan AD, Follenfant M, et al. Toxicity testing of atracurium. *Br J Anaesth* 1983;55:27S–9S.
5. Frank M, Flynn PJ, Hughes R. Atracurium in obstetric anaesthesia. A preliminary report. *Br J Anaesth*. 1983;55:113S-114S.
6. Flynn PJ, Frank M, Hughes R. Use of atracurium in caesarean section. *Br J Anaesth*. 1984;56:599-604.
7. Flynn PJ, Frank M, Hughes R. Evaluation of atracurium in caesarian section using train-of-four responses (abstract). *Anesthesiology*. 1982;57:A286.
8. Baraka A, Jaude CA. Atracurium in a parturient with atypical cholinesterase. *Br J Anaesth*. 1984;56:930-931.
9. Thomas D, Windsor JPW. Prolonged sedation and paralysis in a pregnant patient. Delivery of an infant with a normal Apgar score. *Anaesthesia*. 1985;40:465-467.
10. Mitchell SZ, Freilich JD, Brant D, Flynn M. Anesthetic management of pheochromocytoma resection during pregnancy. *Anesth Analg*. 1987;66:478-480.
11. Hardy PAJ. Atracurium and bradycardia. *Anaesthesia*. 1985;40:504-505.
12. Stuart JC, Kan AF, Rowbottom SJ, et al. Acid aspiration prophylaxis for emergency caesarean section. *Anaesthesia*. 1996;51:415-421.
13. Biehl D, Palahniuk RJ. Update on obstetrical anaesthesia. *Can Anaesth Soc J*. 1986;33:238-245.
14. Mouw RJC, Hermans J, Brandenburg HCR, Kanhai HHH. Effects of pancuronium or atracurium on the anemic fetus during and directly after

intrauterine transfusion (IUT): a double blind randomized study (abstract). *Am J Obstet Gynecol*. 1997;176:S18.

15. Bernstein HH, Chitkara U, Plosker H, et al. Use of atracurium besylate to arrest fetal activity during intrauterine intravascular transfusions. *Obstet Gynecol*. 1988;72:813-816.
16. Fan SZ, Huang FY, Lin SY, et al. Intrauterine neuromuscular blockade in fetus. *Acta Anaesth Sin*. 1990;28:31-34.
17. Spigset O. Anaesthetic agents and excretion in breast milk. *Acta Anaesthesiol Scand*. 1994;38:94-103.

ATROPINE

Autonomic/Antidote (Anticholinergic—Antimuscarinic)

PREGNANCY RECOMMENDATION: Human Data Suggest Low Risk

BREASTFEEDING RECOMMENDATION: Probably Compatible

PREGNANCY SUMMARY

From the combined data of the CPP, MMSS, and Group Health Cooperative of Puget Sound, a total of 879 first-trimester exposures to atropine were reported. There were 30 (3.4%) major anomalies described, and no pattern to the defects was seen. Further data from the CPP reported a total of 71 (3.1%) major birth anomalies in 2,323 first-trimester exposures to parasympatholytic agents as a group, and again, no pattern was seen. The drug will cross the placenta, so fetal exposure will occur. Animal reproduction studies have not been conducted. Using this agent during pregnancy should be based on the pros and cons of the mother's clinical need for diagnosis and to assess treatment options versus any potential fetal risk that might occur from exposure. Use of atropine and atropine-like drugs can affect the appearance of FHR monitor tracing by decreasing the variability and increasing the baseline, both consistent with parasympathetic blockage.

BREASTFEEDING SUMMARY

According to the manufacturer, trace amounts of atropine can be found in human breast milk. Specific amounts are not available, so it is not known whether it may affect a nursing infant. Although neonates are particularly sensitive to anticholinergic agents, no adverse effects have been reported in nursing infants whose mothers were taking atropine. Breastfeeding while using this drug should be based on the mother's clinical need for treatment versus any potential infant risks that might occur. If used, the infant should be monitored for the most common reported adult side effects of dry mouth and blurred vision (both leading to irritability) and increased heart rate. Because of the drug's anticholinergic effects, there is the possibility of interfering with breast milk production in the early stages of breastfeeding, as well as decreasing breast milk supply with long-term use. However, the approved uses of this drug suggest short-term episodes.

References

1. Nishimura H, Tanimura T. *Clinical Aspects of the Teratogenicity of Drugs*. American Elsevier; 1976:63.
2. Kivalo I, Saarikoski S. Placental transmission of atropine at full-term pregnancy. *Br J Anaesth*. 1977;49:1017-1021.
3. Kanto J, Virtanen R, Iisalo E, et al. Placental transfer and pharmacokinetics of atropine after a single maternal intravenous and intramuscular administration. *Acta Anaesth Scand*. 1981;25:85-88.
4. Onnen I, Barrier G, d'Athis P, et al. Placental transfer of atropine at the end of pregnancy. *Eur J Clin Pharmacol*. 1979;15:443-446.
5. Piper JM, Baum C, Kennedy DL, Price P. Maternal use of prescribed drugs associated with recognized fetal adverse drug reactions. *Am J Obstet Gynecol*. 1988;159:1173-1177.
6. Hellman LM, Fillisti LP. Analysis of the atropine test for placental transfer in gravidas with toxemia and diabetes. *Am J Obstet Gynecol*. 1965;91:797-805.
7. Roodenburg PJ, Wladimiroff JW, Van Weering HK. Effect of maternal intravenous administration of atropine (0.5 mg) on fetal breathing and heart pattern. *Contrib Gynecol Obstet*. 1979;6:92-97.
8. Heinonen OP, Slone D, Shapiro S. *Birth Defects and Drugs in Pregnancy*. Publishing Sciences Group; 1977.
9. Diaz DM, Diaz SF, Marx GF. Cardiovascular effects of glycopyrrolate and belladonna derivatives in obstetric patients. *Bull NY Acad Med*. 1980;56:245-248.
10. Roper RE, Salem MG. Effects of glycopyrrolate and atropine combined with antacid on gastric acidity. *Br J Anaesth*. 1981;53:1277-1280.
11. Abboud T, Raya J, Sadri S, et al. Fetal and maternal cardiovascular effects of atropine and glycopyrrolate. *Anesth Analg*. 1983;62:426-430.
12. Siebert JR, Barr M Jr, Jackson JG, Benjamin DR. Ebstein's anomaly and extracardiac defects. *Am J Dis Child*. 1989;143:570-572.
13. Stewart JJ. Gastrointestinal drugs. In: Wilson JT, ed. *Drugs in Breast Milk*. ADIS Press; 1981:65-71.
14. Renou P, Warwick N, Wood C. Autonomic control of fetal heart rate. *Am J Obstet Gynecol*. 1969;105:949-953.
15. Schifferli P, Caldeyro-Barcia R. Effects of atropine and beta adrenergic drugs on the heart rate of the human fetus. In: Boreus L, ed. *Fetal Pharmacology*. Raven Press; 1973:259-279.

ATROPINE OPHTHALMIC

Ophthalmic/Autonomic (Anticholinergic—Topical)

PREGNANCY RECOMMENDATION: No Human Data and No Relevant Animal Data

BREASTFEEDING RECOMMENDATION: Probably Compatible

PREGNANCY SUMMARY

No reports describing the use of atropine ophthalmic in human pregnancy have been located. Atropine appears to cross the placenta following use by injection. Therefore, because the drug is absorbed systemically following ophthalmic use, fetal exposure is possible. However, the overall amount is likely to be very limited. Therefore, the absence of human pregnancy experience prevents a complete assessment of the embryofetal risk. Animal reproduction studies with this ophthalmic formulation have not been conducted. Using this drug during pregnancy should be based on the pros and cons of the mother's clinical need for treatment versus any potential fetal risk that might occur from exposure. Use of atropine and atropine-like drugs can affect the appearance of FHR monitor tracing by decreasing the variability and increasing the baseline, both consistent with parasympathetic blockage. If used during pregnancy, consider placing pressure over the tear duct in the corner of the eye for at least 1 minute, and then remove any excess solution with absorbent tissue to decrease the amount of drug reaching the systemic circulation even further.

BREASTFEEDING SUMMARY

No reports describing the use of atropine ophthalmic during human lactation have been located. The manufacturer states that atropine has been found in breast milk following the injection of atropine. Therefore, because the drug is absorbed systemically following ophthalmic use, exposure to a breastfed infant is possible. However, the overall amount is likely to be very limited. Breastfeeding while using this drug should be based on the mother's clinical need for treatment versus any potential infant risks that might occur. If used, the infant should be monitored for the most common reported adult systemic side effects of nausea, dizziness, and headache (all leading to irritability), dry mouth, tachycardia, and lethargy. Because of the drug's anticholinergic effects, there is the possibility of interfering with breast milk production in the early stages of breastfeeding, as well as decreasing breast milk supply with long-term use. A method to decrease some systemic absorption with ophthalmic use is described above in the Pregnancy Summary.

References

1. Prescribing Information. Atropine ophthalmic. Akorn, Inc; 2019.
2. Renou P, Warwick N, Wood C. Autonomic control of fetal heart rate. *Am J Obstet Gynecol*. 1969;105:949-953.
3. Schifferli P, Caldeyro-Barcia R. Effects of atropine and beta adrenergic drugs on the heart rate of the human fetus. In: Boreus L, ed. *Fetal Pharmacology*. Raven Press; 1973:259-279.

AURANOFIN

Immunologic (Gold Compound)

PREGNANCY RECOMMENDATION: No Human Data—Animal Data Suggest Low Risk

BREASTFEEDING RECOMMENDATION: Probably Compatible

PREGNANCY SUMMARY

No reports describing the use of auranofin in human pregnancy have been located. Because of rapid metabolism, the drug itself will not cross the placenta. However, gold has been shown to cross with other gold-containing compounds. Therefore, some fetal exposure will likely occur. Therefore, the absence of human pregnancy experience prevents a complete assessment of the embryofetal risk. Animal studies did not show any embryofetal toxicity or teratogenicity in two species at doses of more than 10 times the RHD. Using this drug during pregnancy should be based on the pros and cons of the mother's clinical need for treatment versus any potential fetal risk that might occur from exposure.

BREASTFEEDING SUMMARY

No reports describing the use of auranofin during human lactation have been located. Intact auranofin has not been detected in blood and, therefore, would not be excreted into breast milk. However, gold released from auranofin will likely be found in breast milk, as seen with other gold-containing compounds. The manufacturer recommends that breastfeeding not occur during treatment with auranofin. Nevertheless, breastfeeding while using this drug should be based on the mother's clinical need for treatment versus any potential infant risks that might occur. If used, the infant should be monitored for the most common reported adult side effects of nausea, abdominal pain, and pruritus (all leading to irritability), diarrhea, rash, and various laboratory abnormalities (see PI).

Reference

1. Prescribing Information. Ridaura. Prometheus Laboratories; 2017.

AVACINCAPTAD PEGOL

Ophthalmic (Intravitreal—Complement C5 Inhibitor)

PREGNANCY RECOMMENDATION: No Human Data—Animal Data Suggest Low Risk

BREASTFEEDING RECOMMENDATION: Probably Compatible

PREGNANCY SUMMARY

No reports describing the use of avacincaptad pegol in human pregnancy have been located. Though placental transfer may be possible, fetal exposure is probably negligible. However, the absence of human pregnancy experience prevents a complete assessment of the embryofetal risk. Animal studies did not show any embryofetal toxicity in two species at doses less than 10 times the RHOD, though drug administration occurred daily for 12 to 13 days (normal human dosing is once every 3-4 weeks). Using this drug during pregnancy should be based on the pros and cons of the mother's clinical need for treatment versus any potential fetal risk that might occur from exposure.

BREASTFEEDING SUMMARY

It is not known if avacincaptad pegol is excreted into human breast milk. The amount of the drug that might be excreted into breast milk is likely to be clinically insignificant. However, further study is needed. Breastfeeding while using this drug should be based on the mother's clinical need for treatment versus any potential infant risks that might occur. Because the drug is used intravitreal, adverse systemic adult side effects were not reported.

Reference

1. Prescribing Information. Izervay. Iveric Bio, Inc; 2024.

AVACOPAN

Miscellaneous (Complement Inhibitor)

PREGNANCY RECOMMENDATION: No Human Data—Animal Data Suggest Potential Risk

BREASTFEEDING RECOMMENDATION: Potential Toxicity

PREGNANCY SUMMARY

No reports describing the use of avacopan in human pregnancy have been located. Avacopan and its active metabolite probably cross the placenta, so some fetal exposure will probably occur. Therefore, the absence of human pregnancy experience prevents a complete assessment of the embryofetal risk. Animal data found some embryofetal toxicity in one species. Using this drug during pregnancy should be based on the pros and cons of the mother's clinical need for treatment versus any potential fetal risk that might occur from exposure. In addition, hypertension was seen in 18% of patients in the clinical trials.

BREASTFEEDING SUMMARY

No reports describing the use of avacopan during human lactation have been located. Avacopan and its active metabolite are likely present in breast milk, so some infant exposure will probably occur. Breastfeeding while using this drug should be based on the mother's clinical need for treatment. If used, the infant should be monitored for the most common reported adult side effects of nausea, headache, and abdominal pain (all leading to irritability), diarrhea, lethargy, vomiting, rash, and hypertension.

Reference

1. Prescribing Information. Tavneos. ChemoCentryx; 2021.

AVALGLUCOSIDASE ALFA

Genetic/Endocrine (Enzyme)

PREGNANCY RECOMMENDATION: No Human Data—Animal Data Suggest Low Risk

BREASTFEEDING RECOMMENDATION: Probably Compatible

PREGNANCY SUMMARY

No reports describing the use of avalglucosidase alfa in human pregnancy have been located. Based on likely limited placental transfer, fetal exposure is probably negligible. However, the absence of human pregnancy experience prevents a complete assessment of the embryofetal risk. Animal data did not show any embryofetal toxicity. Uncontrolled Pompe disease during pregnancy has been associated with worsening respiratory and musculoskeletal symptoms in some women. Therefore, using this drug during pregnancy should be based on the pros and cons of the mother's clinical need for treatment versus any potential fetal risk that might occur from exposure. There is a pregnancy and lactation exposure registry that monitors outcomes in women using this drug. Health care providers and women who are pregnant or lactating and using this drug are encouraged to call 1-800-745-4447, extension 15500.

BREASTFEEDING SUMMARY

No reports describing the use of avalglucosidase alfa during human lactation have been located. It is unlikely to be excreted into breast milk. However, because it is primarily a protein, if the drug were to be ingested through breastfeeding, it would probably be digested in the infant's gastrointestinal tract and not be absorbed. Breastfeeding while using this drug should be based on the mother's clinical need for treatment. If used, the infant should be monitored for the most common reported adult side effects of headache, nausea, arthralgia, myalgia, and pruritus (all leading to irritability), lethargy, diarrhea, and vomiting. Health care providers (and women who are lactating using this drug) are encouraged to contact 1-800-745-4447 extension 15500. Another hydrolytic lysosomal glycogen-specific enzyme replacement, alglucosidase alfa, was found in human breast milk (see Alglucosidase Alfa).

Reference

1. Prescribing Information. Nexviazyme NGPT. Genzyme; 2021.

AVANAFIL

Men's Health (Phosphodiesterase-5 Enzyme Inhibitor)

PREGNANCY RECOMMENDATION: *Contraindicated

BREASTFEEDING RECOMMENDATION: *Contraindicated

PREGNANCY SUMMARY

No reports describing the use of avanafil in human pregnancy have been located. *The drug is not indicated for use in women. However, avanafil would probably cross the placenta, so fetal exposure could occur. The absence of human pregnancy experience prevents a complete assessment of any embryofetal risk. Animal studies did not cause any embryofetal toxicity in two species at doses of less than 10 times the RHD.

BREASTFEEDING SUMMARY

No reports describing the use of avanafil during human lactation have been located. *The drug is not indicated for use in women. Nevertheless, the drug would probably be found in breast milk, so some infant exposure could occur. If, for some reason, the drug were to be used while breastfeeding, the infant should be monitored for the most common reported adult side effects of headache and back pain (both leading to irritability), flushing, and nasal congestion.

Reference

1. Prescribing Information. Stendra. Vivus, Inc; 2020.

AVAPRITINIB

Antineoplastic (Tyrosine Kinase Inhibitor)

PREGNANCY RECOMMENDATION: No Human Data—Animal Data Suggest Potential Risk

BREASTFEEDING RECOMMENDATION: Potential Toxicity

PREGNANCY SUMMARY

No reports describing the use of avapritinib in human pregnancy have been located. The drug probably crosses the placenta in small amounts. Therefore, the absence of human pregnancy experience prevents a complete assessment of the embryofetal risk. Animal studies found avapritinib to have both fetotoxic and teratogenic effects. Based on these animal data and its mechanism of action, the manufacturer recommends that women with reproductive potential who are taking avapritinib use effective contraception during treatment and for at least 6 weeks after the last dose. They also recommend that males with female partners of reproductive potential use effective contraception during treatment and for 6 weeks after the last dose. Nevertheless, using this drug during pregnancy should be based on the pros and cons of the mother's clinical need for treatment versus any potential fetal risk that might occur from exposure.

BREASTFEEDING SUMMARY

Avapritinib will probably enter human breast milk in small amounts. Due to concerns regarding potential adverse effects for a breastfed infant, the manufacturer recommends that women not breastfeed while being treated with avapritinib and for at least 2 weeks after the last dose. However, breastfeeding while using this drug should be based on the mother's clinical need for treatment. If used, the infant should be monitored for the most common reported adult side effects of nausea and abdominal pain (both leading to irritability), edema, vomiting, lethargy, diarrhea, constipation, and rash.

Reference

1. Prescribing Information. Ayvakit. Blueprint Medicines Corporation; 2020.

AVATROMBOPAG

Hematologic (Thrombopoietin Receptor Agonist)

PREGNANCY RECOMMENDATION: No Human Data—Animal Data Suggest Potential Risk

BREASTFEEDING RECOMMENDATION: Potential Toxicity

PREGNANCY SUMMARY

No reports describing the use of avatrombopag in human pregnancy have been located. Some amount of the drug will probably cross the placenta, so fetal exposure will likely occur. Therefore, the absence of human pregnancy experience prevents a complete assessment of the embryofetal risk. Animal studies did show some embryofetal toxicity in one species at 10 times the RHD. Using this drug during pregnancy should be based on the pros and cons of the mother's clinical need for treatment versus any potential fetal risk that might occur from exposure.

BREASTFEEDING SUMMARY

No reports describing the use of avatrombopag during breastfeeding have been located. The drug will probably appear in breast milk, so some infant exposure will likely occur. However, due to a concern for potential serious adverse effects that might be seen in a breastfed infant, the manufacturer recommends that women not breastfeed while being treated with this drug and for at least 2 weeks after the last dose. Nevertheless, breastfeeding while using this drug should be based on the mother's clinical need for treatment versus any potential infant risks that might occur. If used, the infant should be monitored for the most common reported adult side effects of nausea, headache, arthralgia, and abdominal pain (all leading to irritability), fatigue (lethargy), fever, and peripheral edema.

Reference

1. Prescribing Information. Doptelet. Sobi, Inc; 2021.

AVELUMAB

Antineoplastic (Programmed Cell Death Ligand 1 Blocking Monoclonal Antibody)

PREGNANCY RECOMMENDATION: No Human Data and No Relevant Animal Data

BREASTFEEDING RECOMMENDATION: Probably Compatible

PREGNANCY SUMMARY

No reports describing the use of avelumab during human pregnancy have been located. As an IgG antibody, it likely crosses the placenta, especially during the second half of pregnancy, so some fetal exposure will probably occur. However, the absence of human pregnancy experience prevents a complete assessment of the embryofetal risk. No animal reproduction studies have been conducted. Regarding reproduction, the main function of the PD-L1/PD-1 pathway is to preserve pregnancy by maintaining maternal immune tolerance to a fetus. In the mouse model, blocking this signal during pregnancy resulted in an increase in fetal loss. Based on the drug's mechanism of action, the manufacturer recommends that women with reproductive potential use effective contraception during treatment and for 1 month after the last dose. Nevertheless, using this drug during pregnancy should be based on the pros and cons of the mother's clinical need for treatment versus any potential fetal risk that might occur from exposure. There is a registry for women who are pregnant and have cancer. For more information, women and health care providers are encouraged to contact the Cancer and Pregnancy Registry at 1-877-635-4499.

BREASTFEEDING SUMMARY

No reports describing the use of avelumab during human lactation have been located. It is known that IgG antibodies can be found in human breast milk, but are not found in the neonatal or infant circulation. Additionally, if any IgG antibodies were to be ingested through breastfeeding, they would probably be digested in the infant's gastrointestinal tract and not be absorbed. Regardless, based on the drug's mechanism of action and the concern for potential serious adverse effects that might be seen in a breastfed infant, the manufacturer recommends that women not breastfeed while being treated with this drug and for at least 1 month after the last dose. Nevertheless, breastfeeding while using this drug should be based on the mother's clinical need for treatment versus any potential infant risks that might occur. If used, the infant should be monitored for the most common reported adult side effects of nausea, musculoskeletal pain, abdominal pain, and headache (all leading to irritability), diarrhea, fatigue (lethargy), decreased appetite, peripheral edema, and rash.

Reference

1. Prescribing Information. Bavencio. EMD Serono; 2020.

AXATILIMAB

Immunologic (Monoclonal Antibody—Colony Stimulating Factor-1 Receptor Antagonist)

PREGNANCY RECOMMENDATION: No Human Data and No Relevant Animal Data

BREASTFEEDING RECOMMENDATION: Probably Compatible

PREGNANCY SUMMARY

No reports describing the use of axatilimab during human pregnancy have been located. As an IgG antibody, the drug will likely cross the placenta, so some fetal exposure will probably occur. However, the absence of human pregnancy experience prevents a complete assessment of the embryofetal risk. Animal reproduction and fertility studies have not been conducted. Based on the drug's mechanism of action, the manufacturer recommends that women with reproductive potential use effective contraception during treatment and for 30 days after the last dose. Nevertheless, using this drug during pregnancy should be based on the pros and cons of the mother's clinical need for treatment versus any potential fetal risk that might occur from exposure.

BREASTFEEDING SUMMARY

No reports describing the use of axatilimab during human lactation have been located. It is known that IgG antibodies can be found in human breast milk, but are not found in the neonatal or infant circulation. Additionally, if any IgG antibodies were to be ingested through breastfeeding, they would probably be digested in the infant's gastrointestinal tract and not be absorbed. However, due to a concern for potential serious adverse effects that might be seen in a breastfed infant, the manufacturer recommends that women not breastfeed while being treated with this drug and for at least 30 days after the last dose. Nevertheless, breastfeeding while using this drug should be based on the mother's clinical need for treatment versus any potential infant risks that might occur. If used, the infant should be monitored for the most common reported adult side effects of headache, nausea, and musculoskeletal pain (all leading to irritability), fatigue (lethargy), various infections, diarrhea, cough, fever, and various laboratory abnormalities (See PI).

Reference

1. Prescribing Information. Niktimvo. Incyte Corp; 2024.

A

AXITINIB

Antineoplastic (Tyrosine Kinase Inhibitor)

PREGNANCY RECOMMENDATION: No Human Data—Animal Data Suggest Potential Risk

BREASTFEEDING RECOMMENDATION: Potential Toxicity

PREGNANCY SUMMARY

No reports describing the use of axitinib in human pregnancy have been located. The drug will probably cross the placenta, so some fetal exposure will likely occur. Therefore, the absence of human pregnancy experience prevents a complete assessment of the embryofetal risk. Animal studies did show embryofetal toxicity with malformations (cleft palate) in one species at doses of less than 10 times the RHD. Based on the drug's mechanism of action and findings in the animal studies, the manufacturer recommends that women with reproductive potential use effective contraception during treatment. They also recommend that males with female partners of reproductive potential use effective contraception during treatment. Nevertheless, using this drug during pregnancy should be based on the pros and cons of the mother's clinical need for treatment versus any potential fetal risk that might occur from exposure. During the clinical trials, up to 40% of treated patients developed hypertension, 11% developed proteinuria, and 22% developed elevated liver enzymes. If these findings were to all occur in a pregnant patient using this drug in the second half of gestation, it would be very difficult to differentiate this from HELLP syndrome (hemolysis, elevated liver enzymes, and low platelets). There is a registry for women who are pregnant and have cancer. For more information, women and health care providers are encouraged to contact the Cancer and Pregnancy Registry at 1-877-635-4499.

BREASTFEEDING SUMMARY

No reports describing the use of axitinib during human lactation have been located. The drug will probably be found in breast milk, so some infant exposure will likely occur. Due to a concern for potential serious adverse effects that might be seen in a breastfed infant, the manufacturer recommends that women not breastfeed while being treated with this drug. Nevertheless, breastfeeding while using this drug should be based on the mother's clinical need for treatment versus any potential infant risks that might occur. If used, the infant should be monitored for the most common reported adult side effects of nausea (leading to irritability), diarrhea, fatigue (lethargy), vomiting, hypertension, and various laboratory abnormalities (see PI).

Reference

1. Prescribing Information. Inlyta. Pfizer Laboratories; 2021.

AZACITIDINE

Antineoplastic (Pyrimidine Nucleoside Analogue)

PREGNANCY RECOMMENDATION: Limited Human Data—Animal Data Suggest Risk

BREASTFEEDING RECOMMENDATION: Potential Toxicity

PREGNANCY SUMMARY

One case report was located that described the use of azacitidine at 30 weeks' gestation. The infant was delivered prematurely and overall did well with no identified adverse events seen in the infant related to the drug. The drug will probably cross the placenta, so some fetal exposure will likely occur. Therefore, this limited human pregnancy experience prevents a complete assessment of the embryofetal risk. Animal studies did show some embryotoxicity with teratogenicity in two species at doses of less than the RHD. However, the drug in both species was administered intraperitoneally, whereas use in humans is subcutaneous (SC) or IV. It is not possible to determine if this administration location makes a difference in pregnant animals. Based on animal studies and the drug's mechanism of action, the manufacturer recommends that women with reproductive potential use effective contraception during treatment and for 6 months after the last dose. They also recommend that males with female partners of reproductive potential use effective contraception during treatment and for 3 months after the last dose. Regardless, using this drug during pregnancy should be based on the pros and cons of the mother's clinical need for treatment versus any potential fetal risk that might occur from exposure. There is a registry for women who are pregnant and have cancer. For more information, women and health care providers are encouraged to contact the Cancer and Pregnancy Registry at 1-877-635-4499.

BREASTFEEDING SUMMARY

No reports describing the use of azacitidine during human lactation have been located. The drug will probably be found in human breast milk, so some infant exposure will likely occur. However, due to a concern for potential serious adverse effects that might be seen in a breastfed infant, the manufacturer recommends that women not breastfeed while being treated with this drug and for at least 1 week after the last dose. Nevertheless, breastfeeding while using this drug should be based on the mother's clinical need for treatment versus any potential infant risks that might occur. If used, the infant should be monitored for the most common reported adult side effects of nausea (leading to irritability), diarrhea, fever, vomiting, and various laboratory abnormalities (see PI)

References

1. Prescribing Information. Vidaza. Celgene Corp; 2022.
2. Mahdi AJ, Gosrani D, Chakraborty M, et al. Successful molecular targeted treatment of AML in pregnancy with azacitidine and sorafenib with no adverse fetal outcome. *Br J Haematol*. 2018;180:603-604.

AZATHIOPRINE

Immunologic (Antimetabolite)

PREGNANCY RECOMMENDATION: **Human Data Suggest Potential Risk (Third Trimester) (Maternal Benefit May Outweigh Any Embryofetal Risk)**

BREASTFEEDING RECOMMENDATION: **Probably Compatible**

PREGNANCY SUMMARY

Numerous case reports and series have been located that describe the use of azathioprine during human pregnancy. Of the few that describe the use of the drug in the first trimester, no unusual increase in the number of major birth anomalies has been seen. A few neonates have been described as having decreased immune status when the drug was used up to birth. In addition, the FDA recently sent out an alert that the use of thiopurines, including azathioprine, during pregnancy can increase the risk for intrahepatic cholestasis of pregnancy. The drug crosses the placenta, so some fetal exposure will occur. Animal data did show some embryofetal toxicity with malformations in two species at doses of less than 10 times the RHD. Using this drug during pregnancy should be based on the pros and cons of the mother's clinical need for treatment versus any potential fetal risk that might occur from exposure. In summary, however, the evidence suggests that the maternal benefit of treatment may outweigh the potential risk to the fetus and newborn in many instances.

BREASTFEEDING SUMMARY

Six studies were located that describe the use of azathioprine during human lactation. A total of 22 women had breast milk levels analyzed for mercaptopurine (the active metabolite) following maternal doses of about 75 mg/d up to 150 mg/d. Concentrations ranged from undetectable (LLQ of 1 ng/mL) up to about 50 ng/mL. The calculated RIDs were all less than 1%. There were 14 infants who had blood levels drawn for mercaptopurine following exposure to azathioprine through breast milk. The drug was not detected in the serum of any of the infants (LLQ of about 1 ng/mL for some analyses). Breastfeeding while using this drug should be based on the mother's clinical need for treatment versus any potential infant risks that might occur. If used, the infant should be monitored for the most common reported adult side effects of nausea, dizziness, myalgia, and abdominal cramps (all leading to irritability), diarrhea, lethargy, alopecia, decreased appetite (monitor infant growth), rash, fever, and various laboratory abnormalities (see PI).

References

1. Sarrikoski S, Seppala M. Immunosuppression during pregnancy. Transmission of azathioprine and its metabolites from the mother to the fetus. *Am J Obstet Gynecol*. 1973;115:1100-1106.
2. Mercaptopurine. In: Sweetman SC, ed. *Martindale. The Complete Drug Reference*. 34th ed. Pharmaceutical Press; 2005:567-568.
3. Tuchmann-Duplessis H, Mercier-Parot L. Foetopathes therapeutiques: production experimentale de malformations des membres. *Union Med Can*. 1968;97:283-288. As cited in Shepard TH. *Catalog of Teratogenic Agents*. 6th ed. Johns Hopkins University Press; 1989:63.
4. Product information. Azathioprine. Amneal Pharmaceuticals; 2017.
5. Gillibrand PN. Systemic lupus erythematosus in pregnancy treated with azathioprine. *Proc R Soc Med*. 1966;59:834.
6. Board JA, Lee HM, Draper DA, Hume DM. Pregnancy following kidney homotransplantation from a non-twin: report of a case with concurrent administration of azathioprine and prednisone. *Obstet Gynecol*. 1967;29:318-323.
7. Kaufmann JJ, Dignam W, Goodwin WE, et al. Successful, normal childbirth after kidney homotransplantation. *JAMA*. 1967;200:338-341.
8. Anonymous. Eleventh annual report of human renal transplant registry. *JAMA*. 1973;216:1197.
9. Nolan GH, Sweet RL, Laros RK, Roure CA. Renal cadaver transplantation followed by successful pregnancies. *Obstet Gynecol*. 1974;43:732-738.
10. Sharon E, Jones J, Diamond H, Kaplan D. Pregnancy and azathioprine in systemic lupus erythematosus. *Am J Obstet Gynecol*. 1974;118:25-27.
11. Cote CJ, Meuwissen HJ, Pickering RJ. Effects on the neonate of prednisone and azathioprine administered to the mother during pregnancy. *J Pediatr*. 1974;85:324-328.
12. Erkman J, Blythe JG. Azathioprine therapy complicated by pregnancy. *Obstet Gynecol*. 1972;40:708-709.
13. Price HV, Salaman JR, Laurence KM, Langmaid H. Immunosuppressive drugs and the foetus. *Transplantation*. 1976;21:294-298.
14. The Registration Committee of the European Dialysis and Transplant Association. Successful pregnancies in women treated by dialysis and kidney transplantation. *Br J Obstet Gynaecol*. 1980;87:839-845.

15. Golby M. Fertility after renal transplantation. *Transplantation*. 1930;10:201-207.
16. Rabau-Friedman E, Mashiach S, et al. Association of hypoparathyroidism and successful pregnancy in kidney transplant recipient. *Obstet Gynecol*. 1982;59:126-128.
17. Myers RL, Schmid R, Newton JJ. Childbirth after liver transplantation. *Transplantation*. 1980;29:432.
18. Williams PF, Johnstone M. Normal pregnancy in renal transplant recipient with history of eclampsia and intrauterine death. *BMJ*. 1982;285:1535.
19. Westney LS, Callender CO, Stevens J, et al. Successful pregnancy with sickle cell disease and renal transplantation. *Obstet Gynecol*. 1984;63:752-755.
20. Ogburn PL Jr, Kitzmiller JL, Hare JW, et al. Pregnancy following renal transplantation in class T diabetes mellitus. *JAMA*. 1986;255:911-915.
21. Marushak A, Weber T, Bock J, et al. Pregnancy following kidney transplantation. *Acta Obstet Gynecol Scand*. 1986;65:557-559.
22. Key TC, Resnik R, Dittrich HC, Reisner LS. Successful pregnancy after cardiac transplantation. *Am J Obstet Gynecol*. 1989;160:367-371.
23. Davison JM, Lindheimer MD. Pregnancy in renal transplant recipients. *J Reprod Med*. 1982;27:613-621.
24. Symington GR, Mackay IR, Lambert RP. Cancer and teratogenesis: infrequent occurrence after medical use of immunosuppressive drugs. *Aust NZ J Med*. 1977;7:368-372.
25. Alstead EM, Ritchie JK, Lennard-Jones JE, et al. Safety of azathioprine in pregnancy in inflammatory bowel disease. *Gastroenterology*. 1990;99:443-446.
26. Haugen G, Fauchald P, Sødal G, et al. Pregnancy outcome in renal allograft recipients: influence of ciclosporin A. *Eur J Obstet Gynecol Reprod Biol*. 1991;39:25-29.
27. Kossoy LR, Herbert CM III, Wentz AC. Management of heart transplant recipients: guidelines for the obstetrician-gynecologist. *Am J Obstet Gynecol*. 1988;159:490-499.
28. Cararach V, Carmona F, Monleón FJ, Andreu J. Pregnancy after renal transplantation: 25 years experience in Spain. *Br J Obstet Gynaecol*. 1993;100:122-125.
29. Sturgiss SN, Davison JM. Perinatal outcome in renal allograft recipients: prognostic significance of hypertension and renal function before and during pregnancy. *Obstet Gynecol*. 1991;78:573-577.
30. Sturgiss SN, Davison JM. Effect of pregnancy on long-term function of renal allografts. *Am J Kidney Dis*. 1992;19:167-172.
31. Laifer SA, Darby MJ, Scantlebury VP, et al. Pregnancy and liver transplantation. *Obstet Gynecol*. 1990;76:1083-1088.
32. Zaballos J, Perez-Cerda F, Riaño D, et al. Anesthetic management of liver transplantation in a pregnant patient with fulminant hepatitis. *Transplant Proc*. 1991;23:1994-1995.
33. Ville Y, Fernandez H, Samuel D, et al. Pregnancy in liver transplant recipients: course and outcome in 19 cases. *Am J Obstet Gynecol*. 1993;168:896-902.
34. Kirk EP. Organ transplantation and pregnancy. A case report and review. *Am J Obstet Gynecol*. 1991;164:1629-1634.
35. Nishimura H, Tanimura T. *Clinical Aspects of the Teratogenicity of Drugs*. American Elsevier; 1976:106-107.
36. Williamson RA, Karp LE. Azathioprine teratogenicity: review of the literature and case report. *Obstet Gynecol*. 1981;58:247-250.
37. Burleson RL, Sunderji SG, Aubry RH, et al. Renal allotransplantation during pregnancy. Successful outcome for mother, child, and kidney. *Transplantation*. 1983;36:334.
38. Leb DE, Weisskopf B, Kanovitz BS. Chromosome aberrations in the child of a kidney transplant recipient. *Arch Intern Med*. 1971;128:441-444.
39. DeWitte DB, Buick MK, Cyran SE, Maisels MJ. Neonatal pancytopenia and severe combined immunodeficiency associated with antenatal administration of azathioprine and prednisone. *J Pediatr*. 1984;105:625-628.
40. Davison JM, Dellagrammatikas H, Parkin JM. Maternal azathioprine therapy and depressed haemopoiesis in the babies of renal allograft patients. *Br J Obstet Gynaecol*. 1985;92:233-239.
41. Scott JR. Fetal growth retardation associated with maternal administration of immunosuppressive drugs. *Am J Obstet Gynecol*. 1977;128:668-676.
42. Pirson Y, Van Lierde M, Ghysen J, et al. Retardation of fetal growth in patients receiving immunosuppressive therapy. *N Engl J Med*. 1985;313:328.
43. Zerner J, Doil KL, Drewry J, Leeber DA. Intrauterine contraceptive device failures in renal transplant patients. *J Reprod Med*. 1981;26:99-102.
44. Moretti ME, Verjee Z, Ito S, Koren G. Breast-feeding during maternal use of azathioprine. *Ann Pharmacother*. 2006;40:2269-2272.
45. Gardiner SJ, Gearry RB, Roberts RI, et al. Comment: breast-feeding during maternal use of azathioprine. *Ann Pharmacother*. 2007;41:719-720.
46. Moretti ME, Verjee Z, Ito S, Koren G. Reply. Comment: breast-feeding during maternal use of azathioprine. *Ann Pharmacother*. 2007;41:720.

AZELASTINE

Antihistamine (Intranasal)

PREGNANCY RECOMMENDATION: No Human Data—Animal Data Suggest Low Risk

BREASTFEEDING RECOMMENDATION: Probably Compatible

PREGNANCY SUMMARY

No reports describing the use of azelastine in human pregnancy have been located. The drug and active metabolite will probably cross the placenta, so some fetal exposure will likely occur. However, the systemic bioavailability after intranasal use is only about 40%, so the overall exposure is very limited. Nevertheless, the absence of human pregnancy experience prevents a complete assessment of the embryofetal risk. Animal studies did not show any embryofetal toxicity in three species at doses of less than 10 times the MRHDID. Using this drug during pregnancy should be based on the pros and cons of the mother's clinical need for treatment versus any potential fetal risk that might occur from exposure.

BREASTFEEDING SUMMARY

No reports describing the use of azelastine during human lactation have been located. The drug and its active metabolite will probably be found in breast milk, so some infant exposure will likely occur. However, the systemic bioavailability after intranasal use is only about 40%. Breastfeeding while using this drug should be based on the mother's clinical need for treatment versus any potential infant risks that might occur. If used, the infant should be monitored for the most common reported adult side effects of nausea, headache, and dizziness (all leading to irritability), fatigue (lethargy), somnolence, and dry mouth. Some antihistamines have been reported to decrease prolactin levels. Nevertheless, the amount of drug that might be seen systemically in a breastfeeding mother following intranasal use is likely to be small with minimal effect on the overall prolactin level.

Reference

1. Prescribing Information. Azelastine nasal. LGM Pharma; 2020.

AZELASTINE OPHTHALMIC

Ophthalmic/Antihistamine (Topical)

PREGNANCY RECOMMENDATION: No Human Data—Animal Data Suggest Low Risk

BREASTFEEDING RECOMMENDATION: Probably Compatible

PREGNANCY SUMMARY

No reports describing the use of azelastine ophthalmic in human pregnancy have been located. The drug and active metabolite will probably cross the placenta, so some fetal exposure will likely occur. However, the systemic levels obtained following topical ocular use are very low, so the overall exposure is negligible. Nevertheless, the absence of human pregnancy experience prevents a complete assessment of the embryofetal risk. Animal studies did not show any embryofetal toxicity in three species at doses of less than 10 times the maximum recommended human intranasal dose. When drug levels in animals are compared to levels seen with topical ocular use, exposures are more than 25,000 times the maximum recommended human oral dose (MRHOD). Using this drug during pregnancy should be based on the pros and cons of the mother's clinical need for treatment versus any potential fetal risk that might occur from exposure.

BREASTFEEDING SUMMARY

No reports describing the use of azelastine ophthalmic during human lactation have been located. The drug and its active metabolite will probably be found in breast milk, so some infant exposure will likely occur. However, the systemic levels obtained following topical ocular use are very low and would probably be clinically insignificant. Breastfeeding while using this drug should be based on the mother's clinical need for treatment versus any potential infant risks that might occur. If used, the infant should be monitored for the most common reported adult side effects of nausea, headache, and dizziness (all leading to irritability), fatigue (lethargy), somnolence, and dry mouth. Some antihistamines have been reported to decrease prolactin levels. Nevertheless, the amount of drug that might be seen systemically in a breastfeeding mother following topical ophthalmic use is likely to be extremely small, with minimal effect on the overall prolactin level.

Reference

1. Prescribing Information. Azelastine ophthalmic. Sun Pharmaceuticals Industries; 2019.

AZFICEL-T

Dermatologic (Autologous Cell Product)

PREGNANCY RECOMMENDATION: No Human Data but Probably Compatible

BREASTFEEDING RECOMMENDATION: Probably Compatible

PREGNANCY SUMMARY

No reports describing the use of azficel-T in human pregnancy have been located. The cells will not cross the placenta, so fetal exposure will not occur. Nevertheless, the absence of human pregnancy experience prevents a complete assessment of the embryofetal risk. Because it is an autologous product that is obtained from the patient by skin biopsy, reproduction studies in animals have not been conducted. Using this product during pregnancy should be based on the woman's overall needs.

BREASTFEEDING SUMMARY

No reports describing the use of azficel-T during human lactation have been located. Because the cells are injected intradermally, they should not be found in the systemic circulation, and therefore, would not be present in breast milk. Moreover, the product is made from the patient's own cells and would not be expected to harm a nursing infant. Using this product while breastfeeding should be based on the woman's overall needs.

Reference

1. Prescribing Information. Laviv. Fibrocell Technologies; 2019.

AZILSARTAN MEDOXOMIL

Antihypertensive (Angiotensin II Receptor Blocker)

PREGNANCY RECOMMENDATION: Human Data Suggest Risk (Second and Third Trimesters)

BREASTFEEDING RECOMMENDATION: Potential Toxicity

PREGNANCY SUMMARY

No reports describing the use of azilsartan in human pregnancy have been located. Though the data are small, first-trimester exposure to other ARB drugs has not been shown to significantly increase the risk for congenital anomalies. In addition, no pattern to the anomalies has been identified. However, numerous case reports and reviews have reported that the use of ARBs, in the second half of pregnancy, can, in some cases, produce severe fetal renal dysfunction. This can lead to anomalies related to longstanding oligohydramnios and fetal/neonatal death. There are cases, however, where the process reverses itself when the drug is discontinued. These findings are similar to those seen with ACE inhibitors. Azilsartan actually carries a boxed warning for these risks. The drug will probably cross the placenta, so some fetal exposure will likely occur. Animal studies did show some embryofetal toxicity in two species at doses of less than 10 times the RHD. Women of reproductive age using azilsartan medoxomil should be informed of these risks, so that they can closely monitor if pregnancy transpires. If a positive pregnancy test occurs, she and her health care providers can modify treatment (if possible) so that the drug is not used in the second or third trimesters. For treating hypertension in pregnancy, ACOG recommends nifedipine and labetalol as first-line agents.

BREASTFEEDING SUMMARY

No reports describing the use of azilsartan during human lactation have been located. The drug will probably be found in human breast milk, so some infant exposure will likely occur. Due to a concern for potential serious adverse effects that might be seen in a breastfed infant, the manufacturer recommends that women not breastfeed while being treated with this drug. Nevertheless, breastfeeding while using this drug should be based on the mother's clinical need for treatment versus any potential infant risks that might occur. If used, the infant should be monitored for the most common reported adult side effects of nausea and dizziness (both leading to irritability), diarrhea, fatigue (lethargy), and cough.

References

1. Prescribing Information. Edarbi. Arbor Pharmaceuticals; 2016.
2. Polifka JE. Is there an embryopathy associated with first-trimester exposure to angiotensin-converting enzyme inhibitors and angiotensin receptor antagonists? A critical review of the evidence. *Birth Defects Res A Clin Mol Teratol*. 2012;94:576-598.

AZITHROMYCIN

Antibacterial (Macrolide)

PREGNANCY RECOMMENDATION: Human Data Suggest Low Risk

BREASTFEEDING RECOMMENDATION: Probably Compatible

PREGNANCY SUMMARY

Several studies have been located that describe the use of azithromycin during human pregnancy. From more than 800 first-trimester exposures, the congenital anomaly rate was about 4.1%, but no pattern to the defects was seen. The drug has also been used to treat various infections during pregnancy in the second and third trimesters, and no adverse fetal effects were described from this use. The drug crosses the placenta, so some fetal exposure will occur. Animal data did not show any embryofetal toxicity or teratogenicity in two species at doses of less than 10 times the RHD based on BSA. Using this agent during pregnancy should be based on the pros and cons of the mother's clinical need for treatment versus any potential fetal risk that might occur from exposure. Azithromycin was found to prolong the QT interval in some patients in the clinical trials.

BREASTFEEDING SUMMARY

A few studies describing the use of azithromycin during human lactation were located. From a total of about 50 lactating women, the drug was detected in nearly every sample. The drug concentrations in breast milk ranged from about 0.5 to 3 mcg/mL. The issue with these analyses is that the drug has a long elimination half-life, where it may take time to reach a steady state, making it difficult to fully determine total infant exposure. Overall, most calculated RIDs were less than 10%, but in some cases, it may be higher. The manufacturer reports a warning for a risk of producing infantile hypertrophic pyloric stenosis with the use of azithromycin up to 6 weeks of age. However, the data on this potential risk has not fully confirmed this finding. Breastfeeding while using this drug should be based on the mother's clinical need for treatment versus any potential infant risks that might occur. If used, the infant should be monitored for the most common reported adult side effects of nausea and abdominal pain (both leading to irritability), diarrhea, and vomiting.

References

1. Prescribing Information. Zithromax. Pfizer Laboratories; 2018.
2. Ramsey PS, Vaules MB, Vasdev GM, et al. Maternal and transplacental pharmacokinetics of azithromycin. *Am J Obstet Gynecol.* 2003;188:714-718.
3. Heikkinen T, Laine K, Neuvonen PJ, Ekblad U. The transplacental transfer of the macrolide antibiotics erythromycin, roxithromycin and azithromycin. *Br J Obstet Gynaecol.* 2000;107:770-775.
4. Edwards M, Rainwater K, Carter S, et al. Comparison of azithromycin and erythromycin for Chlamydia cervicitis in pregnancy (abstract). *Am J Obstet Gynecol.* 1994;170:419.
5. Bush MR, Rosa C. Azithromycin and erythromycin in the treatment of cervical chlamydial infection during pregnancy. *Obstet Gynecol.* 1994;84:61-63.
6. Rosenn M, Macones GA, Silverman N. A randomized trial of erythromycin and azithromycin for the treatment of chlamydia infection in pregnancy (abstract). *Am J Obstet Gynecol.* 1996;174:410.
7. Wehbeh H, Ruggiero R, Ali Y, et al. A randomized clinical trial of a single dose of azithromycin in the treatment of chlamydia among pregnant women (abstract). *Am J Obstet Gynecol.* 1996;174:361.
8. Wehbeh HA, Ruggeirio RM, Shahem S, Lopez G, Ali Y. Single-dose azithromycin for chlamydia in pregnant women. *J Reprod Med.* 1998;43:509-514.
9. Ogasawara KK, Goodwin TM. Efficacy of azithromycin in reducing lower genital ureaplasma colonization in women at risk for preterm delivery (abstract). *Am J Obstet Gynecol.* 1997;176:S57.
10. Choi EK, Pai H. Azithromycin therapy for scrub typhus during pregnancy. *Clin Infect Dis.* 1998;27:1538-1539.
11. Wilton LV, Pearce GL, Martin RM, et al. The outcomes of pregnancy in women exposed to newly marketed drugs in general practice in England. *Br J Obstet Gynaecol.* 1998;105:882-889.
12. Tellem R, Shechtman S, Arnon J, et al. Pregnancy outcome after gestational exposure to the new macrolides: a prospective controlled cohort study (abstract). *Reprod Toxicol.* 2005;20:484.
13. Sarkar M, Woodland C, Koren G, Einarson A. Pregnancy outcome following gestational exposure to azithromycin. *BMC Pregnancy Childbirth.* 2006;6:18.
14. Cooper WO, Hernandez-Diaz S, Arbogast PG, et al. Antibiotics potentially used in response to bioterrorism and the risk of major congenital malformations. *Paediatr Perinat Epidemiol.* 2009;23:18-28.
15. Cerar D, Karner P, Avsic-Zupanc T, Strle F. Azithromycin for acute Q fever in pregnancy. *Wien Klin Wochenschr.* 2009;121:469-472.
16. Wawer MJ, Sewankambo NK, Serwadda D, et al; The Rakai Project Study Group. Control of sexually transmitted disease for AIDS prevention in Uganda: a randomised community trial. *Lancet.* 1999;353:525-535.
17. Gray RH, Wabwire-Mangen F, Kigozi G, et al. Randomized trial of presumptive sexually transmitted disease therapy during pregnancy in Rakai, Uganda. *Am J Obstet Gynecol.* 2001;185:1209-1217.
18. Kigozi GG, Brahmbhatt H, Wabwire-Mangen F, et al. Treatment of *Trichomonas* in pregnancy and adverse outcomes of pregnancy: a subanalysis of a randomized trial in Rakai, Uganda. *Am J Obstet Gynecol.* 2003;189:1398-1400.
19. Bar-Oz B, Diav-Citrin O, Shechtman S, et al. Pregnancy outcome after gestational exposure to the new macrolides: a prospective multi-center observational study. *Eur J Obstet Gynecol Reprod Biol.* 2008;141:31-34.
20. Bar-Oz B, Weber-Schoendorfer C, Berlin M, et al. The outcomes of pregnancy in women exposed to the new macrolides in the first trimester: a prospective, multicentre, observations study. *Drug Saf.* 2012;35:589-598.
21. Hauth JC, Cliver S, Hodgkins P, et al. Mid-trimester metronidazole and azithromycin did not prevent preterm birth in women at increased risk: a double-blind trial. *Am J Obstet Gynecol.* 2001;185(6 suppl):S86.
22. van den Broek NR, White SA, Goodall M, et al. The APPLe study: a randomized, community-based, placebo-controlled trial of azithromycin for the prevention of preterm birth, with meta-analysis. *PLoS Med.* 2009;6:e100091.
23. Sorensen HT, Skriver MV, Pedersen L, et al. Risk of infantile hypertrophic pyloric stenosis after maternal postnatal use of macrolides. *Scand J Infect Dis.* 2003;35:104-106.
24. Kelsey JJ, Moser LR, Jennings JC, Munger MA. Presence of azithromycin breast milk concentrations: a case report. *Am J Obstet Gynecol.* 1994;170:1375-1376.
25. Goldstein LH, Berlin M, Tsur L, et al. The safety of macrolides during lactation. *Breastfeed Med.* 2009;4:157-200.

AZTREONAM

Antibacterial (Monobactam)

PREGNANCY RECOMMENDATION: Limited Human Data—Animal Data Suggest Low Risk

BREASTFEEDING RECOMMENDATION: Probably Compatible

PREGNANCY SUMMARY

A few reports have described the therapeutic use of aztreonam during human pregnancy. Most exposures were in the second or third trimesters. No adverse fetal effects were described. The drug crosses the placenta, so some fetal exposure will occur. However, this limited human pregnancy experience prevents a complete assessment of the embryofetal risk. Animal data did not show any embryofetal toxicity or malformations in two species at doses of less than 10 times the RHD. Using this drug during pregnancy should be based on the pros and cons of the mother's clinical need for treatment versus any potential fetal risk that might occur from exposure. If the drug is indicated, it should not be withheld because of pregnancy.

BREASTFEEDING SUMMARY

Two studies were located that describe the use of aztreonam during human lactation. A total of about 22 women were evaluated following a single 1,000 mg IV or IM dose. Drug levels in breast milk ranged from about 0.2 to 1 mcg/mL. The calculated RIDs were all 1% or less. The mean adult plasma level following a 1,000 mg dose is about 90 mcg/mL. The manufacturer recommends that patients consider not nursing while this drug is administered. However, breastfeeding while using this drug should be based on the mother's clinical need for treatment versus any potential infant risks that might occur. If used, the infant should be monitored for the most common reported adult side effects of nausea, pruritus, and abdominal cramps (all leading to irritability), diarrhea, flushing, rash, vomiting, and various laboratory abnormalities (see PI).

References

1. Prescribing Information. Azactam. E. R. Squibb & Sons; 2017.
2. Furuhashi T, Kato I, Igarashi Y, Nakayoshi H. Toxicity study of azthreonam: fertility study in rats. *Chemotherapy*. 1985;33:190-202. As cited in Shepard TH. *Catalog of Teratogenic Agents*. 6th ed. Johns Hopkins University Press; 1989:66.
3. Furuhashi T, Ushida K, Sato K, Nakayoshi H. Toxicity study on azthreonam: teratology study in rats. *Chemotherapy*. 1985;33:203-218. As cited in Shepard TH. *Catalog of Teratogenic Agents*. 6th ed. Johns Hopkins University Press; 1989:66.
4. Furuhashi T, Ushida K, Kakei A, Nakayoshi H. Toxicity study on azthreonam: perinatal and postnatal study in rats. *Chemotherapy*. 1985;33:219-231. As cited in Shepard TH. *Catalog of Teratogenic Agents*. 6th ed. Johns Hopkins University Press; 1989:66.
5. Singhvi SM, Ita CE, Shaw JM, et al. Distribution of aztreonam into fetuses and milk of rats. *Antimicrob Agents Chemother*. 1984;26:132-135.
6. Hayashi R, Devlin RG, Frantz M, Stern M. Concentration of aztreonam in body fluids in mid-pregnancy (abstract). *Clin Pharmacol Ther*. 1984;35:246.
7. Ito K, Hirose R, Tamaya T, et al. Pharmacokinetic and clinical studies on aztreonam in the perinatal period. *Jpn J Antibiot*. 1990;43:719-726.
8. Matsuda S, Oh K, Hirayama H. Transplacental transfer and clinical application of aztreonam. *Jpn J Antibiot*. 1990;43:700-705.
9. Obata I, Yamato T, Hayashi S, et al. Pharmacokinetic study of aztreonam transfer from mother to fetus. *Jpn J Antibiot*. 1990;43:70-80.
10. Cho N, Fukunaga K, Kunii K, Kobayashi I. Studies on aztreonam in the perinatal period. *Jpn J Antibiot*. 1990;43:706-718.
11. Nau H. Clinical pharmacokinetics in pregnancy and perinatology. II. Penicillins. *Dev Pharmacol Ther*. 1987;10:174-198.
12. Cook V, Allen S, Summersgill J, Gall S. The pharmacokinetics of aztreonam during pregnancy (abstract). *Am J Obstet Gynecol*. 1994;170:420.
13. Itakura A, Kurauchi O, Mizutani S, et al. The levels of aztreonam in the cord bloods and tissues after administration to pregnant women. *Jpn J Antibiot*. 1995;48:749-753.
14. Fleiss PM, Richwald GA, Gordon J, et al. Aztreonam in human serum and breast milk. *Br J Clin Pharmacol*. 1985;19:509-511.

B

BACITRACIN

Antibacterial

PREGNANCY RECOMMENDATION: Limited Human Data—No Relevant Animal Data

BREASTFEEDING RECOMMENDATION: Probably Compatible

PREGNANCY SUMMARY

The Collaborative Perinatal Project reported 18 patients with first-trimester exposure (route of administration not specified) to bacitracin, and no association with newborn malformations was found. When used topically or ophthalmically, a clinically insignificant amount of the drug may reach the fetal circulation. A greater fetal exposure would probably occur if administered intramuscularly (IM), but again, the amount reaching the fetus would probably be small. Therefore, this limited human pregnancy experience prevents a complete assessment of the embryofetal risk. Animal reproduction studies have not been performed. Using this drug during pregnancy should be based on the pros and cons of the mother's clinical need for treatment versus any potential fetal risk that might occur from exposure.

BREASTFEEDING SUMMARY

No reports describing the use of bacitracin during human lactation have been located. When administered topically or ophthalmically, a clinically insignificant amount of the drug may be found in breast milk. When administered IM, a limited amount of the drug may be excreted into breast milk. Nevertheless, because it is a polypeptide, if the drug were to be ingested through breastfeeding, it would probably be digested in the infant's gastrointestinal tract and not be absorbed. Breastfeeding while using this drug should be based on the mother's clinical need for treatment. If used, the infant should be monitored for the most common reported adult side effects of nausea (leading to irritability), vomiting, and rash.

References

1. Prescribing Information. Bacitracin. Pharmacia & Upjohn; 2018.
2. Heinonen OP, Slone D, Shapiro S. *Birth Defects and Drugs in Pregnancy*. Publishing Sciences Group; 1983:297, 301.

BACLOFEN

Miscellaneous (Skeletal Muscle Relaxant)

PREGNANCY RECOMMENDATION: Limited Human Data—No Relevant Animal Data

BREASTFEEDING RECOMMENDATION: Probably Compatible

PREGNANCY SUMMARY

In a study from the European Network of Teratogen Information Services (ENTIS—6 European teratogen information centers and 16 French pharmacovigilance centers), baclofen exposure during the first trimester was reported in 134 patients, with 5 (3.7%) anomalies identified. This rate falls within the expected range for major anomalies in pregnancy of 2% to 4%. There was no pattern to the five anomalies. However, the authors reported an anomaly rate of only about 1% in 400 controls, so this comparison was significant. We also identified 19 case reports involving 21 deliveries with first-trimester exposure to baclofen. Of these, 13 births were exposed to intrathecal baclofen and 8 to oral baclofen (four with daily doses of ≤40 mg and four with daily doses of 80-160 mg). No anomalies were reported. None of the neonates demonstrated any signs of withdrawal postdelivery when exposed to the drug intrathecally or with oral doses of 40 mg/day or less. All four neonates exposed to daily dosages of 80 to 160 mg exhibited signs of withdrawal. All four neonates were successfully treated with baclofen tapers and did well. The drug crosses the placenta, so fetal exposure will occur. However, this limited human pregnancy experience still prevents a complete assessment of the embryofetal risk. Animal reproduction studies only showed embryofetal toxicity at doses of more than 10 times the maximum recommended human dose (MRHD) that were also associated with maternal toxicity. Using this drug during pregnancy should be based on the pros and cons of the mother's clinical need for treatment versus any potential fetal risk that might occur from exposure. Lastly, the drug has been associated with seizures following acute or abrupt withdrawal in patients using the drug chronically.

BREASTFEEDING SUMMARY

Three studies were located that analyzed baclofen levels in breast milk: with intrathecal use, after a single 20 mg oral dose, and in a patient receiving 80 mg orally per day. The breast milk levels were low, ranging from 0.6 ng/mL (with intrathecal use) to 380 ng/mL (with a mother taking 80 mg/d orally). In the highest-dose exposure, it was determined that the infant would receive a daily dose of about 0.05 mg/kg of the drug or about 4% of the maternal weight-adjusted dose. Three other case reports describe infants exposed to baclofen during breastfeeding, and no adverse effects related to the drug were noted. Thus, small amounts of the drug are excreted into breast milk, but levels are low and probably not clinically significant. Breastfeeding while using this drug should be based on the mother's clinical need for treatment. If used, the infant should be monitored for the most common reported adult side effects of somnolence, lethargy, and irritability.

References

1. Prescribing Information. Baclofen. Metacel Pharmaceuticals, LLC; 2019.
2. Balakirouchenane D, Khoudour N, Couchana L, et al. Pharmacokinetics of baclofen in a full-term newborn after intrauterine exposure: a case report. *Neonatology*. 2021;118:624-627.
3. Bernard N, Beghin D, Huttel E, et al. Pregnancy outcome after in utero exposure to baclofen: an ENTIS collaborative study. *Birth Defects Res*. 2014;100:525.
4. Delhaas EM, Verhagen J. Pregnancy in a quadriplegic patient treated with continuous intrathecal baclofen infusion to manage her severe spasticity. Case report. *Paraplegia*. 1992;30:527-528.
5. Munoz FC, Marco DG, Perez AV, Camacho MM. Pregnancy outcome in a woman exposed to continuous intrathecal baclofen infusion. *Ann Pharmacother*. 2000;34:956.
6. Engrand N, Van de Perre P, Vilain G, Benhamou D. Intrathecal baclofen for severe tetanus in a pregnant woman. *Eur J Anaesthesiol*. 2001;18:261-263.
7. Roberts AG, Graves CR, Konrad PE, et al. Intrathecal baclofen pump implantation during pregnancy. *Neurology*. 2003;61:1156-1157.
8. Dalton CM, Keenan E, Jarrett L, et al. The safety of baclofen in pregnancy: intrathecal therapy in multiple sclerosis. *Mult Scler*. 2008;14:571-572.
9. Ali Sakr Esa W, Toma I, Tetzlaff JE, Barsoum S. Epidural analgesia in labor for a woman with an intrathecal baclofen pump. *Int J Obstet Anesth*. 2009;18:64-66.
10. DeVries-Rio M, Warren D, Delaney G, et al. Intrathecal baclofen and pregnancy: implications for clinical care. *Can J Neurosci Nurs*. 2009;31:21-24.
11. Morton CM, Rosenow J, Wong C, Kirschner KL. Intrathecal baclofen administration during pregnancy: a case series and focused clinical review. *PM R*. 2009;1:1025-1029.
12. Tandon SS, Hoskins I, Azhar S. Intrathecal baclofen pump—a viable therapeutic option in pregnancy. *Obstet Med*. 2010;3:119-120.
13. Mendez-Lucena C, Chacon Pena J, Garcia-Moreno JM. Intrathecal baclofen for dystonia treatment during pregnancy: a case report. *Neurologia*. 2016;31:131-132.
14. Hara T, Nakajima M, Sugano H, et al. Pregnancy and breastfeeding during intrathecal baclofen therapy—a case study and review. *NMC Case Rep J*. 2018;25:65-68.
15. Ratnayaka BDM, Dhaliwal H, Watkin S. Neonatal convulsions after withdrawal of baclofen. *BMJ*. 2001;323:85.
16. Moran LR, Almeida PG, Worden S, Huttner KM. Intrauterine baclofen exposure: a multidisciplinary approach. *Pediatrics*. 2004;114:e267-e269.
17. Weatherby SJM, Woolner P, Clarke CE. Pregnancy in stiff-limb syndrome. *Mov Disord*. 2004;19:852-854.
18. Goldkamp J, Blaskiewicz R, Myles T. Stiff person syndrome and pregnancy. *Obstet Gynecol*. 2011;118:454-457.
19. Duncan SD, Devlin LA. Use of baclofen for withdrawal in a preterm infant. *J Perinatol*. 2013;33:327-328.
20. Freeman EH, Delaney RM. Neonatal baclofen withdrawal: a report of an infant presenting with severe feeding difficulties. *J Pediatr Nurs*. 2016;31:346-349.
21. Mousigian MA, Rosenblum SA, Knierbein EEN, Daunter AK. Neonatal baclofen withdrawal following intrauterine exposure. *J Pediatr Rehabil Med*. 2022;15:389-394.
22. Eriksson G, Swahn C-G. Concentrations of baclofen in serum and breast milk from a lactating woman. *Scand J Clin Lab Invest*. 1981;41:185-187.
23. Lin HH, Barton N, Wiegand TJ. Baclofen distribution into breast milk—a potential for toxicity? *J Med Toxicol*. 2014;10:86. Abstract.

BALOXAVIR MARBOXIL

Antiviral (Endonuclease Inhibitor)

PREGNANCY RECOMMENDATION: No Human Data—Animal Data Suggest Low Risk

BREASTFEEDING RECOMMENDATION: Probably Compatible

PREGNANCY SUMMARY

No reports describing the use of baloxavir marboxil in human pregnancy have been located. The drug will probably cross the placenta, so some fetal exposure will likely occur. Therefore, the absence of human pregnancy experience prevents a complete assessment of the embryofetal risk. Animal studies did not show any embryofetal toxicity. Using this drug during pregnancy should be based on the pros and cons of the mother's clinical need for treatment versus any potential fetal risk that might occur from exposure.

B

BREASTFEEDING SUMMARY

No reports describing the use of baloxavir marboxil during human lactation have been located. The drug will probably be found in breast milk, so some infant exposure will likely occur. Breastfeeding while using this drug should be based on the mother's clinical need for treatment. If used, the infant should be monitored for the most common reported adult side effects of nausea and headache (both leading to irritability), diarrhea, and sinusitis.

Reference

1. Prescribing Information. Xofluza. Genentech USA, Inc; 2023.

BALSALAZIDE

Gastrointestinal

PREGNANCY RECOMMENDATION: Human Data Suggest Low Risk

BREASTFEEDING RECOMMENDATION: Probably Compatible

PREGNANCY SUMMARY

Data from published cohort studies, case reports, and a meta-analysis have not shown an increased risk for birth anomalies or poor pregnancy outcome in pregnant patients exposed to mesalamine, the active metabolite for balsalazide (see Mesalamine). A limited amount of the drug will probably cross the placenta, but fetal exposure is probably clinically insignificant. Animal studies did not show any embryofetal toxicity. Using this drug during pregnancy should be based on the pros and cons of the mother's clinical need for treatment versus any potential fetal risk that might occur from exposure.

BREASTFEEDING SUMMARY

No reports describing the use of balsalazide during human lactation have been located. In studies on mesalamine, the active metabolite of balsalazide, only small amounts are absorbed into the systemic circulation (see Mesalamine). Mesalamine has been detected in human breast milk at levels from non-detectable to 0.5 mg/L. Based on these concentrations, the relative infant dose (RID) is only about 0.1%. Breastfeeding while using this drug should be based on the mother's clinical need for treatment. If used, the infant should be monitored for the most common reported adult side effects of nausea, headache, abdominal pain, and arthralgia (all leading to irritability), diarrhea, vomiting, and respiratory infection.

Reference

1. Prescribing Information. Balsalazide. Salix Pharmaceuticals; 2022.

BARICITINIB

Immunologic (Kinase Inhibitor)

PREGNANCY RECOMMENDATION: Limited Human Data—Animal Data Suggest Low Risk

BREASTFEEDING RECOMMENDATION: Potential Toxicity

PREGNANCY SUMMARY

Published data on a limited number of patients with pregnancy exposure to baricitinib did not show an increased risk for fetal malformations. The spontaneous abortion rate was higher than expected, but many of these patients were also exposed to methotrexate or combinations of other antirheumatic drugs. Baricitinib most likely will cross the placenta, so some fetal exposure will probably occur. Therefore, this limited human pregnancy experience prevents a complete assessment of the embryofetal risk. Animal studies did not show any increased risk for embryofetal toxicity. Using this drug during pregnancy should be based on the pros and cons of the mother's clinical need for treatment versus any potential fetal risk that might occur from exposure. There is a pregnancy exposure registry that monitors pregnancy outcomes in women using this drug. Health care providers and patients are encouraged to call Eli Lilly and Company at 1-800-545-5979.

BREASTFEEDING SUMMARY

No reports describing the use of baricitinib during human lactation have been located. The drug will probably be found in breast milk. However, due to the concern for potential serious adverse effects that might be seen in a breastfed infant, the manufacturer recommends that women not breastfeed while being treated with this drug and for at least 4 days after the last dose. Nevertheless, breastfeeding while using this drug should be based on the mother's clinical need for treatment. If used, the infant should be monitored for the most common reported adult side effects of nausea, headache, and abdominal pain (all leading to irritability), upper respiratory tract infection, urinary tract infection, and various laboratory abnormalities (see Prescribing Information [PI]).

References

1. Prescribing Information. Olumiant. Eli Lilly; 2022.
2. Bergamini B, Seneschal J, Meyers KJ, et al. Pregnancy outcomes in patients exposed to baricitinib in clinical trials and during post-marketing surveillance. *Br J Dermatol*. 2023 August/online ahead of print.
3. Costanzo G, Firinu D, Losa F, et al. Baricitinib exposure during pregnancy in rheumatoid arthritis. *Ther Adv Musculoskelet Dis*. 2020;12:1-3.

BASILIXIMAB

Immunologic (Monoclonal Antibody)

PREGNANCY RECOMMENDATION: *No Human Data—Animal Data Suggest Low Risk

BREASTFEEDING RECOMMENDATION: Probably Compatible

PREGNANCY SUMMARY

No reports describing the use of basiliximab in human pregnancy have been located. As an immunoglobulin G (IgG) antibody, it likely crosses the placenta, especially during the second half of pregnancy, so some fetal exposure will probably occur. Therefore, the absence of human pregnancy experience prevents a complete assessment of the embryofetal risk. Animal studies did not show any embryofetal toxicity. Based on the drug's mechanism of action, the manufacturer recommends that women with reproductive potential use effective contraception during treatment and for 4 months after the last dose. *Nevertheless, the use of this drug during pregnancy is not likely to occur because it is used twice as an induction immunosuppressant in patients receiving a renal transplant.

BREASTFEEDING SUMMARY

No reports describing the use of basiliximab during human lactation have been located. It is known that IgG antibodies can be found in human breast milk but are not found in the neonatal or infant circulation. Additionally, if any IgG antibodies were to be ingested through breastfeeding, they would probably be digested in the infant's gastrointestinal tract and not be absorbed. Breastfeeding while using this drug should be based on the mother's clinical need for treatment. If used, the infant should be monitored for the most common reported adult side effects of nausea, headache, and abdominal pain (all leading to irritability), diarrhea, vomiting, constipation, fever, peripheral edema, and various laboratory abnormalities (see PI).

Reference

1. Prescribing Information. Simulect. Novartis Pharmaceuticals; 2016.

BAZEDOXIFENE AND CONJUGATED ESTROGENS

CONTRACEPTIVE

SEE ORAL CONTRACEPTIVES

BECLOMETHASONE

Respiratory (Corticosteroid—Asthma—Inhaler/Nasal/Topical)

PREGNANCY RECOMMENDATION: Human Data Suggest Low Risk

BREASTFEEDING RECOMMENDATION: Probably Compatible

PREGNANCY SUMMARY

Three studies were located that specifically evaluated the risk for major birth anomalies with first-trimester use of inhaled beclomethasone in patients with asthma. The rate of major anomalies in more than 450 cases was 3.7%, which falls within the expected rate. In two other large studies evaluating the risk of major anomalies in more than 14,000 pregnant patients using inhaled corticosteroids, the rate overall was about 5.6%. However, no pattern was seen with the anomalies, and the

(continued)

B

severity of disease and coexposure to other drugs could increase the risk. Specific information regarding the number of cases with beclomethasone inhalation in these large studies was not provided. Data on the risk for birth anomalies with the use of beclomethasone nasal spray were limited, but fetal exposure to the drug is lower with intranasal use than that seen with inhalation use. The drug will probably cross the placenta, but the overall amount is likely to be minimal. Animal studies did show embryofetal toxicity with malformations in two species with doses less than 10 times the recommended human dose (RHD), but were not seen in a third species with doses more than 10 times the RHD. Women who are pregnant and have taken asthma medications during pregnancy are encouraged to contact MotherToBaby Pregnancy Studies at 877-311-8972. The most recent American College of Obstetricians and Gynecologists (ACOG) publication on asthma in pregnancy (published in 2008—reaffirmed in 2020) and the 2023 Global Initiative for Asthma (GINA) guidelines state that the advantages of actively treating asthma in pregnancy markedly outweigh the potential risks of the medications. Inhaled corticosteroids are usually the first-line treatment for mild to moderate persistent asthma in pregnancy. Listed alternative treatments include cromolyn, theophylline, or leukotriene receptor antagonists. However, ACOG recommends long-acting β_2-agonists as the preferred add-on drug when pregnant patients are not controlled with inhaled corticosteroids. The reasoning for this is that long-acting inhaled β_2-agonists have been shown to be more effective as an add-on treatment in nonpregnant patients; whereas, theophylline has more side effects and requires serum monitoring, and there are minimal data on the leukotriene receptor antagonists in human pregnancy.

BREASTFEEDING SUMMARY

No reports describing the use of beclomethasone during human lactation have been located. The drug may be found in breast milk, but the levels are likely to be negligible. Breastfeeding while using this drug should be based on the mother's clinical need for treatment versus any potential infant risks that might occur. If used, the infant should be monitored for the most common reported adult side effects of headache (leading to irritability) and upper respiratory tract infection.

References

1. Joint Committee of the American College of Obstetricians and Gynecologists (ACOG) and the American College of Allergy, Asthma, and Immunology (ACAAI). Position statement: the use of newer asthma and allergy medications during pregnancy. *Ann Allergy Asthma Immunol*. 2000;84:475-480.
2. Prescribing Information. QVAR. Teva Pharmaceuticals USA; 2021.
3. Brown HM, Storey G. Treatment of allergy of the respiratory tract with beclomethasone dipropionate steroid aerosol. *Postgrad Med J*. 1975;51(suppl 4):59-64.
4. Greenberger PA, Patterson R. Beclomethasone dipropionate for severe asthma during pregnancy. *Ann Intern Med*. 1983;98:478-480.
5. Dombrowski MP, Schatz M, Wise R, et al.; for the National Institute of Child Health and Human Development Maternal-Fetal Medicine Units Network, and the National Heart, Lung, and Blood Institute. Randomized trial of inhaled beclomethasone dipropionate versus theophylline for moderate asthma during pregnancy. *Am J Obstet Gynecol*. 2004;190:737-744.
6. Namazy J, Schatz M, Long L, et al. Use of inhaled steroids by pregnant asthmatic women does not reduce intrauterine growth. *J Allergy Clin Immunol*. 2004;113:427-432.
7. Rahimi R, Nikfar S, Abdollahi M. Meta-analysis finds use of inhaled corticosteroids during pregnancy safe: a systematic meta-analysis review. *Hum Exp Toxicol*. 2006;25:447-452.
8. Murphy VE, Fittock RJ, Zarzycki PK, et al. Metabolism of synthetic steroids by the human placenta. *Placenta*. 2007;28:39-46.
9. de Aguiar MM, da Silva HJ, Rizzo JA, et al. Inhaled beclomethasone in pregnancy asthmatic women—a systematic review. *Allergol Immunopathol*. 2014;42:493-499.
10. American College of Obstetricians and Gynecologists—Asthma in Pregnancy. ACOG Practice Bulletin No. 90. *Obstet Gynecol*. *2008*;111:457-464. Reaffirmed 2020.

BEDAQUILINE

Anti-Infective (Antituberculosis)

PREGNANCY RECOMMENDATION: Limited Human Data—Animal Data Suggest Low Risk

BREASTFEEDING RECOMMENDATION: Probably Compatible

PREGNANCY SUMMARY

A case report described the use of bedaquiline and linezolid in a pregnant woman with drug-resistant tuberculosis. Treatment was started at 36 weeks' gestation, and the infant was delivered at 39 weeks with no complications. No abnormalities were noted in the child at birth and for 2 years after delivery. The drug will probably cross the placenta, so some fetal exposure will likely occur. Therefore, this limited human experience prevents a complete assessment of the embryofetal risk. Animal studies did not show any embryofetal toxicity. In 2013, the US Centers for Disease Control and Prevention (CDC) recommendations for multidrug-resistant tuberculosis in pregnancy stated that bedaquiline could be considered for use in pregnancy when treatment options were limited. Using this drug during pregnancy should be based on the pros and cons of the mother's clinical need for treatment versus any potential fetal risk that might occur from exposure. The drug can also prolong the QT interval.

B

BREASTFEEDING SUMMARY

No reports describing the use of bedaquiline during human lactation have been located. The drug will probably be found in breast milk, so some infant exposure will likely occur. Breastfeeding while using this drug should be based on the mother's clinical need for treatment. If used, the infant should be monitored for the most common reported adult side effects of nausea, headache, arthralgia, chest pain, and abdominal pain (all leading to irritability) and elevated liver function tests.

References

1. Prescribing Information. Sirturo. Janssen Products, LP; 2021.
2. Centers for Disease Control and Prevention. Provisional CDC guidelines for the use and safety monitoring of bedaquiline fumarate (Sirturo) for the treatment of multidrug-resistant tuberculosis. *MMWR Recomm Rep*. 2013; 62:1-12.
3. Jaspard M, Elefany-Amoura E, Melonio I, et al. Bedaquiline and linezolid for extensively drug-resistant tuberculosis in pregnant women. *Emerg Infect Dis*. 2017;23:1731-1732.

BELANTAMAB MAFODOTIN

Antineoplastic (Monoclonal Antibody)

PREGNANCY RECOMMENDATION: *Contraindicated

BREASTFEEDING RECOMMENDATION: *Contraindicated

PREGNANCY SUMMARY

No reports describing the use of belantamab mafodotin in human or animal pregnancies have been located. Therefore, the absence of human pregnancy experience prevents a complete assessment of the embryofetal risk. Because it is an antibody of the IgG class, it probably crosses the placenta. The drug is composed of three components: the antibody, a protease-resistant linker, and a microtubule inhibitor (monomethylauristatin F [MMAF]). *Because MMAF specifically targets actively dividing cells, leading to cell death, the manufacturer recommends that the drug not be used during pregnancy. However, there could be clinical cases where a pregnant woman with advanced multiple myeloma might consider treatment based on the gestational age and an in-depth discussion of the pros and cons. The manufacturer also recommends effective contraception for women of childbearing age while receiving this treatment and for 4 months after the last dose. They also recommend that males with female partners of reproductive potential use effective contraception during treatment and for 6 months after the last dose. Belantamab mafodotin can cause serious ocular toxicity and may also produce thrombocytopenia. There is a registry for women who are pregnant and have cancer. For more information, women and health care providers are encouraged to contact the Cancer and Pregnancy Registry at 1-877-635-4499.

BREASTFEEDING SUMMARY

Belantamab mafodotin probably enters breast milk. However, if used while breastfeeding, newborn effects from the antibody portion would most likely be negligible due to probable digestion of the antibody in the infant's gastrointestinal tract. *However, absorption of the microtubule inhibitor MMAF by itself is possible. Based on the mechanism of action of MMAF and the significant risk for serious adverse side effects, the manufacturer recommends that pregnant women not breastfeed while being treated with this drug and for up to 3 months after the last dose.

Reference

1. Prescribing Information. Blenrep. GlaxoSmithKline Research Triangle Park; 2020.

BELATACEPT

Immunologic (Fc Antibody Fragment—Selective T-Cell Costimulation Blocker)

PREGNANCY RECOMMENDATION: Limited Human Data—Animal Data Suggest Low Risk

BREASTFEEDING RECOMMENDATION: Probably Compatible

PREGNANCY SUMMARY

A case series of 13 patients with 17 pregnancies on belatacept during the first trimester and continuing through gestation reported 14 live births with no identified anomalies and 3 (17.6%) spontaneous abortions. Of the 14 deliveries, 6 (43%) were preterm (34-36 weeks' gestation), but the reason for preterm delivery was not fully supplied. Because it is the Fc

(*continued*)

B

portion of an antibody, the drug will probably cross the placenta, so some fetal exposure will likely occur. Therefore, this limited human experience prevents a complete assessment of the embryofetal risk. Animal reproduction studies did not show any embryofetal toxicity. Using this drug during pregnancy should be based on the pros and cons of the mother's clinical need for treatment versus any potential fetal risk that might occur from exposure. There is a pregnancy exposure registry that monitors pregnancy outcomes in women using this drug. Health care providers are encouraged to call the Transplant Pregnancy Registry International at 1-877-955-6877. If belatacept is used in combination with mycophenolate mofetil, then use may be contraindicated (see Mycophenolate).

BREASTFEEDING SUMMARY

A case series reported eight patients who breastfed following delivery. The patients were on belatacept during the pregnancy and continued postdelivery. No complications or reports of newborn difficulties were described. It is known that IgG antibodies can be found in human breast milk, but are not found in the neonatal or infant circulation. Additionally, if any IgG antibodies were to be ingested through breastfeeding, they would probably be digested in the infant's gastrointestinal tract and not be absorbed. Breastfeeding while using this drug should be based on the mother's clinical need for treatment. If used, the infant should be monitored for the most common reported adult side effects of nausea and headache (both leading to irritability), diarrhea, vomiting, constipation, pyrexia, peripheral edema, cough, and various laboratory abnormalities (see PI). If used in combination with mycophenolate mofetil, breastfeeding may be contraindicated (see Mycophenolate).

References

1. Prescribing Information. Nulojix. Bristol-Myers Squibb; 2021.
2. Coscia L, Cohen D, Dube GK, et al. Outcomes with belatacept exposure during pregnancy in kidney transplant recipients: a case series. *Transplantation*. 2023;107:2047-2054.
3. Combs J, Kagan A, Boelkins M, et al. Belatacept during pregnancy in renal transplant recipients: two case reports. *Am J Transplant*. 2018;18:2079-2082.
4. Kintmalm GB, Gunby RT. Successful pregnancy in a liver transplant recipient on belatacept. *Liver Transpl*. 2020;26:1193-1194.

BELIMUMAB

Immunologic (Monoclonal Antibody)

PREGNANCY RECOMMENDATION: Limited Human Data—Animal Data Suggest Low Risk

BREASTFEEDING RECOMMENDATION: Probably Compatible

PREGNANCY SUMMARY

Several studies and case reports on the use of belimumab during human pregnancy have been located. Some patients are included in more than one publication, but to fully reconcile this is not possible. The data primarily come from the clinical trials, the belimumab pregnancy registry, the World Health Organization Pharmacovigilance database (VigiBase), and the EudraVigilance database. Over 400 belimumab exposures were described, and the rates of reported birth anomalies ranged from 1% to 20%. However, there were no patterns to the anomalies; some would not be caused by a drug, and some anomalies could be genetic (or family history) in origin. In addition, all of the studies were compounded by the fact that the patients had significant medical issues related to systemic lupus erythematosus and were often on numerous other medications during the first trimester, many of which are known to cause poor pregnancy outcomes (such as methotrexate). Finally, poor outcomes may be disproportionately reported to some of these databases compared with normal outcomes. Because the drug is an IgG antibody, it should not cross the placenta in any clinically significant amount during the first trimester. Belimumab has been shown to cross the placenta at the end of pregnancy, which would be expected. Nevertheless, this human pregnancy experience still prevents a complete assessment of the embryofetal risk. The manufacturer states that if prevention of pregnancy is warranted, then women with reproductive potential should use effective contraception during treatment with belimumab and for 1 week after the last dose. There is a belimumab pregnancy exposure registry that monitors pregnancy outcomes in women using this drug. Health care providers are encouraged to call 1-877-311-8972.

BREASTFEEDING SUMMARY

Two reports describing the use of belimumab during human lactation have been located. In both cases, the breastfed infants did well with no reported adverse reactions. The breast milk levels were low, at about 1/200 to 1/500 of those found in the maternal serum. This verifies that the drug, as an IgG antibody, can be found in breast milk. However, as an IgG antibody, it would likely be digested in the infant's gastrointestinal tract and not be absorbed. Breastfeeding while using this drug should be based on the mother's clinical need for treatment. If used, the infant should be monitored for the most common reported adult side effects of nausea, headache, and

B

extremity pain (all leading to irritability), diarrhea, pyrexia, insomnia, and nasopharyngitis.

References

1. Prescribing Information. Benlysta. Glaxo Smith Klein LLC; 2023.
2. Bitter H, Warren DJ, Bolstad N, et al. Transplacental passage of belimumab during pregnancy and follow-up of a child exposed in utero. *Ann Rheum Dis*. 2023;82:577-579.
3. Petri M, Landy H, Clowse MEB, et al. Belimumab use during pregnancy: a summary of birth defects and pregnancy loss from belimumab clinical trials, a pregnancy registry and postmarketing reports. *Ann Rheum Dis*. 2023;82:217-225.
4. Juliao P, Wurst K, Pimenta JM, et al. Belimumab use during pregnancy: interim results of the belimumab pregnancy registry. *Birth Defects Res*. 2023; 115:188-204.
5. Dernoncourt A, Liabeuf S, Bennis Y, et al. Fetal and neonatal adverse drug reactions associated with biologics taken during pregnancy with autoimmune diseases: insights from an analysis of the World Health Organization Pharmacovigilance database (VigiBase). *BioDrugs*. 2023;37:73-87.
6. Ghalandari N, Crijns HJMJ, Bergman JEH, et al. Reported congenital malformations after exposure to non-tumor necrosis factor inhibitor biologics: a retrospective comparative study in EudraVigilance. *Br J Clin Pharmacol*. 2022;88:5378-5388.
7. Ghalandari N, Crijns HJMJ, Dolhain RJEM, et al. Dilemma of belimumab therapy (dis) continuation during pregnancy: results of a retrospective study in EudraVigilance. *Lupus*. 2023;32:189-197.
8. Danve A, Perry L, Deodhar A. Use of belimumab throughout pregnancy to treat active systemic lupus erythematosus-a case report. *Semin Arthritis Rheum*. 2014;44:195-197.
9. Emmi G, Silvestri E, Squatrito D. Favorable pregnancy outcome in a patient with systemic lupus erythematosus treated with belimumab: a confirmation report. *Semin Arthritis Rheum*. 2016;25:e26-e27.
10. Kumthekar A, Danve A, Deodhar A. Use of belimumab throughout 2 consecutive pregnancies with systemic lupus erythematosus. *J Rheumatol*. 2017; 44:1416-1417.
11. Bitter H, Bendvold AN, Ostensen ME. Lymphocyte changes and vaccination response in a child exposed to belimumab during pregnancy. *Ann Rheum Dis*. 2018;77:1692-1693.
12. Kao JH, Lan TY, Lu CH, et al. Pregnancy outcomes in patients treated with belimumab: report from real-world experience. *Semin Arthritis Rheum*. 2021;51:963-968.
13. Lai Y, Li B, Huang J, et al. Different pregnancy outcomes in patients with systemic lupus erythematosus treated with belimumab. *Lupus*. 2023;31: 149-154.
14. Nakai T, Ikeda Y, Yamaguchi K, et al. A case report of two systemic lupus erythematosus pregnancies with early placental exposure to belimumab: case report with review. *Mod Rheumatol Case Rep*. 2023;7:82-86.
15. Wei SR, Zhu ZZ, Xu J, Mo HY. Favorable pregnancy outcomes in two patients with systemic lupus erythematosus treated with belimumab. *Int J Rheum Dis*. 2023;26:154-156.
16. Saito J, Yakuwa N, Ishizuka T, et al. Belimumab concentrations in maternal serum and breast milk during breastfeeding and the safety assessment of the infant: a case study. *Breastfeed Med*. 2020;15:475-457.

BELINOSTAT

Antineoplastic (Histone Deacetylase Inhibitor)

PREGNANCY RECOMMENDATION: **No Human Data and No Relevant Animal Data**

BREASTFEEDING RECOMMENDATION: **Potential Toxicity**

PREGNANCY SUMMARY

No reports describing the use of belinostat in human pregnancy have been located. Based on likely placental transfer, some fetal exposure will probably occur. Therefore, the absence of human pregnancy experience prevents a complete assessment of the embryofetal risk. Animal reproduction studies have not been performed. Based on the drug's mechanism of action, the manufacturer recommends that women with reproductive potential use effective contraception during treatment and for 6 months after the last dose. They also recommend that males with female partners of reproductive potential use effective contraception during treatment and for 3 months after the last dose. Nevertheless, using this drug during pregnancy should be based on the pros and cons of the mother's clinical need for treatment versus any potential fetal risk that might occur from exposure. Women who are pregnant and have cancer are encouraged to contact the Cancer and Pregnancy Registry at 1-877-635-4499.

BREASTFEEDING SUMMARY

No reports describing the use of belinostat during human lactation have been located. The drug will probably be found in breast milk, so some infant exposure will likely occur. Due to the concern for potential serious adverse effects that might be seen in a breastfed infant, the manufacturer recommends that women not breastfeed while being treated with this drug and for at least 2 weeks after the last dose. Nevertheless, breastfeeding while using this drug should be based on the mother's clinical need for treatment. If used, the infant should be monitored for the most common reported adult side effects of nausea (leading to irritability), vomiting, pyrexia, lethargy, and anemia.

Reference

1. Prescribing Information. Beleodaq. Acrotech Biopharma, Inc; 2023.

BELUMOSUDIL

Immunologic (Kinase Inhibitor)

PREGNANCY RECOMMENDATION: **No Human Data—Animal Data Suggest Risk**

BREASTFEEDING RECOMMENDATION: **Potential Toxicity**

B

PREGNANCY SUMMARY

No reports describing the use of belumosudil in human pregnancy have been located. Belumosudil will likely cross the placenta, so some fetal exposure will probably occur. Therefore, the absence of human pregnancy experience prevents a complete assessment of embryofetal risk. Embryofetal toxicity with malformations was observed in animal studies. Based on animal studies and the drug's mechanism of action, the manufacturer recommends that women with reproductive potential use effective contraception during treatment and for 1 week after the last dose. They also recommend that males with female partners of reproductive potential use effective contraception during treatment and for 1 week after the last dose. Nevertheless, using this drug during pregnancy should be based on the pros and cons of the mother's clinical need for treatment versus any potential fetal risk that might occur from exposure. Hypertension was reported in up to 21% of patients treated with this drug in the clinical trials.

BREASTFEEDING SUMMARY

No reports describing the use of belumosudil during human lactation have been located. The drug will likely be found in breast milk, so some infant exposure will probably occur. Based on animal studies and the drug's mechanism of action, the manufacturer recommends that women not breastfeed while being treated with this drug and for at least 1 week after the last dose. Nevertheless, breastfeeding while using this drug should be based on the mother's clinical need for treatment. If used, the infant should be monitored for the most common reported adult side effects of nausea, abdominal pain, musculoskeletal pain, and headache (all leading to irritability), infections, diarrhea, cough, edema, hypertension, and various laboratory abnormalities (see PI).

Reference

1. Prescribing Information. Rezurock. Kadmon Pharmaceuticals; 2022.

BELZUTIFAN

Antineoplastic (HIF-2alpa Inhibitor)

PREGNANCY RECOMMENDATION: No Human Data—Animal Data Suggest Potential Risk

BREASTFEEDING RECOMMENDATION: Potential Toxicity

PREGNANCY SUMMARY

No reports describing the use of belzutifan in human pregnancy have been located. The drug will likely cross the placenta, so fetal exposure will probably occur. Therefore, the absence of human pregnancy experience prevents a complete assessment of the embryofetal risk. Embryofetal toxicity was observed in animals. Based on the animal studies, the manufacturer recommends that women with reproductive potential use effective contraception during treatment and for 1 week after the last dose. They also recommend that males with female partners of reproductive potential use effective contraception during treatment and for 1 week after the last dose. Nevertheless, using this drug during pregnancy should be based on the pros and cons of the mother's clinical need for treatment versus any potential fetal risk that might occur from exposure. Elevated glucose levels were reported in 34% of patients treated with this drug in the clinical trials. Therefore, if used during pregnancy, glucose levels should be monitored. In addition, hypertension was reported in up to 13% of patients treated with this drug in clinical trials. There is a registry for women who are pregnant and have cancer. For more information, women and health care providers are encouraged to contact the Cancer and Pregnancy Registry at 1-877-635-4499.

BREASTFEEDING SUMMARY

No reports describing the use of belzutifan during human lactation have been located. The drug will likely be found in breast milk, so infant exposure will probably occur. Because of the potential for serious adverse effects that might be seen in a breastfed infant, the manufacturer recommends that women not breastfeed while taking this medication and for 1 week after the last dose. Nevertheless, breastfeeding while using this drug should be based on the mother's clinical need for treatment. If used, the infant should be monitored for the most common reported adult side effects of nausea and headache (both leading to irritability), lethargy, elevated glucose, and other laboratory abnormalities (see PI).

Reference

1. Prescribing Information. Welireg. Merck Sharp & Dohme; 2022.

B

BEMPEDOIC ACID

Antilipemic

PREGNANCY RECOMMENDATION: No Human Data—Animal Data Suggest Low Risk

BREASTFEEDING RECOMMENDATION: Potential Toxicity

PREGNANCY SUMMARY

No reports describing the use of bempedoic acid in human pregnancy have been located. Some amount of the drug will probably cross the placenta. Therefore, the absence of human pregnancy experience prevents a complete assessment of the embryofetal risk. Because bempedoic acid decreases cholesterol synthesis and other substances derived from cholesterol, the manufacturer recommends that the drug be discontinued prior to conception or as soon as pregnancy is recognized unless the benefits of therapy outweigh the potential risk to the fetus. Women who are pregnant and have taken bempedoic acid at any time during pregnancy are encouraged to contact the Bempedoic Acid Pregnancy Surveillance Program at 1-833-377-7633.

BREASTFEEDING SUMMARY

No reports describing the use of bempedoic acid during human lactation have been located. The drug will probably be found in breast milk, but in small amounts. Because of the concern for decreased cholesterol synthesis, the manufacturer recommends that women not breastfeed during treatment with this drug. However, breastfeeding while using this drug should be based on the mother's clinical need for treatment. If used, the infant should be monitored for the most common reported adult side effects of muscle pain, back pain, and abdominal pain (all leading to irritability) and upper respiratory tract infections.

Reference

1. Prescribing Information. Nexletol. Esperion Therapeutics, Inc; 2021.

BENAZEPRIL

Antihypertensive (Angiotensin—Converting Enzyme Inhibitor)

PREGNANCY RECOMMENDATION: Contraindicated (Second and Third Trimesters)

BREASTFEEDING RECOMMENDATION: Probably Compatible

PREGNANCY SUMMARY

Two case reports describing the use of benazepril to treat hypertension in pregnancy with first-trimester exposure were located. Both described the presence of severe oligohydramnios and other findings related to low amniotic fluid levels in the late second trimester. Each patient discontinued the drug, one at 24 weeks' gestation and the other at 27 weeks' gestation, and the findings reversed. Both infants were delivered at term with no abnormalities noted. No other studies specific to benazepril use in pregnancy were found. Regarding angiotensin-converting enzyme (ACE) inhibitors in general, use during the second and third trimesters of pregnancy has been associated with fetal renal toxicity, as stated by the boxed warning for this drug. Numerous cases of severe oligohydramnios leading to findings of limb contractures, craniofacial deformation, and pulmonary hypoplasia with neonatal death have been reported. These fetal renal effects are often permanent, but if the drug is discontinued as soon as possible, they can be reversible in some cases. However, ACE inhibitors should not be used in the second and third trimesters, if at all possible. Regarding first-trimester exposure to ACE inhibitors in general, there was some concern about teratogenicity, especially cardiac and central nervous system. However, 2 large studies of more than 4,450 first-trimester exposures to ACE inhibitors did not find any increased risks for anomalies compared with other pregnant patients with hypertension on treatment with other antihypertensive agents or on no treatment at all. Therefore, the final summary determined that the use of ACE inhibitors in the first trimester did not increase the risk for fetal malformations compared with other pregnant women with hypertension. Benazepril and its active metabolite, benazeprilat, will cross the placenta, so fetal exposure will occur. However, this limited human pregnancy experience with benazepril prevents a complete assessment of the embryofetal risk. Animal reproduction studies did not show any embryofetal toxicity. Women of reproductive age using benazepril should be informed of these risks so that they can closely monitor if pregnancy transpires. If a positive pregnancy test occurs, she and her health care providers can modify treatment (if possible) so that the drug is not used in the second or third trimesters. For treating hypertension in pregnancy, ACOG recommends nifedipine and labetalol as first-line agents.

B

BREASTFEEDING SUMMARY

Benazepril and benazeprilat are excreted into human breast milk. Nine lactating women were given benazepril, and the peak breast milk concentration about 1 hour after drug administration was 0.9 ng/mL, whereas the peak milk level of benazeprilat (its active metabolite) was 2 ng/mL. The RID was less than 0.14%. These results are consistent with the data from other ACE inhibitors (see Captopril and Enalapril) that have been found in low amounts in breast milk and have no adverse effects in nursing infants. Breastfeeding while using this drug should be based on the mother's clinical need for treatment. If used, the infant should be monitored for the most common reported adult side effects of headache (leading to irritability) and cough.

References

1. Prescribing Information. Lotensin. Validus Pharmaceuticals, LLC; 2019.
2. American College of Obstetricians and Gynecologists—Chronic Hypertension in Pregnancy. ACOG Practice Bulletin No. 203. *Obstet Gynecol*. 2019;133:e26-e50.
3. American College of Obstetricians and Gynecologists—Gestational Hypertension and Preeclampsia. ACOG Practice Bulletin No. 222. *Obstet Gynecol*. 2020;135:e237-e260.
4. Chisholm CA, Chescheir NC, Kennedy M. Reversible oligohydramnios in a pregnancy with angiotensin-converting enzyme inhibitor exposure. *Am J Perinatol*. 1997;14:511-513.
5. Muller PR, James A. Pregnancy with prolonged fetal exposure to an angiotensin-converting enzyme inhibitor. *J Perinatol*. 2002;22:582-584.
6. Barr M Jr. Teratogen update: angiotensin-converting enzyme inhibitors. *Teratology*. 1994;50:399-409.
7. Shotan A, Widerhorn J, Hurst A, Elkayam U. Risks of angiotensin-converting enzyme inhibition during pregnancy: experimental and clinical evidence, potential mechanisms, and recommendations for use. *Am J Med*. 1994;96:451-456.
8. Cooper WO, Hernandez-Diaz S, Arbogast PG, et al. Major congenital malformations after first-trimester exposure to ACE inhibitors. *N Engl J Med*. 2006;354:2443-2451.
9. Bateman BT, Patorno E, Desai RJ, et al. Angiotensin-converting enzyme inhibitors and the risk of congenital malformations. *Obstet Gynecol*. 2017;129:174-184.
10. Li DK, Yang C, Andrade S, et al. Maternal exposure to angiotensin converting enzyme inhibitors in the first trimester and risk of malformations in offspring: a retrospective cohort study. *BMJ*. 2011;343:d5931(1-10).
11. Kaiser G, Ackerman R, Dieterle W, Fleiss PM. Benazepril and benazeprilat in human plasma and breast milk (abstract). *Eur J Clin Pharmacol*. 1989;36(suppl):A303. As cited by National Library of Medicine LactMed database, September 7, 2013.

BENDAMUSTINE

Antineoplastic (Alkylating Agent)

PREGNANCY RECOMMENDATION: *No Human Data—Animal Data Suggest Risk

BREASTFEEDING RECOMMENDATION: Potential Toxicity

PREGNANCY SUMMARY

No reports describing the use of bendamustine in human pregnancy have been located. Based on likely placental transfer, some fetal exposure will probably occur. Therefore, the absence of human pregnancy experience prevents a complete assessment of the embryofetal risk. Animal studies did show embryofetal toxicity. Based on the animal studies and the drug's mechanism of action, the manufacturer recommends that women with reproductive potential use effective contraception during treatment and for 6 months after the last dose. They also recommend that males with female partners of reproductive potential use effective contraception during treatment and for 3 months after the last dose. Nevertheless, using this drug during pregnancy should be based on the pros and cons of the mother's clinical need for treatment versus any potential fetal risk that might occur from exposure. *However, other agents in this drug class may be teratogenic in human pregnancy, and combined with the animal data, strongly suggest that bendamustine should not be given in the first trimester, if at all possible. A position statement from the National Study Commission on Cytotoxic Exposure is discussed in the monograph for cyclophosphamide (see Cyclophosphamide). Women who are pregnant and have cancer are encouraged to contact the Cancer and Pregnancy Registry at 1-877-635-4499.

BREASTFEEDING SUMMARY

No reports describing the use of bendamustine during human lactation have been located. The drug will likely be found in breast milk, so some infant exposure will probably occur. Due to the concern for potential serious adverse effects that might be seen in a breastfed infant, the manufacturer recommends that women not breastfeed while being treated with this drug and for at least 1 week after the last dose. Nevertheless, breastfeeding while using this drug should be based on the mother's clinical need for treatment. If used, the infant should be monitored for the most common reported adult side effects of nausea and headache (both leading to irritability), diarrhea, lethargy, vomiting, constipation, rash, pyrexia, and various laboratory abnormalities (see PI).

Reference

1. Prescribing Information. Treanda. Teva Pharmaceuticals USA, Inc; 2019.

B

BENDROFLUMETHIAZIDE

Cardiovascular (Thiazide Diuretic)

PREGNANCY RECOMMENDATION: Limited Human Data—Animal Data Suggest Low Risk

BREASTFEEDING RECOMMENDATION: Probably Compatible

PREGNANCY SUMMARY

The Collaborative Perinatal Project reported on 13 first-trimester exposures to bendroflumethiazide, but specific outcome data for this drug alone were not supplied. There were 206 total first-trimester exposures to all thiazide diuretics, and 12 (5.8%) major malformations were identified. However, no specific pattern was seen, and many of the patients were on other drugs at the time. There were 1,156 exposures (anytime during the pregnancy) to bendroflumethiazide, and only 20 (1.7%) newborns with malformations were described. The drug was also used in a large number of patients after 30 weeks' gestation in an attempt to prevent preeclampsia and eclampsia, and no fetal adverse effects were noted. The drug will probably cross the placenta, so fetal exposure will likely occur. Therefore, this limited human pregnancy experience (especially first-trimester exposure) prevents a complete assessment of the embryofetal risk. Animal studies did not show any embryofetal toxicity in two animal species. Using this drug during pregnancy should be based on the pros and cons of the mother's clinical need for treatment versus any potential fetal risk that might occur from exposure.

BREASTFEEDING SUMMARY

In the past, bendroflumethiazide was used to suppress lactation. The drug can decrease maternal prolactin levels, and therefore, theoretically, might affect the initiation of breastfeeding. However, there are no data on whether the drug is found in breast milk. The drug will probably be excreted into breast milk (as seen with chlorothiazide); therefore, infant exposure will likely occur. Breastfeeding while using this drug should be based on the mother's clinical need for treatment. If used, the infant should be monitored for the most common reported adult side effects of nausea, headache, abdominal cramping, and pruritus (all leading to irritability), vomiting, diarrhea, rash, and constipation.

References

1. Prescribing Information. Corzide. Pfizer, Inc; 2023.
2. Heinonen OP, Slone D, Shapiro S. *Birth Defects and Drugs in Pregnancy*. Publishing Sciences Group; 1983:372-3733, 441.
3. Cuadros A, Tatum HJ. The prophylactic and therapeutic use of bendroflumethiazide in pregnancy. *Am J Obstet Gynecol*. 1964;89:891-897.
4. Stevens AC, Keysser CH, Kulesza JS, et al. Preclinical safety evaluation of the nadolol/bendroflumethiazide combination in mice, rats, and dogs. *Fundam Appl Toxicol*. 1984;4:360-369.
5. Healy M. Suppressing lactation with oral diuretics. *Lancet*. 1961;1:1353-1354.
6. Gezelle HD, Dhont M, Thiery M, Parewyck E. Puerperal lactation suppression and prolactin. *Acta Obstet Gynecol Scand*. 1979;58:469-472.

BENRALIZUMAB

Respiratory (Antiasthmatic—Monoclonal Antibody)

PREGNANCY RECOMMENDATION: Limited Human Data—Animal Data Suggest Low Risk

BREASTFEEDING RECOMMENDATION: Probably Compatible

PREGNANCY SUMMARY

Two case reports describing the use of benralizumab in human pregnancy were located. Both patients did well. The first delivered a healthy child at term with no reported anomalies, who was still progressing normally at 1 year of age. The newborn's eosinophil count was zero at delivery and did not become detectable until 7 months of age. Birth information was not supplied in the second case. In addition, drug levels in both infants at birth were not supplied. As an IgG antibody, benralizumab likely crosses the placenta, so some fetal exposure will probably occur. However, the limited human pregnancy experience prevents a complete assessment of the embryofetal risk. Animal studies did not show any embryofetal toxicity. Using this drug during pregnancy should be based on the pros and cons of the mother's clinical need for treatment versus any potential fetal risk that might occur from exposure. There is a pregnancy exposure registry that monitors pregnancy outcomes in women using this drug. Health care providers are encouraged to call the Fasenra Pregnancy Exposure Registry at 1-877-311-8972.

B

BREASTFEEDING SUMMARY

No reports describing the use of benralizumab during human lactation have been located. It is known that IgG antibodies can be found in breast milk, but are not found in the neonatal or infant circulation. Additionally, if any IgG antibodies were to be ingested through breastfeeding, they would probably be digested in the infant's gastrointestinal tract and not be absorbed. Breastfeeding while using this drug should be based on the mother's clinical need for treatment. If used, the infant should be monitored for the most common reported adult side effects of headache (leading to irritability) and pharyngitis.

References

1. Prescribing Information. Fasenra. AstraZeneca Pharmaceuticals, LP; 2021.
2. Manetz S, Maric I, Brown T, et al. Successful pregnancy in the setting of eosinophil depletion by benralizumab. *J Allergy Clin Immunol Pract*. 2021;9: 1405-1407.e3.
3. Saco T, Tabatabaian F. Breathing for two: a case of severe eosinophilic asthma during pregnancy treated with benralizumab. *Ann Allergy Asthma Immunol*. 2018;121:s92.

BENZNIDAZOLE

Anti-Infective (Antiprotozoal)

PREGNANCY RECOMMENDATION: Limited Human Data—Animal Data Suggest Potential Risk

BREASTFEEDING RECOMMENDATION: Probably Compatible

PREGNANCY SUMMARY

Limited human data specific to birth anomalies from exposure to benznidazole have been reported. One case report and one case series describe five pregnancies with exposure to benznidazole at the time of conception or in the first trimester, and no anomalies were identified at delivery. A sixth case report describes using benznidazole at 32 weeks' gestation to treat a woman with HIV who developed encephalitis due to Chagas disease. The treatment was effective, and the newborn had no issues. The drug probably crosses the placenta, so some fetal exposure will likely occur. However, this limited human pregnancy experience prevents a complete assessment of the embryofetal risk. Animal studies did show embryofetal toxicity. From a clinical standpoint, most patients (including newborns) are asymptomatic when infected with Chagas disease in the early stages. However, long-term effects from chronic disease over time can be significant. The World Health Organization considers Chagas disease a "neglected tropical disease." The risk of perinatal transmission of Chagas disease during gestation is estimated to be about 5%. While the benefits of treating an asymptomatic mother during pregnancy are not clear, identifying and treating an infected newborn could be crucial. However, because of the potential for adverse fetal effects seen in animal studies, the manufacturer recommends that women with reproductive potential use effective contraception during treatment with benznidazole and for 5 days after the last dose. Nevertheless, decisions to treat during pregnancy should be based on fully informed consent, with pros and cons discussed.

BREASTFEEDING SUMMARY

A study of 12 lactating women found that benznidazole was excreted into human breast milk but at low levels (range of 6%-17% of the recommended daily dose for pediatric patients with Chagas disease). None of the neonates demonstrated any adverse effects during or after study treatment. In addition, the presence of *Trypanosoma cruzi* was not found in the breast milk of 21 lactating women. The presence of *Trypanosoma cruzi* in breast milk is theoretically possible with cracked/bleeding nipples; however, Chagas disease is not a reason to avoid breastfeeding. The manufacturer, however, recommends that women not breastfeed while being treated with this drug due to the concern for potential serious adverse effects that might be seen in a breastfed infant exposed to benznidazole. Nevertheless, if the drug is used while breastfeeding, the infant should be monitored for the most common reported side effects of abdominal pain, headache, nausea, and pruritus (all leading to irritability), vomiting, decreased appetite (monitor infant weight), and rash.

References

1. Prescribing Information. Benznidazole. Exeltis USA, Inc; 2017.
2. Correa VR, Barbosa FG, de Melo Junio CA, et al. Uneventful benznidazole treatment of acute Chagas disease during pregnancy: a case report. *Rev Soc Bras Med Trop*. 2014;47:397-400.
3. Vazquez C, Garcia-Vazquez E, Carrilero B, et al. Pregnancy and Chagas disease: benznidazole's impact on pregnancy and newborns: a report of four cases. *Am J Trop Med Hyg*. 2020;102:1075-1077.
4. Bisio M, Altcheh J, Lattner J, et al. Benznidazole treatment of chagasic encephalitis in a pregnant woman with AIDS. *Emerg Infect Dis*. 2013;19: 1490-1492.
5. Livingston EG, Duggal R, Dotters-Katz S. Screening for Chagas disease during pregnancy in the United States—a literature review. *Trop Med Infect Dis*. 2021;6(4):202-215.
6. Garcia-Bournissen F, Moroni S, Masrson ME, et al. Limited infant exposure to benznidazole through breast milk during maternal treatment for Chagas disease. *Arch Dis Child*. 2015;100:90-94.
7. Bittencourt AL, Sadigursky M, Da Silva AA, et al. Evaluation of Chagas disease transmission through breast-feeding. *Mem Inst Oswaldo Cruz*. 1988; 83(1):37-39.
8. Campos R, Pinto PL, Moreira AA, et al. Experimental study on the transmission of Chagas disease by milk. *Rev Hosp Clin Fac Med Sao Paulo*. 1988;43: 146-147.
9. Ferreira CS, Martinho PC, Amato Neto V, Cruz RR. Pasteurization of human milk to prevent transmission of Chagas disease. *Rev Inst Med Trop Sao Paula*. 2001;43:161-162.

BENZOCAINE

Anesthetic (Topical)

PREGNANCY RECOMMENDATION: Limited Human Data—No Relevant Animal Data

BREASTFEEDING RECOMMENDATION: Probably Compatible

PREGNANCY SUMMARY

The Collaborative Perinatal Project reported on 47 patients with first-trimester exposure. Five (10.6%) newborns were identified with malformations, though no specific pattern was noted, and coexposures to other drugs were not described. From these data, no evidence of an association with large categories of major or minor malformations or with individual defects was found. Based on likely placental transfer, some fetal exposure may occur, but the amount overall should be negligible. However, the absence of human pregnancy experience prevents a complete assessment of the embryofetal risk. Animal reproduction studies have not been performed. There are numerous over-the-counter (OTC) products that contain benzocaine, which suggests a wide use of this anesthetic. Though there is no evidence that topical use of this drug is associated with any aspect of adverse embryofetal development, the best medical course would be to avoid use of benzocaine on mucous membranes or damaged skin during pregnancy (if possible). Methemoglobinemia has been reported with various anesthetic drugs, including benzocaine, and the US Food and Drug Administration (FDA) distributed a warning letter on this potential risk in May 2018.

BREASTFEEDING SUMMARY

No reports describing the use of benzocaine during human lactation have been located. The drug will probably be found in breast milk; however, the amount should be negligible. Nevertheless, because methemoglobinemia (though rare) is a serious and even fatal disorder, it is not recommended that benzocaine be applied to the breast or nipple of a nursing mother.

References

1. Prescribing Information. Benzocaine. Bellus Medical; 2017.
2. Guay J. Methemoglobinemia related to local anesthetics: a summary of 242 episodes. *Anesth Analg*. 2009;108:837-845.
3. FDA warning letter regarding the risk of methemoglobinemia and benzocaine. May 2018. https://www.fda.gov/files/drugs/published/FDA-Letter-Regarding-Benzocaine.pdf
4. Heinonen OP, Slone D, Shapiro S. *Birth Defects and Drugs in Pregnancy*. Publishing Sciences Group; 1983:357-360.

BENZPHETAMINE

Central Nervous System (Anorexiant)

PREGNANCY RECOMMENDATION: *Contraindicated

BREASTFEEDING RECOMMENDATION: *Contraindicated

PREGNANCY SUMMARY

No reports describing the use of benzphetamine in human pregnancy have been located. The drug will likely cross the placenta, so some fetal exposure will probably occur. Therefore, the absence of human pregnancy experience prevents a complete assessment of the embryofetal risk. Animal reproduction studies have not been performed. The drug is a controlled substance, Schedule III. *Because of its close relationship to amphetamines, the manufacturer states that this drug is contraindicated for use during pregnancy. Additionally, anorectic drugs are not indicated for use during pregnancy.

BREASTFEEDING SUMMARY

No reports describing the use of benzphetamine during lactation have been located. The drug will likely be found in breast milk, so some infant exposure will probably occur. *Benzphetamine is chemically and pharmacologically related to the amphetamines. In addition, anorectic drugs are not indicated during breastfeeding. As such, it is contraindicated during breastfeeding (see Amphetamines).

Reference

1. Prescribing Information. Benzphetamine hydrochloride. Pharmacia & Upjohn Company LLC; 2023.

B

BENZTROPINE

Autonomic (Anticholinergic)

PREGNANCY RECOMMENDATION: Limited Human Data—No Relevant Human Data

BREASTFEEDING RECOMMENDATION: Potential Toxicity

PREGNANCY SUMMARY

A few publications have reported the use of benztropine in pregnancy. The largest was the Michigan Medicaid Surveillance Study, which identified 84 first-trimester exposures with 4 (4.8%) anomalies, 3 of which were cardiac. The other publications involve seven pregnancies that did not report findings regarding first-trimester exposure. Based on likely placental transfer, some fetal exposure will probably occur. Therefore, this limited human pregnancy experience prevents a complete assessment of the embryofetal risk. Use of atropine and atropine-like drugs can affect the appearance of the fetal heart rate (FHR) monitor tracing by decreasing the variability and increasing the baseline, both consistent with parasympathetic blockage. In addition, transient increases in the FHR were seen during contractions.

BREASTFEEDING SUMMARY

No reports describing the use of benztropine during human lactation have been located. The drug will probably be found in breast milk, so some infant exposure will likely occur. Breastfeeding while using this drug should be based on the mother's clinical need for treatment. If used, the infant should be monitored for the most common reported adult side effects of nausea and headache (both leading to irritability), somnolence, constipation, flushing, and dry mouth. Because of the drug's anticholinergic effects, there is the possibility of interfering with breast milk production in the early stages of breastfeeding, as well as overall breast milk supply with long-term use.

References

1. Prescribing Information. Cogentin. Merck Sharp & Dohme; 2022.
2. Heinonen OP, Slone D, Shapiro S. *Birth Defects and Drugs in Pregnancy*. Publishing Sciences Group; 1983:346, 353.
3. Falterman CG, Richardson CJ. Small left colon syndrome associated with maternal ingestion of psychotropic drugs. *J Pediatr*. 1980;97:308-310.
4. Gossell-Williams M, Fletcher H, Zeisel SH. Unexpected depletion in plasma choline and phosphatidylcholine concentrations in a pregnant woman with bipolar affective disorder being treated with lithium, haloperidol and benztropine: a case report. *J Med Case Rep*. 2008;2:55(1-4).

BENZYL ALCOHOL

Anti-Infective (Topical)/Preservative

PREGNANCY RECOMMENDATION: *Limited Human Data—Animal Data Suggest Low Risk

BREASTFEEDING RECOMMENDATION: *Probably Compatible (Topically)/Potential Toxicity (Intravenous)

PREGNANCY SUMMARY

One case report of first-trimester exposure to benzyl alcohol did not identify any fetal or newborn malformations or complications. The drug will likely cross the placenta, so some fetal exposure will probably occur. Therefore, this limited human pregnancy experience prevents a complete assessment of the embryofetal risk. Animal reproduction studies did not show any embryofetal toxicity. Benzyl alcohol has been associated with serious and possibly fatal reactions in neonates, including "gasping syndrome" when consumed orally. Gasping syndrome is central nervous system depression with metabolic acidosis, leading to gasping respirations. This syndrome has primarily been seen with blood levels that are more than 20 times those that were found following systemic absorption with topical use. However, systemic levels might be higher if benzyl alcohol is administered through injection (as a multidose drug vial preservative). *Therefore, it is recommended that benzyl alcohol containing injectable products not be used during pregnancy, if possible.

BREASTFEEDING SUMMARY

No reports describing exposure to benzyl alcohol during human lactation have been located. The drug will probably be found in breast milk. However, plasma concentrations are very low following systemic absorption with topical use. In addition, the plasma amount that might be found after benzyl alcohol is administered through injection (as a preservative found in some multidose drug vials) is also likely to be small. Nevertheless, "gasping syndrome" is still a potential risk, so use in neonates (especially preterm newborns) is not recommended. *Therefore, using injectable drug alternatives (that do not contain benzyl alcohol) would be recommended while breastfeeding.

References

1. Prescribing Information. Ulesfia. Cerecor; 2019.
2. Centers for Disease Control and Prevention. Neonatal deaths associated with use of benzyl alcohol—United States. *MMWR*. 1982;31:290-291.
3. Nair B. Final report on the safety assessment of benzyl alcohol, benzoic acid, and sodium benzoate. *Int J Toxicol*. 2001;20(suppl 3):23-50.
4. Craig DB, Habib GG. Flaccid paraparesis following obstetrical epidural anesthesia: possible role of benzyl alcohol. *Anesth Analg*. 1977;56:219-221.
5. Moll S. A low-molecular-weight heparin preparation contraindicated during pregnancy. *Am J Obstet Gynecol*. 2001;184:1046.
6. Anderson CW, Ng KJ, Andresen B, Cordero L. Benzyl alcohol poisoning in a premature newborn infant. *Am J Obstet Gynecol*. 1984;148:344-346.

BEPOTASTINE BESILATE OPHTHALMIC

Ophthalmic (Antihistamine)

PREGNANCY RECOMMENDATION: No Human Data—Animal Data Suggest Low Risk

BREASTFEEDING RECOMMENDATION: Probably Compatible

PREGNANCY SUMMARY

No reports describing the use of bepotastine besilate ophthalmic solution in human pregnancy have been located. The drug will probably cross the placenta, but the amount should be negligible due to low serum concentrations following ophthalmic use. Nevertheless, the absence of human pregnancy experience prevents a complete assessment of the embryofetal risk. Animal reproduction studies did not show any embryofetal toxicity. Using this drug during pregnancy should be based on the pros and cons of the mother's clinical need for treatment versus any potential fetal risk that might occur from exposure. If used during pregnancy, consider placing pressure over the tear duct in the corner of the eye for at least 1 minute, and then remove any excess solution with absorbent tissue to decrease the amount of drug reaching the systemic circulation even further.

BREASTFEEDING SUMMARY

No reports describing the use of bepotastine besilate ophthalmic solution during human lactation have been located. The amount of drug that may be found in breast milk is probably clinically insignificant based on low plasma levels following systemic absorption with ophthalmic use. Breastfeeding while using this drug should be based on the mother's clinical need for treatment. If used, the infant should be monitored for the most common reported adult side effects of headache (leading to irritability) and nasopharyngitis. A method to decrease some systemic absorption with ophthalmic use is described above in the Pregnancy Summary.

Reference

1. Prescribing Information. Bepreve. Bausch & Lomb; 2018.

BERDAZIMER

Dermatologic (Topical Skin Product—Antiviral)

PREGNANCY RECOMMENDATION: No Human Data and No Relevant Animal Data

BREASTFEEDING RECOMMENDATION: Probably Compatible

PREGNANCY SUMMARY

No reports describing the use of berdazimer in human pregnancy have been located. Though placental transfer may be possible, fetal exposure is probably negligible. However, the absence of human pregnancy experience prevents a complete assessment of the embryofetal risk. Animal studies used the drug orally, and comparisons with what might be absorbed systemically following topical use could not be made. Using this drug during pregnancy should be based on the pros and cons of the mother's clinical need for treatment versus any potential fetal risk that might occur from exposure.

BREASTFEEDING SUMMARY

It is not known if berdazimer is excreted into human breast milk. Based on the low plasma levels found following systemic absorption, the total drug amount found in breast milk is likely to be negligible. Breastfeeding while using this drug should be based on the mother's clinical need for treatment versus any potential infant risks that might occur. Because the drug is used topically, adverse systemic adult reactions were not reported. Do not apply the gel on or near the nipple area.

Reference

1. Prescribing Information. Zelsuvmi. LNHC, Inc; 2024.

B

BEROTRALSTAT

Hematologic/Immunologic (Kallikrein Inhibitor)

PREGNANCY RECOMMENDATION: No Human Data—Animal Data Suggest Low Risk

BREASTFEEDING RECOMMENDATION: Probably Compatible

PREGNANCY SUMMARY

No reports describing the use of berotralstat in human pregnancy have been located. Some amount of the drug most likely crosses the placenta, but fetal exposure is probably minimal. However, the absence of human pregnancy experience prevents a complete assessment of the embryofetal risk. Animal data did not show fetotoxic effects. The drug should not be used in treating acute attacks of angioedema. In addition, doses higher than the recommended dose have been associated with prolongation of the cardiac QT interval.

BREASTFEEDING SUMMARY

Berotralstat probably enters breast milk, but the amount is most likely negligible. If the clinical decision is to use this drug while breastfeeding, the infant should be monitored for the most common reported adult side effects of abdominal and/or back pain (leading to irritability), vomiting, diarrhea, and gastroesophageal reflux.

Reference

1. Prescribing Information. Orladeyo. BioCryst Pharmaceuticals, Inc; 2020.

BESIFLOXACIN OPHTHALMIC

Ophthalmic (Antibacterial—Flouroquinolone)

PREGNANCY RECOMMENDATION: No Human Data—Animal Data Suggest Low Risk

BREASTFEEDING RECOMMENDATION: Probably Compatible

PREGNANCY SUMMARY

No reports describing the use of besifloxacin ophthalmic suspension in human pregnancy have been located. The drug will probably cross the placenta, but the amount should be negligible due to low serum concentrations following ophthalmic use. Nevertheless, the absence of human pregnancy experience prevents a complete assessment of the embryofetal risk. Animal reproduction studies did not show any embryofetal toxicity. Using this drug during pregnancy should be based on the pros and cons of the mother's clinical need for treatment versus any potential fetal risk that might occur from exposure. If used during pregnancy, consider placing pressure over the tear duct in the corner of the eye for at least 1 minute, and then remove any excess solution with absorbent tissue to decrease the amount of drug reaching the systemic circulation even further.

BREASTFEEDING SUMMARY

No reports describing the use of besifloxacin ophthalmic suspension during human lactation have been located. The drug will probably be excreted into breast milk. However, the amount is probably clinically insignificant based on low plasma levels following systemic absorption with ophthalmic use. Breastfeeding while using this drug should be based on the mother's clinical need for treatment. Systemic adult adverse reactions were not reported due to the low plasma levels seen with ophthalmic use. A method to decrease some systemic absorption with ophthalmic use is described above in the Pregnancy Summary.

Reference

1. Prescribing Information. Besivance. Bausch & Lomb; 2018.

β-CAROTENE

Vitamin (Fat Soluble)

PREGNANCY RECOMMENDATION: Compatible

BREASTFEEDING RECOMMENDATION: Compatible

B

PREGNANCY SUMMARY

There is no known embryofetal risk from the use of this vitamin in pregnancy when taking normal doses. A single case describing the use of β-carotene in human pregnancy reported a patient taking the vitamin for treating skin lesions caused by porphyria. She was on high doses at the time of conception, but discontinued the treatment at about 4 to 5 weeks' gestation. The β-carotene level was elevated, but the vitamin A level was low-normal at 2 weeks after her last dose. She delivered a healthy term infant with no malformations or complications identified. This vitamin will likely cross the placenta, so some fetal exposure will probably occur. However, the limited data on excess use of this vitamin prevent a complete assessment of the embryofetal risk.

BREASTFEEDING SUMMARY

Although there are no reports describing the use of β-carotene during human lactation, this vitamin is considered to be compatible with breastfeeding (see Vitamin A). The vitamin does appear in breast milk. The effects of excess intake of this vitamin during breastfeeding are unknown.

References

1. Beta carotene (oral route) description and brand names. 2023. www.mayoclinic.org/drugs-supplements /beta-carotene-oral-route/description/drg 20066795
2. Nishimura H, Tanimura T. *Clinical Aspects of the Teratogenicity of Drugs*. Elsevier; 1978:252.
3. Polifka JE, Dolan CR, Donlan MA, Friedman JM. Clinical teratology counseling and consultation report: high dose β-carotene use during early pregnancy. *Teratology*. 1996;54:103-107.
4. Johnson EJ, Qin H, Krinsky NI, Russell R. β-Carotene isomers in human serum, breast milk and buccal mucosa cells after continuous oral doses of all-trans and 9-cis β-carotene. *J Nutr*. 1997;127:1993-1999.

BETAMETHASONE

Corticosteroid (Glucocorticoid)

PREGNANCY RECOMMENDATION: Human Data Suggest Compatible (Late Second and Early Third Trimesters)

BREASTFEEDING RECOMMENDATION: Probably Compatible (Short-Term Use)

PREGNANCY SUMMARY

No reports linking the use of betamethasone with human birth defects have been located. Numerous studies have been published since the early 1970s regarding the use of betamethasone and the reduction of respiratory distress syndrome in preterm newborns (especially those <32 weeks' gestation). In addition, several studies have reported a lower rate of intraventricular hemorrhage and periventricular leukomalacia, as well as improved survival in extremely premature newborns exposed to antenatal betamethasone compared with those who had no exposure. These antenatal exposures, however, can produce maternal hyperglycemia. Lastly, several studies regarding long-term follow-up of exposed infants show that, overall, there are no adverse effects seen in cognitive, psychosocial, and physical development. The drug crosses the placenta, so fetal exposure will occur. Therefore, this limited first-trimester human pregnancy experience prevents a complete assessment of the embryofetal risk. Animal studies did show some embryofetal toxicity and malformations in one species with IM doses of less than 10 times the RHD used in obstetrics. This was not seen in another species with IM doses of more than 10 times the RHD used in obstetrics. Using this drug during pregnancy should be based on the pros and cons of the mother's clinical need for treatment versus any potential fetal risk that might occur from exposure.

BREASTFEEDING SUMMARY

No reports describing the use of betamethasone during human lactation have been located. The drug will probably be found in breast milk, so infant exposure will likely occur. Betamethasone is one of the more potent glucocorticoid corticosteroids, and if possible, the use of less-potent alternatives is recommended. However, breastfeeding while using this drug should be based on the mother's clinical need for treatment versus any potential infant risks that might occur. If used, the infant should be monitored for the most common reported adult side effects of myopathy and gastritis (both leading to irritability), infections, bruising, edema, flushing, and hyperglycemia.

A few studies have suggested that antenatal betamethasone exposure may delay lactogenesis in some patients.

References

1. Banks BA, Cnaan A, Morgan MA, et al.; The North American Thyrotropin-Releasing Hormone Study Group. Multiple courses of antenatal corticosteroids and outcome of premature neonates. *Am J Obstet Gynecol*. 1999;181:709-717.
2. French NP, Hagan R, Evans SF, et al. Repeated antenatal corticosteroids: size at birth and subsequent development. *Am J Obstet Gynecol*. 1999;180: 114-121.
3. Abbasi S, Hirsch D, Davis J, et al. Effect of single versus multiple courses of antenatal corticosteroids on maternal and neonatal outcome. *Am J Obstet Gynecol*. 2000;182:1243-1249.

B

4. Taeusch HW Jr. Glucocorticoid prophylaxis for respiratory distress syndrome: a review of potential toxicity. *J Pediatr*. 1975;87:617-623.
5. Johnson JWC, Mitzner W, London WT, et al. Betamethasone and the rhesus fetus: multisystemic effects. *Am J Obstet Gynecol*. 1979;133:677-684.
6. Ballard PL, Granberg P, Ballard RA. Glucocorticoid levels in maternal and cord serum after prenatal betamethasone therapy to prevent respiratory distress syndrome. *J Clin Invest*. 1975;56:1548-1554.
7. Levitz M, Jansen V, Dancis J. The transfer and metabolism of corticosteroids in the perfused human placenta. *Am J Obstet Gynecol*. 1978;132:363-366.
8. Liggins GC, Howie RN. A controlled trial of antepartum glucocorticoid treatment for prevention of the respiratory distress syndrome in premature infants. *Pediatrics*. 1972;50:515-525.
9. Gluck L. Administration of corticosteroids to induce maturation of fetal lung. *Am J Dis Child*. 1976;130:976-978.
10. Ballard RA, Ballard PL. Use of prenatal glucocorticoid therapy to prevent respiratory distress syndrome: a supporting view. *Am J Dis Child*. 1976;130: 982-987.
11. Mead PB, Clapp JF III. The use of betamethasone and timed delivery in management of premature rupture of the membranes in the preterm pregnancy. *J Reprod Med*. 1977;19:3-7.
12. Block MF, Kling OR, Crosby WM. Antenatal glucocorticoid therapy for the prevention of respiratory distress syndrome in the premature infant. *Obstet Gynecol*. 1977;50:186-190.
13. Ballard RA, Ballard PL, Granberg JP, Sniderman S. Prenatal administration of betamethasone for prevention of respiratory distress syndrome. *J Pediatr*. 1979;94:97-101.
14. Nochimson DJ, Petrie RH. Glucocorticoid therapy for the induction of pulmonary maturity in severely hypertensive gravid women. *Am J Obstet Gynecol*. 1979;133:449-451.
15. Eggers TR, Doyle LW, Pepperell RJ. Premature labour. *Med J Aust*. 1979; 1:213-216.
16. Doran TA, Swyer P, MacMurray B, et al. Results of a double-blind controlled study on the use of betamethasone in the prevention of respiratory distress syndrome. *Am J Obstet Gynecol*. 1980;136:313-320.
17. Schutte MF, Treffers PE, Koppe JG, Breur W. The influence of betamethasone and orciprenaline on the incidence of respiratory distress syndrome in the newborn after preterm labour. *Br J Obstet Gynaecol*. 1980;87:127-131.
18. Dillon WP, Egan EA. Aggressive obstetric management in late second-trimester deliveries. *Obstet Gynecol*. 1981;58:685-690.
19. Johnson DE, Munson DP, Thompson TR. Effect of antenatal administration of betamethasone on hospital costs and survival of premature infants. *Pediatrics*. 1981;68:633-637.
20. Bishop EH. Acceleration of fetal pulmonary maturity. *Obstet Gynecol*. 1981;58(suppl):48S-51S.
21. Ballard PL, Ballard RA. Corticosteroids and respiratory distress syndrome: status 1979. *Pediatrics*. 1979;63:163-165.
22. Gamsu HR, Mullinger BM, Donnai P, Dash CH. Antenatal administration of betamethasone to prevent respiratory distress syndrome in preterm infants: report of a UK multicentre trial. *Br J Obstet Gynaecol*. 1989;96: 401-410.
23. Eggers TR, Doyle LW, Pepperell RJ. Premature rupture of the membranes. *Med J Aust*. 1979;1:209-213.
24. Garite TJ, Freeman RK, Linzey EM, Braly PS, Dorchester WL. Prospective randomized study of corticosteroids in the management of premature rupture of the membranes and the premature gestation. *Am J Obstet Gynecol*. 1981;141:508-515.
25. Garite TJ. Premature rupture of the membranes: the enigma of the obstetrician. *Am J Obstet Gynecol*. 1985;151:1001-1005.
26. Nelson LH, Meis PJ, Hatjis CG, et al. Premature rupture of membranes: a prospective, randomized evaluation of steroids, latent phase, and expectant management. *Obstet Gynecol*. 1985;66:55-58.
27. Simpson GF, Harbert GM Jr. Use of β-methadone in management of preterm gestation with premature rupture of membranes. *Obstet Gynecol*. 1985;66:168-175.
28. Kuhn RJP, Speirs AL, Pepperell RJ, et al. Betamethasone, albuterol, and threatened premature delivery: benefits and risks. *Obstet Gynecol*. 1982;60: 403-408.
29. Schmidt PL, Sims ME, Strassner HT, et al. Effect of antepartum glucocorticoid administration upon neonatal respiratory distress syndrome and perinatal infection. *Am J Obstet Gynecol*. 1984;148:178-186.
30. Morales WJ, Angel JL, O'Brien WF, Knuppel RA. Use of ampicillin and corticosteroids in premature rupture of membranes: a randomized study. *Obstet Gynecol*. 1989;73:721-726.
31. Ballard PL, Ballard RA, Granberg JP, et al. Fetal sex and prenatal betamethasone therapy. *J Pediatr*. 1980;97:451-454.
32. Avery ME, Aylward G, Creasy R, et al. Update on prenatal steroid for prevention of respiratory distress: report of a conference—September 26-28, 1985. *Am J Obstet Gynecol*. 1986;155:2-5.
33. Khoury MJ, Marks JS, McCarthy BJ, Zaro SM. Factors affecting the sex differential in neonatal mortality: the role of respiratory distress syndrome. *Am J Obstet Gynecol*. 1985;151:777-782.
34. Turrentine MA, Dupras-Wilson P, Wilkins IA. A retrospective analysis of the effect of antenatal steroid administration on the incidence of respiratory distress syndrome in preterm twin pregnancies. *Am J Perinatol*. 1996;13:351-354.
35. Papageorgiou AN, Desgranges MF, Masson M, et al. The antenatal use of betamethasone in the prevention of respiratory distress syndrome: a controlled double-blind study. *Pediatrics*. 1979;63:73-79.
36. Bielawski D, Hiatt IM, Hegyi T. Betamethasone-induced leukaemoid reaction in pre-term infant. *Lancet*. 1978;1:218-219.
37. Hoff DS, Mammel MC. Suspected betamethasone-induced leukemoid reaction in a premature infant. *Pharmacotherapy*. 1997;17:1031-1034.
38. Ferguson JE, Hensleigh PA, Gill P. Effects of betamethasone on white blood cells in patients with premature rupture of the membranes and preterm labor. *Am J Obstet Gynecol*. 1984;150:439-441.
39. Catanzarite VA, McHargue AM, Sandberg EC, Dyson DC. Respiratory arrest during therapy for premature labor in a patient with myasthenia gravis. *Obstet Gynecol*. 1984;64:819-822.
40. Gonen R, Samberg I, Sharf M. Hypertensive crisis associated with ritodrine infusion and betamethasone administration in premature labor. *Eur J Obstet Gynecol Reprod Biol*. 1982;13:129-132.
41. Waffarn F, Siassi B, Cabal LA, Schmidt PL. Effect of antenatal glucocorticoids on clinical closure of the ductus arteriosus. *Am J Dis Child*. 1983;137:336-338.
42. Wasserstrum N, Huhta JC, Mari G, et al. Betamethasone and the human fetal ductus arteriosus. *Obstet Gynecol*. 1989;74:897-900.
43. Ballard PL. Combined hormonal treatment and lung maturation. *Semin Perinatol*. 1984;8:283-292.
44. Dorr HG, Versmold HT, Sippell WG, et al. Antenatal betamethasone therapy: effects on maternal, fetal, and neonatal mineralocorticoids, glucocorticoids, and progestins. *J Pediatr*. 1986;108:990-993.
45. Bradley BS, Kumar SP, Mehta PN, Ezhuthachan SG. Neonatal cushingoid syndrome resulting from serial courses of antenatal betamethasone. *Obstet Gynecol*. 1994;83:869-872.
46. McKenna DS, Wittber GM, Nagaraja HN, Samuels P. The effects of repeated doses of antenatal corticosteroids on maternal adrenal function. *Am J Obstet Gynecol*. 2000;183:669-673.
47. Helal KJ, Gordon MC, Lightner CR, Barth WH Jr. Adrenal suppression induced by betamethasone in women at risk for premature delivery. *Obstet Gynecol*. 2000;96:287-290.
48. Terrone DA, Rinehart BK, Rhodes PG, et al. Multiple courses of betamethasone to enhance fetal lung maturation do not suppress neonatal adrenal response. *Am J Obstet Gynecol*. 1999;180:1349-1353.
49. MacArthur BA, Howie RN, Dezoete JA, Elkins J. Cognitive and psychosocial development of 4-year-old children whose mothers were treated antenatally with betamethasone. *Pediatrics*. 1981;68:638-643.
50. MacArthur BA, Howie RN, Dezoete JA, Elkins J. School progress and cognitive development of 6-year-old children whose mothers were treated antenatally with betamethasone. *Pediatrics*. 1982;70:99-105.
51. Schmand B, Neuvel J, Smolders-de Haas H, et al. Psychological development of children who were treated antenatally with corticosteroids to prevent respiratory distress syndrome. *Pediatrics*. 1990;86:58-64.
52. Smolders-de Haas H, Neuvel J, Schmand B, et al. Physical development and medical history of children who were treated antenatally with corticosteroids to prevent respiratory distress syndrome: a 10- to 12-year follow-up. *Pediatrics*. 1990;85:65-70.
53. Doyle LW, Kitchen WH, Ford GW, et al. Effects of antenatal steroid therapy on mortality and morbidity in very low birth weight infants. *J Pediatr*. 1986; 108:287-292.
54. Doyle LW, Kitchen WH, Ford GW, et al. Antenatal steroid therapy and 5-year outcome of extremely low birth weight infants. *Obstet Gynecol*. 1989;73:743-746.
55. Baud O, Foix-L'Helias L, Kaminski M, et al. Antenatal glucocorticoid treatment and cystic periventricular leukomalacia in very premature infants. *N Engl J Med*. 1999;341:1190-1196.
56. Fanaroff AA, Hack M. Periventricular leukomalacia—prospects for prevention. *N Engl J Med*. 1999;341:1229-1231.
57. Leviton A, Dammann O, Allred EN, et al.; for the Developmental Epidemiology Network Investigators. Antenatal corticosteroids and cranial ultrasonographic abnormalities. *Am J Obstet Gynecol*. 1999;181:1007-1017.

58. Ment LR, Oh W, Ehrenkranz RA, Philip AGS, Duncan CC, Makuch RW. Antenatal steroids, delivery mode, and intraventricular hemorrhage in preterm infants. *Am J Obstet Gynecol*. 1995;172:795-800.
59. Garland JS, Buck R, Leviton A. Effect of maternal glucocorticoid exposure on risk of severe intraventricular hemorrhage in surfactant-treated preterm infants. *J Pediatr*. 1995;126:272-279.
60. Chen B, Basil JB, Schefft GL, et al. Antenatal steroids and intraventricular hemorrhage after premature rupture of membranes at 24-28 weeks' gestation. *Am J Perinatol*. 1997;14:171-176.
61. Canterino JC, Verma U, Visintainer PF, et al. Antenatal steroids and neonatal periventricular leukomalacia. *Obstet Gynecol*. 2001;97:135-139.
62. Ville Y, Vincent Y, Tordjman N, et al. Effect of betamethasone on the fetal heart rate pattern assessed by computerized cardiotocography in normal twin pregnancies. *Fetal Diagn Ther*. 1995;10:301-306.
63. Senat MV, Minoui S, Multon O, et al. Effect of dexamethasone and betamethasone on fetal heart rate variability in preterm labour: a randomised study. *Br J Obstet Gynaecol*. 1998;105:749-755.
64. Yunis KA, Bitar FF, Hayek P, et al. Transient hypertrophic cardiomyopathy in the newborn following multiple doses of antenatal corticosteroids. *Am J Perinatol*. 1999;16:17-21.

BETAMETHASONE TOPICAL/OPHTHALMIC/NASAL

Corticosteroid (Glucocorticoid)

PREGNANCY RECOMMENDATION: Limited Human Data—No Relevant Animal Data

BREASTFEEDING RECOMMENDATION: Probably Compatible (Short-Term Use)

PREGNANCY SUMMARY

Betamethasone topical ointment use in pregnancy was located in two publications, reporting on three patients. One exposure was in the second trimester, and two were in the third trimester; all three delivered healthy newborns with no reported complications or anomalies. One case report with the use of betamethasone ophthalmic solution in the third trimester was also located. The infant was delivered about 4 weeks later and was healthy with no reported anomalies. Lastly, a case of iatrogenic Cushing syndrome was diagnosed in a 23-week pregnant woman who used the nasal spray chronically for 5 months (including first-trimester exposure). It was determined that she was using about 10 mg of betamethasone per week. The drug was eventually discontinued, and the Cushing syndrome resolved. She delivered at term a healthy newborn with no reported anomalies or complications. Betamethasone crosses the placenta with IM usage and will probably cross with these external products, but the amount of systemic absorption is unknown. With short-term usage, the amount is likely to be clinically insignificant. However, with chronic use, fetal effects can occur (as seen in the nasal spray case discussed above). Therefore, this limited human pregnancy experience prevents a complete assessment of the embryofetal risk. Betamethasone has not been studied in animals using the topical, ophthalmic/otic, or nasal spray applications. It did show some embryofetal toxicity and malformations in one species with IM doses of less than 10 times the RHD used in obstetrics. This was not seen in another species with IM doses of more than 10 times the RHD used in obstetrics. Using these drugs during pregnancy should be based on the pros and cons of the mother's clinical need for treatment versus any potential fetal risk that might occur from exposure.

BREASTFEEDING SUMMARY

One case report of a breastfeeding woman using topical betamethasone was located. The betamethasone ointment was later changed to clobetasol ointment; however, the infant had no reported complications during the treatment process. No reports describing the use of betamethasone ophthalmic/otic or the nasal spray during human lactation have been located. The drug will probably be found in breast milk. However, the overall amount of betamethasone absorbed systemically with these products in short-term usage is probably clinically insignificant. Nevertheless, long-term usage should probably be avoided if at all possible. Betamethasone is one of the more potent glucocorticoid corticosteroids, and if possible, the use of less-potent alternatives is recommended. However, breastfeeding while using this drug should be based on the mother's clinical need for treatment versus any potential infant risks that might occur. If used, the infant should be monitored for the most common reported adult side effects of myopathy and gastritis (both leading to irritability), infections, bruising, edema, flushing, and hyperglycemia.

References

1. Prescribing Information. Diprolene. Merck & Company, Inc; 2021.
2. Prescribing Information. Vistamethasone. Martindale Pharma; 2020.
3. Prescribing Information. Betamethasone nasal spray. LGM Pharma; 2020.
4. Ballard PL, Granberg P, Ballard RA. Glucocorticoid levels in maternal and cord serum after prenatal betamethasone therapy to prevent respiratory distress syndrome. *J Clin Invest*. 1975;56:1548-1554.
5. Levitz M, Jansen V, Dancis J. The transfer and metabolism of corticosteroids in the perfused human placenta. *Am J Obstet Gynecol*. 1978;132:363-366.
6. Normand F, Armingaud P, Esteve E. Dyshidrosis and acral purpura during polymorphic dermatitis in pregnancy: 2 cases. *Ann Dermatol Venereol*. 2001;128:531-533.
7. Valeyrie L, Lebrun-Vignes B, Bodak N, et al. Pemphigoid gestationis: treatment by topical class I corticosteroid. *Ann Dermatol Venereol*. 2001;128:638-640.
8. Sugita K, Mizumoto K, Kato N, Zako M. Early resolution of subretinal fluid without high-dose corticosteroids in a pregnant patient with Vogt-Koyanagi-Harada disease: a case report. *J Ophthalmic Inflamm Infect*. 2015;5:20.
9. Scutelnicu A, Panaitescu AM, Ciobanu AM, et al. Iatrogenic Cushing's syndrome as a consequence of nasal use of betamethasone spray during pregnancy. *Acta Endocrinol (Buchar)*. 2020;16:511-517.
10. Westermann L, Hugel R, Meier M, et al. Glucocorticosteroid-resistant pemphigoid gestationis: successful treatment with adjuvant immunoadsorption. *J Dermatol*. 2012;39:168-171.

B

BETAXOLOL

Antihypertensive (Cardioselective β_1-Blocker)

PREGNANCY RECOMMENDATION: Limited Human Data—Animal Data Suggest Low Risk

BREASTFEEDING RECOMMENDATION: Potential Toxicity

PREGNANCY SUMMARY

One study reported the outcomes of 22 women treated with betaxolol for mild to moderate hypertension during pregnancy. Treatment was begun at a mean gestational age of about 31 weeks. At delivery, no fetal anomalies or complications were seen in the 23 infants (one set of twins). The drug crosses the placenta, so fetal exposure will occur. Therefore, this limited human pregnancy experience prevents a complete assessment of the embryofetal risk. Animal studies did not show any embryofetal toxicity. For treating hypertension in pregnancy, ACOG recommends nifedipine and labetalol as first-line agents. Some β-blockers may cause intrauterine growth restriction (IUGR). However, IUGR is also associated with hypertensive disorders in pregnancy. Although growth restriction is a serious concern, the benefits of maternal therapy with β-blockers, in some cases, might outweigh the risks to the fetus and must be judged on a case-by-case basis.

BREASTFEEDING SUMMARY

No reports have been located that describe the use of betaxolol during human lactation. Betaxolol is excreted into human breast milk in quantities sufficient to produce β-blockade in a nursing infant. Therefore, breastfeeding while using this drug should be based on the mother's clinical need for treatment. If used, the infant should be monitored for the most common reported adult side effects of bradycardia, lethargy, and dyspnea.

References

1. Prescribing Information. Betaxolol. Epic Pharma LLC; 2016.
2. ACOG Practice Bulletin No. 203: chronic hypertension in pregnancy. *Obstet Gynecol*. 2019;133:e26-e50.
3. Morselli PL, Boutroy MJ, Bianchetti G, et al. Placental transfer and perinatal pharmacokinetics of betaxolol. *Eur J Clin Pharmacol*. 1990;38:477-483.
4. Boutroy MJ, Morselli PL, Bianchetti G, et al. Betaxolol: a pilot study of its pharmacological and therapeutic properties in pregnancy. *Eur J Clin Pharmacol*. 1990;38:535-539.

BETAXOLOL OPHTHALMIC

Ophthalmic (Antiglaucoma)

PREGNANCY RECOMMENDATION: No Human Data—Animal Data Suggest Low Risk

BREASTFEEDING RECOMMENDATION: Probably Compatible

PREGNANCY SUMMARY

No reports describing the use of betaxolol ophthalmic suspension in human pregnancy have been located. The drug will cross the placenta, but the amount following ophthalmic use is likely to be clinically insignificant. However, the absence of human pregnancy experience prevents a complete assessment of the embryofetal risk. Animal reproduction studies did not show any embryofetal toxicity. If used during pregnancy, consider placing pressure over the tear duct in the corner of the eye for at least 1 minute, and then remove any excess solution with absorbent tissue to decrease the amount of drug reaching the systemic circulation even further.

BREASTFEEDING SUMMARY

No reports describing the use of betaxolol ophthalmic suspension in human lactation have been located. Plasma concentrations of betaxolol after ocular administration have not been reported. The drug is excreted into breast milk following oral administration (see Betaxolol). Although plasma concentrations should be very low after ocular use, there is the potential for adverse effects in a nursing infant. Therefore, breastfeeding while using this ophthalmic drug should be based on the mother's clinical need for treatment. If used, the infant should be monitored for the most common reported adult side effects of bradycardia, lethargy, and dyspnea. A method to decrease some systemic absorption with ophthalmic use is described above in the Pregnancy Summary.

References

1. Prescribing Information. Betaxolol. Epic Pharma LLC; 2016.

B

BETHANECHOL

Autonomic (Cholinergic)

PREGNANCY RECOMMENDATION: Limited Human Data—No Relevant Animal Data

BREASTFEEDING RECOMMENDATION: Probably Compatible (Possibly Hold Breastfeeding)

PREGNANCY SUMMARY

No reports describing the use of bethanechol in human pregnancy with verified outcome data have been located. The drug will probably cross the placenta, so some fetal exposure will likely occur. Therefore, the absence of human pregnancy experience prevents a complete assessment of the embryofetal risk. Animal reproduction studies have not been performed. Using this drug during pregnancy should be based on the pros and cons of the mother's clinical need for treatment versus any potential fetal risk that might occur from exposure.

BREASTFEEDING SUMMARY

No reports describing the use of bethanechol during human lactation have been located. The drug will probably be found in breast milk, so some infant exposure will likely occur. Breastfeeding while using this drug should be based on the mother's clinical need for treatment. If used, the infant should be monitored for the most common reported adult side effects of nausea and headache (both leading to irritability), diarrhea, lacrimation, sweating, and excess salivation.

References

1. Prescribing Information. Bethanechol. Amneal Pharmaceuticals LLC; 2022.
2. Heinonen OP, Slone D, Shapiro S. *Birth Defects and Drugs in Pregnancy*. Publishing Sciences Group; 1983:346.

BETRIXABAN

Hematologic (Anticoagulant)

PREGNANCY RECOMMENDATION: No Human Data—Animal Data Suggest Low Risk

BREASTFEEDING RECOMMENDATION: Potential Toxicity

PREGNANCY SUMMARY

No reports describing the use of betrixaban in human pregnancy have been located. Based on likely placental transfer, some fetal exposure will probably occur. However, the absence of human pregnancy experience prevents a complete assessment of the embryofetal risk. Animal studies did not show any embryofetal toxicity. Using this drug during pregnancy should be based on the pros and cons of the mother's clinical need for treatment versus any potential fetal risk that might occur from exposure. There is a potential risk for spinal and epidural hematomas associated with these types of neuraxial anesthesia in patients using this drug.

BREASTFEEDING SUMMARY

No reports describing the use of betrixaban during human lactation have been located. Some of the drug probably enters breast milk, so infant exposure will likely occur. Breastfeeding while using this drug should be based on the mother's clinical need for treatment. If used, the infant should be monitored for the most common reported adult side effect of bleeding.

Reference

1. Prescribing Information. Bevyxxa. Portola Pharmaceuticals, Inc; 2020.

BEVACIZUMAB

Antineoplastic (Monoclonal Antibody—Vascular Endothelial Growth Factor Inhibitor)

PREGNANCY RECOMMENDATION: Limited Human Data—Animal Data Suggest Potential Risk

BREASTFEEDING RECOMMENDATION: Probably Compatible

B

PREGNANCY SUMMARY

A total of 11 case studies regarding 20 pregnancies have been located describing first-trimester exposure to intravitreal bevacizumab. Of these, 15 patients delivered at term, and 1 delivered preterm (for severe preeclampsia), and no fetal anomalies or complications related to the drug were identified. The remaining four pregnancies were first-trimester spontaneous abortions. No reports describing the use of intravascular (IV) bevacizumab in human pregnancy have been located. Vascular endothelial growth factor (VEGF) is important for the developing fetus, especially in the first trimester. However, monoclonal antibodies are not expected to cross the placenta until after the first trimester. As an IgG antibody, it likely crosses the placenta during the second half of gestation, so some fetal exposure will probably occur. Therefore, this limited human pregnancy experience prevents a complete assessment of the embryofetal risk. Animal studies did show embryofetal toxicity in one species. Based on these animal studies and the drug's mechanism of action, the manufacturer recommends that women with reproductive potential use effective contraception during treatment and for 6 months after the last dose. Nevertheless, using this drug during pregnancy should be based on the pros and cons of the mother's clinical need for treatment versus any potential fetal risk that might occur from exposure. Women who are pregnant and have cancer are encouraged to contact the Cancer and Pregnancy Registry at 1-877-635-4499.

BREASTFEEDING SUMMARY

No reports describing the IV use of bevacizumab during human lactation have been located. Two women were using intravitreal bevacizumab while breastfeeding, and breast milk samples did not have detectable levels. Another patient breastfed while being treated with intravitreal injections, and no infant adverse effects were identified. However, it is known that IgG antibodies can be found in human breast milk (especially if administered IV), but are not found in the neonatal or infant circulation. Additionally, if any IgG antibodies were to be ingested through breastfeeding, they would probably be digested in the infant's gastrointestinal tract and not be absorbed. However, due to the concern for potential serious adverse effects that might be seen in a breastfed infant, the manufacturer recommends that women not breastfeed while being treated with this drug and for at least 6 months after the last dose. Nevertheless, breastfeeding while using this drug should be based on the mother's clinical need for treatment. If used, the infant should be monitored for the most common reported adult side effects of headache and back pain (both leading to irritability), epistaxis, and dry skin.

References

1. Prescribing Information. Avastin. Genentech, Inc; 2022.
2. Avery RL, Castellarin AA, Steinle NC, et al. Systemic pharmacokinetics and pharmacodynamics of intravitreal aflibercept, bevacizumab, and ranibizumab. *Retina*. 2017;37:1847-1858.
3. Rosen E, Rubowitz A, Ferencz JR. Exposure to verteporfin and bevacizumab therapy for choroidal neovascularization secondary to punctate inner choroidopathy during pregnancy. *Eye (Lond)*. 2009;23:1479.
4. Petrou P, Georgalas I, Giavaras G, et al. Early loss of pregnancy after intravitreal bevacizumab injection. *Acta Ophthalmol*. 2010;88:e136.
5. Wu Z, Huang J, Sadda S. Inadvertent use of bevacizumab to treat choroidal neovascularization during pregnancy: a case report. *Ann Acad Med Singapore*. 2010;39:143-145.
6. Tarantola RM, Folk JC, Boldt HC, Mahajan VB. Intravitreal bevacizumab during pregnancy. *Retina*. 2010;30:1405-1411.
7. Introini U, Casalino G, Cardani A, et al. Intravitreal bevacizumab for a subfoveal myopic choroidal neovascularization in the first trimester of pregnancy. *J Ocul Pharmacol Ther*. 2012;28:553-555.
8. Gomez LI, de Santiago Rodriguez MA, Follana NI, et al. Neovascular membrane and pregnancy treatment with bevacizumab. *Arch Soc Esp Oftalmol*. 2013;88:453-454.
9. Sullivan L, Kelly SP, Glenn A, et al. Intravitreal bevacizumab injection in unrecognized early pregnancy. *Eye*. 2014;28:492-494.
10. Polizzi S, Ferrara G, Restaino S, et al. Inadvertent use of bevacizumab in pregnant woman with diabetes mellitus type 1. *J Basic Clin Physiol Pharmacol*. 2015;26:161-163.
11. Polizzi S, Mahajan VB. Intravitreal anti-VEGF injections in pregnancy: case series and review of literature. *J Ocul Pharmacol Ther*. 2015;31:605-610.
12. Sarmad A, Lip PL. Intravitreal anti-vascular endothelial growth factor in early pregnancy and the complex management of advance diabetic retinopathy and maculopathy during pregnancy. *Acta Ophthalmol*. 2016;94:e812-e813.
13. Kianersi F, Ghanbari H, Naderi Beni Z, Naderi Beni A. Intravitreal vascular endothelial growth factor (VEGF) inhibitor injection in patient during pregnancy. *J Drug Assess*. 2021;10:7-9.
14. McFarland TJ, Rhoads AD, Hartzell M, et al. Bevacizumab levels in breast milk after long-term intravitreal injections. *Retina*. 2015;35:1670-1673.

BEXAGLIFLOZIN

Antidiabetic (Sodium-Glucose Cotransportor-2 [SGLT2] Inhibitor)

PREGNANCY RECOMMENDATION: No Human Data—Animal Data Suggest Potential Risk

BREASTFEEDING RECOMMENDATION: Potential Toxicity

PREGNANCY SUMMARY

No reports describing the use of bexagliflozin in human pregnancy have been located. The drug will probably cross the placenta, so some fetal exposure will likely occur. Therefore, the absence of human pregnancy experience prevents a complete

B

assessment of the embryofetal risk. Animal studies did not demonstrate any embryofetal toxicity. However, because of the findings in rats administered the drug postnatally (regarding possible kidney injury), the manufacturer recommends that the drug not be used in the second and third trimesters of pregnancy. Nevertheless, using this drug during pregnancy should be based on the pros and cons of the mother's clinical need for treatment versus any potential fetal risk that might occur from exposure. Fetal renal status can be monitored by perinatal ultrasound. In addition, postmarketing surveillance has detected an increase in the incidence of necrotizing fasciitis of the perineum (Fournier gangrene) in both men and women with diabetes.

BREASTFEEDING SUMMARY

No reports describing the use of bexagliflozin in human lactation have been located. The drug will probably be found in breast milk, so some infant exposure will likely occur. Because of the findings in rats administered the drug postnatally (regarding possible renal injury), the manufacturer recommends that women not breastfeed while using this drug. However, breastfeeding should be based on the mother's clinical need for treatment. If the drug is used, the infant should be monitored for the most common reported adult side effects of mycotic infections, urinary tract infections, and increased urination frequency.

Reference

1. Prescribing Information. Brenzavvy. TheracosBio, LLC; 2023.

BEXAROTENE

Antineoplastic (Retinoid)

PREGNANCY RECOMMENDATION: *Contraindicated (First Trimester)/No Human Data-Animal Data Suggest Potential Risk (Second and Third Trimesters)

BREASTFEEDING RECOMMENDATION: Potential Toxicity

PREGNANCY SUMMARY

No reports describing the use of bexarotene in human pregnancy have been located. The drug will probably cross the placenta, so some fetal exposure will likely occur. Therefore, the absence of human pregnancy experience prevents a complete assessment of the embryofetal risk. Animal studies did show embryofetal toxicity with malformations in one species. The drug carries a boxed warning for being a teratogen similar to other retinoid drugs in its class. *Based on the animal studies and the drug's mechanism of action, the manufacturer recommends that women with reproductive potential use two reliable forms of effective contraception for at least 1 month prior to therapy, during treatment, and for at least 1 month after the last dose. They also state that pregnancy tests should be performed every month. For males with female partners of reproductive potential, they recommend that condoms be used during treatment and for at least 1 month after the last dose. Nevertheless, using this drug after the first trimester in some clinical settings should be based on the pros and cons of the mother's clinical need for treatment versus any potential fetal risk that might occur from exposure. Women who are pregnant and have cancer are encouraged to contact the Cancer and Pregnancy Registry at 1-877-635-4499.

BREASTFEEDING SUMMARY

No reports describing the use of bexarotene during human lactation have been located. The drug will probably appear in breast milk, so some infant exposure will likely occur. Breastfeeding while using this drug should be based on the mother's clinical need for treatment. If used, the infant should be monitored for the most common reported adult side effects of nausea and headache (both leading to irritability), peripheral edema, rash, and various laboratory abnormalities (see PI).

Reference

1. Prescribing Information. Targretin. Ligand Pharmaceuticals, Inc; 2017.

BEZLOTOXUMAB

Antidote (Monoclonal Antibody)

PREGNANCY RECOMMENDATION: No Human Data and No Relevant Animal Data

BREASTFEEDING RECOMMENDATION: Probably Compatible

B

PREGNANCY SUMMARY

No reports describing the use of bezlotoxumab in human pregnancy have been located. As an IgG antibody, it likely crosses the placenta, so some fetal exposure will probably occur. Therefore, the absence of human pregnancy experience prevents a complete assessment of the embryofetal risk. Animal reproduction studies have not been conducted. Using this agent during pregnancy should be based on the pros and cons of the mother's clinical need for treatment versus any potential fetal risk that might occur from exposure.

BREASTFEEDING SUMMARY

No reports describing the use of bezlotoxumab during human lactation have been located. It is known that IgG antibodies can be found in human breast milk, but are not found in the neonatal or infant circulation. Additionally, if any IgG antibodies were to be ingested through breastfeeding, they would probably be digested in the infant's gastrointestinal tract and not be absorbed. Breastfeeding while using this drug should be based on the mother's clinical need for treatment. If used, the infant should be monitored for the most common reported adult side effects of nausea and headache (both leading to irritability) and pyrexia.

Reference

1. Prescribing Information. Zinplava. Merck Sharpe & Dohme; 2023.

BICTEGRAVIR/EMTRICITABINE/TENOFOVIR

Antiretroviral

PREGNANCY RECOMMENDATION: Limited Human Data for the Combination—Animal Data Suggest Low Risk for Bictegravir/Human Data Suggest Low Risk for Tenofovir/Emtricitabine

BREASTFEEDING RECOMMENDATION: *Contraindicated

PREGNANCY SUMMARY

All three drugs cross the human placenta. There are a few limited reports on the use of bictegravir in human pregnancy, and the available data are reassuring. Human data from the Antiretroviral Pregnancy Registry (APR) for emtricitabine and tenofovir suggest that these drugs are compatible for use in pregnancy. Animal data did not show any embryofetal toxicity for all three drug components. This combination drug has the potential for causing a severe acute exacerbation of hepatitis B (in patients coinfected with HIV-1 and hepatitis B virus [HBV]) when emtricitabine and/or tenofovir are discontinued. This risk could occur with the discontinuation of this combination drug. In order to decrease the perinatal transmission of HIV-1 to the neonate, this drug should not be withheld if a pregnant woman is infected with HIV-1 and has an approved indication for use. There is a pregnancy exposure registry that monitors pregnancy outcomes in patients using this drug during gestation. Health care providers are encouraged to call APR at 1-800-258-4263.

BREASTFEEDING SUMMARY

Emtricitabine has been found in human breast milk. Bictegravir and tenofovir are also probably excreted into human breast milk, so infant exposure would likely occur for all three drugs. *However, the current CDC recommendation is that mothers infected with HIV should not breastfeed their infants in order to reduce the risk of postnatal transmission of the virus to the neonate. In a clinical setting where a mother is not infected with HIV (or in cases where the HIV viral load is negative), the drug by itself is probably compatible.

References

1. Prescribing Information. Biktarvy. Gilead Sciences, Inc; 2021.
2. Pencole L, Le MP, Bouchet-Crivat F, et al. Placental transfer of the integrase strand inhibitors cabotegravir and bictegravir in the ex-vivo human cotyledon perfusion model. *AIDS*. 2020;34:2145-2149.
3. Le MP, Ferre VM, Mazy F, et al. Bictegravir pharmacokinetics in a late-presenting HIV-1-infected pregnant woman: a case report. *J Antimicrob Chemother*. 2022;77:851-853.
4. Bukkems VE, Hidalgo-Tenorio C, Garcia C, et al. First pharmacokinetics data of bictegravir in pregnant women living with HIV. *AIDS*. 2021;35:2405-2410.
5. Nissim O, Lazenby GB. The use of integrase strand transfer inhibitors to treat HIV in pregnancy. *J Midwifery Womens Health*. 2021;66:403-406.
6. Zash R, Makhema J, Shapiro RL. Neural-tube defects with dolutegravir treatment from the time of conception. *N Engl Med*. 2018;379:979-981.
7. van de Nen NS, Posniak AL, Levi JA, et al. Analysis of pharmacovigilance databases for dolutegravir safety in pregnancy. *Clin Inf Dis*. 2020;70:2599-2606.

B

BIMATOPROST OPHTHALMIC

Ophthalmic (Prostaglandin Agonist)

PREGNANCY RECOMMENDATION: No Human Data—Animal Data Suggest Low Risk

BREASTFEEDING RECOMMENDATION: Probably Compatible

PREGNANCY SUMMARY

No reports describing the use of bimatoprost ophthalmic in human pregnancy have been located. The drug will probably cross the placenta, but fetal exposure is probably negligible. Nevertheless, the absence of human pregnancy experience prevents a complete assessment of the embryofetal risk. Animal studies did not show any embryofetal toxicity. Prostaglandin $F_{2\alpha}$ (a similar prostaglandin agonist) can produce uterine contractions and has been used in treating postpartum hemorrhage. However, the blood levels that may be seen with ophthalmic use of bimatoprost are probably clinically insignificant. If used during pregnancy, consider placing pressure over the tear duct in the corner of the eye for at least 1 minute, and then remove any excess solution with absorbent tissue to decrease the amount of drug reaching the systemic circulation even further.

BREASTFEEDING SUMMARY

No reports describing the use of bimatoprost ophthalmic solution during human lactation have been located. The drug may appear in breast milk, but the amount is probably clinically insignificant. Breastfeeding while using this drug should be based on the mother's clinical need for treatment. Adverse systemic reactions in adults have not been reported. A method to decrease some systemic absorption with ophthalmic use is described above in the Pregnancy Summary.

References

1. Prescribing Information. Lumigan. Allergan; 2017.
2. Prescribing Information. Latisse. Allergan; 2021.

BIMEKIZUMAB

Dermatologic/Immunologic (Monoclonal Antibody—Interleukin 17A and Interleukin 17F Antagonist)

PREGNANCY RECOMMENDATION: No Human Data—Animal Data Suggest Low Risk

BREASTFEEDING RECOMMENDATION: Probably Compatible

PREGNANCY SUMMARY

No reports describing the use of bimekizumab in human pregnancy have been located. As an IgG antibody, the drug will likely cross the placenta, so some fetal exposure will probably occur. However, the absence of human pregnancy experience prevents a complete assessment of the embryofetal risk. Animal reproduction studies did not show any embryofetal toxicity or malformations in one species at doses of more than 10 times the RHD. Using this drug during pregnancy should be based on the pros and cons of the mother's clinical need for treatment versus any potential fetal risk that might occur from exposure. The manufacturer states that because the drug interferes with the immune response, the administration of live vaccines should be delayed in newborns for a minimum of 4 months after birth. There is a pregnancy exposure registry that monitors pregnancy outcomes in patients using this drug during gestation. Health care providers are encouraged to call the Organization of Teratology Information Specialists (OTIS) Autoimmune Diseases Study at 1-877-311-8972

BREASTFEEDING SUMMARY

No reports describing the use of bimekizumab during human lactation have been located. It is known that IgG antibodies can be found in human breast milk, but are not found in the neonatal or infant circulation. Additionally, if any IgG antibodies were to be ingested through breastfeeding, they would probably be digested in the infant's gastrointestinal tract and not be absorbed. Breastfeeding while using this drug should be based on the mother's clinical need for treatment. If used, the infant should be monitored for the most common reported adult side effects of headaches and abdominal pain (both leading to irritability) and upper respiratory infections.

Reference

1. Prescribing Information. Bimzelx. UCB, Inc; 2023.

B

BINIMETINIB

Antineoplastic (Kinase Inhibitor)

PREGNANCY RECOMMENDATION: No Human Data and No Relevant Animal Data

BREASTFEEDING RECOMMENDATION: Potential Toxicity

PREGNANCY SUMMARY

No reports describing the use of binimetinib in human pregnancy have been located. The drug will likely cross the placenta, so some fetal exposure will probably occur. Therefore, the absence of human pregnancy experience prevents a complete assessment of the embryofetal risk. The drug was found to cause embryofetal toxicity in animals, but the doses used also caused maternal toxicity. Based on animal studies and the drug's mechanism of action, the manufacturer recommends that women with reproductive potential use effective contraception during treatment and for 1 month after the last dose. However, using this drug during pregnancy should be based on the pros and cons of the mother's clinical need for treatment versus any potential fetal risk that might occur from exposure. Women who are pregnant and have cancer are encouraged to contact the Cancer and Pregnancy Registry at 1-877-635-4499.

BREASTFEEDING SUMMARY

No reports describing the use of binimetinib during human lactation have been located. The drug will probably be found in breast milk, so some infant exposure will likely occur. Due to the concern for potential serious adverse effects that might be seen in a breastfed infant, the manufacturer recommends that women not breastfeed while being treated with this drug and for at least 3 days after the last dose. Nevertheless, breastfeeding while using this drug should be based on the mother's clinical need for treatment. If used, the infant should be monitored for the most common reported adult side effects of nausea and abdominal pain (both leading to irritability), diarrhea, lethargy, and vomiting.

Reference

1. Prescribing Information. Mektovi. Array BioPharma, Inc; 2019.

BIRCH TRITERPENES

Dermatologic (Topical Skin Product)

PREGNANCY RECOMMENDATION: No Human Data—Animal Data Suggest Low Risk

BREASTFEEDING RECOMMENDATION: Probably Compatible

PREGNANCY SUMMARY

No human data specific to birch triterpenes have been reported. Though placental transfer is possible, fetal exposure is probably minimal because of the topical use of the drug and low plasma levels seen following systemic absorption. However, the absence of human pregnancy experience prevents a complete assessment of the embryofetal risk. Animal data did not show any embryofetal toxicity in one species, even when administered orally. Using this drug during pregnancy should be based on the pros and cons of the mother's clinical need for treatment versus any potential fetal risk that might occur from exposure.

BREASTFEEDING SUMMARY

It is not known if birch triterpenes are excreted into human breast milk. Some triterpenes may be found in breast milk, but the overall amounts are likely to be clinically insignificant. Breastfeeding while using this drug should be based on the mother's clinical need for treatment. Because the drug is used topically, adverse systemic adult reactions were not reported.

Reference

1. Prescribing Information. Filsuvez. Amryt Pharmaceuticals DAC; 2023.

B

BISACODYL

Gastrointestinal (Stimulant)

PREGNANCY RECOMMENDATION: No Human Data and No Relevant Animal Data

BREASTFEEDING RECOMMENDATION: Probably Compatible

PREGNANCY SUMMARY

No reports describing the use of bisacodyl in human pregnancy have been located. The drug will probably cross the placenta, but fetal levels are probably negligible due to poor systemic absorption. However, the absence of human pregnancy experience prevents a complete assessment of the embryofetal risk. Animal reproduction studies have not been performed. Using this drug during pregnancy should be based on the pros and cons of the mother's clinical need for treatment versus any potential fetal risk that might occur from exposure.

BREASTFEEDING SUMMARY

Eight lactating women received bisacodyl for several days, and all tested breast milk samples were negative (lower limit of detection 1 ng/mL). The drug could be excreted into breast milk, but the low systemic blood levels that occur with oral or rectal use probably limit excretion significantly. Breastfeeding while using this drug should be based on the mother's clinical need for treatment.

References

1. Prescribing Information. Bisacodyl. Major Pharmaceuticals; 2019.
2. Friedrich C, Richter E, Trommeshauser D, et al. Absence of excretion of the active moiety of bisacodyl and sodium picosulfate into human breast milk: an open-label, parallel-group multiple-dose study in healthy lactating women. *Drug Metab Pharmacokinet*. 2011;26:458-464.

BISMUTH SUBSALICYLATE

Gastrointestinal (Antidiarrheal/Dyspepsia)

PREGNANCY RECOMMENDATION: Limited Human Data—No Relevant Animal Data

BREASTFEEDING RECOMMENDATION: Potential Toxicity

PREGNANCY SUMMARY

Limited reports describing the use of bismuth subsalicylate in human pregnancy have been located. The Collaborative Perinatal Project reported on 15 exposures to bismuth subgallate and bismuth subcarbonate in the first trimester, and no major malformations were identified. There were 144 exposures (anytime during the pregnancy) to bismuth subgallate and 5 (3.5%) newborns with malformations were described. The salicylate portion of the drug will cross the placenta, so some fetal exposure will occur. The bismuth portion, if it crosses, will likely be clinically insignificant. Therefore, this limited human pregnancy experience prevents a complete assessment of the embryofetal risk. No animal reproduction studies have been located. Acetylsalicylic acid (ASA or aspirin) is a strong prostaglandin inhibitor of platelets and decreases platelet function. ASA also has strong anti-inflammatory activity. Salicylic acid (salicylate by itself) is a weak inhibitor of this prostaglandin pathway and, therefore, has minimal antiplatelet and anti-inflammatory activity. Therefore, it appears that the presence of the acetyl moiety is required to suppress platelet function. Using this drug during pregnancy should be based on the pros and cons of the mother's clinical need for treatment versus any potential fetal risk that might occur from exposure.

BREASTFEEDING SUMMARY

No reports describing the use of bismuth subsalicylate during human lactation have been located. Because the bismuth portion is poorly absorbed systemically, any amount that might be found in breast milk will likely be clinically insignificant. Salicylates, however, are excreted in breast milk and are eliminated more slowly from breast milk than from plasma with breast milk to plasma ratios rising from about 0.05 at 3 hours to about 0.34 at 12 hours. However, breast milk concentrations are still low. There has been concern about using salicylates during pregnancy but these are different than acetylsalicylate. The antiplatelet and anti-inflammatory effects are minimal with salicylates (the acetyl moiety is required). Breastfeeding while using this drug should be based on the mother's clinical need for treatment. If used, the infant should be monitored for the most common reported adult side effects of headache and irritability.

B

References

1. Bismuth Subsalicylate. 2023. www.dailymed.nlm.nih.gov/dailymed/druginfo.cfm
2. European Agency for the Evaluation of Medicinal Products. Bismuth subnitrate, bismuth subcarbonate, bismuth subgallate, bismuth subsalicylate. April 1997. Accessed 2023. www.ema.europa.eu/bismuth
3. O'Brien JR. Effects of salicylates on human platelets. *Lancet*. 1968;1:779-783.
4. Weiss HJ, Aledort ML, Shaul I. The effect of salicylates on the haemostatic properties of platelets in man. *J Clin Invest*. 1968;47:2169-2180.
5. Heinonen OP, Slone D, Shapiro S. *Birth Defects and Drugs in Pregnancy*. Publishing Sciences Group; 1983:385, 497.
6. Findlay JWA, DeAngelis RL, Kearney MF, et al. Analgesic drugs in breast milk and plasma. *Clin Pharmacol Ther*. 1981;29:625-633.

BISOPROLOL

Antihypertensive (Cardioselective β_1-Blocker)

PREGNANCY RECOMMENDATION: Limited Human Data—Animal Data Suggest Low Risk

BREASTFEEDING RECOMMENDATION: Potential Toxicity

PREGNANCY SUMMARY

An observational cohort study reported on 339 pregnancies with first-trimester exposure to bisoprolol compared with 678 nonhypertensive controls. There were no significant differences between the groups in terms of spontaneous abortions or major congenital malformations. However, there were higher rates of preterm birth and reduced birth weights in the bisoprolol-exposed group (which may have been caused by the presence of hypertension). Five case reports described six first-trimester exposures to bisoprolol for various cardiac conditions. All of the patients were on several other medications, and the five delivered infants had no reported anomalies. One newborn was found to have bilateral cleft lip and palate, hypertelorism, frontal bossing, and bilateral asymmetric hypoplasia of the toes. The pregnant mother also used naproxen and sumatriptan in the first trimester. Bisoprolol probably crosses the placenta, so some fetal exposure will likely occur. Therefore, the data regarding the risk of teratogenicity are very reassuring, but further studies are needed for confirmation. Animal studies did not show an increased risk for teratogenicity. For treating hypertension in pregnancy, ACOG recommends nifedipine and labetalol as first-line agents. Some β-blockers may cause IUGR. However, IUGR is also associated with hypertensive disorders in pregnancy. Although growth restriction is a serious concern, the benefits of maternal therapy with β-blockers, in some cases, might outweigh the risks to the fetus and must be judged on a case-by-case basis.

BREASTFEEDING SUMMARY

Bisoprolol was used by a breastfeeding woman starting 6 days postpartum. Bisoprolol levels were not detected in breast milk samples 11 to 18 days after drug initiation. However, the drug might be found in breast milk in some cases. Therefore, breastfeeding while using this drug should be based on the mother's clinical need for treatment. If used, the infant should be monitored for the most common reported adult side effects of nausea (leading to irritability), bradycardia, hypotension, diarrhea, and lethargy.

References

1. Prescribing Information. Bisoprolol fumarate. Unichem Pharmaceuticals; 2018.
2. Hoeltzenbein M, Fietz AK, Kayser, et al. Pregnancy outcome after first trimester exposure to bisoprolol: an observational cohort study. *J Hypertens*. 2018; 36:2109-2117.
3. Miyawaki N, Toyota T, Higasa K, et al. Successful pregnancy and delivery in a young-onset hypertrophic cardiomyopathy patient with a novel double-base substitution in the MYN7 gene. *J Cardiol Cases*. 2022;27:8-11.
4. Gluszak M, Borowiecka E, Borowiecka-Elwertowska A, Barcz E. Acute heart failure due to myocarditis in the first trimester of pregnancy. *Ginekol Pol*. 2013; 84:476-479.
5. Cozzolino M, Perelli F, Corioni S, et al. Successful obstetric management of arrhythmogenic right ventricular cardiomyopathy. *Gynecol Obstet Invest*. 2014;78:266-271.
6. Sawant RD, Freeman LJ, Stanley KPS, McKelvey A. Pregnancy and treatment outcome in a patient with left ventricular non-compaction. *Eur J Heart Fail*. 2013;15:592-595.
7. Kajantie E, Somer M. Bilateral cleft lip and palate, hypertelorism and hypoplastic toes. *Clin Dysmorphol*. 2004;13:195-196.
8. Kayser A, Beck E, Hoeltzenbein M, et al. Neonatal effects of intrauterine metoprolol/bisoprolol exposure during the second and third trimester: a cohort study with two comparison groups. *J Hypertens*. 2020;38:354-361.
9. Kubota K, Inai K, Shimada E, Shinohara T. Alpha/beta and beta-blocker exposure in pregnancy and the risk of neonatal hypoglycemia and small for gestational age. *Circ J*. 2023;87:569-577.
10. Khurana R, Bin Jardan YA, Wilkie J, Brocks DR. Breast milk concentrations of amiodarone, desethyl amiodarone, and bisoprolol following short -term drug exposure: two case reports. *J Clin Pharmacol*. 2014;54:828-831.

BIVALIRUDIN

Hematologic (Anticoagulant)

PREGNANCY RECOMMENDATION: No Human Data—Animal Data Suggest Low Risk (Maternal Benefit May Outweigh Embryofetal Risk)

BREASTFEEDING RECOMMENDATION: Probably Compatible

B

PREGNANCY SUMMARY

No reports describing the use of bivalirudin in human pregnancy have been located. The drug is not likely to cross the placenta; however, because it consists of a protein, it is not known whether some fetal exposure could occur. Nevertheless, the absence of human pregnancy experience prevents a complete assessment of the embryofetal risk. Animal studies did not show any embryofetal toxicity. Using this drug during pregnancy should be based on the pros and cons of the mother's clinical need for treatment versus any potential fetal risk that might occur from exposure. The drug is also to be used in combination with aspirin, so if used during pregnancy, this would also need to be considered (see Aspirin).

BREASTFEEDING SUMMARY

No reports describing the use of bivalirudin during human lactation have been located. The drug is not expected to be found in breast milk at levels that would be clinically indicated. However, it is a polypeptide, so some infant exposure might occur. Nevertheless, because it is a polypeptide, if the drug were to be ingested through breastfeeding, it would probably be digested in the infant's gastrointestinal tract and not be absorbed. Breastfeeding while using this drug should be based on the mother's clinical need for treatment. If used, the infant should be monitored for the most common reported adult side effects of headache (leading to irritability), thrombocytopenia, bleeding, and pyrexia. Lastly, the drug is to be used in combination with aspirin, so if used while breastfeeding this will also need to be considered (see Aspirin).

Reference

1. Prescribing Information. Angiomax. The Medicines Company; 2016.

BLACK WIDOW SPIDER ANTIVENIN

Antidote (Antivenom)

PREGNANCY RECOMMENDATION: Limited Human Data—No Relevant Animal Data

BREASTFEEDING RECOMMENDATION: Probably Compatible

PREGNANCY SUMMARY

Three case reports of patients who received black widow spider antivenin during pregnancy were located. One use occurred at 16 weeks' gestation, another at 22 weeks, and the third at 38 weeks' gestation. Two patients delivered healthy newborns at term. The third patient did well after treatment, was discharged, but the delivery information was not supplied. The antivenin is not likely to cross the placenta in clinically significant amounts. However, this limited human pregnancy experience prevents a complete assessment of the embryofetal risk. Animal reproduction studies have not been performed. Using this antivenin during pregnancy should be based on the pros and cons of the mother's clinical need for treatment versus any potential fetal risk that might occur from exposure.

BREASTFEEDING SUMMARY

No reports describing the use of black widow spider antivenin during human lactation have been located. The antivenin is not likely to be found in breast milk. However, if any of the globulins were to be ingested through breastfeeding, because they are proteins, they would probably be digested in the infant's gastrointestinal tract and not be absorbed. Using this antivenin while breastfeeding should be based on the mother's clinical need for treatment.

References

1. Prescribing Information. Antivenin—*Latrodectus mactans*. Merck Sharp & Dohme; 2023.
2. Russell FE, Marcus P, Streng JA. Black widow envenomation during pregnancy: report of a case. *Toxicon*. 1979;17:188-189.
3. Handel CC, Izquierdo LA, Curet LB. Black widow spider (*Latrodectus mactans*) bite during pregnancy. *West J Med*. 1994;160:261-262.
4. Sherman RP, Groll JM, Gonzalez DI, Aerts MA. Black widow spider (*Latrodectus mactans*) envenomation in a term pregnancy. *Curr Surg*. 2000;57:346-348.

BLEOMYCIN

Antineoplastic (Glycopeptide Antibiotic)

PREGNANCY RECOMMENDATION: Limited Human Data—Animal Data Suggest Risk

BREASTFEEDING RECOMMENDATION: Potential Toxicity

B

PREGNANCY SUMMARY

No reports describing the use of bleomycin during the first trimester have been located. One study described the use of bleomycin, doxorubicin, vinblastine, and dacarbazine in 44 pregnancies complicated by various stages of Hodgkin lymphoma. The study stated that there were four with first-trimester exposures, but these four began treatment at 12, 13, 16, and 16 weeks' gestation. No reported congenital anomalies were identified in these 44 cases, and all of the infants appeared to be developing normally, years after birth. More than 15 other cases of exposure to bleomycin used in the second and third trimesters of pregnancy have been reported, and no malformations or major neonatal complications were described. A limited amount of the drug may cross the placenta, so some fetal exposure may occur, especially in the second half of gestation. Therefore, this limited first-trimester human pregnancy experience prevents a complete assessment of the embryofetal risk. Animal studies did show embryofetal in one species and teratogenicity in another species at doses of less than 10 times the RHD. Using this drug during pregnancy should be based on the pros and cons of the mother's clinical need for treatment versus any potential fetal risk that might occur from exposure. There is a registry for women who are pregnant and have cancer. For more information, women and health care providers are encouraged to contact the Cancer and Pregnancy Registry at 1-877-635-4499.

BREASTFEEDING SUMMARY

No reports describing the use of bleomycin during human lactation have been located. A limited amount of the drug may be found in breast milk, so some infant exposure will likely occur. The manufacturer recommends that the drug not be used during breastfeeding. Nevertheless, breastfeeding while using this drug should be based on the mother's clinical need for treatment versus any potential infant risks that might occur. If used, the infant should be monitored for the most common reported adult side effects of pruritus, dizziness, and abdominal pain (all leading to irritability), diarrhea, lethargy, alopecia, vomiting, decreased appetite, cough, bruising, and rash.

References

1. Prescribing Information. Bleomycin. Hospira; 2018.
2. Bornstein RS, Hungerford DA, Haller G, Engstrom PF, Yarbro JW. Cytogenetic effects of bleomycin therapy in man. *Cancer Res*. 1971;31:2004-2007.
3. Ortega J. Multiple agent chemotherapy including bleomycin of non-Hodgkin's lymphoma during pregnancy. *Cancer*. 1977;40:2829-2835.
4. Falkson HC, Simson IW, Falkson G. Non-Hodgkin's lymphoma in pregnancy. *Cancer*. 1980;45:1679-1682.
5. Haerr RW, Pratt AT. Multiagent chemotherapy for sarcoma diagnosed during pregnancy. *Cancer*. 1985;56:1028-1033.
6. Raffles A, Williams J, Costeloe K, Clark P. Transplacental effects of maternal cancer chemotherapy: case report. *Br J Obstet Gynaecol*. 1989;96:1099-1100.
7. Malone JM, Gershenson DM, Creasy RK, et al. Endodermal sinus tumor of the ovary associated with pregnancy. *Obstet Gynecol*. 1986;68(suppl):86S-89S.
8. Rodriguez JM, Haggag M. VACOP-B chemotherapy for high grade non-Hodgkin's lymphoma in pregnancy. *Clin Oncol*. 1995;7:319-320.
9. Anselmo AP, Cavalieri E, Maurizi Enrici R, et al. Hodgkin's disease during pregnancy: diagnostic and therapeutic management. *Fetal Diagn Ther*. 1999;14:102-105.
10. Han JY, Nava-Ocampo AA, Kim TJ, et al. Pregnancy outcome after prenatal exposure to bleomycin, etoposide and cisplatin for malignant ovarian germ cell tumors: report of 2 cases. *Reprod Tox*. 2005;19:557-561.
11. Sanchez M, Pellicer B, del Puig Cozar M, et al. Hodgkin lymphoma in pregnancy: a case report. *Clin Adv Hematol Oncol*. 2013;11:533-536.
12. Gershenson DM. Menstrual and reproductive function after treatment with combination chemotherapy for malignant ovarian germ cell tumors. *J Clin Oncol*. 1988;6:270-275.
13. Moshe Y, Bentur OS, Lishner M, Avivi L. The management of Hodgkin lymphomas in pregnancies. *Eur J Haematol*. 2017;99:385-391.
14. Aviles A, Nambo MJ, Neri N. Treatment of early stages Hodgkin lymphoma during pregnancy. *Mediterr J Hematol Infect Dis*. 2018;10:e2018006.
15. Martin RH, Ernst S, Rademaker A, et al. Chromosomal abnormalities in sperm from testicular cancer patients before and after chemotherapy. *Hum Genet*. 1997;99:214-218.

BLINATUMOMAB

Antineoplastic (Monoclonal Antibody—Bispecific T-Cell Engager)

PREGNANCY RECOMMENDATION: No Human Data and No Relevant Animal Data

BREASTFEEDING RECOMMENDATION: Probably Compatible

PREGNANCY SUMMARY

No reports describing the use of blinatumomab in human pregnancy have been located. As an IgG antibody, it likely crosses the placenta, so some fetal exposure will probably occur. Therefore, the absence of human pregnancy experience prevents a complete assessment of the embryofetal risk. Animal reproduction studies have not been performed. However, based on the drug's mechanism of action, the manufacturer recommends that women with reproductive potential use effective contraception during treatment and for 48 hours after the last dose. Nevertheless, using this drug during pregnancy should be based on the pros and cons of the mother's clinical need for treatment versus any potential fetal risk that might occur from exposure. Some drug preparations come with the preservative benzyl alcohol, which has been associated with serious and

B

possibly fatal reactions in neonates, including "gasping syndrome" when consumed orally in large quantities. The amount of benzyl alcohol that might pass to the fetus with these preservative preparations is likely to be small, but preservative-free preparations are recommended if used during pregnancy. Lastly, due to the drug's mechanism of action, if used during gestation, there is a theoretical risk that the neonate could have B-cell depletion, so it is recommended that this be evaluated postdelivery. Women who are pregnant and have cancer are encouraged to contact the Cancer and Pregnancy Registry at 1-877-635-4499.

BREASTFEEDING SUMMARY

No reports describing the use of blinatumomab during human lactation have been located. It is known that IgG antibodies can be found in human breast milk, but are not found in the neonatal or infant circulation. Additionally, if any IgG antibodies were to be ingested through breastfeeding, they would probably be digested in the infant's gastrointestinal tract and not be absorbed. Nevertheless, due to the concern for potential serious adverse effects that might be seen in a breastfed infant, the manufacturer recommends that women not breastfeed while being treated with this drug and for at least 48 hours after the last dose. Regardless, breastfeeding while using this drug should be based on the mother's clinical need for treatment. If used, the infant should be monitored for the most common reported adult side effects of headache (leading to irritability), pyrexia, peripheral edema, anemia, neutropenia, and thrombocytopenia.

References

1. Prescribing Information. Blincyto. Amgen, Inc; 2023.
2. Nair B. Final report on the safety assessment of benzyl alcohol, benzoic acid, and sodium benzoate. *Int J Toxicol*. 2001;20(suppl 3):23-50.

BORTEZOMIB

Antineoplastic (Proteasome Inhibitor)

PREGNANCY RECOMMENDATION: No Human Data—Animal Data Suggest Potential Risk

BREASTFEEDING RECOMMENDATION: Potential Toxicity

PREGNANCY SUMMARY

No reports describing the use of bortezomib in human pregnancy have been located. The drug will probably cross the placenta, so some fetal exposure will likely occur. Therefore, the absence of human pregnancy experience prevents a complete assessment of the embryofetal risk. Animal reproduction studies showed embryofetal toxicity in one animal species. Based on animal studies and the drug's mechanism of action, the manufacturer recommends that women with reproductive potential use effective contraception during treatment and for 7 months after the last dose. They also recommend that males with female partners of reproductive potential use effective contraception during treatment and for 4 months after the last dose. Nevertheless, using this drug during pregnancy should be based on the pros and cons of the mother's clinical need for treatment versus any potential fetal risk that might occur from exposure. Women who are pregnant and have cancer are encouraged to contact the Cancer and Pregnancy Registry at 1-877-635-4499.

BREASTFEEDING SUMMARY

No reports describing the use of bortezomib during human lactation have been located. The drug will probably be found in breast milk, so some infant exposure will likely occur. Due to the concern for potential serious adverse effects that might be seen in a breastfed infant, the manufacturer recommends that women not breastfeed while being treated with this drug and for at least 2 months after the last dose. However, breastfeeding while using this drug should be based on the mother's clinical need for treatment. If used, the infant should be monitored for the most common reported adult side effects of nausea and neuralgia (both leading to irritability), diarrhea, lethargy, pyrexia, vomiting, constipation, decreased appetite, rash, and various laboratory abnormalities (see PI).

Reference

1. Prescribing Information. Velcade. Takeda Pharmaceuticals America, Inc; 2022.

BOSENTAN

Cardiovascular (Vasodilator)

PREGNANCY RECOMMENDATION: Limited Human Data—Animal Data Suggest Potential Risk

BREASTFEEDING RECOMMENDATION: Probably Compatible

B

PREGNANCY SUMMARY

Five case reports that describe first-trimester exposure to bosentan were located. All five patients had significant pulmonary hypertension, and all delivered healthy infants with no fetal anomalies identified (four preterm and one term). The drug will probably cross the placenta, so some fetal exposure will likely occur. Therefore, this limited human pregnancy experience prevents a complete assessment of the embryofetal risk. Animal studies did show embryofetal toxicity in one species. Based on these animal studies and the drug's mechanism of action, the manufacturer recommends that women with reproductive potential use effective nonhormonal contraception during treatment and for 1 month after the last dose. In addition, based on the animal studies, the drug carries a boxed warning for an increased risk of embryofetal toxicity. Nevertheless, using this drug during pregnancy should be based on the pros and cons of the mother's clinical need for treatment versus any potential fetal risk that might occur from exposure.

BREASTFEEDING SUMMARY

Two reports describing the use of bosentan during human lactation were located. Both infants did well with no reported adverse reactions. One report found that levels in breast milk samples for bosentan were very low at about 49 ng/mL. The daily infant dosage ranged from about 0.3 to 0.6 mcg/kg/d with a RID of only 0.24%. However, due to the concern for potential serious adverse effects that might be seen in a breastfed infant, the manufacturer recommends that women not breastfeed while being treated with this drug. Nevertheless, breastfeeding while using this drug should be based on the mother's clinical need for treatment. If used, the infant should be monitored for the most common reported adult side effects of headache, nausea, and abdominal pain (all leading to irritability), diarrhea, vomiting, rash, and peripheral edema.

References

1. Prescribing Information. Tracleer. Actelion Pharmaceuticals; 2022.
2. Molelekwa V, Akhter P, McKenna P, et al. Eisenmenger's syndrome in a 27 week pregnancy—management with bosentan and sildenafil. *Ir Med J*. 2005;98:87-88.
3. Elliot CA, Stewart P, Webster VJ, et al. The use of iloprost in early pregnancy in patients with pulmonary hypertension. *Eur Respir J*. 2005;26:168-173.
4. Streit M, Speich R, Fischler M, Ulrich S. Successful pregnancy in pulmonary arterial hypertension associated with systemic lupus erythematosus: a case report. *J Med Case Rep*. 2009;3:7255.
5. Tokgoz HC, Kaymaz C, Poci N, et al. A successful cesarean delivery without fetal or maternal morbidity in an Eisenmenger patient with cor triatriatum sinistrum, double-orifice mitral valve, large ventricular septal defect, and single ventricle who was under long-term bosentan treatment. *Turk Kardiyol Dem Ars*. 2017;45:184-188.
6. Amann U, Wentzell N, Kollhorst B, Haug U. Prescribing of endothelin receptor antagonists and riociguat in women of childbearing age in a large German claims database study. *Reprod Toxicol*. 2023;119:108415(1-7).
7. Nauwelaerts N, Ceulemans M, Deferm N, et al. Case report: bosentan and sildenafil exposure in human milk—a contribution from the concePTION project. *Front Pharmacol*. 2022;13:e1-e2.

BOSUTINIB

Antineoplastic (Tyrosine Kinase Inhibitor)

PREGNANCY RECOMMENDATION: Limited Human Data—Animal Data Suggest Potential Risk

BREASTFEEDING RECOMMENDATION: Potential Toxicity

PREGNANCY SUMMARY

A brief report of the Pfizer safety database described four patients with exposure to bosutinib during pregnancy that delivered at term and no fetal anomalies or complications were found. The drug will probably cross the placenta, so some fetal exposure will likely occur. Therefore, this limited human pregnancy experience prevents a complete assessment of the embryofetal risk. Animal reproduction studies reported embryofetal toxicity. Based on these animal studies and the drug's mechanism of action, the manufacturer recommends that women with reproductive potential use effective contraception during treatment and for 2 weeks after the last dose. Nevertheless, using this drug during pregnancy should be based on the pros and cons of the mother's clinical need for treatment versus any potential fetal risk that might occur from exposure. Women who are pregnant and have cancer are encouraged to contact the Cancer and Pregnancy Registry at 1-877-635-4499.

BREASTFEEDING SUMMARY

No reports describing the use of bosutinib during human lactation have been located. The drug will probably be found in breast milk, so infant exposure will likely occur. Due to the concern for potential serious adverse effects that might be seen in a breastfed infant, the manufacturer recommends that women not breastfeed while being treated with this drug and for at least 2 weeks after the last dose. Nevertheless, breastfeeding while using this drug should be based on the mother's clinical need for treatment. If used, the infant should be monitored for the most common reported adult side effects of nausea, abdominal pain, and headache (all leading to irritability), diarrhea, lethargy, vomiting, pyrexia, rash, and various laboratory abnormalities (see PI).

References

1. Prescribing Information. Bosulif. Pfizer Laboratories; 2023.
2. Cortes JE, Gambacorti-Passerini C, Deininger M, et al. Pregnancy outcomes in patients treated with bosutinib. *Int J Hematol Oncol*. 2020;9:IJH25(1-9).

BOTULINUM TOXIN TYPE A AND TYPE B

Toxins (Botulinum)

PREGNANCY RECOMMENDATION: Limited Human Data—Animal Data Suggest Low Risk

BREASTFEEDING RECOMMENDATION: Probably Compatible

PREGNANCY SUMMARY

An analysis of data from the Allergan Global Safety Database described a total of 195 prospective pregnancies resulting in 197 newborns. Most of these exposures occurred preconception or in the first trimester (before pregnancy was known). After eliminating 13 elective terminations, there were 32 (17.4%) spontaneous abortions and 152 live births. Of the live births, there was one major and two minor anomalies (2.0%). These rates fall within the expected range for spontaneous abortion and birth defects in the United States. In addition, a few other cases have been reported, and no major birth defects or complications were described. Botulinum toxin type A has not been detected in the systemic circulation following IM or intradermal administration. However, it has been found in breast milk (see description below in the Breastfeeding Summary), which suggests that some of the toxin may enter the maternal bloodstream in some cases. Regardless, based on the very low levels detected, any amount that may be present at the maternal/fetal interface would likely lead to negligible amounts that cross. Animal reproduction studies did not produce any embryofetal toxicity or teratogenicity in one species using single injections with doses less than 10 times the RHD. All other animal studies used multiple injections over a short time period. Using this drug during pregnancy should be based on the pros and cons of the mother's clinical need for treatment versus any potential fetal risk that might occur from exposure.

BREASTFEEDING SUMMARY

Two reports have been located that have evaluated breast milk for the presence of botulinum toxin type A in seven breastfeeding women. In two women, the toxin was not detected (lower limit of detection 46 pg/mL for these two patients). In the other five women, the toxin was detected with a peak level of 747 pg/mL in one mother's breast milk and 422 pg/mL in the second mother's breast milk. The other three cases had peak levels all below 50 pg/mL. Using the highest peak level obtained, the infant would receive about 112 ng/kg/d. However, because these toxins are large proteins, if they were to be ingested through breastfeeding, they would probably be digested in the infant's gastrointestinal tract and not be absorbed. Therefore, breastfeeding while using this drug should be based on the mother's clinical need for treatment versus any potential infant risks that might occur. If used, the infant should be monitored for the most common reported adult side effects of headache (leading to irritability), cough, flu-like symptoms, sweating, and weakness (lethargy).

References

1. Anonymous. Botulinum toxin. *Consensus Statement*. 1990;8:1-20.
2. Tsui JKC. Botulinum toxin as a therapeutic agent. *Pharmacol Ther*. 1996; 72:13-24.
3. Product information. Botox. Allergan; 2018.
4. Product information. Botox cosmetic. Allergan; 2017.
5. Hart LG, Dixon RL, Long JP, Mackay B. Studies using *Clostridium botulinum* toxin—type A. *Toxicol Appl Pharmacol*. 1965;7:84-89.
6. St. Clair EH, DiLiberti JH, O'Brien ML. Observations of an infant born to a mother with botulism. *J Pediatr*. 1975;87:658.
7. CDC. Wound botulism—California 1995. *MMWR*. 1995;44:889-892.
8. Polo JM, Martin J, Berciano J. Botulism and pregnancy. *Lancet*. 1996;348:195.
9. Robin L, Herman D, Redett R. Botulism in a pregnant woman. *N Engl J Med*. 1996;335:823-824.
10. Robinson AY, Grogan PM. OnabotulinumtoxinA successfully used as migraine prophylaxis during pregnancy: a case report. *Headache*. 2014;179: e703-e704.
11. Garza JJ, Downard CD, Clayton N, et al. *Clostridium botulinum* toxin inhibits myometrial activity in vitro: possible application on the prevention of preterm labor after fetal surgery. *J Pediatr Surg*. 2003;38:511-513.
12. Hooft N, Schmidt ES, Bremner RM. Achalasia in pregnancy: botulinum toxin A injection of lower esophageal sphincter. *Case Rep Surg*. 2015;2015:328970.
13. Jain P, Jain M, Jain S. Subcutaneous injection of botulinum toxin-A in postherpetic neuralgia during pregnancy. *Ann Indian Acad Neurol*. 2017;20:430.
14. Trivedi MK, Kroumpouzos G, Murase JE. A review of the safety of cosmetic procedures during pregnancy and lactation. *Int J Womens Dermatol*. 2017; 3:6-10.

BREMELANOTIDE

Miscellaneous (Melanocortin Receptor Agonist)

PREGNANCY RECOMMENDATION: Limited Human Data—No Relevant Animal Data

BREASTFEEDING RECOMMENDATION: Probably Compatible

B

PREGNANCY SUMMARY

Limited human data on the use of bremelanotide in human pregnancy have been reported. The drug will probably cross the placenta, so some fetal exposure will likely occur. In the clinical trials of more than 1,000 patients using this drug for up to 12 months, 7 pregnancies were reported. Of these, one was a spontaneous abortion (14%—expected rate 15%-20%), one was lost to follow-up, and five had full-term births with no reported major anomalies. No relevant animal data have been reported. The manufacturer does recommend that women use effective contraception while using this drug and to discontinue any use if pregnancy is suspected. The drug can also transiently increase blood pressure. There is a pregnancy exposure registry that monitors pregnancy outcomes in women using this drug. Health care providers are encouraged to call the Vyleesi Pregnancy Exposure Registry at 1-877-411-2510.

BREASTFEEDING SUMMARY

Bremelanotide probably enters breast milk in a limited amount. However, because it is a heptapeptide, if the drug were to be ingested through breastfeeding, it probably would be digested in the infant's gastrointestinal tract and not be absorbed. Breastfeeding while using this drug should be based on the mother's clinical need for treatment. If used, the infant should be monitored for the most common reported adult side effects of nausea and headache (both leading to irritability) and flushing.

Reference

1. Prescribing Information. Vyleesi. AMAG Pharmaceuticals, Inc; 2019.

BRENTUXIMAB VEDOTIN

Antineoplastic (Monoclonal Antibody Conjugate)

PREGNANCY RECOMMENDATION: No Human Data—Animal Data Suggest Potential Risk

BREASTFEEDING RECOMMENDATION: Potential Toxicity

PREGNANCY SUMMARY

No reports describing the use of brentuximab vedotin in human pregnancy have been located. As an IgG antibody, the drug will likely cross the placenta, so some fetal exposure will probably occur. In addition, monomethyl auristatin E (the active portion of the antineoplastic) will also probably cross the placenta, so some fetal exposure to this agent will also occur. Therefore, the absence of human pregnancy experience prevents a complete assessment of the embryofetal risk. Animal reproduction studies did show embryofetal toxicity in one species. Based on these animal studies and the drug's mechanism of action, the manufacturer recommends that women with reproductive potential use effective contraception during treatment and for 2 months after the last dose. They also recommend that males with female partners of reproductive potential use effective contraception during treatment and for 4 months after the last dose. Nevertheless, using this drug during pregnancy should be based on the pros and cons of the mother's clinical need for treatment versus any potential fetal risk that might occur from exposure. Women who are pregnant and have cancer are encouraged to contact the Cancer and Pregnancy Registry at 1-877-635-4499.

BREASTFEEDING SUMMARY

No reports describing the use of brentuximab vedotin during human lactation have been located. It is known that IgG antibodies can be found in human breast milk, but are not found in the neonatal or infant circulation. Additionally, if any IgG antibodies were to be ingested through breastfeeding, they would probably be digested in the infant's gastrointestinal tract and not be absorbed. However, monomethyl auristatin E, the cell-killing component, will also likely be found in breast milk and might be systemically absorbed. Therefore, the manufacturer recommends that women not breastfeed while being treated with brentuximab vedotin. Nevertheless, breastfeeding while using this drug should be based on the mother's clinical need for treatment. If used, the infant should be monitored for the most common reported adult side effects of nausea, neuropathy, and abdominal pain (all leading to irritability), diarrhea, lethargy, alopecia, vomiting, constipation, pyrexia, and various laboratory abnormalities (see PI).

Reference

1. Prescribing Information. Adcetris. Seagen, Inc; 2023.

B

BREXANOLONE

Mental Health (Antidepressant)

PREGNANCY RECOMMENDATION: *Contraindicated

BREASTFEEDING RECOMMENDATION: Probably Compatible

PREGNANCY SUMMARY

No reports describing the use of brexanolone in human pregnancy have been located. The drug will probably cross the placenta, so some fetal exposure will likely occur. Therefore, the absence of human pregnancy experience prevents a complete assessment of the embryofetal risk. Animal studies did show some embryofetal toxicity in one species at doses less than 10 times the RHD. *However, based on the drug's FDA approval, it is currently only to be used for treating postpartum depression. Therefore, it is contraindicated for use during an ongoing pregnancy. There is a pregnancy exposure registry that monitors pregnancy outcomes in women using this drug. Health care providers are encouraged to call the National Pregnancy Registry for Antidepressants at 1-844-405-6185.

BREASTFEEDING SUMMARY

One report describing the use of brexanolone during human lactation has been located. Pharmacokinetic properties were evaluated in 12 healthy lactating women. The mean concentrations of brexanolone in breast milk during treatment ranged from about 47 to 125 ng/mL. This fell to less than 10 ng/mL by 36 hours after the treatment was completed. The RID was about 1.3%. In addition, the drug is meant to be administered IV. Oral absorption is poor at less than 5%. Breastfeeding while using this drug should be based on the mother's clinical need for treatment. If used, the infant should be monitored for the most common reported adult side effects of somnolence, dry mouth, and flushing.

References

1. Prescribing Information. Zulresso. Sage Therapeutics; 2022.
2. Wald J, Henningsson A, Hanze E, et al. Allopregnanolone concentrations in breast milk and plasma from healthy volunteers receiving brexanolone injection, with population pharmacokinetic modeling of potential relative infant dose. *Clin Pharmacokinet*. 2022,61:1307-1319.

BREXPIPRAZOLE

Mental Health (Atypical Antipsychotic)

PREGNANCY RECOMMENDATION: No Human Data—Animal Data Suggest Low Risk

BREASTFEEDING RECOMMENDATION: Potential Toxicity

PREGNANCY SUMMARY

No reports describing the use of brexpiprazole in human pregnancy have been located. The drug will probably cross the placenta, so some fetal exposure will likely occur. Therefore, the absence of human pregnancy experience prevents a complete assessment of the embryofetal risk. Animal reproduction studies did not show any embryofetal toxicity or teratogenicity. Using this drug during pregnancy should be based on the pros and cons of the mother's clinical need for treatment versus any potential fetal risk that might occur from exposure. The manufacturer states that use of the drug in the third trimester could lead to extrapyramidal and/or withdrawal symptoms in newborns postdelivery. There is also a pregnancy exposure registry that monitors pregnancy outcomes in women using this drug. Health care providers are encouraged to call the National Pregnancy Registry for Atypical Antipsychotics at 1-866-961-2388.

BREASTFEEDING SUMMARY

No reports describing the use of brexpiprazole during human lactation have been located. The drug will probably be found in breast milk, so some infant exposure will likely occur. Breastfeeding while using this drug should be based on the mother's clinical need for treatment. If used, the infant should be monitored for the most common reported adult side effects of irritability and somnolence.

Reference

1. Prescribing Information. Rexulti. Otsuka Pharmaceutical Company; 2023.

B

BRIGATINIB

Antineoplastic (Tyrosine Kinase Inhibitor)

PREGNANCY RECOMMENDATION: No Human Data—Animal Data Suggest Potential Risk

BREASTFEEDING RECOMMENDATION: Potential Toxicity

PREGNANCY SUMMARY

No reports describing the use of brigatinib in human pregnancy have been located. Some amount of the drug will probably cross the placenta, so fetal exposure will likely occur. However, the absence of human pregnancy experience prevents a complete assessment of the embryofetal risk. Animal studies showed embryofetal toxicity and teratogenicity. Based on the animal studies and the drug's mechanism of action, the manufacturer recommends that women with reproductive potential use effective contraception during treatment and for 4 months after the last dose. They also recommend that males with female partners of reproductive potential use effective contraception during treatment and for 3 months after the last dose. However, using this drug during pregnancy should be based on the pros and cons of the mother's clinical need for treatment versus any potential fetal risk that might occur from exposure. In the clinical trials, the drug caused hypertension and hyperglycemia in 32% and 56% of the participants, respectively. There is a registry for women who are pregnant and have cancer. For more information, women and health care providers are encouraged to contact the Cancer and Pregnancy Registry at 1-877-635-4499.

BREASTFEEDING SUMMARY

No reports describing the use of brigatinib during human lactation have been located. Some amount of the drug probably enters breast milk, so infant exposure will likely occur. However, due to the concern for potential serious adverse effects in a breastfed infant, the manufacturer recommends that women not breastfeed while being treated with brigatinib and for at least 1 week after the last dose. Nevertheless, breastfeeding while using this drug should be based on the mother's clinical need for treatment. If used, the infant should be monitored for the most common reported adult side effects of nausea, headache, and myalgia (all leading to irritability), diarrhea, vomiting, rash, lethargy, cough, and hypertension.

Reference

1. Prescribing Information. Alunbrig. Takeda Pharmaceutical Company Limited; 2020.

BRILLIANT BLUE G

Ophthalmic (Diagnostic Agent)

PREGNANCY RECOMMENDATION: No Human Data and No Relevant Animal Data

BREASTFEEDING RECOMMENDATION: Probably Compatible

PREGNANCY SUMMARY

No reports describing the use of brilliant blue G ophthalmic solution in human pregnancy have been located. Based on intravitreal use and lack of any systemic absorption of the dye, fetal exposure is probably nonexistent. However, the absence of human pregnancy experience prevents a complete assessment of the embryofetal risk. Animal reproduction studies have not been conducted. Using this drug during pregnancy should be based on the pros and cons of the mother's clinical need for treatment versus any potential fetal risk that might occur from exposure.

BREASTFEEDING SUMMARY

No reports describing the use of brilliant blue G ophthalmic solution during human lactation have been located. The drug will probably not be found in breast milk, so infant exposure is likely to be nonexistent. Breastfeeding while using this drug should be based on the mother's clinical need for treatment. Because it is used intravitreal with negligible systemic absorption, adult adverse reactions have not been evaluated.

Reference

1. Prescribing Information. TissueBlue. Dutch Ophthalmic USA; 2019.

B

BRIMONIDINE OPHTHALMIC

Ophthalmic (Antiglaucoma)

PREGNANCY RECOMMENDATION: Limited Human Data—Animal Data Suggest Low Risk

BREASTFEEDING RECOMMENDATION: Probably Compatible

PREGNANCY SUMMARY

A case report described a pregnancy in a patient with open-angle glaucoma who was treated with brimonidine ophthalmic solution and latanoprost during the first trimester. This drug therapy was then discontinued, but treatment with brimonidine, dorzolamide, and timolol was restarted in the third trimester. She delivered at term a newborn with no identified anomalies or complications. The drug will probably cross the placenta, but fetal exposure is likely to be negligible following ocular use. Nevertheless, this limited human pregnancy experience prevents a complete assessment of the embryofetal risk. Animal reproduction studies did not show any embryofetal toxicity. Using this drug during pregnancy should be based on the pros and cons of the mother's clinical need for treatment versus any potential fetal risk that might occur from exposure. If used during pregnancy, consider placing pressure over the tear duct in the corner of the eye for at least 1 minute, and then remove any excess solution with absorbent tissue to decrease the amount of drug reaching the systemic circulation even further.

BREASTFEEDING SUMMARY

One report has described the use of brimonidine ophthalmic solution during human lactation. The ophthalmic drugs of brimonidine, dorzolamide, and timolol were administered during breastfeeding, and no adverse effects in the neonate were identified. The drug might be found in breast milk after ocular use, but the amount is likely to be negligible and not clinically significant. Breastfeeding while using this drug should be based on the mother's clinical need for treatment. If used, the infant should be monitored for the most common reported adult side effects of headache (leading to irritability) and oral dryness. A method to decrease some systemic absorption with ophthalmic use is described above in the Pregnancy Summary.

References

1. Prescribing Information. Alphagan. Allergan; 2018.
2. Johnson SM, Martinez M, Freedman S. Management of glaucoma in pregnancy and lactation. *Surv Ophthalmol*. 2001;45:449-454.

BRINZOLAMIDE OPHTHALMIC

Ophthalmic (Antiglaucoma)

PREGNANCY RECOMMENDATION: No Human Data—Animal Data Suggest Low Risk

BREASTFEEDING RECOMMENDATION: Probably Compatible

PREGNANCY SUMMARY

No reports describing the use of brinzolamide ophthalmic in human pregnancy have been located. The drug will probably cross the placenta, but fetal exposure is likely to be negligible following ocular use. However, the absence of human pregnancy experience prevents a complete assessment of the embryofetal risk. Animal reproduction studies did not show any embryofetal toxicity. The manufacturer states that the drug is not recommended for use during pregnancy and that women with reproductive potential should use effective contraception during treatment. Nevertheless, using this drug during pregnancy should be based on the pros and cons of the mother's clinical need for treatment versus any potential fetal risk that might occur from exposure. If used during pregnancy, consider placing pressure over the tear duct in the corner of the eye for at least 1 minute, and then remove any excess solution with absorbent tissue to decrease the amount of drug reaching the systemic circulation even further.

BREASTFEEDING SUMMARY

No reports describing the use of brinzolamide ophthalmic during human lactation have been located. The drug might be found in breast milk after ocular use, but the amount is likely to be negligible and not clinically significant. The manufacturer states that the drug is not recommended for use during lactation. Nevertheless, breastfeeding while using this drug should be based on the mother's clinical need for treatment. If used, the infant should be monitored for the most common reported adult side effects of headache (leading to irritability), oral dryness, and lethargy. A method to decrease some systemic absorption with ophthalmic use is described above in the Pregnancy Summary.

Reference

1. Prescribing Information. Azopt. Novartis Pharmaceuticals Canada; 2023.

B

BRIVARACETAM

Central Nervous System (Antiseizure)

PREGNANCY RECOMMENDATION: Limited Human Data—Animal Data Suggest Low Risk

BREASTFEEDING RECOMMENDATION: Probably Compatible

PREGNANCY SUMMARY

Three case reports describe six pregnancies and seven newborns (one set of twins) with first-trimester exposure to brivaracetam. All of the pregnancies delivered at term with no reported major malformations or complications. The drug will cross the placenta, so fetal exposure will occur (a cord blood to maternal serum ratio of about 1.1). Nevertheless, this limited human pregnancy experience prevents a complete assessment of the embryofetal risk. Animal studies did not show any embryofetal toxicity. Using this drug during pregnancy should be based on the pros and cons of the mother's clinical need for treatment versus any potential fetal risk that might occur from exposure. There is a pregnancy exposure registry that monitors pregnancy outcomes in women using anticonvulsant drugs during pregnancy. Health care providers are encouraged to call the North American Antiepileptic Drug Pregnancy Registry at 1-888-233-2334.

BREASTFEEDING SUMMARY

Two reports described three patients (with one set of twins, so four newborns) who used brivaracetam while breastfeeding. The four neonates did well with no reported complications. The mean breast milk to maternal serum concentration ratio was about 0.71. Infant serum levels ranged from undetectable to 0.25 ng/mL. This demonstrates that the drug can be found in breast milk with absorption by the infant. However, further cases of infants exposed to this drug while breastfeeding are needed. Breastfeeding while using this drug should be based on the mother's clinical need for treatment. If used, the infant should be monitored for the most common reported adult side effects of nausea (leading to irritability), vomiting, sedation, and lethargy.

References

1. Prescribing Information. Briviact. UCB, Inc; 2023.
2. Landmark CJ, Rektorli L, Burns ML, et al. Pharmacokinetic data on brivaracetam, lacosamide and perampanel during pregnancy and lactation. *Epileptic Disord.* 2021;23:426-431.
3. Paolini SL, Pilato M, Rajasekaran V, et al. Outcomes in three cases after brivaracetam treatment during pregnancy. *Acta Neurol Scand.* 2020;141:438-441.
4. Navarro CE. A healthy outcome of a pregnant woman with drug-resistant juvenile myoclonic epilepsy treated with brivaracetam. *Neurol Sci.* 2023;44:753-755.

BRODALUMAB

Dermatologic (Monoclonal Antibody—Antipsoriatic)

PREGNANCY RECOMMENDATION: No Human Data—Animal Data Suggest Low Risk

BREASTFEEDING RECOMMENDATION: Probably Compatible

PREGNANCY SUMMARY

No reports describing the use of brodalumab during human pregnancy have been located. As an IgG antibody, it likely crosses the placenta, so some fetal exposure will probably occur. Therefore, the absence of human pregnancy experience prevents a complete assessment of the embryofetal risk. Animal reproduction studies did not show any embryofetal toxicity. Using this drug during pregnancy should be based on the pros and cons of the mother's clinical need for treatment versus any potential fetal risk that might occur from exposure.

BREASTFEEDING SUMMARY

No reports describing the use of brodalumab during human lactation have been located. It is known that IgG antibodies can be found in human breast milk, but are not found in the neonatal or infant circulation. Additionally, if any IgG antibodies were to be ingested through breastfeeding, they would probably be digested in the infant's gastrointestinal tract and not be absorbed. Breastfeeding while using this drug should be based on the mother's clinical need for treatment. If used, the infant should be monitored for the most common reported adult side effects of arthralgia, headache, oropharyngeal pain, nausea, and myalgia (all leading to irritability), lethargy, diarrhea, and neutropenia.

Reference

1. Prescribing Information. Siliq. Bausch health US, LLC; 2020.

B

BROLUCIZUMAB

Ophthalmic (Monoclonal Antibody—Vascular Endothelial Growth Factor Inhibitor)

PREGNANCY RECOMMENDATION: No Human Data—Animal Data Suggest Potential Risk

BREASTFEEDING RECOMMENDATION: Probably Compatible

PREGNANCY SUMMARY

No reports describing the use of brolucizumab in human pregnancy have been located. As an IgG antibody, it likely crosses the placenta, so some fetal exposure will probably occur. However, systemic blood levels are low following intravitreal injection. Nevertheless, the absence of human pregnancy experience prevents a complete assessment of the embryofetal risk. Animal reproduction studies did show embryofetal toxicity in one animal species. Based on these animal studies and the drug's mechanism of action, the manufacturer recommends that women with reproductive potential use effective contraception during treatment and for 1 month after the last dose. Regardless, using this drug during pregnancy should be based on the pros and cons of the mother's clinical need for treatment versus any potential fetal risk that might occur from exposure.

BREASTFEEDING SUMMARY

No reports describing the use of brolucizumab during human lactation have been located. It is known that IgG antibodies can be found in human breast milk, but are not found in the neonatal or infant circulation. Additionally, if any IgG antibodies were to be ingested through breastfeeding, they would probably be digested in the infant's gastrointestinal tract and not be absorbed. However, due to the concern for potential serious adverse effects that might be seen in a breastfed infant, the manufacturer recommends that women not breastfeed while being treated with this drug and for at least 1 month after the last dose. Nevertheless, breastfeeding while using this drug should be based on the mother's clinical need for treatment. Though the drug is absorbed into the circulation, plasma levels are low, so adverse systemic drug reactions were not reported.

Reference

1. Prescribing Information. Beovu. Novartis Pharmaceuticals Corp; 2022.

BROMFENAC OPHTHALMIC

Ophthalmic (Nonsteroidal Anti-Inflammatory)

PREGNANCY RECOMMENDATION: No Human Data and No Relevant Animal Data

BREASTFEEDING RECOMMENDATION: Probably Compatible

PREGNANCY SUMMARY

No reports describing the use of bromfenac ophthalmic solution in human pregnancy have been located. The drug will probably cross the placenta; however, the amount of fetal exposure is likely to be clinically insignificant. Nevertheless, the absence of human pregnancy experience prevents a complete assessment of the embryofetal risk. Animal reproduction studies were not relevant. Using this drug during pregnancy should be based on the pros and cons of the mother's clinical need for treatment versus any potential fetal risk that might occur from exposure. If used during pregnancy, consider placing pressure over the tear duct in the corner of the eye for at least 1 minute, and then remove any excess solution with absorbent tissue to decrease the amount of drug reaching the systemic circulation even further.

BREASTFEEDING SUMMARY

No reports describing the use of bromfenac ophthalmic solution during human lactation have been located. The drug may be found in breast milk, but the levels would probably be clinically insignificant. Moreover, other nonsteroidal anti-inflammatory drugs (NSAIDs) are compatible with breastfeeding, even when given orally (see Ibuprofen). Breastfeeding while using this drug should be based on the mother's clinical need for treatment. If used, the infant should be monitored for the most common reported adult systemic side effect of headache (leading to irritability). A method to decrease some systemic absorption with ophthalmic use is described above in the Pregnancy Summary.

Reference

1. Prescribing Information. BromSite. Sun Pharmaceutical Industries; 2018.

B

BROMOCRIPTINE

Endocrine/Metabolic (Dopamine Agonist)

PREGNANCY RECOMMENDATION: Human Data Suggest Compatible

BREASTFEEDING RECOMMENDATION: *Contraindicated

PREGNANCY SUMMARY

From three large studies (the manufacturer, a large literature review, and the Michigan Medicaid Surveillance Study) plus follow-up cases, more than 2,500 first-trimester exposures to bromocriptine were reported. The major birth anomaly rate was about 3.5% with no pattern seen in the identified malformations. This rate falls within the expected rate of 2% to 4% for anomalies in the United States. The spontaneous abortion rate was about 11%. Bromocriptine does not appear to pose a significant risk to the fetus. The drug will probably cross the placenta, so fetal exposure will likely occur. Animal reproduction studies did not show any embryofetal toxicity or teratogenicity in three species (two with doses <10 times the RHD and one with >10 times the RHD). Using this drug during pregnancy should be based on the pros and cons of the mother's clinical need for treatment versus any potential fetal risk that might occur from exposure.

BREASTFEEDING SUMMARY

In the past, bromocriptine was used for the prevention of physiologic breast engorgement postdelivery. *However, this practice was stopped in the United States in 1994 due to increased risks for stroke, seizures, and cardiovascular events (some that lead to maternal death). One study did analyze breast milk for the presence of bromocriptine in 14 women taking 2.5 mg daily. The drug was not found in all breast milk samples (lower limit of detection 200 pg/mL). A few studies have been reported where successful breastfeeding has occurred while taking bromocriptine, but in most cases, breastfeeding had already been established. In addition, no adverse effects were reported in the breastfed infants. The manufacturer recommends that the drug not be used during lactation. However, in the rare circumstance where it might be indicated in a patient with established breastfeeding, the infant should be monitored for the most common reported adult side effects of nausea, headache, dizziness, and abdominal pain (all leading to irritability), diarrhea, lethargy, vomiting, and somnolence.

References

1. Prescribing Information. Bromocriptine mesylate. Paddock Laboratories; 2015.
2. Turkalj I, Braun P, Krupp P. Surveillance of bromocriptine in pregnancy. *JAMA*. 1982;247:1589-1591.
3. Konopka P, Raymond JP, Merceron RE, Seneze J. Continuous administration of bromocriptine in the prevention of neurological complications in pregnant women with prolactinomas. *Am J Obstet Gynecol*. 1983;146:935-938.
4. Canales ES, Garcia IC, Ruiz JE, Zarate A. Bromocriptine as prophylactic therapy in prolactinoma during pregnancy. *Fertil Steril*. 1981;36:524-526.
5. Bergh T, Nillius SJ, Larsson SG, Wide L. Effects of bromocriptine-induced pregnancy on prolactin-secreting pituitary tumors. *Acta Endocrinol*. 1981; 98:333.
6. Yuen BH, Cannon W, Sy L, Booth J, Burch P. Regression of pituitary microadenoma during and following bromocriptine therapy: persistent defect in prolactin regulation before and throughout pregnancy. *Am J Obstet Gynecol*. 1982;142:634-639.
7. Maeda T, Ushiroyama T, Okuda K, et al. Effective bromocriptine treatment of a pituitary macroadenoma during pregnancy. *Obstet Gynecol*. 1983;61:117-121.
8. Hammond CB, Haney AF, Land MR, et al. The outcome of pregnancy in patients with treated and untreated prolactin-secreting pituitary tumors. *Am J Obstet Gynecol*. 1983;147:148-157.
9. Cundy T, Grundy EN, Melville H, Sheldon J. Bromocriptine treatment of acromegaly following spontaneous conception. *Fertil Steril*. 1984;42:134-136.
10. Randall S, Laing I, Chapman AJ, et al. Pregnancies in women with hyperprolactinaemia: obstetric and endocrinological management of 50 pregnancies in 37 women. *Br J Obstet Gynaecol*. 1982;89:20-33.
11. Andersen AN, Starup J, Tabor A, et al. The possible prognostic value of serum prolactin increment during pregnancy in hyperprolactinaemic patients. *Acta Endocrinol*. 1983;102:1-5.
12. Van Roon E, van der Vijver JCM, Gerretsen G, et al. Rapid regression of a suprasellar extending prolactinoma after bromocriptine treatment during pregnancy. *Fertil Steril*. 1981;36:173-177.
13. Crosignani P, Ferrari C, Mattei AM. Visual field defects and reduced visual acuity during pregnancy in two patients with prolactinoma: rapid regression of symptoms under bromocriptine: case reports. *Br J Obstet Gynaecol*. 1984;91:821-823.
14. Hurault-Delarue C, Montastruc JL, Beau AB, et al. Pregnancy outcome in women exposed to dopamine agonists during pregnancy: a pharmacoepidemiology study in EFEMERIS database. *Arch Gynecol Obstet*. 2014;290: 263-270.
15. Saraiva J, Gomes L, Paiva S, et al. Giant macroprolactinoma and pregnancy. *Arq Bras Endocrinol Metab*. 2013;57:558-561.
16. Thorbert G, Akerlund M. Inhibition of lactation by cyclofenil and bromocriptine. *Br J Obstet Gynaecol*. 1983;90:739-742.
17. Committee on Drugs, American Academy of Pediatrics. The transfer of drugs and other chemicals into human milk. *Pediatrics*. 2001;108:77689.

BROMPHENIRAMINE

Antihistamine

PREGNANCY RECOMMENDATION: Limited Human Data—No Relevant Animal Data

BREASTFEEDING RECOMMENDATION: Probably Compatible

B

PREGNANCY SUMMARY

From 4 publications, a total of at least 371 first-trimester exposures to brompheniramine reported 17 anomalies (4.6%). This rate could be as low as 3.6%. The studies all varied regarding the types of anomalies (some being minor), and most patients, if not all, were using other drugs at the same time. Brompheniramine will probably cross the placenta, so fetal exposure will likely occur. Therefore, this human pregnancy experience still prevents a complete assessment of the embryofetal risk. In general, antihistamines are considered low risk in pregnancy. Animal reproduction studies have not been located. In the United States, brompheniramine is no longer available as a single drug product. It is only available in combination with other drugs, such as acetaminophen, phenylephrine, and pseudoephedrine. Using this drug during pregnancy should be based on the pros and cons of the mother's clinical need for treatment versus any potential fetal risk that might occur from exposure.

BREASTFEEDING SUMMARY

No reports describing the use of brompheniramine during human lactation have been located. The drug will probably be found in breast milk, so some infant exposure will likely occur. Breastfeeding while using this drug (in combination with other included ingredients) should be based on the mother's clinical need for treatment. If used, the infant should be monitored for the most common reported adult side effects of nausea and headache (leading to irritability), somnolence, diarrhea, vomiting, and dry mouth.

References

1. Prescribing Information. Dimetapp. Foundation Consumer Brands, LLC; 2023.
2. Heinonen OP, Slone D, Shapiro S. *Birth Defects and Drugs in Pregnancy*. Publishing Sciences Group; 1983:322-325.
3. Jick H, Holmes LB, Hunter JR, et al. First-trimester drug use and congenital disorders. *JAMA*. 1981;246:343-346.
4. Aselton P, Jick H, Milunsky A, et al. First-trimester drug use and congenital disorders. *Obstet Gynecol*. 1985;65:451-455.
5. Seto A, Einarson T, Korne G. Evaluation of brompheniramine safety in pregnancy. *Reprod Toxicol*. 1993;7:393-395.

BUDESONIDE

Respiratory (Corticosteroid—Asthma—Inhalation/Nasal)

PREGNANCY RECOMMENDATION: Human Data Suggest Low Risk

BREASTFEEDING RECOMMENDATION: Probably Compatible

PREGNANCY SUMMARY

In a large study from the Swedish Medical Birth Registry of 2,014 infants exposed in the first trimester to inhaled budesonide, the rate of congenital malformations was 3.8%. This was not different from the expected rate of the general population of 3.5%. In addition, the incidence of orofacial clefts was also not increased. In a second large study, 2,113 infants were exposed to the intranasal product, and the rate of anomalies was 4.5%. Again, this was not different from the general population rate of 3.5%. The rate of orofacial clefts was also not elevated. However, cardiac defects were higher than expected. This has not been universally seen in other studies. Several other series and case reports have not shown an increase in birth anomalies with the use of inhaled or intranasal budesonide. The drug will likely cross the placenta, so fetal exposure will probably occur. Animal studies did show embryofetal toxicity in one species at doses less than 10 times the maximum recommended human daily inhaled dose (MRHDID). Poorly controlled asthma can increase the risk for IUGR, preterm birth, and other pregnancy complications. Therefore, asthma treatment during pregnancy is recommended. Women who are pregnant and have taken asthma medications during pregnancy are encouraged to contact MotherToBaby Pregnancy Studies at 877-311-8972. The most recent ACOG publication on asthma in pregnancy (published in 2008—reaffirmed in 2020) and the 2023 GINA guidelines state that the advantages of actively treating asthma in pregnancy markedly outweigh the potential risks of the medications. Inhaled corticosteroids are usually the first-line treatment for mild to moderate persistent asthma in pregnancy. Listed alternative treatments include cromolyn, theophylline, or leukotriene receptor antagonists. However, ACOG recommends long-acting β_2-agonists as the preferred add-on drug when pregnant patients are not controlled with inhaled corticosteroids. The reasoning for this is that long-acting inhaled β_2-agonists have been shown to be more effective as an add-on treatment in nonpregnant patients, whereas theophylline has more side effects and requires serum monitoring, and there are minimal data on the leukotriene receptor antagonists in human pregnancy.

BREASTFEEDING SUMMARY

Budesonide was evaluated in eight breastfeeding women being treated for asthma (four with a 200 mcg dose and four with a 400 mcg dose treated twice daily). The peak drug levels were 168 and 335 pg/mL for the 200 and 400 mcg doses, respectively. The RIDs were calculated to be less than 1%. Four of the infants had blood levels evaluated, and budesonide was not detected in any infant (lower level of detection of about 17 pg/mL). No studies have been located regarding infant

B

exposure to budesonide nasal spray. Breastfeeding while using this drug should be based on the mother's clinical need for treatment versus any potential infant risks that might occur. If used, the infant should be monitored for the most common reported adult side effects of nausea and headache (both leading to irritability), fatigue (lethargy), and cough.

References

1. Quick reference from the Working Group on Managing Asthma During Pregnancy: recommendations for pharmacologic treatment—update 2004. National Institutes of Health (NIH Publication No. 05-3279). Accessed September 2013. https://www.nhlbi.nih.gov/files/docs/astpreg_qr.pdf
2. Product Information. Pulmicort turbuhaler. AstraZeneca; 2016.
3. Product Information. Rhinocort. Johnson & Johnson Consumer; 2016.
4. Kihlstrom I, Lundberg C. Teratogenicity study of the new glucocorticosteroid budesonide in rabbits. *Arzneimittelforschung*. 1987;37:43-46.
5. Kallen B, Rydhstroem H, Aberg A. Congenital malformations after the use of inhaled budesonide in early pregnancy. *Obstet Gynecol*. 1999;93:392-395.
6. Norjavaara E, Gerhardsson de Verdier M. Normal pregnancy outcomes in a population-based study including 2968 pregnant women exposed to budesonide. *J Allergy Clin Immunol*. 2003;111:736-742.
7. Kallen BAJ, Olausson PO. Maternal drug use in early pregnancy and infant cardiovascular defect. *Reprod Toxicol*. 2003;17:255-261.
8. Namazy J, Schatz M, Long L, et al. Use of inhaled steroids by pregnant asthmatic women does not reduce intrauterine growth. *J Allergy Clin Immunol*. 2004;113:427-432.
9. Rahimi R, Nikfar S, Abdollahi M. Meta-analysis finds use of inhaled corticosteroids during pregnancy safe: a systematic meta-analysis review. *Hum Exp Toxicol*. 2006;25:447-452.
10. Murphy VE, Fittock RJ, Zarzycki PK, et al. Metabolism of synthetic steroids by the human placenta. *Placenta*. 2007;28:39-46.
11. Falt A, Bengtsson T, Kennedy BM, et al. Exposure of infants to budesonide through breast milk of asthmatic mothers. *J Allergy Clin Immunol*. 2007;120:798-802.
12. Asthma in pregnancy. ACOG Practice Bulletin No. 90. American College of Obstetricians and Gynecologists. *Obstet Gynecol*. 2008;111:457-464. Reaffirmed 2020.

BUDESONIDE

Gastrointestinal (Corticosteroid—Ulcerative Colitis—Oral/Rectal)

PREGNANCY RECOMMENDATION: Limited Human Data—Animal Data Suggest Risk

BREASTFEEDING RECOMMENDATION: Probably Compatible

PREGNANCY SUMMARY

No studies have been located that have evaluated the risk for birth anomalies with oral or rectal budesonide. A few large studies with the inhalation or nasal spray budesonide products have not shown any elevated risk for teratogenicity compared with the general population. In addition, no consistently elevated risk for specific organ defects has been found in these studies. The drug will likely cross the placenta, so some fetal exposure will probably occur. Animal studies did show embryofetal toxicity in two species at doses less than 10 times the MRHDID. Therefore, using this drug during pregnancy should be based on the pros and cons of the mother's clinical need for treatment versus any potential fetal risk that might occur from exposure. Poorly controlled ulcerative colitis can increase the risk for IUGR, preterm birth, and other pregnancy complications. Therefore, the benefits of treatment may outweigh any potential fetal risks that might occur from use of this medication.

BREASTFEEDING SUMMARY

Studies evaluating the use of the oral and rectal forms of budesonide during human lactation have not been located. Budesonide was evaluated in eight breastfeeding women being treated for asthma with peak drug levels of up to 335 pg/mL for the 800 mg daily dose. The RIDs were calculated to be less than 1% with inhalation use. The manufacturer states that plasma levels with the oral medication could be up to 10 times higher than that of levels seen with inhalation use. This could make the RID much higher. Plasma levels with the rectal product are much lower. In addition, budesonide was not detected in the blood of newborns who were exposed to breast milk from inhalation use. Therefore, the risk to an exposed infant by way of the oral or rectal products is likely to be very small. Breastfeeding while using this drug should be based on the mother's clinical need for treatment versus any potential infant risks that might occur. If used, the infant should be monitored for the most common reported adult side effects of nausea, abdominal pain, arthralgia, and headache (all leading to irritability), fatigue (lethargy), and constipation.

References

1. Prescribing Information. Uceris. Salix Pharmaceuticals; 2020.
2. Falt A, Bengtsson T, Kennedy BM, et al. Exposure of infants to budesonide through breast milk of asthmatic mothers. *J Allergy Clin Immunol*. 2007;120:798-802.

BUMETANIDE

Cardiovascular (Loop Diuretic)

PREGNANCY RECOMMENDATION: Limited Human Data—Animal Data Suggest Low Risk

BREASTFEEDING RECOMMENDATION: Probably Compatible

B

PREGNANCY SUMMARY

In a surveillance study of Michigan Medicaid recipients involving 229,101 completed pregnancies, 44 newborns had been exposed to bumetanide during the first trimester. Two (4.5%) major birth defects were observed, both of which were cardiovascular defects. Based on likely placental transfer, some fetal exposure will probably occur. However, this limited human pregnancy experience prevents a complete assessment of the embryofetal risk. Animal reproduction studies did not show any embryofetal toxicity. Using this drug during pregnancy should be based on the pros and cons of the mother's clinical need for treatment versus any potential fetal risk that might occur from exposure.

BREASTFEEDING SUMMARY

No reports describing the use of bumetanide during human lactation have been located. The drug will probably be found in breast milk, so some infant exposure will likely occur. The manufacturer recommends that women not breastfeed when using this drug. Nevertheless, breastfeeding while using this drug should be based on the mother's clinical need for treatment. If used, the infant should be monitored for the most common reported adult side effects of myalgia, nausea, headache, abdominal pain, and pruritus (all leading to irritability), vomiting, rash, and various electrolyte abnormalities (see PI). There have also been some concerns that the drug could suppress lactation in the early stages of breastfeeding.

Reference

1. Prescribing Information. Bumetanide. Hospira; 2018.

BUPRENORPHINE

Pain (Opioid Agonist-Antagonist)

PREGNANCY RECOMMENDATION: **Human Data Suggest Low Risk (First Trimester)/*Human Data Suggest Risk (Third Trimester)**

BREASTFEEDING RECOMMENDATION: ***Probably Compatible**

PREGNANCY SUMMARY

Buprenorphine was compared with methadone in a large study involving 13,360 Medicaid beneficiaries (from 2000 to 2018) who were dispensed the drugs in the first trimester. The rate of any birth anomaly in the buprenorphine group was 5.1% in 9,514 patients versus a 6.1% rate in the methadone group of 3,846 patients. This 1% difference was significant. In addition, there was a lower risk for cardiac, central nervous system, urinary tract, and limb defects, but a higher risk for gastrointestinal malformations with buprenorphine use compared with methadone. In a second large study, 82,901 pregnant patients who filled two or more prescriptions for opioid drugs in the first trimester (exposed group) were compared with 2,697,355 pregnant patients without this exposure. The rate of birth anomalies was 4.1% in the exposed group versus 3.7% in the unexposed group. The most commonly prescribed opioid drugs were hydrocodone, oxycodone, and codeine. Specific details for buprenorphine were not provided. No difference was seen in categories of specific malformations, other than a slightly increased risk for oral clefts. Numerous other reviews and cohorts evaluating the risk of birth anomalies and first-trimester use of opioid drugs have found some associations with various birth defect categories, but no specific pattern has been identified. Buprenorphine and its three active metabolites cross the placenta, so fetal exposure will occur for all of these substances. Animal studies did find some embryofetal toxicity (but not teratogenicity) in two species at doses of less than 10 times the RHD. The drug has the potential for producing dependence, resulting in misuse. *In addition, with chronic use during pregnancy and near delivery, neonatal opioid withdrawal syndrome can occur in infants postdelivery. Buprenorphine is classified as a Schedule III controlled substance, and its morphine milligram equivalents (MME) is about 30 to 40. ACOG recommends that both buprenorphine and methadone should be considered as options for treating opioid use disorder during pregnancy.

BREASTFEEDING SUMMARY

Numerous studies have shown that buprenorphine and the three active metabolites can be found in breast milk. Levels overall are low. Calculated RIDs are usually about 3% to less than 1% overall. The drug and its active metabolites have also been detected in infant serum after exposure through breastfeeding. Levels are often not detected, but in some cases, infant blood levels have been reported as high as 5 ng/mL. *Several studies have shown a lower rate of neonatal opioid withdrawal syndrome with breastfeeding (in cases where a mother was using buprenorphine through most of the pregnancy up to delivery). It is not known whether these small amounts help minimize the symptoms of this disorder. Breastfeeding is recommended for infants of mothers who were taking buprenorphine to manage opioid use disorder during pregnancy, unless there are other illicit drugs being used or other contraindications. If used, the infant should be monitored for the most common reported

B

adult side effects of headache and nausea (both leading to irritability), somnolence, lethargy, constipation, and peripheral edema. Signs or symptoms of withdrawal should be assessed if breastfeeding is abruptly discontinued.

References

1. Committee on Obstetric Practice. Committee Opinion No. 711: opioid use and opioid use disorder in pregnancy. *Obstet Gynecol*. 2017;130:e81-e94.
2. Prescribing Information. Buprenorphine. Actavis Pharma; 2018.
3. Marquet P, Chevrel J, Lavignasse P, et al. Buprenorphine withdrawal syndrome in a newborn. *Clin Pharmacol Ther*. 1997;62:569-571.
4. Celleno D, Costantino P, Emanuelli M, et al. Epidural analgesia during and after cesarean delivery: comparison of five opioids. *Reg Anesth*. 1991;16:79-83.
5. Cohen S, Amar D, Pantuck CB, et al. Epidural patient-controlled analgesia after cesarean section: buprenorphine-0.015% bupivacaine with epinephrine versus fentanyl-0.015% bupivacaine with and without epinephrine. *Anesth Analg*. 1992;74:226-230.
6. Cohen S, Amar D, Pantuck CB, et al. Adverse effects of epidural 0.03% bupivacaine during analgesia after cesarean section. *Anesth Analg*. 1992;75:753-756.
7. Lehmann KA, Stern S, Breuker KH. Obstetrical peridural anesthesia with bupivacaine and buprenorphine: a randomized double-blind study in comparison with untreated controls. *Anaesthesist*. 1992;41:414-422.
8. Roy S, Basu RK. Role of sublingual administration of tablet buprenorphine hydrochloride on relief of labour pain. *J Indian Med Assoc*. 1992;90:151-153.
9. Jones HE, Johnson RE, Jasinski DR, et al. Buprenorphine versus methadone in the treatment of pregnant opioid dependent patients: effects on the neonatal abstinence syndrome (PROMISE Study). *Drug Alcohol Depend*. 2005;79:1-10.
10. Jones HE, Kaltenback K, Heil SH, et al. Neonatal abstinence syndrome after methadone or buprenorphine exposure (MOTHER Study). *N Engl J Med*. 2010;363:2320-2331.
11. Meyer MC, Johnston AM, Crocker AM, Heil SH. Methadone and buprenorphine for opioid dependence during pregnancy: a retrospective cohort study. *J Addict Med*. 2015;9:81-86.
12. Hirose M, Hosokawa T, Tanaka Y. Extradural buprenorphine suppresses breast feeding after caesarean section. *Br J Anaesth*. 1997;79:120-121.
13. Celebioglu B. Extradural buprenorphine and breast feeding after caesarean section. *Br J Anaesth*. 1998;80:271.
14. O'Connor AB, Collett A, Alto WA, O'Brien LM. Breastfeeding rates and the relationship between breastfeeding and neonatal abstinence syndrome in women maintained on buprenorphine during pregnancy. *J Midwifery Womens Health*. 2013;58:383-388.
15. Welle-Strand GK, Skurtveit S, Jansson LM, et al. Breastfeeding reduces the need for withdrawal treatment in opioid-exposed infants. *Acta Paediatr*. 2013;102:1060-1066.
16. Gower S, Bartu A, Ilett KF, et al. The wellbeing of infants exposed to buprenorphine via breast milk at 4 weeks of age. *J Hum Lact*. 2014;30:217-223.
17. Suarez EA, Bateman BT, Straub L, et al. First trimester use of buprenorphine or methadone and the risk of congenital malformations. *JAMA Intern Med*. 2024;184:242-251.
18. Bateman BT, Hernandez-Diaz S, Straub L, et al. Association of first trimester prescription opioid use with congenital malformations in the offspring: population based cohort. *BMJ*. 2021;372:n012.

BUPROPION

Mental Health (Antidepressant)

PREGNANCY RECOMMENDATION: Human Data Suggest Low Risk

BREASTFEEDING RECOMMENDATION: Potential Toxicity

PREGNANCY SUMMARY

Numerous studies have been located that describe the use of bupropion during human pregnancy. Data from the United Healthcare database and the International Bupropion Pregnancy Registry reported a total of more than 1,980 first-trimester exposures. Excluding first-trimester elective terminations, the rate of birth anomalies was 2.6%. Numerous other studies and case reports have also not shown an elevated risk for birth anomalies. However, some studies have described a slightly elevated risk for congenital heart defects, though this finding has not been universal in all evaluations. Animal studies did not show any clear evidence of teratogenicity in two species (one with doses <10 times the RHD and one with doses >10 times the RHD). Using this drug during pregnancy should be based on the pros and cons of the mother's clinical need for treatment versus any potential fetal risk that might occur from exposure. There is a pregnancy exposure registry that monitors pregnancy outcomes in women using antidepressant drugs. Health care providers are encouraged to call the National Pregnancy Registry for Antidepressants at 1-844-405-6185.

BREASTFEEDING SUMMARY

Numerous studies have been located that have evaluated the use of bupropion during human lactation. A total of 16 cases of breastfeeding demonstrated that bupropion and its three active metabolites are found in breast milk. Maternal doses ranged from 150 to 450 mg/d, and bupropion breast milk levels ranged from 4 to about 190 ng/mL. The calculated RIDs for two of the studies involving 14 mother/infant pairs ranged from 2% to about 5%. A few studies also analyzed blood levels for bupropion in infants exposed to the drug through breastfeeding. Bupropion was not detected in three cases. In a fourth case, an infant of about 6 months of age was evaluated following a seizure while being exposed to escitalopram and bupropion through breastfeeding. Bupropion was detected in the infant's blood, but at a low level that could not be quantified. Hydroxybupropion was found at levels of 11.2 and 17.1 ng/mL. Urine has also been evaluated in infants exposed to bupropion through breastfeeding. In two cases, the drug was not detected (lower limit of quantification 10 ng/mL). Bupropion was detected in the urine of the third infant at a level of 41 ng/mL. The manufacturer states that providers should exercise caution if bupropion is used during breastfeeding. Breastfeeding while using this drug should be based on the mother's clinical need for treatment versus any potential infant risks that might occur. If used, the infant

B

should be monitored for the most common reported adult side effects of nausea, headache, and dizziness (all leading to irritability), vomiting, constipation, rash, elevated heart rate, sweating, tremor, and insomnia.

References

1. Weintraub M, Evan P. Bupropion: a chemically and pharmacologically unique antidepressant. *Hosp Form*. 1989;24:254-259.
2. Prescribing Information. Wellbutrin SR. GlaxoSmithKline; 2017.
3. Earhart AD, Patrikeeva S, Wang X, et al. Transplacental transfer and metabolism of bupropion. *J Matern Fetal Neonatal Med*. 2010;23:409-416.
4. Wang X, Abdelrahman DR, Zharikova OL, et al. Bupropion metabolism by human placenta. *Biochem Pharmacol*. 2010;79:1684-1690.
5. Fokina VM, West H, Oncken C, et al. Bupropion therapy during pregnancy: the drug and its major metabolites in umbilical cord plasma and amniotic fluid. *Am J Obstet Gynecol*. 2016;215:497.e1-497.e7.
6. Chun-Fai-Chan B, Koren G, Fayez I, et al. Pregnancy outcome of women exposed to bupropion during pregnancy: a prospective comparative study. *Am J Obstet Gynecol*. 2005;192:932-936.
7. Einarson TR, Einarson A. Newer antidepressants in pregnancy and rates of major malformations: a meta-analysis of prospective comparative studies. *Pharmacoepidemiol Drug Saf*. 2005;14:823-827.
8. The Bupropion Pregnancy Registry. Final Report, 1 September 1997 through 31 March 2008. GlaxoSmithKline; August 2008.
9. Cole JA, Modell JG, Haight BR, et al. Bupropion in pregnancy and the prevalence of congenital malformations. *Pharmacoepidemiol Drug Saf*. 2007;16:474-484.
10. Thyagarajan V, Clifford CR, Wurst KE, et al. Bupropion therapy in pregnancy and the occurrence of cardiovascular malformations in infants. *Pharmacoepidemiol Drug Saf*. 2012;21:1240-1242.
11. Einarson A, Choi J, Einarson TR, Koren G. Incidence of major malformations in infants following antidepressant exposure in pregnancy: results of a large prospective cohort study. *Can J Psychiatry*. 2009;54:242-246.
12. Alwan S, Reefhuis J, Botto LD, et al.; The National Birth Defects Prevention Study. Maternal use of bupropion and risk for congenital heart defects. *Am J Obstet Gynecol*. 2010;203:52.e1-52.e6.
13. Louik C, Kerr S, Mitchell AA. First-trimester exposure to bupropion and risk of cardiac malformations. *Pharmacoepidemiol Drug Saf*. 2014;23:1066-1075.
14. Figueroa R. Use of antidepressants during pregnancy and risk of attention-deficit/hyperactivity disorder in the offspring. *J Dev Behav Pediatr*. 2010;31:641-648.
15. Fokina VM, Xu M, Rytting E, et al. Pharmacokinetics of bupropion and its pharmacologically active metabolites in pregnancy. *Drug Metab Dispos*. 2016;44:1832-1838.
16. Hendrick V, Suri R, Gitlin MJ, Ortiz-Portillo E. Bupropion use during pregnancy: a systematic review. *Prim Care Companion CNS Disord*. 2017;19:pii .17r02160.
17. De Long NE, Barra NG, Hardy DB, Holloway AC. Is it safe to use smoking cessation therapeutics during pregnancy? *Expert Opin Drug Saf*. 2014;13(12):1721-1731.
18. Coleman T, Chamberlain C, Davey MA, et al. Pharmacological interventions for promoting smoking cessation during pregnancy. *Cochrane Database Syst Rev*. 2015;12:CDo10078.
19. Berard A, Zhao JP, Sheehy O. Success of smoking cessation interventions during pregnancy. *Am J Obstet Gynecol*. 2016;215:611.e1-611.e8.
20. Nanovskaya TN, Oncken C, Fokina VM, et al. Bupropion sustained release for pregnant smokers: a randomized, placebo-controlled trial. *Am J Obstet Gynecol*. 2017;216:420.e1-420.e9.
21. Briggs GG, Samson JH, Ambrose PJ, Schroeder DH. Excretion of bupropion in breast milk. *Ann Pharmacother*. 1993;27:431-433.
22. Baab S, Peindl K, Piontek C, Wisner K. Serum bupropion levels in 2 breast-feeding mother-infant pairs. *J Clin Psychiatry*. 2002;63:910-911.
23. Haas JS, Kaplan CP, Barenboim DJ III, Benowitz NL. Bupropion in breast milk: an exposure assessment for potential treatment to prevent post-partum tobacco use. *Tob Control*. 2004;13:52-56.
24. Chaudron LH, Schoenecker CJ. Bupropion and breastfeeding: a case of a possible infant seizure. *J Clin Psychiatry*. 2004;65:881-882.
25. Neuman G, Colantonio D, Delaney S, et al. Bupropion and escitalopram during lactation. *Ann Pharmacother*. 2014;48:928-931.
26. Davis MF, Miller HS, Nolan PE Jr. Bupropion levels in breast milk for 4 mother-infant pairs: more answers to lingering questions. *J Clin Psychiatry*. 2009;70:297-298.
27. Wisner KL, Perel JM, Findling RL. Antidepressant treatment during breast-feeding. *Am J Psychiatry*. 1996;153:1132-1137.
28. Committee on Drugs, American Academy of Pediatrics. The transfer of drugs and other chemicals into human milk. *Pediatrics*. 2001;108:776-789.

BUROSUMAB

Genetic (Monoclonal Antibody)

PREGNANCY RECOMMENDATION: No Human Data—Animal Data Suggest Low Risk

BREASTFEEDING RECOMMENDATION: Probably Compatible

PREGNANCY SUMMARY

No reports describing the use of burosumab in human pregnancy have been located. As an IgG antibody, it likely crosses the placenta, so some fetal exposure will probably occur. Therefore, the absence of human pregnancy experience prevents a complete assessment of the embryofetal risk. Animal reproduction studies did not show any embryofetal toxicity. Using this drug during pregnancy should be based on the pros and cons of the mother's clinical need for treatment versus any potential fetal risk that might occur from exposure. There is a pregnancy exposure registry that monitors pregnancy outcomes in women using this drug. Health care providers are encouraged to call Kyowa Kirin at 1-844-768-3544.

BREASTFEEDING SUMMARY

No reports describing the use of burosumab during human lactation have been located. It is known that IgG antibodies can be found in human breast milk, but are not found in the neonatal or infant circulation. Additionally, if any IgG antibodies were to be ingested through breastfeeding, they would probably be digested in the infant's gastrointestinal tract and not be absorbed. Breastfeeding while using this drug should be based on the mother's clinical need for treatment. If used, the infant should be monitored for the most common reported adult side effects of headache, extremity pain, and abdominal pain (all leading to irritability), pyrexia, vomiting, cough, constipation, and rash.

Reference

1. Prescribing Information. Crysvita. Kyowa Kirin, Inc; 2023.

B

BUSPIRONE

Mental Health (Antianxiety)

PREGNANCY RECOMMENDATION: Limited Human Data—Animal Data Suggest Low Risk

BREASTFEEDING RECOMMENDATION: Potential Toxicity

PREGNANCY SUMMARY

A few studies on the use of buspirone during human pregnancy were located. In combined data from the Massachusetts General Hospital National Pregnancy Registry for Psychiatric Medications, Michigan Medicaid recipients—FDA, and pregnancies exposed to newly marketed drugs in England, a total of 127 pregnancies were exposed to buspirone, and 2 (1.6%) anomalies were reported. In addition, two case reports were also identified with mothers using buspirone in the first trimester, and no fetal anomalies were reported. The drug will likely cross the placenta, so some fetal exposure will probably occur. Though these data are reassuring, this limited human pregnancy experience still prevents a complete assessment of the embryofetal risk. Animal reproduction studies did not show any embryofetal toxicity. Using this drug during pregnancy should be based on the pros and cons of the mother's clinical need for treatment versus any potential fetal risk that might occur from exposure.

BREASTFEEDING SUMMARY

One case report of breastfeeding exposure to buspirone was located. The infant was also exposed to venlafaxine, and no adverse reactions were identified in the infant. It appears that buspirone can increase serum prolactin levels, but this should not adversely affect lactation. The drug will likely be found in breast milk, so some infant exposure will probably occur. Breastfeeding while using this drug should be based on the mother's clinical need for treatment. If used, the infant should be monitored for the most common reported adult side effects of nausea and headache (both leading to irritability), insomnia, and lethargy.

References

1. Prescribing Information. Buspirone. Actavis Pharma; 2018.
2. Freeman MP, Szpunar MJ, Kobylski LA, et al. Pregnancy outcomes after first-trimester exposure to buspirone: prospective longitudinal outcomes from the MGH National Pregnancy Registry for Psychiatric Medications. *Arch Womens Ment Health*. 2022;25:923-928.
3. Wilton LV, Pearce GL, Martin RM, et al. The outcomes of pregnancy in women exposed to newly marketed drugs in general practice in England. *Br J Obstet Gynaecol*. 1998;105:882-889.
4. Seifritz E, Holsboer-Trachsler E, Haberthur F, et al. Unrecognized pregnancy during citalopram treatment. *Am J Psychiatry*. 1993;150:1428-1429.
5. Brent NB, Wisner KL. Fluoxetine and carbamazepine concentrations in a nursing mother/infant pair. *Clin Pediatr*. 1998;37:41-44.
6. Newport DJ, Ritchie JC, Knight BT, et al. Venlafaxine in human breastmilk and nursing infant plasma. Determination of exposure. *J Clin Psychiatry*. 2009;70:1304-1310.
7. Gomez-Gil E, Navines R, Martinez De Osaba MJ, et al. Hormonal responses to the 5-HT1a agonist buspirone in remitted endogenous depressive patients after long-term imipramine treatment. *Psychoneuroendocrinology*. 2010;35:481-489.
8. Navines R, Gomez-Gil E, Matin-Santos R, et al. Hormonal response to buspirone is not impaired in major depression. *Hum Psychopharmacol*. 2007;22:389-395.
9. Maskall DD, Zis AP, Lam RW, et al. Prolactin response to buspirone challenge in the presence of dopaminergic blockade. *Biol Psychiatry*. 1995;38:235-239.

BUSULFAN

Antineoplastic (Alkylating Agent)

PREGNANCY RECOMMENDATION: Limited Human Data—Animal Data Suggest Risk

BREASTFEEDING RECOMMENDATION: Potential Toxicity

PREGNANCY SUMMARY

Numerous case reports and series were located that describe the use of busulfan in about 50 pregnant patients. Of these, about 30 involved first-trimester exposure. There were five newborns with major anomalies described, and all involved different organ systems. Some reports described IUGR, but this was not universally seen. The drug (and the **dimethylacetamide (DMA) solvent**) will probably cross the placenta, so some fetal exposure will likely occur. Animal studies did show embryofetal toxicity with malformations in three species, but dosing was not provided. Based on these animal studies, the manufacturer recommends that women with reproductive potential use effective contraception during treatment and for 1 week after the last dose. They also recommend that males with female partners of reproductive potential use effective contraception during treatment and for 1 week after the last dose. Nevertheless, using this drug during pregnancy should be

B

based on the pros and cons of the mother's clinical need for treatment versus any potential fetal risk that might occur from exposure. There is a registry for women who are pregnant and have cancer. For more information, women and health care providers are encouraged to contact the Cancer and Pregnancy Registry at 1-877-635-4499.

BREASTFEEDING SUMMARY

One study was located that described an infant who had no reported issues while exposed to busulfan through breastfeeding over a 5-week period. No breast milk or infant samples were obtained. The drug (and the DMA solvent) will probably be found in breast milk, so some infant exposure will likely occur. The manufacturer recommends that breastfeeding not occur when busulfan is used. Nevertheless, breastfeeding while using this drug should be based on the mother's clinical need for treatment versus any potential infant risks that might occur. If used, the infant should be monitored for the most common reported adult side effects of nausea, abdominal pain, headache, and anxiety (all leading to irritability), diarrhea, vomiting, decreased appetite (monitor infant growth), insomnia, pyrexia, and various laboratory abnormalities (see PI).

References

1. Prescribing Information. Myleran. Aspen Global; 2019.
2. Nicholson HO. Cytotoxic drugs in pregnancy: review of reported cases. *J Obstet Gynaecol Br Commonw*. 1968;75:307-312.
3. Lee RA, Johnson CE, Hanlon DG. Leukemia during pregnancy. *Am J Obstet Gynecol*. 1962;84:455-458.
4. Diamond I, Anderson MM, McCreadie SR. Transplacental transmission of busulfan (Myleran) in a mother with leukemia: production of fetal malformation and cytomegaly. *Pediatrics*. 1960;25:85-90.
5. Abramovici A, Shaklai M, Pinkhas J. Myeloschisis in a six weeks embryo of a leukemic woman treated by busulfan. *Teratology*. 1978;18:241-246.
6. Gililland J, Weinstein L. The effects of cancer chemotherapeutic agents on the developing fetus. *Obstet Gynecol Surv*. 1983;38:6-13.
7. Ozumba BC, Obi GO. Successful pregnancy in a patient with chronic myeloid leukemia following therapy with cytotoxic drugs. *Int J Gynecol Obstet*. 1992;38:49-53.
8. Boros SJ, Reynolds JW. Intrauterine growth retardation following third-trimester exposure to busulfan. *Am J Obstet Gynecol*. 1977;129:111-112.
9. Dugdale M, Fort AT. Busulfan treatment of leukemia during pregnancy. *JAMA*. 1967;199:131-133.
10. Zuazu J, Julia A, Sierra J, et al. Pregnancy outcome in hematologic malignancies. *Cancer*. 1991;67:703-709.
11. Dobbing J. Pregnancy and leukaemia. *Lancet*. 1977;1:1155.
12. Wiebe VJ, Sipila PEH. Pharmacology of antineoplastic agents in pregnancy. *Crit Rev Oncol Hematol*. 1994;16:75-112.
13. Gebhart E, Schwanitz G, Hartwich G. Chromosomal aberrations during busulfan therapy. *Dtsch Med Wochenschr*. 1974;99:52-56.
14. Galton DAG, Till M, Wiltshaw E. Busulfan: summary of clinical results. *Ann NY Acad Sci*. 1958;68:967-973.
15. Schilsky RL, Lewis BJ, Sherins RJ, Young RC. Gonadal dysfunction in patients receiving chemotherapy for cancer. *Ann Intern Med*. 1980;93:109-114.
16. Shalev O, Rahav G, Milwidsky A. Reversible busulfan-induced ovarian failure. *Eur J Obstet Gynecol Reprod Biol*. 1987;26:239-242.
17. Bounameaux T, Durenne JM. A case of leukemia in a lactating female: effect of treatment with busulfan on the infant. *Ann Soc Belge Med Trop*. 1964;44:381-383.

BUTALBITAL

Central Nervous System (Barbiturate)

PREGNANCY RECOMMENDATION: Human Data Suggest Potential Risk (First and Third Trimesters)—No Relevant Animal Data

BREASTFEEDING RECOMMENDATION: Potential Toxicity

PREGNANCY SUMMARY

A total of 1,236 first-trimester exposures to butalbital were reported in combined data from the Collaborative Perinatal Project and the Michigan Medicaid FDA databases. There were 57 (4.6%) newborns identified with major or minor malformations. However, no specific pattern was noted, and coexposures to other drugs occurred. In a publication from the National Birth Defects Prevention Study, 73 self-reported periconceptional butalbital exposure cases were reported. The drug was associated with a significant increase in cardiac malformations, including tetralogy of Fallot, pulmonary valve stenosis, and secundum type atrial septal defect. However, self-reported recall history can be flawed (in some cases, the interview occurred up to 3 years after the patient's first-trimester time period); verification of actual drug use, the dosage, and exact timing of use during the first trimester cannot be confirmed; and recall may be affected by whether or not a mother delivered a newborn with an anomaly. Lastly, neonatal withdrawal has been described in a newborn shortly after delivery in a case where the mother took a combination drug of butalbital, caffeine, and acetaminophen for the last 2 months of the pregnancy. The drug will probably cross the placenta, so some fetal exposure will likely occur. Therefore, further study in the use of butalbital during human pregnancy is needed in order to provide a complete assessment of the embryofetal risk, especially in the area of cardiac anomalies. Animal reproduction studies have not been conducted. Using this drug during pregnancy should be based on the pros and cons of the mother's clinical need for treatment versus any potential fetal risk that might occur from exposure. The drug has the potential for the development of tolerance and misuse. It is classified as a Schedule III controlled substance. ACOG recommends against the use of products containing butalbital because of increased risks for overuse with headache, tolerance, and no significant analgesia.

B

BREASTFEEDING SUMMARY

No published studies describing the use of butalbital during human lactation have been located. An abstract reported on a breastfeeding newborn that had lethargy, vomiting, and poor feeding in a mother using a drug combination of butalbital, acetaminophen, and caffeine. The neonate's symptoms were thought to be caused by the butalbital. The drug will probably be excreted into breast milk, so some infant exposure will likely occur. Other barbiturates are known to be found in breast milk. Breastfeeding while using this drug should be based on the mother's clinical need for treatment. If used, the infant should be monitored for the most common reported adult side effects of nausea and abdominal pain (both leading to irritability), sedation, vomiting, and shortness of breath.

References

1. Prescribing Information. Butalbital, acetaminophen, caffeine. Actavis Pharma, Inc; 2017.
2. Headaches in Pregnancy and Postpartum. Clinical Practice Guideline No. 3. American College of Obstetricians and Gynecologists. *Obstet Gynecol.* 2021;139:944-972.
3. Heinonen OP, Slone D, Shapiro S. *Birth Defects and Drugs in Pregnancy.* Publishing Sciences Group; 1983:336-337.
4. Browne ML, Van Zutphen AR, Botto LD, et al. Maternal butalbital use and selected defects in the national birth defects prevention study. *Headache.* 2014;54:54-66.
5. Ostrea EM. Neonatal withdrawal from intrauterine exposure to butalbital. *Am J Obstet Gynecol.* 1982;143:597-599.
6. Vohra V, Marraffa JM. Maternal use of acetaminophen-butalbital-caffeine product resulting in neonate butalbital exposure through breast milk. *Clin Toxicol.* 2019;57:549. [Abstract].

BUTENAFINE

Dermatologic (Antifungal—Topical)

PREGNANCY RECOMMENDATION: No Human Data and No Relevant Animal Data

BREASTFEEDING RECOMMENDATION: Probably Compatible

PREGNANCY SUMMARY

No reports describing the use of butenafine in human pregnancy have been located. The drug will probably cross the placenta; however, due to its topical use and low systemic absorption, fetal exposure is likely negligible. However, the absence of human pregnancy experience prevents a complete assessment of the embryofetal risk. Animal reproduction studies were not relevant. Using this drug during pregnancy should be based on the pros and cons of the mother's clinical need for treatment versus any potential fetal risk that might occur from exposure.

BREASTFEEDING SUMMARY

No reports describing the use of butenafine during human lactation have been located. Due to the topical use of the drug and low plasma levels seen following systemic absorption, infant exposure is likely negligible. Breastfeeding while using this drug should be based on the mother's clinical need for treatment. Due to the topical use of the drug, systemic adverse drug reactions were not recorded. Use of this topical agent around the nipple area should not occur during lactation.

Reference

1. Prescribing Information. Mentax. Mylan Pharmaceuticals, Inc; 2018.

BUTORPHANOL

Pain (Analgesic/Opioid)

PREGNANCY RECOMMENDATION: Limited Human Data—Animal Data Suggest Low Risk

BREASTFEEDING RECOMMENDATION: Probably Compatible

PREGNANCY SUMMARY

No reports describing the use of butorphanol in human pregnancy during the first trimester have been located. The drug crosses the term placenta, so some fetal exposure will occur. Therefore, the absence of first-trimester exposure in human pregnancy prevents a complete assessment of the embryofetal risk. Numerous studies have analyzed the use of this drug as an analgesic during term labor, with results that are about equal to other available narcotic choices. Butorphanol may also decrease shivering associated with epidural anesthesia and decrease morphine-induced pruritus after cesarean delivery. Lastly, a sinusoidal-like FHR pattern may occur in some cases when the drug is administered during labor. A true sinusoidal

B

FHR pattern is very rare and concerning and is associated with severe chronic fetal anemia or severe acute intrapartum asphyxia. It is defined as: (1) a stable baseline with regular oscillations; (2) oscillation amplitude of 5 to 15 beats per minute, rarely greater; (3) frequency of two to five cycles per minute as long-term variability; (4) flat absent short-term variability; (5) the sinusoidal oscillation is above and below the baseline; and (6) no areas of normal FHR patterns, such as accelerations. With the change in FHR monitor definitions, variability is now described as a whole and is not broken down into short-term or long-term variability. However, a true sinusoidal pattern is somewhat of an exception to these new definitions. The sinusoidal-like FHR patterns seen with butorphanol and other narcotics administered intrapartum demonstrate the uniform sine wave (long-term variability) pattern, but some short-term variability is usually present in the waveform itself; the pattern begins abruptly shortly after drug administration; and a normal FHR pattern (with accelerations, etc) was present prior to administration, and develops again as the drug wears off, usually within 1 to 2 hours (unless the drug is readministered). A true sinusoidal pattern will not resolve prior to delivery unless the severe fetal anemia is corrected by an intrauterine transfusion. Using this drug during pregnancy should be based on the pros and cons of the mother's clinical need for treatment versus any potential fetal risk that might occur from exposure. The drug (because it is an opioid) carries a boxed warning for an increased risk of misuse, addiction, life-threatening respiratory depression, and neonatal opioid withdrawal syndrome. The drug is classified as a Schedule IV controlled substance.

BREASTFEEDING SUMMARY

Butorphanol was found to be excreted into breast milk with a calculated total infant dose of about 4 mcg/L of breast milk. The maximum amount of drug that might be consumed by an exclusively breastfed infant is about 0.1% of the maternal weight-adjusted dose. In addition, the drug is poorly absorbed orally and actually is not available in this format in the United States. Therefore, this amount is probably clinically insignificant. Another study did not report any adverse infant effects in 22 mothers who breastfed while receiving butorphanol. Lastly, some narcotic drugs have been found to increase serum prolactin levels, but this should not adversely affect breastfeeding. Breastfeeding while using this drug should be based on the mother's clinical need for treatment. If used, the infant should be monitored for the most common reported adult side effects of nausea and pruritus (both leading to irritability), somnolence, lethargy, respiratory depression, and vomiting.

References

1. Prescribing Information. Butorphanol. NovaPlus; 2023.
2. Pittman KA, Smyth RD, Losada M, et al. Human perinatal distribution of butorphanol. *Am J Obstet Gynecol*. 1980;138:797-800.
3. Maduska AL, Hajghassemali M. A double-blind comparison of butorphanol and meperidine in labour: maternal pain relief and effect on the newborn. *Can Anaesth Soc J*. 1978;25:398-404.
4. Quilligan EJ, Keegan KA, Donahue MJ. Double-blind comparison of intravenously injected butorphanol and meperidine in parturients. *Int J Gynaecol Obstet*. 1980;18:363-367.
5. Hodgkinson R, Huff RW, Hayashi RH, Husain FJ. Double-blind comparison of maternal analgesia and neonatal neurobehavior following intravenous butorphanol and meperidine. *J Int Med Res*. 1979;7:224-230.
6. Atkinson BD, Truitt LJ, Rayburn WF, et al. Double-blind comparison of intravenous butorphanol (Stadol) and fentanyl (Sublimaze) for analgesia during labor. *Am J Obstet Gynecol*. 1994;171:993-998.
7. Hunt CO, Naulty JS, Malinow AM, et al. Epidural butorphanol-bupivacaine for analgesia during labor and delivery. *Anesth Analg*. 1989;68:323-327.
8. Nelson KE, Eisenach JC. Intravenous butorphanol, meperidine, and their combination relieve pain and distress in women in labor. *Anesthesiology*. 2005;102:1008-1013.
9. Garrity K, Jang A, Wagner S. Butorphanol use in laboring patients with preeclampsia or chronic hypertension. *Pregnancy Hypertens*. 2016;6:288-290.
10. Juneja M, Ackerman WE III, Heine MF, et al. Butorphanol for the relief of shivering associated with extradural anesthesia in parturients. *J Clin Anesth* 1992;4:390-393.
11. Wu Z, Kong M, Wang N, et al. Intravenous butorphanol administration reduces intrathecal morphine-induced pruritus after cesarean delivery: a randomized, double-blind, placebo-controlled study. *J Anesth*. 2012;26: 752-757.
12. Angel JL, Knuppel RA, Lake M. Sinusoidal fetal heart rate pattern associated with intravenous butorphanol administration: a case report. *Am J Obstet Gynecol*. 1984;149:465-467.
13. Welt SI. Sinusoidal fetal heart rate and butorphanol administration. *Am J Obstet Gynecol*. 1985;152:362-363.
14. Hatjis CG, Meis PJ. Sinusoidal fetal heart rate pattern associated with butorphanol administration. *Obstet Gynecol*. 1986;67:377-380.
15. Modanlou HD, Freeman RK. Sinusoidal fetal heart rate pattern: its definition and clinical significance. *Am J Obstet Gynecol*. 1982;142:1033.
16. American College of Obstetricians & Gynecologists. Intrapartum fetal heart rate monitoring: nomenclature, interpretation, and general management principles. Practice Bulletin No. 106. July 2009.
17. Tolis G, Dent R, Guyda H. Opiates, prolactin, and the dopamine receptor. *J Clin Endocrinol Metab*. 1978;47:200-203.

C

CABAZITAXEL

Antineoplastic (Microtubule Inhibitor)

PREGNANCY RECOMMENDATION: *Contraindicated

BREASTFEEDING RECOMMENDATION: *Contraindicated

PREGNANCY SUMMARY

No reports describing the use of cabazitaxel in human pregnancy have been located. The drug will probably cross the placenta, so some fetal exposure will likely occur. Therefore, the absence of human pregnancy experience prevents a complete assessment of the embryofetal risk. *However, based on the drug's approved use, it is contraindicated for use in women. Animal data showed embryofetal toxicity at exposures much less than the maximum recommended human dose (MRHD). Based on these animal studies, the manufacturer recommends that males with female partners of reproductive potential use effective contraception during treatment and for 3 months after the last dose. There is a registry for women who are pregnant and have cancer. For more information, women and health care providers are encouraged to contact the Cancer and Pregnancy Registry at 1-877-635-4499.

BREASTFEEDING SUMMARY

No reports describing the use of cabazitaxel during human lactation have been located. The drug would likely be found in breast milk, so some infant exposure would probably occur. *However, based on the drug's approved use, it is contraindicated for use in women. If, for some reason, the drug were to be used off-label in a lactating woman, the infant should be monitored for the most common reported adult side effects of nausea and back pain (both leading to irritability), fatigue (lethargy), diarrhea, vomiting, and various laboratory abnormalities (see Prescribing Information [PI]).

Reference

1. Prescribing Information. *Jevtana*. Sanofi-Aventis US; 2021.

CABERGOLINE

Endocrine/Metabolic (Prolactin Inhibition)

PREGNANCY RECOMMENDATION: Human Data Suggest Low Risk

BREASTFEEDING RECOMMENDATION: Contraindicated

PREGNANCY SUMMARY

Elevated prolactin levels can lead to infertility. Cabergoline is used to lower prolactin levels, and by doing so, many women conceive. Therefore, there are numerous studies totaling more than 600 pregnancy outcomes while on cabergoline at the time of conception and into the first trimester. The major birth anomaly rate falls within the expected 2% to 4% rate in the United States, and no pattern to the reported anomalies has been identified. The drug will probably cross the placenta, so some fetal exposure will likely occur. Animal studies did show some embryofetal toxicity in one species at doses of less than the recommended human dose (RHD), but this was not seen in two other species with doses more than 10 times the RHD. Using this drug during pregnancy should be based on the pros and cons of the mother's clinical need for treatment versus any potential fetal risk that might occur from exposure. The drug should not be used in patients with hypertension (including hypertension related to pregnancy), unless it is felt that the benefits outweigh the potential risks.

BREASTFEEDING SUMMARY

No reports describing the use of cabergoline regarding whether the drug is excreted into breast milk were located. A few reports have described newborns exposed to the drug during lactation with no reported infant complications. Although it is not an approved indication, cabergoline suppresses lactation because it inhibits prolactin release from the anterior pituitary gland. This action is similar to that of bromocriptine, another prolactin-inhibiting agent. A number of studies have reported the successful response rate of lactation suppression when cabergoline is administered postpartum. The manufacturer states that cabergoline should not be used to suppress physiologic lactation because of the known toxicities associated with bromocriptine (hypertension, stroke, and seizures) when used for this purpose. If cabergoline is used while a mother is nursing, the infant should be monitored for hypertension, along with the most common reported adult side effects of headache, dizziness, and nausea (all leading to irritability), and constipation.

References

1. Colao A, di Sarno A, Pivonello R, et al. Dopamine receptor agonists for treating prolactinomas. *Expert Opin Investig Drugs*. 2002;11:787-800.
2. Robert E, Musatti L, Piscitelli G, et al. Pregnancy outcome after treatment with the ergot derivative, cabergoline. *Reprod Toxicol*. 1996;10:333-737.
3. Product information. *Cabergoline*. Apotex; 2017.
4. Beltrame D, Longo M, Mazue G. Reproductive toxicity of cabergoline in mice, rats, and rabbits. *Reprod Toxicol*. 1996;10:471-483.
5. Negishi H, Koide SS. Prevention and termination of pregnancy in rats by cabergoline, a dopamine agonist. *J Reprod Fertil*. 1997;109:103-107.
6. Ferrari C, Paracchi A, Mattei AM, et al. Cabergoline in the long-term therapy of hyperprolactinemic disorders. *Acta Endocrinol*. 1992;126:489-494.
7. Jones TH, Fraser RB. Cabergoline treated hyperprolactinaemia results in pregnancy in a bromocriptine intolerant patient after seventeen years of infertility. *Br J Obstet Gynaecol*. 1994;101:349-350.
8. Ciccarelli E, Grottoli S, Razzore P, et al. Long-term treatment with cabergoline, a new long-lasting ergoline derivative, in idiopathic or tumorous hyperprolactinaemia and outcome of drug-induced pregnancy. *J Endocrinol Invest*. 1997;20:547-551.
9. Ricci E, Parazzini F, Motta T, et al. Pregnancy outcome after cabergoline treatment in early weeks of gestation. *Reprod Toxicol*. 2002;16:791-793.
10. Scott M, Chowdhury M. Pregnancy in Parkinson's disease: unique case report and review of the literature. *Mov Disord*. 2005;20:1078-1079.
11. Schlechte JA. Update in pituitary 2010. *J Clin Endocrinol Metab*. 2011; 96:1-8.
12. Colao A, Abs R, Barcena DG, et al. Pregnancy outcomes following cabergoline treatment: extended results from a 12 year observational study. *Clin Endocrinol (Oxf)*. 2008;68:66-71.
13. Ono M, Miki N, Amano K, et al. Individualized high dose cabergoline therapy for hyperprolactinemic infertility in women with micro-and macroprolactinomas. *J Clin Endocrinol Metab*. 2010;95:2672-2679.
14. Lebbe M, Hubinont C, Bernard P, et al. Outcome of 100 pregnancies initiated under treatment with cabergoline in hyperprolactinaemic women. *Clin Endocrinol (Oxf)*. 2010;73:236-242.
15. Woo I, Ehsanipoor RM. Cabergoline therapy for Cushing disease throughout pregnancy. *Obstet Gynecol*. 2013;122:485-487.
16. Hurault-Delarue C, Montastruc JL, Beau AB, et al. Pregnancy outcome in women exposed to dopamine agonists during pregnancy: a pharmacoepidemiology study in EFEMERIS database. *Arch Gynecol Obstet*. 2014;290: 263-270.
17. Araujo B, Belo S, Carvalho D. Pregnancy and tumor outcomes in women with prolactinoma. *Exp Clin Endocrinol Diabetes*. 2017;125:642-648.
18. Sek KS, Deepak DS, Lee KO. Use of cabergoline for the management of persistent Cushing's disease in pregnancy. *BMJ Case Rep*. 2017;2017: bcr-2016-217855.
19. Melis GB, Gambacciani M, Paoletti AM, et al. Dose-related prolactin inhibitory effect of the new long-acting dopamine receptor agonist cabergoline in normal cycling, puerperal, and hyperprolactinemic women. *J Clin Endocrinol Metab*. 1987;65:541-545.
20. Melis GB, Mais V, Paoletti AM, et al. Prevention of puerperal lactation by a single oral administration of the new prolactin-inhibiting drug, cabergoline. *Obstet Gynecol*. 1988;71:311-314.
21. Giorda G, de Vincentiis S, Motta T, et al. Cabergoline versus bromocriptine in suppression of lactation after cesarean delivery. *Gynecol Obstet Invest*. 1991;31:93-96.
22. Rolland R, Piscitelli G, Ferrari C, et al; the European Multicentre Study Group for Cabergoline in Lactation Inhibition. Single dose cabergoline versus bromocriptine in inhibition of puerperal lactation: randomised, double blind, multicentre study. *Br Med J*. 1991;302:1367-1371.
23. Caballero-Gordo A, Lopez-Nazareno N, Calderay M, et al. Oral cabergoline. Single-dose inhibition of puerperal lactation. *J Reprod Med*. 1991;36: 717-721.
24. Ferrari C, Piscitelli G, Grosignani PG. Cabergoline: a new drug for the treatment of hyperprolactinaemia. *Hum Reprod*. 1995;10:1647-1652.

CABOTEGRAVIR AND RILPIVIRINE

Antiretroviral (Non-Nucleoside Reverse Transcriptase Inhibitor)

PREGNANCY RECOMMENDATION: Limited Human Data—Animal Data Suggests Low Risk

BREASTFEEDING RECOMMENDATION: *Contraindicated

PREGNANCY SUMMARY

No reports describing the use of the combination product cabotegravir/rilpivirine or cabotegravir by itself in human pregnancy have been located. As of the end of 2020, over 390 exposures to rilpivirine during the first trimester and over 170 exposures in the second/third trimester have been reported to the Antiretroviral Pregnancy Registry. The prevalence of birth anomalies from first-trimester exposure was only 1.3%. Both drugs will likely cross the placenta, so some fetal exposure will probably occur. Therefore, the absence of human pregnancy experience with cabotegravir prevents a complete assessment of the embryofetal risk. Animal studies did not show any embryofetal toxicity. Using this drug during pregnancy should be based on the pros and cons of the mother's clinical need for treatment versus any potential fetal risk that might occur from exposure. Cabotegravir/rilpivirine can be detected in the systemic circulation for up to 12 months after the last injection. The manufacturer recommends that cabotegravir/rilpivirine levels be monitored closely during pregnancy because oral rilpivirine may have lower levels during gestation. Women who are pregnant and have taken cabotegravir/rilpivirine at any time during pregnancy are encouraged to contact the Antiretroviral Pregnancy Registry at 1-800-258-4263.

C

BREASTFEEDING SUMMARY

No reports describing the use of cabotegravir/rilpivirine during human lactation have been located. Both drugs will likely be excreted into breast milk, so infant exposure will probably occur. *For patients not on therapy or those without viral load suppression during pregnancy (at a minimum of throughout the third trimester) and at delivery, replacement milk is recommended.

References

1. Prescribing Information. *Cabenuva*. Viiv Healthcare; 2021.
2. The U.S. Department of Health and Human Services Panel on treatment of HIV during pregnancy and prevention of perinatal transmission. *Recommendations for the use of antiretroviral drugs during pregnancy and interventions to reduce perinatal HIV transmission in the United States*. Accessed January 5, 2023. https://clinicalinfo.hiv.gov/en/guidelines/perinatal

CABOZANTINIB

Antineoplastic (Tyrosine Kinase Inhibitor)

PREGNANCY RECOMMENDATION: No Human Data—Animal Data Suggest Risk

BREASTFEEDING RECOMMENDATION: Potential Toxicity

PREGNANCY SUMMARY

No reports describing the use of cabozantinib in human pregnancy have been located. The drug will probably cross the placenta, so some fetal exposure will likely occur. Therefore, the absence of human pregnancy experience prevents a complete assessment of the embryofetal risk. Animal studies did show embryofetal toxicity with malformations in two animal species. Based on these animal studies and the drug's mechanism of action, the manufacturer recommends that women with reproductive potential use effective contraception during treatment and for 4 months after the last dose. However, using this drug during pregnancy should be based on the pros and cons of the mother's clinical need for treatment versus any potential fetal risk that might occur from exposure. In the clinical trials, up to 36% of patients developed hypertension, and 7% were found to have proteinuria (this could mimic preeclampsia). There is a registry for women who are pregnant and have cancer. For more information, women and health care providers are encouraged to contact the Cancer and Pregnancy Registry at 1-877-635-4499.

BREASTFEEDING SUMMARY

No reports describing the use of cabozantinib during human lactation have been located. Some amount of the drug will likely be found in breast milk, so infant exposure will probably occur. Therefore, due to a concern for potential serious adverse effects that might be seen in a breastfed infant, the manufacturer recommends that women not breastfeed while being treated with this drug and for at least 4 months after the last dose. Nevertheless, breastfeeding while using this drug should be based on the mother's clinical need for treatment versus any potential infant risks. If used, the infant should be monitored for the most common reported adult side effects of nausea (leading to irritability), fatigue (lethargy), vomiting, diarrhea, decreased appetite, and hypertension.

Reference

1. Prescribing Information. *Cometriq*. Exelixis; 2019.

CALASPARGASE PEGOL

Antineoplastic (Enzyme)

PREGNANCY RECOMMENDATION: No Human Data and No Relevant Animal Data

BREASTFEEDING RECOMMENDATION: Probably Compatible

PREGNANCY SUMMARY

No reports describing the use of calaspargase pegol in human pregnancy have been located. Because the drug consists of a large protein, it is not known whether some fetal exposure will occur. However, the absence of human pregnancy experience prevents a complete assessment of the embryofetal risk. Animal reproduction studies have not been performed. Because of the mechanism of action, the manufacturer recommends that females of reproductive potential use effective nonhormonal contraception during treatment with this drug and for 3 months after the last dose. Nevertheless, using this drug during pregnancy should be based on the pros and cons of the mother's clinical need for treatment versus any potential fetal risk that might occur from exposure.

BREASTFEEDING SUMMARY

It is not known if calaspargase pegol is excreted into human breast milk. The drug and its components will probably not appear in breast milk, or the levels would be negligible. Furthermore, if ingested through breastfeeding, the enzyme is a protein, and it most likely would be digested in the infant's gastrointestinal tract and not be absorbed. However, the manufacturer recommends that women not breastfeed their infant if treated with this drug and for 3 months after the last dose. Nevertheless, breastfeeding while using calaspargase pegol should be based on the mother's clinical need for treatment. If used, the infant should be monitored for the most common reported adult side effects of pancreatitis and abnormal clotting studies.

C

Reference

1. Prescribing Information. *Asparlas*. Servier Pharmaceutical, LLC; 2018.

CALCIFEDIOL

Vitamin

PREGNANCY RECOMMENDATION: Human Data Suggest Compatible

BREASTFEEDING RECOMMENDATION: Compatible

See Vitamin D.

CALCIPOTRIENE

Dermatologic (Topical/Antipsoriatic)

PREGNANCY RECOMMENDATION: No Human Data—Animal Data Suggest Low Risk

BREASTFEEDING RECOMMENDATION: Probably Compatible

PREGNANCY SUMMARY

No reports describing the use of calcipotriene in human pregnancy have been located. The drug may cross the placenta with topical use, but the overall amount is likely to be clinically insignificant. However, the absence of human pregnancy experience prevents a complete assessment of the embryofetal risk. Animal data did not show any embryofetal toxicity or malformations in two species at doses of less than 10 times the recommended human therapeutic dose (RHTD). Some embryofetal toxicity was seen, but in doses of more than 10 times the RHTD. Using this drug during pregnancy should be based on the pros and cons of the mother's clinical need for treatment versus any potential fetal risk that might occur from exposure.

BREASTFEEDING SUMMARY

No reports describing the use of calcipotriene during human lactation have been located. The drug may be found in breast milk, but the overall amount is likely to be clinically insignificant. Breastfeeding while using this drug should be based on the mother's clinical need for treatment versus any potential infant risks that might occur. Because of the topical use of the drug, systemic side effects were not reported.

Reference

1. Prescribing Information. *Dovonex cream/ointment*. LEO Pharma, Inc; 2019.

CALCITONIN SALMON

Endocrine (Calcium Regulation Hormone)

PREGNANCY RECOMMENDATION: Limited Human Data—Animal Data Suggest Low Risk

BREASTFEEDING RECOMMENDATION: Probably Compatible

C

PREGNANCY SUMMARY

Five case reports were located describing the use of calcitonin salmon during human pregnancy. In two cases, the administration occurred at about 10 weeks of gestation, one a single dose and the other continued throughout the pregnancy. The other three occurred in the third trimester. All newborns were healthy at delivery with no reported anomalies. The drug does not appear to cross the placenta. However, if any drug does cross, this would likely occur during the second half of pregnancy, but the amount would probably be negligible. Regardless, this limited human pregnancy experience prevents a complete assessment of the embryofetal risk. Animal studies did not show any embryofetal toxicity or teratogenicity in two species at doses of less than 10 times the RHD. The manufacturer states that the drug is not indicated for use in females with reproductive potential due to limited clinical information. Nevertheless, using this drug during pregnancy should be based on the pros and cons of the mother's clinical need for treatment versus any potential fetal risk that might occur from exposure (especially since it does not appear to cross the placenta).

BREASTFEEDING SUMMARY

One report describing the use of calcitonin salmon during human lactation has been located. The drug was being administered to a postpartum woman who was also receiving various doses of azathioprine, prednisone, warfarin, calcitriol, and acetaminophen. She nursed for about 12 months. Her infant was evaluated at 15 months of age and was found to have normal growth and development. Calcitonin and procalcitonin are normal constituents of human breast milk. However, because it is a polypeptide, if the drug were to be ingested through breastfeeding, it would probably be digested in the infant's gastrointestinal tract and not be absorbed. The manufacturer states that the drug is not indicated for use in lactating females because of a lack of studies and the possibility of decreasing serum prolactin levels. Nevertheless, breastfeeding while using this drug should be based on the mother's clinical need for treatment versus any potential infant risks that might occur. If used, the infant should be monitored for the most common reported adult side effects of back pain, arthralgia, and headache (all leading to irritability). In addition, no studies have been located that have shown calcitonin salmon lowers prolactin levels in lactating women.

References

1. Prescribing Information. *Miacalcin*. Mylan Pharmaceuticals Inc; 2021.
2. Kovarik J, Woloszczuk W, Linkesch W, et al. Calcitonin in pregnancy. *Lancet*. 1980;1:199-200.
3. Schnatz PF, Curry SL. Primary hyperparathyroidism in pregnancy: evidence-based management. *Obstet Gynecol Surv*. 2002;57:365-376.
4. Turek T, Wigton A. Calcitonin for phantom limb pain in a pregnant woman. *Am J Health Syst Pharm*. 2012;69:2149-2152.
5. Krysiak R, Wilk M, Okopien B. Recurrent pancreatitis induced by hyperparathyroidism in pregnancy. *Arch Gynecol Obstet*. 2011;284:531-534.
6. Fromm GA, Labarrere CA, Ramirez J, et al. Hypercalcaemia in pregnancy in a renal transplant recipient with secondary hyperparathyroidism—case report. *Br J Obstet Gynaecol*. 1990;97:1049-1053.
7. Murray JA, Newman 3rd WA, Dacus JV. Hyperparathyroidism in pregnancy: diagnostic dilemma? *Obstet Gynecol Surv*. 1997;52:202-205.
8. Horjus C, Groot I, Telting D, et al. Cinacalcet for hyperparathyroidism in pregnancy and puerperium. *J Pediatr Endocrinol Metab*. 2009;22:741-749.
9. Moretti ME, Verjee Z, Ito S, Koren G. Breast-feeding during maternal use of azathioprine. *Ann Pharmacother*. 2006;40:2269-2271.
10. Ballard O, Morrow AL. Human milk composition: nutrients and bioactive factors. *Pediatr Clin North Am*. 2013;60:49-74.
11. Koldovsky O. Hormones in milk. *Vitam Horm*. 1995;50:77-149.

CALCITRIOL

Vitamin

PREGNANCY RECOMMENDATION: Limited Human Data—Animal Data Suggests Potential Risk

BREASTFEEDING RECOMMENDATION: Probably Compatible

PREGNANCY SUMMARY

The manufacturer cited a case of mild hypercalcemia during the first 2 days of life in an infant who was exposed to a maternal oral dose during pregnancy that was about 10 to 21 times the MRHD. The hypercalcemia resolved in the neonate by the third day of life. Overall, there is no evidence that recommended doses of vitamin D during pregnancy are harmful. The vitamin probably crosses the placenta, so some fetal exposure will likely occur. Therefore, the absence of human pregnancy experience prevents a complete assessment of the embryofetal risk. Animal studies did show some potential teratogenicity in one species at doses of less than 10 times the RHD. Using this drug during pregnancy should be based on the pros and cons of the mother's clinical need for treatment versus any potential fetal risk that might occur from exposure.

BREASTFEEDING SUMMARY

Five reports were located that describe the use of calcitriol during human lactation in six newborns. No calcitriol blood levels were obtained, but no complications were reported in the nursing newborns. Taking an appropriate dose of calcitriol while breastfeeding is probably not harmful to a nursing infant. Breastfeeding while using this drug should be based on the mother's clinical need for treatment. If used, the infant should be monitored for the most common reported adult side effects of headache, nausea, and muscle/bone/abdominal pain (all leading to irritability), lethargy, and somnolence. If used chronically while breastfeeding, it is recommended that infant calcium levels be monitored.

References

1. Prescribing Information. *Rocaltrol*. Validus Pharmaceuticals; 2021.
2. Cundy T, Haining SA, Guilland-Cumming DF, et al. Remission of hypoparathyroidism during lactation: evidence for a physiological role for prolactin in the regulation of vitamin D metabolism. *Clin Endocrinol (Oxf)*. 1987;26:667-674.
3. Caplan RH, Wickus GG. Reduced calcitriol requirements for treating hypoparathyroidism during lactation. a case report. *J Reprod Med*. 1993;38:914-918.
4. Callies F, Arlt W, Scholz HJ, et al. Management of hypoparathyroidism during pregnancy—report of twelve cases. *Eur J Endocrinol*. 1998;139:284-289.
5. Moretti ME, Verjee Z, Ito S, et al. Breast-feeding during maternal use of azathioprine. *Ann Pharmacother*. 2006;40:2269-2272.
6. Shulman D. Subcutaneous infusion of rhPTH(1-43) during pregnancy and nursing in a woman with autosomal dominant hypoparathyroidism 1. *J Endocr Soc*. 2022;6:bvac031.

C

CALCIUM CARBONATE

Gastrointestinal/Nutrient (Antacid—Mineral)

PREGNANCY RECOMMENDATION: Compatible (With Recommended Use)

BREASTFEEDING RECOMMENDATION: Compatible (With Recommended Use)

PREGNANCY SUMMARY

Sufficient maternal calcium intake is important to ensure adequate mineralization of the fetal skeleton. The American College of Obstetricians and Gynecologists (ACOG) recommends a maximum daily dose of 2,500 mg of calcium in pregnancy. No studies have been performed on calcium use in the first trimester and the risk for teratogenicity. Calcium is part of a normal diet and is found in prenatal vitamins, and therefore, would not be considered a teratogen. A number of studies have evaluated calcium supplementation with calcium carbonate to prevent or reduce the risk of hypertensive disorders in pregnancy (gestational hypertension and preeclampsia). Although many of these studies reported a reduction in hypertensive disorders, two large studies did not find this association. Excess calcium intake can lead to an increased risk for kidney stones, constipation, and decrease the gastrointestinal absorption of iron and zinc. In addition, excessive ingestion of calcium carbonate has been associated with three published cases of milk-alkali syndrome in pregnancy. Milk-alkali syndrome is a disorder of severe hypercalcemia caused by excess intake of calcium (usually antacids), often in conjunction with high dietary intake, usually to treat acid indigestion. It is characterized by elevated blood calcium levels, metabolic alkalosis, and acute renal injury. Patients present with confusion, tremors, psychosis, nausea, vomiting, polyuria, and pruritus. If untreated, this disorder can lead to renal failure and death. Calcium crosses the placenta.

BREASTFEEDING SUMMARY

The recommended daily allowance (RDA) for calcium during lactation is about 1,300 mg/d. Calcium is excreted into breast milk. No specific studies have analyzed breastfeeding for adverse effects with calcium supplementation. However, this mineral is part of a normal diet and is needed for normal development and sustenance. Therefore, normal dosages are considered compatible during pregnancy.

References

1. Prescribing Information. *Calcium Carbonate*. Numerous Suppliers; 2023.
2. Care AD. The placental transfer of calcium. *J Dev Physiol*. 1991;15:253-257.
3. Belizan JM, Villar J, Zalazar A, et al. Preliminary evidence of the effect of calcium supplementation on blood pressure in normal pregnant women. *Am J Obstet Gynecol*. 1983;146:175-180.
4. Villar J, Repke J, Belizan JM, et al. Calcium supplementation reduces blood pressure during pregnancy: results of a randomized controlled clinical trial. *Obstet Gynecol*. 1987;70:317-322.
5. Repke JT, Villar J, Anderson C, et al. Biochemical changes associated with blood pressure reduction induced by calcium supplementation during pregnancy. *Am J Obstet Gynecol*. 1989;160:684-690.
6. Villar J, Repke JT. Calcium supplementation during pregnancy may reduce preterm delivery in high-risk patients. *Am J Obstet Gynecol*. 1990;163:1124-1131.
7. Belizan JM, Villar J, Gonzalez L, et al. Calcium supplementation to prevent hypertensive disorders of pregnancy. *N Engl J Med*. 1991;325:1399-1405.
8. Sanchez-Ramos L, Briones DK, Kaunitz AM, et al. Prevention of pregnancy-induced hypertension by calcium supplementation in angiotensin II-sensitive patients. *Obstet Gynecol*. 1994;84:349-353.
9. Carroli G, Duley L, Belizan JM, et al. Calcium supplementation during pregnancy: a systematic review of randomised controlled trials. *Br J Obstet Gynaecol*. 1994;101:753-758.
10. Sanchez-Ramos L, Adair CD, Kaunitz AM, et al. Calcium supplementation in mild preeclampsia remote from term: a randomized double-blind clinical trial. *Obstet Gynecol*. 1995;85:915-918.
11. Bucher HC, Guyatt GH, Cook RJ, et al. Effect of calcium supplementation on pregnancy-induced hypertension and preeclampsia—a meta-analysis of randomized controlled trials. *JAMA*. 1996;275:1113-1117.
12. Lopez-Jaramillo P, Delgado F, Jacome P, et al. Calcium supplementation and risk of preeclampsia in Ecuadorian pregnant teenagers. *Obstet Gynecol*. 1997;90:162-167.
13. Boggess KA, Samuel L, Schmucker BC, et al. A randomized controlled trial of the effect of third-trimester calcium supplementation on maternal hemodynamic function. *Obstet Gynecol*. 1997;90:157-161.
14. Levine RJ, Hauth JC, Curet LB, et al. Trial of calcium to prevent preeclampsia. *N Engl J Med*. 1997;337:69-76.

15. Villar J, Abdel-Aleem H, Merialdi M, et al; on behalf of the World Organization Calcium Supplementation for the Prevention for Preeclampsia Trial Group. World Health Organization randomized trial of calcium supplementation among low calcium intake pregnant women. *Am J Obstet Gynecol*. 2006;194:639-649.
16. Ullian ME, Linas SL. The milk-alkali syndrome in pregnancy—case report. *Miner Electrolyte Metab*. 1988;14:208-210.
17. Kleinman GE, Rodriquez H, Good MC, et al. Hypercalcemic crisis in pregnancy associated with excessive ingestion of calcium carbonate antacid (milk-alkali syndrome): successful treatment with hemodialysis. *Obstet Gynecol*. 1991;78:496-499.
18. Picolos MK, Sims CR, Mastrobattista JM, et al. Milk-alkali syndrome in pregnancy. *Obstet Gynecol*. 2004;104:1201-1204.
19. Neville MC. Calcium secretion into milk. *J Mammary Gland Biol Neoplasia*. 2005;10:119-128.

C

CAMPHOR

Anesthetic (Topical)

PREGNANCY RECOMMENDATION: Limited Human Data—Animal Data Suggest Low Risk

BREASTFEEDING RECOMMENDATION: Probably Compatible

PREGNANCY SUMMARY

Camphor is toxic and potentially a fatal poison if taken orally in sufficient quantities. Four cases of fetal exposure after accidental ingestion, including a case of fetal death and neonatal respiratory failure, have been reported. No reports linking the use of topically applied camphor with congenital defects have been located. Camphor crosses the placenta, so fetal exposure will occur. Therefore, this limited human pregnancy experience prevents a complete assessment of the embryofetal risk. Animal studies did not show any embryofetal toxicity with oral exposure, but amounts used were not described. Using this drug during pregnancy should be based on the pros and cons of the mother's clinical need for treatment versus any potential fetal risk that might occur from exposure.

BREASTFEEDING SUMMARY

No reports were located that describe the use of topical camphor during human lactation. If found systemically, the drug will probably be found in breast milk, so some infant exposure could occur. However, in most cases, the amount of drug that is absorbed from a limited area should be minimal. It is recommended that use on large areas or on or around the nipple be avoided (especially with un-intact skin), if possible. Breastfeeding while using this drug should be based on the mother's clinical need for treatment versus any potential infant risks that might occur. Due to the topical use of this drug, systemic side effects were not assessed.

References

1. Weiss J, Catalano P. Camphorated oil intoxication during pregnancy. *Pediatrics*. 1973;52:713-714.
2. Figgs J, Hamilton R, Homel S, et al. Camphorated oil intoxication in pregnancy. report of a case. *Obstet Gynecol*. 1965;25:255-258.
3. Blackman WB, Curry HB. Camphor poisoning: report of case occurring during pregnancy. *J Fla Med Assoc*. 1957;43:99.
4. Jacobziner H, Raybin HW. Camphor poisoning. *Arch Pediatr*. 1962;79:28.
5. Rabl W, Katzgraber F, Steinlechner M. Camphor ingestion for abortion (case report). *Forensic Sci Int* 1997;89:137–40.
6. Heinonen OP, Slone D, Shapiro S. *Birth Defects and Drugs in Pregnancy*. Publishing Sciences Group; 1977.

CANAGLIFLOZIN

Antidiabetic (SGLT2 Inhibitor)

PREGNANCY RECOMMENDATION: No Human Data—Animal Data Suggest Potential Risk

BREASTFEEDING RECOMMENDATION: Potential Toxicity

PREGNANCY SUMMARY

No reports describing the use of canagliflozin in human pregnancy have been located. Based on ex vivo human placenta perfusion studies, the drug crosses the placenta. Therefore, the absence of human pregnancy experience prevents a complete assessment of the embryofetal risk. Animal studies found potential renal issues of increased kidney weight and renal pelvic and tubular dilation in one species when the drug was administered at a time of development that corresponded to human kidney development. Nevertheless, using this drug during pregnancy should be based on the pros and cons of the mother's clinical need for treatment versus any potential fetal risk that might occur from exposure. ACOG recommends that insulin be used for types 1 and 2 diabetes during pregnancy and, if diet therapy alone is not successful, for gestational diabetes.

BREASTFEEDING SUMMARY

No reports describing the use of canagliflozin during human lactation have been located. The drug will likely be found in breast milk, so some infant exposure will probably occur. Because of the potential fetal/infant renal issues seen in animal studies, the manufacturer recommends that a decision be made to either discontinue the drug or stop breastfeeding. Nevertheless, if breastfeeding occurs, the infant should be monitored for the most common reported adult side effects of urinary tract infection and mycotic infections.

References

1. Prescribing Information. *Invokana*. Janssen Pharmaceuticals; 2019.
2. Gestational Diabetes Mellitus. ACOG Practice Bulletin No. 190. American College of Obstetricians and Gynecologists. *Obstet Gynecol*. 2018;131: e49-e64.
3. Pregestational Diabetes Mellitus. ACOG Practice Bulletin No. 201. American College of Obstetricians and Gynecologists. *Obstet Gynecol*. 2018;132: e228-e248.
4. Kuoni S, Steiner R, Saleh L, et al. Safety assessment of the SGLT2 inhibitors empagliflozin, dapagliflozin and canagliflozin during pregnancy: an *ex vivo* human placenta perfusion and *in vitro* study. *Biomed Pharmacother*. 2024;171:116177.

CANAKINUMAB

Immunologic (Monoclonal Antibody)

PREGNANCY RECOMMENDATION: Limited Human Data—Animal Data Suggest Low Risk

BREASTFEEDING RECOMMENDATION: Probably Compatible

PREGNANCY SUMMARY

Eight publications were located that reported the use of canakinumab during human pregnancy and also described the overall outcome. Of 23 total pregnancies, 21 were exposed at the time of conception/first trimester. Two (9.5%) were spontaneously aborted (one at 6 weeks' and the other at 16 weeks' gestation) and the remaining 19 delivered healthy newborns at term or near term with no reported anomalies or complications that might be related to the drug. There were two pregnancies with third-trimester exposure and both delivered infants with no observed anomalies or complications. A systematic review of interleukin (IL)-1 blocking drugs (canakinumab and anakinra) found no major obstetrical or neonatal complications and could probably be safely used in treating pregnancies with inflammatory conditions. On the other hand, in an analysis of data from the World Health Organization Pharmacovigilance Database (VigiBase), there was a possible association for an increased signal risk for musculoskeletal malformations and immune system disorders with the use of canakinumab during pregnancy. However, spontaneous reporting safety profile databases have numerous limitations. They are biased toward the reporting of pregnancy complications and poor outcomes rather than normal outcomes. They can also lack clinical details and have missing information, including drug dosages, duration of use, and specific timing of drug exposure during pregnancy. Therefore, they cannot report the incidence of adverse events or provide a measure of risk. These databases can primarily provide information on whether or not a significant disproportionality exists in the reporting frequency of specific adverse events. Canakinumab crosses the placenta at term, so some fetal exposure will occur. However, this limited human pregnancy experience still prevents a complete assessment of the embryofetal risk. Animal studies did not show any embryofetal toxicity or teratogenicity in two species at doses of more than 10 times the RHD. Using this drug during pregnancy should be based on the pros and cons of the mother's clinical need for treatment versus any potential fetal risk that might occur from exposure.

BREASTFEEDING SUMMARY

Five studies were located that describe the use of canakinumab during human lactation. A total of 10 infants were exposed to breast milk in mothers who were being treated with canakinumab, and none of the infants were reported to have any complications related to the drug. In one study, the drug was found in breast milk at very low levels of 3.8 to 22.8 ng/mL with a calculated relative infant dose (RID) of less than 0.1%. In this same study, the mother continued to take canakinumab, receiving further doses at 2 weeks and 4 months postdelivery, and she continued to breastfeed. The infant's blood was analyzed at 6 months of age and canakinumab was not detected. In a second study, the milk level for canakinumab postdelivery was undetected, but the lower limit of detection for this particular study was 500 ng/mL. It is known that immunoglobulin G (IgG) antibodies can be found in human breast milk (as reported in one study earlier), but are not found in the neonatal or infant circulation. Additionally, if any IgG antibodies were to be ingested through breastfeeding, they would probably be digested in the infant's gastrointestinal tract and not be absorbed (consistent with the same study mentioned earlier). Nevertheless, breastfeeding while using this drug should be based on the mother's clinical need for treatment versus any potential infant risks that might occur. If used, the infant should be monitored for the most common reported adult side effects of nausea, headache, abdominal pain, and musculoskeletal pain (all leading to irritability), diarrhea, and nasopharyngitis.

References

1. Prescribing Information. *Ilaris*. Novartis Pharmaceuticals; 2020.
2. Egawa M, Imai K, Mori M, et al. Placental transfer of canakinumab in a patient with Muckle-Wells Syndrome. *J Clin Immunol*. 2017;37:339-341.
3. Bosshard N, Zbinden A, Eriksson KK, Forger F. Rituximab and canakinumab use during lactation: no detectable serum levels in breastfed infants. *Rheumatol Ther*. 2021;8:1043-1048.

4. Weber E, Millet A, Beghin D, et al. Safety of canakinumab during pregnancy: seven new cases. *Rheumatology*. 2022;61:e229-e231.
5. Hansmann S, Ambjoernsen K, Koitschev A, et al. IL-1 inhibition in Muckle-Wells-Syndrome: withdrawal resulting in rapid deterioration of hearing loss. *Pediatr Rheumatol*. 2015;13(suppl 1):28.
6. Youngstein T, Hoffmann P, Gui A, et al. International multi-centre study of pregnancy outcomes with interleukin-1 inhibitors. *Rheumatology*. 2017;56: 2012-2018.
7. Gunn JL, Waller R, O-Neil L, David J. Canakinumab use during pregnancy for the treatment of systemic onset juvenile idiopathic arthritis and refractory macrophage activation syndrome. *Rheumatology*. 2018;57(suppl 3): key075.345.
8. Babaoglu H, Varan O, Kucuk H, et al. Effectiveness of canakinumab in colchicine- and anakinra-resistant or -intolerant adult familial Mediterranean fever patients: a single-center real-life study. *J Clin Rheumatol*. 2020;26:7-13.
9. Ilgen U, Eyupoglu S, Yayla ME, Kucuksahin O. Fetal exposure to canakinumab: a report of three pregnancies. *Clin Rheumatol*. 2022;41:1261-1263.
10. Brien ME, Gaudreault V, Hughes K, et al. A systematic review of the safety of blocking the IL-1 system in human pregnancy. *J Clin Med*. 2021;11:225. doi:10.3390/jcm11010225
11. Dernoncourt A, Liabeuf S, Bennis Y, et al. Fetal and neonatal adverse reactions associated with biologics taken during pregnancy by women with autoimmune diseases: insights from an analysis of the World Health Organization Pharmacovigilance Database (VigiBase). *Biodrugs*. 2023;37:73-87.

CANDESARTAN CILEXETIL

Antihypertensive (ARB—Angiotensin II Receptor Blocker)

PREGNANCY RECOMMENDATION: Human Data Suggest Risk (Second and Third Trimesters)

BREASTFEEDING RECOMMENDATION: Probably Compatible

PREGNANCY SUMMARY

Though the data are small, first-trimester exposure to candesartan and other angiotensin II receptor blockers (ARBs) has not been shown to significantly increase the risk for congenital anomalies. However, numerous case reports and reviews have reported that the use of ARBs, including candesartan, in the second half of pregnancy can, in some cases, produce severe fetal renal dysfunction. This can lead to anomalies related to longstanding oligohydramnios and fetal/neonatal death. There are cases, however, where the process reverses itself when the drug is discontinued. These findings are similar to those seen with angiotensin-converting enzyme (ACE) inhibitors. The drug actually carries a boxed warning for these risks. The drug will probably cross the placenta, so some fetal exposure will likely occur. Animal studies did not show any embryofetal toxicity in two species at doses of less than and more than 10 times the MRHD. However, in one species, there was some embryofetal toxicity when used in the second half of gestation. Women of reproductive age using candesartan should be informed of these risks, so that they can closely monitor if pregnancy transpires. If a positive pregnancy test occurs, she and her health care providers can modify treatment (if possible) so that the drug is not used in the second or third trimesters. For treating hypertension in pregnancy, ACOG recommends nifedipine and labetalol as first-line agents.

BREASTFEEDING SUMMARY

One report that evaluated the use of candesartan during human lactation was located. Breast milk samples were analyzed in three women, and the maximum milk level was 3.78 ng/mL. The RID was calculated to be about 0.1%. Two of the newborns had serum levels checked, and candesartan was not detected (lower limit of detection for the test was 0.2 ng/mL). These findings are consistent with the molecular weight (MW), suggesting that the drug will be found in breast milk, but the very high plasma protein binding should limit excretion. The manufacturer recommends not breastfeeding if the drug is used, or that the drug be discontinued while breastfeeding. Nevertheless, breastfeeding while using this drug should be based on the mother's clinical need for treatment versus any potential infant risks that might occur. If used, the infant should be monitored for the most common reported adult side effects of headache, dizziness, and back pain (all leading to irritability), cough, and hyperkalemia.

References

1. Product information. *Atacand*. AstraZeneca Pharmaceuticals; 2016.
2. Hinsberger A, Wingen AM, Hoyer PF. Angiotensin-II-receptor inhibitors in pregnancy. *Lancet*. 2001;357:1620.
3. Cox RM, Anerson JM, Cox P. Defective embryogenesis with angiotensin II receptor antagonists in pregnancy. *Br J Obstet Gynaecol*. 2003;110: 1038-1040.
4. Schaefer C. Angiotensin II-receptor-antagonists: further evidence of fetotoxicity but not teratogenicity. *Birth Defects Res (Part A)*. 2003;67:591-594.
5. Alwan S, Polifka JE, Friedman JM. Angiotensin II receptor antagonist treatment during pregnancy. *Birth Defects Res (Part A)*. 2005;73:123-130.
6. Vendemmia M, Garcia-Meric P, Rizzotti A, et al. Fetal and neonatal consequences of antenatal exposure to type 1 angiotensin II receptor-antagonists. *J Matern Fetal Neonatal Med*. 2005;19:137-140.
7. Bald M, Holder M, Zieger M, et al. Increased renal echogenicity in a preterm neonate: question. *Pediatr Nephrol*. 2005;20:1664-1665.
8. Bald M, Holder M, Zieger M, et al. Increased renal echogenicity in a preterm neonate: answer. *Pediatr Nephrol*. 2005;20:1666-1668.
9. Velazquez-Armenta EY, Han JY, Choi JS, et al. Angiotensin II receptor blockers in pregnancy: a case report and systematic review of the literature. *Hypertens Pregnancy*. 2007;26:51-66.
10. Munk PS, von Brandis P, Larsen AI. Reversible fetal renal failure after maternal treatment with candesartan: a case report. *Reprod Toxicol*. 2010;29: 381-382.
11. Porta M, Hainer JW, Jansson SO, et al; DIRECT Study Group. Exposure to candesartan during the first trimester of pregnancy in type 1 diabetes: experience from the Placebo-Controlled DIabetic REtinopathy Candesartan Trials. *Diabetologia*. 2011;54:1298-1303.
12. Polifka JE. Is there an embryopathy associated with first-trimester exposure to angiotensin-converting enzyme inhibitors and angiotensin receptor antagonists? A critical review of the evidence. *Birth Defects Res (Part A)*. 2012;94:576-598.
13. Coberger ED, Jensen BP, Dalrymple JM. Transfer of candesartan into human breast milk. *Obstet Gynecol*. 2019;134(3):481-484. doi:10.1097/AOG.0000000000003446 PMID; 31403599

CANGRELOR

Hematologic (Antiplatelet)

PREGNANCY RECOMMENDATION: No Human Data—Animal Data Suggest Risk/Maternal Benefit May Outweigh Any Embryofetal Risk

BREASTFEEDING RECOMMENDATION: Probably Compatible

PREGNANCY SUMMARY

No reports describing the use of cangrelor in human pregnancy have been located. The animal data suggest a moderate risk, but the absence of human pregnancy data prevent an assessment of the embryofetal risk. The characteristics of the drug suggest that clinically significant amounts will not cross the placenta. Moreover, the maternal benefit appears to outweigh the risk, so the drug should not be withheld because of pregnancy.

BREASTFEEDING SUMMARY

No reports describing the use of cangrelor during human lactation have been located. Based on the drug's pharmacological parameters, clinically significant amounts will not be excreted into breast milk. Moreover, a mother would be unable to breastfeed when the drug is given because it is used during percutaneous coronary intervention. Thus, a mother could nurse her infant after the procedure with no risk to the infant.

Reference

1. Prescribing Information. *Kengreal*. The Medicines Company; 2022.

CANNABIDIOL

Central Nervous System (Antiseizure)

PREGNANCY RECOMMENDATION: No Human Data—Animal Data Suggest Low Risk

BREASTFEEDING RECOMMENDATION: Potential Toxicity

PREGNANCY SUMMARY

No reports describing the use of cannabidiol in human pregnancy have been located. The drug will probably cross the placenta, so some fetal exposure will likely occur. Therefore, the absence of human pregnancy experience prevents a complete assessment of the embryofetal risk. Animal studies did not show any embryofetal toxicity in one species at doses of less than 10 times the RHD. The drug did cause some embryofetal toxicity in a second species at doses of less than 10 times the RHD, but this dose also caused maternal toxicity. Using this drug during pregnancy should be based on the pros and cons of the mother's clinical need for treatment versus any potential fetal risk that might occur from exposure. Cannabidiol does not appear to produce dependence or withdrawal. There is a pregnancy exposure registry that monitors pregnancy outcomes in women using antiseizure drugs. Health care providers are encouraged to call the North American Antiepileptic Drug Pregnancy Registry at 1-888-233-2334.

BREASTFEEDING SUMMARY

No reports regarding the use of cannabidiol during human lactation have been located. One study that evaluated breast milk levels of cannabidiol in 50 women who reported using cannabis found cannabidiol levels ranging from about 1 to 9 ng/mL. This shows that cannabidiol can be found in breast milk. However, there is no way to accurately quantify the maternal dose (because cannabis use can take place in many forms—smoking, vaping, inhalation, oral, etc). Cannabidiol, the drug by itself, will probably be excreted into breast milk, so some infant exposure will likely occur. Breastfeeding while using this drug should be based on the mother's clinical need for treatment versus any potential infant risks that might occur. If used, the infant should be monitored for the most common reported adult side effects of somnolence, decreased appetite, diarrhea, elevated liver function tests, fatigue (lethargy), rash, insomnia, and poor-quality sleep.

Reference

1. Prescribing Information. *Epidiolex*. Greenwich Biosciences; 2020.

C

CAPECITABINE

Antineoplastic (Antimetabolite Pyrimidine Analogue)

PREGNANCY RECOMMENDATION: Limited Human Data—Animal Data Suggest Risk

BREASTFEEDING RECOMMENDATION: Potential Toxicity

PREGNANCY SUMMARY

Two case reports of capecitabine use during pregnancy were located. Both involved the use of the drug at conception and in the first trimester. One patient was also receiving lapatinib and temozolomide, and the other patient received temozolomide only. Both delivered neonates (one at 32 weeks' gestation and the other at term) with no reported anomalies. The drug will probably cross the placenta, so some fetal exposure will likely occur. However, this limited human pregnancy experience prevents a complete assessment of the embryofetal risk. Animal studies did show embryofetal toxicity in two species (one with birth anomalies) at doses less than 10 times the RHD. Therefore, using this drug during pregnancy should be based on the pros and cons of the mother's clinical need for treatment versus any potential fetal risk that might occur from exposure (see also Fluorouracil).

BREASTFEEDING SUMMARY

No reports describing the use of capecitabine during human lactation have been located. However, one study was found that evaluated numerous breast milk samples for 5-fluorouracil (5-FU) in a lactating mother. None of the samples had any detectable 5-FU (lower limit of detection at 65 ng/mL). However, some capecitabine and 5-FU will likely be found in breast milk. Therefore, further breast milk testing is required. The manufacturer recommends that women not breastfeed while using this drug. Nevertheless, breastfeeding while using this drug should be based on the mother's clinical need for treatment versus any potential infant risks that might occur. If used, the infant should be monitored for the most common reported adult side effects of nausea and abdominal pain (both leading to irritability), diarrhea, fatigue (lethargy), vomiting, and elevated bilirubin levels.

References

1. Prescribing Information. *Xeloda*. Genentech; 2022.
2. Castellanos MI, Childress KJ, Ramirez M, Venkatramani R. Fetal exposure to capecitabine and temozolomide during the first trimester: a case report. *J Gynecol Obstet Hum Reprod*. 2020;49:101881.
3. Sharma A, Nguyen HS, Lozen A, et al. Brain metastases from breast cancer during pregnancy. *Surg Neurol Int*. 2016;7(suppl 23):S603-S606.
4. Cardonick E, Usmani A, Ghaffar S. Perinatal outcomes of a pregnancy complicated by cancer, including neonatal follow-up after in utero exposure to chemotherapy: results of an international registry. *Am J Clin Oncol*. 2010;33:221-228.
5. Peccatori FA, Giovannetti E, Pistilli B, et al. "The only thing I know is that I know nothing": 5-fluorouracil in human milk. *Ann Oncol*. 2012;23:543-544.

CAPIVASERTIB

Antineoplastic (Kinase Inhibitor)

PREGNANCY RECOMMENDATION: No Human Data—Animal Data Suggest Potential Risk

BREASTFEEDING RECOMMENDATION: Potential Toxicity

PREGNANCY SUMMARY

No reports describing the use of capivasertib in human pregnancy have been located. The drug will likely cross the placenta, so some fetal exposure will probably occur. Therefore, the absence of human pregnancy experience prevents a complete assessment of the embryofetal risk. Animal studies did show embryofetal toxicity with malformations in one species at doses of less than 10 times the RHD. Based on these animal studies and the drug's mechanism of action, the manufacturer recommends that women with reproductive potential use effective contraception during treatment and for 1 month after the last dose. They also recommend that males with female partners of reproductive potential use effective contraception during treatment and for 4 months after the last dose. Nevertheless, using this drug during pregnancy should be based on the pros and cons of the mother's clinical need for treatment versus any potential fetal risk that might occur from exposure. In the clinical trials, up to 18% of patients developed hyperglycemia. Therefore, if used, maternal glucose levels need to be monitored. There is a registry for women who are pregnant and have cancer. For more information, women and health care providers are encouraged to contact the Cancer and Pregnancy Registry at 1-877-635-4499.

BREASTFEEDING SUMMARY

No reports describing the use of capivasertib during human lactation have been located. The drug will likely be found in breast milk, so some infant exposure will probably occur. Due to a concern for potential serious adverse effects that might be seen in a breastfed infant, the manufacturer recommends that women not breastfeed while being treated with this drug. Nevertheless, breastfeeding while using this drug should be based on the mother's clinical need for treatment versus any potential infant risk that might occur. If used, the infant should be monitored for the most common reported adult side effects of nausea and stomatitis (both leading to irritability), diarrhea, fatigue (lethargy), vomiting, elevated glucose levels, and other various laboratory abnormalities (see PI).

C

Reference

1. Prescribing Information. *Truqap*. AstraZeneca; 2023.

CAPLACIZUMAB

Hematologic (Nanobody)

PREGNANCY RECOMMENDATION: Limited Human Data—Animal Data Suggest Low Risk

BREASTFEEDING RECOMMENDATION: Probably Compatible

PREGNANCY SUMMARY

Four case reports of the use of caplacizumab during human pregnancy were located. In two cases, the drug was administered in the third trimester shortly (a few days and 3 weeks) before delivery, and both newborns overall did well. A third case involved the administration of caplacizumab in the first trimester of a twin gestation. A missed abortion was noted, but it is unknown whether this missed abortion occurred prior to or after the initiation of the caplacizumab. The fourth case described the use of the drug starting at about 19 weeks' gestation in a complicated pregnancy. Caplacizumab was reportedly found in the amniotic fluid and fetal blood after the 20-week pregnancy was terminated for poor fetal prognosis, with severe intrauterine growth restriction (IUGR), oligohydramnios, and placental hydrops. Measured caplacizumab levels were low at about 50 ng/mL (or about 5-10 times lower than maternal levels). Two other publications discussed the use of the drug in a total of five postpartum patients without any reported adverse sequela. Based on the drug's structure, in that it does not contain the Fc region of an immunoglobulin, it should not cross the placenta. However, the one report above suggests that caplacizumab can cross, though it is unknown if the placental hydrops played a role in the passage. In addition, the levels obtained were very low. Nevertheless, this limited human pregnancy experience prevents a complete assessment of the embryofetal risk. Animal studies did not show any embryofetal toxicity or malformations in one species at doses of more than 10 times the RHD. Using this drug during pregnancy should be based on the pros and cons of the mother's clinical need for treatment versus any potential fetal risk that might occur from exposure.

BREASTFEEDING SUMMARY

No reports describing the use of caplacizumab during human lactation have been located. It is known that IgG antibodies (and antibody fragments) can be found in human breast milk but are not found in the neonatal or infant circulation. Additionally, if any antibodies were to be ingested through breastfeeding, they would probably be digested in the infant's gastrointestinal tract and not be absorbed. Breastfeeding while using this drug should be based on the mother's clinical need for treatment versus any potential infant risks that might occur. If used, the infant should be monitored for the most common reported adult side effects of headache (leading to irritability), epistaxis, and gingival bleeding.

References

1. Prescribing Information. *Cablivi*. Ablynx US; 2022.
2. Kuhne L, Volker LA, Hagmann H, et al. First use of the anti-VWF nanobody caplacizumab to treat iTTP in pregnancy. *Br J Haematol*. 2022;196:e30-e33.
3. Odetola O, Martin KA, Dreyer M, et al. A safe and effective use of caplacizumab in pregnancy-related acquired thrombotic thrombocytopenia purpura. *Br J Haematol*. 2023:202:879-882.
4. Schimmer RR, Sutter T, Bachofner A, et al. Successful management of refractory immune-medicated thrombotic thrombocytopenia purpura during pregnancy and delivery using the anti-VWF nanobody caplacizumab. 2024;204:1994-1998.
5. Jacob G, Dhaliwal A, Chaudhary V. An interesting case of refractory thrombotic thrombocytopenia purpura in the first trimester of a twin pregnancy. *Cureus*. 2023;15:e47153.
6. Bruzzese A, Vigna E, Martino EA, et al. Safety and efficacy of caplacizumab in a case of thrombotic thrombocytopenia purpura in the postpartum period. *Blood Coagul Fibrinolysis*. 2023;34:215-217.
7. Beranger N, Coppo P, Tsatsaris V, et al. Management and follow-up of pregnancy-onset thrombotic thrombocytopenia purpura: the French experience. *Blood Advances*. 2024;8:183-193.

C

CAPMATINIB

Antineoplastic (Kinase Inhibitor)

PREGNANCY RECOMMENDATION: No Human Data—Animal Data Suggest Risk

BREASTFEEDING RECOMMENDATION: Potential Toxicity

PREGNANCY SUMMARY

No reports describing the use of capmatinib in human pregnancy have been located. Based on likely placental transfer, some fetal exposure will probably occur. However, the absence of human pregnancy experience prevents a complete assessment of the embryofetal risk. Animal studies showed fetotoxicity and teratogenicity. Due to the findings from these animal studies and the drug's mechanism of action, the manufacturer recommends that women with reproductive potential use effective contraception during treatment and for 1 week after the last dose. They also recommend that males with female partners of reproductive potential use effective contraception during treatment and for 1 week after the last dose. However, using this drug during pregnancy should be based on the pros and cons of the mother's clinical need for treatment versus any potential fetal risk that might occur from exposure.

BREASTFEEDING SUMMARY

No reports describing the use of capmatinib during human lactation have been located. Some amount of the drug will likely enter breast milk, so infant exposure will probably occur. However, due to the concern for potential serious side effects in a breastfed infant, the manufacturer recommends that women not breastfeed while being treated with capmatinib and for at least 1 week after the last dose. Nevertheless, breastfeeding while using this drug should be based on the mother's clinical need for treatment. If used, the infant should be monitored for the most common reported adult side effects of nausea (leading to irritability), edema, lethargy, vomiting, dyspnea, and decreased appetite.

Reference

1. Prescribing Information. *Tabrecta*. Novartis Pharmaceuticals Corporation; 2022.

CAPREOMYCIN

Antibacterial (Antituberculosis)

PREGNANCY RECOMMENDATION: Limited Human Data—Animal Data Suggest Potential Risk

BREASTFEEDING RECOMMENDATION: Probably Compatible

PREGNANCY SUMMARY

Two patients have been reported with first-trimester exposure to capreomycin (along with several other drugs), and neither had any identified anomalies. A long-term follow-up report on these cases (4-5 years of age) did not show any significant issues. A third exposure occurred at about 26 weeks of gestation, and again the child did well. The drug will probably cross the placenta, so some fetal exposure will likely occur. Therefore, this limited human pregnancy experience prevents a complete assessment of the embryofetal risk. Animal studies did show some embryofetal toxicity with malformations in one species. Using this drug during pregnancy should be based on the pros and cons of the mother's clinical need for treatment versus any potential fetal risk that might occur from exposure.

BREASTFEEDING SUMMARY

Two patients have been reported to use capreomycin during lactation, one who used the drug throughout gestation and postdelivery, and the other only postpartum. At follow-up ages of 4.6 and 5.1 years, neither was showing any significant abnormalities. Some amount of the drug may be found in breast milk, but capreomycin is poorly absorbed orally (<1% of a dose). Therefore, any amount that may be found in breast milk is likely to be clinically insignificant. Breastfeeding while using this drug should be based on the mother's clinical need for treatment versus any potential infant risks that might occur. If used, the infant should be monitored for the most common reported adult side effects of abdominal pain (leading to irritability), diarrhea, rash, nephrotoxicity, and cranial nerve VIII injury.

References

1. Prescribing Information. *Capastat*. Hisun Pharmaceuticals, Inc; 2023.
2. Lessnau KDKL, Qarah S. Multidrug-resistant tuberculosis in pregnancy: case report and review of the literature. *Chest*. 2003;123:953-956.
3. Shin S, Guerra D, Rich M, et al. Treatment of multidrug-resistant tuberculosis during pregnancy: a report of 7 cases. *Clin Infect Dis*. 2003;36:996-1003.
4. Drobac PC, Castillo HD, Sweetland A, et al. Treatment of multidrug-resistant tuberculosis during pregnancy: long-term follow-up of 6 children with intrauterine exposure to second-line agents. *Clin Infect Dis*. 2005;40:1689-1692.

CAPTOPRIL

Antihypertensive (ACE—Angiotensin-I-Converting Enzyme Inhibitor)

PREGNANCY RECOMMENDATION: Contraindicated (Second and Third Trimesters)

BREASTFEEDING RECOMMENDATION: Probably Compatible

C

PREGNANCY SUMMARY

Though the data are small, first-trimester exposure to captopril has not been shown to significantly increase the risk for congenital anomalies. One study did not show an increased risk, while the second one did. However, no pattern to the anomalies was identified. However, numerous case reports and reviews have reported that the use of ACE inhibitors, including captopril, in the second half of pregnancy can, in some cases, produce severe fetal renal dysfunction. This can lead to anomalies related to longstanding oligohydramnios and fetal/neonatal death. There are cases, however, where the process reverses itself when the drug is discontinued. These findings are similar to those seen with ARBs. The drug actually carries a boxed warning for these risks. The drug appears to cross the placenta, so fetal exposure will occur. Animal studies did not show any embryofetal toxicity in three species at doses of more than 10 times the MRHD. Women of reproductive age using captopril should be informed of these risks, so that they can closely monitor if pregnancy transpires. If a positive pregnancy test occurs, she and her health care providers can modify treatment (if possible) so that the drug is not used in the second or third trimesters. For treating hypertension in pregnancy, ACOG recommends nifedipine and labetalol as first-line agents.

BREASTFEEDING SUMMARY

Captopril was found to be excreted into human breast milk in a study of 11 women taking the drug at 300 mg/d. The average maximum breast milk level was 4.7 ng/mL, and the calculated RID was only 0.014%. The manufacturer recommends not breastfeeding if the drug is used, or that the drug be discontinued while breastfeeding. Nevertheless, breastfeeding while using this drug should be based on the mother's clinical need for treatment versus any potential infant risks that might occur. If used, the infant should be monitored for the most common reported adult side effects of headache, pruritus, and arthralgia (all leading to irritability), cough, rash, hypotension, and tachycardia.

References

1. Product information. *Captopril*. Apotex Corp; 2017.
2. Broughton Pipkin F, Turner SR, Symonds EM. Possible risk with captopril in pregnancy: some animal data. *Lancet*. 1980;1:1256.
3. Broughton Pipkin F, Symonds EM, Turner SR. The effect of captopril (SQ14,225) upon mother and fetus in the chronically cannulated ewe and in the pregnant rabbit. *J Physiol*. 1982;323:415-422.
4. Keith IM, Will JA, Weir EK. Captopril: association with fetal death and pulmonary vascular changes in the rabbit. *Proc Soc Exp Biol Med*. 1982;170:378-383.
5. Lumbers ER, Kingsford NM, Menzies RI, et al. Acute effects of captopril, an angiotensin-converting enzyme inhibitor, on the pregnant ewe and fetus. *Am J Physiol*. 1992;262(5 pt 2):R754-R760.
6. Binder ND, Faber JJ. Effects of captopril on blood pressure, placental blood flow and uterine oxygen consumption in pregnant rabbits. *J Pharmacol Exp Ther*. 1992;260:294-299.
7. Carey RM, Cutler J, Friedewald W, et al. The 1984 report of the Joint National Committee on detection, evaluation, and treatment of high blood pressure. *Arch Intern Med*. 1984;144:1045-1046.
8. Lindheimer MD, Katz AI. Hypertension in pregnancy. *N Engl J Med*. 1985;313:675-680.
9. Lip GYH, Churchill D, Beevers M, et al. Angiotensin-converting-enzyme inhibitors in early pregnancy. *Lancet*. 1997;350:1446-1447.
10. Duminy PC, Burger PT. Fetal abnormality associated with the use of captopril during pregnancy. *S Afr Med J*. 1981;60:805.
11. Broude AM. Fetal abnormality associated with captopril during pregnancy. *S Afr Med J*. 1982;61:68.
12. Kaler SG, Patrinos ME, Lambert GH, et al. Hypertrichosis and congenital anomalies associated with maternal use of minoxidil. *Pediatrics*. 1987;79:434-436.
13. Owen J, Hauth JC. Polyarteritis nodosa in pregnancy: a case report and brief literature review. *Am J Obstet Gynecol*. 1989;160:606-607.
14. Guignard JP, Burgener F, Calame A. Persistent anuria in a neonate: a side effect of captopril? (abstract). *Int J Pediatr Nephrol*. 1981;2:133.
15. Millar JA, Wilson PD, Morrison N. Management of severe hypertension in pregnancy by a combined drug regimen including captopril: case report. *NZ Med J*. 1983;96:796-798.
16. Boutroy MJ, Vert P, Hurault de Ligny B, et al. Captopril administration in pregnancy impairs fetal angiotensin converting enzyme activity and neonatal adaptation. *Lancet*. 1984;2:935-936.
17. Rothberg AD, Lorenz R. Can captopril cause fetal and neonatal renal failure? *Pediatr Pharmacol (New York)*. 1984;4:189-192.
18. Coen G, Cugini P, Gerlini G, et al. Successful treatment of long-lasting severe hypertension with captopril during a twin pregnancy. *Nephron*. 1985;40:498-500.
19. Knott PD, Thorpe SS, Lamont CAR. Congenital renal dysgenesis possibly due to captopril. *Lancet*. 1989;1:451.
20. Smith AM. Are ACE inhibitors safe in pregnancy? *Lancet*. 1989;2:750-751.
21. Fiocchi R, Lijnen P, Fagard R, et al. Captopril during pregnancy. *Lancet*. 1984;2:1153.
22. Caraman PL, Miton A, Hurault de Ligny B, et al. Grossesses sous captopril. *Therapie*. 1984;39:59-63.
23. Plouin PF, Tchobroutsky C. Angiotensin converting-enzyme inhibition during human pregnancy: fifteen cases. *Presse Méd*. 1985;14:2175-2178.
24. Ducret F, Pointet PH, Lauvergeon B, et al. Grossesse sous inhibiteur de l'enzyme de conversion. *Presse Méd*. 1985;14:897.
25. Barr M. Fetal effects of angiotensin converting enzyme inhibitor (abstract). *Teratology*. 1990;41:536.
26. Pryde PG, Nugent CE, Sedman AB, et al. ACE inhibitor fetopathy (abstract). *Am J Obstet Gynecol*. 1992;166:348.
27. Kreft-Jais C, Plouin P-F, Tchobroutsky C, et al. Angiotensin-converting enzyme inhibitors during pregnancy: a survey of 22 patients given captopril and nine given enalapril. *Br J Obstet Gynaecol*. 1988;95:420-422.
28. Piper JM, Ray WA, Rosa FW. Pregnancy outcome following exposure to angiotensin-converting enzyme inhibitors. *Obstet Gynecol*. 1992;80:429-432.
29. Hanssens M, Keirse MJNC, Vankelecom F, et al. Fetal and neonatal effects of treatment with angiotensin-converting enzyme inhibitors in pregnancy. *Obstet Gynecol*. 1991;78:128-135.
30. Rosa FW, Bosco LA, Graham CF, et al. Neonatal anuria with maternal angiotensin-converting enzyme inhibition. *Obstet Gynecol*. 1989;74:371-374.
31. Barr M Jr, Cohen MM Jr. ACE inhibitor fetopathy and hypocalvaria: the kidney-skull connection. *Teratology*. 1991;44:485-495.
32. Brent RL, Beckman DA. Angiotensin-converting enzyme inhibitors, an embryopathic class of drugs with unique properties: information for clinical teratology counselors. *Teratology*. 1991;43:543-546.
33. Martin RA, Jones KL, Mendoza A, et al. Effect of ACE inhibition on the fetal kidney: decreased renal blood flow. *Teratology*. 1992;46:317-321.

34. Easterling TR, Carr DB, Davis C, et al. Low-dose, short-acting, angiotensin-converting enzyme inhibitors as rescue therapy in pregnancy. *Obstet Gynecol.* 2000;96:956-961.
35. Cooper WO, Hernandez-Diaz S, Arbogast PG, et al. Major congenital malformations after first-trimester exposure to ACE inhibitors. *N Engl J Med.* 2006;354:2443-2451.
36. Friedman JM. ACE inhibitors and congenital anomalies. *N Engl J Med.* 2006; 354:2498-2500.
37. Scialli AR, Lione A. ACE inhibitors and major congenital malformations. *N Engl J Med.* 2006;355:1280.
38. Cooper WO, Ray WA. Reply—ACE inhibitors and major congenital malformations. *N Engl J Med.* 2006;355:1281.
39. Barr M Jr. Teratogen update: angiotensin-converting enzyme inhibitors. *Teratology.* 1994;50:399-409.
40. Shotan A, Widerhorn J, Hurst A, et al. Risks of angiotensin-converting enzyme inhibition during pregnancy: experimental and clinical evidence, potential mechanisms, and recommendations for use. *Am J Med.* 1994;96:451-456.
41. Robillard JE, Nakamura KT, Matherne GP, et al. Renal hemodynamics and functional adjustments to postnatal life. *Semin Perinatol.* 1988;12:143-150.
42. Guignard JP, Gouyon JB. Adverse effects of drugs on the immature kidney. *Biol Neonate.* 1988;53:243-252.
43. Polifka JE. Is there an embryopathy associated with first-trimester exposure to angiotensin-converting enzyme inhibitors and angiotensin receptor antagonists? A critical review of the evidence. *Birth Defects Res (Part A).* 2012;94:576-598.
44. Devlin RG, Fleiss PM. Selective resistance to the passage of captopril into human milk. *Clin Pharmacol Ther.* 1980;27:250.
45. Devlin RG, Fleiss PM. Captopril in human blood and breast milk. *J Clin Pharmacol.* 1981;21:110-113.

CARBACHOL OPHTHALMIC

Ophthalmic/Autonomic (Parasympathomimetic—Cholinergic)

PREGNANCY RECOMMENDATION: No Human Data and No Relevant Animal Data

BREASTFEEDING RECOMMENDATION: Probably Compatible

PREGNANCY SUMMARY

No reports describing the use of carbachol ophthalmic in human pregnancy have been located. The drug will probably cross the placenta, so some fetal exposure will likely occur. Therefore, the absence of human pregnancy experience prevents a complete assessment of the embryofetal risk. Animal studies have not been conducted. Using this drug during pregnancy should be based on the pros and cons of the mother's clinical need for treatment versus any potential fetal risk that might occur from exposure. Because the drug is only administered intraocularly, the levels in the systemic circulation are probably low. If used during pregnancy, consider placing pressure over the tear duct in the corner of the eye for at least 1 minute, and then remove any excess solution with absorbent tissue to decrease the amount of drug reaching the systemic circulation even further.

BREASTFEEDING SUMMARY

No reports describing the use of carbachol ophthalmic during human lactation have been located. The MW suggests that the drug will be found in breast milk. However, because it is only administered by intraocular injection, it is unlikely that clinically significant amounts would be excreted into milk. In addition, a method to further decrease some systemic absorption with ophthalmic use is described above in the Pregnancy Summary.

Reference

1. Prescribing Information. *Miostat.* Alcon Laboratories; 2019.

CARBAMAZEPINE

Central Nervous System (Antiseizure)

PREGNANCY RECOMMENDATION: Human Data Suggest Risk (Maternal Benefit May Outweigh Embryo–Fetal Risk)

BREASTFEEDING RECOMMENDATION: Probably Compatible

PREGNANCY SUMMARY

Numerous studies have evaluated the use of carbamazepine in human pregnancy. Using the summary data from a meta-analysis plus two other large studies, a total of 101 (6.4%) major birth anomalies were described in 1,587 first-trimester exposures. Some of these defects involved cardiovascular anomalies and neural tube defects. Based on multiple case reports of neural tube defects with carbamazepine exposures, there appears to be an increased risk for this anomaly. Some reports describe this risk as high as 1%. The drug has also been associated with facial defects, nail hypoplasia, and other subtle anomalies seen with other antiseizure medications. Another confounder is that many of these patients have seizures during pregnancy while on therapy, and it is difficult to separate this factor from the overall pregnancy outcome. The drug crosses the placenta, so some fetal exposures will occur. Some embryofetal toxicity with malformations was seen in one species, but at doses of more than 10 times the RHD. Although pregnant women should be advised of these potential adverse outcomes with carbamazepine use, if the drug is required during pregnancy, it should not be withheld because the benefits of preventing seizures outweigh the potential fetal harm. Therefore, using this drug during pregnancy should be based on the pros and cons of the mother's clinical need for treatment versus any potential fetal risk that might occur from exposure.

BREASTFEEDING SUMMARY

Numerous studies have been published that confirm that carbamazepine and the active metabolite, the epoxide, are found in breast milk. When treating patients for seizures, many are on combination therapies. These other drugs can sometimes affect the metabolism of carbamazepine, which can lead to higher or lower blood levels. However, more than 100 breastfeeding patients have had their breast milk evaluated. Patients have been assessed while on monotherapy, as well as in combination with other anticonvulsants (and other drugs). Maternal drug dosages have mostly varied from about 4 mg/kg/d to about 15 mg/kg/d. Breast milk levels for carbamazepine have also varied, with most studies reporting values ranging from undetectable to 7 mcg/mL. Carbamazepine itself is pharmacologically inactive. Therefore, the more important assessment is the levels related to the epoxide metabolite (the active drug). The epoxide levels have been evaluated in more than 70 patients, reporting values ranging from undetectable to 4 mcg/mL. RIDs in nearly all cases were less than 10%. Several infants exposed to breast milk from a mother using carbamazepine have had serum levels obtained. Many of these were found to be below the level of detection for both carbamazepine and the epoxide. Levels that were recorded ranged from about 0.5 to 2 mcg/mL for carbamazepine, and less than 1 mcg/mL for the epoxide. Lastly, regarding the effects on breastfeeding infants exposed to breast milk from mothers using carbamazepine, over 50 infants have been described. Over half of these had no reported complications. In the others, the primary reported issue was poor eating with lower weight gain, followed by sedation and jaundice (some of which might have been caused by other factors unrelated to carbamazepine). A study of 199 children was evaluated at 3 years of age for cognitive outcome who had been breastfed while their mothers were taking a single antiepileptic drug (carbamazepine, lamotrigine, phenytoin, or valproate). The mean adjusted IQ score for exposed children was 99, whereas the mean adjusted IQ score of nonbreastfed infants was 98. The manufacturer recommends to avoid breastfeeding when a mother is taking carbamazepine. Nevertheless, breastfeeding while using this drug should be based on the mother's clinical need for treatment versus any potential infant risks that might occur. If used, the infant should be monitored for the most common reported adult side effects of headache and dizziness (both leading to irritability), sedation, decreased appetite, and rash.

References

1. Product information. *Tegretol*. Novartis Pharmaceuticals; 2020.
2. Pynnonen S, Kanto J, Sillanpae M, et al. Carbamazepine: placental transport, tissue concentrations in the foetus and newborns, and level in milk. *Acta Pharmacol Toxicol*. 1977;41:244-253.
3. Rane A, Bertilsson L, Palmer L. Disposition of placentally transferred carbamazepine (Tegretol) in the newborn. *Eur J Clin Pharmacol*. 1975;8:283-284.
4. Nau H, Kuhnz W, Egger HJ, et al. Anticonvulsants during pregnancy and lactation: transplacental, maternal and neonatal pharmacokinetics. *Clin Pharmacokinet*. 1982;7:508-543.
5. Hiilesmaa VK. Evaluation of placental function in women on antiepileptic drugs. *J Perinat Med*. 1983;11:187-192.
6. Rosa F. Holoprosencephaly and antiepileptic exposures. *Teratology*. 1995; 51:230.
7. Geigy Pharmaceuticals. Tegretol in epilepsy. In: *Monograph 319-80950*. Ciba-Geigy; 1978:18-19.
8. McMullin GP. Teratogenic effects of anticonvulsants. *Br Med J*. 1971;4:430.
9. Pynnonen S, Sillanpae M. Carbamazepine and mothers milk. *Lancet*. 1975; 2:563.
10. Lander CM, Edwards VE, Endie MJ, et al. Plasma anticonvulsant concentrations during pregnancy. *Neurology*. 1977;27:128-131.
11. Nakane Y, Okuma T, Takahashi R, et al. Multi-institutional study on the teratogenicity and fetal toxicity to antiepileptic drugs: a report of a collaborative study group in Japan. *Epilepsia*. 1980;21:633-680.
12. Janz D. The teratogenic risk of antiepileptic drugs. *Epilepsia*. 1975;16:159-169.
13. Meyer JG. Teratogenic risk of anticonvulsants and the effects on pregnancy and birth. *Eur Neurol*. 1979;10:179-190.
14. Niebyl JR, Blake DA, Freeman JM, et al. Carbamazepine levels in pregnancy and lactation. *Obstet Gynecol*. 1979;53:139-140.
15. Hicks EP. Carbamazepine in two pregnancies. *Clin Exp Neurol*. 1979;16:269-275.
16. Thomas D, Buchanan N. Teratogenic effects of anticonvulsants. *J Pediatr*. 1981;99:163.
17. Niesen M, Froscher W. Finger-and toenail hypoplasia after carbamazepine monotherapy in late pregnancy. *Neuropediatrics*. 1985;16:167-168.
18. Jacobson SJ, Jones K, Johnson K, et al. Prospective multicentre study of pregnancy outcome after lithium exposure during first trimester. *Lancet*. 1992; 339:530-533.
19. Hiilesmaa VK, Teramo K, Granstrom ML, et al. Fetal head growth retardation associated with maternal antiepileptic drugs. *Lancet*. 1981;2:165-167.
20. Hiilesmaa VK, Bardy A, Teramo K. Obstetric outcome in women with epilepsy. *Am J Obstet Gynecol*. 1985;152:499-504.
21. Gaily E, Kantola-Sorsa E, Granstrom M-L. Intelligence of children of epileptic mothers. *J Pediatr*. 1988;113:677-684.
22. Jones KL, Lacro RV, Johnson KA, et al. Pattern of malformations in the children of women treated with carbamazepine during pregnancy. *N Engl J Med*. 1989;320:1661-1666.
23. Vestermark V, Vestermark S. Teratogenic effect of carbamazepine. *Arch Dis Child*. 1991;66:641-642.
24. Janz D. Antiepileptic drugs and pregnancy: altered utilization patterns and teratogenesis. *Epilepsia*. 1982;23(suppl 1):S53-S63.
25. Paulson GW, Paulson RB. Teratogenic effects of anticonvulsants. *Arch Neurol*. 1981;38:140-143.
26. Jones KL, Johnson KA, Adams J, et al. Teratogenic effects of carbamazepine. *N Engl J Med*. 1989;321:1481.
27. Rosa FW. Spina bifida in infants of women treated with carbamazepine during pregnancy. *N Engl J Med*. 1991;324:674-677.
28. Teratogenesis with carbamazepine. *Lancet*. 1991;337:1316-1317.
29. Hughes RL. Spina bifida in infants of women taking carbamazepine. *N Engl J Med*. 1991;325:664.
30. Hesdorffer DC, Hauser WA. Spina bifida in infants of women taking carbamazepine. *N Engl J Med*. 1991;325:664.
31. Rosa F. Spina bifida in infants of women taking carbamazepine. *N Engl J Med*. 1991;325:664-665.
32. Oakeshott P, Hunt GM. Carbamazepine and spina bifida. *Br Med J*. 1991; 303:651.
33. Hernandez-Diaz S, Werler MM, Walker AM, et al. Folic acid antagonists during pregnancy and the risk of birth defects. *N Engl J Med*. 2000;343: 1608-1614.
34. Hernandez-Diaz S, Werler MM, Walker AM, et al. Neural tube defects in relation to use of folic acid antagonists during pregnancy. *Am J Epidemiol*. 2001;153:981-988.

C

35. Ornoy A, Cohen E. Outcome of children born to epileptic mothers treated with carbamazepine during pregnancy. *Arch Dis Child*. 1996;75:517-520.
36. Wide K, Winbladh B, Tomson T, et al. Psychomotor development and minor anomalies in children exposed to antiepileptic drugs in utero: a prospective population-based study. *Dev Med Child Neurol*. 2000;42:87-92.
37. Wide K, Winbladh B, Tomson T, et al. Body dimensions of infants exposed to antiepileptic drugs in utero: observations spanning 25 years. *Epilepsia*. 2000;41:854-861.
38. Jick SS, Terris BZ. Anticonvulsants and congenital malformations. *Pharmacotherapy*. 1997;17:561-564.
39. Arpino C, Brescianini S, Robert E, et al. Teratogenic effects of antiepileptic drugs: use of an international database on malformations and drug exposure (MADRE). *Epilepsia*. 2000;41:1436-1443.
40. Canger R, Battino D, Canevini MP, et al. Malformations in offspring of women with epilepsy: a prospective study. *Epilepsia*. 1999;40:1231-1236.
41. Holmes LB, Harvey EA, Coull BA, et al. The teratogenicity of anticonvulsant drugs. *N Engl J Med*. 2001;344:1132-1138.
42. Almgren M, Kallen B, Lavebratt C. Population-based study of antiepileptic drug exposure *in utero*—influence on head circumference in newborns. *Seizure*. 2009;18:672-675.
43. Scolnik D, Nulman I, Rovet J, et al. Neurodevelopment of children exposed in utero to phenytoin and carbamazepine monotherapy. *JAMA*. 1994;271:767-770.
44. Jeret JS. Neurodevelopment after in utero exposure to phenytoin and carbamazepine. *JAMA*. 1994;272:850.
45. Loring DW, Meador KJ, Thompson WO. Neurodevelopment of children exposed in utero to phenytoin and carbamazepine. *JAMA*. 1994;272:850-851.
46. Koren G. Neurodevelopment of children exposed in utero to phenytoin and carbamazepine. *JAMA*. 1994;272:851.
47. Meador KJ, Baker GA, Browning N, et al; for the NEAD Study Group. Fetal antiepileptic drug exposure and cognitive outcomes at age 6 years (NEAD study): a prospective observational study. *Lancet Neurol*. 2013;12:244-252.
48. Diav-Citrin O, Shechtman S, Arnon J, et al. Is carbamazepine teratogenic? A prospective controlled study of 210 pregnancies. *Neurology*. 2001;57:321-324.
49. Matalon S, Shechtman S, Goldzweig G, et al. The teratogenic effect of carbamazepine: a meta-analysis of 1255 exposures. *Reprod Toxicol*. 2002;16:9-17.
50. Lindhout D, Höppener RJEA, Meinardi H. Teratogenicity of antiepileptic drug combinations with special emphasis on epoxidation (of carbamazepine). *Epilepsia*. 1984;25:77-83.
51. Koren G. Comment on antiepileptics and antipsychotics. *Teratology*. 2002;66:273.
52. Little BB, Santos-Ramos R, Newell JF, et al. Megadose carbamazepine during the period of neural tube closure. *Obstet Gynecol*. 1993;82:705-708.
53. *The Lamotrigine Pregnancy Registry: final report: 1 September 1992 through 31 March 2010*. GlaxoSmithKline; 2010.
54. Al-Shammri S, Guberman A, Hsu E. Neuroblastoma and fetal exposure to phenytoin in a child without dysmorphic features. *Can J Neurol Sci*. 1992;19:243-245.
55. Markestad T, Ulstein M, Strandjord RE, et al. Anticonvulsant drug therapy in human pregnancy: effects on serum concentrations of vitamin D metabolites in maternal and cord blood. *Am J Obstet Gynecol*. 1984;150:254-258.
56. Kok TH, Taitz LS, Bennett MJ, et al. Drowsiness due to clemastine transmitted in breast milk. *Lancet*. 1982;1:914-915.
57. Wisner KL, Perel JM. Serum levels of valproate and carbamazepine in breastfeeding mother-infant pairs. *J Clin Psychopharmacol*. 1998;18:167-169.
58. Brent NB, Wisner KL. Fluoxetine and carbamazepine concentrations in a nursing mother/infant pair. *Clin Pediatr (Phila)*. 1998;37:41-44.
59. Meador KJ, Baker GA, Browning N, et al; for the NEAD Study Group. Effects of breastfeeding in children of women taking antiepileptic drugs. *Neurology*. 2010;75:1954-1960.
60. American Academy of Pediatrics Committee on Drugs. The transfer of drugs and other chemicals into human milk. *Pediatrics*. 2001;108:776-789.

CARBIDOPA

Central Nervous System (Anti-Parkinson)

PREGNANCY RECOMMENDATION: Limited Human Data—Animal Data Suggest Risk

BREASTFEEDING RECOMMENDATION: Probably Compatible

PREGNANCY SUMMARY

Several case reports and series were found describing the use of carbidopa/levodopa treatment during the first trimester. A total of 14 pregnancies were described, with 2 (14%) spontaneous abortions and 12 healthy infants with no reported anomalies. The drug probably crosses the placenta, so fetal exposure will likely occur. Because carbidopa is administered with levodopa, animal reproduction studies have evaluated the combination. In one species, some embryofetal toxicity was seen at doses less than 10 times the RHD, and in a second species, some teratogenicity was seen at doses less than 10 times the RHD (for the levodopa component). No embryofetal toxicity or teratogenicity was seen in a third species at doses of more than 10 times the RHD. Using this drug during pregnancy should be based on the pros and cons of the mother's clinical need for treatment versus any potential fetal risk that might occur from exposure.

BREASTFEEDING SUMMARY

A few studies describing the use of carbidopa during human lactation have been located. In all cases, the drug was administered with levodopa. Levodopa was analyzed in one study and found to be excreted into breast milk (see Levodopa), but carbidopa levels were not assessed. None of the breastfed infants appeared to have any problems when exposed to carbidopa. The drug will probably be found in breast milk, so some infant exposure will likely occur. Breastfeeding while using this drug should be based on the mother's clinical need for treatment versus any potential infant risks that might occur. If used, the infant should be monitored for the most common reported adult side effects of dyspepsia, muscle cramps, back pain, and pruritus (all leading to irritability), diarrhea, vomiting, and rash. Because the combination product contains levodopa that is converted into dopamine, this could lead to a decrease in prolactin and potentially cause lactation suppression.

References

1. Product information. *Sinemet*. Merck Sharp & Dohme; 2018.
2. Product information. *Stalevo*. Novartis Pharmaceuticals; 2016.
3. Kitchin KT, DiStefano V. L-Dopa and brown fat hemorrhage in the rat pup. *Toxicol Appl Pharmacol*. 1976;38:251-263.
4. Seybold VS, Miller JW, Lewis PR. Investigation of a dopaminergic mechanism for regulating oxytocin release. *J Pharmacol Exp Ther*. 1978;207:605-610.
5. Vickers S, Stuart EK, Bianchine JR, et al. Metabolism of carbidopa [L-(-)-α-hydrazino-3,4-dihydroxy-α-methylhydrocinnamic acid monohydrate], an

aromatic amino acid decarboxylase inhibitor, in the rat, dog, rhesus monkey, and man. *Drug Metab Dispos*. 1974;2:9-22.
6. Merchant CA, Cohen G, Mytilineou C, et al. Human transplacental transfer of carbidopa/levodopa. *J Neural Transm Park Dis Dement Sect*. 1995;9:239-242.
7. Cook DG, Klawans HL. Levodopa during pregnancy. *Clin Neuropharmacol*. 1985;8:93-95.
8. Golbe LI. Parkinson's disease and pregnancy. *Neurology*. 1987;37:1245-1249.
9. Ball MC, Sagar HJ. Levodopa in pregnancy. *Mov Disord*. 1995;10:115.
10. Nomoto M, Kaseda S, Iwata S, et al. Levodopa in pregnancy. *Mov Disord*. 1997;12:261.
11. Watanabe T, Matsubara S, Baba Y, et al. Successful management of pregnancy in a patient with Segawa disease: case report and literature review. *J Obstet Gynaecol Res*. 2009;35:562-564.
12. Lindh J. Short episode of seizures in a newborn of mother treated with levodopa/carbidopa/entacapone and bromocriptine. *Mov Disord*. 2007;22:1515.
13. Serikawa S, Shimohata T, Akashi M, et al. Successful twin pregnancy is a patient with parkin-associated autosomal recessive juvenile parkinsonism. *BMC Neurol*. 2011;17(11):72.
14. Ward VD. Anaesthesia for caesarean section in a patient with Parkinson's disease. *Int J Obstet Anesth*. 2018;34:99-102.

C

CARBINOXAMINE

Antihistamine

PREGNANCY RECOMMENDATION: Limited Human Data and No Relevant Animal Data

BREASTFEEDING RECOMMENDATION: *Contraindicated

PREGNANCY SUMMARY

The Collaborative Perinatal Project reported two first-trimester exposures to carbinoxamine, but no information was supplied on whether either of these two cases involved fetal anomalies. Decades of published data on antihistamine drugs as a group have not identified a drug-related increased risk for fetal malformations, spontaneous abortion, or adverse maternal/fetal outcomes. Carbinoxamine will probably cross the placenta, so some fetal exposure will likely occur. Therefore, this limited human pregnancy experience prevents a complete assessment of the embryofetal risk. Animal reproduction studies have not been performed. Using this drug during pregnancy should be based on the pros and cons of the mother's clinical need for treatment versus any potential fetal risk that might occur from exposure.

BREASTFEEDING SUMMARY

No reports describing the use of carbinoxamine during human lactation have been located. The drug will probably be found in breast milk, so infant exposure will likely occur. *Due to postmarketing reports of deaths in infants under the age of 2 exposed to carbinoxamine by oral administration, the manufacturer recommends that the drug not be used while breastfeeding. The Federal Register report from 2006 described 21 cases of infant death under the age of 2 extending back to 1983. However, they also stated that in most of these cases, other active ingredients or other clinical factors aside from the drug could also have been responsible for the death. Nevertheless, due to the extensive number of other available antihistamines, an alternative is recommended for use if needed in a lactating mother.

References

1. Prescribing Information. *Carbinoxamine*. Aytu Therapeutics, LLC; 2021.
2. Heinonen OP, Slone D, Shapiro S. *Birth Defects and Drugs in Pregnancy*. Wright PSB; 1983:323.
3. Food and Drug Administration. Carbinoxamine products: enforcement action dates. *Fed Regist*. 2006;71:33462.
4. Centers for Disease Control and Prevention. Infant deaths associated with cough and cold medications—two states, 2005. *MMWR Morb Mortal Wkly Rep*. 2007;56:1-4.

CARBOPLATIN

Antineoplastic (Alkylating Agent—Platinum Compound)

PREGNANCY RECOMMENDATION: Limited Human Data—Animal Data Suggest Potential Risk

BREASTFEEDING RECOMMENDATION: Potential Toxicity

PREGNANCY SUMMARY

Several case reports and a review describing the use of carboplatin during pregnancy were located. Overall, there were 11 pregnancies with second-trimester (*n* = 8) and third-trimester (*n* = 3) exposure, and overall, they did well. No fetal malformations were seen in 10 cases. Clubfoot was seen in the remaining pregnancy, but this patient had a family history of clubfoot. No first-trimester exposure cases were located. The drug crosses the placenta, so fetal exposure will

(*continued*)

C

occur. Therefore, the absence of human pregnancy experience prevents a complete assessment of the embryofetal risk. Animal studies did show embryofetal toxicity with malformations in one species at doses of less than 10 times the RHD. The manufacturer recommends that women avoid becoming pregnant while taking this drug. Nevertheless, using this drug during pregnancy should be based on the pros and cons of the mother's clinical need for treatment versus any potential fetal risk that might occur from exposure. There is a registry for women who are pregnant and have cancer. For more information, women and health care providers are encouraged to contact the Cancer and Pregnancy Registry at 1-877-635-4499.

BREASTFEEDING SUMMARY

Two studies that demonstrated the presence of carboplatin in breast milk were located. The peak levels in the two patients were 900 and 350 ng/mL. Because carboplatin is administered on a weekly basis (in some cases) or every 4 weeks (in other therapy programs), daily weight-adjusted values are difficult to interpret. However, RIDs could exceed 10% in some clinical scenarios. The manufacturer recommends that breastfeeding be avoided while using this drug. Nevertheless, breastfeeding while using this drug should be based on the mother's clinical need for treatment versus any potential infant risks that might occur. If used, the infant should be monitored for the most common reported adult side effects of nausea, abdominal pain, and peripheral neuropathies (all leading to irritability), diarrhea, alopecia, vomiting, ototoxicity, and various laboratory abnormalities (see PI).

References

1. Product information. *Carboplatin*. Accord Healthcare; 2017.
2. Kai S, Kohmura H, Ishikawa K, et al. Teratogenic effects of carboplatin, an oncostatic drug, administered during the early organogenetic period in rats. *J Toxicol Sci*. 1989;14:115-130.
3. Leslie KK. Chemotherapy and pregnancy. *Clin Obstet Gynecol*. 2002;45:153-164.
4. Koc ON, McFee M, Reed E, et al. Detection of platinum-DNA adducts in cord blood lymphocytes following in utero platinum exposure. *Eur J Cancer*. 1994;30A:716-717.
5. Henderson CE, Elia G, Garfinkel D, et al. Platinum chemotherapy during pregnancy for serous cystadenocarcinoma of the ovary. *Gynecol Oncol*. 1993;49:92-94.
6. Shamkhani H, Anderson LM, Henderson CE, et al. DNA adducts in human and patas monkey maternal and fetal tissues induced by platinum drug chemotherapy. *Reprod Toxicol*. 1994;8:207-216.
7. Méndez LE, Mueller A, Salom E, et al. Paclitaxel and carboplatin chemotherapy administered during pregnancy for advanced epithelial ovarian cancer. *Obstet Gynecol*. 2003;102:1200-1202.
8. Hudson CN, Slevin ML, Tebbutt H. Successful pregnancy after treatment of stage III bilateral ovarian dysgerminoma. *Br J Obstet Gynaecol*. 1995;102:1015-1016.
9. Lawal AH, Lynch CB. Borderline ovarian cancer, bilateral surgical castration, chemotherapy and a normal delivery after ovum donation and in vitro fertilisation-embryo transfer. *Br J Obstet Gynaecol*. 1996;103:931-932.
10. Schilder JM, Thompson AM, DePriest PD, et al. Outcome of reproductive age women with stage 1A or 1C invasive epithelial ovarian cancer treated with fertility-sparing therapy. *Gynecol Oncol*. 2002;87:1-7.
11. Chiarelli AM, Marrett LD, Darlington GA. Pregnancy outcomes in females after treatment for childhood cancer. *Epidemiology*. 2000;11:161-166.
12. Seiden MV, Spitzer TR, McAfee S, et al. Successful pregnancy after high-dose cyclophosphamide, carboplatinum, and taxol with peripheral blood stem cell transplant in a young woman with ovarian cancer. *Gynecol Oncol*. 2001;83:412-414.
13. Tabata T, Nishiura K, Tanida K, et al. Carboplatin chemotherapy in a pregnant patient with undifferentiated ovarian carcinoma: case report and review of the literature. *Int J Gynecol Cancer*. 2008;18:181-184.
14. Mir O, Berveiller P, Ropert S, et al. Use of platinum derivatives during pregnancy. *Cancer*. 2008;113:3069-3074.
15. Azim HA Jr, Scarfone G, Peccatori FA. Carboplatin and weekly paclitaxel for the treatment of advanced non-small cell lung cancer (NSCLC) during pregnancy. *J Thorac Oncol*. 2009;4:559-560.
16. Chun KC, Kim DY, Kim JH, et al. Neoadjuvant chemotherapy with paclitaxel plus platinum followed by radical surgery in early cervical cancer during pregnancy: three case reports. *Jpn J Clin Oncol*. 2010;40:694-698.
17. Gottschalk I, Berg C, Harbeck N, et al. Fetal renal insufficiency following trastuzumab treatment for breast cancer in pregnancy: case report and review of the current literature. *Breast Cancer (Basel)*. 2011;6:475-478.
18. Smith ER, Borowsky ME, Jain VD. Intraperitoneal chemotherapy in a pregnant woman with ovarian cancer. *Obstet Gynecol*. 2013;122:481-483.
19. Griffin SJ, Milla M, Baker TE, et al. Transfer of carboplatin and paclitaxel into breast milk. *J Hum Lact*. 2012;28:457-459.

CARBOPROST

Miscellaneous (Prostaglandin)

PREGNANCY RECOMMENDATION: *Contraindicated (in an Ongoing Pregnancy)

BREASTFEEDING RECOMMENDATION: Probably Compatible (Hold Breastfeeding)

PREGNANCY SUMMARY

No reports describing the outcomes of human pregnancies following the use of carboprost in the first trimester. The drug will probably cross the placenta, so some fetal exposure will likely occur. Therefore, the absence of human pregnancy experience prevents a complete assessment of the embryofetal risk. Animal studies did show embryofetal toxicity in two species at doses less than 10 times the RHD. *However, the drug is contraindicated for use in an ongoing pregnancy. It is approved for use following delivery for treating postpartum hemorrhage. The drug should be used with caution in patients with pulmonary disease (eg, asthma) and in patients with hypertension.

C

BREASTFEEDING SUMMARY

No reports describing the use of carboprost during human lactation have been located. The drug will probably be found in breast milk, so some infant exposure will likely occur. However, this treatment would likely be limited to a short time period in treating a patient with postpartum hemorrhage, when breastfeeding might be limited. However, due to a concern for potential serious adverse effects that might be seen in a breastfed infant, the manufacturer recommends that women not breastfeed while being treated with this drug and for at least 6 hours after the last dose. Breastfeeding could also be held. If the clinical decision is to use this drug while breastfeeding, the infant should be monitored for the most common reported adult side effects of nausea, headache, and muscular pain (all leading to irritability), vomiting, diarrhea, and flushing.

References

1. Product information. *Hemabate*. Pharmacia and Upjohn; 2020.
2. Arnon J, Ornoy A. Clinical teratology counseling and consultation case report: outcome of pregnancy after failure of early induced abortions. *Teratology*. 1995;52:126-127.
3. Pastuszak AL, Schuler L, Speck-Martins CE, et al. Use of misoprostol during pregnancy and Möbius syndrome in infants. *N Engl J Med*. 1998;338:1881-1885.

CARFILZOMIB

Antineoplastic (Proteosome Inhibitor)

PREGNANCY RECOMMENDATION: No Human Data—Animal Data Suggest Potential Risk

BREASTFEEDING RECOMMENDATION: Potential Toxicity

PREGNANCY SUMMARY

No reports describing the use of carfilzomib in human pregnancy have been located. A limited amount of the drug may cross the placenta, so some fetal exposure might occur. Therefore, the absence of human pregnancy experience prevents a complete assessment of the embryofetal risk. Animal data did show some embryofetal toxicity in one species at doses less than 10 times the RHD. Based on animal studies and the drug's mechanism of action, the manufacturer recommends that women with reproductive potential avoid becoming pregnant during treatment with this drug. Nevertheless, using this drug during pregnancy should be based on the pros and cons of the mother's clinical need for treatment versus any potential fetal risk that might occur from exposure. There is a registry for women who are pregnant and have cancer. For more information, women and health care providers are encouraged to contact the Cancer and Pregnancy Registry at 1-877-635-4499.

BREASTFEEDING SUMMARY

No reports describing the use of carfilzomib during human lactation have been located. The drug may be found in breast milk, so some infant exposure might occur. The manufacturer recommends that the drug be discontinued or breastfeeding be stopped if used during lactation. Nevertheless, breastfeeding while using this drug should be based on the mother's clinical need for treatment versus any potential infant risks that might occur. If used, the infant should be monitored for the most common reported adult side effects of nausea and abdominal pain (both leading to irritability), diarrhea, fatigue (lethargy), fever, and various laboratory abnormalities (see PI).

Reference

1. Prescribing Information. *Kyprolis*. Onyx Pharmaceuticals; 2022.

CARGLUMIC ACID

Endocrine/Metabolic (Hyperammonemia)

PREGNANCY RECOMMENDATION: Limited Human Data—Animal Data Suggest Low Risk/remove / (Maternal Benefit May Outweigh Embryo–Fetal Risk)

BREASTFEEDING RECOMMENDATION: Probably Compatible

PREGNANCY SUMMARY

One report was located that described the use of carglumic acid in human pregnancy. A patient with partial *N*-acetylglutamate synthase (NAGS) deficiency used carglumic acid throughout two separate pregnancies (conception through delivery), giving birth at term in both cases with no reported fetal anomalies or complications. The drug will probably cross the

(*continued*)

placenta, so some fetal exposure will likely occur. However, this limited human pregnancy experience prevents a complete assessment of the embryofetal risk. Animal studies did not show any embryofetal toxicity in two species. Using this drug during pregnancy should be based on the pros and cons of the mother's clinical need for treatment versus any potential fetal risk that might occur from exposure.

BREASTFEEDING SUMMARY

One report describing the use of carglumic acid during human lactation has been located. The mother took carglumic acid throughout the pregnancy and breastfed postdelivery with no reported complications or issues. Drug levels were not tested in breast milk. The drug will probably be excreted into breast milk. However, due to a concern for potential serious adverse effects that might be seen in a breastfed infant, the manufacturer recommends that women not breastfeed while being treated with this drug. Nevertheless, breastfeeding while using this drug should be based on the mother's clinical need for treatment versus any potential infant risks that might occur. If used, the infant should be monitored for the most common reported adult side effects of headache and abdominal pain (both leading to irritability), diarrhea, vomiting, fever, infections, and anemia.

References

1. Prescribing Information. *Carbaglu*. Orphan Europe; 2019.
2. Haidar LA, Pachnis P, Gotway GK, et al. Partial N-acetyl glutamate synthase deficiency presenting as postpartum hyperammonemia: diagnosis and subsequent pregnancy management. *JIMD Reports*. 2023;64:403-409.

CARIPRAZINE

Mental Health (Atypical Antipsychotic)

PREGNANCY RECOMMENDATION: No Human Data—Animal Data Suggest Potential Risk

BREASTFEEDING RECOMMENDATION: Potential Toxicity

PREGNANCY SUMMARY

No reports describing the use of cariprazine in human pregnancy have been located. The drug will probably cross the placenta, so some fetal exposure will likely occur. Therefore, the absence of human pregnancy experience prevents a complete assessment of the embryofetal risk. Use of antipsychotic drugs near delivery has been reported to cause withdrawal and/or extrapyramidal symptoms in neonates, presenting with hypertonia, hypotonia, tremor, agitation, somnolence, respiratory issues, and feeding dysfunction. Animal studies did show embryofetal toxicity with malformations in one species at doses less than 10 times the RHD. Using this drug during pregnancy should be based on the pros and cons of the mother's clinical need for treatment versus any potential fetal risk that might occur from exposure. There is a pregnancy exposure registry that monitors pregnancy outcomes in women using atypical antipsychotic drugs. Health care providers are encouraged to contact the National Pregnancy Registry for Atypical Antipsychotics at 1-866-961-2388.

BREASTFEEDING SUMMARY

No reports describing the use of cariprazine during human lactation have been located. The drug and its active metabolites will probably be found in breast milk, so some infant exposure will likely occur. Drugs that are partial dopamine receptor agonists may affect breast milk supply. Breastfeeding while using this drug should be based on the mother's clinical need for treatment versus any potential infant risks that might occur. If used, the infant should be monitored for the most common reported adult side effects of nausea (leading to irritability), somnolence, vomiting, and extrapyramidal symptoms.

References

1. Prescribing Information. *Vraylar*. Allergan; 2022.
2. Naughton S, O'Hara K, Nelson J, Keightley P. Aripiprazole, brexpiprazole, and cariprazine can affect milk supply: advice to breastfeeding mothers. *Australas Psychiatry*. 2023;31:201-204.

CARISOPRODOL

Pain (Muscle Relaxant)

PREGNANCY RECOMMENDATION: Limited Human Data—No Relevant Animal Data

BREASTFEEDING RECOMMENDATION: Probably Compatible

PREGNANCY SUMMARY

In the combined data from the Collaborative Perinatal Project, Michigan Medicaid, US Food and Drug Administration (FDA) data, and two case reports, a total of 439 pregnancies with first-trimester exposure to carisoprodol and meprobamate have been reported. There were 23 (5.2%) birth anomalies identified. However, no specific pattern was noted, and coexposures to other drugs were not described. The drug will probably cross the placenta, so some fetal exposure will likely occur. However, this limited human pregnancy experience still prevents a complete assessment of the embryofetal risk. Animal studies have not been conducted with carisoprodol, but for meprobamate, no significant embryofetal toxicity was shown (see Meprobamate). Using this drug during pregnancy should be based on the pros and cons of the mother's clinical need for treatment versus any potential fetal risk that might occur from exposure.

BREASTFEEDING SUMMARY

Three studies have been located that demonstrate the presence of carisoprodol and meprobamate in human breast milk. In one study of a mother using 2,100 mg/d of carisoprodol, the breast milk levels for carisoprodol and meprobamate were 0.9 and 11.6 mcg/mL, respectively. The calculated RID was about 4.1%. In a second study of a mother who was using 2,800 mg/d, the peak carisoprodol and meprobamate levels obtained were 1.4 and 17.1 mcg/mL, respectively. The calculated RID was about 6.9%. A third study found carisoprodol and meprobamate (qualitatively) in the breast milk of a mother who was thought to be abusing carisoprodol. One of the studies evaluated the infant's serum levels for the drug and active metabolite, but concentrations were below the level of detection. The drug, therefore, does get excreted into breast milk. Breastfeeding while using this drug should be based on the mother's clinical need for treatment versus any potential infant risks that might occur. If used, the infant should be monitored for the most common reported adult side effects of headache and dizziness (both leading to irritability), somnolence, and lethargy.

References

1. Prescribing Information. *Soma*. Meda Pharmaceuticals; 2019.
2. Heinonen OP, Slone D, Shapiro S. *Birth Defects and Drugs in Pregnancy*. Wright PSB; 1983:360.
3. Nordeng H, Zahlsen K, Spigset O. Transfer of carisoprodol to breast milk. *Ther Drug Monit*. 2001;23:298-300.
4. Briggs GG, Ambrose PJ, Nageotte MP, et al. High-dose carisoprodol during pregnancy and lactation. *Ann Pharmacother*. 2008;42:898-901.
5. Bailey DN, Briggs JR. Carisoprodol: an unrecognized drug of abuse. *Am J Clin Pathol*. 2002;117:396-400.

CARMUSTINE

Antineoplastic (Alkylating Agent)

PREGNANCY RECOMMENDATION: Limited Human Data—Animal Data Suggest Risk

BREASTFEEDING RECOMMENDATION: Potential Toxicity

PREGNANCY SUMMARY

Two case reports were located that described the use of carmustine in human pregnancy. One occurred in the first trimester and the other in the second trimester. Both infants were delivered with no identified anomalies and did well. The drug will probably cross the placenta, so some fetal exposure will likely occur. However, this limited human pregnancy experience prevents a complete assessment of the embryofetal risk. Animal studies did show embryofetal toxicity and malformations in two species at doses of less than 10 times the RHD. Based on animal studies and the drug's mechanism of action, the manufacturer recommends that women with reproductive potential use effective contraception during treatment and for 6 months after the last dose. They also recommend that males with female partners of reproductive potential use effective contraception during treatment and for 3 months after the last dose. Nevertheless, using this drug during pregnancy should be based on the pros and cons of the mother's clinical need for treatment versus any potential fetal risk that might occur from exposure.

BREASTFEEDING SUMMARY

No reports describing the use of carmustine during lactation have been located. The drug will probably be excreted into breast milk, so some infant exposure will likely occur. However, due to a concern for potential serious adverse effects that might be seen in a breastfed infant, the manufacturer recommends that women not breastfeed while being treated with this drug. Nevertheless, breastfeeding while using this drug should be based on the mother's clinical need for treatment versus any potential infant risks that might occur. If used, the infant should be monitored for the most common reported adult side effects of nausea and abdominal pain (both leading to irritability), diarrhea, vomiting, pulmonary issues, and various laboratory abnormalities (see PI).

References

1. Prescribing Information. *BICNU*. Heritage Pharmaceuticals; 2018.

2. Benardete EA, Kriegstein AR. Increase excitability and decreased sensitivity to GABA in an animal model of dysplastic cortex. *Epilepsia*. 2002;43:970-982.
3. Schapira DV, Chudley AE. Successful pregnancy following continuous treatment with combination chemotherapy before conception and throughout pregnancy. *Cancer*. 1984;54:800-803.
4. DiPaola RS, Goodin S, Ratzell M, et al. Chemotherapy for metastatic melanoma during pregnancy. *Gynecol Oncol*. 1997;66:526-530.
5. Blatt J, Mulvihill JJ, Ziegler JL, et al. Pregnancy outcome following cancer chemotherapy. *Am J Med*. 1980;69:828-832.
6. Green DM, Zevon MA, Lowrie G, et al. Congenital anomalies in children of patients who received chemotherapy for cancer in childhood and adolescence. *N Engl J Med*. 1991;325:141-146.
7. Bierman PJ, Bagin RG, Jagannath S, et al. High dose chemotherapy followed by autologous hematopoietic rescue in Hodgkin's disease: long-term follow-up in 128 patients. *Ann Oncol*. 1993;4:767-773.
8. Brice P, Pautier P, Marolleau JP, et al. Pregnancy after autologous bone marrow transplantation for malignant lymphomas. *Nouv Rev Fr Hematol*. 1994; 36:387-388.
9. Chiarelli AM, Marrett LD, Darlington GA. Pregnancy outcomes in females after treatment for childhood cancer. *Epidemiology*. 2000;11:161-166.
10. Green DM, Whitton JA, Stovall M, et al. Pregnancy outcome of female survivors of childhood cancer: a report from the Childhood Cancer Survivor study. *Am J Obstet Gynecol*. 2002;187:1070-1080.

CARTEOLOL OPHTHALMIC

Ophthalmic/Autonomic (Topical—β-Adrenergic Antagonist)

PREGNANCY RECOMMENDATION: No Human Data and No Relevant Animal Data

BREASTFEEDING RECOMMENDATION: Probably Compatible

PREGNANCY SUMMARY

No reports describing the use of carteolol ophthalmic in human pregnancy have been located. The drug will probably cross the placenta; however, because of the topical ocular use, fetal exposure is probably negligible. Nevertheless, the absence of human pregnancy experience prevents a complete assessment of the embryofetal risk. No relevant animal studies have been conducted. Using this drug during pregnancy should be based on the pros and cons of the mother's clinical need for treatment versus any potential fetal risk that might occur from exposure. If used during pregnancy, consider placing pressure over the tear duct in the corner of the eye for at least 1 minute, and then remove any excess solution with absorbent tissue to decrease the amount of drug reaching the systemic circulation even further.

BREASTFEEDING SUMMARY

No reports describing the use of carteolol ophthalmic during human lactation have been located. The drug will likely be found in breast milk, but the amount following topical ocular use is likely to be negligible. Breastfeeding while using this drug should be based on the mother's clinical need for treatment versus any potential infant risks that might occur. If used, the infant should be monitored for the most common reported adult side effects of nausea, dizziness, and headache (all leading to irritability), insomnia, bradycardia, and decreased blood pressure. A method to further decrease some systemic absorption with ophthalmic use is described above in the Pregnancy Summary.

Reference

1. Prescribing Information. *Carteolol*. Sandoz; 2021.

CARVEDILOL

Autonomic (α/β-Adrenergic Antagonist)

PREGNANCY RECOMMENDATION: Limited Human Data—Animal Data Suggest Low Risk

BREASTFEEDING RECOMMENDATION: Probably Compatible

PREGNANCY SUMMARY

Three case reports describing the use of carvedilol at the time of conception and continuing to delivery were located. All three delivered healthy newborns with no reported anomalies. Use of carvedilol was not found to be associated with small-for-gestational-age newborns in two small studies (total of 45 pregnancies). However, it was associated with neonatal hypoglycemia when used near the time of delivery. The drug will probably cross the placenta, so some fetal exposure will likely occur. Therefore, this limited human pregnancy experience prevents a complete assessment of the embryofetal risk. Animal studies did not show any embryofetal toxicity or teratogenicity in two species at doses of less than 10 times the RHD. Using this drug during pregnancy should be based on the pros and cons of the mother's clinical need for treatment versus any potential fetal risk that might occur from exposure.

BREASTFEEDING SUMMARY

No reports describing the use of carvedilol in human lactation have been located. The drug will probably be found in breast milk, so some infant exposure will likely occur. Breastfeeding while using this drug should be based on the mother's clinical need for treatment versus any potential infant risks that might occur. If used, the infant should be monitored for the most common reported adult side effects of dizziness (leading to irritability), diarrhea, fatigue (lethargy), slow heart rate, and hyperglycemia.

References

1. Prescribing Information. *Coreg*. GlaxoSmithKline; 2020.
2. Muller PR, James A. Pregnancy with prolonged fetal exposure to an angiotensin-converting enzyme inhibitor. *J Perinatol*. 2002;22:582-584.
3. Fadol AP, Lech T, Bickford C, Yusef SW. Pregnancy in a patient with cancer and heart failure: challenges and complexities. *J Adv Pract Oncol*. 2012;3: 85-93.
4. Inoue W, Motoki H, Yoshie K, Kuwahara K. Successful management of a pregnant patient with Danon cardiomyopathy. *Intern Med*. 2024;63: 681-686.
5. Tanaka K, Tanaka H, Kamiya C, et al. Beta-blockers and fetal growth restriction in pregnant women with cardiovascular disease. *Circ J*. 2016;80: 2221-2226.
6. Kubota K, Inai K, Shimada E, Shinohara T. α/β- and β-blocker exposure in pregnancy and the risk of neonatal hypoglycemia and small for gestational age. *Circ J*. 2023;87:569-577.

C

CASANTHRANOL

Gastrointestinal/Dietary Supplement (Laxative)

PREGNANCY RECOMMENDATION: Limited Human Data—No Relevant Animal Data

BREASTFEEDING RECOMMENDATION: *Probably Compatible

PREGNANCY SUMMARY

Between the Collaborative Perinatal Project and the Michigan Medicaid Surveillance Study, 117 first-trimester exposures to casanthranol were reported, with 6 (5.1%) newborns identified who had malformations. No specific pattern was seen in the anomalies, and coexposures to other drugs were not described. In the Collaborative Perinatal Project alone, for anytime use during pregnancy, there were a total of 109 patients with 3 (2.8%) newborns found to have anomalies. Based on likely placental transfer, some fetal exposure may occur. However, the amount overall should be minimal due to poor systemic absorption from the gastrointestinal tract. Nevertheless, this limited human pregnancy experience prevents a complete assessment of the embryofetal risk. No animal reproduction studies have been located. Using this supplement during pregnancy should be based on the pros and cons of the mother's clinical need for treatment versus any potential fetal risk that might occur from exposure. The supplement was FDA-approved for treating constipation until 2002, when this was removed for a lack of safety and efficacy evidence. It is now only available as an over-the-counter supplement.

BREASTFEEDING SUMMARY

No reports describing the use of casanthranol in human lactation have been located. The anthranol glycosides will probably be found in breast milk, but the poor absorption from the gastrointestinal tract should limit infant exposure. Per the manufacturer, casanthranol is excreted into human breast milk. Back in 2001, the American Academy of Pediatrics classified casanthranol as compatible with breastfeeding. *However, today other alternatives might be available.

References

1. Prescribing Information. *Casanthranol*. Selleck, USA; 2022.
2. Food and Drug Administration. Status of certain additional over-the-counter drug category II and III active ingredients. *Fed Regist*. 2002;67:31125.
3. Heinonen OP, Slone D, Shapiro S. *Birth Defects and Drugs in Pregnancy*. Wright PSB; 1983:385,442.
4. American Academy of Pediatrics Committee on Drugs. The transfer of drugs and other chemicals into human milk. *Pediatrics*. 2001;108:776-789.

CASCARA SAGRADA

Gastrointestinal/Dietary Supplement (Laxative)

PREGNANCY RECOMMENDATION: Limited Human Data—No Relevant Animal Data

BREASTFEEDING RECOMMENDATION: Potential Toxicity

C

PREGNANCY SUMMARY

The Collaborative Perinatal Project reported 53 first-trimester exposures to cascara, with 3 (5.7%) newborns identified who had malformations. No specific pattern was seen in the two cases, and coexposures to other drugs were not described. For anytime use during the pregnancy, there were a total of 188 pregnant patients, with 7 (3.7%) newborns that had anomalies. Based on likely placental transfer, some fetal exposure may occur, but the overall amount is unknown. Therefore, this limited human pregnancy experience prevents a complete assessment of the embryofetal risk. No animal reproduction studies have been located. Using this supplement during pregnancy should be based on the pros and cons of the mother's clinical need for treatment versus any potential fetal risk that might occur from exposure. The supplement was FDA-approved for treating constipation until 2002, when it was removed due to a lack of safety and efficacy evidence. It is now only available as an over-the-counter supplement.

BREASTFEEDING SUMMARY

One study evaluated the presence of cascara sagrada in the breast milk of 10 lactating women. The supplement was detected in five of the samples (with a test sensitivity of 1.1 mg/mL). With a more sensitive test, additional samples may have been positive. This study also reported that 10 of 22 breastfed infants had loose stools after their mothers took cascara. However, another study reported no loose stools in 142 newborns after their mothers took the supplement. Back in 2001, the American Academy of Pediatrics classified cascara sagrada as compatible with breastfeeding. However, today other alternatives might be available.

References

1. Prescribing Information. *Cascara Sagrada*. Monterey Bay Herb Company; 2022.
2. Food and Drug Administration. Status of certain additional over-the-counter drug category II and III active ingredients. *Fed Regist*. 2002;67:31125.
3. Heinonen OP, Slone D, Shapiro S. *Birth Defects and Drugs in Pregnancy*. Wright PSB; 1983:385,442.
4. Tyson RM, Shrader EA, Perlman HH. Drugs transmitted through breast milk: Part I: laxatives. *J Pediatr*. 1937;11:824-832.
5. Duncan AS. Standardized senna as a laxative in the puerperium: a clinical assessment. *Br Med J*. 1957;1:439-441.
6. American Academy of Pediatrics Committee on Drugs. The transfer of drugs and other chemicals into human milk. *Pediatrics*. 2001;108:776-789.

CASIMERSEN

Genetic (Antisense Oligonucleotide)

PREGNANCY RECOMMENDATION: No Human Data and No Relevant Animal Data

BREASTFEEDING RECOMMENDATION: Probably Compatible

PREGNANCY SUMMARY

No reports describing the use of casimersen in human pregnancy have been located. Placental transfer is likely to be clinically insignificant. However, the absence of human pregnancy experience prevents a complete assessment of the embryofetal risk. Animal reproduction studies have not been performed. Duchenne Muscular Dystrophy (DMD) is primarily seen in males (X-linked recessive genetic disorder). Females with severe DMD who are of reproductive age potential are exceedingly rare. Using this drug during pregnancy should be based on the pros and cons of the mother's clinical need for treatment versus any potential fetal risk that might occur from exposure.

BREASTFEEDING SUMMARY

No reports describing the use of casimersen during human lactation have been located. Excretion of the drug into breast milk is likely to be clinically insignificant. Breastfeeding while using this drug should be based on the mother's clinical need for treatment. If used, the infant should be monitored for the most common reported adult side effects of headache, arthralgia, and oropharyngeal pain (all leading to irritability), upper respiratory tract infection, cough, and pyrexia.

Reference

1. Prescribing Information. *Amondys 45*. Sarepta Therapeutics; 2021.

CASPOFUNGIN

Anti-Infective (Antifungal)

PREGNANCY RECOMMENDATION: No Human Data—Animal Data Suggest Risk

BREASTFEEDING RECOMMENDATION: Probably Compatible

C

PREGNANCY SUMMARY

No reports describing the use of caspofungin in human pregnancy have been located. A limited amount of the drug may cross the placenta, so some fetal exposure might occur. Therefore, the absence of human pregnancy experience prevents a complete assessment of the embryofetal risk. Animal studies did show some embryofetal toxicity in two species at doses less than 10 times the RHD. Using this drug during pregnancy should be based on the pros and cons of the mother's clinical need for treatment versus any potential fetal risk that might occur from exposure.

BREASTFEEDING SUMMARY

No reports describing the use of caspofungin during human lactation have been located. A limited amount of the drug may be excreted into breast milk. However, less than 1% of an oral dose is absorbed orally, so infant exposure is likely to be clinically insignificant. Breastfeeding while using this drug should be based on the mother's clinical need for treatment versus any potential infant risks that might occur. If used, the infant should be monitored for the most common reported adult side effects of diarrhea, fever, elevated liver function tests, and rash.

Reference

1. Prescribing Information. *Caspofungin*. Mylan Institutional; 2021.

CASTOR OIL

Gastrointestinal (Laxative)

PREGNANCY RECOMMENDATION: Human Data Suggest Potential Risk

BREASTFEEDING RECOMMENDATION: Potential Toxicity

PREGNANCY SUMMARY

Overall, castor oil has not been studied with first-trimester use in regard to embryofetal toxicity or teratogenicity. The primary components of the drug (ricinoleic, linoleic, and α-linolenic acids) cross the placenta, so some fetal exposure will occur. Therefore, the absence of human pregnancy experience prevents a complete assessment of the embryofetal risk. One report was located that described an infant with multiple anomalies that was exposed to the toxin, ricin, through the use of castor seed at the time of conception and during the first 2 months of gestation. By report, no other drugs were taken during pregnancy. Although this report of multiple congenital defects attributed to castor seeds early in gestation requires confirmation, castor beans/seeds should be avoided during pregnancy. Castor oil has been used since ancient times to induce labor. However, studies on the efficacy for this indication and fetal/newborn safety have been mixed, with most larger analyses not showing benefit. The mechanism of action of castor oil's oxytocic effect is not fully known. It is thought to be related to systemic absorption of ricinoleic acid that activates EP3 and EP4 prostaglandin receptors in smooth muscle cells (found in the uterus), leading to contractions. In more recent times, the use of castor oil as an oxytocic agent has declined, probably because of the availability of safer and more physiologic agents. As for castor oil, the limited human data offer no documented benefits for the mother or fetus. Thus, castor oil (as a laxative or for other purposes before term pregnancy) should be used with caution. Its use at term should only be on the advice of a health care provider.

BREASTFEEDING SUMMARY

No reports describing the use of castor oil during human lactation have been located. Linoleic and α-linolenic acids are essential fatty acids (both unsaturated) that are absorbed systemically and found in human breast milk. The MWs of linoleic and α-linolenic acids are 280 and 278, respectively. Some ricinoleic acid (also unsaturated with an MW of 298) is also absorbed systemically. Therefore, ricinoleic acid (the primary component of castor oil) is also probably found in breast milk. Therefore, diarrhea in the nursing infant is a potential complication. Other laxatives that are considered safe for use while breastfeeding (eg, osmotic laxatives that are minimally absorbed systemically) are recommended as first-line agents.

References

1. Nabors GG. Castor oil as an adjunct to induction of labor: critical re-evaluation. *Am J Obstet Gynecol*. 1958;75:36-38.
2. Gattuso JM, Kamm MA. Adverse effects of drugs used in the management of constipation and diarrhoea. *Drug Saf*. 1994;10:47-65.
3. Mauhoub ME, Khalifa MM, Jaswal OB, et al. "Ricin syndrome." A possible new teratogenic syndrome associated with ingestion of castor oil seed in early pregnancy: a case report. *Ann Trop Paediatr*. 1983;3:57-61.
4. Ernst E. Herbal medicinal products during pregnancy: are they safe? *Br J Obstet Gynaecol*. 2002;109:227-235.
5. Mathie JG, Dawson BH. Effect of castor oil, soap enema, and hot bath on the pregnant human uterus near term: a tocographic study. *Br Med J*. 1959;1:1162-1165.
6. McFarlin BL, Gibson MH, O'Rear J, et al. A national survey of herbal preparation use by nurse-midwives for labor stimulation. *J Nurse Midwifery*. 1999;44:205-216.
7. Davis L. The use of castor oil to stimulate labor in patients with premature rupture of membranes. *J Nurse Midwifery*. 1984;29:366-370.
8. Harris M, Nye M. Self-administration of castor oil. *Mod Midwife*. 1994;4:29-30.
9. Summers L. Methods of cervical ripening and labor induction. *J Nurse Midwifery*. 1997;42:71-85.
10. Garry D, Figueroa R, Guillaume J, et al. Use of castor oil in pregnancies at term. *Altern Ther Health Med*. 2000;6:77-79.

11. Lippert TH, Mueck AO. Labour induction with alternative drugs? *J Obstet Gynaecol*. 2002;22:343.
12. Kelly AJ, Kavanagh J, Thomas J. Castor oil, bath and/or enema for cervical priming and induction of labour. *Cochrane Database Syst Rev*. 2002;(2):CD003099. doi:10.1002/14651858.CD003099
13. Tenore JL. Methods for cervical ripening and induction of labor. *Am Fam Physician*. 2003;67:2123-2128.
14. Mitri F, Hofmeyr GJ, Van Gelderen CJ. Meconium during labor—self-medication and other associations. *S Afr Med J*. 1987;71:431-433.
15. Steingrub JS, Lopez T, Teres D, et al. Amniotic fluid embolism associated with castor oil ingestion. *Crit Care Med*. 1988;16:642-643.
16. Sicuranza GB, Figueroa R. Uterine rupture associated with castor oil ingestion. *J Matern Fetal Neonatal Med*. 2003;13:133-134.
17. Tendulkar S. Local lubrication in labour. *Indian Med J*. 1967;61:176.
18. Benakappa DG, Shivananda MR, Benakappa AD. Breast-feeding practices in rural Karnataka (India) with special reference to lactation failure. *Acta Peadiatr Jpn*. 1989;31:391-398.

CEDAZURIDINE/DECITABINE

Antineoplastic

PREGNANCY RECOMMENDATION: Limited Human Data—No Relevant Animal Data

BREASTFEEDING RECOMMENDATION: Potential Toxicity

PREGNANCY SUMMARY

No reports describing the use of cedazuridine/decitabine in human pregnancy have been located. Based on likely placental transfer for both drugs, fetal exposure will probably occur. There is one case report of possible teratogenic effects in a patient potentially exposed to decitabine in the first trimester. Based on the reported pregnancy dating in the manuscript, the patient received her last treatment of decitabine about 2 to 3 weeks prior to conception. The fetus was found to have holoprosencephaly, midface anomalies (hypotelorism, arhinia, cleft lip and palate) and rocker-bottom feet. Genetic testing was not performed. These anomalies are commonly seen with trisomy 13 and other genetic abnormalities; however, teratogenicity cannot fully be ruled out. Animal data for decitabine did show fetotoxic effects at levels below the RHD, but with intraperitoneal injections. Significant myelosuppression was seen in more than 50% of adult patients treated with this drug. Because of the risk for myelosuppression in both a pregnant mother and her fetus and the potential fetal anomaly risks seen in animal studies for decitabine, the manufacturer recommends that women with reproductive potential use effective contraception while being treated with cedazuridine/decitabine and for 6 months after the final dose. They also advise that males with female partners of reproductive potential also use effective contraception during treatment and for 3 months after the final dose.

BREASTFEEDING SUMMARY

Cedazuridine and decitabine probably enter breast milk. Because of the potential for serious myelosuppression seen in adults treated with cedazuridine/decitabine, the manufacturer recommends that women not breastfeed during treatment or for 2 weeks after the final dose. However, if the clinical decision is to breastfeed while using this drug, the infant should be monitored for the most common reported adult side effects of headache, myalgias, and arthralgias (all leading to irritability), myelosuppression, lethargy, diarrhea, constipation, decreased appetite, and rash.

References

1. Prescribing Information. *Inqovi*. Otsuka Pharmaceutical Co., Ltd, Taiho Oncology, Inc; 2020.
2. Lee BS, Sathar J, Ong TC. Teratogenic effect of decitabine in a pregnant patient with acute myeloid leukemia: a case report. *Hematol Transfus Cell Ther*. 2022;44(3):429-432.

CEFACLOR

Antibacterial (Cephalosporin)

PREGNANCY RECOMMENDATION: Human Data Suggest Potential Risk—Animal Data Suggest Low Risk

BREASTFEEDING RECOMMENDATION: Compatible

PREGNANCY SUMMARY

In a surveillance study of Michigan Medicaid recipients, 1,325 newborns were exposed to cefaclor during the first trimester, and 75 (5.7%) major birth defects were observed (53 expected). The data for total defects, cardiovascular, and oral clefts were suggestive of an association between cefaclor and congenital anomalies, but other factors, such as the mother's disease, may be involved. Numerous evaluations of other cephalosporin drugs have not found an increased risk for birth

C

anomalies. The drug will probably cross the placenta, so some fetal exposure will likely occur. Therefore, further analysis regarding safety is necessary. Animal studies did not demonstrate any embryofetal toxicity or malformations in three animal species. Using this drug during pregnancy should be based on the pros and cons of the mother's clinical need for treatment versus any potential fetal risk that might occur from exposure.

BREASTFEEDING SUMMARY

Cefaclor is excreted into breast milk, but in low concentrations. One study evaluated breast milk levels in two patients who received a 250 mg dose. The drug was not detected in the milk for one patient, and levels of 150 to 190 ng/mL were seen in the other patient up to 4 hours after the dose, but were undetectable at 5 hours. Following a single 500 mg oral dose, peak breast milk levels ranged from 180 to 350 ng/mL. Only trace amounts of the antibiotic could be measured at 1 and 6 hours. Even though these levels are low, modification of bowel flora is possible. Breastfeeding while using this drug should be based on the mother's clinical need for treatment versus any potential infant risks that might occur. If used, the infant should be monitored for the most common reported adult side effects of nausea and pruritus (both leading to irritability), hypersensitivity reactions, diarrhea, vomiting, rash, and eosinophilia.

References

1. Prescribing Information. *Cefaclor*. Avadel Pharmaceuticals; 2019.
2. Takase Z, Shirafuji H, Uchida M. Clinical and laboratory studies of cefaclor in the field of obstetrics and gynecology. *Chemotherapy (Tokyo)*. 1979; 27(suppl):666-672.

CEFADROXIL

Antibacterial (Cephalosporin)

PREGNANCY RECOMMENDATION: Human Data Suggest Low Risk

BREASTFEEDING RECOMMENDATION: Compatible

PREGNANCY SUMMARY

In the Michigan Medicaid FDA evaluation, 722 newborns had been exposed to cefadroxil during the first trimester. A total of 27 (3.7%) major birth defects were observed (30 expected). The drug does cross the placenta, so some fetal exposure will occur. These data do not support an association between the drug and congenital birth defects. Animal studies did not show any embryofetal toxicity or malformations in two species at doses of more than 10 times the RHD. Using this drug during pregnancy should be based on the pros and cons of the mother's clinical need for treatment versus any potential fetal risk that might occur from exposure.

BREASTFEEDING SUMMARY

Three studies have shown that cefadroxil is excreted into breast milk in low concentrations. The peak breast milk level following a single 500-mg oral dose was about 0.9 mcg/mL, which occurred at 5 to 6 hours after dosing. The peak breast milk level following a 1-g oral dose was about 2.4 mcg/mL at 6 to 7 hours after dosing. In all three of the above studies, the drug was not found in the breast milk for the first hour after a dose. Although the above breast milk levels are low, the use of this drug could modify infant bowel flora. Breastfeeding while using this drug should be based on the mother's clinical need for treatment versus any potential infant risks that might occur. If used, the infant should be monitored for the most common reported adult side effects of nausea, pruritus, arthralgia, and abdominal pain (all leading to irritability), diarrhea, fever, and rash.

References

1. Prescribing Information. *Cefadroxil*. Aurobindo Pharma; 2021.
2. Takase Z, Shirafuji H, Uchida M. Experimental and clinical studies of cefadroxil in the treatment of infections in the field of obstetrics and gynecology. *Chemotherapy (Tokyo)*. 1980;28(suppl 2):424-431.
3. Kafetzi DA, Siafas CA, Georgakopoulos PA, et al. Passage of cephalosporins and amoxicillin into the breast milk. *Acta Paediatr Scand*. 1981;70:285-288.
4. Matsuda S. Transfer of antibiotics into maternal milk. *Biol Res Pregnancy Perinatol*. 1984;5:57-60.

CEFAZOLIN

Antibacterial (Cephalosporin)

PREGNANCY RECOMMENDATION: Limited Human Data—Animal Data Suggest Low Risk

BREASTFEEDING RECOMMENDATION: Compatible

C

PREGNANCY SUMMARY

A limited number of cases describing the use of cefazolin in human pregnancy have not shown an increased risk for adverse outcomes. No detectable teratogenic risk with cephalosporin antibiotics was found in a large 2001 study (see Cephalexin). Cephalosporins are usually considered safe to use during pregnancy (see other cephalosporins for published human experience). The drug crosses the placenta, so some fetal exposure will occur. However, further analysis regarding first-trimester safety is needed. Animal studies did not demonstrate any embryofetal toxicity or malformations in three species at doses of less than 10 times the RHD. Using this drug during pregnancy should be based on the pros and cons of the mother's clinical need for treatment versus any potential fetal risk that might occur from exposure.

BREASTFEEDING SUMMARY

Cefazolin has been found in human breast milk. So, some infant exposure will occur. Most breast milk levels were low (some were undetectable). However, the use of cephalosporins can modify infant bowel flora. Breastfeeding while using this drug should be based on the mother's clinical need for treatment versus any potential infant risks that might occur. If used, the infant should be monitored for the most common reported adult side effects of nausea, pruritus, and abdominal pain (all leading to irritability), diarrhea, vomiting, rash, and allergic reactions. The use of cephalosporins in pediatrics is generally considered compatible with breastfeeding.

References

1. Prescribing Information. *Cefazolin*. Baxter Healthcare; 2019.
2. Dekel A, Elian I, Gibor Y, et al. Transplacental passage of cefazolin in the first trimester of pregnancy. *Eur J Obstet Gynecol Reprod Biol*. 1980;10:303-307.
3. Bernard B, Barton L, Abate M, et al. Maternal-fetal transfer of cefazolin in the first twenty weeks of pregnancy. *J Infect Dis*. 1977;136:377-382.
4. Cho N, Ito T, Saito T, et al. Clinical studies on cefazolin in the field of obstetrics and gynecology. *Chemotherapy (Tokyo)*. 1970;18:770-777.
5. von Kobyletzki D, Reither K, Gellen J, et al. Pharmacokinetic studies with cefazolin in obstetrics and gynecology. *Infection*. 1974;2(suppl):60-67.
6. Brown CEL, Christmas JT, Bawdon RE. Placental transfer of cefazolin and piperacillin in pregnancies remote from term complicated by Rh isoimmunization. *Am J Obstet Gynecol*. 1990;163:938-943.
7. Sanchez-Ramos L, McAlpine KJ, Adair CD, et al. Pyelonephritis in pregnancy: once-a-day ceftriaxone versus multiple doses of cefazolin. *Am J Obstet Gynecol*. 1995;172:129-133.
8. Yoshioka H, Cho K, Takimoto M, et al. Transfer of cefazolin into human milk. *J Pediatr*. 1979;94:151-152.
9. American Academy of Pediatrics Committee on Drugs. The transfer of drugs and other chemicals into human milk. *Pediatrics*. 2001;108:776-789.

CEFDINIR

Antibacterial (Cephalosporin)

PREGNANCY RECOMMENDATION: No Human Data—Animal Data Suggest Low Risk

BREASTFEEDING RECOMMENDATION: Probably Compatible

PREGNANCY SUMMARY

No reports describing the use of cefdinir in human pregnancy have been located. Numerous evaluations of other cephalosporin drugs have not found an increased risk for birth anomalies. The drug will probably cross the placenta, so some fetal exposure will likely occur. Therefore, the absence of human pregnancy experience prevents a complete assessment of the embryofetal risk. Animal studies did not find any embryofetal toxicity or malformations in two species. Using this drug during pregnancy should be based on the pros and cons of the mother's clinical need for treatment versus any potential fetal risk that might occur from exposure.

BREASTFEEDING SUMMARY

According to the manufacturer, cefdinir was not found in human breast milk following a single dose of 600 mg. However, in some instances, the drug will probably be found in breast milk, so some infant exposure will likely occur. In general, cephalosporin drugs are considered acceptable for use in nursing mothers. Breastfeeding while using this drug should be based on the mother's clinical need for treatment versus any potential infant risks that might occur. If used, the infant should be monitored for the most common reported adult side effects of nausea and pruritus (both leading to irritability), hypersensitivity reactions, diarrhea, vomiting, and rash.

Reference

1. Prescribing Information. *Cefdinir*. Aurobindo Pharma; 2021.

C

CEFDITOREN

Antibacterial (Cephalosporin)

PREGNANCY RECOMMENDATION: No Human Data—Animal Data Suggest Low Risk

BREASTFEEDING RECOMMENDATION: Probably Compatible

PREGNANCY SUMMARY

No reports describing the use of cefditoren in human pregnancy have been located. Numerous evaluations of other cephalosporin drugs have not found an increased risk for birth anomalies. Some amount of the drug will probably cross the placenta, so fetal exposure will likely occur. Therefore, the absence of human pregnancy experience prevents a complete assessment of the embryofetal risk. Animal studies did not find any embryofetal toxicity or malformations in two species. Using this drug during pregnancy should be based on the pros and cons of the mother's clinical need for treatment versus any potential fetal risk that might occur from exposure.

BREASTFEEDING SUMMARY

No reports describing the use of cefditoren during human lactation have been located. Some amount of the drug might be found in breast milk, so infant exposure may occur. In general, cephalosporin drugs are considered acceptable for use in nursing mothers. Breastfeeding while using this drug should be based on the mother's clinical need for treatment versus any potential infant risks that might occur. If used, the infant should be monitored for the most common reported adult side effects of nausea and pruritus (both leading to irritability), hypersensitivity reactions, diarrhea, vomiting, and rash.

Reference

1. Prescribing Information. *Spectracef*. Vansen Pharma; 2018.

CEFEPIME

Antibacterial (Cephalosporin)

PREGNANCY RECOMMENDATION: No Human Data—Animal Data Suggest Low Risk

BREASTFEEDING RECOMMENDATION: Probably Compatible

PREGNANCY SUMMARY

No reports describing the use of cefepime in human pregnancy have been located. Cephalosporins are usually considered safe to use during pregnancy (see other cephalosporins for published human experience). The drug crosses the placenta at low levels, so some fetal exposure will occur. Therefore, the absence of human pregnancy experience prevents a complete assessment of the embryofetal risk. Animal studies did not demonstrate any embryofetal toxicity or malformations in three species at doses of less than 10 times the RHD. Using this drug during pregnancy should be based on the pros and cons of the mother's clinical need for treatment versus any potential fetal risk that might occur from exposure.

BREASTFEEDING SUMMARY

According to the manufacturer, cefepime is excreted into human breast milk at low concentrations (0.5 mcg/mL), so some newborn exposure will occur. In spite of this low dose, modification of bowel flora may occur. Breastfeeding while using this drug should be based on the mother's clinical need for treatment versus any potential infant risks that might occur. If used, the infant should be monitored for the most common reported adult side effects of nausea, pruritus, and abdominal pain (all leading to irritability), diarrhea, vomiting, rash, and allergic reactions. The use of cephalosporins in pediatrics is generally considered compatible with breastfeeding.

References

1. Prescribing Information. *Maxipime*. Hospira; 2021.
2. Ozyuncu O, Nemutlu E, Katlan D, et al. Maternal and fetal blood levels of moxifloxacin, levofloxacin, cefepime and cefoperazone. *Int J Antimicrob Agents*. 2010;36:175-178.

C

CEFEPIME/ENMETAZOBACTAM

Antibacterial (Cephalosporin)

PREGNANCY RECOMMENDATION: No Human Data—Animal Data Suggest Low Risk

BREASTFEEDING RECOMMENDATION: Probably Compatible

PREGNANCY SUMMARY

No reports describing the use of cefepime/enmetazobactam in human pregnancy have been located. Numerous evaluations of other cephalosporin drugs have not found an increased risk for birth anomalies. Cefepime crosses the placenta, so some fetal exposure will occur. For enmetazobactam, some of the drug will probably cross the placenta, so fetal exposure will also likely occur. However, the absence of human pregnancy experience prevents a complete assessment of the embryofetal risk. Animal studies did not demonstrate any embryofetal toxicity or malformations in three species at doses of less than 10 times the RHD for cefepime and in two species at doses of less than 10 times the RHD for enmetazobactam. Using this drug during pregnancy should be based on the pros and cons of the mother's clinical need for treatment versus any potential fetal risk that might occur from exposure.

BREASTFEEDING SUMMARY

No reports describing the use of cefepime/enmetazobactam during human lactation have been located. The manufacturer states that cefepime is found in human breast milk in low concentrations, so some newborn exposure will occur. For enmetazobactam, some of this drug will also be found in breast milk. In general, cephalosporin drugs are considered acceptable for use in nursing mothers. Breastfeeding while using this drug should be based on the mother's clinical need for treatment versus any potential infant risks that might occur. If used, the infant should be monitored for the most common reported adult side effects of nausea and pruritus (both leading to irritability), hypersensitivity reactions, diarrhea, vomiting, and rash. Because some infant exposure will occur, modification of bowel flora can occur.

References

1. Prescribing Information. *Exblifep*. Allecra Therapeutics SAS; 2024.
2. Ozyuncu O, Nemutlu E, Katlan D, et al. Maternal and fetal blood levels of moxifloxacin, levofloxacin, cefepime and cefoperazone. *Int J Antimicrob Agents*. 2010;36:175-178.

CEFIDEROCOL

Antibacterial (Cephalosporin)

PREGNANCY RECOMMENDATION: No Human Data—Animal Data Suggest Low Risk

BREASTFEEDING RECOMMENDATION: Probably Compatible

PREGNANCY SUMMARY

No human data specific to birth anomalies from exposure to cefiderocol have been reported. Placental transfer of the drug would not be expected. However, the absence of human pregnancy experience prevents a complete assessment of the embryofetal risk. Animal data did not show any embryofetal toxicity. Numerous studies have analyzed the potential risk for embryofetal malformations with the use of cephalosporin drugs in general during pregnancy, and no drug-associated risks have been found.

BREASTFEEDING SUMMARY

Cefiderocol will most likely not be found in human breast milk, or the expected amount would be negligible. However, breastfeeding while using this drug should be based on the mother's clinical need for treatment.

Reference

1. Prescribing Information. *Fetroja*. Shionogi & Co., Ltd; 2019.

C

CEFIXIME

Antibacterial (Cephalosporin)

PREGNANCY RECOMMENDATION: Limited Human Data—Animal Data Suggest Low Risk

BREASTFEEDING RECOMMENDATION: Probably Compatible

PREGNANCY SUMMARY

Limited human pregnancy data regarding the use of this drug during the first trimester have been located. Data do not suggest embryofetal risk. Cephalosporins are usually considered safe to use during pregnancy (see other cephalosporins for published human experience). The drug crosses the placenta at low levels, so some fetal exposure will occur. Therefore, the absence of human pregnancy experience prevents a complete assessment of the embryofetal risk. Animal studies did not demonstrate any embryofetal toxicity or malformations in two species at doses of less than 10 times the RHD. Using this drug during pregnancy should be based on the pros and cons of the mother's clinical need for treatment versus any potential fetal risk that might occur from exposure.

BREASTFEEDING SUMMARY

No reports describing the use of cefixime during human lactation have been located. Low concentrations of other cephalosporins have been found in breast milk. Therefore, the presence of cefixime in breast milk should be expected. Modification of bowel flora can occur when antibacterial drugs are ingested through breastfeeding. Breastfeeding while using this drug should be based on the mother's clinical need for treatment versus any potential infant risks that might occur. If used, the infant should be monitored for the most common reported adult side effects of nausea, pruritus, and abdominal pain (all leading to irritability), diarrhea, vomiting, rash, and allergic reactions. The use of cephalosporins in pediatrics is generally considered compatible with breastfeeding.

References

1. Prescribing Information. *Suprax*. Lupin Limited; 2016.
2. Ozyuncu O, Beksac MS, Nemutlu E, et al. Maternal blood and amniotic fluid levels of moxifloxacin, levofloxacin and cefixime. *J Obstet Gynecol*. 2010;36:484-487.
3. Wilton LV, Pearce GL, Martin RM, et al. The outcomes of pregnancy in women exposed to newly marketed drugs in general practice in England. *Br J Obstet Gynaecol*. 1998;105:882-889.
4. Ramus RM, Sheffield JS, Mayfield JA, et al. A randomized trial that compared oral cefixime and intramuscular ceftriaxone for the treatment of gonorrhea in pregnancy. *Am J Obstet Gynecol*. 2001;185:629-632.
5. Wawer MJ, Sewankambo NK, Serwadda D, et al; Rakai Project Study Group. Control of sexually transmitted disease for AIDS prevention in Uganda: a randomised community trial. *Lancet*. 1999;353:525-535.
6. Gray RH, Wabwire-Mangen F, Kigozi G, et al. Randomized trial of presumptive sexually transmitted disease therapy during pregnancy in Rakai, Uganda. *Am J Obstet Gynecol*. 2001;185:1209-1217.
7. Kigozi GG, Brahmbhatt H, Wabwire-Mangen F, et al. Treatment of *Trichomonas* in pregnancy and adverse outcomes of pregnancy: a subanalysis of a randomized trial in Rakai, Uganda. *Am J Obstet Gynecol*. 2003;189:1398-1400.

CEFOTAXIME

Antibacterial (Cephalosporin)

PREGNANCY RECOMMENDATION: Limited Human Data—Animal Data Suggest Low Risk

BREASTFEEDING RECOMMENDATION: Compatible

PREGNANCY SUMMARY

There is limited human pregnancy data with cefotaxime. No detectable teratogenic risk with cephalosporin antibiotics was found in a large 2001 study (see Cephalexin). Cephalosporins are usually considered safe to use during pregnancy (see other cephalosporins for published human experience). The drug crosses the placenta at low levels, so some fetal exposure will occur. Therefore, this limited human pregnancy experience prevents a complete assessment of the embryofetal risk. Animal studies did not demonstrate any embryofetal toxicity or malformations in three species at doses of less than 10 times the RHD. Using this drug during pregnancy should be based on the pros and cons of the mother's clinical need for treatment versus any potential fetal risk that might occur from exposure.

BREASTFEEDING SUMMARY

Cefotaxime was evaluated in 24 lactating women. In 19 women, a dose of 1 g was administered. In seven cases, the drug was not detected (lower limit of quantification (LLQ) of 100 ng/mL). In the other 12, low levels were found (highest value of 520 ng/mL). In five other women, a dose of 2 g was administered. In all cases, the drug was found in breast milk with a range of 0.3 to 1.6 mcg/mL (calculated RIDs all <1%). Modification of bowel flora can occur when antibacterial drugs are ingested through breastfeeding. Breastfeeding while using this drug should be based on the mother's clinical need for treatment versus any potential infant risks that might occur. If used, the infant should be monitored for the most common reported adult side effects of nausea, pruritus, and abdominal pain (all leading to irritability), diarrhea, vomiting, rash, and allergic reactions. The use of cephalosporins in pediatrics is generally considered compatible with breastfeeding.

References

1. Prescribing Information. *Cefotaxime*. Wockhardt; 2017.
2. Kafetzis DA, Lazarides CV, Siafas CA, et al. Transfer of cefotaxime in human milk and from mother to foetus. *J Antimicrob Chemother*. 1980;6(suppl A):135-141.
3. Maberry MC, Trimmer KJ, Bawdon RE, et al. Antibiotic concentration in maternal blood, cord blood and placental tissue in women with chorioamnionitis. *Gynecol Obstet Invest*. 1992;33:185-186.
4. Kafetzis DA, Siafas CA, Georgakopoulos PA, et al. Passage of cephalosporins and amoxicillin into the breast milk. *Acta Paediatr Scand*. 1981;70:285-288.
5. Takase Z, Fujiwara M, Kohmoto Y, et al. Study of cefotaxime in the perinatal period. *Jpn J Antibiot*. 1982;35:1893-1897.
6. Matsuda S. Transfer of antibiotics into maternal milk. *Biol Res Pregnancy Perinatol*. 1984;5:57-60.
7. American Academy of Pediatrics Committee on Drugs. The transfer of drugs and other chemicals into human milk. *Pediatrics*. 2001;108:776-789.

CEFOTETAN

Antibacterial (Cephalosporin)

PREGNANCY RECOMMENDATION: Limited Human Data—Animal Data Suggest Low Risk

BREASTFEEDING RECOMMENDATION: Compatible

PREGNANCY SUMMARY

There is limited human pregnancy data with cefotetan. No detectable teratogenic risk with cephalosporin antibiotics was found in a large 2001 study (see Cephalexin). Cephalosporins are usually considered safe to use during pregnancy (see other cephalosporins for published human experience). The drug crosses the placenta at low levels, so some fetal exposure will occur. Therefore, this limited human pregnancy experience prevents a complete assessment of the embryofetal risk. Animal studies did not demonstrate any embryofetal toxicity or malformations in two species at doses of more than 10 times the RHD. Using this drug during pregnancy should be based on the pros and cons of the mother's clinical need for treatment versus any potential fetal risk that might occur from exposure.

BREASTFEEDING SUMMARY

Cefotetan was evaluated in 14 lactating women. In nine women, a dose of 1 g was administered. The drug was found in breast milk with a peak level of about 0.5 mcg/mL. In the other five cases, a dose of 2 g was administered. The drug was found in breast milk (highest value of 590 ng/mL). The calculated RIDs were all less than 1%. Modification of bowel flora can occur when antibacterial drugs are ingested through breastfeeding. Breastfeeding while using this drug should be based on the mother's clinical need for treatment versus any potential infant risks that might occur. If used, the infant should be monitored for the most common reported adult side effects of nausea, pruritus, and abdominal pain (all leading to irritability), diarrhea, vomiting, rash, and allergic reactions. The use of cephalosporins in pediatrics is generally considered compatible with breastfeeding.

References

1. Prescribing Information. *Cefotetan*. Fresenius Kabi USA; 2018.
2. Bergogne-Berezin E, Berthelot O, Ravina JH, et al. Study of placental transfer of cefotetan (abstract). Program and Abstracts at : 25th Interscience Conference on Antimicrobial Agents and Chemotherapy; September 29–October 2, 1985:144; Minneapolis, MN.
3. Takase Z, Fujiwara M, Kawamoto Y, et al. Laboratory and clinical studies of cefotetan (YM09330) in the field of obstetrics and gynecology (English abstract). *Chemotherapy (Tokyo)*. 1982;30(suppl 1):869-881.
4. Motomura R, Teramoto C, Souda Y, et al. Fundamental and clinical study of cefotetan (YM09330) in the field of obstetrics and gynecology (English abstract). *Chemotherapy (Tokyo)*. 1982;30(suppl 1):882-887.
5. Cho N, Fukunaga K, Kunii K. Fundamental and clinical studies on cefotetan (YM09330) in the field of obstetrics and gynecology (English abstract). *Chemotherapy (Tokyo)*. 1982;30(suppl 1):832-842.
6. Novelli A, Mazzei T, Ciuffi M, et al. The penetration of intramuscular cefotetan disodium into human extra-vascular fluid and maternal milk secretion. *Chemotherapy*. 1983;2:337-342.
7. Matsuda S. Transfer of antibiotics into maternal milk. *Biol Res Pregnancy Perinatol*. 1984;5:57-60.

CEFOXITIN

Antibacterial (Cephalosporin)

PREGNANCY RECOMMENDATION: Limited Human Data—Animal Data Suggest Low Risk

BREASTFEEDING RECOMMENDATION: Compatible

PREGNANCY SUMMARY

There are limited human pregnancy data with cefoxitin. No detectable teratogenic risk with cephalosporin antibiotics was found in a large 2001 study (see Cephalexin). Cephalosporins are usually considered safe to use during pregnancy (see other cephalosporins for published human experience). The drug crosses the placenta at low levels, so some fetal exposure will occur. Therefore, this limited human pregnancy experience prevents a complete assessment of the embryofetal risk. Animal studies did not demonstrate any embryofetal toxicity or malformations in two species at doses of more than 10 times the RHD. Using this drug during pregnancy should be based on the pros and cons of the mother's clinical need for treatment versus any potential fetal risk that might occur from exposure.

BREASTFEEDING SUMMARY

Cefoxitin was evaluated in 65 lactating women. In numerous cases, the drug was not detected. In those cases where the drug was found, levels were usually low. In one case, following a 1-g intravenous (IV) dose, a peak breast milk level of 5.6 mcg/mL was found, suggesting a RID of just over 5%. All the other calculated RIDs were 1.5% or less. Modification of bowel flora can occur when antibacterial drugs are ingested through breastfeeding. Breastfeeding while using this drug should be based on the mother's clinical need for treatment versus any potential infant risks that might occur. If used, the infant should be monitored for the most common reported adult side effects of nausea, pruritus, and abdominal pain (all leading to irritability), diarrhea, vomiting, rash, and allergic reactions. The use of cephalosporins in pediatrics is generally considered compatible with breastfeeding.

References

1. Prescribing Information. *Cefoxitin*. Fresenius Kabi USA; 2023.
2. Bergone-Berezin B, Kafe H, Berthelot G, et al. Pharmacokinetic study of cefoxitin in bronchial secretions. Presented at: The 10th International Congress of Chemotherapy; September 18–23, 1977; Zurich, Switzerland. American Society for Microbiology; 1978.
3. Aokawa H, Minagawa M, Yamamiohi K, et al. Studies on cefoxitin. *Chemotherapy (Tokyo)*. 1977;(suppl):394.
4. Matsuda S, Tanno M, Kashiwakura S, et al. Basic and clinical studies on cefoxitin. *Chemotherapy (Tokyo)*. 1977;(suppl):396.
5. Berthelot G, Bergogne-Berezin B, Morel O, et al. Cefoxitin: pharmacokinetic study in bronchial secretions-transplacental diffusion (abstract No. 80). Paper presented at: 10th International Congress of Chemotherapy; September 18-23, 1977; Zurich, Switzerland.
6. Mashimo K, Mihashi S, Fukaya I, et al. New drug symposium IV. Cefoxitin. *Chemotherapy (Tokyo)*. 1978;26:114-119.
7. Matsuda S, Tanno M, Kashiwakura T, et al. Laboratory and clinical studies on cefoxitin in the field of obstetrics and gynecology. *Chemotherapy (Tokyo)*. 1978;26(suppl 1):460-467.
8. Cho N, Ubhara K, Suigizaki K, et al. Clinical studies of cefoxitin in the field of obstetrics and gynecology. *Chemotherapy (Tokyo)*. 1978;26(suppl 1): 468-475.
9. Seiga K, Minagawa M, Yamaji K, et al. Study on cefoxitin. *Chemotherapy (Tokyo)*. 1978;26(suppl 1):491-501.
10. Takase Z, Shirafuji H, Uchida M. Clinical and laboratory studies on cefoxitin in the field of obstetrics and gynecology. *Chemotherapy (Tokyo)*. 1978; 26(suppl 1):502-505.
11. Bergogne-Berezin B, Lambert-Zeohovsky N, Rouvillois JL. Placental transfer of cefoxitin (abstract No.314). Paper presented at: 18th Interscience Conference on Antimicrobial Agents and Chemotherapy; October 1-4, 1978; Atlanta, GA.
12. Brogden RN, Heel RC, Speight TM, et al. Cefoxitin: a review of its antibacterial activity, pharmacological properties and therapeutic use. *Drugs*. 1979;17:1-37.
13. Dubois M, Delapierre D, Demonty J, et al. Transplacental and mammary transfer of cefoxitin (abstract No. 118). Paper presented at: 11th International Congress of Chemotherapy and 19th Interscience Conference on Antimicrobial Agents and Chemotherapy; October 1-5, 1979; Boston, MA.
14. Bergogne-Berezin B, Morel O, Kafe H, et al. Pharmacokinetic study of cefoxitin in man: diffusion into the bronchi and transfer across the placenta. *Therapie*. 1979;34:345-354.
15. Roex AJM, van Loenen AC, Puyenbroek JI, et al. Secretion of cefoxitin in breast milk following short-term prophylactic administration in caesarean section. *Eur J Obstet Gynecol Reprod Biol*. 1987;25:299-302.
16. American Academy of Pediatrics Committee on Drugs. The transfer of drugs and other chemicals into human milk. *Pediatrics*. 2001;108:776-789.

CEFPODOXIME

Antibacterial (Cephalosporin)

PREGNANCY RECOMMENDATION: Limited Human Data—Animal Data Suggest Low Risk

BREASTFEEDING RECOMMENDATION: Probably Compatible

PREGNANCY SUMMARY

One report describing the use of cefpodoxime in human pregnancy was located. Cefpodoxime and/or azithromycin were used to treat 241 pregnant women diagnosed with chlamydia and/or gonorrhea. Concurrent patient-partner treatment was provided to 45 of these women, and they were less likely to have a repeat infection. However, no information was provided on the pregnancy outcome. Numerous evaluations of other cephalosporin drugs have not found an increased risk for birth anomalies. The drug will probably cross the placenta, so some fetal exposure will likely occur. However, this limited human pregnancy experience prevents a complete assessment of the embryofetal risk. Animal studies did not find any embryofetal toxicity or malformations in two species. Using this drug during pregnancy should be based on the pros and cons of the mother's clinical need for treatment versus any potential fetal risk that might occur from exposure.

C

BREASTFEEDING SUMMARY

According to the manufacturer, cefpodoxime was measured in the milk of three lactating women. At 4 hours after an oral 200 mg dose, levels were 0%, 2%, and 6% of the concomitant maternal serum levels, and at 6 hours were 0%, 9%, and 16%. These levels would suggest that the RID would be less than 10%. In general, cephalosporin drugs are considered acceptable for use in nursing mothers. Breastfeeding while using this drug should be based on the mother's clinical need for treatment versus any potential infant risks that might occur. If used, the infant should be monitored for the most common reported adult side effects of nausea and pruritus (both leading to irritability), hypersensitivity reactions, diarrhea, vomiting, and rash.

References

1. Prescribing Information. *Cefpodoxime*. Aurobindo Pharma; 2022.
2. Mmeje O, Coleman JS. Concurrent patient-partner treatment in pregnancy: an alternative to expedited partner therapy? *Sex Transm Dis*. 2012; 39:665-670.

CEFPROZIL

Antibacterial (Cephalosporin)

PREGNANCY RECOMMENDATION: No Human Data—Animal Data Suggest Low Risk

BREASTFEEDING RECOMMENDATION: Compatible

PREGNANCY SUMMARY

No reports describing the use of cefprozil in human pregnancy have been located. Numerous evaluations of other cephalosporin drugs have not found an increased risk for birth anomalies. The drug will probably cross the placenta, so some fetal exposure will likely occur. Therefore, the absence of human pregnancy experience prevents a complete assessment of the embryofetal risk. Animal studies did not find any embryofetal toxicity or malformations in three species. Using this drug during pregnancy should be based on the pros and cons of the mother's clinical need for treatment versus any potential fetal risk that might occur from exposure.

BREASTFEEDING SUMMARY

One study was located that evaluated cefprozil in nine lactating women. The milk concentrations following a 1-g oral dose ranged from 0.25 to 3.4 mcg/mL. This would result in a maximum RID of about 3.8%. In general, cephalosporin drugs are considered acceptable for use in nursing mothers. Breastfeeding while using this drug should be based on the mother's clinical need for treatment versus any potential infant risks that might occur. If used, the infant should be monitored for the most common reported adult side effects of nausea and pruritus (both leading to irritability), hypersensitivity reactions, diarrhea, vomiting, and rash.

References

1. Prescribing Information. *Cefprozil*. Aurobindo Pharma; 2021.
2. Shyu WC, Shah VR, Campbell DA, et al. Excretion of cefprozil into human breast milk. *Antimicrob Agents Chemother*. 1992;36:938-941.

CEFTAROLINE FOSAMIL

Antibacterial (Cephalosporin)

PREGNANCY RECOMMENDATION: No Human Data—Animal Data Suggest Low Risk

BREASTFEEDING RECOMMENDATION: Probably Compatible

PREGNANCY SUMMARY

No reports describing the use of ceftaroline fosamil in human pregnancy have been located. Numerous evaluations of other cephalosporin drugs have not found an increased risk for birth anomalies. The drug will probably cross the placenta, so some fetal exposure will likely occur. Therefore, the absence of human pregnancy experience prevents a complete assessment of the embryofetal risk. Animal studies did not show any embryofetal toxicity or malformations in two species. Using this drug during pregnancy should be based on the pros and cons of the mother's clinical need for treatment versus any potential fetal risk that might occur from exposure.

C

BREASTFEEDING SUMMARY

No reports describing the use of ceftaroline fosamil during human lactation have been located. Some of the drug will likely be excreted into breast milk. In general, cephalosporin drugs are considered acceptable for use in nursing mothers. Breastfeeding while using this drug should be based on the mother's clinical need for treatment versus any potential infant risks that might occur. If used, the infant should be monitored for the most common reported adult side effects of nausea and pruritus (both leading to irritability), hypersensitivity reactions, diarrhea, vomiting, and rash.

Reference

1. Prescribing Information. *Teflaro*. Allergan; 2021.

CEFTAZIDIME

Antibacterial (Cephalosporin)

PREGNANCY RECOMMENDATION: Limited Human Data—Animal Data Suggest Low Risk

BREASTFEEDING RECOMMENDATION: Compatible

PREGNANCY SUMMARY

There is limited human pregnancy data with ceftazidime. No detectable teratogenic risk with cephalosporin antibiotics was found in a large 2001 study (see Cephalexin). Cephalosporins are usually considered safe to use during pregnancy (see other cephalosporins for published human experience). The drug crosses the placenta at low levels, so some fetal exposure will occur. Therefore, this limited human pregnancy experience prevents a complete assessment of the embryofetal risk. Animal studies did not demonstrate any embryofetal toxicity or malformations in two species at doses of more than 10 times the RHD. Using this drug during pregnancy should be based on the pros and cons of the mother's clinical need for treatment versus any potential fetal risk that might occur from exposure.

BREASTFEEDING SUMMARY

Ceftazidime levels were evaluated in breast milk in 11 lactating women administered 2 g IV every 8 hours. The drug was detected in all samples with a mean level of 3.9 mcg/mL. The calculated RID was less than 1%. In general, cephalosporin drugs are considered acceptable for use in nursing mothers. Modification of bowel flora can occur when antibacterial drugs are ingested through breastfeeding. Breastfeeding while using this drug should be based on the mother's clinical need for treatment versus any potential infant risks that might occur. If used, the infant should be monitored for the most common reported adult side effects of nausea and pruritus (both leading to irritability), hypersensitivity reactions, diarrhea, vomiting, and rash.

References

1. Prescribing Information. *Ceftazidime*. Sagent Pharmaceuticals; 2020.
2. Cho N, Suzuki H, Mitsukawa M, et al. Fundamental and clinical evaluation of ceftazidime in the field of obstetrics and gynecology (English abstract). *Chemotherapy (Tokyo)*. 1983;31(suppl 3):772-782.
3. Giamarellou H, Gazis J, Petrikkos G, et al. A study of cefoxitin, moxalactam, and ceftazidime kinetics in pregnancy. *Am J Obstet Gynecol*. 1983;147:914-919.
4. Jørgensen NP, Walstad RA, Molne K. The concentrations of ceftazidime and thiopental in maternal plasma, placental tissue and amniotic fluid in early pregnancy. *Acta Obstet Gynecol Scand*. 1987;66:29-33.
5. Nathorst-Boos J, Philipson A, Hedman A, et al. Renal elimination of ceftazidime during pregnancy. *Am J Obstet Gynecol*. 1995;172:163-166.
6. Blanco JD, Jorgensen JH, Castaneda YS, et al. Ceftazidime levels in human breast milk. *Antimicrob Agents Chemother*. 1983;23:479-480.
7. American Academy of Pediatrics Committee on Drugs. The transfer of drugs and other chemicals into human milk. *Pediatrics*. 2001;108:776-789.

CEFTIBUTEN

Antibacterial (Cephalosporin)

PREGNANCY RECOMMENDATION: No Human Data—Animal Data Suggest Low Risk

BREASTFEEDING RECOMMENDATION: Probably Compatible

PREGNANCY SUMMARY

No reports describing the use of ceftibuten in the first trimester during human pregnancy have been located. Numerous evaluations of other cephalosporin drugs have not found an increased risk for birth anomalies. The drug will probably cross the placenta, so some fetal exposure will likely occur. Therefore, the absence of human pregnancy experience prevents a complete assessment of the embryofetal risk. One study reported the successful use of ceftibuten in treating urinary tract

(*continued*)

infections during pregnancy, but specific birth outcomes were not provided. Animal studies did not show any embryofetal toxicity or malformations in two species. Using this drug during pregnancy should be based on the pros and cons of the mother's clinical need for treatment versus any potential fetal risk that might occur from exposure.

C

BREASTFEEDING SUMMARY

One report was located that evaluated the use of ceftibuten in six lactating women. The drug was not identified in the breast milk from all six patients (the lower limits of detection for the test were 1 mcg/mL). However, some of the drug may be found in milk with a more sensitive test. In general, cephalosporin drugs are considered acceptable for use in nursing mothers. Breastfeeding while using this drug should be based on the mother's clinical need for treatment versus any potential infant risks that might occur. If used, the infant should be monitored for the most common reported adult side effects of nausea and pruritus (both leading to irritability), hypersensitivity reactions, diarrhea, vomiting, and rash.

References

1. Prescribing Information. *Cedax*. Pernix Therapeutics; 2018.
2. Krcmery S, Hromec J, Demesova D. Treatment of lower urinary tract infection in pregnancy. *Int J Antimicrob Agents*. 2001;17:279-282.
3. Barr WH, Lin C-C, Radwanski E, et al. The Pharmacokinetics of ceftibuten in humans. *Diagn Microbiol Infect Dis*. 1991;14:93-100.

CEFTOBIPROLE MEDOCARIL

Antibacterial (Cephalosporin)

PREGNANCY RECOMMENDATION: No Human Data—Animal Data Suggest Low Risk

BREASTFEEDING RECOMMENDATION: Probably Compatible

PREGNANCY SUMMARY

No reports describing the use of ceftobiprole medocaril in human pregnancy have been located. Available data from other cephalosporins used during pregnancy, over several decades, have not established a drug-associated risk for major birth anomalies, spontaneous abortion, or other adverse fetal outcomes. The drug will likely cross the placenta, so some fetal exposure will probably occur. Therefore, the absence of human pregnancy experience prevents a complete assessment of the embryofetal risk. Animal studies did not show any embryofetal toxicity in two species at doses of less than 10 times the RHD. Using this drug during pregnancy should be based on the pros and cons of the mother's clinical need for treatment versus any potential fetal risk that might occur from exposure.

BREASTFEEDING SUMMARY

No reports describing the use of ceftobiprole medocaril during human lactation have been located. The drug will likely be found in breast milk, so some infant exposure will probably occur. The cephalosporin class of drugs is considered safe for use while breastfeeding, though there is always a risk for disrupting the infant's gastrointestinal flora, leading to thrush or diarrhea. Breastfeeding while using this drug should be based on the mother's clinical need for treatment versus any potential infant risk that might occur. If used, the infant should be monitored for the most common reported side effects of nausea and headache (both leading to irritability), vomiting, rash, and diarrhea.

Reference

1. Prescribing Information. *Zevtera*. Basilea Pharmaceuticals International; 2024.

CEFTRIAXONE

Antibacterial (Cephalosporin)

PREGNANCY RECOMMENDATION: Limited Human Data—Animal Data Suggest Low Risk

BREASTFEEDING RECOMMENDATION: Compatible

PREGNANCY SUMMARY

In a surveillance study of Michigan Medicaid recipients, 60 newborns were exposed to ceftriaxone during the first trimester. Four (6.7%) major birth defects were observed. Of these, three cardiovascular defects (one expected) were noted. This has not been seen with any other cephalosporin. No anomalies were observed in five other categories of defects (oral clefts, spina bifida, polydactyly, limb reduction defects, and hypospadias) for which specific data were available. A possible association between ceftriaxone and cardiovascular defects is suggested, but other factors, such as the mother's disease, concurrent drug use, and chance, may be involved. Several other studies using this drug in the second and third trimesters did not produce any adverse effects. Numerous evaluations of other cephalosporin drugs have not found an increased risk for birth anomalies (see Cephalexin). The drug will cross the placenta, so some fetal exposure will occur. Therefore, further analysis regarding safety is necessary. Animal studies did not demonstrate any embryofetal toxicity or malformations in three animal species (two at doses of >10 times the RHD and one species at doses <10 times the RHD). Using this drug during pregnancy should be based on the pros and cons of the mother's clinical need for treatment versus any potential fetal risk that might occur from exposure.

C

BREASTFEEDING SUMMARY

Ceftriaxone was evaluated in human breast milk in 20 lactating women who received a 1-g IV or intramuscular (IM) dose. The peak breast milk level was about 0.7 mcg/mL. The calculated RID was less than 1%. In general, cephalosporin drugs are considered acceptable for use in nursing mothers. Modification of bowel flora can occur when antibacterial drugs are ingested through breastfeeding. Breastfeeding while using this drug should be based on the mother's clinical need for treatment versus any potential infant risks that might occur. If used, the infant should be monitored for the most common reported adult side effects of nausea and pruritus (both leading to irritability), hypersensitivity reactions, diarrhea, vomiting, and rash.

References

1. Prescribing Information. *Ceftriaxone*. Sagent Pharmaceuticals; 2022.
2. Kafetzis DA, Brater DC, Fanourgakis JE, et al. Placental and breast-milk transfer of ceftriaxone (C). Presented at: 22nd Interscience Conference on Antimicrobial Agents in Chemotherapy; October 4–6, 1982; Miami, FL. Academic Press; 1983:155.
3. Kafetzis DA, Brater DC, Fanourgakis JE, et al. Ceftriaxone distribution between maternal blood and fetal blood and tissues at parturition and between blood and milk postpartum. *Antimicrob Agents Chemother*. 1983;23:870-873.
4. Cho N, Kunii K, Fukunago K, et al. Antimicrobial activity, pharmacokinetics and clinical studies of ceftriaxone in obstetrics and gynecology. Presented at: 13th International Congress on Chemotherapy; August 28 to September 2, 1983; Vienna, Austria. Excerpta Medica; 1984:100,64-66.
5. Graber H, Magyar T. Pharmacokinetics of ceftriaxone in pregnancy. *Am J Med*. 1984;77:117-118.
6. Bourget P, Fernandez H, Quinquis V, et al. Pharmacokinetics and protein binding of ceftriaxone during pregnancy. *Antimicrob Agents Chemother*. 1993; 37:54-59.
7. Sanchez-Ramos L, McAlpine KJ, Adair CD, et al. Pyelonephritis in pregnancy: once-a-day ceftriaxone versus multiple doses of cefazolin. *Am J Obstet Gynecol*. 1995;172:129-133.
8. Lang R, Shalit I, Segal J, et al. Maternal and fetal and tissue levels of ceftriaxone following preoperative prophylaxis in emergency cesarean section. *Chemotherapy*. 1993;39:77-81.
9. Cavenee MR, Farris JR, Spalding TR, et al. Treatment of gonorrhea in pregnancy. *Obstet Gynecol*. 1993;81:33-38.
10. Deger R, Ludmir J. Neisseria sicca endocarditis complicating pregnancy. A case report. *J Reprod Med*. 1992;37:473-475.
11. Wing DA, Hendershott CM, Debuque L, et al. Outpatient treatment of acute pyelonephritis in pregnancy afte4 24 weeks. *Obstet Gynecol*. 1999;94: 683-688.
12. Kaplan YC, Keskin-Arsian E, Acar S, et al. Teicoplanin use during breastfeeding. *Breastfeed Med*. 2017;12:124.
13. American Academy of Pediatrics Committee on Drugs. The transfer of drugs and other chemicals into human milk. *Pediatrics*. 2001;108:776-789.

CEFUROXIME

Antibacterial (Cephalosporin)

PREGNANCY RECOMMENDATION: Limited Human Data—Animal Data Suggest Low Risk

BREASTFEEDING RECOMMENDATION: Compatible

PREGNANCY SUMMARY

In a surveillance study of Michigan Medicaid recipients and data from three teratogen information services, a total of 240 first-trimester pregnancy exposures to ceftriaxone were located. Of these, there were six (2.5%) major anomalies identified, and no pattern to the defects was noted. The drug will cross the placenta, so some fetal exposure will occur. However, this limited human pregnancy experience still prevents a complete assessment of the embryofetal risk. A few other studies have reported the successful use of this drug in the second and third trimesters, with no serious adverse effects noted. Animal studies did not show any embryofetal toxicity or malformations in two species (at doses of <10 times the RHD in one species and at doses of >10 times the RHD in the other species). Cephalosporins are usually considered safe to use during pregnancy. Using this drug during pregnancy should be based on the pros and cons of the mother's clinical need for treatment versus any potential fetal risk that might occur from exposure.

BREASTFEEDING SUMMARY

Cefuroxime was evaluated in human breast milk in 18 lactating women who received doses that varied from 500 mg to 2,250 mg/d (some orally and some by IV or IM). The peak breast milk level obtained was 1.45 mcg/mL. All of the calculated RIDs were 2% or less. In general, cephalosporin drugs are considered acceptable for use in nursing mothers. Modification of bowel flora can occur when antibacterial drugs are ingested through breastfeeding. Breastfeeding while using this drug should be based on the mother's clinical need for treatment versus any potential infant risks that might occur. If used, the infant should be monitored for the most common reported adult side effects of nausea and pruritus (both leading to irritability), hypersensitivity reactions, diarrhea, vomiting, and rash.

C

References

1. Prescribing Information. *Cefuroxime Axetil*. Aurobindo Pharma; 2019.
2. Craft I, Mullinger BM, Kennedy MRK. Placental transfer of cefuroxime. *Br J Obstet Gynaecol*. 1981;88:141-145.
3. Bousfield P, Browning AK, Mullinger BM, et al. Cefuroxime: potential use in pregnant women at term. *Br J Obstet Gynaecol*. 1981;88:146-149.
4. Bergogne-Berezin E, Pierre J, Even P, et al. Study of penetration of cefuroxime into bronchial secretions and of its placental transfer. *Therapie*. 1980;35:677-684.
5. Tzingounis V, Makris N, Zolotas J, et al. Cefuroxime prophylaxis in caesarean section. *Pharmatherapeutica*. 1982;3:140-142.
6. Coppi G, Berti MA, Chehade A, Franchi I, Magro B. A study of the transplacental transfer of cefuroxime in humans. *Curr Ther Res*. 1982;32:712-716.
7. Bousefield PF. Use of cefuroxime in pregnant women at term. *Res Clin Forums*. 1984;6:53-58.
8. Holt DE, Fisk NM, Spencer JAD, de Louvlis J, Hurley R, Harvey D. Transplacental transfer of cefuroxime in uncomplicated pregnancies and those complicated by hydrops or changes in amniotic fluid volume. *Arch Dis Child*. 1993;68:54-57.
9. De Leeuw JW, Roumen FJ, Bouckaert PX, Cremers HM, Vree TB. Achievement of therapeutic concentrations of cefuroxime in early preterm gestations with premature rupture of the membranes. *Obstet Gynecol*. 1993;81:255-260.
10. Berkovitch M, Segal-Socher I, Greenberg R, et al. First trimester exposure to cefuroxime: a prospective cohort study. *Br J Clin Pharmacol*. 2000;50:161-165.
11. Faro S, Pastorek JG II, Plauche WC, Korndorffer FA, Aldridge KE. Short-course parenteral antibiotic therapy for pyelonephritis in pregnancy. *South Med J*. 1984;77:455-457.
12. Benyamini L, Merlob P, Stahl B, et al. The safety of amoxicillin/clavulanic acid and cefuroxime during lactation. *Ther Drug Monit*. 2005;27:499-502.

CELECOXIB

Pain (Nonsteroidal Anti-inflammatory Drug)

PREGNANCY RECOMMENDATION: Human Data Suggest Risk (Second Half of Gestation)

BREASTFEEDING RECOMMENDATION: Probably Compatible

PREGNANCY SUMMARY

A population-based pregnancy registry (*n* = 36,387) was developed by linking three databases in Quebec. There were 93 infants (8.8%) with any congenital defect in 1,056 mothers who had filled prescriptions for nonsteroidal anti-inflammatory drugs (NSAIDs) in the first trimester. In the controls, there were 2,478 infants (7%) with any anomaly in 35,331 mothers who had not filled such a prescription. The adjusted odds ratio (OR) was 2.21 (95% confidence interval [CI] 1.72-2.85). However, about 90 of these exposures were associated to celecoxib and no significant difference was seen. In a study involving the Danish birth registry, 46 (4.2%) total congenital anomalies were seen in 1,106 pregnancies with probable NSAID usage compared with 564 (3.3%) anomalies in 17,259 control pregnancies. This rate was not significantly different. Specific data on the type of NSAID was not provided. This study also did not show any increased risks for low birth weight or preterm delivery. There was a higher risk for spontaneous abortion, but the reported rates were only 1.4% in the NSAID group and 1.1% in the control group. The drug will probably cross the placenta, so fetal exposure will likely occur. Animal studies did show embryofetal toxicity and/or malformations in two species at doses of less than 10 times the RHD. In addition, NSAIDs can cause premature stricture or closure of the fetal ductus arteriosus when used in the latter portion of gestation. In some instances, this can produce pulmonary hypertension in the neonate. These drugs have also been reported to produce fetal renal dysfunction leading to oligohydramnios when used after 20 weeks' gestation (see Indomethacin). Therefore, if possible, use between 20 and 30 weeks' gestation should be limited, and if possible, no usage after 30 weeks' gestation. If used more than a few days continuously after 20 weeks' gestation, an ultrasound to evaluate amniotic fluid volume is suggested. If celecoxib is used in pregnancy for the treatment of rheumatoid arthritis, health care professionals are encouraged to call the toll-free number (877-311-8972) for information about patient enrollment in the Organization of Teratology Information Specialists (OTIS) Rheumatoid Arthritis study.

BREASTFEEDING SUMMARY

Celecoxib has been shown to be excreted into human breast milk in a few studies. In three studies, a total of 12 mothers received daily doses of 200 mg, and the highest breast milk level obtained was 330 ng/mL. Breast milk levels overall ranged from undetectable to 330 ng/mL. The calculated RIDs in these studies were 1.4%, 0.3%, and 0.23%. Plasma concentrations of celecoxib (maternal dose of 200 mg/d) were below the limit of detection (10 ng/mL) in two infants. Breastfeeding while using this drug should be based on the mother's clinical need for treatment versus any potential infant risks that might occur. If used, the infant should be monitored for the most common reported adult side effects of nausea, headache, and abdominal pain (all leading to irritability), diarrhea, vomiting, and rash.

C

References

1. Tassinari MS, Cook JC, Hunt ME. NSAIDs and development toxicity. *Birth Defects Res (Part B)*. 2003;68:3-4.
2. Levin DL. Effects of inhibition of prostaglandin synthesis on fetal development, oxygenation, and the fetal circulation. *Semin Perinatol*. 1980;4:35-44.
3. Van Marter LJ, Leviton A, Allred EN, et al. Persistent pulmonary hypertension of the newborn and smoking and aspirin and nonsteroidal antiinflammatory drug consumption during pregnancy. *Pediatrics*. 1996;97:658-663.
4. Fuchs F. Prevention of prematurity. *Am J Obstet Gynecol*. 1976;126:809-820.
5. Powell JG, Cochrane RL. The effects of a number of non-steroidal anti-inflammatory compounds on parturition in the rat. *Prostaglandins*. 1982;23:469-488.
6. Matt DW, Borzelleca JF. Toxic effects on the female reproductive system during pregnancy, parturition, and lactation. In: Witorsch RJ, ed. *Reproductive Toxicology*. 2nd ed. Raven Press; 1995:175-193.
7. Dawood MY. Nonsteroidal antiinflammatory drugs and reproduction. *Am J Obstet Gynecol*. 1993;169:1255-1265.
8. Product information. *Celebrex*. G.D. Searle LLC Division of Pfizer; 2021.
9. Hausman N, Beharry KD, Nishihara KC, et al. Effect of the antenatal administration of celecoxib during the second and third trimesters of pregnancy on prostaglandin, cytokine, and nitric oxide levels in rabbits. *Am J Obstet Gynecol*. 2003;189:1737-1743.
10. Hausman N, Beharry K, Nishihara K, et al. Response of fetal prostanoids, nitric oxide, and ductus arteriosus to the short-and long-term antenatal administration of celecoxib, a selective cyclo-oxygenase-2 inhibitor, in the pregnant rabbit. *Am J Obstet Gynecol*. 2003;189:1744-1750.
11. Nielsen GL, Sorensen HT, Larsen H, et al. Risk of adverse birth outcome and miscarriage in pregnant users of non-steroidal anti-inflammatory drugs: population based observational study and case-control study. *Br Med J*. 2001;322:266-270.
12. Ericson A, Kallen BAJ. Nonsteroidal anti-inflammatory drugs in early pregnancy. *Reprod Toxicol*. 2001;15:371-373.
13. Li DK, Liu L, Odouli R. Exposure to non-steroidal anti-inflammatory drugs during pregnancy and risk of miscarriage: population based cohort study. *Br Med J*. 2003;327:368-371.
14. Ofori B, Oraichi D, Blais L, et al. Risk of congenital anomalies in pregnant users of non-steroidal anti-inflammatory drugs: a nested case-control study. *Birth Defects Res (Part B)*. 2006;77:268-279.
15. Slattery MM, Friel AM, Healy DG, et al. Uterine relaxant effects of cyclooxygenase-2 inhibitors in vitro. *Obstet Gynecol*. 2001;98:563-569.
16. Stika CS, Gross GA, Leguizamon G, et al. A prospective randomized safety trial of celecoxib for treatment of preterm labor. *Am J Obstet Gynecol*. 2002;187:653-660.
17. Borna S, Saeidi FM. Celecoxib versus magnesium sulfate to arrest preterm labor: randomized trial. *J Obstet Gynaecol Res*. 2007;33:631-634.
18. Nakhai-Pour HR, Broy P, Sheehy O, et al. Use of nonaspirin nonsteroidal anti-inflammatory drugs during pregnancy and the risk of spontaneous abortion. *CMAJ*. 2011;183:1713-1720.
19. Knoppert DC, Stempak D, Baruchel S, et al. Celecoxib in human milk: a case report. *Pharmacotherapy*. 2003;23:97-100.
20. Hale TW, McDonald R, Boger J. Transfer of celecoxib into human milk. *J Hum Lact*. 2004;20:397-403.
21. Gardiner SJ, Doogue MP, Zhang M, et al. Quantification of infant exposure to celecoxib through breast milk. *Br J Clin Pharmacol*. 2005;61:101-104.

CEMIPLIMAB

Antineoplastic (Monoclonal Antibody—PD-1 Receptor Blocker)

PREGNANCY RECOMMENDATION: No Human Data—Animal Data Suggest Potential Risk

BREASTFEEDING RECOMMENDATION: Potential Toxicity

PREGNANCY SUMMARY

No reports describing the use of cemiplimab in human pregnancy have been located. As an IgG antibody, it likely crosses the placenta, especially during the second half of gestation, so some fetal exposure will probably occur. Therefore, the absence of human pregnancy experience prevents a complete assessment of the embryofetal risk. Animal reproduction studies have not been conducted. However, in a murine model, blockage of the programmed cell death protein 1 (PD-1) receptor led to an increase in fetal loss. Based on the mechanism of action of cemiplimab, the manufacturer recommends that women with reproductive potential use effective contraception during treatment and for 4 months after the last dose. Nevertheless, using this drug during pregnancy should be based on the pros and cons of the mother's clinical need for treatment versus any potential fetal risk that might occur from exposure. There is a registry for women who are pregnant and have cancer. For more information, women and health care providers are encouraged to contact the Cancer and Pregnancy Registry at 1-877-635-4499.

BREASTFEEDING SUMMARY

No reports describing the use of cemiplimab during human lactation have been located. It is known that IgG antibodies can be found in human breast milk but are not found in the neonatal or infant circulation. Additionally, if any IgG antibodies were to be ingested through breastfeeding, they would probably be digested in the infant's gastrointestinal tract and not be absorbed. However, due to a concern for potential serious adverse effects that might be seen in a breastfed infant, the manufacturer recommends that women not breastfeed while being treated with this drug and for at least 4 months after the last dose. Nevertheless, breastfeeding while using this drug should be based on the mother's clinical need for treatment versus any potential infant risks that might occur. If used, the infant should be monitored for the most common reported adult side effects of nausea, musculoskeletal pain, and peripheral neuropathy (all leading to irritability), diarrhea, fatigue (lethargy), alopecia, vomiting, decreased appetite, and rash.

Reference

1. Prescribing Information. *Libtayo*. Regeneron Pharmaceuticals; 2023.

C

CENEGERMIN OPTHALMIC

Ophthalmic (Topical—Human Nerve Growth Factor)

PREGNANCY RECOMMENDATION: No Human Data and No Relevant Animal Data

BREASTFEEDING RECOMMENDATION: Probably Compatible

PREGNANCY SUMMARY

No reports describing the use of cenegermin in human pregnancy have been located. The drug may cross the placenta in the second half of gestation; however, because of the topical ocular use of the drug and negligible blood levels seen following systemic absorption, the amount of drug would likely be clinically insignificant. Animal studies did show some embryofetal toxicity with malformations but at doses above 200 times the maximum recommended human ophthalmic dose (MRHOD). Using this drug during pregnancy should be based on the pros and cons of the mother's clinical need for treatment versus any potential fetal risk that might occur from exposure. If used during pregnancy, consider placing pressure over the tear duct in the corner of the eye for at least 1 minute, and then remove any excess solution with absorbent tissue to decrease the amount of drug reaching the systemic circulation even further.

BREASTFEEDING SUMMARY

No reports describing the use of cenegermin in human lactation have been located. Due to negligible systemic absorption following topical ocular use, any breast milk levels would likely be clinically insignificant. Furthermore, because the drug is a protein, if any were to be ingested through breastfeeding, it would probably be digested in the infant's gastrointestinal tract and not be absorbed. Breastfeeding while using this drug should be based on the mother's clinical need for treatment versus any potential infant risks that might occur. Because of negligible plasma absorption, systemic side effects were not reported. A method to decrease some systemic absorption with ophthalmic use is described above in the Pregnancy Summary.

Reference

1. Prescribing Information. *Oxervate*. Dompe Farmaceeutici; 2019.

CENOBAMATE

Mental Health (Antiseizure)

PREGNANCY RECOMMENDATION: No Human Data—Animal Data Suggest Low Risk

BREASTFEEDING RECOMMENDATION: Probably Compatible

PREGNANCY SUMMARY

No reports describing the use of cenobamate in human pregnancy have been located. The drug probably crosses the placenta, so some fetal exposure will likely occur. Therefore, the absence of human pregnancy experience prevents a complete assessment of the embryofetal risk. Animal studies did not show any embryofetal toxicity when administered at doses that did not produce maternal toxicity. The drug is a controlled substance (Schedule V) and has risks for misuse when used for nonmedical reasons. Drug dependence can also occur, leading to withdrawal symptoms of insomnia, decreased appetite, decreased mood, and amnesia. Cenobamate has been shown to shorten the cardiac QT interval. There is a pregnancy exposure registry that monitors pregnancy outcomes in women exposed to antiepileptic drugs. Health care providers are encouraged to call the North American Antiepileptic Drug Pregnancy Registry by calling 1-888-233-2334.

BREASTFEEDING SUMMARY

Cenobamate probably enters breast milk. Breastfeeding while using this drug should be based on the mother's clinical need for treatment. If used, the infant should be monitored for the most common reported adult side effects of nausea and headache (both leading to irritability), sedation, and constipation.

Reference

1. Prescribing Information. *Xcopri*. SK Life Science, Inc; 2019.

C

CENTRUROIDES IMMUNE F(AB')$_2$ (EQUINE)

Antidote (Scorpion)

PREGNANCY RECOMMENDATION: No Human Data and No Relevant Animal Data/Maternal Benefit May Outweigh Any Embryofetal Risk

BREASTFEEDING RECOMMENDATION: Probably Compatible

PREGNANCY SUMMARY

No reports describing the use of *Centruroides* antivenom in human pregnancy have been located. Because the antivenom does not contain the Fc portion of the equine immune globulins, transplacental transfer should be negligible. However, the absence of human pregnancy experience prevents a complete assessment of the embryofetal risk. Animal reproduction studies have not been conducted. The maternal benefit probably outweighs any unknown embryofetal risk, so if indicated, the antivenom should not be withheld because of pregnancy.

BREASTFEEDING SUMMARY

No reports describing the use of *Centruroides* antivenom during human lactation have been located. The high MWs of these immune fragments suggest that they will not be excreted into breast milk. However, it is known that antibodies can be found in human breast milk but are not found in the neonatal or infant circulation. Additionally, if any of these immunoglobulin fragments were to be ingested through breastfeeding, they would probably be digested in the infant's gastrointestinal tract and not be absorbed. Breastfeeding while using this drug should be based on the mother's clinical need for treatment versus any potential infant risks that might occur. Use of the antivenom should not be withheld if clinically needed in a lactating woman.

Reference

1. Prescribing Information. *Anascorp*. Rare Disease Therapeutics; 2022.

CEPHALEXIN

Antibacterial (Cephalosporin)

PREGNANCY RECOMMENDATION: Human Data Suggest Potential Risk—Animal Data Suggest Low Risk

BREASTFEEDING RECOMMENDATION: Compatible

PREGNANCY SUMMARY

In a surveillance study of Michigan Medicaid recipients, 3,613 newborns were exposed to cephalexin during the first trimester, and 176 (4.9%) major birth defects were observed (145 expected). The data for total defects, cardiovascular, and oral clefts were suggestive of an association between cephalexin and congenital anomalies, but no pattern was seen, and other factors, such as the mother's disease, may be involved. Opposing data for this finding were seen in a Hungarian case-control surveillance study of congenital abnormalities that examined the association between cephalosporins (cephalexin, cefaclor, cefamandole, cefoperazone, cefotaxime, ceftibuten, and cefuroxime) and birth defects. Cases were drawn from 22,865 pregnant women who had fetuses or newborn infants with congenital abnormalities. Matched controls were obtained from pregnant women who had infants without defects. Most of the case women were treated with cephalexin. No detectable teratogenic risk was found. Evaluations of other cephalosporin drugs have not found an increased risk for birth anomalies. The drug crosses the placenta, so some fetal exposure will likely occur. Therefore, further analysis regarding safety is necessary. Animal studies did not demonstrate any embryofetal toxicity or malformations in two animal species at doses of less than 10 times the RHD. Although some data suggest an association with congenital malformations, cephalosporins are usually considered safe to use during pregnancy. Using this drug during pregnancy should be based on the pros and cons of the mother's clinical need for treatment versus any potential fetal risk that might occur from exposure.

BREASTFEEDING SUMMARY

Cephalexin was evaluated in human breast milk in nine lactating women who received doses that varied from 500 mg to 2,000 mg/d orally. The peak breast milk level obtained was 1 mcg/mL. All of the calculated RIDs were 1.5% or less. In general, cephalosporin drugs are considered acceptable for use in nursing mothers. Modification of bowel flora can occur when antibacterial drugs are ingested through breastfeeding. Breastfeeding while using this drug should be based on the mother's clinical need for treatment versus any potential infant risks that might occur. If used, the infant should be monitored for the most common reported adult side effects of nausea and pruritus (both leading to irritability), hypersensitivity reactions, diarrhea, vomiting, and rash.

C

References

1. Product information. *Keflex*. Pragma Pharmaceuticals; 2018.
2. Paterson ML, Henderson A, Lunan CB, et al. Transplacental transfer of cephalexin. *Clin Med*. 1972;79:22-24.
3. Creatsas G, Pavlatos M, Lolis D, et al. A study of the kinetics of cephapirin and cephalexin in pregnancy. *Curr Med Res Opin*. 1980;7:43-46.
4. Hirsch HA. Behandlung von harnwegsinfektionen in gynakologic und geburtshilfe mit cephalexin. *Int J Clin Pharmacol*. 1969;2(suppl):121-123.
5. Brumfitt W, Pursell R. Double-blind trial to compare ampicillin, cephalexin, co-trimoxazole, and trimethoprim in treatment of urinary infection. *Br Med J*. 1972;2:673-676.
6. Mizuno S, Metsuda S, Mori S. Clinical evaluation of cephalexin in obstetrics and gynaecology. Presented at: Symposium on the Clinical Evaluation of Cephalexin, Royal Society of Medicine; June 2 and 3, 1969; London.
7. Guttman D. Cephalexin in urinary tract infections-preliminary results. Presented at: Symposium on the Clinical Evaluation of Cephalexin, Royal Society of Medicine; June 2 and 3, 1969; London.
8. Soto RF, Fesbre F, Cordido A, et al. Ensayo con cefalexina en el tratamiento de infecciones urinarias en pacientes embarazadas. *Rev Obstet Ginecol Venez*. 1972;32:637-641.
9. Campbell-Brown M, McFadyen IR. Bacteriuria in pregnancy treated with a single dose of cephalexin. *Br J Obstet Gynaecol*. 1983;90:1054-1059.
10. Jakobi P, Neiger R, Merzbach D, et al. Single-dose antimicrobial therapy in the treatment of asymptomatic bacteriuria in pregnancy. *Am J Obstet Gynecol*. 1987;156:1148-1152.
11. Pfau A, Sacks TG. Effective prophylaxis for recurrent urinary tract infections during pregnancy. *Clin Infect Dis*. 1992;14:810-814.
12. Wing DA, Hendershott CM, Debuque L, et al. Outpatient treatment of acute pyelonephritis in pregnancy afte4 24 weeks. *Obstet Gynecol*. 1999;94:683-688.
13. Czeizel AE, Rockenbauer M, Sorensen HT, et al. Use of cephalosporins during pregnancy and in the presence of congenital abnormalities: a population-based, case-control study. *Am J Obstet Gynecol*. 2001;184:1289-1296.
14. Kafetzis D, Siafas C, Georgakopoulos P, et al. Passage of cephalosporins and amoxicillin into the breast milk. *Acta Paediatr Scand*. 1981;70:285-288.
15. Ilett KF, Hackett LP, Ingle B, et al. Transfer of probenecid and cephalexin into breast milk. *Ann Pharmacother*. 2006;40:986-989.

CERITINIB

Antineoplastic (Tyrosine Kinase Inhibitor)

PREGNANCY RECOMMENDATION: Limited Human Data—Animal Data Suggest Risk

BREASTFEEDING RECOMMENDATION: Potential Toxicity

PREGNANCY SUMMARY

One case report was located of a patient diagnosed with metastatic non–small cell lung carcinoma prior to pregnancy. She was eventually started on ceritinib at about 31 weeks' gestation and delivered at 36 weeks' gestation, a healthy newborn, other than familial polydactyly. The drug will probably cross the placenta, so some fetal exposure will likely occur. Therefore, this limited human pregnancy experience prevents a complete assessment of the embryofetal risk. Animal studies did show some embryofetal toxicity with malformations in two species at doses less than 10 times the RHD. Therefore, based on these animal studies and the drug's mechanism of action, the manufacturer recommends that women with reproductive potential use effective contraception during treatment and for 6 months after the last dose. They also recommend that males with female partners of reproductive potential use effective contraception during treatment and for 3 months after the last dose. Nevertheless, using this drug during pregnancy should be based on the pros and cons of the mother's clinical need for treatment versus any potential fetal risk that might occur from exposure. In the clinical trials, the drug was found to produce hyperglycemia in 13% of the patients; therefore, glucose monitoring should occur if used during pregnancy. Use of this drug has also been associated with prolongation of the QT interval. There is a registry for women who are pregnant and have cancer. For more information, women and health care providers are encouraged to contact the Cancer and Pregnancy Registry at 1-877-635-4499.

BREASTFEEDING SUMMARY

No reports describing the use of ceritinib during human lactation have been located. The drug will likely appear in breast milk, so some infant exposure will probably occur. Due to a concern for potential serious adverse effects that might be seen in a breastfed infant, the manufacturer recommends that women not breastfeed while being treated with this drug and for at least 2 weeks after the last dose. Nevertheless, breastfeeding while using this drug should be based on the mother's clinical need for treatment versus any potential infant risks that might occur. If used, the infant should be monitored for the most common reported adult side effects of nausea and abdominal pain (both leading to irritability), diarrhea, fatigue (lethargy), vomiting, and decreased appetite.

References

1. Prescribing Information. *Zykadia*. Novartis Pharmaceuticals; 2021.
2. Boudy AS, Grausz N, Selleret L, et al. Use of tyrosine kinase inhibitors during pregnancy for oncogenic-driven advanced non-small cell lung carcinoma. *Lung Cancer*. 2021;161:68-75.

C

CERLIPONASE ALFA

Lysosomal Exopeptidase Enzyme

PREGNANCY RECOMMENDATION: No Human Data and No Relevant Animal Data

BREASTFEEDING RECOMMENDATION: Probably Compatible

PREGNANCY SUMMARY

No reports describing the use of cerliponase alfa in human pregnancy have been located. The drug most likely does not cross the placenta; therefore, fetal exposure is probably nonexistent or extremely limited. However, the absence of human pregnancy experience prevents a complete assessment of the embryofetal risk. Animal studies have not been performed.

BREASTFEEDING SUMMARY

No reports describing the use of cerliponase alfa during human lactation have been located. The drug most likely will not appear in breast milk. Furthermore, because it is an enzyme, if any drug were to be present in breast milk, it would most likely be digested in the infant's gastrointestinal tract and not be absorbed. Breastfeeding while using this drug should be based on the mother's clinical need for treatment. If used, the infant should be monitored for the most common reported adult side effects of headache (leading to irritability), pyrexia, and vomiting.

Reference

1. Prescribing Information. *Brineura*. BioMarin Pharmaceutical Inc; 2017.

CERTOLIZUMAB PEGOL

Immunologic (Immunomodulator)

PREGNANCY RECOMMENDATION: Limited Human Data Suggest Low Risk

BREASTFEEDING RECOMMENDATION: Probably Compatible

PREGNANCY SUMMARY

Several studies have been located that describe the use of certolizumab pegol during human pregnancy. The largest study involved a pharmacovigilance database that reported more than 500 exposures to the drug. From more than 450 live births, the congenital anomaly rate was only 1.7%. A few other studies with smaller numbers have also not shown an increased risk for birth defects. In 2011, the World Congress of Gastroenterology stated, "Certolizumab pegol in pregnancy is considered to be low risk and compatible with use during conception and pregnancy in women." The drug has been shown to cross the placenta in the third trimester at delivery in low levels. Therefore, some fetal exposure can occur. Animal reproduction studies using a rodent antimurine tumor necrosis factor alpha (TNFα) pegylated Fab' fragment, similar to certolizumab pegol, did not cause any embryofetal toxicity or malformations at doses of less than 10 times the RHD. Using this drug during pregnancy should be based on the pros and cons of the mother's clinical need for treatment versus any potential fetal risk that might occur from exposure. If certolizumab is used in pregnancy, health care professionals are encouraged to call the toll-free number 1-877-311-8972 for information about patient enrollment in the Organization of Teratology Information Specialists (OTIS) study and pregnancy registry.

BREASTFEEDING SUMMARY

Certolizumab pegol was evaluated in 34 lactating women. In 18 (53%) cases, the drug was not detected in several breast milk samples. Of the 16 cases that did have a breast milk sample positive for the drug, the highest level obtained was less than 1% of the maternal dose. In one of the studies, pegol was also analyzed in 137 milk samples, and none of the cases came back as positive. A total of 10 infants had blood levels analyzed for certolizumab pegol, and in 9 cases, the drug was not detected. In the tenth case, a positive blood level was found, but it was difficult to determine if this result was related to the presence of leftover transplacental transfer. It is known that IgG antibodies can be found in human breast milk, but are not found in the neonatal or infant circulation. Additionally, if any IgG antibodies or fragments were to be ingested through breastfeeding, they would probably be digested in the infant's gastrointestinal tract and not be absorbed. Breastfeeding while using this drug should be based on the mother's clinical need for treatment versus any potential infant risks that might occur. If used, the infant should be monitored for the most common reported adult side effects of infections and rash.

References

1. Mahadevan U, Cucchiara S, Hyams JS, et al. The London position statement of the World Congress of Gastroenterology on biological therapy for IBD with the European Crohn's and Colitis Organization: pregnancy and pediatrics. *Am J Gastroenterol*. 2011;106:214-223.

C

2. Khanna D, McMahon M, Furst DE. Safety of tumor necrosis factor-α antagonists. *Drug Saf.* 2004;27:307-324.
3. Gotestam Skorpen C, Hoeltzenbein M, Tincani A, et al. The EULAR points to consider for use of antirheumatic drugs before pregnancy, and during pregnancy and lactation. *Ann Rheum Dis.* 2016;75:795-810.
4. Product information. *Cimzia.* UCB; 2022.
5. Mahadevan U, Wolf DC, Dubinsky M, et al. Placental transfer of anti-tumor necrosis factor agents in pregnant patients with inflammatory bowel disease. *Clin Gastroenterol Hepatol.* 2013;11:286-292.
6. Marriette X, Forger F, Abraham B, et al. Lack of placental transfer of certolizumab pegol during pregnancy: results from CRIB, a prospective, postmarketing, pharmacokinetic study. *Ann Rheum Dis.* 2018;77:228-233.
7. Marchioni RM, Lichtenstein GR. Tumor necrosis factor-α inhibitor therapy and fetal risk: a systematic literature review. *World J Gastroenterol.* 2013;19:2591-2602.
8. Gisbert JP, Chaparro M. Safety of anti-TNF agents during pregnancy and breastfeeding in women with inflammatory bowel disease. *Am J Gastroenterol.* 2013;108:1426-1438.
9. Seirafi M, de Vroey B, Amiot A, et al. Factors associated with pregnancy outcome in anti-TNF treated women with inflammatory bowel disease. *Aliment Pharmacol Ther.* 2014;40:363-373.
10. Bazzani C, Scrivo R, Andreoli L, et al. Prospectively-followed pregnancies in patients with inflammatory arthritis taking biological drugs: an Italian multicenter study. *Clin Exp Rheumatol.* 2015;33:688-693.
11. Weber-Schoendorfer C, Oppermann M, Wacker E, et al. Pregnancy outcome after TNF-α inhibitor therapy during the first trimester: a prospective multicenter cohort study. *Br J Clin Pharmacol.* 2015;80:727-729.
12. Clowse MEB, Scheuerle AE, Chambers C, et al. Pregnancy outcomes after exposure to certolizumab pegol: updated results from a pharmacovigilance safety database. *Arthritis Rheumatol.* 2018;70:1399-1407. doi:10.1002/art.40508.
13. Wieringa JW, Driessen GJ, Van Der Woude CJ. Pregnant women with inflammatory bowel disease: the effects of biologicals on pregnancy, outcome of infants, and the developing immune system. *Expert Rev Gastroenterol Hepatol.* 2018;12:811-818.
14. Matro R, Martin CF, Wolf DC, et al. Detection of biologic agents in breast milk and implications for infection, growth, and development in infants born to women with inflammatory bowel disease: results from the PIANO registry (abstract). *Gastroenterology.* 2015;148:S141.
15. Clowse ME, Forger F, Hwang C, et al. Minimal to no transfer of certolizumab pegol into breast milk: results from CRADLE, a prospective, postmarketing, multicentre, pharmacokinetic study. *Ann Rheum Dis.* 2017;76:1890-1896.
16. Matro R, Martin CF, Wolf D, et al. Exposure concentrations of infants breastfed by women receiving biologic therapies for inflammatory bowel diseases and effects of breastfeeding on infections and development. *Gastroenterology.* 2018;155:696-704. doi:10.1053/j.gastro.2018.05.040

CETIRIZINE

Antihistamine (H_1 Receptor Antagonist)

PREGNANCY RECOMMENDATION: Limited Human Data—Animal Data Suggest Low Risk

BREASTFEEDING RECOMMENDATION: Compatible

PREGNANCY SUMMARY

Several studies have examined the use of cetirizine in human pregnancy. Of 230 first-trimester exposures, a total of 4 (1.7%) major anomalies were identified. No pattern to the defects was noted. The drug will probably cross the placenta, so some fetal exposure will likely occur. Cetirizine was not found to cause any embryofetal toxicity or malformations in three species at doses of more than 10 times the RHD. Although cetirizine appears unlikely to be a major human teratogen, an oral first-generation agent, such as chlorpheniramine or tripelennamine, should be considered if antihistamine therapy during pregnancy (especially in the first trimester) is required. Cetirizine is considered an acceptable alternative if a first-generation agent was not tolerated. Using this drug during pregnancy should be based on the pros and cons of the mother's clinical need for treatment versus any potential fetal risk that might occur from exposure.

BREASTFEEDING SUMMARY

A few studies have reported the use of cetirizine during human lactation. From a total of more than 270 lactating women, the drug was found in breast milk in low quantities, which is consistent with the MW. A few other studies have reported cetirizine use for effects on the infant, and overall, no adverse events related to the drug exposure were seen. However, as with any antihistamine, sedation is a possibility. Breastfeeding while using this drug should be based on the mother's clinical need for treatment versus any potential infant risks that might occur. If used, the infant should be monitored for the most common reported adult side effects of dizziness and abdominal pain (both leading to irritability), vomiting, fatigue (lethargy), and somnolence.

References

1. Mazzotta P, Loebstein R, Koren G. Treating allergic rhinitis in pregnancy: safety considerations. *Drug Saf.* 1999;20:361-375.
2. Horak F, Stubner UP. Comparative tolerability of second generation antihistamines. *Drug Saf.* 1999;20:385-401.
3. Position Statement of a Joint Committee of the American College of Obstetricians and Gynecologists and the American College of Allergy, Asthma and Immunology. The use of newer asthma and allergy medications during pregnancy. *Ann Allergy Asthma Immunol.* 2000;84:475-480.
4. Product information. *Zyrtec.* Johnson & Johnson Consumer, McNeil Consumer Health Care Division; 2018.
5. Einarson A, Bailey B, Jung G, et al. Prospective controlled study of hydroxyzine and cetirizine in pregnancy. *Ann Allergy Asthma Immunol.* 1997;78:183-186.
6. Schatz M, Petitti D. Antihistamines and pregnancy. *Ann Allergy Asthma Immunol.* 1997;78:157-159.
7. Wilton LV, Pearce GL, Martin RM, et al. The outcomes of pregnancy in women exposed to newly marketed drugs in general practice in England. *Br J Obstet Gynaecol.* 1998;105:882-889.
8. Einarson A, Levichek Z, Einarson TR, Koren G. The antiemetic effect of cetirizine during pregnancy. *Ann Pharmacother.* 2000;34:1486-1487.
9. Weber-Schoendorfer C, Schaefer C. The safety of cetirizine during pregnancy—a prospective observational cohort study. *Reprod Toxicol.* 2008;26:19-23.
10. Westermann L, Hugel R, Meier M, et al. Glucocorticosteroid-resistant pemphigoid gestationis: successful treatment with adjuvant immunoadsorption. *J Dermatol.* 2012;39:168-171.
11. Gashlin LZ, Sullo D, Lawrence RA, Rosen-Carole C. Treatment of narcolepsy with sodium oxybate while breastfeeding: a case report. *Breastfeed Med.* 2016;11:261-263.

C

CETIRIZINE OPHTHALMIC

Antihistamine (H_1 Receptor Antagonist)

PREGNANCY RECOMMENDATION: No Human Data—Animal Data Suggest Low Risk

BREASTFEEDING RECOMMENDATION: Probably Compatible

PREGNANCY SUMMARY

No studies have been located that have evaluated the use of cetirizine ophthalmic during human pregnancy. Several studies have examined the use of cetirizine in human pregnancy. Of 230 first-trimester exposures, a total of 4 (1.7%) major anomalies were identified. No pattern to the defects was noted. The drug will probably cross the placenta, so some fetal exposure will likely occur. Therefore, the absence of human pregnancy experience prevents a complete assessment of the embryofetal risk. Cetirizine was not found to cause any embryofetal toxicity or malformations in three species at doses of more than 10 times the RHD. Using this drug during pregnancy should be based on the pros and cons of the mother's clinical need for treatment versus any potential fetal risk that might occur from exposure. If used during pregnancy, consider placing pressure over the tear duct in the corner of the eye for at least 1 minute, and then remove any excess solution with absorbent tissue to decrease the amount of drug reaching the systemic circulation even further.

BREASTFEEDING SUMMARY

No studies have been located that describe the use of cetirizine ophthalmic during human lactation. Several studies have been performed that evaluated the use of oral cetirizine during breastfeeding. From a total of more than 270 lactating women, the drug was found in breast milk in low quantities, which is consistent with the MW. A few other studies have reported cetirizine use for effects on the infant, and overall, no adverse events related to the drug exposure were seen. However, with the low levels of systemic absorption found following ocular use, the amount of exposure to a breastfeeding infant with ophthalmic use is likely to be clinically insignificant. Breastfeeding while using this drug should be based on the mother's clinical need for treatment versus any potential infant risks that might occur. A method to decrease some systemic absorption with ophthalmic use is described above in the Pregnancy Summary.

Reference

1. Prescribing Information. *Zerviate*. Eyevance Pharmaceuticals, LLC; 2020.

CETUXIMAB

Antineoplastic (Monoclonal Antibody—EGFR Antagonist)

PREGNANCY RECOMMENDATION: No Human Data—Animal Data Suggest Risk

BREASTFEEDING RECOMMENDATION: Probably Compatible

PREGNANCY SUMMARY

No reports describing the use of cetuximab in human pregnancy have been located. As an IgG antibody, it likely crosses the placenta, especially during the second half of pregnancy, so some fetal exposure will probably occur. Therefore, the absence of human pregnancy experience prevents a complete assessment of the embryofetal risk. Animal studies did show some embryofetal toxicity in one species at doses less than 10 times the RHD. In addition, in the mouse model, EGFR is critically important in the reproductive process involving implantation, placental development, and embryofetal survival. Therefore, blockage of this receptor may increase the risk for fetal loss and poor pregnancy outcome. Based on the drug's mechanism of action, the manufacturer recommends that women with reproductive potential use effective contraception during treatment and for 2 months after the last dose. Nevertheless, using this drug during pregnancy should be based on the pros and cons of the mother's clinical need for treatment versus any potential fetal risk that might occur from exposure. There is a registry for women who are pregnant and have cancer. For more information, women and health care providers are encouraged to contact the Cancer and Pregnancy Registry at 1-877-635-4499.

BREASTFEEDING SUMMARY

No reports describing the use of cetuximab during lactation have been located. It is known that IgG antibodies can be found in human breast milk, but are not found in the neonatal or infant circulation. Additionally, if any IgG antibodies were to be ingested through breastfeeding, they would probably be digested in the infant's gastrointestinal tract and not be absorbed. However, due to a concern for potential serious adverse effects that might be seen in a breastfed infant, the manufacturer recommends that women not breastfeed while being treated with this drug and for at least 2 months after the last dose. Nevertheless, breastfeeding while using this drug should be based on the mother's clinical need for treatment versus any potential infant risks that might occur. If used, the infant should be monitored for the most common reported adult side effects of headache and pruritus (both leading to irritability), diarrhea, rash, and infections.

Reference

1. Prescribing Information. *Erbitux*. ImClone; 2019.

CEVIMELINE

Autonomic (Cholinergic)

PREGNANCY RECOMMENDATION: No Human Data and No Relevant Animal Data

BREASTFEEDING RECOMMENDATION: Probably Compatible

PREGNANCY SUMMARY

No reports describing the use of cevimeline in human pregnancy have been located. The drug will probably cross the placenta, so some fetal exposure will likely occur. Therefore, the absence of human pregnancy experience prevents a complete assessment of the embryofetal risk. Animal studies did show some embryofetal toxicity in one species at a dose less than 10 times the MRHD, but this dose also caused maternal toxicity. Using this drug during pregnancy should be based on the pros and cons of the mother's clinical need for treatment versus any potential fetal risk that might occur from exposure.

BREASTFEEDING SUMMARY

No reports describing the use of cevimeline during human lactation have been located. The drug will probably be found in breast milk, so some infant exposure will likely occur. Breastfeeding while using this drug should be based on the mother's clinical need for treatment versus any potential infant risks that might occur. If used, the infant should be monitored for the most common reported adult side effects of nausea, abdominal pain, headache, and dizziness (all leading to irritability), diarrhea, vomiting, and rash.

Reference

1. Prescribing Information. *Cevimeline*. Sun Pharmaceutical Industries; 2019.

CHENODIOL

Gastrointestinal (Gallstone Dissolution Agent)

PREGNANCY RECOMMENDATION: *Contraindicated

BREASTFEEDING RECOMMENDATION: *Contraindicated

PREGNANCY SUMMARY

No reports on the use of chenodiol during human pregnancy have been located. The drug will probably cross the placenta, so some fetal exposure will likely occur. Therefore, the absence of human pregnancy experience prevents a complete assessment of the embryofetal risk. Animal studies did show some embryofetal toxicity in two species at doses of less than 10 times the RHD. The drug has a potential for hepatotoxicity and also a poor response rate in some patients. Therefore, the manufacturer states that the drug is contraindicated for use during pregnancy. *Based on the approved use for the drug in patients who are poor surgical candidates because of disease and age, the use of the drug during pregnancy is very limited.

BREASTFEEDING SUMMARY

No reports describing the use of chenodiol during human lactation have been located. The drug will probably be found in breast milk, so some infant exposure will likely occur. *Based on the approved use for the drug in patients who are poor surgical candidates because of disease and age, using the drug during breastfeeding is very limited. If used, the infant should be monitored for the most common reported adult side effects of nausea and abdominal pain (both leading to irritability), diarrhea, and vomiting.

References

1. Product information. *Chenodiol*. LGM Pharma Solutions, LLC; 2022.
2. Kitao T, Kamishita S, Yoshikawa H, Sakaguchi M. Teratogenicity studies of chenodeoxycholic acid in rats. *Yakuri to Chiryo*. 1982;10:3887-3901. As cited in Shepard TH. *Catalog of Teratogenic Agents*. 6th ed. Johns Hopkins University Press; 1989:127.
3. Takahashi H, Miyashita T, Tozuka K. Effects of chenodeoxycholic acid, administered in the organogenetic period, on the pre-and post-natal development of rat's and mouse's offsprings. *Oyo Yakuri (Pharmacometrics)*. 1978;15:1047-1055.
4. McSherry CK, Morrissey KP, Swarm RL, et al. Chenodeoxycholic acid induced liver injury in pregnant and neonatal baboons. *Ann Surg*. 1976;184:490-499.

5. Celle G, Cavanna M, Bocchini R, Robbiano L. Chenodeoxycholic acid (CDCA) versus ursodeoxycholic acid (UDCA): a comparison of their effects in pregnant rats. *Arch Int Pharmacodyn Ther*. 1980;246:149-158.
6. Sprinkle DJ, Hassan AS, Subbiah MTR. Effect of chenodeoxycholic acid feeding during gestation in the rat on bile acid metabolism and liver morphology. *Proc Soc Exp Biol Med*. 1984;175:386-397.
7. Heywood R, Palmer AK, Foll CV, Lee MR. Pathological changes in fetal rhesus monkey induced by oral chenodeoxycholic acid. *Lancet*. 1973;2:1021.
8. Allan RN, Thistle JL, Hofmann AF, Carter JA. Lithocholate metabolism during chemotherapy for gallstone dissolution. 1. Serum levels of sulphated and unsulphated lithocholates. *Gut*. 1976;17:405-412.

CHLORAL HYDRATE

Central Nervous System (Sedative/Hypnotic)

PREGNANCY RECOMMENDATION: Limited Human Data—No Relevant Animal Data

BREASTFEEDING RECOMMENDATION: Potential Toxicity

PREGNANCY SUMMARY

The Collaborative Perinatal Project reported 71 first-trimester exposures to chloral hydrate, with 7 (9.9%) identified major birth anomalies. For anytime use during pregnancy, there were 9 (2.5%) major anomalies seen in 358 exposures. No pattern to the congenital defects was identified. The drug crosses the placenta, so fetal exposure will occur. However, this limited human pregnancy experience prevents a complete assessment of the embryofetal risk. Animal reproduction studies have not been located. Using this drug during pregnancy should be based on the pros and cons of the mother's clinical need for treatment versus any potential fetal risk that might occur from exposure. The drug carries a risk for misuse, dependence, and withdrawal. It is classified as a Schedule IV drug.

BREASTFEEDING SUMMARY

Chloral hydrate and the active metabolite (trichloroethanol) have both been found in human breast milk. One study analyzed 50 lactating women who received a rectal dose of 1.3 g of chloral hydrate. The peak breast milk levels for the drug were about 10 mcg/mL, and for the metabolite were about 40 mcg/mL (both within the first hour after use). The calculated RID using the peak level for chloral hydrate was about 8%. However, the calculated RID for trichloroethanol could be as high as 30%. Based on these values, the drug should be used with caution in a breastfeeding infant, especially due to the longer half-life of the active metabolite. Breastfeeding while using this drug should be based on the mother's clinical need for treatment versus any potential infant risks that might occur. If used, the infant should be monitored for the most common reported adult side effects of nausea, headache, and abdominal pain (all leading to irritability), diarrhea, vomiting, somnolence, and sedation.

References

1. Product information. *Chloralum*. Remedy Makers; 2011.
2. Bernstine JB, Meyer AE, Hayman HB. Maternal and fetal blood estimation following the administration of chloral hydrate during labor. *J Obstet Gynecol Br Emp*. 1954;61:683-685.
3. Heinonen OP, Slone D, Shapiro S. *Birth Defects and Drugs in Pregnancy*. Publishing Sciences Group; 1977.
4. Bernstine JB, Meyer AE, Bernstine RL. Maternal blood and breast milk estimation following the administration of chloral hydrate during the puerperium. *J Obstet Gynecol Br Emp*. 1956;63:228-231.
5. Lacey JH. Dichloralphenazone and breast milk. *Br Med J*. 1971;4:684.
6. American Academy of Pediatrics Committee on Drugs. The transfer of drugs and other chemicals into human milk. *Pediatrics*. 2001;108:776-789.

CHLORAMPHENICOL

Antibacterial

PREGNANCY RECOMMENDATION: Limited Human Data—No Relevant Animal Data

BREASTFEEDING RECOMMENDATION: Potential Toxicity

PREGNANCY SUMMARY

The Collaborative Perinatal Project reported 98 first-trimester exposures to chloramphenicol with 5 (5.1%) major anomalies described. There were 348 exposures anytime during gestation, with 8 (2.3%) major birth defects identified. There was no pattern to the anomalies noted. A few other cases have reported the use of chloramphenicol during the first trimester with no increased risk identified for congenital anomalies. Several studies have also reported the use of chloramphenicol in the

(*continued*)

C

second and third trimesters of pregnancy with no identified major adverse newborn effects noted. The drug crosses the placenta, so fetal exposure will occur. Therefore, this limited human pregnancy experience prevents a complete assessment of the embryofetal risk. Animal reproduction studies have not been located. Using this drug during pregnancy should be based on the pros and cons of the mother's clinical need for treatment versus any potential fetal risk that might occur from exposure. There is also a potential risk for gray baby syndrome (see Breastfeeding Summary).

BREASTFEEDING SUMMARY

Chloramphenicol has been studied during human lactation. A total of 21 women were administered doses ranging from 500 to 2,000 mg. The highest peak level recorded was about 6.1 mcg/mL. Several RIDs were calculated, and all were about 3%. None were above 10%. "Gray baby syndrome" is a disorder seen in newborns (especially premature) that can be fatal. The cases seem to occur with high newborn blood levels of the drug. Symptoms start with abdominal distension, followed by pallid cyanosis, then vasomotor collapse with decreased respirations leading to death. Most occur with the use of the drug shortly after birth. It does not appear that this disorder could occur with the amount of drug exposure that might occur through breastfeeding. However, if the clinical decision is to use this drug while breastfeeding, the infant should be monitored for these symptoms along with nausea (leading to irritability), vomiting, rash, and blood dyscrasias.

References

1. Oberheuser F. Praktische Erfahrungen mit Medikamenten in der Schwangerschaft. *Therapiewoche*. 1971;31:2200. As reported in Manten A. Antibiotic drugs. In: Dukes MNG, ed. *Meyler's Side Effects of Drugs*: Volume VIII. American Elsevier; 1975:604.
2. Sutherland JM. Fatal cardiovascular collapse of infants receiving large amounts of chloramphenicol. *AMA J Dis Child*. 1959;97:761-767.
3. Weiss CV, Glazko AJ, Weston JK. Chloramphenicol in the newborn infant. A physiologic explanation of its toxicity when given in excessive doses. *N Engl J Med*. 1960;262:787-794.
4. Schwarz RH, Crombleholme WR. Antibiotics in pregnancy. *South Med J*. 1979;72:1315-1318.
5. Product information. *Chloramphenicol Sodium Succinate*. Fresenius Kabi USA; 2019.
6. Scott WC, Warner RF. Placental transfer of chloramphenicol (Chloromycetin). *JAMA*. 1950;142:1331-1332.
7. Ross S, Burke RG, Sites J, et al. Placental transmission of chloramphenicol (Chloromycetin). *JAMA*. 1950;142:1361.
8. Heinonen OP, Slone D, Shapiro S. *Birth Defects and Drugs in Pregnancy*. Publishing Sciences Group; 1977.
9. Schiffman P, Samet CM, Fox L, et al. Typhoid fever in pregnancy-with probable typhoid hepatitis. *NY State J Med*. 1977;77:1778-1779.
10. Cunningham FG, Morris GB, Mickal A. Acute pyelonephritis of pregnancy: a clinical review. *Obstet Gynecol*. 1973;42:112-117.
11. Ravid R, Roaff R. On the possible teratogenicity of antibiotic drugs administered during pregnancy. In: Klingberg MA, Abramovici H, Chemke J, eds. *Drugs and Fetal Development*. Plenum Press; 1972:505-510.
12. Markley KC, Levine AB, Chan Y. Rocky Mountain spotted fever in pregnancy. *Obstet Gynecol*. 1998;91:860.
13. Smadel JE, Woodward TE, Ley HL Jr, Lewthwaite R. Chloramphenicol (Chloromycetin) in the treatment of Tsutsugamushi disease (scrub typhus). *J Clin Invest*. 1949;28:1196-1215.
14. Prochazka J, Havelka J, Hejzlar M. Excretion of chloramphenicol by human milk. *Cas Lek Cesk*. 1964;103:378-380.
15. Havelka J, Hejzlar M, Popov V, et al. Excretion of chloramphenicol in human milk. *Chemotherapy*. 1968;13:204-211.
16. American Academy of Pediatrics Committee on Drugs. The transfer of drugs and other chemicals into human milk. *Pediatrics*. 2001;108:776-789.
17. Update: drugs in breast milk. *Med Lett Drugs Ther*. 1979;21:21-24.
18. Havelka J, Frankova A. Contribution to the question of side effects of chloramphenicol therapy in newborns. *Cesk Pediatr*. 1972;21:31-33.

CHLORCYCLIZINE

Antihistamine (H_1 Antagonist)

PREGNANCY RECOMMENDATION: Limited Human Data—No Relevant Animal Data

BREASTFEEDING RECOMMENDATION: Probably Compatible

PREGNANCY SUMMARY

The Collaborative Perinatal Project reported first-trimester exposure to 113 antihistamine drugs (of which 13 were chlorcyclizine). Four (3.5%) newborns with anomalies were identified, but specific data on chlorcyclizine were not provided. In a second study regarding over 800 first-trimester exposures to antihistamine drugs, no increased risk for birth anomalies was found. Meclizine and cyclizine were the most commonly used. Specific numbers on chlorcyclizine were not provided. The drug will probably cross the placenta, so some fetal exposure will likely occur. Therefore, this limited human pregnancy experience prevents a complete assessment of the embryofetal risk. Animal studies did not provide relevant data because all dosing was more than 10 times the RHD. Using this drug during pregnancy should be based on the pros and cons of the mother's clinical need for treatment versus any potential fetal risk that might occur from exposure.

BREASTFEEDING SUMMARY

No reports describing the use of chlorcyclizine during human lactation have been located. The drug will probably be found in breast milk, so some infant exposure will likely occur. Breastfeeding while using this drug should be based on the mother's clinical need for treatment versus any potential infant risks that might occur. If used, the infant should be monitored for the most common reported adult side effects of dizziness and dry mouth (both leading to irritability), somnolence, and constipation. Because of the drug's anticholinergic effects, there is the possibility of interfering with breast milk production in the early stages of breastfeeding, as well as decreasing milk supply with long-term use.

References

1. Prescribing Information. *Chlorcyclizine*. Magna Pharmaceutical; 2020.
2. Heinonen OP, Slone D, Shapiro S. *Birth Defects and Drugs in Pregnancy*. Wright PSB; 1983:324.
3. Yerushalmy J, Milkovich L. Evaluation of the teratogenic effect of meclizine in man. *Am J Obstet Gynecol*. 1965;93:553-562.

C

CHLORDIAZEPOXIDE

Central Nervous System (Benzodiazepine)

PREGNANCY RECOMMENDATION: Human Data Suggest Potential Risk (First and Third Trimesters)

BREASTFEEDING RECOMMENDATION: Potential Toxicity

PREGNANCY SUMMARY

In combined data from the Collaborative Perinatal Project and the Michigan Medicaid surveillance study, a total of 1,045 first-trimester exposures were reported. Of these, 55 (5.3%) major anomalies were identified (42 expected). However, no pattern to the congenital defects was found. Also, from the Collaborative Perinatal Project, there were 740 anytime exposures with 13 (1.8%) major anomalies identified. There have been other studies with smaller numbers that have suggested an increased risk for anomalies in general. However, a recent review analyzed 12 studies and concluded that benzodiazepine drugs as a class were not associated with an increased risk for congenital defects. The drug crosses the placenta, so fetal exposure will occur. Animal studies did not show any increased risk for embryofetal toxicity or malformations in one species at doses of more than 10 times the RHD. Using this drug during pregnancy should be based on the pros and cons of the mother's clinical need for treatment versus any potential fetal risk that might occur from exposure. Continuous use during gestation has resulted in neonatal withdrawal, and depression of the newborn may occur if chlordiazepoxide is used close to birth. Consequently, if the maternal condition requires the use of this drug during pregnancy, the lowest possible dose should be taken. Moreover, abrupt discontinuance of chlordiazepoxide should be avoided due to an increased risk for seizures. The drug carries a boxed warning for an increased risk of profound sedation, respiratory depression, coma, and death with concomitant use with opioid drugs. Chlordiazepoxide is classified as a Schedule IV controlled substance.

BREASTFEEDING SUMMARY

No reports describing the use of chlordiazepoxide during human lactation have been located. The drug will probably be found in breast milk, so some infant exposure will likely occur. Breastfeeding while using this drug should be based on the mother's clinical need for treatment versus any potential infant risks that might occur. If used, the infant should be monitored for the most common reported adult side effects of dizziness and nausea (both leading to irritability), somnolence, drowsiness, rash, and peripheral edema. Because the drug and its active metabolites have long elimination half-lives, use of an alternative drug might be indicated (see Temazepam).

References

1. Product information. *Chlordiazepoxide*. Solco Healthcare US; 2017.
2. Milkovich L, van den Berg BJ. Effects of prenatal meprobamate and chlordiazepoxide hydrochloride on human embryonic and fetal development. *N Engl J Med*. 1974;291:1268-1271.
3. Rothman KJ, Fyler DC, Golblatt A, Kreidberg MB. Exogenous hormones and other drug exposures of children with congenital heart disease. *Am J Epidemiol*. 1979;109:433-439.
4. Crombie DL, Pinsent RJ, Fleming DM, et al. Fetal effects of tranquilizers in pregnancy. *N Engl J Med*. 1975;293:198-199.
5. Hartz SC, Heinonen OP, Shapiro S, et al. Antenatal exposure to meprobamate and chlordiazepoxide in relation to malformations, mental development, and childhood mortality. *N Engl J Med*. 1975;292:726-728.
6. Bracken MB, Holford TR. Exposure to prescribed drugs in pregnancy and association with congenital malformations. *Obstet Gynecol*. 1981;58:336-344.
7. American Academy of Pediatrics Committee on Drugs. Psychotropic drugs in pregnancy and lactation. *Pediatrics*. 1982;69:241-244.
8. Heinonen OP, Slone D, Shapiro S. *Birth Defects and Drugs in Pregnancy*. Publishing Sciences Group; 1977:336-337.
9. Bergman U, Rosa FW, Baum C, et al. Effects of exposure to benzodiazepine during fetal life. *Lancet*. 1992;340:694-696.
10. Athinarayanan P, Pierog SH, Nigam SK, Glass L. Chlordiazepoxide withdrawal in the neonate. *Am J Obstet Gynecol*. 1976;124:212-213.
11. Decancq HG Jr, Bosco JR, Townsend EH Jr. Chlordiazepoxide in labour: its effect on the newborn infant. *J Pediatr*. 1965;67:836-840.
12. Mark PM, Hamel J. Librium for patients in labor. *Obstet Gynecol*. 1968; 32:188-194.
13. Stirrat GM, Edington PT, Berry DJ. Transplacental passage of chlordiazepoxide. *Br Med J*. 1974;2:729.
14. Duckman S, Spina T, Attardi M, Meyer A. Double-blind study of chlordiazepoxide in obstetrics. *Obstet Gynecol*. 1964;24:601-605.
15. Kanto JH. Use of benzodiazepines during pregnancy, labour and lactation, with particular reference to pharmacokinetic considerations. *Drugs*. 1982; 23:354-380.
16. Bitnun S. Possible effect of chlordiazepoxide on the fetus. *Can Med Assoc J*. 1969;100:351.
17. Bellantuono C, Tofani S, Di Sciascio G, Santone G. Benzodiazepine exposure in pregnancy and risk of major malformations: a critical overview. *Gen Hosp Psychiatry*. 2013;35:3-8.

C

CHLORHEXIDINE

Anti-infective (Antiseptic/Disinfectant)

PREGNANCY RECOMMENDATION: Limited Human Data (First Trimester) Human Data Suggest Low Risk (Second and Third Trimesters)

BREASTFEEDING RECOMMENDATION: Probably Compatible

PREGNANCY SUMMARY

No reports describing the use of chlorhexidine during the first trimester were located. One case was listed in the Collaborative Perinatal Project data, but the outcome of this single case was not presented. A number of studies have documented the safety and possible effectiveness of vaginal disinfection with chlorhexidine prior to delivery, primarily to prevent colonization of newborns with group B streptococci. In addition, application to the groin and perineum, to the abdomen prior to cesarean section, and whole body washing have also been effective in preventing fetal and maternal infection in some instances, though these findings are not universal. No adverse effects in the newborns were observed. If found in the systemic circulation, this antiseptic can probably cross the placenta. However, based on the low systemic absorption with topical use (and even vaginal use), the overall amount is likely to be clinically insignificant. Animal studies did not show any embryofetal toxicity or malformations in one species. Using this topical agent during pregnancy should be based on the pros and cons of the mother's clinical need for treatment versus any potential fetal risk that might occur from exposure.

BREASTFEEDING SUMMARY

No reports describing the excretion of chlorhexidine into human breast milk have been located. This antiseptic could be found in breast milk, but the low systemic levels seen following topical use are very low. Therefore, the overall amount is likely to be clinically insignificant. As a general precaution, the mother's nipples should be rinsed thoroughly with water if chlorhexidine is used on them as a disinfectant, even though absorption of the agent from the gastrointestinal tract is poor. Breastfeeding while using this cleanser should be based on the mother's clinical need for treatment versus any potential infant risks that might occur. Due to the topical use of this antiseptic, systemic side effects have not been evaluated.

References

1. Multipurpose spermicides. *Lancet*. 1992;340:211-213.
2. Gilman MR, De Salva SJ. Teratology studies of benzethonium chloride, cetyl pyridinium chloride and chlorhexidine in rats (Abstract). *Toxicol Appl Pharmacol*. 1979;48:A35.
3. Vorherr H, Ulrich JA, Messer RH, Hurwitz EB. Antimicrobial effect of chlorhexidine on bacteria of groin, perineum and vagina. *J Reprod Med*. 1980; 24:153-157.
4. Christensen KK, Christensen P, Dykes AK, et al. Chlorhexidine for prevention of neonatal colonization with group B streptococci. I. In vitro effect of chlorhexidine on group B streptococci. *Eur J Obstet Gynecol Reprod Biol*. 1983;16:157-165.
5. Dykes AK, Christensen KK, Christensen P, Kahlmeter G. Chlorhexidine for prevention of neonatal colonization with group B streptococci. II. Chlorhexidine concentrations and recovery of group B streptococci following vaginal washing in pregnant women. *Eur J Obstet Gynecol Reprod Biol*. 1983;16:167-172.
6. Christensen KK, Christensen P. Chlorhexidine for prevention of neonatal colonization with GBS. *Antibiot Chemother*. 1985;35:296-302.
7. Christensen KK, Christensen P, Dykes AK, Kahlmeter G. Chlorhexidine for prevention of neonatal colonization with group B streptococci. III. Effect of vaginal washing with chlorhexidine before rupture of the membranes. *Eur J Obstet Gynecol Reprod Biol*. 1985;19:231-236.
8. Christensen KK, Dykes AK, Christensen P. Reduced colonization of newborns with group B streptococci following washing of the birth canal with chlorhexidine. *J Perinat Med*. 1985;13:239-243.
9. Easmon CSF. Group B streptococcus. *Infect Control*. 1986;7(suppl 2):135-137.
10. Dykes AK, Christensen KK, Christensen P. Chlorhexidine for prevention of neonatal colonization with group B streptococci. IV. Depressed puerperal carriage following vaginal washing with chlorhexidine during labour. *Eur J Obstet Gynecol Reprod Biol*. 1987;24:293-297.
11. Burman LG, Christensen P, Christensen K, et al; The Swedish Chlorhexidine Study Group. Prevention of excess neonatal morbidity associated with group B streptococci by vaginal chlorhexidine disinfection during labour. *Lancet*. 1992;340:65-69.
12. Burman LG, Tullus K. Vaginal chlorhexidine disinfection during labour. *Lancet*. 1992;340:791-792.
13. Lindemann R, Henrichsen T, Svenningsen L, Hjelle K. Vaginal chlorhexidine disinfection during labour. *Lancet*. 1992;340:792.
14. Henrichsen T, Lindemann R, Svenningsen L, Hjelle K. Prevention of neonatal infections by vaginal chlorhexidine disinfection during labour. *Acta Paediatr*. 1994;83:923-926.
15. Kollée LAA, Speyer I, van Kuijck MAP, et al. Prevention of group B streptococci transmission during delivery by vaginal application of chlorhexidine gel. *Eur J Obstet Gynecol Reprod Biol*. 1989;31:47-51.
16. Vorherr H, Vorherr UF, Moss JC. Comparative effectiveness of chlorhexidine, povidone-iodine, and hexachlorophene on the bacteria of the perineum and groin of pregnant women. *Am J Infect Control*. 1988;16:178-181.
17. Brown TR, Ehrlich CE, Stehman FB, et al. A clinical evaluation of chlorhexidine gluconate spray as compared with iodophor scrub for preoperative skin preparation. *Surg Gynecol Obstet*. 1984;158:363-366.
18. Sanderson PJ, Haji TC. Transfer of group B streptococci from mothers to neonates: effect of whole body washing of mothers with chlorhexidine. *J Hosp Infect*. 1985;6:257-264.
19. Frost L, Pedersen M, Seiersen E. Changes in hygienic procedures reduce infection following caesarean section. *J Hosp Infect*. 1989;13:143-148.
20. Sweeten KM, Ericksen NL, Blanco JD. Chlorhexidine versus sterile water vaginal wash during labor to prevent peripartum infection. *Am J Obstet Gynecol*. 1997;176:426-430.
21. Rouse DJ, Hauth JC, Andrews WW, et al. Chlorhexidine vaginal irrigation for the prevention of peripartal infection: a placebo-controlled randomized clinical trial. *Am J Obstet Gynecol*. 1997;176:617-622.
22. Elfast RA. Chlorhexidine prophylaxis at labor. Prevention of sudden infant death? *Lakartidningen*. 1993;90:3771-3772.
23. Eriksen NL, Blanco JD. Chlorhexidine versus sterile water vaginal wash during labor to prevent peripartum infection (Abstract). *Am J Obstet Gynecol*. 1995;172:304.
24. Vorherr H, Vorherr UF, Mehta P, et al. Antimicrobial effect of chlorhexidine and povidone-iodine on vaginal bacteria. *J Infect*. 1984;8:195-199.
25. Nilsson G, Larsson L, Christensen KK, et al. Chlorhexidine for prevention of neonatal colonization with group B streptococci. V. Chlorhexidine concentrations in blood following vaginal washing during delivery. *Eur J Obstet Gynecol Reprod Biol*. 1989;31:221-226.
26. Feldman R, van Oppen C, Noorduyn A. Vaginal chlorhexidine disinfection during labour. *Lancet*. 1992;340:791.
27. Goldenberg RL, McClure EM, Saleem S. A review of studies with chlorhexidine applied directly to the umbilical cord. *Am J Perinatol*. 2013;30:699-701.

C

CHLOROQUINE

Anti-Infective (Antimalarial/Amebicide)

PREGNANCY RECOMMENDATION: Limited Human Data—No Relevant Animal Data (Maternal Benefit Probably Outweighs Any Embryofetal Risk)

BREASTFEEDING RECOMMENDATION: Probably Compatible

PREGNANCY SUMMARY

A few studies were located that described the use of chloroquine during the first trimester of human pregnancy. A total of 176 cases were found, with only 2 (1.1%) major malformations identified. Numerous other studies were located that reported improved pregnancy outcomes when used in active malaria cases. The drug crosses the placenta, so fetal exposure will occur. However, the fetal levels are not likely to prevent congenital malaria. Animal studies showed embryofetal toxicity and malformations but at doses well above 10 times the RHD. Therefore, this limited human pregnancy experience of first-trimester exposure prevents a complete assessment of the embryofetal risk. Regardless, the maternal and fetal benefit of preventing and treating malaria far outweighs the risk, if any, to the embryo/fetus. The drug should be used cautiously in patients with glucose-6-phosphate dehydrogenase (G6PD) deficiency.

BREASTFEEDING SUMMARY

Several studies have evaluated the use of chloroquine during human lactation. The drug was found in breast milk in every case. Some levels may be compromised because the drug was used during pregnancy, and with the long elimination half-life, transplacental contribution cannot be ruled out based on when the blood was obtained postdelivery. However, there are several cases when the drug was first administered postpartum that resulted in positive breast milk levels. Most calculated RIDs were less than 10%, but a few were higher. Regardless, no adverse effects in infants have been identified. Furthermore, the reported breast milk levels are insufficient to provide adequate infant protection against malaria. Due to a concern for potential serious adverse effects that might be seen in a breastfed infant, the manufacturer recommends that women not breastfeed while being treated with this drug. Nevertheless, breastfeeding while using this drug should be based on the mother's clinical need for treatment versus any potential infant risks that might occur. If used, the infant should be monitored for the most common reported adult side effects of nausea, tinnitus, headache, myopathy, and abdominal pain (all leading to irritability), diarrhea, vomiting, rash, and various laboratory abnormalities (see PI).

References

1. Product information. *Chloroquine Phosphate*. Rising Pharmaceuticals; 2018.
2. Gilles HM, Lawson JB, Sibelas M, et al. Malaria, anaemia and pregnancy. *Ann Trop Med Parasitol*. 1969;63:245-263.
3. Diro M, Beydoun SN. Malaria in pregnancy. *South Med J*. 1982;75:959-962.
4. Malaria in pregnancy. *Lancet*. 1983;2:84-85.
5. Strang A, Lachman E, Pitsoe SB, et al. Malaria in pregnancy with fatal complications: case report. *Br J Obstet Gynaecol*. 1984;91:399-403.
6. Ross JB, Garatsos S. Absence of chloroquine induced ototoxicity in a fetus. *Arch Dermatol*. 1974;109:573.
7. Lewis R, Lauresen NJ, Birnbaum S. Malaria associated with pregnancy. *Obstet Gynecol*. 1973;42:698-700.
8. Udalova LD. The effect of chloroquine on the embryonal development of rats. *Pharmacol Toxicol (Russian)*. 1967;2:226-228. As cited in Shepard TH. *Catalog of Teratogenic Agents*. 6th ed. Johns Hopkins University Press; 1989:140-141.
9. Akintonwa A, Gbajumo SA, Biola Mabadeje AF. Placental and milk transfer of chloroquine in humans. *Ther Drug Monit*. 1988;10:147-149.
10. Centers for Disease Control. Recommendations for the prevention of malaria among travelers. *MMWR Recomm Rep*. 1990;39:1-10.
11. World Health Organization. Practical chemotherapy of malaria. *WHO Tech Rep Ser*. 1990;805:1-141.
12. Subramanian D, Moise KJ Jr, White AC Jr. Imported malaria in pregnancy: report of four cases and review of management. *Clin Infect Dis*. 1992;15:408-413.
13. Hart CW, Naunton RF. The ototoxicity of chloroquine phosphate. *Arch Otolaryngol*. 1964;80:407-412.
14. Wolfe MS, Cordero JF. Safety of chloroquine in chemosuppression of malaria during pregnancy. *Br Med J*. 1985;290:1466-1467.
15. Klinger G, Morad Y, Westall CA, et al. Ocular toxicity and antenatal exposure to chloroquine or hydroxychloroquine for rheumatic diseases. *Lancet*. 2001;358:813-814.
16. Edstein MD, Veenendaal JR, Newman K, Hyslop R. Excretion of chloroquine, dapsone and pyrimethamine in human milk. *Br J Clin Pharmacol*. 1986;22:733-735.
17. American Academy of Pediatrics Committee on Drugs. The transfer of drugs and other chemicals into human milk. *Pediatrics*. 2001;108:776-789.

CHLOROTHIAZIDE

Cardiovascular (Diuretic—Thiazide)

PREGNANCY RECOMMENDATION: Limited Human Data—Animal Data Suggest Low Risk

BREASTFEEDING RECOMMENDATION: Probably Compatible

C

PREGNANCY SUMMARY

Most studies that evaluated chlorothiazide use in human pregnancy described administration in the second and third trimesters in treating preeclampsia and other medical conditions. From two large databases that studied drug use in pregnancy and the risk for birth defects (Collaborative Perinatal Project and the Michigan Medicaid Surveillance Study), there were a total of 83 pregnancies with first-trimester exposure to chlorothiazide, and 4 (4.8%) birth defects were found (3-4 expected). For hydrochlorothiazide, there were 674 first-trimester exposures with 31 (4.6%) major congenital anomalies (27 expected). No pattern to the anomalies was found. For anytime use in pregnancy (most of which were after the first trimester), there were more than 12,850 exposures with 232 (1.8%) major birth anomalies identified. The drug crosses the placenta, so some fetal exposure will occur. Therefore, this limited human pregnancy experience suggests that the use of this drug in the first trimester, overall, is low risk. Animal studies did not show any embryofetal toxicity in three species at doses of less than 10 times the RHD (in two) and more than 10 times the RHD (in one). However, a full evaluation of birth anomalies may not have been conducted. Diuretics are not recommended for the treatment of gestational hypertension or preeclampsia because of the maternal hypovolemia characteristic of this disease. Other risks to the fetus or newborn include hypoglycemia, thrombocytopenia, hyponatremia, and hypokalemia. Using this drug during pregnancy should be based on the pros and cons of the mother's clinical need for treatment versus any potential fetal risk that might occur from exposure.

BREASTFEEDING SUMMARY

One study was located that evaluated human breast milk for chlorothiazide. In 11 lactating women, chlorothiazide was not detected in any of the breast milk samples following a single dose of 500 mg (LLQ of 1 mcg/mL). The drug may have been present in breast milk, but in the nanogram per milliliter range. Assuming a breast milk level of 900 ng/mL, a theoretically calculated RID in this case would be less than 2%. Due to a concern for potential serious adverse effects that might be seen in a breastfed infant, the manufacturer recommends that women not breastfeed while being treated with this drug. Nevertheless, breastfeeding while using this drug should be based on the mother's clinical need for treatment versus any potential infant risks that might occur. If used, the infant should be monitored for the most common reported adult side effects of nausea, headache, dizziness, and abdominal cramps (all leading to irritability), diarrhea, vomiting, lethargy, hypotension, and rash.

References

1. Product information. *Diuril*. Salix Pharmaceuticals; 2017.
2. Garnet J. Placental transfer of chlorothiazide. *Obstet Gynecol*. 1963;21:123-125.
3. Beermann B, Fahraeus L, Groschinsky-Grind M, Lindstrom B. Placental transfer of hydrochlorothiazide. *Gynecol Obstet Invest*. 1980;11:45-48.
4. Mulley BA, Parr GD, Pau WK, et al. Placental transfer of chlorthalidone and its elimination in maternal milk. *Eur J Clin Pharmacol*. 1978;13:129-131.
5. Finnerty FA Jr, Buchholz JH, Tuckman J. Evaluation of chlorothiazide (Diuril) in the toxemias of pregnancy: analysis of 144 patients. *JAMA*. 1958;166:141-144.
6. Zuspan FP, Bell JD, Barnes AC. Balance-ward and double-blind diuretic studies during pregnancy. *Obstet Gynecol*. 1960;16:543-549.
7. Sears RT. Oral diuretics in pregnancy toxaemia. *Br Med J*. 1960;2:148.
8. Assoli NS. Renal effects of hydrochlorothiazide in normal and toxemic pregnancy. *Clin Pharmacol Ther*. 1960;1:48-52.
9. Tatum H, Waterman EA. The prophylactic and therapeutic use of the thiazides in pregnancy. *GP*. 1961;24:101-105.
10. Flowers CE, Grizzle JE, Easterling WE, Bonner OB. Chlorothiazide as a prophylaxis against toxemia of pregnancy. *Am J Obstet Gynecol*. 1962;84:919-929.
11. Weseley AC, Douglas GW. Continuous use of chlorothiazide for prevention of toxemia of pregnancy. *Obstet Gynecol*. 1962;19:355-358.
12. Finnerty FA Jr. How to treat toxemia of pregnancy. *GP*. 1963;27:116-121.
13. Fallis NE, Plauche WC, Mosey LM, Langford HG. Thiazide versus placebo in prophylaxis of toxemia of pregnancy in primigravid patients. *Am J Obstet Gynecol*. 1964;88:502-504.
14. Landesman R, Aguero O, Wilson K, LaRussa R, Campbell W, Penaloza O. The prophylactic use of chlorthalidone, a sulfonamide diuretic, in pregnancy. *J Obstet Gynaecol Br Commonw*. 1965;72:1004-1010.
15. Cuadros A, Tatum H. The prophylactic and therapeutic use of bendroflumethiazide in pregnancy. *Am J Obstet Gynecol*. 1964;89:891-897.
16. Finnerty FA Jr, Bepko FJ Jr. Lowering the perinatal mortality and the prematurity rate: the value of prophylactic thiazides in juveniles. *JAMA*. 1966;195:429-432.
17. Kraus GW, Marchese JR, Yen SSC. Prophylactic use of hydrochlorothiazide in pregnancy. *JAMA*. 1966;198:1150-1154.
18. Gray MJ. Use and abuse of thiazides in pregnancy. *Clin Obstet Gynecol*. 1968;11:568-578.
19. Heinonen OP, Slone D, Shapiro S. *Birth Defects and Drugs in Pregnancy*. Publishing Sciences Group; 1977.
20. Watt JD, Philipp EE. Oral diuretics in pregnancy toxemia. *Br Med J*. 1960;1:1807.
21. Lindheimer MD, Katz AI. Sodium and diuretics in pregnancy. *N Engl J Med*. 1973;288:891-894.
22. Lammintausta R, Erkkola R, Eronen M. Effect of chlorothiazide treatment of renin-aldosterone system during pregnancy. *Acta Obstet Gynecol Scand*. 1978;57:389-392.
23. Sibai BM, Grossman RA, Grossman HG. Effects of diuretics on plasma volume in pregnancies with long-term hypertension. *Am J Obstet Gynecol*. 1984;150:831-835.
24. Christianson R, Page EW. Diuretic drugs and pregnancy. *Obstet Gynecol*. 1976;48:647-652.
25. Shoemaker ES, Grant NF, Madden JD, MacDonald PC. The effect of thiazide diuretics on placental function. *Tex Med*. 1973;69:109-115.
26. Lakin N, Zeytinoglu J, Younger M, White P. Effect of chlorothiazide on insulin requirements of pregnant diabetic women. *JAMA*. 1960;173:353-354.
27. Esbenshade JH Jr, Smith RT. Thiazides and pregnancy: a study of carbohydrate tolerance. *Am J Obstet Gynecol*. 1965;92:270-271.
28. Senior B, Slone D, Shapiro S, et al. Benzothiadiazides and neonatal hypoglycaemia. *Lancet*. 1976;2:377.
29. Menzies DN. Controlled trial of chlorothiazide in treatment of early pre-eclampsia. *Br Med J*. 1964;1:739-742.
30. Harley JD, Robin H, Robertson SEJ. Thiazide-induced neonatal haemolysis? *Br Med J*. 1964;1:696-697.
31. Goldman JA, Neri A, Ovadia J, et al. Effect of chlorothiazide on intravenous glucose tolerance in pregnancy. *Am J Obstet Gynecol*. 1969;105:556-560.
32. Rodriguez SU, Leikin SL, Hiller MC. Neonatal thrombocytopenia associated with ante-partum administration of thiazide drugs. *N Engl J Med*. 1964;270:881-884.
33. Leikin SL. Thiazide and neonatal thrombocytopenia. *N Engl J Med*. 1964;271:161.
34. Prescott LF. Neonatal thrombocytopenia and thiazide drugs. *Br Med J*. 1964;1:1438.
35. Jones JE, Reed JF Jr. Renal vein thrombosis and thrombocytopenia in the newborn infant. *J Pediatr*. 1965;67:681-682.
36. Karpatkin S, Strick N, Karpatkin MB, Siskind GW. Cumulative experience in the detection of antiplatelet antibody in 234 patients with idiopathic

thrombocytopenic purpura, systemic lupus erythematosus and other clinical disorders. *Am J Med*. 1972;52:776-785.
37. Finnerty FA Jr, Assoli NS. Thiazide and neonatal thrombocytopenia. *N Engl J Med*. 1964;271:160-161.
38. Jerkner K, Kutti J, Victoria L. Platelet counts in mothers and their newborn infants with respect to antepartum administration of oral diuretics. *Acta Med Scand*. 1973;194:473-475.
39. Pritchard JA, Walley PJ. Severe hypokalemia due to prolonged administration of chlorothiazide during pregnancy. *Am J Obstet Gynecol*. 1961;81:1241-1244.
40. Alstatt LB. Transplacental hyponatremia in the newborn infant. *J Pediatr*. 1965;66:985-988.
41. Anderson GG, Hanson TM. Chronic fetal bradycardia: possible association with hypokalemia. *Obstet Gynecol*. 1974;44:896-898.
42. Crosland D, Flowers C. Chlorothiazide and its relationship to neonatal jaundice. *Obstet Gynecol*. 1963;22:500-504.
43. Minkowitz S, Soloway HB, Hall JE, Yermakov V. Fatal hemorrhagic pancreatitis following chlorothiazide administration in pregnancy. *Obstet Gynecol*. 1964;24:337-342.
44. Werthmann MW Jr, Krees SV. Excretion of chlorothiazide in human breast milk. *J Pediatr*. 1972;81:781-783.
45. Drugs in breast milk. *Med Lett Drugs Ther*. 1976;16:25-27.
46. Dailey JW. Anticoagulant and cardiovascular drugs. In: Wilson JT, ed. *Drugs in Breast Milk*. ADIS Press; 1981:61-64.
47. Miller ME, Cohn RD, Burghart PH. Hydrochlorothiazide disposition in a mother and her breast-fed infant. *J Pediatr*. 1982;101:789-791.
48. Healy M. Suppressing lactation with oral diuretics. *Lancet*. 1961;1:1353-1354.
49. Catz CS, Giacoia GP. Drugs and breast milk. *Pediatr Clin North Am*. 1972;19:151-166.
50. American Academy of Pediatrics Committee on Drugs. The transfer of drugs and other chemicals into human milk. *Pediatrics*. 2001;108:776-789.

CHLORPHENIRAMINE

Antihistamine

PREGNANCY RECOMMENDATION: Human Data Suggest Low Risk

BREASTFEEDING RECOMMENDATION: Probably Compatible

PREGNANCY SUMMARY

From four publications, a total of 1,421 first-trimester exposures to chlorpheniramine were reported, and 64 (4.5%) major anomalies were identified (57 expected). For anytime use, there were 82 (2.1%) major anomalies seen in 3,931 exposures. No pattern to the congenital defects was found. The drug will probably cross the placenta, so fetal exposure will likely occur. In general, antihistamines are considered low risk in pregnancy. Animal reproduction studies have not been located. Using this drug during pregnancy should be based on the pros and cons of the mother's clinical need for treatment versus any potential fetal risk that might occur from exposure.

BREASTFEEDING SUMMARY

No reports describing the use of chlorpheniramine during human lactation have been located. The drug will probably be excreted into breast milk, so some infant exposure will likely occur. Some antihistamines, with prolonged usage, may interfere with prolactin production, which could then lead to a decrease in milk supply. Breastfeeding while using this drug should be based on the mother's clinical need for treatment. If used, the infant should be monitored for the most common reported adult side effects of nausea and headache (leading to irritability), somnolence, diarrhea, and vomiting.

References

1. Product information. *Chlorpheniramine*. L&R Distributors; 2020.
2. Heinonen OP, Slone D, Shapiro S. *Birth Defects and Drugs in Pregnancy*. Publishing Sciences Group; 1977.
3. Nelson MM, Forfar JO. Associations between drugs administered during pregnancy and congenital abnormalities of the fetus. *Br Med J*. 1971;1:523-527.
4. Golbus MS, Koerper MA, Hall BD. Failure to diagnose osteopetrosis *in utero*. *Lancet*. 1976;2:1246.
5. Black RA, Hill DA. Over-the-counter medications in pregnancy. *Am Fam Physician*. 2003;67:2517-2524.
6. Das BP, Joshi M, Pant CR. An overview of over the counter drugs in pregnancy and lactation. *Kathmandu Univ Med J (KUMJ)*. 2006;4:545-551.
7. Li Q, Mitchell AA, Werler MM, et al. Assessment of antihistamine use in early pregnancy and birth defects. *J Allergy Clin Immunol Pract*. 2013;1(6):666-674.
8. Ito S, Blajchman A, Stephenson M, Eliopoulos C, Koren G. Prospective follow-up of adverse reactions in breast-fed infants exposed to maternal medication. *Am J Obstet Gynecol*. 1993;168:1393-1399.

CHLORPROMAZINE

Mental Health (Antipsychotic—Phenothiazine)

PREGNANCY RECOMMENDATION: Limited Human Data—Animal Data Suggest Potential Risk

BREASTFEEDING RECOMMENDATION: Potential Toxicity

C

PREGNANCY SUMMARY

A few studies have been located that described the use of chlorpromazine during the first trimester of pregnancy. A total of 235 cases were identified, with 9 (3.8%) major anomalies identified (9-10 expected). There were also 284 exposures at any time during gestation, with 8 (2.8%) major defects identified. There were no patterns to the anomalies that were reported. A few literature reviews have also not found an increased risk for teratogenicity with the use of the phenothiazine class of drugs. The drug will cross the placenta, so fetal exposure will occur. However, this limited human pregnancy experience still prevents a complete assessment of the embryofetal risk. Animal studies did show some embryofetal toxicity in one species at doses less than 10 times the RHD. Use near delivery has been associated with some newborn depression and also extrapyramidal signs in a few neonates. Using this drug during pregnancy should be based on the pros and cons of the mother's clinical need for treatment versus any potential fetal risk that might occur from exposure.

BREASTFEEDING SUMMARY

Several studies have evaluated chlorpromazine in human breast milk. The drug has been found in several samples, but the levels of the drug do not seem to correlate with maternal dosage. In several samples, the drug was not detected. In others, the two highest levels obtained were 290 and 272 ng/mL. In both cases, the RIDs were less than 4%. Most reports describe no adverse effects in infants while breastfeeding during maternal use. There are occasional reports of drowsiness. In addition, there was a report that two children had a decline in developmental scores when their mothers were using both chlorpromazine and haloperidol. Therefore, this combination should be used with caution. Due to a concern for potential serious adverse effects that might be seen in a breastfed infant, the manufacturer recommends that women not breastfeed while being treated with this drug. Nevertheless, breastfeeding while using this drug should be based on the mother's clinical need for treatment versus any potential infant risks that might occur. If used, the infant should be monitored for the most common reported adult side effects of nausea and dizziness (both leading to irritability), lethargy, constipation, insomnia, and uncontrolled movements. The drug has also been associated with hyperprolactinemia, but this should not adversely affect breastfeeding.

References

1. Product information. *Chlorpromazine Hydrochloride*. Sandoz; 2018.
2. Ullberg S, Lindquist NG, Sjostrand SE. Accumulation of chorio-retinotoxic drugs in the foetal eye. *Nature*. 1970;227:1257-1258.
3. Franchi G, Gianni AM. Chlorpromazine distribution in maternal and fetal tissues and biological fluids. *Acta Anaesthesiol (Padava)*. 1957;8:197-207.
4. Moya F, Thorndike V. Passage of drugs across the placenta. *Am J Obstet Gynecol*. 1962;84:1778-1798.
5. O'Donoghue SEF. Distribution of pethidine and chlorpromazine in maternal, foetal and neonatal biological fluids. *Nature*. 1971;229:124-125.
6. Hammond JE, Toseland PA. Placental transfer of chlorpromazine. *Arch Dis Child*. 1970;45:139-140.
7. Drugs and the fetal eye. *Lancet*. 1971;1:122.
8. Karp M, Lamb VE, Benaron HBW. The use of chlorpromazine in the obstetric patient: a preliminary report. *Am J Obstet Gynecol*. 1955;69:780-785.
9. Benaron HBW, Dorr EM, Roddick WJ, et al. The use of chlorpromazine in the obstetric patient: a preliminary report: I. In the treatment of nausea and vomiting of pregnancy. *Am J Obstet Gynecol*. 1955;69:776-779.
10. Sullivan CL. Treatment of nausea and vomiting of pregnancy with chlorpromazine: a report of 100 cases. *Postgrad Med*. 1957;22:429-432.
11. Harer WB. Chlorpromazine in normal labor. *Obstet Gynecol*. 1956;8:1-9.
12. Lindley JE, Rogers SF, Moyer JH. Analgesic-potentiation effect of chlorpromazine during labor; a study of 2093 patients. *Obstet Gynecol*. 1957;10:582-586.
13. Bryans CI Jr, Mulherin CM. The use of chlorpromazine in obstetrical analgesia. *Am J Obstet Gynecol*. 1959;77:406-411.
14. Christhilf SM Jr, Monias MB, Riley RA Jr, Sheehan JC. Chlorpromazine in obstetric analgesia. *Obstet Gynecol*. 1960;15:625-629.
15. Rodgers CD, Wickard CP, McCaskill MR. Labor and delivery without terminal anesthesia. A report of the use of chlorpromazine. *Obstet Gynecol*. 1961;17:92-95.
16. Hill RM, Desmond MM, Kay JL. Extrapyramidal dysfunction in an infant of a schizophrenic mother. *J Pediatr*. 1966;69:589-595.
17. Ayd FJ Jr. Phenothiazine therapy during pregnancy-effects on the newborn infant. *Int J Drug Ther Newslett*. 1968;3:39-40.
18. Tamer A, McKay R, Arias D, et al. Phenothiazine-induced extrapyramidal dysfunction in the neonate. *J Pediatr*. 1969;75:479-480.
19. Levy W, Wisniewski K. Chlorpromazine causing extrapyramidal dysfunction in newborn infant of psychotic mother. *NY State J Med*. 1974;74:684-685.
20. O'Connor M, Johnson GH, James DI. Intrauterine effect of phenothiazines. *Med J Aust*. 1981;1:416-417.
21. Falterman CG, Richardson J. Small left colon syndrome associated with maternal ingestion of psychotropic drugs. *J Pediatr*. 1980;97:308-310.
22. Kris EB, Carmichael DM. Chlorpromazine maintenance therapy during pregnancy and confinement. *Psychiatr Q*. 1957;31:690-695.
23. Kris EB. Children born to mothers maintained on pharmacotherapy during pregnancy and postpartum. *Recent Adv Biol Psychiatry*. 1962;4:180-187.
24. Kris EB. Children of mothers maintained on pharmacotherapy during pregnancy and postpartum. *Curr Ther Res*. 1965;7:785-789.
25. Sobel DE. Fetal damage due to ECT, insulin coma, chlorpromazine, or reserpine. *Arch Gen Psychiatry*. 1960;2:606-611.
26. Ayd FJ Jr. Children born of mothers treated with chlorpromazine during pregnancy. *Clin Med*. 1964;71:1758-1763.
27. Loke KH, Salleh R. Electroconvulsive therapy for the acutely psychotic pregnant patient: a review of 3 cases. *Med J Malaysia*. 1983;38:131-133.
28. Slone D, Siskind V, Heinonen OP, et al. Antenatal exposure to the phenothiazines in relation to congenital malformations, perinatal mortality rate, birth weight, and intelligence quotient score. *Am J Obstet Gynecol*. 1977;128:486-488.
29. Rumeau-Rouquette C, Goujard J, Huel G. Possible teratogenic effect of phenothiazines in human beings. *Teratology*. 1976;15:57-64.
30. O'Leary JL, O'Leary JA. Nonthalidomide ectromelia: report of a case. *Obstet Gynecol*. 1964;23:17-20.
31. Levin RM, Amsterdam JD, Winokur A, Wein AJ. Effects of psychotropic drugs on human sperm motility. *Fertil Steril*. 1981;36:503-506.
32. Platt JE, Friedhoff AJ, Broman SH, et al. Effects of prenatal exposure to neuroleptic drugs on children's growth. *Neuropsychopharmacology*. 1988;1:205-212.
33. Ergenekon E, Atalay Y, Tunaoglu S, Koc E. Transient heart block in a newborn due to maternal antipsychotic treatment during pregnancy. *Eur J Pediatr*. 2000;159:137-138.
34. Ananth J. Congenital malformations with psychopharmacologic agents. *Compr Psychiatry*. 1975;16:437-445.
35. Elia J, Katz IR, Simpson GM. Teratogenicity of psychotherapeutic medications. *Psychopharmacol Bull*. 1987;23:531-586.
36. Blacker KH, Weinstein BJ, Ellman GL. Mothers milk and chlorpromazine. *Am J Psychol*. 1962;114:178-179.
37. Wiles DH, Orr MW, Kolakowska T. Chlorpromazine levels in plasma and milk of nursing mothers. *Br J Clin Pharmacol*. 1978;5:272-273.
38. American Academy of Pediatrics Committee on Drugs. The transfer of drugs and other chemicals into human milk. *Pediatrics*. 2001;108:776-789.

C

CHLORTHALIDONE

Cardiovascular (Diuretic)

PREGNANCY RECOMMENDATION: Limited Human Data—Animal Data Suggest Low Risk

BREASTFEEDING RECOMMENDATION: Probably Compatible

PREGNANCY SUMMARY

The Collaborative Perinatal Project reported 20 patients with 2 (10%) newborns identified who had malformations. However, no specific pattern was noted between the two birth defects, and coexposures to other drugs were not described. For anytime exposure to chlorthalidone during pregnancy, there were 33 (2.5%) major anomalies in 1,310 exposures. The drug will cross the placenta, so some fetal exposure will occur. However, this limited human pregnancy experience still prevents a complete assessment of the embryofetal risk. Animal studies did not show any embryofetal toxicity or malformations in two species at doses of more than 10 times the RHD. In general, diuretics are not recommended for the treatment of hypertension in pregnancy. Using this drug during pregnancy should be based on the pros and cons of the mother's clinical need for treatment versus any potential fetal risk that might occur from exposure.

BREASTFEEDING SUMMARY

Chlorthalidone has been shown to be excreted into human breast milk. In one study that evaluated seven lactating women, milk levels 3 days after delivery ranged from 90 to 860 ng/mL, with a mean of about 365 ng/mL. The calculated RID was about 6%. Due to a concern for potential serious adverse effects that might be seen in a breastfed infant, the manufacturer recommends that women not breastfeed while being treated with this drug. Nevertheless, breastfeeding while using this drug should be based on the mother's clinical need for treatment versus any potential infant risks that might occur. If used, the infant should be monitored for the most common reported adult side effects of nausea, dizziness, and abdominal cramps (all leading to irritability), diarrhea, vomiting, rash, and hyperglycemia.

References

1. Product information. *Chlorthalidone*. Nivagen Pharmaceuticals; 2018.
2. Mulley BA, Parr GD, Pau WK, et al. Placental transfer of chlorthalidone and its elimination in maternal milk. *Eur J Clin Pharmacol*. 1978;17:129-131.
3. Reiher KH. Suppression of lactation by stimulation of diuresis. *Zentralbl Gynakol*. 1963;85:188-190.
4. Vercruysse J. Inhibition of lactation. Comparative study of an estro-androgen and of a diuretic. *Brux Med*. 1966;46:1258-1266.
5. Heinonen OP, Slone D, Shapiro S. *Birth Defects and Drugs in Pregnancy*. Wright PSB; 1983:373,441.

CHLORZOXAZONE

Pain (Muscle Relaxant)

PREGNANCY RECOMMENDATION: Limited Human Data—No Relevant Animal Data

BREASTFEEDING RECOMMENDATION: Probably Compatible

PREGNANCY SUMMARY

In a surveillance study of Michigan Medicaid recipients, 12 (3.9%) major birth defects were identified in 305 first-trimester exposures of combined data from 1980 to 1992. No specific pattern was noted for the anomalies, and coexposures to other drugs were not described. The drug will probably cross the placenta, so some fetal exposure will likely occur. However, this limited human pregnancy experience prevents a complete assessment of the embryofetal risk. Animal reproduction studies have not been conducted. Using this drug during pregnancy should be based on the pros and cons of the mother's clinical need for treatment versus any potential fetal risk that might occur from exposure.

BREASTFEEDING SUMMARY

No reports describing the use of chlorzoxazone during human lactation have been located. The drug will probably be found in breast milk, so some infant exposure will likely occur. Breastfeeding while using this drug should be based on the mother's clinical need for treatment versus any potential infant risks that might occur. If used, the infant should be monitored for the most common reported adult side effects of nausea and dizziness (both leading to irritability), vomiting, somnolence, and rash.

Reference

1. Prescribing Information. *Chlorzoxazone*. Solubiomix; 2018.

C

CHOLECALCIFEROL

Vitamin

PREGNANCY RECOMMENDATION: Compatible

BREASTFEEDING RECOMMENDATION: Compatible

See Vitamin D.

CHOLESTYRAMINE

Antilipemic

PREGNANCY RECOMMENDATION: Human Data Suggest Low Risk

BREASTFEEDING RECOMMENDATION: Compatible

PREGNANCY SUMMARY

Only a few reports have been located that describe the use of cholestyramine in about eight patients in the first trimester. No fetal anomalies were identified. In addition, the drug is not systemically absorbed following oral use, so it will not be at the placental interface to cross. Fetal exposure will not occur, so teratogenicity related directly to the drug is not possible. However, long-term use can decrease maternal absorption of the fat-soluble vitamins (A, D, E, and K), and deficiencies in some of these at the time of organogenesis can lead to fetal harm. The drug has been used in treating pruritus associated with intrahepatic cholestasis of pregnancy (ICP) for years. This disease, by itself, can lead to poor pregnancy outcomes, despite treatment with cholestyramine. Vitamin K deficiency can lead to bleeding, and in theory, could lead to a deficiency in the fetus that results in bleeding. Because there is little benefit to lowering cholesterol levels during pregnancy, and ICP can be treated with ursodiol, using this drug during pregnancy should be based on the pros and cons of the mother's clinical need for treatment versus any potential fetal risk that might occur from exposure.

BREASTFEEDING SUMMARY

No reports describing the use of cholestyramine during human lactation have been located. The drug is not absorbed systemically; therefore, it should not be found in human milk. However, long-term use of the drug can decrease the absorption of the fat-soluble vitamins (A, D, E, and K). Therefore, supplementation for some of these might be needed if used for a long time while breastfeeding.

References

1. Product information. *Questran*. Par Pharmaceutical; 2018.
2. Koda S, Anabuki K, Miki T, et al. Reproductive studies on cholestyramine. *Kiso to Rinsho*. 1982;16:2040-2094. As cited in Shepard TH. *Catalog of Teratogenic Agents*. 7th ed. Johns Hopkins University Press; 1992:90.
3. Innis SM. Effect of cholestyramine administration during pregnancy in the rat. *Am J Obstet Gynecol*. 1983;146:13-16.
4. Lutz EE, Margolis AJ. Obstetric hepatosis: treatment with cholestyramine and interim response to steroids. *Obstet Gynecol*. 1969;33:64-71.
5. Heikkinen J, Maentausta O, Ylostalo P, Janne O. Serum bile acid levels in intrahepatic cholestasis of pregnancy during treatment with phenobarbital or cholestyramine. *Eur J Obstet Gynecol Reprod Biol*. 1982;14:153-162.
6. Shaw D, Frohlich J, Wittmann BAK, Willms M. A prospective study of 18 patients with cholestasis of pregnancy. *Am J Obstet Gynecol*. 1982;142:621-625.
7. Schorr-Lesnick B, Lebovics E, Dworkin B, Rosenthal WS. Liver disease unique to pregnancy. *Am J Gastroenterol*. 1991;86:659-670.
8. Sadler LC, Lane M, North R. Severe fetal intracranial haemorrhage during treatment with cholestyramine for intrahepatic cholestasis of pregnancy. *Br J Obstet Gynaecol*. 1995;102:169-170.
9. Jenkins JK, Boothby LA. Treatment of itching associated with intrahepatic cholestasis of pregnancy. *Ann Pharmacother*. 2002;36:1462-1465.
10. Kondrackiene J, Beuers U, Kupcinskas L. Efficacy and safety of ursodeoxycholic acid versus cholestyramine in intrahepatic cholestasis of pregnancy. *Gastroenterology*. 2005;129:894-901.
11. Sentilhes L, Verspyck E, Pia P, Marpeau L. Fetal death in a patient with intrahepatic cholestasis of pregnancy. *Obstet Gynecol*. 2006;107:458-460.
12. Fedorkow DM, Persaud D, Nimrod CA. Inflammatory bowel disease: a controlled study of late pregnancy outcome. *Am J Obstet Gynecol*. 1989;160:998-1001.
13. Rosa F. Anti-cholesterol agent pregnancy exposure outcomes. Presented at: 7th International Organization for Teratogen Information Services; April 1994; Woods Hole, MA.

CHOLIC ACID

Gastrointestinal (Bile Acid)

PREGNANCY RECOMMENDATION: No Human Data and No Relevant Animal Data

BREASTFEEDING RECOMMENDATION: Probably Compatible

PREGNANCY SUMMARY

No reports describing the use of cholic acid during human pregnancy have been located. Endogenous cholic acid crosses the placenta. Therefore, because cholic acid, the drug, is identical to endogenous cholic acid, it will also cross and fetal exposure will occur. However, the absence of human pregnancy experience prevents a complete assessment of the embryofetal risk. Animal reproduction studies have not been conducted. Using this drug during pregnancy should be based on the pros and cons of the mother's clinical need for treatment versus any potential fetal risk that might occur from exposure. There is a registry that monitors pregnancy outcomes in women taking this drug during pregnancy (COCOA Registry [ChOlbam: Child and mOther's heAlth]). Health care providers can enroll patients by calling 1-844-202-6262.

BREASTFEEDING SUMMARY

No reports describing the use of cholic acid during human lactation have been located. Endogenous cholic acid is known to be found in human breast milk, and therefore, this oral formulation should also be excreted into breast milk. To what extent this drug will increase the normal amount of cholic acid in breast milk is unknown. Breastfeeding while using this drug should be based on the mother's clinical need for treatment versus any potential infant risks that might occur. If used, the infant should be monitored for the most common reported adult side effects of nausea, malaise, peripheral neuropathy, and abdominal pain (all leading to irritability), diarrhea, and jaundice.

Reference

1. Product information. *Cholbam*. Manchester Pharmaceuticals; 2017.

CHOLINE C 11

Radiopharmaceutical

PREGNANCY RECOMMENDATION: *Contraindicated

BREASTFEEDING RECOMMENDATION: *Contraindicated

PREGNANCY SUMMARY

No reports describing the use of choline C 11 in human pregnancy have been located. The drug will probably cross the placenta, but the rapid clearance should limit fetal exposure. However, the absence of human pregnancy experience prevents a complete assessment of the embryofetal risk. No animal studies have been conducted. All radiopharmaceuticals have the potential to cause harm depending on the stage of fetal development and the magnitude of the radiation dose. *Nevertheless, this radioactive diagnostic agent is not indicated for use in females.

BREASTFEEDING SUMMARY

No reports describing the use of choline C 11 during human lactation have been located. The drug will probably be excreted into breast milk, but the rapid clearance should limit infant exposure. The manufacturer recommends that women should be advised to avoid the use of choline C 11 while breastfeeding. *However, this radioactive diagnostic agent is not indicated for use in females.

Reference

1. Prescribing Information. *Choline C 11 injection*. Mayo Clinic PET Radiochemistry Facility; 2012.

CHONDROITIN

Dietary Supplement

PREGNANCY RECOMMENDATION: No Human Data—No Relevant Animal Data

BREASTFEEDING RECOMMENDATION: Probably Compatible

PREGNANCY SUMMARY

No reports describing the use of chondroitin during human pregnancy have been located. It is possible that a minimal amount of the supplement will cross the placenta, so some fetal exposure may occur. Therefore, the absence of human

(*continued*)

C

pregnancy experience prevents a complete assessment of the embryofetal risk. The amount of chondroitin used in animal studies cannot be compared to the amount used in human consumption. Moreover, the lack of standardization prevents knowing the exact dose taken. The oral bioavailability depends on the MW of the product used, and this may not be known from the product's package insert or label and may not be consistent from product to product. However, chondroitin is an endogenous substance widely found in human tissues, so the embryo/fetus must synthesize it during development. Therefore, it is difficult to assess the overall risk with planned or inadvertent use of chondroitin during gestation.

BREASTFEEDING SUMMARY

No reports describing the use of chondroitin during human lactation have been located. Chondroitin is normally found in human breast milk, with one study reporting an average concentration of about 230 mcg/mL. The MW of the glycosaminoglycans in chondroitin supplements would suggest that most will not be excreted into breast milk. With the low oral bioavailability of the drug following maternal use, combined with minimal excretion into breast milk, followed by the likely low oral bioavailability from the infant's gastrointestinal tract with breastfeeding, the overall amount of exposure is probably negligible. If some chondroitin were to be excreted into breast milk, it is unknown how much this might increase the chondroitin level above what is naturally found in human breast milk. Therefore, the use of chondroitin during lactation is probably compatible.

References

1. Chondroitin. *PDR health*. Accessed March 20, 2006. http://www.pdrhealth.com/drug_info/nmdrugprofiles/nutsupdrugs/cho_0071.shtml
2. Kamei T. The teratogenic effect of excessive chondroitin sulfate in the DDN strain of mice. *Med Biol*. 1961;60:126-129. As cited in Shepard TH. *Catalog of Teratogenic Agents*. 10th ed. The Johns Hopkins University Press; 2001: 107-108.
3. Hamada Y. Studies on anti-atherosclerotic agents. IX. Teratological studies of sodium chondroitin polysulfate. *Oyo Yakuri*. 1972;6:589-594. As cited in Shepard TH. *Catalog of Teratogenic Agents*. 10th ed. The Johns Hopkins University Press; 2001:107.
4. Coppa GV, Gabrielli O, Buzzega D, et al. Composition and structure elucidation of human milk glycosaminoglycans. *Glycobiology*. 2011;21:295-303.

CHORAMBUCIL

Antineoplastic (Alkylating Agent)

PREGNANCY RECOMMENDATION: Limited Human Data—Animal Data Suggest Potential Toxicity

BREASTFEEDING RECOMMENDATION: Potential Toxicity

PREGNANCY SUMMARY

A few case reports were located that described the use of chlorambucil during human pregnancy. With first-trimester exposure, unilateral renal agenesis and a cardiac defect were reported along with a few normal outcomes. The drug will probably cross the placenta, so some fetal exposure will likely occur. However, this limited human pregnancy experience prevents a complete assessment of the embryofetal risk. Animal studies did show some embryofetal toxicity with malformations in one species at doses of less than 10 times the RHD. Using this drug during pregnancy should be based on the pros and cons of the mother's clinical need for treatment versus any potential fetal risk that might occur from exposure. There is a registry for women who are pregnant and have cancer. For more information, women and health care providers are encouraged to contact the Cancer and Pregnancy Registry at 1-877-635-4499.

BREASTFEEDING SUMMARY

No reports describing the use of chlorambucil during lactation have been located. The drug will probably be found in breast milk, so some infant exposure will likely occur. However, due to a concern for potential serious adverse effects that might be seen in a breastfed infant, the manufacturer recommends that women not breastfeed while being treated with this drug. Nevertheless, breastfeeding while using this drug should be based on the mother's clinical need for treatment versus any potential infant risks that might occur. If used, the infant should be monitored for the most common reported adult side effects of nausea and abdominal pain (both leading to irritability), diarrhea, lethargy, vomiting, rash, and various laboratory abnormalities (see PI).

References

1. Product information. *Leukeran*. Aspen Global; 2019.
2. Sokal JE, Lessmann EM. Effects of cancer chemotherapeutic agents on the human fetus. *JAMA*. 1960;172:1765-1771.
3. Jacobs C, Donaldson SS, Rosenberg SA, Kaplan HS. Management of the pregnant patient with Hodgkin's disease. *Ann Intern Med*. 1981;95:669-675.
4. Shotton D, Monie IW. Possible teratogenic effect of chlorambucil on a human fetus. *JAMA*. 1963;186:74-75.
5. Steege JF, Caldwell DS. Renal agenesis after first trimester exposure to chlorambucil. *South Med J*. 1980;73:1414-1415.

6. Thompson J, Conklin KA. Anesthetic management of a pregnant patient with scleroderma. *Anesthesiology*. 1983;59:69-71.
7. Rugh R, Skaredoff L. Radiation and radiomimetic chlorambucil and the fetal retina. *Arch Ophthalmol*. 1965;74:382-393. As cited by Schardein JL. *Chemically Induced Birth Defects*. 3rd ed. Marcel Dekker; 2000:581-582.
8. Ali R, Kimya Y, Koksal N, et al. Pregnancy in chronic lymphocytic leukemia: experience with fetal exposure to chlorambucil. *Leuk Res*. 2009;33:567-569.
9. Lawler SD, Lele KP. Chromosomal damage induced by chlorambucil and chronic lymphocytic leukemia. *Scand J Haematol*. 1972;9:603-612.

CICLESONIDE

Respiratory (Oral/Nasal Inhalation—Corticosteroid)

PREGNANCY RECOMMENDATION: Limited Human Data—No Relevant Animal Data

BREASTFEEDING RECOMMENDATION: Probably Compatible

PREGNANCY SUMMARY

No reports describing the first-trimester use of ciclesonide in human pregnancy have been located. A single case report of ciclesonide use (along with numerous other medications) at 34 weeks' gestation in a mother diagnosed with COVID-19 acute respiratory distress was found. She delivered a few days later, and the child did well. The drug may cross the placenta, but blood levels are likely to be clinically insignificant. However, this limited human pregnancy experience prevents a complete assessment of the embryofetal risk. Animal studies did not show any embryofetal toxicity in one species when the drug was administered orally, but did show embryofetal toxicity with malformations in another species upon subcutaneous (SC) administration. The approved use for the drug is oral/nasal inhalation. Using this drug during pregnancy should be based on the pros and cons of the mother's clinical need for treatment versus any potential fetal risk that might occur from exposure. Women who are pregnant and have taken asthma medications during pregnancy are encouraged to contact MotherToBaby Pregnancy Studies at 877-311-8972. The most recent ACOG publication on asthma in pregnancy (published in 2008—reaffirmed in 2020) and the 2023 Global Initiative for Asthma (GINA) guidelines state that the advantages of actively treating asthma in pregnancy markedly outweigh the potential risks of the medications. Inhaled corticosteroids are usually the first-line treatment for mild to moderate persistent asthma in pregnancy. Listed alternative treatments include cromolyn, theophylline, or leukotriene receptor antagonists. However, ACOG recommends long-acting β_2-agonists as the preferred add-on drug when pregnant patients are not controlled with inhaled corticosteroids. The reasoning for this is that long-acting inhaled β_2-agonists have been shown to be more effective as an add-on treatment in nonpregnant patients; whereas, theophylline has more side effects and requires serum monitoring and there are minimal data on the leukotriene receptor antagonists in human pregnancy.

BREASTFEEDING SUMMARY

No reports describing the use of ciclesonide during human lactation have been located. The drug may be found in breast milk; however, due to the very poor oral absorption of the drug (<1%) and numerous other pK factors, any amount would likely be clinically insignificant. Breastfeeding while using this drug should be based on the mother's clinical need for treatment versus any potential infant risks that might occur. If used, the infant should be monitored for the most common reported adult side effects of headache, arthralgia, and back pain (all leading to irritability), sinusitis, and nasopharyngitis.

References

1. Prescribing Information. *Alvesco*. Covis Pharma; 2019.
2. American College of Obstetricians and Gynecologists. ACOG practice bulletin No. 90: asthma in pregnancy. *Obstet Gynecol*. 2008;111:457-464.
3. Global Initiative for Asthma. *Global safety for asthma management and prevention, 2023*. Update July 2023. www.ginasthma.org
4. Chinen Y, Kinjyo Y, Mekaru K, et al. Critical respiratory failure in pregnancy complicated with COVID-19: a case report. *Case Rep Womens Health*. 2021;30:e00309.

CICLOPIROX

Anti-Infective (Antifungal—Topical)

PREGNANCY RECOMMENDATION: No Human Data—Animal Data Suggest Low Risk

BREASTFEEDING RECOMMENDATION: Probably Compatible

C

PREGNANCY SUMMARY

No reports describing the use of ciclopirox in human pregnancy have been located. The drug will probably cross the placenta, but the overall amount is likely to be clinically insignificant. However, the absence of human pregnancy experience prevents a complete assessment of the embryofetal risk. Animal studies did not show any embryofetal toxicity or malformations in four different animal species. Using this drug during pregnancy should be based on the pros and cons of the mother's clinical need for treatment versus any potential fetal risk that might occur from exposure.

BREASTFEEDING SUMMARY

No reports describing the use of ciclopirox during human lactation have been located. The amount of the drug that may be found in breast milk is likely to be clinically insignificant. Breastfeeding while using this drug should be based on the mother's clinical need for treatment versus any potential infant risks that might occur. Due to the topical use of the drug, systemic side effects were not reported.

Reference

1. Prescribing Information. *Ciclopirox*. Glenmark Pharmaceuticals; 2018.

CIDOFOVIR

Antiviral (Cytomegalovirus)

PREGNANCY RECOMMENDATION: No Human Data and No Relevant Animal Data *(Maternal Benefit May Outweigh Embryo–Fetal Risk)

BREASTFEEDING RECOMMENDATION: *Contraindicated

PREGNANCY SUMMARY

No reports describing the use of cidofovir during human pregnancy have been located. The drug will probably cross the placenta, so some fetal exposure will likely occur. Therefore, the absence of human pregnancy experience prevents a complete assessment of the embryofetal risk. Animal studies did show embryofetal toxicity in two species at doses of less than 10 times the RHD, but they were administered the drug daily for up to 10 to 12 days. Normal dosing in humans is a dose every other week. Using this drug during pregnancy should be based on the pros and cons of the mother's clinical need for treatment versus any potential fetal risk that might occur from exposure. *The use of cidofovir after the first trimester in a pregnant woman living with HIV with sight-threatening cytomegalovirus (CMV) retinitis should be considered. If used, the patient's renal function needs to be monitored closely (boxed warning).

BREASTFEEDING SUMMARY

No reports describing the use of cidofovir during human lactation have been located. Some of the drug will likely be found in breast milk. *However, the only approved indication for using this drug (currently) is in the treatment of CMV retinitis in patients infected with HIV type 1 (HIV-1). Because HIV-1 can be transmitted in breast milk, breastfeeding is not recommended in developed countries where there are available, affordable milk substitutes.

References

1. Product information. *Cidofovir*. Heritage Pharmaceuticals; 2018.
2. Brown ZA, Watts DH. Antiviral therapy in pregnancy. *Clin Obstet Gynecol*. 1990;33:276-289.
3. de Martino M, Tovo P-A, Pezzotti P, et al. HIV-1 transmission through breast-milk: appraisal of risk according to duration of feeding. *AIDS*. 1992; 6:991-997.
4. Van de Perre P. Postnatal transmission of human immunodeficiency virus type 1: the breast-feeding dilemma. *Am J Obstet Gynecol*. 1995;173: 483-487.

CILOSTAZOL

Hematologic (Antiplatelet)

PREGNANCY RECOMMENDATION: Limited Human Data—Animal Data Suggest Risk

BREASTFEEDING RECOMMENDATION: Potential Toxicity

C

PREGNANCY SUMMARY

One report describing the use of cilostazol during human pregnancy was located. Cilostazol was used along with numerous other drugs to treat a 24-week pregnant woman with polymorphic ventricular tachycardia. Treatment was unsuccessful, and she underwent an emergency cesarean section, delivering a very premature newborn that was limp and apneic, with multiple bruises noted. It is unknown if the bruising had any relationship to the cilostazol. The drug and active metabolites will probably cross the placenta, so some fetal exposure will likely occur. Therefore, this limited human pregnancy experience prevents a complete assessment of the embryofetal risk. Animal studies did show embryofetal toxicity with malformations in two species at doses less than 10 times the RHD. Using this drug during pregnancy should be based on the pros and cons of the mother's clinical need for treatment versus any potential fetal risk that might occur from exposure.

BREASTFEEDING SUMMARY

No reports describing the use of cilostazol during human lactation have been located. The drug will probably be found in breast milk, so some infant exposure will likely occur. Due to a concern for potential serious adverse effects that might be seen in a breastfed infant, the manufacturer recommends that women not breastfeed while being treated with this drug. Nevertheless, breastfeeding while using this drug should be based on the mother's clinical need for treatment versus any potential infant risks that might occur. If used, the infant should be monitored for the most common reported adult side effects of headache (leading to irritability), diarrhea, and tachycardia.

References

1. Prescribing Information. *Cilostazol*. Teva Pharmaceuticals USA; 2017.
2. Burrows K, Fox J, Biblo LA, Roth JA. Pregnancy and short-coupled torsades de pointes. *Pacing Clin Electrophysiol*. 2013;36:e77-e79.

CIMETIDINE

Gastrointestinal (Antisecretory)

PREGNANCY RECOMMENDATION: Human Data Suggest Low Risk

BREASTFEEDING RECOMMENDATION: Probably Compatible

PREGNANCY SUMMARY

Several studies have evaluated cimetidine and the H_2 inhibitor group as a whole, and increased risks have not been identified. The rate of birth anomalies from nearly 800 first-trimester exposures is about 4%, but no pattern to the defects has been shown. In addition, a meta-analysis involving nearly 2,400 patients and a second large study of nearly 1,150 first-trimester exposures have not shown an increased risk for congenital malformation with the use of H_2 blockers. The drug crosses the placenta, so some fetal exposure will occur. Animal studies did not show any embryofetal toxicity or teratogenicity in two species, one at doses of less than 10 times the RHD and the other at more than 10 times the RHD. Using this drug during pregnancy should be based on the pros and cons of the mother's clinical need for treatment versus any potential fetal risk that might occur from exposure.

BREASTFEEDING SUMMARY

From two studies, cimetidine was analyzed in a total of 13 lactating women. The drug was found in human breast milk with peak levels of about 6 mcg/mL. However, the calculated RIDs were less than 10% in most cases. No adverse effects in infants have been reported. Due to a concern for potential serious adverse effects that might be seen in a breastfed infant, the manufacturer recommends that women not breastfeed while being treated with this drug. Nevertheless, breastfeeding while using this drug should be based on the mother's clinical need for treatment versus any potential infant risks that might occur. If used, the infant should be monitored for the most common reported adult side effects of nausea, headache, dizziness, and abdominal pain (all leading to irritability), diarrhea, lethargy, and rash. The drug has also been shown to increase prolactin levels, but this should not adversely affect breastfeeding.

References

1. Product information. *Tagamet*. Medtech Products; 2019.
2. Finkelstein W, Isselbacher KJ. Cimetidine. *N Engl J Med*. 1978;299:992-996.
3. Pinelli F, Trivulzio S, Colombo R, et al. Antiprostatic effect of cimetidine in rats. *Agents Actions*. 1987;22:197-201.
4. Sawyer D, Conner CS, Scalley R. Cimetidine: adverse reactions and acute toxicity. *Am J Hosp Pharm*. 1981;38:188-197.
5. Anand S, Van Thiel DH. Prenatal and neonatal exposure to cimetidine results in gonadal and sexual dysfunction in adult males. *Science*. 1982;21:493-494.
6. Parker S, Udani M, Gavaler JS, Van Thiel DH. Pre-and neonatal exposure to cimetidine but not ranitidine adversely affects adult sexual functioning of male rats. *Neurobehav Toxicol Teratol*. 1984;6:313-318.
7. Parker S, Schade RR, Pohl CR, et al. Prenatal and neonatal exposure of male rat pups to cimetidine but not ranitidine adversely affects subsequent adult sexual functioning. *Gastroenterology*. 1984;86:675-680.
8. Walker TF, Bott JH, Bond BC. Cimetidine does not demasculinize male rat offspring exposed in utero. *Fundam Appl Toxicol*. 1987;8:188-197.
9. Shapiro BH, Hirst SA, Babalola GO, Bitar MS. Prospective study on the sexual development of male and female rats perinatally exposed to maternally administered cimetidine. *Toxicol Lett*. 1988;44:315-329.

C

10. Dicke JM, Johnson RF, Henderson GI, et al. A comparative evaluation of the transport of H_2-receptor antagonists by the human and baboon placenta. *Am J Med Sci*. 1988;295:198-206.
11. Schenker S, Dicke J, Johnson RF, et al. Human placental transport of cimetidine. *J Clin Invest*. 1987;80:1428-1434.
12. Howe JP, McGowan WAW, Moore J, et al. The placental transfer of cimetidine. *Anaesthesia*. 1981;36:371-375.
13. McGowan WAW. Safety of cimetidine in obstetric patients. *J R Soc Med*. 1979; 72:902-907.
14. Johnston JR, Moore J, McCaughey W, et al. Use of cimetidine as an oral antacid in obstetric anesthesia. *Anesth Analg*. 1983;62:720-726.
15. Knott PD, Thorpe SS, Lamont CAR. Congenital renal dysgenesis possibly due to captopril. *Lancet*. 1989;1:451.
16. Corazza GR, Gasbarrini G, Di Nisio Q, Zulli P. Cimetidine (Tagamet) in peptic ulcer therapy during pregnancy: a report of three cases. *Clin Trials J*. 1982; 19:91-93.
17. Glade G, Saccar CL, Pereira GR. Cimetidine in pregnancy: apparent transient liver impairment in the newborn. *Am J Dis Child*. 1980;134:87-88.
18. Zulli P, DiNisio Q. Cimetidine treatment during pregnancy. *Lancet*. 1978; 2:945-946.
19. Husemeyer RP, Davenport HT. Prophylaxis for Mendelson's syndrome before elective caesarean sections. A comparison of cimetidine and magnesium trisilicate mixture regimens. *Br J Obstet Gynaecol*. 1980;87:565-570.
20. Pickering BG, Palahniuk RJ, Cumming M. Cimetidine premedication in elective caesarean section. *Can Anaesth Soc J*. 1980;27:33-35.
21. Dundee JW, Moore J, Johnston JR, McCaughey W. Cimetidine and obstetric anaesthesia. *Lancet*. 1981;2:252.
22. McCaughey W, Howe JP, Moore J, Dundee JW. Cimetidine in elective caesarean section. Effect on gastric acidity. *Anaesthesia*. 1981;36:167-172.
23. Crawford JS. Cimetidine in elective caesarean section. *Anaesthesia*. 1981; 36:641-642.
24. McCaughey W, Howe JP, Moore J, Dundee JW. Cimetidine in elective caesarean section. *Anaesthesia*. 1981;36:642.
25. Hodgkinson R, Glassenberg R, Joyce TH III, et al. Safety and efficacy of cimetidine and antacid in reducing gastric acidity before elective cesarean section. *Anesthesiology*. 1982;57:A408.
26. Ostheimer GW, Morrison JA, Lavoie C, et al. The effect of cimetidine on mother, newborn and neonatal neurobehavior. *Anesthesiology*. 1982;57: A405.
27. Hodgkinson R, Glassenberg R, Joyce TH III, et al. Comparison of cimetidine (Tagamet) with antacid for safety and effectiveness in reducing gastric acidity before elective cesarean section. *Anesthesiology*. 1983;59:86-90.
28. Qvist N, Storm K. Cimethidine pre-anesthetic: a prophylactic method against Mendelson's syndrome in cesarean section. *Acta Obstet Gynecol Scand*. 1983;62:157-159.
29. Okasha AS, Motaweh MM, Bali A. Cimetidine–antacid combination as premedication for elective caesarean section. *Can Anaesth Soc J*. 1983;30: 593-597.
30. Frank M, Evans M, Flynn P, Aun C. Comparison of the prophylactic use of magnesium trisilicate mixture B.P.C., sodium citrate mixture or cimetidine in obstetrics. *Br J Anaesth*. 1984;56:355-362.
31. McAuley DM, Halliday HL, Johnston JR, et al. Cimetidine in labour: absence of adverse effect on the high–risk fetus. *Br J Obstet Gynaecol*. 1985; 92:350-355.
32. Johnston JR, McCaughey W, Moore J, Dundee JW. Cimetidine as an oral antacid before elective caesarean section. *Anaesthesia*. 1982;37:26-32.
33. Johnston JR, McCaughey W, Moore J, Dundee JW. A field trial of cimetidine as the sole oral antacid in obstetric anaesthesia. *Anaesthesia*. 1982; 37:33-38.
34. Thorburn J, Moir DD. Antacid therapy for emergency caesarean section. *Anaesthesia*. 1987;42:352-355.
35. Howe JP, Dundee JW, Moore J, McCaughey W. Cimetidine: has it a place in obstetric anaesthesia? *Anaesthesia*. 1980;35:421-422.
36. Koren G, Zemlickis DM. Outcome of pregnancy after first trimester exposure to H2 receptor antagonists. *Am J Perinatol*. 1991;8:37-38.
37. Magee LA, Inocencion G, Kamboj L, et al. Safety of first trimester exposure to histamine H_2 blockers: a prospective cohort study. *Dig Dis Sci*. 1996;41:1145-1149.
38. Kallen B. Delivery outcome after the use of acid-suppressing drugs in early pregnancy with special reference to omeprazole. *Br J Obstet Gynaecol*. 1998;105:877-881.
39. Ruigomez A, Rodriguez LAG, Cattaruzzi C, et al. Use of cimetidine, omeprazole, and ranitidine in pregnant women and pregnancy outcomes. *Am J Epidemiol*. 1999;150:476-481.
40. Dehlink E, Yen E, Leichtner AM, et al. First evidence of a possible association between gastric acid suppression during pregnancy and childhood asthma: a population-based register study. *Clin Exp Allergy*. 2009;39:246-253.
41. Garbis H, Elefant E, Diav-Citrin O, et al. Pregnancy outcome after exposure to ranitidine and other H2-blockers—a collaborative study of the European Network of Teratology Information Services. *Reprod Toxicol*. 2005;453-458.
42. Smallwood RA, Berlin RG, Castagnoli N, et al. Safety of acid-suppressing drugs. *Dig Dis Sci*. 1995;40(suppl):63S-80S.
43. Broussard CN, Richter JE. Treating gastro-oesophageal reflux disease during pregnancy and lactation. What are the safest therapy options? *Drug Saf*. 1998;19:325-337.
44. Katz PO, Castell DO. Gastroesophageal reflux disease during pregnancy. *Gastroenterol Clin North Am*. 1998;27:153-167.
45. Richter JE. Gastroesophageal reflux disease during pregnancy. *Gastroenterol Clin North Am*. 2003;32:235-261.
46. Richter JE. Review article: the management of heartburn in pregnancy. *Aliment Pharmacol Ther*. 2005;22:749-757.
47. Gill SK, O'Brien L, Koren G. The safety of histamine 2 (H2) blockers in pregnancy: a meta-analysis. *Dig Dis Sci*. 2009;54:1835-1838.
48. Matok I, Gorodischer R, Koren G, et al. The safety of H_2-blockers use during pregnancy. *J. Clin Pharmacol*. 2010;50:81-87.
49. Somogyi A, Gugler R. Cimetidine excretion into breast milk. *Br J Clin Pharmacol*. 1979;7:627-629.
50. Oo CY, Kuhn RJ, Desai N, McNamara PJ. Active transport of cimetidine into human milk. *Clin Pharmacol Ther*. 1995;58:548-555.
51. American Academy of Pediatrics Committee on Drugs. The transfer of drugs and other chemicals into human milk. *Pediatrics*. 2001;108:776-789.

CINACALCET

Miscellaneous (Calcimimetic)

PREGNANCY RECOMMENDATION: Limited Human Data—Animal Data Suggest Low Risk

BREASTFEEDING RECOMMENDATION: Probably Compatible

PREGNANCY SUMMARY

Several case reports have been located that describe the use of cinacalcet during human pregnancy. In the few that had first-trimester use, no birth anomalies have been described. Most of the exposures have been in the second and third trimester, and in several cases, the neonates had abnormal calcium levels postbirth (though these were all treated without any prolonged issues noted). The drug will probably cross the placenta, so some fetal exposure will likely occur. However, this limited human pregnancy experience prevents a complete assessment of the embryofetal risk. Animal studies did not show any teratogenicity or embryofetal toxicity (in the absence of maternal toxicity) in two species at doses of less than 10 times the RHD. Using this drug during pregnancy should be based on the pros and cons of the mother's clinical need for treatment versus any potential fetal risk that might occur from exposure. There is a pregnancy exposure registry that monitors pregnancy outcomes in women using this drug. Health care providers are encouraged to call Amgen's Pregnancy Surveillance Program at 1-800-772-6436.

C

BREASTFEEDING SUMMARY

No reports describing the use of cinacalcet during human lactation have been located. The drug will likely be found in breast milk. Due to a concern for potential serious adverse effects that might be seen in a breastfed infant, the manufacturer recommends that women not breastfeed while being treated with this drug. Nevertheless, breastfeeding while using this drug should be based on the mother's clinical need for treatment versus any potential infant risks that might occur. If used, the infant should be monitored for the most common reported adult side effects of nausea (leading to irritability), diarrhea, and vomiting. The drug has been safely used in neonates.

References

1. Product information. *Sensipar*. Amgen; 2019.
2. Nadarasa K, Bailey M, Chahal H, et al. The use of cinacalcet in pregnancy to treat a complex case of parathyroid carcinoma. *Endocrinol Diabetes Metab Case Rep*. 2014;2014:140056.
3. Horton WB, Stumpf MM, Coppock JD, et al. Gestational primary hyperparathyroidism due to ectopic parathyroid adenoma: case report and literature review. *J Endocr Soc*. 2017;1:1150-1155.
4. Horjus C, Groot I, Telting D, et al. Cinacalcet for hyperparathyroidism in pregnancy and puerperium. *J Pediatr Endocrinol Metab*. 2009;22:741-749.
5. Edling KL, Korenman SG, Janzen C, et al. A pregnant dilemma: primary hyperthyroidism due to parathyromatosis in pregnancy. *Endocr Pract*. 2013;6:1-15.
6. Vera L, Oddo S, Di Lorgi N, et al. Primary hyperparathyroidism in pregnancy treated with cinacalcet: a case report and review of the literature. *J Med Case Rep*. 2016;10:361.
7. Rey E, Jacob CE, Koolian M, Morin F. Hypercalcemia in pregnancy—a multifaceted challenge: case reports and literature review. *Clin Case Rep*. 2016;4:1001-1008.
8. Garcia IG, Fradejas MR, Macias Mdlos AM, et al. Primary hyperparathyroidism in pregnancy treated with cinacalcet: a case report. *J Obstet Gynaecol*. 2018;38:132-134.
9. Refardt J, Farina P, Hoesli I, Meter C. Hypercalcemic crisis in third trimenon: evaluating the optimal treatment strategy. *Gynecol Endocrinol*. 2018;34:833-836.

CIPAGLUCOSIDASE ALFA

Genetic (Lysosomal Glycogen-Specific α-Glucosidase Enzyme)

PREGNANCY RECOMMENDATION: No Human Data—Animal Data Suggest Low Risk

BREASTFEEDING RECOMMENDATION: Probably Compatible

PREGNANCY SUMMARY

No reports describing the use of cipaglucosidase alfa in human pregnancy have been located. The drug will not likely cross the placenta, especially during the first half of gestation. Miglustat (a drug that is administered in combination with this enzyme) most likely will cross the placenta, so fetal exposure to the drug will probably occur (see Miglustat). However, the absence of human pregnancy experience prevents a complete assessment of the embryofetal risk. Animal data did show some embryofetal toxicity in one species at doses less than 10 times the RHD (for miglustat). The doses for cipaglucosidase were more than 10 times the RHD. Based on animal studies, the manufacturer recommends that women with reproductive potential use effective contraception during treatment and for 2 months after the last dose. Nevertheless, using this drug during pregnancy should be based on the pros and cons of the mother's clinical need for treatment versus any potential fetal risk that might occur from exposure.

BREASTFEEDING SUMMARY

No reports describing the use of cipaglucosidase alfa during human lactation have been located. This large protein drug would not be expected to be found in human breast milk. Additionally, if any of this protein were to be ingested through breastfeeding, it would probably be digested in the infant's gastrointestinal tract and not be absorbed. However, the drug is administered along with miglustat, which will probably be found in breast milk. No lactation data on miglustat currently exists. Therefore, due to a concern for potential serious adverse effects that might be seen in a breastfed infant exposed to both of these drugs, the manufacturer recommends that women not breastfeed while being treated with this drug. Nevertheless, breastfeeding while using this drug should be based on the mother's clinical need for treatment versus any potential infant risk that might occur. If used, the infant should be monitored for the most common reported adult side effects of nausea, headache, and abdominal pain (all leading to irritability), diarrhea, fatigue (lethargy), and fever.

Reference

1. Prescribing Information. *Pombiliti*. Amicus Therapeutics; 2023.

C

CIPROFLOXACIN

Antibacterial (Fluoroquinolone)

PREGNANCY RECOMMENDATION: Human Data Suggest Potential Risk (First Trimester)

BREASTFEEDING RECOMMENDATION: Potential Toxicity

PREGNANCY SUMMARY

The use of ciprofloxacin has been reported in numerous studies in human pregnancy. Some of the data are difficult to separate out, but of 583 first-trimester exposures, there were 11 (1.8%) major anomalies identified. Several other studies analyzing fluoroquinolones as a group have reported birth anomaly rates of around 4% to 5%, but no pattern has been identified. The drug crosses the placenta, so fetal exposure will occur. Animal studies did not show any embryofetal toxicity or teratogenicity in three species, but doses were lower than the RHD. Higher doses led to maternal toxicity. Overall, the use of ciprofloxacin during human gestation does not appear to be associated with an increased risk of major congenital malformations. However, a causal relationship with some of the birth defects cannot be excluded. Because of this, the use of ciprofloxacin during pregnancy, especially during the first trimester, should be used with caution. Additionally, the FDA has added warnings to all fluoroquinolones for the risk of disabling and potentially permanent effects involving the tendons, muscles, joints, nerves, and central nervous system. At this time, fluoroquinolones should be reserved for those who do not have alternative treatment options.

BREASTFEEDING SUMMARY

A total of three studies regarding the use of ciprofloxacin during human lactation were located. From these, a total of 12 lactating women were administered doses ranging from 500 mg to 1,500 mg in a 24-hour period. The drug was found in all breast milk samples, with a peak value of 3.75 mcg/mL. The three calculated RIDs ranged from about 2% to about 7% (using peak values), and all of the analyses showed that the total infant dose was well below what would normally be administered to an infant (10-40 mg/kg, daily). Due to a concern for potential serious adverse effects that might be seen in a breastfed infant, the manufacturer recommends that women not breastfeed while being treated with this drug. Nevertheless, breastfeeding while using this drug should be based on the mother's clinical need for treatment versus any potential infant risks that might occur. If used, the infant should be monitored for the most common reported adult side effects of nausea (leading to irritability), diarrhea, vomiting, rash, and elevated liver function tests. Because of the boxed warning and a potential increased risk for tendon and joint dysfunction, using this drug for more complicated infections might be warranted.

References

1. Norrby SR, Lietman PS. Safety and tolerability of fluoroquinolones. *Drugs*. 1993;45(suppl 3):59-64.
2. Schaefer C, Amoura-Elefant E, Vial T, et al. Pregnancy outcome after prenatal quinolone exposure: evaluation of a case registry of the European Network of Teratology Information Services (ENTIS). *Eur J Obstet Gynecol Reprod Biol*. 1996;69:83-89.
3. U.S. Food and Drug Administration. *FDA approves safety labeling changes for fluoroquinolones*. Accessed May 24, 2016. http://www.fda.gov/Drugs/DrugSafety/InformationbyDrugClass/ucm500325.htm
4. Product information. *Ciprofloxacin*. Aurobindo Pharma; 2018.
5. Polachek H, Holcberg G, Sapir G, et al. Transfer of ciprofloxacin, ofloxacin and levofloxacin across the perfused human placenta in vitro. *Eur J Obstet Gynecol Reprod Biol*. 2005;122:61-65.
6. Bomford JAL, Ledger JC, O'Keeffe BJ, Reiter CH. Ciprofloxacin use during pregnancy. *Drugs*. 1993;45(suppl 3):461-462.
7. Berkovitch M, Pastuszak A, Gazarian M, et al. Safety of the new quinolones in pregnancy. *Obstet Gynecol*. 1994;84:535-538.
8. Koul PA, Wani JI, Wahid A. Ciprofloxacin for multiresistant enteric fever in pregnancy. *Lancet*. 1995;346:307-308.
9. Leung D, Venkatesan P, Boswell T, et al. Treatment of typhoid in pregnancy. *Lancet*. 1995;346:648.
10. Pastuszak A, Andreou R, Schick B, et al. New postmarketing surveillance data supports a lack of association between quinolone use in pregnancy and fetal and neonatal complications. *Reprod Toxicol*. 1995;9:584.
11. Skannal DG, Dungy-Poythress LJ, Miodovnik M, First MR. Pregnancy in a combined liver and kidney transplant recipient with type 1 primary hyperoxaluria. *Obstet Gynecol*. 1995;86:641-643.
12. Baroncini A, Calzolari E, Calabrese O, Zanetti A. First-trimester exposure to ciprofloxacin (abstract). *Teratology*. 1996;53:24A.
13. Wilton LV, Pearce GI, Mann RD. A comparison of ciprofloxacin, norfloxacin, ofloxacin, azithromycin, and cefixime examined by observational cohort studies. *Br J Clin Pharmacol*. 1996;41:277-284.
14. Ludlam H, Wreghitt TG, Thornton S, et al. Q fever in pregnancy. *J Infect*. 1997;34:75-78.
15. Loebstein R, Addis A, Ho E, et al. Pregnancy outcome following gestational exposure to fluoroquinolones: a multicenter prospective controlled study. *Antimicrob Agents Chemother*. 1998;42:1336-1339.
16. Wogelius P, Norgaard M, Gislum M, et al. Further analysis of the risk of adverse birth outcome after maternal use of fluoroquinolones. *Int J Antimicrob Agents*. 2005;26:323-326.
17. Cooper WO, Hernandez-Diaz S, Arbogast PG, et al. Antibiotics potentially used in response to bioterrorism and the risk of major congenital malformations. *Paediatr Perinat Epidemiol*. 2009;23:18-28.
18. Giamarellou H, Kolokythas E, Petrikkos G, et al. Pharmacokinetics of three newer quinolones in pregnant and lactating women. *Am J Med*. 1989; 87(suppl 5A):49S-51S.
19. Cover DL, Mueller BA. Ciprofloxacin penetration into human breast milk: a case report. *Ann Pharmacother*. 1990;24:703-704.
20. Gardner DK, Gabbe SG, Harter C. Simultaneous concentrations of ciprofloxacin in breast milk and in serum in mother and breast-fed infant. *Clin Pharm*. 1992;11:352-354.
21. Harmon T, Burkhart G, Applebaum H. Perforated pseudomembranous colitis in the breast-fed infant. *J Pediatr Surg*. 1992;27:744-746.
22. Lumbiganon P, Pengsaa K, Sookpranee T. Ciprofloxacin in neonates and its possible effect on the teeth. *Pediatr Infect Dis J*. 1991;10:619-620.
23. American Academy of Pediatrics Committee on Drugs. The transfer of drugs and other chemicals into human milk. *Pediatrics*. 2001;108:776-789.

CIPROFLOXACIN OPHTHALMIC

Ophthalmic/Antibacterial (Topical—Quinolone)

PREGNANCY RECOMMENDATION: No Human Data—Animal Data Suggest Low Risk

BREASTFEEDING RECOMMENDATION: Probably Compatible

C

PREGNANCY SUMMARY

No reports describing the use of ciprofloxacin ophthalmic in human pregnancy have been located. The drug will probably cross the placenta, but the amount that would occur with ocular use is likely to be clinically insignificant. However, the absence of human pregnancy experience prevents a complete assessment of the embryofetal risk. Animal studies did not show any embryofetal toxicity or teratogenicity in two species at doses less than 10 times the RHD. Using this drug during pregnancy should be based on the pros and cons of the mother's clinical need for treatment versus any potential fetal risk that might occur from exposure. If used during pregnancy, consider placing pressure over the tear duct in the corner of the eye for at least 1 minute, and then remove any excess solution with absorbent tissue to decrease the amount of drug reaching the systemic circulation even further.

BREASTFEEDING SUMMARY

No reports describing the use of ciprofloxacin ophthalmic during human lactation have been located. Ciprofloxacin has been found in breast milk. But the amount seen with ocular use is likely to be clinically insignificant. Breastfeeding while using this drug should be based on the mother's clinical need for treatment versus any potential infant risks that might occur. Due to very low blood levels seen with topical ocular use, systemic adverse reactions were not recorded. A method to decrease some systemic absorption with ophthalmic use is described above in the Pregnancy Summary.

References

1. Prescribing Information. *Ciprofloxacin Ophthalmic*. Altaire Pharmaceuticals; 2019.
2. Polachek H, Holcberg G, Sapir G, et al. Transfer of ciprofloxacin, ofloxacin and levofloxacin across the perfused human placenta in vitro. *Eur J Obstet Gynecol Reprod Biol*. 2005;122:61-65.
3. Giamarellou H, Kolokythas E, Petrikkos G, et al. Pharmacokinetics of three newer quinolones in pregnant and lactating women. *Am J Med*. 1989; 87(suppl 5A):49S-51S.
4. Cover DL, Mueller BA. Ciprofloxacin penetration into human breast milk: a case report. *Ann Pharmacother*. 1990;24:703-704.
5. Gardner DK, Gabbe SG, Harter C. Simultaneous concentrations of ciprofloxacin in breast milk and in serum in mother and breast-fed infant. *Clin Pharm*. 1992;11:352-354.

CISPLATIN

Antineoplastic (Alkylating—Platinum-Based)

PREGNANCY RECOMMENDATION: Limited Human Data—Animal Data Suggest Risk

BREASTFEEDING RECOMMENDATION: Potential Toxicity

PREGNANCY SUMMARY

One case report describes the use of cisplatin in the first trimester, and no anomalies were identified. In a second study, there were 14 women who reported having used combination chemotherapies at around the time of conception, and with the long elimination half-life of cisplatin, some embryos were probably exposed. No anomalies were described at delivery. Several other case reports exist involving the successful use of the drug in the second and third trimesters without any adverse effects related to the drug being identified. The drug crosses the placenta, so some fetal exposure will occur. However, this limited human pregnancy experience prevents a complete assessment of the embryofetal risk. Animal studies did show embryofetal toxicity with malformations in two species at doses less than 10 times the RHD; however, they were administered daily for several days, which is different than how it is used in human administration. Based on animal studies and the drug's mechanism of action, the manufacturer recommends that women with reproductive potential use effective contraception during treatment and for 1 week after the last dose. They also recommend that males with female partners of reproductive potential use effective contraception during treatment and for 1 week after the last dose. Nevertheless, using this drug during pregnancy should be based on the pros and cons of the mother's clinical need for treatment versus any potential fetal risk that might occur from exposure. Nevertheless, using this drug during pregnancy should be based on the pros and cons of the mother's clinical need for treatment versus any potential fetal risk that might occur from exposure. The primary unknown concern with the use of this drug is the long-term effects of platinum, which can be found in a person's system for many months (if not longer) once the chemotherapy treatment protocol is complete. There is a registry for women who are pregnant and have cancer. For more information, women and health care providers are encouraged to contact the Cancer and Pregnancy Registry at 1-877-635-4499.

C

BREASTFEEDING SUMMARY

Several case reports have been located that describe the use of cisplatin during human breastfeeding. Of 11 lactating women, the drug was detected in 8 with a peak level of about 5.5 mcg/mL. The remaining values ranged from about 7 to 800 ng/mL. However, the drug level in human breast milk did not appear to correlate with the maternal dose administered. In addition, some studies analyzed cisplatin levels and others just platinum levels. The calculated RIDs were all under 10% except for one. Due to a concern for potential serious adverse effects that might be seen in a breastfed infant, the manufacturer recommends that women not breastfeed while being treated with this drug. Nevertheless, breastfeeding while using this drug should be based on the mother's clinical need for treatment versus any potential infant risks that might occur. If used, the infant should be monitored for the most common reported adult side effects of nausea and abdominal pain (both leading to irritability), vomiting, diarrhea, lethargy, alopecia, decreased appetite, and various laboratory abnormalities (see PI). The primary concern is whether or not platinum by itself is harmful or if it has any long-term effects. Regardless, the infant's exposure would come through oral exposure, where the drug is poorly absorbed.

References

1. Product information. *Cisplatin*. West-Ward Pharmaceuticals; 2018.
2. Diwan BA, Anderson LM, Ward JM, et al. Transplacental carcinogenesis by cisplatin in F344/NCr rats: promotion of kidney tumors by postnatal administration of sodium barbital. *Toxicol Appl Pharmacol*. 1995;132:115-121.
3. Giurgiovich AJ, Diwan BA, Lee KB, Anderson LM, Rice JM, Poirier MC. Cisplatin-DNA adduct formation in maternal and fetal rat tissues after transplacental cisplatin exposure. *Carcinogenesis*. 1996;17:1665-1669.
4. Kinkead T, Flores C, Carboni AA, et al. Short term effects of cis-platinum on male reproduction, fertility and pregnancy outcome. *J Urol*. 1992;147:201-206.
5. Jacobs AJ, Marchevsky A, Gordon RE, et al. Oat cell carcinoma of the uterine cervix in a pregnant woman treated with cis-diamminedichloroplatinum. *Gynecol Oncol*. 1980;9:405-410.
6. Malone JM, Gershenson DM, Creasy RK, et al. Endodermal sinus tumor of the ovary associated with pregnancy. *Obstet Gynecol*. 1986;68(suppl):86S-89S.
7. Raffles A, Williams J, Costeloe K, Clark P. Transplacental effects of maternal cancer chemotherapy: case report. *Br J Obstet Gynaecol*. 1989;96:1099-1100.
8. Malfetano JH, Goldkrand JW. Cis-platinum combination chemotherapy during pregnancy for advanced epithelial ovarian carcinoma. *Obstet Gynecol*. 1990;75:545-547.
9. King LA, Nevin PC, Williams PP, Carson LF. Treatment of advanced epithelial ovarian carcinoma in pregnancy with cisplatin-based chemotherapy. *Gynecol Oncol*. 1991;41:78-80.
10. Buller RE, Darrow V, Manetta A, et al. Conservative surgical management of dysgerminoma concomitant with pregnancy. *Obstet Gynecol*. 1992;79:887-890.
11. Henderson CE, Elia G, Garfinkel D, et al. Platinum chemotherapy during pregnancy for serous cystadenocarcinoma of the ovary. *Gynecol Oncol*. 1993;49:92-94.
12. Giacalone P-L, Laffargue F, Benos P, et al. Cis-platinum neoadjuvant chemotherapy in a pregnant woman with invasive carcinoma of the uterine cervix. *Br J Obstet Gynaecol*. 1996;103:932-934.
13. Tomlinson MW, Treadwell MC, Deppe G. Platinum based chemotherapy to treat recurrent Sertoli-Leydig cell ovarian carcinoma during pregnancy. *Eur J Gynaecol Oncol*. 1997;18:44-46.
14. Janne PA, Rodriguez-Thompson D, Metcalf DR, et al. Chemotherapy for a patient with advanced non-small-cell lung cancer during pregnancy: a case report and a review of chemotherapy treatment during pregnancy. *Oncology*. 2001;61:175-183.
15. Ferrandina G, Distefano M, Testa A, et al. Management of an advance ovarian cancer at 15 weeks of gestation: case report and literature review. *Gynecol Oncol*. 2005;97:693-696.
16. Motegi M, Takakura S, Takano H, et al. Adjuvant chemotherapy in a pregnant woman with endodermal sinus tumor the ovary. *Obstet Gynecol*. 2007;109:537-540.
17. Kim JH, Kim HS, Sung CW, et al. Docetaxel, gemcitabine, and cisplatin administered for non-small cell lung cancer during the first and second trimester of an unrecognized pregnancy. *Lung Cancer*. 2008;59:270-273.
18. Rouzi AA, Sahly NN, Sahly NF, Alahwal MS. Cisplatinum and docetaxel for ovarian cancer in pregnancy. *Arch Gynecol Obstet*. 2009;280:823-825.
19. Gershenson DM. Menstrual and reproductive function after treatment with combination chemotherapy for malignant ovarian germ cell tumors. *J Clin Oncol*. 1988;6:270-275.
20. Bakri Y, Pedersen P, Nassar M. Normal pregnancy after curative multiagent chemotherapy for choriocarcinoma with brain metastases. *Acta Obstet Gynecol Scand*. 1991;70:611-613.
21. Green DM, Zevon MA, Lowrie G, et al. Congenital anomalies in children of patients who received chemotherapy for cancer in childhood and adolescence. *N Engl J Med*. 1991;325:141-146.
22. Bower M, Fife K, Holden L, et al. Chemotherapy for ovarian germ cell tumours. *Eur J Cancer*. 1996;32A:593-597.
23. Rubery ED. Return of fertility after curative chemotherapy for disseminated teratoma of testis. *Lancet*. 1983;1:186.
24. Egan PC, Costanza ME, Dodion P, et al. Doxorubicin and cisplatin excretion into human milk. *Cancer Treat Rep*. 1985;69:1387-1389.
25. De Vries EGE, Van Der Zee AGJ, Uges DRA, Sleijfer DTH. Excretion of platinum into breast milk. *Lancet*. 1989;1:497.
26. Ben-Baruch G, Menczer J, Goshen R, et al. Cisplatin excretion in human milk. *J Natl Cancer Inst*. 1992;84:451-452.

CITALOPRAM

Mental Health (Antidepressant—SSRI)

PREGNANCY RECOMMENDATION: Human Data Suggest Risk (Third Trimester)

BREASTFEEDING RECOMMENDATION: Potential Toxicity

PREGNANCY SUMMARY

Numerous studies have reported the use of citalopram during human pregnancy. In the combined data of about 280 first-trimester exposures, there were 9 (3.2%) major anomalies identified. No pattern to the defects was seen. In a large study of more than 2,500 first-trimester exposures to citalopram, no increased risk for cardiac anomalies was seen. In three large literature reviews, no increased risk for teratogenicity was found for the selective serotonin reuptake inhibitor (SSRI) drugs as a whole, except for possibly paroxetine. The drug will cross the placenta, so fetal exposure will occur. Regarding third-trimester use, several studies were located that described neonates who showed signs of withdrawal (apnea, tremor, feeding difficulties, vomiting, hypotonia, hypertonia, and cyanosis) postdelivery, and some were reported to have seizures. Using this drug during pregnancy should be based on the pros and cons of the mother's clinical need for treatment versus any potential fetal risk that might occur from exposure. There is a pregnancy exposure registry that monitors pregnancy outcomes in women using antidepressant drugs. Health care providers are encouraged to call the National Pregnancy Registry for Antidepressants at 1-844-405-6185.

C

BREASTFEEDING SUMMARY

Numerous studies have evaluated citalopram use during human breastfeeding. A total of about 60 women have been studied, and the drug was found in nearly every provided sample. The levels ranged from about 40 ng/mL to about 450 ng/mL. Most of the calculated RIDs ranged from about 2.5% to 9%, but a few exceeded 10%. However, infant serum levels have also been studied in nearly 40 newborns. The infant levels ranged from undetectable to about 13 ng/mL. These levels were only about 1% to about 10% the maternal values. Breastfeeding while using this drug should be based on the mother's clinical need for treatment versus any potential infant risks that might occur. If used, the infant should be monitored for the most common reported adult side effects of nausea, dizziness, and headache (all leading to irritability), lethargy, drowsiness, sweating, constipation, and rash. A few reports exist of newborns showing signs of withdrawal postdelivery.

References

1. Product information. *Celexa*. Allergan USA; 2019.
2. Shuey DL, Sadler TW, Lauder JM. Serotonin as a regulator of craniofacial morphogenesis: site specific malformations following exposure to serotonin uptake inhibitors. *Teratology*. 1992;46:367-378.
3. Heikkinen T, Ekblad U, Laine K. Transplacental transfer of citalopram, fluoxetine and their primary demethylated metabolites in isolated perfused human placenta. *BJOG*. 2002;109:1003-1008.
4. Hendrick V, Stowe ZN, Altshuler LL, et al. Placental passage of antidepressant medications. *Am J Psychiatry*. 2003;160:993-996.
5. Heikkinen T, Ekblad U, Kero P, et al. Citalopram in pregnancy and lactation. *Clin Pharmacol Ther*. 2002;72:184-191.
6. Seifritz E, Holsboer-Trachsler E, Haberthur F, et al. Unrecognized pregnancy during citalopram treatment. *Am J Psychiatry*. 1993;150:1428-1429.
7. Nordeng H, Lindemann R, Perminov KV, Reikvam A. Neonatal withdrawal syndrome after *in utero* exposure to selective serotonin reuptake inhibitors. *Acta Paediatr*. 2001;90:288-291.
8. Zeskind PS, Stephens LE. Maternal selective serotonin reuptake inhibitor use during pregnancy and newborn neurobehavior. *Pediatrics*. 2004;113:368-375.
9. Hendrick V, Smith LM, Suri R, et al. Birth outcomes after prenatal exposure to antidepressant medication. *Am J Obstet Gynecol*. 2003;188:812-815.
10. DeMyer W. Brain, midline caves. In: Buyse ML, ed. *Birth Defects Encyclopedia*. Blackwell Scientific Publications; 1990:238.
11. Sanz EJ, De-las-Cuevas C, Kiuru A, Edwards R. Selective serotonin reuptake inhibitors in pregnant women and neonatal withdrawal syndrome: a database analysis. *Lancet*. 2005;365:482-487.
12. Moses-Kolko EL, Bogen D, Perel J, et al. Neonatal signs after late in utero exposure to serotonin reuptake inhibitors. *JAMA*. 2005;293:2372-2383.
13. Oberlander TF, Warburton W, Misri S, et al. Neonatal outcomes after prenatal exposure to selective serotonin reuptake inhibitor antidepressants and maternal depression using population-based linked health data. *Arch Gen Psychiatry*. 2006;63:898-906.
14. Levinson-Castiel R, Merlob P, Linder N, et al. Neonatal abstinence syndrome after in utero exposure to selective serotonin reuptake inhibitors in term infants. *Arch Pediatr Adoles Med*. 2006;160:173-176.
15. Sivojelezova A, Shuhaiber S, Sarkissian L, et al. Citalopram use in pregnancy: prospective comparative evaluation of pregnancy and fetal outcome. *Am J Obstet Gynecol*. 2005;193:2004-2009.
16. Rahimi R, Nikfar S, Abdollahi M. Pregnancy outcomes following exposure to serotonin reuptake inhibitors: a meta-analysis of clinical trials. *Reprod Toxicol*. 2006;22:571-575.
17. Alwan S, Reefhuis J, Rasmussen S, et al. Maternal use of selective serotonin reuptake inhibitors and risk for birth defects (abstract). *Birth Defects Res (Part A)*. 2005;73:291.
18. Ericson A, Kallen B, Wiholm BE. Delivery outcome after the use of antidepressants in early pregnancy. *Eur J Clin Pharmacol*. 1999;55:503-508.
19. Kallen B, Olausson PO. Antidepressant drugs during pregnancy and infant congenital heart defect. *Reprod Toxicol*. 2006;21:221-222.
20. Kallen BAJ, Olausson PO. Maternal use of selective serotonin re-uptake inhibitors in early pregnancy and infant congenital malformations. *Birth Defects Res (Part A)*. 2007;79:301-308.
21. Berard A, Ramos E, Rey E, et al. First trimester exposure to paroxetine and risk of cardiac malformations in infants: the importance of dosage. *Birth Defects Res (Part B)*. 2007;80:18-27.
22. Ferreira E, Carceller AM, Agogue C, et al. Effects of selective serotonin reuptake inhibitors and venlafaxine during pregnancy in term and preterm neonates. *Pediatrics*. 2007;119:52-59.
23. Bellantuono C, Migliarese G, Gentile S. Serotonin reuptake inhibitors in pregnancy and the risk of major malformations: a systematic review. *Hum Psychopharmacol Clin Exp*. 2007;22:121-128.
24. Chambers CD, Hernandez-Diaz S, Van Marter LJ, et al. Selective serotonin-reuptake inhibitors and risk of persistent pulmonary hypertension of the newborn. *N Engl J Med*. 2006;354:579-587.
25. Alwan S, Reefhuis J, Rasmussen SA, et al; National Birth Defects Prevention Study. Use of selective serotonin-reuptake inhibitors in pregnancy and the risk of birth defects. *N Engl J Med*. 2007;356:2684-2692.
26. Louik C, Lin AE, Werler MM, et al. First-trimester use of selective serotonin-reuptake inhibitors and the risk of birth defects. *N Engl J Med*. 2007;356:2675-2683.
27. Greene MF. Teratogenicity of SSRIs—serious concern or much ado about little? *N Engl J Med*. 2007;356:2732-2733.
28. Einarson A, Choi J, Einarson TR, Koren G. Incidence of major malformations in infants following antidepressant exposure in pregnancy: results of a large prospective cohort study. *Can J Psychiatry*. 2009;54:242-246.
29. Nordeng H, van Gelder HJ, Spigset O, et al. Pregnancy outcome after exposure to antidepressants and the role of maternal depression: results from the Norwegian mother and child cohort study. *J Clin Psychopharmacol*. 2012;32:186-194.
30. Spigset O, Carleborg L, Ohman R, Norstrom A. Excretion of citalopram in breast milk. *Br J Clin Pharmacol*. 1997;44:295-298.
31. Jensen PN, Olesen OV, Bertelsen A, Linnet K. Citalopram and desmethylcitalopram concentrations in breast milk and in serum of mother and infant. *Ther Drug Monit*. 1997;19:236-239.
32. Rampono J, Kristensen JH, Hackett LP, et al. Citalopram and demethylcitalopram in human milk; distribution, excretion and effects in breast fed infants. *Br J Clin Pharmacol*. 2000;50:263-268.
33. Schmidt K, Olesen OV, Jensen PN. Citalopram and breast-feeding: serum concentration and side effects in the infant. *Biol Psychiatry*. 2000;47:164-165.
34. Lee A, Woo J, Ito S. Frequency of infant adverse events that are associated with citalopram use during breast-feeding. *Am J Obstet Gynecol*. 2004;190:218-221.
35. Berle JO, Steen VM, Aamo TO, et al. Breastfeeding during maternal antidepressant treatment with serotonin reuptake inhibitors: infant exposure, clinical symptoms, and cytochrome P450 genotypes. *J Clin Psychiatry*. 2004;65:1228-1234.
36. Marshall AM, Nommsen-Rivers LA, Hernandez LI, et al. Serotonin transport and metabolism in the mammary gland modulates secretory activation and involution. *J Clin Endocrinol Metab*. 2010;95:837-846.
37. Edwards JG, Anderson I. Systematic review and guide to selection of selective serotonin reuptake inhibitors. *Drugs*. 1999;57:507-533.

C

CLADRIBINE

Antineoplastic (Antimetabolite)

PREGNANCY RECOMMENDATION: Limited Human Data—Animal Data Suggest Risk

BREASTFEEDING RECOMMENDATION: Potential Toxicity

PREGNANCY SUMMARY

Two studies have reported the use of cladribine in the treatment of multiple sclerosis around the time of pregnancy. No confirmed pregnancy outcome data could be found in cases with confirmed use during the first trimester. A total of about 18 exposures to cladribine within the 6 months prior to the last menstrual period (LMP) were described, and there was 1 major anomaly identified. Six months was chosen due to the potential for genotoxicity. However, with an elimination half-life of about 5.5 hours, the drug would be mostly cleared from the patient's system within about 28 to 33 hours (5 to 6 half-lives). Another case report described the use of cladribine in treating a pregnant woman with hairy cell leukemia at about 32 weeks' gestation. She delivered a healthy newborn at term. The drug will probably cross the placenta, so some fetal exposure will likely occur. However, this limited human pregnancy experience prevents a complete assessment of the embryofetal risk. Animal studies did show some embryofetal toxicity in two species at doses of less than 10 times the RHD. Based on animal studies and the drug's mechanism of action, the manufacturer recommends that women with reproductive potential use effective contraception during treatment. Nevertheless, using this drug during pregnancy should be based on the pros and cons of the mother's clinical need for treatment versus any potential fetal risk that might occur from exposure.

BREASTFEEDING SUMMARY

A total of three women have had breast milk evaluated while using cladribine. In all three cases, the drug was found in breast milk. The calculated average RIDs ranged from about 2.3% to 4.7%. Due to a concern for potential serious adverse effects that might be seen in a breastfed infant, the manufacturer recommends that women not breastfeed while being treated with this drug. Nevertheless, breastfeeding while using this drug should be based on the mother's clinical need for treatment versus any potential infant risks that might occur. If used, the infant should be monitored for the most common reported adult side effects of nausea and headache (both leading to irritability), diarrhea, fatigue (lethargy), fever, rash, and decreased appetite.

References

1. Robak T. Current treatment options in hairy cell leukemia and hairy cell leukemia variant. *Cancer Treat Rev*. 2006;32:365-376.
2. Product information. *Cladribine*. Mylan Institutional; 2018.
3. Alothman A, Sparling TG. Managing hairy cell leukemia in pregnancy. *Ann Intern Med*. 1994;120:1048-1049.
4. Orlowski RZ. Successful pregnancy after cladribine therapy for hairy cell leukemia. *Leuk Lymphoma*. 2004;45:187-188.
5. Daver N, Nazha A, Kantarjian HM, et al. Treatment of hairy cell leukemia during pregnancy: are purine analogues and rituximab viable therapeutic options. *Clin Lymphoma Myeloma Leuk*. 2013;13:86-89.

CLARITHROMYCIN

Antibacterial (Macrolide)

PREGNANCY RECOMMENDATION: Human Data Suggest Low Risk

BREASTFEEDING RECOMMENDATION: Probably Compatible

PREGNANCY SUMMARY

From several studies, there were 6 (1.8%) major anomalies found in 328 first-trimester exposures to clarithromycin in the first trimester of pregnancy. Other studies on the macrolide antibiotics as a group have reported congenital birth defect rates between 3% and 4%. In addition, no pattern to the anomalies has been identified. The drug appears to cross the placenta, so some fetal exposure will likely occur. Animal studies showed embryofetal toxicity in three species, but in one, the dose was more than 10 times the RHD, and in another, maternal toxicity occurred. In a fourth species, no embryofetal toxicity was seen at doses of less than 10 times the RHD. Using this drug during pregnancy should be based on the pros and cons of the mother's clinical need for treatment versus any potential fetal risk that might occur from exposure.

BREASTFEEDING SUMMARY

The drug has been studied in human lactation. In 12 women who were administered 250 mg twice a day, the drug was found in every sample, with a peak level obtained of about 0.85 mcg/mL. The calculated RID was about 1.8%. In a separate case report, a lactating woman was administered one 500 mg dose, resulting in a peak breast milk level of about

3.7 mcg/mL. This resulted in a RID of about 6.2%. The calculated RID using the average milk level was only 1.2%. In earlier studies, there was a concern that the use of clarithromycin during breastfeeding increased the risk for hypertrophic pyloric stenosis in the infant. However, two meta-analyses did not find this association. Breastfeeding while using this drug should be based on the mother's clinical need for treatment versus any potential infant risks that might occur. If used, the infant should be monitored for the most common reported adult side effects of dizziness and abdominal pain (both leading to irritability), diarrhea, vomiting, and rash. In addition, any antibacterial drug can alter the newborn's normal gastrointestinal tract flora.

References

1. Product information. *Clarithromycin*. Estreno Pharmaceuticals; 2019.
2. Witt A, Sommer EM, Cichna M, et al. Placental transfer of clarithromycin surpasses other macrolide antibiotics. *Am J Obstet Gynecol*. 2003;188: 816-819.
3. Schick B, Hom M, Librizzi R, Donnenfeld A. Pregnancy outcome following exposure to clarithromycin (abstract). Abstracts presented at: Ninth International Conference of the Organization of Teratology Information Services; May 2–4, 1996; Salt Lake City, UT. *Reprod Toxicol*. 1996;10:162.
4. Escobar LF, Weaver DD. Charge association. In: Buyse ML, ed. *Birth Defects Encyclopedia: Vol. 1*. Center for Birth Defects Information Services; 1990:308-309.
5. Einarson A, Phillips E, Mawji F, et al. A prospective controlled multicentre study of clarithromycin in pregnancy. *Am J Perinatol*. 1998;15:523-525.
6. Bar-Oz B, Diav-Citrin O, Shechtman S, et al. Pregnancy outcome after gestational exposure to the new macrolides: a prospective multi-center observational study. *Eur J Obstet Gynecol Reprod Biol*. 2008;141:31-34.
7. Bar-Oz B, Weber-Schoendorfer C, Berlin M, et al. The outcomes of pregnancy in women exposed to the new macrolides in the first trimester: a prospective, multicentre, observational study. *Drug Saf*. 2012;35:589-598.
8. -Jacoby EB, Porter KB. *Helicobacter pylori* infection and persistent hyperemesis gravidarum. *Am J Perinatol*. 1999;16:85-88.
9. Tellem R, Shechtman S, Arnon J, et al. Pregnancy outcome after gestational exposure to the new macrolides: a prospective controlled cohort study (abstract). *Reprod Toxicol*. 2005;20:484.
10. Sorensen HT, Skriver MV, Pedersen L, et al. Risk of infantile hypertrophic pyloric stenosis after maternal postnatal use of macrolides. *Scand J Infect Dis*. 2003;35:104-106.
11. Sedimayr TH, Peters F, Raasch W, Kees F. Clarithromycin, a new macrolide antibiotic: effectiveness in puerperal infections and pharmacokinetics in breast milk. *Geburtshilfe Frauenheilkd*. 1993;53:488-491.
12. Goldstein LH, Berlin M, Tsur L, et al. The safety of macrolides during lactation. *Breastfeed Med*. 2009;4:157-200.

CLASCOTERONE

Androgen Receptor Inhibitor (Topical Skin Product)

PREGNANCY RECOMMENDATION: *No Human Data—Animal Data Suggest Low Risk

BREASTFEEDING RECOMMENDATION: Probably Compatible

PREGNANCY SUMMARY

No reports describing the use of clascoterone in human pregnancy have been located. The drug will probably cross the placenta; however, fetal exposure is probably negligible. Animal data, overall, did not show any embryofetal toxicity, even when administered subcutaneously. However, the absence of human pregnancy experience prevents a complete assessment of the embryofetal risk. *Based on drug indication, use during pregnancy is uncertain.

BREASTFEEDING SUMMARY

Clascoterone probably enters breast milk. However, because the drug is for topical use with low plasma levels found following systemic absorption, the total drug amount found in breast milk is likely to be negligible. Breastfeeding while using clascoterone should be based on the mother's clinical need for treatment.

Reference

1. Prescribing Information. *Winlevi*. Sun Pharmaceuticals Industries, Ltd; 2020.

CLAVULANATE POTASSIUM

Anti-Infective (β-Lactamase Inhibitor)

PREGNANCY RECOMMENDATION: Human Data Suggest Low Risk

BREASTFEEDING RECOMMENDATION: Probably Compatible

PREGNANCY SUMMARY

Two studies were located that described the use of clavulanic acid with amoxicillin in the first trimester. Of 714 exposures, there were 27 (3.8%) major anomalies. No pattern to the defects was identified. Combination antibiotics with clavulanate

(*continued*)

C

have been used in the second and third trimesters for preterm premature rupture of the membranes and other infections without any major adverse reactions related to the drug being reported. The drug crosses the placenta, so some fetal exposure will occur. Animal studies did not show any embryofetal toxicity in two species at doses of less than 10 times the RHD. Using this drug during pregnancy should be based on the pros and cons of the mother's clinical need for treatment versus any potential fetal risk that might occur from exposure.

BREASTFEEDING SUMMARY

No reports describing maternal milk levels for clavulanate potassium have been located. A few studies have evaluated infant response to the combination of clavulanic acid with other antibiotics; no major adverse reactions were reported. The drug, in combination with ampicillin, can alter infant bowel flora, leading to diarrhea. Breastfeeding while using this drug should be based on the mother's clinical need for treatment versus any potential infant risks that might occur. If used, the infant should be monitored for the most common reported adult side effects of nausea, headache, pruritus, and abdominal pain (all leading to irritability), diarrhea, and rash.

References

1. Product information. *Amoxicillin and Clavulanate Potassium*. Micro Labs; 2019.
2. Baldwin JA, Schardein JL, Koshima Y. Reproduction studies of BRL14151K and BRL25000. I. Teratology studies in rats. *Chemotherapy (Tokyo)*. 1983;31(suppl 2):238-251.
3. Baldwin JA, Schardein JL, Koshima Y. Reproduction studies of BRL14151K and BRL25000. II. Peri-and post-natal studies in rats. *Chemotherapy (Tokyo)*. 1983;31(suppl 2):252-262.
4. Hirakawa T, Suzuki T, Sano Y, et al. Reproduction studies of BRL14151K and BRL25000. III. Fertility studies in rats. *Chemotherapy (Tokyo)*. 1983;31(suppl 2):263-272.
5. James PA, Hardy TL, Koshima Y. Reproduction studies of BRL 25000. IV. Teratology in pig. *Chemotherapy (Tokyo)*. 1983;31(suppl 2):274-279.
6. Tasker TCG, Cockburn A, Jackson D, et al. Safety of ticarcillin/potassium clavulanate. *J Antimicrob Chemother*. 1986;17:225-232.
7. Matsuda S, Tanno M, Kashiwagura T, Seida A. Fundamental and clinical studies on BRL25000 (clavulanic acid-amoxicillin) in the field of obstetrics and gynecology. *Chemotherapy (Tokyo)*. 1982;30(suppl 2):538-547.
8. Takase Z, Shirafuji H, Uchida M. Clinical and laboratory studies on BRL25000 (clavulanic acid-amoxicillin) in the field of obstetrics and gynecology. *Chemotherapy (Tokyo)*. 1982;30(suppl 2):579-586.
9. Fortunato SJ, Bawdon RE, Swan KF, et al. Transfer of Timentin (ticarcillin and clavulanic acid) across the in vitro perfused human placenta: comparison with other agents. *Am J Obstet Gynecol*. 1992;167:1595-1599.
10. Matsuda S. Augmentin treatment in obstetrics and gynaecology. In: Leigh DA, Robinson OPW, eds. *Augmentin: Proceedings of an International Symposium, Montreux, Switzerland. July 1981*. Excerpta Medica; 1982:179-191.
11. Mayer HO, Jeschek H, Kowatsch A. Augmentin in the treatment of urinary tract infection in pregnant women and pelvic inflammatory disease. In: Croydon EAP, Michel MF, eds. *Proceedings of the European Symposium on Augmentin, Scheveningen, June 1982*. Excerpta Medica; 1983:207-217.
12. Pedler SJ, Bint AJ. Comparative study of amoxicillin-clavulanic acid and cephalexin in the treatment of bacteriuria during pregnancy. *Antimicrob Agents Chemother*. 1985;27:508-510.
13. Kenyon SL, Taylor DJ, Tarnow-Mordi W; ORACLE Collaborative Group. Broad-spectrum antibiotics for preterm, prelabour rupture of fetal membranes: the ORACLE I randomised trial. *Lancet*. 2001;357:979-988.
14. Lovett SM, Weiss JD, Diogo MJ, et al. A prospective, double-blind, randomized, controlled clinical trial of ampicillin-sulbactam for preterm premature rupture of membranes in women receiving antenatal corticosteroid therapy. *Am J Obstet Gynecol*. 1997;176:1030-1038.
15. Berkovitch M, Diav-Citrin O, Greenberg R, et al. First-trimester exposure to amoxycillin/clavulanic acid: a prospective, controlled study. *Br J Clin Pharmacol*. 2004;58:298-302.
16. Campbell AC, McLeay JC, Passmore CM. The excretion of ampicillin in breast milk and its effect on the suckling infant (Abstract). *Br J Clin Pharmacol*. 1991;31:230.
17. Benyamini L, Merlob P, Stahl B, et al. The safety of amoxicillin/clavulanic acid and cefuroxime during lactation. *Ther Drug Monit*. 2005;27:499-502.
18. Cherif F, Aidli S, Kastalli S, et al. Drug induced urticaria via breastfeeding (Abstract). *Fundam Clin Pharmacol*. 2009;23(suppl 1):203. doi:10.1111/j.1472-8206.2009.00689.x.

CLEMASTINE

Antihistamine (H_1 Antagonist)

PREGNANCY RECOMMENDATION: Human Data Suggest Compatible

BREASTFEEDING RECOMMENDATION: Potential Toxicity

PREGNANCY SUMMARY

In a surveillance study of Michigan Medicaid recipients, 1,617 newborns had been exposed to clemastine during the first trimester. A total of 71 (4.4%) major birth defects were found (68 expected). However, no specific pattern was noted, and coexposures to other drugs were not described. A second study, regarding data from the Swedish Medical Birth Registry, reported on a total of 18,197 births from women who used antihistamine drugs (for nausea and vomiting of pregnancy or for allergy treatment) during early pregnancy out of 403,545 delivered infants. There were 1,230 pregnant women who used clemastine in the antihistamine group. The birth anomaly rate in the antihistamine group was 3.17%; this was no different from the 3.16% rate for the entire population. Specific data on the patients who were only using clemastine was not provided. In addition, the birth anomaly rate in the clemastine group when the drug was only used for allergy treatment was 3.20%. Again, this was no different from the 3.16% birth anomaly rate of the entire population, but again, specific numbers were not described. The drug will probably cross the placenta, so some fetal exposure will likely occur. Animal studies did not show any embryofetal toxicity or teratogenicity in two species at doses of more than 10 times the RHD. Using this drug during pregnancy should be based on the pros and cons of the mother's clinical need for treatment versus any potential fetal risk that might occur from exposure.

C

BREASTFEEDING SUMMARY

In one case report, clemastine was found to be excreted into human breast milk with a mean level of about 5 to 10 ng/mL at 20 hours after the last dose. The maternal plasma level was 20 ng/mL. The drug could not be detected in the infant's plasma. The calculated RID was 4.5%. The 10-week-old girl developed drowsiness, irritability, refusal to feed, neck stiffness, and a high-pitched cry 12 hours after the mother began taking the antihistamine at a dose of 1 mg twice daily. She was also taking phenytoin and carbamazepine. Symptoms in the baby resolved within 24 hours after the drug was stopped. It is unknown if these symptoms were related to clemastine or to the combination of drugs. Breastfeeding while using this drug should be based on the mother's clinical need for treatment versus any potential infant risks that might occur. If used, the infant should be monitored for the most common reported adult side effects of nausea, headache, and dizziness (all leading to irritability), sedation, diarrhea, lethargy, vomiting, dry mouth, and rash. Because of the drug's anticholinergic effects, there is the possibility of interfering with milk production in the early stages of breastfeeding, as well as decreasing milk supply with long-term use.

References

1. Prescribing Information. *Clemastine Fumarate*. Teva Pharmaceuticals USA; 2018.
2. Kallen B. Use of antihistamine drugs in early pregnancy and delivery outcome. *J Matern Fetal Neonatal Med*. 2002;11:146-152.
3. Kok TH, Taitz LS, Bennett MJ, Holt DW. Drowsiness due to clemastine transmitted in breast milk. *Lancet*. 1982;139(8277):914-915.

CLEVIDIPINE

Antihypertensive (Calcium Channel Blocker)

PREGNANCY RECOMMENDATION: No Human Data—Animal Data Suggest Risk

BREASTFEEDING RECOMMENDATION: Potential Toxicity

PREGNANCY SUMMARY

No reports describing the use of clevidipine in human pregnancy have been located. The drug will probably cross the placenta, so some fetal exposure will likely occur. Therefore, the absence of human pregnancy experience prevents a complete assessment of the embryofetal risk. Animal studies did show embryofetal toxicity in two species at doses less than 10 times the RHD. Using this drug during pregnancy should be based on the pros and cons of the mother's clinical need for treatment versus any potential fetal risk that might occur from exposure. However, for treating hypertension in pregnancy, ACOG recommends nifedipine (also a calcium channel blocker) and labetalol as first-line agents. Some β-blockers may cause IUGR. However, IUGR is also associated with hypertensive disorders in pregnancy. Although growth restriction is a serious concern, the benefits of maternal therapy with β-blockers, in some cases, might outweigh the risks to the fetus and must be judged on a case-by-case basis.

BREASTFEEDING SUMMARY

No reports describing the use of clevidipine during human lactation have been located. The drug will probably be found in breast milk, so some infant exposure will likely occur. Breastfeeding while using this drug should be based on the mother's clinical need for treatment versus any potential infant risks that might occur. If used, the infant should be monitored for the most common reported adult side effects of nausea and headache (both leading to irritability) and vomiting.

References

1. Prescribing Information. *Cleviprex*. Fresenius Kabi Austria GmbH; 2018.
2. American College of Obstetricians and Gynecologists. ACOG practice bulletin No. 203: chronic hypertension in pregnancy. *Obstet Gynecol*. 2019; 133:e26-e50.

CLIDINIUM

Autonomic (Anticholinergic)

PREGNANCY RECOMMENDATION: Limited Human Data—Animal Data Suggest Low Risk

BREASTFEEDING RECOMMENDATION: *Potential Toxicity

PREGNANCY SUMMARY

The Collaborative Perinatal Project reported first-trimester exposure to anticholinergic drugs in 2,323 patients, with 114 (4.9%) newborns identified who had malformations. However, no specific pattern was noted, and coexposures to other drugs were not described. Of these, only four used clidinium. The drug will probably cross the placenta, so some fetal exposure will likely

(continued)

C

occur. Therefore, the absence of human pregnancy experience prevents a complete assessment of the embryofetal risk. Animal studies for clidinium did not show any embryofetal toxicity in two species. Clidinium is only available in combination with chlordiazepoxide (an antianxiety medication—see Chlordiazepoxide). Using this drug during pregnancy should be based on the pros and cons of the mother's clinical need for treatment versus any potential fetal risk that might occur from exposure.

BREASTFEEDING SUMMARY

No reports describing the use of clidinium during human lactation have been located. The drug will probably be found in breast milk, so some infant exposure will likely occur. *However, the drug is only available in combination with chlordiazepoxide (an antianxiety medication). Therefore, breastfeeding while using this product should be based on the mother's clinical need for treatment versus any potential infant risks that might occur. If used, the infant should be monitored for the most common reported adult side effects of nausea and blurry vision (both leading to irritability), sedation, dry mouth, constipation, and rash. Because of the drug's anticholinergic effects, there is the possibility of interfering with breast milk production in the early stages of breastfeeding, as well as, decreasing breast milk supply with long-term use.

References

1. Prescribing Information. *Librax*. Aurobinda Pharma, Ltd; 2023.
2. Heinonen OP, Slone D, Shapiro S. *Birth Defects and Drugs in Pregnancy*. Wright PSB; 1983:347.

CLINDAMYCIN

Antibacterial (Lincosamide)

PREGNANCY RECOMMENDATION: Limited Human Data—Animal Data Suggest Low Risk

BREASTFEEDING RECOMMENDATION: Potential Toxicity

PREGNANCY SUMMARY

The Michigan Medicaid Surveillance study reported 647 first-trimester exposures to clindamycin, and 31 (4.8%) congenital anomalies were identified. No pattern to the defects was seen and no specific organ structure had elevated rates. Use of the drug has been reported in the second and third trimesters without any adverse effects related to the drug described. The drug crosses the placenta, so some fetal exposure will occur. Animal studies did not show any embryofetal toxicity or teratogenicity in two species at doses of less than 10 times the RHD. In a recent review of antibiotics in pregnancy, clindamycin was one of the drugs considered safe and effective in pregnancy. Using this drug during pregnancy should be based on the pros and cons of the mother's clinical need for treatment versus any potential fetal risk that might occur from exposure.

BREASTFEEDING SUMMARY

Several studies have been located that described the use of clindamycin during human lactation. A total of 26 lactating women were evaluated and the drug was found in every breast milk sample. Several calculated RIDs were obtained, and all were under 10% (the highest being about 9.1%). The drug has the potential to alter the gastrointestinal flora of the newborn if exposed to the drug through breastfeeding. One infant was found to have bloody stools when exposed to clindamycin and gentamicin from breastfeeding. Nevertheless, breastfeeding while using this drug should be based on the mother's clinical need for treatment versus any potential infant risks that might occur. If used, the infant should be monitored for the most common reported adult side effects of nausea, joint pain, and pruritus (all leading to irritability), vomiting, rash, and diarrhea.

References

1. Weinstein AJ, Gibbs RS, Gallagher M. Placental transfer of clindamycin and gentamicin in term pregnancy. *Am J Obstet Gynecol*. 1976;124:688-691.
2. Philipson A, Sabath LD, Charles D. Erythromycin and clindamycin absorption and elimination in pregnant women. *Clin Pharmacol Ther*. 1976;19:68-77.
3. Rehu M, Jahkola M. Prophylactic antibiotics in caesarean section: effect of a short preoperative course of benzyl penicillin or clindamycin plus gentamicin on postoperative infectious morbidity. *Ann Clin Res*. 1980;12:45-48.
4. Product information. *Clindamycin*. Sagent Pharmaceuticals; 2018.
5. Philipson A, Sabath LD, Charles D. Transplacental passage of erythromycin and clindamycin. *N Engl J Med*. 1973;288:1219-1221.
6. Gilstrap LC III, Bawdon RE, Burris J. Antibiotic concentration in maternal blood, cord blood, and placental membranes in chorioamnionitis. *Obstet Gynecol*. 1988;72:124-125.
7. Muanda FT, Sheehy O, Berard A. Use of antibiotics during pregnancy and the risk of major congenital malformations: a population based cohort study. *Br J Clin Pharmacol*. 2017;83:2557-2571.
8. McGregor JA, French JI, Seo K. Adjunctive clindamycin therapy for preterm labor: results of a double-blind, placebo-controlled trial. *Am J Obstet Gynecol*. 1991;165:867-875.
9. Ugwumadu A, Manyonda I, Reid F, Hay P. Effect of oral clindamycin on late miscarriage and preterm delivery in asymptomatic women with abnormal vaginal flora and bacterial vaginosis: a randomised controlled trial. *Lancet*. 2003;361:983-988.
10. Vermeulen GM, Bruinse HW. Prophylactic administration of clindamycin 2% vaginal cream to reduce the incidence of spontaneous preterm birth in women with an increased recurrence risk: a randomized placebo-controlled double-blind trial. *Br J Obstet Gynaecol*. 1999;106:652-657.
11. Kekki M, Turki T, Pelkonen J, et al. Vaginal clindamycin in preventing preterm birth and peripartal infections in asymptomatic women with bacterial vaginosis: a randomized, controlled trial. *Obstet Gynecol*. 2001;97:643-648.
12. Kurkinen-Raty M, Vuopala S, Koskela M, et al. A randomized controlled trial of vaginal clindamycin for early pregnancy bacterial vaginosis. *Br J Obstet Gynaecol*. 2000;107:1427-1432.
13. Lamont RF, Duncan SLB, Mandal D, Bassett P. Intravaginal clindamycin to reduce preterm birth in women with abnormal genital tract flora. *Obstet Gynecol*. 2003;101:516-522.

14. Bookstaver PB, Bland CM, Griffin B, et al. A review of antibiotic use in pregnancy. *Pharmacotherapy*. 2015;35:1052-1062.
15. Smith JA, Morgan JR, Rachlis AR, Papsin FR. Clindamycin in human breast milk. *Can Med Assoc J*. 1975;112:806.
16. Mann CF. Clindamycin and breast-feeding. *Pediatrics*. 1980;66:1030-1031.
17. American Academy of Pediatrics Committee on Drugs. The transfer of drugs and other chemicals into human milk. *Pediatrics*. 2001;108:776-789.
18. Wear CD, Towers CT, Brown MS, et al. Transplacental passage of clindamycin from mother to neonate. *J Perinatol*. 2016;36:960-961.

CLOBAZAM

Central Nervous System (Antiseizure)

PREGNANCY RECOMMENDATION: Limited Human Data—Animal Data Suggest Risk

BREASTFEEDING RECOMMENDATION: Potential Toxicity

PREGNANCY SUMMARY

There is limited information on the effects of clobazam use during human pregnancy. Nearly all studies have described the use of clobazam in combination therapy with other drugs, including other anticonvulsants. In one study that described the use of clobazam and lamotrigine in the first trimester, there was 1 neural tube defect (NTD) in 13 pregnancies (the other 12 had no identified anomalies). Overall, no pattern to any anomalies with the use of clobazam has been described, but again, the numbers are small. The drug crosses the placenta, so fetal exposure will occur. However, this limited human pregnancy experience prevents a complete assessment of the embryofetal risk. Animal studies did show embryofetal toxicity with malformations in two species at doses of less than the RHD. Using this drug during pregnancy should be based on the pros and cons of the mother's clinical need for treatment versus any potential fetal risk that might occur from exposure. The drug is a Schedule IV controlled substance and has the risk for dependence, misuse, and withdrawal. It carries a boxed warning for increased risks of profound sedation, respiratory depression, coma, and death with concomitant use with opioid drugs. There is a pregnancy exposure registry that monitors pregnancy outcomes in women using antiseizure drugs. Health care providers are encouraged to call the North American Antiepileptic Drug Pregnancy Registry at 1-888-233-2334.

BREASTFEEDING SUMMARY

Clobazam and the active metabolite have been shown to be excreted into human breast milk according to the manufacturer. This was also described in a review article. The calculated RIDs in these reports were less than 10%, but prolonged use of the drug during breastfeeding could result in higher infant levels. Due to a concern for potential serious adverse effects that might be seen in a breastfed infant, the manufacturer recommends that women not breastfeed while being treated with this drug. Nevertheless, breastfeeding while using this drug should be based on the mother's clinical need for treatment versus any potential infant risks that might occur. If used, the infant should be monitored for the most common reported adult side effects of somnolence, sedation, lethargy, constipation, and pyrexia.

References

1. Brodie MJ, Dichter MA. Established antiepileptic drugs. *Seizure*. 1997;6:159-174.
2. Product information. *Onfi*. Lundbeck Pharmaceuticals; 2018.
3. Pundey SK, Gupta S. Neuroembryopathic effect of clobazam in rat: a histological study. *Nepal Med Coll J*. 2005;7:10-12.
4. Nandakumaran M, Rey E, Helou A, et al. Materno-fetal placental transfer of clobazam and norclobazam in late gestation. *Dev Pharmacol Ther*. 1982;4(suppl 1):135-143.
5. Feely M, Gibson J. Intermittent clobazam for catamenial epilepsy: tolerance avoided. *J Neurol Neurosurg Psychiatry*. 1984;47:1279-1282.
6. Kulaga S, Sheehy O, Zargarzadeh AH, et al. Antiepileptic drug use during pregnancy: perinatal outcomes. *Seizure*. 2011;20:667-672.
7. *The Lamotrigine Pregnancy Registry: final report: 1 September 1992 through 31 March 2010*. GlaxoSmithKline; 2010.
8. Thomas SV, Jose M, Divakaran S, Sankara Sarma S. Malformation risk of antiepileptic drug exposure during pregnancy in women with epilepsy: results from a pregnancy registry in South India. *Epilepsia*. 2017;58:274-281.
9. Trivedi M, Jose M, Philip RM, et al. Spontaneous fetal loss in women with epilepsy: prospective data from pregnancy registry in India. *Epilepsy Res*. 2018;146:50-53.
10. Bar-Oz B, Nulman I, Koren G, Ito S. Anticonvulsants and breast feeding—a clinical review. *Paediatr Drugs*. 2000;2:113-126.
11. Hägg S, Spigset O. Anticonvulsant use during lactation. *Drug Saf*. 2000;22:425-440.

CLOBETASOL

Corticosteroid (Topical)

PREGNANCY RECOMMENDATION: Limited Human Data—No Relevant Animal Data

BREASTFEEDING RECOMMENDATION: Potential Toxicity

C

PREGNANCY SUMMARY

A few case reports have described the use of topical clobetasol during the second and third trimesters of human pregnancy for treating pemphigoid gestationis and other dermatoses. No adverse effects were described. The drug will probably cross the placenta, so some fetal exposure will likely occur. However, the amount that is absorbed systemically with topical use is not known. Therefore, this limited human pregnancy experience prevents a complete assessment of the embryofetal risk. Animal studies have not been conducted with any of the topical preparations. Using this drug during pregnancy should be based on the pros and cons of the mother's clinical need for treatment versus any potential fetal risk that might occur from exposure.

BREASTFEEDING SUMMARY

One case report of the use of topical clobetasol during human lactation was located. A nursing woman was being treated for pemphigoid gestationis and was eventually administered clobetasol ointment. She responded well and continued breastfeeding throughout treatment. Her infant was developing normally at 8 weeks of age and beyond. The drug will probably be found in breast milk, but the amount is unknown with topical use. Breastfeeding while using this drug should be based on the mother's clinical need for treatment versus any potential infant risks that might occur. If used, the infant should be monitored for the most common reported adult side effects of pruritus (leading to irritability), edema, nasopharyngitis, and upper respiratory tract infection. In addition, it is not recommended for use on or near the nipple area.

References

1. Prescribing Information. *Clobetasol (ointment)*. Alembic Pharmaceuticals, Inc; 2024.
2. Prescribing Information. *Clobex (lotion/shampoo)*. Galderma Laboratories; 2018.
3. Mairos JS, Veca CP, Ribeiro V. Herpes gestationis. *Acta Medica Portuguesa*. 2004;17:107-109.
4. Orsini G, Loizzi P, Morelli L, et al. Severe form of herpes gestationis. *Minerva Ginecol*. 2003;55:271-274.
5. de la Rosa Carrillo D. Vegetating Darier's disease during pregnancy. *Acta Derm Venereol*. 2006;86:259-260.
6. Elmuradi S, Ojeda D, Stoopler ET. Oral pemphigus vulgaris in pregnancy. *J Obstet Gynaecol Can*. 2015;36:951.
7. Westermann L, Hugel R, Meier M, et al. Glucocorticosteroid-resistant pemphigoid gestationis: successful treatment with adjuvant immunoadsorption. *J Dermatol*. 2012;39:168-171.

CLOFARABINE

Antineoplastic (Antimetabolite Purine Nucleoside)

PREGNANCY RECOMMENDATION: No Human Data—Animal Data Suggest Risk

BREASTFEEDING RECOMMENDATION: Potential Toxicity

PREGNANCY SUMMARY

No reports describing the use of clofarabine in human pregnancy have been located. The drug will probably cross the placenta, so some fetal exposure will likely occur. Therefore, the absence of human pregnancy experience prevents a complete assessment of the embryofetal risk. The drug was found to cause embryofetal toxicity with malformations in two animal species at doses of less than 10 times the RHD. The manufacturer recommends that women avoid becoming pregnant when using this drug. Nevertheless, using this drug during pregnancy should be based on the pros and cons of the mother's clinical need for treatment versus any potential fetal risk that might occur from exposure.

BREASTFEEDING SUMMARY

No reports describing the use of clofarabine during human lactation have been located. The drug will probably be found in breast milk, so some infant exposure will likely occur. The drug can be absorbed orally with a bioavailability of about 58%. The manufacturer recommends that women not breastfeed while using this drug. Nevertheless, breastfeeding while using this drug should be based on the mother's clinical need for treatment versus any potential infant risks that might occur from exposure. If used, the infant should be monitored for the most common reported adult side effects of nausea, headache, and pruritus (all leading to irritability), diarrhea, fatigue (lethargy), vomiting, rash, fever, and flushing.

Reference

1. Prescribing Information. *Clolar*. Sanofi-Aventis U.S.; 2020.

CLOMIPHENE

Reproductive (Ovulation Induction)

PREGNANCY RECOMMENDATION: *Contraindicated

BREASTFEEDING RECOMMENDATION: Potential Toxicity

PREGNANCY SUMMARY

Numerous case reports and small series have been located that describe the use of clomiphene during the first trimester of pregnancy. Several have reported birth anomalies, and others have not. In one review, the percentage of congenital anomalies after clomiphene use was no greater than in the normal population. Similarly, another study involving 1,034 pregnancies after clomiphene-induced ovulation found no association with the incidence or type of malformation. The drug will probably cross the placenta, so some fetal exposure will likely occur. *However, the approved use of this drug is to induce ovulation, and therefore, it is not approved for use during pregnancy. Patients requiring the use of clomiphene for ovulation induction should be cautioned that each new course of the drug should be started only after pregnancy has been excluded.

BREASTFEEDING SUMMARY

One case of clomiphene use in a lactating woman was located. The mean breast milk level was about 300 ng/mL, with a peak value of 583 ng/mL. These resulted in calculated RIDs of about 2.2% and 4.3%, respectively. Several studies have evaluated the use of clomiphene to suppress lactation, and most have shown some improved effect. The drug can also decrease prolactin levels. Using this drug to induce ovulation while breastfeeding would not be common, but these decisions cannot be made by the individual patient. If the clinical decision is to use this drug while breastfeeding, the infant should be monitored for the most common reported adult side effects of headache, abdominal pain, dizziness, and blurred vision (all leading to irritability), vomiting, diarrhea, flushing, and insomnia.

References

1. Product information. *Clomiphene*. Par Pharmaceuticals; 2017.
2. Shepard TH. *Catalog of Teratogenic Agents*. 6th ed. Johns Hopkins University Press; 1989:158-159.
3. Dziadek M. Preovulatory administration of clomiphene citrate to mice causes fetal growth retardation and neural tube defects (exencephaly) by an indirect maternal effect. *Teratology*. 1993;47:263-273.
4. Barrett C, Hakim C. Anencephaly, ovulation stimulation, subfertility, and illegitimacy. *Lancet*. 1973;2:916-917.
5. Dyson JL, Kohler HG. Anencephaly and ovulation stimulation. *Lancet*. 1973;1:1256-1257.
6. Field B, Kerr C. Ovulation stimulation and defects of neural tube closure. *Lancet*. 1974;2:1511.
7. Sandler B. Anencephaly and ovulation stimulation. *Lancet*. 1973;2:379.
8. Biale Y, Leventhal H, Altaras M, Ben-Aderet N. Anencephaly and clomiphene-induced pregnancy. *Acta Obstet Gynecol Scand*. 1978;57:483-484.
9. Asch RH, Greenblatt RB. Update on the safety and efficacy of clomiphene citrate as a therapeutic agent. *J Reprod Med*. 1976;17:175-180.
10. Harlap S. Ovulation induction and congenital malformations. *Lancet*. 1976;2:961.
11. James WH. Clomiphene, anencephaly, and spina bifida. *Lancet*. 1977;1:603.
12. Ahlgren M, Kallen B, Rannevik G. Outcome of pregnancy after clomiphene therapy. *Acta Obstet Gynecol Scand*. 1976;55:371-375.
13. Elwood JM. Clomiphene and anencephalic births. *Lancet*. 1974;1:31.
14. Czeizel A. Ovulation induction and neural tube defects. *Lancet*. 1989;2:167.
15. Cuckle H, Wald N. Ovulation induction and neural tube defects. *Lancet*. 1989;2:1281.
16. Cornel MC, Ten Kate LP, Graham Dukes MN, et al. Ovulation induction and neural tube defects. *Lancet*. 1989;1:1386.
17. Cornel MC, Ten Kate LP, Te Meerman GJ. Ovulation induction, in-vitro fertilisation, and neural tube defects. *Lancet*. 1989;2:1530.
18. Kurachi K, Aono T, Minagawa J, Miyake A. Congenital malformations of newborn infants after clomiphene-induced ovulation. *Fertil Steril*. 1983;40:187-189.
19. Mills JL, Simpson JL, Rhoads GG, et al. Risk of neural tube defects in relation to maternal fertility and fertility drug use. *Lancet*. 1990;336:103-104.
20. Rosa F. Ovulation induction and neural tube defects. *Lancet*. 1990;336:1327.
21. Mills JL. Clomiphene and neural-tube defects. *Lancet*. 1991;337:853.
22. Van Loon K, Besseghir K, Eshkol A. Neural tube defects after infertility treatment: a review. *Fertil Steril*. 1992;58:875-884.
23. Shoham Z, Zosmer A, Insler V. Early miscarriage and fetal malformations after induction of ovulation (by clomiphene citrate and/or human menotropins), in vitro fertilization, and gamete intrafallopian transfer. *Fertil Steril*. 1991;55:1-11.
24. Werler MM, Louik C, Shapiro S, Mitchell AA. Ovulation induction and risk of neural tube defects. *Lancet*. 1994;344:445-446.
25. Greenland S, Ackerman DL. Clomiphene citrate and neural tube defects: a pooled analysis of controlled epidemiologic studies and recommendations for future studies. *Fertil Steril*. 1995;64:936-941.
26. Miles PA, Taylor HB, Hill WC. Hydatidiform mole in a clomiphene related pregnancy: a case report. *Obstet Gynecol*. 1971;37:358-359.
27. Schneiderman CI, Waxman B. Clomid therapy and subsequent hydatidiform mole formation: a case report. *Obstet Gynecol*. 1972;39:787-788.
28. Wajntraub G, Kamar R, Pardo Y. Hydatidiform mole after treatment with clomiphene. *Fertil Steril*. 1974;25:904-905.
29. Berman P. Congenital abnormalities associated with maternal clomiphene ingestion. *Lancet*. 1975;2:878.
30. Drew AL. Letter to the editor. *Dev Med Child Neurol*. 1974;16:276.
31. Hack M, Brish M, Serr DM, et al. Outcome of pregnancy after induced ovulation. Follow-up of pregnancies and children born after clomiphene therapy. *JAMA*. 1972;220:1329-1333.
32. Ylikorkala O. Congenital anomalies and clomiphene. *Lancet*. 1975;2:1262-1263.
33. Laing IA, Steer CR, Dudgeon J, Brown JK. Clomiphene and congenital retinopathy. *Lancet*. 1981;2:1107-1108.
34. Ford WDA, Little KET. Fetal ovarian dysplasia possibly associated with clomiphene. *Lancet*. 1981;2:1107.
35. Kistner RW. Induction of ovulation with clomiphene citrate. *Obstet Gynecol Surv*. 1965;20:873-899.
36. Goldfarb AF, Morales A, Rakoff AE, Protos P. Critical review of 160 clomiphene-related pregnancies. *Obstet Gynecol*. 1968;31:342-345.
37. Oakely GP, Flynt IW. Increased prevalence of Down's syndrome (mongolism) among the offspring of women treated with ovulation-inducing agents. *Teratology*. 1972;5:264.
38. Singhi M, Singhi S. Possible relationship between clomiphene and neural tube defects. *J Pediatr*. 1978;93:152.
39. Mor-Joseph S, Anteby SO, Granat M, et al. Recurrent molar pregnancies associated with clomiphene citrate and human gonadotropins. *Am J Obstet Gynecol*. 1985;151:1085-1086.
40. Bishai R, Arbour L, Lyons C, Koren G. Intrauterine exposure to clomiphene and neonatal persistent hyperplastic primary vitreous. *Teratology*. 1999;60:143-145.
41. Dickey RP, Taylor SN, Curole DN, et al. Incidence of spontaneous abortion in clomiphene pregnancies. *Hum Reprod*. 1996;11:2623-2628.
42. Haring DAJP, Cornel MC, Van der Linden JC, et al. Acardius acephalus after induced ovulation: a case report. *Teratology*. 1993;47:257-262.
43. Martinez-Roman S, Torres PJ, Puerto B. Acardius acephalus after ovulation induction by clomiphene. *Teratology*. 1995;51:231-232.
44. Sceusa DK, Klein PE. Ultrasound diagnosis of an acardius acephalic monster in a quintuplet pregnancy. *JDMS*. 1990;2:109-112. As cited by Martinez-Roman S, Torres PJ, Puerto B. Acardius acephalus after ovulation induction by clomiphene. *Teratology*. 1995;51:231-232.
45. Melamed I, Bujanover Y, Hammer J, Spirer Z. Hepatoblastoma in an infant born to a mother after hormonal treatment for sterility. *N Engl J Med*. 1982;307:820.
46. Zuckerman H, Carmel S. The inhibition of lactation by clomiphene. *J Obstet Gynaecol Br Commonw*. 1973;80:822-823.
47. Kalir R, David MP, Kraicer PF. Clomiphene citrate in suppression of puerperal lactation. *Am J Obstet Gynecol*. 1975;122:570-572.
48. Weinstein D, Ben-David M, Polishuk WZ. Serum prolactin and the suppression of lactation. *Br J Obstet Gynaecol*. 1976;83:679-682.

49. Canales ES, Lasso P, Soria J, Zarate A. Effect of clomiphene on prolactin secretion and lactation in puerperal women. *Br J Obstet Gynaecol*. 1977; 84:758-759.
50. Masala A, Delitala G, Lo Dico G, et al. Effect of clomiphene on release of prolactin induced by mechanical breast emptying in women post partum. *J Endocrinol*. 1977;74:501-502.
51. Masala A, Delitala G, Alagna S, et al. Clomiphene and puerperal lactation. *Panminerva Med*. 1978;20:1613.

CLOMIPRAMINE

Mental Health (Antidepressant/Tricyclic)

PREGNANCY RECOMMENDATION: Limited Human Data—Animal Data Suggest Low Risk

BREASTFEEDING RECOMMENDATION: Probably Compatible

PREGNANCY SUMMARY

Two studies were located that analyzed the effects of antidepressants on pregnancy. It is difficult to separate clomipramine use and first-trimester exposure risk in these reports. In one of these studies, there was an association between clomipramine and cardiac defects. However, it was not determined if this could be related to the disease state of the mother. This potential association needs further study. Numerous case reports have described newborn withdrawal in infants with long-term clomipramine exposure near the time of delivery. These symptoms include hypertonia, hypotonia, lethargy, seizures, tremor, and other neurologic findings, and in many cases, treatment for a few weeks was required. In these cases, there were a few first-trimester exposures, and no birth anomalies were found. Although the data are very limited, no long-term effects of in utero exposure to clomipramine have been observed. The drug crosses the placenta, so fetal exposure will occur. However, this limited human pregnancy experience prevents a complete assessment of the embryofetal risk. Animal studies did not show any embryofetal toxicity or teratogenicity in two species at doses of less than 10 times the RHD. Using this drug during pregnancy should be based on the pros and cons of the mother's clinical need for treatment versus any potential fetal risk that might occur from exposure. Because the approved use for the drug is in treating obsessive-compulsive disorder, use in the last trimester might be altered in some patients. There is a pregnancy exposure registry that monitors pregnancy outcomes in women using antidepressant drugs. Health care providers are encouraged to call the National Pregnancy Registry for Antidepressants at 1-844-405-6185.

BREASTFEEDING SUMMARY

Clomipramine has been evaluated in human lactation in a few breastfeeding women. Several breast milk samples were provided from a total of four lactating women. The drug was found in every sample. Levels ranged from 60 ng/mL to 624 ng/mL. Using mean values, all the calculated RIDs were less than 3%. Using the peak value, the calculated RID was about 5%. Infant blood levels have also been analyzed in eight newborns who were exposed to clomipramine through breastfeeding. The drug was detected in two cases at levels that ranged from about 3 ng/mL to 45 ng/mL. In the other six infants, the drug was not detected, but in four cases, the LLQ was 10 ng/mL, and in the fifth infant, it was 50 ng/mL (and therefore, may have been below these thresholds). In the sixth case, the drug was not detected in the infant's blood, and the LLQ was 0.1 ng/mL. A few studies have also reported on infant effects, and overall, no adverse reactions have been consistently described. The drug has been shown to increase prolactin levels, but this should not adversely affect breastfeeding. Breastfeeding while using this drug should be based on the mother's clinical need for treatment versus any potential infant risks that might occur. If used, the infant should be monitored for the most common reported adult side effects of nausea, visual disturbances, headache, dizziness, and abdominal pain (all leading to irritability), fatigue (lethargy), constipation, somnolence, tremor, and sweating.

References

1. Product information. *Clomipramine Hydrochloride*. Sandoz; 2018.
2. McElhatton PR, Garbis HM, Elefant E, et al. The outcome of pregnancy in 689 women exposed to therapeutic doses of antidepressants. A collaborative study of the European Network of Teratology Information Services (ENTIS). *Reprod Toxicol*. 1996;10:285-294.
3. Kallen BAJ, Olausson PO. Maternal drug use in early pregnancy and infant cardiovascular defect. *Reprod Toxicol*. 2003;17:255-261.
4. Kallen B, Olausson PO. Antidepressant drugs during pregnancy and infant congenital heart defect. *Reprod Toxicol*. 2006;21:221-222.
5. Ben Muza A, Smith CS. Neonatal effects of maternal clomipramine therapy. *Arch Dis Child*. 1979;54:405.
6. Ostergaard GZ, Pedersen SE. Neonatal effects of maternal clomipramine treatment. *Pediatrics*. 1982;69:233-234.
7. Cowe L, Lloyd DJ, Dawling S. Neonatal convulsions caused by withdrawal from maternal clomipramine. *Br Med J*. 1982;284:1837-1838.
8. Schimmell MS, Katz EZ, Shaag Y, et al. Toxic neonatal effects following maternal clomipramine therapy. *J Toxicol Clin Toxicol*. 1991;29:479-484.
9. Singh S, Gulati S, Narang A, Bhakoo ON. Non-narcotic withdrawal syndrome in a neonate due to maternal clomipramine therapy. *J Pediatr Child Health*. 1990;26:110.
10. Bromiker R, Kaplan M. Apparent intrauterine fetal withdrawal from clomipramine hydrochloride. *JAMA*. 1994;272:1722-1723.
11. Bloem BR, Lammers GJ, Roofthooft DWE, et al. Clomipramine withdrawal in newborns. *Arch Dis Child Fetal Neonatal Ed*. 1999;81:F77.
12. Nulman I, Rovet J, Stewart DE, et al. Child development following exposure to tricyclic antidepressants or fluoxetine throughout fetal life: a prospective, controlled study. *Am J Psychiatry*. 2002;159:1889-1895.
13. Wisner KL, Perel JM, Findling RL. Antidepressant treatment during breastfeeding. *Am J Psychiatry*. 1996;153:1132-1137.
14. Yoshida K, Smith B, Craggs M, Kumar RC. Investigation of pharmacokinetics and of possible adverse effects in infants exposed to tricyclic antidepressants in breast-milk. *J Affect Disord*. 1997;43:225-237.

C

CLOMOCYCLINE

Antibacterial (Tetracycline)

PREGNANCY RECOMMENDATION: ***Contraindicated (Second and Third Trimesters)**

BREASTFEEDING RECOMMENDATION: **Potential Toxicity**

PREGNANCY SUMMARY

No reports describing the use of clomocycline in human pregnancy have been located. The drug will probably cross the placenta, so some fetal exposure will likely occur. Therefore, the absence of human pregnancy experience prevents a complete assessment of the embryofetal risk. *Studies on tetracycline showed that use of the drug in the second and third trimesters could produce discolored teeth and bone, as well as bone stippling (see Tetracycline). Using this drug during pregnancy should be based on the pros and cons of the mother's clinical need for treatment versus any potential fetal risk that might occur from exposure.

BREASTFEEDING SUMMARY

No reports describing the use of clomocycline during human lactation have been located. Based on the MW, the drug will likely be found in breast milk. Breastfeeding while using this drug should be based on the mother's clinical need for treatment versus any potential infant risks that might occur. If used, the infant should be monitored for the most common reported adult side effects of nausea and abdominal pain (both leading to irritability), diarrhea, vomiting, constipation, decreased appetite, and rash.

Reference

1. Prescribing Information. *Clomocycline*. MedKoo Biosciences, Inc; 2021.

CLONAZEPAM

Mental Health (Antiseizure)

PREGNANCY RECOMMENDATION: **Limited Human Data—Animal Data Suggest Potential Risk**

BREASTFEEDING RECOMMENDATION: **Probably Compatible (Short-Term Use)**

PREGNANCY SUMMARY

The use of clonazepam has been reported in human pregnancy in several studies. Though specific numbers for clonazepam are low, of about 150 first-trimester exposures, there were 7 major anomalies (4.7%) (6 expected). No specific pattern was seen. Other studies have evaluated for any adverse newborn effects when exposed near the time of delivery. Some cases of withdrawal symptoms were located, but this was not a universal finding. The drug crosses the placenta, so fetal exposure will occur. However, this limited human pregnancy experience prevents a complete assessment of the embryofetal risk. Animal studies did show embryofetal toxicity in one species at doses of less than 10 times the RHD, but not in a second species. In a third species, no embryofetal toxicity was seen at doses of more than 10 times the RHD. The effectiveness of the drug in long-term use (more than 9 weeks) has not been evaluated. The manufacturer recommends that the drug not be used in the first trimester for treating panic disorder. Nevertheless, using this drug during pregnancy should be based on the pros and cons of the mother's clinical need for treatment versus any potential fetal risk that might occur from exposure. The drug can lead to dependence, addiction, and withdrawal. Withdrawal symptoms can occur in newborns postbirth when used near delivery. The drug is classified as a Schedule IV controlled substance. There is a pregnancy exposure registry that monitors pregnancy outcomes in women using antiseizure drugs. Health care providers are encouraged to call the North American Antiepileptic Drug Pregnancy Registry at 1-888-233-2334.

BREASTFEEDING SUMMARY

Several case reports have described the use of clonazepam during human lactation. The drug was found in every breast milk sample provided by five breastfeeding women. The breast milk levels ranged from about 4 ng/mL to 45 ng/mL. The calculated RIDs were all less than 2.5% Clonazepam has also been analyzed for infant blood levels. In a total of 14 infants, 10 did not have detectable levels (LLQ ranged from 5-14 ng/mL). In the other four cases, the infant's blood levels ranged from about 5 to 22 ng/mL. In one case, the level was only about 10% of the maternal level. In a second case, the infant's level was about 40% of the maternal serum level. Several reports have described some adverse effects in breastfed newborns (eg, drowsiness, tremors, decreased appetite, laziness, etc), but there are many infants without any reported issues.

Due to a concern for potential serious adverse effects that might be seen in a breastfed infant, the manufacturer recommends that women not breastfeed while being treated with this drug. Nevertheless, breastfeeding while using this drug should be based on the mother's clinical need for treatment versus any potential infant risks that might occur. If used, the infant should be monitored for the most common reported adult side effects of headache, dizziness, arthralgias, and abdominal pain (all leading to irritability), somnolence, tremors, constipation, and rash.

C

References

1. Product information. *Clonazepam*. Mylan Pharmaceuticals; 2018.
2. Hiilesmaa VK, Bardy A, Teramo K. Obstetric outcome in women with epilepsy. *Am J Obstet Gynecol*. 1985;152:499-504.
3. Canger R, Battino D, Canevini MP, et al. Obstetrical and neonatal outcome following clonazepam use during pregnancy: a case series. *Psychother Psychosom*. 2001;70:158-162.
4. Eros E, Czeizel AE, Rockenbauer M, et al. A population-based case-control teratology study of nitrazepam, medazepam, tofisopam, alprazolam, and clonazepam treatment during pregnancy. *Eur J Obstet Gynecol Reprod Biol*. 2002;101:147-154.
5. Lin AE, Peller AJ, Westgate MN, et al. Clonazepam use in pregnancy and the risk of malformations. *Birth Defects Res (Part A)*. 2004;70:534-536.
6. *The Lamotrigine Pregnancy Registry: final report: 1 September 1992 through 31 March 2010*. GlaxoSmithKline; 2010.
7. Fisher JB, Edgren BE, Mammel MC, Coleman JM. Neonatal apnea associated with maternal clonazepam therapy: a case report. *Obstet Gynecol*. 1985;66(suppl):34S-35S.
8. Haeusler MC, Hoellwarth ME, Holzer P. Paralytic ileus in a fetus-neonate after maternal intake of benzodiazepine. *Prenat Diagn*. 1995;15:1165-1167.
9. Almgren M, Kallen B, Lavebratt C. Population-based study of antiepileptic drug exposure *in utero*—influence on head circumference in newborns. *Seizure*. 2009;18:672-675.
10. Veroniki AA, Rios P, Cogo E, et al. Comparative safety of antiepileptic drugs for neurological development in children exposed during pregnancy and breast feeding: a systematic review and network meta-analysis. *BMJ Open*. 2017;7(7):e017248.
11. Andrade C. Adverse pregnancy outcomes associated with gestational exposure to antiepileptic drugs. *J Clin Psychiatry*. 2018;79:18f12467.
12. Soderman P, Matheson I. Clonazepam in breast milk. *Eur J Pediatr*. 1988;147:212-213.
13. Misri S, Corral M, Wardrop AA, Kendrick K. Quetiapine augmentation in lactation: a series of case reports. *J Clin Psychopharmacol*. 2006;26:508-511.
14. Kelly LE, Poon S, Madadi P, Koren G. Neonatal benzodiazepines exposure during breastfeeding. *J Pediatr*. 2012;161:448-451.

CLONIDINE

Antihypertensive (Central Acting α-Agonist)

PREGNANCY RECOMMENDATION: Limited Human Data—Animal Data Suggest Risk

BREASTFEEDING RECOMMENDATION: Potential Toxicity

PREGNANCY SUMMARY

From two studies, a total of 71 pregnancies were exposed to clonidine in the first trimester, and of these, 3 (4,2%) congenital anomalies were described. No pattern to the defects was seen. The drug will cross the placenta, so some fetal exposure will occur. However, this limited human pregnancy experience prevents a complete assessment of the embryofetal risk. The drug was found to cause some embryofetal toxicity in two species at doses of less than 10 times the RHD. Using this drug during pregnancy should be based on the pros and cons of the mother's clinical need for treatment versus any potential fetal risk that might occur from exposure.

BREASTFEEDING SUMMARY

Three studies were located that evaluated breast milk levels for clonidine. In a total of 13 lactating women, the drug was found in every breast milk sample. The levels ranged from 0.6 ng/mL to more than 3 ng/mL. The calculated RIDs using mean values ranged from about 4% to 9.8%. If peak values were used, several RIDs would exceed 10%. Infant blood levels have also been analyzed following exposure to the drug from breastfeeding and appear to be about 50% of the maternal serum concentrations. Breastfeeding while using this drug should be based on the mother's clinical need for treatment versus any potential infant risks that might occur. If used, the infant should be monitored for the most common reported adult side effects of nausea, headache, blurred vision, and dizziness (all leading to irritability), fatigue (lethargy), constipation, and decreased heart rate and blood pressure. There are a few case reports of infants who appeared to have some adverse reactions when exposed to clonidine through breastfeeding. If an alternative antihypertensive agent can be used by the mother, this would be recommended.

References

1. Product information. *Clonidine*. Amneal Pharmaceuticals NY; 2019.
2. Hartikainen-Sorri A-L, Heikkinen JE, Koivisto M. Pharmacokinetics of clonidine during pregnancy and nursing. *Obstet Gynecol*. 1987;69:598-600.
3. Boutroy MJ, Gisonna CR, Legagneur M. Clonidine: placental transfer and neonatal adaption. *Early Hum Dev*. 1988;17:275-286.
4. Turnbull AC, Ahmed S. Catapres in the treatment of hypertension in pregnancy, a preliminary study. In: *Catapres in Hypertension*. Symposium of the Royal College of Surgeons; 1970:237-245.
5. Johnston CI, Aickin DR. The control of high blood pressure during labour with clonidine. *Med J Aust*. 1971;2:132.
6. Raftos J, Bauer GE, Lewis RG, et al. Clonidine in the treatment of severe hypertension. *Med J Aust*. 1973;1:786-793.
7. Horvath JS, Phippard A, Korda A, et al. Clonidine hydrochloride—a safe and effective antihypertensive agent in pregnancy. *Obstet Gynecol*. 1985;66:634-638.
8. Horvath JS, Korda A, Child A, et al. Hypertension in pregnancy: a study of 142 women presenting before 32 weeks' gestation. *Med J Aust*. 1985;143:19-21.
9. Ng-Wing Tin L, Frelon JH, Beaute Y, et al. Clonidine et traitement de l'hypertension arterielle de la femme enceinte. *Rev Fr Gynécol Obstét*. 1986;81:563-566.
10. Ng-Wing-Tin L, Frelon JH, Hardy F, Bazin C. Clonidine et traitement des urgences hypertensives de la femme enceinte. *Rev fr Gynécol Obstét*. 1987;82:519-522.

11. Lubbe WF. Treatment of hypertension in pregnancy. *J Cardiovasc Pharmacol*. 1990;16(suppl 7):S110-S113.
12. Kaaja R, Hiilesmaa V, Holma K, Jarvenpaa A-L. Maternal antihypertensive therapy with beta-blockers associated with poor outcome in very-low birth-weight infants. *Int J Gynecol Obstet*. 1992;38:195-199.
13. Maina A, Arrotta M, Cicogna L, et al. Transdermal clonidine in the treatment of severe hyperemesis. A pilot randomized control trial: CLONEMESI. *BJOG*. 2014;121:1556-1562.
14. Le Polain B, De Kock M, Scholtes JL, Van Lierde M. Clonidine combined with sufentanil and bupivacaine with adrenaline for obstetric analgesia. *Br J Anaesth*. 1993;71:657-660.
15. O'Meara ME, Gin T. Comparison of 0.125% bupivacaine with 0.125% bupivacaine and clonidine as extradural analgesia in the first stage of labour. *Br J Anaesth*. 1993;71:651-656.
16. Gautier PE, De Kock M, Fanard L, et al. Intrathecal clonidine combined with sufentanil for labor analgesia. *Anesthesiology*. 1998;88:651-656.
17. Mercier FJ, Dounas M, Bouaziz H, et al. The effect of adding a minidose of clonidine to intrathecal sufentanil for labor analgesia. *Anesthesiology*. 1998;89:594-601.
18. Dashe JS, Jackson GL, Olscher DA, et al. Opioid detoxification in pregnancy. *Obstet Gynecol*. 1998;92:854-858.
19. Bunjes R, Schaefer C, Holzinger D. Clonidine and breast-feeding. *Clin Pharm*. 1993;12:178-179.
20. Sevrez C, Lavocat MP, Mounier G, et al. Transplacental or breast milk intoxication to clonidine: a case of neonatal hypotonia and drowsiness. *Arch Pediatr*. 2014;21:198-200.

CLOPIDOGREL

Hematologic (Antiplatelet)

PREGNANCY RECOMMENDATION: Limited Human Data—Animal Data Suggest Low Risk (Maternal Benefit May Outweigh Embryofetal Risk)

BREASTFEEDING RECOMMENDATION: Probably Compatible

PREGNANCY SUMMARY

Numerous case reports were located that described the use of clopidogrel in human pregnancy. There were six with first-trimester exposure, five without any identified anomalies, and one with a ventricular septal defect (VSD). An additional five cases reported use in the second and third trimesters, and all did well without any adverse events related to the drug. The drug will probably cross the placenta, so some fetal exposure will likely occur. However, this limited human pregnancy experience prevents a complete assessment of the embryofetal risk. Animal studies did not show any embryofetal toxicity or teratogenicity in two species at doses of more than 10 times the RHD. The known benefits to a woman with acute coronary syndrome or a myocardial infarction appear to outweigh the unknown embryofetal risks of using this drug. If a patient's condition requires clopidogrel, the treatment should not be withheld because of pregnancy.

BREASTFEEDING SUMMARY

No reports describing the use of clopidogrel during human lactation have been located. The drug will probably be found in breast milk, so some infant exposure will likely occur. Due to a concern for potential serious adverse effects that might be seen in a breastfed infant, the manufacturer recommends that women not breastfeed while being treated with this drug. Nevertheless, breastfeeding while using this drug should be based on the mother's clinical need for treatment versus any potential infant risks that might occur. If used, the infant should be monitored for the most common reported adult side effects of bruising and bleeding.

References

1. Product information. *Plavix*. Bristol-Myers Squibb/Sanofi Pharmaceuticals; 2018.
2. Klinzing P, Markert UR, Liesaus K, Peiker G. Case report: successful pregnancy and delivery after myocardial infarction and essential thrombocythemia treated with clopidogrel. *Clin Exp Obstet Gynecol*. 2001;28:215-216.
3. Boztosun B, Olcay A, Avci A, Kirma C. Treatment of acute myocardial infarction in pregnancy with coronary artery balloon angioplasty and stenting: use of tirofiban and clopidogrel. *Int J Cardiol*. 2008;127:413-416.
4. Al-Aqeedi RF, Al-Nabti AD. Drug-eluting stent implantation for acute myocardial infarction during pregnancy with use of glycoprotein IIb/IIIa inhibitor. *J Invasive Cardiol*. 2008;20:E146-E149.
5. Cuthill JA, Young S, Greer IA, Oldroyd K. Anaesthetic considerations in a parturient with critical coronary artery disease and a drug-eluting stent presenting for caesarean section. *Int J Obstet Anesth*. 2005;14:167-171.
6. Arimura T, Mitsutake R, Miura S, et al. Acute myocardial infarction associated with pregnancy successfully treated with percutaneous coronary intervention. *Intern Med*. 2009;48:1383-1386.
7. Santiago-Diaz P, Arrebola-Moreno AL, Ramirez-Hernandez JA, Melgares-Moreno R. Use of antiplatelet drugs during pregnancy. *Rev Exp Cardiol*. 2009;62:1197-1198.
8. De Santis M, De Luca C, Mappa I, et al. Clopidogrel treatment during pregnancy: a case report and a review of the literature. *Intern Med*. 2011;50:1769-1773.
9. Myers GR, Hoffman MK, Marshall ES. Clopidogrel use throughout pregnancy in a patient with a drug-eluting coronary stent. *Obstet Gynecol*. 2011;118:32-33.
10. Reilly CR, Cuesta-Fernandez A, Kayaleh OR. Successful gestation and delivery using clopidogrel for secondary stroke prophylaxis: a case report and literature review. *Arch Gynecol Obstet*. 2014;290:591-594.
11. Babic Z, Gabric ID, Pintaric H. Successful primary percutaneous coronary intervention in the first trimester of pregnancy. *Catheter Cardiovasc Interv*. 2011;77:522-525.
12. Jaiswal A, Rashid M, Balek M, Park C. Acute myocardial infarction during pregnancy: a clinical checkmate. *Indian Heart J*. 2013;65:464-468.
13. Duarte FP, O'Neill P, Centeno MJ, et al. Myocardial infarction in the 31st week of pregnancy—case report. *Rev Bras Anestesiol*. 2011;61:225-231.

C

CLORAZEPATE

Mental Health (Benzodiazepine)

PREGNANCY RECOMMENDATION: Limited Human Data Suggest Potential Risk (Especially Third Trimester)—Animal Data Suggest Low Risk

BREASTFEEDING RECOMMENDATION: Potential Toxicity

PREGNANCY SUMMARY

Three reports describing the use of clorazepate during human pregnancy were located. One report described multiple severe anomalies in an infant exposed to clorazepate during the first trimester, starting around the fifth week of gestation. However, it is unknown if any of these anomalies had any connection to clorazepate exposure; no other anomalies like this have been reported with clorazepate use. From the Lamotrigine Pregnancy Registry, two prospectively enrolled pregnancies with first-trimester exposure to clorazepate and lamotrigine (with or without other anticonvulsants) resulted in one fetal death and one spontaneous abortion. The third report involved a massive clorazepate overdose at about 39 weeks' gestation. Newborn nordiazepam and oxazepam blood levels postdelivery were markedly elevated and remained elevated (consistent with the long elimination half-lives) until enterodialysis with activated charcoal was performed. This limited human pregnancy experience; however, prevents a complete assessment of the embryofetal risk. The active metabolites of the drug cross the placenta. Benzodiazepine use during the second half of pregnancy can lead to changes in the fetal heart monitor tracing with a decrease/absence in variability and loss of accelerations that can be prolonged (long elimination half-life consistent with the overdose case described earlier). In addition, if used during labor, neonatal depression can occur immediately postbirth. The drug is a Schedule IV controlled substance and has a risk for producing physical and psychological dependence. Abrupt withdrawal has been associated with producing seizures. There is a pregnancy exposure registry that monitors pregnancy outcomes in women using antiseizure drugs. Health care providers are encouraged to call the North American Antiepileptic Drug Pregnancy Registry at 1-888-233-2334.

BREASTFEEDING SUMMARY

Following a single 20-mg clorazepate dose administered IM to seven women during labor, low concentrations of nordiazepam, the active metabolite, were found in milk at 2 days with little change by 4 days. The drug was found to accumulate in the neonate's blood. Other benzodiazepines accumulate in human breast milk, and adverse effects in the nursing infant have been reported (see Diazepam). Breastfeeding while using this drug should be based on the mother's clinical need for treatment versus any potential infant risks that might occur. Because of clorazepate's long elimination half-life, using an alternate drug is suggested. However, if used, the infant should be monitored for the most common reported adult side effects of nausea, headache, and dizziness (all leading to irritability), sleepiness, lethargy, tremor, and rash.

References

1. Prescribing Information. *Clorazepate Dipotassium*. Ranbaxy Pharmaceuticals; 2012.
2. Guerre-Millo M, Rey E, Challier JC, et al. Transfer in vitro of three benzodiazepines across the human placenta. *Eur J Clin Pharmacol*. 1979;15:171-173.
3. Rey E, Giraux P, d'Athis P, et al. Pharmacokinetics of the placental transfer and distribution of clorazepate and its metabolite nordiazepam in the feto-placental unit and in the neonate. *Eur J Clin Pharmacol*. 1979;15:181-185.
4. Patel DA, Patel AR. Clorazepate and congenital malformations. *JAMA*. 1980;244:135-136.
5. *The Lamotrigine Pregnancy Registry: final report: 1 September 1992 through 31 March 2010*. GlaxoSmithKline; 2010.
6. Malgorn G, Leboucher B, Harry P, et al. Benzodiazepine poisoning in a neonate: clinical and toxicokinetic evaluation following enterodialysis with activated charcoal. *Arch Pediatr*. 2004;11:819-821.

CLOTRIMAZOLE

Anti-Infective (Antifungal)

PREGNANCY RECOMMENDATION: Human Data Suggest Low Risk

BREASTFEEDING RECOMMENDATION: Probably Compatible

PREGNANCY SUMMARY

Clotrimazole use during the first trimester has been evaluated in several studies involving more than 3,000 cases. Though the overall rate of birth defects is near 4%, no pattern to the anomalies was seen. In addition, exposure to numerous other drugs occurred. If the drug is found in the systemic circulation, it will likely cross the placenta, so fetal exposure would occur.

However, with the low systemic exposure following intravaginal and topical skin use, the amount of any fetal exposure is likely to be negligible. Animal studies did show some embryofetal toxicity in three species, but at doses well above 10 times the RHD. Using this drug during pregnancy should be based on the pros and cons of the mother's clinical need for treatment versus any potential fetal risk that might occur from exposure.

C

BREASTFEEDING SUMMARY

No reports of the use of clotrimazole during human lactation have been located. If the drug is found in the systemic circulation, it will probably be found in human breast milk, and infant exposure could occur. Regardless, the systemic absorption of clotrimazole from the skin and vagina is minimal. Therefore, any amount is likely to be clinically insignificant. Breastfeeding while using this drug should be based on the mother's clinical need for treatment versus any potential infant risks that might occur. If used, the infant should be monitored for the most common reported adult side effects of nausea and abdominal pain (both leading to irritability), vomiting, and pruritus.

References

1. Product information. *Lotrimin*. Schering; 2000.
2. Rosa FW, Baum C, Shaw M. Pregnancy outcomes after first-trimester vaginitis drug therapy. *Obstet Gynecol*. 1987;69:751-755.
3. Czeizel AE, Toth M, Rockenbauer M. No teratogenic effect after clotrimazole therapy during pregnancy. *Epidemiology*. 1999;10:437-440.
4. Kragie L, Turner SD, Patten CJ, et al. Assessing pregnancy risks of azole antifungals using a high throughput aromatase inhibition assay. *Endocr Res*. 2002;28:129-140.
5. Harada N. Genetic analysis of human placental aromatase deficiency. *J Steroid Biochem Mol Biol*. 1993;44:331-340.
6. Daniel S, Rotem R, Koren G, et al. Vaginal antimycotics and the risk for spontaneous abortions. *Am J Obstet Gynecol*. 2018;218:601.e1-601.e7.
7. Tan CG, Good CS, Milne LJR, Loudon JDO. A comparative trial of six-day therapy with clotrimazole and nystatin in pregnant patients with vaginal candidiasis. *Postgrad Med*. 1974;50(suppl 1):102-105.
8. Frerich W, Gad A. The frequency of Candida infections in pregnancy and their treatment with clotrimazole. *Curr Med Res Opin*. 1977;4:640-644.
9. Haram K, Digranes A. Vulvovaginal candidiasis in pregnancy treated with clotrimazole. *Acta Obstet Gynecol Scand*. 1978;57:453-455.
10. Svendsen E, Lie S, Gunderson TH, et al. Comparative evaluation of miconazole, clotrimazole and nystatin in the treatment of candidal vulvo-vaginitis. *Curr Ther Res*. 1978;23:666-672.
11. Patel VM, Schwartz RA, Lambert WC. Topical antiviral and antifungal medications in pregnancy: a review of safety profiles. *J Eur Acad Dermatol Venereol*. 2017;31:1440-1446.
12. Rotem R, Fishman B, Daniel S, et al. Risk of major congenital malformations following first-trimester exposure to vaginal azoles used for treating vulvovaginal candidiasis: a population-based retrospective cohort study. *BJOG*. 2018;125:1550-1556.

CLOZAPINE

Mental Health (Antipsychotic)

PREGNANCY RECOMMENDATION: Limited Human Data—Animal Data Suggest Low Risk (Maternal Benefit May Outweigh Any Fetal Risk)

BREASTFEEDING RECOMMENDATION: Potential Toxicity

PREGNANCY SUMMARY

Several case reports were located that described first-trimester exposure to clozapine. No birth anomalies were described in about 20 cases. The drug crosses the placenta, so some fetal exposure will occur. However, the absence of human pregnancy experience prevents a complete assessment of the embryofetal risk. Animal studies did not show any embryofetal toxicity in two species at doses of less than 10 times the RHD. Because clozapine is indicated for severe, debilitating mental disease, the benefits to the mother appear to outweigh the unknown embryofetal risk. However, there is a risk of extrapyramidal and/or withdrawal symptoms in the newborn if the drug is used in the third trimester near delivery. Because of the limited human pregnancy experience with atypical antipsychotics, the ACOG does not recommend the routine use of these agents in pregnancy, but a risk-benefit assessment may indicate that such use is appropriate. There is a pregnancy exposure registry that monitors pregnancy outcomes in women using atypical antipsychotic drugs. Health care providers are encouraged to contact the National Pregnancy Registry for Atypical Antipsychotics at 1-866-961-2388.

BREASTFEEDING SUMMARY

Clozapine has been found in breast milk in one patient who was on 50 mg/d that increased to 100 mg/d. Though the breast milk concentration to maternal plasma level was 3 to 4 times higher, the maximum breast milk level obtained was about 116 ng/mL, resulting in a calculated RID of less than 1.5%. A total of eight infants have been described in the literature regarding any adverse effects in infants related to breastfeeding exposure to clozapine. Of these, five cases had no adverse effects reported. In the other three, there was one with speech delay that was corrected by age 5, one infant with sedation, and one with agranulocytosis (unsure if this was related to the drug exposure). More studies are needed regarding the use of this drug while breastfeeding. The drug does not appear to affect prolactin blood levels. Due to a concern for potential serious adverse effects that might be seen in a breastfed infant, the manufacturer recommends that women not breastfeed while being treated with this drug. Nevertheless, breastfeeding while using this drug

C

should be based on the mother's clinical need for treatment versus any potential infant risks that might occur. If used, the infant should be monitored for the most common reported adult side effects of nausea, headache, and dizziness (all leading to irritability), sedation, tremor, fever, constipation, and cardiovascular reactions.

References

1. Product information. *Clozaril*. HLS Therapeutics (USA); 2018.
2. American College of Obstetricians and Gynecologists. ACOG practice bulletin No. 92: use of psychiatric medications during pregnancy and lactation. *Obstet Gynecol*. 2008;111:1001-1019.
3. Althuler LL, Cohen L, Szuba MP, et al. Pharmacologic management of psychiatric illness during pregnancy: dilemmas and guidelines. *Am J Psychiatry*. 1996;153:592-606.
4. Koren G, Cohn T, Chitayat D, et al. Use of atypical antipsychotics during pregnancy and the risk of neural tube defects in infants. *Am J Psychiatry*. 2002;159:136-137.
5. Barnas C, Bergant A, Hummer M, et al. Clozapine concentrations in maternal and fetal plasma, amniotic fluid, and breast milk. *Am J Psychiatry*. 1994; 151:945.
6. Walderman MD, Safferman AZ. Pregnancy and clozapine. *Am J Psychiatry*. 1993;150:168-169.
7. Lieberman J, Safferman AZ. Clinical profile of clozapine: adverse reactions and agranulocytosis. In: Lapierre Y, Jones B, eds. *Clozapine in Treatment Resistant Schizophrenia: A Scientific Update*. Royal Society of Medicine; 1992. As cited in Walderman MD, Safferman AZ. Pregnancy and clozapine. Am J Psychiatry. 1993;150:168-169.
8. Di Michele V, Ramenghi LA, Sabatino G. Clozapine and lorazepam administration in pregnancy. *Eur Psychiatry*. 1996;11:214.
9. McKenna K, Koren G, Tetelbaum M, et al. Pregnancy outcome of women using atypical antipsychotic drugs: a prospective comparative study. *J Clin Psychiatry*. 2005;66:444-449.
10. Shao P, Ou J, Peng M, et al. Effects of clozapine and other atypical antipsychotics on infants development who were exposed to as fetus: a post-hoc analysis. *PLoS One*. 2014;10:e0123373.
11. Dev VJ, Krupp P. Adverse event profile and safety of clozapine. *Rev Contemp Pharmacother*. 1995;6:197-208. As cited in Clozapine. National Library of Medicine LactMed Database; 2013.
12. Mendhekar D. Possible delayed speech acquisition with clozapine therapy during pregnancy and lactation. *J Neuropsychiatry Clin Neurosci*. 2007;19: 196-197.
13. American Academy of Pediatrics Committee on Drugs. The transfer of drugs and other chemicals into human milk. *Pediatrics*. 2001;108:776-789.

COBICISTAT

Antiretroviral (CYP3A Inhibitor)

PREGNANCY RECOMMENDATION: Limited Human Data—Animal Data Suggest Low Risk

BREASTFEEDING RECOMMENDATION: *Contraindicated

PREGNANCY SUMMARY

Numerous reports regarding the use of cobicistat during human pregnancy were located. No adverse effects related to the drug were noted, but the studies primarily evaluated the effect of the drug and pregnancy on various antiretroviral drug levels. The drug crosses the placenta, so some fetal exposure will occur. Therefore, this limited human pregnancy experience prevents a complete assessment of the embryofetal risk. Animal studies did not show any embryofetal toxicity in two species at doses of less than 10 times the RHD. Using this drug during pregnancy should be based on the pros and cons of the mother's clinical need for treatment versus any potential fetal risk that might occur from exposure. If a pregnant woman is taking this drug, health care providers are encouraged to register her by calling the Antiretroviral Pregnancy Registry at 1-800-258-4263.

BREASTFEEDING SUMMARY

No reports describing the use of cobicistat during human lactation have been located. Some of the drug will likely be found in breast milk. *However, the current Centers for Disease Control and Prevention recommendation is that mothers infected with HIV should NOT breastfeed their infants in order to reduce the risk of postnatal transmission of the virus to the neonate. In a clinical setting where a mother is not infected with HIV (or in cases where the HIV viral load is negative), the drug by itself is probably compatible. If used, the infant should be monitored for the most common reported adult side effects of jaundice and rash.

References

1. Prescribing Information. *Tybost*. Gilead Sciences; 2020.
2. Rimawi BH, Johnson E, Rajakumar A, et al. Pharmacokinetics and placental transfer of elvitegravir, dolutegravir, and other antiretrovirals during pregnancy. *Antimicrob Agents Chemother*. 2017;61:e02213-16.

COBIMETINIB

Antineoplastic (Kinase Inhibitor)

PREGNANCY RECOMMENDATION: No Human Data—Animal Data Suggest Potential Risk

BREASTFEEDING RECOMMENDATION: Potential Toxicity

C

PREGNANCY SUMMARY

No reports describing the use of cobimetinib in human pregnancy have been located. A limited amount of the drug may cross the placenta, so some fetal exposure might occur. Therefore, the absence of human pregnancy experience prevents a complete assessment of the embryofetal risk. Animal studies did show some embryofetal toxicity with malformations in one species at doses less than 10 times the RHD. Based on animal studies and the drug's mechanism of action, the manufacturer recommends that women with reproductive potential use effective contraception during treatment and for 2 weeks after the last dose. Nevertheless, using this drug during pregnancy should be based on the pros and cons of the mother's clinical need for treatment versus any potential fetal risk that might occur from exposure. In the clinical trials, 26% of patients on cobimetinib and vemurafenib had a decrease in left ventricular ejection fraction (LVEF). In patients who were only on vemurafenib, 19% had a decrease in LVEF. Patients should have a baseline LVEF obtained prior to drug initiation. There is a registry for women who are pregnant and have cancer. For more information, women and health care providers are encouraged to contact the Cancer and Pregnancy Registry at 1-877-635-4499.

BREASTFEEDING SUMMARY

No reports describing the use of cobimetinib during human lactation have been located. A limited amount of the drug may be found in breast milk. Due to a concern for potential serious adverse effects that might be seen in a breastfed infant, the manufacturer recommends that women not breastfeed while being treated with this drug and for at least 2 weeks after the last dose. However, breastfeeding while using this drug should be based on the mother's clinical need for treatment versus any potential infant risks that might occur. If used, the infant should be monitored for the most common reported adult side effects of nausea (leading to irritability), diarrhea, vomiting, fever, and various laboratory abnormalities (see PI).

Reference

1. Prescribing Information. *Cotellic*. Genentech; 2020.

CODEINE

Pain (Opioid)

PREGNANCY RECOMMENDATION: Human Data Suggest Risk (Third Trimester)

BREASTFEEDING RECOMMENDATION: *Potential Toxicity

PREGNANCY SUMMARY

Three large studies were located that evaluated the use of codeine in pregnancy and the risk for birth anomalies. The individual rates for major defects were 4.9%, 5.7%, and 2.4%. Combined data identified 447 (4.5%) major anomalies in 9,896 pregnancies. Though this rate is slightly elevated when compared with the upper limit for birth defects in the general population, no pattern to the anomalies was seen. In addition, many patients had other confounding drug use and maternal disease states that required this analgesic in the first trimester, which may have played a role. The drug crosses the placenta, so some fetal exposure will occur. Therefore, these data suggest that the use of this drug in the first trimester is low risk. Animal studies did show some embryofetal toxicity in three species at doses of less than 10 times the RHD. Using this drug during pregnancy should be based on the pros and cons of the mother's clinical need for treatment versus any potential fetal risk that might occur from exposure. Codeine has a morphine milli-equivalence of about 10% to 15%. It has the potential for dependence, misuse, and withdrawal, and is a Schedule II controlled substance. The drug carries a boxed warning for children for an increased risk of death in ultrarapid codeine metabolizers that convert more of the drug into morphine. This is caused by cytochrome P450 2D6 (CYP2D6) gene polymorphisms that are seen in about 5% of the population. In addition, chronic codeine use throughout pregnancy can lead to an increased risk for neonatal opioid withdrawal syndrome postdelivery.

BREASTFEEDING SUMMARY

Codeine has been studied in about 10 lactating women. Breast milk levels are low, ranging from about 70 ng/mL to 550 ng/mL. The morphine levels ranged from about 8 to 20 ng/mL. Calculated RIDs were less than 3%, but codeine-6-glucuronide was not analyzed, so this could be higher. Infant blood levels were also evaluated in 11 newborns. Concentrations were low, ranging from about 0.8 ng/mL to 4.5 ng/mL. Several other studies have reported cases where newborns showed signs of withdrawal postdelivery with apnea spells, cyanosis, drowsiness, lethargy, and decreased heart rate. However, there are numerous other reports where infants displayed no adverse reactions. Breastfeeding while using this drug should be based on the mother's clinical need for treatment versus any potential infant risks that might occur. If used, the infant should be monitored for the most common reported adult side effects of nausea and dizziness (both leading to irritability), drowsiness, sedation, lethargy, sweating, and vomiting. Some opioid drugs can increase prolactin levels, but this should not adversely

C

affect breastfeeding. *The primary concern with codeine involves the ultrarapid metabolizers, where a newborn could be exposed to or produce more morphine, leading to greater adverse effects. Therefore, using an alternative (if possible) would minimize this risk.

References

1. Shepard TH. *Catalog of Teratogenic Agents*. 10th ed. The Johns Hopkins University Press; 2001:127.
2. Schardein JL. *Chemically Induced Birth Defects*. 3rd ed. Marcel Dekker; 2000:140.
3. Heinonen OP, Slone D, Shapiro S. *Birth Defects and Drugs in Pregnancy*. Publishing Sciences Group; 1977.
4. Bracken MB, Holford TR. Exposure to prescribed drugs in pregnancy and association with congenital malformations. *Obstet Gynecol*. 1981;58:336-344.
5. Saxen I. Associations between oral clefts and drugs taken during pregnancy. *Int J Epidemiol*. 1975;4:37-44.
6. Saxen I. Epidemiology of cleft lip and palate: an attempt to rule out chance correlations. *Br J Prev Soc Med*. 1975;29:103-110.
7. Rothman KJ, Fyler DC, Goldblatt A, Kreidberg MB. Exogenous hormones and other drug exposures of children with congenital heart disease. *Am J Epidemiol*. 1979;109:433-439.
8. Broussard CS, Rasmussen SA, Reefhuis J, et al; National Birth Defects Prevention Study. Maternal treatment with opioid analgesics and risk for birth defects. *Am J Obstet Gynecol*. 2011;204:314-317.
9. Nezvalova-Henriksen K, Spigset O, Nordeng H. Effects of codeine on pregnancy outcome: results from a large population-based cohort study. *Eur J Clin Pharmacol*. 2011;67:1253-1261.
10. Gill AC, Oei J, Lewis NL, et al. Strabismus in infants of opiate-dependent mothers. *Acta Paediatr*. 2003;92:379-385.
11. Bonica JJ. *Principles and Practice of Obstetric Analgesia and Anesthesia*. FA Davis; 1967:245.
12. Van Leeuwen G, Guthrie R, Stange F. Narcotic withdrawal reaction in a newborn infant due to codeine. *Pediatrics*. 1965;36:635-636.
13. Mangurten HH, Benawra R. Neonatal codeine withdrawal in infants of nonaddicted mothers. *Pediatrics*. 1980;65:159-160.
14. Khan K, Chang J. Neonatal abstinence syndrome due to codeine. *Arch Dis Child*. 1997;76:F59-F60.
15. Creanga AA, Sabel JC, Ko JY, et al. Maternal drug use and its effect on neonates—a population-based study in Washington state. *Obstet Gynecol*. 2012;119:924-933.
16. Kwit NT, Hatcher RA. Excretion of drugs in milk. *Am J Dis Child*. 1935; 49:900-904.
17. Horning MG, Stillwell WG, Nowlin J, et al. Identification and quantification of drugs and drug metabolites in human breast milk using GC–MS–COM methods. *Mod Probl Paediatr*. 1975;15:73-79.
18. Drugs in breast milk. *Med Lett Drugs Ther*. 1974;16:25-27.
19. Meny RG, Naumburg EG, Alger LS, et al. Codeine and the breastfed neonate. *J Hum Lact*. 1993;9:237-240.
20. Koren G, Cairns J, Chitayat D, et al. Pharmacogenetics of morphine poisoning in a breastfed neonate of a codeine-prescribed mother. *Lancet*. 2006;368:704.
21. Madadi P, Ross CJD, Hayden MR, et al. Pharmacogenetics of neonatal opioid toxicity following maternal use of codeine during breastfeeding: a case-control study. *Clin Pharmacol Ther*. 2009;85:31-35.
22. Madadi P, Shirazi F, Walter FG, Koren G. Establishing causality of CNS depression in breastfed infants following maternal codeine use. *Paediatr Drugs*. 2008;10:399-404.
23. US Food and Drug Administration. FDA Drug Safety Communication: FDA restrics use of prescription codeine pain and cough medicines and tramadol pain medicines in children; recommends against use in breastfeeding women. April 17, 2017. Accessed November 3, 2025. https://www.fda.gov/drugs/drug-safety-and-availability/fda-drug-safety-communication-fda-restricts-use-prescription-codeine-pain-and-cough-medicines-and
24. Willmann S, Edginton AN, Coboeken K, et al. Risk to the breast-fed neonate from codeine treatment to the mother: a quantitative mechanistic modeling study. *Clin Pharmacol Ther*. 2009;86:634-643.
25. Madadi P, Moretti M, Djokanovic N, et al. Guidelines for maternal codeine use during breastfeeding. *Can Fam Physician*. 2009;55:1077-1078.

COLCHICINE

Antigout

PREGNANCY RECOMMENDATION: Limited Human Data—Animal Data Suggest Risk

BREASTFEEDING RECOMMENDATION: Probably Compatible

PREGNANCY SUMMARY

Numerous case reports and small studies have evaluated the use of colchicine during human pregnancy, and the risk of embryofetal harm appears to be low. The drug crosses the placenta, so some fetal exposure will occur. However, this limited human pregnancy experience still prevents a complete assessment of the embryofetal risk. Animal studies did show some teratogenicity in two species at doses of less than 10 times the RHD. Using this drug during pregnancy should be based on the pros and cons of the mother's clinical need for treatment versus any potential fetal risk that might occur from exposure.

BREASTFEEDING SUMMARY

Three studies were located that evaluated colchicine during human breastfeeding in six lactating women. The drug was found in breast milk in every patient. The highest breast milk level obtained was 31 ng/mL. The calculated RIDs using the peak levels were about 2.5%, 9%, and more than 10%. In one case, infant urine levels were analyzed, and the drug was not detected (LLQ of 5 ng/mL). Lastly, more than 100 follow-up cases of infants exposed to colchicine have not reported any adverse effects in infants. Breastfeeding while using this drug should be based on the mother's clinical need for treatment versus any potential infant risks that might occur. If used, the infant should be monitored for the most common reported adult side effects of abdominal and throat pain (both leading to irritability), diarrhea, and vomiting.

References

1. Berenstadt M, Welsz B, Cuckle H, et al. Chromosomal abnormalities and birth defects among couples with colchicine treated familial Mediterranean fever. *Am J Obstet Gynecol*. 2005;193:1513-1516.
2. Diav-Citrin O, Shechtman S, Schwartz V, et al. Pregnancy outcome after in utero exposure to colchicine. *Am J Obstet Gynecol*. 2010;203:144.e1-144.e8.
3. Ben-Chetrit E, Ben-Chetrit A, Berkun Y, Ben-Chetrit E. Pregnancy outcomes in women with familial Mediterranean fever receiving colchicine: is amniocentesis justified? *Arthritis Care Res*. 2010;62:143-148.
4. Product information. *Colchicine*. West-Ward Pharmaceuticals; 2018.
5. Shepard TH. *Catalog of Teratogenic Agents*. 6th ed. Johns Hopkins University Press; 1989:164-166.

6. Sokal JE, Lessmann EM. Effects of cancer chemotherapeutic agents on the human fetus. *JAMA*. 1960;172:1765-1772.
7. Cohen MM, Levy M, Eliakim M. A cytogenetic evaluation of long-term colchicine therapy in the treatment of familial Mediterranean fever (FMF). *Am J Med Sci*. 1977;274:147-152.
8. Levy M, Yaffe C. Testicular function in patients with familial Mediterranean fever on long-term colchicine treatment. *Fertil Steril*. 1978;29:667-668.
9. Zemer D, Pras M, Sohar E, Gafni J. Colchicine in familial Mediterranean fever. *N Engl J Med*. 1976;294:170-171.
10. Milunsky JM, Milunsky A. Breast-feeding during colchicine therapy for familial Mediterranean fever. *J Pediatr*. 1991;119:164.
11. Ben-Chetrit E, Scherrmann JM, Levy M. Colchicine in breast milk of patients with familial Mediterranean fever. *Arthritis Rheum*. 1996;39:1213-1217.
12. Guillonneau M, Aigrain EJ, Galliot M, et al. Colchicine is excreted at high concentrations in human breast milk. *Eur J Obstet Gynecol Reprod Biol*. 1995;61:177-178.
13. Ehrenfeld M, Brzezinski A, Levy M, Eliakim M. Fertility and obstetric history in patients with familial Mediterranean fever on long-term colchicine therapy. *Br J Obstet Gynaecol*. 1987;94:1186-1191.
14. Shimoni Y, Shalev E. Pregnancy and complicated familial Mediterranean fever. *Int J Gynaecol Obstet*. 1990;33:165-169.
15. Rabinovitch O, Zemer D, Kukia E, et al. Colchicine treatment in conception and pregnancy: two hundred thirty-one pregnancies in patients with familial Mediterranean fever. *Am J Reprod Immunol*. 1992;28:245-246.
16. Mordel N, Birkenfeld A, Rubinger D, et al. Successful full-term pregnancy in familial Mediterranean fever complicated with amyloidosis: case report and review of the literature. *Fetal Diagn Ther*. 1993;8:129-134.
17. Ditkoff EC, Sauer MV. Successful pregnancy in familial Mediterranean fever patient following assisted reproduction. *J Assist Reprod Genet*. 1996;13:684-685.
18. Michael O, Goldman RD, Koren G; Motherisk Team. Safety of colchicine during pregnancy. *Can Fam Physician*. 2003;49:967-969.
19. Ben-Chetrit E, Berkun Y, Ben-Chetrit E, Ben-Chetrit A. The outcome of pregnancy in the wives of men with familial Mediterranean fever treated with colchicine. Semin *Arthritis Rheum*. 2004;34:549-552.
20. Cerquaglia C, Diaco M, Nucera G, et al. Pharmacological and clinical basis of treatment of familial Mediterranean fever (FMF) with colchicine or analogues: an update. *Curr Drug Targets Inflamm Allergy*. 2005;4:117-124.
21. Tutuncu L, Atasoyu EM, Evrenkaya R, Mungen E. Familial Mediterranean fever-related nephrotic syndrome and successful full-term pregnancy. *Arch Med Res*. 2006;37:178-180.
22. Ofir D, Levy A, Wiznitzer A, et al. Familial Mediterranean fever during pregnancy: an independent risk factor for preterm delivery. *Eur J Obstet Gynecol Reprod Biol*. 2008;141:115-118.
23. Cerquaglia C, Verrecchia E, Fonnesu C, et al. Female reproductive dysfunction in familial Mediterranean fever patients with and without colchicine treatment. *Clin Exp Rheumatol*. 2010;28(4 suppl 60):S101.
24. Amoura Z, Schermann JM, Weclisler B, et al. Transplacental passage of colchicine in familial Mediterranean fever. *J Rheumatol*. 1944;21:383.
25. Salesi M, Karimifar M, Salimi F, Mahzouni P. A case of granulomatous mastitis with erythema nodosum and arthritis. *Rheumatol Int*. 2011;31:1093-1095.
26. Cestari AN, Botelho Vieira Filho JP, Yonenaga Y, et al. A case of human reproductive abnormalities possibly induced by colchicine treatment. *Rev Bras Biol*. 1965;25:253-256.
27. Ferreira NR, Buoniconti A. Trisomy after colchicine therapy. *Lancet*. 1968; 2:1304.
28. Walker FA. Trisomy after colchicine therapy. *Lancet*. 1969;1:257-258.
29. Timson J. Trisomy after colchicine therapy. *Lancet*. 1969;1:370.
30. Hoefnagel D. Trisomy after colchicine therapy. *Lancet*. 1969;1:1160.
31. Ferreira NR, Frota-Pessoa O. Trisomy after colchicine therapy. *Lancet*. 1969;1: 1160-1161.
32. Yu TF, Gutman AB. Efficacy of colchicine prophylaxis in gout. Prevention of recurrent gouty arthritis over a mean period of five years in 208 gouty subjects. *Ann Intern Med*. 1961;55:179-192.
33. Goldfinger SE. Colchicine for familial Mediterranean fever: possible adverse effects. *N Engl J Med*. 1974;290:56.
34. Poffenbarger PL, Brinkley BR. Colchicine for familial Mediterranean fever: possible adverse effects. *N Engl J Med*. 1974;290:56.
35. Merlin HE. Azoospermia caused by colchicine—a case report. *Fertil Steril*. 1972;23:180-181.
36. Bremer WJ, Paulsen CA. Colchicine and testicular function in man. *N Engl J Med*. 1976;294:1384-1385.
37. Haimov-Kochman R, Ben-Chetrit E. The effect of colchicine treatment on sperm production and function: a review. *Hum Reprod*. 1998;13:360-362.
38. American Academy of Pediatrics Committee on Drugs. The transfer of drugs and other chemicals into human milk. *Pediatrics*. 2001;108:776-789.

COLESTIPOL

Antilipemic

PREGNANCY RECOMMENDATION: No Human Data—Animal Data Suggest Low Risk

BREASTFEEDING RECOMMENDATION: Probably Compatible

PREGNANCY SUMMARY

No reports describing the use of colestipol in human pregnancy have been located. The drug will not cross the placenta in any clinically significant amount. However, the absence of human pregnancy experience prevents a complete assessment of the embryofetal risk. Animal studies did not show any embryofetal toxicity in two species. Prolonged use of colestipol may result in reduced intestinal absorption of the fat-soluble vitamins A, D, E, and K. Using this drug during pregnancy should be based on the pros and cons of the mother's clinical need for treatment versus any potential fetal risk that might occur from exposure.

BREASTFEEDING SUMMARY

No reports describing the use of colestipol during human lactation have been located. Though the MW of the drug is small enough to be found in breast milk, the complex made with binding to intraintestinal bile acids is not absorbed systemically. Therefore, infant exposure should not occur. Prolonged use of colestipol, however, may result in decreased maternal absorption of the fat-soluble vitamins A, D, E, and K.

Reference

1. Prescribing Information. *Colestipol Hydrochloride*. Greenstone; 2018.

C

COLESEVELAM

Antilipemic (Bile Acid–Binding Molecule)

PREGNANCY RECOMMENDATION: Limited Human Data Suggest Low Risk

BREASTFEEDING RECOMMENDATION: Compatible

PREGNANCY SUMMARY

One report described five cases of familial hypercholesterolemia in pregnancy that were treated with colesevelam before conception. Two women stopped the therapy prior to 4 weeks' gestation, but the other three continued throughout gestation. All five newborns were delivered at term with no identified anomalies or complications. The drug does not cross the placenta because it is not absorbed systemically. Animal studies did not show any embryofetal toxicity or teratogenicity in two species at doses of greater than 10 times the MRHD. Using this drug during pregnancy should be based on the pros and cons of the mother's clinical need for treatment versus any potential fetal risk that might occur from exposure. The effect of colesevelam on the absorption of vitamins and other nutrients from the gastrointestinal tract in pregnant women has not been studied. However, a deficiency of fat-soluble vitamins (A, D, E, and K) is a potential complication if colesevelam is used during pregnancy. To prevent this potential risk, the manufacturer recommends that oral vitamins containing vitamin K be taken at least 4 hours before colesevelam dosing.

BREASTFEEDING SUMMARY

No reports describing the use of colesevelam during human lactation have been located. The drug is not absorbed systemically after oral administration, so a nursing infant will not be exposed via breast milk. However, maternal deficiency of fat-soluble vitamins, especially vitamin K, is a theoretical complication with the use of colesevelam. Therefore, this potentially could result in lower fat-soluble vitamin concentrations in breast milk. However, this has not been studied or reported.

References

1. Prescribing Information. *Colesevelam*. Ascend Laboratories; 2018.
2. Eapen DJ, Valiani K, Reddy S, Sperling L. Management of familial hypercholesterolemia during pregnancy: case series and discussion. *J Clin Lipidol*. 2012;6:88-91.

COLISTIMETHATE

Antibacterial (Polypeptide)

PREGNANCY RECOMMENDATION: Limited Human Data—Animal Data Suggest Potential Risk

BREASTFEEDING RECOMMENDATION: Probably Compatible

PREGNANCY SUMMARY

No reports describing the use of colistimethate in human pregnancy have been located. The drug crosses the placenta at the end of gestation, so some fetal exposure will occur. Passage across the placenta in the first trimester is unknown. Therefore, the absence of early human pregnancy experience prevents a complete assessment of the embryofetal risk. Animal studies did show some embryofetal toxicity with teratogenicity (talipes varus) in one species at doses less than 10 times the MRHD. Using this drug during pregnancy should be based on the pros and cons of the mother's clinical need for treatment versus any potential fetal risk that might occur from exposure.

BREASTFEEDING SUMMARY

Colistimethate was administered to 20 women postdelivery at various doses, and colistin was detected in breast milk at average peak levels of 165 to 215 ng/mL. Therefore, colistin is found in breast milk following an injection of colistimethate. However, colistin is not absorbed from the gastrointestinal tract. In addition, because it is a polypeptide consisting of 10 amino acids, if the drug were to be ingested through breastfeeding, it would probably be digested in the infant's gastrointestinal tract. Breastfeeding while using this drug should be based on the mother's clinical need for treatment versus any potential infant risks that might occur.

References

1. Prescribing Information. *Colistimethate*. Par Pharmaceuticals; 2018.
2. MacAulay MA, Charles D. Placental transmission of colistimethate. *Clin Pharmacol Ther*. 1967;8:578-586.
3. Borderon E, Soutoul JH, Borderon JC, et al. Excretion of antibiotics in human milk. *Med Mal Infect*. 1975;5:373-376.

C

COLLAGENASE (*CLOSTRIDIUM HISTOLYTICUM*)

Dermatologic

PREGNANCY RECOMMENDATION: Human Data Suggest Low Risk

BREASTFEEDING RECOMMENDATION: Compatible

PREGNANCY SUMMARY

No reports describing the use of collagenase *Clostridium histolyticum* in human pregnancy have been located. The drug is not likely to cross the placenta; however, because it consists of two large proteins, it is not known whether some fetal exposure could occur in the second half of gestation. Regardless, administration during pregnancy would only occur in Dupuytren contracture, and systemic levels were not seen with this usage. Animal studies did not show any embryofetal toxicity in one species at doses of more than 10 times the RHD. Using this drug during pregnancy should be based on the pros and cons of the mother's clinical need for treatment versus any potential fetal risk that might occur from exposure. Almost all patients treated with collagenase *Clostridium histolyticum* develop antiproduct antibodies after treatment. The clinical significance of these antibodies on a developing fetus is not known.

BREASTFEEDING SUMMARY

No reports describing the use of collagenase *Clostridium histolyticum* during human lactation have been located. The MWs of collagenase AUX-1 and collagenase AUX-II suggest that the proteins will not be found in breast milk. In addition, there is a lack of systemic absorption with injection into a Dupuytren contracture; the extremely short elimination and they are proteins and likely to be digested (if present) by the infant's gastrointestinal tract (and not absorbed) if any amount were still present, it would be clinically insignificant.

Reference

1. Product information. *Xiaflex*. Endo Pharmaceuticals; 2016.

CONIVAPTAN

Endocrine/Metabolic (Vasopressin Receptor Antagonist)

PREGNANCY RECOMMENDATION: No Human Data—Animal Data Suggest Potential Risk

BREASTFEEDING RECOMMENDATION: Potential Toxicity

PREGNANCY SUMMARY

No reports describing the use of conivaptan in human pregnancy have been located. The drug will probably cross the placenta, so some fetal exposure will likely occur. Therefore, the absence of human pregnancy experience prevents a complete assessment of the embryofetal risk. Animal studies did show some embryofetal toxicity in one species at doses less than the RHD. Using this drug during pregnancy should be based on the pros and cons of the mother's clinical need for treatment versus any potential fetal risk that might occur from exposure.

BREASTFEEDING SUMMARY

No reports describing the use of conivaptan during human lactation have been located. The drug will probably be found in breast milk, so some infant exposure will likely occur. Due to a concern for potential serious adverse effects that might be seen in a breastfed infant, the manufacturer recommends that women not breastfeed while being treated with this drug. Nevertheless, breastfeeding while using this drug should be based on the mother's clinical need for treatment versus any potential infant risks that might occur. If used, the infant should be monitored for the most common reported adult side effects of headache (leading to irritability), fever, hypokalemia, and hypotension.

Reference

1. Prescribing Information. *Vaprisol*. Cumberland Pharmaceuticals; 2018.

C

COPANLISIB

Antineoplastic (Kinase Inhibitor)

PREGNANCY RECOMMENDATION: No Human Data and No Relevant Animal Data

BREASTFEEDING RECOMMENDATION: Potential Toxicity

PREGNANCY SUMMARY

No reports describing the use of copanlisib in human pregnancy have been located. Some amount of the drug will probably cross the placenta, so fetal exposure will likely occur. However, the absence of human pregnancy experience prevents a complete assessment of the embryofetal risk. Animal studies showed embryofetal toxicity and teratogenicity, but all treatment doses caused maternal toxicity. Based on the animal studies and the drug's mechanism of action, the manufacturer recommends that women with reproductive potential use effective contraception during treatment and for 1 month after the last dose. They also recommend that males with female partners of reproductive potential use effective contraception during treatment and for 1 month after the last dose. However, using this drug during pregnancy should be based on the pros and cons of the mother's clinical need for treatment versus any potential fetal risk that might occur from exposure. In the clinical trials, the drug caused hypertension and hyperglycemia in 26% and 41% of the participants, respectively.

BREASTFEEDING SUMMARY

No reports describing the use of copanlisib during human lactation have been located. Some of the drug probably enters breast milk, so infant exposure will likely occur. However, due to the concern for potential serious adverse effects in a breastfed infant, the manufacturer recommends that women not breastfeed while being treated with copanlisib and for at least 1 month after the last dose. Nevertheless, breastfeeding while using this drug should be based on the mother's clinical need for treatment. If used, the infant should be monitored for the most common reported adult side effects of nausea (leading to irritability), diarrhea, lethargy, hypertension, and lower respiratory tract infection.

Reference

1. Prescribing Information. *Aliqopa*. Bayer Healthcare Pharmaceuticals, Inc; 2017.

COPPER CU 64 DOTATATE

Radiopharmaceutical Agent

PREGNANCY RECOMMENDATION: No Human Data and No Relevant Animal Data (Maternal Benefit May Outweigh Embryo–Fetal Risk)

BREASTFEEDING RECOMMENDATION: Potential Toxicity (Hold Breastfeeding)

PREGNANCY SUMMARY

No reports describing the use of Copper Cu 64 dotatate in human pregnancy have been located. A limited amount of the drug may cross the placenta, primarily in the second half of the pregnancy. Animal studies have not been performed. However, the absence of human pregnancy experience prevents a complete assessment of the embryofetal risk. Because this diagnostic agent is radioactive, there could be a potential for fetal harm based on the fetal stage of development and the magnitude of the radiation dose. However, based on the clinical situation (and gestational age), a maternal benefit may outweigh the embryofetal risk in some cases.

BREASTFEEDING SUMMARY

Copper Cu 64 dotatate is probably excreted into human breast milk in limited amounts. The manufacturer recommends that breastfeeding be interrupted for 12 hours after the agent is administered to minimize radiation exposure to the infant.

Reference

1. Prescribing Information. *Detectnet*. Curium US LLC; 2020.

CORTICOTROPIN

Immunologic (Corticosteroid-Stimulating Hormone)

PREGNANCY RECOMMENDATION: Limited Human Data-No Relevant Animal Data

BREASTFEEDING RECOMMENDATION: Probably Compatible

C

PREGNANCY SUMMARY

The Collaborative Perinatal Project reported first-trimester exposure to corticotropin in six patients, and none of the newborns had any identifiable malformations. The drug will probably not cross the placenta, so fetal exposure is unlikely to occur. However, it is unknown what may cross the placenta regarding the other porcine pituitary peptides that may be present. Therefore, the limited human pregnancy experience prevents a complete assessment of the embryofetal risk. Animal reproduction studies have not been located. Corticosteroids have been suggested to cause human malformations, but this has not been confirmed (see Hydrocortisone). Because corticotropin stimulates the release of endogenous corticosteroids, this relationship should be considered when prescribing the drug to women in their reproductive years.

BREASTFEEDING SUMMARY

No reports describing the use of corticotropin during human lactation have been located. The drug will not likely be found in breast milk. Additionally, if any of the corticotropin hormone were to be ingested through breast milk, because it is a protein, it would likely be digested in the infant's gastrointestinal tract and not be absorbed. It is unknown whether any other peptides from the porcine pituitary, that may be found in corticotropin, will be excreted into breast milk. But again, they would likely also be digested in the infant's gastrointestinal tract and not be absorbed. The use of this agent during breastfeeding is probably compatible.

References

1. Prescribing Information. *Acthar gel*. Mallinckrodt; 2024.
2. Heinonen OP, Slone D, Shapiro S. *Birth Defects and Drugs in Pregnancy*. Wright PSB; 1983:391.

CORTISONE

Corticosteroid

See Hydrocortisone.

COSYNTROPIN

Endocrine/Diagnostic (Corticosteroid-Stimulating Hormone)

PREGNANCY RECOMMENDATION: Limited Human Data-No Relevant Animal Data

BREASTFEEDING RECOMMENDATION: Probably Compatible

PREGNANCY SUMMARY

No reports describing the use of cosyntropin in the first trimester of human pregnancy have been located. The drug has been used in the third trimester for diagnostic purposes of possible adrenocortical insufficiency and in one study to potentially increase fetal lung maturity in a group of preterm gestations, with no reported adverse events described. The drug will probably not cross the placenta, so fetal exposure is unlikely to occur. Therefore, this limited human pregnancy experience prevents a complete assessment of the embryofetal risk. Animal reproduction studies have not been located. Using this agent during pregnancy should be based on the pros and cons of the mother's clinical need for diagnosis and to assess treatment options versus any potential fetal risk that might occur from exposure.

BREASTFEEDING SUMMARY

No reports describing the use of cosyntropin during human lactation have been located. The drug will not likely be found in breast milk. Additionally, if any amount of the drug were to be ingested through breast milk, because it is a protein, it would likely be digested in the infant's gastrointestinal tract and not be absorbed. The use of this agent during breastfeeding is probably compatible.

References

1. Prescribing Information. *Cosyntropin*. Sandoz, Inc; 2019.

2. Klimek R, Milewicz S. Reduction of RDS mortality in newborns after administration of synthetic ACTH to the mothers. *Ginekol Pol*. 1983;54:341-343.
3. Johnstone FD, Campbell S. Adrenal response in pregnancy to long-acting tetracosactin. *J Obstet Gynaecol Br Commonw*. 1974;81:363-367.
4. Simmer HH, Tulchinsky D, Gold EM, et al. On the regulation of estrogen production by cortisol and ACTH in human pregnancy at term. *Am J Obstet Gynecol*. 1974;119:283-296.
5. Aral K, Kuwabara Y, Okinaga S. The effect of adrenocorticotropic hormone and dexamethasone, administered to the fetus in utero, upon maternal and fetal estrogens. *Am J Obstet Gynecol*. 1972;113:316-322.
6. Popert AJ. Pregnancy and adrenocortical hormones. Some aspects of their interaction in rheumatic diseases. *Br Med J*. 1962;2:967-972.

C

COUMARIN DERIVATIVES

Anticoagulant

See Warfarin

CRISABOROLE

Dermatologic (Topical)

PREGNANCY RECOMMENDATION: No Human Data—Animal Data Suggest Low Risk

BREASTFEEDING RECOMMENDATION: Probably Compatible

PREGNANCY SUMMARY

No reports describing the use of crisaborole in human pregnancy have been located. The drug will probably cross the placenta, so some fetal exposure may occur. However, the overall amount with topical use is likely to be small. Nevertheless, the absence of human pregnancy experience prevents a complete assessment of the embryofetal risk. Animal studies did not show any embryofetal toxicity or malformations in two species. Using this drug during pregnancy should be based on the pros and cons of the mother's clinical need for treatment versus any potential fetal risk that might occur from exposure.

BREASTFEEDING SUMMARY

No reports describing the use of crisaborole during human lactation have been located. The drug may be found in breast milk, but the overall levels are likely to be small. Breastfeeding while using this drug should be based on the mother's clinical need for treatment versus any potential infant risks that might occur. Because the drug is used topically, systemic side effects were not evaluated.

Reference

1. Prescribing Information. *Eucrisa*. Pfizer, Inc; 2020.

CRIZANLIZUMAB

Hematologic (Monoclonal Antibody)

PREGNANCY RECOMMENDATION: No Human Data—Animal Data Suggest Potential Risk

BREASTFEEDING RECOMMENDATION: Probably Compatible

PREGNANCY SUMMARY

No reports describing the use of crizanlizumab in human pregnancy have been located. As an IgG antibody, it likely crosses the placenta, especially during the second half of pregnancy, so some fetal exposure will probably occur. Therefore, the absence of human pregnancy experience prevents a complete assessment of the embryofetal risk. Animal studies did show some embryofetal toxicity in one species. Using this drug during pregnancy should be based on the pros and cons of the mother's clinical need for treatment versus any potential fetal risk that might occur from exposure.

BREASTFEEDING SUMMARY

No reports describing the use of crizanlizumab during human lactation have been located. It is known that IgG antibodies can be found in human breast milk, but are not found in the neonatal or infant circulation. Additionally, if any IgG antibodies were to be ingested through breastfeeding, they would probably be digested in the infant's gastrointestinal tract and not be absorbed. Breastfeeding while using this drug should be based on the mother's clinical need for treatment versus any potential infant risks that might occur. If used, the infant should be monitored for the most common reported adult side effects of nausea, arthralgia, and back pain (all leading to irritability) and fever.

Reference

1. Prescribing Information. *Adakveo*. Novartis Pharmaceuticals Corp; 2019.

C

CRIZOTINIB

Antineoplastic (Tyrosine Kinase Inhibitor)

PREGNANCY RECOMMENDATION: Limited Human Data—Animal Data Suggest Potential Risk

BREASTFEEDING RECOMMENDATION: Potential Toxicity

PREGNANCY SUMMARY

Two case reports of the use of crizotinib during the second trimester of human pregnancy were located. Preterm delivery occurred in both cases (26 and 30 weeks' gestation), and both infants did well, other than issues related to prematurity. No malformations were noted. In a third study, a patient treated with crizotinib for metastatic Anaplastic Lymphoma Kinase (ALK)-positive lung cancer had egg retrieval performed, followed by a successful surrogate twin delivery. No birth anomalies were noted. The drug appears to cross the placenta, though levels are low overall. However, this limited human pregnancy experience prevents a complete assessment of the embryofetal risk. Animal studies did show some embryofetal toxicity in one species at doses less than 10 times the RHD. Based on these animal studies and the drug's mechanism of action, the manufacturer recommends that women with reproductive potential use effective contraception during treatment and for 45 days after the last dose. They also recommend that males with female partners of reproductive potential use effective contraception during treatment and for 90 days after the last dose. Nevertheless, using this drug during pregnancy should be based on the pros and cons of the mother's clinical need for treatment versus any potential fetal risk that might occur from exposure. Use of this drug has also been associated with prolongation of the QT interval. There is a registry for women who are pregnant and have cancer. For more information, women and health care providers are encouraged to contact the Cancer and Pregnancy Registry at 1-877-635-4499.

BREASTFEEDING SUMMARY

No reports describing the use of crizotinib during human lactation have been located. The drug will probably be found in breast milk, so some infant exposure will likely occur. Due to a concern for potential serious adverse effects that might be seen in a breastfed infant, the manufacturer recommends that women not breastfeed while being treated with this drug and for at least 45 days after the last dose. Nevertheless, breastfeeding while using this drug should be based on the mother's clinical need for treatment versus any potential infant risks that might occur. If used, the infant should be monitored for the most common reported adult side effects of nausea, headache, neuropathy, abdominal pain, and dizziness (all leading to irritability), diarrhea, fatigue (lethargy), vomiting, edema, decreased appetite, rash, fever, and various laboratory abnormalities (see PI).

References

1. Prescribing Information. *Xalkori*. Pfizer Laboratories; 2020.
2. Eliesen GAM, van den Broek P, van den Heuvel JJ, et al. Editor's highlight: placental disposition and effects of crizotinib: an *ex vivo* study in the isolated dual-side perfused human cotyledon. *Toxicol Sci*. 2017;157:500-509.
3. Roelofsen D, van Hove H, Bukkems V, et al. Predicting fetal exposure of crizotinib during pregnancy: combining human *ex vivo* placenta perfusion data with physiologically-based pharmacokinetic modeling. *Toxicol in Vitro*. 2022;85:105471.
4. Jensen KH, Persson G, Storgaard L, et al. Antineoplastic treatment with crizotinib during pregnancy: a case report. *Acta Oncol*. 2019;58:121-122.
5. Padrao E, Melo C, Fernandes G, Magalhaes A. Lung cancer in pregnancy—report of a case treated with crizotinib. *Pulmonology*. 2018;24:205-207.
6. Su HI, Connell MW, Bazhenova LA. Ovarian stimulation in young adult cancer survivors on targeted cancer therapies. *Fertil Steril*. 2016;106:1475-1482.
7. Nieves I, Mota PC, Hespanhol VP. Lung cancer during pregnancy: an unusual case. *Rev Port Pneumol*. 2014;20:46-49.
8. Bellido C, Barbero P, Forcen L, et al. Lung adenocarcinoma during pregnancy: clinical case and literature review. *J Matern Fetal Neonatal Med*. 2019;32:3300-3302.

CROFELEMER

Gastrointestinal (Antidiarrheal)

PREGNANCY RECOMMENDATION: No Human Data—Animal Data Suggest Low Risk

BREASTFEEDING RECOMMENDATION: Probably Compatible

PREGNANCY SUMMARY

No reports describing the use of crofelemer in human pregnancy have been located. The drug probably does not cross the placenta, so any fetal exposure would likely be clinically insignificant. However, the absence of human pregnancy experience

(*continued*)

C

prevents a complete assessment of the embryofetal risk. Animal studies did not show any embryofetal toxicity in one animal species. Using this drug during pregnancy should be based on the pros and cons of the mother's clinical need for treatment versus any potential fetal risk that might occur from exposure.

BREASTFEEDING SUMMARY

No reports describing the use of crofelemer during human lactation have been located. The drug is not likely to be found in breast milk, especially at any level that would be clinically significant. Breastfeeding while using this drug should be based on the mother's clinical need for treatment versus any potential infant risks that might occur. If used, the infant should be monitored for the most common reported adult side effects of nausea and back pain (both leading to irritability), cough, flatulence, and elevated bilirubin levels.

Reference

1. Prescribing Information. *Mytesi*. Napo Pharmaceuticals; 2018.

CROMOLYN SODIUM

Respiratory/Gastrointestinal (Mast Cell Stabilizer)

PREGNANCY RECOMMENDATION: Human Data Suggest Low Risk

BREASTFEEDING RECOMMENDATION: Probably Compatible

PREGNANCY SUMMARY

Several studies have reported the use of cromolyn sodium in the first trimester of human pregnancy. From a total of over 670 exposures, 18 (2.7%) major anomalies were identified. No pattern to the anomalies was seen. The drug may cross the placenta; however, most levels would likely be clinically insignificant due to low systemic absorption of the oral, nasal spray, and inhalation products. Animal studies did not show any embryofetal toxicity or malformations in three species at doses of more than 10 times the RHD. Using this drug during pregnancy should be based on the pros and cons of the mother's clinical need for treatment versus any potential fetal risk that might occur from exposure.

BREASTFEEDING SUMMARY

No reports describing the use of cromolyn sodium during lactation have been located. The drug may be found in breast milk, but the low systemic levels following oral, nasal spray, and inhalation use, along with the short elimination half-life, should greatly limit infant exposure. Breastfeeding while using this drug should be based on the mother's clinical need for treatment versus any potential infant risks that might occur. If used, the infant should be monitored for the most common reported adult side effects of nausea and abdominal cramping (both leading to irritability, vomiting, diarrhea, edema, rash, and cough).

References

1. Product information. *Cromolyn Sodium solution*. Wallace Pharmaceuticals; 2015.
2. Product information. *Cromolyn Sodium spray*. Bausch & Lomb; 2017.
3. Dykes MHM. Evaluation of an antiasthmatic agent cromolyn sodium (Aarane, Intal). *JAMA*. 1974;227:1061-1062.
4. Greenberger P, Patterson R. Safety of therapy for allergic symptoms during pregnancy. *Ann Intern Med*. 1978;89:234-237.
5. Weinstein AM, Dubin BD, Podleski WK, et al. Asthma and pregnancy. *JAMA*. 1979;241:1161-1165.
6. Pratt WR. Allergic diseases in pregnancy and breast feeding. *Ann Allergy Asthma Immunol*. 1981;47:355-360.
7. Mawhinney H, Spector SL. Optimum management of asthma in pregnancy. *Drugs*. 1986;32:178-187.
8. Niebyl JR. *Drug Use in Pregnancy*. Lea & Febiger; 1982:53.
9. Cox JSG, Beach JE, Blair AMJN, Clarke AJ. Disodium cromoglycate (Intal). *Adv Drug Res*. 1970;5:135-136. As cited in Shepard TH. *Catalog of Teratogenic Agents*. 6th ed. Johns Hopkins University Press; 1989:174.
10. Shepard TH. *Catalog of Teratogenic Agents*. 6th ed. Johns Hopkins University Press; 1989:174.
11. Wilson J. Use of sodium cromoglycate during pregnancy: results on 296 asthmatic women. *Acta Therap*. 1982;8(suppl):45-51.
12. Blaiss MS; National Institute of Health. Management of asthma during pregnancy. *Allergy Asthma Proc*. 2004;25:375-379.
13. National Heart, Lung, and Blood Institute; National Asthma Education and Prevention Program Asthma and Pregnancy Working Group. NAEPP expert panel report. Managing asthma during pregnancy: recommendations for pharmacologic treatment-2004 update. J Allergy Clin Immunol. 2005 Jan;115(1):34-46.

CROMOLYN SODIUM OPHTHALMIC

Ophthalmic (Mast Cell Stabilizer)

PREGNANCY RECOMMENDATION: No Human Data—Animal Data Suggest Low Risk

BREASTFEEDING RECOMMENDATION: Probably Compatible

C

PREGNANCY SUMMARY

No reports describing the use of cromolyn sodium ophthalmic in human pregnancy have been located. The drug may cross the placenta; however, any levels would likely be clinically insignificant. Nevertheless, the absence of human pregnancy experience prevents a complete assessment of the embryofetal risk. Animal studies did not show any malformations or embryofetal toxicity in three species. Using this drug during pregnancy should be based on the pros and cons of the mother's clinical need for treatment versus any potential fetal risk that might occur from exposure. If used during pregnancy, consider placing pressure over the tear duct in the corner of the eye for at least 1 minute, and then remove any excess solution with absorbent tissue to decrease the amount of drug reaching the systemic circulation even further.

BREASTFEEDING SUMMARY

No reports describing the use of cromolyn sodium ophthalmic during lactation have been located. The drug may be found in breast milk, but any levels would likely be clinically insignificant. Breastfeeding while using this drug should be based on the mother's clinical need for treatment versus any potential infant risks that might occur. If used, the infant should be monitored for the most common reported adult side effects of edema, rash, and cough. A method to decrease some systemic absorption with ophthalmic use is described above in the Pregnancy Summary.

Reference

1. Prescribing Information. *Cromolyn Sodium Ophthalmic solution*. Akorn; 2019.

CROVALIMAB

Hematologic (Monoclonal Antibody—Complement C5 Inhibitor)

PREGNANCY RECOMMENDATION: No Human Data—Animal Data Suggest Low Risk

BREASTFEEDING RECOMMENDATION: Probably Compatible

PREGNANCY SUMMARY

No reports describing the use of crovalimab in human pregnancy have been located. As an IgG antibody, it likely crosses the placenta, especially during the second half of pregnancy, so some fetal exposure will probably occur. Therefore, the absence of human pregnancy experience prevents a complete assessment of the embryofetal risk. Animal reproduction studies did not show any embryofetal toxicity or malformations in one species at doses of more than 10 times the RHD. Using this drug during pregnancy should be based on the pros and cons of the mother's clinical need for treatment versus any potential fetal risk that might occur from exposure.

BREASTFEEDING SUMMARY

No reports describing the use of crovalimab during human lactation have been located. It is known that IgG antibodies can be found in human breast milk, but are not found in the neonatal or infant circulation. Additionally, if any IgG antibodies were to be ingested through breastfeeding, they would probably be digested in the infant's gastrointestinal tract and not be absorbed. Regardless, due to a concern for potential serious adverse effects that might be seen in a breastfed infant, the manufacturer recommends that women not breastfeed while being treated with this drug and for at least 9 months after the last dose. Nevertheless, breastfeeding while using this drug should be based on the mother's clinical need for treatment. If used, the infant should be monitored for the most common reported adult side effects of various infections.

Reference

1. Prescribing Information. *Piasky*. Genentech; 2024.

CYCLOBENZAPRINE

Pain (Muscle Relaxant)

PREGNANCY RECOMMENDATION: Human Data Suggest Potential Risk—Animal Data Suggest Low Risk

BREASTFEEDING RECOMMENDATION: Potential Toxicity

C

PREGNANCY SUMMARY

In a surveillance study of Michigan Medicaid recipients, there were 713 first-trimester exposures to cyclobenzaprine. A total of 36 (5.0%) major birth defects were observed (29 expected). However, no specific pattern to the anomalies was noted, and coexposures to other drugs occurred but were not described. A case report described the use of cyclobenzaprine at 34 weeks' gestation, and no adverse effects were described in the delivered infant. A second case report described a patient who was using cyclobenzaprine and acetaminophen in the last few weeks of gestation, and the delivered infant developed persistent pulmonary hypertension (PPH) due to premature closure of the ductus arteriosus. It is not known if the PPH was caused by the cyclobenzaprine, and this newborn medical condition has not been further reported in conjunction with cyclobenzaprine exposure. Combined data from the National Birth Defects Prevention Study and the Birth Defect Study to Evaluate Pregnancy Exposures found 51 (0.15%) self-reported periconceptional exposures (defined as 1 month prior to conception to 3 months of completed pregnancy) to cyclobenzaprine out of 33,615 cases of infants with anomalies. These were compared with 9 (0.07%) cyclobenzaprine-exposed in 13,110 control patients. The drug was found to be associated with a significant increase in cardiac malformations involving atrial septal defects, pulmonary valve stenosis, coarctation of the aorta, and transposition of the great vessels. In addition, there was a significant increase in the risk for cleft lip and palate and anorectal atresia/stenosis. However, self-reported recall history can be flawed (in some cases, the interview occurred up to 3 years after the patient's first trimester); verification of actual drug use, dosage, and exact timing of use during the first trimester cannot be confirmed; and recall may be affected by whether or not a mother delivered a newborn with an anomaly. The drug will probably cross the placenta, so some fetal exposure will likely occur. Animal studies did not show any embryofetal toxicity or teratogenicity in three species at doses of more than 10 times the RHD. Using this drug during pregnancy should be based on the pros and cons of the mother's clinical need for treatment versus any potential fetal risk that might occur from exposure. It is recommended that the drug only be used for a short duration, up to 2 to 3 weeks.

BREASTFEEDING SUMMARY

One study evaluated the transfer of cyclobenzaprine in two lactating mothers. One mother was taking 5 mg daily, and the other mother was using 20 mg daily. Based on peak breast milk levels, the maximum calculated weight-adjusted RID is about 1.3%. A second case report from the US Poison Control Centers described a 16-day-old infant who was hospitalized for bradycardia, hypotension, and respiratory arrest. The mother was breastfeeding and using cyclobenzaprine and oxycodone. This combination could have been the cause. Breastfeeding while using this drug should be based on the mother's clinical need for treatment versus any potential infant risks that might occur. If used, the infant should be monitored for the most common reported adult side effects of nausea, dizziness, headache, and abdominal pain (all leading to irritability), diarrhea, lethargy, and somnolence. Cyclobenzaprine should be used with caution by a lactating mother if other sedating drugs are being simultaneously administered (ie, opioids, benzodiazepines, etc).

References

1. Prescribing Information. *Cyclobenzaprine*. Unichem; 2020.
2. Moreira A, Barbin C, Martinez H, et al. Maternal use of cyclobenzaprine (Flexeril) may induce ductal closure and persistent pulmonary hypertension in neonates. *J Matern Fetal Neonatal Med*. 2014;27:1177-1179.
3. Wong JW, Chin JM, Schlueter RJ. Shingles in pregnancy: an elusive case of left upper quadrant abdominal pain. *Hawaii J Med Public Health*. 2018;77:179-182.
4. Fisher SC, Howley MM, Tran EI, et al. Maternal cyclobenzaprine exposure and risk of birth defects in the National Birth Defects Prevention Study (1997-2011) and Birth Defects Study to Evaluate Pregnancy Exposures (2014-2018). *Pharmacoepidemiol Drug Saf*. 2023;32:855-862.
5. Burra B, Datta P, Rewers-Felkins K, et al. Transfer of cyclobenzaprine into human milk and subsequent infant exposure. *J Hum Lact*. 2019;35:559-562.
6. Beauchamp GA, Hendrickson RG, Horowitz BZ, Spyker DA. Exposures through breast milk: an analysis of exposure and information calls to the U.S. Poison Centers, 2001-2017. *Breastfeed Med*. 2019;14:508-512.

CYCLOPENTOLATE OPHTHALMIC

Ophthalmic (Topical—Anticholinergic)

PREGNANCY RECOMMENDATION: No Human Data and No Relevant Animal Data

BREASTFEEDING RECOMMENDATION: Probably Compatible

PREGNANCY SUMMARY

No reports describing the use of cyclopentolate ophthalmic in human pregnancy have been located. The drug may cross the placenta, but the amount is probably clinically insignificant. However, the absence of human pregnancy experience prevents a complete assessment of the embryofetal risk. Animal reproduction studies have not been located. Using this drug during pregnancy should be based on the pros and cons of the mother's clinical need for treatment versus any potential fetal risk that might occur from exposure. If used during pregnancy, consider placing pressure over the tear duct in the corner of the eye for at least 1 minute, and then remove any excess solution with absorbent tissue to decrease the amount of drug reaching the systemic circulation even further.

BREASTFEEDING SUMMARY

No reports describing the use of cyclopentolate ophthalmic during human lactation have been located. The drug may be found in breast milk, but the amount is probably clinically insignificant. Breastfeeding while using this drug should be based on the mother's clinical need for treatment versus any potential infant risks that might occur. Systemic side effects with normal ocular use have not been reported. Anticholinergic drugs can affect breast milk production in the early stages of breastfeeding, as well as decrease breast milk supply with long-term use. However, the amount of exposure with topical ocular use is not likely to have this effect. A method to further decrease some systemic absorption with ophthalmic use is described above in the Pregnancy Summary.

C

References

1. Prescribing Information. *Cyclogyl*. Alcon Laboratories; 2018.
2. Lahdes K, Huupponen R, Kaila T, et al. Plasma concentration and ocular effects of cyclopentolate after ocular application of three formulations. *Br J Clin Pharmacol*. 1993;35:479-483.

CYCLOPHOSPHAMIDE

Antineoplastic (Alkylating Agent)

PREGNANCY RECOMMENDATION: Limited Human Data—Animal Data Suggest Risk

BREASTFEEDING RECOMMENDATION: Potential Toxicity

PREGNANCY SUMMARY

Numerous case reports have been located that describe the use of cyclophosphamide during pregnancy. First-trimester exposure has occurred unplanned in the majority of cases. Several cases describe multiple birth anomalies, but the amount of drug exposure, coexposure to other drugs, and the timing of exposure vary. There are a few first-trimester exposures that describe normal outcomes. Many other case reports describe the use of the drug in the second and third trimesters, with most newborn outcomes being good. The drug appears to cross the placenta, so some fetal exposure will occur. Therefore, this limited human pregnancy experience prevents a complete assessment of the embryofetal risk. Animal studies did show embryofetal toxicity in four species at doses of less than 10 times the RHD; however, the drug was administered daily for several days. Based on animal studies and the drug's mechanism of action, the manufacturer recommends that women with reproductive potential use effective contraception during treatment and for 1 year after the last dose. They also recommend that males with female partners of reproductive potential use effective contraception during treatment and for 4 months after the last dose. Nevertheless, using this drug during pregnancy should be based on the pros and cons of the mother's clinical need for treatment versus any potential fetal risk that might occur from exposure. The drug has been found to have cardiotoxic effects and can prolong the QT interval. Cyclophosphamide solution for IV use contains alcohol. A 50 mg/kg injection contains about 0.155 g/kg of ethanol. For a 75 kg patient, that would be 11.625 g of alcohol. A 12-ounce beer at 5% ethanol per volume contains about 14 g of alcohol. The 50 mg/kg dose is usually divided and administered over 2 to 5 days. Therefore, this "beer" would be spread out over 2 to 5 days. There is a registry for women who are pregnant and have cancer. For more information, women and health care providers are encouraged to contact the Cancer and Pregnancy Registry at 1-877-635-4499.

BREASTFEEDING SUMMARY

A few studies have been located that describe the use of cyclophosphamide during human lactation. In one case, a mother received about 2,800 mg daily for 4 days in preparation for a stem cell transplantation. The peak breast milk level was about 40.8 mcg/mL, and the calculated RID was about 4.8%. In a few other studies, lactating women received doses every 2 to 3 weeks, and breast milk levels ranged from about 1 to 18 mcg/mL. In these studies, the two active metabolites (aldophosphamide and phosphoramide mustard) were not analyzed; therefore, infant exposure is likely higher. Due to a concern for potential serious adverse effects that might be seen in a breastfed infant, the manufacturer recommends that women not breastfeed while being treated with this drug and for at least 1 week after the last dose. Nevertheless, breastfeeding while using this drug should be based on the mother's clinical need for treatment versus any potential infant risks that might occur. If used, the infant should be monitored for the most common reported adult side effects of nausea and abdominal cramps (both leading to irritability), diarrhea, lethargy, alopecia, vomiting, fever, and various laboratory abnormalities (see PI).

References

1. Greenberg LH, Tanaka KR. Congenital anomalies probably induced by cyclophosphamide. *JAMA*. 1964;188:423-426.
2. Toledo TM, Harper RC, Moser RH. Fetal effects during cyclophosphamide and irradiation therapy. *Ann Intern Med*. 1971;74:87-91.
3. Coates A. Cyclophosphamide in pregnancy. *Aust N Z J Obstet Gynaecol*. 1970;10:33-34.
4. Murray CL, Reichert JA, Anderson J, Twiggs LB. Multimodal cancer therapy for breast cancer in the first trimester of pregnancy. *JAMA*. 1984;252:2607-2608.

C

5. Sweet DL, Kinzie J. Consequences of radiotherapy and antineoplastic therapy for the fetus. *J Reprod Med.* 1976;17:241-246.
6. Kirshon B, Wasserstrum N, Willis R, et al. Teratogenic effects of first-trimester cyclophosphamide therapy. *Obstet Gynecol.* 1988;72:462-464.
7. Zemlickis D, Lishner M, Erlich R, Koren G. Teratogenicity and carcinogenicity in a twin exposed in utero to cyclophosphamide. *Teratogenesis Carcinog Mutagen.* 1993;13:139-143.
8. Enns GM, Roeder E, Chan RT, et al. Apparent cyclophosphamide (Cytoxan) embryopathy: a distinct phenotype? *Am J Med Genet.* 1999;86:237-241.
9. Lacher MJ, Geller W. Cyclophosphamide and vinblastine sulfate in Hodgkin's disease during pregnancy. *JAMA.* 1966;195:486-488.
10. Lergier JE, Jimenez E, Maldonado N, Veray F. Normal pregnancy in multiple myeloma treated with cyclophosphamide. *Cancer.* 1974;34:1018-1022.
11. Garcia V, Miguel JS, Borrasca AL. Doxorubicin in the first trimester of pregnancy. *Ann Intern Med.* 1981;94:547.
12. Lowenthal RM, Funnell CF, Hope DM, et al. Normal infant after combination chemotherapy including teniposide for Burkitt's lymphoma in pregnancy. *Med Pediatr Oncol.* 1982;10:165-169.
13. Daly H, McCann SR, Hanratty TD, Temperley IJ. Successful pregnancy during combination chemotherapy for Hodgkin's disease. *Acta Haematol (Basel).* 1980;64:154-156.
14. Pizzuto J, Aviles A, Noriega L, et al. Treatment of acute leukemia during pregnancy: presentation of nine cases. *Cancer Treat Rep.* 1980;64:679-683.
15. Sears HF, Reid J. Granulocytic sarcoma: local presentation of a systemic disease. *Cancer.* 1976;37:1808-1813.
16. Falkson HC, Simson IW, Falkson G. Non-Hodgkin's lymphoma in pregnancy. *Cancer.* 1980;45:1679-1682.
17. Webb GA. The use of hyperalimentation and chemotherapy in pregnancy: a case report. *Am J Obstet Gynecol.* 1980;137:263-266.
18. Gililland J, Weinstein L. The effects of cancer chemotherapeutic agents on the developing fetus. *Obstet Gynecol Surv.* 1983;38:6-13.
19. Weed JC Jr, Roh RA, Mendenhall HW. Recurrent endodermal sinus tumor during pregnancy. *Obstet Gynecol.* 1979;54:653-656.
20. Kim DS, Park MI. Maternal and fetal survival following surgery and chemotherapy of endodermal sinus tumor of the ovary during pregnancy: a case report. *Obstet Gynecol.* 1989;73:503-507.
21. Malfetano JH, Goldkrand JW. Cis-platinum combination chemotherapy during pregnancy for advanced epithelial ovarian carcinoma. *Obstet Gynecol.* 1990;75:545-547.
22. Schleuning M, Clemm C. Chromosomal aberrations in a newborn whose mother received cytotoxic treatment during pregnancy. *N Engl J Med.* 1987;317:1666-1667.
23. Haerr RW, Pratt AT. Multiagent chemotherapy for sarcoma diagnosed during pregnancy. *Cancer.* 1985;56:1028-1033.
24. Turchi JJ, Villasis C. Anthracyclines in the treatment of malignancy in pregnancy. *Cancer.* 1988;61:435-440.
25. Okun DB, Groncy PK, Sieger L, Tanaka KR. Acute leukemia in pregnancy: transient neonatal myelosuppression after combination chemotherapy in the mother. *Med Pediatr Oncol.* 1979;7:315-319.
26. Ortega J. Multiple agent chemotherapy including bleomycin of non-Hodgkin's lymphoma during pregnancy. *Cancer.* 1977;40:2829-2835.
27. Hardin JA. Cyclophosphamide treatment of lymphoma during third trimester of pregnancy. *Obstet Gynecol.* 1972;39:850-851.
28. Khurshid M, Saleem M. Acute leukaemia in pregnancy. *Lancet.* 1978;2:534-535.
29. Yankowitz J, Kuller JA, Thomas RL. Pregnancy complicated by Goodpasture syndrome. *Obstet Gynecol.* 1992;79:806-808.
30. Barry C, Davis S, Garrard P, Ferguson IT. Churg-Strauss disease: deterioration in a twin pregnancy. Successful outcome following treatment with corticosteroids and cyclophosphamide. *Br J Obstet Gynaecol.* 1997;104:746-747.
31. Mavrommatis CG, Daskalakis GJ, Papageorgiou IS, et al. Non-Hodgkin's lymphoma during pregnancy—case report. *Eur J Obstet Gynecol Reprod Biol.* 1998;79:95-97.
32. Dayoan ES, Dimen LL, Boylen CT. Successful treatment of Wegener's granulomatosis during pregnancy: a case report and review of the medical literature. *Chest.* 1998;113:836-838.
33. Cuvier C, Espie M, Extra JM, Marty M. Vinorelbine in pregnancy. *Eur J Cancer.* 1997;33:168-169.
34. Giacalone PL, Laffargue F, Benos P. Chemotherapy for breast carcinoma during pregnancy. *Cancer.* 1999;86:2266-2272.
35. Nicholson HO. Cytotoxic drugs in pregnancy: review of reported cases. *J Obstet Gynaecol Br Commonw.* 1968;75:307-312.
36. Dobbing J. Pregnancy and leukaemia. *Lancet.* 1977;1:1155.
37. Schilsky RL, Lewis BJ, Sherins RJ, Young RC. Gonadal dysfunction in patients receiving chemotherapy for cancer. *Ann Intern Med.* 1980;93:109-114.
38. Stewart BH. Drugs that cause and cure male infertility. *Drug Ther.* 1975;5:42-48.
39. Schwartz PE, Vidone RA. Pregnancy following combination chemotherapy for a mixed germ cell tumor of the ovary. *Gynecol Oncol.* 1981;12:373-378.
40. Bacon C, Kernahan J. Successful pregnancy in acute leukaemia. *Lancet.* 1975;2:515.
41. Qureshji MA, Pennington JH, Goldsmith HJ, Cox PE. Cyclophosphamide therapy and sterility. *Lancet.* 1972;2:1290-1291.
42. George CRP, Evans RA. Cyclophosphamide and infertility. *Lancet.* 1972;1:840-841.
43. Sherins RJ, DeVita VT Jr. Effect of drug treatment for lymphoma on male reproductive capacity. *Ann Intern Med.* 1973;79:216-220.
44. Lendon M, Palmer MK, Hann IM, et al. Testicular histology after combination chemotherapy in childhood for acute lymphoblastic leukaemia. *Lancet.* 1978;2:439-441.
45. Uldall PR, Feest TG, Morley AR, et al. Cyclophosphamide therapy in adults with minimal-change nephrotic syndrome. *Lancet.* 1972;2:1250-1253.
46. Card RT, Holmes IH, Sugarman RG, et al. Successful pregnancy after high dose chemotherapy and marrow transplantation for treatment of aplastic anemia. *Exp Hematol.* 1980;8:57-60.
47. Deeg HJ, Kennedy MS, Sanders JE, et al. Successful pregnancy after marrow transplantation for severe aplastic anemia and immunosuppression with cyclosporine. *JAMA.* 1983;250:647.
48. Javaheri G, Lifchez A, Valle J. Pregnancy following removal of and long-term chemotherapy for ovarian malignant teratoma. *Obstet Gynecol.* 1983;61:8S-9S.
49. Rustin GJS, Booth M, Dent J, et al. Pregnancy after cytotoxic chemotherapy for gestational trophoblastic tumours. *Br Med J.* 1984;288:103-106.
50. Lee RB, Kelly J, Elg SA, Benson WL. Pregnancy following conservative surgery and adjunctive chemotherapy for stage III immature teratoma of the ovary. *Obstet Gynecol.* 1989;73:853-855.
51. Hinkes E, Plotkin D. Reversible drug-induced sterility in a patient with acute leukemia. *JAMA.* 1973;223:1490-1491.
52. Russell JA, Powles RL, Oliver RTD. Conception and congenital abnormalities after chemotherapy of acute myelogenous leukaemia in two men. *Br Med J.* 1976;1:1508.
53. Evenson DP, Arlin Z, Welt S, et al. Male reproductive capacity may recover following drug treatment with the L-10 protocol for acute lymphocytic leukemia. *Cancer.* 1984;53:30-36.
54. Tolchin SF, Winkelstein A, Rodnan GP, et al. Chromosome abnormalities from cyclophosphamide therapy in rheumatoid arthritis and progressive systemic sclerosis (scleroderma). *Arthritis Rheum.* 1974;17:375-382.
55. Gershenson DM. Menstrual and reproductive function after treatment with combination chemotherapy for malignant ovarian germ cell tumors. *J Clin Oncol.* 1988;6:270-275.
56. Watson AR, Rance CP, Bain J. Long term effects of cyclophosphamide on testicular function. *Br Med J.* 1985;291:1457-1460.
57. Selevan SG, Lindbohm M-L, Hornung RW, Hemminki K. A study of occupational exposure to antineoplastic drugs and fetal loss in nurses. *N Engl J Med.* 1985;313:1173-1178.
58. Selevan SG, Hornung RW. Antineoplastic drugs and spontaneous abortion in nurses. *N Engl J Med.* 1986;314:1050-1051.
59. Kalter H. Antineoplastic drugs and spontaneous abortion in nurses. *N Engl J Med.* 1986;314:1048-1049.
60. Mulvihill JJ, Stewart KR. Antineoplastic drugs and spontaneous abortion in nurses. *N Engl J Med.* 1986;314:1049.
61. Chabner BA. Antineoplastic drugs and spontaneous abortion in nurses. *N Engl J Med.* 1986;314:1049-1050.
62. Zellmer WA. Antineoplastic drugs and spontaneous abortion in nurses. *N Engl J Med.* 1986;314:1050.
63. Wiernik PH, Duncan JH. Cyclophosphamide in human milk. *Lancet.* 1971;1:912.
64. Amato D, Niblett JS. Neutropenia from cyclophosphamide in breast milk. *Med J Aust.* 1977;1:383-384.
65. Durodola JI. Administration of cyclophosphamide during late pregnancy and early lactation: a case report. *J Natl Med Assoc.* 1979;71:165-166.
66. American Academy of Pediatrics Committee on Drugs. The transfer of drugs and other chemicals into human milk. *Pediatrics.* 2001;108:776-789.

CYCLOSERINE

Antibacterial (Antituberculosis)

PREGNANCY RECOMMENDATION: Limited Human Data—Animal Data Suggest Low Risk (Maternal Risk May Outweigh Embryo–Fetal Risk)

BREASTFEEDING RECOMMENDATION: Probably Compatible

PREGNANCY SUMMARY

A total of four cases were located that described first-trimester exposure to cycloserine. No fetal anomalies were noted at the time of delivery. Use of the drug has also been reported in the second and third trimesters in a few patients, with no adverse effects related to the drug being reported. The drug crosses the placenta, so some fetal exposure will occur. However, this limited human pregnancy experience prevents a complete assessment of the embryofetal risk. Animal studies did not show any embryofetal toxicity or teratogenicity in one species at doses of less than 10 times the RHD. Using this drug during pregnancy should be based on the pros and cons of the mother's clinical need for treatment versus any potential fetal risk that might occur from exposure. However, the drug should not be withheld because of pregnancy if the maternal condition requires the antibiotic.

BREASTFEEDING SUMMARY

Two studies were located that evaluated the use of cycloserine during human lactation in several patients. The drug was found in breast milk with levels that ranged from about 5 to 20 mcg/mL. A maximum calculated RID was about 20%. However, if the drug is needed by the mother, then breastfeeding should not prevent its use. If the clinical decision is to use this drug while breastfeeding, the infant should be monitored for the most common reported adult side effects of headache and paresthesia (both leading to irritability), rash, and drowsiness.

References

1. Product information. *Seromycin*. Purdue GMP Center; 2011.
2. Heinonen OP, Slone D, Shapiro S. *Birth Defects and Drugs in Pregnancy*. Publishing Sciences Group; 1977:297.
3. American Thoracic Society. Medical Section of the American Lung Association: treatment of tuberculosis and tuberculosis infection in adults and children. *Am Rev Respir Dis*. 1986;134:355-363.
4. Lessnau KD, Qarah S. Multidrug-resistant tuberculosis in pregnancy: a case report and review of the literature. *Chest*. 2003;123:953-956.
5. Takashima T, Danno K, Tamura Y, et al. Treatment outcome of patients with multidrug-resistant pulmonary tuberculosis during pregnancy. *Kekkaku*. 2006;81:413-418.
6. Morton RF, McKenna MH, Charles E. Studies on the absorption, diffusion, and excretion of cycloserine. *Antibiot Annu*. 1955;3:169-172. As cited by Snider DE Jr, Powell KE. Should women taking antituberculosis drugs breast-feed? *Arch Intern Med*. 1984;144:589-590.
7. Vorherr H. Drug excretion in breast milk. *Postgrad Med*. 1974;56:97-104. As cited by Snider DE Jr, Powell KE. Should women taking antituberculosis drugs breast-feed? *Arch Intern Med*. 1984;144:589-590.

CYCLOSPORINE

Immunologic (Immunosuppressant)

PREGNANCY RECOMMENDATION: Limited Human Data—Animal Data Suggest Potential Toxicity

BREASTFEEDING RECOMMENDATION: Probably Compatible

PREGNANCY SUMMARY

Numerous cases reports and small studies have been located that describe the use of cyclosporine in the first trimester of pregnancy. Of 56 pregnancies, 9 (16%) spontaneous abortions occurred. There were 2 (4.3%) major anomalies seen in the remaining 47 pregnancies. The drug crosses the placenta, so some fetal exposure will occur. However, this limited human pregnancy experience prevents a complete assessment of the embryofetal risk. The drug was found to cause some embryofetal toxicity in two species at doses less than 10 times the RHD, but maternal toxicity also occurred. When used as an immunosuppressant, the disease process itself makes these pregnancies high risk and subject to numerous potential problems, of which the most common is growth restriction. This latter problem is probably related to the mother's disease rather than to her drug therapy, but a contribution from cyclosporine cannot be excluded. Additionally, because cyclosporine is dissolvable in ethanol, the medical product contains ethanol (about 15% by volume in the solution and about 12% in the

(*continued*)

C

soft gel capsules). However, even with maximum daily doses, the total amount of ethanol consumed is less than 1 mL/d, which is then distributed throughout the maternal bloodstream. Therefore, any amount at the placental interface is probably clinically insignificant. Using this drug during pregnancy should be based on the pros and cons of the mother's clinical need for treatment versus any potential fetal risk that might occur from exposure. If cyclosporine is used in pregnancy for the treatment of rheumatoid arthritis or psoriasis, health care professionals are encouraged to call 1-877-311-8,972 for information about patient enrollment in the OTIS Rheumatoid Arthritis study.

BREASTFEEDING SUMMARY

Several studies have been located evaluating the use of cyclosporine during human lactation. Nearly 30 women were tested, and all but one had detectable levels in breast milk. The highest recorded level was about 570 ng/mL. All of the calculated RIDs were 5% or less. The drug was also tested in the blood of 19 infants whose mothers were using cyclosporine during breastfeeding. Of these, 16 had undetectable levels (LLQ ranging from 3 to 30 ng/mL). The three cases with positive infant blood levels had values of 21, 30, and 131 ng/mL. These findings may occur based on the oral bioavailability from the infant's gastrointestinal tract. However, due to a concern for potential serious adverse effects that might be seen in a breastfed infant, the manufacturer recommends that women not breastfeed while being treated with this drug. Nevertheless, breastfeeding while using this drug should be based on the mother's clinical need for treatment versus any potential infant risks that might occur. If used, the infant should be monitored for the most common reported adult side effects of nausea, dizziness, headache, and abdominal pain (all leading to irritability), diarrhea, fatigue (lethargy), vomiting, fever, and cough.

References

1. Product information. *Neoral*. Novartis Pharmaceuticals; 2017.
2. Christopher V, Al-Chalabi T, Richardson PD, et al. Pregnancy outcome after liver transplantation: a single-center experience of 71 pregnancies in 45 recipients. *Liver Transpl*. 2006;12:1138-1143.
3. Lewis GJ, Lamont CAR, Lee HA, Slapak M. Successful pregnancy in a renal transplant recipient taking cyclosporin A. *Br Med J*. 1983;286:603.
4. Flechner SM, Katz AR, Rogers AJ, et al. The presence of cyclosporine in body tissues and fluids during pregnancy. *Am J Kidney Dis*. 1985;5:60-63.
5. Burrows DA, O'Neil TJ, Sorrells TL. Successful twin pregnancy after renal transplant maintained on cyclosporine A immunosuppression. *Obstet Gynecol*. 1988;72:459-461.
6. Lowenstein BR, Vain NW, Perrone SV, et al. Successful pregnancy and vaginal delivery after heart transplantation. *Am J Obstet Gynecol*. 1988;158:589-590.
7. Ziegenhagen DJ, Grombach G, Dieckmann M, et al. Pregnancy under cyclosporine administration after renal transplantation. *Dtsch Med Wochenschr*. 1988;113:260-263.
8. Klintmalm G, Althoff P, Appleby G, Segerbrandt E. Renal function in a newborn baby delivered of a renal transplant patient taking cyclosporine. *Transplantation*. 1984;38:198-199.
9. Grischke E, Kaufmann M, Dreikorn K, et al. Successful pregnancy after kidney transplantation and cyclosporin A. *Geburtshilfe Frauenheilkd*. 1986;46:176-179.
10. Pikrell MD, Sawers R, Michael J. Pregnancy after renal transplantation: severe intrauterine growth retardation during treatment with cyclosporin A. *Br Med J*. 1988;296:825.
11. Calne RY, Brons IGM, Williams PF, et al. Successful pregnancy after paratopic segmental pancreas and kidney transplantation. *Br Med J*. 1988;296:1709.
12. Pujals JM, Figueras G, Puig JM, et al. Osseous malformation in baby born to woman on cyclosporin. *Lancet*. 1989;1:667.
13. Al-Khader AA, Absy M, Al-Hasani MK, et al. Successful pregnancy in renal transplant recipients treated with cyclosporine. *Transplantation*. 1988;45:987-988.
14. Sims CJ, Porter KB, Knuppel RA. Successful pregnancy after a liver transplant. *Am J Obstet Gynecol*. 1989;161:532-533.
15. Deeg HJ, Kennedy MS, Sanders JE, et al. Successful pregnancy after marrow transplantation for severe aplastic anemia and immunosuppression with cyclosporine. *JAMA*. 1983;250:647.
16. Kossoy LR, Herbert CM III, Wentz AC. Management of heart transplant recipients: guidelines for the obstetrician—gynecologist. *Am J Obstet Gynecol*. 1988;159:490-499.
17. Lau RJ, Scott JR. Pregnancy following renal transplantation. *Clin Obstet Gynecol*. 1985;28:339-350.
18. Tauscher AE, Fleischer AB Jr, Phelps KC, Feldman SR. Psoriasis and pregnancy. *J Cutan Med Surg*. 2002;6:561-570.
19. Lebwohl M. A clinician's paradigm in the treatment of psoriasis. *J Am Acad Dermatol*. 2005;53:S59-S69.
20. Thiagarajan (Munoz-Flores) KD, Easterling T, Davis C, Bond EF. Breast-feeding by a cyclosporin-treated mother. *Obstet Gynecol*. 2001;97:816-818.
21. Moretti ME, Sgro M, Johnson DW, et al. Cyclosporin excretion into breast milk. *Transplantation*. 2003;75:2144-2146.
22. American Academy of Pediatrics Committee on Drugs. The transfer of drugs and other chemicals into human milk. *Pediatrics*. 2001;108:776-789.

CYCLOSPORINE OPHTHALMIC

Ophthalmic/Immunologic (Immunosuppressant)

PREGNANCY RECOMMENDATION: Human Data Suggest Low Risk

BREASTFEEDING RECOMMENDATION: Probably Compatible

PREGNANCY SUMMARY

One case report was located that described the use of cyclosporine ophthalmic in a woman at 36 weeks' gestation. She delivered shortly thereafter, and no adverse fetal effects were noted. Since the drug is not detected systemically with ophthalmic use, any amount that may be in the systemic circulation that could cross should be clinically insignificant. Though further studies reporting the use of this ophthalmic drug during pregnancy would be beneficial, the drug is low risk because of the lack of any measurable systemic absorption. No relevant animal studies have been conducted with this drug. If used during pregnancy, consider placing pressure over the tear duct in the corner of the eye for at least 1 minute, and then remove any excess solution with absorbent tissue to theoretically decrease the amount of drug reaching the systemic circulation even further.

C

BREASTFEEDING SUMMARY

No reports describing the use of cyclosporine ophthalmic during human lactation have been located. Because the drug was not detected systemically with ocular use, any amount that might be found in breast milk would be clinically insignificant. The drug was found in human breast milk in patients with oral use of the drug, but in most cases, cyclosporine was not found in the infant's blood. Breastfeeding while using this drug should be based on the mother's clinical need for treatment versus any potential infant risks that might occur. Due to the lack of vascular drug absorption with ocular use, systemic side effects were not analyzed. A method to further reduce systemic concentrations, if they occur at all, is described above in the Pregnancy Summary.

Reference

1. Product information. *Restasis*. Allergan; 2017.

CYPROHEPTADINE

Antihistamine/Antiserotonin

PREGNANCY RECOMMENDATION: Limited Human Data—Animal Data Suggest Low Risk

BREASTFEEDING RECOMMENDATION: Probably Compatible

PREGNANCY SUMMARY

From the Michigan Medicaid FDA data and several case reports, a total of about 292 first-trimester exposures to cyproheptadine were found and 12 (4.1%) major anomalies were described (12 expected). No pattern to the anomalies was identified. The drug will probably cross the placenta, so some fetal exposure will likely occur. However, this limited human pregnancy experience prevents a complete assessment of the embryofetal risk. Animal studies did not show any embryofetal toxicity or teratogenicity in three species at doses of more than 10 times the RHD. Using this drug during pregnancy should be based on the pros and cons of the mother's clinical need for treatment versus any potential fetal risk that might occur from exposure.

BREASTFEEDING SUMMARY

No reports describing the use of cyproheptadine during human lactation have been located. The drug will probably be found in breast milk, so some infant exposure will likely occur. Chronic use of cyproheptadine will lower serum prolactin levels, and it has been used in the management of galactorrhea. No studies have been found, however, that evaluated its potential to interfere with the normal human lactation process. Because of the increased sensitivity of newborns to antihistamines and the potential for adverse reactions, the manufacturer considers cyproheptadine to be contraindicated in nursing mothers. Nevertheless, breastfeeding while using this drug should be based on the mother's clinical need for treatment versus any potential infant risks that might occur. If used, the infant should be monitored for the most common reported adult side effects of nausea, dizziness, and blurred vision (all leading to irritability), diarrhea, vomiting, rash, sedation, and decreased appetite (monitor growth).

References

1. Product information. *Cyproheptadine*. Actavis Pharma; 2018.
2. Sadovsky E, Pfeifer Y, Polishuk WZ, Sulman FG. A trial of cyproheptadine in habitual abortion. *Isr J Med Sci*. 1972;8:623-625.
3. Sadovsky E, Pfeifer Y, Sadovsky A, Sulman FG. Prevention of hypothalamic habitual abortion by Periactin. *Harefuah*. 1970;78:332-334. As cited in Anonymous. References and reviews. *JAMA*. 1970;212:1253.
4. Pfeifer Y, Sadovsky E, Sulman FG. Prevention of serotonin abortion in pregnant rats by five serotonin antagonists. *Obstet Gynecol*. 1969;33:709-714.
5. Shepard TH. *Catalog of Teratogenic Agents*. 8th ed. Johns Hopkins University Press; 1995:121-122.
6. Kasperlik-Zaluska A, Migdalska B, Hartwig W, et al. Two pregnancies in a woman with Cushing's syndrome treated with cyproheptadine. *Br J Obstet Gynaecol*. 1980;87:1171-1173.
7. Khir ASM, How J, Bewsher PD. Successful pregnancy after cyproheptadine treatment for Cushing's disease. *Eur J Obstet Gynecol Reprod Biol*. 1982;13:343-347.
8. Aron DC, Schnall AM, Sheeler LR. Cushing's syndrome and pregnancy. *Am J Obstet Gynecol*. 1990;162:244-252.
9. Griffith DN, Ross EJ. Pregnancy after cyproheptadine treatment for Cushing's disease. *N Engl J Med*. 1981;305:893-894.
10. Czeizel AE, Mosonyi A. Monitoring of early human fetal development in women exposed to large doses of chemicals. *Environ Mol Mutagen*. 1997;30:240-244.
11. Wortsman J, Soler NG, Hirschowitz J. Cyproheptadine in the management of the galactorrhea-amenorrhea syndrome. *Ann Intern Med*. 1979;90:923-925.

C

CYSTEAMINE

Genetic (Cystine-Depleting Agent)

PREGNANCY RECOMMENDATION: Limited Human Data—Animal Data Suggest Potential Risk

BREASTFEEDING RECOMMENDATION: Potential Toxicity

PREGNANCY SUMMARY

One report describing the use of cysteamine during human pregnancy was located. The patient was on cysteamine at the time of conception through to delivery at about 32 weeks' gestation, resulting in a healthy newborn with no reported anomalies. Several other reports describe 12 to 15 patients (some duplication of patients may exist) who were on cysteamine at the time of conception, with the drug being discontinued in the early first trimester following pregnancy confirmation. None of the delivered newborns were reported to have birth anomalies. In these studies, nearly 50% of the patients developed preeclampsia. The drug will probably cross the placenta, so some fetal exposure will likely occur. Therefore, this limited human pregnancy experience prevents a complete assessment of the embryofetal risk. Lastly, placental cystine crystals have been found on pathology in a patient with cystinosis who had high blood cystine levels. The significance of this is unknown. Animal studies did show embryofetal toxicity with malformations in one species. Using this drug during pregnancy should be based on the pros and cons of the mother's clinical need for treatment versus any potential fetal risk that might occur from exposure.

BREASTFEEDING SUMMARY

No reports describing the use of cysteamine during human lactation have been located. The drug will probably be found in breast milk, so some infant exposure will likely occur. Breastfeeding while using this drug should be based on the mother's clinical need for treatment versus any potential infant risks that might occur. If used, the infant should be monitored for the most common reported adult side effects of nausea and abdominal pain (both leading to irritability), diarrhea, lethargy, vomiting, fever, and rash.

References

1. Prescribing Information. *Cystagon*. Mylan Pharmaceuticals, Inc; 2021.
2. Haase M, Morgera S, Bamberg C, et al. Successful pregnancies in dialysis patients including those suffering from cystinosis and familial Mediterranean fever. *J Nephrol*. 2006;19:677-681.
3. Kuczborska K, Gozdowska J, Lewandowska D, et al. Therapeutic problems and pregnancy in a patient with infantile nephropathic cystinosis: a case report. *Transplant Proc*. 2019;51:545-547.
4. Blakey H, Proudfoot-Jones J, Knox E, Lipkin G. Pregnancy in women with cystinosis. *Clin Kidney J*. 2019;12:855-858.
5. Servais A, Janssen MCH, Blakey H, et al. Pregnancy in cystinosis patients with chronic kidney disease: a European case series. *J Inherit Metab Dis*. 2022;45: 963-968.
6. Reiss RE, Kuwabara T, Smith ML, Gahl WA. Successful pregnancy despite placental crystals in a woman with nephropathic cystinosis. *N Engl J Med*. 1988;319:223-226.
7. Besouw MTP, Kremer JAM, Janssen MCH, Levtchenko EN. Fertility status in male cystinosis patients treated with cysteamine. *Fertil Steril*. 2010;93: 1880-1883.
8. Veys KR, D'Hauwers KW, van Dongen AJCM, et al. First successful conception induced by male cystinosis patient. *JIMD Rep*. 2018;38:1-6.

CYSTEAMINE OPHTHALMIC

Ophthalmic/Genetic (Topical—Cystine-Depleting)

PREGNANCY RECOMMENDATION: No Human Data and No Relevant Animal Data

BREASTFEEDING RECOMMENDATION: Probably Compatible

PREGNANCY SUMMARY

No reports describing the use of cysteamine ophthalmic in human pregnancy have been located. The drug may cross the placenta, but the amount is likely to be clinically insignificant. However, the absence of human pregnancy experience prevents a complete assessment of the embryofetal risk. No relevant animal studies have been conducted. Using this drug during pregnancy should be based on the pros and cons of the mother's clinical need for treatment versus any potential fetal risk that might occur from exposure. If used during pregnancy, consider placing pressure over the tear duct in the corner of the eye for at least 1 minute, and then remove any excess solution with absorbent tissue to decrease the amount of drug reaching the systemic circulation even further.

C

BREASTFEEDING SUMMARY

No reports describing the use of cysteamine ophthalmic during human lactation have been located. The drug may be found in breast milk, but the overall amount is probably clinically insignificant. Breastfeeding while using this drug should be based on the mother's clinical need for treatment versus any potential infant risks that might occur. If used, the infant should be monitored for the most common reported adult side effects of nausea and abdominal pain (both leading to irritability), diarrhea, lethargy, vomiting, fever, and rash. A method to decrease some systemic absorption with ophthalmic use is described above in the Pregnancy Summary.

Reference

1. Prescribing Information. *Cystadrops*. Recordati Rare Diseases; 2021.

CYTARABINE

Antineoplastic (Antimetabolite)

PREGNANCY RECOMMENDATION: Limited Human Data—Animal data Suggest Risk

BREASTFEEDING RECOMMENDATION: Potential Toxicity (Hold Breastfeeding)

PREGNANCY SUMMARY

Numerous case reports describing the use of cytarabine during human pregnancy have been located. Of about 8 to 10 first-trimester exposures, 2 anomalies were described that both involved limb abnormalities. Use in the second and third trimesters has reported a few cases in newborns delivered with hematologic abnormalities that were transient in most cases, except for one with pancytopenia. The drug will probably cross the placenta, so some fetal exposure will likely occur. However, this limited human pregnancy experience prevents a complete assessment of the embryofetal risk. Animal studies did show fetal malformations in two species (dosages not supplied). Intrathecal use should have lower systemic exposure when compared with IV or IM administration. Using this drug during pregnancy should be based on the pros and cons of the mother's clinical need for treatment versus any potential fetal risk that might occur from exposure. There is a registry for women who are pregnant and have cancer. For more information, women and health care providers are encouraged to contact the Cancer and Pregnancy Registry at 1-877-635-4499.

BREASTFEEDING SUMMARY

No reports describing the use of cytarabine during human lactation have been located. The drug will probably be found in breast milk, so some infant exposure will likely occur. The amount of drug found in breast milk with intrathecal use should be minimal. In addition, oral bioavailability is only 20%, so infant systemic exposure from breastfeeding should be decreased. However, due to a concern for potential serious adverse effects that might be seen in a breastfed infant, the manufacturer recommends that women not breastfeed while being treated with this drug. Nevertheless, breastfeeding while using this drug should be based on the mother's clinical need for treatment versus any potential infant risks that might occur. If used, the infant should be monitored for the most common reported adult side effects of nausea, headache, pruritus, and abdominal pain (all leading to irritability), diarrhea, alopecia, vomiting, decreased appetite (monitor growth), rash, and various laboratory abnormalities (see PI). Because of the short elimination half-life, breastfeeding could also be held for 12 to 15 hours (>5 half-lives).

References

1. Product information. *Cytarabine*. Mylan Institutional; 2018.
2. Pawliger DF, McLean FW, Noyes WD. Normal fetus after cytosine arabinoside therapy. *Ann Intern Med*. 1971;74:1012.
3. Au-Yong R, Collins P, Young JA. Acute myeloblastic leukemia during pregnancy. *Br Med J*. 1972;4:493-494.
4. Raich PC, Curet LB. Treatment of acute leukemia during pregnancy. *Cancer*. 1975;36:861-862.
5. Gokal R, Durrant J, Baum JD, Bennett MJ. Successful pregnancy in acute monocytic leukaemia. *Br J Cancer*. 1976;34:299-302.
6. Sears HF, Reid J. Granulocytic sarcoma: local presentation of a systemic disease. *Cancer*. 1976;37:1808-1813.
7. Durie BGM, Giles HR. Successful treatment of acute leukemia during pregnancy. *Arch Intern Med*. 1977;137:90-91.
8. Lilleyman JS, Hill AS, Anderton KJ. Consequences of acute myelogenous leukemia in early pregnancy. *Cancer*. 1977;40:1300-1303.
9. Moreno H, Castleberry RP, McCann WP. Cytosine arabinoside and 6-thioguanine in the treatment of childhood acute myeloblastic leukemia. *Cancer*. 1977;40:998-1004.
10. Newcomb M, Balducci L, Thigpen JT, Morrison FS. Acute leukemia in pregnancy: successful delivery after cytarabine and doxorubicin. *JAMA*. 1978;239:2691-2692.
11. Manoharan A, Leyden MJ. Acute non-lymphocytic leukaemia in the third trimester of pregnancy. *Aust N Z J Med*. 1979;9:71-74.
12. Pizzuto J, Aviles A, Noriega L, et al. Treatment of acute leukemia during pregnancy: presentation of nine cases. *Cancer Treat Rep*. 1980;64:679-683.
13. Colbert N, Najman A, Gorin NC, et al. Acute leukaemia during pregnancy: favourable course of pregnancy in two patients treated with cytosine arabinoside and anthracyclines. *Nouv Presse Med*. 1980;9:175-178.
14. Tobias JS, Bloom HJG. Doxorubicin in pregnancy. *Lancet*. 1980;1:776.
15. Taylor G, Blom J. Acute leukemia during pregnancy. *South Med J*. 1980;73:1314-1315.
16. Dara P, Slater LM, Armentrout SA. Successful pregnancy during chemotherapy for acute leukemia. *Cancer*. 1981;47:845-846.
17. Plows CW. Acute myelomonocytic leukemia in pregnancy: report of a case. *Am J Obstet Gynecol*. 1982;143:41-43.
18. De Souza JJL, Bezwoda WR, Jetham D, Sonnendecker EWW. Acute leukaemia in pregnancy: a case report and discussion on modern management. *S Afr Med J*. 1982;62:295-296.
19. Feliu J, Juarez S, Ordonez A, et al. Acute leukemia and pregnancy. *Cancer*. 1988;61:580-584.
20. Volkenandt M, Buchner T, Hiddemann W, Van De Loo J. Acute leukaemia during pregnancy. *Lancet*. 1987;2:1521-1522.

21. Maurer LH, Forcier RJ, McIntyre OR, Benirschke K. Fetal group C trisomy after cytosine arabinoside and thioguanine. *Ann Intern Med*. 1971;75:809-810.
22. Lowenthal RM, Marsden KA, Newman NM, et al. Normal infant after treatment of acute myeloid leukaemia in pregnancy with daunorubicin. *Aust N Z J Med*. 1978;8:431-432.
23. O'Donnell R, Costigan C, O'Donnell LG. Two cases of acute leukaemia in pregnancy. *Acta Haematol*. 1979;61:298-300.
24. Doney KC, Kraemer KG, Shepard TH. Combination chemotherapy for acute myelocytic leukemia during pregnancy: three case reports. *Cancer Treat Rep*. 1979;63:369-371.
25. Cantini E, Yanes B. Acute myelogenous leukemia in pregnancy. *South Med J*. 1984;77:1050-1052.
26. Alegre A, Chunchurreta R, Rodrigueq-Alarcon J, et al. Successful pregnancy in acute promyelocytic leukemia. *Cancer*. 1982;49:152-153.
27. Hamer JW, Beard MEJ, Duff GB. Pregnancy complicated by acute myeloid leukaemia. *N Z Med J*. 1979;89:212-213.
28. Schleuning M, Clemm C. Chromosomal aberrations in a newborn whose mother received cytotoxic treatment during pregnancy. *N Engl J Med*. 1987; 317:1666-1667.
29. Wagner VM, Hill JS, Weaver D, Baehner RL. Congenital abnormalities in baby born to cytarabine treated mother. *Lancet*. 1980;2:98-99.
30. Schafer AI. Teratogenic effects of antileukemic chemotherapy. *Arch Intern Med*. 1981;141:514-515.
31. Russell JA, Powles RL, Oliver RTD. Conception and congenital abnormalities after chemotherapy of acute myelogenous leukaemia in two men. *Br Med J*. 1976;1:1508.
32. Lendon M, Palmer MK, Hann IM, et al. Testicular histology after combination chemotherapy in childhood for acute lymphoblastic leukaemia. *Lancet*. 1978;2:439-441.
33. Lilleyman JS. Male fertility after successful chemotherapy for lymphoblastic leukaemia. *Lancet*. 1979;2:1125.
34. Matthews JH, Wood JK. Male fertility during chemotherapy for acute leukemia. *N Engl J Med*. 1980;303:1235.
35. Nicholson HO. Cytotoxic drugs in pregnancy: review of reported cases. *J Obstet Gynaecol Br Commonw*. 1968;75:307-312.
36. Dobbing J. Pregnancy and leukaemia. *Lancet*. 1977;1:1155.

D

DABIGATRAN ETEXILATE

Hematologic (Anticoagulant—Thrombin Inhibitor)

PREGNANCY RECOMMENDATION: *Contraindicated

BREASTFEEDING RECOMMENDATION: Potential Toxicity

PREGNANCY SUMMARY

No reports describing the use of dabigatran etexilate in the first trimester of human pregnancy have been located. A few cases of use in the later stages of pregnancy have not described any adverse fetal effects. Based on ex vivo placental perfusion data, dabigatran crosses the placenta, so some fetal exposure will occur. However, this limited human pregnancy experience prevents a complete assessment of the embryofetal risk. Animal studies did show some embryofetal toxicity in two species at doses of less than 10 times the recommended human dose (RHD). Using this drug during pregnancy should be based on the pros and cons of the mother's clinical need for treatment versus any potential fetal risk that might occur from exposure. *Because the drug appears to cross the placenta, this could theoretically affect fetal coagulation. Therefore, other anticoagulants, such as the low-molecular-weight heparins, appear to be a better choice in pregnancy.

BREASTFEEDING SUMMARY

One study evaluating dabigatran etexilate in human lactation was located. In two mothers, breast milk samples were evaluated, and the drug was detected at low levels with a peak concentration of about 53 ng/mL. The calculated relative infant dose (RID) was less than 1%. Infant levels have not been analyzed, but based on the mean oral bioavailability of only 5%, any infant systemic absorption from these low levels would likely be clinically insignificant. However, there is no information on the four glucuronide active metabolites, but they are probably also excreted in breast milk. The effect of this exposure on a nursing infant is unknown. Until such data are available, use of other anticoagulants, such as low-molecular-weight heparins, should be considered. If the clinical decision is to use this drug while breastfeeding, the infant should be monitored for the most common reported adult side effects of nausea (leading to irritability), bruising, and bleeding.

References

1. Prescribing Information. *Pradaxa*. Boehringer Ingelheim Pharmaceuticals; 2021.
2. Huisman MV. Further issues with new oral anticoagulants. *Curr Pharm Des*. 2010;16:3487-3489.
3. *An open label, non-randomised, phase II study to determine if dabigatran and its metabolites are detectable in breast milk following oral administration to non-breastfeeding mothers*. Accessed October 27, 2018. https://www.clinicaltrialsregister.eu/ctr-search/trial/2014-004249-29/results
4. Ayuk P, Kampouraki E, Truemann A, et al. Investigation of dabigatran secretion into breast milk: implications for oral thromboprophylaxis in postpartum women. *Am J Hematol*. 2020;95:E10-E13.
5. Daei M, Khalili H, Heidari Z. Direct oral anticoagulant safety during breastfeeding: a narrative review. *Eur J Clin Pharmacol*. 2021;77:1465-1471.

DABRAFENIB

Antineoplastic (BRAF Kinase Inhibitor)

PREGNANCY RECOMMENDATION: No Human Data—Animal Data Suggest Potential Risk

BREASTFEEDING RECOMMENDATION: Potential Toxicity

PREGNANCY SUMMARY

No reports describing the use of dabrafenib in human pregnancy have been located. The drug will probably cross the placenta, so some fetal exposure will likely occur. Therefore, the absence of human pregnancy experience prevents a complete assessment of the embryofetal risk. Animal studies did show embryofetal toxicity with malformations in one species at

(*continued*)

doses less than 10 times the RHD. Based on these animal studies and the drug's mechanism of action, the manufacturer recommends that women with reproductive potential use effective nonhormonal contraception during treatment and for 2 weeks after the last dose. They also recommend that males with female partners of reproductive potential use effective contraception during treatment and for 2 weeks after the last dose. Nevertheless, using this drug during pregnancy should be based on the pros and cons of the mother's clinical need for treatment versus any potential fetal risk that might occur from exposure. In the clinical trials, a decrease of more than 10% in the left ventricular ejection fraction was seen in 6% of the treated patients. There is a pregnancy registry for women who are pregnant and have cancer. For more information, women who are pregnant and have cancer and health care providers are encouraged to contact the Cancer and Pregnancy Registry at 1-877-635-4499.

BREASTFEEDING SUMMARY

No reports describing the use of dabrafenib during human lactation have been located. The drug will likely be found in breast milk, so some infant exposure will probably occur. Due to the concern for potential serious adverse effects that might be seen in a breastfed infant, the manufacturer recommends that women not breastfeed while being treated with this drug and for at least 2 weeks after the last dose. Nevertheless, breastfeeding while using this drug should be based on the mother's clinical need for treatment. If used, the infant should be monitored for the most common reported adult side effects of nausea, arthralgia, and abdominal pain (all leading to irritability), diarrhea, alopecia, vomiting, fever, cough, rash, and various laboratory abnormalities (see Prescribing Information [PI]).

Reference

1. Prescribing Information. *Tafinlar*. Novartis Pharmaceuticals; 2022.

DACARBAZINE

Antineoplastic (Alkylating Agent)

PREGNANCY RECOMMENDATION: Limited Human Data—Animal Data Suggest Potential Risk

BREASTFEEDING RECOMMENDATION: Potential Toxicity

PREGNANCY SUMMARY

Several studies regarding the use of dacarbazine during human pregnancy have been located. More than 170 pregnancies have been described, with most exposures occurring in the second and third trimesters of pregnancy. A few first-trimester exposures have been reported, and no major birth anomalies have been described. The drug will probably cross the placenta, so some fetal exposure will likely occur. However, this limited human pregnancy experience prevents a complete assessment of the embryofetal risk. Using this drug during pregnancy should be based on the pros and cons of the mother's clinical need for treatment versus any potential fetal risk that might occur from exposure. There is a registry for women who are pregnant and have cancer. For more information, women and health care providers are encouraged to contact the Cancer and Pregnancy Registry at 1-877-635-4499.

BREASTFEEDING SUMMARY

One study was located that described breastfeeding in a woman who was being treated for Hodgkin lymphoma with dacarbazine, along with bleomycin, vinblastine, and doxorubicin. Drug levels were not analyzed. However, the study did show an alteration in the breast milk microbial population and metabolic profile. Regardless, no adverse effects were reported in the infant. Due to a concern for potential serious adverse effects that might be seen in a breastfed infant, the manufacturer recommends that women not breastfeed while being treated with this drug. Nevertheless, breastfeeding while using this drug should be based on the mother's clinical need for treatment versus any potential infant risks that might occur. If used, the infant should be monitored for the most common reported adult side effects of nausea, headache, and abdominal pain (all leading to irritability), diarrhea, alopecia, vomiting, fever, decreased appetite (monitor infant growth), and rash.

References

1. Prescribing Information. *Dacarbazine*. Hospira, Inc; 2021.
2. Zemlickis D, Lishner M, Degendorfer P, et al. Fetal outcome after in utero exposure to cancer chemotherapy. *Arch Intern Med*. 1992;152:573-576.
3. Anselmo AP, Cavalier E, Maurizi Enrici R, et al. Hodgkin's disease during pregnancy: diagnostic and therapeutic management. *Fetal Diagn Ther*. 1999;14:102-105.
4. Green DM, Zevon MA, Lowries G, et al. Congenital anomalies in children of patients who received chemotherapy for cancer in childhood and adolescence. *N Engl J Med*. 1991;325:141-146.
5. Green DM, Whitton JA, Stovall M, et al. Pregnancy outcome of female survivors of childhood cancer: a report from the Childhood Cancer Survivor study. *Am J Obstet Gynecol*. 2002;187:1070-1080.

6. Sanchez M, Pellicer B, del Puig Cozar M, et al. Hodgkin lymphoma in pregnancy: a case report. *Clin Adv Hematol Oncol*. 2013;11:533-536.
7. Moshe Y, Bentur OS, Lishner M, et al. The management of Hodgkin lymphomas in pregnancies. *Eur J Haematol*. 2017;99:385-391.
8. Kantrowitz-Gordon I, Hays K, Kayode O, et al. Pharmacokinetics of dacarbazine (DTIC) in pregnancy. *Cancer Chemother Pharmacol*. 2018;81:455-460.
9. Aviles A, Nambo MJ, Neri N. Treatment of early stages Hodgkin lymphoma during pregnancy. *Mediterr J Hematol Infect Dis*. 2018;10:e2018006.
10. Van Driessche F, Perez CA. Hodgkin lymphoma in pregnancy: achieving the best outcome for both mother and infant. *Clin Adv Hematol Oncol*. 2013;11:537-538.
11. Urbaniak C, McMillan A, Angelini M, et al. Effect of chemotherapy on the microbiota and metabolome of human milk, a case report. *Microbiome*. 2014;2:24.

DACLIZUMAB

Immunologic (Monoclonal Antibody)

PREGNANCY RECOMMENDATION: Limited Human Data—Animal Data Suggest Low Risk

BREASTFEEDING RECOMMENDATION: Probably Compatible

PREGNANCY SUMMARY

One report describing the use of daclizumab in human pregnancy was located. The data come from the clinical trials. Of 24 pregnancies with exposure to daclizumab at less than 6 months prior to gestation or during pregnancy, there were 20 live births with 1 anomaly (5%) and 4 spontaneous abortions (17%). As an immunoglobulin G (IgG) antibody, it likely crosses the placenta, especially during the second half of pregnancy, so some fetal exposure will probably occur. Therefore, this limited human pregnancy experience prevents a complete assessment of the embryofetal risk. No embryofetal toxicity was seen in one animal species at a dose of more than 10 times the RHD. Using this drug during pregnancy should be based on the pros and cons of the mother's clinical need for treatment versus any potential fetal risk that might occur from exposure.

BREASTFEEDING SUMMARY

No reports describing the use of daclizumab during human lactation have been located. It is known that IgG antibodies can be found in human breast milk, but are not found in the neonatal or infant circulation. Additionally, if any IgG antibodies were to be ingested through breastfeeding, they would probably be digested in the infant's gastrointestinal tract and not be absorbed. Breastfeeding while using this drug should be based on the mother's clinical need for treatment. If used, the infant should be monitored for the most common reported adult side effects of upper respiratory tract infection, rash, and elevated liver function tests.

References

1. Prescribing Information. *Zinbryta*. Biogen, Inc; 2020.
2. Gold R, Stefoski D, Selmaj K, et al. Pregnancy experience: nonclinical studies and pregnancy outcomes in the daclizumab clinical study program. *Neurol Ther*. 2016;5:169-182.

DACOMITINIB

Antineoplastic (Epidermal Growth Factor Receptor Kinase Inhibitor)

PREGNANCY RECOMMENDATION: No Human Data—Animal Data Suggest Potential Risk

BREASTFEEDING RECOMMENDATION: Potential Toxicity

PREGNANCY SUMMARY

No reports describing the use of dacomitinib in human pregnancy have been located. The drug will probably cross the placenta, so some fetal exposure will likely occur. Therefore, the absence of human pregnancy experience prevents a complete assessment of the embryofetal risk. Animal studies did show embryofetal toxicity with malformations in one species at doses less than 10 times the RHD. Based on these animal studies and the drug's mechanism of action, the manufacturer recommends that women with reproductive potential use effective contraception during treatment and for 17 days after the last dose. Nevertheless, using this drug during pregnancy should be based on the pros and cons of the mother's clinical need for treatment versus any potential fetal risk that might occur from exposure. There is a pregnancy registry for women who are pregnant and have cancer. For more information, women who are pregnant and have cancer and health care providers are encouraged to contact the Cancer and Pregnancy Registry at 1-877-635-4499.

BREASTFEEDING SUMMARY

No reports describing the use of dacomitinib during human lactation have been located. The drug will likely be found in breast milk, so some infant exposure will probably occur. Due to the concern for potential serious adverse effects that might be seen in a breastfed infant, the manufacturer recommends that women not breastfeed while being treated with this drug and for at least 2 weeks after the last dose. Nevertheless, breastfeeding while using this drug should be based on the mother's clinical need for treatment. If used, the infant should be monitored for the most common reported adult side effects of nausea and pruritus (both leading to irritability), diarrhea, alopecia, vomiting, cough, rash, decreased appetite, and various laboratory abnormalities (see PI).

Reference

1. Prescribing Information. *Vizimpro*. Pfizer Laboratories; 2020.

DACTINOMYCIN

Antineoplastic (Antimitotic Antibacterial)

PREGNANCY RECOMMENDATION: Limited Human Data—Animal Data Suggest Risk

BREASTFEEDING RECOMMENDATION: Potential Toxicity

PREGNANCY SUMMARY

No reports describing the use of dactinomycin in the first trimester of pregnancy have been located. The drug has been reported in a few pregnancies in the second and third trimesters without any adverse fetal effects described. A limited amount of the drug may cross the placenta (especially in the third trimester), so some fetal exposure may occur. Therefore, this limited human pregnancy experience prevents a complete assessment of the embryofetal risk. Animal studies did show embryofetal toxicity with malformations in three species at doses of less than 10 times the RHD. Based on animal studies and the drug's mechanism of action, the manufacturer recommends that women with reproductive potential use effective contraception during treatment and for 6 months after the last dose. They also recommend that males with female partners of reproductive potential use effective contraception during treatment and for 3 months after the last dose. Nevertheless, using this drug during pregnancy should be based on the pros and cons of the mother's clinical need for treatment versus any potential fetal risk that might occur from exposure. There is a registry for women who are pregnant and have cancer. For more information, women and health care providers are encouraged to contact the Cancer and Pregnancy Registry at 1-877-635-4499.

BREASTFEEDING SUMMARY

No reports describing the use of dactinomycin during human lactation have been located. A limited amount of the drug may be found in human breast milk, so some infant exposure may occur. Due to a concern for potential serious adverse effects that might be seen in a breastfed infant, the manufacturer recommends that women not breastfeed while being treated with this drug and for at least 2 weeks after the last dose. Nevertheless, breastfeeding while using this drug should be based on the mother's clinical need for treatment versus any potential infant risks that might occur. If used, the infant should be monitored for the most common reported adult side effects of nausea and abdominal pain (both leading to irritability), fatigue (lethargy), alopecia, vomiting, rash, fever, and various laboratory abnormalities (see PI).

References

1. Prescribing Information. *Dactinomycin*. Mylan Institutional; 2018.
2. Ross GT. Congenital anomalies among children born of mothers receiving chemotherapy for gestational trophoblastic neoplasms. *Cancer*. 1976;37:1043-1047.
3. Walden PAM, Bagshawe KD. Pregnancies after chemotherapy for gestational trophoblastic tumours. *Lancet*. 1979;2:1241.
4. Schwartz PE, Vidone RA. Pregnancy following combination chemotherapy for a mixed germ cell tumor of the ovary. *Gynecol Oncol*. 1981;12:373-378.
5. Pastorfide GB, Goldstein DP. Pregnancy after hydatidiform mole. *Obstet Gynecol*. 1973;42:67-70.
6. Rustin GJS, Booth M, Dent J, et al. Pregnancy after cytotoxic chemotherapy for gestational trophoblastic tumours. *Br Med J*. 1984;288:103-106.
7. Evenson DP, Arlin Z, Welt S, et al. Male reproductive capacity may recover following drug treatment with the L-10 protocol for acute lymphocytic leukemia. *Cancer*. 1984;53:30-36.
8. Sivanesaratnam V, Sen DK. Normal pregnancy after successful treatment of choriocarcinoma with cerebral metastases: a case report. *J Reprod Med*. 1988;33:402-403.
9. Lee RB, Kelly J, Elg SA, et al. Pregnancy following conservative surgery and adjunctive chemotherapy for stage III immature teratoma of the ovary. *Obstet Gynecol*. 1989;73:853-855.
10. Bakri YN, Pedersen P, Nassar M. Normal pregnancy after curative multiagent chemotherapy for choriocarcinoma with brain metastases. *Acta Obstet Gynecol Scand*. 1991;70:611-613.
11. Green DM, Zevon MA, Lowrie G, et al. Congenital anomalies in children of patients who received chemotherapy for cancer in childhood and adolescence. *N Engl J Med*. 1991;325:141-146.
12. Byrne J, Nicholson HS, Mulvihill JJ. Absence of birth defects in offspring of women treated with dactinomycin. *N Engl J Med*. 1992;326:137.
13. Nicholson HO. Cytotoxic drugs in pregnancy: review of reported cases. *J Obstet Gynaecol Br Commonw*. 1968;75:307-312.
14. Gililland J, Weinstein L. The effects of cancer chemotherapeutic agents on the developing fetus. *Obstet Gynecol Surv*. 1983;38:6-13.
15. Haerr RW, Pratt AT. Multiagent chemotherapy for sarcoma diagnosed during pregnancy. *Cancer*. 1985;56:1028-1033.
16. Weed JC Jr, Roh RA, Mendenhall HW. Recurrent endodermal sinus tumor during pregnancy. *Obstet Gynecol*. 1979;54:653-656.
17. Kim DS, Park MI. Maternal and fetal survival following surgery and chemotherapy of endodermal sinus tumor of the ovary during pregnancy: a case report. *Obstet Gynecol*. 1989;73:503-507.
18. Kim DS, Moon H, Lee JA, et al. Anticancer drugs during pregnancy: are we able to discard them? *Am J Obstet Gynecol*. 1992;166:265.
19. Dobbing J. Pregnancy and leukaemia. *Lancet*. 1977;1:1155.
20. Gershenson DM. Menstrual and reproductive function after treatment with combination chemotherapy for malignant ovarian germ cell tumors. *J Clin Oncol*. 1988;6:270-275.

DALBAVANCIN

Antibacterial (Lipoglycopeptide)

PREGNANCY RECOMMENDATION: Limited Human Data—Animal Data Suggest Potential Risk

BREASTFEEDING RECOMMENDATION: Probably Compatible

D

PREGNANCY SUMMARY

One case report was located that described the use of dalbavancin in treating a pregnant woman with multidrug-resistant endocarditis. Treatment occurred for 4 weeks in the third trimester up to delivery. The child had no reported complications or anomalies. Dalbavancin will likely have negligible placental transfer, so fetal exposure will probably be clinically insignificant. However, this limited human pregnancy experience prevents a complete assessment of the embryofetal risk. Animal studies did show embryofetal toxicity in one species at doses less than 10 times the RHD. Using this drug during pregnancy should be based on the pros and cons of the mother's clinical need for treatment versus any potential fetal risk that might occur from exposure.

BREASTFEEDING SUMMARY

One report describing the use of dalbavancin during human lactation was located. A lactating mother developed a multidrug-resistant, methicillin-resistant Staphylococcus aureus infection associated with nipple blebs at 6 months postpartum. She continued to breastfeed (through pumping) while being treated for several weeks with dalbavancin, and the infection resolved. There were no reports of any adverse effects seen in the infant. A limited amount of drug may be excreted into breast milk. However, the drug is poorly absorbed orally, and because the drug partially consists of a peptide, if any drug were to be ingested through breastfeeding, it would probably be partially digested in the infant's gastrointestinal tract and not be absorbed. Therefore, any possible exposure to this drug during breastfeeding is likely to be clinically insignificant. Breastfeeding while using this drug should be based on the mother's clinical need for treatment. If used, the infant should be monitored for the most common reported adult side effects of headache and nausea (both leading to irritability) and diarrhea.

References

1. Prescribing Information. *Dalvance*. Durata Therapeutics; 2020.
2. Steele JM, Seabury RW, Hale CM, et al. Unsuccessful treatment of methicillin-resistant Staphylococcus aureus endocarditis with dalbavancin. *J Clin Pharm Ther*. 2018;43:101-103.
3. Mitchell KB, Eglash A, Bamberger ET. Mammary dysbiosis and nipple blebs treated with intravenous daptomycin and dalbavancin. *J Hum Lact*. 2020;36:365-368.

DALFAMPRIDINE

Central Nervous System (Potassium Channel Blocker—Multiple Sclerosis)

PREGNANCY RECOMMENDATION: No Human Data—Animal Data Suggest Potential Risk

BREASTFEEDING RECOMMENDATION: Potential Toxicity

PREGNANCY SUMMARY

No reports describing the use of dalfampridine in human pregnancy have been located. The drug will probably cross the placenta, so some fetal exposure will likely occur. Therefore, the absence of human pregnancy experience prevents a complete assessment of the embryofetal risk. Animal studies did not show any teratogenicity in two species at doses of less than 10 times the RHD, despite maternal toxicity. However, when administered from before conception, through gestation, and through lactation, there was some decreased pup survival at about 1.5 times the RHD. Using this drug during pregnancy should be based on the pros and cons of the mother's clinical need for treatment versus any potential fetal risk that might occur from exposure.

BREASTFEEDING SUMMARY

No reports describing the use of dalfampridine during human lactation have been located. The drug will probably be excreted into human breast milk, so some infant exposure will likely occur. However, due to a concern for potential serious adverse effects that might be seen in a breastfed infant, the manufacturer recommends that women not breastfeed while being treated with this drug. Nevertheless, breastfeeding while using this drug should be based on the mother's clinical need for treatment versus any potential infant risks that might occur. If used, the infant should be monitored for the most common reported adult side effects of nausea, headache, dizziness, and back pain (all leading to irritability), insomnia, constipation, and urinary tract infection (1).

Reference

1. Prescribing Information. *Ampyra*. Acorda Therapeutics; 2017.

D

DALTEPARIN

Hematologic (Anticoagulant—Low-Molecular-Weight Heparin)

PREGNANCY RECOMMENDATION: Human Data Suggest Compatible

BREASTFEEDING RECOMMENDATION: Compatible

PREGNANCY SUMMARY

Several reports have been located that describe the use of dalteparin in human pregnancy. Most of these exposures have occurred in the second and third trimesters. No adverse effects related to the drug were described. The drug does not cross the placenta, so fetal exposure will not occur. Animal studies did not show any embryofetal toxicity in two species at doses of less than 10 times the RHD. The use of dalteparin during pregnancy appears to present no more fetal or newborn risk than that from standard, unfractionated heparin. Multidose vials of dalteparin contain the preservative benzyl alcohol, which is fully discussed below in the Breastfeeding Summary.

BREASTFEEDING SUMMARY

In three reports, low-molecular-weight heparin was not detected in human breast milk, consistent with the MW. Breastfeeding while using this drug should be based on the mother's clinical need for treatment versus any potential infant risks that might occur. However, because dalteparin is poorly absorbed orally, if any of the drug were to be found in breast milk, the effect on the infant would be clinically insignificant. Thus, the risk to a nursing infant from ingestion of dalteparin from breast milk appears to be negligible. Therefore, exposure to a breastfeeding newborn is not likely. Multidose vials of dalteparin contain the preservative benzyl alcohol, which has been associated with serious and possibly fatal reactions in neonates, including "gasping syndrome" when consumed orally. However, benzyl alcohol is rapidly metabolized to benzoic acid in the liver and then binds to glycine and is excreted as hippuric acid. In addition, this syndrome has usually been seen in neonatal exposures of about 100 to 400 mg/kg/d. The concentration of benzyl alcohol in the multidose vials is 14 mg/mL. One milliliter of the multidose vial is 25,000 international units (IU) of the drug. If a pregnant or breastfeeding woman were to inject 10,000 IU/d, this would amount to about 6 mg (or ~0.9 mg/kg/d). Therefore, any risk of benzyl alcohol exposure is negligible. In addition, the drug is supplied in numerous single-dose syringes that do not contain benzyl alcohol.

References

1. Prescribing Information. *Fragmin*. Pfizer Laboratories Div Pfizer; 2018.
2. Nelson-Piercy C. Low molecular weight heparin for obstetric thromboprophylaxis. *Br J Obstet Gynaecol*. 1994;101:6-8.
3. Forestier F, Solé Y, Aiach M, et al. Absence of transplacental passage of Fragmin (Kabi) during the second and the third trimesters of pregnancy. *Thromb Haemost*. 1992;67:180-181.
4. Harenberg J, Leber G, Zimmermann R, et al. Prevention of thromboembolism with low-molecular weight heparin in pregnancy. *Geburtshilfe Frauenheilkd*. 1987;47:15-18.
5. De Boer K, Heyboer H, ten Cate JW, et al. Low molecular weight heparin treatment in a pregnant woman with allergy to standard heparins and heparinoid. *Thromb Haemost*. 1989;61:148.
6. Melissari E, Parker CJ, Wilson NV, et al. Use of low molecular weight heparin in pregnancy. *Thromb Haemost*. 1992;68:652-656.
7. Shefras J, Farquharson RG. Bone density studies in pregnant women receiving heparin. *Eur J Obstet Gynecol Reprod Biol*. 1996;65:171-174.
8. Wahlberg TB, Kher A. Low molecular weight heparin as thromboprophylaxis in pregnancy. *Haemostasis*. 1994;24:55-56.
9. Manoharan A. Use of low molecular weight heparin during pregnancy. *J Clin Pathol*. 1994;47:94-95.
10. Rasmussen C, Wadt J, Jacobsen B. Thromboembolic prophylaxis with low molecular weight heparin during pregnancy. *Int J Gynecol Obstet*. 1994;47:121-125.
11. Anand SS, Brimble S, Ginsberg JS. Management of iliofemoral thrombosis in a pregnant patient with heparin resistance. *Arch Intern Med*. 1997;157:815-816.
12. Pettila V, Kaaja R, Leinonen P, et al. Thromboprophylaxis with low molecular weight heparin (dalteparin) in pregnancy. *Thromb Res*. 1999;96:275-282.
13. Rey E, Rivard GE. Prophylaxis and treatment of thromboembolic diseases during pregnancy with dalteparin. *Int J Gynecol Obstet*. 2000;71:19-24.
14. Bates SM, Greer IA, Middeldorp S, et al. VTE, thrombophilia, antithrombotic therapy, and pregnancy: antithrombotic therapy and prevention of thrombosis, 9th ed: American College of Chest Physicians Evidence-Based Clinical Practice Guidelines. *Chest*. 2012;141(2 suppl):e691S-e736S.
15. Lindhoff-Last E, Willeke A, Thalhammer C, et al. Hirudin treatment in a breastfeeding woman. *Lancet*. 2000;355:467-468.
16. Richter C, Sitzmann J, Lang P, et al. Excretion of low molecular weight heparin in human milk. *Br J Clin Pharmacol*. 2001;52:708-710.
17. Nair B. Final report on the safety assessment of benzyl alcohol, benzoic acid, and sodium benzoate. *Int J Toxicol*. 2001;20(suppl 3):23-50.

DANAZOL

Reproductive Health/Miscellaneous (Androgen—Immunomodulator)

PREGNANCY RECOMMENDATION: *Contraindicated

BREASTFEEDING RECOMMENDATION: *Contraindicated

D

PREGNANCY SUMMARY

A number of reports have described the inadvertent use of danazol during human gestation, resulting in female virilization with clitoral hypertrophy, labial fusion, and ambiguous genitalia, and so on. It appears that this risk primarily occurs when exposure goes beyond 8 weeks of gestation. These findings also confirm that the drug crosses the placenta, so fetal exposure occurs. There are also numerous reports of no major birth anomalies when exposure occurs at the time of conception, followed by abrupt danazol discontinuation. Animal studies did show some embryofetal toxicity in one species at doses of less than 10 times the RHD. Because danazol is used to treat endometriosis, frequently in an infertile woman, a barrier (nonhormonal) contraception method is recommended to prevent accidental use during conception. *The drug is approved for use in treating endometriosis and fibrocystic breast disease, which would not be indicated during pregnancy. The only exception that would need a combined informed conference between the patient and her health care providers would be in treating hereditary angioedema. However, numerous options of other medications are available for this disorder. The drug carries a boxed warning for a contraindication for use during pregnancy.

BREASTFEEDING SUMMARY

No reports describing the use of danazol during human lactation have been located. Due to a concern for potential serious adverse effects that might be seen in a breastfed infant, the manufacturer recommends that women not breastfeed while being treated with this drug. *The drug is approved for use in treating endometriosis and fibrocystic breast disease, which would not be indicated while breastfeeding. The only exception that would need a combined informed conference between the patient and her health care providers would be in treating hereditary angioedema. However, numerous options of other medications are available for this disorder.

References

1. Prescribing Information. *Danazol*. Teva Pharmaceuticals USA; 2018.
2. Duck SC, Katayama KP. Danazol may cause female pseudohermaphroditism. *Fertil Steril*. 1981;35:230-231.
3. Castro-Magana M, Cheruvanky T, Collipp PJ, et al. Transient adrenogenital syndrome due to exposure to danazol in utero. *Am J Dis Child*. 1981;135:1032-1034.
4. Peress MR, Kreutner AK, Mathur RS, et al. Female pseudohermaphroditism with somatic chromosomal anomaly in association with in utero exposure to danazol. *Am J Obstet Gynecol*. 1982;142:708-709.
5. Schwartz RP. Ambiguous genitalia in a term female infant due to exposure to danazol in utero. *Am J Dis Child*. 1982;136:474.
6. Wentz AC. Adverse effects of danazol in pregnancy. *Ann Intern Med*. 1982;96:672-673.
7. Shaw RW, Farquhar JW. Female pseudohermaphroditism associated with danazol exposure in utero. Case report. *Br J Obstet Gynecol*. 1984;91:386-389.
8. Rosa FW. Virilization of the female fetus with maternal danazol exposure. *Am J Obstet Gynecol*. 1984;149:99-100.
9. Kingsbury AC. Danazol and fetal masculinization: a warning. *Med J Aust*. 1985;143:410-411.
10. Quagliarello J, Greco MA. Danazol and urogenital sinus formation in pregnancy. *Fertil Steril*. 1985;43:939-942.
11. Brunskill PJ. The effects of fetal exposure to danazol. *Br J Obstet Gynaecol*. 1992;99:212-215.
12. Daniell JF, Christianson C. Combined laparoscopic surgery and danazol therapy for pelvic endometriosis. *Fertil Steril*. 1981;35:521-525.
13. Fayez JA, Collazo LM, Vernon C. Comparison of different modalities of treatment for minimal and mild endometriosis. *Am J Obstet Gynecol*. 1988;159:927-932.
14. Butler L, Wilson E, Belisle S, et al. Collaborative study of pregnancy rates following danazol therapy of stage I endometriosis. *Fertil Steril*. 1984;41:373-376.
15. Dmowski WP, Cohen MR. Antigonadotropin (danazol) in the treatment of endometriosis. Evaluation of posttreatment fertility and three-year follow-up data. *Am J Obstet Gynecol*. 1978;130:41-48.
16. Money J, Mathews D. Prenatal exposure to virilizing progestins: an adult follow-up study of twelve women. *Arch Sex Behav*. 1982;11:73-83.

DANICOPAN

Hematologic (Small Molecule Complement Factor D Inhibitor)

PREGNANCY RECOMMENDATION: No Human Data—Animal Data Suggest Low Risk

BREASTFEEDING RECOMMENDATION: Potential Toxicity

PREGNANCY SUMMARY

No reports describing the use of danicopan in human pregnancy have been located. The drug will likely cross the placenta, so some fetal exposure will probably occur. Therefore, the absence of human pregnancy experience prevents a complete assessment of the embryofetal risk. Animal studies did not show any embryofetal toxicity or malformations in two species at doses of more than 10 times the RHD. Using this drug during pregnancy should be based on the pros and cons of the mother's clinical need for treatment versus any potential fetal risk that might occur from exposure. The drug does carry a boxed warning for an increased risk of serious infections caused by encapsulated bacteria, including Neisseria meningitidis, Streptococcus pneumonia, and Haemophilus influenzae type B.

BREASTFEEDING SUMMARY

No reports describing the use of danicopan during human lactation have been located. The drug will likely be found in breast milk, so some infant exposure will probably occur. Due to a concern for potential serious adverse effects that might be seen in a breastfed infant, including infections with encapsulated bacteria (see boxed warning above in Pregnancy

Summary), the manufacturer recommends that women not breastfeed while being treated with this drug and for at least 3 days after the last dose. However, breastfeeding while using this drug should be based on the mother's clinical need for treatment versus any potential infant risk that might occur. If used, the infant should be monitored for the most common reported adult side effect of headache (leading to irritability).

Reference

1. Prescribing Information. *Velsipity*. Pfizer, Inc; 2023.

D

DANTROLENE

Pain (Muscle Relaxant) Muscle Relaxant

PREGNANCY RECOMMENDATION: Limited Human Data—Animal Data Suggest Risk (Maternal Benefit May Outweigh Any Embryofetal Risk for Malignant Hyperthermia)

BREASTFEEDING RECOMMENDATION: Potential Toxicity (Hold Breastfeeding)

PREGNANCY SUMMARY

Dantrolene has been used intravenously (IV) in a limited number of pregnant patients shortly before delivery. No fetal or newborn adverse effects have been described. No data are available for longer-term use and exposure with the oral agent. No reports have been located regarding first-trimester exposure to the drug. The drug crosses the placenta, so fetal exposure will occur. Therefore, this limited human pregnancy experience prevents a complete assessment of the embryofetal risk. Animal studies did show some embryofetal toxicity in two species at doses of less than 10 times the RHD. Using this drug during pregnancy should be based on the pros and cons of the mother's clinical need for treatment versus any potential fetal risk that might occur from exposure. However, because malignant hyperthermia can be fatal, treatment of a pregnant woman with this disorder may outweigh any potential embryofetal risk.

BREASTFEEDING SUMMARY

Dantrolene has been shown to be excreted into human breast milk. A pregnant woman developed malignant hyperthermia associated with anesthesia used during a cesarean delivery. Postdelivery, she was treated with IV dantrolene for 3 days. The peak breast milk level was about 1.2 mcg/mL obtained on the second day. The breast milk level on the fourth day (about 35 hours after the last dose) was 50 ng/mL. The estimated elimination half-life from breast milk was about 9 hours. Due to a concern for potential serious adverse effects that might be seen in a breastfed infant, the manufacturer recommends that women not breastfeed while being treated with this drug. An alternative option would be to hold breastfeeding for about 2 days after the last dantrolene dose. This would ensure that the exposure of the nursing infant would be negligible. No data are available for breastfeeding with the use of the oral agent.

References

1. Prescribing Information. *Dantrolene sodium*. Impax Generics; 2017.
2. Nagaoka T, Osuka F, Hatano M. Reproductive studies of dantrolene. Teratogenicity study in rabbits. *Clinical Report*. 1977;11:2212-2217. As cited in Shepard TH. Catalog of Teratogenic Agents. 6th ed. Johns Hopkins University Press; 1989:549.
3. Nagaoka T, Osuka F, Shigemura T, et al. Reproductive test of dantrolene. Teratogenicity test on rats. *Clinical Report*. 1977;11:2218-2230. As cited in Shepard TH. Catalog of Teratogenic Agents. 6th ed. Johns Hopkins University Press; 1989:549.
4. Morison DH. Placental transfer of dantrolene. *Anesthesiology*. 1983;59:265.
5. Glassenberg R, Cohen H. Intravenous dantrolene in a pregnant malignant hyperthermia susceptible (MHS) patient (abstract). *Anesthesiology*. 1984;61:A404.
6. Shime J, Gare D, Andrews J, et al. Dantrolene in pregnancy: lack of adverse effects on the fetus and newborn infant. *Am J Obstet Gynecol*. 1988;159:831-834.
7. Cupryn JP, Kennedy A, Byrick RJ. Malignant hyperthermia in pregnancy. *Am J Obstet Gynecol*. 1984;150:327-328.
8. Khalil SN, Williams JP, Bourke DL. Management of a malignant hyperthermia susceptible patient in labor with 2-chloroprocaine epidural anesthesia. *Anesth Analg*. 1983;62:119-121.
9. Kaplan RF, Kellner KR. More on malignant hyperthermia during delivery. *Am J Obstet Gynecol*. 1985;152:608-609.
10. Sorosky JI, Ingardia CJ, Botti JJ. Diagnosis and management of susceptibility to malignant hyperthermia in pregnancy. *Am J Perinatol*. 1989;6:46-48.
11. Sessler DI. Malignant hyperthermia. *J Pediatr*. 1986;109:9-14.
12. Fricker RM, Hoerauf KH, Drewe J, et al. Secretion of dantrolene into breast milk after acute therapy of a suspected malignant hyperthermia crisis during cesarean section. *Anesthesiology*. 1998;89:1023-1025.

DAPAGLIFLOZIN

Antidiabetic (Sodium Glucose Cotransporter 2 Inhibitor)

PREGNANCY RECOMMENDATION: No Human Data—Animal Data Suggest Potential Risk

BREASTFEEDING RECOMMENDATION: Potential Toxicity

D

PREGNANCY SUMMARY

No reports describing the use of dapagliflozin in human pregnancy have been located. The drug was shown to cross the placenta through ex vivo human placental perfusion analysis with a maximum fetal to maternal blood level of about 67%. So fetal exposure appears to occur. Therefore, the absence of human pregnancy experience prevents a complete assessment of the embryofetal risk. Embryofetal toxicity was observed in one animal species at doses more than 10 times the maximum recommended human dose (MRHD) during the period of renal development that corresponds to the late second and third trimester of human renal development. Due to this finding, the manufacturer does not recommend the use of empagliflozin during the second and third trimesters of pregnancy. Nevertheless, using this drug during pregnancy should be based on the pros and cons of the mother's clinical need for treatment versus any potential fetal risk that might occur from exposure. In addition, fetal renal status can be monitored by perinatal ultrasound.

BREASTFEEDING SUMMARY

No reports describing the use of dapagliflozin during human lactation have been located. The drug will probably be found in breast milk, so some infant exposure will likely occur. Because renal toxicity was observed in animal studies corresponding to the late second and third trimesters of human pregnancy, the manufacturer does not recommend the use of empagliflozin while breastfeeding. Nevertheless, breastfeeding while using this drug should be based on the mother's clinical need for treatment. If used, the infant should be monitored for the most common reported adult side effects of urinary tract and genital mycotic infections.

References

1. Prescribing Information. *Farxiga*. AstraZeneca Pharmaceuticals; 2019.
2. Kuoni S, Muller D, Simoes-Wust AP, Steiner R. Simultaneous LC-MS/MS quantification of SGLT2 inhibitors and antipyrine in medium and tissue from human ex vivo placental perfusions. *J Chromatogr B Analyt Biomed Life Sci*. 2023;1228:123841.
3. Kuoni S, Steiner R, Saleh L, et al. Safety assessment of the SGLT2 inhibitors empagliflozin, dapagliflozin, and canagliflozin during pregnancy: an ex vivo human placenta perfusion and in vitro study. *Biomed Pharmacother*. 2023;171:116177.

DAPRODUSTAT

Hematologic (Hypoxia Inducible Factor Inhibitor)

PREGNANCY RECOMMENDATION: No Human Data—Animal Data Suggest Low Risk

BREASTFEEDING RECOMMENDATION: Potential Toxicity

PREGNANCY SUMMARY

No reports describing the use of daprodustat in human pregnancy have been located. The drug will likely cross the placenta, so some fetal exposure will probably occur. Therefore, the absence of human pregnancy experience prevents a complete assessment of the embryofetal risk. Animal studies did not show any embryofetal toxicity. Using this drug during pregnancy should be based on the pros and cons of the mother's clinical need for treatment versus any potential fetal risk that might occur from exposure. In the clinical trials, an increase in hypertension and thrombotic events (arterial and venous) were seen.

BREASTFEEDING SUMMARY

No reports describing the use of daprodustat during human lactation have been located. The drug will likely be excreted into breast milk, so some infant exposure will probably occur. Due to the concern for potential serious adverse effects that might be seen in a breastfed infant, the manufacturer recommends that women not breastfeed while being treated with this drug and for at least 1 week after the last dose. Nevertheless, breastfeeding while using this drug should be based on the mother's clinical need for treatment. If used, the infant should be monitored for the most common reported adult side effects of abdominal pain (leading to irritability), hypertension, and thrombotic events.

Reference

1. Prescribing Information. *Jesduvroq*. GlaxoSmithKline; 2023.

DAPSONE

Antibacterial/Dermatologic (Leprostatic—Anti-Inflammatory)

PREGNANCY RECOMMENDATION: Limited Human Data—No Relevant Animal Data (Maternal Benefit May Outweigh Any Embryofetal Risk—Leprosy)

BREASTFEEDING RECOMMENDATION: Potential Toxicity

PREGNANCY SUMMARY

Several studies describing the use of dapsone during human pregnancy were located. Of a total of about 70 first-trimester exposures (from case reports and small series), there were 2 (2.9%) major birth defects described. Use of the drug in the second and third trimesters has also been reported without any serious newborn outcomes described, other than hemolytic anemia. The drug crosses the placenta, so fetal exposure will occur. However, this limited human pregnancy experience prevents a complete assessment of the embryofetal risk. Animal reproduction and fertility studies have not been located. Using the oral drug during pregnancy should be based on the pros and cons of the mother's clinical need for treatment versus any potential fetal risk that might occur from exposure. Using the topical agent is less likely to cause any significant fetal complications, due to much lower serum concentrations. However, this has not been analyzed in human pregnancy. In addition, the approved use for topical dapsone is in treating acne (which can probably be temporarily avoided in most pregnancies). Hemolytic anemia can occur with the use of dapsone, especially in patients with glucose-6-phosphate dehydrogenase (G6PD) deficiency.

BREASTFEEDING SUMMARY

Dapsone and its primary metabolite, monoacetyldapsone, have been found in breast milk. The calculated RIDs can range from about 2% to about 15%. The drug has also been found in infant blood with a combined concentration (dapsone and the metabolite) of about 640 ng/mL, which is about 25% of the mean maternal blood concentration seen with oral use. A case of newborn hemolytic anemia was located with exposure through breastfeeding. No evaluation for G6PD deficiency was performed. Due to a concern for potential serious adverse effects that might be seen in a breastfed infant, the manufacturer recommends that women not breastfeed while being treated with this drug. Nevertheless, breastfeeding while using this drug should be based on the mother's clinical need for treatment versus any potential infant risks that might occur. If used, the infant should be monitored for the most common reported adult side effects of nausea, headache, dizziness, and abdominal pain (all leading to irritability), vomiting, decreased appetite (monitor growth), rash, fever, insomnia, and anemia. The risk for hemolytic anemia is higher for neonates than for adults. The use of the topical agent is less likely to cause any significant newborn complications due to much lower blood levels. However, this has not been evaluated in human pregnancy, and the approved use of topical dapsone is in treating acne.

References

1. Information. *Dapsone*. Alvogen; 2019.
2. Griciute L, Tomatis L. Carcinogenicity of dapsone in mice and rats. *Int J Cancer*. 1980;25:123-129.
3. Hocking DR. Neonatal haemolytic disease due to dapsone. *Med J Aust*. 1968;1:1130-1131.
4. Diamond WJ. Herpes gestationis. *S Afr Med J*. 1976;50:739-740.
5. Sanders SW, Zone JJ, Foltz RL, et al. Hemolytic anemia induced by dapsone transmitted through breast milk. *Ann Intern Med*. 1982;96:465-466.
6. Sills ES, Mabie WC. A refractory case of herpes gestationis. *J Tenn Med Assoc*. 1992;85:559-560.
7. Kirtschig G, Collier PM, Emmerson RW, et al. Severe case of pemphigoid gestationis with unusual target antigen. *Br J Dermatol*. 1994;131:108-111.
8. Tuffanelli DL. Successful pregnancy in a patient with dermatitis herpetiformis treated with low-dose dapsone. *Arch Dermatol*. 1982;118:876.
9. Maurus JN. Hansen's disease in pregnancy. *Obstet Gynecol*. 1978;52:22-25.
10. Duncan ME. An historical and clinical review of the interaction of leprosy and pregnancy: a cycle to be broken. *Soc Sci Med*. 1993;37:457-472.
11. Bhargava P, Kuldeep CM, Mathur NK. Antileprosy drugs, pregnancy and fetal outcome. *Int J Lepr Other Mycobact Dis*. 1996;64:457.
12. Lyde CB. Pregnancy in patients with Hansen disease. *Arch Dermatol*. 1997;133:623-627.
13. Thornton YS, Bowe ET. Neonatal hyperbilirubinemia after treatment of maternal leprosy. *South Med J*. 1989;82:668.
14. Sturchler D. Malaria prophylaxis in travelers: the current position. *Experientia*. 1984;40:1357-1362.
15. Brown GV. Chemoprophylaxis of malaria. *Med J Aust*. 1986;144:696-702.
16. Anonymous. Prevention of malaria in pregnancy and early childhood. *Br Med J*. 1984;289:1296-1297.
17. Greenwood AM, Armstrong JRM, Byass P, et al. Malaria chemoprophylaxis, birth weight and child survival. *Trans R Soc Trop Med Hyg*. 1992;86:483-485.
18. Greenwood AM, Menendez C, Todd J, et al. The distribution of birth weights in Gambian women who received malaria chemoprophylaxis during their first pregnancy and in control women. *Trans R Soc Trop Med Hyg*. 1994;88:311-312.
19. Menendez C, Todd J, Alonso PL, et al. Malaria chemoprophylaxis, infection of the placenta and birth weight in Gambian primigravidae. *J Trop Med Hyg*. 1994;97:244-248.
20. Kahn G. Dapsone is safe during pregnancy. *J Am Acad Dermatol*. 1985;13:838-839.
21. Spracklen FHN, Monteagudo FSE. Malaria prophylaxis. *S Afr Med J*. 1986;70:316.
22. Luzzi GA, Peto TEA. Adverse effects of antimalarials. An update. *Drug Saf*. 1993;8:295-311.
23. Keuter M, van Eijk A, Hoogstrate M, et al. Comparison of chloroquine, pyrimethamine and sulfadoxine, and chlorproguanil and dapsone as treatment for falciparum malaria in pregnant and non-pregnant women, Kakamega district, Kenya. *Br Med J*. 1990;301:466-470.
24. Harpey J-P, Darbois Y, Lefebvre G. Teratogenicity of pyrimethamine. *Lancet*. 1983;2:399.
25. Connelly RT, Lourwood DL. Pneumocystis carinii pneumonia prophylaxis during pregnancy. *Pharmacotherapy*. 1994;14:424-429.
26. American College of Obstetricians and Gynecologists. Human immunodeficiency virus infections in pregnancy. *Educational Bulletin No. 232*. January 1997.
27. Erstad BL. Dapsone-induced methemoglobinemia and hemolytic anemia. *Clin Pharm*. 1992;11:800-805.
28. Wan J, Imadojemu S, Werth VP. Management of rheumatic and autoimmune blistering disease in pregnancy and postpartum. *Clin Dermatol*. 2016;34:344-352.
29. Ozturk Z, Tatliparmak A. Leprosy treatment during pregnancy and breastfeeding: a case report and brief review of literature. *Dermatol Ther*. 2017;30:e12414.
30. Tang ASO, Yeo ST, Teh YC, et al. The mystery of "saturation gap": a case of dapsone-induced methaemoglobinemia in a pregnant mother with leprosy. *Oxf Med Case Reports*. 2019;2019(1):omy111.
31. Spracklen FHN. Malaria 1984. Part I. Malaria prophylaxis. *S Afr Med J*. 1984;65:1037-1041.
32. Dreisbach JA. Sulphone levels in breast milk of mothers on sulphone therapy. *Lepr Rev*. 1952;23:101-106.
33. Edstein MD, Veenendaal JR, Newman K, et al. Excretion of chloroquine, dapsone and pyrimethamine in human milk. *Br J Clin Pharmacol*. 1986;22:733-735.
34. Committee on Drugs, American Academy of Pediatrics. The transfer of drugs and other chemicals into human milk. *Pediatrics*. 2001;108:776-789.

DAPTOMYCIN

Antibacterial

PREGNANCY RECOMMENDATION: Limited Human Data—Animal Data Suggest Low Risk

BREASTFEEDING RECOMMENDATION: Probably Compatible

D

PREGNANCY SUMMARY

No reports describing the use of daptomycin in the first trimester of human pregnancy have been located. Five case reports were located where pregnant women were treated with a course of daptomycin during the early second trimester, third trimester, and peripartum. No reported complications from using the drug were reported in the exposed fetuses/newborns. The drug may cross the placenta, more so in the second half of pregnancy, so some fetal exposure may occur. Therefore, this limited human pregnancy experience prevents a complete assessment of the embryofetal risk. Animal studies did not show any embryofetal toxicity in two animal species at doses less than 10 times the RHD. Using this drug during pregnancy should be based on the pros and cons of the mother's clinical need for treatment versus any potential fetal risk that might occur from exposure.

BREASTFEEDING SUMMARY

Several studies have been located that describe the use of daptomycin during breastfeeding. In one case, the drug levels in breast milk ranged from 121 to 330 ng/mL. The breast milk to maternal plasma ratios ranged from 0.002 to 0.006, and the estimated RID was about 0.5%. In another case, the maximum breast milk level of the drug during lactation was 44.7 ng/mL with a breast milk to plasma ratio of about 0.001. Lastly, a lactating mother was treated for several weeks with daptomycin and dalbavancin, and the infection resolved. There were no reports of any adverse effects seen in the infant or in the other two cases discussed earlier. Because it is a peptide consisting of 13 amino acids, if any drug were to be ingested through breastfeeding, some of it would likely be digested in the infant's gastrointestinal tract and not be absorbed. Breastfeeding while using this drug should be based on the mother's clinical need for treatment. If used, the infant should be primarily monitored for gastrointestinal side effects of nausea and abdominal pain (both leading to irritability), diarrhea, and vomiting.

References

1. Prescribing Information. *Cubicin*. Merck Sharp & Dohme; 2022.
2. Cunha BA, Hamid N, Kessler H, et al. Daptomycin cure after cefazolin treatment failure of methicillin-sensitive Staphylococcus aureus (MSSA) tricuspid valve acute bacterial endocarditis from a peripherally inserted central catheter (PICC) line. *Heart Lung*. 2005;34:442-447.
3. Shea K, Hilburger E, Baroco A, Oldfield E. Successful treatment of vancomycin-resistant Enterococcus faecium pyelonephritis with daptomycin during pregnancy. *Ann Pharmacother*. 2008;42:722-725.
4. Stroup JS, Wagner J, Badzinski T. Use of daptomycin in a pregnant patient with Staphylococcus aureus endocarditis. *Ann Pharmacother*. 2010;44:746-749.
5. Klibanov OM, Vickery S, Nortey C. Successful treatment of infective panniculitis with daptomycin in a pregnant, morbidly obese patient. *Ann Pharmacother*. 2014;48:652-655.
6. Nguyen LN, Lopes C, Folk JJ. Vertebral osteomyelitis in pregnancy from a methicillin-resistant Staphylococcus aureus vulvar abscess: a case report. *J Reprod Med*. 2015;60:362-364.
7. Cesari E, Roda G, Visconti GL, et al. Daptomycin excretion into human milk. *Br J Clin Pharmacol*. 2018;84:394-395.
8. Dei Cas M, Casagni E, Gambaro V, et al. Determination of daptomycin in human plasma and breast milk by UPLC/MS-MS. *J Chromatogr B Analyt Technol Biomed Life Sci*. 2019;1116:38-43.
9. Buitrago MI, Crompton JA, Bertolami S, et al. Extremely low excretion of daptomycin into breast milk of a nursing mother with methicillin-resistant Staphylococcus aureus pelvic inflammatory disease. *Pharmacotherapy*. 2009;29:347-351.
10. Mitchell KB, Eglash A, Bamberger ET. Mammary dysbiosis and nipple blebs treated with intravenous daptomycin and dalbavancin. *J Hum Lact*. 2020;36:365-368.

DARATUMUMAB

Antineoplastic (Monoclonal Antibody)

PREGNANCY RECOMMENDATION: No Human Data and No Relevant Animal Data

BREASTFEEDING RECOMMENDATION: Probably Compatible

PREGNANCY SUMMARY

No reports describing the use of daratumumab in human pregnancy have been located. As an IgG antibody, it likely crosses the placenta, especially during the second half of pregnancy, so some fetal exposure will probably occur. Therefore, the absence of human pregnancy experience prevents a complete assessment of the embryofetal risk. No animal reproduction

(*continued*)

studies with daratumumab have been located. Based on the drug's mechanism of action, the manufacturer recommends that women with reproductive potential use effective contraception during treatment and for 3 months after the last dose. Nevertheless, using this drug during pregnancy should be based on the pros and cons of the mother's clinical need for treatment versus any potential fetal risk that might occur from exposure.

D

BREASTFEEDING SUMMARY

No reports describing the use of daratumumab during human lactation have been located. It is known that IgG antibodies can be found in human breast milk but are not found in the neonatal or infant circulation. Additionally, if any IgG antibodies were to be ingested through breastfeeding, they would probably be digested in the infant's gastrointestinal tract and not be absorbed. However, due to the concern for potential serious adverse effects that might be seen in a breastfed infant, the manufacturer recommends that women not breastfeed when on this medication, especially if they are on other treatments, such as those in the thalidomide class of drugs. Nevertheless, breastfeeding while using this drug as monotherapy should be based on the mother's clinical need for treatment. If used, the infant should be monitored for the most common reported adult side effects of nausea and neuropathy (both leading to irritability), fatigue (lethargy), cough, fever, vomiting, and various laboratory abnormalities (see PI).

Reference

1. Prescribing Information. *Darzalex*. Janssen Biotech; 2023.

DARBEPOETIN ALFA

Hematologic (Hematopoietic)

PREGNANCY RECOMMENDATION: Human Data Suggest Low Risk (Maternal Benefit May Outweigh Any Embryofetal Risk)

BREASTFEEDING RECOMMENDATION: Probably Compatible

PREGNANCY SUMMARY

One case report of first-trimester exposure to darbepoetin alfa in human pregnancy was located. The drug was discontinued during the latter part of the first trimester with a pregnancy confirmation of twins. It was later restarted at about 18 weeks' gestation. She ultimately delivered at about 33 weeks' gestation, and no fetal malformations or complications were described other than prematurity. A total of seven other case reports described the use of darbepoetin alfa in eight pregnancies where the drug was first initiated in the mid-second to mid-third trimesters. All the pregnancies delivered healthy newborns with no reported anomalies or complications other than prematurity. The drug is not likely to cross the placenta in any clinically significant amount. The experience with epoetin alfa (see Epoetin Alfa) further suggests that darbepoetin does not represent a significant embryo or fetal risk. Because anemia and the need for frequent blood transfusions present significant risks to the mother and fetus, the benefits derived from darbepoetin may outweigh any potential fetal risks in some clinical situations. Animal studies did show a slight increased risk for embryofetal toxicity in one species at doses less than 10 times the RHD. Therefore, using this drug during pregnancy should be based on the pros and cons of the mother's clinical need for treatment. There is a pregnancy exposure registry that monitors pregnancy outcomes in women using this drug. Health care providers are encouraged to call the Amgen Pregnancy Surveillance Program at 1-800-7726436-2510. Lastly, the drug was found to cause hypertension in up to 40% of patients in the clinical trials.

BREASTFEEDING SUMMARY

No reports describing the use of darbepoetin alfa in human lactation have been located. The drug will not likely be found in breast milk. In addition, if any amount of the drug were to be ingested through breastfeeding, because it consists of a protein, it would probably be digested in the infant's gastrointestinal tract and not be absorbed. Furthermore, erythropoietin is a normal component of human breast milk. Therefore, any risk to a nursing infant from ingestion of the drug is likely to be nonexistent.

References

1. Prescribing Information. *Aranesp*. Amgen; 2021.
2. Malek A, Sager R, Eckardt KU, et al. Lack of transport of erythropoietin across the human placenta as studied by an in vitro perfusion system. *Pflugers Arch*. 1994;427:157-161.
3. Schneider H, Malek A. Lack of permeability of the human placenta for erythropoietin. *J Perinat Med*. 1995;23:71-76.
4. Reisenberger K, Egarter C, Kapiotis S, et al. Transfer of erythropoietin across the placenta perfused in vitro. *Obstet Gynecol*. 1997;89:738-742.
5. Tamaki S, Shinoda K, Matsumoto T, et al. Successful perinatal management of a dichorionic diamniotic twin pregnancy in an anaemic kidney transplant patient treated with darbepoetin alfa: a case report. *J Obstet Gynaecol*. 2020;40:427-429.
6. Morton A, Dalzell F, Isbel N, Prado T. Pregnancy outcome in a renal transplant recipient with residual mild tertiary hyperparathyroidism. *Br J Obstet Gynaecol*. 2005;112:124-125.
7. Goshom J, Youell TD. Darbepoetin alfa treatment for post-renal transplantation anemia during pregnancy. *Am J Kidney Dis*. 2005;46:e81-e86.

8. Sobito-Jarek L, Popowska-Drojecka J, Muszytowski M, et al. Anemia treatment with darbepoetin alpha in pregnant female with chronic renal failure: report of two cases. *Adv Med Sci*. 2006;51:309-311.
9. Ghosh A, Ayers KJ. Darbepoetin alfa for treatment of anaemia in a case of chronic renal failure during pregnancy—case report. *Clin Exp Obstet Gynecol*. 2007;34:193-194.
10. Maccio A, Madeddu C, Chessa P, et al. Use of erythropoiesis stimulating agents for the treatment of anaemia and related fatigue in a pregnant woman with HbH disease. *Br J Haematol*. 2009;146:335-337.
11. Cannas G, Dubreuil L, Fichez A, et al. Delayed severe hemolytic transfusion reaction during pregnancy in a woman with beta-thalassemia intermediate: successful outcome after eculizumab administration. *Am J Case Rep*. 2021;22:e931107-1-e931107-6.
12. Morton A. Low haptoglobin and a positive direct antiglobulin test without haemolysis in pregnancy. *Obstetric Med*. 2022;15:280-282.

D

DARIDOREXANT

Central Nervous System (Depressant—Orexin Receptor Antagonist)

PREGNANCY RECOMMENDATION: No Human Data—Animal Data Suggest Low Risk

BREASTFEEDING RECOMMENDATION: Probably Compatible

PREGNANCY SUMMARY

No reports describing the use of daridorexant in human pregnancy have been located. Daridorexant is likely to cross the placenta, so some fetal exposure will probably occur. Therefore, the absence of human pregnancy experience prevents a complete assessment of embryofetal risk. Animal data did not show any embryofetal toxicity. Using this drug during pregnancy should be based on the pros and cons of the mother's clinical need for treatment versus any potential fetal risk that might occur from exposure. There is a pregnancy exposure registry that monitors pregnancy outcomes in women exposed to daridorexant during pregnancy. For more information, health care providers or patients are encouraged to contact 833-400-9611.

BREASTFEEDING SUMMARY

No reports describing the use of daridorexant during human lactation have been located. The drug will likely be found in breast milk, so some infant exposure will probably occur. Breastfeeding while using this drug should be based on the mother's clinical need for treatment. If used, the infant should be monitored for the most common reported adult side effects of headache (leading to irritability) and somnolence or lethargy.

Reference

1. Prescribing Information. *Quviviq*. Idorsia Pharmaceuticals US, Inc; 2023.

DARIFENACIN

Urinary (Anticholinergic)

PREGNANCY RECOMMENDATION: No Human Data—Animal Data Suggest Low Risk

BREASTFEEDING RECOMMENDATION: Probably Compatible

PREGNANCY SUMMARY

No reports describing the use of darifenacin in human pregnancy have been located. The drug will probably cross the placenta, so some fetal exposure will likely occur. Therefore, the absence of human pregnancy experience prevents a complete assessment of the embryofetal risk. Animal reproduction studies did not show any embryofetal toxicity or malformations in two animal species. Using this drug during pregnancy should be based on the pros and cons of the mother's clinical need for treatment versus any potential fetal risk that might occur from exposure. Lastly, muscarinic antagonists are like parasympathetic blocking agents, which can alter the appearance of the fetal heart monitor tracing by causing an elevation of the baseline rate and decreasing variability.

BREASTFEEDING SUMMARY

No reports describing the use of darifenacin during human lactation have been located. The drug will probably be found in breast milk, so some infant exposure will likely occur. The effect of exposure on a nursing infant is unknown. Because of the drug's anticholinergic effects, there is the possibility of interfering with breast milk production in the early stages of breastfeeding, as well as decreasing breast milk supply with long-term use. Therefore, breastfeeding while using this drug should be based on the mother's clinical need for treatment. If used, the infant should be monitored for the most common reported adult side effects of headache and nausea (both leading to irritability), constipation, and urinary tract infection.

Reference

1. Prescribing Information. *Darifenacin*. Novartis; 2020.

D

DAROLUTAMIDE

Antineoplastic (Androgen Receptor Antagonist)

PREGNANCY RECOMMENDATION: *Contraindicated

BREASTFEEDING RECOMMENDATION: *Contraindicated

PREGNANCY SUMMARY

No reports describing the use of darolutamide in human pregnancy have been located. Based on likely placental transfer, fetal exposure would probably occur. However, the absence of human pregnancy experience prevents a complete assessment of the embryofetal risk. Animal studies have not been performed. Due to the potential for fetal harm based on the mechanism of action, the manufacturer recommends that males with female partners of reproductive potential use effective contraception while on this drug and for 1 week after the last dose. *Based on the drug indication, it should not be used in females.

BREASTFEEDING SUMMARY

Darolutamide probably enters breast milk; however, *based on the drug indication, it should not be used while breastfeeding.

Reference

1. Prescribing Information. *Nubeqa*. Orion Corporation, Orion Pharma, for Bayer Healthcare Pharmaceuticals, Inc; 2019.

DARUNAVIR

Antiretroviral (Protease Inhibitor)

PREGNANCY RECOMMENDATION: Limited Human Data—Animal Data Suggest Low Risk (Maternal Benefit May Outweigh Any Embryofetal Risk)

BREASTFEEDING RECOMMENDATION: *Contraindicated

PREGNANCY SUMMARY

Several reports have described the use of darunavir in human pregnancy. The number of cases with first-trimester exposure to this specific antiretroviral drug is small, but overall, there did not appear to be any increased risk for major congenital anomalies or pregnancy complications. The drug crosses the placenta, so fetal exposure will occur. However, this limited human pregnancy experience with darunavir prevents a complete assessment of the embryofetal risk. Animal studies did not show any embryofetal toxicity or teratogenicity in three species at doses of less than 10 times the RHD. In order to decrease the perinatal transmission of HIV-1 to the neonate, this drug should not be withheld if a pregnant woman is infected with HIV-1 with a positive viral load and is a candidate for this drug's usage. There is a pregnancy exposure registry that monitors pregnancy outcomes in patients using this drug during gestation. Health care providers are encouraged to call the Antiretroviral Pregnancy Registry (APR) at 1-800-258-4263.

BREASTFEEDING SUMMARY

One report describing the use of darunavir during lactation has been located. The drug was found in human breast milk at low levels. The calculated RIDs were all less than 1%. *However, the current Centers for Disease Control and Prevention recommendation is that mothers infected with HIV should not breastfeed their infants in order to reduce the risk of postnatal transmission of the virus to the neonate. In a clinical setting where a mother is not infected with HIV (or in cases where the HIV viral load is negative), the drug by itself is probably compatible.

References

1. Prescribing Information. *Prezista*. Janssen Products; 2019.
2. Ripamonti D, Cattaneo D, Cortinovis M, et al. Transplacental passage of ritonavir-boosted darunavir in two pregnant women. *Int J STD Aids*. 2009;20:215-216.

3. Furco A, Gosrani B, Nicholas S, et al. Successful use of darunavir, etravirine, enfuvirtide and tenofovir/emtricitabine in pregnant woman with multiclass HIV resistance. *AIDS*. 2009;23:434-435.
4. Pinnetti C, Tamburrini E, Ragazzoni E, et al. Decreased plasma levels of darunavir/ritonavir in a vertically infected pregnant woman carrying multiclass-resistant HIV type-1. *Antivir Ther*. 2010;15:127-129.
5. Sued O, Lattner J, Gun A, et al. Use of darunavir and enfuvirtide in a pregnant woman. *Int J STD Aids*. 2008;19:866-867.
6. Pacanowski J, Bollens D, Poirier JM, et al. Efficacy of darunavir despite low plasma trough levels during late pregnancy in an HIV-hepatitis C virus-infected patient. *AIDS*. 2009;23:1923-1924.
7. Antiretroviral Pregnancy Registry Steering Committee. *Antiretroviral Pregnancy Registry International Interim Report for 1 January 1989 through 31 July 2009*. Registry Coordinating Center; 2009. Accessed May 29, 2010. www.apregistry.com
8. CDC. Public Health Service Task Force recommendations for the use of antiretroviral drugs in pregnant women infected with HIV-1 for maternal health and for reducing perinatal HIV-1 transmission in the United States. *MMWR*. 1998;47:RR-2.
9. Fassett M, Kramer F, Stek A. Treatment with protease inhibitors in pregnancy is not associated with an increased incidence of gestational diabetes (abstract). *Am J Obstet Gynecol*. 2000;182:S97.
10. Carpenter CCJ, Fischi MA, Hammer SM, et al. Antiretroviral therapy for HIV infection in 1996. *JAMA*. 1996;276:146-154.
11. Minkoff H, Augenbraun M. Antiretroviral therapy for pregnant women. *Am J Obstet Gynecol*. 1997;176:478-489.
12. Minkoff H. Human immunodeficiency virus infection in pregnancy. *Obstet Gynecol*. 2003;101:797-810.
13. Panel on Antiretroviral Guidelines for Adults and Adolescents. *Guidelines for the Use of Antiretroviral Agents in HIV-1-Infected Adults and Adolescents*. Department of Health and Human Services; December 1, 2009:1-161. Accessed September 17, 2010:60, 96-98.
14. Panel on Treatment of HIV-Infected Pregnant Women and Prevention of Perinatal Transmission. *Recommendations for Use of Antiretroviral Drugs in Pregnant HIV-1-Infected Women for Maternal Health and Interventions to Reduce Perinatal HIV Transmission in the United States*. May 24, 2010:1-117. Accessed September 17, 2010:30, 39-44 (Table 5).
15. Pope R Jr, Kashuba A. Darunavir for use in pregnant women with HIV. *Expert Rev Clin Pharmacol*. 2017;10:1317-1327.
16. Murtagh R, Else LJ, Kuan KB, et al. Therapeutic drug monitoring of darunavir/ritonavir in pregnancy. *Antivir Ther*. 2019; 24(3):229-233.
17. Brown ZA, Watts DH. Antiviral therapy in pregnancy. *Clin Obstet Gynecol*. 1990;33:276-289.
18. De Martino M, Tovo P-A, Pezzotti P, et al. HIV-1 transmission through breast-milk: appraisal of risk according to duration of feeding. *AIDS*. 1992; 6:991-997.
19. Van de Perre P. Postnatal transmission of human immunodeficiency virus type 1: the breast feeding dilemma. *Am J Obstet Gynecol*. 1995;173:483-487.
20. Aebi-Popp K, Kahlert CR, Crisinel PA, et al. Transfer of antiretroviral drugs into breastmilk: a prospective study from the Swiss Mother and Child HIV Cohort Study. *J Antimicrob Chemother*. 2022;77:3436-3442.

D

DASATINIB

Antineoplastic (Tyrosine Kinase Inhibitor)

PREGNANCY RECOMMENDATION: Limited Human Data Animal Data Suggest Risk

BREASTFEEDING RECOMMENDATION: Potential Toxicity

PREGNANCY SUMMARY

A few studies analyzing the use of dasatinib in human pregnancy were located. From a few case reports and patients reported to the manufacturer (both biased to reporting of abnormal cases), a total of about 25 pregnancies with first-trimester exposure were described. Of these, there were 19 normal infants without any identified anomalies and 6 cases with major birth defects. One study has shown that the drug crosses the placenta, so fetal exposure will occur. However, this limited human pregnancy experience prevents a complete assessment of the embryofetal risk. Animal studies did show embryofetal toxicity in two species at doses of less than the RHD. Using this drug during pregnancy should be based on the pros and cons of the mother's clinical need for treatment versus any potential fetal risk that might occur from exposure. In the clinical trials, the drug caused left ventricular dysfunction and prolongation of the QT interval in about 2% of the patients. There is a registry for women who are pregnant and have cancer. For more information, women and health care providers are encouraged to contact the Cancer and Pregnancy Registry at 1-877-635-4499.

BREASTFEEDING SUMMARY

One report described the use of dasatinib during human lactation. A woman with chronic myeloid leukemia received dasatinib during pregnancy and while breastfeeding, and no adverse reactions were reported in the infant. The drug will probably be found in breast milk, so some infant exposure will likely occur. Due to a concern for potential serious adverse effects that might be seen in a breastfed infant, the manufacturer recommends that women not breastfeed while being treated with this drug. Nevertheless, breastfeeding while using this drug should be based on the mother's clinical need for treatment versus any potential infant risks that might occur. If used, the infant should be monitored for the most common reported adult side effects of nausea and musculoskeletal pain (both leading to irritability), diarrhea, rash, peripheral edema, and myelosuppression.

References

1. Prescribing Information. *Sprycel*. E.R. Squib & Sons; 2019.
2. Conchon M, Sanabani SS, Serpa M, et al. Successful pregnancy and delivery in a patient with chronic myeloid leukemia while on dasatinib therapy. *Adv Hematol*. 2010;2010:136252.
3. Cortes J, O'Brien S, Ault P, et al. Pregnancy outcomes among patients with chronic myeloid leukemia treated with dasatinib. *Blood*. 2008;112:Abstract No. 3230. As cited by Conchon M, Sanabani SS, Serpa M, et al. Successful pregnancy and delivery in a patient with chronic myeloid leukemia while on dasatinib therapy. Adv Hematol. 2010;2010:136252.
4. Berveiller P, Andreoli A, Mir O, et al. A dramatic fetal outcome following transplacental transfer of dasatinib. *Anti-Cancer Drugs*. 2012;23:754-757.
5. Cortes JE, Abruzzese E, Chelysheva E, et al. The impact of dasatinib on pregnancy outcomes. *Am J Hematol*. 2015;90:1111-1115.

6. Barkoulas T, Hall PD. Experience with dasatinib and nilotinib use in pregnancy. *J Oncol Pharm Practice*. 2018;24:121-128.
7. Alizadeh H, Jaafar H, Kajtar B. Outcome of 3 pregnancies in a patient with chronic myeloid leukemia who received 3 types of tyrosine kinase inhibitors each in different pregnancy: follow-up of the case with a review of published reports. *Ann Saudi Med*. 2015;35:468-471.

D

DASIGLUCAGON

Miscellaneous (Antihypoglycemic Agent)

PREGNANCY RECOMMENDATION: No Human Data—Animal Data Suggest Low Risk (Maternal Benefit May Outweigh Embryofetal Risk)

BREASTFEEDING RECOMMENDATION: Probably Compatible

PREGNANCY SUMMARY

No reports describing the use of dasiglucagon in human pregnancy have been located. Dasiglucagon is not likely to cross the placenta, so any fetal exposure would probably be clinically insignificant. However, the absence of human pregnancy experience prevents a complete assessment of the embryofetal risk. Animal data did not show any embryofetal toxicity. Using this drug during pregnancy should be based on the pros and cons of the mother's clinical need for treatment versus any potential fetal risk that might occur from exposure.

BREASTFEEDING SUMMARY

No reports describing the use of dasiglucagon during human lactation have been located. It is not likely to be excreted into breast milk. However, because it is a peptide, if the drug were to be ingested through breastfeeding, it would probably be digested in the infant's gastrointestinal tract and not be absorbed. Breastfeeding while using this drug should be based on the mother's clinical need for treatment. If used, the infant should be monitored for the most common reported adult side effects of nausea and headache (both leading to irritability), diarrhea, and vomiting.

Reference

1. Prescribing Information. *Zegalogue*. Zealand Pharma A/S; 2021.

DAUNORUBICIN

Antineoplastic (Anthracycline Cytotoxic Antibiotic)

PREGNANCY RECOMMENDATION: Limited Human Data—Animal Data Suggest Potential Risk

BREASTFEEDING RECOMMENDATION: Potential Toxicity

PREGNANCY SUMMARY

Several case reports and series have described human pregnancies with exposure to daunorubicin. Of the three first-trimester exposures, no major anomalies were described. However, several cases of neonatal anemia or neutropenia were reported. The drug crosses the placenta, so fetal exposure will occur. Therefore, this limited human pregnancy experience prevents a complete assessment of the embryofetal risk. Animal studies did show embryofetal toxicity with teratogenicity in one species at doses less than the RHD. These doses also caused severe maternal toxicity. Based on animal studies and the drug's mechanism of action, the manufacturer recommends that women with reproductive potential use effective contraception during treatment and for 6 months after the last dose. They also recommend that males with female partners of reproductive potential use effective contraception during treatment and for 6 months after the last dose. Nevertheless, using this drug during pregnancy should be based on the pros and cons of the mother's clinical need for treatment versus any potential fetal risk that might occur from exposure. In the clinical trials, the drug was found to cause cardiotoxicity similar to other anthracycline antineoplastic agents. Daunorubicin in combination with cytarabine also caused copper toxicity, and if used, this should be monitored closely. There is a registry for women who are pregnant and have cancer. For more information, women and health care providers are encouraged to contact the Cancer and Pregnancy Registry at 1-877-635-4499.

BREASTFEEDING SUMMARY

No reports describing the use of daunorubicin during lactation have been located. The drug will probably be found in human breast milk, so some infant exposure will likely occur. However, due to a concern for potential serious adverse effects that might be seen in a breastfed infant, the manufacturer recommends that women not breastfeed while being treated with this drug and for at least 2 weeks after the last dose. Nevertheless, breastfeeding while using this drug should be based on the mother's clinical need for treatment versus any potential infant risks that might occur. If used, the infant should be monitored for the most common reported adult side effects of nausea, headache, musculoskeletal pain, and abdominal pain (all leading to irritability), diarrhea, fatigue (lethargy), vomiting, decreased appetite (monitor growth), rash, and peripheral edema.

References

1. Ali S, Jones GL, Culligan DJ, et al. British Committee for Standards in Haematology. Guidelines for the diagnosis and management of acute myeloid leukaemia in pregnancy. *Br J Haematol*. 2015;170:487-495.
2. Prescribing Information. *Daunorubicin*. West-Ward Pharmaceuticals; 2018.
3. Sears HF, Reid J. Granulocytic sarcoma: local presentation of a systemic disease. *Cancer*. 1976;37:1808-1813.
4. Lilleyman JS, Hill AS, Anderton KJ. Consequences of acute myelogenous leukemia in early pregnancy. *Cancer*. 1977;40:1300-1303.
5. Colbert N, Najman A, Gorin NC, et al. Acute leukaemia during pregnancy: favourable course of pregnancy in two patients treated with cytosine arabinoside and anthracyclines. *Nouv Presse Med*. 1980;9:175-178.
6. Tobias JS, Bloom HJG. Doxorubicin in pregnancy. *Lancet*. 1980;1:776.
7. Sanz MA, Rafecas FJ. Successful pregnancy during chemotherapy for acute promyelocytic leukemia. *N Engl J Med*. 1982;306:939.
8. Alegre A, Chunchurreta R, Rodriguez-Alarcon J, et al. Successful pregnancy in acute promyelocytic leukemia. *Cancer*. 1982;49:152-153.
9. Gililland J, Weinstein L. The effects of cancer chemotherapeutic agents on the developing fetus. *Obstet Gynecol Surv*. 1983;38:6-13.
10. Feliu J, Juarez S, Ordonez A, et al. Acute leukemia and pregnancy. *Cancer*. 1988;61:580-584.
11. Volkenandt M, Buchner T, Hiddemann W, et al. Acute leukaemia during pregnancy. *Lancet*. 1987;2:1521-1522.
12. Turchi JJ, Villasis C. Anthracyclines in the treatment of malignancy in pregnancy. *Cancer*. 1988;61:435-440.
13. Schleuning M, Clemm C. Chromosomal aberrations in a newborn whose mother received cytotoxic treatment during pregnancy. *N Engl J Med*. 1987;317:1666-1667.
14. Gokal R, Durrant J, Baum JD, et al. Successful pregnancy in acute monocytic leukaemia. *Br J Cancer*. 1976;34:299-302.
15. Lowenthal RM, Marsden KA, Newman NM, et al. Normal infant after treatment of acute myeloid leukaemia in pregnancy with daunorubicin. *Aust NZ J Med*. 1978;8:431-432.
16. O'Donnell R, Costigan C, O'Connell LG. Two cases of acute leukaemia in pregnancy. *Acta Haematol*. 1979;61:298-300.
17. Hamer JW, Beard MEJ, Duff GB. Pregnancy complicated by acute myeloid leukaemia. *NZ Med J*. 1979;89:212-213.
18. Doney KC, Kraemer KG, Shepard TH. Combination chemotherapy for acute myelocytic leukemia during pregnancy: three case reports. *Cancer Treat Rep*. 1979;63:369-371.
19. Okun DB, Groncy PK, Sieger L, et al. Acute leukemia in pregnancy: transient neonatal myelosuppression after combination chemotherapy in the mother. *Med Pediatr Oncol*. 1979;7:315-319.
20. Cantini E, Yanes B. Acute myelogenous leukemia in pregnancy. *South Med J*. 1984;77:1050-1052.
21. Morishita S, Imai A, Kawabata I, et al. Acute myelogenous leukemia in pregnancy: fetal blood sampling and early effects of chemotherapy. *Int J Gynecol Obstet*. 1994;44:273-277.
22. Nicholson HO. Cytotoxic drugs in pregnancy: review of reported cases. *J Obstet Gynaecol Br Commonw*. 1968;75:307-312.
23. Dobbing J. Pregnancy and leukaemia. *Lancet*. 1977;1:1155.
24. Russell JA, Powles RL, Oliver RTD. Conception and congenital abnormalities after chemotherapy of acute myelogenous leukaemia in two men. *Br Med J*. 1976;1:1508.
25. Matthews JH, Wood JK. Male fertility during chemotherapy for acute leukemia. *N Engl J Med*. 1980;303:1235.
26. Estiu M. Successful pregnancy in leukaemia. *Lancet*. 1977;1:433.

DAXIBOTULINUMTOXINA

Central Nervous System (Neuromuscular Blocker Agent/Toxin)

PREGNANCY RECOMMENDATION: No Human Data—Animal Data Suggest Low Risk

BREASTFEEDING RECOMMENDATION: Probably Compatible

PREGNANCY SUMMARY

No reports describing the use of daxibotulinumtoxinA in human pregnancy have been located. Because it most likely will not cross the placenta, fetal exposure is expected to be nonexistent. However, if the administration is done incorrectly, systemic exposure is possible. Therefore, the absence of human pregnancy experience prevents a complete assessment of the embryofetal risk. Animal data did not show any embryofetal toxicity. Using this drug during pregnancy should be based on the pros and cons of the mother's clinical need for treatment versus any potential fetal risk that might occur from exposure. However, based on drug indication, use during pregnancy is not recommended.

BREASTFEEDING SUMMARY

No reports describing the use of daxibotulinumtoxinA during human lactation have been located. The lack of systemic absorption should limit infant exposure. However, if any toxin were to be ingested through breastfeeding, because it is a polypeptide, it would probably be digested in the infant's gastrointestinal tract and not be absorbed. Breastfeeding while using this drug should be based on the mother's clinical need for treatment. If used, the infant should be monitored for the most common reported adult side effect of headache (leading to irritability).

Reference

1. Prescribing Information. *Daxxify*. Revance Therapeutics, Inc; 2022.

DECITABINE

Antineoplastic (Pyrimidine Nucleoside Analogue)

PREGNANCY RECOMMENDATION: Limited Human Data—Animal Data Suggest Potential Risk

BREASTFEEDING RECOMMENDATION: Potential Toxicity

D

PREGNANCY SUMMARY

One case of first-trimester exposure to decitabine was located that resulted in numerous major fetal anomalies. The pregnancy was terminated in the mid-second trimester. The drug probably crosses the placenta, so some fetal exposure will likely occur. Therefore, this single human pregnancy case report prevents a complete assessment of the embryofetal risk. Animal studies did show embryofetal toxicity with teratogenicity in two species at doses of less than the RHD. However, the drug was administered intraperitoneally over a few days, so comparison with IV use is difficult. Based on animal studies and the drug's mechanism of action, the manufacturer recommends that women with reproductive potential use effective contraception during treatment and for 6 months after the last dose. They also recommend that males with female partners of reproductive potential use effective contraception during treatment and for 3 months after the last dose. Nevertheless, using this drug during pregnancy should be based on the pros and cons of the mother's clinical need for treatment versus any potential fetal risk that might occur from exposure. There is a registry for women who are pregnant and have cancer. For more information, women and health care providers are encouraged to contact the Cancer and Pregnancy Registry at 1-877-635-4499.

BREASTFEEDING SUMMARY

No reports describing the use of decitabine during human lactation have been located. The drug will probably be found in human breast milk, so some infant exposure will likely occur. Due to a concern for potential serious adverse effects that might be seen in a breastfed infant, the manufacturer recommends that women not breastfeed while being treated with this drug and for at least 1 week after the last dose. Nevertheless, breastfeeding while using this drug should be based on the mother's clinical need for treatment versus any potential infant risks that might occur. If used, the infant should be monitored for the most common reported adult side effects of anemia, neutropenia, thrombocytopenia, and pyrexia.

Reference

1. Prescribing Information. *Decitabine*. Astex Pharmaceuticals, Inc; 2020.

DEFERASIROX

Chelating Agent

PREGNANCY RECOMMENDATION: Limited Human Data—Animal Data Suggest Potential Risk

BREASTFEEDING RECOMMENDATION: Potential Toxicity

PREGNANCY SUMMARY

Four case studies describing the use of deferasirox in human pregnancy were located. A total of 12 pregnancies were reported with inadvertent exposure at conception. Deferasirox was discontinued with pregnancy confirmation ranging from 6 to 22 weeks' gestation. All 12 pregnancies delivered healthy newborns at or near term with no reported anomalies or complications. In one other study, 15 women with beta-thalassemia were reported to have 19 pregnancies with first-trimester exposure to iron-chelating agents. Of these 15 women, 12 were on single-agent therapy and 3 were on double-agent therapy (thus, 4 were using deferasirox, 9 deferoxamine, and 5 deferiprone). The spontaneous loss rate was 21%, but of the remaining deliveries, no fetal anomalies were reported. However, information regarding specific pregnancy outcomes based on each individual drug was not supplied. The drug will probably cross the placenta, so some fetal exposure will likely occur. However, this limited human pregnancy experience prevents a complete assessment of the embryofetal risk. Animal studies found some embryofetal toxicity in one species at doses less than 10 times the RHD. Using this drug during pregnancy should be based on the pros and cons of the mother's clinical need for treatment versus any potential fetal risk that might occur from exposure.

BREASTFEEDING SUMMARY

One abstract was located that described the use of deferasirox during human lactation. A patient with beta-thalassemia was started on the drug shortly after birth. The breast milk drug level was undetectable (<0.1 ng/mL) when analyzed 2 hours after a treatment dose. This would suggest that transfer into breast milk is very limited; however, a single case with one sample evaluated cannot confirm that the drug will not be found in breast milk. Further study is indicated. However, due to the concern for potential serious adverse effects that might be seen in a breastfed infant, the manufacturer recommends that women not breastfeed while being treated with this drug. Nevertheless, breastfeeding while using this drug should be based on the mother's clinical need for treatment. If used, the infant should be monitored for the most common reported adult side effects of nausea and abdominal pain (both leading to irritability), vomiting, diarrhea, rash, and elevated serum creatinine levels.

References

1. Prescribing Information. *Exjade*. Novartis Pharmaceutical; 2021.
2. Vini D, Servos P, Drosou M. Normal pregnancy in a patient with β-thalassemia major receiving iron chelation therapy with deferasirox (Exjade). *Eur J Haematol*. 2011;86:274-275.
3. Anastasi S, Lisi R, Abbate G, et al. Absence of teratogenicity of deferasirox treatment during pregnancy in a thalassemic patient. *Pediatr Endocrinol Rev*. 2011; 8(suppl 2):345-347.
4. Ricchi P, Costantini S, Spasiano A, et al. A case of well-tolerated and safe deferasirox administration during the first trimester of a spontaneous pregnancy in an advanced maternal age thalassemic patient. *Acta Haematol*. 2011;125:222-224.
5. Diamantidis MD, Neokleous N, Agapidou A, et al. Iron chelation therapy of transfusion-dependent β-thalassemia during pregnancy in the era of novel drugs: is deferasirox toxic? *Int J Hematol*. 2016;103:537-544.
6. Fozza C, Asara MA, Vacca N, et al. Pregnancy outcome among women with Beta-Thalassemia Major in North Sardinia. *Acta Haematol*. 2017;138: 166-167.
7. Giampreti A, Mattioli F, Faraoni L, et al. Lactation in beta thalassemia major: is deferasirox compatible? The first case with clinical data and breastmilk concentrations. *Clin Toxicol (Abstract)*. 2018;56:539.

DEFERIPRONE

Chelating Agent

PREGNANCY RECOMMENDATION: Limited Human Data—Animal Data Suggest Risk

BREASTFEEDING RECOMMENDATION: Potential Toxicity

PREGNANCY SUMMARY

Two studies were found that reported the use of deferiprone in human pregnancy. One reported exposure to the drug from conception through 20 weeks' gestation. The newborn was delivered prematurely but did well with no reported anomalies or adverse issues related to the drug treatment. In the other study, 15 women with beta-thalassemia were reported to have 19 pregnancies with first-trimester exposure to iron-chelating agents. Of these 15 women, 12 were on single-agent therapy and 3 were on double-agent therapy (thus, 5 were using deferiprone, 9 deferoxamine, and 4 deferasirox). The spontaneous loss rate was 21%, but of the remaining deliveries, no fetal anomalies were reported. However, information regarding specific pregnancy outcomes based on each individual drug was not supplied. The drug will probably cross the placenta, so some fetal exposure will likely occur. However, this limited human pregnancy experience prevents a complete assessment of the embryofetal risk. Animal studies did show embryofetal toxicity in two species at doses less than 10 times the MRHD. Based on these animal studies, the manufacturer recommends that women avoid getting pregnant while receiving this drug. However, using this drug during pregnancy should be based on the pros and cons of the mother's clinical need for treatment versus any potential fetal risk that might occur from exposure.

BREASTFEEDING SUMMARY

No reports describing the use of deferiprone during human lactation have been located. The drug is probably actively transported into breast milk by binding to lactoferrin, allowing for transfer to the infant through breastfeeding. Because of this, the manufacturer recommends that women not breastfeed while using this drug and for 2 weeks after the last dose. However, breastfeeding while using this drug should be based on the mother's clinical need for treatment. If used, the infant should be monitored for the most common reported adult side effects of nausea, arthralgia, and abdominal pain (all leading to irritability), vomiting, elevated liver function tests, and neutropenia.

References

1. Prescribing Information. *Ferriprox*. Chiesi Pharmaceuticals, Inc; 2023.
2. Ahmad MF, Zakaria NZ, Arsad N, et al. A case of post-splenectomy transfusion-dependent homozygous beta-thalassemia major complicated with myocardial siderosis and osteoporosis and usage of iron-chelating therapy with deferiprone in pregnancy. *Horm Mol Biol Clin Investig*. 2019;39: 2019005.
3. Fozza C, Asara MA, Vacca N, et al. Pregnancy outcome among women with Beta-Thalassemia Major in North Sardinia. *Acta Haematol*. 2017; 138:166-167.
4. Asmari M, Waqas M, Ibrahim AE, et al. Microscale thermophoresis and molecular modelling to explore the chelating drug transportation in the milk to infant. *Molecules*. 2022;27:4604(1-8).

D

DEFEROXAMINE

Antidote/Chelating

PREGNANCY RECOMMENDATION: **Limited Human Data—Animal Data Suggest Potential Risk**

BREASTFEEDING RECOMMENDATION: **Potential Toxicity**

PREGNANCY SUMMARY

Several case reports and small series have been located that describe the use of deferoxamine during pregnancy. Of these, at least 15 first-trimester exposures occurred, and no birth anomalies were described at delivery. In an additional 25 plus cases, exposures to the drug were in the second or third trimesters, and no adverse effects related to the drug were reported. The drug will probably cross the placenta, so some fetal exposure will likely occur. However, this limited human pregnancy experience prevents a complete assessment of the embryofetal risk. Animal studies did show some embryofetal toxicity in two species at doses of less than 10 times the RHD (in one species, there was maternal toxicity noted). Based on animal studies, the manufacturer recommends that women with reproductive potential use effective contraception during treatment and for 1 month after the last dose. Nevertheless, using this drug during pregnancy should be based on the pros and cons of the mother's clinical need for treatment versus any potential fetal risk that might occur from exposure. Alternatives to this drug are deferasirox and deferiprone.

BREASTFEEDING SUMMARY

One study was located that described the use of deferoxamine in a breastfeeding mother. Breast milk levels for the drug were not obtained, but the breast milk iron levels were decreased on average by about 3-fold from the normal expected range. No adverse effects were reported in three infants exposed to deferoxamine through breastfeeding. The drug will probably be excreted into breast milk. However, the drug is poorly absorbed orally, so any infant exposure through breast milk will likely result in very low infant systemic levels. Regardless, due to a concern for potential serious adverse effects that might be seen in a breastfed infant, the manufacturer recommends that women not breastfeed while being treated with this drug and for at least 1 week after the last dose. Nevertheless, breastfeeding while using this drug should be based on the mother's clinical need for treatment versus any potential infant risks that might occur. If used, the infant should be monitored for the most common reported adult side effects of nausea, headache, dizziness, and abdominal pain (all leading to irritability), diarrhea, lethargy, fever, rash, and low serum iron (monitor levels).

References

1. Singer ST, Vichinsky EP. Deferoxamine treatment during pregnancy: is it harmful? *Am J Hematol*. 1999;60:24-26.
2. Domingo JL. Developmental toxicity of metal chelating agents. *Reprod Toxicol*. 1998;12:499-510.
3. Prescribing Information. *Desferal*. Pfizer, Inc; 2023.
4. Thomas RM, Skalicka AE. Successful pregnancy in transfusion-dependent thalassaemia. *Arch Dis Child*. 1980;55:572-574.
5. Rayburn WF, Donn SM, Wulf ME. Iron overdose during pregnancy: successful therapy with deferoxamine. *Am J Obstet Gynecol*. 1983;147:717-718.
6. Blanc P, Hryhorczuk D, Danel I. Deferoxamine treatment of acute iron intoxication in pregnancy. *Obstet Gynecol*. 1984;64:12S-14S.
7. Van Ameyde KJ, Tenenbein M. Whole bowel irrigation during pregnancy. *Am J Obstet Gynecol*. 1989;160:646-647.
8. Lacoste H, Goyert GL, Goldman LS, et al. Acute iron intoxication in pregnancy: case report and review of the literature. *Obstet Gynecol*. 1992;80:500-501.
9. Strom RL, Schiller P, Seeds AE, et al. Fatal iron poisoning in a pregnant female: case report. *Minn Med*. 1976;59:483-489.
10. Surbek DV, Glanzmann R, Nars PW, et al. Pregnancy and lactation in homozygous β-thalassemia major. *J Perinat Med*. 1998;26:240-243.
11. Pafumi C, Zizza G, Caruso S, et al. Pregnancy outcome in transfusion-dependent thalassemic woman. *Ann Hematol*. 2000;79:571-573.

DEFIBROTIDE

Hematologic (Thrombolytic)

PREGNANCY RECOMMENDATION: **No Human Data—Animal Data Suggest Risk**

BREASTFEEDING RECOMMENDATION: **Probably Compatible**

PREGNANCY SUMMARY

No reports describing the use of defibrotide in human pregnancy have been located. The drug will probably not cross the placenta, but if any exposure does occur, it would likely be clinically insignificant. However, the absence of human pregnancy experience prevents a complete assessment of the embryofetal risk. Animal data did show embryofetal toxicity in two animal species, but all doses also caused maternal toxicity. Using this drug during pregnancy should be based on the pros and cons of the mother's clinical need for treatment versus any potential fetal risk that might occur from exposure.

BREASTFEEDING SUMMARY

No reports describing the use of defibrotide during human lactation have been located. The drug will likely not be excreted into breast milk. In addition, because it is an oligonucleotide, if the drug were to be ingested through breastfeeding, it would probably be partially digested in the infant's gastrointestinal tract and not be absorbed. Breastfeeding while using this drug should be based on the mother's clinical need for treatment. If used, the infant should be monitored for the most common reported adult side effects of nausea (leading to irritability), vomiting, diarrhea, and nosebleeds.

Reference

1. Prescribing Information. *Defitelio*. Jazz Pharmaceuticals; 2023.

D

DEFLAZACORT

Corticosteroid

PREGNANCY RECOMMENDATION: No Human Data and No Relevant Animal Data

BREASTFEEDING RECOMMENDATION: Probably Compatible

PREGNANCY SUMMARY

No reports describing the use of deflazacort in human pregnancy have been located. The drug will probably cross the placenta as seen with other corticosteroids, so some fetal exposure will likely occur. Therefore, the absence of human pregnancy experience prevents a complete assessment of the embryofetal risk. Studies in humans with other corticosteroids suggest that there may be an increased risk for orofacial clefts, though this has not been seen universally. The risk of orofacial clefts might increase from a baseline of 1 per 1,000 infants to 3 to 5 per 1,000 infants. Elevated glucose levels have been reported in patients treated with this drug. Therefore, if used during pregnancy, glucose levels should be monitored.

BREASTFEEDING SUMMARY

No reports describing the use of deflazacort or its active metabolite during human lactation have been located, but other corticosteroids are found in human breast milk. Breastfeeding while using this drug should be based on the mother's clinical need for treatment. If used, the infant should be monitored for the most common reported adult side effects of increased weight gain, increased appetite, upper respiratory tract infection, cough, hirsutism, and nasopharyngitis.

References

1. Prescribing Information. *Emflaza*. Marathon Pharmaceuticals; 2019.
2. Yun BH, Joo DJ, Seo SK, et al. Effect of deflazacort on pregnancy outcome in kidney transplant patients: should we change the immunosuppressant before conception? *BMC Nephrol*. 2019;20:161-169.

DEHYDROEPIANDROSTERONE

Miscellaneous/Dietary Supplement

PREGNANCY RECOMMENDATION: *Contraindicated (FDA-Approved Product)/Limited Human Data-No Relevant Animal Data (Dietary Supplement)

BREASTFEEDING RECOMMENDATION: *Contraindicated (FDA-Approved Product)/Potential Toxicity (Dietary Supplement)

PREGNANCY SUMMARY

No reports investigating the potential teratogenic effects from the use of dehydroepiandrosterone (DHEA) in human pregnancy have been located. DHEA and its active metabolite, DHEA sulfate (DHEA-S), are intermediates in the biosynthesis of androgens and estrogens. DHEA and DHEA-S most likely cross the placenta, but the fetal adrenal gland also produces DHEA and DHEA-S, and this is the primary producer of these hormones during gestation. However, most DHEA and DHEA-S are converted into estrogens by the placenta. The animal reproduction data (with the supplement) suggest that DHEA and/or DHEA-S may cause embryofetal risks, including virilization of the external genitalia in female fetuses. However, normal dosing of the supplement is not known for determining the amount of animal exposure that occurred. *The approved DHEA vaginal product is contraindicated during pregnancy because its approved use is in menopausal women. Any risk for use of the supplement during human gestation is unknown.

BREASTFEEDING SUMMARY

No reports describing the use of the DHEA vaginal product during human lactation have been located. In addition, no reports on the use of the supplement during human lactation have been found. Estrogens have been associated with decreased breast milk production (see Ethinyl Estradiol). Because DHEA and DHEA-S are converted to estrogens (and androgens), this could be a theoretical concern. *The approved DHEA vaginal product is contraindicated during breastfeeding because its approved use is in menopausal women. Any risk for use of the supplement during human lactation is unknown.

D

References

1. Kroboth PD, Salek FS, Pittenger AL, et al. DHEA and DHEA-S: a review. *J Clin Pharmacol*. 1999;39:327-348.
2. Cohen H, Cohen M. DHAS half-life in pregnancy, its prognostic value in high risk pregnancies. *J Steroid Biochem*. 1977;8:381-383.
3. Harper MJ. Estrogenic effects of dehydroepiandrosterone and its sulfate in rats. *Endocrinology*. 1969;84:229-235.
4. Goldman AS. Virilization of the external genitalia of the female rat fetus by dehydroepiandrosterone. *Endocrinology*. 1970;87:432-435.
5. Kirchner DL, Mercieca MD, Crowell JA, Levine BS. Developmental toxicity of dehydroepiandrosterone (DHEA) in rats and rabbits. *Teratology*. 1998;57:243.
6. Gandelman R, Simon NG, McDermott NJ. Prenatal exposure to testosterone and its precursors influences morphology and later behavioral responsiveness to testosterone of female mice. *Physiol Behav*. 1979;23:23-26.
7. de Catanzaro D, MacNiven E, Ricciuti F. Comparison of the adverse effects of adrenal and ovarian steroids on early pregnancy in mice. *Psychoneuroendocrinology*. 1991;16:525-536.
8. Kaaks R, Berrino F, Key T, et al. Serum sex steroids in premenopausal women and breast cancer risk within the European Prospective Investigation into Cancer and Nutrition (EPIC). *J Natl Cancer Inst*. 2005;97:755-765.
9. Atkinson G, Campbell DJ, Cawood ML, et al. Steroids in human intrauterine fluids of early pregnancy. *Clin Endocrinol (Oxf)*. 1996;44:435-440.
10. Barad D, Gleicher N. Effect of dehydroepiandrosterone on oocyte and embryo yields, embryo grade and cell number in IVF. *Hum Reprod*. 2006;21:2845-2849.
11. Barad D, Brill H, Gleicher N. Update on the use of dehydroepiandrosterone supplementation among women with diminished ovarian function. *J Assist Reprod Genet*. 2007;24:629-634.
12. Oladapo OT, Fawole B. Treatments for suppression of lactation. *Cochrane Database Syst Rev*. 2009;(1):CD005937.
13. Prescribing Information. *Prasterone*. Myriel Pharmaceuticals, LLC; 2020.

DELAFLOXACIN

Antibacterial (Fluoroquinolone)

PREGNANCY RECOMMENDATION: No Human Data—Animal Data Suggest Potential Risk

BREASTFEEDING RECOMMENDATION: Potential Toxicity

PREGNANCY SUMMARY

No reports describing the use of delafloxacin in human pregnancy have been located. The drug will probably cross the placenta, so fetal exposure will likely occur. However, the absence of human pregnancy experience prevents a complete assessment of embryofetal risk. Animal studies did not show any embryofetal toxicity at doses that did not cause maternal toxicity. Using this drug during pregnancy should be based on the pros and cons of the mother's clinical need for treatment versus any potential fetal risk that might occur from exposure.

BREASTFEEDING SUMMARY

No reports describing the use of delafloxacin during human lactation have been located. The drug will probably enter breast milk, so infant exposure will likely occur. Breastfeeding should be based on the mother's clinical need for treatment. If used, the infant should be monitored for the most common reported adult side effects of headache and nausea (both leading to irritability), diarrhea, vomiting, and elevated liver transaminases.

Reference

1. Prescribing Information. *Baxdela*. Melinta Therapeutics, Inc; 2019.

DEMECLOCYCLINE

Antibacterial (Tetracycline)

PREGNANCY RECOMMENDATION: *Contraindicated

BREASTFEEDING RECOMMENDATION: *Contraindicated

PREGNANCY SUMMARY

Several studies evaluating the use of demeclocycline during human pregnancy have been located. From 90 first-trimester exposures, 5 (5.6%) major anomalies were described, but no pattern to the defects was seen. For anytime exposure, there were 6 (2.1%) malformations in 280 cases. The drug will cross the placenta, so fetal exposure will occur. Therefore, this limited human pregnancy experience prevents a complete assessment of the embryofetal risk. Animal studies did show some embryofetal toxicity in two species, but dosing was not supplied. *Tetracycline drugs have a risk for producing stable calcium complexes (bone stippling) that may affect bone growth and stability. This class of drugs can also permanently discolor teeth. This has usually been found with long-term exposures during gestation. With other available antibacterial drug choices, the need for demeclocycline use during pregnancy is very limited.

D

BREASTFEEDING SUMMARY

A total of 45 women using demeclocycline during human lactation have been identified. The drug was found in most samples, with a peak reported level of 1.4 mcg/mL. Using this value, the maximum RID would be near 5%. The other calculated RIDs were less than 3%. *Due to a concern for potential serious adverse effects that might be seen in a breastfed infant (including tooth discoloration), the manufacturer recommends that women not breastfeed while being treated with this drug. This has been suggested by other experts in the field. However, when the data are examined closely, the risk of tooth discoloration is thought to be negligible with short-term use (7-10 days). Breastfeeding while using this drug should be based on the mother's clinical need for treatment versus any potential infant risks that might occur. If used, the infant should be monitored for the most common reported adult side effects of nausea (leading to irritability), diarrhea, vomiting, decreased appetite (monitor growth), and rash. With the availability of other antibacterial choices, the need for demeclocycline is probably limited.

Reference

1. Prescribing Information. *Demeclocycline*. LGM Pharma; 2020.
2. Heinonen OP, Slone D, Shapiro S. *Birth Defects and Drugs in Pregnancy*. Wright PSB; 1983:301, 435.

DENOSUMAB

Bone Health (Antiosteoporosis)

PREGNANCY RECOMMENDATION: *Contraindicated

BREASTFEEDING RECOMMENDATION: *Contraindicated/Probably Compatible

PREGNANCY SUMMARY

No reports describing the use of denosumab during human pregnancy have been located. Several studies have been published regarding the use of denosumab in treating pregnancy/lactation-associated osteoporosis with good results. However, this usage occurred after pregnancy and breastfeeding had been completed. As an IgG antibody, it likely crosses the placenta, especially during the second half of gestation, so some fetal exposure will probably occur. Therefore, the absence of human pregnancy experience prevents a complete assessment of the embryofetal risk. Animal studies did not show any embryofetal toxicity or teratogenicity in one species when treated during organogenesis at doses of more than 10 times the RHD. *Based on the primary approved use of the drug in treating osteoporosis in postmenopausal women, the drug would be contraindicated for use during pregnancy. However, using this drug during pregnancy for treating bone loss in women with breast cancer should be based on the pros and cons of the mother's clinical need for treatment versus any potential fetal risk that might occur from exposure.

BREASTFEEDING SUMMARY

No reports describing the use of denosumab during human lactation have been located. However, it is known that IgG antibodies can be found in human breast milk, but are not found in the neonatal or infant circulation. Additionally, if any IgG antibodies were to be ingested through breastfeeding, they would probably be digested in the infant's gastrointestinal tract and not be absorbed. Due to a concern for potential serious adverse effects that might be seen in a breastfed infant, the manufacturer recommends that women not breastfeed while being treated with this drug. *Based on the primary approved use of the drug in treating osteoporosis in postmenopausal women, the drug would be contraindicated for use during breastfeeding. However, using this drug during lactation for treating bone loss in women with breast cancer should be based on the mother's clinical need for treatment versus any potential infant risks that might occur. If used, the infant should be monitored for the most common reported adult side effects of bone, extremity, and musculoskeletal pain, and arthralgia (all leading to irritability).

Reference

1. Prescribing Information. *Prolia*. Amgen; 2023.

DEOXYCHOLIC ACID

Dermatologic (Fat Cytolytic)

PREGNANCY RECOMMENDATION: *No Human Data—Animal Data Suggest Potential Risk

BREASTFEEDING RECOMMENDATION: *Probably Compatible

D

PREGNANCY SUMMARY

No reports describing the use of deoxycholic acid injection during human pregnancy have been located. The drug is a natural bile acid component that is sequestered in the enterohepatic circulation loop. The drug probably crosses the placenta, so some fetal exposure will likely occur. Therefore, the absence of human pregnancy experience prevents a complete assessment of the embryofetal risk. The primary issue is whether an elevation of deoxycholic acid above normal endogenous levels over a period of possibly 6 months is harmful. The animal data showed low risk in one species, but embryofetal toxicity in a second species occurred at doses less than 10 times the RHD. However, maternal toxicity was seen with all doses in this second species, and the frequency of animal injections compared with human dosage was not supplied. *Nevertheless, the approved indication for use in treating submental fat can probably be delayed until after pregnancy and lactation are completed.

BREASTFEEDING SUMMARY

No reports describing the use of deoxycholic acid injection during human lactation have been located. Endogenous deoxycholic acid is found in human breast milk, and some amount of the substance likely be excreted into breast milk. Therefore, this injectable product will also likely be found in breast milk, so some infant exposure will probably occur. *Nevertheless, the approved indication for use in treating submental fat can probably be delayed until after pregnancy and lactation are completed. If the clinical decision is to use this drug while breastfeeding, the infant should be monitored for the most common reported adult side effects of various pains (leading to irritability) and flushing.

Reference

1. Prescribing Information. *Kybella*. Allergan Pharmaceuticals; 2020.

DESFLURANE

Anesthetic (General)

PREGNANCY RECOMMENDATION: Limited Human Data—No Relevant Animal Data

BREASTFEEDING RECOMMENDATION: Probably Compatible

PREGNANCY SUMMARY

No studies describing the use of desflurane in the first trimester of human pregnancy have been located. Several studies have described the use of the drug for anesthesia at the time of delivery, and no adverse newborn effects were described. The drug has been shown to cross the placenta at delivery, so fetal/newborn exposure will occur at that time. Desflurane will also probably cross the placenta throughout gestation. Therefore, the absence of the first-trimester human pregnancy experience prevents a complete assessment of the embryofetal risk. Animal data did show some embryofetal toxicity in two species (no teratogenicity), but dosing occurred daily for 10 to 13 days. Human exposure (in the majority of cases) would occur only once. Using this anesthetic agent during pregnancy should be based on the pros and cons of the mother's clinical need versus any potential fetal risk that might occur from exposure. Desflurane is one of the anesthetic agents that can increase the risk for malignant hyperthermia. Desflurane's potency is only about 20% of the potency of isoflurane, which is also an anesthetic agent that can increase the risk for malignant hyperthermia.

BREASTFEEDING SUMMARY

No reports analyzing human breast milk levels for desflurane have been located. Although desflurane has been administered during labor and delivery, the effects of this exposure on an infant that begins nursing shortly after birth have not been described. The drug is probably excreted into breast milk, but with the short elimination half-life, overall breast milk exposure is probably limited. In addition, the extent of drug absorption from oral exposure is not known. Using a mean elimination half-life of about 8 minutes, the drug should be completely gone from the maternal circulation in less than an hour. Therefore, a mother should be able to breastfeed within an hour of recovery following maternal surgery where this anesthetic agent was used. If used, the infant can be monitored for the most common reported adult side effects of nausea (leading to irritability), vomiting, and cough.

References

1. Friedman JM. Teratogen update: anesthetic agents. *Teratology*. 1988; 37:69-77.
2. Eger EI II. Desflurane animal and human pharmacology: aspects of kinetics, safety, and MAC. *Anesth Analg*. 1992;75:S3-S9.
3. Prescribing Information. *Desflurane*. Sandoz; 2020.
4. Trevor AJ, Miller RD. General anesthetics. In: Katzung BG, ed. *Basic and Clinical Pharmacology*. 8th ed. McGraw-Hill; 2001:426.
5. Kanto J. Risk-benefit assessment of anaesthetic agents in the puerperium. *Drug Saf*. 1991;6:285-301.
6. Wallace DH, Armstrong A, Darras A, et al. The effect of desflurane or low-dose enflurane on uterine tone at cesarean delivery: placental transfer and recovery (abstract). *Anesthesiology*. 1993;79:A1019.
7. Abboud TK, Zhu J, Richardson M, et al. Desflurane: a new volatile anesthetic for cesarean section. Maternal and neonatal effects. *Acta Anaesthesiol Scand*. 1995;39:723-726.
8. Abboud TK, Swart F, Zhu J, et al. Desflurane analgesia for vaginal delivery. *Acta Anaethesiol Scan*. 1995;39:259-261.
9. Sessler DI, Badgwell JM. Exposure of postoperative nurses to exhaled anesthetic gases. *Anesth Analg*. 1998;87:1083-1088.
10. Byhahn C, Lischke V, Westphal K. Occupational exposure in the hospital to laughing gas and the new inhalation anesthetics desflurane and sevoflurane. *Dtsch Med Wochenschr*. 1999;134:137-141.
11. Ho JT, Feldman JM. High-dose desflurane for tocolysis during intrapartum myelomeningocele repair in a patient with post-adriamycin cardiomyopathy. *A&A Case Reports*. 2016;7:49-52.
12. Olutoye OA, Baker BW, Belfort MA, et al. Food and Drug Administration warning on anesthesia and brain development: implications for obstetric and fetal surgery. *Am J Obstet Gynecol*. 2018;218:98-102.
13. Spigset O. Anaesthetic agents and excretion in breast milk. *Acta Anaesthesiol Scand*. 1994;38:94-103.

DESIPRAMINE

Antidepressant (Tricyclic)

PREGNANCY RECOMMENDATION: Limited Human Data (First Trimester)/Human Data Suggest Risk (Third Trimester)

BREASTFEEDING RECOMMENDATION: Probably Compatible

PREGNANCY SUMMARY

The Collaborative Perinatal Project reported first-trimester exposure to desipramine in 31 patients, with 1 (3.2%) newborn identified who had a major malformation. The drug will probably cross the placenta, so some fetal exposure will likely occur. Therefore, this limited human pregnancy experience prevents a complete assessment of the embryofetal risk. When used near delivery, neonatal withdrawal symptoms occur, including irritability, tremors, tachycardia, and rapid respirations. Animal reproduction studies have not been located. Using this drug during pregnancy should be based on the pros and cons of the mother's clinical need for treatment versus any potential fetal risk that might occur from exposure. There is a pregnancy exposure registry that monitors pregnancy outcomes in women using antidepressant drugs. Health care providers are encouraged to call the National Pregnancy Registry for Antidepressants at 1-844-405-6185.

BREASTFEEDING SUMMARY

One study was located that analyzed desipramine levels in human breast milk. The peak reported concentration was about 340 ng/mL. The calculated RID was well below 1%. In another study, four infants had blood levels evaluated for the presence of desipramine following exposure through breastfeeding. The drug was not detected in any of the infants (lower limit of quantification (LLQ) was 25 ng/mL in two infants and 10 ng/mL in the other two infants). No adverse effects have been reported in infants with exposure through breastfeeding, though the numbers are small. The drug has been found to elevate prolactin levels, but this should not adversely affect breastfeeding. Breastfeeding while using this drug should be based on the mother's clinical need for treatment versus any potential infant risks that might occur. If used, the infant should be monitored for the most common reported adult side effects of nausea, abdominal pain, anxiety, and paresthesia (all leading to irritability), vomiting, constipation, insomnia, and rash.

References

1. Yonkers KA, Wisner KL, Stewart DE, et al. The management of depression during pregnancy: a report from the American Psychiatric Association and the American College of Obstetricians and Gynecologists. *Obstet Gynecol*. 2009;114:703-713.
2. Webster PA. Withdrawal symptoms in neonates associated with maternal antidepressant therapy. *Lancet*. 1973;2:318-319.
3. Product Information. *Desipramine Hydrochloride*. Amneal Pharmaceuticals; 2018.
4. McElhatton PR, Garbis HM, Elefant E, et al. The outcome of pregnancy in 689 women exposed to therapeutic doses of antidepressants: a collaborative study of the European Network of Teratology Information Services (ENTIS). *Reprod Toxicol*. 1996;10:285-294.
5. Levin RM, Amsterdam JD, Winokur A, et al. Effects of psychotropic drugs on human sperm motility. *Fertil Steril*. 1981;36:503-506.
6. Nulman I, Rovet J, Stewart DE, et al. Child development following exposure to tricyclic antidepressants or fluoxetine throughout fetal life: a prospective, controlled study. *Am J Psychiatry*. 2002;159:1889-1895.
7. Sovner R, Orsulak PJ. Excretion of imipramine and desipramine in human breast milk. *Am J Psychiatry*. 1979;136:451-452.
8. Erickson SH, Smith GH, Heidrich F. Tricyclics and breast-feeding. *Am J Psychiatry*. 1979;136:1483.
9. Stancer HC, Reed KL. Desipramine and 2-hydroxydesipramine in human breast milk and the nursing infant's serum. *Am J Psychiatry*. 1986;143:1597-1600.
10. Wisner KL, Perel JM, Findling RL. Antidepressant treatment during breastfeeding. *Am J Psychiatry*. 1996;153:1132-1137.
11. Committee on Drugs, American Academy of Pediatrics. The transfer of drugs and other chemicals into human milk. *Pediatrics*. 2001;108:776-789.

D

DESLORATADINE

Antihistamine

PREGNANCY RECOMMENDATION: Human Data and Animal Data Suggest Low Risk

BREASTFEEDING RECOMMENDATION: Probably Compatible

PREGNANCY SUMMARY

One study evaluating the risk of desloratadine use in human pregnancy was located. The Danish Nationwide Registries compared desloratadine pregnancy exposures with an equal number of patients who used loratadine during pregnancy. Of 1,674 first-trimester exposures to desloratadine, there were 76 (4.5%) major anomalies versus 71 (4.2%) major anomalies in 1,674 loratadine-exposed pregnancies. The risk for spontaneous abortion was 256 in 2,749 pregnancies (9.3%) with desloratadine exposure versus 230 in 2,749 pregnancies (8.4%) with loratadine exposure (P = .2). The preterm delivery rate was also not different, 5.6% for desloratadine and 6.6% with loratadine. In the early 2000s there was a report that the use of loratadine (and desloratadine) produced an increased risk for hypospadias. However, several large follow-up studies did not confirm this finding. The drug will likely cross the placenta, so some fetal exposure will probably occur. Animal studies did not find any embryofetal toxicity or malformations in two animal species at doses less than 10 times the RHD. Using this drug during pregnancy should be based on the pros and cons of the mother's clinical need for treatment versus any potential fetal risk that might occur from exposure.

BREASTFEEDING SUMMARY

Although there are no reports describing the use of desloratadine during human lactation, the parent compound (loratadine) has been studied. Both loratadine and desloratadine are excreted into human breast milk. In one study evaluating loratadine use in six lactating women, the RID following a 40 mg dose was only 0.46%. Breastfeeding while using this drug should be based on the mother's clinical need for treatment. If used, the infant should be monitored for the most common reported adult side effects of nausea and myalgia (both leading to irritability), fatigue (lethargy), and somnolence.

References

1. 1.Prescribing Information. *Desloratadine*. Sun Pharma; 2020.
2. Andersson NW, Poulsen HE, Andersen JT. Desloratadine use during pregnancy and risk of adverse fetal outcomes: a nationwide cohort study. *J Allergy Clin Immunol Pract*. 2020;8:1598-1605.
3. Kallen B, Olausson PO. Monitoring of maternal drug use and infant congenital malformations. Does loratadine cause hypospadias? *Int J Risk Safety Med*. 2002;14:115-119.
4. Kallen B, Olausson PO. No increased risk of infant hypospadias after maternal use of loratadine in early pregnancy. *Int J Med Sci*. 2006;3:106-107.
5. Pedersen L, Norgaard M, Rothman KJ, Sorensen HT. Loratadine during pregnancy and hypospadias. *Epidemiol*. 2008;19:359-360.
6. Schwarz EB, Moretti ME, Nayak S, Koren G. Risk of hypospadias in offspring of women using loratadine during pregnancy: a systematic review and meta-analysis. *Drug Safety*. 2008;31:775-788.
7. Hilbert J, Radwanski E, Affrime MB, et al. Excretion of loratadine in human breastmilk. *J Clin Pharmacol*. 1988;28:234-239.

DESMOPRESSIN

Miscellaneous (Antidiuretic Hormone)

PREGNANCY RECOMMENDATION: Limited Human Data- Animal Data Suggest Low Risk

BREASTFEEDING RECOMMENDATION: Compatible

PREGNANCY SUMMARY

Several reports have described the use of desmopressin during human pregnancy in treating diabetes insipidus. No drug-related adverse effects were observed in the newborns. In a total of about 30 first-trimester exposures, 1 (3.3%) major birth anomaly was described. However, desmopressin is not likely to cross the placenta in clinically significant amounts. Therefore, fetal exposure is thought to be negligible. Animal studies did not show any embryofetal toxicity or teratogenicity in two species at doses of more than 10 times the RHD. The drug can cause severe hyponatremia, but this risk is higher with the injectable form, for which it carries a boxed warning. Using this drug during pregnancy should be based on the pros and cons of the mother's clinical need for treatment versus any potential fetal risk that might occur from exposure.

BREASTFEEDING SUMMARY

One patient using the desmopressin nasal spray for treating diabetes insipidus had milk arginine vasopressin levels analyzed. Breast milk concentrations increased about 50% from the background level; however, these amounts were very low (baseline level of 1 pg/mL increasing to 1.5 pg/mL). This would suggest that this change is clinically insignificant. No studies regarding the use of the IV, subcutaneous (SC) and oral formulations have been located. An additional factor is that the drug is an octapeptide, and if it were to be ingested through breastfeeding, it would probably be somewhat digested in the infant's gastrointestinal tract and not be absorbed. Breastfeeding while using this drug should be based on the mother's clinical need for treatment versus any potential infant risks that might occur. If used, the infant should be monitored for the most common reported adult side effects of nausea, headache, dizziness, and abdominal pain (all leading to irritability), flushing, decreased urine output, and hyponatremia.

References

1. Prescribing Information. *Desmopressin acetate*. Teva Parenteral Medicines; 2019.
2. Hamai Y, Fujii T, Nishina H, et al. Differential clinical courses of pregnancies complicated by diabetes insipidus which does, or does not, pre-date the pregnancy. *Hum Reprod*. 1997;12:1816-1818.
3. Ray JG. DDAVP use during pregnancy: an analysis of its safety for mother and child. *Obstet Gynecol Surv*. 1998;53:450-455.
4. Briet JW. Diabetes insipidus, Sheehan's syndrome and pregnancy. *Eur J Obstet Gynecol*. 1998;77:201-203.
5. Choi HS, Kim YH, Kim CS, et al. Diabetes insipidus presenting with oligohydramnios and polyuria during pregnancy. *J Nippon Med Sch*. 2018;85:191-193.
6. Hime MC, Richardson JA. Diabetes insipidus and pregnancy. *Obstet Gynecol Surv*. 1978;33:375-379.
7. Hadi HA, Mashini IS, Devoe LD. Diabetes insipidus during pregnancy complicated by preeclampsia. A case report. *J Reprod Med*. 1985;30:206-208.
8. Kallen BA, Carlsson SS, Bemgtsson BKA. Diabetes insipidus and sue of desmopressin (Minirin) during pregnancy. *Eur J Endocrinol*. 1995;132:144-146.
9. Hanson RS, Powrie RO, Larson L. Diabetes insipidus in pregnancy: a treatable cause of oligohydramnios. *Obstet Gynecol*. 1007;89:816-817.

D

DESVENLAFAXINE

Mental Health (Serotonin-Norepinephrine Reuptake Inhibitor (SNRI))

PREGNANCY RECOMMENDATION: Limited Human Data (First Trimester) - Animal Data Suggest Low Risk/Human Data Suggest Potential Risk (Third Trimester)

BREASTFEEDING RECOMMENDATION: Potential Toxicity

PREGNANCY SUMMARY

No reports describing the use of desvenlafaxine in human pregnancy have been located. However, desvenlafaxine is the major active metabolite of venlafaxine. There are several publications describing the use of venlafaxine in human pregnancy. A recent systematic review found that first-trimester use of venlafaxine (n = 3,186) did not increase the risk for major congenital malformations. However, the American College of Obstetricians and Gynecologists (ACOG) state that the use of antidepressants, including desvenlafaxine, during pregnancy increases the risk for persistent pulmonary hypertension and transient neonatal adaptation syndrome when used near delivery. Desvenlafaxine crosses the placenta, so fetal exposure will occur. Animal data did not find any embryofetal toxicity or teratogenicity in two species at doses of less than and more than 10 times the RHD. Using this drug during pregnancy should be based on the pros and cons of the mother's clinical need for treatment versus any potential fetal risk that might occur from exposure. There is a pregnancy exposure registry that monitors pregnancy outcomes in women exposed to antidepressants during pregnancy. For more information, health care providers or patients are encouraged to contact the National Pregnancy Registry for Antidepressants at 844-405-6185. Exposure in the latter part of pregnancy has been associated with a neonatal withdrawal syndrome postdelivery that can include irritability, tremors, excessive crying, apnea, and even seizures. ACOG states that untreated and undertreated mental health disorders should be considered an exposure. Pregnancy and lactation alone should not be a reason to withhold or discontinue mental health medications.

BREASTFEEDING SUMMARY

Two studies were located that describe the use of desvenlafaxine during human lactation. The drug was found in all breast milk samples. Using mean breast milk levels, calculated RIDs were about 7% to 8%. However, infant serum levels were also analyzed in these cases. The infant serum levels were only about 2% to 5% of the maternal blood levels obtained. The drug may elevate serum prolactin levels in a few patients, but this should not adversely affect breastfeeding. Breastfeeding while using this drug should be based on the mother's clinical need for treatment versus any potential infant risks that might occur. If used, the infant should be monitored for the most common reported adult side effects of nausea (leading to irritability), somnolence, sweating, decreased appetite (monitor infant growth), and constipation.

References

1. Product information. *Pristiq Extended Release*. Wyeth Pharmaceuticals; 2019.
2. Rampono J, Simmer K, Ilett KF, et al. Placental transfer of SSRI and SNRI antidepressants and effects on the neonate. *Pharmacopsychiatry*. 2009;42:95-100.
3. Ilett KF, Hackett LP, Dusci LJ, et al. Distribution and excretion of venlafaxine and O-desmethylvenlafaxine in human milk. *Br J Clin Pharmacol*. 1998;45:459-462.

4. Ilett KF, Kristensen JH, Hackett LP, et al. Distribution of venlafaxine and its O-desmethyl metabolite in human milk and their effects in breastfed infants. *Br J Clin Pharmacol*. 2002;53:17-22.
5. Newport DJ, Ritchie JC, Knight BT, et al. Venlafaxine in human breast milk and nursing infant plasma: determination of exposure. *J Clin Psychiatry*. 2009;70:1304-1310.
6. Ilett KF, Watt F, Hackett LP, et al. Assessment of infant dose through milk in a lactating woman taking amisulpride and desvenlafaxine for treatment-resistant depression. *Ther Drug Monit*. 2010;32:704-707.
7. Rampono J, Teoh S, Hackett LP, et al. Estimation of desvenlafaxine transfer into milk and infant exposure during its use in lactating women with postnatal depression. *Arch Womens Ment Health*. 2011;14:49-53.
8. Preskorn S, Patroneva A, Silman H, et al. Comparison of the pharmacokinetics of venlafaxine extended release and desvenlafaxine in extensive and poor cytochrome P450 2D6 metabolizers. *J Clin Psychopharmacol*. 2009;29:39-43.
9. Keightley P, Schmidt Sotomayor N, O'Hara K, et al. Lurasidone in lactation: a case study with laboratory and clinical outcomes. *Aust N Z J Psychiatry*. 2020;54:1035-1036.

DEUCRAVACITINIB

Dermatologic (Kinase Inhibitor)

PREGNANCY RECOMMENDATION: No Human Data—Animal Data Suggest Low Risk

BREASTFEEDING RECOMMENDATION: Probably Compatible

PREGNANCY SUMMARY

No reports describing the use of deucravacitinib in human pregnancy have been located. Some amount of the drug will probably cross the placenta, so fetal exposure will likely occur. However, the absence of human pregnancy experience prevents a complete assessment of the embryofetal risk. Animal studies did not show any embryofetal toxicity. Using this drug during pregnancy should be based on the pros and cons of the mother's clinical need for treatment versus any potential fetal risk that might occur from exposure. There is a pregnancy exposure registry that monitors pregnancy outcomes in women using this drug. Health care providers are encouraged to call 1-800-721-5072.

BREASTFEEDING SUMMARY

No reports describing the use of deucravacitinib during human lactation have been located. Some of the drug probably enters breast milk, so infant exposure will likely occur. Breastfeeding while using this drug should be based on the mother's clinical need for treatment. If used, the infant should be monitored for the most common reported adult side effects of upper respiratory tract infection, rash, and several laboratory abnormalities (see PI).

Reference

1. Prescribing Information. *Sotyktu*. Bristol-Myers Squibb Company; 2022.

DEURUXOLITINIB

Antineoplastic (Janus Kinase Inhibitor)

PREGNANCY RECOMMENDATION: No Human Data—Animal Data Suggest Potential Risk

BREASTFEEDING RECOMMENDATION: Potential Toxicity

PREGNANCY SUMMARY

No reports describing the use of deuruxolitinib in human pregnancy have been located. The drug will likely cross the placenta, so some fetal exposure will probably occur. Therefore, the absence of human pregnancy experience prevents a complete assessment of the embryofetal risk. Animal studies did show embryofetal toxicity with malformations in one species at doses of less than 10 times the RHD. In a second species, there was embryofetal toxicity at doses less than the RHD, but this dose also caused maternal toxicity. Based on animal studies and the drug's mechanism of action, the manufacturer recommends that women with reproductive potential use effective contraception during treatment with this drug. Nevertheless, using this drug during pregnancy should be based on the pros and cons of the mother's clinical need for treatment versus any potential fetal risk that might occur from exposure. In the first trimester, an informed decision should be made based on the need for treating the alopecia versus postponing treatment. There is a registry for women who are pregnant and have used this drug. For more information, women and health care providers are encouraged to contact the Leqselvi Pregnancy Registry at 1-800-818-4555.

BREASTFEEDING SUMMARY

No reports describing the use of deuruxolitinib during human lactation have been located. The drug will likely be found in breast milk, so some infant exposure will probably occur. Due to a concern for potential serious adverse effects that might be seen in a breastfed infant, the manufacturer recommends that women not breastfeed while being treated with this drug and for at least 1 day after the last dose. Nevertheless, breastfeeding while using this drug should be based on the mother's clinical need for treatment versus any potential infant risk that might occur. If used, the infant should be monitored for the most common reported adult side effects of headache (leading to irritability), fatigue (lethargy), rash, elevated creatine phosphokinase (CPK) levels, and other various laboratory abnormalities.

Reference

1. Prescribing Information. *Leqselvi*. Sun Pharmaceutical Industries, Inc; 2024.

D

DEUTETRABENAZINE

Central Nervous System (Vesicular Monoamine Transporter 2 Inhibitor)

PREGNANCY RECOMMENDATION: No Human Data—Animal Data Suggest Potential Risk

BREASTFEEDING RECOMMENDATION: Potential Toxicity

PREGNANCY SUMMARY

No reports describing the use of deutetrabenazine in human pregnancy have been located. The drug and its active metabolites will probably cross the placenta, so fetal exposure will likely occur. However, the absence of human pregnancy experience prevents a complete assessment of embryofetal risk. Animal studies did show some embryofetal toxicity in one species (but not a second species) at doses of less than 10 times the RHD. Using this drug during pregnancy should be based on the pros and cons of the mother's clinical need for treatment versus any potential fetal risk that might occur from exposure.

BREASTFEEDING SUMMARY

No reports describing the use of deutetrabenazine during human lactation have been located. The drug and its active metabolites will probably enter breast milk, so infant exposure will likely occur. Breastfeeding should be based on the mother's clinical need for treatment. If used, the infant should be monitored for the most common reported adult side effects of somnolence, diarrhea, and lethargy.

Reference

1. Prescribing Information. *Austedo*. Teva Neuroscience, Inc; 2022.

DEXAMETHASONE

Corticosteroid (Glucocorticoid)

PREGNANCY RECOMMENDATION: Human Data Suggest Low Risk (Late Second and Early Third Trimesters)

BREASTFEEDING RECOMMENDATION: Probably Compatible (Short-Term Use)

PREGNANCY SUMMARY

Dexamethasone is a corticosteroid with potency similar to betamethasone. No reports linking the use of dexamethasone with human birth defects have been located. In one study describing first-trimester use, 2 (3.6%) major anomalies were seen in 55 exposures (2 expected). Neither was a cleft lip or palate. Numerous studies have been published since the early 1970s regarding the use of corticosteroids and the reduction of respiratory distress syndrome in preterm newborns (especially those <32 weeks' gestation). In addition, several studies have reported a lower rate of intraventricular hemorrhage and periventricular leukomalacia, as well as improved survival in extremely premature newborns exposed to antenatal corticosteroids compared with those that had no exposure. Dexamethasone and betamethasone are the two primary corticosteroids used in this process. These antenatal exposures, however, can produce maternal hyperglycemia. Lastly, several studies regarding long-term follow-up of exposed infants show that, overall, there are no adverse effects seen in cognitive, psychosocial, and physical development. The drug crosses the placenta, so fetal exposure will occur. Therefore, this limited first-trimester human pregnancy experience prevents a complete assessment of the embryofetal risk. Animal studies did show some embryofetal toxicity and malformations in one species with intramuscular (IM) doses of less than 10 times the RHD (as used

(continued)

in obstetrics). This was not seen in another species with IM doses less than 10 times the RHD. Using this drug during pregnancy should be based on the pros and cons of the mother's clinical need for treatment versus any potential fetal risk that might occur from exposure.

D

BREASTFEEDING SUMMARY

No reports describing the use of dexamethasone during human lactation have been located. The drug will probably be found in breast milk, so infant exposure will likely occur. Dexamethasone is one of the more potent glucocorticoid corticosteroids, and if possible, the use of less potent alternatives is recommended. However, breastfeeding while using this drug should be based on the mother's clinical need for treatment versus any potential infant risks that might occur. If used, the infant should be monitored for the most common reported adult side effects of headache, nausea, myopathy, and gastritis (all leading to irritability), infections, bruising, edema, flushing, insomnia, and hyperglycemia. A few studies have suggested that antenatal dexamethasone may delay lactogenesis in some patients.

References

1. Osathanondh R, Tulchinsky D, Kamali H, et al. Dexamethasone levels in treated pregnant women and newborn infants. *J Pediatr*. 1977;90:617-620.
2. Levitz M, Jansen V, Dancis J. The transfer and metabolism of corticosteroids in the perfused human placenta. *Am J Obstet Gynecol*. 1978;132:363-366.
3. Carmichael SL, Shaw GM. Maternal corticosteroid use and risk of selected congenital anomalies. *Am J Med Genet*. 1999;86:242-244.
4. Reck G, Nowostawski, Bredwoldt M. Plasma levels of free estriol and cortisol under ACTH and dexamethasone during late pregnancy. *Acta Endocrinol*. 1977; 84:86-87.
5. Kauppilla A. ACTH levels in maternal, fetal and neonatal plasma after short term prenatal dexamethasone therapy. *Br J Obstet Gynaecol*. 1977;84: 128-134.
6. Warren JC, Cheatum SG. Maternal urinary estrogen excretion: effect of adrenal suppression. *J Clin Endocrinol*. 1967;27:436-438.
7. Caspi I, Schreyer P, Weinraub Z, et al. Changes in amniotic fluid lecithin-sphingomyelin ratio following maternal dexamethasone administration. *Am J Obstet Gynecol*. 1975;122:327-331.
8. Spellacy WN, Buhi WC, Riggall FC, et al. Human amniotic fluid lecithin/sphingomyelin ratio changes with estrogen or glucocorticoid treatment. *Am J Obstet Gynecol*. 1973;115:216-218.
9. Caspi E, Schreyer P, Weinraub Z, et al. Prevention of the respiratory distress syndrome in premature infants by antepartum glucocorticoid therapy. *Br J Obstet Gynaecol*. 1976;83:187-193.
10. Ballard RA, Ballard PL. Use of prenatal glucocorticoid therapy to prevent respiratory distress syndrome. *Am J Dis Child*. 1976;130:982-987.
11. Thornfeldt RE, Franklin RW, Pickering NA, et al. The effect of glucocorticoids on the maturation of premature lung membranes: preventing the respiratory distress syndrome by glucocorticoids. *Am J Obstet Gynecol*. 1978;131:143-148.
12. Ballard PL, Ballard RA. Corticosteroids and respiratory distress syndrome: status 1979. *Pediatrics*. 1979;63:163-165.
13. Taeusch HW Jr, Frigoletto F, Kitzmiller J, et al. Risk of respiratory distress syndrome after prenatal dexamethasone treatment. *Pediatrics*. 1979;63:64-72.
14. Caspi E, Schreyer P, Weinraub Z, et al. Dexamethasone for prevention of respiratory distress syndrome: multiple perinatal factors. *Obstet Gynecol*. 1981;57:41-47.
15. Bishop EH. Acceleration of fetal pulmonary maturity. *Obstet Gynecol*. 1981;58(suppl):48S-51S.
16. Farrell PM, Engle MJ, Zachman RD, et al. Amniotic fluid phospholipids after maternal administration of dexamethasone. *Am J Obstet Gynecol*. 1983;145:484-490.
17. Ruvinsky ED, Douvas SG, Roberts WE, et al. Maternal administration of dexamethasone in severe pregnancy-induced hypertension. *Am J Obstet Gynecol*. 1984;149:722-726.
18. Avery ME. The argument for prenatal administration of dexamethasone to prevent respiratory distress syndrome. *J Pediatr*. 1984;104:240.
19. Sepkowitz S. Prenatal corticosteroid therapy to prevent respiratory distress syndrome. *J Pediatr*. 1984;105:338-339.
20. Avery ME. Prenatal corticosteroid therapy to prevent respiratory distress syndrome (reply). *J Pediatr*. 1984;105:339.
21. Levy DL. Maternal administration of dexamethasone to prevent RDS. *J Pediatr*. 1984;105:339.
22. Eggers TR, Doyle LW, Pepperell RJ. Premature rupture of the membranes. *Med J Aust*. 1979;1:209-213.
23. Garite TJ, Freeman RK, Linzey EM, et al. Prospective randomized study of corticosteroids in the management of premature rupture of the membranes and the premature gestation. *Am J Obstet Gynecol*. 1981;141:508-515.
24. Garite TJ. Premature rupture of the membranes: the enigma of the obstetrician. *Am J Obstet Gynecol*. 1985;151:1001-1005.
25. Curet LB, Morrison JC, Rao AV. Antenatal therapy with corticosteroids and postpartum complications. *Am J Obstet Gynecol*. 1985;152:83-84.
26. Otero L, Conlon C, Reynolds P, et al. Neonatal leukocytosis associated with prenatal administration of dexamethasone. *Pediatrics*. 1981;68:778-780.
27. Anday EK, Harris MC. Leukemoid reaction associated with antenatal dexamethasone administration. *J Pediatr*. 1982;101:614-616.
28. Schatz M, Patterson R, Zeitz S, et al. Corticosteroid therapy for the pregnant asthmatic patient. *JAMA*. 1975;233:804-807.
29. Jenssen H, Wright PB. The effect of dexamethasone therapy in prolonged pregnancy. *Acta Obstet Gynecol Scand*. 1977;56:467-473.
30. Navot D, Rozen E, Sadovsky E. Effect of dexamethasone on amniotic fluid absorbance in Rh-sensitized pregnancy. *Br J Obstet Gynaecol*. 1982;89: 456-458.
31. Yin CS, Scott JR. Unsuccessful treatment of fetal immunologic thrombocytopenia with dexamethasone. *Am J Obstet Gynecol*. 1985;152:316-317.
32. David M, Forest MG. Prenatal treatment of congenital adrenal hyperplasia resulting from 21-hydroxylase deficiency. *J Pediatr*. 1984;105:799-803.
33. Evans MI, Chrousos GP, Mann DW, et al. Pharmacologic suppression of the fetal adrenal gland in utero. *JAMA*. 1985;253:1015-1020.
34. Taeusch HW Jr. Glucocorticoid prophylaxis for respiratory distress syndrome: a review of potential toxicity. *J Pediatr*. 1975;87:617-623.
35. Johnson JWC, Mitzner W, London WT, et al. Betamethasone and the rhesus fetus: multisystemic effects. *Am J Obstet Gynecol*. 1979;133:677-684.
36. Wong YC, Beardsmore CS, Silverman M. Antenatal dexamethasone and subsequent lung growth. *Arch Dis Child*. 1982;57:536-538.
37. Collaborative Group on Antenatal Steroid Therapy. Effects of antenatal dexamethasone administration in the infant: long-term follow-up. *J Pediatr*. 1984;104:259-267.

DEXAMETHASONE INTRAOCULAR SUSPENSION

Ophthalmic/Corticosteroid

PREGNANCY RECOMMENDATION: Limited Human Data—Animal Data Suggest Potential Risk

BREASTFEEDING RECOMMENDATION: Probably Compatible

PREGNANCY SUMMARY

A single case report described the use of intraocular ophthalmic dexamethasone in pregnancy. A pregnant patient presented with markedly decreased vision secondary to ocular toxoplasmosis. She refused systemic therapy and was treated intravitreally with dexamethasone and clindamycin in the late first trimester. Four weeks later, she was treated with a second intraocular course. Her vision returned to normal. A full-term infant was born without evidence of teratogenicity or toxoplasmosis. The drug may cross the placenta, but the very low blood levels seen following systemic absorption with intraocular use suggest that the amount would be clinically insignificant. However, the absence of human pregnancy experience prevents a complete assessment of the embryofetal risk. The animal reproduction data suggest risk, but the plasma drug concentrations are very low, and the levels were not compared. Using this drug during pregnancy should be based on the pros and cons of the mother's clinical need for treatment versus any potential fetal risk that might occur from exposure.

BREASTFEEDING SUMMARY

No reports describing the intraocular use of dexamethasone ophthalmic suspension during human lactation have been located. The drug may be found in breast milk, but the very low systemic plasma concentrations seen with intraocular application suggest that any amount excreted would probably be clinically insignificant. Breastfeeding while using this drug should be based on the mother's clinical need for treatment. Because of the intraocular usage, systemic adverse reactions were not analyzed.

References

1. Prescribing Information. *Dexycu*. Icon Bioscience, Inc; 2020.
2. Osathanondh R, Tulchinsky D, Kamali H, et al. Dexamethasone levels in treated pregnant women and newborn infants. *J Pediatr*. 1977;90:617-620.
3. Levitz M, Jansen V, Dancis J. The transfer and metabolism of corticosteroids in the perfused human placenta. *Am J Obstet Gynecol*. 1978;132:363-366.
4. Martinez CE, Zhang D, Conway MD, et al. Successful management of ocular toxoplasmosis during pregnancy using combined intraocular clindamycin and dexamethasone with systemic sulfadiazine. *Int Ophthalmol*. 1999; 22:85-88.

DEXAMETHASONE OPHTHALMIC IMPLANT

Ophthalmic/Corticosteroid

PREGNANCY RECOMMENDATION: Limited Human Data—Animal Data Suggest Potential Risk

BREASTFEEDING RECOMMENDATION: Probably Compatible

PREGNANCY SUMMARY

Two case series describing the use of dexamethasone intravitreal implants in human pregnancy were located. A total of eight pregnant patients with diabetic macular edema or choroidal neovascularization received the implants in the second or early third trimester of pregnancy. No complications occurred, and all eight delivered healthy newborns with no reported anomalies. The drug may cross the placenta, but the very low blood levels seen following systemic absorption suggest that the amount would be clinically insignificant. However, the absence of human pregnancy experience prevents a complete assessment of the embryofetal risk. The animal reproduction data suggest risk, but the plasma drug concentrations are very low, and the levels were not compared. Using this drug during pregnancy should be based on the pros and cons of the mother's clinical need for treatment versus any potential fetal risk that might occur from exposure.

BREASTFEEDING SUMMARY

No reports describing the use of the dexamethasone ophthalmic implant during human lactation have been located. The drug may be found in breast milk, but the very low systemic plasma concentrations seen with the implant suggest that any amount excreted would probably be clinically insignificant. Breastfeeding while using this drug should be based on the mother's clinical need for treatment. Because of the intravitreal usage, systemic adverse reactions were not analyzed.

References

1. Prescribing Information. *Ozurdex*. Allergan; 2020.
2. Osathanondh R, Tulchinsky D, Kamali H, et al. Dexamethasone levels in treated pregnant women and newborn infants. *J Pediatr*. 1977;90:617-620.
3. Levitz M, Jansen V, Dancis J. The transfer and metabolism of corticosteroids in the perfused human placenta. *Am J Obstet Gynecol*. 1978;132:363-366.
4. Concillado M, Lund-Andersen H, Mathiesen ER, et al. Dexamethasone intravitreal implant for diabetic macular edema during pregnancy. *Am J Ophthalmol*. 2016;165:7-15.
5. Capuano V, Serra R, Oubraham H, et al. Dexamethasone intravitreal implant for choroidal neovascularization during pregnancy. *Retin Cases Brief Rep*. 2019;13(4):300-307.
6. Hodzic-Hadzibegovic D, Ba-Ali S, Valerius M, Lund-Andersen H. Quantification of fluid resorption from diabetic macular oedema with foveal serous detachment after dexamethasone intravitreal implant (Ozurdex) in a pregnant diabetic. *Acta Ophthalmol*. 2017;95:324-325.

D

DEXAMETHASONE OPHTHALMIC TOPICAL

Ophthalmic/Corticosteroid (Topical)

PREGNANCY RECOMMENDATION: Limited Human Data—Animal Data Suggest Potential Risk

BREASTFEEDING RECOMMENDATION: Probably Compatible

PREGNANCY SUMMARY

No reports describing the use of topical dexamethasone ophthalmic in human pregnancy have been located. The drug may cross the placenta, but the very low blood levels seen following systemic absorption with topical use suggest that the amount would be clinically insignificant. However, the absence of human pregnancy experience prevents a complete assessment of the embryofetal risk. The animal data suggest risk; however, systemic blood levels of dexamethasone were not reported. Using this drug during pregnancy should be based on the pros and cons of the mother's clinical need for treatment versus any potential fetal risk that might occur from exposure. If used during pregnancy, consider placing pressure over the tear duct in the corner of the eye for at least 1 minute, and then remove any excess solution with absorbent tissue to decrease the amount of drug reaching the systemic circulation even further.

BREASTFEEDING SUMMARY

No reports describing the use of dexamethasone ophthalmic suspension during human lactation have been located. The drug will probably be excreted into breast milk. Although not specified, the plasma concentrations are probably very low and should be clinically insignificant. The amount in circulation can be decreased even further by using the method described above in the Pregnancy Summary.

References

1. Prescribing Information. *Maxidex*. Novartis; 2022.
2. Osathanondh R, Tulchinsky D, Kamali H, et al. Dexamethasone levels in treated pregnant women and newborn infants. *J Pediatr*. 1977;90:617-620.
3. Levitz M, Jansen V, Dancis J. The transfer and metabolism of corticosteroids in the perfused human placenta. *Am J Obstet Gynecol*. 1978;132:363-366.

DEXBROMPHENIRAMINE

Antihistamine (Histamine H1 Antagonist)

PREGNANCY RECOMMENDATION: Limited Human Data—No Relevant Animal Data

BREASTFEEDING RECOMMENDATION: Probably Compatible

PREGNANCY SUMMARY

From one publication, 14 first-trimester exposures to dexbrompheniramine were reported. One infant with a major or minor malformation was identified. The type of malformation was not reported. In addition, simultaneous use with other drugs was not provided. The drug will probably cross the placenta, so fetal exposure will likely occur. However, this limited human pregnancy experience prevents a complete assessment of the embryofetal risk. Animal reproduction studies have not been located. Using this drug during pregnancy should be based on the pros and cons of the mother's clinical need for treatment versus any potential fetal risk that might occur from exposure.

BREASTFEEDING SUMMARY

One report of a breastfed infant with exposure to dexbrompheniramine (and also ephedrine) during human lactation was located. The infant was about 11 weeks of age and was reported to have sleep issues and irritability. No breast milk or infant drug levels were obtained, and it is unknown if the infant's symptoms were related to one or both drugs or just random. Dexbrompheniramine will probably be found in breast milk, so some infant exposure will likely occur. Breastfeeding while using this drug should be based on the mother's clinical need for treatment. If used, the infant should be monitored for the most common reported adult side effects of nausea and headache (leading to irritability), somnolence, diarrhea, vomiting, and dry mouth.

References

1. Prescribing Information. *Dexbrompheniramine*. Poly Pharmaceuticals, Inc; 2023.
2. Heinonen OP, Slone D, Shapiro S. *Birth Defects and Drugs in Pregnancy*. Publishing Sciences Group; 1983:323.
3. Mortimer EA Jr. Drug toxicity from breast milk? *Pediatrics*. 1977;60:780-781.

DEXCHLORPHENIRAMINE

Antihistamine (Histamine H1 Antagonist)

PREGNANCY RECOMMENDATION: Human Data Suggest Low Risk

BREASTFEEDING RECOMMENDATION: Probably Compatible

PREGNANCY SUMMARY

In a surveillance study of Michigan Medicaid recipients involving 229,101 completed pregnancies conducted between 1985 and 1992, 1,080 newborns had been exposed to dexchlorpheniramine during the first trimester. A total of 50 (4.6%) major birth defects were observed (43 expected). However, based on different categories of birth anomalies, the data did not support an association between the drug and congenital birth defects. Based on likely placental transfer, some fetal exposure will probably occur. Animal reproduction studies have not been located for dexchlorpheniramine. Using this drug during pregnancy should be based on the pros and cons of the mother's clinical need for treatment versus any potential fetal risk that might occur from exposure.

BREASTFEEDING SUMMARY

No reports describing the use of dexchlorpheniramine during human lactation have been located (see also Chlorpheniramine). The manufacturer states that the drug is excreted into breast milk. Breastfeeding while using this drug should be based on the mother's clinical need for treatment. If used, the infant should be monitored for the most common reported adult side effects of nausea and headache (leading to irritability), somnolence, diarrhea, vomiting, and dry mouth.

References

1. Prescribing Information. *Dexchlorpheniramine*. Foxland Pharmaceuticals; 2020.
2. Ferreres-Garcia K, de Leon-Luis J, Seoane E, et al. A case study of anaphylaxis in a pregnant woman. *Ginecol Obstet Mex*. 2014;82:188-193.

DEXLANSOPRAZOLE

Gastrointestinal (Proton Pump Inhibitor)

PREGNANCY RECOMMENDATION: No Human Data—Animal Data Suggest Low Risk

BREASTFEEDING RECOMMENDATION: Probably Compatible

PREGNANCY SUMMARY

No reports describing the use of dexlansoprazole in human pregnancy have been located. The drug will probably cross the placenta, so some fetal exposure will likely occur. Therefore, the absence of human pregnancy experience prevents a complete assessment of the embryofetal risk. A meta-analysis of proton pump inhibitors in pregnancy compared 1,530 exposed patients with 133,410 not exposed. There was no increased risk for major congenital malformations, spontaneous abortion, or preterm birth. Animal studies did not show any embryofetal toxicity in two species at doses of greater than 10 times the RHD. Using this drug during pregnancy should be based on the pros and cons of the mother's clinical need for treatment versus any potential fetal risk that might occur from exposure.

BREASTFEEDING SUMMARY

No reports describing the use of dexlansoprazole during human lactation have been located. The drug will probably be found in breast milk, so some infant exposure will likely occur. Breastfeeding while using this drug should be based on the mother's clinical need for treatment. If used, the infant should be monitored for the most common reported adult side effects of nausea and abdominal pain (both leading to irritability), diarrhea, vomiting, and upper respiratory infection.

References

1. Prescribing Information. *Dexilant*. Takeda Pharmaceuticals America; 2020.
2. Gill SK, O'Brien L, Einarson TR, Koren G. The safety of proton pump inhibitors (PPIs) in pregnancy: a meta-analysis. *Am J Gastroenterol*. 2009;104:1541-1545.

D

DEXMEDETOMIDINE

Central Nervous System (Sedative)

PREGNANCY RECOMMENDATION: Limited Human Data—Animal Data Suggest Potential Risk

BREASTFEEDING RECOMMENDATION: Probably Compatible

PREGNANCY SUMMARY

The human pregnancy experience with dexmedetomidine is limited to short-term use immediately before or during cesarean delivery. No fetal/newborn adverse effects have been described. The drug appears to cross the placenta at term, as seen in an ex vivo placental perfusion study. Therefore, this limited first-trimester human pregnancy experience prevents a complete assessment of the embryofetal risk. Animal studies did show some embryofetal toxicity in two species at doses of less than the RHD; however, the drug was administered daily for almost 2 weeks. The approved use in humans is for only 24 hours. However, there are a few studies in humans that have described using the drug in severe intensive care unit (ICU) cases for more than 24 hours. In this clinical setting, an informed decision-making process should occur if use for more than 24 hours is needed.

BREASTFEEDING SUMMARY

Three studies analyzing dexmedetomidine use during human lactation were located. In a total of 15 lactating women, the drug was not detected in the breast milk in 3 cases (LLQ of 3 pg/mL). In the remaining 12 cases, the peak breast milk level at the conclusion of drug administration was 594 pg/mL in one breast milk sample. Dexmedetomidine was undetectable in all samples at 24 hours after the last infusion dose concluded. Furthermore, oral bioavailability is poor, so infant absorption from the low concentration found in breast milk is likely to be clinically insignificant. With the short elimination half-life, if there is any newborn concern regarding exposure, breastfeeding can be held for 10 to 12 hours (five to six half-lives). Breastfeeding while using this drug should be based on the mother's clinical need for treatment versus any potential infant risks that might occur. If used, the infant should be monitored for the most common reported adult side effect of irritability.

References

1. Sia AT, Sng BL. Intravenous dexmedetomidine for obstetric anaesthesia and analgesia: converting a challenge into an opportunity? *Int J Obstet Anesth*. 2009;18:204-206.
2. Prescribing Information. *Precedex*. Hospira; 2019.
3. Ala-Kokko TI, Pienimäki P, Lampela E, et al. Transfer of clonidine and dexmedetomidine across the isolated perfused human placenta. *Acta Anaesthesiol Scand*. 1997;41:313-319.
4. Neumann MM, Davio MB, Macknet MR, et al. Dexmedetomidine for awake fiberoptic intubation in a parturient with spinal muscular atrophy type III for cesarean delivery. *Int J Obstet Anesth*. 2009;18:403-407.
5. Abu-Halaweh SA, Al Oweidi AKS, Abu-Malooh H, et al. Intravenous dexmedetomidine infusion for labour analgesia in patient with preeclampsia. *Eur J Anaesthesiol*. 2009;26:86-87.
6. Palanisamy A, Klickovich RJ, Ramsay M, et al. Intravenous dexmedetomidine as an adjunct for labor analgesia and cesarean delivery anesthesia in a parturient with a tethered spinal cord. *Int J Obstet Anesth*. 2009;18:258-261.
7. Sia AT, Kwek K, Yeo GS. The in vitro effects of clonidine and dexmedetomidine on human myometrium. *Int J Obstet Anesth*. 2005;14:104-107.
8. Yu M, Han C, Jiang X, et al. Effect and placental transfer of dexmedetomidine during caesarean section under general anaesthesia. *Basic Clin Pharmacol Toxicol*. 2015;117:204-208.
9. Handlogten KS, Sharpe EE, Brost BC, et al. Dexmedetomidine and mannitol for awake craniotomy in a pregnant patient. *Anesth Analg*. 2015;120:1099-1103.
10. Yousef AA, Salem HA, Moustafa MZ. Effect of mini-dose epidural dexmedetomidine in elective cesarean section using combined spinal-epidural anesthesia: a randomized double-blinded controlled study. *J Anesth*. 2015;29:708-714.
11. Dodd SE, Hunter Guevara LR, Datta P, et al. Dexmedetomidine levels in breast milk: analysis of breast milk expressed during and after awake craniotomy. *Breastfeed Med*. 2021;16:919-921.
12. Wang Y, Fang X, Liu C, et al. Impact of intraoperative infusion and postoperative PCIA of dexmedetomidine on early breastfeeding after elective cesarean section: a randomized double-blind controlled trial. *Drug Des Devel Ther*. 2020;14:1083-1093.
13. Zhao W, Ma L, Wang J, et al. Retrospective comparison of the safety and effectiveness of dexmedetomidine versus standard of care before and during cesarean delivery in a maternity unit in Zhengzhou, China. *Med Sci Monit*. 2020;26:e925709.
14. Ozaki M, Takeda J, Tanaka K, et al. Safety and efficacy of dexmedetomidine for long-term sedation in critically ill patients. *J Anesth*. 2013;28:38-50.

DEXMETHYLPHENIDATE

Central Nervous System (Stimulant)

PREGNANCY RECOMMENDATION: No Human Data—Animal Data Suggest Low Risk

BREASTFEEDING RECOMMENDATION: Probably Compatible

PREGNANCY SUMMARY

No reports describing the use of dexmethylphenidate in human pregnancy have been located. The drug will probably cross the placenta, so some fetal exposure will likely occur. Therefore, the absence of human pregnancy experience prevents a complete assessment of the embryofetal risk. Numerous studies have been conducted with methylphenidate, and the primary concern might be an increased risk for preterm birth (see Methylphenidate). Animal studies did not find any embryofetal toxicity in two animal species at doses less than 10 times the MRHD. Using this drug during pregnancy should be based on the pros and cons of the mother's clinical need for treatment versus any potential fetal risk that might occur from exposure. Dexmethylphenidate was found to cause an increase in blood pressure during the clinical trials. The drug also carries a boxed warning for an increased risk of drug dependence. It is classified as a Schedule II drug.

D

BREASTFEEDING SUMMARY

No reports describing the use of dexmethylphenidate during human lactation have been located. The drug will probably be found in breast milk, so some infant exposure will likely occur. However, if it is similar to methylphenidate, the exposure is probably very small. Studies on methylphenidate (see Methylphenidate) during lactation have shown relatively low levels in breast milk with an RID of less than 1%. Breastfeeding while using this drug should be based on the mother's clinical need for treatment. If used, the infant should be monitored for the most common reported adult side effects of nausea, headache, and anxiety (all leading to irritability) and decreased appetite.

Reference

1. Prescribing Information. *Focalin*. Novartis; 2023.

DEXRAZOXANE

Antidote

PREGNANCY RECOMMENDATION: No Human Data—Animal Data Suggest Risk (Maternal Benefit May Outweigh Embryofetal Risk)

BREASTFEEDING RECOMMENDATION: Potential Toxicity

PREGNANCY SUMMARY

No reports describing the use of dexrazoxane in human pregnancy have been located. The drug will probably cross the placenta, so some fetal exposure will likely occur. Therefore, the absence of human pregnancy experience prevents a complete assessment of the embryofetal risk. Animal data showed embryofetal toxicity in two animal species at doses equal to or below the MRHD. Maternal toxicity also occurred at these doses. The manufacturer recommends that women with reproductive potential use highly effective contraception during treatment. However, dexrazoxane is intended to protect the patient from doxorubicin-induced cardiomyopathy. Therefore, using this drug during pregnancy should be based on the pros and cons of the mother's clinical need for treatment versus any potential fetal risk that might occur from exposure.

BREASTFEEDING SUMMARY

No reports describing the use of dexrazoxane during human lactation have been located. The drug will probably be found in breast milk, so some infant exposure will likely occur. The manufacturer recommends that women not breastfeed while using this drug. Nevertheless, breastfeeding should be based on the mother's clinical need for treatment. If used, the infant should be monitored for the most common reported adult side effects of nausea and abdominal pain (both leading to irritability), diarrhea, vomiting, and decreased appetite.

Reference

1. Prescribing Information. *Zinecard*. Pfizer; 2020.

DEXTROAMPHETAMINE

Central Nervous System (Stimulant)

(SEE AMPHETAMINE)

DEXTROMETHORPHAN

Respiratory (Antitussive)

PREGNANCY RECOMMENDATION: Human Data Suggest Low Risk

BREASTFEEDING RECOMMENDATION: Probably Compatible

D

PREGNANCY SUMMARY

Combined data from a few studies described 13 (2.7%) major anomalies in 487 first-trimester exposures. For anytime use in one large study, there were 15 (2.6%) major birth defects in 580 pregnancies. The drug probably crosses the placenta, so some fetal exposure will likely occur. Animal studies did not describe any increased risk for embryofetal toxicity or malformations, but dosing was not supplied. Using this drug during pregnancy should be based on the pros and cons of the mother's clinical need for treatment versus any potential fetal risk that might occur from exposure. The drug has been around for over 65 years and has been commonly used during pregnancy. Dextromethorphan is the enantiomer (mirror image) of the opioid drug, levomethorphan, but has negligible analgesic effects.

BREASTFEEDING SUMMARY

A total of 28 women were evaluated that were using dextromethorphan during lactation. The drug and the active metabolite (dextrorphan) were found in breast milk samples with peak levels of about 4 and 18 mcg/mL, respectively. Using peak values for both drugs, the calculated RID was still less than 1%. In eight cases, infant serum was tested. Seven of these had undetectable concentrations. The drug was detected in the eighth case, but at low levels. Breastfeeding while using this drug should be based on the mother's clinical need for treatment versus any potential infant risks that might occur. If used, the infant should be monitored for the most common reported adult side effects of nausea, dizziness, and abdominal pain (all leading to irritability) and drowsiness. Some over-the-counter (OTC) products may contain ethanol, so choosing one without alcohol is recommended.

References

1. Brent RL. Studies of the fetal effects of dextromethorphan in ovo. *Teratology*. 1999;60:57-58. (Originally published as an untitled letter to the editor: Pediatr Res. 1998;44:415-416.)
2. Polifka JE, Shepard TH. Studies of the fetal effects of dextromethorphan in ovo. *Teratology*. 1999;60:56-57. (Originally published as an untitled letter to the editor: Pediatr Res. 1998;44:415.)
3. Andaloro VJ, Monaghan DT, Rosenquist TH. Dextromethorphan and other N-methyl-D-aspartate receptor antagonists are teratogenic in the avian embryo model. *Pediatr Res*. 1998;43:1-7.
4. Brent RL, Shepard TH, Polifka JE. Response to Dr. Rosenquist's comments pertaining to the paper by Andaloro et al ('98) "Dextromethorphan and other N-methyl-D-aspartate receptor antagonists are teratogenic in the avian embryo model" and letters to the editor by Polifka JE and Shepard TH ('98) and Brent RL ('98). *Teratology*. 1999;60:61-62.
5. Rosenquist TH. Studies of the fetal effects of dextromethorphan in ovo. *Teratology*. 1999;60:56-60. (Originally published as an untitled author's response: Pediatr Res. 1998;44:416-417.)
6. Jacqz-Aigrain E, Cresteil T. Cytochrome P450-dependent metabolism of dextromethorphan: fetal and adult studies. *Dev Pharmacol Ther*. 1992;18:161-168.
7. Heinonen OP, Slone D, Shapiro S. *Birth Defects and Drugs in Pregnancy*. Publishing Sciences Group; 1977.
8. Chasnoff IJ, Diggs G, Schnoll SH. Fetal alcohol effects and maternal cough syrup abuse. *Am J Dis Child*. 1981;135:968.
9. Robinson HB Jr, Tross K. Agenesis of the cloacal membrane. A probable teratogenic anomaly. *Perspect Pediatr Pathol*. 1984;8:79-96.
10. Aselton P, Jick H, Milunsky A, et al. First-trimester drug use and congenital disorders. *Obstet Gynecol*. 1985;65:451-455.
11. Martinez-Frias ML, Rodriguez-Pinilla E. Epidemiologic analysis of prenatal exposure to cough medicines containing dextromethorphan: no evidence of human teratogenicity. *Teratology*. 2001;63:38-41.
12. Rayburn WF. OTC drugs and pregnancy. *Perinatol Neonatol*. 1984;8:21-27.
13. Berglund F, Flodh H, Lundborg P, et al. Drug use during pregnancy and breast-feeding. A classification system for drug information. *Acta Obstet Gynecol Scand Suppl*. 1984;126:1-55.
14. Onnis A, Grella P. *The Biochemical Effects of Drugs in Pregnancy*. Vol 2. Ellis Horwood Limited; 1984:62-63.
15. Clark SL. Asthma in pregnancy. National Asthma Education Program Working Group on Asthma and Pregnancy, National Institutes of Health, National Heart, Lung, and Blood Institute. *Obstet Gynecol*. 1993;82:1036-1040.
16. Report of the Working Group on Asthma and Pregnancy. Executive summary: management of asthma during pregnancy. *J Allergy Clin Immunol*. 1994;93:139-162.
17. Koren G, Pastuszak A, Ito S. Drugs in pregnancy. *N Engl J Med*. 1998;338:1128-1137.
18. Einarson A, Lyszkiewicz D, Koren G. The safety of dextromethorphan in pregnancy: results of a controlled study. *Chest*. 2001;119:466-469.

DIATRIZOATE

Diagnostic (Radiopaque Contrast)

PREGNANCY RECOMMENDATION: Limited Human Data—Animal Data Suggest Low Risk

BREASTFEEDING RECOMMENDATION: Probably Compatible

PREGNANCY SUMMARY

Numerous case reports and series were located that have described the use of diatrizoate during human pregnancy. Essentially all of these have involved the use of the diagnostic agent with amniography. No fetal/newborn adverse effects overall were reported in these studies. The contrast agent appears to cross the placenta, so some fetal exposure will occur. However, the absence of first-trimester human pregnancy experience prevents a complete assessment of the embryofetal risk. Animal studies did not appear to show any embryofetal toxicity or malformations in two species. Using diatrizoate during pregnancy should be based on the pros and cons of the mother's clinical need for diagnosis versus any potential fetal risk that might occur from exposure. The guidelines of the Contrast Media Safety Committee of the European Society of Urogenital Radiology recommend that iodinated contrast media may be used in pregnancy if such use is essential. However, neonatal thyroid function should be checked during the first week of life.

BREASTFEEDING SUMMARY

Two case reports were located that describe the use of diatrizoate during human lactation. Breast milk samples were analyzed for iodine levels. In one case, the breast milk sample was negative for iodine (LLQ of 2 mcg/mL). In the second case, the total milk iodine after 24 hours was 31 mg, which was well below 1% of the maternal dose of 93 g. Additionally, the drug has negligible oral bioavailability. Therefore, if any amount of the contrast agent were to be found in breast milk, the amount absorbed (if any) would be clinically insignificant. If the clinical decision is to use this diagnostic agent while breastfeeding, the infant should be monitored for the most common reported adult side effects of nausea (leading to irritability), vomiting, and flushing.

References

1. Prescribing Information. *Hypaque sodium*. Amersham Health; 2006.
2. Prescribing Information. *Cystografin*. Bracco Diagnostics; 2006.
3. Webb JAW, Thomsen HS, Morcos SK. The use of iodinated and gadolinium contrast media during pregnancy and lactation. *Eur Radiol*. 2005;15:1234-1240.
4. McLain CR Jr. Amniography studies of the gastrointestinal motility of the human fetus. *Am J Obstet Gynecol*. 1963;86:1079-1087.
5. McLain CR Jr. Amniography, a versatile diagnostic procedure in obstetrics. *Obstet Gynecol*. 1964;23:45-50.
6. McLain CR Jr. Amniography for diagnosis and management of fetal death in utero. *Obstet Gynecol*. 1965;26:233-236.
7. Ferris EJ, Shapiro JH, Spira J. Roentgenologic aspects of intrauterine transfusion. *JAMA*. 1966;196:127-128.
8. Wiltchik SG, Schwarz RH, Emich JP Jr. Amniography for placental localization. *Obstet Gynecol*. 1966;28:641-645.
9. Misenhimer HR. Fetal hemorrhage associated with amniocentesis. *Am J Obstet Gynecol*. 1966;94:1133-1135.
10. Blumberg ML, Wohl GT, Wiltchik S, et al. Placental localization by amniography. *AJR*. 1967;100:688-697.
11. Berner HW Jr. Amniography, an accurate way to localize the placenta. *Obstet Gynecol*. 1967;29:200-206.
12. Creasman WT, Lawrence RA, Thiede HA. Fetal complications of amniocentesis. *JAMA*. 1968;204:949-952.
13. Bottorff MK, Fish SA. Amniography. *S Med J*. 1971;64:1203-1206.
14. Morrison JC, Boyd M, Friedman BI, et al. The effects of Renografin-60 on the fetal thyroid. *Obstet Gynecol*. 1973;42:99-103.
15. Rodesch F, Camus M, Ermans AM, et al. Adverse effect of amniofetography on fetal thyroid function. *Am J Obstet Gynecol*. 1976;126:723-726.
16. FitzJohn TP, Williams DG, Laker MF, et al. Intravenous urography during lactation. *Br J Radiol*. 1982;55:603-605.
17. Committee on Drugs, American Academy of Pediatrics. The transfer of drugs and other chemicals into human milk. *Pediatrics*. 2001;108:776-789.

DIAZEPAM

Central Nervous System (Sedative)

PREGNANCY RECOMMENDATION: Human Data Suggest Potential Risk

BREASTFEEDING RECOMMENDATION: Potential Toxicity

PREGNANCY SUMMARY

Numerous studies have been published describing the use of diazepam during human pregnancy. In reviews and meta-analyses, benzodiazepine drugs as a group have not been associated with an overall risk for teratogenicity. Several studies suggested an increased risk for cleft lip and palate, as well as inguinal hernia with diazepam use. However, these risks have not been confirmed. Several analyses looking specifically at diazepam use in the first trimester have shown congenital anomaly rates that fall within the expected range, and others have shown an increased risk, but no pattern to the defects has been seen. The drug crosses the placenta, so fetal exposure will occur. In addition, because of the long elimination half-lives of diazepam and nordiazepam, use in the latter part of gestation can adversely affect the appearance of the fetal heart rate (FHR) tracing by producing prolonged decreased variability. Continuous use during gestation has resulted in neonatal withdrawal, and a dose-related syndrome is apparent if diazepam is used close to delivery. Diazepam has the potential for producing dependence, tolerance, and misuse that can produce withdrawal symptoms upon discontinuation (after longer use). Acute discontinuation of the drug can produce seizures in some patients. It is a Schedule IV controlled substance. Consequently, if the maternal condition requires the use of diazepam during pregnancy, the lowest possible dose for the shortest amount of time should be followed.

BREASTFEEDING SUMMARY

Diazepam and its active metabolite, nordiazepam, have been found in human breast milk in several studies. The drug was found in the breast milk of all 18 lactating women. The calculated RIDs for diazepam were all under 10%, but if nordiazepam is added, then the total RID exceeds 10% in many cases. The breast milk levels of nordiazepam were higher than diazepam in most cases. Infant blood has also been analyzed in four cases where exposure to the drug was through breastfeeding. Blood levels were in the low therapeutic range for adults in two cases. (Therapeutic range in adults is 100 ng/mL to 2 mcg/mL.) Because of the long elimination half-lives for diazepam and nordiazepam, the drugs may accumulate in breastfed infants. Due to a concern for potential serious adverse effects that might be seen in a breastfed infant, the manufacturer recommends that women not breastfeed while being treated with this drug. Several other benzodiazepine drugs are available, and many have shorter elimination half-lives. Therefore, if possible, an alternative can be used if the mother clinically needs benzodiazepine treatment (see Triazolam).

References

1. Prescribing Information. *Diazepam*. Genetech; 2018.
2. Erkkola R, Kanto J, Sellman R. Diazepam in early human pregnancy. *Acta Obstet Gynecol Scand*. 1974;53:135-138.
3. Kanto J, Erkkola R, Sellman R. Accumulation of diazepam and N-demethyldiazepam in the fetal blood during labor. *Ann Clin Res*. 1973; 5:375-379.
4. Idanpaan-Heikkila JE, Jouppila PI, Puolakka JO, et al. Placental transfer and fetal metabolism of diazepam in early human pregnancy. *Am J Obstet Gynecol*. 1971;109:1011-1016.
5. Mandelli M, Morselli PL, Nordio S, et al. Placental transfer of diazepam and its disposition in the newborn. *Clin Pharmacol Ther*. 1975;17:564-572.
6. Gamble JAS, Moore J, Lamke H, et al. A study of plasma diazepam levels in mother and infant. *Br J Obstet Gynaecol*. 1977;84:588-591.
7. Haram K, Bakke DM, Johannessen KH, et al. Transplacental passage of diazepam during labor: influence of uterine contractions. *Clin Pharmacol Ther*. 1978;24:590-599.
8. Bakke OM, Haram K, Lygre T, et al. Comparison of the placental transfer of thiopental and diazepam in caesarean section. *Eur J Clin Pharmacol*. 1981;21: 221-227.
9. Haram K, Bakke OM. Diazepam as an induction agent for caesarean section: a clinical and pharmacokinetic study of fetal drug exposure. *Br J Obstet Gynaecol*. 1980;87:506-512.
10. Kanto JH. Use of benzodiazepines during pregnancy, labour and lactation, with particular reference to pharmacokinetic considerations. *Drugs*. 1982; 23:354-380.
11. Bakke OM, Haram K. Time-course of transplacental passage of diazepam: influence of injection-delivery interval on neonatal drug concentrations. *Clin Pharmacokinet*. 1982;7:353-362.
12. Jauniaux E, Jurkovic D, Lees C, et al. In-vivo study of diazepam transfer across the first trimester human placenta. *Hum Reprod*. 1996;11:889-892.
13. Jorgensen NP, Thurmann-Nielsen E, Walstad RA. Pharmacokinetics and distribution of diazepam and oxazepam in early pregnancy. *Acta Obstet Gynecol Scand*. 1988;67:493-497.
14. Lee JN, Chen SS, Richens A, et al. Serum protein binding of diazepam in maternal and foetal serum during pregnancy. *Br J Clin Pharmacol*. 1982;14: 551-554.
15. Ridd MJ, Brown KF, Nation RL, et al. Differential transplacental binding of diazepam: causes and implications. *Eur J Clin Pharmacol*. 1983;24:595-601.
16. Rivas F, Hernandez A, Cantu JM. Acentric craniofacial cleft in a newborn female prenatally exposed to a high dose of diazepam. *Teratology*. 1984;30: 179-180.
17. Safra JM, Oakley GP Jr. Association between cleft lip with or without cleft palate and prenatal exposure to diazepam. *Lancet*. 1975;2:478-480.
18. Saxen I. Epidemiology of cleft lip and palate: an attempt to rule out chance correlations. *Br J Prev Soc Med*. 1975;29:103-110.
19. Saxen I. Associations between oral clefts and drugs taken during pregnancy. *Int J Epidemiol*. 1975;4:37-44.
20. Saxen I, Saxen L. Association between maternal intake of diazepam and oral clefts. *Lancet*. 1975;2:498.
21. Safra MJ, Oakley GP Jr. Valium: an oral cleft teratogen? *Cleft Palate J*. 1976; 13:198-200.
22. Czeizel A. Diazepam, phenytoin, and etiology of cleft lip and/or cleft palate. *Lancet*. 1976;1:810.
23. Rosenberg L, Mitchell AA, Parsells JL, et al. Lack of relation of oral clefts to diazepam use during pregnancy. *N Engl J Med*. 1983;309:1282-1285.
24. Shiono PH, Mills JL. Oral clefts and diazepam use during pregnancy. *N Engl J Med*. 1984;311:919-920.
25. Lakos P, Czeizel E. A teratological evaluation of anticonvulsant drugs. *Acta Paediatr Acad Sci Hung*. 1977;18:145-153.
26. Entman SS, Vaughn WK. Lack of relation of oral clefts to diazepam use in pregnancy. *N Engl J Med*. 1984;310:1121-1122.
27. Rosenberg L, Mitchell AA. Lack of relation of oral clefts to diazepam use in pregnancy. *N Engl J Med*. 1984;310:1122.
28. Bracken MB, Holford TR. Exposure to prescribed drugs in pregnancy and association with congenital malformations. *Obstet Gynecol*. 1981;58:336-344.
29. Rothman KJ, Fyler DC, Goldblatt A, et al. Exogenous hormones and other drug exposures of children with congenital heart disease. *Am J Epidemiol*. 1979;109:433-439.
30. Istvan EJ. Drug-associated congenital abnormalities. *Can Med Assoc J*. 1970; 103:1394.
31. Ringrose CAD. The hazard of neurotrophic drugs in the fertile years. *Can Med Assoc J*. 1972;106:1058.
32. Fourth Annual Report of the New Zealand Committee on Adverse Drug Reactions. *NZ Med J*. 1969;70:118-122.
33. Laegreid L, Olegard R, Walstrom J, et al. Teratogenic effects of benzodiazepine use during pregnancy. *J Pediatr*. 1989;114:126-131.
34. Bergman U, Rosa FW, Baum C, et al. Effects of exposure to benzodiazepine during fetal life. *Lancet*. 1992;340:694-696.
35. Courtens W, Vamos E, Hainaut M, et al. Moebius syndrome in an infant exposed in utero to benzodiazepines. *J Pediatr*. 1992;121:833-834.
36. Czeizel AE, Mosonyi A. Monitoring of early human fetal development in women exposed to large doses of chemicals. *Environ Mol Mutagen*. 1997;30: 240-244.
37. Dolovich LR, Addis A, Vaillancourt JMR, et al. Benzodiazepine use in pregnancy and major malformations or oral cleft: meta-analysis of cohort and case-controlled studies. *Br Med J*. 1998;317:839-843.
38. Game E, Bergman U. Benzodiazepine use in pregnancy and major malformations or oral clefts. *Br Med J*. 1999;319:918.
39. Cates C. Pooled results are sensitive to zero transformation used. *Br Med J*. 1999;319:918-919.
40. Khan KS, Wukes C, Gee H. Quality of primary studies must influence inferences made from meta-analyses. *Br Med J*. 1999;319:919.
41. Ornoy A, Arnon J, Shechtman S, et al. Is benzodiazepine use during pregnancy really teratogenic? *Reprod Toxicol*. 1998;12:511-515.
42. Greenblatt DJ, Shader RI. Effect of benzodiazepines in neonates. *N Engl J Med*. 1975;292:649.
43. Modif M, Brinkman CR, Assali NS. Effects of diazepam on uteroplacental and fetal hemodynamics and metabolism. *Obstet Gynecol*. 1973;41:364-368.
44. Toaff ME, Hezroni J, Toaff R. Effect of diazepam on uterine activity during labor. *Isr J Med Sci*. 1977;13:1007-1009.
45. Shannon RW, Fraser GP, Aitken RG, et al. Diazepam in preeclamptic toxaemia with special reference to its effect on the newborn infant. *Br J Clin Pract*. 1972;26:271-275.
46. Yeh SY, Paul RIT, Cordero L, et al. A study of diazepam during labor. *Obstet Gynecol*. 1974;43:363-373.
47. Kasturilal D, Shetti RN. Role of diazepam in the management of eclampsia. *Curr Ther Res*. 1975;18:627-630.
48. Eliot BW, Hill JG, Cole AP, Hailey DM. Continuous pethidine/diazepam infusion during labor and its effects on the newborn. *Br J Obstet Gynaecol*. 1975;82:126-131.
49. Lean TH, Retnam SS, Sivasamboo R. Use of benzodiazepines in the management of eclampsia. *J Obstet Gynaecol Br Commonw*. 1968;75:856-862.
50. Scanlon JW. Effect of benzodiazepines in neonates. *N Engl J Med*. 1975; 292:649.
51. Gillberg C. "Floppy infant syndrome" and maternal diazepam. *Lancet*. 1977; 2(8031):244.
52. Haram K. "Floppy infant syndrome" and maternal diazepam. *Lancet*. 1977; 310(8038):612-613.
53. Speight AN. Floppy-infant syndrome and maternal diazepam and/or nitrazepam. *Lancet*. 1977;1:878.
54. Rementeria JL, Bhatt K. Withdrawal symptoms in neonates from intrauterine exposure to diazepam. *J Pediatr*. 1977;90:123-126.
55. Thearle MJ, Dunn PM. Exchange transfusions for diazepam intoxication at birth followed by jejunal stenosis. *Proc R Soc Med*. 1973;66:13-14.
56. Backes CR, Cordero L. Withdrawal symptoms in the neonate from presumptive intrauterine exposure to diazepam: report of case. *J Am Osteopath Assoc*. 1980;79:584-585.
57. Cree JE, Meyer J, Hailey DM. Diazepam in labour: its metabolism and effect on the clinical condition and thermogenesis of the newborn. *Br Med J*. 1973;4:251-255.
58. McAllister CB. Placental transfer and neonatal effects of diazepam when administered to women just before delivery. *Br J Anaesth*. 1980;52:423-427.
59. Owen JR, Irani SF, Blair AW. Effect of diazepam administered to mothers during labour on temperature regulation of neonate. *Arch Dis Child*. 1972;47: 107-110.
60. Scher J, Hailey DM, Beard RW. The effects of diazepam on the fetus. *J Obstet Gynaecol Br Commonw*. 1972;79:635-638.
61. Van Geijn HP, Jongsma HW, Doesburg WH, et al. The effect of diazepam administration during pregnancy or labor on the heart rate variability of the newborn infant. *Eur J Obstet Gynaecol Reprod Biol*. 1980;10:187-201.
62. Birger M, Homberg R, Insler V. Clinical evaluation of fetal movements. *Int J Gynaecol Obstet*. 1980;18:377-382.
63. Einarson A, Selby P, Koren G. Abrupt discontinuation of psychotropic drugs during pregnancy: fear of teratogenic risk and impact on counseling. *J Psychiatry Neurosci*. 2001;26:44-48.
64. Van Geijn HP, Kenemans P, Vise T, et al. Pharmacokinetics of diazepam and occurrence in breast milk. Paper presented at: Proceedings of the Sixth International Congress of Pharmacology, Helsinki, Finland, 1975:514.

65. Hill RM, Nowlin J, Lertratanangkoon K, et al. The identification and quantification of drugs in human breast milk. *Clin Res*. 1974;22:77A.
66. Cole AP, Hailey DM. Diazepam and active metabolite in breast milk and their transfer to the neonate. *Arch Dis Child*. 1975;50:741-742.
67. Patrick MJ, Tilstone WJ, Reavey P. Diazepam and breast-feeding. *Lancet*. 1972;1:542-543.
68. Catz CS. Diazepam in breast milk. *Drug Ther*. 1973;3:72-73.
69. Wesson DR, Camber S, Harkey M, et al. Diazepam and desmethyldiazepam in breast milk. *J Psychoactive Drugs*. 1985;17:55-56.
70. Committee on Drugs, American Academy of Pediatrics. The transfer of drugs and other chemicals into human milk. *Pediatrics*. 2001;108: 776-789.

DIAZOXIDE

Miscellaneous (Antihypoglycemic)

PREGNANCY RECOMMENDATION: Limited Human Data—Animal Data Suggest Risk

BREASTFEEDING RECOMMENDATION: Potential Toxicity

PREGNANCY SUMMARY

One case report was located that described the use of diazoxide starting at the end of the second trimester of pregnancy. A healthy newborn was delivered with no adverse reactions related to the drug. The drug was found to cross the placenta, so fetal exposure will occur. However, this limited human pregnancy experience prevents a complete assessment of the embryofetal risk. Animal studies did show embryofetal toxicity and malformations in two species, but dosing was not provided. Using this drug during pregnancy should be based on the pros and cons of the mother's clinical need for treatment versus any potential fetal risk that might occur from exposure.

BREASTFEEDING SUMMARY

One study was located that described the use of diazoxide during human lactation. The mother had been treated since the age of 4 for a chronic medical condition that produced hypoglycemia. Her daily dosage was 150 to 175 mg/d. The peak and trough levels were 3.1 and 0.7 mcg/mL. The calculated RID overall was less than 10%. Due to a concern for potential serious adverse effects that might be seen in a breastfed infant, the manufacturer recommends that women not breastfeed while being treated with this drug. Nevertheless, breastfeeding while using this drug should be based on the mother's clinical need for treatment (one of these being chronic disorders that produce hypoglycemia) versus any potential infant risks that might occur. If used, the infant should be monitored for the most common reported adult side effects of nausea, headache, and abdominal pain (all leading to irritability), diarrhea, vomiting, weakness (lethargy), rash, and hyperglycemia.

References

1. Prescribing Information. *Proglycem*. Teva Pharmaceuticals USA; 2019.
2. Saito J, Kawasaki H, Adachi N, et al. Diazoxide during pregnancy and lactation: drug levels in maternal serum, cord blood, breast milk, and infant serum: a case report. *Gynecol Endocrinol*. 2022;38:528-530.

DICHLORPHENAMIDE

Miscellaneous (Carbonic Anhydrase Inhibitor)

PREGNANCY RECOMMENDATION: No Human Data and No Relevant Animal Data

BREASTFEEDING RECOMMENDATION: Potential Toxicity

PREGNANCY SUMMARY

No reports describing the use of dichlorphenamide in human pregnancy have been located. The drug will probably cross the placenta, so some fetal exposure will likely occur. Therefore, the absence of human pregnancy experience prevents a complete assessment of the embryofetal risk. Animal studies did show embryofetal toxicity in one species at doses of more than 10 times the MRHD. Using this drug during pregnancy should be based on the pros and cons of the mother's clinical need for treatment versus any potential fetal risk that might occur from exposure. The drug did cause metabolic acidosis in some patients during the clinical trials. Therefore, if prolonged use occurs, serum bicarbonate status should be evaluated.

BREASTFEEDING SUMMARY

No reports describing the use of dichlorphenamide during human lactation have been located. The drug will probably be found in breast milk, so some infant exposure will likely occur. Breastfeeding while using this drug should be based on the mother's clinical need for treatment. If used, the infant should be monitored for the most common reported adult side effects of nausea and paresthesia (both leading to irritability) and lethargy. The drug did cause metabolic acidosis in some patients during the clinical trials. Therefore, if prolonged use occurs, serum bicarbonate status should be evaluated.

D

Reference

1. Prescribing Information. *Keveyis*. Xeris Pharmaceuticals, Inc; 2023.

DICLOFENAC

Pain (Nonsteroidal Anti-Inflammatory Drug)

PREGNANCY RECOMMENDATION: Human Data Suggest Risk (Second and Third Trimester)

BREASTFEEDING RECOMMENDATION: Probably Compatible

PREGNANCY SUMMARY

Numerous studies were located that described the use of diclofenac in the first trimester. Of about 190 pregnancies, there were 5 (2.6%) major anomalies identified. However, many studies described the risk of premature closure of the ductus arteriosus when used in the third trimester. This can lead to pulmonary hypertension in the newborn and other neonatal complications. Use in the second half of gestation has also been associated with a decrease in fetal urine production, leading to oligohydramnios. The drug crosses the placenta, so fetal exposure will occur. However, this limited human pregnancy experience prevents a complete assessment of the embryofetal risk. Animal studies did not show any teratogenicity in three species at doses of less than 10 times the RHD. However, these doses caused maternal toxicity, and with this, there was some embryofetal toxicity. Using this drug during pregnancy should be based on the pros and cons of the mother's clinical need for treatment versus any potential fetal risk that might occur from exposure. If possible, avoid use in the second half of gestation or limit use to a minimal number of doses.

BREASTFEEDING SUMMARY

Three studies were located that described the use of diclofenac during human lactation. In 12 cases, the drug was not detected (LLQ in six cases was 100 ng/mL, and in the other six was 10 ng/mL). In one case, the drug was detected at a level of 100 ng/mL (mother's daily dose of 150 mg). The calculated RID was less than 1%. Breastfeeding while using this drug should be based on the mother's clinical need for treatment versus any potential infant risks that might occur. If used, the infant should be monitored for the most common reported adult side effects of nausea, headache, and dizziness (all leading to irritability), vomiting, constipation, and insomnia.

References

1. Levin DL. Effects of inhibition of prostaglandin synthesis on fetal development, oxygenation, and the fetal circulation. *Semin Perinatol*. 1980;4:35-44.
2. Van Marter LJ, Leviton A, Allred EN, et al. Persistent pulmonary hypertension of the newborn and smoking and aspirin and nonsteroidal antiinflammatory drug consumption during pregnancy. *Pediatrics*. 1996;97:658-663.
3. Matt DW, Borzelleca JF. Toxic effects on the female reproductive system during pregnancy, parturition, and lactation. In Witorsch RJ, ed. *Reproductive Toxicology*. 2nd ed. Raven Press; 1995:175-193.
4. Dawood MY. Nonsteroidal antiinflammatory drugs and reproduction. *Am J Obstet Gynecol*. 1993;169:1255-1265.
5. Product Information. *Diclofenac Potassium*. Sandoz; 2019.
6. Siu SSN, Yeung JHK, Lau TK. A study on placental transfer of diclofenac in first trimester of human pregnancy. *Hum Reprod*. 2000;15:2423-2425.
7. Royburt M, Peled Y, Kaplan B, et al. Non-traumatic rupture of kidney in pregnancy—case report and review. *Acta Obstet Gynecol Scan*. 1994;73:663-667.
8. Nielsen GL, Sorensen HT, Larsen H, et al. Risk of adverse birth outcome and miscarriage in pregnant users of non-steroidal anti-inflammatory drugs: population based observational study and case-control study. *Br Med J*. 2001;322:266-270.
9. Ericson A, Kallen BAJ. Nonsteroidal anti-inflammatory drugs in early pregnancy. *Reprod Toxicol*. 2001;15:371-375.
10. Li DK, Liu L, Odouli R. Exposure to non-steroidal anti-inflammatory drugs during pregnancy and risk of miscarriage: population based cohort study. *Br Med J*. 2003;327:368-371.
11. Tassinari MS, Cook JC, Hurtt ME. NSAIDs and developmental toxicity. *Birth Defects Res (Part B)*. 2003;68:3-4.
12. Kallen BAJ, Olausson PO. Maternal drug use in early pregnancy and infant cardiovascular defect. *Reprod Toxicol*. 2003;17:255-261.
13. Ofori B, Oraichi D, Blais L, et al. Risk of congenital anomalies in pregnant users of non-steroidal anti-inflammatory drugs: a nested case-control study. *Birth Defects Res (Part B)*. 2006;77:268-279.
14. Adverse Drug Reactions Advisory Committee. Premature closure of the fetal ductus arteriosus after maternal use of non-steroidal anti-inflammatory drugs. *Med J Aust*. 1998;169:270-271.
15. Zenker M, Klinge J, Kruger C, et al. Severe pulmonary hypertension in a neonate caused by premature closure of the ductus arteriosus following maternal treatment with diclofenac: a case report. *J Perinat Med*. 1998;26:231-234.
16. Rein AJJT, Nadjari M, Elchalal U, et al. Contraction of the fetal ductus arteriosus induced by diclofenac. *Fetal Diagn Ther*. 1999;14:24-25.
17. Mas C, Menahem S. Premature in utero closure of the ductus arteriosus following maternal ingestion of sodium diclofenac. *Aust NZ J Obstet Gynaecol*. 1999;39:106-107.
18. Siu KL, Lee WH. Maternal diclofenac sodium ingestion and severe neonatal pulmonary hypertension. *J Paediatr Child Health*. 2004;40:152-153.
19. Cassina M, De Santis M, Cesari E, et al. First trimester diclofenac exposure and pregnancy outcome. *Reprod Toxicol*. 2010;30:401-404.
20. Anderson PO. Medication use while breast feeding a neonate. *Neonatal Pharmacol Q*. 1993;2:3-14.
21. Goldsmith DP. Neonatal rheumatic disorders. View of the pediatrician. *Rheum Dis Clin North Am*. 1989;15:287-305.
22. Needs CJ, Brooks PM. Antirheumatic medication during lactation. *Br J Rheumatol*. 1985;24:291-297.

DICLOFENAC OPHTHALMIC

Ophthalmic (Nonsteroidal Anti-Inflammatory Drug)

PREGNANCY RECOMMENDATION: No Human Data—Animal Data Suggest Low Risk

BREASTFEEDING RECOMMENDATION: Probably Compatible

D

PREGNANCY SUMMARY

No reports describing the use of diclofenac ophthalmic solution in human pregnancy have been located. The drug can cross the placenta, but fetal exposure with ophthalmic use is probably clinically insignificant. However, the absence of human pregnancy experience prevents a complete assessment of the embryofetal risk. Animal studies did not show any embryofetal toxicity or malformations in three animal species at doses much greater than 10 times the recommended human ophthalmic dose. Using this drug during pregnancy should be based on the pros and cons of the mother's clinical need for treatment versus any potential fetal risk that might occur from exposure. If used during pregnancy, consider placing pressure over the tear duct in the corner of the eye for at least 1 minute, and then remove any excess solution with absorbent tissue to further decrease any amount of drug reaching the systemic circulation. Nonsteroidal anti-inflammatory drugs (NSAIDs) have been associated with premature closure of the fetal ductus arteriosus, especially when used in the second half of gestation. However, with negligible to no systemic absorption following ophthalmic use, this effect is not likely to occur.

BREASTFEEDING SUMMARY

No reports describing the use of diclofenac ophthalmic during human lactation have been located. Due to the negligible systemic absorption with ophthalmic use, if any drug were to be present in breast milk, it would likely be clinically insignificant. Breastfeeding while using this drug should be based on the mother's clinical need for treatment. A method to further reduce any possible systemic drug concentration is described above in the Pregnancy Summary.

Reference

1. Prescribing Information. *Voltaren ophthalmic*. Novartis Pharmaceutical; 2022.

DICLOXACILLIN

Antibiotic (Penicillin)

PREGNANCY RECOMMENDATION: Limited Human Data—Probably Compatible

BREASTFEEDING RECOMMENDATION: Compatible

PREGNANCY SUMMARY

In two large group studies (the Michigan Medicaid Surveillance study and the Group Health Cooperative of Puget Sound), there were 132 first-trimester exposures to dicloxacillin, with 3 (2.3%) reported anomalies. The Collaborative Perinatal Project reported 3,546 first-trimester exposures to all penicillin derivatives, and 88 (2.5%) were found to have major malformations. For the use of all penicillin derivatives at any time during pregnancy, 7,171 exposures were recorded with 119 (1.7%) fetal malformations identified. Data specific to dicloxacillin was not provided. In all three analyses, no evidence was found to suggest a relationship to large categories of major or minor malformations or to individual defects. Dicloxacillin crosses the placenta, but levels are lower in concentration compared with other penicillin derivatives. Animal studies did not show any embryofetal toxicity or malformations. Although the reported experience with dicloxacillin is limited, all penicillins are considered low risk in pregnancy.

BREASTFEEDING SUMMARY

Two reports describing the use of dicloxacillin during human lactation were located. Both manuscripts found that the drug was found in breast milk with reported levels of about 50 ng/mL up to 300 ng/mL. One study determined that the average daily infant dosage was 8 mcg/kg, resulting in a calculated RID of only about 0.03%. Breastfeeding while using this drug should be based on the mother's clinical need for treatment. If used, the infant should be monitored for the most common reported infant side effects of diarrhea, rash, and possible allergic reactions.

References

1. Prescribing Information. *Dicloxacillin*. Teva Pharmaceuticals; 2022.
2. MacAulay M, Berg S, Charles D. Placental transfer of dicloxacillin at term. *Am J Obstet Gynecol*. 1968;102:1162-1168.
3. Depp R, Kind A, Kirby W, et al. Transplacental passage of methicillin and dicloxacillin into the fetus and amniotic fluid. *Am J Obstet Gynecol*. 1970;107:1054-1057.
4. Heinonen OP, Slone D, Shapiro S. *Birth Defects and Drugs in Pregnancy*. Publishing Sciences Group; 1983:301,435.
5. Aselton P, Jick H, Milunsky A, et al. First-trimester drug use and congenital disorders. *Obstet Gynecol*. 1985;65:451-455.
6. Matsuda S. Transfer of antibiotics into maternal milk. *Biol Res Pregnancy Perinatol*. 1984;5:57-60.
7. Muysson M, Datta P, Rewers-Felkins K, et al. Transfer of dicloxacillin into human milk. *Breastfeed Med*. 2020;15:715-717.

D

DICYCLOMINE

Autonomic (Antimuscarinic)

PREGNANCY RECOMMENDATION: Human Data Suggest Compatible

BREASTFEEDING RECOMMENDATION: Probably Compatible

PREGNANCY SUMMARY

From two large databases (the Collaborative Perinatal Project and the Michigan Medicaid Surveillance study), a total of 1,666 first-trimester exposures to dicyclomine were described. There were 63 (3.8%) major anomalies identified. No pattern to the anomalies was seen. In addition, this drug was part of Bendectin back in the late 1950s to mid-1970s. This drug was used by hundreds of thousands of pregnant women in the first trimester with no proven teratogenicity. The drug will probably cross the placenta, so some fetal exposure will likely occur. Animal studies did not show any embryofetal toxicity in two species at doses of more than 10 times the RHD. Using this drug during pregnancy should be based on the pros and cons of the mother's clinical need for treatment versus any potential fetal risk that might occur from exposure.

BREASTFEEDING SUMMARY

The manufacturer described one case of a woman who was administered a 20 mg dose of dicyclomine while breastfeeding. The milk was tested 2 hours later, where a concentration of 131 ng/mL was detected. This would calculate to a RID of about 6.9%. Anticholinergic drugs can decrease serum prolactin levels, and this can lead to a decrease in breast milk production in some patients. Due to a concern for potential serious adverse effects that might be seen in a breastfed infant, the manufacturer recommends that women not breastfeed while being treated with this drug. Nevertheless, breastfeeding while using this drug should be based on the mother's clinical need for treatment versus any potential infant risks that might occur. If used, the infant should be monitored for the most common reported adult side effects of nausea, dizziness, asthenia, and blurred vision (all leading to irritability) and somnolence.

References

1. Friedman JM, Little BB, Brent RL, et al. Potential human teratogenicity of frequently prescribed drugs. *Obstet Gynecol*. 1990;75:594-599.
2. Prescribing Information. *Dicyclomine hydrochloride*. Actavis Pharma; 2019.
3. Gibson JP, Staples RE, Larson EJ, et al. Teratology and reproduction studies with an antinauseant. *Toxicol Appl Pharmacol*. 1968;13:439-447.
4. Heinonen OP, Slone D, Shapiro S. *Birth Defects and Drugs in Pregnancy*. Publishing Sciences Group; 1977.
5. Nelson MM, Forfar JO. Associations between drugs administered during pregnancy and congenital abnormalities of the fetus. *Br Med J*. 1971;1:523-527.

DIETHYLPROPION

Central Nervous System (Stimulant/Anorexiant)

PREGNANCY RECOMMENDATION: Limited Human Data—Animal Data Suggest Low Risk

BREASTFEEDING RECOMMENDATION: Potential Toxicity

PREGNANCY SUMMARY

A few studies have been located that describe the use of diethylpropion during human pregnancy. Two of these described weight loss in pregnant women using this drug, which occurred in nearly half the women. The publications stated that there were no adverse fetal effects seen. In two others, about 50 patients used the drug in the first trimester, and no anomalies were reported. In a final paper, there were 12 anomalies seen in 1,232 patients who used the drug during pregnancy. Of these, 271 exposures were in the first trimester, but the study did not state whether all

12 newborns with birth defects were in the first trimester group. The drug will probably cross the placenta, so some fetal exposure will likely occur. Therefore, this limited human pregnancy experience prevents a complete assessment of the embryofetal risk. Animal studies did not show any embryofetal toxicity or malformations in one species at doses of less than 10 times the RHD. Weight loss therapy during pregnancy is not recommended. However, using this drug during pregnancy should be based on the pros and cons of the mother's clinical need for treatment versus any potential fetal risk that might occur from exposure.

D

BREASTFEEDING SUMMARY

No reports describing the use of diethylpropion during human lactation have been located. The drug will likely be found in breast milk, so infant exposure will probably occur. The manufacturer states that diethylpropion is excreted into breast milk. Breastfeeding while using this drug should be based on the mother's clinical need for treatment. If used, the infant should be monitored for the most common reported adult side effects of nausea, headache, anxiety, and abdominal pain (all leading to irritability), hypertension, tachycardia, diarrhea, vomiting, decreased appetite, and rash.

References

1. Prescribing Information. *Diethylpropion hydrochloride*. KVK-Tech; 2020.
2. Schardein JL. *Drugs as Teratogens*. CRC Press; 1976:73-75.
3. Silverman M, Okun R. The use of an appetite suppressant (diethylpropion hydrochloride) during pregnancy. *Curr Ther Res*. 1971;13:648-653.
4. Bunde CA, Leyland HM. A controlled retrospective survey in evaluation of teratogenicity. *J New Drugs*. 1965;5:193-198.

DIFELIKEFALIN

Miscellaneous (κ Opioid Receptor Agonist)

PREGNANCY RECOMMENDATION: No Human Data—Animal Data Suggest Low Risk

BREASTFEEDING RECOMMENDATION: Probably Compatible

PREGNANCY SUMMARY

No reports describing the use of difelikefalin in human pregnancy have been located. Some amount of the drug will likely cross the placenta, so fetal exposure will probably occur. Therefore, the absence of human pregnancy experience prevents a complete assessment of embryofetal risk. Animal data did not show embryofetal toxicity. Using this drug during pregnancy should be based on the pros and cons of the mother's clinical need for treatment versus any potential fetal risk that might occur from exposure.

BREASTFEEDING SUMMARY

No reports describing the use of difelikefalin during human lactation have been located. Some amount of the drug will likely be found in breast milk, so infant exposure will probably occur. Breastfeeding while using this drug should be based on the mother's clinical need for treatment. If used, the infant should be monitored for the most common reported adult side effects of headache and nausea (both leading to irritability), diarrhea, elevated potassium levels, and sleep dysfunction.

Reference

1. Prescribing Information. *Korsuva*. Vifor (International); 2021.

DIFLUNISAL

Pain (NSAID)

PREGNANCY RECOMMENDATION: Human Data Suggest Risk in the Second Half of Gestation

BREASTFEEDING RECOMMENDATION: Probably Compatible

PREGNANCY SUMMARY

In a surveillance study of Michigan Medicaid recipients, 258 newborns had been exposed to diflunisal during the first trimester. A total of 19 (7.4%) major birth defects were observed. However, no specific pattern to the anomalies was identified, and in six specific defect categories, the observed versus expected ratios were not elevated. Several studies have looked at

(*continued*)

NSAIDs as a group and have found mixed results regarding embryofetal toxicity and malformations. Overall, their use does not appear to significantly increase the risk for birth defects or preterm delivery. Constriction of the ductus arteriosus in utero is a pharmacologic consequence arising from the use of prostaglandin synthesis inhibitors during pregnancy. Persistent pulmonary hypertension of the newborn may occur if these agents are used in the third trimester close to birth. These drugs have also been shown to inhibit labor and prolong pregnancy in humans (see Indomethacin). Use of NSAIDs has been associated with oligohydramnios when used in the second half of gestation. The drug will likely cross the placenta, so some fetal exposure will probably occur. Therefore, this limited human pregnancy experience prevents a complete assessment of the embryofetal risk. Animal studies showed some embryofetal toxicity in one animal species at doses of less than 10 times the RHD. Using this drug during pregnancy should be based on the pros and cons of the mother's clinical need for treatment versus any potential fetal risk that might occur from exposure.

D

BREASTFEEDING SUMMARY

According to the manufacturer, diflunisal is found in breast milk. The amount present in breast milk is only 2% to 7% of the maternal plasma levels. These percentages would result in a calculated maximum RID of below 10% in most clinical scenarios but could reach as high as 15% with chronic use (more than 10 days) using a dose of 500 mg twice a day. Breastfeeding while using this drug should be based on the mother's clinical need for treatment. If used, the infant should be monitored for the most common reported adult side effects of nausea, headache, and abdominal pain (all leading to irritability), diarrhea, insomnia, vomiting, and rash.

References

1. Prescribing Information. *Diflunisal*. Merck, Sharpe, & Dohme; 2021.
2. Nielsen GL, Sorensen HT, Larsen H, et al. Risk of adverse birth outcome and miscarriage in pregnant users of non-steroidal anti-inflammatory drugs: population based observational study and case-control study. *Br Med J*. 2001;322:266-270.
3. Ericson A, Kallen BAJ. Nonsteroidal anti-inflammatory drugs in early pregnancy. *Reprod Toxicol*. 2001;15:371-375.
4. Li DK, Liu L, Odouli R. Exposure to non-steroidal anti-inflammatory drugs during pregnancy and risk of miscarriage: population based cohort study. *Br Med J*. 2003;327:368-371.
5. Tassinari MS, Cook JC, Hurtt ME. NSAIDs and developmental toxicity. *Birth Defects Res (Part B)*. 2003;68:3-4.
6. Levin DL. Effects of inhibition of prostaglandin synthesis on fetal development, oxygenation, and the fetal circulation. *Semin Perinatol*. 1980;4:35-44.
7. Van Marter LJ, Leviton A, Allred EN, et al. Persistent pulmonary hypertension of the newborn and smoking and aspirin and nonsteroidal anti-inflammatory drug consumption during pregnancy. *Pediatrics*. 1996;97:658-663.
8. Fuchs F. Prevention of prematurity. *Am J Obstet Gynecol*. 1976;126:809-820.

DIFLUPREDNATE OPHTHALMIC

Ophthalmic/Corticosteroid

PREGNANCY RECOMMENDATION: No Human Data and No Relevant Animal Data

BREASTFEEDING RECOMMENDATION: Probably Compatible

PREGNANCY SUMMARY

No reports describing the use of difluprednate ophthalmic solution in human pregnancy have been located. The drug theoretically can cross the placenta, but fetal exposure is probably clinically insignificant due to nonquantifiable systemic absorption following ophthalmic use. However, the absence of human pregnancy experience prevents a complete assessment of the embryofetal risk. Animal studies showed embryofetal toxicity and malformations in two species, but the drug was administered subcutaneously. Using this drug during pregnancy should be based on the pros and cons of the mother's clinical need for treatment versus any potential fetal risk that might occur from exposure. If used during pregnancy, consider placing pressure over the tear duct in the corner of the eye for at least 1 minute, and then remove any excess solution with absorbent tissue to further decrease any amount of drug reaching the systemic circulation.

BREASTFEEDING SUMMARY

No reports describing the use of difluprednate ophthalmic during human lactation have been located. Due to the negligible systemic absorption with ophthalmic use, if any drug were to be present in breast milk, it would likely be clinically insignificant. Breastfeeding while using this drug should be based on the mother's clinical need for treatment. A method to further reduce any possible systemic drug concentration is described above in the Pregnancy Summary.

Reference

1. Prescribing Information. *Durezol*. Amneal Pharmaceuticals, Inc; 2021.

DIGITALIS

Cardiac Glycoside

SEE DIGOXIN

D

DIGITOXIN

Cardiac Glycoside

SEE DIGOXIN

DIGOXIN

Cardiovascular (Cardiac Glycoside)

PREGNANCY RECOMMENDATION: Limited Human Data (First Trimester)/Human Data Suggest Low Risk (Second and Third Trimesters)

BREASTFEEDING RECOMMENDATION: Probably Compatible

PREGNANCY SUMMARY

From the Collaborative Perinatal Project, the Michigan Medicaid Surveillance study, and the Group Health Cooperative of Puget Sound, there were 3 (1.3%) major birth anomalies described in 228 patients with first-trimester exposure. Numerous studies have been located where digoxin has been used to treat fetal arrhythmias and cardiac failure without any reported major fetal or newborn adverse reactions. The drug crosses the placenta, so fetal exposure will occur. However, this limited human pregnancy experience prevents a complete assessment of the embryofetal risk. Animal reproduction and fertility studies have not been located. Using this drug during pregnancy should be based on the pros and cons of the mother's clinical need for treatment versus any potential fetal risk that might occur from exposure. Digitoxin was recently removed from the US market, but is still available in Canada and Europe.

BREASTFEEDING SUMMARY

Several studies have been located that describe the use of digoxin during human lactation. For digoxin, a total of 30 women have had breast milk levels analyzed while using this drug. Digoxin was not detected in a couple of cases (LLQ of 100 pg/mL), but was found in most samples. The peak level in a mother taking 0.75 mg/d was 1.9 ng/mL. Several RIDs were calculated, and all were under 4%. In three cases, infant blood levels were evaluated. For two of these, the drug was not detected (LLQ of 100 pg/mL) in mothers using 0.25 mg/d. In the third case, the newborn had a cord blood level of 600 pg/mL and on day 7 had a value of 200 pg/mL. The mother used 0.25 mg/d during pregnancy and while breastfeeding. With an elimination half-life of about 2 days, some of this drug found on day 7 may still be related to transplacental passage. Breastfeeding while using this drug should be based on the mother's clinical need for treatment versus any potential infant risks that might occur. If used, the infant should be monitored for the most common reported adult side effects of nausea and blurred vision (both leading to irritability), diarrhea, vomiting, and decreased appetite (monitor growth).

References

1. Marzo A, Lo Cicero G, Brina A, et al. Preliminary data on the pharmacokinetics of digoxin in pregnancy. *Boll Soc Ital Biol Sper*. 1980;56:219-223.
2. Luxford AME, Kellaway GSM. Pharmacokinetics of digoxin in pregnancy. *Eur J Clin Pharmacol*. 1983;25:117-121.
3. Shepard TH. *Catalog of Teratogenic Agents*. 3rd ed. Johns Hopkins University Press; 1980:116-117.
4. Saarikoski S. Placental transfer and fetal uptake of 3H-digoxin in humans. *Br J Obstet Gynaecol*. 1976;83:879-884.
5. Okita GT, Plotz EF, Davis ME. Placental transfer of radioactive digitoxin in pregnant women and its fetal distribution. *Circ Res*. 1956;4:376-380.
6. Rogers MC, Willserson JT, Goldblatt A, et al. Serum digoxin concentrations in the human fetus, neonate and infant. *N Engl J Med*. 1972;287:1010-1013.
7. Chan V, Tse TF, Wong V. Transfer of digoxin across the placenta and into breast milk. *Br J Obstet Gynaecol*. 1978;85:605-609.
8. Allonen H, Kanto J, Lisalo E. The foeto-maternal distribution of digoxin in early human pregnancy. *Acta Pharmacol Toxicol*. 1976;39:477-480.
9. Finley JP, Waxman MB, Wong PY, et al. Digoxin excretion in human milk. *J Pediatr*. 1979;94:339-340.
10. Soyka LF. Digoxin: placental transfer, effects on the fetus, and therapeutic use in the newborn. *Clin Perinatol*. 1975;2:23-35.
11. Padeletti L, Porciani MC, Scimone G. Placental transfer of digoxin (beta-methyl-digoxin) in man. *Int J Clin Pharmacol Biopharm*. 1979;17:82-83.
12. Lingman G, Ohrlander S, Ohlin P. Intrauterine digoxin treatment of fetal paroxysmal tachycardia: case report. *Br J Obstet Gynaecol*. 1980;87:340-342.
13. Kerenyi TD, Gleicher N, Meller J, et al. Transplacental cardioversion of intrauterine supraventricular tachycardia with digitalis. *Lancet*. 1980;2:393-394.
14. Harrigan JT, Kangos JJ, Sikka A, et al. Successful treatment of fetal congestive heart failure secondary to tachycardia. *N Engl J Med*. 1981;304:1527-1529.
15. Diro M, Beydoun SN, Jaramillo B, et al. Successful pregnancy in a woman with a left ventricular cardiac aneurysm: a case report. *J Reprod Med*. 1983;28:559-563.
16. Heaton FC, Vaughan R. Intrauterine supraventricular tachycardia: cardioversion with maternal digoxin. *Obstet Gynecol*. 1982;60:749-752.

17. Simpson PC, Trudinger BJ, Walker A, et al. The intrauterine treatment of fetal cardiac failure in a twin pregnancy with an acardiac, acephalic monster. *Am J Obstet Gynecol*. 1983;147:842-844.
18. Spinnato JA, Shaver DC, Flinn GS, et al. Fetal supraventricular tachycardia: in utero therapy with digoxin and quinidine. *Obstet Gynecol*. 1984;64:730-735.
19. Bortolotti U, Milano A, Mazzucco A, et al. Pregnancy in patients with a porcine valve bioprosthesis. *Am J Cardiol*. 1982;50:1051-1054.
20. Rotmensch HH, Rotmensch S, Elkayam U. Management of cardiac arrhythmias during pregnancy: current concepts. *Drugs*. 1987;33:623-633.
21. Tamari I, Eldar M, Rabinowitz B, et al. Medical treatment of cardiovascular disorders during pregnancy. *Am Heart J*. 1982;104:1357-1363.
22. Dumesic DA, Silverman NH, Tobias S, et al. Transplacental cardioversion of fetal supraventricular tachycardia with procainamide. *N Engl J Med*. 1982;307:1128-1131.
23. Gleicher N, Elkayam U. Cardiac problems in pregnancy. II. Fetal aspects: advances in intrauterine diagnosis and therapy. *JAMA*. 1984;252:78-80.
24. Golichowski AM, Caldwell R, Hartsough A, et al. Pharmacologic cardioversion of intrauterine supraventricular tachycardia. A case report. *J Reprod Med*. 1985;30:139-144.
25. Reece EA, Romero R, Santulli T, et al. In utero diagnosis and management of fetal tachypnea. A case report. *J Reprod Med*. 1985;30:221-224.
26. Weiner CP, Thompson MIB. Direct treatment of fetal supraventricular tachycardia after failed transplacental therapy. *Am J Obstet Gynecol*. 1988;158:570-573.
27. Sherman JL Jr, Locke RV. Transplacental neonatal digitalis intoxication. *Am J Cardiol*. 1960;6:834-837.
28. Weaver JB, Pearson JF. Influence of digitalis on time of onset and duration of labour in women with cardiac disease. *Br Med J*. 1973;3:519-520.
29. Ho PC, Chen TY, Wong V. The effect of maternal cardiac disease and digoxin administration on labour, fetal weight and maturity at birth. *Aust NZ J Obstet Gynaecol*. 1980;20:24-27.
30. Levy M, Granit L, Laufer N. Excretion of drugs in human milk. *N Engl J Med*.1977;297:789.
31. Loughnan PM. Digoxin excretion in human breast milk. *J Pediatr*. 1978;92:1019-1020.
32. Aselton P, Jick H, Milunsky A, et al. First-trimester drug use and congenital anomalies. *Obstet Gynecol*. 1986;65:451-455.

DIGOXIN IMMUNE FAB

Antidote

PREGNANCY RECOMMENDATION: Limited Human Data—No Relevant Animal Data (Maternal Benefit May Outweigh Any Embryofetal Risk)

BREASTFEEDING RECOMMENDATION: Probably Compatible

PREGNANCY SUMMARY

No reports describing the use of digoxin immune Fab in the first trimester have been located. There was a case report that described the use of digoxin immune Fab in treating a woman with severe preeclampsia in the third trimester. Several other studies have followed, showing an improved outcome in this patient population, especially if they are positive for an endogenous digitalis-like factor. No drug-induced adverse effects were observed in the fetuses or newborns. The drug will likely not cross the placenta. However, this limited human pregnancy experience (especially first-trimester use) prevents a complete assessment of the embryofetal risk. Animal reproduction studies have not been conducted. Using this drug during pregnancy should be based on the pros and cons of the mother's clinical need for treatment versus any potential fetal risk that might occur from exposure. In cases of digoxin overdose, the maternal benefits of therapy should take priority over any potential embryofetal risk.

BREASTFEEDING SUMMARY

No reports describing the use of digoxin immune Fab during human lactation have been located. It is doubtful that any clinically significant amounts would be excreted into breast milk. Additionally, if any of this antibody fragment were to be ingested through breastfeeding, it would probably be digested in the infant's gastrointestinal tract and not be absorbed. Breastfeeding while using this drug should be based on the mother's clinical need for treatment.

References

1. Prescribing Information. *Digifab*. BTG International; 2021.
2. Goodlin RC. Antidigoxin antibodies in eclampsia. *N Engl J Med*. 1988;318:518-519.
3. Adair CD, Buckalew V, Taylor K, et al. Elevated endoxin-like factor complicating a multifetal second trimester pregnancy: treatment with digoxin-binding immunoglobulin. *Am J Nephrol*. 1996;16:529-531.
4. Adair CD, Luper A, Rose JC, et al. The hemodynamic effects of intravenous digoxin-binding fab immunoglobulin in severe preeclampsia: a double-blind, randomized, clinical trial. *J Perinatol*. 2009;29:284-289.
5. Adair CD, Buckalew VM, Kipikasa J, et al. Repeated dosing of digoxin-fragmented antibody in preterm preeclampsia. *J Perinatol*. 2009;29:163-165.
6. Adair CD, Buckalew VM, Graves SW, et al. Digoxin immune fab treatment for severe preeclampsia. *Am J Perinatol*. 2010;27:655-662.
7. Graves SW, Hopoate-Sitake M, Johnson A, et al. PPo87. Deep trial secondary analysis: digoxin immune fab fragment treatment has additional benefits in endogenous digitalis-like factor positive preeclamptic women. *Pregnancy Hypertens*. 2012;2:287-288.
8. Lam GK, Hopoate-Sitake M, Adair CD, et al. Digoxin antibody fragment, antigen binding (Fab), treatment of preeclampsia in women with endogenous digitalis-like factor: a secondary analysis of the DEEP trial. *Am J Obstet Gynecol*. 2013;209:119.e1-119.e6.

DIHYDROCODEINE

Pain (Opioid Agonist)

PREGNANCY RECOMMENDATION: No Human Data - No Relevant Animal Data (First Trimester)/ Human Data Suggest Risk (Third Trimester)

BREASTFEEDING RECOMMENDATION: Potential Toxicity

D

PREGNANCY SUMMARY

No reports describing the use of dihydrocodeine during human pregnancy were located, other than its use in treating pain during parturition. The drug will likely cross the placenta, so some fetal exposure will probably occur. Therefore, the absence of human pregnancy experience prevents a complete assessment of the embryofetal risk. Animal reproduction studies have not been conducted. Using this drug during pregnancy should be based on the pros and cons of the mother's clinical need for treatment versus any potential fetal risk that might occur from exposure. Chronic use of this drug in the third trimester can increase the risk for neonatal abstinence syndrome in the newborn postdelivery. The drug carries a boxed warning for this. In addition, dihydrocodeine is metabolized via the cytochrome P450 2D6 (CYP2D6) enzyme pathway to an active metabolite, dihydromorphine, just as codeine is metabolized to morphine. Some individuals have a genotype variant of this enzyme that results in ultrarapid metabolism. This can lead to higher-than-expected morphine levels that may increase the risk for respiratory depression.

BREASTFEEDING SUMMARY

In the United States, dihydrocodeine is only available in combination with aspirin and caffeine (see Aspirin and Caffeine). No reports describing the use of dihydrocodeine during human lactation have been located. The drug will likely be found in breast milk (consistent with other opioid drugs), so infant exposure will probably occur. Both aspirin and caffeine are excreted into breast milk. Because of the concern for newborn respiratory depression, especially in the presence of ultrarapid metabolizers, the manufacturer recommends that women not breastfeed while using this drug. ACOG states that if codeine (dihydrocodeine) is used postpartum in a nursing mother, the infant should be closely monitored for excessive sedation. If opiate drugs are needed for postpartum pain management in a nursing mother, other options may be better suited.

References

1. Prescribing Information. *Acetaminophen, caffeine, dihydrocodeine*. Sun Pharmaceutical Inductries; 2020.
2. Gasche Y, Daali Y, Fathi M, et al. Codeine intoxication associated with ultrarapid CYP2D6 metabolism. *N Engl J Med*. 2004;351:2827-2831.
3. Ruch WA, Ruch RM. A preliminary report on dihydrocodeine-scopolamine in obstetrics. *Am J Obstet Gynecol*. 1957;74:1125-1127.
4. Myers JD. A preliminary clinical evaluation of dihydrocodeine bitartrate in normal parturition. *Am J Obstet Gynecol*. 1958;75:1096-1100.
5. Purkis IE. Mepazine (pacatal), meperidine, and dihydrocodeine (nadeine) in labour. *Can Anaesth Soc J*. 1060;7:136-148.
6. Sliom CM. Analgesia during labour: a comparison between dihydrocodeine and pethidine. *S Afr Med J*. 1970;44:317-319.
7. Postpartum Pain Management. ACOG Committee Opinion No. 742. *Obstet Gynecol*. 2018;132:e35-e43.

DIHYDROERGOTAMINE

Autonomic (Ergot Alkaloid)

PREGNANCY RECOMMENDATION: Limited Human Data—Animal Data Suggest Risk

BREASTFEEDING RECOMMENDATION: Probably Compatible

PREGNANCY SUMMARY

A few studies describing the use of dihydroergotamine during human pregnancy were located. About 60 first-trimester exposures have been described with no increased risk for major birth anomalies reported. Other reports describe a few cases with exposure in the latter half of gestation to treat hypotension and migraine headaches without any reported fetal adverse reactions. The drug probably crosses the placenta, so some fetal exposure will likely occur. However, this limited human pregnancy experience prevents a complete assessment of the embryofetal risk. Animal studies did show some embryofetal toxicity in two species at doses less than the RHD. However, treatment in these animals was daily for a longer period than is recommended in humans. Using this drug during pregnancy should be based on the pros and cons of the mother's clinical need for treatment versus any potential fetal risk that might occur from exposure. The drug

(continued)

is technically contraindicated for use with other vasoconstricting drugs. Transient hypertension can also occur with use; therefore, it should be avoided in patients with or at risk for hypertension in pregnancy. Lastly, ergotamine has been shown to have oxytocic properties since the early 1900s and can produce a prolonged and marked increase in uterine tone. This could lead to FHR decelerations that might produce fetal hypoxia. It is not known whether a prolonged increase in uterine tone or contractions could occur with the use of dihydroergotamine, but this should be monitored if the drug is used in the latter portion of gestation.

D

BREASTFEEDING SUMMARY

No reports describing the use of dihydroergotamine during human lactation have been located. The drug will probably be found in breast milk, so some infant exposure will likely occur. A related drug, ergotamine, has been found in human breast milk. Due to a concern for potential serious adverse effects that might be seen in a breastfed infant, the manufacturer recommends that women not breastfeed while being treated with this drug and for at least 3 days after the last dose. Regardless, the issue with dihydroergotamine is that oral bioavailability is only 1%. Therefore, any amount that might be orally absorbed from exposure through human breast milk would likely be clinically insignificant. Dihydroergotamine is a member of the same chemical family as bromocriptine, an agent that is used to suppress lactation. Although no specific information has been located proving this effect, ergot alkaloids may hinder lactation by inhibiting prolactin secretion. If the clinical decision is to use this drug while breastfeeding, the infant should be monitored for the most common reported adult side effects of nausea and dizziness (both leading to irritability), vomiting, insomnia, and diarrhea.

References

1. Prescribing Information. *Dihydroergotamine mesylate*. West-Ward Pharmaceuticals; 2018.
2. Prescribing Information. *Dihydroergotamine mesylate*. Oceanside Pharmaceuticals; 2017.
3. Parfitt K, ed. Martindale. *The Complete Drug Reference*. 32nd ed. Pharmaceutical Press; 1999:444-445.
4. Gill RC, Farrar JM. Experiences with di-hydro-ergotamine in the treatment of primary uterine inertia. *J Obstet Gynaecol Br Emp*. 1951;58:79-91.
5. Altman SG, Waltman R, Lubin S, et al. Oxytocic and toxic actions of dihydroergotamine-45. *Am J Obstet Gynecol*. 1952;64:101-109.
6. Heinonen OP, Sloan D, Shapiro S. *Birth Defects and Drugs in Pregnancy*. Publishing Sciences Group; 1977:358-359.
7. Goeschen K, Peters I, Schneider J. Hypotension in pregnancy, a sequela of adrenal cortex insufficiency? *Geburtshilfe Frauenheilkd*. 1987;47:854-858.
8. Goeschen K, Behrens O, Muhlhaus K, et al. Effect of dihydroergotamine (DHE) on fetal hemodynamics. *Z Geburtshilfe Perinatol*. 1989;193:264-267.
9. Seifritz E, Holsboer-Trachsler E, Haberthur F, et al. Unrecognized pregnancy during citalopram treatment. *Am J Psychiatry*. 1993;150:1428-1429.
10. Berard A, Kori S. Dihydroergotamine (DHE) use during gestation and the risk of adverse pregnancy outcomes. *Headache*. 2012;52:1085-1093.
11. Vorherr H. Contraindications to breast-feeding. *JAMA*. 1974;227:676.

DIHYDROTACHYSTEROL

Vitamin

SEE VITAMIN D

DILTIAZEM

Cardiovascular (Calcium Channel Blocker)

PREGNANCY RECOMMENDATION: Limited Human Data—Animal Data Suggest Risk

BREASTFEEDING RECOMMENDATION: Potential Toxicity

PREGNANCY SUMMARY

A few studies describing the use of diltiazem during human pregnancy were located. Four (13%) anomalies have been seen in about 30 first-trimester exposures, but no pattern to the defects was seen, and the numbers are too small to determine a cause-and-effect relationship. In two larger evaluations analyzing calcium channel blocker drugs as a group, no increased risks for congenital anomalies were seen when compared to unexposed pregnancies. About 10% of the cases were exposed to diltiazem, but specific data were not provided. The drug will probably cross the placenta, so fetal exposure will likely occur. However, this limited human pregnancy experience prevents a complete assessment of the embryofetal risk. Animal studies did show embryofetal toxicity with malformations in three species at doses of less than 10 times the RHD. Using this drug during pregnancy should be based on the pros and cons of the mother's clinical need for treatment versus any potential fetal risk that might occur from exposure.

BREASTFEEDING SUMMARY

One case report was located that described the use of diltiazem during human lactation. The peak breast milk level detected was 230 ng/mL with a calculated RID of about 1%. Due to a concern for potential serious adverse effects that might be seen in a breastfed infant, the manufacturer recommends that women not breastfeed while being treated with this drug. Nevertheless, breastfeeding while using this drug should be based on the mother's clinical need for treatment versus any potential infant risks that might occur. If used, the infant should be monitored for the most common reported adult side effects of nausea, headache, and dizziness (all leading to irritability), rash, and peripheral edema.

References

1. Prescribing Information. *Diltiazem*. Oceanside Pharmaceuticals; 2017.
2. Kogan BA, Iwamoto HS. Lower urinary tract function in the sheep fetus: studies of autonomic control and pharmacologic responses of the fetal bladder. *J Urol*. 1989;141:1019-1024.
3. Lubbe WF. Use of diltiazem during pregnancy. *NZ Med J*. 1987;100:121.
4. Magee LA, Schick B, Donnenfeld AE, et al. The safety of calcium channel blockers in human pregnancy: a prospective, multicenter cohort study. *Am J Obstet Gynecol*. 1996;174:823-828.
5. Lacassie HJ, Germain AM, Valdes G, et al. Management of Eisenmenger syndrome in pregnancy with sildenafil and L-arginine. *Obstet Gynecol*. 2004;103:1118-1120.
6. El-Sayed Y, Holbrook RH Jr. Diltiazem (D) for the maintenance tocolysis of preterm labor (PTL): a prospective randomized trial (abstract). *Am J Obstet Gynecol*. 1996;174:468.
7. Weber-Schoendorfer C, Hannemann D, Meister R, et al. The safety of calcium channel blockers during pregnancy: a prospective, multicenter, observational study. *Reprod Toxicol*. 2008;26:24-30.
8. Okada M, Inoue H, Nakamura Y, et al. Excretion of diltiazem in human milk. *N Engl J Med*. 1985;313:992-993.
9. Committee on Drugs, American Academy of Pediatrics. The transfer of drugs and other chemicals into human milk. *Pediatrics*. 2001;108:776-789.

DIMENHYDRINATE

Antihistamine/Antiemetic

PREGNANCY RECOMMENDATION: Human Data Suggest Low Risk

BREASTFEEDING RECOMMENDATION: Probably Compatible

PREGNANCY SUMMARY

In one large study, 8 (2.5%) major fetal anomalies were described in 319 first-trimester exposures to dimenhydrinate. No pattern to the defects was seen. Another study analyzed a group of 266 newborns with major anomalies compared with a group of 266 newborns without anomalies, and the use of dimenhydrinate in the anomaly group was no different from the control group. The drug probably crosses the placenta, so some fetal exposures will likely occur. Animal studies did not show any embryofetal toxicity or teratogenicity in two species at doses of more than 10 times the RHD. Using this drug during pregnancy should be based on the pros and cons of the mother's clinical need for treatment versus any potential fetal risk that might occur from exposure.

BREASTFEEDING SUMMARY

One study was located that described the use of dimenhydrinate in four lactating women. The drug was not detected in two breast milk samples. It was detected in the other two cases with reported levels of 42 and 100 ng/mL. The calculated RID with the higher concentration was about 1%. Due to a concern for potential serious adverse effects that might be seen in a breastfed infant, the manufacturer recommends that women not breastfeed while being treated with this drug. Nevertheless, breastfeeding while using this drug should be based on the mother's clinical need for treatment versus any potential infant risks that might occur. If used, the infant should be monitored for the most common reported adult side effects of headache and blurred vision (both leading to irritability), drowsiness, constipation, and rash.

References

1. Mellin GW, Katzenstein M. Meclozine and fetal abnormalities. *Lancet*. 1963;1:222-223.
2. Watt LO. Oxytocic effects of dimenhydrinate in obstetrics. *Can Med Assoc J*. 1961;84:533-534.
3. Rotter CW, Whitaker JL, Yared J. The use of intravenous Dramamine to shorten the time of labor and potentiate analgesia. *Am J Obstet Gynecol*. 1958:75:1101-1104.
4. Scott RS, Wallace KH, Badley DN, et al. Use of dimenhydrinate in labor. *Am J Obstet Gynecol*. 1962;83:25-28.
5. Humphreys DW. Safe relief of pain during labor with dimenhydrinate. *Clin Med (Winnetka)*. 1962;69:1165-1168.
6. Cooper K. Failure of dimenhydrinate to shorten labor. *Am J Obstet Gynecol*. 1963;86:1041-1043.
7. Harkins JL, Van Praagh IG, Irwin NT. A clinical evaluation of intravenous dimenhydrinate in labor. *Can Med Assoc J*. 1964;91:164-166.
8. Scott RS. The use of intravenous dimenhydrinate in labor. *New Physician*. 1964;13:302-307.
9. Klieger JA, Massart JJ. Clinical and laboratory survey into the oxytocic effects of dimenhydrinate in labor. *Am J Obstet Gynecol*. 1965;92:1-10.
10. Hay TB, Wood C. The effect of dimenhydrinate on uterine contractions. *Aust NZ J Obstet Gynaecol*. 1967;1:81-89.
11. Shephard B, Cruz A, Spellacy W. The acute effects of Dramamine on uterine contractibility during labor. *J Reprod Med*. 1976;16:27-28.
12. Hara GS, Carter RP, Krantz KE. Dramamine in labor: potential boon or a possible bomb? *J Kans Med Soc*. 1980;81:134-136, 155.
13. Gross S, Librach C, Cecutti A. Maternal weight loss associated with hyperemesis gravidarum: a predictor of fetal outcome. *Am J Obstet Gynecol*. 1989;160:906-909.

D

DIMERCAPROL

Chelating Agent (Antidote)

PREGNANCY RECOMMENDATION: Limited Human Data—Animal Data Suggest Potential Risk (Maternal Benefit May Outweigh Any Embryofetal Risk)

BREASTFEEDING RECOMMENDATION: *Contraindicated (Hold Breastfeeding)

PREGNANCY SUMMARY

No reports describing the use of dimercaprol in the first trimester of pregnancy have been located. A few case reports using the drug in the second and third trimesters were found, and no adverse fetal effects were seen related to the drug. Adverse pregnancy outcomes occurred due to the metal intoxication. The drug will probably cross the placenta, so some fetal exposure will likely occur. Therefore, this limited human pregnancy experience prevents a complete assessment of the embryofetal risk. Animal studies did show embryofetal toxicity in one species at doses of less than 10 times the RHD. However, the maternal benefit, and indirect fetal benefit, for treating heavy metal poisonings appears to outweigh any unknown embryofetal risk. Therefore, if indicated, dimercaprol should not be withheld because of pregnancy.

BREASTFEEDING SUMMARY

No reports describing the use of dimercaprol during human lactation have been located. The drug will probably be found in breast milk, so some infant exposure will likely occur. *Because the use of dimercaprol implies poisoning with arsenic, gold, mercury, or lead, these metals will also likely be excreted into breast milk and are toxic to a nursing infant. Therefore, breastfeeding while using this drug is contraindicated. Breastfeeding can be held (pump and discard) until the poisoning is resolved.

References

1. Bailey B. Are there teratogenic risks associated with antidotes used in the acute management of poisoned pregnant women? *Birth Def Res A Clin Mol Teratol*. 2003;67:133-140.
2. Prescribing Information. *BAL*. Akorn; 2017.
3. Domingo JL. Developmental toxicity of metal chelating agents. *Reprod Toxicol*. 1998;12:499-510.
4. Kantor HI, Levin PM. Arsenical encephalopathy in pregnancy with recovery. *Am J Obstet Gynecol*. 1948;56:370-374.
5. Lugo G, Cassady G, Palmisano P. Acute maternal arsenic intoxication with neonatal death. *Am J Dis Child*. 1969;117:328-330.
6. Tait PA, Vora A, James S, et al. Severe congenital lead poisoning in a preterm infant due to a herbal remedy. *Med J Aust*. 2002;177:193-195.
7. Shannon M. Severe lead poisoning in pregnancy. *Ambul Pediatr*. 2003;3:37-39.

DIMETHYL FUMARATE

Immunologic (Neurologic)

PREGNANCY RECOMMENDATION: Limited Human Data—Animal Data Suggest Potential Risk

BREASTFEEDING RECOMMENDATION: Probably Compatible

PREGNANCY SUMMARY

A few studies were located that described the use of dimethyl fumarate in human pregnancy. In about 30 cases, there appears to have been first-trimester exposure, and the studies state that the defect rate was not increased. However, specific numbers were not supplied. The drug probably crosses the placenta, so some fetal exposure likely occurs. However, this limited human pregnancy experience prevents a complete assessment of the embryofetal risk. Animal studies did show embryofetal toxicity in one species at a dose of less than 10 times the RHD. Using this drug during pregnancy should be based on the pros and cons of the mother's clinical need for treatment versus any potential fetal risk that might occur from exposure. There is a pregnancy exposure registry that monitors pregnancy outcomes in women using this drug. Health care providers are encouraged to call the Tecfidera Pregnancy Exposure Registry at 1-800-456-2255.

BREASTFEEDING SUMMARY

Two studies describing the use of dimethyl fumarate during human lactation were located. In three breastfeeding women, the peak breast milk levels for monomethyl fumarate (MMF) ranged from 3.7 to 83.5 ng/mL. Using the peak levels, the calculated RIDs were all less than 1%. Breastfeeding while using this drug should be based on the mother's clinical need for treatment versus any potential infant risks that might occur. If used, the infant should be monitored for the most common reported adult side effects of nausea and abdominal pain (both leading to irritability), diarrhea, and flushing.

References

1. Prescribing Information. *Tecfidera*. Biogen; 2018.
2. Lu E, Wang BW, Alwan S, et al. A review of safety-related pregnancy data surrounding the oral disease-modifying drugs for multiple sclerosis. *CNS Drugs*. 2014;28:89-94.
3. Gold R, Phillips JT, Havrdova E, et al. Delayed-release dimethyl fumarate and pregnancy preclinical studies and pregnancy outcomes from clinical trials and postmarketing experience. *Neurol Ther*. 2015;4:93-194.
4. Ciplea AI, Datta P, Rewers-Felkins K, et al. Dimethyl fumarate transfer into human milk. *Ther Adv Neurol Disord*. 2020;13:1756286420968414.

DINOPROSTONE

Endocrine/Metabolic (Prostaglandin E2)

PREGNANCY RECOMMENDATION: *Contraindicated First Trimester Use in an Ongoing Pregnancy/Compatible for Second Trimester Uterine Evacuation and Cervical Ripening at Delivery

BREASTFEEDING RECOMMENDATION: *Contraindicated

PREGNANCY SUMMARY

No reports describing human pregnancy outcomes following the use of dinoprostone in failed medical abortions have been located. Use of dinoprostone for cervical ripening near term has not been associated with an excess of adverse outcomes for the infant. *However, in the case of dinoprostone, the most common use of the product would be after the first trimester, and therefore, would be contraindicated in an ongoing pregnancy. Animal reproduction studies have not been located. Using this drug during pregnancy after the first trimester should be based on the pros and cons of the mother's clinical need for treatment versus any potential fetal risk that might occur from exposure.

BREASTFEEDING SUMMARY

No reports describing the use of dinoprostone during human lactation have been located. Endogenous prostaglandin E2 is naturally found in breast milk in low quantities. Prostaglandin E2 levels do go up with dinoprostone use, especially with the 20 mg suppositories, but the very short elimination half-life should limit the amount that is found in human breast milk. *However, the approved use for the drug is cervical ripening and evacuation of uterine contents in the second trimester, and therefore is not indicated for use in a breastfeeding mother.

References

1. Prescribing Information. *Cervidil*. Ferring Pharmaceuticals; 2020.
2. Prescribing Information. *Prostin E2*. Pharmacia & Upjohn; 2020.
3. Arnon J, Ornoy A. Clinical teratology counseling and consultation case report: outcome of pregnancy after failure of early induced abortions. *Teratology*. 1995;52:126-127.

DIPHENHYDRAMINE

Antihistamine (First Generation)

PREGNANCY RECOMMENDATION: Human Data Suggest Low Risk

BREASTFEEDING RECOMMENDATION: Probably Compatible

PREGNANCY SUMMARY

Several large studies have evaluated the use of diphenhydramine during human pregnancy. From a total of more than 2,700 first-trimester exposures, 110 (4.0%) major anomalies were described. But no pattern to the defects was seen. Diphenhydramine has been used for decades in pregnancy for treating symptoms of the common cold and seasonal allergies, and even for the promotion of sleep due to its sedating properties, and no major concerns have been identified. The drug crosses the placenta, so some fetal exposure will occur. Animal studies did not show any embryofetal toxicity or teratogenicity in two species at doses of less than 10 times the RHD. Using this drug during pregnancy should be based on the pros and cons of the mother's clinical need for treatment versus any potential fetal risk that might occur from exposure.

BREASTFEEDING SUMMARY

Diphenhydramine is excreted into human breast milk, but levels have not been reported. Therefore, with maternal use, some infant exposure will occur. Due to a concern for potential serious adverse effects that might be seen in a breastfed infant, the manufacturer recommends that women not breastfeed while being treated with this drug. Nevertheless, breastfeeding while using this drug should be based on the mother's clinical need for treatment versus any potential infant risks that might occur. If used, the infant should be monitored for the most common reported adult side effects of abdominal cramps and dizziness (both leading to irritability), sedation, somnolence, vomiting, constipation, and rash. Because it has anticholinergic properties, it could affect breast milk production, but this has not been thoroughly analyzed.

References

1. Schatz M, Petitti D. Antihistamines and pregnancy. *Ann Allergy Asthma Immunol*. 1997;78:157-159.
2. Prescribing Information. *Benadryl*. Johnson & Johnson Consumer, McNeil Consumer Healthcare; 2018.
3. Yoo GD, Axelson JE, Taylor SM, et al. Placental transfer of diphenhydramine in chronically instrumented pregnant sheep. *J Pharm Sci*. 1986;75:685-687.
4. Heinonen OP, Sloan D, Shapiro S. *Birth Defects and Drugs in Pregnancy*. Publishing Sciences Group; 1977.
5. Saxen I. Cleft palate and maternal diphenhydramine intake. *Lancet*. 1974;1:407-408.
6. Nelson MM, Forfar JO. Associations between drugs administered during pregnancy and congenital abnormalities of the fetus. *Br Med J*. 1971; 1:523-527.
7. Aselton P, Jick H, Milunsky A, et al. First-trimester drug use and congenital disorders. *Obstet Gynecol*. 1985;65:451-455.
8. Parkin DE. Probable Benadryl withdrawal manifestations in a newborn infant. *J Pediatr*. 1974;85:580.
9. Halbrecht I, Komlos L, Shabtay F, et al. Triploidy 69, XXX in a stillborn girl. *Clin Genet*. 1973;4:210-212.
10. Nageotte MP, Briggs GG, Towers CV, et al. Droperidol and diphenhydramine in the management of hyperemesis gravidarum. *Am J Obstet Gynecol*. 1996;174:1801-1806.
11. Turcotte V, Ferreira E, Duperron L. Utilité du dropéridol et de la diphenhydramine dans l'hyperemesis gravidarum. *J Soc Obstet Gynaecol Can*. 2001;23:133-139.
12. Kargas GA, Kargas SA, Bruyere HJ Jr, et al. Perinatal mortality due to interaction of diphenhydramine and temazepam. *N Engl J Med*. 1985;313:1417.
13. Hara GS, Carter RP, Krantz KE. Dramamine in labor: potential boon or a possible bomb? *J Kans Med Soc*. 1980;81:134-136, 155.
14. Brost BC, Scardo JA, Newman RB. Diphenhydramine overdose during pregnancy: lessons from the past. *Am J Obstet Gynecol*. 1996;175:1376-1377.
15. O'Brien TE. Excretion of drugs in human milk. *Am J Hosp Pharm*. 1974; 31:844-854.

DIPHENOXYLATE

Gastrointestinal (Antidiarrheal)

PREGNANCY RECOMMENDATION: Limited Human Data—No Relevant Animal Data

BREASTFEEDING RECOMMENDATION: Potential Toxicity

PREGNANCY SUMMARY

The Collaborative Perinatal Project reported no observed malformations with seven first-trimester exposures to diphenoxylate. The Michigan Medicaid US Food and Drug Administration (FDA) database reported 9 (5.2%) major birth defects in 179 newborns with first-trimester exposure (7 expected). However, the anomalies were random with no specific pattern, and therefore, were not thought to be caused by the drug. One other case report with first-trimester exposure delivered a healthy term infant with no fetal malformations identified. Two other cases were identified in the literature that described newborns with multiple anomalies; however, the exposures were beyond the susceptible stages of development for the identified defects and were not considered causative. The drug will likely cross the placenta, so some fetal exposure will probably occur. Therefore, this limited human pregnancy experience prevents a complete assessment of the embryofetal risk. Animal studies did show some embryofetal toxicity (no teratogenicity) in three animal species, but at doses of more than 10 times the RHD. Using this drug during pregnancy should be based on the pros and cons of the mother's clinical need for treatment versus any potential fetal risk that might occur from exposure. Diphenoxylate has the potential for dependence and overuse and is classified as a Schedule V controlled substance.

BREASTFEEDING SUMMARY

No reports describing the use of diphenoxylate during human lactation have been located. It is available in the United States only combined with atropine (see also Atropine). The drug will likely be found in breast milk, so some infant exposure will probably occur. Breastfeeding while using this drug should be based on the mother's clinical need for treatment. If used, the infant should be monitored for the most common reported adult side effects of nausea, headache, and abdominal pain (all leading to irritability), sedation, and vomiting. Because of the drug's potential for dependence, prolonged use during lactation is not recommended.

References

1. Prescribing Information. *Lomotil*. G.D. Searle LLC Division of Pfizer; 2020.
2. Heinonen OP, Slone D, Shapiro S. *Birth Defects and Drugs in Pregnancy*. Publishing Sciences Group; 1983:287.
3. Gomez-Lobo V, Landy HJ, Matsumoto C, et al. Pregnancy in an intestinal transplant recipient. *Obstet Gynecol*. 2012;120:497-500.
4. Siebert JR, Barr M Jr, Jackson JC, et al. Ebstein's anomaly and extracardiac defects. *Am J Dis Child*. 1989;143:570-572.
5. Ho CK, Kaufman RL, McAlister WH. Congenital malformations. *Am J Dis Child*. 1975;129:714-716.

DIPHTHERIA/TETANUS TOXOIDS/ACELLULAR PERTUSSIS VACCINE ADSORBED

SEE VACCINE, TETANUS TOXOID/REDUCED DIPHTHERIA TOXOID/ACELLULAR PERTUSSIS ADSORBED

D

DIPYRIDAMOLE

Hematologic (Antiplatelet)

PREGNANCY RECOMMENDATION: Limited Human Data—Animal Data Suggest Low Risk

BREASTFEEDING RECOMMENDATION: Probably Compatible

PREGNANCY SUMMARY

Numerous studies have been located that describe the use of dipyridamole during human pregnancy. Most of these exposures have occurred in the second and third trimesters. Of the few first-trimester uses, a couple of infants with major anomalies were described, but the mothers were also on warfarin. The described defects were consistent with warfarin use. The drug probably crosses the placenta, so some fetal exposure will likely occur. However, this limited human pregnancy experience prevents a complete assessment of the embryofetal risk. Using this drug during pregnancy should be based on the pros and cons of the mother's clinical need for treatment versus any potential fetal risk that might occur from exposure. Because dipyridamole is used as an adjunct with warfarin, warfarin use in the first trimester should be avoided, if possible (see Warfarin). Therefore, the use of dipyridamole in the first trimester should be rare.

BREASTFEEDING SUMMARY

Dipyridamole was reported to be found in human breast milk by the manufacturer, but details were not provided. However, this suggests that some infant exposure will occur. The effect of this exposure on a nursing infant is unknown. Breastfeeding while using this drug should be based on the mother's clinical need for treatment versus any potential infant risks that might occur. If used, the infant should be monitored for the most common reported adult side effects of abdominal cramps, headache, and dizziness (all leading to irritability) and rash.

References

1. Product information. *Persantine*. Boehringer Ingelheim Pharmaceuticals; 2018.
2. Tejani N. Anticoagulant therapy with cardiac valve prosthesis during pregnancy. *Obstet Gynecol*. 1973;42:785-793.
3. Del Bosque MR. Dipyridamole and anticoagulants in the management of pregnant women with cardiac valvular prosthesis. *Ginecol Obstet Mex*. 1973;33:191-198.
4. Littler WA, Bonnar J, Redman CWG, et al. Reduced pulmonary arterial compliance in hypertensive patients. *Lancet*. 1973;1:1274-1278.
5. Biale Y, Lewenthal H, Gueron M, et al. Caesarean section in patient with mitral-valve prosthesis. *Lancet*. 1977;1:907.
6. Taguchi K. Pregnancy in patients with a prosthetic heart valve. *Surg Gynecol Obstet*. 1977;145:206-208.
7. Ahmad R, Rajah SM, Mearns AJ, et al. Dipyridamole in successful management of pregnant women with prosthetic heart valve. *Lancet*. 1976;2:1414-1415.
8. Biale Y, Cantor A, Lewenthal H, et al. The course of pregnancy in patients with artificial heart valves treated with dipyridamole. *Int J Gynaecol Obstet*. 1980;18:128-132.
9. Salazar E, Zajarias A, Gutierrez N, et al. The problem of cardiac valve prostheses, anticoagulants, and pregnancy. *Circulation*. 1984;70(suppl 1):I169-I177.
10. Lauchkner W, Schwarz R, Retzke U. Cardiovascular action of dipyridamole in advanced pregnancy. *Zentralbl Gynaekol*. 1981;103:220-227.
11. Beaufils M, Uzan S, Donsimoni R, et al. Prevention of pre-eclampsia by early antiplatelet therapy. *Lancet*. 1985;1:840-842.
12. Beaufils M, Uzan S, Donsimoni R, et al. Prospective controlled study of early antiplatelet therapy in prevention of preeclampsia. *Adv Nephrol*. 1986;15:87-94.
13. Wallenburg HCS, Rotmans N. Prevention of recurrent idiopathic fetal growth retardation by low-dose aspirin and dipyridamole. *Am J Obstet Gynecol*. 1987;157:1230-1235.
14. Uzan S, Beaufils M, Bazin B, et al. Idiopathic recurrent fetal growth retardation and aspirin-dipyridamole therapy. *Am J Obstet Gynecol*. 1989;160:763.
15. Wallenburg HCS, Rotmans N. Idiopathic recurrent fetal growth retardation and aspirin-dipyridamole therapy. Reply. *Am J Obstet Gynecol*. 1989;160:763-764.
16. Wallenburg HCS, Rotmans N. Prophylactic low-dose aspirin and dipyridamole in pregnancy. *Lancet*. 1988;1:939.
17. Capetta P, Airoldi ML, Tasca A, et al. Prevention of pre-eclampsia and placental insufficiency. *Lancet*. 1986;1:919.
18. Romero R, Lockwood C, Oyarzun E, et al. Toxemia: new concepts in an old disease. *Semin Perinatol*. 1988;12:302-323.
19. van Vliet EO, Askie LA, Mol BW, et al. Antiplatelet agents and the prevention of spontaneous preterm birth: a systematic review and meta-analysis. *Obstet Gynecol*. 2017;129:327-336.

DISOPYRAMIDE

Cardiovascular (Antiarrhythmic)

PREGNANCY RECOMMENDATION: Limited Human Data - Animal Data Suggest Potential Risk

BREASTFEEDING RECOMMENDATION: Probably Compatible

D

PREGNANCY SUMMARY

Several case reports have been located that describe the use of disopyramide during human pregnancy. Two of these reported the use of the drug throughout pregnancy, and both delivered healthy newborns with no reported anomalies. A total of 6 other case reports involving 12 delivered pregnancies were located that described the use of disopyramide in the second and third trimesters or at delivery. No adverse maternal or infant effects were noted. The drug crosses the placenta, so some fetal exposure will occur. However, this limited human pregnancy experience prevents a complete assessment of the embryofetal risk. Animal studies showed embryofetal toxicity in one species at doses of less than 10 times the RHD, but not in a second species at doses of more than 10 times the RHD. Using this drug during pregnancy should be based on the pros and cons of the mother's clinical need for treatment versus any potential fetal risk that might occur from exposure. The drug carries a boxed warning for an increased risk of cardiovascular mortality. It has also been shown to prolong the QT interval and widen the QRS complex.

BREASTFEEDING SUMMARY

A total of five case reports were located that described the use of disopyramide during human lactation. The drug and the active metabolite N-monodesalkyl disopyramide (NMD) were found in most breast milk samples. In two women, both the drug and NMD were measured, and the combined levels using the peak concentrations resulted in calculated RIDs of 18% and 13%. Average values of the drugs in breast milk would produce RIDs closer to 10%. When only disopyramide was measured, the calculated RIDs using peak levels were 2.6% and 6.7%. However, in four of these five cases, infant serum levels were measured. In two, levels were not detected (LLQ of 450 and 500 ng/mL). In the remaining two infants, serum levels for the drugs were only about 7.5% and 12.5% of the maternal concentrations. Because of these low infant serum levels, use of disopyramide is probably compatible with breastfeeding. Nevertheless, breastfeeding while using this drug should be based on the mother's clinical need for treatment versus any potential infant risks that might occur. If used, the infant should be monitored for the most common reported adult side effects of nausea, headache, myalgias, blurred vision, and dizziness (all leading to irritability), fatigue (lethargy), and constipation.

References

1. Prescribing Information. *Norpace*. G. D. Searle LLC Division of Pfizer; 2023.
2. Shaxted EJ, Milton PJ. Disopyramide in pregnancy: a case report. *Curr Med Res Opin*. 1979;6:70-72.
3. Ellsworth AJ, Horn JR, Raisys VA, et al. Disopyramide and N-monodesalkyl disopyramide in serum and breast milk. *Drug Intell Clin Pharm*. 1989;23:56-57.
4. Tadmor OP, Keren A, Rosenak D, et al. The effect of disopyramide on uterine contractions during pregnancy. *Am J Obstet Gynecol*. 1990;162:482-486.
5. MacKintosh D, Buchanan N. Excretion of disopyramide in human breast milk. *Br J Clin Pharmacol*. 1985;19:856-857.
6. Leonard RF, Braun TE, Levy AM. Initiation of uterine contractions by disopyramide during pregnancy. *N Engl J Med*. 1978;299:84-85.
7. Stokes IM, Evans J, Stone M. Myocardial infarction and cardiac arrest in the second trimester followed by assisted vaginal delivery under epidural analgesia at 38 weeks gestation. Case report. *Br J Obstet Gynaecol*. 1984;91:197-198.
8. Abbi M, Kriplani A, Singh B. Preterm labor and accidental hemorrhage after disopyramide therapy in pregnancy; A case report. *J Reprod Med*. 1999;44:653-655.
9. Barnett DB, Hudson SA, McBurney A. Disopyramide and its N-monodesalkyl metabolite in breast milk. *Br J Clin Pharmacol*. 1982;14:310-312.
10. Hoppu K, Neuvonen PJ, Korte T. Disopyramide and breast feeding. *Br J Clin Pharmacol*. 1986;21:553.
11. Wakaumi M, Tsuruoka S, Sakamoto K, et al. Pilsicainide in breast milk from a mother: comparison with disopyramide and propafenone. *Br J Clin Pharmacol*. 2004;59:120-121.

DISULFIRAM

Miscellaneous (Alcohol Antagonist)

PREGNANCY RECOMMENDATION: Limited Human Data—No Relevant Animal Data

BREASTFEEDING RECOMMENDATION: Potential Toxicity

PREGNANCY SUMMARY

The Michigan Medicaid Surveillance study reported 1 (4%) major anomaly in 25 first-trimester exposures to the drug. Numerous other case reports and small series have been published that describe about 38 other pregnancies. Several normal newborns were reported, along with many that had major birth defects, some of which could be drug exposure-based. However, case reports are often biased toward the reporting of abnormal outcomes. The drug most likely crosses the placenta, so some fetal exposure will probably occur. However, this limited human pregnancy experience prevents a complete assessment of the embryofetal risk. Animal reproduction studies have not been located. Using this drug during pregnancy should be based on the pros and cons of the mother's clinical need for treatment versus any potential fetal risk that might occur from exposure.

BREASTFEEDING SUMMARY

No reports describing the use of disulfiram during human lactation have been located. The drug will probably be found in breast milk, so some infant exposure will likely occur. Due to a concern for potential serious adverse effects that might be seen in a breastfed infant, the manufacturer recommends that women not breastfeed while being treated with this drug. Breastfeeding while using this drug should be based on the mother's clinical need for treatment versus any potential infant risks that might occur. However, alcohol use during breastfeeding is not recommended, and if a deterrent is needed, other options for abstaining from alcohol use might be considered.

References

1. Prescribing Information. *Disulfiram*. Teva Pharmaceuticals USA; 2020.
2. Shepard TH. *Catalog of Teratogenic Agents*. 6th ed. Johns Hopkins University Press; 1989:239-240.
3. Favre-Tissot M, Delatour P. Psychopharmacologie et teratogenese a propos du sulfirame: essal experimental. *Ann Med Psychol*. 1965;1:735-740. As cited in Shepard TH. Catalog of Teratogenic Agents. 6th ed. Johns Hopkins University Press, 1989:239-240.
4. Nora AH, Nora JJ, Blu J. Limb-reduction anomalies in infants born to disulfiram-treated alcoholic mothers. *Lancet*. 1977;2:664.
5. Hamon B, Soyez C, Jonville AP, et al. Grossesse chez les malades traitées par le disulfirame. *Press Med*. 1991;20:1092.
6. Gardner RJM, Clarkson JE. A malformed child whose previously alcoholic mother had taken disulfiram. *NZ Med J*. 1981;93:184-186. As cited in Reitnauer PJ, Callanan NP, Farber RA, Aylsworth AS. Prenatal exposure to disulfiram implicated in the cause of malformations in discordant monozygotic twins. Teratology. 1997;56:358-362.
7. Dehaene P, Titran M, Dubois D. Syndrome de Pierre Robin et malformations cardiaques chez un nouveau-ne. *Presse Med*. 1984;13:1394-1395. As cited in Reitnauer PJ, Callanan NP, Farber RA, Aylsworth AS. Prenatal exposure to disulfiram implicated in the cause of malformations in discordant monozygotic twins. Teratology. 1997;56:358-362.
8. Helmbrecht GD, Hoskins IA. First trimester disulfiram exposure: report of two cases. *Am J Perinatol*. 1993;10:5-7.
9. Reitnauer PJ, Callanan NP, Farber RA, et al. Prenatal exposure to disulfiram implicated in the cause of malformations in discordant monozygotic twins. *Teratology*. 1997;56:358-362.
10. Johnson KA, Jones KL, Chambers CC, et al. The effect of disulfiram on the unborn baby (abstract). *Teratology*. 1991;43:438.

DOBUTAMINE

Cardiovascular (Inotropic Agent)

PREGNANCY RECOMMENDATION: Limited Human Data—Animal Data Suggest Low Risk

BREASTFEEDING RECOMMENDATION: Probably Compatible

PREGNANCY SUMMARY

Only a few case reports exist that describe the use of dobutamine during human pregnancy. All of these occurred in the second or third trimester. No adverse effects for the fetus related to the drug were described. The drug will probably cross the placenta, but overall fetal exposure is likely to be very small (2-minute elimination half-life and high plasma protein binding). Therefore, this limited human pregnancy experience prevents a complete assessment of the embryofetal risk. Animal studies did not show any embryofetal toxicity or teratogenicity in two species at doses of less than 10 times the RHD. Using this drug during pregnancy should be based on the pros and cons of the mother's clinical need for treatment versus any potential fetal risk that might occur from exposure.

BREASTFEEDING SUMMARY

No reports describing the use of dobutamine during human lactation have been located. The drug will probably be found in human breast milk, so some infant exposure might occur. However, the amount should be limited due to the high plasma protein binding and the 2-minute elimination half-life. Furthermore, it is only used for a few hours in most instances, and therefore, holding breastfeeding is an option. Based on the elimination half-life, dobutamine should be out of the maternal system by 30 minutes after the drug is discontinued.

References

1. Prescribing Information. *Dobutamine*. Hospira; 2018.
2. Stokes IM, Evans J, Stone M. Myocardial infarction and cardiac arrest in the second trimester followed by assisted vaginal delivery under epidural analgesia at 38 weeks gestation. Case report. *Br J Obstet Gynaecol*. 1984;91:197-198.
3. Graves C, Wheeler T, Troiano N. The effect of dobutamine hydrochloride on ventricular function and oxygen transport in patients with severe preeclampsia (abstract). *Am J Obstet Gynecol*. 1996;174:332.
4. Cho FN. Management of pregnant women with cardiac diseases at potential risk of thromboembolism—experience and review. *Int J Cardiol*. 2009;136:229-232.

DOCETAXEL

Antineoplastic (Antimitotic)

PREGNANCY RECOMMENDATION: Limited Human Data—Animal Data Suggest Risk

BREASTFEEDING RECOMMENDATION: Potential Toxicity

D

PREGNANCY SUMMARY

Several case reports describing the use of docetaxel during human pregnancy were located. Docetaxel use was always in combination with other antineoplastics. A total of 10 cases were described, and overall, the newborns in every case (except one) did well with no reported adverse effects related to the drug combinations. In one case, multiple congenital anomalies were found, but exposure was in the third trimester. There was one exposure in the first trimester (pregnancy unknown) and one treated at 12 weeks of gestation, both without any congenital defects identified. The others were all treated in the second and third trimesters. The drug appears to cross the placenta in low amounts, so some fetal exposure will likely occur. However, this limited human pregnancy experience prevents a complete assessment of the embryofetal risk. Animal data did show some embryofetal toxicity in two species (no teratogenicity), at doses less than the RHD, but treatment occurred daily for 10 to 13 days. Human exposure (in the majority of cases) would occur only once every 21 days. It is not possible to correlate this difference. Using this drug during pregnancy should be based on the pros and cons of the mother's clinical need for treatment versus any potential fetal risk that might occur from exposure. The product contains 276 mg of alcohol per milliliter. To put this into perspective, one of the larger doses for docetaxel is 115 mg/m2. On average, a 70 kg person has a body surface area (BSA) of about 1.73/m2, which suggests a treatment of about 200 mg of docetaxel. This would require about 20 mL of docetaxel (10 mg/mL). This 20 mL would contain about 5,520 mg of alcohol. A standard drink in the United States is 0.6 fl oz, which is 14 g (14,000 mg) of alcohol. The amount of alcohol to be administered is about 40% of one 12-oz (5% alcohol) beer or one 5-oz (12%) wine. Some docetaxel products do not contain alcohol.

BREASTFEEDING SUMMARY

No reports describing the use of docetaxel during human lactation have been reported. The drug will probably be found in breast milk, so some infant exposure will likely occur. Due to a concern for potential serious adverse effects that might be seen in a breastfed infant, the manufacturer recommends that women not breastfeed while being treated with this drug and for at least 1 week after the last dose. Nevertheless, breastfeeding while using this drug should be based on the mother's clinical need for treatment versus any potential infant risks that might occur. If used, the infant should be monitored for the most common reported adult side effects of nausea, myalgia, and neuropathy (all leading to irritability), diarrhea, alopecia, vomiting, decreased appetite (monitor growth), rash, and various laboratory abnormalities (see PI).

References

1. Prescribing Information. *Taxotere*. Sanofi-Aventis; 2019.
2. Berveiller P, Vinot C, Mir O, et al. Comparative transplacental transfer of taxanes using the human perfused cotyledon placental model. *Am J Obstet Gynecol*. 2012;207:514.e1-514.e7.
3. De Santis M, Lucchese A, De Carlos S, et al. Metastatic breast cancer in pregnancy: first case of chemotherapy with docetaxel. *Eur J Cancer Care (Engl)*. 2000;9:235-237.
4. Nieto Y, Santisteban M, Armendia JM, et al. Docetaxel administered during pregnancy for inflammatory breast carcinoma. *Clin Breast Cancer*. 2006;6:533-534.
5. Potluri V, Lewis D, Burton GV. Chemotherapy with taxanes in breast cancer during pregnancy: case report and review of the literature. *Clin Breast Cancer*. 2006;7;167-170.
6. Gainford MC, Clemons M. Breast cancer in pregnancy: are taxanes safe? *Clin Oncol (R Coll Radiol)*. 2006;18:159.
7. Sekar R, Stone PR. Trastuzumab use for metastatic breast cancer in pregnancy. *Obstet Gynecol*. 2007;110:507-510.
8. Kim JH, Kim HS, Sung CW, et al. Docetaxel, gemcitabine, and cisplatin administered for non-small cell lung cancer during the first and second trimester of an unrecognized pregnancy. *Lung Cancer*. 2008;59:270-273.
9. Rouzi AA, Sahly NN, Sahly NF, et al. Cisplatinum and docetaxel for ovarian cancer in pregnancy. *Arch Gynecol Obstet*. 2009;280:823-825.
10. Yates R, Zhang J. Lung cancer in pregnancy: an unusual case of complete response to chemotherapy. *Cureus*. 2015;7:e440.
11. Aktoz F, Yalcin AC, Yuzdemir HS, et al. Treatment of massive liver metastasis of breast cancer during pregnancy: first report of a complete remission with trastuzumab and review of the literature. *J Matern Fetal Neonatal Med*. 2018;33:1-6.

DOCUSATE CALCIUM

Gastrointestinal (Laxative)

SEE DOCUSATE SODIUM

DOCUSATE POTASSIUM

Gastrointestinal (Laxative)

SEE DOCUSATE SODIUM

DOCUSATE SODIUM

Gastrointestinal (Laxative)

PREGNANCY RECOMMENDATION: Human Data Suggest Compatible

BREASTFEEDING RECOMMENDATION: Compatible

D

PREGNANCY SUMMARY

From four large population studies, a total of 1,054 pregnancies were exposed to docusate sodium in the first trimester, with 15 (1.4%) major anomalies identified. In addition, no pattern was seen in the anomalies that occurred. Furthermore, the drug is so poorly absorbed systemically that measurable levels cannot be detected. Therefore, these data do not support an association between the drug and congenital birth defects. Animal reproduction studies have not been conducted. Using this drug during pregnancy should be based on the pros and cons of the mother's clinical need for treatment versus any potential fetal risk that might occur from exposure.

BREASTFEEDING SUMMARY

A combination of docusate sodium and dihydroxyanthraquinone was given to 35 postpartum breastfeeding women. One infant developed diarrhea, but the relationship between the symptom and the laxative is unknown. Because the drug is not systemically absorbed to any measurable level, it will not likely be found in breast milk. However, studies on this have not been conducted. Breastfeeding while using this drug should be based on the mother's clinical need for treatment. If used, the infant should be monitored for the most common reported adult side effects of nausea and abdominal pain (both leading to irritability), diarrhea, and vomiting.

References

1. Prescribing Information. *Docusate sodium*. American Health Pkg; 2023.
2. Heinonen OP, Slone D, Shapiro S. *Birth Defects and Drugs in Pregnancy*. Publishing Sciences Group; 1983: 385, 442.
3. Jick H, Holmes LB, Hunter JR, et al. First-trimester drug use and congenital disorders. *JAMA*. 1981;246:343-346.
4. Aselton P, Jich H, Milunsky A, et al. First-trimester drug use and congenital disorders. *Obstet Gynecol*. 1985;65:451-455.
5. Schindler AM. Isolated neonatal hypomagnesaemia associated with maternal overuse of stool softener. *Lancet*. 1984;2:822.
6. Greenhalf JO, Leonard HSD. Laxatives in the treatment of constipation in pregnant and breast-feeding mothers. *Practitioner*. 1973;210:259-263.

DOFETILIDE

Cardiovascular (Antiarrhythmic)

PREGNANCY RECOMMENDATION: No Human Data—Animal Data Suggest Risk (Maternal Benefit May Outweigh Embryo–Fetal Risk)

BREASTFEEDING RECOMMENDATION: Potential Toxicity

PREGNANCY SUMMARY

No reports describing the use of dofetilide in human pregnancy have been located. The drug will probably cross the placenta, so some fetal exposure will likely occur. Therefore, the absence of human pregnancy experience prevents a complete assessment of the embryofetal risk. Animal data showed embryofetal toxicity and malformations in two species at doses less than 10 times the RHD. Using this drug during pregnancy should be based on the pros and cons of the mother's clinical need for treatment versus any potential fetal risk that might occur from exposure. In some clinical cases, the maternal benefit may outweigh the fetal risk. The drug can prolong the QT interval, and it has a boxed warning for serious ventricular arrhythmias.

BREASTFEEDING SUMMARY

No reports describing the use of dofetilide during human lactation have been located. The drug will probably be found in breast milk, so some infant exposure will likely occur. The effect of this exposure on a nursing infant is unknown. Breastfeeding while using this drug should be based on the mother's clinical need for treatment. If used, the infant should be monitored for the most common reported adult side effects of nausea, headache, and dizziness (all leading to irritability), diarrhea, and rash.

Reference

1. Prescribing Information. *Dofetilide*. Pfizer; 2023.

D

DOLASETRON

Gastrointestinal (Antiemetic)

PREGNANCY RECOMMENDATION: No Human Data—Animal Data Suggest Low Risk

BREASTFEEDING RECOMMENDATION: Probably Compatible

PREGNANCY SUMMARY

No reports describing the use of dolasetron in human pregnancy have been located. The drug will probably cross the placenta, so some fetal exposure will likely occur. Therefore, the absence of human pregnancy experience prevents a complete assessment of the embryofetal risk. Animal studies did not show any embryofetal toxicity in two species. Using this drug during pregnancy should be based on the pros and cons of the mother's clinical need for treatment versus any potential fetal risk that might occur from exposure. The drug has been shown to prolong the QT interval.

BREASTFEEDING SUMMARY

No reports describing the use of dolasetron during human lactation have been located. The drug will likely be excreted into breast milk. Breastfeeding while using this drug should be based on the mother's clinical need for treatment. If used, the infant should be monitored for the most common reported adult side effects of headache and abdominal pain (both leading to irritability), fatigue (lethargy), and diarrhea.

Reference

1. Prescribing Information. *Anzemet*. Validus Pharmaceuticals; 2020.

DOLUTEGRAVIR

Antiretroviral (Integrase Strand Transfer Inhibitor)

PREGNANCY RECOMMENDATION: Human Data Suggested Low Risk (Maternal Benefit May Outweigh Any Embryofetal Risk)

BREASTFEEDING RECOMMENDATION: *Contraindicated

PREGNANCY SUMMARY

Several reports have been located that describe the use of dolutegravir in human pregnancy. There was an initial study of 426 first-trimester exposures to the drug, and 4 (0.94%) neural tube defects (NTDs) occurred. However, several follow-up studies have occurred with nearly 2,000 first-trimester exposures, and this risk was no longer found when compared with other pregnancies of women infected with HIV. The overall risk for major anomalies does not appear to be increased above the human baseline risk. The drug crosses the placenta, so some fetal exposure will occur. Animal studies did not show any embryofetal toxicity or teratogenicity in two species at doses of more than 10 times the RHD. In order to decrease the risk for perinatal transmission of HIV-1 to the neonate, this drug should not be withheld if a pregnant woman is infected with HIV-1, especially if she has a positive viral load or is failing her current treatment regimen, and she is a candidate for this drug's usage.

BREASTFEEDING SUMMARY

Dolutegravir has been evaluated in numerous lactating women. A total of 37 women, all treated with 50 mg daily, had positive breast milk levels for the drug. Using the peak values, the maximum calculated RIDs were less than 5%. *However, the current Centers for Disease Control and Prevention recommendation is that mothers infected with HIV should not breastfeed their infants in order to reduce the risk of postnatal transmission of the virus to the neonate. In a clinical setting where a mother is not infected with HIV (or in cases where the HIV viral load is negative), the drug by itself is probably compatible.

References

1. Prescribing Information. *Tivicay*. ViiV Healthcare; 2018.
2. Rimawi BH, Johnson E, Rajakumar A, et al. Pharmacokinetics and placental transfer for elvitegravir, dolutegravir, and other antiretrovirals during pregnancy. *Antimicrob Agents Chemother*. 2017;61;e02213-e02216.
3. Zash R, Jacobson DL, Diseko M, et al. Comparative safety of dolutegravir-based or efavirenz-based antiretroviral treatment started during pregnancy in Botswana: an observational study. *Lancet Glob Health*. 2018;6:e804-e810.
4. Zash R, Makhema J, Shapiro RL. Neural-tube defects with dolutegravir treatment from the time of conception. *N Engl J Med*. 2018;379:979-981.
5. Zash R, Holmes L, Diseko M, et al. Neural-tube defects antiretroviral treatment regimens in Botswana. *N Engl J Med*. 2019;381:827-840.
6. Bornhede R, Soeria-Atmadja S, Westling K, et al. Dolutegravir in pregnancy-effects on HIV-positive women and their infants. *Eur J Clin Microbiol Infect Dis*. 2018;37:495-500.

7. Vannappagari V, Thorne C, for APR and EPPICC. Pregnancy and neonatal outcomes following prenatal exposure to dolutegravir. *J Acquir Immune Defic Syndr*. 2019;81(4):371-378.
8. Kobbe R, Schalkwijk S, Dunay G, et al. Dolutegravir in breast milk and maternal and infant plasma during breastfeeding. *AIDS*. 2016;30:2731-2735.
9. Department of Health and Human Services. *Recommendations for the use of antiretroviral drugs during pregnancy and interventions to reduce perinatal HIV transmission in the United States*. Infant feeding for individuals with HIV in the United States; 2023. https://clinicalinfo.hiv.go
10. Chinula L, Ziemba L, Brummel S, et al. Efficacy and safety of three antiretroviral therapy regimens started in pregnancy up to 50 weeks post partum: a multicentre, open-label, randomised, controlled, phase 3 trial. *Lancet HIV*. 2023;10:e363-e374.

D

DONANEMAB

Central Nervous System (Monoclonal Antibody—Alzheimer Disease)

PREGNANCY RECOMMENDATION: No Human Data and No Relevant Animal Data

BREASTFEEDING RECOMMENDATION: Probably Compatible

PREGNANCY SUMMARY

No reports describing the use of donanemab in human pregnancy have been located. As an IgG antibody, it likely crosses the placenta, especially during the second half of pregnancy, so some fetal exposure will probably occur. Therefore, the absence of human pregnancy experience prevents a complete assessment of the embryofetal risk. Animal reproduction and fertility studies have not been conducted. Using this drug during pregnancy should be based on the pros and cons of the mother's clinical need for treatment versus any potential fetal risk that might occur from exposure. Alzheimer disease is very rare in women of childbearing age. In addition, using donanemab requires numerous brain magnetic resonance imaging (MRI) scans to monitor for the development of amyloid-related imaging abnormalities (ARIA). The drug carries a boxed warning for this risk. Therefore, this factor also needs to be considered if using this drug during pregnancy is an option.

BREASTFEEDING SUMMARY

No reports describing the use of donanemab during human lactation have been located. It is known that IgG antibodies can be found in human breast milk, but are not found in the neonatal or infant circulation. Additionally, if any IgG antibodies were to be ingested through breastfeeding, they would probably be digested in the infant's gastrointestinal tract and not be absorbed. Nevertheless, breastfeeding while using this drug should be based on the mother's clinical need for treatment. If used, the infant should be monitored for the most common reported adult side effect of headache (leading to irritability).

Reference

1. Prescribing Information. *Kisunla*. Eli Lilly; 2024.

DONEPEZIL

Central Nervous System (Acetylcholinesterase Inhibitor)

PREGNANCY RECOMMENDATION: No Human Data—Animal Data Suggest Potential Risk

BREASTFEEDING RECOMMENDATION: Potential Toxicity

PREGNANCY SUMMARY

No reports describing the use of donepezil in human pregnancy have been located. The drug and its active metabolites will probably cross the placenta, so some fetal exposure will likely occur. Therefore, the absence of human pregnancy experience prevents a complete assessment of the embryofetal risk. Animal studies did show some embryofetal toxicity in one species at doses less than 10 times the RHD. Using this drug during pregnancy should be based on the pros and cons of the mother's clinical need for treatment versus any potential fetal risk that might occur from exposure.

BREASTFEEDING SUMMARY

No reports describing the use of donepezil during human lactation have been located. The drug and its active metabolites will probably be found in breast milk, so some infant exposure will likely occur. Breastfeeding while using this drug should be based on the mother's clinical need for treatment. If used, the infant should be monitored for the most common reported adult side effects of nausea and myalgia (both leading to irritability), diarrhea, fatigue (lethargy), vomiting, insomnia, and decreased appetite.

Reference

1. Prescribing Information. *Donepezil*. Hisun Pharmaceuticals USA; 2020.

DOPAMINE

Cardiovascular (Inotropic Agent)

PREGNANCY RECOMMENDATION: Limited Human Data—Animal Data Suggest Low Risk

BREASTFEEDING RECOMMENDATION: Probably Compatible

D

PREGNANCY SUMMARY

Only a few case reports exist that describe the use of dopamine during human pregnancy. All of these occurred in the second or third trimester. No adverse effects for the fetus related to the drug were described. The drug will probably cross the placenta, but overall fetal exposure is likely to be very small (2-minute elimination half-life). Therefore, this limited human pregnancy experience prevents a complete assessment of the embryofetal risk. Animal studies did not show any embryofetal toxicity or teratogenicity in two species at doses of less than 10 times the RHD. Using this drug during pregnancy should be based on the pros and cons of the mother's clinical need for treatment versus any potential fetal risk that might occur from exposure.

BREASTFEEDING SUMMARY

No reports describing the use of dopamine during human lactation have been located. The drug may be found in human breast milk, but the overall amount is likely to be small (due to the 2-minute elimination half-life). Because it is only indicated for life-threatening situations, it is doubtful if any lactation reports will occur. In addition, breastfeeding should not prevent treatment with this drug. Based on the elimination half-life, dopamine should be out of the maternal system by 30 minutes after the drug is discontinued.

References

1. Prescribing Information. *Dopamine oral*. Deseret Biologicals; 2018.
2. Prescribing Information. *Dopamine injection*. Hospira; 2018.
3. Fishburne JI Jr, Dormer KJ, Payne GG, et al. Effects of amrinone and dopamine on uterine blood flow and vascular responses in the gravid baboon. *Am J Obstet Gynecol*. 1988;158:829-837.
4. Clark RB, Brunner JA III. Dopamine for the treatment of spinal hypotension during cesarean section. *Anesthesiology*. 1980;53:514-517.
5. Gerstner G, Grunberger W. Dopamine treatment for prevention of renal failure in patients with severe eclampsia. *Clin Exp Obstet Gynecol*. 1980; 7:219-222.
6. Nasu K, Yoshimatsu J, Anai T, et al. Low-dose dopamine in treating acute renal failure caused by preeclampsia. *Gynecol Obstet Invest*. 1996;42:140-141.
7. Kirshon B, Lee W, Mauer MB, et al. Effects of low-dose dopamine therapy in the oliguric patient with preeclampsia. *Am J Obstet Gynecol*. 1988;159: 604-607.
8. Leduc L, Kirshon B, Diaz SF, et al. Intrathecal morphine analgesia and low-dose dopamine for oliguria in severe maternal pulmonary hypertension—a case report. *J Reprod Med*. 1990;35:727-729.

DORAVIRINE

Antiretroviral (Non-Nucleoside Reverse Transcriptase Inhibitor)

PREGNANCY RECOMMENDATION: No Human Data—Animal Data Suggest Low Risk (Maternal Benefit May Outweigh Embryofetal Risk)

BREASTFEEDING RECOMMENDATION: *Contraindicated

PREGNANCY SUMMARY

No reports describing the use of doravirine in human pregnancy have been located. The drug will cross the placenta, so some fetal exposure will occur. Therefore, the absence of human pregnancy experience prevents a complete assessment of the embryofetal risk. Animal studies did not show any embryofetal toxicity in two species at doses less than 10 times the RHD. In order to decrease the perinatal transmission of HIV-1 to the neonate, this drug should not be withheld if a pregnant woman is infected with HIV-1 with a positive viral load and she is a candidate for this drug's usage. There is a pregnancy exposure registry that monitors pregnancy outcomes in patients using this drug during gestation. Health care providers are encouraged to call the APR at 1-800-258-4263. Doravirine is not indicated for use in treating HIV-2.

BREASTFEEDING SUMMARY

No reports describing the use of doravirine during human lactation have been located. The drug will likely be found in breast milk. *However, the current Centers for Disease Control and Prevention recommendation is that mothers infected with HIV should not breastfeed their infants in order to reduce the risk of postnatal transmission of the virus to the neonate. In a clinical setting where a mother is not infected with HIV (or in cases where the HIV viral load is negative), the drug by itself is probably compatible.

References

1. Prescribing Information. *Pifeltro*. Merck Sharp & Dohme; 2020.
2. Le, MP, Pencole L, Peytavin G, et al. Placental transfer of doravirine, a recent HIV-1 NNRTI in the ex vivo human cotyledon perfusion model. *J Antimicrob Chemother*. 2021;76:2364-2367.
3. Bukkems VE, van Hove H, Roelofsen D, et al. Prediction of maternal and fetal doravirine exposure by integrating physiologically based pharmacokinetic modeling and human placenta perfusion experiments. *Clin Pharmacokinet*. 2022;61:1129-1141.

D

DORIPENEM

Antibacterial

PREGNANCY RECOMMENDATION: No Human Data—Animal Data Suggest Low Risk

BREASTFEEDING RECOMMENDATION: Probably Compatible

PREGNANCY SUMMARY

No reports describing the use of doripenem in human pregnancy have been located. The drug will probably cross the placenta, so some fetal exposure will likely occur. Therefore, the absence of human pregnancy experience prevents a complete assessment of the embryofetal risk. Animal studies did not show any embryofetal toxicity in two species at doses less than 10 times the RHD. Using this drug during pregnancy should be based on the pros and cons of the mother's clinical need for treatment versus any potential fetal risk that might occur from exposure.

BREASTFEEDING SUMMARY

No reports describing the use of doripenem during human lactation have been located. The drug will probably be found in breast milk, so some infant exposure will likely occur. Breastfeeding while using this drug should be based on the mother's clinical need for treatment. If used, the infant should be monitored for the most common reported adult side effects of nausea and headache (both leading to irritability), diarrhea, and rash.

Reference

1. Prescribing Information. *Doribax*. Shionogi & Co. Ltd; 2020.

DORNASE ALFA

Respiratory (Enzyme)

PREGNANCY RECOMMENDATION: No Human Data—Animal Data Suggest Low Risk

BREASTFEEDING RECOMMENDATION: Probably Compatible

PREGNANCY SUMMARY

One case report describing the use of dornase alfa in human pregnancy was located. The drug, along with alteplase, was administered to the intrapleural space at about 28 weeks' gestation to treat a pregnant patient with a complicated parapneumonic effusion. The treatment was well tolerated, and no complications occurred. Delivery information was not provided. The drug will not likely cross the placenta in any clinically significant amount. However, this limited human pregnancy experience prevents a complete assessment of the embryofetal risk. Animal studies did not find any embryofetal toxicity in two species administered doses of more than 10 times the RHD. Using this drug during pregnancy should be based on the pros and cons of the mother's clinical need for treatment versus any potential fetal risk that might occur from exposure.

BREASTFEEDING SUMMARY

No reports describing the use of dornase alfa during human lactation have been located. The drug is not expected to be found in breast milk. Because the enzyme is a natural constituent of the mother's circulation, the risk to a nursing infant from a mother's use is thought to be clinically insignificant.

References

1. Prescribing Information. *Pulmozyme*. Genentech; 2021.
2. Amariei D, Tran BC, Yao R, et al. Intrapleural alteplase and dornase in a pregnant woman with complicated parapneumonic effusion. *Ann Thorac Surg*. 2019;108:e293-e294.

D

DORZOLAMIDE OPHTHALMIC

Ophthalmic (Carbonic Anhydrase Inhibitor)

PREGNANCY RECOMMENDATION: Limited Human Data—Animal Data Suggest Low Risk

BREASTFEEDING RECOMMENDATION: Probably Compatible

PREGNANCY SUMMARY

One case report of dorzolamide use in the first trimester of human pregnancy was located. The patient had glaucoma and was on dorzolamide and timolol throughout the first and third trimesters. She delivered a healthy newborn with no reported anomalies. Two other case reports were found that describe the use of the drug in the second and third trimesters. Both delivered healthy neonates with no reported complications. The drug would likely cross the placenta, so some fetal exposure is possible. However, the systemic blood levels with ophthalmic use are very low and are probably clinically insignificant. However, this limited human pregnancy experience prevents a complete assessment of the embryofetal risk. Animal studies did not show any embryofetal toxicity. Using this drug during pregnancy should be based on the pros and cons of the mother's clinical need for treatment versus any potential fetal risk that might occur from exposure. If used during pregnancy, consider placing pressure over the tear duct in the corner of the eye for at least 1 minute, and then remove any excess solution with absorbent tissue to decrease the amount of drug reaching the systemic circulation even further.

BREASTFEEDING SUMMARY

One case report was found that described the use of dorzolamide during human lactation. The patient breastfed for several months, and no adverse events were reported in the infant. The breast milk was not analyzed for the presence of the drug. Though the pharmacokinetics suggest that the drug will be found in breast milk, the very low systemic blood levels seen with ophthalmic use suggest that the total amount excreted would probably be clinically insignificant. Breastfeeding while using this drug should be based on the mother's clinical need for treatment. Because of the poor absorption with ophthalmic use, systemic side effects were not reported. The amount in circulation can be decreased even further by using the method described above in the Pregnancy Summary.

References

1. Prescribing Information. *Dorzolamide*. Bausch & Lomb; 2020.
2. Mendez-Hernandez C, Garcia-Feijoo J, Saenz-Frances F, et al. Topical intraocular pressure therapy effects on pregnancy. *Clin Ophthalmol*. 2012;6:1629-1632.
3. Colas-Tomas T, Lopez TE. Ex-PRESS mini-shunt implanted in a pregnant patient with iridocorneal endothelial syndrome. *Eur J Ophthalmol*. 2019;30:NP25-NP28.
4. Johnson SM, Martinez M, Freedman S. Management of glaucoma in pregnancy and lactation. *Sur Ophthalmol*. 2001;45:449-454.

DOSTARLIMAB

Antineoplastic (Monoclonal Antibody)

PREGNANCY RECOMMENDATION: No Human Data—No Relevant Animal Data

BREASTFEEDING RECOMMENDATION: Probably Compatible

PREGNANCY SUMMARY

No reports describing the use of dostarlimab in human pregnancy have been located. As an IgG antibody, dostarlimab is likely to cross the placenta, so some fetal exposure will probably occur. Therefore, the absence of human pregnancy experience prevents a complete assessment of the embryofetal risk. Animal studies have not been conducted. Based on the drug's mechanism of action, the manufacturer recommends that women with reproductive potential who are taking dostarlimab use effective contraception during treatment and for at least 4 months after the last dose. Nevertheless, using this drug during pregnancy should be based on the pros and cons of the mother's clinical need for treatment versus any potential fetal risk that might occur from exposure.

BREASTFEEDING SUMMARY

No reports describing the use of dostarlimab during human lactation have been located. It is known that IgG antibodies can be found in human breast milk, but are not found in the neonatal or infant circulation. Additionally, if any IgG antibodies were to be ingested through breastfeeding, they would probably be digested in the infant's gastrointestinal tract and not be absorbed. Regardless, due to the concern for potential serious adverse effects that might be seen in a breastfed infant, the manufacturer recommends that women not breastfeed while taking dostarlimab and for 4 months after the last dose. Nevertheless, breastfeeding while using this drug should be based on the mother's clinical need for treatment. If used, the infant should be monitored for the most common reported adult side effects of nausea (leading to irritability), lethargy, anemia, diarrhea, and constipation.

Reference

1. Prescribing Information. *Jemperli*. GlaxoSmithKline; 2021.

D

DOXAPRAM

Respiratory (Stimulant)

PREGNANCY RECOMMENDATION: No Human Data—Animal Data Suggest Low Risk

BREASTFEEDING RECOMMENDATION: Probably Compatible

PREGNANCY SUMMARY

No reports describing the use of doxapram in human pregnancy have been located. The drug will probably cross the placenta, so some fetal exposure will likely occur. Therefore, the absence of human pregnancy experience prevents a complete assessment of the embryofetal risk. Animal studies did not show any embryofetal toxicity in one species at doses less than 10 times the RHD. Using this drug during pregnancy should be based on the pros and cons of the mother's clinical need for treatment versus any potential fetal risk that might occur from exposure. Lastly, the drug is supplied as multidose vials that contain the preservative, benzyl alcohol. Benzyl alcohol has been associated with serious and possibly fatal reactions in neonates, including "gasping syndrome" when consumed orally. However, benzyl alcohol is rapidly metabolized to benzoic acid in the liver and then binds to glycine and is excreted as hippuric acid. Therefore, any fetal exposure is likely to be clinically insignificant.

BREASTFEEDING SUMMARY

No reports describing the use of doxapram during human lactation have been located. The drug will probably be found in breast milk, so some infant exposure will likely occur. Breastfeeding while using this drug should be based on the mother's clinical need for treatment. One study was found where 83 newborns were given doxapram postdelivery compared to 83 neonates treated with normal resuscitation efforts. The doxapram group had a slightly lower pH drop with no rise in PCO2 at 10 minutes after birth. It is uncertain whether this difference was significant. However, none of the 83 infants were reported to have any complications related to the administered doxapram. The drug is supplied as multidose vials that contain the preservative, benzyl alcohol. Benzyl alcohol has been associated with serious and possibly fatal reactions in neonates, including "gasping syndrome" when consumed orally. However, benzyl alcohol is rapidly metabolized to benzoic acid in the liver and then binds to glycine and is excreted as hippuric acid. Therefore, exposure to benzyl alcohol by way of breastfeeding is not likely to have any clinical significance to a neonate; whereas exposure to the drug directly administered to the newborn would need to be monitored.

References

1. Prescribing Information. *Dopram*. West-Ward Pharmaceuticals; 2020.
2. Nair B. Final report on the safety assessment of benzyl alcohol, benzoic acid, and sodium benzoate. *Int J Toxicol*. 2001;20(suppl 3):23-50.
3. Gupta PK, Moore J. The use of doxapram in the newborn. *J Obstet Gynaecol Br Commonw*. 1973;80:1002-1006.

DOXAZOSIN

Autonomic (Sympatholytic)

PREGNANCY RECOMMENDATION: Limited Human Data—Animal Data Suggest Low Risk

BREASTFEEDING RECOMMENDATION: Probably Compatible

PREGNANCY SUMMARY

One case report of first-trimester exposure to doxazosin in human pregnancy was located. The patient was on the drug at conception and continued the drug after pregnancy confirmation. She delivered at term a healthy newborn with no reported anomalies. Five other case reports describe the use of doxazosin in six pregnancies, starting the drug in the second or third trimesters to treat hypertension. The patients all responded well and delivered at term or near term, and no fetal or newborn complications related to the drug were reported. The drug appears to cross the placenta with a fetal level of about 80%

(*continued*)

of the maternal level. Therefore, fetal exposure will occur. However, this limited human pregnancy experience prevents a complete assessment of the embryofetal risk. Animal studies did not find any embryofetal toxicity in two species at doses of less than 10 times the RHD. Using this drug during pregnancy should be based on the pros and cons of the mother's clinical need for treatment versus any potential fetal risk that might occur from exposure.

D

BREASTFEEDING SUMMARY

Two case reports regarding the use of doxazosin during human lactation were located. In one case, no drug was identified in breast milk (the lower limit of detection for the test used was 25 ng/mL). In the second case, a maximum breast milk drug level of 4.2 ng/mL was reported. The estimated maximum RID was calculated to be about 0.09%. Therefore, the drug can be found in breast milk, but levels are very low and probably not clinically significant. Breastfeeding while using this drug should be based on the mother's clinical need for treatment. If used, the infant should be monitored for the most common reported adult side effects of headache and dizziness (both leading to irritability), fatigue (lethargy), and hypotension.

References

1. Prescribing Information. *Doxazosin*. Roering Pfizer; 2021.
2. Versmissen J, Koch BC, Roofthooft DW, et al. Doxazosin treatment of phaeochromocytoma during pregnancy: placental transfer and disposition in breast milk. *Br J Clin Pharmacol*. 2016;82:568-569.
3. Chu PY, Burks ML, Solorzano CC, Bao S. Robotic paraganglioma resection in a pregnant patient. *AACE Clin Case Rep*. 2020;6:3197-3200.
4. Yasui M, Hattori Y, Uemura K, et al. Pheochromocytoma during pregnancy—2 case reports. *Nihon Hinyokika Gakkai Zasshi*. 2016;107:245-250.
5. Giampaolino P, Della Corte L, Formisano C, et al. Pheochromocytoma in third trimester pregnancy. *Gynecol Endocrin*. 2018;34:1016-1018.
6. Marques P, Tufton N, Bhattacharya S, et al. Hypertension due to a deoxycorticosterone-secreting adrenal tumour diagnosed during pregnancy. *Endocrinol Diabetes Metab Case Rep*. 2019;18-0164(1-5).
7. Bettencourt AR, Alves C. Perioperative management of a patient with secreting paraganglioma undergoing cesarean section. *Case Rep Anesthesiol*. 2022:9065324(1-3).
8. Jensen BP, Dalrymple JM, Begg EJ. Transfer of doxazosin into breast milk. *J Hum Lact*. 2013;29:150-153.

DOXEPIN

Antidepressant (Tricyclic)

PREGNANCY RECOMMENDATION: Limited Human Data (First Trimester)/Human Data Suggest Risk (Third Trimester)

BREASTFEEDING RECOMMENDATION: Potential Toxicity

PREGNANCY SUMMARY

Several studies have been located that describe the use of doxepin during human pregnancy. The Michigan Medicaid Surveillance study reported 118 first-trimester exposures with 12 (10.2%) major malformations described. However, no pattern to the defects was seen, and these patients had exposures to other drugs. Other studies analyzing antidepressant use as a group in human pregnancy have not shown an increased risk for anomalies. The drug probably crosses the placenta, so some fetal exposure will likely occur. Therefore, this limited human pregnancy experience prevents a complete assessment of the embryofetal risk. Animal studies did not show any embryofetal toxicity in two species at doses of less than 10 times the RHD. In these studies, the level of nordoxepin was less than 10 times in one species and more than 10 times the RHD in the second. When used near term, a neonatal withdrawal syndrome can occur, showing irritability, restlessness, tremor, vomiting, poor tone, constant crying, apnea, and cyanosis.

BREASTFEEDING SUMMARY

Three studies have been located that describe the use of doxepin during human pregnancy. In three women, the drug and metabolite (nordoxepin) were found in all breast milk samples. The calculated RIDs were all less than 4%. In these three cases, the infant's blood levels were evaluated. In two cases, the drug levels were low, but in the third, the nordoxepin blood level was similar to the maternal blood level. Due to a concern for potential serious adverse effects that might be seen in a breastfed infant, the manufacturer recommends that women not breastfeed while being treated with this drug. Nevertheless, breastfeeding while using this drug should be based on the mother's clinical need for treatment versus any potential infant risks that might occur. If used, the infant should be monitored for the most common reported adult side effects of nausea (leading to irritability), sedation, and somnolence. Because of the sedating effect and higher levels of active metabolite in breast milk, other alternatives may be indicated.

References

1. Yonkers KA, Wisner KL, Stewart DE, et al. The management of depression during pregnancy: a report from the American Psychiatric Association and the American College of Obstetricians and Gynecologists. *Obstet Gynecol*. 2009;114:703-713.
2. Prescribing Information. *Doxepin*. Amneal Pharmaceuticals NY; 2019.
3. Owaki Y, Momiyama H, Onodera N. Effects of doxepin hydrochloride administered to pregnant rats upon the fetuses and their postnatal development.

Oyo Yakuri. 1971;5:913-924. As cited in Shepard TH. Catalog of Teratogenic Agents. 6th ed. Johns Hopkins University Press, 1989:243.
4. Owaki Y, Momiyama H, Onodera N. Effects of doxepin hydrochloride administered to pregnant rabbits upon the fetuses. *Oyo Yakuri*. 1971;5:905-912. As cited in Shepard TH. Catalog of Teratogenic Agents. 6th ed. Johns Hopkins University Press, 1989:243.
5. McElhatton PR, Garbis HM, Elefant E, et al. The outcome of pregnancy in 689 women exposed to therapeutic doses of antidepressants. A collaborative study of the European Network of Teratology Information Services (ENTIS). *Reprod Toxicol*. 1996;10:285-294.
6. Falterman CG, Richardson CJ. Small left colon syndrome associated with maternal ingestion of psychotropic drugs. *J Pediatr*. 1980;97:308-310.
7. Nulman I, Rovet J, Stewart DE, et al. Child development following exposure to tricyclic antidepressants or fluoxetine throughout fetal life: a prospective, controlled study. *Am J Psychiatry*. 2002;159:1889-1895.
8. Matheson I, Pande H, Alertsen AR. Respiratory depression caused by N-desmethyldoxepin in breast milk. *Lancet*. 1985;2:1124.
9. Kemp J, Ilett KF, Booth J, et al. Excretion of doxepin and N-desmethyldoxepin in human milk. *Br J Clin Pharmacol*. 1985;20:497-499.
10. Frey OR, Scheidt P, von Brenndorff AI. Adverse effects in a newborn infant breast-fed by a mother treated with doxepin. *Ann Pharmacother*. 1999;33:690-693.

D

DOXORUBICIN

Antineoplastic (Anthracycline Cytotoxic Antibiotic)

PREGNANCY RECOMMENDATION: Limited Human Data—Animal Data Suggest Risk

BREASTFEEDING RECOMMENDATION: Potential Toxicity

PREGNANCY SUMMARY

Numerous case reports and small series evaluating the use of doxorubicin during human pregnancy were located. More than 20 cases have been reported, including about 7 with first-trimester exposure. Nearly all of the patients were on multiple antineoplastic agents treating various malignancies. Of these seven first-trimester cases, two ended in spontaneous abortions, and four infants were delivered without any birth defects described and were doing well. In the seventh case, the infant had an imperforate anus with a rectovaginal fistula that was later repaired. Of the remaining reported cases, all exposures were in the second and third trimesters with no major adverse effects related to the drug noted. The drug appears to cross the placenta (though levels may be low), so some fetal exposure will occur. Therefore, this limited human pregnancy experience prevents a complete assessment of the embryofetal risk. Animal studies did show some embryofetal toxicity with malformations in two species at doses of less than 10 times the RHD. Multiple daily doses did occur in these animal studies, so correlations to human exposure are not possible. Based on these animal studies and the drug's mechanism of action, the manufacturer recommends that women with reproductive potential use effective contraception during treatment and for 6 months after the last dose. They also recommend that males with female partners of reproductive potential use effective contraception during treatment and for 3 months after the last dose. Nevertheless, using this drug during pregnancy should be based on the pros and cons of the mother's clinical need for treatment versus any potential fetal risk that might occur from exposure. The drug carries a boxed warning for an increased risk of cardiomyopathy and other risks. There is a registry for women who are pregnant and have cancer. For more information, women and health care providers are encouraged to contact the Cancer and Pregnancy Registry at 1-877-635-4499.

BREASTFEEDING SUMMARY

Three studies were located (involving four lactating women) that evaluated human breast milk for doxorubicin. The drug was found in the breast milk in all four cases. In two women, both doxorubicin and doxorubicinol were studied, and the calculated RID using peak values for both drug concentrations was about 3% and 14%. In the other two cases, using peak breast milk levels for doxorubicin only (doxorubicinol was not analyzed), the calculated RIDs were about 1.9% and 2.6%. Infant serum levels have not been evaluated. Due to a concern for potential serious adverse effects that might be seen in a breastfed infant, the manufacturer recommends that women not breastfeed while being treated with this drug and for at least 10 days after the last dose. Nevertheless, breastfeeding while using this drug should be based on the mother's clinical need for treatment versus any potential infant risks that might occur. If used, the infant should be monitored for the most common reported adult side effects of nausea (leading to irritability), vomiting, diarrhea, alopecia, and various laboratory abnormalities (see PI).

References

1. Product information. *Doxorubicin*. BluePoint Laboratories; 2018.
2. Roboz J, Gleicher N, Wu K, et al. Does doxorubicin cross the placenta? *Lancet*. 1979;2:1382-1383.
3. D'Incalci M, Broggini M, Buscaglia M, et al. Transplacental passage of doxorubicin. *Lancet*. 1983;1:75.
4. Karp GI, Von Oeyen P, Valone F, et al. Doxorubicin in pregnancy: possible transplacental passage. *Cancer Treat Rep*. 1983;67:773-777.
5. Soininen SK, Repo JK, Karttunen V, et al. Human placental cell and tissue uptake of doxorubicin and its liposomal formulations. *Toxcol Lett*. 2015;239:108-114.
6. Khursid M, Saleem M. Acute leukaemia in pregnancy. *Lancet*. 1978;2:534-535.
7. Newcomb M, Balducci L, Thigpen JT, et al. Acute leukemia in pregnancy: successful delivery after cytarabine and doxorubicin. *JAMA*. 1978;239:2691-2692.
8. Hassenstein E, Riedel H. Zur teratogenitat von Adriamycin ein fallbericht. *Geburtshilfe Frauenheilkd*. 1978;38:131-133.
9. Cervantes F, Rozman C. Adriamycina y embarazo. *Sangre (Barc)*. 1980;25:627.
10. Pizzuto J, Aviles A, Noriega L, et al. Treatment of acute leukemia during pregnancy: presentation of nine cases. *Cancer Treat Rep*. 1980;64:679-683.
11. Tobias JS, Bloom HJG. Doxorubicin in pregnancy. *Lancet*. 1980;1:776.
12. Garcia V, San Miguel J, Borrasca AL. Doxorubicin in the first trimester of pregnancy. *Ann Intern Med*. 1981;94:547.

13. Garcia V, San Miguel IJ, Borrasca AL. Adriamycin and pregnancy. *Sangre (Barc)*. 1981;26:129.
14. Dara P, Slater LM, Armentrout SA. Successful pregnancy during chemotherapy for acute leukemia. *Cancer*. 1981;47:845-846.
15. Lowenthal RM, Funnell CF, Hope DM, et al. Normal infant after combination chemotherapy including teniposide for Burkitt's lymphoma in pregnancy. *Med Pediatr Oncol*. 1982;10:165-169.
16. Webb GA. The use of hyperalimentation and chemotherapy in pregnancy: a case report. *Am J Obstet Gynecol*. 1980;137:263-266.
17. Gililland J, Weinstein L. The effects of cancer chemotherapeutic agents on the developing fetus. *Obstet Gynecol Surv*. 1983;38:6-13.
18. Murray CL, Reichert JA, Anderson J, et al. Multimodal cancer therapy for breast cancer in the first trimester of pregnancy. A case report. *JAMA*. 1984;252:2607-2608.
19. Haerr RW, Pratt AT. Multiagent chemotherapy for sarcoma diagnosed during pregnancy. *Cancer*. 1985;56:1028-1033.
20. Turchi JJ, Villasis C. Anthracyclines in the treatment of malignancy in pregnancy. *Cancer*. 1988;61:435-440.
21. Giacalone PL, Laffargue F, Benos P. Chemotherapy for breast carcinoma during pregnancy. *Cancer*. 1999;86:2266-2272.
22. Nakajima W, Ishida A, Takahashi M, et al. Good outcome for infant of mother treated with chemotherapy for Ewing sarcoma at 25-30 weeks' gestation. *J Pediatr Hematol Oncol*. 2004;26:308-311.
23. Lam MSH. Treatment of Burkitt's lymphoma during pregnancy. *Ann Pharmacother*. 2006;40:2048-2052.
24. Dobbing J. Pregnancy and leukaemia. *Lancet*. 1977;1:1155.
25. Lendon M, Palmer MK, Hann IM, et al. Testicular histology after combination chemotherapy in childhood for acute lymphoblastic leukaemia. *Lancet*. 1978;2:439-441.
26. Schilsky RL, Lewis BJ, Sherins RJ, et al. Gonadal dysfunction in patients receiving chemotherapy for cancer. *Ann Intern Med*. 1980;93:109-114.
27. Rustin GJS, Booth M, Dent J, et al. Pregnancy after cytotoxic chemotherapy for gestational trophoblastic tumours. *Br Med J*. 1984;288:103-106.
28. Gershenson DM. Menstrual and reproductive function after treatment with combination chemotherapy for malignant ovarian germ cell tumors. *J Clin Oncol*. 1988;6:270-275.
29. Egan PC, Costanza ME, Dodion P, et al. Doxorubicin and cisplatin excretion into human milk. *Cancer Treat Rep*. 1985;69:1387-1389.
30. Committee on Drugs, American Academy of Pediatrics. The transfer of drugs and other chemicals into human milk. *Pediatrics*. 2001;108:776-789.

DOXYCYCLINE

Antibacterial (Tetracycline)

PREGNANCY RECOMMENDATION: Limited Human Data—Animal Data Suggest Risk

BREASTFEEDING RECOMMENDATION: Potential Toxicity

PREGNANCY SUMMARY

One study analyzed a large number of newborns with birth defects (18,515) versus a control group of newborns with no anomalies (32,804). Doxycycline was used in 56 (0.3%) participants in the anomaly group and 63 participants (0.19%) in the control group. This difference was significant, but the use of the drug was anytime during the pregnancy. In another small study, there were no reported congenital defects in 43 newborns exposed to doxycycline in the first trimester. The drug crosses the placenta, so some fetal exposure will occur. Therefore, this limited human pregnancy experience prevents a complete assessment of the embryofetal risk. Animal studies did show some embryofetal toxicity with malformations in two species at doses of less than 10 times the RHD. Using this drug during pregnancy should be based on the pros and cons of the mother's clinical need for treatment versus any potential fetal risk that might occur from exposure. Treatment for 7 to 14 days in the second and third trimesters is thought to be low risk.

BREASTFEEDING SUMMARY

Several studies have been located that have analyzed human breast milk for the presence of doxycycline. A total of 46 lactating women were studied following doses of 100 and 200 mg/d. Doxycycline was found in all the samples tested. Using mean breast milk levels, all calculated RIDs were less than 10%. However, if peak values were used, some RIDs were greater than 10%. No studies evaluating infant serum levels were located. Breastfeeding while using this drug should be based on the mother's clinical need for treatment versus any potential infant risks that might occur. If used, the infant should be monitored for the most common reported adult side effects of nausea (leading to irritability), diarrhea, vomiting, decreased appetite, and rash.

References

1. Morganti G, Ceccarelli G, Ciaffi EG. Comparative concentrations of a tetracycline antibiotic in serum and maternal milk. *Antibiotica*. 1968;6:216-223.
2. Prescribing Information. Doxycycline. Mylan Pharmaceuticals, Inc. 2019.

DOXYLAMINE

Antihistamine (Antiemetic)

PREGNANCY RECOMMENDATION: Human Data Suggest Compatible

BREASTFEEDING RECOMMENDATION: Probably Compatible

PREGNANCY SUMMARY

From two large databases (the Collaborative Perinatal Project and the Group Health Cooperative of Puget Sound), a total of 5,003 first-trimester exposures to doxylamine were described. There were 83 (1.7%) major anomalies identified. No pattern to the anomalies was seen. Two large meta-analyses of more than 15 studies each did not show any increased risk for congenital birth defects. In fact, one study showed that the drug actually reduced the risk of birth defects, possibly related to better maternal nutrition intake due to less vomiting. Lastly, this drug was part of Bendectin from 1956 to 1983. It was used by hundreds of thousands of pregnant women in the first trimester with no proven teratogenicity. The drug will probably cross the placenta, so some fetal exposure will likely occur. Animal studies did not show any embryofetal toxicity in two species at doses of less than 10 times the RHD. Using this drug during pregnancy should be based on the pros and cons of the mother's clinical need for treatment versus any potential fetal risk that might occur from exposure. Before the FDA changed the drug classification regarding drugs and their effects on pregnancy, doxylamine was labeled Category A (one of the only true drugs with this classification). Other Category A drugs were vitamins, replacement hormones, and so on.

BREASTFEEDING SUMMARY

No reports describing the use of doxylamine or the fixed combination of doxylamine/pyridoxine (vitamin B6) during human lactation have been located. Both components of the fixed combination, however, are available as single agents. Pyridoxine (Vitamin B6) is excreted into breast milk but presents no risk to a nursing infant (see Vitamin B6). Doxylamine will also probably be excreted into breast milk, so some infant exposure to this drug will likely occur. Breastfeeding while using this drug should be based on the mother's clinical need for treatment versus any potential infant risks that might occur. If used, the infant should be monitored for the most common reported adult side effects of dizziness, headaches, and blurred vision (all leading to irritability), sedation, somnolence, and constipation.

References

1. Prescribing Information. *Diclegis*. Duchesnay USA; 2018.
2. Gibson JP, Staples RE, Larson EJ, et al. Teratology and reproduction studies with an antinauseant. *Toxicol Appl Pharmacol*. 1968;13:439-447.
3. Sturman G, Freeman P, Bailey AR, et al. Loss of skeletal integrity in rat fetuses from dams treated with histamine H1 antagonists. *Agents Actions*. 1993;38:C185-C187.
4. Tyl RW, Price CJ, Marr MC, et al. Developmental toxicity evaluation of Bendectin in CD rats. *Teratology*. 1988;37:539-552.
5. McClure HM. Research and development studies relative to the experimental induction of oral facial malformation in the Rhesus monkey. No. 1 DE52452 Final report, May 1975–July 1981, August 1982. As cited in Brent RL. Bendectin: review of the medical literature of a comprehensively studied human nonteratogen and the most prevalent tortogen-litigen. *Reprod Toxicol*. 1995;9:337-349.
6. Hendrickx AG, Cukierski M, Prahalada S, et al. Evaluation of Bendectin embryotoxicity in nonhuman primates: I. Ventricular septal defects in prenatal macaques and baboon. *Teratology*. 1985;32:179-189.
7. Hendrickx AG, Cukierski M, Prahalada S, et al. Evaluation of Bendectin embryotoxicity in nonhuman primates: II. Double-blind study in term cynomolgus monkeys. *Teratology*. 1985;32:191-194.
8. Korcok M. The Bendectin debate. *Can Med Assoc J*. 1980;123:922-928.
9. Soverchia G, Perri PF. Two cases of malformations of a limb in infants of mothers treated with an antiemetic in a very early phase of pregnancy. *Pediatr Med Chir*. 1981;3:97-99.
10. Donaldson GL, Bury RG. Multiple congenital abnormalities in a newborn boy associated with maternal use of fluphenazine enanthate and other drugs during pregnancy. *Acta Paediatr Scand*. 1982;71:335-338.
11. Grodofsky MP, Wilmott RW. Possible association of use of Bendectin during early pregnancy and congenital lung hypoplasia. *N Engl J Med*. 1984;311:732.
12. Fisher JE, Nelson SJ, Allen JE, et al. Congenital cystic adenomatoid malformation of the lung. A unique variant. *Am J Dis Child*. 1982;136:1071-1074.
13. Bracken MB, Berg A. Bendectin (Debendox) and congenital diaphragmatic hernia. *Lancet*. 1983;1:586.
14. Golding J, Vivian S, Baldwin JA. Maternal anti-nauseants and clefts of lip and palate. *Human Toxicol*. 1983;2:63-73.
15. Robison LL, Buckley JD, Daigle AE, et al. Maternal drug use and risk of childhood nonlymphoblastic leukemia among offspring: an epidemiologic investigation implicating marijuana (a report from the Childrens Cancer Study Group). *Cancer*. 1989;63:1904-1911.
16. Heinonen OP, Slone D, Shapiro S. *Birth Defects and Drugs in Pregnancy*. Publishing Sciences Group; 1977:474-475.
17. Ohga K, Yamanaka R, Kinumaki H, et al. Bendectin (Debendox) and congenital diaphragmatic hernia. *Lancet*. 1983;1:930.
18. Eskenazi B, Bracken MB. Bendectin (Debendox) as a risk factor for pyloric stenosis. *Am J Obstet Gynecol*. 1982;144:919-924.
19. Zierler S, Rothman KJ. Congenital heart disease in relation to maternal use of Bendectin and other drugs in early pregnancy. *N Engl J Med*. 1985;313:347-352.
20. Bendectin and pyloric stenosis. *FDA Drug Bull*. 1983;13:14-15.
21. Mitchell AA, Schwingl PJ, Rosenberg L, et al. Birth defects in relation to Bendectin use in pregnancy. II. Pyloric stenosis. *Am J Obstet Gynecol*. 1983;147:737-742.
22. Aselton P, Jick H, Chentow SJ, et al. Pyloric stenosis and maternal Bendectin exposure. *Am J Epidemiol*. 1984;120:251-256.
23. Sieber WK. Pyloric stenosis. In: Buyse ML, ed. *Birth Defects Encyclopedia*. Vol. 2. Blackwell Scientific Publications; 1990:1448.
24. Holmes LB. Teratogen update: bendectin. *Teratology*. 1983;27:277-281.
25. Aselton P, Jick H, Milunsky A, et al. First-trimester drug use and congenital malformations. *Obstet Gynecol*. 1985;65:451-455.
26. Milkovich L, van den Berg BJ. An evaluation of the teratogenicity of certain antinauseant drugs. *Am J Obstet Gynecol*. 1976;125:244-248.
27. Shapiro S, Heinonen OP, Siskind V, et al. Antenatal exposure to doxylamine succinate and dicyclomine hydrochloride (Bendectin) in relation to congenital malformations, perinatal mortality rate, birth weight, intelligence quotient score. *Am J Obstet Gynecol*. 1977;128:480-485.
28. Rothman KJ, Flyer DC, Goldblatt A, et al. Exogenous hormones and other drug exposures of children with congenital heart disease. *Am J Epidemiol*. 1979;109:433-439.
29. Bunde CA, Bowles DM. A technique for controlled survey of case records. *Curr Ther Res*. 1963;5:245-248.
30. Gibson GT, Collen DP, McMichael AJ, et al. Congenital anomalies in relation to the use of doxylamine/dicyclomine and other antenatal factors: an ongoing prospective study. *Med J Aust*. 1981;1:410-414.
31. Correy JF, Newman NM. Debendox and limb reduction deformities. *Med J Aust*. 1981;1:417-418.
32. Clarke M, Clayton DG. Safety of Debendox. *Lancet*. 1981;2:659-660.
33. Harron DWG, Griffiths K, Shanks RG. Debendox and congenital malformations in Northern Ireland. *Br Med J*. 1980;4:1379-1381.
34. Smithells RW, Sheppard S. Teratogenicity testing in humans: a method demonstrating safety of Bendectin. *Teratology*. 1978;17:31-35.
35. Morelock S, Hingson R, Kayne H, et al. Bendectin and fetal development: a study at Boston City Hospital. *Am J Obstet Gynecol*. 1982;142:209-213.
36. Cordero JF, Oakley GP, Greenberg F, et al. Is Bendectin a teratogen? *JAMA*. 1981;245:2307-2310.
37. Mitchell AA, Rosenberg L, Shapiro S, et al. Birth defects related to Bendectin use in pregnancy: I. Oral clefts and cardiac defects. *JAMA*. 1981;245:2311-2314.
38. Fleming DM, Knox JDE, Crombie DL. Debendox in early pregnancy and fetal malformation. *Br Med J*. 1981;283:99-101.

39. Greenberg G, Inman WHW, Weatherall JAC, et al. Maternal drug histories and congenital abnormalities. *Br Med J*. 1977;2:853-856.
40. Aselton PJ, Jick H. Additional follow-up of congenital limb disorders in relation to Bendectin use. *JAMA*. 1983;250:33-34.
41. McCredie J, Kricker A, Elliott J, et al. The innocent bystander: doxylamine/dicyclomine/pyridoxine and congenital limb defects. *Med J Aust*. 1984;140:525-527.
42. Brent RR. The Bendectin saga: another American tragedy [editorial]. *Teratology*. 1983;27:283-286.
43. Hughes DT, Cavanagh N. Chromosomal studies on children with phocomelia, exposed to Debendox during early pregnancy. *Lancet*. 1983;2:399.
44. David TJ. Debendox does not cause the Poland anomaly. *Arch Dis Child*. 1982;57:479-480.
45. Shiono PH, Klebanoff MA. Bendectin and human congenital malformations. *Teratology*. 1989;40:151-155.
46. Einarson TR, Leeder JS, Koren G. A method for meta-analysis of epidemiological studies. *Drug Intell Clin Pharm*. 1988;22:813-824.
47. McKeigue PM, Lamm SH, Linn S, et al. Bendectin and birth defects: I. A meta-analysis of the epidemiologic studies. *Teratology*. 1994;50:27-37.
48. Brent RL. Bendectin: review of the medical literature of a comprehensively studied human nonteratogen and the most prevalent tortogen-litigen. *Reprod Toxicol*. 1995;9:337-349.
49. Newman SA. Bendectin—birth defects controversy. *JAMA*. 1990;264:569.
50. Skolnick A. Bendectin—birth defects controversy [reply]. *JAMA*. 1990;264:569-570.
51. Scialli AR. Editor's note. *Reprod Toxicol*. 1999;13:239.
52. Newman SA. Dr. Brent and scientific debate. *Reprod Toxicol*. 1999;13:241-244.
53. Brent RL. Response to Dr. Stuart Newman's commentary on an article entitled "Bendectin: review of the medical literature of a comprehensively studied human nonteratogen and the most prevalent tortogen-litigen". *Reprod Toxicol*. 1999;13:245-253.
54. Newman SA. Response to Dr. Brent's commentary on "Dr. Brent and scientific debate". *Reprod Toxicol*. 1999;13:255-260.
55. Boneva RS, Moore CA, Botto L, et al. Nausea during pregnancy and congenital heart defects: a population-based case-control study. *Am J Epidemiol*. 1999;149:717-725.
56. Ornstein M, Einarson A, Koren G. Bendectin/Diclectin for morning sickness: a Canadian follow-up of an American tragedy. *Reprod Toxicol*. 1995;9:1-6.
57. Kutcher JS, Engle A, Firth J, et al. Bendectin and birth defects II: ecological analyses. *Birth Defects Res (Part A)*. 2003;67:88-97.
58. Brent R. Bendectin and birth defects: hopefully, the final chapter. *Birth Defects Res (Part A)*. 2003;67:79-87.
59. Koren G, Clark S, Hankins GDV, et al. Effectiveness of delayed-release doxylamine and pyridoxine for nausea and vomiting of pregnancy: a randomized placebo-controlled trial. *Am J Obstet Gynecol*. 2010;203:571.e1-571.e7.

DRONABINOL

Gastrointestinal (Antiemetic)

PREGNANCY RECOMMENDATION: Limited Human Data—Animal Data Suggest Low Risk

BREASTFEEDING RECOMMENDATION: *Contraindicated/Probably Compatible

PREGNANCY SUMMARY

Only one case report has described the use of dronabinol in human pregnancy. The patient was on the drug at conception, and it was continued up to delivery. A healthy newborn with no anomalies was reported. The drug probably crosses the placenta, so some fetal exposure will likely occur. Therefore, this limited human pregnancy experience prevents a complete assessment of the embryofetal risk. Animal studies did not show any embryofetal toxicity or teratogenicity in two species at doses of less than 10 times the RHD. Dronabinol can produce dependence, leading to misuse. It is classified as a Schedule III controlled substance. Using this drug during pregnancy should be based on the pros and cons of the mother's clinical need for treatment versus any potential fetal risk that might occur from exposure.

BREASTFEEDING SUMMARY

No reports describing the use of dronabinol during human lactation have been located. The drug will probably be found in breast milk, so some infant exposure will likely occur. *If the drug is needed in treating anorexia with weight loss in patients with AIDS, then breastfeeding is not recommended because of the risk for HIV transmission to the neonate. If needed in treating nausea and vomiting related to cancer chemotherapy, then using this drug should be based on the mother's clinical need for treatment versus any potential infant risks that might occur. If used, the infant should be monitored for the most common reported adult side effects of abdominal pain and dizziness (both leading to irritability), vomiting, and somnolence.

References

1. Product information. *Dronabinol*. Actavis Pharma; 2018.
2. Farooq MU, Ducommun E, Goudreau J. Treatment of a hyperkinetic movement disorder during pregnancy with dronabinol. *Parkinsonism Relat Disord*. 2009;15:249-251.
3. Astley SJ, Little RE. Maternal marijuana use during lactation and infant development at one year. *Neurotoxicol Teratol*. 1990;12:161-168.

DRONEDARONE

Cardiovascular (Antiarrhythmic)

PREGNANCY RECOMMENDATION: No Human Data—Animal Data Suggest Risk

BREASTFEEDING RECOMMENDATION: Potential Toxicity

D

PREGNANCY SUMMARY

No reports describing the use of dronedarone in human pregnancy have been located. The drug will probably cross the placenta, so some fetal exposure will likely occur. Therefore, the absence of human pregnancy experience prevents a complete assessment of the embryofetal risk. Animal data showed embryofetal toxicity and malformations in two animal species at doses less than 10 times the RHD. Based on these animal studies, the manufacturer recommends that women with reproductive potential use effective contraception during treatment with this drug. Nevertheless, using this drug during pregnancy should be based on the pros and cons of the mother's clinical need for treatment versus any potential fetal risk that might occur from exposure. The drug carries a boxed warning for an increased risk of heart failure. Dronedarone can also prolong the QT interval.

BREASTFEEDING SUMMARY

No reports describing the use of dronedarone during human lactation have been located. The drug will probably be found in breast milk, so some infant exposure will likely occur. The effect of this exposure on a nursing infant is unknown. Breastfeeding while using this drug should be based on the mother's clinical need for treatment. If used, the infant should be monitored for the most common reported adult side effects of nausea and abdominal pain (both leading to irritability), vomiting, and diarrhea.

Reference

1. Prescribing Information. *Multaq*. Sanofi-Aventis; 2020.

DROPERIDOL

Antiemetic/Antipsychotic

PREGNANCY RECOMMENDATION: Limited Human Data—Animal Data Suggest Potential Risk

BREASTFEEDING RECOMMENDATION: Potential Toxicity

PREGNANCY SUMMARY

A few studies have evaluated the use of droperidol in treating hyperemesis gravidarum. In more than 140 cases, many of which were in the first trimester, no increased risk for major congenital anomalies or spontaneous abortion was noted. The drug appears to cross the placenta (in low levels), so some infant exposure can occur. However, this limited human pregnancy experience prevents a complete assessment of the embryofetal risk. Animal studies did show some embryofetal toxicity in one species at doses of less than 10 times the RHD. Using this drug during pregnancy should be based on the pros and cons of the mother's clinical need for treatment versus any potential fetal risk that might occur from exposure. The drug carries a boxed warning for an increased risk of cardiac dysfunction due to a prolongation of the QT interval.

BREASTFEEDING SUMMARY

No reports describing the use of droperidol during lactation have been located. The drug will probably be excreted into human breast milk, so some infant exposure will likely occur. Breastfeeding while using this drug should be based on the mother's clinical need for treatment versus any potential infant risks that might occur. If used, the infant should be monitored for the most common reported adult side effects of dizziness and anxiety (both leading to irritability), rash, and somnolence.

References

1. Prescribing Information. *Droperidol*. Hospira; 2020.
2. Zhdanov GG, Ponomarev GM. The concentration of droperidol in the venous blood of the parturients and in the blood of the umbilical cord of neonates. *Anesteziol Reanimatol*. 1980;4:14-16.
3. Smith AM, McNeil WT. Awareness during anesthesia. *Br Med J*. 1969;1:572-573.
4. Pettit GP, Smith GA, McIlroy WL. Droperidol in obstetrics: a double-blind study. *Milit Med*. 1976;141:316-317.
5. Martynshin MYA, Arkhengel'skii AE. Experience in treating early toxicoses of pregnancy with metoclopramide. *Akush Ginekol*. 1981;57:44-45.
6. Nageotte MP, Briggs GG, Towers CV, et al. Droperidol and diphenhydramine in the management of hyperemesis gravidarum. *Am J Obstet Gynecol*. 1996;174:1801-1806.
7. Turcotte V, Ferreira E, Duperron L. Utilité du dropéridol et de la diphenhydramine dans l'hyperemesis gravidarum. *J Soc Obstet Gynaecol Can*. 2001;23:133-139.
8. Ferreira E, Bussieres J-F, Turcotte V, et al. Case-control study comparing droperidol plus diphenhydramine with conventional treatment in hyperemesis gravidarum. *J Pharm Technol*. 2003;19: 349-354.

DROSPIRENONE AND ESTETROL

Contraceptive (Estrogen and Progestin Combination)

SEE ORAL CONTRACEPTIVES

DROXIDOPA

Autonomic (Sympathomimetic)

PREGNANCY RECOMMENDATION: No Human Data—Animal Data Suggest Potential Risk

BREASTFEEDING RECOMMENDATION: Potential Toxicity

D

PREGNANCY SUMMARY

No reports describing the use of droxidopa in human pregnancy have been located. The drug will probably cross the placenta, so some fetal exposure will likely occur. Therefore, the absence of human pregnancy experience prevents a complete assessment of the embryofetal risk. Animal studies did show some embryofetal toxicity in one species at less than 10 times the RHD. Using this drug during pregnancy should be based on the pros and cons of the mother's clinical need for treatment versus any potential fetal risk that might occur from exposure. The drug can produce hypertension, and therefore, blood pressure monitoring should occur (see Norepinephrine).

BREASTFEEDING SUMMARY

No reports describing the use of droxidopa or its active metabolite (norepinephrine) during human lactation have been located. The drug will likely be excreted into breast milk, so some infant exposure will probably occur. Breastfeeding while using this drug should be based on the mother's clinical need for treatment. If used, the infant should be monitored for the most common reported adult side effects of headache, nausea, and dizziness (all leading to irritability), hypertension, and fatigue (lethargy).

Reference

1. Prescribing Information. *Northera*. Chelsea Therapeutics, Inc; 2020.

DULAGLUTIDE

Antidiabetic (Glucagon-Like Peptide-1 Receptor Agonist)

PREGNANCY RECOMMENDATION: Limited Human Data—Animal Data Suggest Low Risk

BREASTFEEDING RECOMMENDATION: Probably Compatible

PREGNANCY SUMMARY

With seven cases of unplanned pregnancies seen during the dulaglutide clinical trials and two other case reports, a total of nine pregnancies with first-trimester exposure have been located. Two pregnancies were electively terminated, but the other seven delivered healthy newborns with no reported anomalies or complications. As an Fc part of an IgG antibody, it likely crosses the placenta, especially during the second half of gestation, so some fetal exposure will probably occur. Therefore, this limited human pregnancy experience prevents a complete assessment of the embryofetal risk. Animal studies did not show any embryofetal toxicity or malformations in two species at doses less than 10 times the RHD. Using this drug during pregnancy should be based on the pros and cons of the mother's clinical need for treatment versus any potential fetal risk that might occur from exposure. ACOG recommends that insulin be used in treating types 1 and 2 diabetes during pregnancy and, if diet therapy alone is not successful, for gestational diabetes.

BREASTFEEDING SUMMARY

No reports describing the use of dulaglutide during human lactation have been located. The drug contains the Fc portion of an IgG antibody, and therefore, might be found in human breast milk. Nevertheless, if any of this drug were to be ingested through breastfeeding, it would probably be digested in the infant's gastrointestinal tract and not be absorbed because it is primarily a protein. Breastfeeding while using this drug should be based on the mother's clinical need for treatment. If used, the infant should be monitored for the most common reported adult side effects of nausea and abdominal pain (both leading to irritability), vomiting, diarrhea, and decreased appetite.

References

1. Prescribing Information. *Trulicity*. Eli Lilly; 2023.
2. Burlina S, Dalfra MG. Caprino R, Lapolla A. A case report on use of dulaglutide in the first weeks of pregnancy in women affected by type 2 diabetes. *Acta Diabetol*. 2023;60:137-138.
3. Alghamdi A, Alsaeddi A, Malki H, Alsaedi A. A case report of a pregnant woman with type 2 diabetes mellitus using dulaglutide during the first trimester of pregnancy. *Cureus*. 2023;15:e44644(1-5).

DULOXETINE

Antidepressant (Selective Serotonin and Norepinephrine Reuptake Inhibitor)

PREGNANCY RECOMMENDATION: Human Data Suggest Low Risk (First Trimester)/Human Data Suggest Potential Risk (Third Trimester)

BREASTFEEDING RECOMMENDATION: Potential Toxicity

PREGNANCY SUMMARY

Several studies have evaluated the use of duloxetine during human pregnancy. In a recent review of nearly 670 pregnancy exposures, no increased risk of major birth anomalies or spontaneous abortion was noted. Many of these had first-trimester exposure. The drug will cross the placenta, so some fetal exposure will occur. Animal studies did show some embryofetal toxicity in two species at doses of less than 10 times the RHD. Duloxetine has been associated with neonatal serotonin syndrome and neonatal behavioral syndrome (withdrawal) postdelivery. There is also a small but increased risk for persistent pulmonary hypertension of the newborn (PPHN) postbirth. Using this drug during pregnancy should be based on the pros and cons of the mother's clinical need for treatment versus any potential fetal risk that might occur from exposure.

BREASTFEEDING SUMMARY

Several studies have been located that have evaluated the use of duloxetine during human lactation. In a total of 10 women on doses that varied from 60 to 90 mg/d, the peak breast milk level was less than 70 ng/mL. Several RIDs were calculated, and all were less than 1%. The drug has been associated with hyperprolactinemia, but this should not adversely affect breastfeeding. Breastfeeding while using this drug should be based on the mother's clinical need for treatment versus any potential infant risks that might occur. If used, the infant should be monitored for the most common reported adult side effects of nausea (leading to irritability), somnolence, decreased appetite (monitor infant growth), and constipation. The long-term effects on neurobehavior and cognitive development from exposure to potent serotonin and norepinephrine reuptake inhibitors (SNRIs) and selective serotonin reuptake inhibitors (SSRIs) during a period of rapid central nervous system (CNS) development have not been adequately studied.

References

1. Prescribing Information. *Cymbalta*. Eli Lilly; 2020.
2. Briggs GG, Ambrose PJ, Ilett KF, et al. Use of duloxetine in pregnancy and lactation. *Ann Pharmacother*. 2009;43:1898-1902.
3. Raskin J, Goldstein DJ, Mallinckrodt CH, et al. Duloxetine in the long-term treatment of major depressive disorder. *J Clin Psychiatry*. 2003;64:1237-1244.
4. Bellantuono C, Migliarese G, Gentile S. Serotonin reuptake inhibitors in pregnancy and the risk of major malformations: a systematic review. *Hum Psychopharmacol Clin Exp*. 2007;22:121-128.
5. Chambers CD, Hernandez-Diaz S, Van Marter LJ, et al. Selective serotonin-reuptake inhibitors and risk of persistent pulmonary hypertension of the newborn. *N Engl J Med*. 2006;354:579-587.
6. Eyal R, Yaeger D. Poor neonatal adaptation after in utero exposure to duloxetine. *Am J Psychiatry*. 2008;165:651.
7. Hoog SL, Cheng Y, Elpers J, et al. Duloxetine and pregnancy outcomes: safety surveillance findings. *Int J Med Sci*. 2013;10:413-419.
8. Andrade C. The safety of duloxetine during pregnancy and lactation. *J Clin Psychiatry*. 2014;75:e1423-e1427.
9. First-trimester pregnancy exposure to venlafaxine or duloxetine and risk of major congenital malformations: a systematic review. *Basic Clin Pharmacol*. 2016;118:32-36.
10. Lobo ED, Loghin C, Knadler M, et al. Pharmacokinetics of duloxetine in breast milk and plasma of healthy postpartum women. *Clin Pharmacokinet*. 2008;47:103-109.
11. Marshall AM, Nommsen-Rivers LA, Hernandez LI, et al. Serotonin transport and metabolism in the mammary gland modulates secretory activation and involution. *J Clin Endocrin Metab*. 2010;95:837-846.
12. American Academy of Pediatrics. Committee on Drugs. The transfer of drugs and other chemicals into human milk. *Pediatrics*. 2001;108:776-789.

DUPILUMAB

Immunologic (Monoclonal Antibody—Immunomodulator)

PREGNANCY RECOMMENDATION: Limited Human Data—Animal Data Suggest Low Risk

BREASTFEEDING RECOMMENDATION: Probably Compatible

PREGNANCY SUMMARY

Several reports were located that describe the use of dupilumab during human pregnancy. No major anomalies were described in about 20 first-trimester exposures. As an IgG antibody, it likely crosses the placenta, especially during the second half of pregnancy, so some fetal exposure will probably occur. However, this limited human pregnancy experience prevents a

(continued)

complete assessment of the embryofetal risk. Animal studies did not show any embryofetal toxicity or teratogenicity in one species at doses of more than 10 times the RHD. Using this drug during pregnancy should be based on the pros and cons of the mother's clinical need for treatment versus any potential fetal risk that might occur from exposure. There is a pregnancy exposure registry that monitors pregnancy outcomes in women using this drug. Health care providers are encouraged to call the Dupixent Pregnancy Exposure Registry at 1-877-311-8972.

D

BREASTFEEDING SUMMARY

A single case was located that described the use of dupilumab during breastfeeding. The drug was detected in the breast milk at a level of about 1.3% of the maternal level. It is known that IgG antibodies can be found in human breast milk, but are not found in the neonatal or infant circulation. Additionally, if any IgG antibodies were to be ingested through breastfeeding, they would probably be digested in the infant's gastrointestinal tract and not be absorbed. Breastfeeding while using this drug should be based on the mother's clinical need for treatment versus any potential infant risks. If used, the infant should be monitored for the most common reported adult side effects of arthralgia, myalgia, dizziness, and oropharyngeal pain (all leading to irritability), insomnia, diarrhea, and eosinophilia.

References

1. Prescribing Information. *Dupixent*. Regeneron Pharmaceuticals, Inc; 2024.
2. Kage P, Simon JC. Treudler R. A case of atopic eczema treated safely with dupilumab during pregnancy and lactation. *J Eur Acad Dermatol Venereol*. 2020;34:e256-e257.
3. Escolà H, Figueras-Nart I, Bonfill-Orti M, et al. Dupilumab for atopic dermatitis during pregnancy and breastfeeding: clinical experience in 13 patients. *J Eur Acad Dermatol Venereol*. 2023;37:e1156-e1160.
4. Hong N, Park SY, Kook HD, et al. Atopic dermatitis treated safely with dupilumab during pregnancy and lactation: a case series of four patients. *Australas J Dermatol*. 2024;65:e100-e103.

DURVALUMAB

Antineoplastic (Monoclonal Antibody)

PREGNANCY RECOMMENDATION: No Human Data—Animal Data Suggest Potential Risk

BREASTFEEDING RECOMMENDATION: Probably Compatible

PREGNANCY SUMMARY

No reports describing the use of durvalumab in human pregnancy have been located. As an IgG antibody, the drug probably crosses the placenta, so some fetal exposure will likely occur. However, the absence of human pregnancy experience prevents a complete assessment of the embryofetal risk. Animal data did show some embryofetal toxicity in one species at doses less than 10 times the RHD. Due to the findings from animal studies and the drug's mechanism of action, the manufacturer recommends that women with reproductive potential use effective contraception during treatment and for at least 3 months after the last dose. Nevertheless, using this drug during pregnancy should be based on the pros and cons of the mother's clinical need for treatment versus any potential fetal risk that might occur from exposure.

BREASTFEEDING SUMMARY

No reports describing the use of durvalumab during human lactation have been located. The drug is likely present in breast milk. However, it is known that IgG antibodies can be found in human breast milk, but are not found in the neonatal or infant circulation. Additionally, if any IgG antibodies were to be ingested through breastfeeding, they would probably be digested in the infant's gastrointestinal tract and not be absorbed. The manufacturer recommends that pregnant women not breastfeed while using this drug and for 3 months after the last dose. However, breastfeeding while using this drug should be based on the mother's clinical need for treatment. If used, the infant should be monitored for the most common reported adult side effects of musculoskeletal pain and nausea (both leading to irritability), lethargy, decreased appetite, peripheral edema, rash, and cough.

Reference

1. Prescribing Information. *Imfinzi*. AstraZeneca Pharmaceuticals, Inc; 2020.

DUVELISIB

Antineoplastics (Kinase Inhibitor)

PREGNANCY RECOMMENDATION: No Human Data—Animal Data Suggest Potential Risk

BREASTFEEDING RECOMMENDATION: Potential Toxicity

D

PREGNANCY SUMMARY

No reports describing the use of duvelisib in human pregnancy have been located. The drug will probably cross the placenta, so some fetal exposure will likely occur. Therefore, the absence of human pregnancy experience prevents a complete assessment of the embryofetal risk. Animal data did show some embryo-fetal toxicity in one species at doses of about 10 times the MRHD, but not in a second species at more than 10 times the MRHD. Based on animal studies and the drug's mechanism of action, the manufacturer recommends that women with reproductive potential use effective contraception during treatment and for 1 month after the last dose. They also recommend that males with female partners of reproductive potential use effective contraception during treatment and for 1 month after the last dose. Nevertheless, using this drug during pregnancy should be based on the pros and cons of the mother's clinical need for treatment versus any potential fetal risk that might occur from exposure.

BREASTFEEDING SUMMARY

No reports describing the use of duvelisib during human lactation have been located. The drug will probably appear in breast milk, so some infant exposure will likely occur. Due to the concern for potential serious adverse effects that might be seen in a breastfed infant, the manufacturer recommends that women not breastfeed while being treated with this drug and for at least 1 month after the last dose. Nevertheless, breastfeeding while using this drug should be based on the mother's clinical need for treatment. If used, the infant should be monitored for the most common reported adult side effects of nausea and musculoskeletal pain (both leading to irritability), diarrhea, fatigue (lethargy), rash, colitis, upper respiratory infection, cough, fever, and various laboratory abnormalities (see PI).

Reference

1. Prescribing Information. *Copiktra*. Secura Bio, Inc; 2021.

E

ECALLANTIDE

Hematologic (Kallikrein Inhibitor)

PREGNANCY RECOMMENDATION: No Human Data—Animal Data Suggest Low Risk

BREASTFEEDING RECOMMENDATION: Probably Compatible

PREGNANCY SUMMARY

No reports describing the use of ecallantide in human pregnancy have been located. Placental transfer is unlikely to be clinically significant, and its short elimination half-life should minimize fetal exposure even further. However, the absence of human pregnancy experience prevents a complete assessment of the embryofetal risk. Animal studies did not show any embryofetal toxicity in two animal species at doses less than 10 times the maximum recommended human dose (MRHD) in the absence of maternal toxicity. Using this drug during pregnancy should be based on the pros and cons of the mother's clinical need for treatment versus any potential fetal risk that might occur from exposure.

BREASTFEEDING SUMMARY

No reports describing the use of ecallantide during human lactation have been located. The drug will not likely be found in breast milk. In addition, because the drug is a protein, if it were to be ingested through breastfeeding, it would probably be digested in the infant's gastrointestinal (GI) tract and not be absorbed. Breastfeeding while using this drug should be based on the mother's clinical need for treatment. If used, the infant should be monitored for the most common reported adult side effects of headache and nausea (both leading to irritability), diarrhea, fever, and nasopharyngitis.

Reference

1. Prescribing Information. Kalbitor. Takeda Pharmaceuticals U.S.A., Inc; 2021.

ECHOTHIOPHATE IODIDE

Ophthalmic (Antiglaucoma)

PREGNANCY RECOMMENDATION: Limited Human Data and No Relevant Animal Data

BREASTFEEDING RECOMMENDATION: Potential Toxicity (Long-Term Use)

PREGNANCY SUMMARY

A case report was located that described the use of echothiophate iodide ophthalmic solution in a pregnant woman for treating glaucoma. The exposure occurred at conception through the first 32 weeks of pregnancy and was then stopped. A healthy, normal, full-term infant was delivered without any reported anomalies. The drug will probably cross the placenta with ophthalmic use, so some fetal exposure will likely occur. Therefore, this limited human pregnancy experience prevents a complete assessment of the embryofetal risk. No animal reproduction studies have been conducted. Using this drug during pregnancy should be based on the pros and cons of the mother's clinical need for treatment versus any potential fetal risk that might occur from exposure. If used, consider placing pressure over the tear duct in the corner of the eye for at least 1 minute, and then remove any excess solution with absorbent tissue to further decrease the amount of drug reaching the systemic circulation.

BREASTFEEDING SUMMARY

No reports describing the use of echothiophate iodide ophthalmic during human lactation have been located. The drug will likely be found in breast milk, so some infant exposure will probably occur. Therefore, breastfeeding while using this drug should be based on the mother's clinical need for treatment. If used, consider placing pressure over the tear duct in the corner of the eye for at least 1 minute, and then remove any excess solution with absorbent tissue to further decrease the amount of drug reaching the systemic circulation. In addition, the infant should be monitored for the most common reported systemic adult side effect of headache (leading to irritability).

References

1. Prescribing Information. Phospholine iodide. Fera Pharmaceuticals; 2021.
2. Birks DA, Prior VJ, Silk E, Whittaker M. Echothiophate iodide treatment of glaucoma in pregnancy. *Arch Ophthal*. 1968;79:283-285.

ECONAZOLE

Anti-Infective (Antifungal/Topical)

PREGNANCY RECOMMENDATION: Limited Human Data—No Relevant Animal Data

BREASTFEEDING RECOMMENDATION: Probably Compatible

PREGNANCY SUMMARY

Two reports reporting the use of topical econazole during human pregnancy describing the overall outcome have been located. In the first study, 117 pregnant patients were treated for vaginal candidiasis with topical econazole, but drug exposure time during gestation was not provided. Of 107 pregnancies with delivery information, no complications or birth anomalies related to the drug were seen. The second study reported data from the Hungarian Case-Control Surveillance of Congenital Abnormalities database involving 2,146,574 deliveries that occurred from 1980 through 1996. Of 22,843 pregnancies with birth anomalies, there were 68 (0.30%) that used econazole compared with 122 (0.32%) that used econazole in 38,151 control pregnancies without any birth anomalies. This comparison was neither significant nor was the number of patients who used econazole in the first trimester. Several other studies have reported the use of econazole to treat vaginal candidiasis during pregnancy, but only provided efficacy data. Based on limited systemic absorption, fetal exposure is likely to be negligible. However, this limited human experience prevents a complete assessment of the embryofetal risk. Animal reproduction studies did show some embryofetal toxicity in three species, but at doses of 10 or more times the recommended human dose (RHD). Using this drug during pregnancy should be based on the pros and cons of the mother's clinical need for treatment versus any potential fetal risk that might occur from exposure.

BREASTFEEDING SUMMARY

No reports describing the use of topical econazole during human lactation have been located. The drug may be found in breast milk, but the amount should be clinically insignificant. Breastfeeding while using this drug should be based on the mother's clinical need for treatment. Because of the topical use, systemic side effects from breastfeeding would not be expected.

References

1. Prescribing Information. Econazole. Mylan Pharmaceuticals; 2018.
2. Goormans E, Beek JM, Declercq JA, et al. Efficacy of econazole in vaginal candidosis during pregnancy. *Curr Med Res Opin*. 1985;9:371-377.
3. Czeizel AE, Kazy Z, Vargha P. A population-based case-control teratological study of vaginal econazole treatment during pregnancy. *Eur J Obstet Gynecol Reprod Biol*. 2003;111:135-140.

ECULIZUMAB

Immunologic (Monoclonal Antibody—Paroxysmal Nocturnal Hemoglobinuria)

PREGNANCY RECOMMENDATION: Limited Human Data—Animal Data Suggest Potential Risk (Maternal Benefit May Outweigh Embryofetal Risk)

BREASTFEEDING RECOMMENDATION: Probably Compatible

PREGNANCY SUMMARY

Numerous publications have been located describing the use of eculizumab during human pregnancy. Over 60 first-trimester exposures have occurred, and no major fetal malformations were described. The premature birth rate was nearly 50%, but this is consistent with paroxysmal nocturnal hemoglobinuria (PNH). Human immunoglobulin G (IgG) antibodies are known to cross the placenta, especially during the second and third trimesters, which suggests that some transfer of eculizumab will occur. However, IgG2 antibodies have been shown to have the least placental transfer of the IgG subtypes. Treatment with eculizumab has been associated with an increased likelihood of fetal survival and decreased maternal complications.

(*continued*)

Regardless, this limited human pregnancy experience still prevents a complete assessment of the embryofetal risk. Animal studies did show some embryofetal toxicity in one species at doses less than 10 times the RHD. Using this drug during pregnancy should be based on the pros and cons of the mother's clinical need for treatment versus any potential fetal risk that might occur from exposure.

BREASTFEEDING SUMMARY

E

Nine reports describing the use of eculizumab in 81 breastfeeding women have been located. Of 49 infants with reported outcomes, only one infant was found to have neutropenia, but this was not attributed to eculizumab. It is known that IgG antibodies can be found in human breast milk, but are not found in the neonatal or infant circulation. Additionally, if any IgG antibodies were to be ingested through breastfeeding, they would probably be digested in the infant's GI tract and not be absorbed. Studies have shown that maternal doses usually produce undetectable levels in breast milk. Breastfeeding while using this drug should be based on the mother's clinical need for treatment versus any potential infant risks that might occur. If used, the infant should be monitored for the most common reported adult side effects of nausea, headache, and abdominal pain (all leading to irritability).

References

1. Ziakas PD, Poulou LS, Pomoni A. Thrombosis in paroxysmal nocturnal hemoglobinuria at a glance: a clinical review. *Curr Vasc Pharmacol.* 2008;6:347-353.
2. Brodsky RA. How I treat paroxysmal nocturnal hemoglobinuria. *Blood.* 2009;113:6522-6527.
3. Danilov AV, Brodsky RA, Craigo S, Smith H, Miller KB. Managing a pregnant patient with paroxysmal nocturnal hemoglobinuria in the era of eculizumab. *Leuk Res.* 2010;34:566-571.
4. Prescribing Information. Soliris. Alexion Pharmaceuticals; 2020.
5. Hillmen P. Eculizumab in paroxysmal nocturnal hemoglobinuria. *N Engl J Med.* 2006;355:2787-2788.
6. Danilov AV, Smith H, Craigo S, et al. Paroxysmal nocturnal hemoglobinuria (PNH) and pregnancy in the era of eculizumab. *Leuk Res.* 2009;33:e4-e5.
7. Kelly R, Arnold L, Richards S, et al. Successful pregnancy outcome in paroxysmal nocturnal haemoglobinuria on long term eculizumab (abstract). *Haematologica.* 2009;94:452.
8. Kelly R, Arnold L, Richards S, et al. The management of pregnancy in paroxysmal nocturnal haemoglobinuria on long term eculizumab. *Br J Haematol.* 2010;149:446-450.
9. Marasca R, Coluccio V, Santachiara R, et al. Pregnancy in PNH: another eculizumab baby. *Br J Haematol.* 2010;150:707-708.
10. Ardissino G, Ossola MW, Baffero GM, et al. Eculizumab for atypical hemolytic uremic syndrome in pregnancy. *Obstet Gynecol.* 2013;122:487-489.
11. Kelly RJ, Hochsmann B, Szer J, et al. Eculizumab in pregnant patients with paroxysmal nocturnal hemoglobinuria. *N Engl J Med.* 2015;373:1032-1039.
12. Hallstensen RF, Bergseth G, Foss S, et al. Eculizumab treatment during pregnancy does not affect the complement system activity of the newborn. *Immunobiology.* 2015;220:452-459.
13. Miyasaka N, Miura O, Kawaguchi T, et al. Pregnancy outcomes of patients with paroxysmal nocturnal hemoglobinuria treated with eculizumab: a Japanese experience and updated review. *Int J Hematol.* 2016;103:703-712.
14. Al-Dosari YM, Al-Zahrani H, Al-Mohareb F, Hashmi S. Pregnancy with paroxysmal nocturnal hemoglobinuria: a case series with review of the literature. *Saudi J Med Sci.* 2021;9:178-189.
15. Manning JE, Anderson RM, Hill A, et al. Pregnancy outcomes in women receiving eculizumab for the management of paroxysmal nocturnal haemoglobinuria. *Obstet Med.* 2022;15:45-49.
16. Servais A, Devillard N, Frémeaux-Bacchi V, et al. Atypical haemolytic uraemic syndrome and pregnancy: outcome with ongoing eculizumab. *Nephrol Dial Transplant.* 2016;31:2122-2130.
17. Gustavsen A, Skattum L, Bergseth G, et al. Effect on mother and child of eculizumab given before caesarean section in a patient with severe antiphospholipid syndrome: a case report. *Medicine (Baltimore).* 2017;96:e6338.
18. Rovere-Querini P, Canti V, Erra R, et al. Eculizumab in a pregnant patient with laboratory onset of catastrophic antiphospholipid syndrome: a case report. *Medicine.* 2018;97:e12584.
19. Burwick RM, Feinberg BB. Eculizumab for the treatment of preeclampsia/HELLP syndrome. *Placenta.* 2013;34:201-203.
20. Alashkar F, Saner FH, Vance C, et al. Pregnancy in classical paroxysmal nocturnal hemoglobinuria and aplastic anemia-paroxysmal nocturnal hemoglobinuria: a high-risk constellation. *Front Med (Lausanne).* 2020;7:543372.
21. Vinogradova M, Kulagin A, Kirsanova T, Shmakov R. Pregnancy outcomes in paroxysmal nocturnal hemoglobinuria depending on the therapeutic approach. *Br J Haematol.* 2017;176(suppl):94-95.
22. Vinogradova MA, Kulagin A, Shmakov R, et al. The pregnancy course and outcomes during targeted therapy of paroxysmal nocturnal hemoglobinuria. *Blood.* 2016;128:2397.
23. Aydin S, Audisio E, Iovino G, et al. Breakthrough hemolysis controlled by eculizumab escalation during pregnancy in paroxysmal nocturnal hemoglobinuria (PNH): a single case report. *Haematologica.* 2017;102(suppl 3):58.
24. Frairia C, Aydin S, Audisio E, et al. Breakthrough hemolysis and thromboembolism controlled by eculizumab during pregnancy in paroxysmal nocturnal hemoglobinuria (PNH): a single institution experience. *HemaSphere.* 2018;2(suppl 2):835-836.
25. Socié G, Caby-Tosi MP, Marantz JL, et al. Eculizumab in paroxysmal nocturnal haemoglobinuria and atypical haemolytic uraemic syndrome: 10-year pharmacovigilance analysis. *Br J Haematol.* 2019;185:297-310.
26. Amisha F, Konda M, Malik P, et al. Clinical-laboratory-genetic profile and outcomes of patients with atypical hemolytic uremic syndrome and restrictive use of eculizumab: a single center experience and a brief review. *Blood.* 2021;138(suppl 1):3159.
27. Fujimoto T, Maeda Y. Eculizumab use throughout pregnancy in two patients with aquaporin-4-positive neuromyelitis optica spectrum disorder. *Clin Exp Neuroimmunol.* 2024;15(3):126-129.
28. Sarris I, Gandhi S, Koumis A, et al. Pregnancy outcome and safety of breastfeeding in two patients with paroxysmal nocturnal haemoglobinuria (PNH) treated with eculizumab. *Arch Dis Child Fetal Neonatal Ed.* 2012;97:43.
29. Ando Y, Kida M, Saika M, et al. Pregnancy and delivery in a PNH patient treated with eculizumab. *Rinsho Ketsueki.* 2014;55:2288-2293.
30. Sharma R, Keyzner A, Liu J, et al. Successful pregnancy outcome in paroxysmal nocturnal hemoglobinuria (PNH) following escalated eculizumab dosing to control breakthrough hemolysis. *Leuk Res Rep.* 2015;4:36-38.

EDARAVONE

Central Nervous System (Amyotrophic Lateral Sclerosis)

PREGNANCY RECOMMENDATION: No Human Data—Animal Data Suggest Potential Risk

BREASTFEEDING RECOMMENDATION: Potential Toxicity

PREGNANCY SUMMARY

No reports describing the use of edaravone in human pregnancy have been located. The drug will probably cross the placenta, so fetal exposure will likely occur. Therefore, the absence of human pregnancy experience prevents a complete assessment of embryofetal risk. Animal studies did show some embryofetal toxicity. Using this drug during pregnancy should be based on the pros and cons of the mother's clinical need for treatment versus any potential fetal risk that might occur from exposure.

BREASTFEEDING SUMMARY

No reports describing the use of edaravone during human lactation have been located. The drug will probably enter breast milk, so infant exposure will likely occur. Breastfeeding should be based on the mother's clinical need for treatment. If used, the infant should be monitored for the most common reported adult side effects of headache (leading to irritability) and rash.

Reference

1. Prescribing Information. Radicava. Mitsubishi Tanabe Pharma Corp; 2017.

EDETATE (ETHYLENEDIAMINETETRAACETIC ACID—EDTA)

Chelating Agent

PREGNANCY RECOMMENDATION: Limited Human Data—Animal Data Suggest Potential Risk (Maternal Benefit May Outweigh Embryofetal Risk)

BREASTFEEDING RECOMMENDATION: *Contraindicated

PREGNANCY SUMMARY

No reports describing the use of EDTA during the first trimester in human pregnancy have been located. Four case reports describing the use of edetate calcium disodium during the third trimester in seven human pregnancies were found. No drug-related complications were described. All seven cases involved lead poisoning; five from pica of lead-based substances, one from a contaminated herbal product that also contained mercury, and one from the use of battery cases as fuel in a living room stove. The drug will probably cross the placenta, so some fetal exposure will likely occur. Therefore, this limited human pregnancy experience prevents a complete assessment of the embryofetal risk. Teratogenicity was observed in one animal species at doses less than 10 times the RHD. The Centers for Disease Control and Prevention (CDC) recommends that pregnant women, particularly in the second and third trimesters, with blood lead levels of 45 to 69 mcg/dL should be considered for chelation therapy. Pregnant women with blood lead levels of 70 mcg/dL or greater should be considered for therapy regardless of trimester. In addition, pregnant patients with encephalopathy should receive treatment regardless of trimester.

BREASTFEEDING SUMMARY

No reports describing the use of EDTA during human lactation have been located. The drug probably will appear in breast milk, but the rapid clearance should limit some excretion. Moreover, edetate is poorly absorbed after oral dosing, at least from the adult GI tract. The risk to a nursing infant from exposure to the drug in breast milk is unknown but is expected to be negligible. However, because the use of edetate implies poisoning with lead, this metal will also be excreted into breast milk and can be toxic to a nursing infant. *The CDC recommends that mothers with blood lead levels of 40 mcg/dL or greater should not initiate breastfeeding and should be advised to pump and discard their breast milk until the levels drop below 40 mcg/dL.

References

1. Schardein JL. Metals. In: *Chemically Induced Birth Defects*. 3rd ed. Marcel Dekker; 2000:879.
2. Bailey B. Are there teratogenic risks associated with antidotes used in the acute management of poisoned pregnant women? *Birth Def Res (Part A)*. 2003;67:133-140.
3. Prescribing Information. Calcium disodium versenate. Medicis Pharmaceutical; 2012.
4. Domingo JL. Developmental toxicity of metal chelating agents. *Reprod Toxicol*. 1998;12:499-510.
5. Angle CR, McIntire MS. Lead poisoning during pregnancy. Fetal tolerance of calcium disodium edetate. *Am J Dis Child*. 1964;108:436-439.
6. Timpo AE, Amin JS, Casalino MB, Yuceoglu AM. Congenital lead intoxication. *J Pediatr*. 1979;94:765-767.
7. Pearl M, Boxi LM. Radiographic findings in congenital lead poisoning. *Radiology*. 1980;136:83-84.
8. Tait PA, Vora A, James S, et al. Severe congenital lead poisoning in a preterm infant due to a herbal remedy. *Med J Aust*. 2002;177:193-195.
9. Shannon M. Severe lead poisoning in pregnancy. *Ambul Pediatr*. 2003;3:37-39.
10. Centers for Disease Control and Prevention (CDC). *Guidelines for the Identification and Management of Lead Exposure in Pregnant and Lactating Women*. CDC; 2010.

EDOXABAN

Hematologic (Anticoagulant—Oral)

PREGNANCY RECOMMENDATION: Limited Human Data—No Relevant Animal Data

BREASTFEEDING RECOMMENDATION: Potential Toxicity

E

PREGNANCY SUMMARY

Limited reports describing the use of edoxaban in human pregnancy have been located. In one study that collected case reports of direct-acting oral anticoagulant exposure during pregnancy from multiple sources, 614 unique pregnancies were identified. Of these, 23 cases were with edoxaban. Excluding elective terminations, of 17 cases with outcome data, there were 16 live births with 1 major anomaly (exposure occurred throughout pregnancy) and 1 spontaneous abortion. The major birth defect was a term infant with lung hypoplasia and congenital renal tubular dysplasia. In another analysis, eight first-trimester exposures were identified, describing seven infants delivered without any identified anomalies and one spontaneous abortion. Some of the drug will likely cross the placenta, so fetal exposure will probably occur. Therefore, this limited human pregnancy experience prevents a complete assessment of the embryofetal risk. In animal studies, embryofetal toxicity was observed in two species, but at doses more than 10 times the RHD. Using this drug during pregnancy should be based on the pros and cons of the mother's clinical need for treatment versus any potential fetal risk that might occur from exposure. The American College of Obstetricians and Gynecologists (ACOG) states that oral direct-acting anticoagulants should be avoided in pregnancy due to insufficient data and the concern for placental transfer producing an indirect effect on fetal blood coagulation. Edoxaban carries a boxed warning of increased risk for spinal/epidural hematoma.

BREASTFEEDING SUMMARY

No reports describing the use of edoxaban during human lactation have been located. The drug may be excreted into breast milk, so some infant exposure will likely occur. ACOG states that oral direct-acting anticoagulants should be avoided while breastfeeding due to the lack of data. If the clinical decision is to use this drug while breastfeeding, the infant should be monitored for the most common reported adult side effects of bleeding, anemia, rash, and abnormal liver function tests.

References

1. Prescribing Information. Savaysa. Daiichi Sankyo; 2021.
2. Sakai M, Ogura J, Yamanoi K, et al. A case pregnancy complicated with ATIII deficiency in a patient who developed severe venous thromboembolism in her fourth pregnancy and had a favourable outcome in her subsequent pregnancy with careful management of anticoagulation therapy including edoxaban. *Case Rep Obstet Gynecol*. 2019;2019:2436828.
3. Beyer-Westendorf J, Tittl L, Bistervels I, et al. Safety of direct oral anticoagulant exposure during pregnancy: a retrospective cohort study. *Lancet Haematol*. 2020;7:e884-e891.
4. Areia AL, Mota-Pinto A. Experience with direct oral anticoagulants in pregnancy—a systematic review. *J Perinat Med*. 2022;50(4):457-461.
5. American College of Obstetricians and Gynecologists' Committee on Practice Bulletins—Obstetrics. ACOG Practice Bulletin No. 196: thromboembolism in pregnancy. *Obstet Gynecol*. 2018;132(1):e1-e17.

EFAVIRENZ

Antiretroviral (Non-Nucleoside Reverse Transcriptase Inhibitor)

PREGNANCY RECOMMENDATION: Human Data Suggest Low Risk (Maternal Benefit May Outweigh Any Embryofetal Risk)

BREASTFEEDING RECOMMENDATION: *Contraindicated

PREGNANCY SUMMARY

From three large studies that involve 4,419 first-trimester exposures to efavirenz, 91 infants (2.1%) with major birth anomalies were identified. No pattern was seen in the anomalies. Prior reports with some antiretroviral drugs suggested an increased risk for neural tube defects, but this was not seen in these large analyses. However, a few recent studies have suggested an increased risk for some neurodevelopmental abnormalities/delay and microcephaly that have been seen in infants exposed to efavirenz in utero. However, these findings have numerous covariables that are difficult to control for. Regardless, these issues require further follow-up. The drug appears to cross the placenta, so fetal exposure will occur. Animal studies did show some embryofetal toxicity and malformations in two species at doses less than 10 times the RHD. In 2023, the updated

US Department of Health and Human Services AIDS Info guidelines for the use of antiretroviral agents during pregnancy recommend that, in most cases, patients continue their regimen during pregnancy if it is tolerated, safe, and effective in suppressing viral replication. The guideline recommends that a discussion and shared decision-making about the known and potential risks, as well as benefits to the mother and fetus, be conducted (acknowledging limited data). This should guide the selection of which antiretroviral agents to use during pregnancy. Additionally, treatment initiation should not be delayed due to concerns about teratogenicity with first-trimester exposure. See the guideline for the most updated information on this subject. If indicated, efavirenz should not be withheld in pregnancy since the expected benefit to the mother with HIV probably outweighs the unknown risk to the fetus. The guidelines note that efavirenz is not associated with an increased risk for congenital anomalies. Providers caring for pregnant patients with HIV and their infants can call the national Perinatal HIV/AIDS hotline (888-448-8765) for free clinical consultation. Additionally, there is a pregnancy exposure registry that monitors pregnancy outcomes in individuals exposed to antiretroviral medications during pregnancy. Health care providers are encouraged to register patients by calling the Antiretroviral Pregnancy Registry (APR) at 1-800-258-4263.

E

BREASTFEEDING SUMMARY

Efavirenz has been found in breast milk and infant blood in mothers using the drug while breastfeeding. Infant plasma levels are low, ranging from 0.4 to 1.5 ng/mL. In 2023, the updated US Department of Health and Human Services AIDS Info guidelines state that using replacement of breast milk through formula or pasteurized donor human breast milk from a milk bank eliminates the risk of postnatal HIV transmission to the infant. Using antiretroviral therapy to achieve and maintain viral suppression during pregnancy and postpartum can decrease the risk for infant transmission to less than 1%, but not zero. *For patients not on therapy for viral load suppression during pregnancy (at a minimum of throughout the third trimester) and at delivery, replacement of breast milk is recommended. Patients on antiretroviral therapy who have a sustained undetectable viral load and who choose to breastfeed or use replacement of breast milk should be supported with this decision. If the clinical decision is to use this drug while breastfeeding, the infant should be monitored for the most common reported adult side effects of dizziness, nausea, and headache (all leading to irritability), rash, fatigue (lethargy), insomnia, and vomiting.

References

1. Prescribing Information. Sustiva. Bristol-Myers Squibb Pharma; 2019.
2. Kreitchmann R, Schalkwijk S, Best B, et al. Efavirenz pharmacokinetics during pregnancy and infant washout. *Antivir Ther.* 2019;24(2):95-103.
3. Cressey TR, Stek A, Capparelli E, et al. Efavirenz pharmacokinetics during the third trimester of pregnancy and postpartum. *J Acquir Immune Defic Syndr.* 2012;59(3):245-252.
4. Antiretroviral Pregnancy Registry Steering Committee. *Antiretroviral Pregnancy Registry Interim Report for 1 January 1989 Through 31 January 2023.* Registry Coordinating Center; 2023.
5. Ford N, Mofenson L, Shubber Z, et al. Safety of efavirenz in the first trimester of pregnancy: an updated systematic review and meta-analysis. *AIDS.* 2014; 28(suppl 2):S123-S131.
6. Sibiude J, Mandelbrot L, Blanche S, et al. Association between prenatal exposure to antiretroviral therapy and birth defects: an analysis of the French Perinatal Cohort Study (ANRS CO1/CO11). *PLoS Med.* 2014;11:e1001635.
7. Mofenson LM, Watts DH. Safety of pediatric HIV elimination: the growing population of HIV- and antiretroviral-exposed but uninfected infants. *PLoS Med.* 2014;11:e1001636.
8. Zash R, Holmes L, Diseko M, et al. Neural-tube defects and antiretroviral treatment regimens in Botswana. *N Engl J Med.* 2019;381:827-840.
9. Mehta UC, van Schalkwyk C, Naidoo P, et al. Birth outcomes following antiretroviral exposure during pregnancy: initial results from a pregnancy exposure registry in South Africa. *South Afr J HIV Med.* 2019;20:971.
10. Martinez de Tejada B; European Pregnancy and Paediatric HIV Cohort Collaboration Study Group. Birth defects after exposure to efavirenz-based antiretroviral therapy at conception/first trimester of pregnancy: a multicohort analysis. *J Acquir Immune Defic Syndr* 2019;80:316-324.
11. Cassidy AR, Williams PL, Leidner J, et al. In utero efavirenz exposure and neurodevelopmental outcomes in HIV-exposed uninfected children in Botswana. *Pediatr Infect Dis J.* 2019;38:828-834.
12. Crowell CS, Williams PL, Yildirim C, et al. Safety of in-utero antiretroviral exposure: neurologic outcomes in children who are HIV-exposed but uninfected. *AIDS.* 2020;34:1377-1387.
13. Williams PL, Yildirim C, Chadwick EG, et al. Association of maternal antiretroviral use with microcephaly in children who are HIV-exposed but uninfected (SMARTT): a prospective cohort study. *Lancet HIV.* 2020;7:e49-e58.
14. Panel on Treatment of HIV During Pregnancy and Prevention of Perinatal Transmission. Recommendations for the use of antiretroviral drugs during pregnancy and interventions to reduce perinatal HIV transmission in the United States. Department of Health and Human Services. Accessed September 24, 2023. https://clinicalinfo.hiv.gov/en/guidelines/perinatal
15. Schneider S, Peltier A, Gras A, et al. Efavirenz in human breast milk, mothers', and newborns' plasma. *J Acquir Immune Defic Syndr.* 2008;48:450-454.
16. Cohan D, Natureeba P, Koss CA, et al. Efficacy and safety of lopinavir/ritonavir versus efavirenz-based antiretroviral therapy in HIV-infected pregnant Ugandan women. *AIDS.* 2015;29:183-191.
17. Oumar AA, Bagayoko-Maiga K, Bahachimi A, et al. Efavirenz and lopinavir levels in HIV-infected women and their nursing infants, in Mali. *J Pharmacol Exp Ther.* 2018;366:479-484.
18. Kapito-Tembo AP, Bauleni A, Wesevich A, et al. Growth and neurodevelopment outcomes in HIV-, tenofovir- and efavirenz-exposed breastfed infants in PMTCT Option B+ program in Malawi. *J Acquir Immune Defic Syndr.* 2021;86:81-90.
19. Chinula L, Ziemba L, Brummel S, et al. Efficacy and safety of three antiretroviral therapy regimens started in pregnancy up to 50 weeks post partum: a multicentre, open-label, randomised, controlled, phase 3 trial. *Lancet HIV.* 2023;10:e363-e374.

EFBEMALENOGRASTIM ALFA

Hematologic (Granulocyte Colony-Stimulating Factor)

PREGNANCY RECOMMENDATION: No Human Data—Animal Data Suggest Low Risk

BREASTFEEDING RECOMMENDATION: Probably Compatible

PREGNANCY SUMMARY

No reports describing the use of efbemalenograstim alfa in human pregnancy have been located. Because of the Fc portions of an IgG2 molecule, the drug will likely cross the placenta, especially during the second half of gestation, so some fetal exposure will probably occur. However, the absence of human pregnancy experience prevents a complete assessment of the embryofetal risk. Animal data did not show any embryofetal toxicity in two species at doses less than 10 times the RHD. Using this drug during pregnancy should be based on the pros and cons of the mother's clinical need for treatment versus any potential fetal risk that might occur from exposure.

E

BREASTFEEDING SUMMARY

No reports describing the use of efbemalenograstim alfa during human lactation have been located. Due to the Fc portions of an IgG2 molecule, the drug might be found in human breast milk. Regardless, it is not likely to be found in the neonatal or infant circulation. Additionally, if any of this recombinant fusion protein were to be ingested through breastfeeding, it would probably be digested in the infant's GI tract and not be absorbed. Breastfeeding while using this drug should be based on the mother's clinical need for treatment versus any potential infant risk that might occur. If used, the infant should be monitored for the most common reported adult side effects of nausea (leading to irritability), anemia, and thrombocytopenia.

Reference

1. Prescribing Information. Ryzneuta. Evive Biotechnology Singapore Pte. Ltd; 2023.

EFGARTIGIMOD ALFA

Central Nervous System (Myasthenia Gravis—Antibody Fragment/Neonatal Fc Receptor Antagonist)

PREGNANCY RECOMMENDATION: No Human Data—Animal Data Suggest Low Risk

BREASTFEEDING RECOMMENDATION: Probably Compatible

PREGNANCY SUMMARY

No reports describing the use of efgartigimod alfa in human pregnancy have been located. As an IgG antibody fragment (the Fc portion), it likely crosses the placenta, especially during the second half of pregnancy. However, because its target is the neonatal Fc receptor itself, levels in the fetus may be minimal. Therefore, the absence of human pregnancy experience prevents a complete assessment of the embryofetal risk. Animal data did not show any embryofetal toxicity. Using this drug during pregnancy should be based on the pros and cons of the mother's clinical need for treatment versus any potential fetal risk that might occur from exposure. The neonatal Fc receptor is an intricate part of the transport system for immunoglobulins across the placenta (see Immunoglobulins in Pregnancy). Therefore, the use of efgartigimod alfa during pregnancy in theory should decrease transplacental passage of all IgG antibodies. Because of this, passive protection of the newborn with immunoglobulins (especially in the third trimester and at delivery) is anticipated to be reduced.

BREASTFEEDING SUMMARY

No reports describing the use of efgartigimod alfa during human lactation have been located. It is known that IgG antibodies can be found in human breast milk, but are not found in the neonatal or infant circulation. Additionally, if any IgG antibodies were to be ingested through breastfeeding, they would probably be digested in the infant's GI tract and not be absorbed. Breastfeeding while using this drug should be based on the mother's clinical need for treatment. If used, the infant should be monitored for the most common reported adult side effects of respiratory tract infections, headache (leading to irritability), and urinary tract infections.

Reference

1. Prescribing Information. Vyvgart. Argenx US; 2022.

EFINACONAZOLE

Anti-Infective (Antifungal—Topical)

PREGNANCY RECOMMENDATION: No Human Data—Animal Data Suggest Low Risk

BREASTFEEDING RECOMMENDATION: Probably Compatible

PREGNANCY SUMMARY

No reports describing the use of efinaconazole in human pregnancy have been located. Placental passage overall is likely to be negligible, but some fetal exposure is possible with extended use. Therefore, the absence of human pregnancy experience prevents a complete assessment of the embryofetal risk. Animal studies did not show any embryofetal toxicity in two animal species despite the administration subcutaneously at doses greater than 10 times the MRHD. Using this drug during pregnancy should be based on the pros and cons of the mother's clinical need for treatment versus any potential fetal risk that might occur from exposure.

E

BREASTFEEDING SUMMARY

No reports describing the use of efinaconazole during human lactation have been located. The drug may be found in breast milk, but levels are likely to be negligible. Breastfeeding while using this drug should be based on the mother's clinical need for treatment. Because of the topical use of the drug, systemic side effects were not reported.

Reference

1. Prescribing Information. Jublia. Bausch Health Companies, Inc; 2022.

EFLAPEGRASTIM

Hematopoietic (Granulocyte Colony-Stimulating Factor)

PREGNANCY RECOMMENDATION: No Human Data—Animal Data Suggest Potential Risk

BREASTFEEDING RECOMMENDATION: Probably Compatible

PREGNANCY SUMMARY

No reports describing the use of eflapegrastim in human pregnancy have been located. Because it contains the Fc portion of an IgG antibody, the drug will likely cross the placenta, so some fetal exposure will probably occur. However, the absence of human pregnancy experience prevents a complete assessment of embryofetal risk. Embryofetal toxicity was observed in one animal species. Using this drug during pregnancy should be based on the pros and cons of the mother's clinical need for treatment versus any potential fetal risk that might occur from exposure.

BREASTFEEDING SUMMARY

No reports describing the use of eflapegrastim during human lactation have been located. It is known that IgG antibodies can be found in human breast milk, but are not found in the neonatal or infant circulation. Additionally, if any IgG antibodies were to be ingested through breastfeeding, they would probably be digested in the infant's GI tract and not be absorbed. Furthermore, the granulocyte colony-stimulating growth factor analogue is a polypeptide consisting of about 175 amino acids, so this would also be digested in the infant's GI tract and not be absorbed. Breastfeeding while using this drug should be based on the mother's clinical need for treatment. If used, the infant should be monitored for the most common reported adult side effects of nausea, myalgia, arthralgia, back pain, headache, and bone pain (all leading to irritability), diarrhea, pyrexia, anemia, rash, and fatigue.

Reference

1. Prescribing Information. Rolvedon. Spectrum Pharmaceuticals, Inc; 2022.

ELACESTRANT

Antineoplastic (Estrogen Receptor Antagonist)

PREGNANCY RECOMMENDATION: *Contraindicated

BREASTFEEDING RECOMMENDATION: *Contraindicated

PREGNANCY SUMMARY

No reports describing the use of elacestrant in human pregnancy have been located. The drug is likely to cross the placenta, so some fetal exposure would probably occur. Animal data showed embryofetal toxicity, but maternal toxicity was also seen.

(continued)

Based on animal studies and the drug's mechanism of action, the manufacturer recommends that women with reproductive potential use effective contraception during treatment and for 1 week after the last dose. They also recommend that males with female partners of reproductive potential use effective contraception during treatment and for 1 week after the last dose. *However, because the drug is only approved for use in postmenopausal women and adult men, it is contraindicated during pregnancy.

E

BREASTFEEDING SUMMARY

No reports describing the use of elacestrant during human lactation have been located. The drug would likely be excreted into breast milk, so some infant exposure would probably occur. Due to the concern for potential serious adverse effects that might be seen in a breastfed infant, the manufacturer recommends that women not breastfeed while being treated with this drug and for at least 1 week after the last dose. *However, because the drug is only approved for use in postmenopausal women and adult men, it is contraindicated during pregnancy and lactation.

Reference

1. Prescribing Information. Orserdu. Stemline Therapies, Inc; 2023.

ELAFIBRANOR

Gastrointestinal (Hepatic—Peroxisome Proliferator–Activated Receptor Agonist)

PREGNANCY RECOMMENDATION: No Human Data—Animal Data Suggest Risk

BREASTFEEDING RECOMMENDATION: Potential Toxicity

PREGNANCY SUMMARY

No reports describing the use of elafibranor in human pregnancy have been located. The drug will likely cross the placenta, so some fetal exposure will probably occur. Therefore, the absence of human pregnancy experience prevents a complete assessment of the embryofetal risk. Animal studies did show embryofetal toxicity in two species at doses of less than 10 times the RHD. Based on these animal studies, the manufacturer recommends that women with reproductive potential use effective contraception during treatment and for 3 weeks after the last dose. Nevertheless, using this drug during pregnancy should be based on the pros and cons of the mother's clinical need for treatment versus any potential fetal risk that might occur from exposure. There is a pregnancy exposure registry that monitors pregnancy outcomes in women using this drug. Health care providers are encouraged to call the Iqirvo Pregnancy Exposure Registry at 1-855-463-5217. Elafibranor was found to cause fractures in 6% of the patients in the clinical trials, which was not seen in the placebo group. The exact cause for this is not fully known.

BREASTFEEDING SUMMARY

No reports describing the use of elafibranor during human lactation have been located. The drug will likely be found in breast milk, so some infant exposure will probably occur. Due to a concern for potential serious adverse effects that might be seen in a breastfed infant, the manufacturer recommends that women not breastfeed while being treated with this drug and for at least 3 weeks after the last dose. Nevertheless, breastfeeding while using this drug should be based on the mother's clinical need for treatment versus any potential infant risk that might occur. If used, the infant should be monitored for the most common reported adult side effects of nausea, abdominal pain, and arthralgia (all leading to irritability), vomiting, rash, diarrhea, and weight loss (monitor infant growth).

Reference

1. Prescribing Information. Iqirvo. Ibsen Biopharmaceuticals, Inc; 2023.

ELAGOLIX

Reproductive Health (Gonadotropin-Releasing Hormone Antagonist)

PREGNANCY RECOMMENDATION: *Contraindicated—No Relevant Animal Data

BREASTFEEDING RECOMMENDATION: Potential Toxicity

PREGNANCY SUMMARY

In the clinical trials, the manufacturer reported 49 pregnancies exposed to elagolix during or just prior to pregnancy. Two (4.1%) major malformations were identified: one infant with a cleft palate, and the second infant with tracheoesophageal fistula. The spontaneous abortion rate was not increased. There were no apparent decreases in birth weights associated with the drug in comparison to the placebo. Elagolix will probably cross the placenta, so some fetal exposure will likely occur. Therefore, this limited human pregnancy experience prevents a complete assessment of the embryofetal risk. *Based on the approved use for the drug, it is contraindicated for use during pregnancy. Animal studies did not show any increased risk for malformations in two species at doses more than 10 times the MRHD, but some embryofetal toxicity occurred in the presence of maternal toxicity. Elagolix can alter menstrual bleeding that may decrease the ability to recognize pregnancy and result in early pregnancy loss. Therefore, the manufacturer recommends that women with reproductive potential use effective contraception during treatment and for 4 weeks after the last dose. There is a pregnancy exposure registry that monitors pregnancy outcomes in women exposed to elagolix during pregnancy. Health care providers or patients are encouraged to contact the registry by calling 1-833-782-7241.

BREASTFEEDING SUMMARY

No reports describing the use of elagolix during human lactation have been located. The drug will probably be excreted into breast milk, so some infant exposure may occur. Breastfeeding while using this drug should be based on the mother's clinical need for treatment. If used, the infant should be monitored for the most common reported adult side effects of nausea, arthralgia, headache, and anxiety (all leading to irritability), insomnia, and sweating.

Reference

1. Prescribing Information. Orilissa. AbbVie; 2023.

ELAPEGADEMASE

Genetic/Immunologic (Enzyme)

PREGNANCY RECOMMENDATION: No Human Data and No Relevant Animal Data (Maternal Benefit May Outweigh Embryofetal Risk)

BREASTFEEDING RECOMMENDATION: Probably Compatible

PREGNANCY SUMMARY

No reports describing the use of elapegademase in human pregnancy have been located. The drug is not likely to cross the placenta; however, because it consists of a protein, it is not known whether some fetal exposure might occur. Two case reports of pregnant women who were treated with pegademase (same class of enzyme replacement therapy) resulted in successful pregnancies and deliveries with no teratogenic effects reported. However, the absence of human pregnancy experience prevents a complete assessment of the embryofetal risk. No animal reproduction studies have been conducted. Because this agent is used for the treatment of a rare, inherited disease that is often fatal, it should not be withheld because of pregnancy.

BREASTFEEDING SUMMARY

No reports describing the use of elapegademase during human lactation have been located. The drug most likely will not appear in breast milk. Furthermore, because it is an enzyme (protein), if any drug were to be present in breast milk, it would probably be digested in the infant's GI tract and not be absorbed. Breastfeeding while using this drug should be based on the mother's clinical need for treatment. If used while breastfeeding, the infant should be monitored for the most common reported adult side effects of cough and vomiting.

Reference

1. Prescribing Information. Revcovi. Chiesi USA, Inc; 2020.

ELBASVIR AND GRAZOPREVIR

Antiviral (Hepatitis C)

PREGNANCY RECOMMENDATION: No Human Data—Animal Data Suggest Low Risk

BREASTFEEDING RECOMMENDATION: Probably Compatible

PREGNANCY SUMMARY

No reports describing the use of elbasvir/grazoprevir in human pregnancy have been located. Some amount of both drugs will probably cross the placenta, so fetal exposure will likely occur. Therefore, the absence of human pregnancy experience prevents a complete assessment of the embryofetal risk. Animal data did not show any embryofetal toxicity. The current guidance for the treatment of hepatitis C recommends that women who become pregnant while taking direct-acting antivirals (DAAs), like elbasvir and grazoprevir, should consult with their physician regarding continuing treatment after discussion about the potential risks and benefits. DAAs, however, are not recommended during pregnancy to reduce mother-to-child transmission. If elbasvir and grazoprevir are administered with ribavirin, this may be contraindicated (see Ribavirin for information regarding contraception during treatment).

E

BREASTFEEDING SUMMARY

No reports describing the use of elbasvir/grazoprevir during human lactation have been located. Both drugs are probably excreted into breast milk in small amounts, so infant exposure will likely occur. Breastfeeding while using this drug should be based on the mother's clinical need for treatment. If used, the infant should be monitored for the most common reported adult side effects of nausea and headache (both leading to irritability) and lethargy. If elbasvir/grazoprevir are administered with ribavirin, see Ribavirin for information regarding lactation during treatment.

References

1. Prescribing Information. Zepatier. Merck Sharp & Dohme, LLC; 2022.
2. AASLD-IDSA. HCV in pregnancy. Accessed February 19, 2023. http://www.hcvguidelines.org/unique-populations/pregnancy

ELETRIPTAN

Central Nervous System (Antimigraine)

PREGNANCY RECOMMENDATION: Limited Human Data—Animal Data Suggest Potential Risk

BREASTFEEDING RECOMMENDATION: Probably Compatible

PREGNANCY SUMMARY

Three studies describing the use of eletriptan during human pregnancy have been located. Two of the studies were from the same author, and some of the patients in the first report are duplicated in the second study. The first study combined data from the Norwegian Mother and Child Cohort Study (findings from two self-administered questionnaires) with data from the Medical Birth Registry of Norway (information provided by health care providers and medical records). In addition, there was an erratum for this paper. The second study combined data from the Medical Birth Registry of Norway with the Norwegian Prescription Database. Because of the unknown number of duplicated patients, only data from the second study will be discussed. A total of 1,210 first-trimester exposures to triptans were identified and compared with 178,565 pregnant patients without triptan use. No increased risk for major congenital malformations was seen with the use of triptans as a group when compared to the non–triptan-exposed pregnant control patients. The third study using data from the Swedish Medical Birth Registry (1,211,670 women) reported 92 (3.3%) major anomalies in 2,777 first-trimester exposures to triptans as a group. Over 98% of the triptans involved sumatriptan, zolmitriptan, and rizatriptan. From these studies, there were 203 first-trimester exposures to eletriptan with 6 (3.0%) major anomalies. A recent meta-analysis, involving six studies (including 2 of the above) with over 4,000 first-trimester exposures to triptans as a group compared with more than a million controls with no triptan exposure, found no increased risk for major anomalies with triptan use. Sumatriptan is the most studied triptan to date (see Sumatriptan). Eletriptan will probably cross the placenta, so some fetal exposure will likely occur. However, this limited human pregnancy experience with eletriptan prevents a complete assessment of the embryofetal risk. Embryofetal toxicity was observed in one animal species at doses less than 10 times the RHD. ACOG suggests the cautious use of triptans, preferably sumatriptan, as second-line therapy for patients uncontrolled by acetaminophen alone or in combination therapy with caffeine or metoclopramide with diphenhydramine. It is also recommended that triptans not be used in pregnant patients with cardiac disease or hypertension due to their possible vasoconstrictive effects. Using this drug during pregnancy should be based on the pros and cons of the mother's clinical need for treatment versus any potential fetal risk that might occur from exposure.

BREASTFEEDING SUMMARY

Two reports that analyzed eletriptan in human breast milk were located. In the first, the maximum concentration of the drug found in breast milk in three lactating patients ranged from 78 to 102 ng/mL. The estimated relative infant dose (RID) was only 0.6% (range 0.3%-0.8%). In the second, the manufacturer evaluated eight lactating women. The mean amount of drug excreted in a 24-hour period was only about 13 mcg. The mean concentration found in breast milk at 24 hours was only 1.7 ng/mL. The active metabolite was not measured in breast milk. The very low concentrations measured suggest that eletriptan is probably compatible with breastfeeding. Breastfeeding while using this drug should be based on the mother's clinical need for treatment. If used, the infant should be monitored for the most common reported adult side effects of headache, chest pain, paresthesia, dizziness, nausea, and skeletal pain (all leading to irritability), fatigue (lethargy), and flushing. ACOG states that using triptans for treating migraine during lactation should be a shared decision-making process. ACOG also suggests avoiding breastfeeding for 24 hours after the use of triptans (except sumatriptan, which is 8-12 hours).

References

1. Prescribing Information. Relpax. Roerig; 2021.
2. Schenker S, Yang Y, Perex A, et al. Sumatriptan (Imitrex) transport by the human placenta. *Proc Soc Exp Biol Med*. 1995;210:213-220.
3. Nezvalova-Henriksen K, Spigset O, Nordeng H. Triptan exposure during pregnancy and the risk of major congenital malformations and adverse pregnancy outcomes: results from the Norwegian Mother Child Cohort Study. *Headache*. 2010;50:563-575.
4. Nezvalova-Henriksen K, Spigset O, Nordeng H. Errata in "Triptan exposure during pregnancy and the risk of major congenital malformations and adverse pregnancy outcomes: results from the Norwegian Mother Child Cohort Study." *Headache*. 2012;52:1319-1320.
5. Nezvalova-Henriksen K, Spigset O, Nordeng H. Triptan safety during pregnancy: a Norwegian population registry study. *Eur J Epidemiol*. 2013;28:759-769.
6. Kallen B, Nilsson E, Otterbald-Olausson P. Delivery outcome after maternal use of drugs for migraine: a register study in Sweden. *Drug Safety*. 2011;34:691-703.
7. Marchenko A, Etwel F, Olutunfese O, et al. Pregnancy outcome following prenatal exposure to triptan medications: a meta-analysis. *Headache*. 2015;55:490-501.
8. Headaches in pregnancy and postpartum: ACOG Clinical Practice Guideline No. 3. *Obstet Gynecol*. 2022;139:944-972.
9. Harris GM, Wood M, Ystrom E, et al. Association of maternal use of triptans during pregnancy with risk of attention-deficit/hyperactivity disorder in offspring. *JAMA Netw Open*. 2022;5(1-14):e2215333.
10. Amundsen S, Nordeng H, Fuskevag OM, et al. Transfer of triptans into human breast milk and estimation of infant drug exposure through breastfeeding. *Basic Clin Pharmacol Toxicol*. 2021;128:795-804.

E

ELEXACAFTOR, TEZACAFTOR, AND IVACAFTOR

Genetic (Cystic Fibrosis Treatment)

PREGNANCY RECOMMENDATION: No Human Data—Animal Data Suggest Low Risk

BREASTFEEDING RECOMMENDATION: Probably Compatible

PREGNANCY SUMMARY

No reports describing the use of elexacaftor, tezacaftor, and ivacaftor in human pregnancy have been located. Some placental transfer is likely to occur for all three drugs. Therefore, the absence of human pregnancy experience prevents a complete assessment of the embryofetal risk. Animal studies did not show embryofetal toxicity for all three drugs. Because cystic fibrosis is a chronic, debilitating genetic disorder, this drug should not be withheld because of pregnancy.

BREASTFEEDING SUMMARY

Elexacaftor, tezacaftor, and ivacaftor are probably excreted into human breast milk. Breastfeeding while using this drug should be based on the mother's clinical need for treatment. If used, the infant should be monitored for the most common reported adult side effects of headache or abdominal pain (both leading to irritability), upper respiratory tract infection, diarrhea, rash, nasal congestion, and rhinorrhea.

Reference

1. Product Information. *Trikafta*. Vertex Pharmaceuticals, Inc; 2019.

ELIGLUSTAT

Genetic (Glucosylceramide Synthase Inhibitor)

PREGNANCY RECOMMENDATION: Limited Human Data—Animal Data Suggest Potential Risk

BREASTFEEDING RECOMMENDATION: Potential Toxicity

PREGNANCY SUMMARY

One publication that reported human pregnancy experience with eliglustat was located. The data came from the clinical trials. Of 16 pregnancies, 13 delivered 14 healthy newborns (one set of twins) with no anomalies identified. The other three pregnancies were early losses. The drug will likely cross the placenta, so some fetal exposure will probably occur. However,

(continued)

this limited human pregnancy experience prevents a complete assessment of the embryofetal risk. Embryofetal toxicity was observed in one animal species at doses less than 10 times the RHD. Poorly controlled Gaucher disease type 1 can lead to pregnancy complications. In addition, pregnancy can exacerbate or produce new manifestations of the disease. Using this drug during pregnancy should be based on the pros and cons of the mother's clinical need for treatment versus any potential fetal risk that might occur from exposure.

E

BREASTFEEDING SUMMARY

No reports describing the use of eliglustat during human lactation have been located. The drug will likely be found in breast milk, so some infant exposure will probably occur. Breastfeeding while using this drug should be based on the mother's clinical need for treatment. If used, the infant should be monitored for the most common reported adult side effects of nausea, headache, and pain (all leading to irritability), fatigue, and diarrhea.

References

1. Prescribing Information. Cerdelga. Genzyme; 2022.
2. Lukina E, Balwani M, Belmatoug N, et al. Pregnancy outcome in women with Gaucher disease type 1 who had unplanned pregnancies during eliglustat clinical trials. *JIMD Rep*. 2021;57:76-84.

ELOSULFASE ALFA

Genetic (Enzyme)

PREGNANCY RECOMMENDATION: Limited Human Data—Animal Data Suggest Potential Risk (Maternal Benefit May Outweigh Embryofetal Risk)

BREASTFEEDING RECOMMENDATION: Probably Compatible

PREGNANCY SUMMARY

One report describing the use of enzyme replacement therapy (ERT) for pregnant women with mucopolysaccharidosis type IVA (MPS-IVA) was identified. The report described the outcomes of four pregnancies treated with ERT, and one of these had received elosulfase alfa. The pregnancy delivered a healthy newborn with no reported anomalies. The drug is not likely to cross the placenta; however, because it consists of a protein, it is not known whether some fetal exposure might occur. Therefore, the absence of human pregnancy experience prevents a complete assessment of the embryofetal risk. Embryofetal toxicity was observed in one animal species at doses less than 10 times the RHD. In patients with MPS type IVA, pregnancy can adversely affect the female's health and increase the risk for adverse outcomes for the mother and fetus. Using this drug during pregnancy should be based on the pros and cons of the mother's clinical need for treatment versus any potential fetal risk that might occur from exposure. There is a Morquio A registry that monitors pregnancy outcomes in women with MPS-IVA who are exposed to elosulfase alfa. For information or enrollment, call 1-800-983-4587.

BREASTFEEDING SUMMARY

No reports describing the use of elosulfase alfa during human lactation have been located. The drug most likely will not appear in breast milk. Furthermore, because it is an enzyme (protein), if any drug were to be present in breast milk, it would probably be digested in the infant's GI tract and not be absorbed. If the clinical decision is to use this drug while breastfeeding, the infant should be monitored for the most common reported adult side effects of headache and abdominal pain (both leading to irritability), fever, vomiting, and lethargy.

References

1. Prescribing Information. Vimizim. BioMarin Pharmaceutical; 2019.
2. Stewart FJ, Bentley A, Burton BK, et al. Pregnancy in patients with mucopolysaccharidosis: a case series. *Mol Genet Metab Rep*. 2016;8:111-115.

ELOTUZUMAB

Antineoplastic (Monoclonal Antibody)

PREGNANCY RECOMMENDATION: *Contraindicated

BREASTFEEDING RECOMMENDATION: Potential Toxicity

PREGNANCY SUMMARY

No reports describing the use of elotuzumab in human pregnancy have been located. As an IgG antibody, elotuzumab likely crosses the placenta, especially in the second half of gestation, so some fetal exposure will probably occur. Therefore, the absence of human pregnancy experience prevents a complete assessment of the embryofetal risk. Animal studies have not been conducted. *Elotuzumab is administered in combination with lenalidomide or pomalidomide, which can cause significant teratogenicity and are contraindicated in pregnancy. See Lenalidomide and Pomalidomide for contraception requirements for women with reproductive potential. If this monoclonal antibody were to be administered without the use of lenalidomide and pomalidomide, then the drug would not necessarily be contraindicated.

E

BREASTFEEDING SUMMARY

No reports describing the use of elotuzumab during human lactation have been located. However, it is known that IgG antibodies can be found in human breast milk but are not found in the neonatal or infant circulation. Additionally, if any IgG antibodies were to be ingested through breastfeeding, they would probably be digested in the infant's GI tract and not be absorbed. However, due to the concern for potential serious adverse effects that might be seen in a breastfed infant, and because the administration of elotuzumab is in combination with lenalidomide or pomalidomide and dexamethasone, the manufacturer recommends that women should not breastfeed during treatment with this drug. (See Lenalidomide, Pomalidomide, and Dexamethasone for additional information.) Nevertheless, breastfeeding while using this drug should be based on the mother's clinical need for treatment. If used, the infant should be monitored for the most common reported adult side effects of peripheral neuropathy (leading to irritability), diarrhea, lethargy, pyrexia, constipation, decreased appetite, and upper respiratory tract infections.

Reference

1. Prescribing Information. Empliciti. Bristol-Myers Squibb; 2022.

ELRANATAMAB

Antineoplastic (Monoclonal Antibody—Anti-BCMA/Anti-CD3 Antibody)

PREGNANCY RECOMMENDATION: **No Human Data and No Relevant Animal Data**

BREASTFEEDING RECOMMENDATION: **Probably Compatible**

PREGNANCY SUMMARY

No reports describing the use of elranatamab in human pregnancy have been located. As an IgG antibody, it likely crosses the placenta, especially during the second half of gestation, so some fetal exposure will probably occur. Therefore, the absence of human pregnancy experience prevents a complete assessment of the embryofetal risk. Animal reproduction and fertility studies have not been conducted with elranatamab. Based on the drug's mechanism of action, the manufacturer recommends that women with reproductive potential use effective contraception during treatment and for 4 months after the last dose. Nevertheless, using this drug during pregnancy should be based on the pros and cons of the mother's clinical need for treatment versus any potential fetal risk that might occur from exposure.

BREASTFEEDING SUMMARY

No reports describing the use of elranatamab during human lactation have been located. It is known that IgG antibodies can be found in human breast milk, but are not found in the neonatal or infant circulation. Additionally, if any IgG antibodies were to be ingested through breastfeeding, they would probably be digested in the infant's GI tract and not be absorbed. Due to a concern for potential serious adverse effects that might be seen in a breastfed infant, the manufacturer recommends that women not breastfeed while being treated with this drug and for at least 4 months after the last dose. Nevertheless, breastfeeding while using this drug should be based on the mother's clinical need for treatment versus any potential infant risks that might occur. If used, the infant should be monitored for the most common reported adult side effects of nausea and musculoskeletal pain (both leading to irritability), diarrhea, rash, fatigue (lethargy), decreased weight (monitor infant growth), cough, upper respiratory infection, fever, and various laboratory abnormalities (see Prescribing Information[PI]).

Reference

1. Prescribing Information. Elrexfio. Pfizer, Inc; 2023.

ELTROMBOPAG

Hematologic (Thrombopoietin Receptor Agonist)

PREGNANCY RECOMMENDATION: Limited Human Data—Animal Data Suggest Potential Risk (Maternal Benefit May Outweigh Embryofetal Risk)

BREASTFEEDING RECOMMENDATION: Potential Toxicity

E

PREGNANCY SUMMARY

Nine publications were located that reported the use of eltrombopag in human pregnancy. A total of 18 pregnancies were described, resulting in 19 newborns (one set of twins). Of these, there were nine cases of first-trimester exposure, and no major malformations were identified. The remaining 11 cases had use in the third trimester and up to delivery with no major pregnancy complications noted. Growth restriction was seen in several neonates, and one had thrombocytosis. The drug will probably cross the placenta, so some fetal exposure will likely occur. However, this limited human pregnancy experience prevents a complete assessment of the embryofetal risk. Embryofetal toxicity was observed in one animal species at doses less than 10 times the human clinical exposure. Based on the animal studies, the manufacturer recommends that women with reproductive potential use effective contraception during treatment and for 1 week after the last dose. Regardless, using this drug during pregnancy should be based on the pros and cons of the mother's clinical need for treatment versus any potential fetal risk that might occur from exposure.

BREASTFEEDING SUMMARY

One report describing the use of eltrombopag during human lactation has been located. The infant had thrombocytosis at birth, which persisted while the mother was breastfeeding. Persistent thrombocytosis may have been associated with eltrombopag in the breast milk. Breast milk drug levels were not obtained. The drug will probably be found in breast milk, so some infant exposure will likely occur. However, eltrombopag also chelates numerous minerals, including calcium, iron, magnesium, and zinc, all of which are found in human breast milk. Therefore, this may further decrease oral absorption by the infant. However, due to a concern for potential serious adverse effects that might be seen in a breastfed infant, the manufacturer recommends that women not breastfeed while being treated with this drug. Nevertheless, breastfeeding while using this drug should be based on the mother's clinical need for treatment versus any potential infant risks that might occur. If used, the infant should be monitored for the most common reported adult side effects of nausea and headache (both leading to irritability), fever, anemia, increased alanine aminotransferase, cough, fatigue (lethargy), and diarrhea.

References

1. Prescribing Information. Promacta. Novartis Pharmaceuticals; 2023.
2. Alkaabi J, Alkindi S, Riyami N, et al. Successful treatment of severe thrombocytopenia with romiplostim in a pregnant patient with systemic lupus erythematosus. *Lupus*. 2012;21:1571-1574.
3. Purushothaman J, Puthumana KJ, Kumar A, et al. A case of refractory immune thrombocytopenia in pregnancy managed with eltrombopag. *Asian J Transfus Sci*. 2016;10:155-158.
4. Favier R, De Carne C, Elefant E, et al. Eltrombopag to treat thrombocytopenia during last month of pregnancy in a woman with MYH9-related disease: a case report. *A&A Practice*. 2018;10:10-12.
5. Suzuki N, Hiraga J, Hariyama Y, et al. A low birth weight infant with no malformations delivered by a primary immune thrombocytopenia patient treated with eltrombopag. *Int J Hematol*. 2018;108:109-111.
6. Ferreira I, Sousa F, Vasco E, et al. Severe immune thrombocytopenia in pregnancy treated with eltrombopag—a case report. *J Gynecol Obstet Hum Reprod*. 2018;47:405-408.
7. Mendicino F, Santoro C, Martino E, et al. Eltrombopag treatment for severe immune thrombocytopenia during pregnancy: a case report. *Blood Coagul Fibrinolysis*. 2021;32:519-521.
8. Michel M, Ruggeri M, Gonzalez-Lopez TJ, et al. Use of thrombopoietin receptor agonists for immune thrombocytopenia in pregnancy: results from a multicenter study. *Blood*. 2020;136:3056-3061.
9. Sammartano V, Santoni A, Defina M, et al. Efficacy and safety of eltrombopag during conception and first trimester of pregnancy in a case of refractory severe immune thrombocytopenia. *Blood Coagul Fibrinolysis*. 2020;31:416-418.
10. Shibata S, Misugi T, Nakane T, et al. Use of eltrombopag for the first trimester pregnancy complicated with refractory idiopathic thrombocytopenic purpura: a case report and literature review. *Cureus*. 2022;14:e22505.
11. Weingarten SJ, Friedman D, Arora A. Eltrombopag use for refractory immune thrombocytopenia in pregnancy: a case report. *Case Rep Womens Health*. 2020;29:e00281.

ELUXADOLINE

Gastrointestinal (μ-Opioid Agonist)

PREGNANCY RECOMMENDATION: No Human Data—Animal Data Suggest Low Risk

BREASTFEEDING RECOMMENDATION: Probably Compatible

PREGNANCY SUMMARY

No reports describing the use of eluxadoline in human pregnancy have been located. Based on likely limited placental transfer, fetal exposure should be minimal. However, the absence of human pregnancy experience prevents a complete assessment of the embryofetal risk. Animal data did not show any embryofetal toxicity in two animal species. Using this drug during pregnancy should be based on the pros and cons of the mother's clinical need for treatment versus any potential fetal risk that might occur from exposure.

E

BREASTFEEDING SUMMARY

No reports describing the use of eluxadoline during human lactation have been located. Some amount of the drug may be found in breast milk, but infant absorption with oral use will likely be negligible. If the clinical decision is to use this drug while breastfeeding, the infant should be monitored for the most common reported adult side effects of nausea and abdominal pain (both leading to irritability) and constipation.

Reference

1. Prescribing Information. Viberzi. Allergan USA, Inc; 2020.

EMAPALUMAB

Antineoplastic (Monoclonal Antibody—Interferon-γ Inhibitor)

PREGNANCY RECOMMENDATION: No Human Data—Animal Data Suggest Low Risk

BREASTFEEDING RECOMMENDATION: Probably Compatible

PREGNANCY SUMMARY

No reports describing the use of emapalumab in human pregnancy have been located. Because it is an antibody of the IgG class, it probably crosses the placenta, especially in the second half of gestation, so some fetal exposure is likely to occur. However, the absence of human pregnancy experience prevents a complete assessment of the embryofetal risk. Animal data did not show any embryofetal toxicity at doses of more than 10 times the RHD. About 40% of patients treated with this medication reported hypertension. Using this drug during pregnancy should be based on the pros and cons of the mother's clinical need for treatment versus any potential fetal risk that might occur from exposure.

BREASTFEEDING SUMMARY

Emapalumab probably enters breast milk. However, it is known that IgG antibodies found in human breast milk are not found in the neonatal or infant circulation. Additionally, if any IgG antibodies were to be ingested through breastfeeding, they would probably be digested in the infant's GI tract and not be absorbed. If the clinical decision is to use this drug during breastfeeding, the infant should be monitored for the most common reported adult side effects of abdominal pain (leading to irritability), infections, hypertension, pyrexia, rash, diarrhea, constipation, and cough.

Reference

1. Prescribing Information. Gamifant. Swedish Orphan Biovitrum AB for Sobi, Inc; 2022.

EMICIZUMAB

Genetic (Monoclonal Antibody—Hemophilia A)

PREGNANCY RECOMMENDATION: No Human Data and No Relevant Animal Data

BREASTFEEDING RECOMMENDATION: Probably Compatible

PREGNANCY SUMMARY

No reports describing the use of emicizumab in human pregnancy have been located. As an IgG antibody, the drug likely crosses the placenta, especially in the second half of gestation, so some fetal exposure will probably occur. However, the absence of human pregnancy experience prevents a complete assessment of the embryofetal risk. Animal reproduction studies have not been performed. The manufacturer recommends that women with reproductive potential use effective

(*continued*)

contraception during treatment with emicizumab. Nevertheless, using this drug during pregnancy should be based on the pros and cons of the mother's clinical need for treatment versus any potential fetal risk that might occur from exposure.

BREASTFEEDING SUMMARY

No reports describing the use of emicizumab during human lactation have been located. The drug is likely present in breast milk. However, it is known that IgG antibodies can be found in human breast milk, but are not found in the neonatal or infant circulation. Additionally, if any IgG antibodies were to be ingested through breastfeeding, they would probably be digested in the infant's GI tract and not be absorbed. Breastfeeding while using this drug should be based on the mother's clinical need for treatment. If used, the infant should be monitored for the most common reported adult side effects of headache and arthralgias (both leading to irritability).

Reference

1. Prescribing Information. Hemlibra. Genetech, Inc; 2021.

EMPAGLIFLOZIN

Antidiabetic (SGLT-2 inhibitor)

PREGNANCY RECOMMENDATION: Limited Human Data—Animal Data Suggest Risk for the Second and Third Trimesters

BREASTFEEDING RECOMMENDATION: Potential Toxicity

PREGNANCY SUMMARY

Two case reports describing the use of empagliflozin in human pregnancy have been located. In both cases, the drug exposure occurred in the first trimester, and healthy newborns were delivered without any reported anomalies. The drug was shown to cross the placenta through ex vivo human placental perfusion analysis with a maximum fetal to maternal blood level of about 38%. So fetal exposure appears to occur. Therefore, this limited human pregnancy experience prevents a complete assessment of the embryofetal risk. Embryofetal toxicity was observed in one animal species at doses more than 10 times the MRHD during the period of renal development that corresponds to the late second and third trimester of human renal development. Due to this finding, the manufacturer does not recommend the use of empagliflozin during the second and third trimesters of pregnancy. Nevertheless, using this drug during pregnancy should be based on the pros and cons of the mother's clinical need for treatment versus any potential fetal risk that might occur from exposure. In addition, fetal renal status can be monitored using perinatal ultrasound.

BREASTFEEDING SUMMARY

One case report regarding the use of empagliflozin during human lactation was located. The drug was used in a patient with glycogen storage disease type Ib, and no adverse reactions were reported. The drug will probably appear in breast milk, so some infant exposure will likely occur. Because renal toxicity was observed in animal studies corresponding to the late second and third trimesters of human pregnancy, the manufacturer does not recommend the use of empagliflozin while breastfeeding. Nevertheless, breastfeeding while using this drug should be based on the mother's clinical need for treatment. If used, the infant should be monitored for the most common reported adult side effects of urinary tract and genital mycotic infections.

References

1. Prescribing Information. Jardiance. Boehringer Ingelheim Pharmaceuticals; 2023.
2. Kuoni S, Muller D, Simoes-Wust AP, Steiner R. Simultaneous LC-MS/MS quantification of SGLT2 inhibitors and antipyrine in medium and tissue from human ex vivo placental perfusions. *J Chromatogr B Analyt Biomed Life Sci*. 2023;1228:123841.
3. Kuoni S, Steiner R, Saleh L, et al. Safety assessment of the SGLT2 inhibitors empagliflozin, dapagliflozin, and canagliflozin during pregnancy: an ex vivo human placenta perfusion and in vitro study. *Biomed Pharmacother*. 2023;171:116177.
4. Formoso G, Ginestra F, Di Dalmazi G, et al. Empagliflozin, metformin, and insulin degludec, during pregnancy: a case report. *Acta Diabetol*. 2018;55: 759-761.
5. Grünert SC, Rosenbaum-Fabian S, Schumann A, et al. Two successful pregnancies and first use of empagliflozin during pregnancy in glycogen storage disease type Ib. *JIMD Rep*. 2022;63:303-308.

EMTRICITABINE

Antiretroviral (Nucleoside Reverse Transcriptase Inhibitor)

PREGNANCY RECOMMENDATION: Human Data Suggest Compatible

BREASTFEEDING RECOMMENDATION: *Contraindicated

PREGNANCY SUMMARY

From two large studies that involve more than 4,900 first-trimester exposures to emtricitabine, the rate of congenital anomalies was 3.3%, which was no different than the unexposed rate. No pattern was seen in the anomalies. The drug appears to cross the placenta, so fetal exposure will occur. Animal studies did not show any embryofetal toxicity or malformations in two species at doses of more than 10 times the RHD. In 2023, the updated US Department of Health and Human Services AIDS Info guidelines for the use of antiretroviral agents during pregnancy recommend that, in most cases, patients continue their regimen during pregnancy, if it is tolerated, safe, and effective in suppressing viral replication. The guideline recommends that a discussion and shared decision-making about the known and potential risks, as well as benefits to the mother and fetus, be conducted (acknowledging limited data). This should guide the selection of which antiretroviral agents to use during pregnancy. Additionally, treatment initiation should not be delayed due to concerns about teratogenicity with first-trimester exposure. See the guideline for the most updated information on this subject. If indicated, efavirenz should not be withheld in pregnancy since the expected benefit to the mother with HIV probably outweighs the unknown risk to the fetus. The guidelines note that efavirenz is not associated with an increased risk for congenital anomalies. Providers caring for pregnant patients with HIV and their infants can call the national Perinatal HIV/AIDS hotline (888-448-8765) for free clinical consultation. Additionally, there is a pregnancy exposure registry that monitors pregnancy outcomes in individuals exposed to antiretroviral medications during pregnancy. Health care providers are encouraged to register patients by calling the APR at 1-800-258-4263.

BREASTFEEDING SUMMARY

Emtricitabine has been found in breast milk with median peak and trough levels of about 680 and 175 ng/mL. Infant blood levels are low, ranging from undetectable to about 25 ng/mL. The RID in one study was calculated to be about 2%. In 2023, the updated US Department of Health and Human Services AIDS Info guidelines state that using replacement of breast milk through formula or pasteurized donor human breast milk from a milk bank eliminates the risk of postnatal HIV transmission to the infant. Using antiretroviral therapy to achieve and maintain viral suppression during pregnancy and postpartum can decrease the risk for infant transmission to less than 1%, but not zero. *For patients not on therapy for viral load suppression during pregnancy (at a minimum of throughout the third trimester) and at delivery, replacement of breast milk is recommended. Patients on antiretroviral therapy who have a sustained undetectable viral load and who choose to breastfeed or use replacement of breast milk should be supported with this decision. If the clinical decision is to use this drug while breastfeeding, the infant should be monitored for the most common reported adult side effects of dizziness, nausea, and headache (all leading to irritability), rash, fatigue (lethargy), insomnia, and vomiting.

References

1. Prescribing Information. Emtriva. Gilead Sciences; 2018.
2. Stek AM, Best BM, Luo W, et al. Effect of pregnancy on emtricitabine pharmacokinetics. *HIV Med*. 2012;13(4):226-235.
3. Flynn PM, Mirochnick M, Shapiro DE, et al. Pharmacokinetics and safety of single-dose tenofovir disoproxil fumarate and emtricitabine in HIV-1-infected pregnant women and their infants. *Antimicrob Agents Chemother*. 2011; 55(12):5914-5922.
4. Mugo NR, Hong T, Celum C, et al. Pregnancy incidence and outcomes among women receiving preexposure prophylaxis for HIV prevention: a randomized clinical trial. *JAMA*. 2014;312:362-371.
5. Williams PL, Crain M, Yildirim C, et al. Congenital anomalies and in utero antiretroviral exposure in human immunodeficiency virus-exposed uninfected infants. *JAMA Pediatr*. 2015;169:45-55.
6. Antiretroviral Pregnancy Registry Steering Committee. *Antiretroviral Pregnancy Registry Interim Report for 1 January 1989 Through 31 January 2023*. Registry Coordinating Center; 2023.
7. Panel on Treatment of HIV During Pregnancy and Prevention of Perinatal Transmission. Recommendations for the use of antiretroviral drugs during pregnancy and interventions to reduce perinatal HIV transmission in the United States. Department of Health and Human Services. Accessed September 24, 2023. https://clinicalinfo.hiv.gov/en/guidelines/perinatal
8. Benabound A, Pruvost A, Coffie PA, et al. Concentrations of tenofovir and emtricitabine in breast milk of HIV-1-infected women in Abidjan, Cote d'Ivoire, in the ANRS 12109 TEmAA study, step 2. *Antimicrob Agents Chemother*. 2011;55:1315-1317.
9. Mugwanya KK, Hendrix CW, Mugo NR, et al. Pre-exposure prophylaxis use by breastfeeding HIV-uninfected women: a prospective short-term study of antiretroviral excretion in breast milk and infant absorption. *PLoS Med*. 2016;13:e1002132.
10. Waitt C, Olagunju A, Nakalema S, et al. Plasma and breast milk pharmacokinetics of emtricitabine, tenofovir and lamivudine using dried blood and breast milk spots in nursing African mother-infant pairs. *J Antimicrob Chemother*. 2018;73:1013-1019.

ENALAPRIL

Antihypertensive (Angiotensin-Converting Enzyme Inhibitor)

PREGNANCY RECOMMENDATION: Contraindicated (Second and Third Trimester)

BREASTFEEDING RECOMMENDATION: Probably Compatible

PREGNANCY SUMMARY

Numerous case reports have described the use of enalapril (confined to the first trimester) with no increase in the incidence of birth anomalies, except for one Tennessee Medicaid study. Use of the drug in the second and third trimesters has been found to cause fetal renal dysfunction. This can lead to severe oligohydramnios, producing pulmonary hypoplasia and compression deformities, which are fatal in some cases. There are reports, however, that this is not universal, and a few reports exist that describe a return of normal infant renal function over time. In some pathology cases, the fetal kidneys were not found to have any definite pathologic abnormalities. Therefore, the primary issue may be the severe oligohydramnios, which is produced by the fetal renal dysfunction when the drug is used in the second and third trimesters. Enalapril crosses the placenta, so fetal exposure will occur. Animal studies did show embryofetal toxicity with malformations in one species at doses less than 10 times the RHD. The drug carries a boxed warning for these fetal risks. It recommends that enalapril be discontinued as soon as possible once pregnancy is detected.

BREASTFEEDING SUMMARY

Limited reports describing the use of enalapril during human lactation have been located. Levels of the drug in breast milk are low, at less than 2 ng/mL in most cases. No adverse effects of angiotensin-converting enzyme (ACE) inhibitors in breast milk have been reported in infants. However, due to the concern for potential serious adverse effects, the manufacturer recommends that women not breastfeed during treatment with this drug. However, the ACOG and American Heart Association (AHA) consider ACE inhibitors low risk for use during breastfeeding. Breastfeeding while using this drug should be based on the mother's clinical need for treatment versus any potential infant risks that might occur. If used, the infant should be monitored for the most common reported adult side effects of dizziness (leading to irritability) and hypotension.

References

1. Valdés G, Marinovic D, Falcón C, et al. Placental alterations, intrauterine growth retardation and teratogenicity associated with enalapril use in pregnant rats. *Biol Neonate*. 1992;61:124-130.
2. Reisenberger K, Egarter C, Sternberger B, et al. Placental passage of angiotensin-converting enzyme inhibitors. *Am J Obstet Gynecol*. 1996;174:1450-1455.
3. Kreft-Jais C, Plouin P-F, Tchobroutsky C, Boutroy M-J. Angiotensin-converting enzyme inhibitors during pregnancy: a survey of 22 patients given captopril and nine given enalapril. *Br J Obstet Gynaecol*. 1988;95:420-422.
4. Schubiger G, Flury G, Nussberger J. Enalapril for pregnancy-induced hypertension: acute renal failure in a neonate. *Ann Intern Med*. 1988;108:215-216.
5. Mehta N, Modi N. ACE inhibitors in pregnancy. *Lancet*. 1989;2:96.
6. Broughton Pipkin F, Baker PN, Symonds EM. ACE inhibitors in pregnancy. *Lancet*. 1989;2:96-97.
7. Smith AM. Are ACE inhibitors safe in pregnancy? *Lancet*. 1989;2:750-751.
8. Baethge BA, Wolf RE. Successful pregnancy with scleroderma renal disease and pulmonary hypertension in a patient using angiotensin converting enzyme inhibitors. *Ann Rheum Dis*. 1989;48:776-778.
9. Scott AA, Purohit DM. Neonatal renal failure: a complication of maternal antihypertensive therapy. *Am J Obstet Gynecol*. 1989;160:1223-1224.
10. Hulton SA, Thomson PD, Cooper PA, et al. Angiotensin-converting enzyme inhibitors in pregnancy may result in neonatal renal failure. *S Afr Med J*. 1990;78:673-676.
11. Rosa FW, Bosco LA, Graham CF, et al. Neonatal anuria with maternal angiotensin-converting enzyme inhibition. *Obstet Gynecol* 1989;74:371-374.
12. Rosa FW, Bosco L. Infant renal failure with maternal ACE inhibition (abstract 92). *Am J Obstet Gynecol* 1991;164:273.
13. Cunniff C, Jones KL, Phillipson J, et al. Oligohydramnios sequence and renal tubular malformation associated with maternal enalapril use. *Am J Obstet Gynecol* 1990;162:187-189.
14. Pryde PG, Nugent CE, Sedman AB, et al. ACE inhibitor fetopathy (abstract). *Am J Obstet Gynecol*. 1992;166:348.
15. Neerhof MG, Shlossman PA, Poll DS, et al. Idiopathic aldosteronism in pregnancy. *Obstet Gynecol*. 1991;78:489-491.
16. Boutroy MJ. Fetal effects of maternally administered clonidine and angiotensin-converting enzyme inhibitors. *Dev Pharmacol Ther*. 1989;13:199-204.
17. Svensson A, Andersch B, Dahlof B. ACE-hammare i samband med graviditet kan medfora risker for fostret. *Lakartidningen*. 1986;83:699-700.
18. Scanferla F, Coli U, Landini S, et al. Treatment of pregnancy-induced hypertension with ACE inhibitor enalapril (abstract). *Clin Exp Hypertens Pregn*. 1987;B6:45.
19. Thorpe-Beeston JG, Armar NA, Dancy M, et al. Pregnancy and ACE inhibitors. *Br J Obstet Gynaecol*. 1993;100:692-693.
20. Lavoratti G, Seracini D, Fiorini P, et al. Neonatal anuria by ACE inhibitors during pregnancy. *Nephron*. 1997;76:235-236.
21. Lip GYH, Churchill D, Beevers M, et al. Angiotensin-converting-enzyme inhibitors in early pregnancy. *Lancet*. 1997;350:1446-1447.
22. Steffensen FH, Nielsen GL, Sorensen HT, et al. Pregnancy outcome with ACE-inhibitor use in early pregnancy. *Lancet*. 1998;351:596.
23. Hanssens M, Keirse MJNC, Vankelecom F, et al. Fetal and neonatal effects of treatment with angiotensin-converting enzyme inhibitors in pregnancy. *Obstet Gynecol*. 1991;78:128-135.
24. Kumar D, Moss G, Primhak R, et al. Congenital renal tubular dysplasia and skull ossification defects similar to teratogenic effects of angiotensin converting enzyme (ACE) inhibitors. *J Med Genet*. 1997;34:541-545.
25. Piper JM, Ray WA, Rosa FW. Pregnancy outcome following exposure to angiotensin-converting enzyme inhibitors. *Obstet Gynecol*. 1992;80:429-432.
26. Barr M Jr, Cohen MM Jr. ACE inhibitor fetopathy and hypocalvaria: the kidney-skull connection. *Teratology*. 1991;44:485-495.
27. Brent RL, Beckman DA. Angiotensin-converting enzyme inhibitors, an embryopathic class of drugs with unique properties: information for clinical teratology counselors. *Teratology*. 1991;43:543-546.
28. Martin RA, Jones KL, Mendoza A, et al. Effect of ACE inhibition on the fetal kidney: decreased renal blood flow. *Teratology*. 1992;46:317-321.
29. Tabacova SA, Kimmel CA. Enalapril: pharmacokinetic/dynamic inferences for comparative developmental toxicity. A review. *Reprod Toxicol*. 2001;15:467-478.
30. Cooper WO, Hernandez-Diaz S, Arbogast PG, et al. Major congenital malformations after first-trimester exposure to ACE inhibitors. *N Engl J Med*. 2006;354:2443-2451.
31. Friedman JM. ACE inhibitors and congenital anomalies. *N Engl J Med*. 2006;354:2498-2500.
32. Scialli AR, Lione A. ACE inhibitors and major congenital malformations. *N Engl J Med*. 2006;355:1280.
33. Cooper WO, Ray WA. Reply—ACE inhibitors and major congenital malformations. *N Engl J Med*. 2006;355:1281.
34. Barr M Jr. Teratogen update: angiotensin-converting enzyme inhibitors. *Teratology*. 1994;50:399-409.
35. Shotan A, Widerhorn J, Hurst A, et al. Risks of angiotensin-converting enzyme inhibition during pregnancy: experimental and clinical evidence, potential mechanisms, and recommendations for use. *Am J Med*. 1994;96:451-456.
36. Robillard JE, Nakamura KT, Matherne GP, et al. Renal hemodynamics and functional adjustments to postnatal life. *Semin Perinatol*. 1988;12:143-150.
37. Guignard J-P, Gouyon J-B. Adverse effects of drugs on the immature kidney. *Biol Neonate*. 1988;53:243-252.
38. Polifka JE. Is there an embryopathy associated with first-trimester exposure to angiotensin-converting enzyme inhibitors and angiotensin receptor

antagonists? A critical review of the evidence. *Birth Defects Res (Part A)*. 2012;94:576-598.
39. Huttunen K, Gronhagen-Riska C, Fyhrquist F. Enalapril treatment of a nursing mother with slightly impaired renal function. *Clin Nephrol*. 1989;31:278.
40. Rush JE, Snyder BA, Barrish A, Hichens M. Comment on Huttunen K, Grönhagen-Riska C and Fyhrquist F, 1989. Enalapril treatment of a nursing mother with slightly impaired renal function. *Clin Nephrol*. 1991;35:234.
41. Redman CWG, Kelly JG, Cooper WD. The excretion of enalapril and enalaprilat in human breast milk. *Eur J Clin Pharmacol*. 1990;38:99.
42. Prescribing Information. Enalapril maleate oral solution. Bionpharma, Inc; 2023.
43. ACOG Practice Bulletin No. 203: chronic hypertension in pregnancy. *Obstet Gynecol*. 2019;133:e26-e50.
44. Heidenreich PA, Bozkurt B, Aguilar D, et al. 2022 AHA/ACC/HFSA guideline for the management of heart failure: a report of the American College of Cardiology/American Heart Association Joint Committee on clinical practice guidelines. *Circulation*. 2022;145:e895-e1032.

E

ENASIDENIB

Antineoplastic (Monoclonal Antibody—Isocitrate Dehydrogenase-2 Inhibitor)

PREGNANCY RECOMMENDATION: No Human Data and No Relevant Animal Data

BREASTFEEDING RECOMMENDATION: Potential Toxicity

PREGNANCY SUMMARY

No reports describing the use of enasidenib in human pregnancy have been located. Some amount of the drug will probably cross the placenta, so fetal exposure will likely occur. However, the absence of human pregnancy experience prevents a complete assessment of the embryofetal risk. Animal studies showed embryofetal toxicity, but treatment doses also caused maternal toxicity. Based on the animal studies and the drug's mechanism of action, the manufacturer recommends that women with reproductive potential use effective contraception during treatment and for 1 month after the last dose. They also recommend that males with female partners of reproductive potential use effective contraception during treatment and for 1 month after the last dose. Nevertheless, using this drug during pregnancy should be based on the pros and cons of the mother's clinical need for treatment versus any potential fetal risk that might occur from exposure.

BREASTFEEDING SUMMARY

No reports describing the use of enasidenib during human lactation have been located. Some amount of the drug probably enters breast milk, so infant exposure will likely occur. However, due to the concern for potential serious adverse effects in a breastfed infant, the manufacturer recommends that women not breastfeed while being treated with enasidenib and for at least 1 month after the last dose. Nevertheless, breastfeeding while using this drug should be based on the mother's clinical need for treatment. If used, the infant should be monitored for the most common reported adult side effects of nausea (leading to irritability), diarrhea, vomiting, and decreased appetite.

Reference

1. Product Information. Idhifa. Celgene Corporation; 2017.

ENCORAFENIB

Antineoplastic (Kinase Inhibitor)

PREGNANCY RECOMMENDATION: No Human Data and No Relevant Animal Data

BREASTFEEDING RECOMMENDATION: Potential Toxicity

PREGNANCY SUMMARY

No reports describing the use of encorafenib in human pregnancy have been located. Based on likely limited placental transfer, fetal exposure is probably small. However, the absence of human pregnancy experience prevents a complete assessment of the embryofetal risk. Embryofetal toxicity was observed in two animal species, but at doses greater than 10 times the RHD and in the presence of maternal toxicity. Nevertheless, based on the animal studies and the drug's mechanism of action, the manufacturer recommends that women with reproductive potential use effective nonhormonal contraception during treatment and for 2 weeks after the last dose. However, using this drug during pregnancy should be based on the pros and cons of the mother's clinical need for treatment versus any potential fetal risk that might occur from exposure. There is a pregnancy registry for women who are pregnant and have cancer. For more information, health care providers and women are encouraged to contact the Cancer and Pregnancy Registry at 1-877-635-4499.

BREASTFEEDING SUMMARY

No reports describing the use of encorafenib during human lactation have been located. Some amount of the drug will likely be found in breast milk, so infant exposure will probably occur. Due to the concern for potential serious adverse effects that might be seen in a breastfed infant, the manufacturer recommends that women not breastfeed while being treated with encorafenib and for at least 2 weeks after the last dose. Nevertheless, breastfeeding while using this drug should be based on the mother's clinical need for treatment. If used, the infant should be monitored for the most common reported adult side effects of nausea, abdominal pain, and arthralgia (all leading to irritability), diarrhea, vomiting, rash, and decreased appetite.

Reference

1. Prescribing Information. Braftovi. Array BioPharma, Inc; 2022.

E

ENFORTUMAB VEDOTIN

Antineoplastic (Monoclonal Antibody Drug Conjugate)

PREGNANCY RECOMMENDATION: No Human Data—Animal Data Suggest Potential Risk

BREASTFEEDING RECOMMENDATION: Potential Toxicity

PREGNANCY SUMMARY

No reports describing the use of enfortumab vedotin in human pregnancy have been located. As an IgG antibody, it likely crosses the placenta during the second half of gestation, so some fetal exposure will probably occur. For unconjugated monomethyl auristatin E (MMAE), fetal exposure is also likely to occur, but the overall amount should be limited. The clinical significance of the amount that may be found in the fetal circulation is unknown. Therefore, the absence of human pregnancy experience prevents a complete assessment of the embryofetal risk. Embryofetal toxicity and malformations were observed in one animal species at doses of about equal to the RHD, but maternal toxicity also occurred. Based on these animal studies and the drug's mechanism of action, the manufacturer recommends that women with reproductive potential use effective contraception during treatment and for 2 months after the last dose. They also recommend that males with female partners of reproductive potential use effective contraception during treatment and for 4 months after the last dose. Nevertheless, using this drug during pregnancy should be based on the pros and cons of the mother's clinical need for treatment versus any potential fetal risk that might occur from exposure. Elevated glucose levels were seen in about 14% of patients during the clinical trials; therefore, if the drug is used, maternal glucose levels should be monitored. There is a registry for women who are pregnant and have cancer. For more information, women are encouraged to contact the Cancer and Pregnancy Registry at 877-635-4499.

BREASTFEEDING SUMMARY

No reports describing the use of enfortumab vedotin during human lactation have been located. It is known that IgG antibodies can be found in human breast milk, but are not found in the neonatal or infant circulation. Additionally, if any IgG antibodies were to be ingested through breastfeeding, they would probably be digested in the infant's GI tract and not be absorbed. Very small amounts of MMAE may also be found in breast milk. The clinical significance of this is unknown. Because of a concern for potential serious adverse effects that might be seen in a breastfed infant, the manufacturer recommends that women not breastfeed during treatment and for at least 3 weeks after the last dose. However, the developmental and health benefits of breastfeeding should be considered along with the mother's clinical need for treatment versus any potential adverse effects for a breastfed infant from the drug or the mother's underlying maternal condition. If used, the infant should be monitored for the most common reported adult side effects of pruritus, nausea, and peripheral neuropathy (all leading to irritability), fatigue (lethargy), decreased appetite, rash, alopecia, diarrhea, and various laboratory abnormalities (see PI).

Reference

1. Prescribing Information. Padcev. Seagen, Inc; 2023.

ENFUVIRTIDE

Antiretroviral (Fusion Inhibitor)

PREGNANCY RECOMMENDATION: *Contraindicated HIV-2/for HIV-1 Human Data and Animal Data Suggest Low Risk

BREASTFEEDING RECOMMENDATION: *Contraindicated

PREGNANCY SUMMARY

The APR reported, for the period January 1989 through January 2023, no birth defects were observed in 24 live births with first-trimester exposure to an enfuvirtide-based regimen. In the second/third trimesters, there were 0 of 16 live births with defects. Eleven other reports involving 20 pregnant women who received enfuvirtide with other antivirals in the second half of pregnancy were also identified. With one set of twins, all 21 delivered newborns did well with no reported anomalies or complications related to the drug. All neonates were HIV negative postdelivery except for one case. The drug does not cross the placenta. Animal studies did not show any embryofetal toxicity in two species. There is a pregnancy exposure registry that monitors pregnancy outcomes in individuals exposed to antiretroviral medicines during pregnancy. Health care providers are encouraged to call the APR at 1-800-258-4263. In 2023, the updated US Department of Health and Human Services AIDS Info guidelines for the use of antiretroviral agents during pregnancy recommend that, in most cases, patients continue their regimen during pregnancy if it is tolerated, safe, and effective in suppressing viral replication. The guideline recommends that a discussion occur to help guide the selection of which antiretrovirals to use during pregnancy. This should involve shared decision-making about the known and potential risks as well as benefits to the mother and fetus, acknowledging limited data. Additionally, treatment initiation should not be delayed due to concerns about teratogenicity with first-trimester exposure. See the guideline for the most updated information on continuing, initiating, or switching regimens during pregnancy, if any potential dosing changes are needed due to pharmacokinetic changes of pregnancy, and recommendations for intrapartum and postpartum management. *The guidelines note that enfuvirtide is not recommended for treatment or prophylaxis in pregnant women with HIV-2.

E

BREASTFEEDING SUMMARY

No reports describing the use of enfuvirtide during human lactation have been located. The drug will probably not be found in breast milk. If any excretion into breast milk were to occur, it is likely to be clinically insignificant. Additionally, as a peptide, it would probably be digested in the infant's GI tract and not absorbed. *In 2023, the updated US Department of Health and Human Services AIDS Info guidelines state that using replacement of breast milk through formula or pasteurized donor human breast milk from a milk bank eliminates the risk of postnatal HIV transmission to the infant. Using antiretroviral therapy to achieve and maintain viral suppression during pregnancy and postpartum can decrease the risk for infant transmission to less than 1% but not zero. For patients not on therapy or those without viral load suppression during pregnancy (at a minimum of throughout the third trimester) and at delivery, replacement of breast milk is recommended. Patients on antiretroviral therapy who have a sustained undetectable viral load and who choose to breastfeed or use replacement of breast milk should be supported with this decision

References

1. Prescribing Information. Fuzeon. Genentech; 2019.
2. Ceccaldi PF, Ferreira C, Gavard L, et al. Placental transfer of enfuvirtide in the ex vivo human placental perfusion model. *Am J Obstet Gynecol*. 2008;198: 433.e1-e2.
3. Brennan-Benson P, Pakianathan M, Rice P, et al. Enfuvirtide prevents vertical transmission of multidrug-resistant HIV-1 in pregnancy but does not cross the placenta. *AIDS*. 2006;20:297-299.
4. Furco A, Gosrani B, Nicholas S, et al. Successful use of darunavir, etravirine, enfuvirtide and tenofovir/emtricitabine in pregnant woman with multiclass HIV resistance. *AIDS*. 2009;23:434-435.
5. Jeantils V, Alloui C, Rodrigues A, et al. Use of enfuvirtide in pregnancy in HIV positive women is seven cases. *Gynecol Obstet Fertil*. 2009;37:396-400.
6. Weizsaecker K, Kurowski M, Hoffmeister B, et al. Pharmacokinetic profile in late pregnancy and cord blood concentration of tipranavir and enfuvirtide. *Int. J STD Aids*. 2011;22:294-295.
7. Antiretroviral Pregnancy Registry Steering Committee. *Antiretroviral Pregnancy Registry Interim Report for 1 January 1989 Through 31 January 2023*. Registry Coordinating Center; 2023.
8. Izurieta P, Kakuda TN, Feys C, et al. Safety and pharmacokinetics of etravirine in pregnant HIV-1-infected women. *HIV Med*. 2011;12(4):257-258.
9. Meyohas MC, Lacombe K, Carbonne B, et al. Enfuvirtide prescription at the end of pregnancy to a multi-treated HIV-infected woman with virological breakthrough. *AIDS*. 2004;18:1966-1968.
10. Cohan D, Feakins C, Wara D, et al. Perinatal transmission of multidrug-resistant HIV-1 despite viral suppression on an enfuvirtide-based treatment regimen. *AIDS*. 2009;19:989-990.
11. Wensing AMJ, Boucher CAB, van Kasteren M, et al. Prevention of mother-to-child transmission of multi-drug resistant HIV-1 using maternal therapy with both enfuvirtide and tipranavir. *AIDS*. 2006;20:1465-1467.
12. Madeddu G, Calia GM, Campus ML, et al. Successful prevention of multidrug resistant HIV mother-to-child transmission with enfuvirtide use in late pregnancy. *Int J STD AIDS*. 2008;19:644-645.
13. Sued O, Lattner J, Patterson P, Abusamra L, et al. Use of darunavir and enfuvirtide in a pregnant woman. *Int J STD AIDS*. 2008;19:866-867.
14. Adeyemo A, Wood C, Govind A. Achieving rapid reduction of HIV-1 viral load in HIV-positive pregnant women close to term—an obstetric/medical emergency: a review of three cases. *Int J STD Aids*. 2013;24:591-592.
15. Shust GF, Jao J, Rodriguez-Caprio G, et al. Salvage regimens containing darunavir, etravirine, raltegravir, or enfuvirtide in highly treatment-experienced perinatally infected pregnant women. *J Pediatric Infect Dis Soc*. 2014;3: 246-250.
16. Panel on Treatment of HIV During Pregnancy and Prevention of Perinatal Transmission. Recommendations for the use of antiretroviral drugs during pregnancy and interventions to reduce perinatal HIV transmission in the United States. Department of Health and Human Services. Accessed November 6, 2023. https://clinicalinfo.hiv.gov/en/guidelines/perinatal

ENOXAPARIN

Hematologic (Anticoagulant)

PREGNANCY RECOMMENDATION: Human Data Suggest Compatible

BREASTFEEDING RECOMMENDATION: Compatible

E

PREGNANCY SUMMARY

Several reports have been located that describe the use of enoxaparin in the first trimester, and no increase in birth anomalies has been identified. Though these numbers are small, the drug does not cross the placenta, so fetal malformation risks should be within the expected rate for the United States. Animal studies did not show any increased risks for teratogenicity. ACOG states that low-molecular-weight heparin (LMWH) is considered low risk and is recommended over unfractionated heparin for the prevention and treatment of venous thromboembolism in pregnancy. Enoxaparin carries a boxed warning regarding an increased risk for spinal and epidural hematomas related to diagnostic and regional anesthesia procedures. Providers should carefully consider the timing of epidural/spinal catheter placement and removal in patients taking enoxaparin, and delay dosing of anticoagulant medications after neuraxial blockage and catheter removal to decrease any potential risk.

BREASTFEEDING SUMMARY

Limited reports describing the use of enoxaparin during human lactation have been located. No reports of any anticoagulant effects in breastfed infants have been reported. The drug will not likely be found in breast milk. If excretion into breast milk does occur, it is likely to be clinically insignificant. Additionally, if ingested through breastfeeding, it has poor absorption from the GI tract and again would be clinically insignificant. ACOG considers LMWH compatible with breastfeeding. Regardless, if used while breastfeeding, the infant should be monitored for the most common reported adult side effects of bleeding, anemia, fever, and peripheral edema.

References

1. Prescribing Information. Lovenox. Sanofi-Aventis U.S; 2022.
2. Nelson-Piercy C. Low molecular weight heparin for obstetric thromboprophylaxis. *Br J Obstet Gynaecol*. 1994;101:6-8.
3. American College of Obstetricians and Gynecologists. ACOG Practice Bulletin No. 196: thromboembolism in pregnancy. *Obstet Gynecol*. 2018;132:e1-e17.
4. Priollet P, Roncato M, Aiach M, et al. Low-molecular-weight heparin in venous thrombosis during pregnancy. *Br J Haematol*. 1986;63:605-606.
5. Gillis S, Shushan A, Eldor A. Use of low molecular weight heparin for prophylaxis and treatment of thromboembolism in pregnancy. *Int J Gynecol Obstet*. 1992;39:297-301.
6. Sturridge F, de Swiet M, Letsky E. The use of low molecular weight heparin for thromboprophylaxis in pregnancy. *Br J Obstet Gynaecol*. 1994;101:69-71.
7. Dulitzki M, Pauzner R, Langevitz P, et al. Low-molecular-weight heparin during pregnancy and delivery: preliminary experience with 41 pregnancies. *Obstet Gynecol*. 1996;87:380-383.
8. Dulitzki M, Seidman DS, Sivan E, et al. Low-molecular-weight heparin in pregnancy and delivery: experience with 24 cases. Society of Perinatal Obstetricians (abstracts). *Am J Obstet Gynecol*. 1995;172:363.
9. Nelson-Piercy C, Letsky EA, de Swiet M. Low-molecular-weight heparin for obstetric thromboprophylaxis: experience of sixty-nine pregnancies in sixty-one women at high risk. *Am J Obstet Gynecol*. 1997;176:1062-1068.
10. Funai EF, Klein SA, Lockwood CJ. Successful pregnancy outcome in a patient with both congenital hypofibrinogenemia and protein S deficiency. *Obstet Gynecol*. 1997;89:858.
11. Casele H, Laifer S. Prospective evaluation of bone density changes in pregnant women on low molecular weight heparin (abstract). *Am J Obstet Gynecol*. 1998;178:S65.
12. Laifer SA, Stiller RJ, Dunston-Boone G, et al. Low-molecular weight heparin for treatment of pulmonary embolism in a pregnant woman. *Thromb Haemost*. 1999;82:1361-1362.
13. Ellison J, Walker ID, Greer IA. Antenatal use of enoxaparin for prevention and treatment of thromboembolism in pregnancy. *Br J Obstet Gynaecol*. 2000;107:1116-1121.
14. Magdelaine A, Verdy E, Coulet F, et al. Deep vein thrombosis during enoxaparin prophylactic treatment in a young pregnant woman homozygous for factor V Leiden and heterozygous for the G127-A mutation in the thrombomodulin gene. *Blood Coagul Fibrinolysis*. 2000;11:761-765.
15. Younis JS, Ohel G, Brenner B, et al. The effect of thrombophylaxis on pregnancy outcome in patients with recurrent pregnancy loss associated with factor V Leiden mutation. *Br J Obstet Gynaecol*. 2000;107:415-419.
16. Schulman S. Long-term prophylaxis in venous thromboembolism: LMWH or oral anticoagulation? *Haemostasis*. 1998;(suppl 3):17-21.
17. Conard J, Horellou MH, Samama MM. Management of pregnancy in women with thrombophilia. *Haemostasis*. 1999;29(suppl 1):98-104.
18. Bates SM. Optimal management of pregnant women with acute venous thromboembolism. *Haemostasis*. 1999;29(suppl 1):107-111.
19. Chan WS, Ray JG. Low molecular weight heparin use during pregnancy: issues of safety and practicality. *Obstet Gynecol Surv*. 1999;54:649-654.
20. Robin F, Lecuru F, Desfeux P, et al. Anticoagulant therapy in pregnancy. *Eur J Obstet Gynecol Reprod Biol*. 1999;83:171-177.
21. Sanson BJ, Lensing AWA, Prins MH, et al. Safety of low-molecular-weight heparin in pregnancy: a systematic review. *Thromb Haemost*. 1999;81:668-672.
22. Ensom MHH, Stephenson MD. Low-molecular-weight heparin in pregnancy. *Pharmacotherapy*. 1999;19:1013-1025.
23. Wolf H, Piek JMJ, van Wijk FH, et al. Administration of low molecular weight heparin within two hours prior to cesarean section increases the prevalence of wound hematoma (abstract). *Am J Obstet Gynecol*. 2000;182:S158.
24. Casele HL, Laifer SA, Woelkers DA, et al. Changes in the pharmacokinetics of the low-molecular-weight heparin enoxaparin sodium during pregnancy. *Am J Obstet Gynecol*. 1999;181:1113-1117.
25. Lee RH, Goodwin TM. Massive subchorionic hematoma associated with enoxaparin. *Obstet Gynecol*. 2006;108:787-789.
26. Brenner B. Enoxaparin use in pregnancy: state of the art. *Womens Health (Lond)*. 2007;3:9-14.

ENSIFENTRINE

Respiratory (COPD—Inhibitor of phosphodiesterase 3 and 4 Enzymes)

PREGNANCY RECOMMENDATION: No Human Data—Animal Data Suggest Low Risk

BREASTFEEDING RECOMMENDATION: Probably Compatible

PREGNANCY SUMMARY

No reports describing the use of ensifentrine in human pregnancy have been located. The drug will likely cross the placenta, so some fetal exposure may occur. However, due to low plasma levels seen with inhalation use, the overall amount is likely to be negligible. Regardless, the absence of human pregnancy experience prevents a complete assessment of the embryofetal risk. Animal studies did not show any embryofetal toxicity or malformations in two species (one above and one below 10 times the maximum recommended human daily inhalation dose (MRHDID)). Using this drug during pregnancy should be based on the pros and cons of the mother's clinical need for treatment versus any potential fetal risk that might occur from exposure.

BREASTFEEDING SUMMARY

No reports describing the use of ensifentrine during human lactation have been located. Based on the low plasma levels seen following inhalation use, the overall amount that may be found in human breast milk is likely to be minimal and probably clinically insignificant. However, breastfeeding while using this drug should be based on the mother's clinical need for treatment versus any potential infant risk that might occur. If used, the infant should be monitored for the most common reported adult side effects of back pain (leading to irritability), diarrhea, and urinary tract infection.

Reference

1. Prescribing Information. Ohtuvayre. Verona Pharma; 2024.

ENTACAPONE

Central Nervous System (Anti-Parkinson)

PREGNANCY RECOMMENDATION: Limited Human Data—Animal Data Suggest Potential Risk

BREASTFEEDING RECOMMENDATION: Potential Toxicity

PREGNANCY SUMMARY

Three case reports with the use of entacapone at the time of conception during human pregnancy were located. One was a set of twins resulting in four newborns. The pregnancies all delivered at term or near term. One of the twins was diagnosed with a small ventricular septal defect. One of the singletons had a seizure about 1 hour postdelivery; the etiology was never determined. Overall, the four neonates did well. A fourth case report was identified where entacapone was started in the second trimester. She delivered at 36 weeks' gestation with no reported complications or anomalies. The drug will likely cross the placenta, so some fetal exposure will probably occur. Therefore, this limited human pregnancy experience prevents a complete assessment of the embryofetal risk. Entacapone is always used with levodopa/carbidopa, and, although the data are very limited, these latter agents do not appear to present a major risk to the human fetus (see Carbidopa and Levodopa). Moreover, conditions requiring the use of levodopa/carbidopa during the childbearing years are relatively uncommon, and thus, the use of entacapone should also be uncommon. Animal studies did not show any embryo-fetal toxicity in one animal species at doses of less than 10 times the MRHD. Using this drug during pregnancy should be based on the pros and cons of the mother's clinical need for treatment versus any potential fetal risk that might occur from exposure.

BREASTFEEDING SUMMARY

No reports describing the use of entacapone during human lactation have been located. The drug will probably appear in breast milk in limited amounts, so some fetal exposure will likely occur. Entacapone is given with levodopa/carbidopa. Levodopa is excreted into breast milk. The use of carbidopa during lactation has also been described. Therefore, a nursing infant will probably be exposed to all three drugs via breast milk. The effects of this multiple exposure on a nursing infant are unknown but warrant further investigation. Breastfeeding while using this drug should be based on the mother's clinical need for treatment. If used, the infant should be monitored for the most common reported adult side effects of nausea, abdominal pain, and dyskinesia (all leading to irritability), diarrhea, and vomiting.

References

1. Prescribing Information. Comtan. Novartis Pharmaceuticals; 2018.
2. Lindh J. Short episode of seizures in a newborn of mother treated with levodopa/carbidopa/entacapone and bromocriptine. *Mod Disord*. 2007;22:1515.
3. Serikawa T, Shimohata T, Akashi M, et al. Successful twin pregnancy in a patient with parkin-associated autosomal recessive juvenile parkinsonism. *BMC Neurol*. 2011;11:72.
4. Tufekcioglu Z, Hanagasi H, Cakmakli GY, et al. Use of anti-Parkinson medication during pregnancy: a case series. *J Neurol*. 2018;265:1922-1929.
5. Basile S, Pinelli S, Garibaldi S, et al. Cathecol-O-methyltransferase inhibitors: another possibly useful pharmacological tool for treating Parkinson's disease in pregnancy? *J Obstet Gynaecol*. 2017;37:381-382.

ENTECAVIR

Antiviral (Hepatitis B)

PREGNANCY RECOMMENDATION: Limited Human Data—Animal Data Suggest Low Risk

BREASTFEEDING RECOMMENDATION: Probably Compatible

E

PREGNANCY SUMMARY

From the APR for the period of January 1989 through January 2023, and a second study, a total of 127 first-trimester exposures to entecavir were reported, with only 2 (1.6%) major anomalies identified. In another study that evaluated cases reported to the US Food and Drug Administration (FDA) Adverse Event Reporting System, there was no increased signal for teratogenicity, but an increased signal for spontaneous abortion was identified. However, these spontaneous reporting safety profile databases have numerous limitations. They are biased toward the reporting of pregnancy complications and poor outcomes rather than normal outcomes. They can also lack clinical details and have missing information, including drug dosages, duration of use, and specific timing of drug exposure during pregnancy. Therefore, they cannot report the incidence of adverse events or provide a measure of risk. These databases can primarily provide whether or not a significant disproportionality exists in the reporting frequency of specific adverse events. Therefore, the risk for spontaneous abortion with first-trimester use of entecavir needs to be analyzed further. The drug will probably cross the placenta, so fetal exposure will likely occur. However, this limited human pregnancy experience prevents a complete assessment of the embryofetal risk. Animal studies did not show any embryofetal toxicity in two species. Using this drug during pregnancy should be based on the pros and cons of the mother's clinical need for treatment versus any potential fetal risk that might occur from exposure. The Advisory Committee on Immunization Practices (ACIP) recommends antiviral therapy in the third trimester of pregnancy when hepatitis B virus (HBV) DNA viral load is more than 200,000, and should be continued until delivery or up to 4 weeks postpartum. Tenofovir disoproxil fumarate is the preferred choice of treatment in pregnancy.

BREASTFEEDING SUMMARY

No reports describing the use of entecavir during human lactation have been located. The drug will probably be found in breast milk, so some infant exposure will likely occur. However, the effect of this exposure on a nursing infant is unknown. All infants born to hepatitis B surface antigen (HBsAg)-positive women should receive the hepatitis B vaccine and hepatitis B immune globulin within 12 hours of birth. HBV infection is not a contraindication to breastfeeding, as long as infants receive postexposure prophylaxis. If entecavir is used while breastfeeding, the infant should be monitored for the most common reported adult side effects of headache, nausea, and dizziness (all leading to irritability), diarrhea, and fatigue (lethargy).

References

1. Prescribing Information. Baraclude. E.R. Squibb & Sons; 2018.
2. Antiretroviral Pregnancy Registry Steering Committee. *Antiretroviral Pregnancy Registry Interim Report for 1 January 1989 Through 31 January 2023*. Registry Coordinating Center; 2023.
3. Kakiuchi T, Takahashi H, Iwane S, et al. Entecavir administration to pregnant Japanese woman with chronic hepatitis B and hepatocellular carcinoma: a case report. *Clin Case Rep*. 2021;9:1752-1758.
4. Yang R, Yin N, Zhao Y, et al. Adverse events during pregnancy associated with entecavir and adefovir: new insights from a real-world analysis of cases reported to FDA adverse event reporting system. *Front Pharmacol*. 2022;12: 772768.
5. Gao X, Duan X, Cai H, et al. Pregnancy outcomes for pregnant women with chronic hepatitis B exposing to entecavir or adefovir dipivoxil therapy before or in early pregnancy. *J Matern Fetal Neonatal Med*. 2022;35:476-480.
6. Cao L, Li S, Dong J, et al. Safety of entecavir antiviral therapy during an accidental pregnancy in patients with chronic hepatitis B. *Biomed Rep*. 2023; 19:72.
7. Schillie S, Vellozzi C, Reingold A, et al. Prevention of Hepatitis B virus infection in the United States: recommendations of the Advisory Committee on Immunization Practices. *MMWR Recomm Rep*. 2019;67:1-31.

ENTRECTINIB

Antineoplastic (Kinase Inhibitor)

PREGNANCY RECOMMENDATION: No Human Data—Animal Data Suggest Potential Risk

BREASTFEEDING RECOMMENDATION: Potential Toxicity

PREGNANCY SUMMARY

No reports describing the use of entrectinib in human pregnancy have been located. A limited amount of the drug will probably cross the placenta, so some fetal exposure may occur. Therefore, the absence of human pregnancy experience prevents a complete assessment of the embryofetal risk. Embryofetal toxicity was observed in one animal species at doses less than 10 times the RHD, but this dose also produced maternal toxicity. Due to the reports in humans with congenital mutations leading to changes in tyrosine kinase signaling, findings from animal studies, and the drug's mechanism of action, the manufacturer recommends that women with reproductive potential use effective contraception during treatment and for 5 weeks after the last dose. They also recommend that males with female partners of reproductive potential use effective contraception during treatment and for 3 months after the last dose. Nevertheless, using this drug during pregnancy should be based on the pros and cons of the mother's clinical need for treatment versus any potential fetal risk that might occur from exposure. The drug may also prolong the cardiac QT interval. There is a registry for women who are pregnant and have cancer. For more information, women and health care providers are encouraged to contact the Cancer and Pregnancy Registry at 1-877-635-4499.

E

BREASTFEEDING SUMMARY

No reports describing the use of entrectinib during human lactation have been located. The drug and its active metabolite will probably be found in breast milk, so some infant exposure may occur. Due to a concern for potential serious adverse effects that might occur in a breastfed infant, the manufacturer recommends that women not breastfeed while being treated with this drug and for at least 7 days after the last dose. Nevertheless, breastfeeding while using this drug should be based on the mother's clinical need for treatment. If used, the infant should be monitored for the most common reported adult side effects of nausea, myalgia, and arthralgia (all leading to irritability), diarrhea, fatigue (lethargy), vomiting, constipation, edema, cough, fever, and various laboratory abnormalities (see PI).

Reference

1. Prescribing Information. Rozlytrek. Genetech, 2023.

ENZALUTAMIDE

Antineoplastic (Antiandrogen)

PREGNANCY RECOMMENDATION: *Contraindicated

BREASTFEEDING RECOMMENDATION: *Contraindicated

PREGNANCY SUMMARY

No reports describing the exposure of enzalutamide during human pregnancy have been located. Based on likely placental transfer, some fetal exposure will probably occur. *However, based on the drug's indication, it is contraindicated for use in women. Animal reproduction studies did show embryofetal toxicity in one animal species at doses less than 10 times the RHD. Due to the findings from these animal studies and the drug's mechanism of action, the manufacturer recommends that males with female partners of reproductive potential use effective contraception during treatment and for at least 3 months after the last dose.

BREASTFEEDING SUMMARY

No reports describing the use of enzalutamide during human lactation have been located. *However, such reports are unlikely because the drug is contraindicated for use in women. Nevertheless, if the drug was used during breastfeeding, a limited amount would probably be found in breast milk.

Reference

1. Prescribing Information. Xtandi. Astellas Pharma US; 2023.

EPCORITAMAB

Antineoplastic (Monoclonal Antibody)

PREGNANCY RECOMMENDATION: No Human Data and No Relevant Animal Data

BREASTFEEDING RECOMMENDATION: Probably Compatible

PREGNANCY SUMMARY

No reports describing the use of epcoritamab in human pregnancy have been located. As an IgG antibody, the drug will likely cross the placenta, so some fetal exposure will probably occur. However, the absence of human pregnancy experience prevents a complete assessment of the embryofetal risk. Animal reproduction studies have not been conducted. However, embryofetal toxicity might occur based on the drug's mechanism of action. Because the drug activates T cells, this could theoretically compromise pregnancy maintenance (especially in the first trimester). In addition, because the drug can deplete B cells, newborns could have a low B-cell count postdelivery. Because of this, the manufacturer recommends that women with reproductive potential who are taking epcoritamab use effective contraception during treatment and for at least 4 months after the last dose. Nevertheless, using this drug during pregnancy should be based on the pros and cons of the mother's clinical need for treatment versus any potential fetal risk that might occur from exposure. If used, the newborn should have B-cell levels evaluated postdelivery.

E

BREASTFEEDING SUMMARY

No reports describing the use of epcoritamab during human lactation have been located. It is known that IgG antibodies can be found in human breast milk, but are not found in the neonatal or infant circulation. Additionally, if any IgG antibodies were to be ingested through breastfeeding, they would probably be digested in the infant's GI tract and not be absorbed. However, due to the potential for adverse effects that might be seen in a breastfed infant, the manufacturer recommends that women should not breastfeed while being treated with epcoritamab and for at least 4 months after the last dose. Nevertheless, breastfeeding while using this drug should be based on the mother's clinical need for treatment. If used, the infant should be monitored for the most common reported adult side effects of musculoskeletal pain, abdominal pain, and nausea (all leading to irritability), cytokine release syndrome, lethargy, diarrhea, pyrexia, and various laboratory abnormalities (see PI).

Reference

1. Prescribing Information. Epkinly. Genmab US, Inc; 2023.

EPHEDRINE

Autonomic (Sympathomimetic—α/β Agonist)

PREGNANCY RECOMMENDATION: **Limited Human Data—Animal Data Suggest Low Risk**

BREASTFEEDING RECOMMENDATION: **Probably Compatible**

PREGNANCY SUMMARY

The Collaborative Perinatal Project reported first-trimester exposure to ephedrine in 373 patients, with 17 (4.6%) newborns identified who had major malformations. However, no specific pattern was noted, and coexposures to other drugs were not described. For anytime use during pregnancy, 873 exposures were recorded, with 14 (1.6%) major malformations identified. From these data, no evidence of an association with large categories of major or minor malformations or with individual defects was found. The 2016 Practice Guidelines for Obstetric Anesthesia support the use of intravenous (IV) ephedrine for treating hypotension during neuraxial anesthesia in pregnancy. The guidelines cite five double-blind, placebo-controlled, randomized trials with reduced maternal hypotension during anesthesia for cesarean delivery when compared to placebo. The drug will cross the placenta, so fetal exposure will occur. However, this limited human pregnancy experience prevents a complete assessment of the embryofetal risk. Animal data did not show any embryofetal toxicity in two species at doses less than 10 times the RHD. Using this drug during pregnancy should be based on the pros and cons of the mother's clinical need for treatment versus any potential fetal risk that might occur from exposure.

BREASTFEEDING SUMMARY

No reports describing the use of ephedrine during human lactation have been located. The drug will probably be found in breast milk, so some infant exposure will likely occur. Breastfeeding while using this drug should be based on the mother's clinical need for treatment versus any potential infant risks that might occur. If used, the infant should be monitored for the most common reported adult side effects of nausea (leading to irritability), vomiting, and tachycardia.

References

1. Prescribing Information. Ephedrine. Par Pharmaceutical; 2022.
2. Hughes SC, Ward MG, Levinson G, et al. Placental transfer of ephedrine does not affect neonatal outcome. *Anesthesiology*. 1985;63:217-219.
3. Griffiths SK, Campbell JP. Placental structure, function and drug transfer. *CEACCP*. 2015;15:84-89.
4. Heinonen OP, Slone D, Shapiro S. *Birth Defects and Drugs in Pregnancy*. Publishing Sciences Group; 1977.
5. Practice Guidelines for Obstetric Anesthesia. An updated report by the American Society of Anesthesiologists Task Force on Obstetric Anesthesia and the Society for Obstetric Anesthesia and Perinatology. *Anesthesiology*. 2016;24:270-230.

6. Desalu I, Kushimo OT. Is ephedrine infusion more effective at preventing hypotension than traditional prehydration during spinal anaesthesia for caesarean section in African parturients? *Int J Obstet Anesth*. 2005; 14:294-299.
7. King SW, Rosen MA. Prophylactic ephedrine and hypotension associated with spinal anesthesia for cesarean delivery. *Int J Obstet Anesth*. 1998; 7:18-22.
8. Loughrey JP, Walsh F, Gardiner J. Prophylactic intravenous bolus ephedrine for elective caesarean section under spinal anaesthesia. *Eur J Anaesthesiol*. 2002; 19:63-68.
9. Ngan Kee WD, Khaw KS, Lee BB, et al. A dose response study of prophylactic intravenous ephedrine for the prevention of hypotension during spinal anesthesia for cesarean delivery. *Anesth Analg*. 2000; 90:1390-1395.
10. Ramin SM, Ramin KD, Cox K, et al. Comparison of prophylactic angiotensin II versus ephedrine infusion for prevention of maternal hypotension during spinal anesthesia. *Am J Obstet Gynecol*. 1994; 171:734-739.
11. Dyer RA, Reed AR, van Dyk D, et al. Hemodynamic effects of ephedrine, phenylephrine, and the coadministration of phenylephrine with oxytocin during spinal anesthesia for elective cesarean delivery. *Anesthesiology*. 2009; 111:753-765.
12. LaPorta RF, Arthur GR, Datta S. Phenylephrine in treating maternal hypotension due to spinal anaesthesia for caesarean delivery: effects on neonatal catecholamine concentrations, acid base status and Apgar scores. *Acta Anaesthesiol Scand*. 1995; 39:901-905.
13. Moran DH, Perillo M, LaPorta RF, et al. Phenylephrine in the prevention of hypotension following spinal anesthesia for cesarean delivery. *J Clin Anesth*. 1991; 3:301-305.
14. Pierce ET, Carr DB, Datta S. Effects of ephedrine and phenylephrine on maternal and fetal atrial natriuretic peptide levels during elective cesarean section. *Acta Anaesthesiol Scand*. 1994; 38:48-51.
15. Prakash S, Pramanik V, Chellani H, et al. Maternal and neonatal effects of bolus administration of ephedrine and phenylephrine during spinal anaesthesia for caesarean delivery: a randomised study. *Int J Obstet Anesth*. 2010; 19:24-30.
16. Saravanan S, Kocarev M, Wilson RC, et al. Equivalent dose of ephedrine and phenylephrine in the prevention of post-spinal hypotension in caesarean section. *Br J Anaesth*. 2006; 96:95-99.

E

EPINASTINE HYDROCHLORIDE

Ophthalmic (Antihistamine)

PREGNANCY RECOMMENDATION: No Human Data and No Relevant Animal Data

BREASTFEEDING RECOMMENDATION: Probably Compatible

PREGNANCY SUMMARY

No reports describing the use of epinastine ophthalmic in human pregnancy have been located. Based on likely placental transfer, some fetal exposure might occur. But the amount is probably clinically insignificant due to its very low systemic absorption. However, the absence of human pregnancy experience prevents a complete assessment of the embryofetal risk. Animal studies using an ophthalmic dose at less than 10 times the maximum recommended ocular human dose have not been conducted. Using this drug during pregnancy should be based on the pros and cons of the mother's clinical need for treatment versus any potential fetal risk that might occur from exposure. If used, consider placing pressure over the tear duct in the corner of the eye for at least 1 minute, and remove any excess solution with absorbent tissue to further decrease the amount of drug reaching the systemic circulation.

BREASTFEEDING SUMMARY

One report describing the use of epinastine during human lactation was located. Seven lactating women were administered 20 mg of epinastine orally once a day for 7 days. The drug was found in breast milk with a maximum dose that an infant might obtain of about 8% of the maternal weight-adjusted dosage. The RID was only about 2.5%, and this study evaluated the oral use of the drug. Any exposure following ophthalmic use would probably be undetectable. Breastfeeding while using this drug should be based on the mother's clinical need for treatment. If used, consider placing pressure over the tear duct in the corner of the eye for at least 1 minute, and remove any excess solution with absorbent tissue to further decrease the amount of drug reaching the systemic circulation.

References

1. Prescribing Information. Elestat. Apotex Corp; 2013.
2. Iwasa C, Zaima K, Metori K, et al. Transfer of epinastine to infants through human breast milk. *Pharmazie*. 2019;74:732-736.

EPINEPHRINE

Autonomic (Sympathomimetic—α/β Agonist)

PREGNANCY RECOMMENDATION: Limited Human Data—Animal Data Suggest Risk (Maternal Benefit May Outweigh Embryofetal Risk)

BREASTFEEDING RECOMMENDATION: Probably Compatible

PREGNANCY SUMMARY

The Collaborative Perinatal Project and Michigan Medicaid data reported first-trimester exposure to epinephrine in 224 patients, with 14 (6.3%) newborns identified who had major malformations. However, no specific pattern was noted, and

(*continued*)

coexposures to other drugs were not described. For anytime use during pregnancy, 508 exposures were recorded, with 11 (2.2%) major malformations identified. The drug will cross the placenta, so fetal exposure will occur. However, this limited human pregnancy experience prevents a complete assessment of the embryofetal risk. Animal studies did show embryofetal toxicity in three species at doses less than 10 times the RHD. Anaphylaxis during pregnancy can cause central nervous system damage and death in the mother and fetus. The treatment of anaphylaxis during pregnancy is similar to the nonpregnant population. Epinephrine is the first-line medication. Similarly, hypotension due to septic shock is a medical emergency and can be fatal if untreated. Life-saving treatment should not be withheld due to concerns of the effects of epinephrine on the fetus. However, while the 2021 Surviving Sepsis Guidelines do not specifically address pregnant patients, norepinephrine is recommended as the first-line vasoactive agent in septic shock, and the maternal benefit likely outweighs any embryofetal risk.

E

BREASTFEEDING SUMMARY

No reports describing the use of epinephrine during human lactation have been located. The drug will probably be found in breast milk, so some infant exposure will likely occur. In addition, epinephrine is poorly absorbed from the GI tract. Epinephrine is the first-line medication of choice for the treatment of anaphylaxis. The treatment of anaphylaxis in breastfeeding should be the same as in nonbreastfeeding patients. If used while breastfeeding, the infant should be monitored for some of the most common reported adult side effects of nervousness and agitation (leading to irritability), tremors, and tachycardia.

References

1. Morgan CD, Sandler M, Panigel M. Placental transfer of catecholamines in vitro and in vivo. *Am J Obstet Gynecol*. 1972;112:1068-1075.
2. Nishimura H, Tanimura T. *Clinical Aspects of the Teratogenicity of Drugs*. Elsevier; 1976:231.
3. Shepard TH. *Catalog of Teratogenic Agents*. 3rd ed. The Johns Hopkins University Press; 1980:134-135.
4. Heinonen OP, Slone D, Shapiro S. *Birth Defects and Drugs in Pregnancy*. Publishing Sciences Group; 1977.
5. Entman SS, Moise KJ. Anaphylaxis in pregnancy. *S Med J*. 1984;77:402.
6. Prescribing Information. Epinephrine. Belcher Pharmaceuticals; 2021.
7. Evans L, Rhodes A, Alhazzani W, et al. Surviving sepsis campaign: international guidelines for management of sepsis and septic Shock 2021. *Crit Care Med*. 2021;49:e1063-e1143.

EPIRUBICIN

Antineoplastic (Anthracycline Topoisomerase Inhibitor)

PREGNANCY RECOMMENDATION: Limited Human Data—Animal Data Suggest Potential Risk

BREASTFEEDING RECOMMENDATION: Potential Toxicity

PREGNANCY SUMMARY

Numerous reports describing the use of epirubicin in human pregnancies have been located. Most exposures included other chemotherapy agents, and most were in the second and third trimesters. Of 89 pregnancies and excluding elective terminations, there were 5 (6%) spontaneous abortions, 3 intrauterine fetal demises, and 1 neonatal death. The remaining 80 pregnancies were live births with no reported anomalies. Some amount of the drug may cross the placenta, so fetal exposure will occur. However, this limited human pregnancy experience prevents a complete assessment of the embryofetal risk. Animal studies did show embryofetal toxicity with malformations in one species at doses less than 10 times the RHD, which did not cause maternal toxicity. Due to the findings from animal studies and the drug's mechanism of action, the manufacturer recommends that women with reproductive potential use effective contraception during treatment and for at least 6 months after the last dose. They also recommend that males with female partners of reproductive potential use effective contraception and condoms during treatment and for at least 3 months and 7 days after the last dose, respectively. Nevertheless, using this drug during pregnancy should be based on the pros and cons of the mother's clinical need for treatment versus any potential fetal risk that might occur from exposure. There is a registry for women who are pregnant and have cancer. For more information, women are encouraged to contact the Cancer and Pregnancy Registry at 877-635-4499.

BREASTFEEDING SUMMARY

No reports describing the use of epirubicin during human lactation have been located. The drug will probably be found in breast milk, so some infant exposure will likely occur. Because of the potential for serious adverse effects that might be seen in a breastfed infant, the manufacturer recommends that women receiving epirubicin should not breastfeed during treatment and for at least 7 days after the last dose. Nevertheless, breastfeeding while using this drug should be based on the mother's clinical need for treatment versus any potential infant risks that might occur. If used, the infant should be monitored for the most common reported adult side effects of nausea (leading to irritability), vomiting, diarrhea, infections, alopecia, rash, lethargy, and various laboratory abnormalities (see PI).

References

1. Prescribing Information. Ellence. Pfizer; 2020.

2. Goldwasser F, Pico JL, Cerrina J, et al. Successful chemotherapy including epirubicin in a pregnant non-Hodgkin's lymphoma patient. *Leuk Lymphoma*. 1995;20:173-176.
3. Muller T, Hofmann J, Steck T. Eclampsia after polychemotherapy for nodal-positive breast cancer during pregnancy. *Eur J Obstet Gynecol Reprod Biol*. 1996;67:197-198.
4. Giacalone PL, Laffargue F, Benos P. Chemotherapy for breast carcinoma during pregnancy. *Cancer*. 1999;86:2266-2272.
5. Ramirez-Torres N, Asbun-Bojalil J, Hernandez-Valencia M. Pregnancy and breast cancer. *Cir* . 2013;81:98-107.
6. Framarino-dei-Malatesta M, Perrone G, Giancotti A, et al. Epirubicin: a new entry in the list of fetal cardiotoxic drugs? Intrauterine death of one fetus in a twin pregnancy. Case report and review of literature. *BMC Cancer*. 2015;15:951.
7. Peccatori FA, Azim HA Jr, Scarfone G, et al. Weekly epirubicin in the treatment of gestational breast cancer (GBC). *Breast Cancer Res Treat*. 2009;115:591-594.
8. Leyder M, Laubach M, Breugelmans M, et al. Specific congenital malformations after exposure to cyclophosphamide, epirubicin and 5-fluorouracil during the first trimester of pregnancy. *Gynecol Obstet Invest*. 2011;71:141-144.
9. Passera S, Contarino V, Scarfone G, et al. Effects of in-utero exposure to chemotherapy on fetal brain growth. *Int J Gynecol Cancer*. 2019 Sep;29(7):1195-1202.
10. Parodi E, Alluto A, Moggio G, et al. Transient ventricular hypocinesia after in utero anthracyclines exposure: a case-report and review of the literature. *J Matern Fetal Neonatal Med*. 2012;25:189-192.
11. Gadducci A, Cosio S, Fanucchi A, Nardini V, Roncella M, Conte PF, Genazzani AR. Chemotherapy with epirubicin and paclitaxel for breast cancer during pregnancy: case report and review of the literature. *Anticancer Res*. 2003;23(6D):5225-5229.
12. Eedarapalli P, Biswas N, Coleman M. Epirubicin for breast cancer during pregnancy: a case report. *J Reprod Med*. 2007;52:730-732.
13. Sharma JB, Pushparaj M, Kumar S, et al. Successful pregnancy outcome with 5-fluorouracil, epirubicin, cyclophosphamide chemotherapy, and hemostatic radiotherapy with abdominal shielding for metastatic invasive intraductal breast carcinoma. *Arch Gynecol Obstet*. 2009;279:415-417.
14. Bodner-Adler B, Bodner K, Zeisler H. Breast cancer diagnosed during pregnancy. *Anticancer Res*. 2007;27:1705-1707.
15. Azim HA Jr, Peccatori FA, Scarfone G, et al. Anthracyclines for gestational breast cancer: course and outcome of pregnancy. *Ann Oncol*. 2008;19:1511-1512.
16. Andreadis C, Charalampidou M, Diamantopoulos N, et al. Combined chemotherapy and radiotherapy during conception and first two trimesters of gestation in a woman with metastatic breast cancer. *Gynecol Oncol*. 2004;95:252-255.

E

EPLONTERSEN

Genetic (Antisense Oligonucleotide)

PREGNANCY RECOMMENDATION: No Human Data—Animal Data Suggest Low Risk

BREASTFEEDING RECOMMENDATION: Probably Compatible

PREGNANCY SUMMARY

No reports describing the use of eplontersen in human pregnancy have been located. It is not likely that any clinically significant amount of the drug will cross the placenta, so fetal exposure is probably negligible. However, the absence of human pregnancy experience prevents a complete assessment of the embryofetal risk. Animal data did not show any embryofetal toxicity in one species at doses more than 10 times the RHD. Using this drug during pregnancy should be based on the pros and cons of the mother's clinical need for treatment versus any potential fetal risk that might occur from exposure. The drug can lower the vitamin A level by as much as 70%. Therefore, normal prenatal vitamin usage throughout pregnancy is needed. If there is any question, vitamin A levels can be monitored. Excess vitamin A levels in pregnancy can be harmful, so using more than a daily prenatal vitamin is not recommended, unless blood levels for vitamin A are below normal.

BREASTFEEDING SUMMARY

No reports describing the use of eplontersen during human lactation have been located. The drug is not likely to be found in breast milk, so infant exposure should be negligible. Furthermore, because it is a nucleotide, if the drug were to be ingested through breastfeeding, it would probably be somewhat digested in the infant's GI tract and not be absorbed. Breastfeeding while using this drug should be based on the mother's clinical need for treatment versus any potential infant risk that might occur. If used, the infant should be monitored for the most common reported adult side effects of vitamin A deficiency and vomiting.

Reference

1. Prescribing Information. Wainua. AstraZeneca; 2023.

EPOETIN ALFA

Hematologic (Erythropoiesis-Stimulating Agent)

PREGNANCY RECOMMENDATION: *Limited Human Data—Animal Data Suggest Potential Risk

BREASTFEEDING RECOMMENDATION: Probably Compatible

PREGNANCY SUMMARY

Numerous reports have been located that described the use of epoetin alfa in the first trimester and continued throughout gestation. In more than 20 cases, no fetal anomalies were identified. However, the drug was used in patients with a history of organ transplant and in patients with severe anemia due to other causes, and this led to several preterm births. *The drug does not cross the placenta, so fetal exposure will not occur. However, this limited human pregnancy experience prevents a complete assessment of the embryofetal risk that might be caused by the medical issues described in the boxed warning. Animal studies did show embryofetal toxicity in one species (but not in a second species) at doses less than 10 times the RHD. Using this drug during pregnancy should be based on the pros and cons of the mother's clinical need for treatment versus any potential fetal risk that might occur from exposure. Epoetin alfa carries a boxed warning regarding increased risk of death, myocardial infarction, stroke, venous thromboembolism, thrombosis of vascular access, and tumor progression or recurrence.

E

BREASTFEEDING SUMMARY

One report describing 19 women who received epoetin alfa while breastfeeding was located. No adverse effects were reported in the infants. Endogenous erythropoietin is present in human breast milk. It is not known if recombinant epoetin alfa is present in breast milk. The high MW suggests that it will not be excreted into breast milk. In addition, this glycoprotein would probably be somewhat digested in the infant's GI tract with minimal amounts absorbed. Multidose vials of epoetin alfa contain the preservative benzyl alcohol, which has been associated with serious and possibly fatal reactions in neonates, including "gasping syndrome" when consumed orally. However, benzyl alcohol is rapidly metabolized to benzoic acid in the liver and then binds to glycine and is excreted as hippuric acid. Therefore, exposure to a breastfeeding newborn is not likely. Nevertheless, using the single-dose vials (that do not contain benzyl alcohol) is recommended if needed. Breastfeeding while using this drug should be based on the mother's clinical need for treatment versus any potential infant risks that might occur. If used, the infant should be monitored for the most common reported adult side effects of nausea, headache, and arthralgia (all leading to irritability), vomiting, pruritus, hypertension, and fever.

References

1. Prescribing Information. Epogen. Amgen; 2024.
2. Yankowitz J, Piraino B, Laifer SA, et al. Erythropoietin in pregnancies complicated by severe anemia of renal failure. *Obstet Gynecol*. 1992;80:485-488.
3. Widness JA, Teramo KA, Clemons GK, et al. Direct relationship of antepartum glucose control and fetal erythropoietin in human type 1 (insulin-dependent) diabetic pregnancy. *Diabetologia*. 1990;33:378-383.
4. Salvesen DR, Brudenell JM, Snijders RJM, et al. Fetal plasma erythropoietin in pregnancies complicated by maternal diabetes mellitus. *Am J Obstet Gynecol*. 1993;168:88-94.
5. Thomas RM, Canning CE, Cotes PM, et al. Erythropoietin and cord blood haemoglobin in the regulation of human fetal erythropoiesis. *Br J Obstet Gynaecol*. 1983;90:795-800.
6. Campbell J, Wathen N, Lewis M, et al. Erythropoietin levels in amniotic fluid and extraembryonic coelomic fluid in the first trimester of pregnancy. *Br J Obstet Gynaecol*. 1992;99:974-976.
7. Zivny J, Kobilkova J, Neuwirt J, et al. Regulation of erythropoiesis in fetus and mother during normal pregnancy. *Obstet Gynecol*. 1982;60:77-81.
8. Malek A, Sager R, Eckardt K-U, et al. Lack of transport of erythropoietin across the human placenta as studied by an in vitro perfusion system. *Pflügers Arch*. 1994;427:157-161.
9. Santolaya-Forgas J, Meyer W, Gauthier D, et al. Transplacental passage of erythropoietin (EPO-Alfa): a case control study. Society of Perinatal Obstetricians (abstract). *Am J Obstet Gynecol*. 1997;176:S83.
10. Reisenberger K, Egarter C, Kapiotis S, et al. Transfer of erythropoietin across the placenta perfused in vitro. *Obstet Gynecol*. 1997;89:738-742.
11. Fujimi S, Hori K, Miijima C, et al. Successful pregnancy and delivery in a patient following rHuEPO therapy and on long-term dialysis (abstract). *J Am Soc Nephrol*. 1990;1:391.
12. Barri YM, Al-Furayh O, Qunibi WY, et al. Pregnancy in women on regular hemodialysis. *Dial Transplant*. 1991;20:652-654, 656, 695.
13. McGregor E, Stewart G, Junor BJR, et al. Successful use of recombinant human erythropoietin in pregnancy. *Nephrol Dial Transplant*. 1991;6:292-293.
14. Gadallah MF, Ahmad B, Karubian F, et al. Pregnancy in patients with chronic ambulatory peritoneal dialysis. *Am J Kidney Dis*. 1992;20:407-410.
15. Hou S, Orlowski J, Pahl M, et al. Pregnancy in women with end-stage renal disease: treatment of anemia and premature labor. *Am J Kidney Dis*. 1993;21:16-22.
16. Barth W Jr, Lacroix L, Goldberg M, et al. Recombinant human erythropoietin (rHEpo) for severe anemia in pregnancies complicated by renal disease. Society of Perinatal Obstetricians (abstract). *Am J Obstet Gynecol*. 1994;170:329.
17. Scott LL, Ramin SM, Richey M, et al. Erythropoietin use in pregnancy: two cases and review of the literature. *Am J Perinatol*. 1995;12:22-24.
18. Amoedo ML, Fernandez E, Borras M, et al. Successful pregnancy in a hemodialysis patient treated with erythropoietin. *Nephron*. 1995;70:262-263.
19. Braga J, Marques R, Branco A, et al. Maternal and perinatal implications of the use of human recombinant erythropoietin. *Acta Obstet Gynecol Scand*. 1996;75:449-453.
20. Pascual J, Liano F, Ortuno J. Pregnancy in an anephric woman. *Am J Obstet Gynecol*. 1995;172:1939.
21. Junca J, Vela D, Orts M, et al. Treating the anaemia of a pregnancy with heterozygous β thalassaemia with recombinant human erythropoietin (r-HuEPO). *Eur J Haematol*. 1995;55:277-278.
22. Harris SA, Payne G Jr, Putman JM. Erythropoietin treatment of erythropoietin-deficient anemia with renal disease during pregnancy. *Obstet Gynecol*. 1996;87:812-814.
23. Lin C-P, Huang M-J, Liu H-J, et al. Successful treatment of acute promyelocytic leukemia in a pregnant Jehovah's Witness with all-trans retinoic acid, rhG-CSF, and erythropoietin. *Am J Hematol*. 1996;51:251-252.
24. Emmerson AJB, Coles HJ, Stern CMM, et al. Double blind trial of recombinant human erythropoietin in preterm infants. *Arch Dis Child*. 1993;68:291-296.
25. Makrydimas G, Lolis D, Lialios G, et al. Recombinant human erythropoietin treatment of postpartum anemia. preliminary results. *Eur J Obstet Gynecol Reprod Biol*. 1998;81:27-31.
26. Nair B. Final report on the safety assessment of benzyl alcohol, benzoic acid, and sodium benzoate. *Int J Toxicol*. 2001;20(suppl 3):23-50.

EPOPROSTENOL

Respiratory (Prostacyclin)

PREGNANCY RECOMMENDATION: Limited Human Data—Animal Data Suggest Low Risk (Maternal Benefit May Outweigh Embryofetal Risk)

BREASTFEEDING RECOMMENDATION: Probably Compatible

PREGNANCY SUMMARY

Numerous case reports and series were identified that describe 38 pregnancies with exposure to epoprostenol in all trimesters. No congenital abnormalities were reported that were attributed to epoprostenol. Three in utero and four postnatal deaths were noted. All remaining live births were delivered preterm due to worsening maternal status. The delivered infants experienced an expected neonatal course related to prematurity. The drug will probably cross the placenta, but the overall amount is likely to be clinically insignificant. However, this limited human pregnancy experience prevents a complete assessment of the embryofetal risk. Animal data did not show any embryofetal toxicity in two species at doses less than 10 times the RHD. Pulmonary hypertension is associated with a very high rate of adverse pregnancy outcomes. The maternal benefit of epoprostenol appears to outweigh any potential risks to the fetus.

BREASTFEEDING SUMMARY

No reports describing the use of epoprostenol during human lactation have been located. The drug may be found in human breast milk, but the overall amounts are likely to be negligible. Breastfeeding while using this drug should be based on the mother's clinical need for treatment versus any potential infant risks that might occur. If used, the infant should be monitored for the most common reported adult side effects of nausea and abdominal pain (both leading to irritability), vomiting, hypotension, bradycardia, and tachycardia.

References

1. Prescribing Information. Veletri. Actelion Pharmaceuticals US, Inc; 2022.
2. Fidler J, Bennett MJ, De Swift M, et al. Treatment of pregnancy hypertension with prostacyclin. *Lancet*. 1980;2:31-32.
3. Lewis PJ, Shepherd GL, Ritter J, et al. Prostacyclin and pre-eclampsia. *Lancet*. 1981;1:559.
4. Belch JJF, Thorburn J, Greer IA, et al. Intravenous prostacyclin in the management of pregnancies complicated by severe hypertension. *Clin Exp Hypertens Preg*. 1985;B4:75-86.
5. Jouppila P, Kirkinen P, Koivula A, et al. Failure of exogenous prostacyclin to change placental and fetal blood flow in preeclampsia. *Am J Obstet Gynecol*. 1985;151:661-665.
6. De Belder AJ, Weston MJ. Epoprostenol infusions in thrombotic microangiopathy of pregnancy. *Lancet*. 1992;339:741-742.
7. Huber W, Schweigart U, Classen M. Epoprostenol and plasmapheresis in complicated HELLP syndrome with pancreatitis. *Lancet*. 1994;343:848.
8. Easterling TR, Ralph DD, Schmucker BC. Pulmonary hypertension in pregnancy: treatment with pulmonary vasodilators. *Obstet Gynecol*. 1999;93:494-498.
9. Badalian SS, Silverman RK, Aubry RH, et al. Twin pregnancy in a woman on long-term epoprostenol therapy for primary pulmonary hypertension. A case report. *J Reprod Med*. 2000;45:149-152.
10. Bildirici I, Shumway JB. Intravenous and inhaled epoprostenol for primary pulmonary hypertension during pregnancy and delivery. *Obstet Gynecol*. 2004;103:1102-1105.
11. Bendayan D, Hod M, Oron G, et al. Pregnancy outcome in patients with pulmonary arterial hypertension receiving prostacyclin therapy. *Obstet Gynecol*. 2005;106:1206-1210.
12. Soditt V, Aring C, Groneck P. Improvement of oxygenation induced by aerosolized prostacyclin in a preterm infant with persistent pulmonary hypertension of the newborn. *Intensive Care Med*. 1997;23:1275-1278.
13. Timofeev J, Ruiz G, Fries M, Driggers RW. Intravenous epoprostenol for management of pulmonary arterial hypertension during pregnancy. *AJP Rep*. 2013;3:71-74.
14. Kawabe A, Nakano K, Aiko Y, et al. Successful management of pregnancy in a patient with systemic lupus erythematosus-associated pulmonary arterial hypertension. *Intern Med*. 2018;57:1655-1659.
15. Valko L, Csosza G, Merei A, et al. Management of acutely decompensated chronic thromboembolic pulmonary hypertension in late pregnancy: a case report. *BMC Pregnancy Childbirth*. 2019;19:365.
16. Daimon A, Kamiya CA, Iwanaga N, et al. Management of pulmonary vasodilator therapy in three pregnancies with pulmonary arterial hypertension. *J Obstet Gynaecol Res*. 2017;43:935-938.
17. Goland S, Tsai F, Habib M, et al. Favorable outcome of pregnancy with an elective use of epoprostenol and sildenafil in women with severe pulmonary hypertension. *Cardiology*. 2010;115:205-208.
18. Garabedian MJ, Hansen WF, Gianferrari EA, et al. Epoprostenol treatment for idiopathic pulmonary arterial hypertension in pregnancy. *J Perinatol*. 2010;30:628-631.
19. Moodley J, Gouws E. A comparative study of the use of epoprostenol and dihydralazine in severe hypertension in pregnancy. *Br J Obstet Gynaecol*. 1992;99:727-730.

EPROSARTAN

Antihypertensive (Angiotensin II Receptor Antagonist)

PREGNANCY RECOMMENDATION: Human Data Suggest Risk in the Second and Third Trimesters—Animal Data Suggest Potential Risk

BREASTFEEDING RECOMMENDATION: Potential Toxicity

PREGNANCY SUMMARY

No reports describing the use of eprosartan in human pregnancy have been located. Based on likely limited placental transfer, some fetal exposure will probably occur. Therefore, the absence of human pregnancy experience prevents a complete assessment of the embryofetal risk. The use of drugs that act on the renin-angiotensin system has been associated with fetal renal dysfunction that, in some cases, can result in permanent renal damage. ACOG recommends the use of labetalol or nifedipine if at all possible. Drugs that act on the renin-angiotensin system are not recommended. In the unusual circumstance where this drug is needed or is being used in the second half of gestation, the pregnancy should be monitored

(*continued*)

closely by perinatal ultrasound to assess fetal renal status and amniotic fluid volume. Nevertheless, adverse fetal renal injury may occur prior to the development of oligohydramnios. The drug carries a boxed warning for this risk. Animal data showed embryofetal toxicity in one species at doses less than 10 times the RHD.

BREASTFEEDING SUMMARY

No reports describing the use of eprosartan during human lactation have been located. The drug will probably be found in breast milk, so some infant exposure will likely occur. Breastfeeding while using this drug should be based on the mother's clinical need for treatment. If used, the infant should be monitored for the most common reported adult side effects of nausea and dizziness (both leading to irritability), lethargy, and constipation.

References

1. Prescribing Information. Teveten. AbbVie, Inc; 2020.
2. American College of Obstetricians and Gynecologists. ACOG Practice Bulletin No. 203: chronic hypertension in pregnancy. *Obstet Gynecol*. 2019;133: e26-e50.

EPTIFIBATIDE

Hematologic (Antiplatelet)

PREGNANCY RECOMMENDATION: **Limited Human Data—Animal Data Suggest Low Risk**

BREASTFEEDING RECOMMENDATION: **Probably Compatible**

PREGNANCY SUMMARY

Two case reports describing the use of eptifibatide in human pregnancies were located. Both patients received eptifibatide as part of the overall treatment for an acute myocardial infarct; one at 8 weeks of gestation and the other in the third trimester. Both patients delivered near term with healthy infants and no reported anomalies. Based on likely placenta transfer, some fetal exposure will probably occur. Therefore, the absence of human pregnancy experience prevents a complete assessment of the embryofetal risk. No embryofetal toxicity was seen in two animal species at doses less than 10 times the MRHD. Using this drug during pregnancy should be based on the pros and cons of the mother's clinical need for treatment versus any potential fetal risk that might occur from exposure.

BREASTFEEDING SUMMARY

No reports describing the use of eptifibatide during human lactation have been located. Because of the indicated uses for eptifibatide, it is doubtful if such reports will be forthcoming. Some amount of the drug may be excreted into breast milk. However, the risk is likely low because it consists of a small peptide that would probably be digested in the infant's GI tract and not be absorbed. Breastfeeding while using this drug should be based on the mother's clinical need for treatment. If used, the infant should be monitored for potential side effects of bruising and bleeding.

References

1. Prescribing Information. Integrilin. Merck Sharp & Dohme Corp; 2021.
2. Al-Aqeedi RF, Al-Nabti AD. Drug-eluting stent implantation for acute myocardial infarction during pregnancy with use of glycoprotein IIb/IIIa inhibitor, aspirin, and clopidogrel. *J Invasive Cardiol*. 2008;20:E146-E149.
3. Bauer MEB, Bauer ST, Rabbani AB, et al. Peripartum management of dual antiplatelet therapy and neuraxial labor analgesia after bare metal stent insertion for acute myocardial infarction. *Anesth Analg*. 2012;115:613-615.

EPTINEZUMAB

Central Nervous System (Monoclonal Antibody—Antimigraine)

PREGNANCY RECOMMENDATION: **No Human Data—Animal Data Suggest Low Risk**

BREASTFEEDING RECOMMENDATION: **Probably Compatible**

PREGNANCY SUMMARY

No reports describing the use of eptinezumab in human pregnancy have been located. As an IgG antibody, it likely crosses the placenta, especially in the second half of gestation, so some fetal exposure will probably occur. Therefore, the absence of human pregnancy experience prevents a complete assessment of the embryofetal risk. Animal studies did not show any embryofetal toxicity in two species at doses of more than 10 times the RHD. Using this drug during pregnancy should be based on the pros and cons of the mother's clinical need for treatment versus any potential fetal risk that might occur from exposure.

BREASTFEEDING SUMMARY

Eptinezumab is likely present in breast milk in small amounts. However, it is known that IgG antibodies can be found in human breast milk but are not found in the neonatal or infant circulation. Additionally, if any IgG antibodies were to be ingested through breastfeeding, they would probably be digested in the infant's GI tract and not be absorbed. If the clinical decision is to use this drug while breastfeeding, the infant should be monitored for the most common reported adult side effects of nasopharyngitis and hypersensitivity reactions.

Reference

1. Prescribing Information. Vyepti. Lundbeck Seattle BioPharmaceuticals, Inc; 2020.

ERAVACYCLINE

Antibacterial (Tetracycline Derivative)

PREGNANCY RECOMMENDATION: Contraindicated—Second and Third Trimesters

BREASTFEEDING RECOMMENDATION: Potential Toxicity

PREGNANCY SUMMARY

No reports describing the use of eravacycline in human pregnancy have been reported. The drug will probably cross the placenta, so some fetal exposure will likely occur. However, the absence of human pregnancy experience prevents a complete assessment of the embryofetal risk. Animal data did show embryofetal toxicity and demonstrated transplacental transfer. Numerous studies on tetracycline drugs have shown a risk for tooth discoloration, tooth enamel hypoplasia, and inhibition of bone growth when used in the second and third trimesters of pregnancy (see Tetracycline). Using this drug during pregnancy should be based on the pros and cons of the mother's clinical need for treatment versus any potential fetal risk that might occur from exposure.

BREASTFEEDING SUMMARY

It is not known if eravacycline is excreted into human breast milk. The drug will probably be found in breast milk, so some infant exposure will likely occur. Tooth discoloration, tooth enamel hypoplasia, and inhibition of bone growth are theoretically possible in an infant if the drug is used during breastfeeding, but the expected maternal treatment time should be short-term. The manufacturer recommends that mothers not breastfeed during treatment and for 4 days after the last dose. Nevertheless, breastfeeding while using this drug should be based on the mother's clinical need for treatment. If used, the infant should be monitored for the most common reported adult side effects of nausea (leading to irritability), vomiting, and diarrhea.

Reference

1. Prescribing Information. Xerava. Tetraphase Pharmaceuticals, Inc; 2018.

ERDAFITINIB

Antineoplastic (Kinase Inhibitor)

PREGNANCY RECOMMENDATION: No Human Data—Animal Data Suggest Potential Risk

BREASTFEEDING RECOMMENDATION: Potential Toxicity

PREGNANCY SUMMARY

No reports describing the use of erdafitinib in human pregnancy have been located. Based on likely placental transfer, some fetal exposure will probably occur. However, the absence of human pregnancy experience prevents a complete assessment of the embryofetal risk. Embryofetal toxicity was observed in one animal species at doses less than 10 times the MRHD. Based on animal

(*continued*)

studies and the drug's mechanism of action, the manufacturer recommends that women with reproductive potential use effective contraception during treatment and for 1 month after the last dose. They also recommend that males with female partners of reproductive potential use effective contraception during treatment and for 1 month after the last dose. Nevertheless, using this drug during pregnancy should be based on the pros and cons of the mother's clinical need for treatment versus any potential fetal risk that might occur from exposure. There is a registry for women who are pregnant and have cancer. For more information, women and health care providers are encouraged to contact the Cancer and Pregnancy Registry at 1-877-635-4499.

E

BREASTFEEDING SUMMARY

No reports describing the use of erdafitinib during human lactation have been located. The drug will likely be found in breast milk, so some infant exposure will likely occur. However, due to the concern for potential serious adverse effects that might be seen in a breastfed infant, the manufacturer recommends that women not breastfeed while being treated with erdafitinib and for at least one month after the last dose. Nevertheless, breastfeeding while using this drug should be based on the mother's clinical need for treatment. If used, the infant should be monitored for the most common reported adult side effects of nausea, abdominal pain, and musculoskeletal pain (all leading to irritability), diarrhea, lethargy, alopecia, vomiting, constipation, decreased appetite, and various laboratory abnormalities (see PI).

Reference

1. Prescribing Information. Balversa. Janssen Products; 2019.

ERENUMAB

Central Nervous System (Antimigraine—Monoclonal Antibody)

PREGNANCY RECOMMENDATION: Limited Human Data—Animal Data Suggest Low Risk

BREASTFEEDING RECOMMENDATION: Probably Compatible

PREGNANCY SUMMARY

Three case report studies describing five pregnancies regarding the use of erenumab in human pregnancy were located. Of these, four were on the drug at the time of conception and/or the first trimester. All were delivered at term with no reported adverse effects or fetal malformations. In the fifth case, erenumab was stopped a month prior to conception, but she reportedly had a spontaneous first-trimester loss. Data from the VigiBase safety reporting system (involving 82 pregnancies with some outcome information) did not show any increased signals for fetal or maternal toxicity. As an IgG antibody, it likely crosses the placenta, especially during the second half of gestation, so some fetal exposure will probably occur. Therefore, this limited human pregnancy experience prevents a complete assessment of the embryofetal risk. Animal data did not show any embryofetal toxicity in one animal species at doses greater than 10 times the RHD. Using this drug during pregnancy should be based on the pros and cons of the mother's clinical need for treatment versus any potential fetal risk that might occur from exposure. There is a pregnancy exposure registry that monitors pregnancy outcomes in women exposed to erenumab during pregnancy. Health care providers and patients are encouraged to call 1-833-244-4083.

BREASTFEEDING SUMMARY

Two case reports describing the use of erenumab during human lactation were located. In one case, the mother used erenumab during the pregnancy and partially breastfed her infant postdelivery. In the other case, the drug was started postdelivery. For both infants, no adverse effects were reported, and both were meeting normal expected milestones. It is known that IgG antibodies can be found in human breast milk, but are not found in the neonatal or infant circulation. Additionally, if any IgG antibodies were to be ingested through breastfeeding, they would probably be digested in the infant's GI tract and not be absorbed. Breastfeeding while using this drug should be based on the mother's clinical need for treatment. If used, the infant should be monitored for the most common reported adult side effect of constipation.

References

1. Prescribing Information. Aimovig. Amgen; 2023.
2. Fofi L, Egeo G, Aurilia C, Barbanti P. Erenumab during pregnancy: a case report in a patient with chronic migraine. *Neurol Sci*. 2021;42:2145-2146.
3. Vig SJ, Garza J, Tao Y. The use of erenumab for migraine prophylaxis during pregnancy: a case report and narrative review. *Headache*. 2022;62:1256-1263.
4. Bonifácio GV, de Carvalho SC, Oliveira R, Gil-Gouveia R. Gestational exposure to erenumab—the outcome of three pregnancies. *Headache*. 2022;62:1218-1221.
5. Noseda R, Bedussi F, Gobbi C, et al. Safety profile of erenumab, galcanezumab and fremanezumab in pregnancy and lactation: analysis of the WHO pharmacovigilance database. *Cephalalgia*. 2021;41:789-798.
6. Noseda R, Bedussi F, Gobbi C, et al. Safety profile of monoclonal antibodies targeting the calcitonin gene-related peptide system in pregnancy: updated analysis in VigiBase®. *Cephalalgia*. 2023;43:e1-e10.
7. Henze T. Erenumab during breastfeeding. *Breastfeed Med*. 2019;14:513-514.

ERGOCALCIFEROL (Vitamin D_2)

Vitamin

PREGNANCY RECOMMENDATION: Compatible

BREASTFEEDING RECOMMENDATION: Compatible

See Vitamin D.

E

ERGOTAMINE

Central Nervous System (Antimigraine)

PREGNANCY RECOMMENDATION: *Contraindicated

BREASTFEEDING RECOMMENDATION: Potential Toxicity

PREGNANCY SUMMARY

From the Collaborative Perinatal Project and the Michigan Medicaid data, a total of 84 first-trimester exposures to ergotamine were reported, with 11 (13.1%) major birth anomalies described. Despite the high percentage rate, no pattern to the anomalies was identified. Numerous other case reports have described birth anomalies with exposure to ergotamine, but several other drugs were also used, and again, no pattern has been noted. The drug has been shown to cross the placenta, so some fetal exposure will occur. Therefore, this limited human pregnancy experience prevents a complete assessment of the embryofetal risk. The drug was found to cause some embryofetal toxicity in three species at doses less than 10 times the RHD, but maternal toxicity also occurred in some evaluations. Ergotamine carries a boxed warning regarding serious and/or life-threatening ischemia when administered with potent CYP3A4 inhibitors like protease inhibitors and macrolide antibiotics. It is felt that the use of ergotamine in small amounts does not appear to cause fetotoxicity. *Nevertheless, ergotamine has been shown to strongly stimulate uterine contractions and therefore should be avoided in pregnancy, if at all possible.

BREASTFEEDING SUMMARY

One report describing the use of ergotamine in 30 women during human lactation has been located. No effect on weight gain in the breastfed infants was noted. The drug will probably be found in breast milk, so some infant exposure will likely occur. Due to the concern for potential serious adverse effects that might be seen in a breastfed infant, the manufacturer recommends that a decision be made whether to discontinue nursing or to discontinue the drug, considering the importance of the drug to the mother. If the clinical decision is to use this drug while breastfeeding, the infant should be monitored for the most common reported adult side effects of dizziness, arm or leg pain, and pruritus (all leading to irritability), vomiting, decreased heart rate, and unstable blood pressure.

References

1. Gill RC, Farrar JM. Experiences with di-hydro-ergotamine in the treatment of primary uterine inertia. *J Obstet Gynaecol Br Emp*. 1951;58:79-91.
2. Altman SG, Waltman R, Lubin S, et al. Oxytocic and toxic actions of dihydroergotamine-45. *Am J Obstet Gynecol*. 1952;64:101-109.
3. Grauwiler J, Schon H. Teratological experiments with ergotamine in mice, rats, and rabbits. *Teratology*. 1973;7:227-236.
4. Schon H, Leist KH, Grauwiler J. Single-day treatment of pregnant rats with ergotamine (abstract). *Teratology*. 1975;11:32A.
5. Greatorex JC, Mantle PG. Effect of rye ergot on the pregnant sheep. *J Reprod Fertil*. 1974;37:33-41.
6. Griffith RW, Grauwiler J, Holdel CH, et al. Toxicologic considerations. In Berde B, Schild HO, eds. *Ergot Alkaloids and Related Compounds. Handbook of Experimental Pharmacology*. Vol. 49. Springer Verlag; 1979:805-851.
7. Foster JB. Migraine-traditional uses of ergot compounds. *Postgrad Med J*. 1976;52(suppl 1):12-14.
8. Massey EW. Migraine during pregnancy. *Obstet Gynecol Surv*. 1977;32: 693-696.
9. Lance JW. The pharmacotherapy of migraine. *Med J Aust*. 1986;144:85-88.
10. Reik L Jr. Headaches in pregnancy. *Semin Neurol*. 1988;8:187-192.
11. Heinonen OP, Sloan D, Shapiro S. *Birth Defects and Drugs in Pregnancy*. Publishing Sciences Group; 1977:358-360.
12. Wainscott G, Sullivan FM, Volans GN, et al. The outcome of pregnancy in women suffering from migraine. *Postgrad Med J*. 1978;54:98-102.
13. Peeden JN Jr, Wilroy RS Jr, Soper RG. Prune perineum. *Teratology*. 1979;20: 233-236.
14. Spranger JW, Schinzel A, Myers T, et al. Cerebroarthrodigital syndrome: a newly recognized formal genesis syndrome in three patients with apparent arthromyodysplasia and sacral agenesis, brain malformation and digital hypoplasia. *Am J Med Genet* 1980;5:13-24.
15. Graham JM Jr, Marin-Padilla M, Hoefnagel D. Jejunal atresia associated with Cafergot ingestion during pregnancy. *Clin Pediatr*. 1983;22:226-228.
16. Au KL, Woo JSK, Wong VCW. Intrauterine death from ergotamine overdosage. *Eur J Obstet Gynecol Reprod Biol*. 1985;19:313-315.
17. Hughes HE, Goldstein DA. Birth defects following maternal exposure to ergotamine, beta blockers, and caffeine. *J Med Genet*. 1988;25:396-399.
18. Verloes A, Emonts P, Dubois M, et al. Paraplegia and arthrogryposis multiplex of the lower extremities after intrauterine exposure to ergotamine. *J Med Genet*. 1990;27:213-214.
19. Czeizel A. Teratogenicity of ergotamine. *J Med Genet*. 1989;26:69-70.
20. de Groot ANJA, van Dongen PWJ, van Roosmalen J, et al. Ergotamine-induced fetal stress: review of side effects of ergot alkaloids during pregnancy. *Eur J Obstet Gynecol Reprod Biol*. 1993;51:73-77.
21. Raymond GV. Teratogen update: ergot and ergotamine. *Teratology*. 1995;51: 344-347.
22. Prescribing Information. Ergomar. TerSera Therapeutics; 2024.
23. Jolivet A, Robyn C, Huraux-Rendu C, et al. Effet de dérivés des alcaloïdes de l'ergot de seigle sur la sécrétion lactée dans le post-partum immédiat [Effect of ergot alkaloid derivatives on milk secretion in the immediate postpartum period]. *J Gynecol Obstet Biol Reprod (Paris)*. 1978;7:129-134.

ERIBULIN

Antineoplastic (Antimicrotubular)

PREGNANCY RECOMMENDATION: No Human Data—Animal Data Suggest Potential Risk

BREASTFEEDING RECOMMENDATION: Potential Toxicity

E

PREGNANCY SUMMARY

No reports describing the use of eribulin in human pregnancy have been located. Some amount of the drug will probably cross the placenta, so fetal exposure will likely occur. Therefore, the absence of human pregnancy experience prevents a complete assessment of the embryofetal risk. Embryofetal and maternal toxicity with malformations were observed in one animal species at doses less than the RHD. Based on animal studies and the drug's mechanism of action, the manufacturer recommends that women with reproductive potential use effective contraception during treatment and for 2 weeks after the last dose. They also recommend that males with female partners of reproductive potential use effective contraception during treatment and for 3.5 months after the last dose. Nevertheless, using this drug during pregnancy should be based on the pros and cons of the mother's clinical need for treatment versus any potential fetal risk that might occur from exposure. There is a registry for women who are pregnant and have cancer. For more information, women and health care providers are encouraged to contact the Cancer and Pregnancy Registry at 1-877-635-4499.

BREASTFEEDING SUMMARY

No reports describing the use of eribulin during human lactation have been located. Some amount of the drug will probably be found in breast milk, so infant exposure will likely occur. The effect of this exposure on a nursing infant is unknown. Due to the concern for potential serious adverse effects that might occur in a breastfed infant, the manufacturer recommends that women not breastfeed while being treated with eribulin and for at least 2 weeks after the last dose. Nevertheless, breastfeeding while using this drug should be based on the mother's clinical need for treatment. If used, the infant should be monitored for the most common reported adult side effects of nausea, abdominal pain, and neuropathy (all leading to irritability), diarrhea, alopecia, vomiting, and various laboratory abnormalities (see PI).

Reference

1. Prescribing Information. Halaven. Eisai; 2022.

ERLOTINIB

Antineoplastic (Tyrosine Kinase Inhibitor)

PREGNANCY RECOMMENDATION: Limited Human Data—Animal Data Suggest Potential Risk

BREASTFEEDING RECOMMENDATION: Potential Toxicity

PREGNANCY SUMMARY

A total of four pregnancies describing the use of erlotinib in the first trimester of human pregnancy were located. All four delivered healthy newborns with no anomalies identified. Four other pregnancies, involving five newborns (one set of twins), were exposed to erlotinib in the early second and early third trimesters. All five neonates did well with no reported complications or anomalies. The drug crosses the placenta, so fetal exposure will occur. However, this limited human pregnancy experience prevents a complete assessment of the embryofetal risk. Embryofetal toxicity was observed in one animal species at doses less than 10 times the RHD, but this dose also caused maternal toxicity. Based on animal studies and the drug's mechanism of action, the manufacturer recommends that women with reproductive potential use effective contraception during treatment and for 2 weeks after the last dose. Nevertheless, using this drug during pregnancy should be based on the pros and cons of the mother's clinical need for treatment versus any potential fetal risk that might occur from exposure. There is a registry for women who are pregnant and have cancer. For more information, women and health care providers are encouraged to contact the Cancer and Pregnancy Registry at 1-877-635-4499.

BREASTFEEDING SUMMARY

No reports describing the use of erlotinib during human lactation have been located. The drug will probably be found in breast milk, so some infant exposure will likely occur. Due to the concern for potential serious adverse effects that may be seen in a breastfed infant, the manufacturer recommends that women not breastfeed while being treated with erlotinib and for at least 2 weeks after the last dose. Nevertheless, breastfeeding while using this drug should be based on the mother's clinical need for treatment. If used, the infant should be monitored for the most common reported adult side effects of nausea, myalgia, and abdominal pain (all leading to irritability), diarrhea, lethargy, alopecia, vomiting, decreased appetite, rash, cough, and various laboratory abnormalities (see PI).

References

1. Prescribing Information. Tarceva. Genentech; 2018.
2. Jovelet C, Seck A, Mir O, et al. Variation in transplacental transfer of tyrosine kinase inhibitors in the human perfused cotyledon model. *Ann Oncol*. 2015;26:1500-1504.
3. Ji Y, Schwartz J, Hartford A, et al. Successful treatment of non-small cell lung cancer with erlotinib throughout pregnancy. *JAMA Oncol*. 2015;1:838-840.
4. Rivas G, Llinas N, Bonilla C, et al. Use of erlotinib throughout pregnancy: a case-report of a patient with metastatic lung adenocarcinoma. *Lung Cancer*. 2012;77:469-472.
5. Zambelli A, Antonio Da Prada G, Fregoni V, et al. Erlotinib administration for advanced non-small cell lung cancer during the first 2 months of unrecognized pregnancy. *Lung Cancer*. 2008;60:455-457.
6. Lee CH, Liam CK, Pang YK, et al. Successful pregnancy with epidermal growth factor receptor tyrosine kinase inhibitor treatment of metastatic lung adenocarcinoma presenting with respiratory failure. *Lung Cancer*. 2011;74:349-351.

ERTAPENEM

Antibacterial (Penem)

PREGNANCY RECOMMENDATION: Limited Human Data—Animal Data Suggest Potential Risk

BREASTFEEDING RECOMMENDATION: Probably Compatible

PREGNANCY SUMMARY

One case report was located that described the use of ertapenem during human pregnancy. The drug was used at about 28 weeks' gestation, was well tolerated, and no adverse effects or anomalies were reported in the newborn. Based on likely placental transfer, some fetal exposure will probably occur. Therefore, this limited human pregnancy experience prevents a complete assessment of the embryofetal risk. Embryofetal toxicity was observed in one animal species at doses less than 10 times the RHD. Using this drug during pregnancy should be based on the pros and cons of the mother's clinical need for treatment versus any potential fetal risk that might occur from exposure.

BREASTFEEDING SUMMARY

According to the manufacturer, ertapenem is excreted into breast milk in low levels. Breast milk levels were tested in five lactating women. The breast milk concentrations for ertapenem ranged from undetectable to 380 pg/mL. Breastfeeding while using this drug should be based on the mother's clinical need for treatment. If used, the infant should be monitored for the most common reported adult side effects of nausea and headache (both leading to irritability), diarrhea, and vomiting.

References

1. Prescribing Information. Invanz. Merck Sharp & Dohme; 2022.
2. Erbin A, Gozdas HT, Guler Y, Canat HL. Urosepsis caused by Kluyvera Ascorbata in a pregnant woman. *J Coll Physicians Surg Pak*. 2020;30:324-326.

ERTUGLIFLOZIN

Antidiabetic (SGLT-2 inhibitor)

PREGNANCY RECOMMENDATION: No Human Data—Animal Data Suggest Potential Risk

BREASTFEEDING RECOMMENDATION: Potential Toxicity

PREGNANCY SUMMARY

No reports describing the use of ertugliflozin in human pregnancy have been located. A limited amount of the drug probably crosses the placenta, so some fetal exposure will likely occur. However, the absence of human pregnancy experience prevents a complete assessment of the embryofetal risk. Animal studies did not demonstrate any embryofetal toxicity. However, because of the findings in rats administered the drug postnatally (regarding possible kidney injury), the manufacturer recommends that the drug not be used in the second and third trimesters of pregnancy. Nevertheless, using this drug during pregnancy should be based on the pros and cons of the mother's clinical need for treatment versus any potential fetal risk that might occur from exposure. In addition, fetal renal status can be monitored by perinatal ultrasound.

BREASTFEEDING SUMMARY

No reports describing the use of ertugliflozin in human lactation have been located. A limited amount of the drug is probably found in breast milk. Because of the findings in rats administered the drug postnatally (regarding possible kidney injury), the manufacturer recommends that women not breastfeed while using this drug. However, breastfeeding should be based on the mother's clinical need for treatment. If the drug is used, the infant should be monitored for the most common reported adult side effects of headache (leading to irritability) and mycotic infections.

Reference

1. Prescribing Information. Steglatro. Merck Sharp & Dohme, LLC; 2022.

E

ERYTHROMYCIN

Antibacterial (Macrolide)

PREGNANCY RECOMMENDATION: Limited Human Data (First Trimester) / Human Data Suggest Low risk (Second and third Trimesters)

BREASTFEEDING RECOMMENDATION: Compatible

PREGNANCY SUMMARY

The use of erythromycin during pregnancy in the second and third trimesters is well reported throughout the literature, and no adverse effects related to the drug have been identified. Data on first-trimester use is more limited. The Collaborative Perinatal Project reported 79 pregnancies with first-trimester exposure to erythromycin, and 5 (6.3%) major anomalies were identified. For anytime use during pregnancy, 230 exposures were recorded with 6 (2.6%) anomalies described. No pattern to the anomalies was found, and no evidence to suggest a relationship to specific categories of major or minor malformations or to individual defects was identified. The Hungarian Case-Control Surveillance of Congenital Abnormalities analysis found 113 (0.5%) cases of first-trimester use of erythromycin in 22,865 newborns delivered with congenital anomalies. This was no different than the 175 (0.5%) first-trimester uses of erythromycin in the 38,151 newborns delivered without any birth defects. Early reports suggested a possible association with erythromycin use during pregnancy and infantile hypertrophic pyloric stenosis. However, later reports did not confirm this association. The drug crosses the placenta at low concentrations, but some fetal exposure will likely occur. Animal studies did not show any embryofetal toxicity in one species at doses less than 10 times the RHD. ACOG recommends erythromycin for preterm premature rupture of the membranes.

BREASTFEEDING SUMMARY

Erythromycin has been found in human breast milk in small amounts, so infant exposures occur. Oral doses of 1,200 mg/d produced peak breast milk levels of about 1.6 mcg/mL, and maternal doses of about 2,000 mg/d produced peak levels of about 3.2 mcg/mL. Calculated RIDs are less than 2.5%. Such small amounts are unlikely to cause any adverse infant effects. Breastfeeding while using this drug should be based on the mother's clinical need for treatment versus any potential infant risks that might occur. If used, the infant should be monitored for the most common reported adult side effects of nausea and abdominal cramps (both leading to irritability), diarrhea, vomiting, and decreased appetite (monitor growth).

References

1. Prescribing Information. Ery-tab. Arbor Pharmaceuticals; 2019.
2. Heilman FR, Herrell WE, Wellman WE, et al. Some laboratory and clinical observations on a new antibiotic, erythromycin (Ilotycin). *Proc Staff Meet Mayo Clin*. 1952;27:285-304.
3. Kiefer L, Rubin A, McCoy JB, et al. The placental transfer of erythromycin. *Am J Obstet Gynecol*. 1955;69:174-177.
4. Philipson A, Sabath LD, Charles D. Transplacental passage of erythromycin and clindamycin. *N Engl J Med*. 1973;288:1219-1220.
5. Fenton LJ, Light IJ. Congenital syphilis after maternal treatment with erythromycin. *Obstet Gynecol*. 1976;47:492-494.
6. Philipson A, Sabath LD, Charles D. Erythromycin and clindamycin absorption and elimination in pregnant women. *Clin Pharmacoal Ther*. 1976;19:68-77.
7. McCormack WM, George H, Donner A, et al. Hepatotoxicity of erythromycin estolate during pregnancy. *Antimicrob Agents Chemother*. 1977;12: 630-635.
8. Jaffe P, Liberman MM, McFadyen I, et al. Incidence of congenital limb-reduction deformities. *Lancet*. 1975;1:526-527.
9. Heinonen OP, Slone D, Shapiro S. *Birth Defects and Drugs in Pregnancy*. Publishing Sciences Group; 1977.
10. Gallagher JC, Ismail MA, Aladjem S. Reduced urinary estriol levels with erythromycin therapy. *Obstet Gynecol*. 1980;56:381-382.
11. Merenstein GB, Todd WA, Brown G, et al. Group B beta-hemolytic streptococcus: randomized controlled treatment study at term. *Obstet Gynecol*. 1980;55:315-318.
12. Easmon CSF, Hastings MJG, Deeley J, et al. The effect of intrapartum chemoprophylaxis on the vertical transmission of group B streptococci. *Br J Obstet Gynaecol*. 1983;90:633-635.
13. Quinn PA, Shewchuk AB, Shuber J, et al. Efficacy of antibiotic therapy in preventing spontaneous pregnancy loss among couples colonized with genital mycoplasmas. *Am J Obstet Gynecol*. 1983;145:239-244.
14. Kass EH, McCormack WM. Genital mycoplasma infection and perinatal morbidity. *N Engl J Med*. 1984;311:258.
15. Czeizel AE, Rockenbauer M, Sørensen HT, et al. A population-based case-control teratologic study of oral erythromycin treatment during pregnancy. *Repro Toxicol*. 1999;13:531-536.
16. Kenyon SL, Taylor DJ, Tarnow-Mordi W; for the ORACLE Collaborative Group. Broad-spectrum antibiotics for preterm, prelabour rupture of fetal membranes: the ORACLE I randomised trial. *Lancet*. 2001;357:979-988.
17. Kallen BAJ, Olausson PO. Maternal drug use in early pregnancy and infant cardiovascular defect. *Reprod Toxicol*. 2003;17:255-261.
18. Mahon BE, Rosenman MB, Kleiman MB. Maternal and infant use of erythromycin and other macrolide antibiotics as risk factors for infantile hypertrophic pyloric stenosis. *J Pediatr*. 2001;139;380-384.

19. Louik C, Werler MM, Mitchell AA. Erythromycin use during pregnancy in relation to pyloric stenosis. *Am J Obstet Gynecol.* 2002;186:288-290.
20. Cooper WO, Ray WA, Griffin MR. Prenatal prescription of macrolide antibiotics and infantile hypertrophic pyloric stenosis. *Obstet Gynecol.* 2002;100:101-106.
21. Sorensen HT, Skriver MV, Pedersen L, et al. Risk of infantile hypertrophic pyloric stenosis after maternal postnatal use of macrolides. *Scand J Infect Dis.* 2003;35:104-106.
22. FitzSimmons J, Callahan C, Shanahan B, et al. Chlamydial infections in pregnancy. *J Reprod Med.* 1986;31:19-22.
23. Black-Payne C, Ahrabi MM, Bocchini JA Jr, et al. Treatment of Chlamydia trachomatis identified with chlamydiazyme during pregnancy: impact on perinatal complications and infants. *J Reprod Med.* 1990;35:362-367.
24. Cohen I, Veille JC, Calkins BM. Improved pregnancy outcome following successful treatment of chlamydial infection. *JAMA.* 1990;263:3160-3163.
25. Magat AH, Alger LS, Nagey DA, et al. Double-blind randomized study comparing amoxicillin and erythromycin for the treatment of Chlamydia trachomatis in pregnancy. *Obstet Gynecol.* 1993:81:745-749.
26. Alary M, Joly J-M, Mondor M, et al. Randomised comparison of amoxicillin and erythromycin in treatment of genital chlamydia infection in pregnancy. *Lancet.* 1994;344:1461-1465.
27. Turrentin MA, Newton ER. Amoxicillin or erythromycin for the treatment of antenatal chlamydial infection: a meta-analysis. *Obstet Gynecol.* 1995;86:1021-1025.
28. Knowles JA. Drugs in milk. *Pediatr Curr.* 1972;21:28-32.
29. Ito S, Blajchman A, Stephenson M, et al. Prospective follow-up of adverse reactions in breast-fed infants exposed to maternal medication. *Am J Obstet Gynecol.* 1993;168:1393-1399.
30. Goldstein LH, Berlin M, Tsur L, et al. The safety of macrolides during lactation. *Breastfeed Med.* 2009;4:157-200.
31. Prelabor rupture of membranes: ACOG practice bulletin, number 217. *Obstet Gynecol.* 2020;135(3):e80-e97.
32. Abdellatif M, Ghozy S, Kamel MG, et al. Association between exposure to macrolides and the development of infantile hypertrophic pyloric stenosis: a systematic review and meta-analysis. *Eur J Pediatr.* 2019;178:301-314.
33. Almaramhy HH, Al-Zalabani AH. The association of prenatal and postnatal macrolide exposure with subsequent development of infantile hypertrophic pyloric stenosis: a systematic review and meta-analysis. *Ital J Pediatr.* 2019;45:20.

E

ESCITALOPRAM

Mental Health (Antidepressant—Selective Serotonin Reuptake Inhibitor)

PREGNANCY RECOMMENDATION: Limited Human Data—Animal Data Suggest Low Risk

BREASTFEEDING RECOMMENDATION: Probably Compatible

PREGNANCY SUMMARY

Limited reports describing the use of escitalopram in human pregnancy have been located. Numerous studies on the use of selective serotonin reuptake inhibitor (SSRI) drugs as a group have been performed that have analyzed for birth anomalies, cardiac anomalies, and other complicated pregnancy outcome issues, and overall, no distinct abnormalities or pregnancy complications have been consistently identified. However, the number of patients in these studies using escitalopram is small. The drug does appear to cross the placenta, so some fetal exposure will occur. However, this limited human pregnancy experience prevents a complete assessment of the embryofetal risk. Animal studies did not show any embryofetal toxicity or malformations in one species at doses less than 10 times the RHD. ACOG recommends the use of SSRIs as first-line treatment of depression and anxiety in women without previous use of an effective medication. SSRIs (as a group) are well studied in pregnancy and are considered to be low risk. Neonatal adaptation syndrome is a group of self-limiting symptoms that have been associated with SSRI exposure near delivery. It is estimated to occur in 10% to 30% of exposed infants. Symptoms include irritability, restlessness, tremors, hyperreflexia, poor sleep, poor feeding, and rarely, seizures. If escitalopram is used during pregnancy, newborns should be monitored for these symptoms. There is a pregnancy exposure registry that monitors pregnancy outcomes in women exposed to antidepressants during pregnancy. For more information, health care providers or patients are encouraged to contact the National Pregnancy Registry for Antidepressants at 1-866-961-2388.

BREASTFEEDING SUMMARY

Several studies have analyzed human breast milk for the presence of escitalopram, and the drug has been detected. Peak levels range from about 20 to 200 ng/mL. All of the calculated RIDs have been less than 10%. In addition, no adverse infant effects have been noted. In one study, infant serum levels were analyzed in eight mother-child pairs. The average maternal serum level was about 24 ng/mL, whereas the infant levels were all less than 5 ng/mL. In three infants, escitalopram was not detected (lower limit of quantification at 1 ng/mL). ACOG recommends that if a mother is stable on a particular medication, such as an SSRI, therapy should not be changed postpartum, as exposure is less from breastfeeding than it was during pregnancy. If the clinical decision is to use this drug while breastfeeding, the infant should be monitored for the most common reported adult side effects of drowsiness, restlessness, irritability, poor feeding, and poor weight gain.

References

1. Prescribing Information. Lexapro. Allergan; 2019.
2. Shuey DL, Sadler TW, Lauder JM. Serotonin as a regulator of craniofacial morphogenesis: site specific malformations following exposure to serotonin uptake inhibitors. *Teratology.* 1992;46:367-378.
3. Oberlander TF, Warburton W, Misri S, et al. Neonatal outcomes after prenatal exposure to selective serotonin reuptake inhibitor antidepressants and maternal depression using population-based linked health data. *Arch Gen Psychiatry.* 2006;63:898-906.
4. Alwan S, Reefhuis J, Rasmussen S, et al. Maternal use of selective serotonin reuptake inhibitors and risk for birth defects (abstract). *Birth Defects Res (Part A).* 2005;73:291.
5. Kallen B, Olausson PO. Antidepressant drugs during pregnancy and infant congenital heart defect. *Reprod Toxicol.* 2006;21:221-222.

6. Kallen BAJ, Olausson PO. Maternal use of selective serotonin re-uptake inhibitors in early pregnancy and infant congenital malformations. *Birth Defects Res (Part A)*. 2007;79:301-308.
7. Gentile S. Escitalopram late in pregnancy and while breast-feeding. *Ann Pharmacother*. 2006;40:1696-1697.
8. Berard A, Ramos E, Rey E, et al. First trimester exposure to paroxetine and risk of cardiac malformations in infants: the importance of dosage. *Birth Defects Res (Part B)*. 2007;80:18-27.
9. Bellantuono C, Migliarese G, Gentile S. Serotonin reuptake inhibitors in pregnancy and the risk of major malformations: a systematic review. *Hum Psychopharmacol Clin Exp*. 2007;22:121-128.
10. Chambers CD, Hernandez-Diaz S, Van Marter LJ, et al. Selective serotonin-reuptake inhibitors and risk of persistent pulmonary hypertension of the newborn. *N Engl J Med*. 2006;354:579-587.
11. Alwan S, Reefhuis J, Rasmussen SA, et al; for the National Birth Defects Prevention Study. Use of selective serotonin-reuptake inhibitors in pregnancy and the risk of birth defects. *N Engl J Med*. 2007;356:2684-2692.
12. Louik C, Lin AE, Werler MM, et al. First-trimester use of selective serotonin-reuptake inhibitors and the risk of birth defects. *N Engl J Med*. 2007;356:2675-2683.
13. Greene MF. Teratogenicity of SSRIs—serious concern or much ado about little? *N Engl J Med*. 2007;356:2732-2733.
14. Einarson A, Choi J, Einarson TR, et al. Incidence of major malformations in infants following antidepressant exposure in pregnancy: results of a large prospective cohort study. *Can J Psychiatry*. 2009;54:242-246.
15. Potts AL, Young KL, Carter BS, et al. Necrotizing enterocolitis associated with in utero and breast milk exposure to the selective serotonin reuptake inhibitor, escitalopram. *J Perinatol*. 2007;27:120-122.
16. Nordeng H, van Gelder HJ, Spigset O, et al. Pregnancy outcome after exposure to antidepressants and the role of maternal depression. *J Clin Psychopharmacol*. 2012;32:186-194.
17. Vitale SG, Lagana AS, Muscatello MR, et al. Psychopharmacotherapy in pregnancy and breastfeeding. *Obstet Gynecol Surv*. 2016;71:721-733.
18. Rampono J, Hackett LP, Kristensen JH, et al. Transfer of escitalopram and its metabolite demethylescitalopram into breast milk. *Br J Clin Pharmacol*. 2006;62:316-322.
19. Castberg I, Spigset O. Excretion of escitalopram in breast milk. *J Clin Psychopharmacol*. 2006;26:536-538.
20. Marshall AM, Nommsen-Rivers LA, Hernandez LI, et al. Serotonin transport and metabolism in the mammary gland modulates secretory activation and involution. *J Clin Endocrin Metab*. 2010;95:837-846.
21. Gorman JR, Kao K, Chambers CD. Breastfeeding among women exposed to antidepressants during pregnancy. *J Hum Lact*. 2012;28:181-188.
22. American College of Obstetricians and Gynecologists. Treatment and management of mental health conditions during pregnancy and postpartum: ACOG Clinical Practice Guideline No. 5. *Obstet Gynecol*. 2023; 141: 1262-1288.
23. Cipriani A, Furukawa TA, Salanti G, et al. Comparative efficacy and acceptability of 21 antidepressant drugs for the acute treatment of adults with major depressive disorder: a systematic review and network meta-analysis. *Lancet*. 2018;39:1357-1366.
24. U.S. Food and Drug Administration. Selective serotonin reuptake inhibitor (SSRI) antidepressant use during pregnancy and reports of a rare heart and lung condition in newborn babies. FDA drug safety communication. Accessed September 27, 2023. https://www.fda.gov/drugs/drug-safety-and-availability/fda-drug-safety-communication-selective-serotonin-reuptake-inhibitor-ssri-antidepressant-use-during
25. Moses-Kolko EL, Bogen D, Perel J, et al. Neonatal signs after late in utero exposure to serotonin reuptake inhibitors: literature review and implications for clinical applications. *JAMA*. 2005;293(19):2372-2383.
26. Sit D, Perel JM, Wisniewski SR, et al. Mother-infant antidepressant levels, maternal depression and perinatal events. *J Clin Psychiatry*. 2011;72:994-1001.

ESLICARBAZEPINE

Central Nervous System (Antiseizure)

PREGNANCY RECOMMENDATION: Limited Human Data—Animal Data Suggest Risk

BREASTFEEDING RECOMMENDATION: Potential Toxicity

PREGNANCY SUMMARY

One report describing the use of eslicarbazepine in human pregnancy has been located. The data come from clinical trials and postmarketing surveys, which totaled 76 pregnancies with some clinical outcome data. Excluding ongoing pregnancies, spontaneous abortions, and therapeutic abortions, from 33 deliveries, 30 resulted in live births without congenital defects, and 3 delivered with anomalies (one with a chromosome 18 abnormality, one with talipes, and one with a congenital knee dislocation thought to be mechanical). The final analysis did not show any increased signals of fetal or maternal toxicity. The drug will probably cross the placenta, so some fetal exposure will likely occur. Therefore, this limited human pregnancy experience prevents a complete assessment of the embryofetal risk. Embryofetal toxicity was observed in three animal species at doses less than the MRHD. Using this drug during pregnancy should be based on the pros and cons of the mother's clinical need for treatment versus any potential fetal risk that might occur from exposure. There is a pregnancy exposure registry that monitors pregnancy outcomes in women exposed to antiepileptic drugs during pregnancy. Women who are taking eslicarbazepine and healthcare providers are encouraged to enroll in the North American Antiepileptic Drug (NAAED) Pregnancy Registry by calling 1-888-233-2334.

BREASTFEEDING SUMMARY

No reports describing the use of eslicarbazepine during human lactation have been located. The manufacturer states that the drug is excreted into human breast milk. Eslicarbazepine is the active metabolite of oxcarbazepine. A few studies have evaluated eslicarbazepine levels in mothers using oxcarbazepine during lactation. Overall, the breast milk concentration of eslicarbazepine is about 50% of the maternal plasma level. The infant levels are about 14% or less of the maternal plasma level. Breastfeeding while using this drug should be based on the mother's clinical need for treatment. If used, the infant should be monitored for the most common reported adult side effects of nausea, dizziness, headache, and blurred vision (all leading to irritability), vomiting, somnolence, and fatigue (lethargy).

References

1. Prescribing Information. Aptiom. Sunovion Pharmaceuticals; 2019.
2. Costa R, Magalhaes LM, Graca J, et al. Eslicarbazepine acetate exposure in pregnant women with epilepsy. *Euro J Epilepsy*. 2018;58:72-74.

3. Bulau P, Paar WD, von Unruh GE. Pharmacokinetics of oxcarbazepine and 10-hydroxy-carbazepine in the newborn child of an oxcarbazepine-treated mother. *Eur J Clin Pharmacol*. 1988;34:311-313.
4. Lutz UC, Wiatr G, Gaertner HJ, Bartels M. Oxcarbazepine treatment during breast-feeding: a case report. *J Clin Psychopharmacol*. 2007;27:730-732.
5. Chen CY, Li X, Ma Ly, et al. In utero oxcarbazepine exposure and neonatal abstinence syndrome: case report and brief review of the literature. *Pharmacotherapy*. 2017;37:e71-e75.

ESMOLOL

Cardiovascular (β-Blocker, Antihypertensive, Antiarrhythmic)

PREGNANCY RECOMMENDATION: Limited Human Data—Animal Data Suggest Low Risk

BREASTFEEDING RECOMMENDATION: Probably Compatible

PREGNANCY SUMMARY

Five case reports describing the use of the drug during human pregnancy have been located. Though no fetal anomalies were identified, use was in the second and third trimesters. Decreased fetal heart rate (FHR) was noted in two pregnancies, one of which required an emergency cesarean section. The drug will probably cross the placenta, so fetal exposure will likely occur. Therefore, the limited human pregnancy experience prevents a complete assessment of the embryofetal risk. Animal studies did not show any embryofetal toxicity in two species at doses of less than 10 times the RHD. Maternal hypotension may occur with esmolol use; therefore, the potential for decreased uterine blood flow and resulting fetal compromise should be considered. In emergencies, where first-line agents fail to treat severe hypertension, ACOG considers esmolol a second-line agent. Using this drug during pregnancy should be based on the pros and cons of the mother's clinical need for treatment versus any potential fetal risk that might occur from exposure.

BREASTFEEDING SUMMARY

No reports describing the use of esmolol during human lactation have been located. The drug will probably be found in breast milk, so some infant exposure will likely occur. Because of the short-term indications for this drug and the fact that it must be given by continuous infusion, the opportunities for use of esmolol while nursing are limited. If the clinical decision is to use this drug while breastfeeding, the infant should be monitored for the most common reported adult side effect of hypotension.

References

1. Prescribing Information. Brevibloc. Baxter Healthcare; 2023.
2. Ostman PL, Chestnut DH, Robillard JE, et al. Transplacental passage and hemodynamic effects of esmolol in the gravid ewe. *Anesthesiology*. 1988;69:738-741.
3. Losasso TJ, Muzzi DA, Cucchiara RF. Response of fetal heart rate to maternal administration of esmolol. *Anesthesiology*. 1991;74:782-784.
4. Ducey JP, Knape KG. Maternal esmolol administration resulting in fetal distress and cesarean section in a term pregnancy. *Anesthesiology*. 1992;77:829-832.
5. Gilson GJ, Knieriem KJ, Smith JF, et al. Short-acting beta-adrenergic blockade and the fetus. A case report. *J Reprod Med*. 1992;37:277-279.
6. Fairley CJ, Clarke JT. Use of esmolol in a parturient with hypertrophic obstructive cardiomyopathy. *Br J Anaesthesia*. 1995;75:801-804.
7. Sanchez-Ramos L, Chami YG, Bass TA, et al. Myocardial infarction during pregnancy: management with transluminal coronary angioplasty and metallic intracoronary stents. *Am J Obstet Gynecol*. 1994;171:1392-1393.
8. American College of Obstetricians and Gynecologists. ACOG Practice Bulletin No. 203: chronic hypertension in pregnancy. *Obstet Gynecol*. 2019;133:e26-e50.

ESOMEPRAZOLE

Gastrointestinal (Proton Pump Inhibitor)

PREGNANCY RECOMMENDATION: Human Data Suggest Low Risk

BREASTFEEDING RECOMMENDATION: Probably Compatible

PREGNANCY SUMMARY

In a study of pregnancy data from Denmark involving 840,968 births, 5,082 were exposed to proton pump inhibitors (PPIs). There were 118 (3.2%) congenital anomalies found in 3,651 delivered newborns with first-trimester exposure. Of this, there were 23 (3.4%) birth defects reported in 668 cases with esomeprazole. No specific pattern to the anomalies was noted. In a 2009 meta-analysis of seven studies, the rate of birth anomalies, spontaneous abortion, and preterm birth was no different in 1,530 pregnancies exposed to PPIs compared with 133,410 births without PPI exposure. Lastly, a 2023 meta-analysis of

(continued)

11 studies again did not find an increased risk for congenital anomalies in 5,619 first-trimester exposures to PPIs. However, specific data for the use of esomeprazole were not provided. The drug appears to cross the placenta, so some fetal exposure will occur. However, this limited human pregnancy experience with esomeprazole prevents a complete assessment of the embryofetal risk. Animal data did not show embryofetal toxicity in two species at doses of more than 10 times the RHD. PPIs are generally considered low risk for use in pregnancy, though some of the data is inconsistent. Using this drug during pregnancy should be based on the pros and cons of the mother's clinical need for treatment versus any potential fetal risk that might occur from exposure.

E

BREASTFEEDING SUMMARY

One case report was located that described the use of esomeprazole during human lactation. The peak breast milk level identified was 19.6 ng/mL. The calculated RID was 1.8%. Breastfeeding while using this drug should be based on the mother's clinical need for treatment versus any potential infant risks that might occur. If used, the infant should be monitored for the most common reported adult side effects of headache and abdominal pain (both leading to irritability) and diarrhea. PPIs have been reported to cause elevated prolactin levels in some patients, leading to gynecomastia, but elevated prolactin levels should not adversely affect breastfeeding.

References

1. Prescribing Information. Nexium. AstraZeneca Pharmaceuticals; 2023.
2. Gill SK, O'Brien L, Einarson TR, et al. The safety of proton pump inhibitors (PPIs) in pregnancy: a meta-analysis. *Am J Gastroenterol*. 2009;104: 1541-1545.
3. Dehlink E, Yen E, Leichtner AM, et al. First evidence of a possible association between gastric acid suppression during pregnancy and childhood asthma: a population-based register study. *Clin Exp Allergy*. 2009;39:246-253.
4. Pasternak B, Hviid A. Use of proton-pump inhibitors in early pregnancy and the risk of birth defects. *N Engl J Med*. 2010;363:2114-2123.
5. Mitchell AA. Proton-pump inhibitors and birth defects—some reassurance, but more needed. *N Engl J Med*. 2010;363:2161-2163.
6. Gomez-Lobo V, Landy HJ, Matsumoto C, et al. Pregnancy in an intestinal transplant recipient. *Obstet Gynecol*. 2012;120:497-500.
7. Anderka M, Mitchell AA, Louik C, et al; the National Birth Defects Prevention Study. Medications used to treat nausea and vomiting of pregnancy and the risk of selected birth defects. *Birth Defects Res A Clin Mol Teratol*. 2012;94:22-30.
8. Erichsen R, Mikkelsen E, Pedersen L, et al. Maternal use of proton pump inhibitors during early pregnancy and the prevalence of hypospadias in male offspring. *Am J Ther*. 2014;21:254-259.
9. Broussard CN, Richter JE. Treating gastro-oesophageal reflux disease during pregnancy and lactation. What are the safest therapy options? *Drug Saf*. 1998;19:325-337.
10. Katz PO, Castell DO. Gastroesophageal reflux disease during pregnancy. *Gastroenterol Clin North Am*. 1998;27:153-167.
11. Ramakrishnan A, Katz PO. Pharmacologic management of gastroesophageal reflux disease. *Curr Treat Options Gastroenterol*. 2002;5:301-310.
12. Richter JE. Gastroesophageal reflux disease during pregnancy. *Gastroenterol Clin N Am*. 2003;32:235-261.
13. Richter JE. Review article: the management of heartburn in pregnancy. *Aliment Pharmacol Ther*. 2005;22:749-757.
14. Li CM, Zhernakova A, Engstrand L, et al. Systematic review with meta-analysis: the risks of proton pump inhibitors during pregnancy. *Aliment Pharmacol Ther*. 2020;51(4):410-420.
15. Peron A, Ripoche E, Picot C, et al. Use of proton pump inhibitors during pregnancy: a systematic review and meta-analysis of congenital malformations. *Reprod Toxicol*. 2023;119:108419.
16. Saito J, Yakuwa N, Sandaiji N, et al. Esomeprazole during pregnancy and lactation: esomeprazole levels in maternal serum, cord blood, breast milk, and the infant's serum. *Breastfeed Med*. 2020;15:598-601.

ESTAZOLAM

Central Nervous System (Benzodiazepine Hypnotic)

PREGNANCY RECOMMENDATION: No Human Data and No Relevant Animal Data

BREASTFEEDING RECOMMENDATION: Potential Toxicity

PREGNANCY SUMMARY

No reports describing the use of estazolam in human pregnancy have been located. Based on likely placental transfer, some fetal exposure will probably occur. Therefore, the absence of human pregnancy experience prevents a complete assessment of the embryofetal risk. Animal reproduction studies have not been conducted. Studies in human pregnancy with other benzodiazepine drugs have not shown a clear association in causing major birth anomalies. The use of benzodiazepine drugs throughout pregnancy has been associated with neonatal withdrawal symptoms, and use near delivery may cause neonatal depression, sedation, and hypotonia at the time of birth. There is a pregnancy exposure registry that monitors pregnancy outcomes in women using psychiatric medications during pregnancy. Health care providers are encouraged to call the National Pregnancy Registry for Psychiatric Medications at 1-866-961-2388. The drug also carries a boxed warning for increased risks from the concomitant use with opioid drugs and the risk for misuse, addiction, and dependence, with a potential for withdrawal reactions. Acute withdrawal from benzodiazepine drugs has been associated with seizures.

BREASTFEEDING SUMMARY

No reports describing the use of estazolam during human lactation have been located. The drug will probably be found in breast milk, so some infant exposure will likely occur. Other benzodiazepine drugs have been found in breast milk. The manufacturer recommends not using estazolam while nursing. However, if the clinical decision is to use this drug during lactation, the infant should be monitored for the most common reported adult side effects of nausea, headache, myalgia, and dizziness (all leading to irritability), somnolence, vomiting, and diarrhea.

Reference

1. Prescribing Information. Estazolam. Activis Pharma, Inc; 2020.

ESTRADIOL

Reproductive Health (Estrogen)

PREGNANCY RECOMMENDATION: *Contraindicated

BREASTFEEDING RECOMMENDATION: Probably Compatible

PREGNANCY SUMMARY

The Collaborative Perinatal Project reported 48 patients with first-trimester exposure to estradiol, and 1 (2.1%) birth anomaly was identified. There appears to be no embryofetal toxicity associated with inadvertent use in early pregnancy. Some estradiol may cross the placenta, so fetal exposure might occur. Animal reproduction studies have not been located. *While estradiol has been used in frozen embryo transfer and endometrial support, routine use of estrogens in pregnancy is contraindicated. This is because the hormone has no indication for use during pregnancy.

BREASTFEEDING SUMMARY

Two studies were located that analyzed human breast milk for estradiol. In one study that used a transdermal patch (50, 75, and 100 mcg) in 18 lactating women, estradiol was not detected in any of the breast milk samples (lower limit of detection 6.8 pg/mL). In a second study using 50 or 100 mg vaginal suppositories in six lactating women, peak breast milk levels ranged from about 100 pg/mL up to 1 ng/mL. Lastly, a third study evaluated infant blood levels in six infants whose mothers were administered estradiol by way of transdermal patches (doses of 50-200 mcg). In four cases, estradiol was not detected (lower limit of detection 2.5 pg/mL). The other two had levels of about 7 pg/mL. Therefore, estradiol was found in breast milk, but levels in both breast milk and the infant are low, especially with transdermal patches. Vaginal suppositories have higher quantities, but again, most levels are still in the picogram range. The use of oral estradiol has not been evaluated. Breastfeeding while using this drug should be based on the mother's clinical need for treatment versus any potential infant risks that might occur. If used, the infant should be monitored for appropriate weight gain and the mother for adequate breast milk production.

References

1. Prescribing Information. Estradiol. Physicians Total Care, Inc; 2010.
2. Heinonen OP, Slone D, Shapiro S. *Birth Defects and Drugs in Pregnancy*. Publishing Sciences Group; 1977.
3. Wiseman RA, Dodds-Smith IC. Cardiovascular birth defects and antenatal exposure to female sex hormones: a reevaluation of some base data. *Teratology* 1984;30:359-370.
4. Wilson JG, Brent RL. Are female sex hormones teratogenic? *Am J Obstet Gynecol*. 1981;141:567-580.
5. Luther ER, Roux J, Popat R, et al. The effect of estrogen priming on induction of labor with prostaglandins. *Am J Obstet Gynecol*. 1980;137:351-357.
6. Mørch NF, Lauritsen MP, Svendsen PF. Estradiol and progesterone levels in early pregnancy after natural, estradiol + progesterone or gonadotrophin stimulated frozen embryo transfer cycle: a randomised controlled trial protocol. *BMJ Open*. 2022;12:e058468.
7. Ghaffari F, Chekini Z, Vesali S. Duration of estradiol supplementation in luteal phase support for frozen embryo transfer in hormone replacement treatment cycles: a randomized, controlled phase III trial. *Arch Gynecol Obstet*. 2022;305:767-775.
8. Nilsson S, Nygren KG, Johansson EDB. Transfer of estradiol to human milk. *Am J Obstet Gynecol*. 1978;132:653-657.
9. Perheentupa A, Ruokonen A, Tapanainen JS. Transdermal estradiol treatment suppresses serum gonadotropins during lactation without transfer into breast milk. *Fertil Steril*. 2004;82:903-907.
10. Pinheiro E, Bogen DL, Hoxha D, Wisner KL. Transdermal estradiol treatment during breastfeeding: maternal and infant serum concentrations. *Arch Womens Ment Health*. 2016;19:409-413.
11. Ball DE, Morrison P. Oestrogen transdermal patches for postpartum depression in lactating mothers: a case report. *Cent Afr J Med*. 1999;45:68-70.
12. Illingworth PJ, Seaton JE, McKinlay C, Reid-Thomas V, McNeilly AS. Low dose transdermal oestradiol suppresses gonadotrophin secretion in breast-feeding women. *Hum Reprod*. 1995;10:1671-1677.
13. Perheentupa A, Critchley HO, Illingworth PJ, McNeilley AS. Enhanced sensitivity to steroid-negative feedback during breast-feeding: low-dose estradiol (transdermal estradiol supplementation) suppresses gonadotropins and ovarian activity assessed by inhibin B. *J Clin Endocrinol Metab*. 2000;85:4280-4286.

ESTROGENS, CONJUGATED

Reproductive Health (Estrogen)

PREGNANCY RECOMMENDATION: *Contraindicated

BREASTFEEDING RECOMMENDATION: Probably Compatible

PREGNANCY SUMMARY

The Collaborative Perinatal Project reported 123 patients with first-trimester exposure to conjugated estrogens, and 6 (4.9%) birth anomalies were identified. No pattern to the anomalies was identified. There appears to be no embryofetal toxicity associated with inadvertent use in early pregnancy. Some conjugated estrogens may cross the placenta, so fetal exposure might occur. Animal reproduction studies have not been located. *However, routine use of conjugated estrogens in pregnancy is contraindicated. This is because the hormone has no indication for use during gestation.

E

BREASTFEEDING SUMMARY

No reports describing the use of conjugated estrogens (and estrone) during human lactation have been located. Estrone is naturally found in human breast milk. Estrogens, as a group, have been associated with decreased breast milk production. If breastfeeding is desired, mothers should consider waiting until breastfeeding is well established (6-8 weeks) prior to the use of estrogens. If the clinical decision is to use this drug while breastfeeding, mothers should monitor for adequate breast milk production and infants for appropriate weight gain.

References

1. Heinonen OP, Slone D, Shapiro S. *Birth Defects and Drugs in Pregnancy*. Publishing Sciences Group, 1977.
2. Wiseman RA, Dodds-Smith IC. Cardiovascular birth defects and antenatal exposure to female sex hormones: a reevaluation of some base data. *Teratology*. 1984;30:359-370.
3. Wilson JG, Brent RL. Are female sex hormones teratogenic? *Am J Obstet Gynecol*. 1981;141:567-580.
4. Hagler S, Schultz A, Hankin H, et al. Fetal effects of steroid therapy during pregnancy. *Am J Dis Child*. 1963;106:586-590.
5. Ho CK, Kaufman RL, McAlister WH. Congenital malformations. Cleft palate, congenital heart disease, absent tibiae, and polydactyly. *Am J Dis Child*. 1975;129:714-716.
6. Price R. Pregnancies using conjugated oestrogen therapy. *Med J Aust*. 1980;2:341-342.
7. Dixon GW, Schlesselman JJ, Ory HW, et al. Ethinyl estradiol and conjugated estrogens as postcoital contraceptives. *JAMA*. 1980;244:1336-1339.
8. Prescribing Information. Premarin. Wyeth Pharmaceuticals LLC; 2018.
9. Gilman AG, Goodman LS, Gilman A, eds. *The Pharmacological Basis of Therapeutics*. 6th ed. MacMillan Publishing Co; 1980:1431.
10. Klinger G, Claussen C, Schroder S. Excretion of ethinyloestradiol sulfonate in the human milk. *Zentralbl Gynaekol*. 1981;103:91-95.
11. Booker DE, Pahl IR. Control of postpartum breast engorgement with oral contraceptives. *Am J Obstet Gynecol*. 1967;98(8):1099-1101.
12. Lonnerdal B, Forsum E, Hambraeus L. Effect of oral contraceptives on composition and volume of breast milk. *Am J Clin Nutr*. 1980;33:816-824.

ESTRONE

Reproductive Health (Estrogen)

See Estrogens, Conjugated.

ESZOPICLONE

Central Nervous System (Hypnotic)

PREGNANCY RECOMMENDATION: Limited Human Data—Animal Data Suggest Low Risk

BREASTFEEDING RECOMMENDATION: Potential Toxicity

PREGNANCY SUMMARY

No reports describing the use of eszopiclone in human pregnancy have been located. Based on likely placental transfer, fetal exposure will probably occur. Therefore, the absence of human pregnancy experience prevents a complete assessment of the embryofetal risk. Eszopiclone is the active component of zopiclone, a sedative/hypnotic that has been available outside the United States. There is a human pregnancy experience with zopiclone. One study reported on the outcome of 31 women with first-trimester exposure to zopiclone, and no major birth anomalies were reported at birth. Animal data did not show any embryofetal toxicity in two animal species. Using this drug during pregnancy should be based on the pros and cons of the mother's clinical need for treatment versus any potential fetal risk that might occur from exposure.

BREASTFEEDING SUMMARY

No reports describing the use of eszopiclone during human lactation have been located. The drug will probably be excreted into breast milk, so some infant exposure will likely occur. Eszopiclone is the active component of zopiclone, a sedative/hypnotic that has been available outside the United States. There is a human pregnancy experience with zopiclone. One study evaluated breast milk levels in three women and found a peak breast milk level of about 55 ng/mL. In a second study with 12 lactating women, the peak breast milk concentration range was 23 to 57 ng/mL with a mean maximum concentration of 34 ng/mL. The overall RID was low at about 1.4%. Breastfeeding while using this drug should be based on the mother's clinical need for treatment. If used, the infant should be monitored for the most common reported adult side effects of headache, anxiety, and dizziness (all leading to irritability), somnolence, and rash.

References

1. Prescribing Information. Lunesta. Sunovion Pharmaceuticals; 2019.
2. Diav-Citrin O, Okotore B, Lucarelli K, et al. Pregnancy outcome following first trimester exposure to zopiclone: a prospective controlled cohort study. *Am J Perinatol*. 1999;16:157-160.
3. Gaillot J, Heusse D, Houghton GW, et al. Pharmacokinetics and metabolism of zopiclone. *Int Pharmacopsychiatry*. 1982;17:76-91.
4. Matheson I, Sasnde HA, Gaillot J. The excretion of zopiclone into breastmilk. *Br J Clin Pharmc*. 1990;30:267-271.

E

ETANERCEPT

Immunologic (Antirheumatic—Tumor Necrosis Factor Inhibitor)

PREGNANCY RECOMMENDATION: Limited Human Data—Animal Data Suggest Low Risk

BREASTFEEDING RECOMMENDATION: Probably Compatible

PREGNANCY SUMMARY

Numerous reports have described the use of etanercept in human pregnancy. These reports included over 1,000 etanercept exposures in all trimesters. No significant adverse effects or increased rate of major malformations attributed to the drug were found. In one study of first-trimester exposure, 5 (3.6%) major anomalies were seen in 140 pregnancies. No specific pattern to the anomalies was found. Etanercept has been shown to cross the placenta in low amounts at term, so fetal exposure will occur in the second half of gestation. Nevertheless, this limited human pregnancy experience prevents a complete assessment of the embryofetal risk. Animal data did not show any embryofetal toxicity in two species at doses greater than 10 times the RHD. ACOG, the American College of Rheumatology, and the British Society for Rheumatology consider tumor necrosis factor (TNF)-α inhibitors to be low risk for use in pregnancy.

BREASTFEEDING SUMMARY

Five reports describing the use of etanercept in 10 lactating women were located. No adverse effects were reported. Etanercept was detected in human breast milk, but most levels were low at 5 ng/mL or less. In one case, the maximum level detected was 75 ng/mL. All of the calculated RIDs were less than 2%. In two infants, serum was tested for etanercept, and levels were undetected despite positive levels in breast milk. Because it is a large protein with over 900 amino acids, if the drug were to be ingested through breastfeeding, it would probably be digested in the infant's GI tract and not be absorbed. ACOG, the American College of Rheumatology, and the British Society for Rheumatology consider TNF-α inhibitors compatible for use in breastfeeding. If used, the infant should be monitored for the most common reported adult side effect of infections.

References

1. Prescribing Information. Enbrel. Immunex; 2023.
2. Sills ES, Perloe M, Tucker MJ, et al. Successful ovulation induction, conception, and normal delivery after chronic therapy with etanercept: a recombinant fusion anti-cytokine treatment for rheumatoid arthritis. *Am J Reprod Immunol*. 2001;46:366-368.
3. Wallace DJ, Weisman MH. The use of etanercept and other tumor necrosis factor-α blockers in infertility: it's time to get serious. *J Rheumatol*. 2003;30:1897-1899.
4. Walsh DJ, Shkrobot LV, Palermo GD, et al. Clinical experience with intravenous immunoglobulin and TNF-A inhibitor therapies for recurrent pregnancy loss. *Ulster Med J*. 2009;70:57-58.
5. Chakravarty EF, Sanchez-Yamamoto D, Bush TM. The use of disease modifying antirheumatic drugs in women with rheumatoid arthritis of childbearing age: a survey of practice patterns and pregnancy outcomes. *J Rheumatol*. 2003;30:241-246.
6. Janssen NM, Genta MS. The effects of immunosuppressive and anti-inflammatory medications on fertility, pregnancy, and lactation. *Arch Intern Med*. 2000;160:610-619.
7. Jarvis B, Faulds D. Etanercept. A review of its use in rheumatoid arthritis. *Drugs*. 1999;57:945-966.
8. Khanna D, McMahon M, Furst DE. Safety of tumour necrosis factor-α antagonists. *Drug Saf*. 2004;27:307-324.
9. Chambers CD, Johnson DL, Jones KL; The OTIS Collaborative Research Group. Pregnancy outcome in women exposed to anti-TNF-alpha medications: the OTIS Rheumatoid Arthritis in Pregnancy study (abstract). *Arthritis Rheum*. 2004;50:S479.
10. Chambers CD, Johnson DL, Jones KL. Safety of anti-TNF-α medications in pregnancy (abstract). *J Am Acad Dermatol*. 2005;52(suppl 1):P196.
11. Hyrich KL, Symmons DPM, Watson KD, et al. Pregnancy outcome in women who were exposed to anti-tumor necrosis factor agents: results from a national population register. *Arthritis Rheum*. 2006;54:2701-2702.
12. Roux CH, Brocq O, Breuil V, et al. Pregnancy in rheumatology patients exposed to anti-tumour necrosis factor (TNF)-α therapy. *Rheumatology*. 2007;46:695-698.
13. Carter JD, Ladhani A, Ricca LR, et al. A safety assessment of tumor necrosis factor antagonists during pregnancy: a review of the Food and Drug Administration database. *J Rheumatol*. 2009;36:635-641.
14. Koren G, Inoue M. Do tumor necrosis factor inhibitors cause malformations in humans? *J Rheumatol*. 2009;36:465-466.
15. Berthelot JM, De Bandt M, Goupille P, et al; on behalf of CRI (Club Rhumatismes et Inflammation). Exposition to anti-TNF drugs during pregnancy: outcome of 15 cases and review of the literature. *Joint Bone Spine*. 2009;76:28-34.
16. Umeda N, Ito S, Hayashi T, et al. A patient with rheumatoid arthritis who had a normal delivery under etanercept treatment. *Inter Med*. 2010;49:187-189.
17. Murashima A, Watanabe N, Ozawa N, et al. Etanercept during pregnancy and lactation in a patient with rheumatoid arthritis: drug levels in maternal serum, cord blood, breast milk and the infant's serum. *Ann Rheum Dis*. 2009;68:1793-1794.

18. Giacuzzo S, Padovan M, Capucci R, et al. Pregnancy outcome of mothers with rheumatic diseases exposed to biological agent during pregnancy: a single-centre study. *Ann Rheum Dis*. 2014;73(suppl 2):414.
19. Weber-Schoendorfer C, Oppermann M, Wacker E, et al. Pregnancy outcome after TNF-α inhibitor therapy during the first trimester: a prospective multicenter cohort study. *Br J Clin Pharmacol*. 2015;80:727-729.
20. Diav-Citrin O, Otcheretianski-Volodarsky A, Schechtman S, et al. Pregnancy outcome following gestational exposure to TNF-α–inhibitors: a prospective, comparative, observational study. *Reprod Toxicol*. 2014;43:78-84.
21. Reggia R, Andreoli L, Bazzani C, et al. Long-term follow-up of children born to mothers with chronic arthritides and exposed to anti-TNF alfa agents during pregnancy and breastfeeding: a case-control study. *Arthritis Rheumatol*. 2015;67(suppl 10):Abstract 2524. http://acrabstracts.org/abstract/longterm-follow-up-of-children-born-to-mothers-with-chronic-arthritides-and-exposed-to-anti-tnf-alfa-agents-during-pregancy-and-breastfeeding-a-case-control-study/
22. Ostensen M, Eigenmann GO. Etanercept in breast milk. *J Rheumatol*. 2004;31:1017-1018.
23. American College of Obstetricians and Gynecologists. ACOG Committee Opinion No. 776: immune modulating therapies in pregnancy and lactation. *Obstet Gynecol*. 2019;133:e287-e295.
24. Russell MD, Dey M, Flint J, et al; BSR Standards, Audit and Guidelines Working Group. British Society for Rheumatology guideline on prescribing drugs in pregnancy and breastfeeding: immunomodulatory anti-rheumatic drugs and corticosteroids. *Rheumatology (Oxford)*. 2023;62:e48-e88.
25. Keeling S, Wolbink GJ. Measuring multiple etanercept levels in the breast milk of a nursing mother with rheumatoid arthritis. *J Rheumatol*. 2010; 37:1551.
26. Bertrand K, Rossi S, Wells A, et al. The concentration of etanercept in human milk and infant outcomes. *J Rheumatol*. 2023;50:712-714.
27. Dall'ara F, Reggia R, Bazzani C, et al. FRI0176 safety of anti-TNF alfa agents during pregnancy and breastfeeding: longterm follow up of exposed children in a case-series of mothers with chronic arthritides. *Ann Rheum Dis*. 2016;75(suppl 2):493.
28. Membrive-Jiménez C, Sánchez-Piedra C, Martínez-González O, et al. Safety and effectiveness of bDMARDs during pregnancy in patients with rheumatic diseases: real-world data from the BIOBADASER registry. *Reumatol Clin (Engl Ed)*. 2023;19:500-506.

ETELCALCETIDE

Endocrine (Tryptophan Hydrolase Inhibitor)

PREGNANCY RECOMMENDATION: No Human Data—Animal Data Suggest Low Risk

BREASTFEEDING RECOMMENDATION: Probably Compatible

PREGNANCY SUMMARY

No reports describing the use of etelcalcetide in human pregnancy have been located. Some amount of the drug will probably cross the placenta, so fetal exposure will likely occur. However, the absence of human pregnancy experience prevents a complete assessment of embryofetal risk. Animal studies did not show any embryofetal toxicity. Using this drug during pregnancy should be based on the pros and cons of the mother's clinical need for treatment versus any potential fetal risk that might occur from exposure.

BREASTFEEDING SUMMARY

No reports describing the use of etelcalcetide during human lactation have been located. Some amount of the drug will probably enter breast milk, so infant exposure will likely occur. Based on the drug being found in animal milk and the drug's mechanism of action, the manufacturer recommends that women not breastfeed when using this drug. However, because it is a heptapeptide, if the drug were to be ingested through breastfeeding, it probably would be digested in the infant's GI tract and not be absorbed. Therefore, breastfeeding should be based on the mother's clinical need for treatment. If used, the infant should be monitored for the most common reported adult side effects of headache and nausea (both leading to irritability), diarrhea, vomiting, and hypocalcemia.

Reference

1. Prescribing Information. Parsabiv. Amgen, Inc; 2017.

ETEPLIRSEN

Central Nervous System (Antisense Oligonucleotide—Duchenne Muscular Dystrophy)

PREGNANCY RECOMMENDATION: No Human Data and No Relevant Animal Data

BREASTFEEDING RECOMMENDATION: Probably Compatible

PREGNANCY SUMMARY

No reports describing the use of eteplirsen in human pregnancy have been located. Placental transfer is likely to be clinically insignificant. However, the absence of human pregnancy experience prevents a complete assessment of the embryofetal risk. Animal reproduction studies have not been performed. Duchenne muscular dystrophy (DMD) is primarily seen in males (X-linked recessive genetic disorder). Females with severe DMD who are of reproductive age potential are exceedingly rare. Using this drug during pregnancy should be based on the pros and cons of the mother's clinical need for treatment versus any potential fetal risk that might occur from exposure.

BREASTFEEDING SUMMARY

No reports describing the use of eteplirsen during human lactation have been located. Excretion of the drug into breast milk is likely to be clinically insignificant. Breastfeeding while using this drug should be based on the mother's clinical need for treatment. If used, the infant should be monitored for the most common reported adult side effects of headache (leading to irritability), rash, cough, and vomiting.

Reference

1. Prescribing Information. Exondys 51. Sarepta Therapeutics, Inc; 2022.

E

ETHACRYNIC ACID

Cardiovascular (Loop Diuretic)

PREGNANCY RECOMMENDATION: Limited Human Data—Animal Data Suggest Low Risk

BREASTFEEDING RECOMMENDATION: Probably Compatible

PREGNANCY SUMMARY

No reports describing the use of ethacrynic acid in the first trimester of human pregnancy were located. Ethacrynic acid has been studied for use in treating preeclampsia and maternal edema in the past. However, diuretics are not recommended for the treatment of gestational hypertension because of the maternal hypovolemic characteristic of this disease. Additionally, it may decrease placental perfusion. The drug will probably cross the placenta, so some fetal exposure will likely occur. However, this limited human pregnancy experience prevents a complete assessment of the embryofetal risk. Animal data did not show teratogenicity in two species at doses of more than 10 times the RHD. Using this drug during pregnancy should be based on the pros and cons of the mother's clinical need for treatment versus any potential fetal risk that might occur from exposure.

BREASTFEEDING SUMMARY

No reports describing the use of ethacrynic acid during human lactation have been located. The drug will likely be found in breast milk, so some infant exposure will probably occur. One study was located where ethacrynic acid was used with some success to decrease or limit the amount of breast milk production postdelivery in six women who did not want to breastfeed. However, no follow-up studies or evaluations for this use have occurred. Breastfeeding while using this drug should be based on the mother's clinical need for treatment versus any potential infant risks that might occur. If used, the infant should be monitored for the most common reported adult side effects of nausea and abdominal pain (both leading to irritability), poor feeding (monitor infant growth), vomiting, diarrhea, and lethargy.

References

1. Wilson AL, Matzke GR. The treatment of hypertension in pregnancy. *Drug Intell Clin Pharm*. 1981;15:21-26.
2. Pitkin RM, Kaminetzky HA, Newton M, et al. Maternal nutrition: a selective review of clinical topics. *Obstet Gynecol*. 1972;40:773-785.
3. Lindheimer MD, Katz AI. Sodium and diuretics in pregnancy. *N Engl J Med*. 1973;288:891-894.
4. Christianson R, Page EW. Diuretic drugs and pregnancy. *Obstet Gynecol*. 1976;48:647-652.
5. Delgado Urdapilleta J, Dominguez Robles H, Villalobos Roman M, et al. Ethacrynic acid in the treatment of toxemia of pregnancy. *Ginecol Obstet Mex*. 1968;23:271-280.
6. Felman D, Theoleyre J, Dupoizat H. Investigation of ethacrynic acid in the treatment of excessive gain in weight and pregnancy arterial hypertension. *Lyon Med*. 1967;217:1421-1428.
7. Sands RX, Vita F. Ethacrynic acid (a new diuretic), pregnancy, and excessive fluid retention. *Am J Obstet Gynecol*. 1968;101:603-609.
8. Kittaka S, Aizawa M, Tokue I, et al. Clinical results in Edecril tablet in the treatment of toxemia of late pregnancy. *Obstet Gynecol (Jpn)*. 1968;36:934-937.
9. Mahon R, Dubecq JP, Baudet E, et al. Use of Edecrine in obstetrics. *Bull Fed Soc Gynecol Obstet Lang Fr*. 1968;20:440-442.
10. Imaizumi S, Suzuoki Y, Torri M, et al. Clinical trial of ethacrynic acid (Edecril) for toxemia of pregnancy. *Jpn J Med Consult New Remedies*. 1969;6:2364-2368.
11. Young BK, Haft JI. Treatment of pulmonary edema with ethacrynic acid during labor. *Am J Obstet Gynecol*. 1970;107:330-331.
12. Harrison KA, Ajabor LN, Lawson JB. Ethacrynic acid and packed-blood-cell transfusion in treatment of severe anaemia in pregnancy. *Lancet*. 1971;1:11-14.
13. Fort AT, Morrison JC, Fisk SA. Iatrogenic hypokalemia of pregnancy by furosemide and ethacrynic acid: two case reports. *J Reprod Med*. 1971;6:21-22.
14. Pico I, Greenblatt RB. Endocrinopathies and infertility. IV. Diabetes insipidus and pregnancy. *Fertil Steril*. 1969;20:384-392.
15. Prescribing Information. Edecrin. Bausch Health US, LLC; 2016.
16. Jones HC. Intrauterine ototoxicity: a case report and review of literature. *J Natl Med Assoc*. 1973;65:201-203.

ETHAMBUTOL

Anti-Infective (Antituberculosis)

PREGNANCY RECOMMENDATION: Limited Human Data—No Relevant Animal Data (Maternal Benefit May Outweigh Embryofetal Risk)

BREASTFEEDING RECOMMENDATION: Probably Compatible

E

PREGNANCY SUMMARY

Two reports describing the use of ethambutol as part of a multidrug regimen in human pregnancy reported 45 pregnancies. Exposure was in all trimesters. No major congenital abnormalities were reported in either study. The drug appears to cross the placenta, so fetal exposure will occur. However, this limited human experience prevents a complete assessment of the embryofetal risk. Animal studies reported teratogenicity in two species, but at very high doses. Using this drug during pregnancy should be based on the pros and cons of the mother's clinical need for treatment versus any potential fetal risk that might occur from exposure. The 2016 guidelines for the treatment of drug-susceptible tuberculosis consider ethambutol as a first-line drug (in addition to isoniazid, rifampin, and pyrazinamide) for the treatment of tuberculosis in pregnancy.

BREASTFEEDING SUMMARY

Ethambutol was reported to be excreted into human breast milk. The breast milk to maternal plasma concentration was about one to one. The calculated RID was less than 1%. The 2016 guidelines in the treatment of drug-susceptible tuberculosis consider ethambutol (and other first-line agents) as compatible with breastfeeding. They note that these drugs may appear in breast milk in small concentrations, but have not been reported to cause adverse effects in the infant.

References

1. Prescribing Information. Myambutol. STI Pharma; 2022.
2. Bobrowitz ID. Ethambutol in pregnancy. *Chest*. 1974;66:20-24.
3. Lewit T, Nebel L, Terracina S, Karman S. Ethambutol in pregnancy: observations on embryogenesis. *Chest*. 1974;66:25-26.
4. Shneerson JM, Francis RS. Ethambutol in pregnancy-foetal exposure. *Tubercle*. 1979;60:167-169.
5. Holdiness MR. Transplacental pharmacokinetics of the antituberculosis drugs. *Clin Pharmacokinet*. 1987;13:125-129.
6. Drobac PC, del Castillo H, Sweetland A, et al. Treatment of multi-drug resistant tuberculosis during pregnancy: long-term follow-up of 6 children with intrauterine exposure to second-line agents. *Clin Infect Dis*. 2005;40:1689-1692.
7. Snider DE Jr, Powell KE. Should women taking antituberculosis drugs breast-feed? *Arch Intern Med*. 1984;144:589-590.
8. Nahid P, Dorman SE, Alipanah N, et al. Official American Thoracic Society/Centers for Disease Control and Prevention/Infectious Diseases Society of America Clinical Practice Guidelines: treatment of drug-susceptible tuberculosis. *Clin Infect Dis*. 2016;63(7):e147-e195.

ETHINYL ESTRADIOL

Reproductive Health (Estrogen)

PREGNANCY RECOMMENDATION: *Contraindicated

BREASTFEEDING RECOMMENDATION: Probably Compatible

PREGNANCY SUMMARY

Ethinyl estradiol (EE) is used frequently in combination with progestins for oral contraception (see Oral Contraceptives). From the Collaborative Perinatal Project and one other small study, 8 (7.9%) birth anomalies were identified in 101 first-trimester exposures. No pattern to the defects was identified. The absolute risk of embryofetal harm after inadvertent exposure early in gestation appears to be low. Use of products containing synthetic estrogens later in pregnancy may be associated with feminization of male fetuses (see Oral Contraceptives). *However, routine use of EE in pregnancy is contraindicated. This is because the hormone has no indication for use during gestation.

BREASTFEEDING SUMMARY

One study was located that analyzed human breast milk for the presence of EE. Four women were administered a daily oral contraceptive that contained 50 mcg of EE, and the remaining four were administered a single dose of 500 mcg of EE. No EE was detected in the breast milk of the 50-mcg dosage group (lower limit of detection 50 pg/mL). In the 500-mcg dosage group, peak EE levels were seen in the 3- and 7-hour samples, with levels of 170 to 300 pg/mL. Breastfeeding while using this drug should be based on the mother's clinical need for treatment versus any potential infant risks that might occur. When used in oral contraceptives, EE has been associated with decreased breast milk production. If breastfeeding is desired, mothers should consider waiting until breastfeeding is well established (6-8 weeks) prior to the use of estrogen-containing oral contraceptives. Additionally, the lowest dose of oral contraceptives should be chosen, and infant weight gain should be monitored, or the use of progestin-only birth control should be considered.

References

1. Heinonen OP, Slone D, Shapiro S. *Birth Defects and Drugs in Pregnancy*. Publishing Sciences Group; 1977.
2. Wiseman RA, Dodds-Smith IC. Cardiovascular birth defects and antenatal exposure to female sex hormones: a reevaluation of some base data. *Teratology*. 1984;30:359-370.
3. Wilson JG, Brent RL. Are female sex hormones teratogenic? *Am J Obstet Gynecol*. 1981;141:567-580.
4. Hagler S, Schultz A, Hankin H, et al. Fetal effects of steroid therapy during pregnancy. *Am J Dis Child*. 1963;106:586-590.
5. Dixon GW, Schlesselman JJ, Ory HW, et al. Ethinyl estradiol and conjugated estrogens as postcoital contraceptives. *JAMA*. 1980;244:1336-1339.
6. Gilman AG, Goodman LS, Gilman A, eds. *The Pharmacological Basis of Therapeutics*. 6th ed. MacMillan Publishing Co; 1980:1431.
7. Klinger G, Claussen C, Schroder S. Excretion of ethinyloestradiol sulfonate in the human milk. *Zentralbl Gynaekol*. 1981;103:91-95.
8. Booker DE, Pahl IR. Control of postpartum breast engorgement with oral contraceptives. *Am J Obstet Gynecol*. 1967 Aug 15;98(8):1099-1101.
9. Lonnerdal B, Forsum E, Hambraeus L. Effect of oral contraceptives on composition and volume of breast milk. *Am J Clin Nutr*. 1980;33:816-824.
10. Prescribing Information. Levonorgestrel and ethinyl estradiol and estradiol. Mylan Pharmaceuticals, Inc; 2023.
11. Nilsson S, Nygren KG, Johansson ED. Ethinyl estradiol in human milk and plasma after oral administration. *Contraception*. 1978;17(2):131-139.

E

ETHIODIZED OIL

Diagnostic

PREGNANCY RECOMMENDATION: *Contraindicated

BREASTFEEDING RECOMMENDATION: Potential Toxicity

PREGNANCY SUMMARY

No reports describing the use of ethiodized oil during human pregnancy have been located. Based on likely placental transfer, some fetal exposure could occur. However, the absence of human pregnancy experience prevents a complete assessment of the embryofetal risk. *The drug is contraindicated for systemic intravascular use. With a pregnancy, hysterosalpingography is also contraindicated because of the potential risk to an implanted embryo. The use of preconceptual ethiodized oil has been assessed regarding iodine levels in the mother, breast milk, and newborn, with elevated levels seen in some cases. This has a theoretical risk for producing maternal and/or fetal thyroid dysfunction, and monitoring may be indicated.

BREASTFEEDING SUMMARY

No reports describing the use of ethiodized oil during human lactation have been located. According to the manufacturer, ethiodized oil is excreted into breast milk. Due to the concern that this may interfere with infant thyroid function, the manufacturer recommends that laboratory thyroid testing be considered in a nursing infant of a mother who is receiving this contrast agent.

References

1. Prescribing Information. Lipiodol. Guerbet LLC; 2023.
2. Li R, Chen W, Liu Y, et al. The impact of preconceptual hysterosalpingography with oil-based contrast on maternal and neonatal iodine status. *Reprod Sci*. 2021;28:2887-2894.

ETHIONAMIDE

Anti-Infective (Antitubercular)

PREGNANCY RECOMMENDATION: Limited Human Data—Animal Data Suggest Risk

BREASTFEEDING RECOMMENDATION: Probably Compatible

PREGNANCY SUMMARY

A total of five reports were located that describe the use of ethionamide in 19 pregnancies (20 neonates, one set of twins). Of these, 10 pregnancies were exposed in the first trimester. Nine infants were delivered healthy, with no malformations identified. The last patient delivered premature twins that both had similar major defects of hydrocephalus, short limbs, and one had a cardiac anomaly. The remaining nine were exposed in the second and third trimesters. The drug will probably

(continued)

cross the placenta, so some fetal exposure will likely occur. However, this limited human pregnancy experience prevents a complete assessment of the embryofetal risk. Animal studies did show embryofetal toxicity with malformations in two species at doses of less than 10 times the RHD, but not in a third species. Ethionamide is a second-line agent for drug-resistant tuberculosis. Due to the risk of untreated drug-resistant tuberculosis to a pregnant woman and her fetus, the mother should be counseled on the known and unknown risks of second-line antituberculosis drugs.

E

BREASTFEEDING SUMMARY

Two reports were located that involve the same two patients. The second study is a 4- to 5-year follow-up of both infants following exposure to ethionamide through breastfeeding after delivery. One child had a mild speech delay, and the other had hyperactivity. Otherwise, both children were progressing well. The drug will probably be found in breast milk, so some infant exposure will likely occur. The effect of this exposure on a nursing infant is unknown. Breastfeeding while using this drug should be based on the mother's clinical need for treatment versus any potential infant risks that might occur. If used, the infant should be monitored for the most common reported adult side effects of nausea and abdominal pain (both leading to irritability), vomiting, diarrhea, excessive salivation, and decreased appetite (monitor infant growth).

References

1. Prescribing Information. Trecator. Wyeth Pharmaceuticals; 2023.
2. Hyman C, Wilson LA. Anti-tuberculosis therapy during pregnancy. *J Med Soc NJ*. 1965;62:291-220.
3. Bhatia JL, Raj B. Normal child birth under ethionamide treatment. *Indian J Chest Dis*. 1966;8:167-170.
4. Potworowska M, Sianozecka E, Szufladowicz R. Ethionamide treatment and pregnancy. *Pol Med J*. 1966;5:1152-1158.
5. Shin S, Guerra D, Rich M, et al. Treatment of multidrug-resistant tuberculosis during pregnancy: a report of 7 cases. *Clin Infect Dis*. 2003;36:996-1003.
6. Drobac PC, Castillo HD, Sweetland A, et al. Treatment of multidrug-resistant tuberculosis during pregnancy: long-term follow-up of 6 children with intrauterine exposure to second-line agents. *Clin Infect Dis*. 2005;40:1689-1692.

ETHOSUXIMIDE

Central Nervous System (Antiseizure)

PREGNANCY RECOMMENDATION: Limited Human Data—No Relevant Animal Data

BREASTFEEDING RECOMMENDATION: Potential Toxicity

PREGNANCY SUMMARY

Multiple reports describing the use of ethosuximide in human pregnancy have been located. These reports include 236 infants exposed to ethosuximide in combination with other anticonvulsants and 13 infants whose mothers received monotherapy. Of these, 18 (7.2%) congenital defects were reported. No specific pattern to the anomalies was identified. The drug crosses the placenta with fetal to maternal levels of about one, so fetal exposure will occur. However, this limited human pregnancy experience prevents a complete assessment of the embryofetal risk. Epilepsy itself (as well as other anticonvulsants) can increase the risk for structural anomalies. Animal reproduction studies have not been located. Using this drug during pregnancy should be based on the pros and cons of the mother's clinical need for treatment versus any potential fetal risk that might occur from exposure. The manufacturer recommends that pregnant patients taking this drug enroll in the NAAED Pregnancy Registry by calling the toll-free number 1-888-233-2334.

BREASTFEEDING SUMMARY

Ethosuximide has been found in breast milk with infant plasma levels of about 30% of maternal levels. Three case reports of five infants describing the use of ethosuximide during human lactation reported sedation, poor suckling, and poor weight gain during 4 weeks of breastfeeding in one infant. The mother was also taking primidone and valproic acid. No adverse reactions were noted in the remaining four infants. Breastfeeding while using this drug should be based on the mother's clinical need for treatment versus any potential infant risks that might occur. If used, the infant should be monitored for drowsiness, poor feeding, and poor weight gain.

References

1. Prescribing Information. Ethosuximide. Pfizer; 2023.
2. Fabro S, Brown NA. Teratogenic potential of anticonvulsants. *N Engl J Med*. 1979;300:1280-1281.
3. The National Institute of Health. Anticonvulsants found to have teratogenic potential. *JAMA*. 1981;241:36.
4. Kuhnz W, Koch S, Jakob S, Hartman A, et al. Ethosuximide in epileptic women during pregnancy and lactation period. Placental transfer, serum concentrations in nursed infants and clinical status. *Br J Clin Pharmacol*. 1984;18:671-677.
5. Tomson T, Villen T. Ethosuximide enantiomers in pregnancy and lactation. *Ther Drug Monit*. 1994;16:621-623.
6. Speidel BD, Meadow SR. Maternal epilepsy and abnormalities of the fetus and newborn. *Lancet*. 1972;2:839-843.
7. Fedrick J. Epilepsy and pregnancy: a report from the Oxford Record Linkage Study. *Br Med J*. 1973;2:442-448.
8. Lowe CR. Congenital malformations among infants born to epileptic women. *Lancet*. 1973;1:9-10.
9. Starreveld-Zimmerman AAE, van der Kolk WJ, Meinardi H, Elshve J. Are anticonvulsants teratogenic? *Lancet*. 1973;2:48-49.
10. Kuenssberg EV, Knox JDE. Teratogenic effect of anticonvulsants. *Lancet*. 1973;2:198.

11. Speidel BD, Meadow SR. Epilepsy, anticonvulsants and congenital malformations. *Drugs*. 1974;8:354-365.
12. Janz D. The teratogenic risk of antiepileptic drugs. *Epilepsia*. 1975;16:159-169.
13. Nakane Y, Okuma T, Takahashi R. Multi-institutional study on the teratogenicity and fetal toxicity of antiepileptic drugs: a report of a collaborative study group in Japan. *Epilepsia*. 1980;21:663-680.
14. Heinonen OP, Slone D, Shapiro S. *Birth Defects and Drugs in Pregnancy*. Publishing Sciences Group; 1977:358-359.
15. Dansky L, Andermann E, Andermann F. Major congenital malformations on the offspring of epileptic patients: genetic and environment risk factors. In: *Epilepsy, Pregnancy and the Child. Proceedings of a Workshop Held in Berlin, September 1980*. Raven Press; 1981.
16. The Lamotrigine Pregnancy Registry. Final report. 1 September 1992 through 31 March 2010. GlaxoSmithKline; 2010.
17. Samren EB, van Duijn CM, Koch S, et al. Maternal use of antiepileptic drugs and the risk of major congenital malformations: a joint European prospective study of human teratogenesis associated with maternal epilepsy. *Epilepsia*. 1992;38:981-990.
18. Koup JR, Rose JQ, Cohen ME. Ethosuximide pharmacokinetics in pregnant patient and her newborn. *Epilepsia*. 1978;19:535.
19. Kaneko S, Sato T, Suzuki K. The levels of anticonvulsants in breast milk. *Br J Clin Pharmacol*. 1979;7:624-626.
20. Horning MG, Stillwell WG, Nowlin J, et al. Identification and quantification of drugs and drug metabolites in human breast milk using GC-MS-COM methods. *Mod Probl Paediatr*. 1975;15:73-79.
21. Patsalos PN, Zugman M, Lake C, James A, Ratnaraj N, Sander JW. Serum protein binding of 25 antiepileptic drugs in a routine clinical setting: a comparison of free non-protein-bound concentrations. *Epilepsia*. 2017;58:1234-1243.
22. Rane A, Tunell R. Ethosuximide in human milk and in plasma of a mother and her nursed infant. *Br J Clin Pharmacol*. 1981;12:855-858.
23. Soderman P, Rane A. Ethosuximide and nursing. *Acta Pharmacol Toxicol (Copenh)*. 1986;59(suppl 5, pt 2):Abstract 513.

E

ETHYNODIOL DIACETATE

Reproductive Health (Progestin)

PREGNANCY RECOMMENDATION: *Contraindicated

BREASTFEEDING RECOMMENDATION: Probably Compatible

PREGNANCY SUMMARY

No reports describing the use of ethynodiol diacetate during the first trimester of human pregnancy have been located. Based on likely placental transfer, some fetal exposure will probably occur. However, the absence of human pregnancy experience prevents a complete assessment of the embryofetal risk. Animal reproduction studies have not been conducted. The absolute risk of embryofetal harm after inadvertent exposure to oral contraceptives early in gestation appears to be low. Use of products containing synthetic progestins later in pregnancy may be associated with masculinization of a female fetus (see Oral Contraceptives). *Therefore, routine use of EE in pregnancy is contraindicated. This is because this synthetic hormone has no indication for use during gestation.

BREASTFEEDING SUMMARY

No reports describing the use of ethynodiol diacetate during human lactation have been located. Unlike estrogen-containing contraceptives, progestin-only contraceptives generally demonstrate no consistent alteration of breast milk composition, volume, or duration of lactation. Both estrogens and progestins cross into human breast milk. Reports of adverse effects are lacking. If breastfeeding is desired, the lowest effective dose of oral contraceptives should be chosen, if possible, and infant weight gain should be monitored (see Oral Contraceptives).

Reference

1. Prescribing Information. Ethynodiol diacetate and ethinyl estradiol. Mylan Pharmaceuticals; 2021.

ETODOLAC

Pain (NSAID)

PREGNANCY RECOMMENDATION: Human Data Suggest Risk in the 2nd Half of Gestation

BREASTFEEDING RECOMMENDATION: Potential Toxicity

PREGNANCY SUMMARY

No reports describing the use of etodolac in human pregnancy have been located. Based on likely placental transfer, some fetal exposure will probably occur. Other nonsteroidal anti-inflammatory drugs (NSAIDs), especially those with long half-lives, have been found to cross the placenta. Therefore, the absence of human pregnancy experience prevents a complete assessment of the embryofetal risk. Animal studies did not confirm any risk of embryofetal toxicity or

(*continued*)

malformations in one animal species. Using this drug during pregnancy should be based on the pros and cons of the mother's clinical need for treatment versus any potential fetal risk that might occur from exposure. NSAIDs are prostaglandin synthesis inhibitors and have been associated with premature closure of the ductus arteriosus in utero if used during the third trimester. This can lead to pulmonary hypertension in the newborn at delivery. Therefore, use during the third trimester is not recommended. In addition, use after 20 weeks gestation can produce oligohydramnios.

BREASTFEEDING SUMMARY

No reports describing the use of etodolac during human lactation have been located. The drug will likely be found in breast milk, so some fetal exposure will probably occur. Other NSAIDs have been found in breast milk, especially those with long elimination half-lives. Due to a lack of studies evaluating etodolac during human lactation and in newborns, the manufacturer recommends using other NSAIDs, such as ibuprofen, if needed. If the clinical decision is to use this drug during lactation, the infant should be monitored for the most common reported adult side effects of nausea and abdominal pain (both leading to irritability), vomiting, diarrhea, and GI bleeding.

Reference

1. Prescribing Information. Etodolac. Taro Pharmaceuticals, USA, Inc; 2021.

ETOMIDATE

Anesthetic

PREGNANCY RECOMMENDATION: Limited Human Data—No Relevant Animal Data

BREASTFEEDING RECOMMENDATION: Probably Compatible

PREGNANCY SUMMARY

Reports describing the use of etomidate during human pregnancy have been limited to women undergoing cesarean section. No reports of use of the drug in the first trimester have been located. Etomidate crosses the placenta, so some fetal exposure will occur. However, the drug levels appear to drop fairly quickly, consistent with the short elimination half-life. Regardless, this limited human pregnancy experience prevents a complete assessment of the embryofetal risk. Animal studies showed some embryofetal toxicity (no teratogenicity) in two species at doses less than 10 times the RHD, but these doses also caused maternal toxicity. Using this drug during pregnancy should be based on the pros and cons of the mother's clinical need for treatment versus any potential fetal risk that might occur from exposure. The use of etomidate for the induction of general anesthesia at or near term does not appear to represent a risk of fetal or newborn harm.

BREASTFEEDING SUMMARY

Etomidate has been found in human breast milk in very small amounts, and levels decline rapidly. One study involving 20 women undergoing cesarean section administered a single IV injection of etomidate 0.3 mg/kg IV dose. Mean colostrum drug concentrations at 30 and 120 minutes after the dose were 79 and 16 ng/mL, respectively. Etomidate was not detected in any sample 4 hours after the dose. Due to the rapid drug level decline, little to no risk to the infant is expected. Breastfeeding may occur as soon as the mother has recovered from anesthesia.

References

1. Friedman JM. Teratogen update: anesthetic agents. *Teratology*. 1988;37:69-77.
2. Prescribing Information. Amidate. Hospira; 2022.
3. Suresh MS, Ahmed AE, Solanki DR, et al. Etomidate pharmacokinetics during cesarean section (abstract). *Anesthesiology*. 1988;65:A388.
4. Gregory MA, Davidson DG. Plasma etomidate levels in mother and fetus. *Anaesthesia*. 1991;46:716-718.
5. Crozier TA, Flamm C, Speer CP, et al. Effects of etomidate on the adrenocortical and metabolic adaptation of the neonate. *Br J Anaesth*. 1993;70:47-53.
6. Esener Z, Sarihasan B, Güven H, et al. Thiopentone and etomidate concentrations in maternal and umbilical plasma, and in colostrum. *Br J Anaesth*. 1992;69:586-588.
7. Reddy BK, Pizer B, Bull PT. Neonatal serum cortisol suppression by etomidate compared with thiopentone, for elective caesarean section. *Eur J Anaesthesia*. 1998;5:171-176.
8. Regaert P, Noorduin H. General anesthesia with etomidate, alfentanil and droperidol for caesarean section. *Acta Anaethesiol Belg*. 1984;35:193-200.
9. Tay SM, Ong BC, Tan SA. Cesarean section in a mother with uncorrected congenital coronary to pulmonary artery fistula. *Can J Anesth*. 1999;46:368-371.
10. Orme RMLE, Grange CS, Ainsworth QP, et al. General anaesthesia using remifentanil for caesarean section in parturients with critical aortic stenosis: a series of four cases. *Int J Obstet Anesth*. 2004;13:83-87.
11. Bilehjani E, Kianfar AA, Toofan M, et al. Anesthesia with etomidate and remifentanil for cesarean section in a patient with severe peripartum cardiomyopathy. *Middle East J Anesthesiol*. 2008;19:1141-1147.
12. Coskun D, Mahli A, Korkmaz S, et al. Anaesthesia for caesarean section in the presence of multivalvular heart disease and severe pulmonary hypertension: a case report. *Cases J*. 2009;2:9383.
13. Duman A, Sarkilar G, Dayioglu M, et al. Use of remifentanil in a patient with Eisenmenger syndrome requiring urgent cesarean section. *Middle East J Anesthesiol*. 2010;20:577-580.
14. Tay SM, Ong BC, Tan SA. Cesarean section in a mother with uncorrected congenital coronary to pulmonary artery fistula. *Can J Anesth*. 1999;46:368-371.

15. Orme RMLE, Grange CS, Ainsworth QP, et al. General anaesthesia using remifentanil for caesarean section in parturients with critical aortic stenosis: a series of four cases. *Int J Obstet Anesth*. 2004;13:83-87.
16. Bilehjani E, Kianfar AA, Toofan M, et al. Anesthesia with etomidate and remifentanil for cesarean section in a patient with severe peripartum cardiomyopathy. *Middle East J Anesthesiol*. 2008;19:1141-1147.
17. Coskun D, Mahli A, Korkmaz S, et al. Anaesthesia for caesarean section in the presence of multivalvular heart disease and severe pulmonary hypertension: a case report. *Cases J*. 2009;2:9383.
18. Duman A, Sarkilar G, Dayioglu M, et al. Use of remifentanil in a patient with Eisenmenger syndrome requiring urgent cesarean section. *Middle East J Anesthesiol*. 2010;20:577-580.

ETOPOSIDE

Antineoplastic (Topoisomerase II Inhibitor)

PREGNANCY RECOMMENDATION: Limited Human Data—Animal Data Suggest Risk

BREASTFEEDING RECOMMENDATION: Potential Toxicity

PREGNANCY SUMMARY

Seven case reports describing the use of etoposide as part of combination chemotherapy in human pregnancy have been located. These reports include eight pregnancies with exposure in second and third trimesters. One pregnancy was a fetal demise at 21 weeks' gestation, followed by a maternal death shortly thereafter. These unfortunate complications were related to the severe maternal disease. The remaining seven cases did well overall, except one neonate had bone marrow suppression. The drug will probably cross the placenta, so some fetal exposure will likely occur. However, this limited pregnancy experience, especially in the first trimester, prevents a complete assessment of the embryofetal risk. Embryofetal toxicity with malformations was observed in two animal species at doses less than 10 times the RHD. Based on these animal studies and the drug's mechanism of action, the manufacturer recommends that women with reproductive potential use effective contraception during treatment and for 6 months after the last dose. They also recommend that males with female partners of reproductive potential use effective contraception during treatment and for 4 months after the last dose. Nevertheless, using this drug during pregnancy should be based on the pros and cons of the mother's clinical need for treatment versus any potential fetal risk that might occur from exposure. There is a registry for women who are pregnant and have cancer. For more information, women are encouraged to contact the Cancer and Pregnancy Registry at 877-635-4499.

BREASTFEEDING SUMMARY

One study describing the use of etoposide as part of a combination chemotherapy treatment during human lactation was located. The peak breast milk concentration identified was about 800 ng/mL. Levels in the infant were not obtained. Breast milk concentrations of etoposide were undetectable within 24 hours of drug administration on each day. The infant had no reported adverse reactions to the exposure. However, due to a concern for potential serious adverse effects that might be seen in a breastfed infant, the manufacturer recommends that women not breastfeed while being treated with this drug. Nevertheless, breastfeeding while using etoposide should be based on the mother's clinical need for treatment. If used, the infant should be monitored for the most common reported adult side effects of nausea and abdominal pain (both leading to irritability), diarrhea, lethargy, vomiting, decreased appetite, and various laboratory abnormalities (see PI).

References

1. Prescribing Information. Etoposide. Accord Healthcare, Inc; 2020.
2. Buller RE, Darrow V, Manetta A, et al. Conservative surgical management of dysgerminoma concomitant with pregnancy. *Obstet Gynecol*. 1992;79:887-890.
3. Murray NA, Acolet D, Deane M, et al. Fetal marrow suppression after maternal chemotherapy for leukaemia. *Arch Dis Child*. 1994;71:F209-F210.
4. Raffles A, Williams J, Costeloe K, et al. Transplacental effects of maternal cancer chemotherapy. Case report. *Br J Obstet Gynaecol*. 1989;96:1099-1100.
5. Brunet S, Sureda A, Mateu R, et al. Full-term pregnancy in a patient diagnosed with acute leukemia treated with a protocol including VP-16. *Med Clin (Barc)*. 1993;100:757-758.
6. Rodriguez JM, Haggag M. VACOP-B chemotherapy for high grade non-Hodgkin's lymphoma in pregnancy. *Clin Oncol (R Coll Radiol)*. 1995;7:319-320.
7. Parrott J, Shilling A, Male HJ, et al. Hemophagocytic lymphohistiocytosis in pregnancy: a case series and review of the current literature. *Case Rep Obstet Gynecol*. 2019;2019:9695367.
8. Reid I, Sharma A, Gogbashian A, et al. Germ cell cancer in pregnancy—successfully treated with chemotherapy and surgery. *Gynecol Oncol Rep*. 2023;47:101185.
9. Segna RA, Mitchell DR, Misas JE. Successful treatment of cervical pregnancy with oral etoposide. *Obstet Gynecol*. 1990;76:945-947.
10. Kusaka M, Tanaka T, Fujimoto S. Local etoposide injection for treatment of tubal pregnancy with cardiac activity. *Int J Fertil Menopausal Stud*. 1994;39:11-13.
11. Azuno Y, Kaku K, Fujita N, et al. Mitoxantrone and etoposide in breast milk. *Am J Hematol*. 1995;48:131-132.

ETRASIMOD

Gastrointestinal (Ulcerative Colitis—Sphingosine 1-Phosphate Receptor Modulator)

PREGNANCY RECOMMENDATION: No Human Data—Animal Data Suggest Risk

BREASTFEEDING RECOMMENDATION: Potential Toxicity

E

PREGNANCY SUMMARY

No reports describing the use of etrasimod in human pregnancy have been located. The drug will likely cross the placenta, so some fetal exposure will probably occur. Therefore, the absence of human pregnancy experience prevents a complete assessment of the embryofetal risk. Animal studies did show embryofetal toxicity with malformations in two species at doses of less than 10 times the RHD. Based on these animal studies, the manufacturer recommends that women with reproductive potential use effective contraception during treatment and for 1 week after the last dose. Nevertheless, using this drug during pregnancy should be based on the pros and cons of the mother's clinical need for treatment versus any potential fetal risk that might occur from exposure. There is a pregnancy exposure registry that monitors pregnancy outcomes in women using this drug. Health care providers are encouraged to call the Velsipity Pregnancy Exposure Registry at 1-800-616-3791. Etrasimod can increase the risk for herpes zoster, and it is recommended that patients be tested for varicella zoster virus (VZV) antibody levels. If negative, it is recommended that a full course of VZV vaccination be administered prior to the use of etrasimod. The drug can also decrease the heart rate and cause atrioventricular conduction delays. Therefore, obtaining an electrocardiogram (ECG) to evaluate for preexisting conduction abnormalities is recommended. Active ulcerative colitis during pregnancy can lead to preterm birth, intrauterine growth restriction, and other poor pregnancy outcomes. Therefore, the benefits of treatment may outweigh any fetal effects that might occur.

BREASTFEEDING SUMMARY

No reports describing the use of etrasimod during human lactation have been located. The drug will likely be found in breast milk, so some infant exposure will probably occur. Breastfeeding while using this drug should be based on the mother's clinical need for treatment versus any potential infant risk that might occur. If used, the infant should be monitored for the most common reported adult side effects of headache and dizziness (both leading to irritability) and elevated liver function tests.

Reference

1. Prescribing Information. Velsipity. Pfizer, Inc; 2023.

ETRAVIRINE

Antiretroviral (Non-Nucleoside Reverse Transcriptase Inhibitor)

PREGNANCY RECOMMENDATION: *Contraindicated HIV-2/for HIV-1 Human Data and Animal Data Suggest Low Risk

BREASTFEEDING RECOMMENDATION: *Contraindicated

PREGNANCY SUMMARY

The APR reported, for the period January 1989 through January 2023, major birth defects were observed in 1 of 73 live births (1.4%) with first-trimester exposure to an etravirine-based regimen. Two other case reports describe an additional four first-trimester pregnancy exposures to etravirine, and all four delivered at term with no reported complications to the drug or anomalies. Overall, there were 58 drug exposures in the second/third trimesters, and no reported birth anomalies were identified. The drug crosses the placenta, so fetal exposure will occur. Animal studies did not show any embryofetal toxicity in two species. There is a pregnancy exposure registry that monitors pregnancy outcomes in women exposed to etravirine during pregnancy. Health care providers are encouraged to call the APR at 1-800-258-4263. In 2023, the updated US Department of Health and Human Services AIDS Info guidelines for the use of antiretroviral agents during pregnancy recommend that, in most cases, patients continue their regimen during pregnancy if it is tolerated, safe, and effective in suppressing viral replication. The guideline recommends that a discussion occur to help guide the selection of which antiretrovirals to use during pregnancy. This should involve shared decision-making about the known and potential risks as well as benefits to the mother and fetus, acknowledging limited data. Additionally, treatment initiation should not be delayed due to concerns about teratogenicity with first-trimester exposure. See the guideline for the most updated information on continuing, initiating, or switching regimens during pregnancy, if any potential dosing changes are needed due to pharmacokinetic changes of pregnancy, and recommendations for intrapartum and postpartum management. *The drug is not to be used in treating HIV-2.

BREASTFEEDING SUMMARY

One abstract was located that evaluated etravirine use during human lactation. The drug was found in breast milk with a maximum median concentration of about 798 ng/mL and a median breast milk to maternal plasma ratio of about 1.1 on day 5 of breastfeeding, which increased to about 3.3 on day 14. In 2023, the updated US Department of Health and

Human Services AIDS Info guidelines state that using replacement of breast milk through formula or pasteurized donor human breast milk from a milk bank eliminates the risk of postnatal HIV transmission to the infant. Using antiretroviral therapy to achieve and maintain viral suppression during pregnancy and postpartum decreases the risk for infant transmission to less than 1% but not zero. *For patients not on therapy or those without viral load suppression during pregnancy (at a minimum of throughout the third trimester) and at delivery, replacement of breast milk is recommended. Patients on antiretroviral therapy who have a sustained undetectable viral load and who choose to breastfeed or use replacement of breast milk should be supported with this decision. If the clinical decision is to use this drug while breastfeeding, the infant should be monitored for the most common reported pediatric side effects of rash and diarrhea.

References

1. Prescribing Information. Intelence. Janssen Products; 2023.
2. Mulligan N, Schalkwijk S, Best BM, et al. Etravirine pharmacokinetics in HIV-infected pregnant women. *Front Pharmacol*. 2016;7:239.
3. Ramgopal M, Osiyemi O, Zorrilla C, et al. Pharmacokinetics of total and unbound etravirine in HIV-1-infected pregnant women. *J Acquir Immune Defic Syndr*. 2016;73:268-274.
4. Calcagna A, Trentini L, Marinaro L, et al. Transplacental passage of etravirine and maraviroc in a multidrug-experienced HIV-infected woman failing on darunavir-based HAART in late pregnancy. *J Antimicrob Chemother*. 2013;68:1938-1939.
5. Izurieta P, Kakuda TN, Feys C, et al. Safety and pharmacokinetics of etravirine in pregnant HIV-1-infected women. *HIV Med*. 2011;12(4):257-258.
6. Furco A, Gosrani B, Nicholas S, et al. Successful use of darunavir, etravirine, enfuvirtide and tenofovir/emtricitabine in pregnant woman with multiclass HIV resistance. *AIDS*. 2009;23:434-435.
7. Antiretroviral Pregnancy Registry Steering Committee. Antiretroviral pregnancy registry interim report for 1 January 1989 through 31 January 2023. Registry Coordinating Center; 2023.
8. Jaworsky D, Thompson C, Yudin MH, et al. Use of newer antiretroviral agents, darunavir and etravirine with or without raltegravir, in pregnancy: a report of two cases. *Antivir Ther*. 2010;15:677-680.
9. Shust GF, Jao J, Rodriguez-Caprio G, et al. Salvage regimens containing darunavir, etravirine, raltegravir, or enfuvirtide in highly treatment-experienced perinatally infected pregnant women. *J Pediatric Infect Dis Soc*. 2014;3:246-250.
10. Panel on Treatment of HIV During Pregnancy and Prevention of Perinatal Transmission. Recommendations for the use of antiretroviral drugs during pregnancy and interventions to reduce perinatal HIV transmission in the United States. Department of Health and Human Services. Accessed November 6, 2023. https://clinicalinfo.hiv.gov/en/guidelines/perinatal
11. Spencer LY, Liu S, Wang CH, et al. Intensive etravirine PK and HIV-1 viral load in breast milk and plasma in HIV+ women receiving HAART (abstract). *Top Antivir Med*. 2014;22:466.

EVEROLIMUS

Antineoplastic/Immunologic (mTOR Kinase Inhibitor)

PREGNANCY RECOMMENDATION: Limited Human Data—Animal Data Suggest Risk

BREASTFEEDING RECOMMENDATION: Potential Toxicity

PREGNANCY SUMMARY

Seven case reports/series were located that describe nine cases of everolimus use in the first trimester of pregnancy. No major anomalies related to the drug were identified in all cases. Six were term deliveries and three were late preterm births. Everolimus crosses the placenta at term, so fetal exposure will occur. However, this limited human pregnancy experience prevents a complete assessment of the embryofetal risk. Embryofetal toxicity was observed in two animal species at doses less than 10 times the RHD. The drug is available under the brand names of Zortress and Afinitor. Zortress is approved for oral use in the prophylaxis of organ rejection, while Afinitor is approved for oral use in the treatment of various cancers. They are noted as not interchangeable. Based on animal studies and the drug's mechanism of action, the manufacturer recommends that women with reproductive potential use effective contraception during treatment and for 8 weeks after the last dose. For Afinitor, the manufacturer also recommends that males with female partners of reproductive potential use effective contraception during treatment and for 4 weeks after the last dose. Regardless, using this drug during pregnancy should be based on the pros and cons of the mother's clinical need for treatment versus any potential fetal risk that might occur from exposure. There is a Transplant Pregnancy Registry International (TPRI) that monitors pregnancies that occur in maternal transplant recipients or fathered by male transplant recipients. The TPRI encourages reporting of pregnancies following solid organ transplantation by contacting them at 1-877-955-6877. There is also a registry for women who are pregnant and have cancer. For more information, women are encouraged to contact the Cancer and Pregnancy Registry at 877-635-4499.

BREASTFEEDING SUMMARY

Two reports describing the use of everolimus during human lactation have been located. The drug was found to be excreted into breast milk, but at low levels. In one case, no drug was detected (lower limit of quantification 0.5 ng/mL). In the second case, everolimus was detected at levels ranging from 45 to 66 pg/mL. However, due to a concern for potential serious adverse effects that might be seen in a breastfed infant, the manufacturer recommends that women not breastfeed while being treated with this drug and for 2 weeks after the last dose. Nevertheless, breastfeeding while using this drug should be based on the mother's clinical need for treatment versus any potential infant risks that might occur. If used, the infant should be monitored for the most common reported adult side effects of nausea (leading to irritability), peripheral edema, constipation, hypertension, anemia, and hyperlipidemia.

References

1. Prescribing Information. Zortress. Novartis Pharmaceuticals; 2023.
2. Prescribing Information. Afinitor. Novartis Pharmaceuticals Corporation; 2022.
3. Yamamura M, Kojima T, Koyama M, et al. Everolimus in pregnancy: case report and literature review. *J Obstet Gynaecol*. 2017;43:1350-1352.
4. Veroux M, Corona D, Veroux P. Pregnancy under everolimus-based immunosuppression. *Trans Int*. 2011;24:e115-e117.
5. Carta P, Caroti L, Zanazzi M. Pregnancy in a kidney transplant patient treated with everolimus. *Am J Kidney Dis*. 2012;60:329.
6. Fiocchi R, D'Elia E, Vittori C, et al. First report of a successful pregnancy in an everolimus-treated heart-transplant patient: neonatal disappearance of immunosuppressive drugs. *Am J Transpl*. 2016;16:1319-1322.
7. Margoles HR, Gomes-Lobo V, Veis JH, et al. Successful maternal and fetal outcome in a kidney transplant patient with everolimus exposure throughout pregnancy: a case report. *Transpl Proceed*. 2014;46:281-283.
8. Carta P, Zanazzi M, Minetti EE. Unplanned pregnancies in kidney transplanted patients treated with everolimus: three case reports. *Transpl Int*. 2015;28:370-372.
9. Kociszewska-Najman B, Szpotanska-Sikorska M, Mazanowska N, et al. Transfer of everolimus into colostrum of a kidney transplant mother. *Ann Transplant*. 2017;22:755-758.

E

EVINACUMAB

Antilipemic (Monoclonal Antibody—Homozygous Familial Hypercholesterolemia)

PREGNANCY RECOMMENDATION: No Human Data—Animal Data Suggest Potential Risk

BREASTFEEDING RECOMMENDATION: Probably Compatible

PREGNANCY SUMMARY

No reports describing the use of evinacumab in human pregnancy have been located. As an IgG antibody, evinacumab will likely cross the placenta, so some fetal exposure will probably occur. Therefore, the absence of human pregnancy experience prevents a complete assessment of the embryofetal risk. Embryofetal toxicity with malformations was observed in animal studies. However, based on animal studies, the manufacturer recommends that women with reproductive potential use effective contraception during treatment and for at least 5 months after the last dose. Nevertheless, using this drug during pregnancy should be based on the pros and cons of the mother's clinical need for treatment versus any potential fetal risk that might occur from exposure. There is a pregnancy exposure registry that monitors pregnancy outcomes in women using this drug. Health care providers are encouraged to call the Evkeeza Pregnancy Exposure Registry at 1-833-385-3392.

BREASTFEEDING SUMMARY

No reports describing the use of evinacumab during human lactation have been located. It is known that IgG antibodies can be found in human breast milk, but are not found in the neonatal or infant circulation. Additionally, if any IgG antibodies were to be ingested through breastfeeding, they would probably be digested in the infant's GI tract and not be absorbed. Breastfeeding while using this drug should be based on the mother's clinical need for treatment. If used, the infant should be monitored for the most common reported adult side effects of nausea (leading to irritability), influenza-like illness, and rhinorrhea.

Reference

1. Prescribing Information. Evkeeza. Regeneron Pharmaceuticals; 2021.

EVOLOCUMAB

Antilipemic (Monoclonal Antibody/PCSK9 Inhibitor)

PREGNANCY RECOMMENDATION: Limited Human Data—Animal Data Suggest Low Risk

BREASTFEEDING RECOMMENDATION: Probably Compatible

PREGNANCY SUMMARY

One report describing the use of evolocumab in human pregnancy was located. The mother had heterozygous familial hypercholesterolemia and was treated at 31 and 35 weeks' gestation. The drug was well tolerated, and no adverse effects were reported in the delivered neonate. As an IgG antibody, the drug will likely cross the placenta, especially during the second half of pregnancy, so some fetal exposure will probably occur. However, this limited human pregnancy experience prevents a complete assessment of the embryofetal risk. Animal data did not show any embryofetal toxicity. Using this drug during pregnancy should be based on the pros and cons of the mother's clinical need for treatment versus any potential fetal risk that might occur from exposure. There is a pregnancy safety study for evolocumab. If the drug is administered during pregnancy, health care providers should report the exposure by calling 1-800-772-6436.

BREASTFEEDING SUMMARY

No reports describing the use of evolocumab during human lactation have been located. It is known that IgG antibodies are excreted into breast milk but are not found in the neonatal or infant circulation. Additionally, if any IgG antibodies were to be ingested through breastfeeding, they would probably be digested in the infant's GI tract and not be absorbed. Breastfeeding while using this drug should be based on the mother's clinical need for treatment. If used, the infant should be monitored for the most common reported adult side effects of back pain (leading to irritability) and upper respiratory tract infection.

References

1. Prescribing Information. Repatha. Amgen; 2021.
2. Suzuki T, Tsurane K, Umemoto T, et al. PCSK9 inhibitor use during pregnancy in a case of familial hypercholesterolemia complicated with coronary artery disease. *J Obstet Gynecol Res*. 2024;50:128-132.

E

EXEMESTANE

Antineoplastic (Aromatase Inhibitor)

PREGNANCY RECOMMENDATION: *Contraindicated

BREASTFEEDING RECOMMENDATION: *Contraindicated

PREGNANCY SUMMARY

No reports describing the use of exemestane in human pregnancy have been located. The drug will probably cross the placenta, so some fetal exposure could occur. *However, the drug is contraindicated for use in premenopausal women. It is indicated for use in postmenopausal women with breast cancer who have been treated with tamoxifen for 2 to 3 years. The drug also prevents the conversion of androgens to estrogen. Because estrogen is required to maintain pregnancy, exemestane is further contraindicated for use during pregnancy. Animal data did show embryofetal toxicity in one animal species at doses less than 10 times the RHD.

BREASTFEEDING SUMMARY

No reports describing the use of exemestane during human lactation have been located. The drug will probably be found in breast milk, so some infant exposure could occur. *However, the drug is contraindicated for use in premenopausal women. Despite this, the manufacturer recommends that women not breastfeed while being treated with exemestane and for at least 1 month after the last dose.

Reference

1. Prescribing Information. Aromasin. Pharmacia & Upjohn Company; 2021.

EZETIMIBE

Antilipemic

PREGNANCY RECOMMENDATION: Limited Human Data—Animal Data Suggest Potential Risk

BREASTFEEDING RECOMMENDATION: Potential Toxicity

PREGNANCY SUMMARY

One case report of exposure to ezetimibe at the time of conception during a human pregnancy was located. The drug was discontinued when the pregnancy was confirmed. She delivered at term a healthy male infant with no reported anomalies. The drug will probably cross the placenta, so some fetal exposure will likely occur. However, this limited human pregnancy experience prevents a complete assessment of the embryofetal risk. Animal data did show embryofetal toxicity in one animal species at doses less than 10 times the RHD. Using this drug during pregnancy should be based on the pros and cons of the mother's clinical need for treatment versus any potential fetal risk that might occur from exposure.

BREASTFEEDING SUMMARY

No reports describing the use of ezetimibe during human lactation have been located. The drug and its active metabolite will probably be found in breast milk, so some fetal exposure will likely occur. There is some thought that women should not breastfeed while being treated with ezetimibe due to possible impaired lipid metabolism. However, breastfeeding while using this drug should be based on the mother's clinical need for treatment. If used, the infant should be monitored for the most common reported adult side effects of extremity pain and arthralgia (both leading to irritability), diarrhea, and upper respiratory tract infection.

E

References

1. Prescribing Information. Zetia. Merck Sharp & Dohme; 2018.
2. Al-Dughaishi T, Al-Waili K, Banerjee Y, et al. Successful direct adsorption of lipoproteins (DALI) apheresis during pregnancy in an Omani woman with homozygous familial hypercholesterolemia. *Open Cardiovasc Med J*. 2015;9:114-117.

F

FACTOR XIII CONCENTRATE (HUMAN)

Hematologic (Antihemophilic)

PREGNANCY RECOMMENDATION: Limited Human Data—No Animal Data (Maternal Benefit May Outweigh Embryofetal Risk)

BREASTFEEDING RECOMMENDATION: Probably Compatible

PREGNANCY SUMMARY

Nine case reports describing the use of Factor XIII in human pregnancy have been located. All pregnancies resulted in healthy newborns with no adverse effects expected or reported. Factor XIII does not cross the placenta but is an endogenous substance that is present in the decidual part of the human placenta. However, this limited human pregnancy experience prevents a complete assessment of the embryofetal risk. No animal studies have been conducted. Congenital Factor XIII deficiency is associated with severe bleeding, impaired wound healing, and, in pregnancy, a high risk of spontaneous abortions. Due to the approved indication for the use of this drug, the mother's clinical need for treatment should outweigh the potential fetal risk that might occur from exposure.

BREASTFEEDING SUMMARY

No reports describing the use of Factor XIII during human lactation have been located. Factor XIII is an endogenous glycoprotein, and excretion into breast milk should not occur. However, even if small amounts were found in breast milk, because it is a glycoprotein, it should be digested in the infant's gastrointestinal tract and have no effect on a nursing infant. Consequently, if a mother with this condition chooses to breastfeed her infant, Factor XIII should not be withheld. If used while breastfeeding, the infant should be monitored for the most commonly reported adult side effects of itching, headache, and joint pain (all leading to irritability) and rash.

References

1. Prescribing Information. Corifact. CSL Behring; 2020.
2. Hsiseh L, Nugent D. Factor XIII deficiency. *Haemophilia*. 2008;14:1190-1200.
3. Karimi M, Bereczky Z, Cohan N, Muszbek L. Factor XIII deficiency. *Semin Thromb Hemost*. 2009;35:426-438.
4. Asahina T, Kobayashi T, Okada Y, et al. Studies on the role of adhesive proteins in maintaining pregnancy. *Horm Res*. 1998;50(suppl 2):37-45.
5. Rodeghiero F, Castaman GC, Di Bona E, et al. Successful pregnancy in a woman with congenital factor XIII deficiency treat with substitutive therapy. *Blut*. 1987;55:45-48.
6. Kobayashi T, Terao T, Kojima T, et al. Congenital factor XIII deficiency with treatment of factor XIII concentrate and normal vaginal delivery. *Gynecol Obstet Invest*. 1990;29:235-238.
7. Burrows RF, Ray JG, Burrows EA. Bleeding risk and reproductive capacity among patients with factor XIII deficiency: a case presentation and review of the literature. *Obstet Gynecol Surv*. 2000;55:103-108.
8. Trigui N, Frère C, D'Ercole C, et al. Molecular characterization of a novel mutation in the factor XIII A subunit gene associated with a severe defect and an adulthood diagnosis. *Haemophilia*. 2007;13(2):221-222.
9. Dargaud Y, de Mazancourt P, Rugeri L, et al. An unusual clinical presentation of factor XIII deficiency and issues relating to the monitoring of factor XIII replacement therapy. *Blood Coagul Fibrinolysis*. 2008;19:447-452
10. Abdel-Samad N. Treatment with recombinant factor XIII (Tretten) in a pregnant woman with factor XIII deficiency. *Am J Case Rep*. 2017;18:436-439.
11. Al-Khabori M, Pathare A, Menegatti M, Peyvandi F. Recombinant factor XIII A-subunit in a patient with factor XIII deficiency and recurrent pregnancy loss. *J Thromb Haemost*. 2018;16(6):1052-1054.
12. Ito Y, Tsuji S, Kasahara M, et al. Successful perinatal management of a woman with congenital factor XIII deficiency using recombinant factor XIII: a case report and literature review. *J Obstet Gynaecol Res*. 2024;50(2):262-265.

FAMCICLOVIR

Antiviral (Herpes Simplex and Varicella Zoster)

PREGNANCY RECOMMENDATION: Limited Human Data—Animal Data Suggest Low Risk

BREASTFEEDING RECOMMENDATION: Probably Compatible

PREGNANCY SUMMARY

Two reports describing the use of famciclovir in human pregnancy during the first trimester were located. One major birth anomaly (3.0%) was seen in 33 pregnancies. The drug will probably cross the placenta, so some fetal exposure will likely occur. However, this limited human pregnancy experience prevents a complete assessment of the embryofetal risk. Animal data did not show any embryofetal toxicity in two species at doses less than 10 times the recommended human dose (RHD). The 2021 Centers for Disease Control and Prevention (CDC) Sexually Transmitted Infections Treatment Guidelines note that data regarding prenatal exposure to famciclovir are limited, but data from animal trials suggest low risk in pregnancy. Regardless, it recommends acyclovir for the treatment of genital herpes during pregnancy as it is believed to be safe for use in all trimesters. There is a pregnancy exposure registry that monitors pregnancy outcomes in women exposed to famciclovir during pregnancy. For more information, health care providers or patients are encouraged to contact Novartis Pharmaceuticals Corporation at 1-888-NOW-NOVA (669-6682).

F

BREASTFEEDING SUMMARY

No studies describing the use of famciclovir during human lactation have been located. The drug will likely be found in breast milk, so some infant exposure will probably occur. Until human data are available, other agents such as acyclovir may be preferred. However, breastfeeding while using this drug should be based on the mother's clinical need for treatment versus any potential infant risks that might occur. If used, the infant should be monitored for the most commonly reported adult side effects of headache and nausea (leading to irritability).

References

1. Prescribing Information. Famciclovir. Apotex; 2019.
2. Wilton LV, Pearce GL, Martin RM, Mackay FJ, Mann RD. The outcomes of pregnancy in women exposed to newly marketed drugs in general practice in England. *Br J Obstet Gynaecol*. 1998;105:882-889.
3. Pasternak B, Hviid A. Use of acyclovir, valacyclovir, and famciclovir in the first trimester of pregnancy and the risk of birth defects. *JAMA*. 2010;304:859-866.
4. Workowski KA, Bachmann LH, Chan PA, et al. Sexually transmitted infections treatment guidelines, 2021. *MMWR Recomm Rep*. 2021;70(4):1-187.

FAMOTIDINE

Gastrointestinal (Histamine H_2 Antagonist)

PREGNANCY RECOMMENDATION: Human Data Suggest Low Risk

BREASTFEEDING RECOMMENDATION: Probably Compatible

PREGNANCY SUMMARY

Several studies have evaluated the use of famotidine in human pregnancy. Of 169 first trimester exposures of famotidine reported from the Swedish Medical Birth Registry, the Michigan Medicaid Data, and the European Network of Teratology, 5 (3%) major anomalies were identified. This is not higher than the expected rate for major birth anomalies. In contrast, a total of 58 (6.6%) major birth defects were reported in 878 first trimester exposures to famotidine from the Soroka Medical Center data from Israel. However, this rate was not significantly different from the 5.3% rate of major birth anomalies seen in the (83,945) pregnancy control population. A meta-analysis of the safety of H_2 blockers in pregnancy overall did not show an increased risk for congenital anomalies. No specific pattern to anomalies has been reported. Famotidine crosses the human placenta, so some fetal exposure will occur. Because of the conflicting data, this human pregnancy experience with famotidine prevents a complete assessment of the embryofetal risk. Animal studies did not show any embryofetal toxicity in two species at doses more than 10 times the RHD. Using this drug during pregnancy should be based on the pros and cons of the mother's clinical need for treatment versus any potential fetal risk that might occur from exposure.

BREASTFEEDING SUMMARY

Two abstracts were located that described the use of famotidine during human lactation. A total of 15 postpartum women were administered total daily doses of 40 mg. Average milk concentrations were about 55 ng/mL with mean peak levels of about 72 ng/mL. Calculated relative infant doses (RIDs) were less than 2%. Breastfeeding while using this drug should be based on the mother's clinical need for treatment versus any potential infant risks that might occur. If used, the infant should be monitored for the most commonly reported adult side effects of headache and dizziness (both leading to irritability), diarrhea, or constipation.

References

1. Prescribing Information. Pepcid. Valeant Pharmaceuticals North America; 2018.
2. Burek JD, Majka JA, Bokelman DL. Famotidine: summary of preclinical safety assessment. *Digestion*. 1985;32(suppl 1):7-14.
3. Shibata M, Kawano K, Shiobara Y, et al. Reproductive studies on famotidine (YM 11170) in rats and rabbits. *Oyo Yakuri*. 1983;26:489-497, 543-578, 831-840. As cited in Shepard TH. *Catalog of Teratogenic Agents*. 6th ed. The Johns Hopkins University Press; 1989:273.

4. Dicke JM, Johnson RF, Henderson GI, et al. A comparative evaluation of the transport of H2-receptor antagonists by the human and baboon placenta. *Am J Med Sci*. 1988;295:198-206.
5. Wang X, Rytting E, Abdelrahman DR, et al. Quantitative determination of famotidine in human maternal plasma, umbilical cord plasma and urine using high-performance liquid chromatography-mass spectrometry. *Biomed Chromatogr*. 2013;27:866-873.
6. Magee LA, Inocencion G, Kamboj L, et al. Safety of first trimester exposure to histamine H2 blockers. A prospective cohort study. *Dig Dis Sci*. 1996;41:1145-1149.
7. Kallen B. Delivery outcome after the use of acid-suppressing drugs in early pregnancy with special reference to omeprazole. *Br J Obstet Gynaecol*. 1998;105:877-881.
8. Garbis H, Elefant E, Diav-Citrin O, et al. Pregnancy outcome after exposure to ranitidine and other H2-blockers—A collaborative study of the European Network of Teratology Information Services. *Reprod Toxicol*. 2005; 453-458.
9. Gill SK, O'Brien L, Koren G. The safety of histamine 2 (H2) blockers in pregnancy: a meta-analysis. *Dig Dis Sci*. 2009;54:1835-1838.
10. Matok I, Gorodischer R, Koren G, et al. The safety of H2-blockers use during pregnancy. *J Clin Pharmacol*. 2010;50:81-7.
11. Courtney TP, Shaw RW, Cedar E, et al. Excretion of famotidine in breast milk. *Br J Clin Pharmacol*. 1988;26:639P.
12. Wang X, Zhan Y, Hankins GD, et al. Pharmacokinetics of famotidine in pregnant women. *Am J Obstet Gynecol*. 2011;204(1):S72-S73.

F

FAM-TRASTUZUMAB DERUXTECAN

Antineoplastic (Monoclonal Antibody and Topoisomerase Inhibitor)

PREGNANCY RECOMMENDATION: No Human Data and No Relevant Animal Data

BREASTFEEDING RECOMMENDATION: Potential Toxicity

PREGNANCY SUMMARY

No reports describing the use of fam-trastuzumab deruxtecan in human pregnancy have been located. Because the monoclonal antibody portion is of the immunoglobulin G (IgG) class, it probably crosses the placenta. In addition, deruxtecan by itself will also probably cross the placenta in limited amounts. Therefore, the absence of human pregnancy experience prevents a complete assessment of the embryofetal risk. In postmarketing reports for human epidermal receptor type 2 (HER2)-directed antibody treatments overall, oligohydramnios and oligohydramnios sequence (pulmonary hypoplasia, skeletal abnormalities, and neonatal death) have been described. The manufacturer recommends effective contraception for women of childbearing age while receiving this treatment and for 7 months after the last dose. They also recommend that males with female partners of reproductive potential use effective contraception during treatment and for 4 months after the last dose. Animal studies have not been performed on this drug. If the clinical decision is to use this drug during gestation for maternal benefit, it is recommended that the pregnancy be followed closely by ultrasound for fetal growth and amniotic fluid volume in the second half of pregnancy. The drug can increase the risk for developing left ventricular dysfunction. Therefore, it is recommended that left ventricular ejection fraction be assessed prior to usage and periodically during treatment. Lastly, it may also lead to severe interstitial lung disease and pneumonitis of which some cases have been fatal.

BREASTFEEDING SUMMARY

Fam-trastuzumab deruxtecan probably enters breast milk in limited amounts. However, if used while breastfeeding, newborn effects from the monoclonal antibody portion would probably be negligible due to likely digestion of the antibody in the infant's gastrointestinal tract. The neonatal effects from exposure to deruxtecan are unknown. Based on the drug's mechanism of action and the potential for newborn toxicity (if infant exposure through breastfeeding were to occur), the manufacturer recommends that women not breastfeed while being treated with this drug and for 7 months after the last dose. Nevertheless, breastfeeding while using this drug should be based on the mother's clinical need for treatment. If used, the infant should be monitored for the most commonly reported adult side effects of nausea and abdominal pain (both leading to irritability), lethargy, decreased appetite, vomiting, diarrhea, constipation, cough, and anemia.

Reference

1. Product Information. Enhertu. Daiichi Sankyo, Inc; 2019.

FARICIMAB

OPHTHALMIC (Vascular Endothelial Growth Factor A and Angiopoietin-2 Inhibitor—Monoclonal Antibody)

PREGNANCY RECOMMENDATION: No Human Data and No Relevant Animal Data

BREASTFEEDING RECOMMENDATION: Probably Compatible

PREGNANCY SUMMARY

No reports describing the use of faricimab in human pregnancy have been located. As an IgG antibody, it can cross the placenta, but based on the low systemic absorption after intravitreal use and the lack of binding to the Fc gamma (Fcg) receptor and the neonatal Fc receptor (FcRn), fetal exposure should be negligible. However, the absence of human pregnancy experience prevents a complete assessment of the embryofetal risk. Embryofetal toxicity was observed in animal studies but after intravenous (IV) administration producing very high systemic exposures. Using this drug during pregnancy should be based on the pros and cons of the mother's clinical need for treatment versus any potential fetal risk that might occur from exposure.

BREASTFEEDING SUMMARY

No reports describing the use of faricimab during human lactation have been located. It is known that IgG antibodies can be found in human breast milk but are not found in the neonatal or infant circulation. Additionally, if any IgG antibodies were to be ingested through breastfeeding, they would probably be digested in the infant's gastrointestinal tract and not be absorbed. Breastfeeding while using this drug should be based on the mother's clinical need for treatment.

Reference

1. Product Information. Vabysmo. Genentech; 2023.

FEBUXOSTAT

Miscellaneous (Antigout)

PREGNANCY RECOMMENDATION: No Human Data—Animal Data Suggest Low Risk

BREASTFEEDING RECOMMENDATION: Probably Compatible

PREGNANCY SUMMARY

No reports describing the use of febuxostat in human pregnancy have been located. The drug will likely cross the placenta, so some fetal exposure will probably occur. Therefore, the absence of human pregnancy experience prevents a complete assessment of the embryofetal risk. Animal studies did not show any embryofetal toxicity in two species at doses more than 10 times the maximum RHD (MRHD). Using this drug during pregnancy should be based on the pros and cons of the mother's clinical need for treatment versus any potential fetal risk that might occur from exposure.

BREASTFEEDING SUMMARY

No reports describing the use of febuxostat during human lactation have been located. The drug will probably be found in breast milk, so some infant exposure will likely occur. Breastfeeding while using this drug should be based on the mother's clinical need for treatment. If used, the infant should be monitored for the most commonly reported adult side effects of nausea and joint pain (both leading to irritability), rash, and liver function abnormalities.

Reference

1. Prescribing Information. Uloric. Takeda Pharmaceuticals America; 2020.

FEDRATINIB

Antineoplastic (Kinase Inhibitor)

PREGNANCY RECOMMENDATION: No Human Data—Animal Data Suggest Potential Risk

BREASTFEEDING RECOMMENDATION: Potential Toxicity

PREGNANCY SUMMARY

No reports describing the use of fedratinib in human pregnancy have been located. Based on likely placental transfer, some fetal exposure will probably occur. Therefore, the absence of human pregnancy experience prevents a complete assessment of the embryofetal risk. Animal studies were shown to cause embryofetal toxicity in one species at doses less than 10 times the RHD. Using this drug during pregnancy should be based on the pros and cons of the mother's clinical need for treatment versus any potential fetal risk that might occur from exposure. There is a registry for women who are pregnant and have cancer. For more information, women and health care providers are encouraged to contact the Cancer and Pregnancy Registry at 1-877-635-4499.

BREASTFEEDING SUMMARY

No reports describing the use of fedratinib during human lactation have been located. The drug will likely be found in breast milk, so some infant exposure will probably occur. Due to the concern for potential serious adverse effects that might be seen in a breastfed infant, the manufacturer recommends that women not breastfeed during treatment and for at least 1 month after the last dose. Nevertheless, breastfeeding while using this drug should be based on the mother's clinical need for treatment. If used, the infant should be monitored for the most commonly reported adult side effects of nausea (leading to irritability), diarrhea, vomiting, and anemia.

Reference

1. Prescribing Information. Inrebic. Celgene; 2023.

F

FELBAMATE

Central Nervous System (Antiseizure)

PREGNANCY RECOMMENDATION: Limited Human Data—Animal Data Suggest Low Risk

BREASTFEEDING RECOMMENDATION: Potential Toxicity

PREGNANCY SUMMARY

The Lamotrigine Pregnancy Registry described two pregnancies exposed in the first trimester to felbamate and lamotrigine. One case was electively terminated, and the other resulted in a live birth without any anomalies. The drug will likely cross the placenta, so fetal exposure will probably occur. Therefore, this limited human pregnancy experience prevents a complete assessment of the embryofetal risk. Animal studies did not show any embryofetal toxicity or malformations in two species (one at less than 10 times the RHD and one at more than 10 times the RHD). Using this drug during pregnancy should be based on the pros and cons of the mother's clinical need for treatment versus any potential fetal risk that might occur from exposure. There is a pregnancy exposure registry that monitors pregnancy outcomes in women exposed to antiepileptic drugs during pregnancy. Health care providers and patients are encouraged to contact the North American Antiepileptic Drug Pregnancy registry at 1-888-233-2334.

BREASTFEEDING SUMMARY

No reports describing the use of felbamate during human lactation have been located. Per the manufacturer, the drug has been detected in human milk. Therefore, due to the concern for potential serious adverse effects (aplastic anemia and liver failure), breastfeeding while using this drug should be based on the mother's clinical need for treatment. If used, the infant should be monitored for the most commonly reported adult side effects of nausea and headache (both leading to irritability), decreased appetite, weight loss, and insomnia.

References

1. Prescribing Information. Felbamate. Amneal Pharmaceuticals LLC; 2022.
2. The Lamotrigine Pregnancy Registry. Final report: 1 September 1992 through 31 March 2010. GlaxoSmithKline. 2010. https://pregnancyregistry.gsk.com > lamotrigine

FELODIPINE

Antihypertensive (Calcium Channel Blocker)

PREGNANCY RECOMMENDATION: Limited Human Data—Animal Data Suggest Potential Risk

BREASTFEEDING RECOMMENDATION: Probably Compatible

PREGNANCY SUMMARY

One case report was located that describes the specific use of felodipine in 3 pregnant patients for treating hypertension. Therapy was started before or during the first trimester in each case. All three delivered term newborns with no identified

(continued)

anomalies. All three neonates were small, with one below the 5th percentile and the others at the 10th and 15th percentiles. Although a contribution from felodipine on newborn size cannot be excluded, the low birth weights were probably secondary to maternal hypertension. In two other prospective, multicenter cohort studies of 377 women that had first trimester exposures to calcium channel blockers, no increase in the risk for major congenital malformations was seen when compared to controls. The drug will probably cross the placenta, so some fetal exposure will likely occur. Therefore, this limited human pregnancy experience prevents a complete assessment of the embryofetal risk. Animal studies did show some embryofetal toxicity, with malformations in one animal species at doses less than 10 times the RHD. Using this drug during pregnancy should be based on the pros and cons of the mother's clinical need for treatment versus any potential fetal risk that might occur from exposure.

F

BREASTFEEDING SUMMARY

No reports describing the use of felodipine during human lactation have been located. The drug will likely be found in breast milk, so some infant exposure will probably occur. Breastfeeding while using this drug should be based on the mother's clinical need for treatment. If used, the infant should be monitored for the most commonly reported adult side effects of headache (leading to irritability), peripheral edema, and cough.

References

1. Prescribing Information. Felodipine. Yiling Pharmaceutical; 2020.
2. Casele HL, Windley KC, Prieto JA, et al. Felodipine use in pregnancy. Report of three cases. *J Reprod Med*. 1997;42:378-381.
3. Magee LA, Schick B, Donnenfeld AE, et al. The safety of calcium channel blockers in human pregnancy: a prospective, multicenter cohort study. *Am J Obstet Gynecol*. 1996;174:823-828.
4. Weber-Schoendorfer C, Hannemann D, Meister R, et al. The safety of calcium channel blockers during pregnancy: a prospective, multicenter, observational study. *Reprod Toxicol*. 2008;26:24-30.

FENOFIBRATE

Antilipemic (Peroxisome Proliferator Receptor-α Agonist)

PREGNANCY RECOMMENDATION: Limited Human Data—Animal Data Suggest Potential Risk

BREASTFEEDING RECOMMENDATION: Potential Toxicity

PREGNANCY SUMMARY

Three case reports describing the use of fenofibrate in human pregnancy have been located. Two infants exposed in the first trimester, where the drug was discontinued upon confirmation of pregnancy, resulted in one healthy newborn with no identified anomalies and a fetal demise at 18 weeks' gestation, 3 weeks after developing acute pancreatitis. A third trimester exposure resulted in a normal, healthy newborn. The drug will probably cross the placenta, so some fetal exposure will likely occur. However, this limited human pregnancy experience prevents a complete assessment of the embryofetal risk. Embryofetal toxicity was not seen at doses about equal to the RHD in two species, but did occur at about 8 to 10 times the RHD (along with maternal toxicity). As with other antilipemic agents, there is likely no benefit from use in otherwise healthy women during gestation. However, fenofibrate may be of benefit in treating or preventing hyperlipidemia-associated pancreatitis. Using this drug during pregnancy should be based on the pros and cons of the mother's clinical need for treatment versus any potential fetal risk that might occur from exposure.

BREASTFEEDING SUMMARY

No reports describing the use of fenofibrate in human lactation have been located. The drug will probably be found in human breast milk, so some infant exposure will likely occur. Due to a concern for potential serious adverse effects that might be seen in a breastfed infant, including impaired lipid metabolism, the manufacturer recommends that women not breastfeed while being treated with this drug and for at least 5 days after the last dose. Nevertheless, breastfeeding while using this drug should be based on the mother's clinical need for treatment versus any potential infant risks that might occur. If used, the infant should be monitored for the most commonly reported adult side effects of nausea (leading to irritability), diarrhea, and elevated liver function tests.

References

1. Prescribing Information. Fenofibrate. AbbVie; 2019.
2. Whitten AE, Lorenz RP, Smith JM. Hyperlipidemia-associated pancreatitis in pregnancy managed with fenofibrate. *Obstet Gynecol*. 2011;117:517-9.
3. Sunman H, Canpolat U, Sahiner L, Aytemir K. Use of fenofibrate during the first trimester of an unplanned pregnancy in a patient with hypertriglyceridemia. *Ann Pharmacother*. 2012;46:e5.
4. Amin J, Poon LCY, Teoh TG, et al. Management of hypertriglyceridaemia-induced acute pancreatitis in pregnancy. *J Matern Fetal Neonatal Med*. 2015;28:954-958.

FENOLDOPAM

Antihypertensive (Dopamine Agonist)

PREGNANCY RECOMMENDATION: No Human Data—Animal Data Suggest Low Risk

BREASTFEEDING RECOMMENDATION: Potential Toxicity

F

PREGNANCY SUMMARY

No reports describing the use of fenoldopam in human pregnancy have been located. The drug will likely cross the placenta, so some fetal exposure is possible. Therefore, the absence of human pregnancy experience prevents a complete assessment of the embryofetal risk. Fenoldopam was studied regarding any vascular responses that might occur with the human umbilical artery. At normal treatment levels, no significant differences were seen. Vasoconstriction was seen with fenoldopam, but at supratherapeutic concentrations. Animal studies did not show any embryofetal toxicity or malformations in two species at doses less than 10 times the RHD. Because it is used for the emergency reduction of severe hypertension, the maternal benefit probably outweighs the unknown fetal risk. However, a rapid reduction of maternal blood pressure could compromise placental perfusion, potentially resulting in fetal hypoxia and subsequent bradycardia. Fetal heart rate monitoring, therefore, is recommended during IV infusions of fenoldopam, if the gestational age warrants monitoring.

BREASTFEEDING SUMMARY

No reports describing the use of fenoldopam during human lactation have been located. The drug will probably be found in breast milk, so some infant exposure is possible. Because of the nature of the drug's indication, opportunities for using fenoldopam during breastfeeding are probably rare. If the clinical decision is to use this drug while breastfeeding, the infant should be monitored for the most commonly reported adult side effects of headache and nausea (leading to irritability), hypotension, and flushing.

References

1. Prescribing Information. Corlopam. Hospira; 2021.
2. Sato N, Tanaka KA, Szlam F, et al. The vasodilatory effects of hydralazine, nicardipine, nitroglycerin, and fenoldopam in the human umbilical artery. *Anesth Analg*. 2003;96:539-544.

FENOPROFEN

Pain (Nonsteroidal Anti-Inflammatory Drug)

PREGNANCY RECOMMENDATION: Human Data Suggest Risk in the Third Trimester

BREASTFEEDING RECOMMENDATION: Probably Compatible

PREGNANCY SUMMARY

In a surveillance study of Michigan Medicaid recipients, 191 newborns had been exposed to fenoprofen during the first trimester. A total of six (3.1%) major birth defects were observed. In addition, no specific pattern to the anomalies was identified. Several studies have looked at nonsteroidal anti-inflammatory drugs (NSAIDs) as a group and have found mixed results regarding embryofetal toxicity and malformations. Overall, their use does not appear to significantly increase the risk for birth defects or preterm delivery. Constriction of the ductus arteriosus in utero is a pharmacologic consequence arising from the use of prostaglandin synthesis inhibitors during pregnancy. Persistent pulmonary hypertension of the newborn may occur if these agents are used in the third trimester close to birth. These drugs have also been shown to inhibit labor and prolong pregnancy, in humans (see Indomethacin). The drug will likely cross the placenta, so some fetal exposure will probably occur. Therefore, this limited human pregnancy experience prevents a complete assessment of the embryofetal risk. Animal studies did not show any embryofetal toxicity or malformations in two species at doses less than 10 times the RHD. Using this drug during pregnancy should be based on the pros and cons of the mother's clinical need for treatment versus any potential fetal risk that might occur from exposure. The drug may also cause oligohydramnios if frequently used after 20 weeks gestation.

BREASTFEEDING SUMMARY

Fenoprofen was found to pass into breast milk (consistent with its molecular weight [MW]). The amount in milk, however, is low at about 1.6% of the maternal plasma levels. This percentage would result in a calculated RID of below 10%. Breastfeeding while using this drug should be based on the mother's clinical need for treatment. If used, the infant should be monitored for the most commonly reported adult side effects of nausea, headache, and abdominal pain (all leading to irritability), diarrhea, insomnia, vomiting, and rash.

References

1. Prescribing Information. Fenoprofen. Xspire Pharma; 2020.
2. Rubin A, Chernish SM, Crabtree R, et al. A profile of the physiological disposition and gastro-intestinal effects of fenoprofen in man. *Curr Med Res Opin*. 1974;2:529-544.
3. Nielsen GL, Sorensen HT, Larsen H, et al. Risk of adverse birth outcome and miscarriage in pregnant users of non-steroidal anti-inflammatory drugs: population based observational study and case-control study. *Br Med J*. 2001;322:266-270.
4. Ericson A, Kallen BAJ. Nonsteroidal anti-inflammatory drugs in early pregnancy. *Reprod Toxicol*. 2001;15:371-375.
5. Li DK, Liu L, Odouli R. Exposure to non-steroidal anti-inflammatory drugs during pregnancy and risk of miscarriage: population based cohort study. *Br Med J*. 2003;327:368-371.
6. Tassinari MS, Cook JC, Hurtt ME. NSAIDs and developmental toxicity. *Birth Defects Res B Dev Reprod Toxicol*. 2003;68:3-4.
7. Levin DL. Effects of inhibition of prostaglandin synthesis on fetal development, oxygenation, and the fetal circulation. *Semin Perinatol*. 1980;4:35-44.
8. Van Marter LJ, Leviton A, Allred EN, et al. Persistent pulmonary hypertension of the newborn and smoking and aspirin and nonsteroidal anti-inflammatory drug consumption during pregnancy. *Pediatrics*. 1996;97:658-663.
9. Fuchs F. Prevention of prematurity. *Am J Obstet Gynecol*. 1976;126:809-820.

FENTANYL

Pain (Opioid)

PREGNANCY RECOMMENDATION: **Human Data Suggest Low Risk in the First Trimester/*Human Data Suggest Risk for Chronic Use**

BREASTFEEDING RECOMMENDATION: **Potential Toxicity**

PREGNANCY SUMMARY

Limited studies have evaluated the use of fentanyl in the first trimester. One case report described the use of the drug throughout pregnancy, and no birth anomalies were identified postdelivery. The infant did experience neonatal opioid withdrawal syndrome (NOWS). Numerous other studies have described the use of fentanyl during labor and delivery in conjunction with epidural anesthesia and with cesarean section, and no major adverse outcomes have been described. The National Birth Defects Prevention Study reported an overall rate of 2.6% for major birth anomalies in patients that filled any opioid prescription in the first trimester. This rate was significantly higher than the 2.0% rate in the unexposed control group, but falls within the expected rate for major birth defects in the United States of 2% to 4%. Separate numbers for fentanyl were not provided. For the opioid exposed group, there was a higher rate for cardiovascular and neural tube defects (NTDs), as well as gastroschisis when compared with the control group. However, self-reported recall history can be flawed (in some cases, the interview occurred up to 3 years after the patient's first trimester); verification of actual drug use, the dosage, and exact timing of use during the first trimester cannot be confirmed; and recall may be affected by whether or not a mother delivered a newborn with an anomaly. A few other large database studies have been conducted that were linked to pharmacy prescriptions filled for opioid drugs. Most showed no higher rate for major anomalies when compared with controls. None of these studies could be controlled for illicit opioid use. Lastly, several studies have identified smaller newborn head circumferences at birth in neonates exposed to opiates chronically throughout gestation. The clinical significance of this is unknown. Fentanyl crosses the placenta. However, this limited human pregnancy experience prevents a complete assessment of the embryofetal risk. Embryofetal toxicity was observed in one animal species at doses less than 10 times the RHD. *Neonatal abstinence syndrome (NAS) or NOWS may occur with prolonged exposure to opioids near delivery. The drug carries a Boxed Warning for risks of misuse, addiction; life-threatening respiratory depression; NOWS; and, when combined with benzodiazepines and other central nervous system (CNS) depressants, profound sedation, coma, and death. The drug is a controlled Schedule II substance.

BREASTFEEDING SUMMARY

Several reports were located that evaluated breast milk samples for the presence of fentanyl that was administered during labor and delivery. In cases of a single epidural injection, the drug was not detected in colostrum (lower limit of quantification [LLQ] 100 pg/mL). When administered IV prior to delivery, the drug was detected in colostrum, as it was with continuous epidural fentanyl administration. In all cases, the calculated RIDs were less than 1%. In addition, the usual dose of fentanyl for an infant is about 1 to 2 mcg/kg IV. The measured amounts of the drug in breast milk were all calculated to be less than 10% of this dosage, plus they were oral. One case of a mother using a transdermal patch for chronic pain had higher milk levels than described earlier. Using the measured level, the amount consumed in 24 hours per kilogram was close to 1 mcg/kg (a normal newborn dose). However, infant blood levels were not detected (LLQ of 100 pg/mL). This may be due to the oral exposure compared with IV usage. Breastfeeding while using this drug should be based on the mother's clinical need for treatment versus any potential infant risks that might occur. If used, the infant should be monitored for the most commonly reported adult side effects of drowsiness, sedation, difficulty feeding, or lethargy.

References

1. Prescribing Information. Duragesic. Janssen Pharmaceutica; 2018.
2. Shannon C, Jauniaux E, Gulbis B, et al. Placental transfer of fentanyl in early human pregnancy. *Hum Reprod*. 1998;13:2317-2320.
3. Rayburn W, Rathke A, Leuschen MP, et al. Fentanyl citrate analgesia during labor. *Am J Obstet Gynecol*. 1989;161:202-206.

4. Carrie LES, O'Sullivan GM, Seegobin R. Epidural fentanyl in labour. *Anaesthesia*. 1981;36:965-969.
5. Johnson ES, Colley PS. Effects of nitrous oxide and fentanyl anesthesia on fetal heart-rate variability intra-and postoperatively. *Anesthesiology*. 1980;52:429-430.
6. Viscomi CM, Hood DD, Melone PJ, Eisenach JC. Fetal heart rate variability after epidural fentanyl during labor. *Anesth Analg*. 1990;71:679-683.
7. Justins DM, Francis D, Houlton PG, Reynolds F. A controlled trial of extradural fentanyl in labour. *Br J Anaesth*. 1982;54:409-413.
8. Milon D, Bentue-Ferrer D, Noury D, et al. Peridural anesthesia for cesarean section employing a bupivacaine-fentanyl combination. *Ann Fr Anesth Reanim*. 1983;2:273-279.
9. Fernando R, Bonello E, Gill P, et al. Neonatal welfare and placental transfer of fentanyl and bupivacaine during ambulatory combined spinal epidural analgesia for labour. *Anaesthesia*. 1997;52:517-524.
10. Benlabed M, Dreizzen E, Ecoffey C, et al. Neonatal patterns of breathing after cesarean section with or without epidural fentanyl. *Anesthesiology*. 1990;73:1110-1113.
11. Halonen PM, Paatero H, Hovorka J, et al. Comparison of two fentanyl doses to improve epidural anaesthesia with 0.5% bupivacaine for caesarean section. *Acta Anaesthesiol Scand*. 1993;37:774-779.
12. Porter J, Bonello E, Reynolds F. Effect of epidural fentanyl on neonatal respiration. *Anesthesiology*. 1998;89:79-85.
13. Bader AM, Fragneto R, Terui K, et al. Maternal and neonatal fentanyl and bupivacaine concentrations after epidural infusion during labor. *Anesth Analg*. 1995;81:829-832.
14. Eisele JH, Wright R, Rogge P. Newborn and maternal fentanyl levels at cesarean section (abstract). *Anesth Analg*. 1982;61:179-180.
15. Lindemann R. Respiratory muscle rigidity in a preterm infant after use of fentanyl during Caesarean section. *Eur J Pediatr*. 1998;157:1012-1013.
16. Regan J, Chambers F, Gorman W, MacSullivan R. Neonatal abstinence syndrome due to prolonged administration of fentanyl in pregnancy. *Br J Obstet Gynaecol*. 2000;107:570-572.
17. Broussard CS, Rasmussen SA, Reefhuis J, et al; National Birth Defects Prevention Study. Maternal treatment with opioid analgesics and risk for birth defects. *Am J Obstet Gynecol*. 2011;204:314-317.
18. Steer PL, Biddle CJ, Marley WS, et al. Concentration of fentanyl in colostrum after an analgesic dose. *Can J Anaesth*. 1992;39:231-235.
19. Committee opinion no. 711: opioid use and opioid use disorder in pregnancy. *Obstet Gynecol*. 2017;130:e81-e94.
20. American College of Obstetricians and Gynecologists' Committee on Practice Bulletins—Obstetrics. ACOG Practice Bulletin No. 209: obstetric analgesia and anesthesia. *Obstet Gynecol*. 2019;133:e208-25.

F

FERRIC MALTOL

Hematologic (Iron Supplement)

PREGNANCY RECOMMENDATION: No Human Data—Animal Data Suggest Low Risk

BREASTFEEDING RECOMMENDATION: Compatible

PREGNANCY SUMMARY

No reports describing the specific use of ferric maltol in human pregnancy have been located. The full supplement is not absorbed systemically as an intact complex. Iron does cross the placenta, more so in the third trimester. Maltol will also probably cross the placenta, but is not expected to cause any adverse fetal effects. Animal studies did not show any embryofetal toxicity. Iron supplementation is often recommended during pregnancy.

BREASTFEEDING SUMMARY

Ferric maltol is not absorbed systemically as an intact complex, so it will not be found in breast milk. Breast milk contains very little iron. Maltol will also probably be found in breast milk but is not expected to cause any adverse newborn effects.

Reference

1. Product Information. Accrufer. Shield TX (UK) Ltd; 2019.

FESOTERODINE

Urinary (Anticholinergic)

PREGNANCY RECOMMENDATION: No Human Data—Animal Data Suggest Low Risk

BREASTFEEDING RECOMMENDATION: Probably Compatible

PREGNANCY SUMMARY

No reports describing the use of fesoterodine in human pregnancy have been located. Based on likely placental transfer, some fetal exposure will probably occur. Therefore, the absence of human pregnancy experience prevents a complete assessment of the embryofetal risk. Animal studies did not show any embryofetal toxicity in two species at doses less than 10 times the RHD. Using this drug during pregnancy should be based on the pros and cons of the mother's clinical need for treatment versus any potential fetal risk that might occur from exposure.

BREASTFEEDING SUMMARY

No reports describing the use of fesoterodine during human lactation have been located. The drug and the active metabolite will probably be found in breast milk, so some infant exposure will likely occur. Anticholinergic drugs can decrease serum prolactin levels and have been known to inhibit lactation in animals, especially with long-term use. Therefore, breastfeeding while using this drug should be based on the mother's clinical need for treatment. If used, the infant should be monitored for the most commonly reported adult side effects of dry mouth and constipation.

References

1. Prescribing Information. Toviaz. Pfizer Laboratories; 2021.
2. Masala A, Alagna S, Devilla L, et al. Muscarinic receptor blockade by pirenzepine: effect on prolactin secretion in man. 1982;5:53-55.
3. Aaron DK, Ely DG, Deweese WP, et al. Reducing milk production in ewes at weaning using restricted feeding and methscopolamine bromide. *J Anim Sci.* 1997;75:1434-1442.

F

FEXINIDAZOLE

Antimicrobial (Antiparasitic)

PREGNANCY RECOMMENDATION: No Human Data—Animal Data Suggest Potential Risk

BREASTFEEDING RECOMMENDATION: Potential Toxicity

PREGNANCY SUMMARY

No reports describing the use of fexinidazole in human pregnancy have been located. Fexinidazole and its two active metabolites will likely cross the placenta, so some fetal exposure will probably occur. Therefore, the absence of human pregnancy experience prevents a complete assessment of the embryofetal risk. Embryofetal toxicity with malformations was observed in animal studies. Human African trypanosomiasis should be treated during pregnancy to decrease the risk for disease progression and decrease the risk for vertical transmission. The manufacturer recommends that providers consider the timing of treatment during pregnancy and consider the benefits of fexinidazole to the mother and potential risks to the fetus. Fexinidazole can also prolong the QT interval.

BREASTFEEDING SUMMARY

No reports describing the use of fexinidazole during human lactation have been located. The drug and its active metabolites will likely be excreted into breast milk, so some infant exposure will probably occur. Breastfeeding while using this drug should be based on the mother's clinical need for treatment. If used, the infant should be monitored for the most commonly reported adult side effects of headache, nausea, back pain, and abdominal pain (all leading to irritability), vomiting, poor sleeping, tremor, decreased appetite (monitor growth), hypocalcemia, and hyperkalemia.

Reference

1. Product Information. Fexinidazole. Sanofi-Aventis US; 2021.

FEXOFENADINE

Antihistamine (Histamine H_1 Antagonist/Second Generation)

PREGNANCY RECOMMENDATION: Limited Human Data—Animal Data Suggest Potential Risk

BREASTFEEDING RECOMMENDATION: Probably Compatible

PREGNANCY SUMMARY

The safety of fexofenadine use in pregnancy was evaluated in the nationwide registry-based data from Denmark. Exposure was based on prescriptions filled at any time ranging from 12 weeks prior to conception up to the late third trimester. Risk comparisons were between fexofenadine and an equal number of cetirizine matched controls. No increased risk for major birth defects, spontaneous abortion, preterm birth, and stillbirth was found. In addition, from a safety study on fexofenadine from England using returned questionnaires, no adverse effects related to the drug were seen in 47 reported pregnancies. However, gestational age of use, dosing, and other information were not provided. The recommendations (from a joint committee involving the American College of Obstetricians and Gynecologists [ACOG] and the American College of Allergy, Asthma, and Immunology) are to use oral first-generation antihistamines (such as chlorpheniramine or hydroxyzine) if antihistamine therapy during pregnancy (especially in the first trimester) is required. Second-generation agents, cetirizine or loratadine, were considered acceptable alternatives (not for the first trimester), if a first-generation antihistamine was not tolerated. The drug appears to cross the placenta, so some fetal exposure will likely occur. Therefore, this limited human pregnancy experience (especially first trimester exposure) prevents a complete assessment of the embryofetal risk. Animal studies did not show any embryofetal toxicity or malformations in three species at doses more (two) and less (one) than 10 times the RHD. However, there was some neonatal toxicity seen in one species at doses less than 10 times the RHD. Using this drug during pregnancy should be based on the pros and cons of the mother's clinical need for treatment versus any potential fetal risk that might occur from exposure.

BREASTFEEDING SUMMARY

No reports describing the use of fexofenadine during human lactation have been located. However, fexofenadine is the major active metabolite of terfenadine. One study on terfenadine use during lactation in four women found a maximum concentration of fexofenadine of about 41 ng/mL in breast milk with a milk to plasma ratio of about 0.13. The calculated maximum RID was only 0.45%. Breastfeeding while using this drug should be based on the mother's clinical need for treatment. If used, the infant should be monitored for the most commonly reported adult side effects of nausea, abdominal pain, headache, extremity pain, and back pain (all leading to irritability), diarrhea, vomiting, and somnolence.

References

1. Prescribing Information. Allegra allergy. Sanofi Consumer Health Inc; 2020.
2. Pinto LSR, Tavares do Vale G, de Lima Moreira F, et al. Direct chiral LC-MS/MS analysis of fexofenadine enantiomers in plasma and urine with application in a maternal-fetal pharmacokinetic study. *J Chromatogr B Analyt Technol Biomed Life Sci*. 2020;1145:122094.
3. Pinto L, Bapat P, de Lime Moreira F, et al. Chiral transplacental pharmacokinetics of fexofenadine: impact of P-glycoprotein inhibitor fluoxetine using the human placental perfusion model. *Pharm Res*. 2021;38:647-655.
4. Andersson NW, Torp-Pedersen C, Andersen JT. Association between fexofenadine use during pregnancy and fetal outcomes. *JAMA Pediatr*. 2020;174:e201316.
5. Craig-McFeely PM, Acharya NV, Shakir SA. Evaluation of the safety of fexofenadine from experience gained in general practice use in England in 1997. *Eur J Clin Pharacol*. 2001;57: 313-320.
6. Joint committee of the American College of Obstetricians and Gynecologists (ACOG) and the American College of Allergy, Asthma and Immunology (ACAAI). Position statement. The use of newer asthma and allergy medications during pregnancy. *Ann Allergy Asthma Immunol*. 2000;84:475-480.
7. Lucas BD, Purdy CY, Scarim SK, et al. Terfenadine pharmacokinetics in breast milk in lactating women. *Clin Pharmacol Ther*. 1995;57:398-402.

FEZOLINETANT

Miscellaneous

PREGNANCY RECOMMENDATION: *Contraindicated

BREASTFEEDING RECOMMENDATION: *Contraindicated

PREGNANCY SUMMARY

No reports describing the use of fezolinetant in human pregnancy have been located. The drug would likely cross the placenta, so some fetal exposure would probably occur. Animal data did not show any embryofetal toxicity. *However, because the drug is approved for use in menopausal women, it is contraindicated for use during pregnancy.

BREASTFEEDING SUMMARY

No reports describing the use of fezolinetant during human lactation have been located. The drug would likely be excreted into breast milk, so some infant exposure would probably occur. *However, because the drug is approved for use in menopausal women, it is contraindicated during pregnancy and lactation.

Reference

1. Product Information. Veozah. Astellas Pharma US Inc; 2023.

FIBRIN SEALANT (HUMAN)

Hematologic (Hemostatic Agent)

PREGNANCY RECOMMENDATION: No Human Data and No Relevant Animal Data

BREASTFEEDING RECOMMENDATION: Probably Compatible

PREGNANCY SUMMARY

No reports describing the use of fibrin sealant in pregnancy have been located. It is likely that this hematologic agent will not cross the placenta in any clinically significant amount, if at all. Therefore, fetal exposure is unlikely. However, the absence of

(*continued*)

human pregnancy experience prevents a complete assessment of the embryofetal risk. No animal reproduction studies have been conducted. Using this drug during pregnancy should be based on the pros and cons of the mother's clinical need for treatment versus any potential fetal risk that might occur from exposure. Fibrin sealant is made from human plasma, so it theoretically could carry the risk of transmitting bloodborne viral infections.

BREASTFEEDING SUMMARY

No reports describing the use of fibrin sealant (human) during human lactation have been located. Infant exposure through breastfeeding should not occur. Additionally, if the drug were to be ingested through breastfeeding, it would probably be digested in the infant's gastrointestinal tract and not be absorbed. Breastfeeding while using this drug should be based on the mother's clinical need for treatment versus any potential infant risks that might occur. Because this agent is applied topically, systemic adverse reactions were not analyzed.

F

References

1. Prescribing Information. Artiss. Baxter Healthcare; 2022.
2. Ben-Rafael Z, Ashkenazi J, Shelef M, et al. The use of fibrin sealant in in vitro fertilization and embryo transfer. *Int J Fertil Menopausal Stud.* 1995;40:303-306.
3. Bar-Hava I, Krissi H, Ashkenazi J, et al. Fibrin glue improves pregnancy rates in women of advanced reproductive age and in patients in whom in vitro fertilization attempts repeatedly fail. *Fertil Steril.* 1999;71:821-824.

FIDAXOMICIN

Antibacterial (Macrolide)

PREGNANCY RECOMMENDATION: Limited Human Data—Animal Data Suggest Low Risk

BREASTFEEDING RECOMMENDATION: Probably Compatible

PREGNANCY SUMMARY

A single case report of fidaxomicin use in the first trimester of human pregnancy was located. A patient with a recurrent *Clostridium difficile* infection was treated with fidaxomicin and vancomycin for 10 days during the first trimester of an unknown pregnancy. She delivered at term, a normal infant with no reported anomalies. Due to poor oral absorption, a negligible amount of drug may cross the placenta, but overall, the levels would likely be clinically insignificant. However, this limited human pregnancy experience prevents a complete assessment of the embryofetal risk. Animal studies did not show any embryofetal toxicity in two species at doses more than 10 times the RHD. Using this drug during pregnancy should be based on the pros and cons of the mother's clinical need for treatment versus any potential fetal risk that might occur from exposure.

BREASTFEEDING SUMMARY

No reports describing the use of fidaxomicin during human lactation have been located. The amount of drug that may be found in breast milk is likely to be clinically insignificant. Breastfeeding while using this drug should be based on the mother's clinical need for treatment. If used, the infant should be monitored for the most commonly reported side effects of nausea and abdominal pain (both leading to irritability), diarrhea, and rash.

References

1. Prescribing Information. Dificid. Merck Sharp & Dohme; 2022.
2. Saeedi BJ, Morison DG, Kraft CS, Dhere T. Fecal microbiota transplant for *Clostridium difficile* infection in a pregnant patient. *Obstet Gynecol.* 2017;129:507-9.

FILGRASTIM

Hematologic (Granulocyte Colony-Stimulating Factor)

PREGNANCY RECOMMENDATION: Limited Human Data—Animal Data Suggest Potential Risk

BREASTFEEDING RECOMMENDATION: Probably Compatible

PREGNANCY SUMMARY

Limited reports describing the use of filgrastim during human pregnancy were found. Excluding two elective terminations, six patients had first trimester exposure that resulted in five infants without major anomalies and one termination for abnormal findings on ultrasound (defects not described). An additional 16 pregnancies received treatment for a median of about 2 months during gestation, resulting in 13 normal newborns without any identified anomalies and 3 spontaneous abortions. However, the exact time during the pregnancy when treatment occurred was not specified. At least seven other exposures to filgrastim that occurred in the second and third trimesters did not describe any drug-related complications. It appears that the drug crosses the placenta at least in the second half of gestation, but amounts are difficult to quantify. However, some fetal exposure likely occurs. Regardless, this limited human pregnancy experience prevents a complete assessment of the embryofetal risk. Embryofetal toxicity was observed in one animal species at doses less than 10 times the RHD, but some maternal toxicity also occurred. Using this drug during pregnancy should be based on the pros and cons of the mother's clinical need for treatment versus any potential fetal risk that might occur from exposure.

F

BREASTFEEDING SUMMARY

Granulocyte colony-stimulating factor (G-CSF) is considered a normal component of breast milk. One case report was located that described the use of filgrastim during human lactation. The patient was administered the drug for the purpose of donation. The G-CSF level was undetectable prior to treatment (LLQ 10 pg/mL). The peak level obtained during therapy was 188 pg/mL. A similar finding was seen in a breastfeeding woman who received lenograstim for the purpose of donation. These levels are very low. Furthermore, filgrastim was administered orally to preterm infants and was found not to be systemically absorbed. This is consistent with the drug being a glycoprotein, in that it would likely be digested in the infant's gastrointestinal tract. Breastfeeding while using this drug should be based on the mother's clinical need for treatment. If the clinical decision is to use this drug while breastfeeding, the infant should be monitored for the most commonly reported adult side effects of pain (leading to irritability), rash, fever, cough, and anemia.

References

1. Prescribing Information. Neupogen. Amgen; 2023.
2. Calhoun DA, Ross C, Christensen RD. Transplacental passage of recombinant human granulocyte colony-stimulating factor in women with an imminent preterm delivery. *Am J Obstet Gynecol*. 1996;174:1306-1311.
3. Calhoun DA, Christensen RD. A randomized pilot trial of administration of granulocyte colony-stimulating factor to women before preterm delivery. *Am J Obstet Gynecol*. 1998;179:766-771.
4. Cavenagh JD, Richardson DS, Cahill MR, et al. Treatment of acute myeloid leukaemia in pregnancy. *Lancet*. 1995;346: 441-442.
5. Lin C-P, Huang M-J, Liu H-J, et al. Successful treatment of acute promyelocytic leukemia in a pregnant Jehovah's Witness with all-trans retinoic acid, rhG-CSF, and erythropoietin. *Am J Hematol*. 1996;51:251-252.
6. Arango HA, Kalter CS, Decesare SL, et al. Management of chemotherapy in a pregnancy complicated by a large neuroblastoma. *Obstet Gynecol*. 1994;84:665-668.
7. Welter K, Boxer LA. Severe chronic neutropenia: pathophysiology and therapy. *Semin Hematol*. 1997;34:267-78.
8. Cavallaro AM, Lilleby K, Majolino I, et al. Three to six year follow-up of normal donors who received recombinant human granulocyte colony-stimulating factor. *Bone Marrow Transplant*. 2000;25:85-89.
9. Sangalli MR, Peek M, McDonald A. Prophylactic granulocyte colony-stimulating factor treatment for acquired chronic severe neutropenia in pregnancy. *Aust N Z J Obstet Gynaecol*. 2001;41:470-471.
10. Cottle TE, Fier CJ, Donadieu J, Kinsey SE. Risk and benefit of treatment of severe chronic neutropenia with granulocyte colony-stimulating factor. *Semin Hematol*. 2002;39:134-140.
11. Dale DC, Cottle TE, Fier CJ, et al. Severe chronic neutropenia: treatment and follow up of patients in the Severe Chronic Neutropenia International Registry. *Am J Hematol*. 2003;72:82-93.
12. Kaida K, Ikegame K, Fujioka T, et al. Kinetics of granulocyte colony-stimulating factor in the human milk of a nursing donor receiving treatment for mobilization of the peripheral blood stem cells. *Acta Haematol*. 2007;118:176-177.
13. Calhoun DA, Maheshwari A, Christensen RD. Recombinant granulocyte colony-stimulating factor administered enterally to neonates is not absorbed. *Pediatrics*. 2003;112:421-423.

FINERENONE

Renal (Nonsteroidal Mineralocorticoid Receptor Antagonist)

PREGNANCY RECOMMENDATION: No Human Data—Animal Data Suggest Potential Risk

BREASTFEEDING RECOMMENDATION: Potential Toxicity

PREGNANCY SUMMARY

No reports describing the use of finerenone in human pregnancy have been located. Finerenone is likely to cross the placenta, so some fetal exposure will probably occur. Therefore, the absence of human pregnancy experience prevents a complete assessment of embryofetal risk. Embryofetal toxicity was observed in animal studies. Using this drug during pregnancy should be based on the pros and cons of the mother's clinical need for treatment versus any potential fetal risk that might occur from exposure.

BREASTFEEDING SUMMARY

No reports describing the use of finerenone during human lactation have been located. The drug will likely appear in breast milk, so some infant exposure will probably occur. Due to the potential for adverse effects that might be seen in a breastfed infant (based on animal studies), the manufacturer recommends that women not breastfeed while taking finerenone or for 1 day after the last dose. Nevertheless, if the clinical decision is to use this drug while breastfeeding, the infant should be monitored for the most commonly reported adult side effects of hyperkalemia, hyponatremia, and hypotension.

Reference

1. Product Information. Kerendia. Bayer Healthcare Pharmaceuticals; 2022.

F

FINGOLIMOD

Immunologic (Sphingosine 1-Phosphate Modulator)

PREGNANCY RECOMMENDATION: Limited Human Data—Animal Data Suggest Potential Risk

BREASTFEEDING RECOMMENDATION: Potential Toxicity

PREGNANCY SUMMARY

In data from the phase II, III, and IV clinical trials, excluding elective terminations, ongoing pregnancies, and lost to follow-up, 37 pregnancies resulted in 9 (24%) spontaneous losses and 28 live births with 1 (3.6%) major anomaly. In a second large study of known outcomes from the Novartis Safety Database (that contains data from the Registry, *PR*egnancy outcomes *I*ntensive *M*onitoring—PRIM database, and other cases outside these two entities reported to Novartis), there were 482 exposures to fingolimod with 19 (3.9%) congenital anomalies. This rate is no different than the expected rate for birth anomalies in the United States, and no pattern to the defects was seen. Use occurred at the time of conception, first trimester, and after the first trimester, but data on what anomalies occurred and what gestational age were not provided. The drug will probably cross the placenta, so some fetal exposure will likely occur. However, this limited human pregnancy experience prevents a complete assessment of the embryofetal risk. Embryofetal toxicity was observed in one species at doses less than 10 times the RHD, but not in another species at doses more than 10 times the RHD. The receptor affected by fingolimod participates in angiogenesis and is known to be involved in vascular formation during embryogenesis. In addition, the drug can prolong the QT interval and also cause atrioventricular blockade. Based on animal studies and the drug's mechanism of action, the manufacturer recommends that women with reproductive potential use effective contraception during treatment and for 2 months after the last dose. Nevertheless, using this drug during pregnancy should be based on the pros and cons of the mother's clinical need for treatment versus any potential fetal risk that might occur from exposure. There is a pregnancy exposure registry that monitors pregnancy outcomes in women exposed to fingolimod during pregnancy. Physicians are encouraged to enroll pregnant patients, or pregnant women may register themselves in the GILENYA Pregnancy Registry by calling 1-877-598-7237.

BREASTFEEDING SUMMARY

No reports describing the use of fingolimod during human lactation have been located. The drug and its active metabolite will probably be found in human breast milk, so some infant exposure will likely occur. Breastfeeding while using this drug should be based on the mother's clinical need for treatment. If used, the infant should be monitored for the most commonly reported adult side effects of back pain and headache (both leading to irritability), diarrhea, cough, and elevated liver function tests.

References

1. Prescribing Information. Gilenya. Novartis Pharmaceuticals; 2023.
2. Schmid G, Guba M, Ischenko I, et al. The immunosuppressant FTY720 inhibits tumor angiogenesis via the sphingosine 1-phosphate receptor 1. *J Cell Biochem*. 2007;101:259-270.
3. Chun J, Hartung H-P. Mechanism of action of oral fingolimod (FTY720) in multiple sclerosis. *Clin Neuropharmacol*. 2010;33:91-101.
4. Karlsson G, Francis G, Koren G, et al. Pregnancy outcomes in the clinical development program of fingolimod in multiple sclerosis. *Neurology*. 2014;82:674-680.
5. Navardi S, Sahraian MA. A case of dextrocardia following maternal exposure to generic Fingolimod during the first trimester of pregnancy. *Mult Scler Relat Disord*. 2018;21:69-70.
6. Geissbuhler Y, Vile J, Koren G, et al. Evaluation of pregnancy outcomes in patients with multiple sclerosis after fingolimod exposure. *Ther Adv Neurol Disord*. 2018;11:1756286418804760.

FISH OIL TRIGLYCERIDES

Nutrition (Caloric and Essential Fatty Acid Emulsion)

PREGNANCY RECOMMENDATION: No Human Data and No Relevant Animal Data

BREASTFEEDING RECOMMENDATION: Probably Compatible

PREGNANCY SUMMARY

No reports describing the specific use of this fish oil triglyceride emulsion in human pregnancy have been located. The product contains essential fatty acids, and most if not all of the lipids found within this emulsion will cross the placenta. Animal studies have not been performed.

BREASTFEEDING SUMMARY

The fatty acids found in fish oil triglycerides will be found in breast milk. Preterm and small-for-gestational-age newborns have poor clearance of the lipid emulsion itself, and this could lead to pulmonary lipid accumulation or fat overload syndrome. Lactating women receiving oral omega-3 fatty acids have been shown to have higher levels of these fatty acids in their milk. However, the amounts of fatty acids absorbed by the infant through breastfeeding alone are not likely to be significantly increased.

Reference

1. Product Information. Omegaven. Fresenius Kabi; 2018.

F

FLAVOXATE

Urinary (Antispasmodic/Anticholinergic)

PREGNANCY RECOMMENDATION: Limited Human Data—Animal Data Suggest Low Risk

BREASTFEEDING RECOMMENDATION: Probably Compatible

PREGNANCY SUMMARY

No studies describing the use of flavoxate in the first trimester of human pregnancy were located. One study was identified that described the use of flavoxate as a tocolytic agent in 66 women with premature labor. No adverse effects were noted in the mothers or fetuses. The active compound of the drug will likely cross the placenta, so some fetal exposure will probably occur. However, this limited human pregnancy experience prevents a complete assessment of the embryofetal risk. Animal data did not show any embryofetal toxicity in two species at doses more than 10 times the RHD. Using this drug during pregnancy should be based on the pros and cons of the mother's clinical need for treatment versus any potential fetal risk that might occur from exposure.

BREASTFEEDING SUMMARY

No reports describing the use of flavoxate during human lactation have been located. The active drug metabolite will likely be found in breast milk, so some infant exposure will probably occur. Anticholinergic drugs can decrease serum prolactin levels and have been known to inhibit lactation in animals, especially with long-term use. Therefore, breastfeeding while using this drug should be based on the mother's clinical need for treatment. If used, the infant should be monitored for the most commonly reported adult side effects of nausea and headache (both leading to irritability) and vomiting.

References

1. Prescribing Information. Flavoxate hydrochloride. Perrigo; 2022.
2. Capra A, Paggi G. Use of flavoxate in the treatment of threatened abortion and threatened premature labor. *Minerva Ginecol*. 1972;24:400-404.
3. Masala A, Alagna S, Devilla L, et al. Muscarinic receptor blockade by pirenzepine: effect on prolactin secretion in man. 1982;5:53-55.
4. Aaron DK, Ely DG, Deweese WP, et al. Reducing milk production in ewes at weaning using restricted feeding and methscopolamine bromide. *J Anim Sci*. 1997;75:1434-1442.

FLECAINIDE

Cardiovascular (Antiarrhythmic)

PREGNANCY RECOMMENDATION: Limited Human Data—Animal Data Suggest Potential Risk (Maternal/Fetal Benefit May Outweigh Risk)

BREASTFEEDING RECOMMENDATION: Probably Compatible

PREGNANCY SUMMARY

Studies evaluating the use of flecainide in the first trimester of human pregnancy have not been located. Numerous studies, reviews, and meta-analyses have described the use of flecainide in several hundred pregnancies in the second and third

(*continued*)

trimesters to treat fetal arrhythmias. The drug has been found to be effective in this treatment process, especially when combined with digoxin. Flecainide crosses the placenta, so some fetal exposure will occur. However, this limited first trimester human pregnancy experience prevents a complete assessment of the embryofetal risk. Embryofetal toxicity was observed in one animal species at doses less than 10 times the RHD. Due to the indication for the use of this drug, the maternal or fetal clinical need for treatment likely outweighs the potential fetal risk that might occur from exposure.

BREASTFEEDING SUMMARY

Three reports were located that described the use of flecainide during human lactation. The drug was detected in the milk in every case with levels that ranged from about 0.1 mcg/mL up to 1.6 mcg/mL (depending on the maternal does). The calculated RIDs (using the worst-case scenario) ranged from about 3% to 7%. However, infant blood levels were analyzed in nine cases and the drug was not detected in every case (LLQ 50 ng/mL in one case—LLQ not stated in the remaining eight cases). Breastfeeding while using this drug should be based on the mother's clinical need for treatment versus any potential infant risks that might occur. If used, the infant should be monitored for the most commonly reported adult side effects of dizziness and blurred vision (both leading to irritability) and shortness of breath.

F

References

1. Prescribing Information. Flecainide acetate. ANI Pharmaceuticals; 2023.
2. Wren C, Hunter S. Maternal administration of flecainide to terminate and suppress fetal tachycardia. *Br Med J*. 1988;296:249.
3. Macphail S, Walkinshaw SA. Fetal supraventricular tachycardia: detection by routine auscultation and successful in-utero management: case report. *Br J Obstet Gynaecol*. 1988;95:1073-1076.
4. Wagner X, Jouglard J, Moulin M, et al. Coadministration of flecainide acetate and sotalol during pregnancy: lack of teratogenic effects, passage across the placenta, and excretion in human breast milk. *Am Heart J*. 1990;119:700-702.
5. Kofinas AD, Simon NV, Sagel H, et al. Treatment of fetal supraventricular tachycardia with flecainide acetate after digoxin failure. *Am J Obstet Gynecol*. 1991;165:630-631.
6. Allan LD, Chita SK, Sharland GK, et al. Flecainide in the treatment of fetal tachycardias. *Br Heart J*. 1991;65:46-48.
7. Bourget P, Pons J-C, Delouis C, et al. Flecainide distribution, transplacental passage, and accumulation in the amniotic fluid during the third trimester of pregnancy. *Ann Pharmacother*. 1994;28:1031-1034.
8. van Engelen AD, Weijtens O, Brenner JI, et al. Management outcome and follow-up of fetal tachycardia. *J Am Coll Cardiol*. 1994;24:1371-1375.
9. Simpson JM, Sharland GK. Fetal tachycardias: management and outcome of 127 consecutive cases. *Heart*. 1998;79:576-581.
10. van Gelder-Hasker MR, de Jong CLD, de Vries JIP, van Geijn HP. The effect of flecainide acetate on fetal heart rate variability: a case report. *Obstet Gynecol*. 1995;86:667-669.
11. Amano K, Harada Y, Shoda T, et al. Successful treatment of supraventricular tachycardia with flecainide acetate: a case report. *Fetal Diagn Ther*. 1997;12:328-331.
12. Jaeggi E, Fouron JC, Drblik SP. Fetal atrial flutter: diagnosis, clinical features, treatment, and outcome. *J Pediatr*. 1998;132:335-339.
13. Vanderhal AL, Cocjin J, Santulli TV, et al. Conjugated hyperbilirubinemia in a newborn infant after maternal (transplacental) treatment with flecainide acetate for fetal tachycardia and fetal hydrops. *J Pediatr*. 1995;126:988-990.
14. Alsaied T, Baskar S, Fares M, et al. First-line antiarrhythmic transplacental treatment for fetal tachyarrhythmia: a systematic review and meta-analysis. *J Am Heart Assoc*. 2017;6(12):e007164.
15. Hill GD, Kovach JR, Saudek DE, et al. Transplacental treatment of fetal tachycardia: a systematic review and meta-analysis. *Prenat Diagn*. 2017;37(11):1076-1083.
16. Qin J, Deng Z, Tang C, et al. Efficacy and safety of various first-line therapeutic strategies for fetal tachycardias: a network meta-analysis and systematic review. *Front Pharmacol*. 2022;13:935455.
17. Regitz-Zagrosek V, Roos-Hesselink JW, Bauersachs J, et al. ESC Scientific Document Group. 2018 ESC Guidelines for the management of cardiovascular diseases during pregnancy. *Eur Heart J*. 2018;39(34):3165-3241.
18. McQuinn RL, Pisani A, Wafa S, et al. Flecainide excretion in human breast milk. *Clin Pharmacol Ther*. 1990;48:262-267.
19. van der Zande JA, Cornette IMJ, Roos-Hesselink JW, Flint RB. Maternal, fetal, neonatal and breastmilk flecainide concentration during maternal therapy and lactation: a case report. *Int Breastfeed J*. 2023;18:21.
20. Pizzoglio V, Auffret M, Vial T, Gouraud A. Follow-up of flecainide breastfed infants. *Fundam Clin Pharmacol*. 2023;37:143-144.
21. Pizzoglio V, Auffret M, Vial T, Gouraud A. Follow-up of breastfed infants exposed to maternal flecainide treatment. *Neurotoxicol Teratol*. 2023;98:30.

FLIBANSERIN

Miscellaneous (Serotonin Receptor Agonist/Antagonist)

PREGNANCY RECOMMENDATION: No Human Data—Animal Data Suggest Low Risk

BREASTFEEDING RECOMMENDATION: Probably Compatible

PREGNANCY SUMMARY

No reports describing the use of flibanserin in human pregnancy have been located. The drug will likely cross the placenta, so some fetal exposure will probably occur. Therefore, the absence of human pregnancy experience prevents a complete assessment of the embryofetal risk. Animal data did not show any embryofetal toxicity in two species at doses less than 10 times the RHD. Using this drug during pregnancy should be based on the pros and cons of the mother's clinical need for treatment versus any potential fetal risk that might occur from exposure.

BREASTFEEDING SUMMARY

No reports describing the use of flibanserin during human lactation have been located. The drug will probably appear in breast milk, so some infant exposure will likely occur. However, due to the concern for potential adverse effects, including sedation, that might be seen in a breastfed infant, the manufacturer recommends that women should not breastfeed during treatment with this drug. Breastfeeding while using this drug should be based on the mother's clinical need for treatment. If used while breastfeeding, the infant should be monitored for the most commonly reported adult side effects of nausea (leading to irritability), sedation, lethargy, and poor sleep.

Reference

1. Product Information. Addyi. Sprout Pharmaceuticals, Inc; 2021.

F

FLORBETABEN F18

Radiopharmaceutical

PREGNANCY RECOMMENDATION: *No Human Data and No Relevant Animal Data

BREASTFEEDING RECOMMENDATION: Hold Breastfeeding

PREGNANCY SUMMARY

No reports describing the use of florbetaben F18 in human pregnancy have been located. This diagnostic agent will likely cross the placenta, so some fetal exposure will probably occur. Therefore, the absence of human pregnancy experience prevents a complete assessment of the embryofetal risk. Animal reproduction studies have not been conducted. All radiopharmaceuticals have the potential to cause fetal harm depending on the stage of development and magnitude of the radiation dose. *Therefore, using this agent during pregnancy should be based on the pros and cons of the mother's clinical need for diagnosis and to assess treatment options versus any potential fetal risk that might occur from exposure.

BREASTFEEDING SUMMARY

No reports describing the use of florbetaben F18 during human lactation have been located. Only about 0.07% of an administered F18 radionucleotide appeared in breast milk after administration. The manufacturer recommends that women should avoid the use of florbetaben F18 while breastfeeding or temporarily interrupt breastfeeding for 24 hours. If interrupted, the mother should pump and discard her breast milk for 24 hours after administration to minimize infant radiation exposure. An alternative is to measure the radioactivity in milk and determine when breastfeeding can safely begin again. This process has been described in reference number 3.

References

1. Prescribing Information. Neuraceq. Life Molecular Imaging LTD; 2023.
2. Leide-Svegborn S, Ahlgren L, Johansson L, et al. Excretion of radionucleotides in human breast milk after nuclear medicine examinations. Biokinetic and dosimetric data and recommendations on breastfeeding interruption. *Eur J Nucl Med Mol Imaging*. 2016;43:808-821.
3. Stabin MG, Breitz HB. Breast milk excretion of radiopharmaceuticals: mechanisms, findings, and radiation dosimetry. *J Nucl Med*. 2000;41:863-873.

FLORBETAPIR F18

Radiopharmaceutical

PREGNANCY RECOMMENDATION: *No Human Data and No Relevant Animal Data

BREASTFEEDING RECOMMENDATION: Hold Breastfeeding

PREGNANCY SUMMARY

No reports describing the use of florbetapir F18 in human pregnancy have been located. The drug will probably cross the placenta, but the rapid clearance should limit fetal exposure. However, the absence of human pregnancy experience prevents a complete assessment of the embryofetal risk. No animal studies have been conducted. *Because all radioactive agents have the potential to cause harm, the clinical decision to use this agent in a pregnant patient will need to be based on the stage of fetal development and the expected radiation exposure.

BREASTFEEDING SUMMARY

No reports describing the use of florbetapir F18 during human lactation have been located. The drug will probably be excreted into breast milk, but the rapid clearance should limit infant exposure. However, the manufacturer recommends that women should be advised to avoid the use of florbetapir F18 while breastfeeding or temporarily interrupt breastfeeding for 24 hours (more than 10 half-lives). If interrupted, the mother should pump and discard her breast milk for this time period to minimize radiation exposure.

Reference

1. Product Information. Amyvid. Eli Lilly and Company; 2019.

FLORTAUCIPIR F18

Radiopharmaceutical

PREGNANCY RECOMMENDATION: *No Human Data and No Relevant Animal Data

BREASTFEEDING RECOMMENDATION: Potential Toxicity (Hold Breastfeeding)

F

PREGNANCY SUMMARY

No reports describing the use of flortaucipir F18 in human pregnancy have been located. The drug will probably cross the placenta, so some fetal exposure will likely occur. However, the absence of human pregnancy experience prevents a complete assessment of the embryofetal risk. No animal studies have been conducted. *Nevertheless, all radiopharmaceutical agents have the potential to cause fetal harm depending on the stage of development and magnitude of the radiation dose. Based on the indication, flortaucipir F18 is not likely to be indicated in females of reproductive age.

BREASTFEEDING SUMMARY

No reports describing the use of flortaucipir F18 during human lactation have been located. The drug will probably be excreted into breast milk, but the rapid clearance should limit infant exposure. However, the manufacturer recommends that women should be advised not to breastfeed for 4 hours after administration to minimize potential radiation exposure to the infant. The mother could be given the option of pumping and discarding her breast milk during this time period.

Reference

1. Product Information. Tauvid. Eli Lilly and Company; 2020.

FLOTUFOLASTAT F 18

Radiopharmaceutical Agent

PREGNANCY RECOMMENDATION: *Contraindicated

BREASTFEEDING RECOMMENDATION: *Contraindicated

PREGNANCY SUMMARY

No reports describing the use of flotufolastat F 18 in human pregnancy have been located. The drug may not cross the placenta, or if it does, only minimal amounts might transfer. Animal studies have not been performed. *However, this radioactive diagnostic agent is not indicated for use in females.

BREASTFEEDING SUMMARY

Flotufolastat F 18 is probably excreted into human breast milk. *However, this radioactive diagnostic agent is not indicated for use in females.

Reference

1. Product Information. Posluma. Blue Earth Diagnostics Ltd; 2023.

FLOXURIDINE

Antineoplastic (Antimetabolite)

PREGNANCY RECOMMENDATION: No Human Data—Animal Data Suggest Risk

BREASTFEEDING RECOMMENDATION: Potential Toxicity

PREGNANCY SUMMARY

No reports describing the use of floxuridine in human pregnancy have been located. The drug will probably cross the placenta, so some fetal exposure will likely occur. Therefore, the absence of human pregnancy experience prevents a complete assessment of the embryofetal risk. Animal data did show embryofetal toxicity with malformations in two species at doses less than 10 times the RHD. Because floxuridine interferes with DNA, RNA, and protein synthesis, use in the first trimester might need to be avoided. There is a registry for women who are pregnant and have cancer. For more information, women are encouraged to contact the Cancer and Pregnancy Registry at 877-635-4499.

BREASTFEEDING SUMMARY

No reports describing the use of floxuridine during human lactation have been located. The drug will probably be found in human breast milk, so some infant exposure will likely occur. Based on the drug's mechanism of action, the manufacturer recommends that women not breastfeed while using this drug. Nevertheless, breastfeeding while using this drug should be based on the mother's clinical need for treatment versus any potential infant risks that might occur. If used, the infant should be monitored for the most commonly reported adult side effects of nausea (leading to irritability), diarrhea, vomiting, stomatitis, and various laboratory abnormalities (see Prescribing Information [PI]).

Reference

1. Prescribing Information. Floxuridine. Hikma Pharmaceuticals USA Inc; 2020.

F

FLUCICLOVINE F18

Radiopharmaceutical

PREGNANCY RECOMMENDATION: *Contraindicated

BREASTFEEDING RECOMMENDATION: *Contraindicated

PREGNANCY SUMMARY

No reports describing the use of fluciclovine F18 in human pregnancy have been located. This diagnostic agent will probably cross the placenta, so fetal exposure could occur. *However, fluciclovine F18 is not indicated for use in females. No animal reproduction studies have been conducted. All radiopharmaceuticals have the potential to cause fetal harm depending on the stage of development and magnitude of the radiation dose.

BREASTFEEDING SUMMARY

No reports describing the use of fluciclovine F18 during human lactation have been located. This diagnostic agent will likely be found in breast milk, so infant exposure could occur. *However, fluciclovine F18 is not indicated for use in females.

Reference

1. Prescribing Information. Axumin. Blue Earth Diagnostics; 2022.

FLUCONAZOLE

Anti-Infective (Antifungal)

PREGNANCY RECOMMENDATION: Human Data Suggest Risk (High Doses in the First Trimester)

BREASTFEEDING RECOMMENDATION: Probably Compatible

PREGNANCY SUMMARY

Several case reports were located that describe a multitude of various craniofacial and skeletal anomalies with first trimester exposure to high doses of fluconazole (more than 400 mg/d). This prompted several other large studies evaluating first trimester exposure with doses less than 400 mg/d. The rate of anomalies was 2.9% in more than 500 exposures, and no pattern to the anomalies was identified. The U.S. Food and Drug Administration (FDA) in 2017 issued a drug safety communication informing the public that chronic, high doses of the antifungal drug fluconazole may be associated with a rare and distinct set of birth defects in infants whose mothers were treated with the drug during the first trimester of pregnancy. This risk does not appear to be associated with a single, low dose of fluconazole 150 mg to treat vaginal yeast infection. The drug will likely cross the placenta, so some fetal exposure will probably occur. In those instances in which continuous, high-dose fluconazole is the only therapeutic choice during the first trimester, the patient should be informed of the potential risk to her fetus. Due to published case reports, the manufacturer recommends that women with reproductive potential who are taking fluconazole 400 to 800 mg/d be advised to use effective contraception during treatment and for at least 1 week after the last dose. Nevertheless, using this drug during pregnancy should be based on the pros and cons of the mother's clinical need for treatment versus any potential fetal risk that might occur from exposure.

BREASTFEEDING SUMMARY

Two reports describing the use of fluconazole during human lactation have been located. The peak milk levels in both cases were 4.1 and 2.9 mcg/mL, which results in an RID of more than 10%. However, the drug is used in neonates, and these milk levels would only represent a maximum of about 10% of the normal newborn dose. No serious infant adverse effects have been reported following the maternal use of fluconazole. Breastfeeding while using this drug should be based on the mother's clinical need for treatment versus any potential infant risks that might occur. If used, the infant should be monitored for the most commonly reported adult side effects of nausea, headache, and abdominal pain (all leading to irritability).

References

1. Prescribing Information. Diflucan. Roerig; 2023.
2. Lee BE, Feinberg M, Abraham JJ, Murthy AR. Congenital malformations in an infant born to a woman treated with fluconazole. *Pediatr Infect Dis J.* 1992;11:1062-1064.
3. Pursley TJ, Blomquist IK, Abraham J, Andersen HF, Bartley JA. Fluconazole-induced congenital anomalies in three infants. *Clin Infect Dis.* 1996;22:336-340.
4. Aleck KA, Bartley DL. Multiple malformation syndrome following fluconazole use in pregnancy: report of an additional patient. *Am J Med Genet.* 1997;72:253-256.
5. Inman W, Pearce G, Wilton L. Safety of fluconazole in the treatment of vaginal candidiasis. A prescription-event monitoring study, with special reference to the outcome of pregnancy. *Eur J Clin Pharmacol.* 1994;46: 115-118.
6. Mastroiacovo P, Mazzone T, Botto LD, et al. Prospective assessment of pregnancy outcomes after first-trimester exposure to fluconazole. *Am J Obstet Gynecol.* 1996;175:1645-1650.
7. Kremery V Jr, Huttova M, Masar O. Teratogenicity of fluconazole. *Pediatr Infect Dis.* 1996;15:841.
8. Wiesinger EC, Mayerhofer S, Wenisch C, et al. Fluconazole in Candida albicans sepsis during pregnancy: case report and review of the literature. *Infection.* 1996;24:263-6.
9. Campomori A, Bonati M. Fluconazole treatment for vulvovaginal candidiasis during pregnancy. *Ann Pharmacother.* 1997;31:118-119.
10. Wilton LV, Pearce GL, Martin RM, et al. The outcomes of pregnancy in women exposed to newly marketed drugs in general practice in England. *Br J Obstet Gynaecol.* 1998;105:882-889.
11. Sanchez JM, Moya G. Fluconazole teratogenicity. *Prenat Diagn.* 1998;18:862-863.
12. Kalish RB, Garry D, Figueroa R. Achalasia with Candida esophagitis during pregnancy. *Obstet Gynecol.* 1999;94:850.
13. Sorensen HT, Nielsen GL, Olesen C, et al. Risk of malformations and other outcomes in children exposed to fluconazole in utero. *Br J Clin Pharmacol.* 1999;48:234-238.
14. Lopez-Rangel E, Van Allen MI. Prenatal exposure to fluconazole: an identifiable dysmorphic phenotype. *Birth Defects Res A Clin Mol Teratol.* 2005;73:919-923.
15. King CT, Rogers PD, Cleary JD, Chapman SW. Antifungal therapy during pregnancy. *Clin Infect Dis.* 1998;27:1151-1160.
16. Bean LM, Jackson JR, Dobak WJ, et al. Intra-amniotic fluconazole therapy for Candida albicans intra-amniotic infection. *Obstet Gynecol.* 2013;121:452-454.
17. Molgaard-Nielsen D, Pasternak B, Hviid A. Use of oral fluconazole during pregnancy and the risk of birth defects. *N Engl J Med.* 2013;369:830-839.
18. Molgaard-Nielsen D, Svanstrom H, Melbye M, et al. Association between use of oral fluconazole during pregnancy and risk of spontaneous abortion and stillbirth. *JAMA Pediatr.* 2016;315:58-67.
19. Schilling CG, Seay RE, Larson TA, Meier KR. Excretion of fluconazole in human breast milk (abstract no. 130). *Pharmacotherapy.* 1993;13:287.
20. Force RW. Fluconazole concentrations in breast milk. *Pediatr Infect Dis J.* 1995;14:235-236.
21. Viscoli C, Castagnola E, Corsini M, et al. Fluconazole therapy in an underweight infant. *Eur J Clin Microbiol Infect Dis.* 1989;8:925-926.
22. Wiest DB, Fowler SL, Garner SS, Simons DR. Fluconazole in neonatal disseminated candidiasis. *Arch Dis Child.* 1991;66:1002.
23. Gurses N, Kalayci AG. Fluconazole monotherapy for Candidal meningitis in a premature infant. *Clin Infect Dis.* 1996;23:645-646.
24. Bodley V, Powers D. Long-term treatment of a breastfeeding mother with fluconazole-resolved nipple pain caused by yeast: a case study. *J Hum Lact.* 1997;13:307-311.
25. Moorhead AM, Amir LH, O'Brien PW, Wong S. A prospective study of fluconazole treatment for breast and nipple thrush. *Breastfeed Rev.* 2011;19:25-29.
26. U.S. Food and Drug Administration. FDA drug safety communication: use of long-term, high-dose Diflucan (fluconazole) during pregnancy may be associated with birth defects in infants. Accessed September 22, 2024. https://www.fda.gov/drugs/drug-safety-and-availability/fda-drug-safety-communicationuse-long-term-high-dose-diflucan-fluconazole-during-pregnancy-may-be#ref

FLUCYTOSINE

Anti-Infective (Antifungal)

PREGNANCY RECOMMENDATION: *Contraindicated (First Trimester)

BREASTFEEDING RECOMMENDATION: Potential Toxicity

PREGNANCY SUMMARY

One case of flucytosine use in the first trimester was located. The patient was treated for cryptococcal meningitis. She ultimately did well and delivered at term a healthy newborn with no reported anomalies. Eight other case reports of pregnant patients treated with flucytosine in combination with other medications during the second and third trimesters were located. One patient underwent an elective abortion. Normal outcomes with no reported malformations or drug complications occurred in the other seven newborns. The drug crosses the placenta, so fetal exposure will occur. In addition, with oral use, 5-fluorouracil (5-FU) will also be present. Therefore, this limited human pregnancy experience prevents a complete assessment of the embryofetal risk. Animal studies did show embryofetal toxicity with malformations in one species at doses less than 10 times the RHD. In two other animal species, no embryofetal toxicity was seen at doses less than 10 times the RHD. Using this drug should be based on the pros and cons of the mother's clinical need for treatment versus any potential fetal risk that might occur from exposure. *The primary concern is using this drug in the first trimester due to the potential plasma levels for 5-FU.

BREASTFEEDING SUMMARY

No reports describing the use of flucytosine during human lactation have been located. The drug will probably appear in breast milk, so infant exposure will likely occur. In addition, with oral use, some 5-FU may also be found in breast milk. Due to the concern for potential serious adverse effects (such as bone marrow suppression) that may occur in a breastfed infant, the manufacturer recommends that a decision should be made whether to discontinue nursing or to discontinue the drug, considering the importance of the drug to the mother. However, if the clinical decision is to use this drug while breastfeeding, the infant should be monitored for the most commonly reported adult side effects of abdominal pain and nausea (both leading to irritability), diarrhea, vomiting, rash, hepatitis, and renal toxicity.

References

1. Prescribing Information. Ancobon. Valeant Pharmaceuticals North America; 2020.
2. Diasio RB, Lakings DE, Bennett JE. Evidence for conversion of 5-fluorocytosine to 5-fluorouracil in humans: possible factor in 5-fluorocytosine clinical toxicity. *Antimicrob Agents Chemother*. 1978;14:903-908.
3. Vermes A, Guchelaar HJ, van Kuilenburg ABP, Dankert J. 5-fluorocytosine-related bone-marrow depression and conversion to fluorouracil: a pilot study. *Fundam Clin Pharmacol*. 2002;16:39-47.
4. Stafford CR, Fisher JF, Fadel HE, et al. Cryptococcal meningitis in pregnancy. *Obstet Gynecol*. 1983;62(3 suppl):35s-37s.
5. Philpot CR, Lo D. Cryptococcal meningitis in pregnancy. *Med J Aust*. 1972;2:1005-1007.
6. Schonebeck J, Segerbrand E. Candida albicans septicaemia during first half of pregnancy successfully treated with 5-fluorocytosine. *Br Med J*. 1973;4:337-338.
7. Curole DN. Cryptococcal meningitis in pregnancy. *J Reprod Med*. 1981;26:317-319.
8. Jones JM, Craig WA. Cryptococcal meningitis: resolution eight months after antifungal therapy. *South Med J*. 1983;76:1567-1569.
9. Chotmongkol V, Siricharoensang S. Cryptococcal meningitis in pregnancy: a case report. *J Med Assoc Thai*. 1991;74:421-422.
10. Chotmongkol V, Sookprasert A. Itraconazole in cryptococcal meningitis in pregnancy: a case report. *J Med Assoc Thai*. 1992;75:606-608.
11. Pereira CA, Fischman O, Colombo AL, et al. Cryptococcal meningitis in pregnancy. Review of the literature. Report of 2 cases. *Rev Inst Med Trop Sao Paulo*. 1993;35:367-371.
12. Chen CP, Wang KG. Cryptococcal meningitis in pregnancy. *Am J Perinatol*. 1996;13:35-36.

F

FLUDARABINE PHOSPHATE

Antineoplastic (DNA Synthesis Inhibitor)

PREGNANCY RECOMMENDATION: Limited Human Data—Animal Data Suggest Risk

BREASTFEEDING RECOMMENDATION: Potential Toxicity

PREGNANCY SUMMARY

One case report on the use of fludarabine during human pregnancy was located. Treatment occurred at 22 weeks' gestation and no congenital malformations were identified. The drug will likely cross the placenta, so some fetal exposure will probably occur. Therefore, this limited human pregnancy experience prevents a complete assessment of the embryofetal risk. Animal studies showed embryofetal toxicity with malformations in two species at doses less than 10 times the RHD. Based on the drug's mechanism of action, the manufacturer recommends that women with reproductive potential use effective contraception during treatment with fludarabine and for at least 6 months after the last dose. They also recommend that males with female partners of reproductive potential use effective contraception during treatment with this drug and for at least 95 days after the last dose. Nevertheless, using this drug during pregnancy should be based on the pros and cons of the mother's clinical need for treatment versus any potential fetal risk that might occur from exposure. There is a registry for women who are pregnant and have cancer. For more information, health care providers and women are encouraged to contact the Cancer and Pregnancy Registry at 1-877-635-4499.

BREASTFEEDING SUMMARY

No reports describing the use of fludarabine during human lactation have been located. The drug will probably be found in breast milk, so some infant exposure will likely occur. Due to the concern for potential serious adverse effects that might be seen in a breastfed infant, the manufacturer recommends that women not breastfeed while being treated with this drug. Nevertheless, breastfeeding while using this drug should be based on the mother's clinical need for treatment. If used, the infant should be monitored for the most commonly reported adult side effects of nausea (leading to irritability), fatigue (lethargy), vomiting, decreased appetite, fever, cough, and various laboratory abnormalities (see PI).

References

1. Prescribing Information. Fludarabine phosphate. Sanofi Healthcare India Private Limited; 2022.
2. Baumgartner AK, Oberhoffer R, Jacobs VR, et al. Reversible foetal cerebral ventriculomegaly and cardiomyopathy under chemotherapy for maternal AML. *Onkologie*. 2009;32:40-43.

FLUMAZENIL

Antidote (Benzodiazepine Receptor Antagonist)

PREGNANCY RECOMMENDATION: Limited Human Data—Animal Data Suggest Low Risk (Maternal Benefit May Outweigh Embryofetal Risk for Overdose)

BREASTFEEDING RECOMMENDATION: Probably Compatible

F

PREGNANCY SUMMARY

No reports describing the use of flumazenil during the first trimester in humans have been located. Two case reports of use in the third trimester did not show any adverse effects in either infant. The drug will probably cross the placenta, so some fetal exposure will likely occur. However, this limited human pregnancy experience prevents a complete assessment of the embryofetal risk. Animal data did not show any embryofetal toxicity or malformations in two species at doses more than 10 times the RHD. If the indication for flumazenil use is to reverse a benzodiazepine overdose, the maternal benefit will likely outweigh any embryofetal risk. Therefore, flumazenil should not be withheld during pregnancy in this clinical scenario. The drug carries a Boxed Warning regarding an increased association with seizures (most likely due to acute benzodiazepine withdrawal).

BREASTFEEDING SUMMARY

No reports describing the use of flumazenil during human lactation have been located. The drug will probably be found in human breast milk, so some infant exposure might occur. Flumazenil is absorbed orally, but following first pass through the liver, only about 15% of a dose is bioavailable. IV flumazenil has been given directly to neonates to reverse the sedative effects of diazepam administered to the mother immediately before delivery. If indicated, flumazenil should not be withheld during lactation. If used while breastfeeding, the infant should be monitored for the most commonly reported adult side effects of nausea and agitation (both leading to irritability), flushing, fatigue (lethargy), and vomiting (1). If there is a concern about infant exposure to the drug through breast milk, because of the very short elimination half-life, withholding breastfeeding for 4 to 5 hours after the last dose would significantly minimize any contact.

References

1. Prescribing Information. Flumazenil. Baxter Healthcare; 2018.
2. Shibata T, Kubota N, Yokoyama H. A pregnant woman with convulsion treated with diazepam, which was reversed with flumazenil just prior to cesarean section [Japanese]. *Masui*. 1994;43:572.
3. Stahl MMS, Saldeen P, Vinge E. Reversal of fetal benzodiazepine intoxication using flumazenil. *Br J Obstet Gynaecol*. 1993;100:185-188.
4. Richard P, Autret E, Bardol J, et al. The use of flumazenil in a neonate. *J Toxicol Clin Toxicol*. 1991;29:137-140.
5. Dixon JC, Speidel BD, Dixon JJ. Neonatal flumazenil therapy reverses maternal diazepam. *Acta Paediatr*. 1998;87:225-226.

FLUNISOLIDE

Respiratory/Corticosteroid (Nasal)

PREGNANCY RECOMMENDATION: Limited Human Data—Animal Data Suggest Risk (Human Data Suggest Low Risk for Inhaled Corticosteroids as a Group)

BREASTFEEDING RECOMMENDATION: Probably Compatible

PREGNANCY SUMMARY

Only one study has been identified that specifically examined the effects of inhaled flunisolide (along with other inhaled corticosteroids [ICSs]) in pregnant patients with asthma. The inhaled steroids and the number of patients were beclomethasone (*N* = 277), fluticasone (*N* = 132), triamcinolone (*N* = 81), budesonide (*N* = 43), and flunisolide (*N* = 25). Compared with the general population, the study found no increased incidence of congenital malformations, small-for-gestational-age infants, or preterm births. Similar findings of no increased risks for major malformations, preterm delivery, low birth weight, and pregnancy-induced hypertension were reported in a meta-analysis of ICSs as a group. The drug will likely cross the placenta, but levels are probably very low and clinically insignificant. However, this limited human pregnancy experience with flunisolide prevents a complete assessment of the embryofetal risk. Animal studies did show embryofetal toxicity including malformations in two species at doses less than 10 times the RHD. Using this drug during pregnancy should be based on the pros and cons of the mother's clinical need for treatment versus any potential fetal risk that might occur from exposure.

BREASTFEEDING SUMMARY

No reports describing the use of flunisolide during human lactation have been located. Because of the poor absorption orally, any possible infant exposure is likely to be clinically insignificant. Breastfeeding while using this drug should be based on the mother's clinical need for treatment. If used, the infant should be monitored for the most commonly reported adult side effect of headache (leading to irritability).

References

1. Prescribing Information. Flunisolide. Bausch & Lomb; 2019.
2. Namazy J, Schatz M, Long L, et al. Use of inhaled steroids by pregnant asthmatic women does not reduce intrauterine growth. *J Allergy Clin Immunol*. 2004;113:427-432.
3. Rahimi R, Nikfar S, Abdollahi M. Meta-analysis finds use of inhaled corticosteroids during pregnancy safe: a systematic meta-analysis review. *Hum Exp Toxicol*. 2006;25:447-452.

F

FLUOCINOLONE

Dermatologic/Corticosteroid (Topical)

PREGNANCY RECOMMENDATION: Limited Human Data—No Relevant Animal Data

BREASTFEEDING RECOMMENDATION: Probably Compatible

PREGNANCY SUMMARY

A large case-control study that evaluated the teratogenic potential of topical corticosteroids involving 1,923,413 total births was conducted by the Hungarian Case-Control Surveillance of Congenital Abnormalities program. Among the 20,830 malformed case infants, 73 (0.35%) used a topical corticosteroid during the first trimester compared with 118 (0.33%) of the 35,727 normal control infants. The number of cases and controls that used topical fluocinolone cream was 16 (0.07%) and 47 (0.13%), respectively. Neither of these comparisons was significant. Topical corticosteroid use in the first trimester did not show an increased risk of congenital abnormalities. A meta-analysis evaluating the effects of topical corticosteroids on pregnancy outcome reviewed 14 studies involving 1,601,515 pregnant women. When compared to no exposure, overall, no association with congenital anomalies, orofacial clefts, or preterm delivery was found with the use of any potent corticosteroid medication. The drug will probably cross the placenta in some cases, but the overall amount will likely be clinically insignificant. However, this limited human pregnancy experience prevents a complete assessment of the embryofetal risk. Animal reproduction studies have not been conducted with fluocinolone. Using this drug during pregnancy should be based on the pros and cons of the mother's clinical need for treatment versus any potential fetal risk that might occur from exposure.

BREASTFEEDING SUMMARY

No reports describing the use of fluocinolone during human lactation have been located. The drug will probably be found in breast milk in some cases; however, the overall amount is probably clinically insignificant with topical use. Breastfeeding while using this drug should be based on the mother's clinical need for treatment. Due to the negligible absorption, systemic side effects were not reported. The drug should not be applied directly on the nipple area during lactation.

References

1. Prescribing Information. Fluocinolone. Cosette Pharmaceuticals; 2020.
2. Czeizel AE, Rockenbauer M. Population-based case-control study of teratogenic potential of corticosteroids. *Teratology*. 1997;56:335-40.
3. Chi CC, Wang SH, Wojnarowska F, et al. Safety of topical corticosteroids in pregnancy. *Cochrane Database Syst Rev*. 2015;2015:CD007346.

FLUOCINOLONE OPHTHALMIC IMPLANT

Ophthalmic/Corticosteroid

PREGNANCY RECOMMENDATION: No Human Data and No Relevant Animal Data

BREASTFEEDING RECOMMENDATION: Probably Compatible

PREGNANCY SUMMARY

No reports describing the use of fluocinolone ophthalmic implant in human pregnancy have been located. Two large studies that evaluated the teratogenic potential of topical corticosteroids used in the first trimester did not show an increased risk

(*continued*)

of congenital abnormalities (see Fluocinolone Topical). The drug will probably cross the placenta if it reaches the systemic circulation, but the overall amount will likely be clinically insignificant. However, the absence of human pregnancy experience prevents a complete assessment of the embryofetal risk. Animal reproduction studies have not been conducted with this implant. Using this drug during pregnancy should be based on the pros and cons of the mother's clinical need for treatment versus any potential fetal risk that might occur from exposure.

BREASTFEEDING SUMMARY

No reports describing the use of fluocinolone ophthalmic implant during human lactation have been located. If fluocinolone reaches the systemic circulation, the drug will probably be found in breast milk. However, systemic absorption is below the limit of quantification, so the amount would likely be clinically insignificant. Breastfeeding while using this drug should be based on the mother's clinical need for treatment. Due to the negligible absorption, systemic side effects were not reported.

F

References

1. Prescribing Information. Iluvien. Alimera Sciences; 2019.
2. Czeizel AE, Rockenbauer M. Population-based case-control study of teratogenic potential of corticosteroids. *Teratology*. 1997;56:335-340.
3. Chi CC, Wang SH, Wojnarowska F, et al. Safety of topical corticosteroids in pregnancy. *Cochrane Database Syst Rev*. 2015;2015:CD007346.

FLUOCINONIDE

Dermatologic/Corticosteroid (Topical)

PREGNANCY RECOMMENDATION: Limited Human Data—No Relevant Animal Data

BREASTFEEDING RECOMMENDATION: Probably Compatible

PREGNANCY SUMMARY

One case report was located that described the use of topical fluocinonide in human pregnancy. The patient was treated in the third trimester for a generalized pustular dermatosis, responded well, and delivered at term a healthy newborn with no identified malformations or complications. A large case-control study that evaluated the teratogenic potential of topical corticosteroids involving 1,923,413 total births was conducted by the Hungarian Case-Control Surveillance of Congenital Abnormalities program. Among the 20,830 malformed case infants, 73 (0.35%) used a topical corticosteroid during the first trimester compared with 118 (0.33%) of the 35,727 normal control infants. This comparison was not significant. Topical corticosteroid use in the first trimester did not show an increased risk of congenital abnormalities. A meta-analysis evaluating the effects of topical corticosteroids on pregnancy outcome reviewed 14 studies involving 1,601,515 pregnant women. When compared to no exposure, overall, no association with congenital abnormalities, orofacial clefts, or preterm delivery was found with the use of any potent corticosteroid medication. The drug will probably cross the placenta in some cases, but the overall amount will likely be clinically insignificant. However, this limited human pregnancy experience prevents a complete assessment of the embryofetal risk. Animal reproduction studies have not been conducted with fluocinonide. Using this drug during pregnancy should be based on the pros and cons of the mother's clinical need for treatment versus any potential fetal risk that might occur from exposure.

BREASTFEEDING SUMMARY

No reports describing the use of fluocinonide during human lactation have been located. The drug will probably be found in breast milk in some cases; however, the overall amount is probably clinically insignificant with topical use. Breastfeeding while using this drug should be based on the mother's clinical need for treatment. Due to the negligible absorption, systemic side effects were not reported. The drug should not be applied directly on the nipple area during lactation.

References

1. Prescribing Information. Vanos. MEDICIS, The Dermatology Company; 2019.
2. Valkova S. Food-induced acute generalized exanthematous pustulosis in a pregnant woman. *Skinmed*. 2006;5:199-201.
3. Czeizel AE, Rockenbauer M. Population-based case-control study of teratogenic potential of corticosteroids. *Teratology*. 1997;56:335-340
4. Chi CC, Wang SH, Wojnarowska F, Kirtschig G, Davies E, Bennett C. Safety of topical corticosteroids in pregnancy. *Cochrane Database Syst Rev*. 2015;2015:CD007346.

FLUORESCEIN

Diagnostic

PREGNANCY RECOMMENDATION: Limited Human Data—Animal Data Suggest Low Risk

BREASTFEEDING RECOMMENDATION: *Potential Toxicity

PREGNANCY SUMMARY

Several reports describing the use of intra-amniotic, IV, or ophthalmic fluorescein during human pregnancy were located. The compound was not found to be associated with a high rate of birth anomalies or complications in pregnancy. However, many of these cases were beyond the first trimester. Fluorescein appears to cross the placenta, so some fetal exposure will likely occur. However, this limited human pregnancy experience prevents a complete assessment of the embryofetal risk. Animal data did not show any embryofetal toxicity in two species. ACOG supports the potential use and safety of fluorescein as an alternative dye for intra-amniotic instillation in cases of equivocal preterm premature rupture of membranes. If ophthalmic fluorescein use is needed during pregnancy, consider placing pressure over the tear duct in the corner of the eye for at least 1 minute and then remove any excess solution with absorbent tissue to decrease the amount of compound that might reach the systemic circulation. Using fluorescein during pregnancy should be based on the pros and cons of the mother's clinical need for treatment versus any potential fetal risk that might occur from exposure.

F

BREASTFEEDING SUMMARY

Two reports describing the use of fluorescein during human lactation have been located. In one case, a lactating mother received fluorescein IV and several milk samples were obtained. The peak milk concentration was 372 ng/mL and the half-life of the compound in milk was about 62 hours. In the second case, fluorescein ophthalmic drops were used, and the peak milk level was 22 ng/mL. *There is concern that if fluorescein is consumed through breast milk, it might cause a phototoxic reaction in infants undergoing phototherapy. Therefore, temporarily withholding breastfeeding in infants undergoing phototherapy should be considered. If the clinical decision is to use this drug while breastfeeding, the infant should be monitored for fluorescein-induced phototoxicity (if undergoing phototherapy) and the most commonly reported adult side effects of nausea and gastrointestinal distress (both leading to irritability), skin and urine discoloration, and vomiting.

References

1. Prescribing Information. AK-FLUOR. Akorn, Inc; 2019.
2. Shekleton P, Fidler J, Grimwade J. A case of benign intracranial hypertension in pregnancy. *Br J Obstet Gynaecol*. 1980;87:345-347.
3. Smith RP. A technic for the detection of rupture of the membranes. A review and preliminary report. *Obstet Gynecol*. 1976;48:172-176.
4. Rodrigues M, Meira D, Batista S, Carrilho MM. Accidental pregnancy exposure to verteporfin: obstetrical and neonatal outcomes: a case report. *Aust NZ J Obstet Gynaecol*. 2009;49:236-237.
5. Lin P, Hahn P, Fekrat S. Peripheral retinal vascular leakage demonstrated by ultra-widefield fluorescein angiography in preeclampsia with HELLP syndrome. *Retina*. 2012;32:1689-1690.
6. Halperin LS, Olk RJ, Soubrane G, Coscas G. Safety of fluorescein angiography during pregnancy. *Am J Ophthalmol*. 1990;109:563-566.
7. Olk RJ, Halperin LS, Soubrane G, Coscas G. Fluorescein angiography—is it safe to use in a pregnant patient? *Eur J Ophthalmol*. 1991;1(2):103-106.
8. Interlandi E, Pellegrini F, Silvestrin C, et al. HELLP syndrome-related hypertensive chorioretinopathy: a multimodal imaging and optical coherence tomography angiography (OCTA) study. *Eur J Ophthalmol*. 2023;33:NP88-NP91.
9. Ireland KE, Rodriguez EI, Acosta OM, Ramsey PS. Intra-amniotic dye alternatives for the diagnosis of preterm prelabor rupture of membranes. *Obstet Gynecol*. 2017;129:1040-1045.
10. Prelabor rupture of membranes: ACOG practice bulletin, number 217. *Obstet Gynecol*. 2020;135:e80-e97.
11. Salem H, Loux JJ, Smith S, Nichols CW. Evaluation of the toxicologic and teratogenic potentials of sodium fluorescein in the rat. *Toxicology*. 1979;12:143-150.
12. Burnett CM, Goldenthal EI. The teratogenic potential in rats and rabbits of D and C Yellow no. 8. *Food Chem Toxicol*. 1986;24:819-823.
13. McEnerney JK, Wong WP, Peyman GA. Evaluation of the teratogenicity of fluorescein sodium. *Am J Ophthalmol*. 1977;84:847-850.
14. Maguire AM, Bennett J. Fluorescein elimination in human breast milk. *Arch Ophthalmol*. 1986;106:718-719.
15. Mattern J, Mayer PR. Excretion of fluorescein into breast milk. *Am J Ophthalmol*. 1990;109:598-599.
16. Kearns GL, Williams BJ, Timmons OD. Fluorescein phototoxicity in a premature infant. *J Pediatr*. 1985;107:796-798.
17. American Academy of Pediatrics Committee on Drugs. The transfer of drugs and other chemicals into human milk. *Pediatrics*. 2001;108:776-789.
18. Anderson PO. Medication use while breast feeding a neonate. *Neonatal Pharmacol Q*. 1993;2:3-14.
19. Mattern J, Mayer PR. Excretion of fluorescein into breast milk. *Am J Ophthalmol*. 1990;109:598-599.
20. Maguire AM, Bennett J. Fluorescein elimination in human breast milk. *Arch Ophthalmol*. 1988;106:718-719.

FLUORODOPA F 18

Radiopharmaceutical Agent

PREGNANCY RECOMMENDATION: *No Human Data and No Relevant Animal Data

BREASTFEEDING RECOMMENDATION: Potential Toxicity (Hold Breastfeeding)

PREGNANCY SUMMARY

No reports describing the use of Fluorodopa F 18 in human pregnancy have been located. The drug will probably cross the placenta, so some fetal exposure will likely occur. Therefore, the absence of human pregnancy experience prevents a complete assessment of the embryofetal risk. Animal studies have not been performed. *Because all radioactive agents have the potential to cause fetal harm, the clinical decision to use this agent in a pregnant patient will need to be based on the stage of fetal development and expected radiation exposure.

BREASTFEEDING SUMMARY

Fluorodopa F 18 will probably be excreted into human breast milk. If the clinical decision is to use this agent in a breastfeeding woman, the manufacturer recommends that breastfeeding be held and that she pumps and discards her breast milk for 24 hours (approximately 12 half-lives) after administration.

Reference

1. Product Information. Fluorodopa F 18. The Feinstein Institutes for Medical Research; 2019.

FLUOROESTRADIOL F 18

Radiopharmaceutical

PREGNANCY RECOMMENDATION: *No Human Data and No Relevant Animal Data

BREASTFEEDING RECOMMENDATION: Potential Toxicity (Hold Breastfeeding)

PREGNANCY SUMMARY

No reports describing the use of fluoroestradiol F 18 in human pregnancy have been located. The drug will probably cross the placenta, so some fetal exposure will likely occur. Therefore, the absence of human pregnancy experience prevents a complete assessment of embryofetal risk. No animal studies have been conducted. *However, all radiopharmaceutical agents have the potential to cause fetal harm depending on the stage of fetal development and magnitude of the radiation dose. Using this agent during pregnancy should be based on the pros and cons of the mother's clinical need for diagnosis and to assess treatment options versus any potential fetal risk that might occur from exposure.

BREASTFEEDING SUMMARY

No reports describing the use of fluoroestradiol F 18 during human lactation have been located. The drug will probably enter breast milk, so infant exposure will likely occur. In order to minimize potential radiation exposure to the infant, women should be given the option of holding breastfeeding, pumping, and discarding the breast milk for a period of 4 hours after fluoroestradiol F 18 administration.

Reference

1. Product Information. Cerianna. Zionexa US Corp; 2022.

FLUOROMETHOLONE

Ophthalmic/Corticosteroid (Topical)

PREGNANCY RECOMMENDATION: Limited Human Data—Animal Data Suggest Potential Risk

BREASTFEEDING RECOMMENDATION: Probably Compatible

PREGNANCY SUMMARY

One case report was located that described the use of fluorometholone during human pregnancy. The patient was treated in the second trimester and delivered at term, a healthy newborn with no reported anomalies or complications. The drug will probably cross the placenta, but the overall amount is likely to be clinically insignificant. However, this limited human pregnancy experience prevents a complete assessment of the embryofetal risk. Animal studies did show embryofetal toxicity in one species at doses less than 10 times the RHD. Using this drug during pregnancy should be based on the pros and cons of the mother's clinical need for treatment versus any potential fetal risk that might occur from exposure. If used during pregnancy, consider placing pressure over the tear duct in the corner of the eye for at least 1 minute and then remove any excess solution with absorbent tissue to decrease the amount of drug reaching the systemic circulation even further.

BREASTFEEDING SUMMARY

No reports describing the use of fluorometholone ophthalmic during human lactation have been located. The drug might be found in breast milk in some cases, but the overall amount is likely to be clinically insignificant. Breastfeeding while using this drug should be based on the mother's clinical need for treatment. Due to low absorption, systemic side effects were not recorded. A method to decrease some systemic absorption with ophthalmic use is described in the above Pregnancy Summary.

References

1. Prescribing Information. Fluorometholone. Allergan Inc; 2018.
2. Abbouda A, Trimboli P, Bruscolini A, et al. A mild Grave's ophthalmopathy during pregnancy. *Semin Ophthalmol*. 2014;29:8-10.

FLUOROURACIL

Antineoplastic (Antimetabolite)

PREGNANCY RECOMMENDATION: Limited Human Data—Animal Data Suggest Risk

BREASTFEEDING RECOMMENDATION: Potential Toxicity

PREGNANCY SUMMARY

A few reports were located that describe first trimester exposure to fluorouracil. Two anomalies (both different) were seen in about 20 cases. Numerous other publications have described the use of the drug in the second and third trimesters. The drug will probably cross the placenta, so some fetal exposure will likely occur. Animal studies showed embryofetal toxicity and/or teratogenicity in four species at doses less than 10 times the RHD. Based on animal studies and the drug's mechanism of action, the manufacturer recommends that women with reproductive potential use effective contraception during treatment and for 3 months after the last dose. They also recommend that males with female partners of reproductive potential use effective contraception during treatment and for 3 months after the last dose. Nevertheless, using this drug during pregnancy should be based on the pros and cons of the mother's clinical need for treatment versus any potential fetal risk that might occur from exposure. There is a registry for women who are pregnant and have cancer. For more information, health care providers are encouraged to contact the Cancer and Pregnancy Registry at 877-635-4499.

BREASTFEEDING SUMMARY

One report describing the use of IV fluorouracil during human lactation was located. The report found the drug was not detected in the mother's milk samples (LLQ 65 ng/mL) despite normal maternal plasma levels. The drug will probably be found in breast milk in some patients, so fetal exposure may occur. In addition, this will likely be variable from patient to patient due to the wide range of oral bioavailability of 5-FU (0% up to 80%). However, due to a concern for potential serious adverse effects that might be seen in a breastfed infant, the manufacturer recommends that women not breastfeed while being treated with this drug. Nevertheless, breastfeeding while using this drug should be based on the mother's clinical need for treatment versus any potential infant risks that might occur. If used, the infant should be monitored for the most commonly reported adult side effects of nausea (leading to irritability), vomiting, decreased appetite (monitor infant growth), bone marrow suppression, cardiac toxicity, shortness of breath, and rash.

References

1. Prescribing Information. Efudex. Bausch Health Companies Inc; 2021.
2. Prescribing Information. Fluorouracil. Accord Healthcare; 2017.
3. Stephens JD, Golbus MS, Miller TR, et al. Multiple congenital anomalies in a fetus exposed to 5-fluorouracil during the first trimester. *Am J Obstet Gynecol*. 1980;137:747-749.
4. Turchi JJ, Villasis C. Anthracyclines in the treatment of malignancy in pregnancy. *Cancer.* 1988;61:435-440.
5. Stadler HE, Knowles J. Fluorouracil in pregnancy: effect on the neonate. *JAMA*. 1971;217:214-215.
6. Cuvier C, Espie M, Extra JM, Marty M. Vinorelbine in pregnancy. *Eur J Cancer.* 1997;33:168-169.
7. Giacalone PL, Laffargue F, Benos P. Chemotherapy for breast carcinoma during pregnancy. *Cancer.* 1999;86:2266-2272.
8. Fisher B, Sherman B, Rockette H, et al. L-Phenylalanine (L-PAM) in the management of premenopausal patients with primary breast cancer. *Cancer.* 1979;44:847-857.
9. Schilsky RL, Lewis BJ, Sherins RJ, Young RC. Gonadal dysfunction in patients receiving chemotherapy for cancer. *Ann Intern Med.* 1980;93:109-114.
10. Gershenson DM. Menstrual and reproductive function after treatment with combination chemotherapy for malignant ovarian germ cell tumors. *J Clin Oncol.* 1988;6:270-275.
11. Song H, Wu P, Wang Y, et al. Pregnancy outcomes after successful chemotherapy for choriocarcinoma and invasive mole: long-term follow-up. *Am J Obstet Gynecol.* 1988;158:538-545.
12. Makoshi Z, Perrott C, Al-Khatani K, Al-Mohaisen F. Chemotherapeutic treatment of colorectal cancer in pregnancy: case report. *J Med Case Reports.* 2015;9:140-5.
13. Paccatori FA, Giovannetti E, Pistilli B, et al. "The only think I know is that I know nothing": 5-fluorouracil in human milk. *Ann Oncol.* 2012;23:543-544.

FLUOROURACIL CREAM

Antineoplastic/Dermatologic (Antimetabolite)

PREGNANCY RECOMMENDATION: Limited Human Data—No Relevant Animal Data

BREASTFEEDING RECOMMENDATION: Probably Compatible

PREGNANCY SUMMARY

One manufacturer reported an infant with cleft lip and palate from a woman who appropriately used topical fluorouracil and a second infant with a ventricular septal defect from a woman who used the drug topically on mucous membranes.

(continued)

However, no series evaluating the use of this drug during pregnancy were located. If found in the systemic circulation, fluorouracil will probably cross the placenta, so some fetal exposure is possible. However, the low systemic absorption with topical use suggests that any placental transfer is likely to be clinically insignificant. Therefore, this limited human pregnancy experience prevents a complete assessment of the embryofetal risk. No animal reproduction studies have been conducted. Using this drug during pregnancy should be based on the pros and cons of the mother's clinical need for treatment versus any potential fetal risk that might occur from exposure.

BREASTFEEDING SUMMARY

No reports with the use of topical fluorouracil during human lactation have been located. One report describing the use of IV fluorouracil during human lactation was located. The report found the drug was not detected in the mother's milk samples (LLQ 65 ng/mL) despite normal maternal plasma levels. The drug might be found in breast milk in some patients, so fetal exposure is theoretically possible. However, systemic absorption of topical 5-FU use is only 6%. Therefore, any amount that might be found in breast milk is likely to be clinically insignificant. Because the drug is applied topically, systemic adverse reactions were not monitored.

Reference

1. Prescribing Information. Efudex. Bausch Health Companies Inc; 2021.

FLUOXETINE

Mental Health (Antidepressant/Selective Serotonin Reuptake Inhibitor)

PREGNANCY RECOMMENDATION: Human Data Suggest Low Risk

BREASTFEEDING RECOMMENDATION: Probably Compatible

PREGNANCY SUMMARY

Numerous studies have evaluated the use of fluoxetine in human pregnancy. Of 11 studies with case reports, the rate of major congenital anomalies was about 4% in nearly 700 first trimester exposures. No pattern to the anomalies was seen. Several other large studies and a meta-analysis involving several thousand exposures to selective serotonin reuptake inhibitors (SSRIs) found no increased risk for congenital anomalies when compared with non-antidepressant drug use controls. The drug crosses the placenta, so some fetal exposure occurs. Embryofetal toxicity was observed in one animal species at doses less than 10 times the RHD. ACOG recommends the use of SSRIs as first-line treatment of depression in women without previous use of an effective medication. SSRIs are well studied in pregnancy and are considered to be low risk. Data suggest that sertraline and escitalopram are preferred first-line SSRIs because of their efficacy and tolerability. Neonatal adaptation syndrome is a group of self-limiting symptoms that have been associated with SSRI exposure during pregnancy near delivery. It is estimated to occur in 10% to 30% of exposed infants. Symptoms include irritability, restlessness, tremors, hyperreflexia, poor sleep, poor feeding and rarely, seizures. Using this drug during pregnancy should be based on the mother's clinical need for treatment versus any potential infant risks that might occur. If used, the infant should be monitored for these symptoms post-delivery. There is a pregnancy exposure registry that monitors pregnancy outcomes in women exposed to antidepressants during pregnancy. For more information, health care providers or patients are encouraged to contact the National Pregnancy Registry for Antidepressants at 1-866-961-2388.

BREASTFEEDING SUMMARY

Numerous studies have evaluated fluoxetine and its active metabolite, norfluoxetine, during human lactation. In 12 studies totaling more than 110 lactating women, fluoxetine and norfluoxetine were both found in breast milk samples, with norfluoxetine usually having higher levels. Measured levels ranged from undetectable up to about 220 ng/mL in most instances. Nearly all calculated RIDs were below 10%. In addition, several studies have analyzed infant blood for the presence of these drugs in 77 infants. In nearly half of the cases, fluoxetine was not detected, but norfluoxetine was found. Infant levels were almost always below 10% of the maternal levels (although a few were higher—the highest being 59%).

Fluoxetine has also been associated with causing elevated prolactin levels, but this should not adversely affect breastfeeding. ACOG recommends that if a mother is stable on psychopharmacotherapy, such as an SSRI, therapy should not be changed postpartum as exposure is less from breastfeeding than during pregnancy. If the clinical decision is to use this drug while breastfeeding, the infant should be monitored for the most commonly reported side effects of drowsiness, restlessness, irritability, poor feeding, and poor weight gain.

References

1. Shuey DL, Sadler TW, Lauder JM. Serotonin as a regulator of craniofacial morphogenesis: site-specific malformations following exposure to serotonin uptake inhibitors. *Teratology.* 1992;46:367-378.
2. Prescribing Information. Fluoxetine. Teva Pharmaceuticals; 2022.
3. Cooper GL. The safety of fluoxetine—an update. *Br J Psychiatry.* 1988;153(suppl 3):77-86.

4. Vedernikov Y, Bolanos S, Bytautiene E, et al. Effect of fluoxetine on contractile activity of pregnant rat uterine rings. *Am J Obstet Gynecol.* 2000;182:296-299.
5. Montero D, de Ceballos ML, Del Rio J. Down-regulation of 3H-imipramine binding sites in rat cerebral cortex after prenatal exposure to antidepressants. *Life Sci.* 1990;46:1619-1626.
6. Stanford MS, Patton JH. In utero exposure to fluoxetine HCl increases hematoma frequency at birth. *Pharmacol Biochem Behav.* 1993;45:959-962.
7. Heikkinen T, Ekblad U, Laine K. Transplacental transfer of citalopram, fluoxetine, and their primary demethylated metabolites in isolated perfused human placenta. *BJOG.* 2002;109:1003-1008.
8. Hendrick V, Stowe ZN, Altshuler LL, et al. Placental passage of antidepressant medications. *Am J Psychiatry.* 2003;160:993-996.
9. Pastuszak A, Schick-Boschetto B, Zuber C, et al. Pregnancy outcome following first-trimester exposure to fluoxetine (Prozac). *JAMA.* 1993;269:2246-228.
10. Jacobson SJ, Jones K, Johnson K, et al. Prospective multicentre study of pregnancy outcome after lithium exposure during first trimester. *Lancet.* 1992;339:530-533.
11. Goldstein DJ, Marvel DE. Psychotropic medications during pregnancy: risk to the fetus. *JAMA.* 1993;270:2177.
12. Nulman I, Koren G. The safety of fluoxetine during pregnancy and lactation. *Teratology.* 1996;53:304-308.
13. Chambers CD, Johnson KA, Dick LM, et al. Birth outcomes in pregnant women taking fluoxetine. *N Engl J Med.* 1996;335:1010-1015.
14. Spencer MJ. Fluoxetine hydrochloride (Prozac) toxicity in a neonate. *Pediatrics.* 1993;92:721-722.
15. Mhanna MJ, Bennet JB II, Izatt SD. Potential fluoxetine chloride (Prozac) toxicity in a newborn. *Pediatrics.* 1997;100:158-9.
16. McElhatton PR, Garbis HM, Elefant E, et al. The outcome of pregnancy in 689 women exposed to therapeutic doses of antidepressants. A collaborative study of the European Network of Teratology Information Services (ENTIS). *Reprod Toxicol.* 1996;10:285-294.
17. Goldstein DJ. Effects of third trimester fluoxetine exposure on the newborn. *J Clin Psychopharmacol.* 1995;15:417-420.
18. Goldstein DJ, Corbin LA, Sundell KL. Effects of first-trimester fluoxetine exposure on the newborn. *Obstet Gynecol.* 1997;89:713-718.
19. Nulman I, Rovet J, Stewart DE, et al. Neurodevelopment of children exposed in utero to antidepressant drugs. *N Engl J Med.* 1997;336:258-262.
20. Wilton LV, Pearce GL, Martin RM, et al. The outcomes of pregnancy in women exposed to newly marketed drugs in general practice in England. *Br J Obstet Gynaecol.* 1998;105:882-889.
21. Gupta S, Masand PS, Rangwani S. Selective serotonin reuptake inhibitors in pregnancy and lactation. *Obstet Gynecol Surv.* 1998;53:733-736.
22. Austin MPV, Mitchell PB. Psychotropic medications in pregnant women: treatment dilemmas. *Med J Aust.* 1998;169:428-431.
23. Addis A, Koren G. Safety of fluoxetine during the first trimester of pregnancy: a meta-analytical review of epidemiological studies. *Psychol Med.* 2000;30:89-94.
24. Brent NB, Wisner KL. Fluoxetine and carbamazepine concentrations in a nursing mother/infant pair. *Clin Pediatr.* 1998;37:41-4.
25. Nordeng H, Lindemann R, Perminov KV, Reikvam A. Neonatal withdrawal syndrome after in utero exposure to selective serotonin reuptake inhibitors. *Acta Paediatr.* 2001;90:288-91.
26. Nulman I, Rovet J, Stewart DE, et al. Child development following exposure to tricyclic antidepressants or fluoxetine throughout fetal life: a prospective, controlled study. *Am J Psychiatry.* 2002;159:1889-1895.
27. Casper RC, Fleisher BE, Lee-Ancajas JC, et al. Follow-up of children of depressed mothers exposed or not exposed to antidepressant drugs during pregnancy. *J Pediatr.* 2003;142:402-408.
28. Zeskind PS, Stephens LE. Maternal selective serotonin reuptake inhibitor use during pregnancy and newborn neurobehavior. *Pediatrics.* 2004;113: 368-375.
29. Hendrick V, Smith LM, Suri R, et al Birth outcomes after prenatal exposure to antidepressant medication. *Am J Obstet Gynecol.* 2003;188:812-815.
30. DeMyer W. Brain, midline caves. In: Buyse ML, ed. *Birth Defects Encyclopedia.* Blackwell Scientific Publications; 1990:238.
31. Hines RN, Adams J, Buck GM, et al. NTP-CERHR expert panel report on the reproductive and developmental toxicity of fluoxetine. *Birth Defects Res B Dev Reprod Toxicol.* 2004;71:193-280.
32. Einarson TR, Einarson A. Newer antidepressants in pregnancy and rates of major malformations: a meta-analysis of prospective comparative studies. *Pharmacoepidemiol Drug Saf.* 2005;14:823-827.
33. Sanz EJ, De-las-Cuevas C, Kiuru A, Edwards R. Selective serotonin reuptake inhibitors in pregnant women and neonatal withdrawal syndrome: a database analysis. *Lancet.* 2005;365:482-487.
34. Moses-Kolko EL, Bogen D, Perel J, et al. Neonatal signs after late in utero exposure to serotonin reuptake inhibitors. *JAMA.* 2005;293:2372-2383.
35. Oberlander TF, Grunau RE, Fitzgerald C, et al. Pain reactivity in 2-month-old infants after prenatal and postnatal selective serotonin reuptake inhibitor medication exposure. *Pediatrics.* 2005;115:411-425.
36. Oberlander TF, Warburton W, Misri S, et al. Neonatal outcomes after prenatal exposure to selective serotonin reuptake inhibitor antidepressants and maternal depression using population-based linked health data. *Arch Gen Psychiatry.* 2006;63:898-906.
37. Levinson-Castiel R, Merlob P, Linder N, et al. Neonatal abstinence syndrome after in utero exposure to selective serotonin reuptake inhibitors in term infants. *Arch Pediatr Adolesc Med.* 2006;160:173-6.
38. Rahimi R, Nikfar S, Abdollahi M. Pregnancy outcomes following exposure to serotonin reuptake inhibitors: a meta-analysis of clinical trials. *Reprod Toxicol.* 2006;22:571-575.
39. Alwan S, Reefhuis J, Rasmussen S, et al. Maternal use of selective serotonin reuptake inhibitors and risk for birth defects (abstract). *Birth Defects Res A Clin Mol Teratol.* 2005;73:291.
40. Diav-Citrin O, Shechtman S, Weinbaum D, et al. Paroxetine and fluoxetine in pregnancy: a multicenter, prospective, controlled study (abstract). *Reprod Toxicol.* 2005;20:459.
41. Ericson A, Kallen B, Wiholm BE. Delivery outcome after the use of antidepressants in early pregnancy. *Eur J Clin Pharmacol.* 1999;55:503-508.
42. Kallen B, Olausson PO. Antidepressant drugs during pregnancy and infant congenital heart defect. *Reprod Toxicol.* 2006;21:221-2.
43. Kallen BAJ, Olausson PO. Maternal use of selective serotonin re-uptake inhibitors in early pregnancy and infant congenital malformations. *Birth Defects Res A Clin Mol Teratol.* 2007;79:301-308.
44. Berard A, Ramos E, Rey E, et al. First trimester exposure to paroxetine and risk of cardiac malformations in infants: the importance of dosage. *Birth Defects Res B Dev Reprod Toxicol.* 2007;80:18-27.
45. Ferreira E, Carceller AM, Agogue C, et al. Effects of selective serotonin reuptake inhibitors and venlafaxine during pregnancy in term and preterm neonates. *Pediatrics.* 2007;119:52-59.
46. Bellantuono C, Migliarese G, Gentile S. Serotonin reuptake inhibitors in pregnancy and the risk of major malformations: a systematic review. *Hum Psychopharmacol Clin Exp.* 2007;22:121-128.
47. Chambers CD, Hernandez-Diaz S, Van Marter LJ, et al. Selective serotonin-reuptake inhibitors and risk of persistent pulmonary hypertension of the newborn. *N Engl J Med.* 2006;354:579-587.
48. Alwan S, Reefhuis J, Rasmussen SA, et al; National Birth Defects Prevention Study. Use of selective serotonin-reuptake inhibitors in pregnancy and the risk of birth defects. *N Engl J Med.* 2007;356:2684-2692.
49. Louik C, Lin AE, Werler MM, et al. First-trimester use of selective serotonin-reuptake inhibitors and the risk of birth defects. *N Engl J Med.* 2007;356:2675-2683.
50. Greene MF. Teratogenicity of SSRIs—serious concern or much ado about little? *N Engl J Med.* 2007;356:2732-2733.
51. Williams SF, Alvarez JR, Pedro HF, Apuzzio JJ. Glutaric aciduria type II and narcolepsy in pregnancy. *Obstet Gynecol.* 2008;111:522-4.
52. Einarson A, Choi J, Einarson TR, Koren G. Incidence of major malformations in infants following antidepressant exposure in pregnancy: results of a large prospective cohort study. *Can J Psychiatry.* 2009;54:242-246.
53. Isenberg KE. Excretion of fluoxetine in human breast milk. *J Clin Psychiatry.* 1990;51:169.
54. Burch KJ, Wells BG. Fluoxetine/norfluoxetine concentrations in human milk. *Pediatrics.* 1992;89:676-677.
55. Lester BM, Cucca J, Andreozzi L, et al. Possible association between fluoxetine hydrochloride and colic in an infant. *J Am Acad Child Adolesc Psychiatr.* 1993;32:1253-1255.
56. Wisner KL, Perel JM, Findling RL. Antidepressant treatment during breast feeding. *Am J Psychiatry.* 1996;153:1132-1137.
57. Taddio A, Ito S, Koren G. Excretion of fluoxetine and its metabolite, norfluoxetine, in human breast milk. *J Clin Pharmacol.* 1996;36:42-47.
58. Yoshida K, Smith B, Craggs M, Channi Kumar R. Fluoxetine in breast-milk and developmental outcome of breast-fed infants. *Br J Psychiatry.* 1998;172:175-179.
59. Kristensen JH, Ilett KF, Hackett LP, et al. Distribution and excretion of fluoxetine and norfluoxetine in human milk. *Br J Clin Pharmacol.* 1999;48:521-527.
60. Chambers CD, Anderson PO, Thomas RG, et al. Weight gain in infants breastfed by mothers who take fluoxetine (abstract). *Pediatrics.* 1999;104:1120-1121.
61. Hale TW, Shum S, Grossberg M. Fluoxetine toxicity in a breastfed infant. *Clin Pediatr.* 2001;40:681-684.

62. Marshall AM, Nommsen-Rivers LA, Hernandez LI, et al. Serotonin transport and metabolism in the mammary gland modulates secretory activation and involution. *J Clin Endocrin Metab*. 2010;95:837-846.
63. Nightingale SL. Fluoxetine labeling revised to identify phenytoin interaction and to recommend against use in nursing mothers. *JAMA*. 1994;271:1067.
64. Edwards JG, Anerson I. Systematic review and guide to selection of selective serotonin reuptake inhibitors. *Drugs*. 1999;57:507-533.
65. Treatment and management of mental health conditions during pregnancy and postpartum: ACOG clinical practice guideline no. 5. *Obstet Gynecol*. 2023; 141:1262-1288.
66. Cipriani A, Furukawa TA, Salanti G, et al. Comparative efficacy and acceptability of 21 antidepressant drugs for the acute treatment of adults with major depressive disorder: a systematic review and network meta-analysis. *Lancet*. 2018;39:1357-1366.
67. U.S. Food and Drug Administration. FDA drug safety communication: selective serotonin reuptake inhibitor (SSRI) antidepressant use during pregnancy and reports of a rare heart and lung condition in newborn babies. Accessed September 27, 2023. https://www.fda.gov/drugs/drug-safety-and-availability/fda-drug-safety-communication-selective-serotonin-reuptake-inhibitor-ssri-antidepressant-use-during
68. Moses-Kolko EL, Bogen D, Perel J, et al. Neonatal signs after late in utero exposure to serotonin reuptake inhibitors: literature review and implications for clinical applications. *JAMA*. 2005;293(19):2372-2383.

FLUPHENAZINE

Mental Health (First-Generation Antipsychotic)

PREGNANCY RECOMMENDATION: Limited Human Data—Animal Data Suggest Potential Risk

BREASTFEEDING RECOMMENDATION: Potential Toxicity

PREGNANCY SUMMARY

Four case reports describing the use of fluphenazine in human pregnancy have been located. Three of the cases had exposure in the first trimester and one of these was found to have multiple anomalies at delivery. In the other three cases, normal appearing newborns were delivered. However, extrapyramidal and/or withdrawal symptoms were seen over the few weeks following delivery. These findings have been reported with other phenothiazine antipsychotic agents. The drug will likely cross the placenta, so fetal exposure will probably occur. This transfer will be higher with intramuscular (IM) usage due to the prolonged elimination half-life. Therefore, this limited human pregnancy experience prevents a complete assessment of the embryofetal risk. Animal studies showed embryofetal toxicity in one species at doses less than 10 times the RHD. No embryofetal toxicity was seen in a second species at doses greater than 10 times the RHD. Using this drug during pregnancy should be based on the pros and cons of the mother's clinical need for treatment versus any potential fetal risk that might occur from exposure.

BREASTFEEDING SUMMARY

No reports describing the use of fluphenazine during human lactation have been located. Based on the MW, the drug will be found in breast milk, but the high plasma protein binding should limit some excretion. Regardless, because other phenothiazines are excreted into milk, passage of fluphenazine into milk should be expected. Breastfeeding while using this drug should be based on the mother's clinical need for treatment versus any potential infant risks that might occur. If used, the infant should be monitored for the most commonly reported adult side effects of upset stomach (leading to irritability), sleepiness, insomnia, and lethargy.

References

1. Prescribing Information. Fluphenazine hydrochloride. Sandoz; 2019.
2. Prescribing Information. Fluphenazine hydrochloride. Fresenius Kabi USA; 2016.
3. Shepard TH. *Catalog of Teratogenic Effects*. 8th ed. The Johns Hopkins University Press; 1995:190-191.
4. Abdel-Hamid HA, Abdel-Rahman MS, Abdel-Rahman SA. Teratogenic effect of diphenylhydantoin and/or fluphenazine in mice. *J Appl Toxicol*. 1996;16:221-225.
5. Moya F, Thorndike V. Passage of drugs across the placenta. *Am J Obstet Gynecol*. 1962;84:1778-1798.
6. Cleary MF. Fluphenazine decanoate during pregnancy. *Am J Psychiatry*. 1977;134:815-816.
7. O'Connor M, Johnson GH, James DI. Intrauterine effect of phenothiazines. *Med J Aust*. 1981;1:416-417.
8. Donaldson GL, Bury RG. Multiple congenital abnormalities in a newborn boy associated with maternal use of fluphenazine enanthate and other drugs during pregnancy. *Acta Paediatr Scand*. 1982;71:335-338.
9. Nath SP, Miller DA, Muraskas JK. Severe rhinorrhea and respiratory distress in a neonate exposed to fluphenazine hydrochloride prenatally. *Ann Pharmacother*. 1996;30:35-37.

FLURANDRENOLIDE

Dermatologic/Corticosteroid

PREGNANCY RECOMMENDATION: No Human Data and No Relevant Animal Data

BREASTFEEDING RECOMMENDATION: Probably Compatible

PREGNANCY SUMMARY

No reports describing the use of flurandrenolide in human pregnancy have been located. A large case-control study that evaluated the teratogenic potential of topical corticosteroids involving 1,923,413 total births was conducted by the Hungarian Case-Control Surveillance of Congenital Abnormalities program. Among the 20,830 malformed case infants, 73 (0.35%) used a topical corticosteroid during the first trimester compared with 118 (0.33%) of the 35,727 normal control infants. This comparison was not significant. Topical corticosteroid use in the first trimester did not show an increased risk of congenital abnormalities. A meta-analysis evaluating the effects of topical corticosteroids on pregnancy outcome reviewed 14 studies involving 1,601,515 pregnant women. When compared to no exposure, overall, no association with congenital abnormalities, orofacial clefts, or preterm delivery was found with the use of any potent corticosteroid medication. The drug will probably cross the placenta in some cases, but the overall amount will likely be clinically insignificant. However, this limited human pregnancy experience prevents a complete assessment of the embryofetal risk. Animal reproduction studies have not been conducted with flurandrenolide. Using this drug during pregnancy should be based on the pros and cons of the mother's clinical need for treatment versus any potential fetal risk that might occur from exposure.

F

BREASTFEEDING SUMMARY

No reports describing the use of flurandrenolide during lactation have been located. The drug will probably be found in breast milk in some cases; however, the overall amount is probably clinically insignificant. Breastfeeding while using this drug should be based on the mother's clinical need for treatment. Due to the negligible absorption, systemic side effects were not reported. The drug should not be applied directly on the nipple area during lactation.

References

1. Prescribing Information. Cordran. Aqua Pharmaceuticals; 2013.
2. Prescribing Information. Cordran Tape. Allergen; 2018.
3. Czeizel AE, Rockenbauer M. Population-based case-control study of teratogenic potential of corticosteroids. *Teratology*. 1997;56:335-340.
4. Chi CC, Wang SH, Wojnarowska F, et al. Safety of topical corticosteroids in pregnancy. *Cochrane Database Syst Rev*. 2015;2015:CD007346.

FLURAZEPAM

Central Nervous System (Benzodiazepine Hypnotic)

PREGNANCY RECOMMENDATION: Limited Human Data - Animal Data Suggest Low Risk

BREASTFEEDING RECOMMENDATION: Potential Toxicity

PREGNANCY SUMMARY

In a surveillance study of Michigan Medicaid recipients, 73 newborns had been exposed to flurazepam during the first trimester. There were four (5.5%) major birth anomalies observed (three expected). No pattern to the anomalies was detected. One other case report described a pregnant woman with first trimester exposure to flurazepam (along with several other drugs). She delivered at term a normal infant with no reported anomalies. Based on likely placental transfer, some fetal exposure will probably occur. Therefore, this limited human pregnancy experience prevents a complete assessment of the embryofetal risk. Studies in human pregnancy with other benzodiazepine drugs have not shown a clear association in causing major birth anomalies. In addition, the use of benzodiazepine drugs throughout pregnancy has been associated with neonatal withdrawal symptoms postdelivery. If used near delivery, neonatal depression, sedation, and hypotonia may occur at the time of birth. There is a pregnancy exposure registry that monitors pregnancy outcomes in women using psychiatric medications during pregnancy. Health care providers are encouraged to call the National Pregnancy Registry for Psychiatric Medications at 1-866-961-2388. The drug also carries a Boxed Warning for increased risks from the concomitant use with opioid drugs and the risk for misuse, addiction, and dependence with a potential for withdrawal reactions. Acute withdrawal from benzodiazepine drugs has been associated with seizures.

BREASTFEEDING SUMMARY

No reports describing the use of flurazepam during human lactation have been located. The drug will be found in breast milk, so some infant exposure (especially the active metabolite) will likely occur. Other benzodiazepine drugs have been found in breast milk. The manufacturer recommends not using flurazepam while nursing. However, if the clinical decision is to use this drug during lactation, the infant should be monitored for the most commonly reported adult side effects of nausea, headache, myalgia, and dizziness (all leading to irritability), somnolence, lethargy, vomiting, and diarrhea.

References

1. Prescribing Information. Flurazepam. Chartwell RX, LLC; 2023.
2. Gentile S. Pharmacologic management of borderline personality disorder in a pregnant woman with a previous history of alcohol addiction: a case report. *Clin Drug Investig*. 2015;35:761-763.

FLURBIPROFEN

Pain (NSAID)

PREGNANCY RECOMMENDATION: Human Data Suggest Risk in Third Trimester

BREASTFEEDING RECOMMENDATION: Probably Compatible

F

PREGNANCY SUMMARY

No reports describing the use of flurbiprofen during human pregnancy have been located. Several studies have looked at NSAIDs as a group and have found mixed results regarding embryofetal toxicity and malformations. Overall, their use does not appear to significantly increase the risk of birth defects or preterm delivery. Constriction of the ductus arteriosus in utero is a pharmacologic consequence arising from the use of prostaglandin synthesis inhibitors during pregnancy. Persistent pulmonary hypertension of the newborn may occur if these agents are used in the third trimester close to birth. These drugs also have been shown to inhibit labor and prolong pregnancy, in humans (see Indomethacin). The drug will likely cross the placenta, so some fetal exposure will probably occur. Therefore, the absence of human pregnancy experience prevents a complete assessment of the embryofetal risk. Animal studies did show embryofetal toxicity but not malformations in three species at doses less than 10 times the RHD. Using this drug during pregnancy should be based on the pros and cons of the mother's clinical need for treatment versus any potential fetal risk that might occur from exposure.

BREASTFEEDING SUMMARY

Two studies that evaluated the use of flurbiprofen during human lactation were located. In the combined data, 22 lactating women had breast milk samples tested after using flurbiprofen. The drug was not detected in the milk of 15 of these mothers. In the remaining seven, the maximum level detected was only 92 ng/mL. The calculated RID from all these patients was 0.5% or less. This is consistent with the combination of the low MW but very high plasma protein binding. Breastfeeding while using this drug should be based on the mother's clinical need for treatment. If used, the infant should be monitored for the most commonly reported adult side effects of nausea, headache, and abdominal pain (all leading to irritability), diarrhea, insomnia, vomiting, and rash.

References

1. Prescribing Information. Flurbiprofen. Pfizer; 2020.
2. Nielsen GL, Sorensen HT, Larsen H, et al. Risk of adverse birth outcome and miscarriage in pregnant users of non-steroidal anti-inflammatory drugs: population based observational study and case-control study. *Br Med J.* 2001;322:266-270.
3. Ericson A, Kallen BAJ. Nonsteroidal anti-inflammatory drugs in early pregnancy. *Reprod Toxicol.* 2001;15:371-375.
4. Li DK, Liu L, Odouli R. Exposure to non-steroidal anti-inflammatory drugs during pregnancy and risk of miscarriage: population based cohort study. *Br Med J.* 2003;327:368-371.
5. Tassinari MS, Cook JC, Hurtt ME. NSAIDs and developmental toxicity. *Birth Defects Res B Dev Reprod Toxicol.* 2003;68:3-4.
6. Levin DL. Effects of inhibition of prostaglandin synthesis on fetal development, oxygenation, and the fetal circulation. *Semin Perinatol.* 1980;4:35-44.
7. Van Marter LJ, Leviton A, Allred EN, et al. Persistent pulmonary hypertension of the newborn and smoking and aspirin and nonsteroidal anti-inflammatory drug consumption during pregnancy. *Pediatrics.* 1996;97:658-663.
8. Fuchs F. Prevention of prematurity. *Am J Obstet Gynecol.* 1976;126:809-820.
9. Cox SR, Forbes KK. Excretion of flurbiprofen into breast milk. *Pharmacotherapy.* 1987;7:211-215.
10. Smith IJ, Hinson JL, Johnson VA, et al. Flurbiprofen in post-partum women: plasma and breast milk disposition. 1989;29:174-184.

FLURBIPROFEN

Ophthalmic (NSAID)

PREGNANCY RECOMMENDATION: No Human Data and No Relevant Animal Data

BREASTFEEDING RECOMMENDATION: Probably Compatible

PREGNANCY SUMMARY

No reports describing the use of flurbiprofen ophthalmic in human pregnancy have been located. Based on likely minimal systemic absorption, fetal exposure is probably clinically insignificant. However, the absence of human pregnancy experience prevents a complete assessment of the embryofetal risk. No relevant animal reproduction studies have been conducted. Using this drug during pregnancy should be based on the pros and cons of the mother's clinical need for treatment versus any potential fetal risk that might occur from possible systemic absorption. If used during pregnancy, consider placing pressure over the tear duct in the corner of the eye for at least 1 minute and then remove any excess solution with absorbent tissue to decrease the amount of drug reaching the systemic circulation even further.

BREASTFEEDING SUMMARY

No reports describing the use of flurbiprofen ophthalmic during human lactation have been located. Per the manufacturer, flurbiprofen was found in human breast milk, but the calculated level of exposure is very low at about 0.1 mg/d. Breastfeeding while using this drug should be based on the mother's clinical need for treatment. However, exposure to this drug during breastfeeding is unlikely because it is used during surgery. A method to decrease some systemic absorption with ophthalmic use is described in the above Pregnancy Summary.

Reference

1. Prescribing Information. Flurbiprofen sodium. AMICI Pharmaceuticals; 2020.

F

FLUTEMETAMOL F18

Radiopharmaceutical

PREGNANCY RECOMMENDATION: *No Human Data and No Relevant Animal Data

BREASTFEEDING RECOMMENDATION: Hold Breastfeeding

PREGNANCY SUMMARY

No reports describing the use of flutemetamol F18 in human pregnancy have been located. The drug will probably cross the placenta, but the rapid clearance should limit fetal exposure. However, the absence of human pregnancy experience prevents a complete assessment of the embryofetal risk. No animal studies have been conducted. *Because all radioactive agents have the potential to cause harm, the clinical decision to use this agent in a pregnant patient will need to be based on the stage of fetal development and the expected radiation exposure.

BREASTFEEDING SUMMARY

No reports describing the use of flutemetamol F18 during human lactation have been located. The drug will probably be excreted into breast milk, but the rapid clearance should limit infant exposure. However, the manufacturer recommends that women should be advised to avoid the use of flutemetamol F18 while breastfeeding or temporarily interrupt breastfeeding for 24 hours (more than 10 half-lives). If interrupted, the mother should pump and discard her breast milk for this time period to minimize radiation exposure.

Reference

1. Product Information. Vizamyl. GE Healthcare, Medi-Physics, Inc; 2019.

FLUTICASONE

Corticosteroid (Respiratory/Nasal)

PREGNANCY RECOMMENDATION: Human Data Suggest Compatible

BREASTFEEDING RECOMMENDATION: Probably Compatible

PREGNANCY SUMMARY

Several large studies totaling more than 6,500 pregnancies did not find an increased risk for congenital anomalies with first trimester exposure to inhaled fluticasone. Fluticasone crosses the placenta at low concentrations, but some fetal exposure can occur. Embryofetal toxicity with malformations were observed in three animal species using subcutaneous (SC) doses less than 10 times the maximum recommended human daily intranasal dose (MRHDID); however, maternal toxicity occurred in all three species. ICSs are recommended for the management of asthma in pregnancy. ACOG recommends that while budesonide is considered the ICS of choice during pregnancy, use of ICSs in women who are previously well controlled by a specific agent prior to pregnancy should continue. Treatment should not be stepped down or discontinued during pregnancy.

BREASTFEEDING SUMMARY

No reports describing the use of fluticasone oral inhalation or nasal spray use during human lactation have been located. The drug might be found in breast milk. However, because of the low systemic concentrations obtained with fluticasone inhalation and nasal use and the drug's poor oral bioavailability, it is doubtful if any clinically significant amounts would be absorbed following ingestion by a nursing infant. Breastfeeding while using this drug should be based on the mother's clinical need for treatment versus any potential infant risks that might occur. If used, the infant should be monitored for the most commonly reported adult side effects of headache and nausea (both leading to irritability), vomiting, and cough.

References

1. Tan KS, Thomson NC. Asthma in pregnancy. *Am J Med*. 2000;109:727-733.
2. Joint Committee of the American College of Obstetrics and Gynecologists (ACOG) and the American College of Allergy, Asthma and Immunology (ACAAI). Position statement. The use of newer asthma and allergy medications during pregnancy. *Ann Allergy Asthma Immunol*. 2000;84:475-480.
3. Prescribing Information. Flovent HFA. GlaxoSmithKline; 2021.
4. Battista MC, Boutin M, Venne P, et al. Maternal inhaled fluticasone propionate intake during pregnancy is detected in neonatal cord blood. *Bioanalysis*. 2016;8:1441-1450.
5. Namazy J, Schatz M, Long L, et al. Use of inhaled steroids by pregnant asthmatic women does not reduce intrauterine growth. *J Allergy Clin Immunol*. 2004;113:427-432.
6. Ellegard EK, Hellgren M, Karlsson NG. Fluticasone propionate aqueous nasal spray in pregnancy rhinitis. *Clin Otolaryngol*. 2001;26:394-400.
7. Murphy VE, Fittock RJ, Zarzycki PK, et al. Metabolism of synthetic steroids by the human placenta. *Placenta*. 2007;28:39-46.
8. Choi JS, Han JY, Kim MY, Velazquez-Armenta EY, Nava-Ocampo AA. Pregnancy outcomes in women using inhaled fluticasone during pregnancy: a case series. *Allergol Immunopathol (Madr)*. 2007;35:239-242.
9. Rahimi R, Nikfar S, Abdollahi M. Meta-analysis finds use of inhaled corticosteroids during pregnancy safe: a systematic meta-analysis review. *Hum Exp Toxicol*. 2006;25:447-452.
10. Cossette B, Beauchesne MF, Forget A, et al. Relative perinatal safety of salmeterol vs formoterol and fluticasone vs budesonide use during pregnancy. *Ann Allergy Asthma Immunol*. 2014;112:459-464.
11. Van Zutphen AR, Bell EM, Browne ML, et al; National Birth Defects Prevention Study. Maternal asthma medication use during pregnancy and risk of congenital heart defects. *Birth Defects Res A Clin Mol Teratol*. 2015;103:951-961.
12. Charlton RA, Snowball JM, Nightingale AL, Davis KJ. Safety of fluticasone propionate prescribed for asthma during pregnancy: a UK population-based cohort study. *J Allergy Clin Immunol Pract*. 2015;3:772-9.
13. Alhussien AH, Alhedaithy RA, Alsaleh SA. Safety of intranasal corticosteroid sprays during pregnancy: an updated review. *Eur Arch Otorhinolaryngol*. 2018;275:325-333.
14. Global Initiative for Asthma. Global strategy for asthma management and prevention. Updated 2023. Accessed August 31, 2023. http://www.ginasthma.org
15. National Heart, Lung, and Blood Institute; National Asthma Education and Prevention Program Asthma and Pregnancy Working Group. NAEPP expert panel report. Managing asthma during pregnancy: recommendations for pharmacologic treatment-2004 update. *J Allergy Clin Immunol*. 2005;115:34-46.
16. American College of Obstetricians and Gynecologists. Asthma in pregnancy: ACOG practice bulletin no. 90. *Obstet Gynecol*. 2008;111:457-464.

FLUTICASONE CREAM/LOTION/OINTMENT

Corticosteroid/Dermatologic (Topical)

PREGNANCY RECOMMENDATION: No Human Data and No Relevant Animal Data

BREASTFEEDING RECOMMENDATION: Probably Compatible

PREGNANCY SUMMARY

No reports describing the use of topical fluticasone in human pregnancy have been located. If present in the systemic circulation, the drug will probably cross the placenta, so some fetal exposure could occur. However, with low systemic bioavailability following topical use, a clinically significant exposure of the embryo or fetus is unlikely. Regardless, the absence of human pregnancy experience prevents a complete assessment of the embryofetal risk. Embryofetal toxicity with malformations was observed in three animal species using SC doses less than 10 times the MRHDID; however, maternal toxicity occurred in all species. Using this drug during pregnancy should be based on the pros and cons of the mother's clinical need for treatment versus any potential fetal risk that might occur from exposure.

BREASTFEEDING SUMMARY

No reports describing the use of topical fluticasone during human lactation have been located. The drug might be found in breast milk. However, because of the low systemic concentrations obtained with topical fluticasone use and the drug's poor oral bioavailability, it is doubtful if any clinically significant amounts would be absorbed following ingestion by a nursing infant. Breastfeeding while using this drug should be based on the mother's clinical need for treatment versus any potential infant risks that might occur. Because of the topical use of the drug, systemic adverse reactions were not evaluated.

References

1. Prescribing Information. Cutivate. G&W Laboratories; 2021.
2. Battista MC, Boutin M, Venne P, et al. Maternal inhaled fluticasone propionate intake during pregnancy is detected in neonatal cord blood. *Bioanalysis*. 2016;8:1441-1450.

FLUVASTATIN

Antilipemic

PREGNANCY RECOMMENDATION: *Contraindicated/Limited Human Data—Animal Data Suggest Potential Risk

BREASTFEEDING RECOMMENDATION: *Contraindicated

PREGNANCY SUMMARY

Five studies and a case report describing the use of fluvastatin in 61 human pregnancies have been located. The case report involved first trimester exposure to numerous drugs (including fluvastatin) and the delivered term newborn had no identified birth anomalies. The other five studies were evaluations of "statin drugs" as a group, so specific details on fluvastatin alone were not available. However, these studies have not found an increased risk for congenital malformations. Some studies have shown an increased risk for spontaneous abortion, but maternal disease also plays a role in this complication. The drug will probably cross the placenta, so some fetal exposure may occur. However, this limited human pregnancy experience prevents a complete assessment of the embryofetal risk. Embryofetal toxicity was observed in one species at doses less than 10 times the RHD. *In 2021, the FDA removed the long-standing contraindication to statin use in all women who are pregnant or who are contemplating pregnancy. The removal was requested because the benefits, which include prevention of serious or fatal events in some clinical settings, may outweigh the potential risk in a small group of very high-risk pregnant patients. Despite this removal, the FDA continues to recommend that most patients stop statin use once they learn they are pregnant.

BREASTFEEDING SUMMARY

No reports describing the use of fluvastatin during human lactation have been located. Some drug will probably be found in human breast milk, so infant exposure may occur. *In 2021, the FDA reaffirmed its warning that postpartum patients should not breastfeed when taking a statin because the medication may pass into breast milk and pose a risk to the baby. If possible, statins should be temporarily held until breastfeeding ends. However, patients requiring ongoing statin treatment should consider not breastfeeding and instead use infant formula or other alternatives. If breastfeeding occurs while statins are administered, the hydrophilic ones (pravastatin, rosuvastatin, and fluvastatin) should theoretically have lower milk levels.

References

1. Prescribing Information. Lescol XL. Novartis Pharmaceuticals; 2020.
2. Seguin J, Samuels P. Fluvastatin exposure during pregnancy. *Obstet Gynecol.* 1999;93:847.
3. Winterfeld U, Allignol A, Panchaud A, et al. Pregnancy outcome following maternal exposure to statins: a multicentre prospective study. *BJOG.* 2013;120:463-471.
4. Ofori B, Rey E, Bérard A. Risk of congenital anomalies in pregnant users of statin drugs. *Br J Clin Pharmacol.* 2007;64:496-509.
5. Edison RJ, Muenke M. Mechanistic and epidemiologic considerations in the evaluation of adverse birth outcomes following gestational exposure to statins. *Am J Med Genet A.* 2004;131:287-298.
6. McGrogan A, Snowball J, Charlton RA. Statins during pregnancy: a cohort study using the General Practice Research Database to investigate pregnancy loss. *Pharmacoepidemiol Drug Saf.* 2017;26:843-852.
7. Bateman BT, Hernandez-Diaz S, Fischer MA, et al. Statins and congenital malformations: cohort study. *BMJ.* 2015;350:h1035.
8. U.S. Food and Drug Administration. FDA requests removal of strongest warning against using cholesterol-lowering statins during pregnancy; still advises most pregnant patients should stop taking statins. 2021. https://www.fda.gov/drugs/drug-safety-and-availability/fda-requests-removal-strongest-warning-against-using-cholesterol-lowering-statins-during-pregnancy

FLUVOXAMINE

Mental Health (Antidepressant/SSRI)

PREGNANCY RECOMMENDATION: Limited Human Data—Animal Data Suggest Potential Risk

BREASTFEEDING RECOMMENDATION: Probably Compatible

PREGNANCY SUMMARY

Numerous studies have evaluated the use of fluvoxamine in human pregnancy. Of three studies, there were 3 (4.6%) major anomalies seen in 65 first trimester exposures to fluvoxamine. Several other large studies including the Motherisk database, the Quebec population-based cohort study, the Swedish Medical Birth registry, two large population-based studies, and a meta-analysis found no increased risk for congenital anomalies in pregnancies exposed to antidepressants when compared with non-antidepressant drug use controls. In these studies, the use of fluvoxamine was low and specific outcomes for this drug were not supplied. The drug will probably cross the placenta, so some fetal exposure will likely occur. However, this limited first trimester human pregnancy exposure data prevent a complete assessment of the embryofetal risk. Embryofetal toxicity was observed in one animal species at doses less than 10 times the RHD. SSRIs are generally recommended for the treatment of obsessive-compulsive disorder. ACOG recommends the use of SSRIs as first-line treatment of depression in women without previous use of an effective medication. SSRIs are well studied in pregnancy and are considered to be low risk. Data suggest that sertraline and escitalopram are preferred first-line SSRIs because of their efficacy and tolerability. Neonatal adaptation syndrome is a group of self-limiting symptoms that have been associated with SSRI exposure during pregnancy near delivery. It is estimated to occur in 10% to 30% of exposed infants. Symptoms include irritability, restlessness,

(continued)

tremors, hyperreflexia, poor sleep, poor feeding, and, rarely, seizures. Using this drug during pregnancy should be based on the mother's clinical need for treatment versus any potential infant risks that might occur. If used, the infant should be monitored for these symptoms post-delivery. There is a pregnancy exposure registry that monitors pregnancy outcomes in women exposed to antidepressants during pregnancy. For more information, health care providers or patients are encouraged to contact the National Pregnancy Registry for Antidepressants at 1-866-961-2388.

BREASTFEEDING SUMMARY

Several studies have evaluated fluvoxamine use during human lactation. In three studies involving nine lactating mothers, the drug was detected in breast milk with levels that ranged from about 15 to 490 pg/mL. The levels were usually higher with higher maternal intake. However, the calculated RIDs were less than 1.5%. In eight cases where infant blood levels were analyzed, in six infants the drug was not detected (LLQ of 1 or 2 ng/mL). In two infants, the drug was detected at 45% the maternal level in one case and less than 10% the maternal level in the second case. Fluvoxamine has also been associated with causing elevated prolactin levels, but this should not adversely affect breastfeeding. ACOG recommends that if a mother is stable on psychopharmacotherapy, such as an SSRI, therapy should not be changed postpartum as exposure is less from breastfeeding than during pregnancy. If the clinical decision is to use this drug while breastfeeding, the infant should be monitored for the most commonly reported side effects of drowsiness, restlessness, irritability, poor feeding, and poor weight gain.

References

1. Shuey DL, Sadler TW, Lauder JM. Serotonin as a regulator of craniofacial morphogenesis: site-specific malformations following exposure to serotonin uptake inhibitors. *Teratology*. 1992;46:367-378.
2. Prescribing Information. Fluvoxamine maleate. Actavis Pharma, Inc; 2023.
3. McElhatton PR, Garbis HM, Elefant E, et al. The outcome of pregnancy in 689 women exposed to therapeutic doses of antidepressants. A collaborative study of the European Network of Teratology Information Services (ENTIS). *Reprod Toxicol*. 1996;10:285-294.
4. Wilton LV, Pearce GL, Martin RM, et al. The outcomes of pregnancy in women exposed to newly marketed drugs in general practice in England. *Br J Obstet Gynaecol*. 1998;105:882-9.
5. Kulin NA, Pastuszak A, Sage SR, et al. Pregnancy outcome following maternal use of the new selective serotonin reuptake inhibitors. A prospective controlled multicenter study. *JAMA*. 1998;279:609-610.
6. Koren G. In reply. Risk of fetal anomalies with exposure to selective serotonin reuptake inhibitors. *JAMA*. 1998;279:1873-1874.
7. Casper RC, Fleisher BE, Lee-Ancajas JC, et al. Follow-up of children of depressed mothers exposed or not exposed to antidepressant drugs during pregnancy. *J Pediatr*. 2003;142:402-408.
8. Einarson TR, Einarson A. Newer antidepressants in pregnancy and rates of major malformations: a meta-analysis of prospective comparative studies. *Pharmacoepidemiol Drug Saf*. 2005;14:823-827.
9. Gentile S. Quetiapine-fluvoxamine combination during pregnancy and while breastfeeding. *Arch Womens Ment Health*. 2006;9:158-159.
10. Hendrick V, Smith LM, Suri R, et al. Birth outcomes after prenatal exposure to antidepressant medication. *Am J Obstet Gynecol*. 2003;188:812-815.
11. DeMyer W. Brain, midline caves. In: Buyse ML, ed. *Birth Defects Encyclopedia*. Blackwell Scientific Publications; 1990:238.
12. Moses-Kolko EL, Bogen D, Perel J, et al. Neonatal signs after late in utero exposure to serotonin reuptake inhibitors. *JAMA*. 2005;293:2372-2383.
13. Oberlander TF, Warburton W, Misri S, et al. Neonatal outcomes after prenatal exposure to selective serotonin reuptake inhibitor antidepressants and maternal depression using population-based linked health data. *Arch Gen Psychiatry*. 2006;63:898-906.
14. Rahimi R, Nikfar S, Abdollahi M. Pregnancy outcomes following exposure to serotonin reuptake inhibitors: a meta-analysis of clinical trials. *Reprod Toxicol*. 2006;22:571-575.
15. Alwan S, Reefhuis J, Rasmussen S, et al. Maternal use of selective serotonin reuptake inhibitors and risk for birth defects (abstract). *Birth Defects Res A Clin Mol Teratol*. 2005;73:291.
16. Kallen B, Olausson PO. Antidepressant drugs during pregnancy and infant congenital heart defect. *Reprod Toxicol*. 2006;21:221-222.
17. Kallen BAJ, Olausson PO. Maternal use of selective serotonin re-uptake inhibitors in early pregnancy and infant congenital malformations. *Birth Defects Res A Clin Mol Teratol*. 2007;79:301-308.
18. Berard A, Ramos E, Rey E, et al. First trimester exposure to paroxetine and risk of cardiac malformations in infants: the importance of dosage. *Birth Defects Res B Dev Reprod Toxicol*. 2007;80:18-27.
19. Ferreira E, Carceller AM, Agogue C, et al. Effects of selective serotonin reuptake inhibitors and venlafaxine during pregnancy in term and preterm neonates. *Pediatrics*. 2007;119:52-59.
20. Bellantuono C, Migliarese G, Gentile S. Serotonin reuptake inhibitors in pregnancy and the risk of major malformations: a systematic review. *Hum Psychopharmacol Clin Exp*. 2007;22:121-128.
21. Chambers CD, Hernandez-Diaz S, Van Marter LJ, et al. Selective serotonin-reuptake inhibitors and risk of persistent pulmonary hypertension of the newborn. *N Engl J Med*. 2006;354:579-587.
22. Alwan S, Reefhuis J, Rasmussen SA, et al; National Birth Defects Prevention Study. Use of selective serotonin-reuptake inhibitors in pregnancy and the risk of birth defects. *N Engl J Med*. 2007;356:2684-2692.
23. Louik C, Lin AE, Werler MM, et al. First-trimester use of selective serotonin-reuptake inhibitors and the risk of birth defects. *N Engl J Med*. 2007;356:2675-2683.
24. Greene MF. Teratogenicity of SSRIs—serious concern or much ado about little? *N Engl J Med*. 2007;356:2732-2733.
25. Einarson A, Choi J, Einarson TR, Koren G. Incidence of major malformations in infants following antidepressant exposure in pregnancy: results of a large prospective cohort study. *Can J Psychiatry*. 2009;54:242-246.
26. Wright S, Dawling S, Ashford JJ. Excretion of fluvoxamine in breast milk. *Br J Clin Pharmacol*. 1991;31:209.
27. Yoshida K, Smith B, Channi Kumar R. Fluvoxamine in breast-milk and infant development. *Br J Clin Pharmacol*. 1997;44:209-213.
28. Hagg S, Granberg K, Carleborg L. Excretion of fluvoxamine into breast milk. *Br J Clin Pharmacol*. 2000;49:286-288.
29. Arnold LM, Suckow RF, Lichtenstein PK. Fluvoxamine concentrations in breast milk and in maternal and infant sera. *J Clin Psychopharmacol*. 2000;20:491-493.
30. Edwards JG, Anerson I. Systematic review and guide to selection of selective serotonin reuptake inhibitors. *Drugs*. 1999;57:507-533.
31. Treatment and management of mental health conditions during pregnancy and postpartum: ACOG clinical practice guideline no. 5. *Obstet Gynecol*. 2023;141:1262-1288.
32. Cipriani A, Furukawa TA, Salanti G, et al. Comparative efficacy and acceptability of 21 antidepressant drugs for the acute treatment of adults with major depressive disorder: a systematic review and network meta-analysis. *Lancet*. 2018;39:1357-1366.
33. U.S. Food and Drug Administration. Selective serotonin reuptake inhibitor (SSRI) antidepressant use during pregnancy and reports of a rare heart and lung condition in newborn babies. FDA drug safety communication. Accessed September 27, 2023. https://www.fda.gov/drugs/drug-safety-and-availability/fda-drug-safety-communication-selective-serotonin-reuptake-inhibitor-ssri-antidepressant-use-during
34. Moses-Kolko EL, Bogen D, Perel J, et al. Neonatal signs after late in utero exposure to serotonin reuptake inhibitors: literature review and implications for clinical applications. *JAMA*. 2005;293(19):2372-2383.

FOLIC ACID

Vitamin (B Vitamin)

PREGNANCY RECOMMENDATION: Human Data Suggest Compatible

BREASTFEEDING RECOMMENDATION: Compatible

F

PREGNANCY SUMMARY

Folic acid is an essential vitamin needed by the fetus for normal development. Numerous studies have evaluated the relationship between folic acid and the risk of NTDs. Over years of study, it has become well established that low levels of this vitamin are associated with this birth anomaly. Folate deficiency has also been suggested to increase the risk of spontaneous abortion, placental abruption, and preterm birth. However, studies have not been conclusive in these pregnancy complications. Rapid transfer of folic acid across the placenta occurs during pregnancy. Per ACOG, all women planning to or could become pregnant should start taking folic acid supplementation (400 mcg/d) at least 1 month before pregnancy and continuing at least through the first trimester. Women at high risk for NTD, including women with a prior pregnancy with NTD, or women with seizure disorders (especially when on certain antiepileptics) should take a higher dose.

BREASTFEEDING SUMMARY

Several reports describing the use of folic acid during human lactation were located. Folic acid is naturally found in breast milk and is known to be excreted into breast milk. It is recommended that breastfeeding women receive 500 mcg of folic acid daily though diet, while breastfeeding. Maternal supplementation with folic acid is recommended for those patients with inadequate nutritional intake. Though not specifically reported, no adverse infant effects would be expected from folic acid supplementation using recommended dosages.

References

1. American Hospital Formulary Service. *Drug Information 1997*. American Society of Health-System Pharmacists; 1997:2809-2811.
2. Herbert V. Recommended dietary intakes (RDI) of folate in humans. *Am J Clin Nutr*. 1987;45:661-670.
3. Frank O, Walbroehl G, Thomson A, et al. Placental transfer: fetal retention of some vitamins. *Am J Clin Nutr*. 1970;23:662-663.
4. Kaminetzky HA, Baker H, Frank O, Langer A. The effects of intravenously administered water-soluble vitamins during labor in normovitaminemic and hypovitaminemic gravidas on maternal and neonatal blood vitamin levels at delivery. *Am J Obstet Gynecol*. 1974;120:697-703.
5. Hill EP, Longo LD. Dynamics of maternal-fetal nutrient transfer. *Fed Proc*. 1980;39:239-244.
6. Baker H, Frank O, Deangelis B, et al. Role of placenta in maternal-fetal vitamin transfer in humans. *Am J Obstet Gynecol*. 1981;141:792-796.
7. Landon MJ, Eyre DH, Hytten FE. Transfer of folate to the fetus. *Br J Obstet Gynaecol*. 1975;82:12-19.
8. Baker H, Frank O, Thomason AD, et al. Vitamin profile of 174 mothers and newborns at parturition. *Am J Clin Nutr*. 1975;28:59-65.
9. Kaminetzky HA, Baker H. Micronutrients in pregnancy. *Clin Obstet Gynecol*. 1977;20:263-280.
10. Dostalova L. Correlation of the vitamin status between mother and newborn during delivery. *Dev Pharmacol Ther*. 1982;4(suppl 1):45-57.
11. Bruinse HW, Berg HVD, Haspels AA. Maternal serum folacin levels during and after normal pregnancy. *Eur J Obstet Gynecol Reprod Biol*. 1985;20:153-158.
12. Chanarin I, Rothman D, Ward A, Perry J. Folate status and requirement in pregnancy. *Br Med J*. 1968;2:390-394.
13. Ball EW, Giles C. Folic acid and vitamin B12 levels in pregnancy and their relation to megaloblastic anemia. *J Clin Pathol*. 1964;17:165-174.
14. Ek J, Magnus EM. Plasma and red blood cell folate during normal pregnancies. *Acta Obstet Gynecol Scand*. 1981;60:247-251.
15. Baker H, Ziffer H, Pasher I, Sobotka H. A Comparison of maternal and foetal folic acid and vitamin B12 at parturition. *Br Med J*. 1958;1:978-979.
16. Avery B, Ledger WJ. Folic acid metabolism in well-nourished pregnant women. *Obstet Gynecol*. 1970;35:616-624.
17. Ek J. Plasma and red cell folate values in newborn infants and their mothers in relation to gestational age. *J Pediatr*. 1980;97:288-292.
18. Baker H, Thind IS, Frank O, et al. Vitamin levels in low-birth-weight newborn infants and their mothers. *Am J Obstet Gynecol*. 1977;129:521-524.
19. Horn E. Iron and folate supplements during pregnancy: supplementing everyone treats those at risk and is cost effective. *Br Med J*. 1988;297:1325, 1327.
20. Hibbard BM. Iron and folate supplements during pregnancy: supplementation is valuable only in selected patients. *Br Med J*. 1988;297:1324, 1326.
21. Chanarin I, MacGibbon BM, O'Sullivan WJ, Mollin DL. Folic-acid deficiency in pregnancy: the pathogenesis of megaloblastic anaemia of pregnancy. *Lancet*. 1959;2:634-639.
22. Gatenby PBB, Lillie EW. Clinical analysis of 100 cases of severe megaloblastic anaemia of pregnancy. *Br Med J*. 1960;2:1111-1114.
23. Pritchard JA, Mason RA, Wright MR. Megaloblastic anemia during pregnancy and the puerperium. *Am J Obstet Gynecol*. 1962;83:1004-1020.
24. Fraser JL, Watt HJ. Megaloblastic anemia in pregnancy and the puerperium. *Am J Obstet Gynecol*. 1964;89:532-534.
25. Hibbard BM. The role of folic acid in pregnancy: with particular reference to anaemia, abruption and abortion. *J Obstet Gynaecol Br Commonw*. 1964;71:529-542.
26. Hibbard BM, Hibbard ED, Jeffcoate TNA. Folic acid and reproduction. *Acta Obstet Gynecol Scand*. 1965;44:375-400.
27. Giles C. An account of 335 cases of megaloblastic anaemia of pregnancy and the puerperium. *J Clin Pathol*. 1966;19:1-11.
28. Streiff RR, Little AB. Folic acid deficiency in pregnancy. *N Engl J Med*. 1967;276:776-779.
29. Pritchard JA, Scott DE, Whalley PJ. Folic acid requirements in pregnancy-induced megaloblastic anemia. *JAMA*. 1969;208:1163-1167.
30. Rothman D. Folic acid in pregnancy. *Am J Obstet Gynecol*. 1970;108:149-175.
31. Solano FX Jr, Councell RB. Folate deficiency presenting as pancytopenia in pregnancy. *Am J Obstet Gynecol*. 1986;154:1117-1118.
32. Leung CF, Lao TT, Chang AMZ. Effect of folate supplement on pregnant women with beta-thalassaemia minor. *Eur J Obstet Gynecol Reprod Biol*. 1989;33:209-213.
33. Laurence KM, James N, Miller MH, et al. Double-blind randomised controlled trial of folate treatment before conception to prevent recurrence of neural-tube defects. *Br Med J*. 1981;282:1509-1511.
34. Smithells RW, Sheppard S, Schorah CJ. Vitamin deficiencies and neural tube defects. *Arch Dis Child*. 1976;51:944-950.
35. Schorah CJ, Smithells RW, Scott J. Vitamin B12 and anencephaly. *Lancet*. 1980;1:880.
36. Nelson MM, Forfar JO. Associations between drugs administered during pregnancy and congenital abnormalities of the fetus. *Br Med J*. 1971;1:523-527.
37. Bower C, Stanley FJ. Dietary folate as a risk factor for neural-tube defects: evidence from a case-control study in Western Australia. *Med J Aust*. 1989;150:613-619.
38. Mann J. Dietary folate and neural-tube defects. *Med J Aust*. 1989;150:609.

39. Mills JL, Rhoads GG, Simpson JL, et al. The absence of a relation between the periconceptional use of vitamins and neural-tube defects. *N Engl J Med.* 1989;321:430-435.
40. Milunsky A, Jick H, Jick SS, et al. Multivitamin/folic acid supplementation in early pregnancy reduces the prevalence of neural tube defects. *JAMA.* 1989;262:2847-2852.
41. Czeizel A, Fritz G. Letter to the editor. *JAMA.* 1989;262:1634.
42. Czeizel AE, Dudás I. Prevention of the first occurrence of neural-tube defects by periconceptional vitamin supplementation. *N Engl J Med.* 1992;327:1832-1835.
43. Rosenberg IH. Editorial. Folic acid and neural-tube defects—time for action? *N Engl J Med.* 1992;327:1875-1877.
44. MRC Vitamin Study Research Group. Prevention of neural tube defects: results of the Medical Research Council vitamin study. *Lancet.* 1991;338:131-137.
45. Centers for Disease Control and Prevention. Use of folic acid for prevention of spina bifida and other neural tube defects—1983-1991. *MMWR Morb Mortal Wkly Rep.* 1991;40:513-516.
46. Centers for Disease Control and Prevention. Recommendations for the use of folic acid to reduce the number of cases of spina bifida and other neural tube defects. *MMWR Morb Mortal Wkly Rep.* 1992;41(RR-14):1-7.
47. Anonymous. Folic acid and neural tube defects. *Lancet.* 1991;338:153-154.
48. Scott JM, Kirke P, O'Broin S, Weir DG. Folic acid to prevent neural tube defects. *Lancet.* 1991;338:505.
49. Lucock MD, Wild J, Hartley R, et al. Vitamins to prevent neural tube defects. *Lancet.* 1991;338:894-895.
50. Steegers-Theunissen RPM, Boers GHJ, Trijbels FJM, Eskes TKAB. Neural-tube defects and derangement of homocysteine metabolism. *N Engl J Med.* 1991;324:199-200.
51. Laurence KM. Folic acid to prevent neural tube defects. *Lancet.* 1991;338:379.
52. Super M, Summers EM, Meylan B. Preventing neural tube defects. *Lancet.* 1991;338:755-756.
53. Kirke PN, Daly LE, Elwood JH; Irish Vitamin Study Group. A randomised trial of low dose folic acid to prevent neural tube defects. *Arch Dis Child.* 1992;67:1442-1446.
54. Martinez-Frias M-L, Rodriguez-Pinilla E. Folic acid supplementation and neural tube defects. *Lancet.* 1992;340:620.
55. Werler MM, Shapiro S, Mitchell AA. Periconceptional folic acid exposure and risk of occurrent neural tube defects. *JAMA.* 1993;269:1257-1261.
56. Oakley GP Jr. Folic acid—preventable spina bifida and anencephaly (editorial). *JAMA.* 1993;269:1292-1293.
57. Holzgreve W, Tercanli S, Pietrzik K. Vitamins to prevent neural tube defects. *Lancet.* 1991;338:639-640.
58. Molloy AM, Kirke P, Hillary I, Weir DG, Scott JM. Maternal serum folate and vitamin B12 concentrations in pregnancies associated with neural tube defects. *Arch Dis Child.* 1985;60:660-665.
59. Yates JRW, Ferguson-Smith MA, Shenkin A, et al. Is disordered folate metabolism the basis for the genetic predisposition to neural tube defects? *Clin Genet.* 1987;31:279-287.
60. Mills JL, Tuomilehto J, Yu KF, et al. Maternal vitamin levels during pregnancies producing infants with neural tube defects. *J Pediatr.* 1992;120:863-871.
61. Holmes LB. Prevention of neural tube defects (editorial). *J Pediatr.* 1992;120:918-919.
62. Glanville NT, Cook HW. Folic acid and prevention of neural tube defects. *Can Med Assoc J.* 1992;146:39.
63. Leeming RJ, Blair JA, Brown SE. Vitamins to prevent neural tube defects. *Lancet.* 1991;338:895.
64. Shepard TH. *Catalog of Teratogenic Agents.* 6th ed. he Johns Hopkins University Press; 1989:285-288.
65. Hibbard ED, Smithells RW. Folic acid metabolism and human embryopathy. *Lancet.* 1965;1:1254.
66. Stone ML. Effects on the fetus of folic acid deficiency in pregnancy. *Clin Obstet Gynecol.* 1968;11:1143-1153.
67. Scott DE, Whalley PJ, Pritchard JA. Maternal folate deficiency and pregnancy wastage. II. Fetal malformation. *Obstet Gynecol.* 1970;36:26-28.
68. Pritchard JA, Scott DE, Whalley PJ, Haling RF Jr. Infants of mothers with megaloblastic anemia due to folate deficiency. *JAMA.* 1970;211:1982-1984.
69. Kitay DZ, Hogan WJ, Eberle B, Mynt T. Neutrophil hypersegmentation and folic acid deficiency in pregnancy. *Am J Obstet Gynecol.* 1969;104:1163-1173.
70. Pritchard JA, Scott DE, Whalley PJ. Maternal folate deficiency and pregnancy wastage. IV. Effects of folic acid supplements, anticonvulsants, and oral contraceptives. *Am J Obstet Gynecol.* 1971;109:341-346.
71. Emery AEH, Timson J, Watson-Williams EJ. Pathogenesis of spina bifida. *Lancet.* 1969;2:909-910.
72. Hall MH. Folates and the fetus. *Lancet.* 1977;1:648-649.
73. Emery AEH. Folates and fetal central-nervous-system malformations. *Lancet.* 1977;1:703.
74. Biale Y, Lewenthal H. Effect of folic acid supplementation on congenital malformations due to anticonvulsive drugs. *Eur J Obstet Gynecol Reprod Biol.* 1984;18:211-216.
75. Hiilesmaa VK, Teramo K, Granstrom M-L, Bardy AH. Serum folate concentrations during pregnancy in women with epilepsy: relation to antiepileptic drug concentrations, number of seizures, and fetal outcome. *Br Med J.* 1983;287:577-579.
76. Hansen DK, Grafton TF. Lack of attenuation of valproic acid-induced effects by folinic acid in rat embryos in vitro. *Teratology.* 1991;43:575-582.
77. Wegner C, Nau H. Alteration of embryonic folate metabolism by valproic acid during organogenesis: implications for mechanism of teratogenesis. *Neurology.* 1992;42(suppl 5):17-24.
78. Dansky LV, Rosenblatt DS, Andermann E. Mechanisms of teratogenesis: folic acid and antiepileptic therapy. *Neurology.* 1992;42(suppl 5):32-42.
79. Delgado-Escueta AV, Janz D. Consensus guidelines: preconception counseling, management, and care of the pregnant woman with epilepsy. *Neurology.* 1992;42(suppl 5):149-160.
80. Kondo A, Morota N, Ihara S, et al Risk factors for the occurrence of spina bifida (a case-control study) and the prevalence rate of spina bifida in Japan. *Birth Defects Res A Clin Mol Teratol.* 2013;97:610-615.
81. Hibbard BM, Jeffcoate TNA. Abruptio placentae. *Obstet Gynecol.* 1966;27:155-167.
82. Stone ML, Luhby AL, Feldman R, et al. Folic acid metabolism in pregnancy. *Am J Obstet Gynecol.* 1967;99:638-648.
83. Whalley PJ, Scott DE, Pritchard JA. Maternal folate deficiency and pregnancy wastage. I. Placental abruption. *Am J Obstet Gynecol.* 1969;105:670-678.
84. Whalley PJ, Scott DE, Pritchard JA. Maternal folate deficiency and pregnancy wastage. III. Pregnancy-induced hypertension. *Obstet Gynecol.* 1970;36:29-31.
85. Martin JD, Davis RE. Serum folic acid activity and vaginal bleeding in early pregnancy. *J Obstet Gynaecol Br Commonw.* 1964;71:400-403.
86. Martin RH, Harper TA, Kelso W. Serum-folic-acid in recurrent abortions. *Lancet.* 1965;1:670-672.
87. Martin JD, Davis RE, Stenhouse N. Serum folate and vitamin B12 levels in pregnancy with particular reference to uterine bleeding and bacteriuria. *J Obstet Gynaecol Br Commonw.* 1967;74:697-701.
88. Streiff RR, Little B. Folic acid deficiency as a cause of uterine hemorrhage in pregnancy. *J Clin Invest.* 1965;44:1102.
89. Whiteside MG, Ungar B, Cowling DC. Iron, folic acid and vitamin B12 levels in normal pregnancy, and their influence on birth-weight and the duration of pregnancy. *Med J Aust.* 1968;1:338-342.
90. Goldenberg RL, Tamura T, Cliver SP, et al. Serum folate and fetal growth retardation: a matter of compliance? *Obstet Gynecol.* 1992;79:719-722.
91. Husain OAN, Rothman D, Ellis L. Folic acid deficiency in pregnancy. *J Obstet Gynaecol Br Commonw.* 1963;70:821-827.
92. Abramowicz M, Kass EH. Pathogenesis and prognosis of prematurity (continued). *N Engl J Med.* 1966;275:938-943.
93. Scott KE, Usher R. Fetal malnutrition: its incidence, causes, and effects. *Am J Obstet Gynecol.* 1966;94:951-963.
94. Varadi S, Abbott D, Elwis A. Correlation of peripheral white cell and bone marrow changes with folate levels in pregnancy and their clinical significance. *J Clin Pathol.* 1966;19:33-36.
95. Averback P. Anencephaly associated with megavitamin therapy. *Can Med Assoc J.* 1976;114:995.
96. Mukherjee MD, Sandstead HH, Ratnaparkhi MV, et al. Maternal zinc, iron, folic acid, and protein nutriture and outcome of human pregnancy. *Am J Clin Nutr.* 1984;40:496-507.
97. Centers for Disease Control and Prevention. Recommendations for use of folic acid to reduce number of spina bifida cases and other neural tube defects. *MMWR Morb Mortal Wkly Rep.* 1992;41(RR-14):1-7. As cited in Anonymous. From the Centers for Disease Control and Prevention. *JAMA.* 1993;269:1233, 1236, 1238.
98. Hibbard BM. Folates and fetal development. *Br J Obstet Gynaecol.* 1993;100:307-309.
99. Folic acid for the prevention of recurrent neural tube defects: ACOG committee opinion: Committee on obstetrics: Maternal and fetal medicine number 120—March 1993.. *Int J Gynecol Obstet.* 1993;42(1):75-77.
100. Metz J. Folate deficiency conditioned by lactation. *Am J Clin Nutr.* 1970;23:843-847.
101. Cooperman JM, Dweck HS, Newman LJ, et al. The folate in human milk. *Am J Clin Nutr.* 1982;36:576-580.

102. Ford JE, Zechalko A, Murphy J, Brooke OG. Comparison of the B vitamin composition of milk from mothers of preterm and term babies. *Arch Dis Child*. 1983;58:367-372.
103. Ek J. Plasma, red cell, and breast milk folacin concentrations in lactating women. *Am J Clin Nutr*. 1983;38:929-935.
104. Ek J, Magnus EM. Plasma and red blood cell folate in breastfed infants. *Acta Paediatr Scand*. 1979;68:239-243.
105. Tamura T, Yoshimura Y, Arakawa T. Human milk folate and folate status in lactating mothers and their infants. *Am J Clin Nutr*. 1980;33:193-197.
106. Thomas MR, Sneed SM, Wei C, et al. The effects of vitamin C, vitamin B6, vitamin B12, folic acid, riboflavin, and thiamine on the breast milk and maternal status of well-nourished women at 6 months postpartum. *Am J Clin Nutr*. 1980;33:2151-2156.
107. Smith AM, Picciano MF, Deering RH. Folate intake and blood concentrations of term infants. *Am J Clin Nutr*. 1985;41:590-598.
108. Sneed SM, Zane C, Thomas MR. The effects of ascorbic acid, vitamin B6, vitamin B12, and folic acid supplementation on the breast milk and maternal nutritional status of low socioeconomic lactating women. *Am J Clin Nutr*. 1981;34:1338-1346.
109. Deodhar AD, Rajalakshmi R, Ramakrishnan CV. Studies on human lactation. Part III. Effect of dietary vitamin supplementation on vitamin contents of breast milk. *Acta Paediatr (Stockholm)*. 1964;53:42-48.
110. Bank MR, Kirksey A, West K, Giacoia G. Effect of storage time and temperature on folacin and vitamin C levels in term and preterm human milk. *Am J Clin Nutr*. 1985;41:235-242.
111. Practice bulletin no. 187: neural tube defects. *Obstet Gynecol*. 2017;130: e279-e290.
112. ACOG committee opinion no. 762: prepregnancy counseling. *Obstet Gynecol*. 2019;133:e78-e89.

FOMEPIZOLE

Antidote

PREGNANCY RECOMMENDATION: Limited Human Data—No Relevant Animal Data (Maternal Benefit May Outweigh Any Embryofetal Risk)

BREASTFEEDING RECOMMENDATION: Hold Breastfeeding

PREGNANCY SUMMARY

One report describing the use of fomepizole during human pregnancy was located. A pregnant woman was treated with fomepizole twice during a pregnancy at 11 weeks' gestation and again 6 weeks later for inhalation of carburetor cleaner. The cleaner contained a mixture of methanol, toluene, methylene chloride, and carbon dioxide. No adverse effects were reported with the treatments. However, she was lost to follow-up and the eventual pregnancy outcome was unknown. The drug will likely cross the placenta, so fetal exposure will probably occur. Therefore, this limited human pregnancy experience prevents a complete assessment of the embryofetal risk. Animal reproduction studies have not been conducted. Because these chemicals can be lethal, the maternal benefits of therapy are great and probably outweigh any potential embryofetal risk.

BREASTFEEDING SUMMARY

No reports describing the use of fomepizole during human lactation have been located. The drug will likely be found in breast milk, so infant exposure will probably occur. The effects of this exposure on a nursing infant are unknown. Breastfeeding while using this drug should be based on the mother's clinical need for treatment. If used, the infant should be monitored for the most commonly reported adult side effects of headache, nausea, and dizziness (all leading to irritability). However, because these chemicals can be lethal, the maternal benefits of therapy are great. Breastfeeding should not prevent the use of fomepizole. Another option would be to hold breastfeeding temporarily (pump and discard the breast milk), at least until the therapy is completed. The time required to fully eliminate the drug is unknown. In addition, the poisons for which the drug would be used are ethylene glycol and methanol. The MW and mean elimination half-life of ethylene glycol are about 62 and 6 hours, respectively. The MW and elimination half-life of methanol are about 32 and 4 hours, respectively. Therefore, these poisons will most likely be found in breast milk. If the mother's blood levels for these poisons become undetectable, then the amount in breast milk is likely to be negligible.

References

1. Prescribing Information. Antizol. Paladin Laboratories (USA); 2020.
2. Belson M, Morghan BW. Methanol toxicity in a newborn. *J Toxicol Clin Toxicol*. 2004;42:673-677.
3. Velez LI, Kulstad E, Shepherd G, Roth B. Inhalational methanol toxicity in pregnancy treated twice with fomepizole. *Vet Hum Toxicol*. 2003;45:28-30.

FONDAPARINUX

Hematologic (Anticoagulant)

PREGNANCY RECOMMENDATION: Limited Human Data—Animal Data Suggest Low Risk

BREASTFEEDING RECOMMENDATION: Probably Compatible

PREGNANCY SUMMARY

In one review, of 10 published reports with 2 additional cases, 67 pregnancies were exposed to fondaparinux for the treatment of previous venous thromboembolism or recurrent pregnancy loss. The exposure occurred in all trimesters with only one anomaly identified. The authors noted that fondaparinux was well tolerated and the rate of pregnancy complications was similar to that observed in the general population. Several other studies were located where fondaparinux was used in treating recurrent pregnancy loss, with results being similar to low-molecular-weight heparin (LMWH). The drug has been shown to cross the placenta in small amounts near delivery, so some fetal exposure is possible. However, this limited human pregnancy experience prevents a complete assessment of the embryofetal risk. Animal data did not show any embryofetal toxicity or teratogenicity in two species at doses more than 10 times the RHD. ACOG and the American Society of Hematology guidelines state that fondaparinux is not recommended as first-line therapy in pregnancy given that it has been shown to cross the placenta and that experience in pregnancy is limited. However, it may be considered in pregnant patients with severe heparin allergy or heparin-induced thrombocytopenia when alternative therapy is unavailable. Using this drug during pregnancy should be based on the pros and cons of the mother's clinical need for treatment versus any potential fetal risk that might occur from exposure. Fondaparinux carries a Boxed Warning regarding an increased risk for spinal and epidural hematomas. Providers should carefully consider the timing of epidural/spinal catheter placement and removal in patients taking fondaparinux, and delay dosing after neuraxial blockade and catheter removal to decrease the risk of complications. Lastly, if the drug is used near delivery and were to cross the placenta, caution should be used with operative vaginal delivery.

BREASTFEEDING SUMMARY

No reports describing the use of fondaparinux during human lactation have been located. The high MW and high plasma protein binding suggest that the drug will not be excreted into breast milk. Additionally, if any oral fondaparinux were to be ingested through breastfeeding, clinically significant absorption is unlikely due to poor oral bioavailability. The American Society of Hematology guidelines consider fondaparinux safe for use in breastfeeding. If used while breastfeeding, the infant should be monitored for the most commonly reported adult side effects of bleeding (bruising of skin, blood in urine or stool) and anemia.

References

1. Prescribing Information. Arixtra. Mylan Institutional; 2020.
2. Lagrange F, Brun J-L, Vergnes MC, et al. Fondaparinux sodium does not cross the placental barrier. Study using the in-vitro human dually perfused cotyledon model. Clin Pharmacokinet 2002;41(suppl 2):47-49.
3. Lagrange F, Vergnes C, Brun JL, et al. Absence of placental transfer of pentasaccharide (Fondaparinux, Arixtra®) in the dually perfused human cotyledon in vitro. *Thromb Haemost*. 2002;87:831-835.
4. Dempfle C-EH. Minor transplacental passage of fondaparinux in vivo. *N Engl J Med*. 2004;350:1914-1915.
5. Wijesiriwardana A, Lees DAR, Lush C. Fondaparinux as anticoagulant in a pregnant woman with heparin allergy. *Blood Coagul Fibrinolysis*. 2006;17:147-148.
6. Mazzolai L, Hohlfeld P, Spertini F, et al. Fondaparinux is a safe alternative in case of heparin intolerance during pregnancy. *Blood*. 2006;108:1569-1570.
7. Harenberg J. Treatment of a woman with lupus and thromboembolism and cutaneous intolerance to heparins using fondaparinux during pregnancy. *Thromb Res*. 2007;119:385-388.
8. Gerhardt A, Zotz RB, Stockschlaeder M, Scharf RE. Fondaparinux is an effective alternative anticoagulant in pregnant women with high risk of venous thromboembolism and intolerance to low-molecular-weight heparins and heparinoids. *Thromb Haemost*. 2007;97:496-497.
9. Winger EE, Reed JL. A retrospective analysis of fondaparinux versus enoxaparin treatment in women with infertility or pregnancy loss. *Am J Reprod Immunol*. 2009;62:253-260.
10. Knol HM, Schultinge L, Erwich JJ, Meijer K. Fondaparinux as an alternative anticoagulant therapy during pregnancy. *J Thromb Haemost*. 2010;8:1876-1879.
11. Ciurzyński M, Jankowski K, Pietrzak B, et al. Use of fondaparinux in a pregnant woman with pulmonary embolism and heparin-induced thrombocytopenia. *Med Sci Monit*. 2011;17:CS56-CS59.
12. Darki A, Kodali PP, McPheters JP, et al. Hypereosinophilic syndrome with cardiac involvement. *Tex Heart Inst J*. 2011;38:163-165.
13. Tanimura K, Ebina Y, Sonoyama A, et al. Argatroban therapy for heparin-induced thrombocytopenia during pregnancy in a woman with hereditary antithrombin deficiency. *J Obstet Gynaecol Res*. 2012;38:749-752.
14. Elsaigh E, Thachil J, Nash MJ, et al. The use of fondaparinux in pregnancy. *Br J Haematol*. 2015;168: 762-764.
15. Buonomo A, Nucera E, De Carolis S, et al. A case of heparin allergy with good tolerability to fondaparinux during pregnancy. *J Investig Allergol Clin Immunol*. 2015;25:229-231.
16. De Carlos S, di Pasquo E, Rossi E, et al. Fondaparinux in pregnancy: could it be a safe option? A review of the literature. *Thromb Res*. 2015;135:1049-1051.
17. Dempfle CE, Koscielny J, Lindhoff-Last E, et al. Fondaparinux pre-, peri-, and/or postpartum for the prophylaxis/treatment of venous thromboembolism (FondaPPP). *Clin Appl Thromb Hemost*. 2021;27:1-8.
18. Winger E, Reed J. Fondaparinux versus enoxaparin treatment in women with infertility or pregnancy loss. *Haematologica*. 2010;95(suppl):2.
19. Guo Z, Liu C, Guo X, Zhang Y, Lin X. Comparison between enoxaparin and fondaparinux sodium on anticoagulant therapy in pregnant patient with recurrent miscarriage. *Contemporary Med*. 2020;26:5-8.
20. Liu H, Wang A, Sang X. Effect of enoxaparin and fondaparinux in anticoagulant therapy for re-pregnant women with recurrent miscarriage. *Chin J Pract Med*. 2021;48:106-109.
21. Yang N, Lin J, Chen Z, et al. Comparison of curative effect of fondaparinux sodium and low molecular weight heparin on recurrent spontaneous abortion. *China Modern Doctor*. 2022;60:55-58.
22. Mu F, Wang M, Huang J, Wang F. Pregnancy outcomes and adverse events in patients with recurrent miscarriage receiving fondaparinux versus low molecular-weight heparin: a meta-analysis. *Eur J Obstet Gynecol Reprod Biol*. 2023;287:29-35.
23. American College of Obstetricians and Gynecologists' Committee on Practice Bulletins—Obstetrics. ACOG practice bulletin no. 196: thromboembolism in pregnancy. *Obstet Gynecol*. 2018;132:e1-e17.
24. Bates SM, Rajasekhar A, Middeldorp S, et al. American Society of Hematology 2018 guidelines for management of venous thromboembolism: venous thromboembolism in the context of pregnancy. *Blood Adv*. 2018;2:3317-3359.

FORMOTEROL

Respiratory (β_2-Agonist)

PREGNANCY RECOMMENDATION: Limited Human Data—Animal Data Suggest Low Risk

BREASTFEEDING RECOMMENDATION: Probably Compatible

PREGNANCY SUMMARY

One study reported three pregnancies in a mother who used a budesonide/formoterol inhaler throughout each gestation. All three newborns had orofacial clefts; however, a genetic cause was not ruled out. Conversely, a post-marketing surveillance study in England reported the outcomes of 28 pregnancies that had first trimester exposure to formoterol (many continuing the drug to delivery), reporting 3 (10.7%) spontaneous abortions and 2 (7.1%) congenital anomalies (one cardiac and one pyloric stenosis). No orofacial clefts occurred. The National Asthma Education and Prevention Program (NAEPP) expert panel reviewed six studies of 1,599 women who had taken β_2 agonists during pregnancy. The panel concluded that β_2 agonists are considered safe for use during pregnancy. Some of the drug may cross the placenta, but the overall amounts are likely to be clinically insignificant. However, this limited human pregnancy experience prevents a complete assessment of the embryofetal risk. Animal data did not show any embryofetal toxicity or teratogenicity in two species at doses more than 10 times the MRHDID. Hyperglycemia may occur in patients treated with formoterol. Therefore, glucose levels should be monitored while on treatment. Formoterol should only be prescribed as additional therapy for those who are taking, but are inadequately controlled on, a long-term asthma control medication, such as an ICS.

F

BREASTFEEDING SUMMARY

No reports describing the use of formoterol during human lactation have been located. The drug may be found in human breast milk, but the amount is likely to be clinically insignificant. The NAEPP expert panel considers β_2-adrenergic agonists compatible with breastfeeding. If the clinical decision is to use this drug while breastfeeding, the infant should be monitored for the most commonly reported adult side effects of nausea and headache (both leading to irritability), diarrhea, insomnia, and vomiting.

References

1. Prescribing Information. Perforomist. Mylan Specialty; 2021.
2. Peterka M, Heringova LH, Sukop A, Peterkova R. Anti-asthma drugs formoterol and budesonide (Symbicort) induce orofacial clefts, gastroschisis and heart septum defects in an in vivo model. *In Vivo*. 2021;35:1451-1460.
3. Wilton LV, Shakir SA. A post-marketing surveillance study of formoterol (Foradil). Its use in general practice in England. *Drug Saf*. 2002;25:213-223.
4. Cossette B, Beauchesne MF, Forget A, et al. Relative perinatal safety of salmeterol vs formoterol and fluticasone vs budesonide use during pregnancy. *Ann Allergy Asthma Immunol*. 2014; 112:459-464.
5. National Heart, Lung, and Blood Institute; National Asthma Education and Prevention Program Asthma and Pregnancy Working Group. NAEPP expert panel report. Managing asthma during pregnancy: recommendations for pharmacologic treatment-2004 update. *J Allergy Clin Immunol*. 2005;115:34-46.
6. Dombrowski MP, Schatz M; ACOG Committee on Practice Bulletins-Obstetrics. ACOG practice bulletin: clinical management guidelines for obstetrician-gynecologists number 90, February 2008: asthma in pregnancy. *Obstet Gynecol*. 2008;111:457-464.

FOSCARNET

Antiviral (Cytomegalovirus Retinitis and Resistant Herpes Simplex Virus)

PREGNANCY RECOMMENDATION: Limited Human Data—Animal Data Suggest Potential Risk

BREASTFEEDING RECOMMENDATION: *Contraindicated (Cytomegalovirus Retinitis)/Potential Toxicity (Resistant Herpes Simplex Virus)

PREGNANCY SUMMARY

Only one report describing the use of foscarnet in human pregnancy has been located. Two pregnancies with outcome data described the use of the drug for complicated resistant herpes simplex virus (HSV) infections in the second trimester in one patient and in the third trimester for the second patient. Both delivered infants that did well with no sequalae noted related to the drug exposure. The drug will probably cross the placenta, so fetal exposure will likely occur. However, this limited human pregnancy experience prevents a complete assessment of the embryofetal risk. No embryofetal toxicity or malformations were observed in two species, but doses were well below the RHD. Using this drug during pregnancy should be based on the pros and cons of the mother's clinical need for treatment versus any potential fetal risk that might occur from exposure. Foscarnet carries a Boxed Warning regarding renal impairment. Therefore, in theory, because the drug likely crosses the placenta, it could affect fetal renal function leading to decreased amniotic fluid volume. Therefore, if the drug is being used, monitoring amniotic fluid volume in the second half of gestation is recommended.

BREASTFEEDING SUMMARY

No reports describing the use of foscarnet during human lactation have been located. Based on the low MW, low plasma protein binding, and long elimination half-life, the drug will probably be excreted into breast milk. Due to a concern for potential serious adverse effects that might be seen in a breastfed infant, the manufacturer recommends that women not breastfeed while being treated with this drug. *In relationship to cytomegalovirus (CMV) retinitis associated with HIV, the CDC does not recommend breastfeeding in patients with HIV, especially active HIV. However, the drug is poorly absorbed with oral use, with an oral bioavailability of 10% or less. If the clinical decision is to use this drug while breastfeeding, in patients with resistant HSV, the infant should be monitored for the most commonly reported adult side effects of nausea and headache (both leading to irritability), fever, diarrhea, vomiting, anemia, and renal dysfunction.

References

1. Prescribing Information. Foscavir. Hospira; 2020.
2. Alvarez-McLeod A, Havlik J, Drew KE. Foscarnet treatment of genital infection due to acyclovir-resistant herpes simplex virus type 2 in a pregnant patient with AIDS: case report. *Clin Infect Dis.* 1999;29:937-938.
3. Watts DH. Antiviral agents. *Obstet Gynecol Clin North Am.* 1992;19:563-585.

F

FOSDENOPTERIN

Miscellaneous (Molybdenum Cofactor)

PREGNANCY RECOMMENDATION: No Human Data and No Relevant Animal Data

BREASTFEEDING RECOMMENDATION: Probably Compatible

PREGNANCY SUMMARY

No reports describing the use of fosdenopterin in human pregnancy have been located. Fosdenopterin will likely cross the placenta, so some fetal exposure will probably occur. Therefore, the absence of human pregnancy experience prevents a complete assessment of the embryofetal risk. No animal reproduction studies have been conducted. Using this drug during pregnancy should be based on the pros and cons of the mother's clinical need for treatment versus any potential fetal risk that might occur from exposure.

BREASTFEEDING SUMMARY

No reports describing the use of fosdenopterin during human lactation have been located. The drug will likely be excreted into breast milk, so some infant exposure will probably occur. Breastfeeding while using this drug should be based on the mother's clinical need for treatment. If used, the infant should be monitored for the most commonly reported adult side effects of pyrexia, viral infections, pneumonia, otitis media, vomiting, cough, and diarrhea.

Reference

1. Product Information. Nulibry. Origin Biosciences, Inc; 2022.

FOSFOMYCIN

Antibiotic (Phosphonic)

PREGNANCY RECOMMENDATION: Limited Human Data—Animal Data Suggest Potential Risk

BREASTFEEDING RECOMMENDATION: Probably Compatible

PREGNANCY SUMMARY

Several reports describing the use of fosfomycin in human pregnancy have been located. Though the total numbers are small, these studies do not indicate an increased risk of congenital anomalies and confirm the safety of fosfomycin use in pregnancy. The drug crosses the placenta, so infant exposure will occur. However, this limited human pregnancy experience prevents a complete assessment of the embryofetal risk. Embryofetal toxicity was observed in one animal species at doses less than 10 times the RHD. ACOG supports the use of fosfomycin for the treatment of asymptomatic bacteriuria and acute cystitis in pregnant women.

BREASTFEEDING SUMMARY

Two lactating women were administered fosfomycin by injection (1-2 g), and the mean milk concentrations were about 4 to 5 mcg/mL (colostrum to plasma and milk to plasma ratios of about 0.07). Fosfomycin bioavailability from the gastrointestinal tract is only 35%. Because the current form of drug administration in the United States is only oral (not IV), this should result in lower breast milk levels with even lower exposures to a breastfeeding infant. The risk to a nursing infant from this exposure is unknown, but modification of the infant's bowel flora could occur. If the clinical decision is to use this drug while breastfeeding, the infant should be monitored for the most commonly reported adult side effects of nausea and headache (both leading to irritability) and diarrhea.

References

1. Prescribing Information. Monurol. Allergan; 2018.
2. Ferreres L, Paz M, Martin G, Gobernado M. New studies on placental transfer of fosfomycin. *Chemotherapy*. 1977;23(suppl 1):175-179.
3. Kirby WMM. Pharmacokinetics of fosfomycin. *Chemotherapy*. 1977; 23(suppl 1):141-151.
4. De Cecco L, Ragni N. Urinary tract infections in pregnancy: Monuril single-dose treatment versus traditional therapy. *Eur Urol*. 1987;13(suppl 1): 108-113.
5. Ragni N. Fosfomycin trometamol single dose versus pipemidic acid 7 days in the treatment of bacteriuria in pregnancy. Clinical report, 29 November 1990. Data on file, Forest Laboratories.
6. Reeves DS. Treatment of bacteriuria in pregnancy with single dose fosfomycin trometamol: a review. *Infection*. 1992;20(suppl 4):S313-S316.
7. Moroni M. Monuril effectiveness and tolerability in the treatment and prevention of urinary tract infections. Clinical report. Data on file, Forest Laboratories.
8. Paladini A, Paladini AA, Balbi C, Carati L. Efficacy and safety of fosfomycin trometamol in the treatment of bacteriuria in pregnancy. Clinical report. Data on file, Forest Laboratories.
9. Ragni N, Pivetta C, Paccagnella F, et al. Urinary tract infections in pregnancy. In: Neu HC, Williams JD, eds. *New Trends in Urinary Tract Infections*. International Symposium Rome 1987. Basel, Switzerland: Karger, 1988:197-206.
10. Zinner S. Fosfomycin trometamol versus pipemidic acid in the treatment of bacteriuria in pregnancy. *Chemotherapy*. 1990;36(suppl 1):50-52.
11. Marone P, Concia E, Catinella M, et al. Fosfomycin trometamol in the treatment of urinary tract infections during pregnancy. A multicenter study. Presented at: 3rd International Congress, Infections in Obstetrics and Gynecology; 1988; Pavia, Italy.
12. Thoumsin H, Aghayan M, Lambotte R. Fosfomycin trometamol versus nitrofurantoin in multiple dose in pregnant women. Preliminary results. *Infection*. 1990;18(suppl 2):S94-S97.
13. Moroni M. Monuril in lower uncomplicated urinary tract infections in adults. *Eur Urol*. 1987;13(suppl 1):101-104.
14. De Andrade J, Mendes Carvalho Lopes C, Carneiro daSilva D, et al. Fosfomycin trometamol single-dose in the treatment of uncomplicated urinary tract infections in cardiac pregnant or non pregnant women. A controlled study. *J Bras Ginec*. 1994;104:345-351.
15. Gobernado M, Perez de Leon A, Santos M, et al. Fosfomycin in the treatment of gynecological infections. *Chemotherapy*. 1977;23(suppl 1):287-292.
16. Wilton LV, Pearce GL, Martin RM, et al. The outcomes of pregnancy in women exposed to newly marketed drugs in general practice in England. *Br J Obstet Gynaecol*. 1998;105:882-889.
17. Mannucci C, Dante G, Miroddi M, et al. Vigilance on use of drugs, herbal products, and food supplements during pregnancy: focus on fosfomycin. *J Matern Fetal Neonatal Med*. 2019;32:125-128.
18. Philipps W, Fietz AK, Meixner K, et al. Pregnancy outcome after first-trimester exposure to fosfomycin for the treatment of urinary tract infection: an observational cohort study. *Infection*. 2020;48:57-64.
19. Konwar M, Gogtay NJ, Ravi R, et al. Evaluation of efficacy and safety of fosfomycin versus nitrofurantoin for the treatment of uncomplicated lower urinary tract infection (UTI) in women—a systematic review and meta-analysis. *J Chemother*. 2022;34:139-148.
20. Benevent J, Araujo M, Beau AB, et al First trimester pregnancy exposure to fosfomycin and risk of major congenital anomaly: a comparative study in the EFEMERIS database. *Infection*. 2023;51:137-146.
21. Fosfomycin and breastfeeding. *Aust Prescr*. 2020;43:113.
22. American College of Obstetricians and Gynecologists. Urinary tract infections in pregnant individuals: clinical consensus no. 4. *Obstet Gynecol*. 2023;142:435-445.

FOSINOPRIL

Antihypertensive (Angiotensin-Converting Enzyme Inhibitor)

PREGNANCY RECOMMENDATION: *Contraindicated (Second and Third Trimesters)

BREASTFEEDING RECOMMENDATION: Probably Compatible

PREGNANCY SUMMARY

No reports describing the use of fosinopril in human pregnancy have been located. Some of the drug may cross the placenta, so fetal exposure will likely occur. However, the absence of human pregnancy experience prevents a complete assessment of the embryofetal risk. Animal data did not show any embryofetal toxicity in two species with doses less than 10 times the RHD in one species and more than 10 times the RHD in the second species. Numerous studies on other angiotensin-converting enzyme (ACE) inhibitors (with use in the first trimester) have found no increase in the incidence of birth anomalies, except for one Tennessee Medicaid study. *However, the use of ACE inhibitor drugs in the second and third trimesters has been found to cause fetal renal dysfunction. This can lead to severe oligohydramnios producing pulmonary hypoplasia and compression deformities, which is fatal in some cases. There are reports, however, that this is not universal and a few reports exist that describe a return of normal infant renal function over time. In some pathology cases, the fetal kidneys were not found to have any definite pathologic abnormalities. Therefore, the primary issue may be the severe oligohydramnios that is produced by the fetal renal dysfunction when the drug is used in the second and third trimesters. The drug carries a Boxed Warning for these fetal risks. It recommends that fosinopril be discontinued as soon as possible once pregnancy is detected.

BREASTFEEDING SUMMARY

No published reports describing the use of fosinopril during human lactation have been located. The drug will probably be found in breast milk, so some infant exposure will likely occur. The manufacturer states that fosinopril can be detected in human milk after a daily dose of 20 mg given for 3 days (levels not reported). No adverse effects of ACE inhibitors in breast milk have been reported in infants. However, due to a concern for potential serious adverse effects that might be seen in a breastfed infant, the manufacturer recommends that women not breastfeed while being treated with this drug. Regardless, ACOG and the American Heart Association (AHA) consider ACE inhibitors compatible for use during breastfeeding. If used while breastfeeding, the infant should be monitored for the most commonly reported adult side effects of dizziness and nausea (both leading to irritability), cough, and vomiting.

References

1. Prescribing Information. Fosinopril sodium. Cipla USA, Inc; 2020.
2. Cooper WO, Hernandez-Diaz S, Arbogast PG, et al. Major congenital malformations after first-trimester exposure to ACE inhibitors. *N Engl J Med.* 2006;354:2443-2451.
3. Friedman JM. ACE inhibitors and congenital anomalies. *N Engl J Med.* 2006;354:2498-2500.
4. Scialli AR, Lione A. ACE inhibitors and major congenital malformations. *N Engl J Med*. 2006;355:1280.
5. Cooper WO, Ray WA. Reply—ACE inhibitors and major congenital malformations. *N Engl J Med*. 2006;355:1281.
6. Barr M Jr. Teratogen update: angiotensin-converting enzyme inhibitors. *Teratology*. 1994;50:399-409.
7. Shotan A, Widerhorn J, Hurst A, Elkayam U. Risks of angiotensin-converting enzyme inhibition during pregnancy: experimental and clinical evidence, potential mechanisms, and recommendations for use. *Am J Med.* 1994;96:451-456.
8. Robillard JE, Nakamura KT, Matherne GP, Jose PA. Renal hemodynamics and functional adjustments to postnatal life. *Semin Perinatol*. 1988;12:143-150.
9. Guignard J-P, Gouyon J-B. Adverse effects of drugs on the immature kidney. *Biol Neonate*. 1988;53:243-252.
10. Brent RL, Beckman DA. Angiotensin-converting enzyme inhibitors, an embryopathic class of drugs with unique properties: information for clinical teratology counselors. *Teratology*. 1991;43:543-6.
11. Polifka JE. Is there an embryopathy associated with first-trimester exposure to angiotensin-converting enzyme inhibitors and angiotensin receptor antagonists? A critical review of the evidence. *Birth Defects Res A Clin Mol Teratol*. 2012;94:576-598.
12. American College of Obstetricians and Gynecologists' Committee on Practice Bulletins—Obstetrics. ACOG practice bulletin no. 203: chronic hypertension in pregnancy. *Obstet Gynecol*. 2019;133:e26-e50.
13. Heidenreich PA, Bozkurt B, Aguilar D, et al. 2022 AHA/ACC/HFSA guideline for the management of heart failure: a report of the American College of Cardiology/American Heart Association Joint Committee on Clinical Practice Guidelines. *Circulation*. 2022;145:e895-e1032.

F

FOSTAMATINIB

Antineoplastic (Tyrosine Kinase Inhibitor)

PREGNANCY RECOMMENDATION: No Human Data—Animal Data Suggest Potential Risk

BREASTFEEDING RECOMMENDATION: Potential Toxicity

PREGNANCY SUMMARY

No reports describing the use of fostamatinib in human pregnancy have been located. The drug will probably cross the placenta, so some fetal exposure will likely occur. Therefore, the absence of human pregnancy experience prevents a complete assessment of the embryofetal risk. Animal studies did show embryofetal toxicity in one species at doses less than 10 times the MRHD. Embryofetal toxicity was seen in one other animal species at doses equal to 10 times the MRHD. Based on these animal studies, the manufacturer recommends that women with reproductive potential use effective contraception during treatment and for 1 month after the last dose. Nevertheless, using this drug during pregnancy should be based on the pros and cons of the mother's clinical need for treatment versus any potential fetal risk that might occur from exposure. Hypertension was reported in clinical trials in up to 28% of patients treated with this drug. If used, blood pressure should be closely monitored.

BREASTFEEDING SUMMARY

No reports describing the use of fostamatinib during human lactation have been found. The drug will probably be found in breast milk, so some infant exposure will likely occur. Due to the concern for potential serious adverse effects that might be seen in a breastfed infant, the manufacturer recommends that women not breastfeed while being treated with this drug and for at least 1 month after the last dose. Nevertheless, breastfeeding while using this drug should be based on the mother's clinical need for treatment. If used, the infant should be monitored for the most commonly reported adult side effects of nausea, abdominal pain, and dizziness (all leading to irritability), diarrhea, elevated blood pressure, abnormal liver tests, and fatigue (lethargy).

Reference

1. Prescribing Information. Tavalisse. Rigel Pharmaceuticals, Inc; 2020.

FOSTEMSAVIR

Antiretroviral

PREGNANCY RECOMMENDATION: No Human Data—Animal Data Suggest Low Risk

BREASTFEEDING RECOMMENDATION: *Contraindicated

PREGNANCY SUMMARY

No reports describing the use of fostemsavir in human pregnancy have been located. Some drug will probably cross the placenta. Animal data did not show fetotoxic effects. However, the absence of human pregnancy experience prevents a complete assessment of the embryofetal risk. There is a pregnancy exposure registry that monitors pregnancy outcome in patients using this drug during gestation. Health care providers are encouraged to call the Antiretroviral Pregnancy Registry (APR) at 1-800-258-4263. In order to decrease the perinatal transmission of HIV-1 to the neonate, this drug should not be withheld if a pregnant woman is infected with HIV-1 with a positive viral load who is failing her current treatment regimen.

BREASTFEEDING SUMMARY

Fostemsavir probably enters breast milk. *However, the current CDC recommendation is that mothers infected with HIV should *not* breastfeed their infants in order to reduce the risk of postnatal transmission of the virus to the neonate. In a clinical setting where a mother is not infected with HIV (or in cases where the HIV viral load is negative), the drug by itself is probably compatible.

Reference

1. Product Information. Rukobia. ViiV Healthcare, GlaxoSmithKline; 2020.

F

FREMANEZUMAB

Central Nervous System (Antimigraine—Monoclonal Antibody)

PREGNANCY RECOMMENDATION: Limited Human Data—Animal Data Suggest Low Risk

BREASTFEEDING RECOMMENDATION: Probably Compatible

PREGNANCY SUMMARY

One study that reported pregnancy exposure to fremanezumab was located. A safety report from the VigiBase system described 94 cases with exposures to erenumab (50), galcanezumab (31), and fremanezumab (13). The final analysis did not show any increased signals of fetal or maternal toxicity. Spontaneous reporting safety profile databases have numerous limitations. They are biased toward the reporting of pregnancy complications and poor outcomes rather than normal outcomes. They can also lack clinical details and have missing information including drug dosages, duration of use, and specific timing of drug exposure during pregnancy. Therefore, they cannot report the incidence of adverse events or provide a measure of risk. These databases can primarily provide whether or not a significant disproportionality exists in the reporting frequency of specific adverse events. As an IgG antibody, it likely crosses the placenta, especially during the second half of gestation, so some fetal exposure will occur. Therefore, this limited human pregnancy experience prevents a complete assessment of the embryofetal risk. Animal studies did not show any embryofetal toxicity in two species at doses less than 10 times the RHD. Using this drug during pregnancy should be based on the pros and cons of the mother's clinical need for treatment versus any potential fetal risk that might occur from exposure. There is a pregnancy exposure registry that monitors pregnancy outcomes in women using this drug during pregnancy. Health care providers are encouraged to register pregnant patients by calling 1-833-927-2605.

BREASTFEEDING SUMMARY

No reports describing the use of fremanezumab during human lactation have been located. It is known that IgG antibodies are excreted into breast milk but are not found in the neonatal or infant circulation. Additionally, if any IgG antibodies were to be ingested through breastfeeding, they would probably be digested in the infant's gastrointestinal tract and not be absorbed. Breastfeeding while using this drug should be based on the mother's clinical need for treatment. If used, the infant should be monitored for the most commonly reported adult side effect of headache (leading to irritability).

References

1. Prescribing Information. AJOVY. Teva Pharmaceuticals USA; 2022.
2. Noseda R, Bedussi F, Gobbi C, et al. Safety profile of erenumab, galcanezumab, and fremanezumab in pregnancy and lactation: analysis of the WHO pharmacovigilance database. *Cephalalgia*. 2021;41:789-798.

FROVATRIPTAN

Central Nervous System (Antimigraine)

PREGNANCY RECOMMENDATION: Limited Human Data—Animal Data Suggest Low Risk

BREASTFEEDING RECOMMENDATION: Probably Compatible

PREGNANCY SUMMARY

No reports describing the use of frovatriptan in human pregnancy have been located. A recent meta-analysis involving six studies with over 4,000 first trimester exposures to triptans as a group and more than a million controls with no triptan exposure did not find any increased risk for major anomalies with triptan use. The triptans in the study were sumatriptan, rizatriptan, naratriptan, zolmitriptan, eletriptan, and almotriptan. A sub-analysis evaluating each of these individual drug's risk for major malformations was not reported. The spontaneous abortion rate was higher in the triptan group at 17.8% compared with the no migraine control group at 8.6%. However, the expected spontaneous abortion rate in the United States is 15% to 20%. Therefore, the spontaneous abortion rate in the no migraine control group is very low. There was no difference in the spontaneous abortion rate between the triptan exposed group and the migraine control group with no triptan use. The preterm delivery rate with triptan use was also not increased when compared with both control groups. Based on likely placental transfer, fetal exposure will probably occur. Therefore, the absence of human pregnancy experience with frovatriptan prevents a complete assessment of the embryofetal risk. Animal studies did not find any embryofetal toxicity in one species at doses much greater than 10 times the RHD.

ACOG recommends the use of acetaminophen as first-line treatment for acute migraine. Alternative options for patients uncontrolled by acetaminophen alone or in combination with caffeine are metoclopramide alone or with diphenhydramine. Secondary treatment with triptans (primarily sumatriptan) may be considered. The most used triptan in pregnancy is sumatriptan. There are limited safety data with other triptans. Triptans are not analgesics. They cause vasoconstriction of cranial vessels and inhibit proinflammatory neuropeptide release. There was also a concern that triptan use during pregnancy might increase the risk of attention-deficit/hyperactivity disorder in exposed children. However, a recent large study did not find this association. It is unknown if triptans cause vasoconstriction of uterine or fetal vasculature. Therefore, using this drug during pregnancy should be based on the pros and cons of the mother's clinical need for treatment versus any potential fetal risk that might occur from exposure.

BREASTFEEDING SUMMARY

No reports describing the use of frovatriptan during human lactation have been located. The drug will probably be found in breast milk, so infant exposure will likely occur. In one study, six other triptans were evaluated during lactation and all six were found in breast milk with estimated RIDs ranging from 0.6% to 5.0% (all less than 10%). Breastfeeding while using this drug should be based on the mother's clinical need for treatment. If used, the infant should be monitored for the most commonly reported adult side effects of headache, chest pain, paresthesia, dizziness, nausea, and skeletal pain (all leading to irritability), fatigue (lethargy), and flushing. ACOG states that using triptans for treating migraine during lactation should be a shared decision-making process. ACOG also suggests avoiding breastfeeding for 24 hours after the use of triptans (except sumatriptan, which is 8-12 hours).

References

1. Prescribing Information. Frova. Endo Pharmaceuticals; 2021.
2. Schenker S, Yang Y, Perex A, et al. Sumatriptan (Imitrex) transport by the human placenta. *Proc Soc Exp Biol Med*. 1995;210:213-220.
3. Marchenko A, Etwel F, Olutunfese O, et al. Pregnancy outcome following prenatal exposure to triptan medications: a meta-analysis. *Headache*. 2015;55:490-501.
4. Headaches in pregnancy and postpartum: ACOG clinical practice guideline no. 3. *Obstet Gynecol*. 2022;139:944-972.
5. Harris GM, Wood M, Ystrom E, et al. Association of maternal use of triptans during pregnancy with risk of attention-deficit/hyperactivity disorder in offspring. *JAMA Netw Open*. 2022;5:e2215333.
6. Amundsen S, Nordeng H, Fuskevag OM, et al. Transfer of triptans into human breast milk and estimation of infant drug exposure through breast feeding. *Basic Clin Pharmacol Toxicol*. 2021;128:795-804.

FRUQUINTINIB

Antineoplastic (Vascular Endothelial Growth Factor Receptor Kinase Inhibitor)

PREGNANCY RECOMMENDATION: No Human Data—Animal Data Suggest Potential Risk

BREASTFEEDING RECOMMENDATION: Potential Toxicity

PREGNANCY SUMMARY

No reports describing the use of fruquintinib in human pregnancy have been located. The drug will likely cross the placenta, so some fetal exposure will probably occur. Therefore, the absence of human pregnancy experience prevents a complete assessment of the embryofetal risk. Animal studies did show embryofetal toxicity with malformations in one species at doses less than 10 times the RHD. Based on animal studies and the drug's mechanism of action, the manufacturer recommends that women with reproductive potential use effective contraception during treatment and for 2 weeks after the last dose.

Nevertheless, using this drug during pregnancy should be based on the pros and cons of the mother's clinical need for treatment versus any potential fetal risk that might occur from exposure. In the clinical trials, up to 49% of patients developed hypertension and 36% developed proteinuria. This combination could appear like or mimic preeclampsia. There is a registry for women who are pregnant and have cancer. For more information, women and health care providers are encouraged to contact the Cancer and Pregnancy Registry at 1-877-635-4499.

BREASTFEEDING SUMMARY

No reports describing the use of fruquintinib during human lactation have been located. The drug will likely be found in breast milk, so some infant exposure will probably occur. Due to a concern for potential serious adverse effects that might be seen in a breastfed infant, the manufacturer recommends that women not breastfeed while being treated with this drug and for at least 2 weeks after the last dose. Nevertheless, breastfeeding while using this drug should be based on the mother's clinical need for treatment versus any potential infant risk that might occur. If used, the infant should be monitored for the most commonly reported adult side effects of nausea and abdominal pain (both leading to irritability), diarrhea, hypertension, proteinuria, infections, and elevated liver function tests.

Reference

1. Prescribing Information. Fruzaqla. Takeda Pharmaceuticals America, Inc; 2023.

FULVESTRANT

Antineoplastic (Estrogen Receptor Antagonist)

PREGNANCY RECOMMENDATION: No Human Data—Animal Data Suggest Risk

BREASTFEEDING RECOMMENDATION: Potential Toxicity

PREGNANCY SUMMARY

No reports describing the use of fulvestrant in human pregnancy have been located. Some of the drug will probably cross the placenta, so fetal exposure will likely occur. However, the absence of human pregnancy experience prevents a complete assessment of the embryofetal risk. Embryofetal toxicity with malformations was observed in two animal species at doses less than 10 times the MRHD. Based on animal studies and the drug's mechanism of action, the manufacturer recommends that women with reproductive potential use effective contraception during treatment and for at least 1 year after the last dose. Nevertheless, using this drug during pregnancy should be based on the pros and cons of the mother's clinical need for treatment versus any potential fetal risk that might occur from exposure. There is a registry for women who are pregnant and have cancer. For more information, women are encouraged to contact the Cancer and Pregnancy Registry at 877-635-4499.

BREASTFEEDING SUMMARY

No reports describing the use of fulvestrant during human lactation have been located. The drug will probably be excreted into breast milk, so some infant exposure will likely occur. However, due to a concern for potential serious adverse effects that might be seen in a breastfed infant, the manufacturer recommends that women not breastfeed while being treated with this drug and for at least 1 year after the last dose. Nevertheless, breastfeeding while using this drug should be based on the mother's clinical need for treatment versus any potential infant risks that might occur. If the clinical decision is to use this drug while breastfeeding, the infant should be monitored for the most commonly reported adult side effects of pain (leading to irritability), abnormal liver function tests, vomiting, poor eating (monitor infant growth), cough, and constipation.

Reference

1. Prescribing Information. Faslodex. AstraZeneca Pharmaceuticals; 2021.

FUROSEMIDE

Cardiovascular (Loop Diuretic)

PREGNANCY RECOMMENDATION: Human Data Suggest Low Risk

BREASTFEEDING RECOMMENDATION: Probably Compatible

PREGNANCY SUMMARY

Available data from published observational studies, case reports, and postmarketing analyses, from decades of use, have not demonstrated a drug-associated risk of major birth defects, miscarriage, or other adverse fetal outcomes with furosemide use during pregnancy, especially with limited use. Increased fetal urine production after maternal furosemide therapy has been observed. Administration of the drug to the mother has been used to assess fetal kidney function by provoking urine production, which is then visualized by ultrasonic analysis. Per the manufacturer, the drug crosses the placenta, so fetal exposure will occur. Embryofetal toxicity was observed in two animal species at doses less than 10 times the RHD (in one species it also caused maternal toxicity). Using this drug during pregnancy should be based on the pros and cons of the mother's clinical need for treatment versus any potential fetal risk that might occur from exposure.

F

BREASTFEEDING SUMMARY

Two reports were located that described the use of furosemide during human lactation. Both were used in the potential management of postpartum hypertension. These studies did not show an increased rate of neonatal complications, nor did furosemide affect the rates of exclusive breastfeeding. Milk levels were not evaluated, but the manufacturer states that the drug is found in breast milk. Breastfeeding while using this drug should be based on the mother's clinical need for treatment versus any potential infant risks that might occur. If used, the infant should be monitored for the most commonly reported adult side effects of nausea, dizziness, headache, and pruritus (all leading to irritability), vomiting, diarrhea, rash, and various laboratory abnormalities (electrolyte imbalance).

References

1. Prescribing Information. Furosemide tablets. West-Ward Pharmaceuticals Corp; 2017.
2. Prescribing Information. Furosemide injection. Hospira, Inc; 2023.
3. Votta RA, Parada OH, Windgrad RH, et al. Furosemide action on the creatinine concentration of amniotic fluid. *Am J Obstet Gynecol.* 1975;123:621-624.
4. Carswell W, Semple PF. The effect of furosemide on uric acid levels in maternal blood, fetal blood and amniotic fluid. *J Obstet Gynaecol Br Commonw.* 1974;81:472-474.
5. Jerkner K, Kutti J, Victorin L. Platelet counts in mothers and their newborn infants with respect to antepartum administration of oral diuretics. *Acta Med Scand.* 1973;194:473-475.
6. Shepard TH. *Catalog of Teratogen Agents.* 9th ed. The Johns Hopkins University Press; 1998:215.
7. Beermann B, Groschinsky-Grind M, Fahraeus L, Lindstroem B. Placental transfer of furosemide. *Clin Pharmacol Ther.* 1978;24:560-562.
8. Wladimiroff JW. Effect of furosemide on fetal urine production. *Br J Obstet Gynaecol.* 1975;82:221-4.
9. Stein WW, Halberstadt E, Gerner R, Roemer E. Effect of furosemide on fetal kidney function. *Arch Gynekol.* 1977;224:114-5.
10. Barrett RJ, Rayburn WF, Barr M Jr. Furosemide (Lasix) challenge test in assessing bilateral fetal hydronephrosis. *Am J Obstet Gynecol.* 1983;147:846-847.
11. Harman CR. Maternal furosemide may not provoke urine production in the compromised fetus. *Am J Obstet Gynecol.* 1984;150:322-323.
12. Pecorari D, Ragni N, Autera C. Administration of furosemide to women during confinement, and its action on newborn infants. *Acta Biomed (Italy).* 1969;40:2-11.
13. Pulle C. Diuretic therapy in monosymptomatic edema of pregnancy. *Minerva Med.* 1965;56:1622-1623.
14. DeCecco L. Furosemide in the treatment of edema in pregnancy. *Minerva Med.* 1965;56:1586-1591.
15. Bocci A, Pupita F, Revelli E, et al. The water-salt metabolism in obstetrics and gynecology. *Minerva Ginecol.* 1965;17:103-110.
16. Sideri L. Furosemide in the treatment of oedema in gynaecology and obstetrics. *Clin Ter.* 1966;39:339-346.
17. Wu CC, Lee TT, Kao SC. Evaluation of new diuretic (furosemide) on pregnant women. A pilot study. *J Obstet Gynecol Republ China.* 1966;5:318-320.
18. Loch EG. Treatment of gestosis with diuretics. *Med Klin.* 1966;61:1512-1515.
19. Buchheit H, Nicolai KH. Influence of furosemide (Lasix) on gestational edemas. *Med Klin.* 1966;61:1515-1518.
20. Tanaka T. Studies on the clinical effect of Lasix in edema of pregnancy and toxemia of pregnancy. *Sanka To Fujinka.* 1966;41:914-920.
21. Merger R, Cohen J, Sadut R. Study of the therapeutic effects of furosemide in obstetrics. *Rev Fr Gynecol.* 1967;62:259-265.
22. Nascimento R, Fernandes R, Cunha A. Furosemide as an accessory in the therapy of the toxemia of pregnancy. *Hospital (Portugal).* 1967;71:137-140.
23. Finnerty FA Jr. Advantages and disadvantages of furosemide in the edematous states of pregnancy. *Am J Obstet Gynecol.* 1969;105:1022-1027.
24. Das Gupta S. Frusemide in blood transfusion for severe anemia in pregnancy. *J Obstet Gynaecol India.* 1970;20:521-525.
25. Kawathekar P, Anusuya SR, Sriniwas P, Lagali S. Diazepam (Calmpose) in eclampsia: a preliminary report of 16 cases. *Curr Ther Res.* 1973;15:845-855.
26. Pianetti F. Our results in the treatment of parturient patients with oedema during the five years 1966-1970. *Atti Accad Med Lomb.* 1973;27:137-140.
27. Azcarte Sanchez S, Quesada Rocha T, Rosas Arced J. Evaluation of a plan of treatment in eclampsia (first report). *Ginecol Obstet Mex.* 1973;34:171-186.
28. Bravo Sandoval J. Management of pre-eclampsia-eclampsia in the third gyneco-obstetrical hospital. *Cir Cirjjands.* 1973;41:487-494.
29. Franck H, Gruhl M. Therapeutic experience with nortensin in the treatment of toxemia of pregnancy. *Munch Med Wochenschr.* 1974;116:521-524.
30. Cornu P, Laffay J, Ertel M, Lemiere J. Resuscitation in eclampsia. *Rev Prat.* 1975;25:809-830.
31. Finnerty FA Jr. Management of hypertension in toxemia of pregnancy. *Hosp Med.* 1975;11:52-65.
32. Saldana-Garcia RH. Eclampsia: maternal and fetal mortality. Comparative study of 80 cases. In VIII World Congress of Gynecology and Obstetrics. *Int Cong Ser.* 1976;396:58-59.
33. Palot M, Jakob L, Decaux J, et al. Arterial hypertensions of labor and the postpartum period. *Rev Fr Gynecol Obstet.* 1979;74:173-176.
34. Clark AD, Sevitt LH, Hawkins DF. Use of furosemide in severe toxaemia of pregnancy. *Lancet.* 1972;1:35-36.
35. Kirshon B, Edwards J, Cotton DB. Gordon's syndrome in pregnancy. *Am J Obstet Gynecol.* 1987;156:1110-1111.
36. Pitkin RM, Kaminetzky HA, Newton M, Pritchard JA. Maternal nutrition: a selective review of clinical topics. *Obstet Gynecol.* 1972;40:773-785.
37. Lindheimer MD, Katz AI. Sodium and diuretics in pregnancy. *N Engl J Med.* 1973;288:891-894.
38. Christianson R, Page EW. Diuretic drugs and pregnancy. *Obstet Gynecol.* 1976;48:647-652.
39. Gant NF, Madden JD, Shteri PK, MacDonald PC. The metabolic clearance rate of dehydroisoandrosterone sulfate. IV. Acute effects of induced hypertension, hypotension, and natriuresis in normal and hypertensive pregnancies. *Am J Obstet Gynecol.* 1976;124:143-148.
40. Sibai BM, Grossman RA, Grossman HG. Effects of diuretics on plasma volume in pregnancies with long-term hypertension. *Am J Obstet Gynecol.* 1984;150:831-835.
41. Cominos DC, van der Walt A, van Rooyen AJ. Suppression of postpartum lactation with furosemide. *S Afr Med J.* 1976;50:251-252.
42. Lopes Perdigao J, Lewey J, Hirshberg A, et al. Furosemide for accelerated recovery of blood pressure postpartum in women with a hypertensive disorder of pregnancy: a randomized controlled trial. *Hypertension.* 2021;77:1517-1524.
43. Emeruwa UN, Azad H, Ona S, et al. Lasix for the prevention of de nova postpartum hypertension: a randomized placebo-controlled trial. (LAPP Trial). *Am J Obstet Gynecol.* 2025;232(1):125.e1-125.e21.

FUTIBATINIB

Antineoplastic (Kinase Inhibitor)

PREGNANCY RECOMMENDATION: No Human Data—Animal Data Suggest Potential Risk

BREASTFEEDING RECOMMENDATION: Potential Toxicity

F

PREGNANCY SUMMARY

No reports describing the use of futibatinib in human pregnancy have been located. Some of the drug will probably cross the placenta, so fetal exposure will likely occur. However, the absence of human pregnancy experience prevents a complete assessment of the embryofetal risk. Animal studies did show embryofetal toxicity. Based on these animal studies and the drug's mechanism of action, the manufacturer recommends that women with reproductive potential use effective contraception during treatment and for 1 week after the last dose. They also recommend that males with female partners of reproductive potential use effective contraception during treatment and for 1 week after the last dose. However, using this drug during pregnancy should be based on the pros and cons of the mother's clinical need for treatment versus any potential fetal risk that might occur from exposure.

BREASTFEEDING SUMMARY

No reports describing the use of futibatinib during human lactation have been located. Some of the drug probably enters breast milk, so infant exposure will likely occur. However, due to the concern for potential serious adverse effects in a breastfed infant, the manufacturer recommends that women not breastfeed while being treated with this drug and for at least 1 week after the last dose. Nevertheless, breastfeeding while using this drug should be based on the mother's clinical need for treatment. If used, the infant should be monitored for the most commonly reported adult side effects of musculoskeletal pain, abdominal pain, arthralgia, and nausea (all leading to irritability), vomiting, decreased appetite (monitor growth), urinary tract infection, and several laboratory abnormalities (see PI).

Reference

1. Product Information. Lytgobi. Taiho Pharmaceutical Company; 2022.

GABAPENTIN

Central Nervous System (Antiseizure/Antineuropathy)

PREGNANCY RECOMMENDATION: Limited Human Data—Animal Data Suggest Risk

BREASTFEEDING RECOMMENDATION: Probably Compatible

PREGNANCY SUMMARY

Numerous reports have been located that describe the use of gabapentin in the first trimester of pregnancy. From these, the overall rate of birth anomalies is about 4% or less (in more than 400 exposures), and no pattern to the anomalies has been identified. In addition, a recent review and meta-analysis evaluated 29 cohort studies through April of 2017 regarding the safety of antiepileptic drugs, and no increased risk for birth anomalies was seen with gabapentin. The drug crosses the placenta, so fetal exposure will occur. However, this limited human pregnancy experience prevents a complete assessment of the embryofetal risk. Embryofetal toxicity was observed in three animal species at doses less than 10 times the maximum recommended human dose (MRHD). Using this drug during pregnancy should be based on the pros and cons of the mother's clinical need for treatment versus any potential fetal risk that might occur from exposure. There is a pregnancy exposure registry that monitors pregnancy outcomes in women exposed to antiepileptic drugs during pregnancy. Women who are taking gabapentin are encouraged to enroll in the North American Antiepileptic Drug (NAAED) Pregnancy Registry by calling 1-888-233-2334.

BREASTFEEDING SUMMARY

Several reports have been located that describe the use of gabapentin during lactation. The drug is found in breast milk with levels ranging from about 1 ng/mL to about 9 ng/mL. From these, the calculated relative infant doses (RIDs) are less than 4%. Infant serum levels have also been assessed in a few cases, with levels ranging from undetectable to about 400 pg/mL. These levels are about 12% or less than maternal levels. No adverse effects were noted in any infants. If the clinical decision is to use this drug while breastfeeding, the infant should be monitored for the most common reported pediatric side effects of nausea (leading to irritability), vomiting, somnolence, and fever.

References

1. Prescribing Information. Gabapentin. ACI Healthcare USA, Inc; 2023.
2. Chambers CD, Kao KK, Felix RJ, et al. Pregnancy outcome in infants prenatally exposed to newer anticonvulsants (abstract). *Birth Defects Res A*. 2005;73:316.
3. Holmes LB, Hernandez-Diaz S. Newer anticonvulsants: lamotrigine, topiramate, and gabapentin. *Birth Defects Res A Clin Mol Teratol*. 2012;94:599-606.
4. Jurgens TP, Schaefer C, May A. Treatment of cluster headache in pregnancy and lactation. *Cephalalgia*. 2009;29:391-400.
5. Dichter MA, Brodie MJ. New antiepileptic drugs. *N Engl J Med*. 1996;334:1583-1590.
6. Mack A. Examination of the evidence for off-label use of gabapentin. *J Managed Care Pharm*. 2003;9:559-568.
7. Ohman I, Vitols S, Tomson T. Pharmacokinetics of gabapentin during delivery, in the neonatal period, and lactation: does a fetal accumulation occur during pregnancy? *Epilepsia*. 2005;46:1621-1624.
8. Rosa F. Holoprosencephaly and antiepileptic exposures. *Teratology*. 1995;51:230.
9. The Lamotrigine Pregnancy Registry. Final report: 1 September 1992 through 31 March 2010. GlaxoSmithKline; 2010.
10. Wilton LV, Pearce GL, Martin RM, et al. The outcomes of pregnancy in women exposed to newly marketed drugs in general practice in England. *Br J Obstet Gynaecol*. 1998;105:882-889.
11. Morrell MJ. The new antiepileptic drugs and women: efficacy, reproductive health, pregnancy, and fetal outcome. *Epilepsia*. 1996;37(suppl 6):S34-S44.
12. Marcus DA. Pregnancy and chronic headache. *Expert Opin Pharmacother*. 2002;3:389-393.
13. Wilton LV, Shakir S. A postmarketing surveillance study of gabapentin as add-on therapy for 3,100 patients in England. *Epilepsia*. 2002;43:983-992.
14. Montouris G. Gabapentin exposure in human pregnancy: results from the gabapentin pregnancy registry. *Epilepsy Behav*. 2003;4:310-317.
15. Morrow J, Russell A, Guthrie E, et al. Malformation risks of antiepileptic drugs in pregnancy: a prospective study from the UK Epilepsy and Pregnancy Register. *J Neurol Neurosurg Psychiatry*. 2006;77:193-198.
16. Guttuso Thomas Jr, Robinson LK, Amankwah KS. Gabapentin use in hyperemesis gravidarum: a pilot study. *Early Hum Dev*. 2010;86:65-66.
17. Almgren M, Kallen B, Lavebratt C. Population-based study of antiepileptic drug exposure in utero—influence on head circumference in newborns. *Seizure*. 2009;18:672-675.
18. Fujii H, Goel A, Bernard N, et al. Pregnancy outcomes following gabapentin use: results of a prospective comparative cohort study. *Neurology*. 2013;80:1565-1570.
19. Goldkamp J, Blaskiewicz R, Myles T. Stiff person syndrome and pregnancy. *Obstet Gynecol*. 2011;118:454-457.
20. Veiby G, Daltveit AK, Engelsen BA, et al. Fetal growth restriction and birth defects with newer and older antiepileptic drugs in pregnancy. *J Neurol*. 2014;261:579-588.
21. Kristensen JH, Ilett KF, Hackett LP, et al. Gabapentin and breastfeeding: a case report. *J Hum Lact*. 2006;22:426-428.
22. Ohman I, Tomson T. Gabapentin kinetics during delivery, in the neonatal period, and during lactation. *Epilepsia*. 2009;50(suppl 10):108.
23. Johannessen SI, Helde G, Brodtkorb E. Levetiracetam concentrations in serum and in breast milk at birth and during lactation. *Epilepsia*. 2005;46:775-777.

24. Veroniki AA, Rios P, Cogo E, et al. Comparative safety of antiepileptic drugs for neurological development in children exposed during pregnancy and breast feeding: a systematic review and network meta-analysis. *BMJ Open*. 2017;7:e017248.

25. Desrochers B, Lavu A, Valencia E, et al. Risks of congenital malformations and neonatal intensive care unit admissions with gabapentin use in pregnancy: a cohort study and scoping review with meta-analysis. *Paediatr Perinat Epidemiol*. 2024;38:486-494.

GADOBENATE DIMEGLUMINE

Diagnostic (Gadolinium-Based Contrast Agent)

PREGNANCY RECOMMENDATION: No Human Data—Animal Data Suggest Low Risk

BREASTFEEDING RECOMMENDATION: Probably Compatible

G

PREGNANCY SUMMARY

No reports describing the use of gadobenate dimeglumine in human pregnancy have been located. One study reported the outcome in 25 pregnancies with exposure to gadopentetate dimeglumine near conception or in the early first trimester. Of these, there were 2 (8%) spontaneous abortions and no major fetal anomalies in 23 live births. In one large retrospective study, there were 397 gadolinium-enhanced magnetic resonance imaging (MRI)-exposed pregnancies (in any trimester). No increased risk for congenital anomalies was found with first-trimester exposure, but there was an increased risk for rheumatologic, inflammatory, or infiltrative skin conditions, as well as stillbirth and neonatal death. A breakdown as to the specific gadolinium-based contrast agent (GBCA) used was not provided. In a second large study, 5,991 pregnancies were identified that had GBCA MRI exposure. The rate of neonatal death and neonatal intensive care unit (NICU) admission was no different between those pregnancies exposed to a GBCA compared with the non-exposed control group. But again, a breakdown as to the specific GBCA used was not provided. The drug will probably cross the placenta, so some fetal exposure will likely occur. Therefore, the absence of human pregnancy experience with this specific GBCA prevents a complete assessment of the embryofetal risk. Animal studies did not show embryofetal toxicity in one species at doses of less than 10 times the recommended human dose (RHD), despite receiving multiple doses. In another species, the diagnostic agent did cause embryofetal toxicity at doses of less than 10 times the RHD, but again, it was administered daily for several days, resulting in an exposure much greater than 10 times the RHD. Gadobenate dimeglumine is a linear GBCA, which releases higher amounts of free gadolinium into the body compared with macrocytic GBCAs. This suggests a theoretical risk for higher gadolinium exposure. Other linear GBCAs are gadodiamide, gadopentetate dimeglumine, and gadoversetamide. The American College of Obstetricians and Gynecologists (ACOG) and the American College of Radiology (ACR) recommend that GBCAs should only be administered to a pregnant woman when the clinical benefits clearly outweigh the unknown risk of fetal exposure. The ACR states that each case should be carefully reviewed with the radiologist and referring physician, with documentation of appropriateness in the medical record, including informed consent.

BREASTFEEDING SUMMARY

No reports describing the use of gadobenate dimeglumine during human lactation have been located. The drug may be excreted into breast milk, so some infant exposure might occur. Gadobenate dimeglumine is a linear GBCA, which releases higher amounts of free gadolinium into the body compared with macrocytic GBCAs. This suggests a theoretical risk for higher gadolinium exposure. However, this agent has been safely used in infants. Furthermore, gadolinium is poorly absorbed from the gastrointestinal tract. Therefore, infant exposure from a single GBCA MRI study is likely to be minimal. ACOG and the ACR agree that due to the very small percentage of GBCA that is excreted into breast milk and absorbed by the infant's gastrointestinal tract, breastfeeding should not be interrupted after gadolinium administration. If the mother is concerned about any potential ill effects to the infant, she might consider expressing and discarding breast milk for 12 hours (>5 half-lives). If used while breastfeeding, the infant should be monitored for the most common reported adult side effects of headache and nausea (both leading to irritability).

References

1. Prescribing Information. Multihance. Bracco Diagnostics; 2024.
2. Oh KY, Roberts VHJ, Schabel MC, et al. Gadolinium chelate contrast material in pregnancy: fetal biodistribution in the nonhuman primate. *Radiology*. 2015;276:110-118.
3. De Santis M, Straface G, Cavaliere AF, et al. Gadolinium periconceptional exposure: pregnancy and neonatal outcome. *Acta Obstet Gynecol Scand*. 2007;86:99-101.
4. Ray JG, Vermeulen MJ, Bharatha A, Montanera WJ, Park AL. Association between MRI exposure during pregnancy and fetal and childhood outcomes. *JAMA*. 2016;316(9):952-961.
5. Winterstein AG, Thai TN, Nduaguba S, et al. Risk of fetal or neonatal death or neonatal intensive care unit admission associated with gadolinium magnetic resonance imaging exposure during pregnancy. *AM J Obstet Gynecol*. 2023;228:465.e1-465.e11.
6. Guidelines for diagnostic imaging during pregnancy and lactation. Committee Opinion No. 723. American College of Obstetricians and Gynecologists. *Obstet Gynecol*. 2017;130:e21006.
7. American College of Radiology. *ACR Manual on Contrast Media*. Accessed February 6, 2024. https://www.acr.org/- /media/ACR/Files/Clinical-Resources/Contrast_Media.pdf
8. Fraum TJ, Ludwig DR, Bashir MR, et al. Gadolinium-based contrast agents: a comprehensive risk assessment. *J Magn Reason Imaging*. 2017;46: 338-353.

GADOBUTROL

Diagnostic (Gadolinium-Based Contrast Agent)

PREGNANCY RECOMMENDATION: No Human Data and No Relevant Animal Data

BREASTFEEDING RECOMMENDATION: Probably Compatible

G

PREGNANCY SUMMARY

No reports describing the use of gadobutrol in human pregnancy have been located. One study reported the outcome in 25 pregnancies with exposure to gadopentetate dimeglumine near conception or in the early first trimester. Of these, there were 2 (8%) spontaneous abortions and no major fetal anomalies in 23 live births. In one large retrospective study, there were 397 gadolinium-enhanced MRI-exposed pregnancies (in any trimester). No increased risk for congenital anomalies was found with first-trimester exposure, but there was an increased risk for rheumatologic, inflammatory, or infiltrative skin conditions, as well as stillbirth and neonatal death. Breakdown as to the specific GBCA used was not provided. In a second large study, 5,991 pregnancies were identified that had GBCA MRI exposure. The rate of neonatal death and NICU admission was no different between those pregnancies exposed to a GBCA compared with the nonexposed control group. But again, a breakdown as to the specific GBCA used was not provided. The drug will probably cross the placenta, so some fetal exposure will likely occur. Therefore, the absence of human pregnancy experience with this specific GBCA prevents a complete assessment of the embryofetal risk. Animal studies did show embryofetal toxicity in one species at doses of less than 10 times the RHD, but this dose was used daily, resulting in a much higher exposure (compared with a single injection used in human diagnostic studies). Gadobutrol is a macrocyclic GBCA, which is more stable, releasing lower amounts of free gadolinium into the body. This suggests a theoretical risk for lower gadolinium exposure. Other macrocyclic GBCAs are gadoterate meglumine and gadoteridol. ACOG and the ACR recommend that GBCAs should only be administered to a pregnant woman when the clinical benefits clearly outweigh the unknown risk of fetal exposure. The ACR states that each case should be carefully reviewed with the radiologist and referring physician, with documentation of appropriateness in the medical record, including informed consent.

BREASTFEEDING SUMMARY

No reports describing the use of gadobutrol during human lactation have been located. The drug may be excreted into breast milk, so some infant exposure might occur. Gadolinium is poorly absorbed from the gastrointestinal tract. Therefore, infant exposure from a single GBCA MRI study is likely to be minimal. Gadobutrol is a macrocyclic GBCA, which is more stable, releasing lower amounts of free gadolinium into the body. This suggests a theoretical risk for lower gadolinium exposure. ACOG and the ACR agree that due to the very small percentage of GBCA that is excreted into breast milk and absorbed by the infant's gastrointestinal tract, breastfeeding should not be interrupted after gadolinium administration. If the mother is concerned about any potential ill effects to the infant, she might consider expressing and discarding breast milk for 12 hours (>5 half-lives). If used while breastfeeding, the infant should be monitored for the most common reported adult side effects of headache and nausea (both leading to irritability).

References

1. Prescribing Information. Gadavist. Bayer Healthcare Pharmaceuticals Inc; 2021.
2. Oh KY, Roberts VHJ, Schabel MC, et al. Gadolinium chelate contrast material in pregnancy: fetal biodistribution in the nonhuman primate. *Radiology*. 2015;276:110-118.
3. De Santis M, Straface G, Cavaliere AF, et al. Gadolinium periconceptional exposure: pregnancy and neonatal outcome. *Acta Obstet Gynecol Scand*. 2007;86:99-101.
4. Ray JG, Vermeulen MJ, Bharatha A, Montanera WJ, Park AL. Association between MRI exposure during pregnancy and fetal and childhood outcomes. *JAMA*. 2016;316(9):952-961.
5. Winterstein AG, Thai TN, Nduaguba S, et al. Risk of fetal or neonatal death or neonatal intensive care unit admission associated with gadolinium magnetic resonance imaging exposure during pregnancy. *AM J Obstet Gynecol*. 2023;228:465.e1-465.e11.
6. Guidelines for diagnostic imaging during pregnancy and lactation. Committee Opinion No. 723. American College of Obstetricians and Gynecologists. *Obstet Gynecol*. 2017;130:e21006.
7. American College of Radiology. *ACR Manual on Contrast Media*. Accessed February 6, 2024. https://www.acr.org/- /media/ACR/Files/Clinical-Resources/Contrast_Media.pdf

GADODIAMIDE

Diagnostic (Gadolinium-Based Contrast Agent)

PREGNANCY RECOMMENDATION: No Human Data—Animal Data Suggest Low Risk

BREASTFEEDING RECOMMENDATION: Probably Compatible

PREGNANCY SUMMARY

No reports describing the use of gadodiamide in human pregnancy have been located. One study reported the outcome in 25 pregnancies with exposure to gadopentetate dimeglumine near conception or in the early first trimester. Of these, there were 2 (8%) spontaneous abortions and no major fetal anomalies in 23 live births. In one large retrospective study, there were 397 gadolinium-enhanced MRI-exposed pregnancies (in any trimester). No increased risk for congenital anomalies was found with first-trimester exposure, but there was an increased risk for rheumatologic, inflammatory, or infiltrative skin conditions, as well as stillbirth and neonatal death. A breakdown as to the specific GBCA used was not provided. In a second large study, 5,991 pregnancies were identified that had GBCA MRI exposure. The rate of neonatal death and NICU admission was no different between those pregnancies exposed to a GBCA compared with the nonexposed control group. But again, a breakdown as to the specific GBCA used was not provided. The drug will probably cross the placenta, so some fetal exposure will likely occur. Therefore, the absence of human pregnancy experience with this specific GBCA prevents a complete assessment of the embryofetal risk. Animal studies did show embryofetal toxicity in one species at doses of less than 10 times the RHD, but gadodiamide was administered over numerous days, resulting in a much greater exposure. No embryofetal toxicity or teratogenicity was seen in another species at doses less than 10 times the RHD, despite the administration of daily doses for several days. Gadodiamide is a linear GBCA, which releases higher amounts of free gadolinium into the body compared with macrocytic GBCAs. This suggests a theoretical risk for higher gadolinium exposure. Other linear GBCAs are gadobenate dimeglumine, gadopentetate dimeglumine, and gadoversetamide. ACOG and the ACR recommend that GBCAs should only be administered to a pregnant woman when the clinical benefits clearly outweigh the unknown risk of fetal exposure. The ACR states that each case should be carefully reviewed with the radiologist and referring physician, with documentation of appropriateness in the medical record, including informed consent.

BREASTFEEDING SUMMARY

No reports describing the use of gadodiamide during human lactation have been located. The drug may be excreted into breast milk, so some infant exposure might occur. Gadodiamide is a linear GBCA, which releases higher amounts of free gadolinium into the body compared with macrocytic GBCAs. This suggests a theoretical risk for higher gadolinium exposure. However, one nursing mother did receive gadodiamide with no reported adverse infant effects. She did withhold breastfeeding for about 6 to 8 hours after the injection, which was more than 4 half-lives. Furthermore, gadolinium is poorly absorbed from the gastrointestinal tract. Therefore, infant exposure from a single GBCA MRI study is likely to be minimal. ACOG and the ACR agree that due to the very small percentage of GBCA that is excreted into breast milk and absorbed by the infant's gastrointestinal tract, breastfeeding should not be interrupted after gadolinium administration. If the mother is concerned about any potential ill effects to the infant, she might consider expressing and discarding breast milk for 12 hours (>5 half-lives). If used while breastfeeding, the infant should be monitored for the most common reported adult side effects of headache and nausea (both leading to irritability).

References

1. Prescribing Information. Omniscan. GE Healthcare; 2021.
2. Oh KY, Roberts VHJ, Schabel MC, et al. Gadolinium chelate contrast material in pregnancy: fetal biodistribution in the nonhuman primate. *Radiology*. 2015;276:110-118.
3. De Santis M, Straface G, Cavaliere AF, et al. Gadolinium periconceptional exposure: pregnancy and neonatal outcome. *Acta Obstet Gynecol Scand*. 2007;86:99-101.
4. Ray JG, Vermeulen MJ, Bharatha A, Montanera WJ, Park AL. Association between MRI exposure during pregnancy and fetal and childhood outcomes. *JAMA*. 2016;316(9):952-961.
5. Winterstein AG, Thai TN, Nduaguba S, et al. Risk of fetal or neonatal death or neonatal intensive care unit admission associated with gadolinium magnetic resonance imaging exposure during pregnancy. *Am J Obstet Gynecol*. 2023;228:465.e1-465.e11.
6. Guidelines for diagnostic imaging during pregnancy and lactation. Committee Opinion No. 723. American College of Obstetricians and Gynecologists. *Obstet Gynecol*. 2017;130:e21006.
7. American College of Radiology. *ACR Manual on Contrast Media*. Accessed February 6, 2024. https://www.acr.org/- /media/ACR/Files/Clinical-Resources/Contrast_Media.pdf
8. Acar S, Keskin-Arslan E, Erol-Coskum H, et al. Gadodiamide use during breastfeeding. *Reprod Toxicol*. 2018;80:59-60.

GADOPENTETATE DIMEGLUMINE

Diagnostic (Gadolinium-Based Contrast Agent)

PREGNANCY RECOMMENDATION: Limited Human Data and No Relevant Animal Data

BREASTFEEDING RECOMMENDATION: Probably Compatible

PREGNANCY SUMMARY

Four reports describing the use of gadopentetate dimeglumine in human pregnancy were located. One study and a case report described the outcome in 26 pregnancies with exposure to gadopentetate dimeglumine near conception or in the

(continued)

early first trimester. Of these, there were 2 (8%) spontaneous abortions and no major fetal anomalies in 24 live births. In two other studies, gadopentetate dimeglumine was used in 13 patients in the second or third trimesters and no reported complications or anomalies were described. In one large retrospective study, there were 397 gadolinium-enhanced MRI-exposed pregnancies (in any trimester). No increased risk for congenital anomalies was reported with first-trimester exposure, but there was an increased risk for rheumatologic, inflammatory, or infiltrative skin conditions, as well as stillbirth and neonatal death. A breakdown as to the specific GBCA used was not provided. In a second large study, 5,991 pregnancies were identified that had GBCA MRI exposure. The rate of neonatal death and NICU admission was no different between those pregnancies exposed to a GBCA compared with the nonexposed control group. But again, a breakdown as to the specific GBCA used was not provided. The drug will probably cross the placenta, so some fetal exposure will likely occur. However, this limited human pregnancy experience with this specific GBCA prevents a complete assessment of the embryofetal risk. Animal studies did show embryofetal toxicity in two species at doses of more than 10 times the RHD. Gadopentetate dimeglumine is a linear GBCA, which releases higher amounts of free gadolinium into the body compared with macrocytic GBCAs. This suggests a theoretical risk for higher gadolinium exposure. Other linear GBCAs are gadobenate dimeglumine, gadodiamide, and gadoversetamide. ACOG and the ACR recommend that GBCAs should only be administered to a pregnant woman when the clinical benefits clearly outweigh the unknown risk of fetal exposure. The ACR states that each case should be carefully reviewed with the radiologist and referring physician, with documentation of appropriateness in the medical record, including informed consent.

G

BREASTFEEDING SUMMARY

Three reports were identified that evaluated breast milk levels in 21 lactating women following the administration of gadopentetate dimeglumine. In 20 women, the maternal dose was 0.1 mmol/kg, and in the 21st patient, the dose was 0.2 mmol/kg. The breast milk levels ranged from about 3.3 to 7.4 nmole/mL. The breast milk level in the patient receiving the higher dose fell within the range of values seen with the lower dose. All of the calculated RIDs were less than 1% of the usual maximal neonatal dose of 0.2 mmol/kg. Gadopentetate dimeglumine is a linear GBCA, which releases higher amounts of free gadolinium into the body compared with macrocytic GBCAs. This suggests a theoretical risk for higher gadolinium exposure. However, gadolinium is poorly absorbed from the gastrointestinal tract. Therefore, infant exposure from a single GBCA MRI study is likely to be minimal. ACOG and the ACR agree that due to the very small percentage of GBCA that is excreted into breast milk and absorbed by the infant's gastrointestinal tract, breastfeeding should not be interrupted after gadolinium administration. If the mother is concerned about any potential ill effects to the infant, she might consider expressing and discarding breast milk for 8 hours (~5 half-lives). If used while breastfeeding, the infant should be monitored for the most common reported adult side effects of headache, nausea, and dizziness (all leading to irritability).

References

1. Prescribing Information. Magnevist. Bayer HealthCare Pharmaceuticals; 2018.
2. Oh KY, Roberts VHJ, Schabel MC, et al. Gadolinium chelate contrast material in pregnancy: fetal biodistribution in the nonhuman primate. *Radiology*. 2015;276:110-118.
3. Barkhof F, Heijboer RJJ, Algra PR. Inadvertent IV administration of gadopentetate dimeglumine during early pregnancy. *AJR Am J Roentgenol*. 1992;158:1171.
4. De Santis M, Straface G, Cavaliere AF, et al. Gadolinium periconceptional exposure: pregnancy and neonatal outcome. *Acta Obstet Gynecol*. 2007;86:99-101.
5. Spencer JA, Tomlinson AJ, Weston MJ, et al. Early report: comparison of breath-hold MR excretory urography, Doppler ultrasound and isotope renography in evaluation of symptomatic hydronephrosis in pregnancy. *Clin Radiol*. 2000;55:446-453.
6. Shoenut JP, Semelka RC, Silverman R, et al. MRI in the diagnosis of Crohn's disease in two pregnant women. *J Clin Gastroenterol*. 1993;17:244-247.
7. Ray JG, Vermeulen MJ, Bharatha A, Montanera WJ, Park AL. Association between MRI exposure during pregnancy and fetal and childhood outcomes. *JAMA*. 2016;316(9):952-961.
8. Winterstein AG, Thai TN, Nduaguba S, et al. Risk of fetal or neonatal death or neonatal intensive care unit admission associated with gadolinium magnetic resonance imaging exposure during pregnancy. *Am J Obstet Gynecol*. 2023;228:465.e1-465.e11.
9. Guidelines for diagnostic imaging during pregnancy and lactation. Committee Opinion No. 723. American College of Obstetricians and Gynecologists. *Obstet Gynecol*. 2017;130:e21006.
10. American College of Radiology. *ACR Manual on Contrast Media*. Accessed February 6, 2024. https://www.acr.org/- /media/ACR/Files/Clinical-Resources/Contrast_Media.pdf
11. Schmiedl U, Maravilla KR, Gerlach R, et al. Excretion of gadopentetate dimeglumine in human breast milk. *AJR Am J Roentgenol*. 1990;154:1305-1306.
12. Rofsky NM, Weinreb JC, Litt AW. Quantitative analysis of gadopentetate dimeglumine excreted in breast milk. *J Magn Reson Imaging*. 1993;3:131-132.
13. Kubik-Huch RA, Gottstein-Aalame NM, Frenzel T, et al. Gadopentetate dimeglumine excretion into human breast milk during lactation. *Radiology*. 2000;216:555-558.

GADOPICLENOL

Diagnostic (Gadolinium-Based Contrast Agent)

PREGNANCY RECOMMENDATION: No Human Data—Animal Data Suggest Potential Risk

BREASTFEEDING RECOMMENDATION: Probably Compatible

PREGNANCY SUMMARY

No reports describing the use of gadopiclenol in human pregnancy have been located. Some amount of the drug will likely cross the placenta, so fetal exposure will probably occur. Therefore, the absence of human pregnancy experience prevents a complete assessment of embryofetal risk. No embryofetal toxicity, despite some maternal toxicity, was observed in animal studies. However, other GBCAs administered to pregnant nonhuman primates and mice during gestation did result in measurable levels in the offspring for at least 7 months and 1 month, respectively. The clinical effect of this is unknown. The manufacturer recommends using this agent only if imaging is essential during pregnancy and cannot be delayed because of the potential risks of gadolinium to the fetus. ACOG recommends that gadolinium-based contrast agents with MRI should be limited during pregnancy and only be used if they significantly improve diagnostic imaging and are expected to improve maternal or fetal outcomes. Similarly, the ACR recommends avoiding routine use of GBCAs during pregnancy and that they should only be used when the significant clinical benefit outweighs the unknown risk.

G

BREASTFEEDING SUMMARY

No reports describing the use of gadopiclenol during human lactation have been located. A limited amount of the drug will likely be excreted into breast milk, so some infant exposure will probably occur. Breastfeeding while using this contrast agent should be based on the mother's clinical need for diagnosis. If used, the infant should be monitored for the most common reported adult side effects of headache, nausea, and dizziness (all leading to irritability). ACOG and the ACR state that breastfeeding does not need to be interrupted after the use of gadolinium.

References

1. Product Information. Elucirem. Guerbet, LLC; 2022.
2. American College of Obstetricians and Gynecologists. Guidelines for diagnostic imaging during pregnancy and lactation. Committee Opinion No. 723. *Obstet Gynecol*. 2017;130:e210-e216.
3. American College of Radiology Committee on Drugs and Contrast Media. Gadolinium pregnancy screening statement. Accessed June 18, 2023. https://www.acr.org/Advocacy/Position-Statements/Gadolinium-Pregnancy-Screening
4. ACR Committee on Drugs and Contrast Media. Administration of contrast media to women who are breastfeeding. *ACR Manual on Contrast Media*. 2023;107-108. Accessed June 18, 2023. https://www.acr.org/Clinical-Resources/Clinical-Tools-and-Reference/Contrast-Manual

GADOTERATE MEGLUMINE

Diagnostic (Gadolinium-Based Contrast Agent)

PREGNANCY RECOMMENDATION: Limited Human Data—Animal Data Suggest Low Risk

BREASTFEEDING RECOMMENDATION: Probably Compatible

PREGNANCY SUMMARY

One report was located that described the use of gadoterate meglumine in a human pregnancy at 27 weeks of gestation. The newborn outcome was not provided. Another study reported the outcome in 25 pregnancies with exposure to gadopentetate dimeglumine near conception or in the early first trimester. Of these, there were 2 (8%) spontaneous abortions and no major fetal anomalies in 23 live births. In one large retrospective study, there were 397 gadolinium-enhanced MRI-exposed pregnancies (in any trimester). No increased risk for congenital anomalies was found with first-trimester exposure, but there was an increased risk for rheumatologic, inflammatory, or infiltrative skin conditions, as well as stillbirth and neonatal death. A breakdown as to the specific GBCA used was not provided. In a second large study, 5,991 pregnancies were identified that had GBCA MRI exposure. The rate of neonatal death and NICU admission was no different between those pregnancies exposed to a GBCA compared with the nonexposed control group. But again, a breakdown as to the specific GBCA used was not provided. Some of this diagnostic agent appears to cross the placenta, so fetal exposure will likely occur. However, this limited human pregnancy experience with this specific GBCA prevents a complete assessment of the embryofetal risk. Animal studies did not show any embryofetal toxicity in two species at doses more than 10 times the RHD, despite daily administration over numerous days. Gadoterate meglumine is a macrocyclic GBCA, which is more stable, releasing lower amounts of free gadolinium into the body. This suggests a theoretical risk for lower gadolinium exposure. Other macrocyclic GBCAs are gadobutrol and gadoteridol. ACOG and ACR recommend that GBCAs should only be administered to a pregnant woman when the clinical benefits clearly outweigh the unknown risk of fetal exposure. The ACR states that each case should be carefully reviewed with the radiologist and referring physician, with documentation of appropriateness in the medical record, including informed consent.

BREASTFEEDING SUMMARY

No reports describing the use of gadoterate meglumine during human lactation have been located. The drug may be excreted into breast milk, so some infant exposure might occur. Gadolinium is poorly absorbed from the gastrointestinal tract. Therefore, infant exposure from a single GBCA MRI study is likely to be minimal. Gadoterate meglumine is a macrocyclic GBCA, which is more stable, releasing lower amounts of free gadolinium into the body. This suggests a theoretical risk for lower gadolinium exposure. ACOG and ACR agree that due to the very small percentage of GBCA that is excreted into breast milk and absorbed by the infant's gastrointestinal tract, breastfeeding should not be interrupted after gadolinium administration. If the mother is concerned about any potential ill effects to the infant, she might consider expressing and discarding breast milk for 8 hours (>5 half-lives). If used while breastfeeding, the infant should be monitored for the most common reported adult side effects of headache and nausea (both leading to irritability).

References

1. Prescribing Information. Dotarem. Guerbet LLC; 2021.
2. Laissy JP, Siauve N, Dossier A, Lancelot E. Transient signal intensity enhancement in the amniotic fluid after administration of a macrocyclic gadolinium chelate to a pregnant woman. *J Magn Reson Imaging*. 2021;54:669-671.
3. Oh KY, Roberts VHJ, Schabel MC, et al. Gadolinium chelate contrast material in pregnancy: fetal biodistribution in the nonhuman primate. *Radiology*. 2015;276:110-118.
4. De Santis M, Straface G, Cavaliere AF, et al. Gadolinium periconceptional exposure: pregnancy and neonatal outcome. *Acta Obstet Gynecol Scand*. 2007;86:99-101.
5. Ray JG, Vermeulen MJ, Bharatha A, Montanera WJ, Park AL. Association between MRI exposure during pregnancy and fetal and childhood outcomes. *JAMA*. 2016;316(9):952-961.
6. Winterstein AG, Thai TN, Nduaguba S, et al. Risk of fetal or neonatal death or neonatal intensive care unit admission associated with gadolinium magnetic resonance imaging exposure during pregnancy. *AM J Obstet Gynecol*. 2023;228:465.e1-465.e11.
7. Guidelines for diagnostic imaging during pregnancy and lactation. Committee Opinion No. 723. American College of Obstetricians and Gynecologists. *Obstet Gynecol*. 2017;130:e21006.
8. American College of Radiology. *ACR Manual on Contrast Media*. Accessed February 6, 2024. https://www.acr.org/- /media/ACR/Files/Clinical-Resources/Contrast_Media.pdf

G

GADOTERIDOL

Diagnostic (Gadolinium-Based Contrast Agent)

PREGNANCY RECOMMENDATION: No Human Data and No Relevant Animal Data

BREASTFEEDING RECOMMENDATION: Probably Compatible

PREGNANCY SUMMARY

No reports describing the use of gadoteridol in human pregnancy have been located. One study reported the outcome in 25 pregnancies with exposure to gadopentetate dimeglumine near conception or in the early first trimester. Of these, there were 2 (8%) spontaneous abortions and no major fetal anomalies in 23 live births. In one large retrospective study, there were 397 gadolinium-enhanced MRI-exposed pregnancies (in any trimester). No increased risk for congenital anomalies was reported with first-trimester exposure, but there was an increased risk for rheumatologic, inflammatory, or infiltrative skin conditions, as well as stillbirth and neonatal death. A breakdown as to the specific GBCA used was not provided. In a second large study, 5,991 pregnancies were identified that had GBCA MRI exposure. The rate of neonatal death and NICU admission was no different between those pregnancies exposed to a GBCA compared with the nonexposed control group. But again, a breakdown as to the specific GBCA used was not provided. The drug will probably cross the placenta, so some fetal exposure will likely occur. Therefore, the absence of human pregnancy experience with this specific GBCA prevents a complete assessment of the embryofetal risk. Animal studies did show embryofetal toxicity in two species at doses of less than 10 times the RHD, but these doses were used daily for 12 days, resulting in a much higher exposure (compared with a single injection used in human diagnostic studies). Gadoteridol is a macrocyclic GBCA, which is more stable, releasing lower amounts of free gadolinium into the body. This suggests a theoretical risk for lower gadolinium exposure. Other macrocyclic GBCAs are gadobutrol and gadoterate meglumine. ACOG and ACR recommend that GBCAs should only be administered to a pregnant woman when the clinical benefits clearly outweigh the unknown risk of fetal exposure. The ACR states that each case should be carefully reviewed with the radiologist and referring physician, with documentation of appropriateness in the medical record, including informed consent.

BREASTFEEDING SUMMARY

No reports describing the use of gadoteridol during human lactation have been located. The drug may be excreted into breast milk, so some infant exposure might occur. Gadolinium is poorly absorbed from the gastrointestinal tract. Therefore, infant exposure from a single GBCA MRI study is likely to be minimal. Gadoteridol is a macrocyclic GBCA, which is more stable, releasing lower amounts of free gadolinium into the body. This suggests a theoretical risk for lower gadolinium exposure. ACOG and ACR agree that due to the very small percentage of GBCA that is excreted into breast milk and absorbed by the infant's gastrointestinal tract, breastfeeding should not be interrupted after gadolinium administration. If the mother is concerned about any potential ill effects to the infant, she might consider expressing and discarding breast milk for 10 hours (>5 half-lives). If used while breastfeeding, the infant should be monitored for the most common reported adult side effects of headache and nausea (both leading to irritability).

References

1. Prescribing Information. Prohance. Bracco Diagnostics; 2021.
2. Oh KY, Roberts VHJ, Schabel MC, et al. Gadolinium chelate contrast material in pregnancy: fetal biodistribution in the nonhuman primate. *Radiology*. 2015;276:110-118.

3. De Santis M, Straface G, Cavaliere AF, et al. Gadolinium periconceptional exposure: pregnancy and neonatal outcome. *Acta Obstet Gynecol Scand.* 2007;86:99-101.
4. Ray JG, Vermeulen MJ, Bharatha A, Montanera WJ, Park AL. Association between MRI exposure during pregnancy and fetal and childhood outcomes. *JAMA.* 2016;316(9):952-961.
5. Winterstein AG, Thai TN, Nduaguba S, et al. Risk of fetal or neonatal death or neonatal intensive care unit admission associated with gadolinium magnetic resonance imaging exposure during pregnancy. *AM J Obstet Gynecol.* 2023;228:465.e1-465.e11.
6. Guidelines for diagnostic imaging during pregnancy and lactation. Committee Opinion No. 723. American College of Obstetricians and Gynecologists. *Obstet Gynecol.* 2017;130:e21006.
7. American College of Radiology. *ACR Manual on Contrast Media.* Accessed February 6, 2024. https://www.acr.org/- /media/ACR/Files/Clinical-Resources/Contrast_Media.pdf

GADOVERSETAMIDE

Diagnostic (Gadolinium-Based Contrast Agent)

PREGNANCY RECOMMENDATION: No Human Data—Animal Data Suggest Low Risk

BREASTFEEDING RECOMMENDATION: Probably Compatible

G

PREGNANCY SUMMARY

No reports describing the use of gadoversetamide in human pregnancy have been located. One study reported the outcome in 25 pregnancies with exposure to gadopentetate dimeglumine near conception or in the early first trimester. Of these, there were 2 (8%) spontaneous abortions and no major fetal anomalies in 23 live births. In one large retrospective study, there were 397 gadolinium-enhanced MRI-exposed pregnancies (in any trimester). No increased risk for congenital anomalies was found with first-trimester exposure, but there was an increased risk for rheumatologic, inflammatory, or infiltrative skin conditions, as well as stillbirth and neonatal death. A breakdown as to the specific GBCA used was not provided. In a second large study, 5,991 pregnancies were identified that had GBCA MRI exposure. The rate of neonatal death and NICU admission was no different between those pregnancies exposed to a GBCA compared with the nonexposed control group. But again, a breakdown as to the specific GBCA used was not provided. The drug will probably cross the placenta, so some fetal exposure will likely occur. Therefore, the absence of human pregnancy experience with this specific GBCA prevents a complete assessment of the embryofetal risk. No embryofetal toxicity or teratogenicity was seen in two species at doses less than 10 times the RHD, despite the administration of daily doses for several days. Gadoversetamide is a linear GBCA, which releases higher amounts of free gadolinium into the body compared with macrocytic GBCAs. This suggests a theoretical risk for higher gadolinium exposure. Other linear GBCAs are gadobenate dimeglumine, gadodiamide, and gadopentetate dimeglumine. ACOG and ACR recommend that GBCAs should only be administered to a pregnant woman when the clinical benefits clearly outweigh the unknown risk of fetal exposure. The ACR states that each case should be carefully reviewed with the radiologist and referring physician, with documentation of appropriateness in the medical record, including informed consent.

BREASTFEEDING SUMMARY

No reports describing the use of gadoversetamide during human lactation have been located. The drug may be excreted into breast milk, so some infant exposure might occur. Gadoversetamide is a linear GBCA, which releases higher amounts of free gadolinium into the body compared with macrocytic GBCAs. This suggests a theoretical risk for higher gadolinium exposure. However, gadolinium is poorly absorbed from the gastrointestinal tract. Therefore, infant exposure from a single GBCA MRI study is likely to be minimal. ACOG and ACR agree that due to the very small percentage of GBCA that is excreted into breast milk and absorbed by the infant's gastrointestinal tract, breastfeeding should not be interrupted after gadolinium administration. If the mother is concerned about any potential ill effects to the infant, she might consider expressing and discarding breast milk for 10 hours (>5 half-lives). If used while breastfeeding, the infant should be monitored for the most common reported adult side effects of headache and nausea (both leading to irritability).

References

1. Prescribing Information. Omniscan. GE Healthcare; 2021.
2. Oh KY, Roberts VHJ, Schabel MC, et al. Gadolinium chelate contrast material in pregnancy: fetal biodistribution in the nonhuman primate. *Radiology.* 2015;276:110-118.
3. De Santis M, Straface G, Cavaliere AF, et al. Gadolinium periconceptional exposure: pregnancy and neonatal outcome. *Acta Obstet Gynecol Scand.* 2007;86:99-101.
4. Ray JG, Vermeulen MJ, Bharatha A, Montanera WJ, Park AL. Association between MRI exposure during pregnancy and fetal and childhood outcomes. *JAMA.* 2016;316(9):952-961.
5. Winterstein AG, Thai TN, Nduaguba S, et al. Risk of fetal or neonatal death or neonatal intensive care unit admission associated with gadolinium magnetic resonance imaging exposure during pregnancy. *AM J Obstet Gynecol.* 2023;228:465.e1-465.e11.
6. Guidelines for diagnostic imaging during pregnancy and lactation. Committee Opinion No. 723. American College of Obstetricians and Gynecologists. *Obstet Gynecol.* 2017;130:e21006.
7. American College of Radiology. *ACR Manual on Contrast Media.* Accessed February 6, 2024. https://www.acr.org/-/media/ACR/Files/Clinical-Resources/Contrast_Media.pdf

GALANTAMINE

Central Nervous System (Cholinesterase Inhibitor)

PREGNANCY RECOMMENDATION: No Human Data—Animal Data Suggest Potential Risk

BREASTFEEDING RECOMMENDATION: Potential Toxicity

G

PREGNANCY SUMMARY

No reports describing the use of galantamine in human pregnancy have been located. Because of its indication, such reports should be rare. The drug will probably cross the placenta, so some fetal exposure would likely occur. Therefore, the absence of human pregnancy experience prevents a complete assessment of the embryofetal risk. Embryofetal toxicity was observed in one animal species at doses less than 10 times the MRHD. Using this drug during pregnancy should be based on the pros and cons of the mother's clinical need for treatment versus any potential fetal risk that might occur from exposure.

BREASTFEEDING SUMMARY

No reports describing the use of galantamine during human lactation have been located. Because of its indication, such reports should be rare. The drug will probably be excreted into breast milk, so some infant exposure would likely occur. If the clinical decision is to use this drug while breastfeeding, the infant should be monitored for the most common reported adult side effects of nausea, dizziness, and headache (all leading to irritability), vomiting, and decreased appetite.

Reference

1. Prescribing Information. Razadyne ER. Janssen Pharmaceuticals, Inc; 2022.

GALCANEZUMAB

Central Nervous System (Antimigraine—Monoclonal Antibody)

PREGNANCY RECOMMENDATION: Limited Human Data—Animal Data Suggest Low Risk

BREASTFEEDING RECOMMENDATION: Probably Compatible

PREGNANCY SUMMARY

Data from the VigiBase safety reporting system (involving 22 pregnancies with some outcome information) did not show any increased signals of fetal or maternal toxicity. As an immunoglobulin G (IgG) antibody, it likely crosses the placenta, especially during the second half of gestation, so some fetal exposure will probably occur. Therefore, this limited human pregnancy experience prevents a complete assessment of the embryofetal risk. Animal data did not show any embryofetal toxicity in two animal species at doses greater than 10 times the RHD. Using this drug during pregnancy should be based on the pros and cons of the mother's clinical need for treatment versus any potential fetal risk that might occur from exposure. There is a pregnancy exposure registry that monitors pregnancy outcomes in women exposed to galcanezumab during pregnancy. Health care providers or patients are encouraged to call 1-833-364-2548.

BREASTFEEDING SUMMARY

Three cases of exposure to galcanezumab during human lactation were reported to the VigiBase safety monitoring program, but specific issues or outcomes were not supplied. It is known that IgG antibodies are excreted into breast milk but are not found in the neonatal or infant circulation. Additionally, if any IgG antibodies were to be ingested through breastfeeding, they would probably be digested in the infant's gastrointestinal tract and not be absorbed. Breastfeeding while using this drug should be based on the mother's clinical need for treatment. No systemic side effects have been reported.

References

1. Prescribing Information. Emgality. Eli Lilly; 2021.
2. Noseda R, Bedussi F, Gobbi C, et al. Safety profile of erenumab, galcanezumab and fremanezumab in pregnancy and lactation: analysis of the WHO pharmacovigilance database. *Cephalalgia*. 2021;41:789-798.
3. Noseda R, Bedussi F, Gobbi C, et al. Safety profile of monoclonal antibodies targeting the calcitonin gene-related peptide system in pregnancy: updated analysis in VigiBase®. *Cephalalgia*. 2023;43:e1-e10.

GALLIUM GA 68 DOTATATE

Diagnostic

PREGNANCY RECOMMENDATION: No Human Data and No Relevant Animal Data/Maternal Benefit May Outweigh Embryofetal Risk

BREASTFEEDING RECOMMENDATION: Potential Toxicity (Hold Breastfeeding)

PREGNANCY SUMMARY

No reports describing the use of gallium Ga 68 dotatate in human pregnancy have been located. Based on likely limited placental transfer, fetal exposure is probably small. However, the absence of human pregnancy experience prevents a complete assessment of the embryofetal risk. Because all radiopharmaceuticals have the potential to cause fetal harm, the clinical decision to use this agent in a pregnant patient will need to be based on the stage of fetal development and expected radiation exposure.

G

BREASTFEEDING SUMMARY

No reports describing the use of gallium Ga 68 dotatate during human lactation have been located. A limited amount of the drug may appear in breast milk. If the clinical decision is to use this agent in a breastfeeding woman, the manufacturer recommends that breastfeeding be withheld and that she pump and discard breast milk for 12 hours after administration.

Reference

1. Product Information. Netspot. Advanced Accelerator Applications USA, Inc; 2021.

GALLIUM GA 68 DOTATOC

Diagnostic

PREGNANCY RECOMMENDATION: No Human Data and No Relevant Animal Data

BREASTFEEDING RECOMMENDATION: Potential Toxicity (Hold Breastfeeding)

PREGNANCY SUMMARY

No reports describing the use of gallium Ga 68 dotatoc in human pregnancy have been located. A limited amount of the drug may cross the placenta. Therefore, the absence of human pregnancy experience prevents a complete assessment of the embryofetal risk. Animal studies have not been performed. Because all radioactive agents have the potential to cause fetal harm, the clinical decision to use this agent in a pregnant patient will need to be based on the stage of fetal development and expected radiation exposure.

BREASTFEEDING SUMMARY

A limited amount of gallium Ga 68 dotatoc may be excreted into human breast milk. If the clinical decision is to use this agent in a breastfeeding woman, the manufacturer recommends that breastfeeding be withheld and that she pump and discard breast milk for 8 hours (~7 half-lives) after administration.

Reference

1. Product Information. Gallium 68 DOTATOC. UIHC—PET Imaging Center 0911Z JPP; 2019.

GALLIUM GA 68 PSMA-11

Diagnostic

PREGNANCY RECOMMENDATION: Contraindicated

BREASTFEEDING RECOMMENDATION: Contraindicated

PREGNANCY SUMMARY

No reports describing the use of gallium Ga 68 prostate-specific membrane antigen (PSMA)-11 in human pregnancy have been located. A limited amount of the drug probably crosses the placenta. Animal studies have not been performed. However, this radioactive diagnostic agent is not indicated for use in females.

BREASTFEEDING SUMMARY

Gallium Ga 68 PSMA-11 is probably excreted into human breast milk; however, this radioactive diagnostic agent is not indicated for use in females.

Reference

1. Product Information. Gallium 68 PSMA-11. UCLA Biomedical Cyclotron Facility; 2020.

G

GALSULFASE

Genetic (Enzyme)

PREGNANCY RECOMMENDATION: **No Human Data—Animal Data Suggest Low Risk**

PREGNANCY SUMMARY

No reports describing the use of galsulfase in human pregnancy have been located. Based on likely negligible placental transfer, fetal exposure is probably clinically insignificant. However, the absence of human pregnancy experience prevents a complete assessment of the embryofetal risk. Animal studies did not show any embryofetal toxicity in two species at doses of more than 10 times the RHD. Using this drug during pregnancy should be based on the pros and cons of the mother's clinical need for treatment versus any potential fetal risk that might occur from exposure.

BREASTFEEDING SUMMARY

No reports describing the use of galsulfase during human lactation have been located. The drug is unlikely to appear in breast milk. Furthermore, because it is an enzyme, if any drug were to be present in breast milk, it would most likely be digested in the infant's gastrointestinal tract and not be absorbed. Breastfeeding while using this drug should be based on the mother's clinical need for treatment. If used, the infant should be monitored for the most common reported adult side effects of headache, ear pain, and abdominal pain (all leading to irritability), rash, and shortness of breath.

Reference

1. Prescribing Information. Naglazyme. BioMarin Pharmaceutical; 2020.

GANAXOLONE

Anticonvulsant (GABA A Receptor Positive Modulator)

PREGNANCY RECOMMENDATION: **No Human Data—Animal Data Suggest Risk**

BREASTFEEDING RECOMMENDATION: **Probably Compatible**

PREGNANCY SUMMARY

No reports describing the use of ganaxolone in human pregnancy have been located. The drug is likely to cross the placenta, so fetal exposure will probably occur. Therefore, the absence of human pregnancy experience prevents a complete assessment of the embryofetal risk. Embryofetal toxicity was observed in animal studies at doses below the MRHD. Nevertheless, using this drug during pregnancy should be based on the pros and cons of the mother's clinical need for treatment versus any potential fetal risk that might occur from exposure. There is a pregnancy exposure registry that monitors pregnancy outcomes in women using antiepileptic drugs. Health care providers and women using this drug are encouraged to call the NAAED Pregnancy Registry at 1-888-233-2334.

BREASTFEEDING SUMMARY

A study in five women using ganaxolone during human lactation has been reported. Milk levels of ganaxolone were about 4 times maternal plasma levels, but the calculated maximum RID was less than 1% of the maternal daily dose. This represented 0.24% of the labeled pediatric dose of 63 mg/kg/d. However, the full effect on breast milk production and breastfed infants is unknown. Breastfeeding while using this drug should be based on the mother's clinical need for treatment. If used, the infant should be monitored for the most common reported adult side effects of somnolence, pyrexia, and salivary hypersecretion.

References

1. Product Information. Ztalmy. Marinus Pharmaceuticals, Inc; 2023.
2. National Organization for Rare Disorders. CDKL5 deficiency disorder. Accessed June 27, 2023. https://rarediseases.org/rare-diseases/cdkl5/

GANCICLOVIR

Antiviral (Anti-Cytomegalovirus)

PREGNANCY RECOMMENDATION: Limited Human Data—Animal Data Suggest Potential Risk

BREASTFEEDING RECOMMENDATION: Potential Toxicity

PREGNANCY SUMMARY

Seven case reports and a safety study describing the use of ganciclovir for maternal or fetal cytomegalovirus (CMV) infection in human pregnancy were located. These reports included one ganciclovir exposure in the first trimester and six pregnancies with ganciclovir exposure in the second and third trimesters. No congenital abnormalities were reported. In the study regarding the safety database, 34 adverse pregnancy outcomes and 4 cases of birth defects with ganciclovir or valganciclovir were identified. No increased risk of adverse pregnancy outcomes or birth defects was observed when compared to acyclovir or valacyclovir. Ganciclovir crosses the placenta, so fetal exposure will occur. However, this limited human pregnancy experience prevents a complete assessment of the embryofetal risk. Embryofetal toxicity was observed in one species without maternal toxicity at doses less than 10 times the RHD. Based on animal studies, the manufacturer recommends that women with reproductive potential use effective contraception during treatment and for 1 month after the last dose. They also recommend that males with female partners of reproductive potential use effective contraception during treatment and for 3 months after the last dose. Nevertheless, using this drug during pregnancy should be based on the pros and cons of the mother's clinical need for treatment versus any potential fetal risk that might occur from exposure. The drug carries a Boxed Warning for an increased risk of hematologic toxicity, impairment of fertility, fetal toxicity, mutagenesis, and carcinogenesis.

BREASTFEEDING SUMMARY

No reports describing the use of ganciclovir during human lactation have been located. The drug will probably be found in breast milk, so some infant exposure will likely occur. However, due to a concern for potential serious adverse effects that might be seen in a breastfed infant, the manufacturer recommends that women not breastfeed while being treated with this drug. Regardless, the drug is poorly absorbed from the gastrointestinal tract, so infant systemic exposure is likely limited. Furthermore, symptomatic infections in infants have been treated with ganciclovir. Breastfeeding while using this drug should be based on the mother's clinical need for treatment versus any potential infant risks that might occur. If used, the infant should be monitored for the most common reported adult side effects of fever, diarrhea, and various laboratory abnormalities (see PI).

References

1. Prescribing Information. Cytovene IV. Genentech; 2018.
2. Puliyanda DP, Silverman NS, Lehman D, et al. Successful use of oral ganciclovir for the treatment of intrauterine cytomegalovirus infection in a renal allograft recipient. *Transpl Infect Dis*. 2005;7:71-74.
3. Henderson GI, Hu ZQ, Yang Y, et al. Ganciclovir transfer by human placenta and its effects on rat fetal cells. *Am J Med Sci*. 1993;306:151-156.
4. Gilstrap LC, Bawdon RE, Roberts SW, et al. The transfer of the nucleoside analog ganciclovir across the perfused human placenta. *Am J Obstet Gynecol*. 1994;170:967-973.
5. Brandy RC, Schleiss MR, Witte DP, et al. Placental transfer of ganciclovir in a woman with acquired immunodeficiency syndrome and cytomegalovirus disease. *Pediatr Infect Dis J*. 2002;21:796-797.
6. DeArmond B. Safety considerations in the use of ganciclovir in immunocompromised patients. *Transplant Proc*. 1991;23(suppl 1):26-29.
7. Revello GM, Percivalle E, Baldanti F, et al. Prenatal treatment of congenital human cytomegalovirus infection by fetal intravascular administration of ganciclovir. *Clin Diagn Virol*. 1993;1:61-67.
8. Miller BW, Howard TK, Goss JA, et al. Renal transplantation one week after conception. *Transplantation*. 1995;60:1353-1354.
9. Pescovitz MD. Absence of teratogenicity of oral ganciclovir used during early pregnancy in a liver transplant recipient. *Transplantation*. 1999;67:758-759.
10. Bergin S, Ferguson W, Corcoran S, et al. Symptomatic primary cytomegalovirus infection in a HIV-positive pregnant woman. *Int J STD AIDS*. 2014;25:1041-1043.
11. Kalogeropoulos S, Zarogianni E, Adonakis G, Kaponis A. Severe CMV pneumonitis and the resulting ARDS in a 28-year-old pregnant woman: a case report. *BMC Infect Dis*. 2023;23:176.
12. Contejean A, Leruez-Ville M, Treluyer JM, et al. Assessing the risk of adverse pregnancy outcomes and birth defects reporting in women exposed to ganciclovir or valganciclovir during pregnancy: a pharmacovigilance study. *J Antimicrob Chemother*. 2023;78:1265-1269.
13. Henderson GI, Hu ZQ, Yang Y, Perez TB, Devi BG, Frosto TA, Schenker S. Ganciclovir transfer by human placenta and its effects on rat fetal cells. *Am J Med Sci*. 1993;306:151-156.
14. Nihi F, Moreira D, Santos Lourenço AC, et al. Testicular effects following in utero exposure to the antivirals acyclovir and ganciclovir in rats. *Toxicol Sci*. 2014;139:220-233.

GANCICLOVIR OPHTHALMIC

Ophthalmic/Antiviral (Topical)

PREGNANCY RECOMMENDATION: No Human Data and No Relevant Animal Data

BREASTFEEDING RECOMMENDATION: Probably Compatible

G

PREGNANCY SUMMARY

No reports describing the use of ganciclovir ophthalmic in human pregnancy have been located. The drug crosses the placenta, but the amount with topical use is likely to be clinically insignificant. However, the absence of human pregnancy experience prevents a complete assessment of the embryofetal risk. No relevant animal studies have been conducted. Using this drug during pregnancy should be based on the pros and cons of the mother's clinical need for treatment versus any potential fetal risk that might occur from exposure. If used during pregnancy, consider placing pressure over the tear duct in the corner of the eye for at least 1 minute, and then remove any excess solution with absorbent tissue to decrease the amount of drug reaching the systemic circulation even further.

BREASTFEEDING SUMMARY

No reports describing the use of ganciclovir ophthalmic during human lactation have been located. The overall amount of drug that might be found in breast milk following ophthalmic use is probably clinically insignificant. Because of the very low systemic levels likely to be found with the use of this drug, adverse reactions have not been reported. A method to decrease some systemic absorption with ophthalmic use is described above in the Pregnancy Summary.

References

1. Prescribing Information. Zirgan. Bausch & Lomb; 2020.
2. Henderson GI, Hu ZQ, Yang Y, et al. Ganciclovir transfer by human placenta and its effects on rat fetal cells. *Am J Med Sci.* 1993;306:151-156.
3. Gilstrap LC, Bawdon RE, Roberts SW, et al. The transfer of the nucleoside analog ganciclovir across the perfused human placenta. *Am J Obstet Gynecol.* 1994;170:967-973.
4. Brandy RC, Schleiss MR, Witte DP, et al. Placental transfer of ganciclovir in a woman with acquired immunodeficiency syndrome and cytomegalovirus disease. *Pediatr Infect Dis J.* 2002;21:796-797.

GATIFLOXACIN OPHTHALMIC

Ophthalmic/Antibacterial (Topical)

PREGNANCY RECOMMENDATION: No Human Data and Animal Data Suggest Low Risk

BREASTFEEDING RECOMMENDATION: Probably Compatible

PREGNANCY SUMMARY

No reports describing the use of gatifloxacin ophthalmic in human pregnancy have been located. Based on the absence of quantifiable systemic plasma concentration following ophthalmic use, fetal exposure is probably clinically insignificant. However, the absence of human pregnancy experience prevents a complete assessment of the embryofetal risk. Animal studies did not cause any embryofetal toxicity at doses higher than 10 times the RHD in two species. Using this drug during pregnancy should be based on the pros and cons of the mother's clinical need for treatment versus any potential fetal risk that might occur from exposure. If used during pregnancy, consider placing pressure over the tear duct in the corner of the eye for at least 1 minute, and then remove any excess solution with absorbent tissue to decrease the amount of drug reaching the systemic circulation even further.

BREASTFEEDING SUMMARY

No reports describing the use of gatifloxacin ophthalmic during human lactation have been located. Based on the absence of a quantifiable systemic plasma concentration following the use of gatifloxacin ophthalmic, infant exposure is likely to be clinically insignificant. Breastfeeding while using this drug should be based on the mother's clinical need for treatment. Because of the lack of measurable systemic levels, adverse reactions have not been reported. A method to decrease some systemic absorption with ophthalmic use is described above in the Pregnancy Summary.

Reference

1. Prescribing Information. Zymaxid. Allergan; 2020.

GEFITINIB

Antineoplastic (Epidermal Growth Factor Receptor [EGFR]—Tyrosine Kinase Inhibitor)

PREGNANCY RECOMMENDATION: Limited Human Data—Animal Data Suggest Potential Risk

BREASTFEEDING RECOMMENDATION: Potential Toxicity

PREGNANCY SUMMARY

Two case reports describing the use of gefitinib in the second and third trimesters of pregnancy were located. No adverse outcomes or birth anomalies were identified. The drug appears to cross the placenta, so some fetal exposure will occur. However, this limited human pregnancy experience prevents a complete assessment of the embryofetal risk. Embryofetal toxicity was observed in one animal species at doses less than 10 times the RHD. Based on animal studies and the drug's mechanism of action, the manufacturer recommends that women with reproductive potential use effective contraception during treatment and for 2 weeks after the last dose. Nevertheless, using this drug during pregnancy should be based on the pros and cons of the mother's clinical need for treatment versus any potential fetal risk that might occur from exposure. There is a registry for women who are pregnant and have cancer. For more information, women are encouraged to contact the Cancer and Pregnancy Registry at 877-635-4499.

BREASTFEEDING SUMMARY

No reports describing the use of gefitinib during human lactation have been located. The drug will probably be found in breast milk, so infant exposure will likely occur. Due to a concern for potential serious adverse effects that might be seen in a breastfed infant, the manufacturer recommends that women not breastfeed while being treated with this drug. Nevertheless, breastfeeding while using this drug should be based on the mother's clinical need for treatment versus any potential infant risks that might occur. If used, the infant should be monitored for the most common reported adult side effects of skin reactions, diarrhea, vomiting, decreased appetite (monitor infant weight), and various laboratory abnormalities (see PI).

References

1. Prescribing Information. Iressa. AstraZeneca Pharmaceuticals; 2023.
2. Lee CH, Liam CK, Pang YK, et al. Successful pregnancy with epidermal growth factor receptor tyrosine kinase inhibitor treatment of metastatic lung adenocarcinoma presenting with respiratory failure. *Lung Cancer*. 2011;74:349-351.
3. Gil S, Goetgheluck J, Paci A, et al. Efficacy and safety of gefitinib during pregnancy: case report and literature review. *Lung Cancer*. 2014;85:481-484.

GEMCITABINE

Antineoplastic (Antimetabolite)

PREGNANCY RECOMMENDATION: Limited Human Data—Animal Data Suggest Risk

BREASTFEEDING RECOMMENDATION: Potential Toxicity

PREGNANCY SUMMARY

Six case reports describing the use of gemcitabine in human pregnancy were located. These reports include one pregnancy with exposure in all trimesters and the remaining five exposures in the second and third trimesters. No congenital abnormalities were reported. The drug will probably cross the placenta, so some fetal exposure will likely occur. However, this limited human pregnancy experience prevents a complete assessment of the embryofetal risk. Embryofetal toxicity with malformations was observed in two animal species at doses less than 10 times the RHD. Based on animal studies and the drug's mechanism of action, the manufacturer recommends that women with reproductive potential use effective contraception during treatment and for 6 months after the last dose. They also recommend that males with female partners of reproductive potential use effective contraception during treatment and for 3 months after the last dose. Nevertheless, using this drug during pregnancy should be based on the pros and cons of the mother's clinical need for treatment versus any potential fetal risk that might occur from exposure. There is a registry for women who are pregnant and have cancer. For more information, women are encouraged to contact the Cancer and Pregnancy Registry at 877-635-4499.

BREASTFEEDING SUMMARY

No reports describing the use of gemcitabine during human lactation have been located. The drug will probably be found in breast milk, so some infant exposure will likely occur. Due to a concern for potential serious adverse effects that might be seen in a breastfed infant, the manufacturer recommends that women not breastfeed while being treated with this drug and for a week after the last dose. Nevertheless, breastfeeding while using this drug should be based on the mother's clinical need for treatment versus any potential infant risks that might occur. If used, the infant should be monitored for the most common reported adult side effects of nausea (leading to irritability), vomiting, fever, hematuria, rash, shortness of breath, edema, and various laboratory abnormalities (see PI).

References

1. Prescribing Information. Gemzar. Eli Lilly; 2019.
2. Eudaly JA, Tizzano JP, Higdon GL, et al. Developmental toxicity of gemcitabine, an antimetabolite oncolytic, administered during gestation to CD-1 mice. *Teratology*. 1993;48:365-381.
3. Kim JH, Kim HS, Sung CW, et al. Docetaxel, gemcitabine, and cisplatin administered for non-small cell lung cancer during the first and second trimester of an unrecognized pregnancy. *Lung Cancer*. 2008;59:270-273.
4. Gurumurthy M, Koh P, Singh R, et al. Metastatic non-small-cell lung cancer and the use of gemcitabine during pregnancy. *J Perinatol*. 2009;29:63-65.
5. Lubner S, Hall B, Gopal DV, et al. A 37 year-old pregnant woman with pancreatic adeno-carcinoma treated with surgery and adjuvant chemotherapy: a case report and literature review. *J Gastrointest Oncol*. 2011;2:258-261.
6. Wiesweg M, Aydin S, Koeninger A, et al. Administration of gemcitabine for metastatic adenocarcinoma during pregnancy: a case report and review of the literature. *AJP Rep*. 2014;4:17-22.
7. Steinberg A, Park D, Parker J, Garvey A, Scigliano E, Strong N. HL-284: first documented use of liposomal doxorubicin in a pregnant patient with Hodgkin lymphoma. *Clin Lymphoma Myeloma Leuk Leukemia*. 2020;S248.
8. Diciolla A, Gianoni M, Fleury M, et al. Gallbladder cancer during pregnancy treated with surgery and adjuvant gemcitabine: a case report and review of the literature. *Front Oncol*. 2022;12:1006387.

G

GEMFIBROZIL

Antilipemic (Fibric Acid)

PREGNANCY RECOMMENDATION: Limited Human Data—Animal Data Suggest Risk

BREASTFEEDING RECOMMENDATION: Potential Toxicity

PREGNANCY SUMMARY

Seven reports describing the use of gemfibrozil in 24 human pregnancies were located. Eleven exposures occurred in the first trimester, with one newborn diagnosed with Pierre Robin syndrome (but this finding was not related to the drug use). The remaining 13 exposures occurred in the second and third trimesters, and one defect, a structural brain anomaly, was described. Again, this anomaly was not related to drug exposure. Gemfibrozil crosses the placenta, so fetal exposure will occur. However, this limited human pregnancy experience prevents a complete assessment of the embryofetal risk. Embryofetal toxicity was observed in two animal species at doses less than 10 times the RHD. Using this drug during pregnancy should be based on the pros and cons of the mother's clinical need for treatment versus any potential fetal risk that might occur from exposure.

BREASTFEEDING SUMMARY

No reports describing the use of gemfibrozil during human lactation have been located. The drug will probably appear in breast milk, so some infant exposure will likely occur. Due to a concern for potential serious adverse effects that might be seen in a breastfed infant, the manufacturer recommends that women not breastfeed while being treated with this drug. Nevertheless, breastfeeding while using this drug should be based on the mother's clinical need for treatment versus any potential infant risks that might occur. If used, the infant should be monitored for the most common reported adult side effects of dyspepsia and abdominal pain (both leading to irritability) and diarrhea.

References

1. Prescribing Information. Gemfibrozil. Pfizer; 2023.
2. Kurtz SM, Fitzgerald JE, Fisken RA, et al. Toxicological studies on gemfibrozil. *Proc R Soc Med*. 1976;69(suppl 2):15-23. As cited in Schardein JL. *Chemically Induced Birth Defects*. 2nd ed. Marcel Dekker; 1993:81.
3. Fitzgerald JE, Petrere JA, De La Iglesia FA. Experimental studies on reproduction with the lipid-regulating agent gemfibrozil. *Fund Appl Toxicol*. 1987;8:454-464. As cited in Shepard TH. *Catalog of Teratogenic Agents*. 7th ed. The Johns Hopkins University Press; 1992:188.
4. Rosa F. Anti-cholesterol agent pregnancy exposure outcomes. Paper presented at the 7th International Organization for Teratogen Information Services; April 1994; Woods Hole, MA.
5. Jaber PW, Wilson BB, Johns DW, et al. Eruptive xanthomas during pregnancy. *J Am Acad Dermatol*. 1992;27:300-302.
6. Saadi HF, Kurlander DJ, Erkins JM, et al. Severe hypertriglyceridemia and acute pancreatitis during pregnancy: treatment with gemfibrozil. *Endocr Pract*. 1999;5:33-36.
7. Morse AN, Whitaker MD. Successful pregnancy in a woman with lipoatrophic diabetes mellitus: a case report. *J Reprod Med*. 2000;45:850-852.
8. Al-Shali K, Wang J, Fellows F, et al. Successful pregnancy outcome in a patient with severe chylomicronemia due to compound heterozygosity for mutant lipoprotein lipase. *Clin Biochem*. 2002;35:125-130.
9. Tsai E, Brown JA, Veldee MY, et al. Potential of essential fatty acid deficiency with extremely low fat diet in lipoprotein lipase deficiency during pregnancy: a case report. *BMC Pregnancy Childbirth*. 2004;4:27.
10. Cao S, Dao N, Roloff K, et al. Pregnancies complicated by familial hypertriglyceridemia: a case report. *AJP Rep*. 2018;8:e362-e364.

GENTAMICIN

Antibiotic (Aminoglycoside)

PREGNANCY RECOMMENDATION: Limited Human Data—Animal Data Suggest Low Risk (Maternal Use May Outweigh Any Fetal Risk)

BREASTFEEDING RECOMMENDATION: Probably Compatible

G

PREGNANCY SUMMARY

First-trimester reports describing the use of gentamicin are limited. In one study that evaluated a large population of infants born with birth anomalies (22,865 cases) compared with a control group of infants born without anomalies (38,151 controls), the rate of aminoglycoside use was 38 cases (0.17%) and 42 controls (0.11%). Of these, gentamicin specifically was used in 19 cases (0.08%) and in 19 controls (0.05%). These comparisons were not clinically significant. Numerous other studies have evaluated the use of gentamicin in pregnancy for treating various infections, with the majority being in the second and third trimesters, or at delivery. No pattern of adverse effects has been described. Ototoxicity, which is known to occur after gentamicin therapy, has not been reported as an effect of in utero exposure. However, eighth cranial nerve toxicity in the fetus is well known following exposure to other aminoglycosides (see Kanamycin and Streptomycin) and could potentially occur with gentamicin. Gentamicin crosses the placenta, so some fetal exposure will occur. Animal data did not show embryofetal toxicity in two species. Using this drug during pregnancy should be based on the pros and cons of the mother's clinical need for treatment versus any potential fetal risk that might occur from exposure. Despite the lack of association, gentamicin carries a Boxed Warning regarding the risk of neurotoxicity, nephrotoxicity, ototoxicity, and fetal harm when aminoglycosides are administered to a pregnant woman.

BREASTFEEDING SUMMARY

Three studies describing the use of gentamicin in more than 15 lactating women were located. Of these, gentamicin was detected in breast milk in every case, with levels ranging from a low of 3 ng/mL, 12 hours after a single maternal dose, to a high of nearly 500 ng/mL following multiple maternal doses. However, gentamicin is poorly absorbed following oral administration. Infant serum levels were not detected in cases of single-dose administration. However, the drug was detected in the blood of some infants following multiple maternal doses. Breastfeeding while using this drug should be based on the mother's clinical need for treatment versus any potential infant risks that might occur. If used, the infant should be monitored for the most common reported pediatric side effects of rash and changes in gastrointestinal flora, such as diarrhea, diaper rash, thrush, and bloody stools.

References

1. Prescribing Information. Gentamicin Sulfate. Fresenius Kabi USA, LLC; 2023.
2. Mallie JP, Coulon G, Billerey C, et al. In utero aminoglycosides-induced nephrotoxicity in rat neonates. *Kidney Int*. 1988;33:36-44.
3. Smaoui H, Mallie J-P, Schaeverbeke M, et al. Gentamicin administered during gestation alters glomerular basement membrane development. *Antimicrob Agents Chemother*. 1993;37:1510-1517.
4. Lelievre-Pegorier M, Euzet S, Merlet-Benichou C. Effect of fetal exposure to gentamicin on phosphate transport in young rat kidney. *Am J Physiol*. 1993;265:F807-F812.
5. Stahlmann R, Chahoud I, Thiel R, et al. The developmental toxicity of three antimicrobial agents observed only in nonroutine animal studies. *Reprod Toxicol*. 1997;11:1-7.
6. Percetto G, Baratta A, Menozzi M. Observations on the use of gentamicin in gynecology and obstetrics. *Minerva Ginecol*. 1969;21:1-10.
7. von Kobyletzki D. Experimental studies on the transplacental passage of gentamicin. Presented at Fifth International Congress on Chemotherapy; 1967; Vienna.
8. von Koblyetzki D, Wahlig H, Gebhardt F. Pharmacokinetics of gentamicin during delivery. In: *Antimicrobial Anticancer Chemotherapy-Proceedings of the Sixth International Congress on Chemotherapy, Tokyo*. 1969;Vol 1:650-652.
9. Yoshioka H, Monma T, Matsuda S. Placental transfer of gentamicin. *J Pediatr*. 1972;80:121-123.
10. Garcia S, Ballard C, Martin C, et al. Perinatal pharmacology of gentamicin. *Clin Res*. 1972;20:252.
11. Daubenfeld O, Modde H, Hirsch H. Transfer of gentamicin to the foetus and the amniotic fluid during a steady state in the mother. *Arch Gynecol*. 1974;217:233-240.
12. Kauffman R, Morris J, Azarnoff D. Placental transfer and fetal urinary excretion of gentamicin during constant rate maternal infusion. *Pediatr Res*. 1975;9:104-107.
13. Weinstein A, Gibbs R, Gallagher M. Placental transfer of clindamycin and gentamicin in term pregnancy. *Am J Obstet Gynecol*. 1976;124:688-691.
14. Creatsas G, Pavlatos M, Lolis D, et al. Ampicillin and gentamicin in the treatment of fetal intrauterine infections. *J Perinat Med*. 1980;8:13-18.
15. Gilstrap LC III, Bawdon RE, Burris J. Antibiotic concentration in maternal blood, cord blood, and placental membranes in chorioamnionitis. *Obstet Gynecol*. 1988;72:124-125.
16. Graham JM, Blanco JD, Oshiro BT, et al. Gentamicin levels in pregnant women with pyelonephritis. *Am J Perinatol*. 1994;11:40-41.
17. Regev RH, Litmanowitz I, Arnon S, et al. Gentamicin serum concentrations in neonates born to gentamicin-treated mothers. *Pediatr Infect Dis J*. 2000;19:890-891.
18. Barak J, Mankuta D, Pak I, et al. Transabdominal amnioinfusion of gentamicin: a pharmacokinetic study of maternal plasma and intraamniotic levels (abstract). *Am J Obstet Gynecol*. 1997;176:S59.
19. Freeman D, Matsen J, Arnold N. Amniotic fluid and maternal and cord serum levels of gentamicin after intra-amniotic instillation in patients with premature rupture of the membranes. *Am J Obstet Gynecol*. 1972;113:1138-1141.
20. Hulton SA, Kaplan BS. Renal dysplasia associated with in utero exposure to gentamicin and corticosteroids. *Am J Med Genet*. 1995;58:91-93.
21. Wing DA, Hendershott CM, Debuque L, et al. A randomized trial of three antibiotic regimens for the treatment of pyelonephritis in pregnancy. *Obstet Gynecol*. 1998;92:249-253.
22. Czeizel AE, Rockenbauer M, Olsen J, et al. A teratological study of aminoglycoside antibiotic treatment during pregnancy. *Scand J Infect Dis*. 2000;32:309-313.
23. L'Hommedieu CS, Nicholas D, Armes DA, et al. Potentiation of magnesium sulfate-induced neuromuscular weakness by gentamicin, tobramycin, and amikacin. *J Pediatr*. 1983;102:629-631.
24. Celiloglu M, Celiker S, Guven H, et al. Gentamicin excretion and uptake from breast milk by nursing infants. *Obstet Gynecol*. 1994;84:263-265.
25. Mann CF. Clindamycin and breast-feeding. *Pediatrics*. 1980;66:1030-1031.

G

GENTAMICIN CREAM

Antibacterial (Aminoglycoside—Topical)

PREGNANCY RECOMMENDATION: No Human Data and No Relevant Animal Data

BREASTFEEDING RECOMMENDATION: Probably Compatible

PREGNANCY SUMMARY

No reports describing the use of gentamicin cream in human pregnancy have been located. The drug can cross the placenta, but the amount that might occur with topical use is likely to be clinically insignificant. However, the absence of human pregnancy experience prevents a complete assessment of the embryofetal risk. No relevant animal studies have been conducted. Using this drug during pregnancy should be based on the pros and cons of the mother's clinical need for treatment versus any potential fetal risk that might occur from exposure.

BREASTFEEDING SUMMARY

No reports describing the use of gentamicin cream during human lactation have been located. If found in the systemic circulation, gentamicin will probably be found in breast milk. However, the poor systemic absorption following topical skin use suggests that the amount is likely to be negligible. Breastfeeding while using this drug should be based on the mother's clinical need for treatment. Because of the topical administration, systemic adverse reactions are unlikely.

Reference

1. Prescribing Information. Gentamicin Cream. AdvaCare Pharma; 2020.

GENTAMICIN OPHTHALMIC

Ophthalmic/Antibacterial (Topical Aminoglycoside)

PREGNANCY RECOMMENDATION: No Human Data and No Relevant Animal Data

BREASTFEEDING RECOMMENDATION: Probably Compatible

PREGNANCY SUMMARY

No reports describing the use of gentamicin ophthalmic in human pregnancy have been located. The drug can cross the placenta, but the amount that might occur with ophthalmic use is likely to be clinically insignificant. However, the absence of human pregnancy experience prevents a complete assessment of the embryofetal risk. No relevant animal studies have been conducted. Using this drug during pregnancy should be based on the pros and cons of the mother's clinical need for treatment versus any potential fetal risk that might occur from exposure. If used during pregnancy, consider placing pressure over the tear duct in the corner of the eye for at least 1 minute, and then remove any excess solution with absorbent tissue to decrease the amount of drug reaching the systemic circulation even further.

BREASTFEEDING SUMMARY

No reports describing the use of gentamicin ophthalmic during human lactation have been located. The drug can probably be excreted into breast milk. However, the absence of quantifiable urine concentrations, following extended ophthalmic use, suggests that the amount is likely to be clinically insignificant. Breastfeeding while using this drug should be based on the mother's clinical need for treatment. Because of the topical administration, systemic adverse reactions are unlikely. A method to decrease some systemic absorption with ophthalmic use is described above in the Pregnancy Summary.

References

1. Prescribing Information. Gentamicin Sulfate. Alcon Laboratories, Inc; 2021.
2. Trope GE, Lawrence JR, Hind VM, Everden A. Systemic absorption of topical and subconjunctival gentamicin. *Br J Ophthalmol*. 1979;63:692-693.

GENTIAN VIOLET

Anti-Infective (Topical—Antifungal/Antibacterial)

PREGNANCY RECOMMENDATION: Limited Human Data—No Relevant Animal Data

BREASTFEEDING RECOMMENDATION: Potential Toxicity

PREGNANCY SUMMARY

One report describing the use of gentian violet in 40 human pregnancies identified 4 (10%) fetal anomalies, but no pattern to the defects was seen. If gentian violet is in the systemic circulation, it will probably cross the placenta, so some fetal exposure might occur. However, the amount of systemic absorption is not known. It is felt that minimal systemic absorption occurs following topical administration on mucocutaneous areas. Regardless, this limited human pregnancy experience prevents a complete assessment of the embryofetal risk. No animal reproduction studies have been conducted. Using this drug during pregnancy should be based on the pros and cons of the mother's clinical need for treatment versus any potential fetal risk that might occur from exposure.

BREASTFEEDING SUMMARY

While the amount of systemic absorption is not known, gentian violet is likely minimally absorbed systemically following topical administration, which should limit excretion into breast milk. However, four reports were located that described the use of gentian violet to treat infants with oral thrush that led to various adverse reactions (oral ulcerations, feeding difficulties, cough, and difficulty breathing). The Academy of Breastfeeding Medicine states that gentian violet (≤0.5%) can be used in the treatment of *Candida* infection for no more than 7 days on the nipple. Because of the topical administration, systemic adverse reactions are rare.

References

1. Prescribing Information. Gentian Violet. Laboratorios Jaloma, S.A. de C.V; 2013.
2. Heinonen OP, Slone D, Shapiro S. *Birth Defects and Drugs in Pregnancy*. Publishing Sciences Group; 1977:302.
3. Björnberg A, Mobacken H. Necrotic skin reactions caused by 1 per cent gentian violet and brilliant green. *Acta Derm Venereol*. 1972;52:55-60.
4. Utter AR. Gentian violet and thrush. *J Hum Lact*. 1992;8:6.
5. Utter AR. Gentian violet treatment for thrush: can its use cause breastfeeding problems. *J Hum Lact*. 1990;6:178-180.
6. Baca D, Drexler C, Cullen E. Obstructive laryngotracheitis secondary to gentian violet exposure. *Clin Pediatr (Phila)*. 2001;40:233-235.
7. Berens P, Eglash A, Malloy M, et al. ABM Clinical Protocol #26: persistent pain with breastfeeding. *Breastfeed Med*. 2016;11:46-53.

GEPIRONE

Mental Health (Antidepressant)

PREGNANCY RECOMMENDATION: No Human Data—Animal Data Suggest Potential Risk

BREASTFEEDING RECOMMENDATION: Probably Compatible

PREGNANCY SUMMARY

No reports describing the use of gepirone in human pregnancy have been located. The drug will probably cross the placenta, so some fetal exposure will likely occur. Therefore, the absence of human pregnancy experience prevents a complete assessment of the embryofetal risk. Animal studies did show some embryofetal toxicity in one species at doses of less than 10 times the RHD. Using this drug during pregnancy should be based on the pros and cons of the mother's clinical need for treatment versus any potential fetal risk that might occur from exposure. The drug is associated with prolonging the QT interval. There is also a pregnancy exposure registry that monitors pregnancy outcomes in women using this drug. Health care providers are encouraged to call the National Pregnancy Registry for Antidepressants at 1-844-405-6185.

BREASTFEEDING SUMMARY

No reports describing the use of gepirone during human lactation have been located. The drug will probably be excreted into breast milk. However, it has poor oral bioavailability (only 15%), which should limit the amount of infant exposure. Breastfeeding while using this drug should be based on the mother's clinical need for treatment. If used, the infant should be monitored for the most common reported adult side effects of nausea, dizziness, and abdominal pain (all leading to irritability), somnolence, sedation, and decreased feeding (monitor infant weight).

Reference

1. Prescribing Information. Exxua. Fabre-Kremer; 2023.

GILTERITINIB

Antineoplastic (Tyrosine Kinase Inhibitor)

PREGNANCY RECOMMENDATION: No Human Data—Animal Data Suggest Potential Risk

BREASTFEEDING RECOMMENDATION: Potential Toxicity

PREGNANCY SUMMARY

No reports describing the use of gilteritinib in human pregnancy have been located. Based on likely limited placental transfer, fetal exposure is probably small. However, the absence of human pregnancy experience prevents a complete assessment of the embryofetal risk. Embryofetal toxicity with malformations was observed in one animal species at doses less than 10 times the RHD. However, this dose also caused maternal toxicity. Based on animal studies and the drug's mechanism of action, the manufacturer recommends that women with reproductive potential use effective contraception during treatment and for 6 months after the last dose. They also recommend that males with female partners of reproductive potential use effective contraception during treatment and for 4 months after the last dose. Nevertheless, using this drug during pregnancy should be based on the pros and cons of the mother's clinical need for treatment versus any potential fetal risk that might occur from exposure. There is a registry for women who are pregnant and have cancer. For more information, women and health care providers are encouraged to contact the Cancer and Pregnancy Registry at 1-877-635-4499.

G

BREASTFEEDING SUMMARY

No reports describing the use of gilteritinib during human lactation have been located. A limited amount of the drug may be found in breast milk, so some infant exposure will likely occur. However, due to the concern for potential serious adverse effects that might be seen in a breastfed infant, the manufacturer recommends that women not breastfeed while being treated with gilteritinib and for at least 2 months after the last dose. Nevertheless, breastfeeding while using this drug should be based on the mother's clinical need for treatment. If used, the infant should be monitored for the most common reported adult side effects of nausea, arthralgia, dizziness, and headache (all leading to irritability), fever, peripheral edema, rash, diarrhea, shortness of breath, cough, constipation, and various laboratory abnormalities (see PI).

Reference

1. Prescribing Information. Xospata. Astellas Pharma US; 2022.

GIVINOSTAT

Genetic (Histone Deacetylase Inhibitor—Duchenne Muscular Dystrophy)

PREGNANCY RECOMMENDATION: No Human Data—Animal Data Suggest Potential Risk (Maternal Benefit May Outweigh Any Embryofetal Risk)

BREASTFEEDING RECOMMENDATION: Potential Toxicity

PREGNANCY SUMMARY

No reports describing the use of givinostat in human pregnancy have been located. The drug will probably cross the placenta, so some fetal exposure will likely occur. Therefore, the absence of human pregnancy experience prevents a complete assessment of the embryofetal risk. Animal reproduction studies did show some embryofetal toxicity in one species at doses of less than 10 times the RHD. Duchenne muscular dystrophy (DMD) is primarily seen in males (X-linked recessive genetic disorder). Females with severe DMD who are of reproductive age potential are exceedingly rare. Using this drug during pregnancy should be based on the pros and cons of the mother's clinical need for treatment versus any potential fetal risk that might occur from exposure. Givinostat is also associated with prolongation of the QT interval.

BREASTFEEDING SUMMARY

No reports describing the use of givinostat during human lactation have been located. The drug will likely be found in human breast milk, so some infant exposure will probably occur. Breastfeeding while using this drug should be based on the mother's clinical need for treatment versus any potential infant risks that might occur. If used, the infant should be monitored for the most common reported adult side effects of nausea and abdominal pain (both leading to irritability), vomiting, diarrhea, fever, elevated triglycerides, and thrombocytopenia.

Reference

1. Prescribing Information. Duvyzat. ITF Therapeutics, LLC; 2024.

GIVOSIRAN

Miscellaneous (Aminolevulinic Acid Synthase 1-Directed Small Interfering RNA)

PREGNANCY RECOMMENDATION: No Human Data and No Relevant Animal Data

BREASTFEEDING RECOMMENDATION: Probably Compatible

PREGNANCY SUMMARY

No reports describing the use of givosiran in human pregnancy have been located. Based on no placental transfer or very negligible transfer, fetal exposure is likely to be clinically insignificant. However, the absence of human pregnancy experience prevents a complete assessment of the embryofetal risk. Animal studies in two species produced maternal toxicity. Using this drug during pregnancy should be based on the pros and cons of the mother's clinical need for treatment versus any potential fetal risk that might occur from exposure.

BREASTFEEDING SUMMARY

No reports describing the use of givosiran during human lactation have been located. The drug will not likely be found in breast milk. However, if some excretion were to occur, it would most likely be digested in the infant's gastrointestinal tract and not be absorbed. If the clinical decision is to use this drug while breastfeeding, the infant should be monitored for the most common reported adult systemic side effects of nausea (leading to irritability).

Reference

1. Prescribing Information. Givlaari. Alnylam Pharmaceuticals; 2023.

G

GLASDEGIB

Antineoplastic (Hedgehog Pathway Inhibitor)

PREGNANCY RECOMMENDATION: No Human Data—Animal Data Suggest Risk

BREASTFEEDING RECOMMENDATION: Potential Toxicity

PREGNANCY SUMMARY

No reports describing the use of glasdegib in human pregnancy have been located. Based on likely placental transfer, some fetal exposure will probably occur. Therefore, the absence of human pregnancy experience prevents a complete assessment of the embryofetal risk. Embryofetal toxicity with malformations was observed in two animal species at doses less than 10 times the RHD. Based on these animal studies and the drug's mechanism of action, the manufacturer recommends that women with reproductive potential use effective contraception during treatment and for 30 days after the last dose. They also recommend that males with female partners of reproductive potential use effective contraception during treatment and for 30 days after the last dose. Nevertheless, using this drug during pregnancy should be based on the pros and cons of the mother's clinical need for treatment versus any potential fetal risk that might occur from exposure. Pregnancy exposures should be reported to Pfizer at 1-800-438-1985. Glasdegib is associated with QT prolongation. It is recommended that the QTc interval be monitored prior to and during treatment. Glasdegib also carries a Boxed Warning regarding the increased risk for embryofetal toxicity.

BREASTFEEDING SUMMARY

No reports describing the use of glasdegib during human lactation have been located. The drug will probably appear in breast milk, so some infant exposure will likely occur. Because of a concern for potential serious adverse effects that might be seen in a breastfed infant, the manufacturer recommends that women not breastfeed while being treated with glasdegib and for at least 30 days after the last dose. Nevertheless, breastfeeding while using this drug should be based on the mother's clinical need for treatment. If used, the infant should be monitored for the most common reported adult side effects of nausea, musculoskeletal pain, and abdominal pain (all leading to irritability), fatigue (lethargy), fever, peripheral edema, shortness of breath, decreased appetite, constipation, rash, and various laboratory abnormalities (see PI).

Reference

1. Prescribing Information. Daurismo. Pfizer Laboratories Div Pfizer; 2023.

GLATIRAMER

Immunologic (Biologic)

PREGNANCY RECOMMENDATION: Limited Human Data—Animal Data Suggest Low Risk

BREASTFEEDING RECOMMENDATION: Probably Compatible

PREGNANCY SUMMARY

Several reports describing the use of glatiramer in all trimesters of human pregnancy were located. From four studies, there were 4 (4.5%) major anomalies in 89 pregnancies with first-trimester exposure, and all four defects were different. In two large reviews evaluating the treatment of multiple sclerosis in pregnancy, no major concerns for embryofetal harm were identified with the use of glatiramer. Placental transfer in the first trimester is unlikely to be clinically significant. However, this limited human pregnancy experience prevents a complete assessment of the embryofetal risk. Animal data did not show any embryofetal toxicity in two species at doses greater than 10 times the RHD. Using this drug during pregnancy should be based on the pros and cons of the mother's clinical need for treatment versus any potential fetal risk that might occur from exposure.

BREASTFEEDING SUMMARY

Limited reports describing the use of glatiramer during human lactation have been located. In 17 healthy lactation volunteers, breast milk levels were not detected in 8 volunteers (lower limit of quantification 50 ng/mL). Low levels were detected in the remaining nine volunteers. If the detected levels are considered to be peak milk levels, then the maximum maternal weight-adjusted dose would be 9%. However, due to poor oral bioavailability, the systemic exposure would be well below 1%. A few studies describing effects on breastfed infants have not reported any adverse effects in the infant. Additionally, because it consists of polypeptides of varying sizes, if the drug were to be ingested through breastfeeding, it would likely be digested in the infant's gastrointestinal tract and not be absorbed. Breastfeeding while using this drug should be based on the mother's clinical need for treatment versus any potential infant risks that might occur. If used, the infant should be monitored for the most common reported adult side effects of chest pain (leading to irritability), rash, and shortness of breath.

References

1. Prescribing Information. Glatiramer Acetate. Mylan Pharmaceuticals Inc; 2024.
2. Weber-Schoendorfer C, Schaefer C. Multiple sclerosis, immunomodulators, and pregnancy outcome: a prospective observational study. *Mult Scler*. 2009;15:1037-1042.
3. Salminen HJ, Leggett H, Boggild M. Glatiramer acetate exposure in pregnancy: preliminary safety and birth outcomes. *J Neurol*. 2010;257:2020-2023.
4. Hellwig K, Gold R. Glatiramer acetate and interferon-beta throughout gestation and postpartum in women with multiple sclerosis. *J Neurol*. 2011;258:502-503.
5. Hellwig K, Haghikia A, Gold R. Multiple sclerosis and pregnancy: experience from a nationwide database in Germany. *Ther Adv Neurol Disord*. 2012;5:247-253.
6. Giannini M, Portaccio E, Ghezzi A, et al. Pregnancy and fetal outcomes after glatiramer acetate exposure in patients with multiple sclerosis: a prospective observational multicentric study. *BMC Neurol*. 2012;12:124.
7. Fragoso YD, Adoni T, Alves-Leon SV, et al. Long-term effects of exposure to disease-modifying drugs in the offspring of mothers with multiple sclerosis: a retrospective chart review. *CNS Drugs*. 2013;27:955-961.
8. Ruuskanen J, Malm H, Airas L. Multiple sclerosis and pregnancy. *Duodecim*. 2013;129:1457-1464.
9. Ghezzi A, Annovazzi P, Portaccio E, et al. Current recommendations for multiple sclerosis treatment in pregnancy and puerperium. *Expert Rev Clin Immunol*. 2013;9:683-691.
10. Lu E, Wang BW, Guimond C, et al. Safety of disease-modifying drugs for multiple sclerosis in pregnancy: current challenges and future considerations for effective pharmacovigilance. *Expert Rev Neurother*. 2013;13:251-261.
11. Herbstritt S, Langer-Gould A, Rockhof M, et al. Glatiramer acetate during early pregnancy: a prospective cohort study. *Mult Scler*. 2016;22:810-816.
12. MacDonald SC, McElrath TF, Hernández-Díaz S. Use and safety of disease-modifying therapy in pregnant women with multiple sclerosis. *Pharmacoepidemiol Drug Saf*. 2019;28:556-560.
13. Nguyen AL, Havrdova EK, Horakova D, et al. Incidence of pregnancy and disease-modifying therapy exposure trends in women with multiple sclerosis: a contemporary cohort study. *Mult Scler Relat Disord*. 2019;28:235-243.
14. Sandberg-Wollheim M, Neudorfer O, Grinspan A, et al. Pregnancy outcomes from the Branded Glatiramer Acetate Pregnancy Database. *Int J MS Care*. 2018;20:9-14.
15. Ciplea AI, Langer-Gould A, Stahl A, et al. Safety of potential breast milk exposure to IFN-β or glatiramer acetate: one-year infant outcomes. *Neurol Neuroimmunol Neuroinfamm*. 2020.
16. Kaplan S, Zeygarnik M, Stern T. Pregnancy, Fetal, and Infant Outcomes Following Maternal Exposure to Glatiramer Acetate During Pregnancy and Breastfeeding. *Drug Saf*. 2022;45:345-357.
17. Ciplea AI, Kurzeja A, Thiel S, et al. Eighteen-month safety analysis of offspring breastfed by mothers receiving glatiramer acetate therapy for relapsing multiple sclerosis—COBRA study. *Mult Scler*. 2022;28:1641-1650.
18. Ciplea AI, Kurzeja A, Thiel S, et al. Safety evaluations of offspring breastfed by mothers receiving glatiramer acetate for relapsing multiple sclerosis. *Mult Scler Relat Disord*. 2023;75:104771.

GLECAPREVIR/PIBRENTASVIR

Antiviral (Hepatitis C)

PREGNANCY RECOMMENDATION: No Human Data—Animal Data Suggest Low Risk

BREASTFEEDING RECOMMENDATION: Probably Compatible

PREGNANCY SUMMARY

No reports describing the use of glecaprevir/pibrentasvir in human pregnancy have been located. Because both drugs probably cross the placenta in limited amounts, a minimal amount of fetal exposure will probably occur. However, the absence of human pregnancy experience prevents a complete assessment of the embryofetal risk. Animal studies did not show any embryofetal toxicity. A risk of developing a reactivation of hepatitis B that can lead to fulminant hepatitis, hepatic failure, and even death can occur with the use of this drug.

BREASTFEEDING SUMMARY

No reports describing the use of glecaprevir/pibrentasvir in human lactation have been located. Minimal amounts of both drugs are probably found in breast milk. Breastfeeding while using this drug should be based on the mother's clinical need for treatment. If used, the infant should be monitored for the most common reported adult side effects of headache and nausea (both leading to irritability), diarrhea, and lethargy.

Reference

1. Product Information. Mavyret. AbbVie, Inc; 2021.

GLIMEPIRIDE

Antidiabetic (Sulfonylurea)

PREGNANCY RECOMMENDATION: Limited Human Data—Animal Data Suggest Low Risk (In the Absence of Hypoglycemia)

BREASTFEEDING RECOMMENDATION: Probably Compatible

G

PREGNANCY SUMMARY

One case report describing the first-trimester use of glimepiride in human pregnancy did not result in any minor or major malformations. In this case, the mother was exposed to seven other drugs in the first trimester (orlistat, simvastatin, ramipril, metformin, aspirin, ciprofloxacin, and thiocolchicoside). The drug will probably cross the placenta, so some fetal exposure will probably occur. However, this limited human pregnancy experience prevents a complete assessment of the embryofetal risk. In animal studies, no embryofetal toxicity was seen in two species at doses of more than 10 times the RHD, in the presence of normal glucose status. Embryofetal toxicity was seen in the presence of maternal hypoglycemia. ACOG and the American Diabetes Association (ADA) recommend that insulin be used for types 1 and 2 diabetes occurring during pregnancy and, if diet therapy alone is not successful, for gestational diabetes. Oral agents such as metformin and glyburide should not be used as first-line agents, as both will likely cross the placenta. Other oral medications and injectable glucose-lowering medications lack safety data. Additionally, due to concerns for adverse neonatal reactions, such as hypoglycemia, the manufacturer recommends that glimepiride be discontinued at least 2 weeks prior to the expected date of delivery.

BREASTFEEDING SUMMARY

No reports describing the use of glimepiride during human lactation have been located. The drug will probably be found in breast milk, so some infant exposure will likely occur. Breastfeeding while using this drug should be based on the mother's clinical need for treatment versus any potential infant risks that might occur. If used, the infant should be monitored for the most common reported adult side effects of headache, nausea, and dizziness (all leading to irritability) and signs of hypoglycemia such as sweating, poor feeding, tremors, lethargy, low tone, seizures, paleness, shortness of breath, and hypothermia.

References

1. Prescribing Information. Glimepiride. Carlsbad Technology, Inc; 2019.
2. Kalyoncu NI, Yaris F, Kadioglu M, et al. Pregnancy outcome following exposure to orlistat, ramipril, glimepiride in a woman with metabolic syndrome. *Saudi Med J*. 2005;26:497-499.
3. ACOG Practice Bulletin No. 190: Gestational Diabetes Mellitus. *Obstet Gynecol*. 2018;131:e49-e64.
4. American Diabetes Association Professional Practice Committee; 15. Management of diabetes in pregnancy: standards of medical care in diabetes—2022. *Diabetes Care*. 2022;45(suppl_1): S232-S243.

GLIPIZIDE

Antidiabetic (Sulfonylurea)

PREGNANCY RECOMMENDATION: Limited Human Data—Animal Data Suggest Low Risk

BREASTFEEDING RECOMMENDATION: Probably Compatible

PREGNANCY SUMMARY

One case report was located of a pregnant patient who took glipizide throughout a pregnancy, delivering a newborn with no identified anomalies. In a second study, four women using hypoglycemic agents, including glipizide (number not specified), did not identify any adverse effects or anomalies in the delivered neonates. Other studies evaluating oral hypoglycemic drugs

(continued)

have not found an association between their use during organogenesis and congenital malformations. Instead, the observed anomalies appear to be related to poor maternal glycemic control. Glipizide likely crosses the placenta, so some fetal exposure will probably occur. However, this limited human pregnancy experience prevents a complete assessment of the embryofetal risk. Animal studies did not find any embryofetal toxicity in two species at doses of less than 10 times the RHD (in one species) and at doses of more than 10 times the RHD (in the second species). ACOG and the ADA recommend that insulin be used for types 1 and 2 diabetes occurring during pregnancy and, if diet therapy alone is not successful, for gestational diabetes. Oral agents such as metformin and glyburide should not be used as first-line agents, as both cross the placenta. Other oral medications and injectable glucose-lowering medications lack safety data. Additionally, due to concerns for adverse neonatal reactions, such as hypoglycemia, the manufacturer recommends that glipizide be discontinued at least 1 month prior to the expected date of delivery.

BREASTFEEDING SUMMARY

G

One report of two women who were taking glipizide postdelivery had undetectable milk trough levels (lower limit of detection of 80 ng/mL). One woman had a peak milk concentration of 200 ng/mL (3 hours after dose). The authors estimated that the maximum theoretical infant dose as a percentage of the weight-adjusted maternal dose was less than 27% for glipizide. Blood glucose levels were normal in both of the exclusively breastfed infants. Breastfeeding while using this drug should be based on the mother's clinical need for treatment versus any potential infant risks that might occur. If used, the infant should be monitored for the most common reported adult side effects of nausea (leading to irritability) and diarrhea and signs of hypoglycemia such as sweating, poor feeding, tremors, lethargy, low tone, seizures, paleness, shortness of breath, and hypothermia.

References

1. Prescribing Information. Glucotrol. Pfizer; 2023.
2. Elliott BD, Schenker S, Langer O, et al. Comparative placental transport of oral hypoglycemic agents in humans: a model of human placental drug transfer. *Am J Obstet Gynecol*. 1994;171:653-660.
3. Onnis A, Grella P. *The Biochemical Effects of Drugs in Pregnancy*. Vol 2. Ellis Horwood Limited; 1984:174-175.
4. Klupa T, Kozek E, Nowak N, et al. The first case report of sulfonylurea use in a woman with permanent neonatal diabetes mellitus due to KCNJ11 mutation during a high-risk pregnancy. *J Clin Endocrinol Metab*. 2010;95:3599-3604.
5. Towner D, Kjos SL, Leung B, et al. Congenital malformations in pregnancies complicated by NIDDM. *Diabetes Care*. 1995;18:1446–1451.
6. ACOG Practice Bulletin No. 190: Gestational Diabetes Mellitus. *Obstet Gynecol*. 2018;131:e49-e64.
7. American Diabetes Association Professional Practice Committee; 15. Management of diabetes in pregnancy: standards of medical care in diabetes—2022. *Diabetes Care*. 2022;45(suppl_1): S232-S243.
8. Feig DS, Briggs GG, Kraemer JM, et al. Transfer of glyburide and glipizide into breast milk. *Diabetes Care*. 2005;28:1851-1855.

GLOFITAMAB

Antineoplastic (Monoclonal Antibody)

PREGNANCY RECOMMENDATION: No Human Data—Animal Data Suggest Potential Risk

BREASTFEEDING RECOMMENDATION: Probably Compatible

PREGNANCY SUMMARY

No reports describing the use of glofitamab in human pregnancy have been located. As an IgG antibody, the drug will likely cross the placenta, so some fetal exposure will probably occur. However, the absence of human pregnancy experience prevents a complete assessment of the embryofetal risk. Animal reproduction studies have not been conducted. However, embryofetal toxicity might occur based on the drug's mechanism of action. Because the drug activates T cells, this could theoretically compromise pregnancy maintenance (especially in the first trimester). In addition, because the drug can deplete B cells, newborns could have a low B cell count postdelivery. Because of this, the manufacturer recommends that women with reproductive potential who are taking glofitamab use effective contraception during treatment and for at least 1 month after the last dose. Nevertheless, using this drug during pregnancy should be based on the pros and cons of the mother's clinical need for treatment versus any potential fetal risk that might occur from exposure. If used, the newborn should have B cell levels evaluated postdelivery.

BREASTFEEDING SUMMARY

No reports describing the use of glofitamab during human lactation have been located. It is known that IgG antibodies can be found in human breast milk, but are not found in the neonatal or infant circulation. Additionally, if any IgG antibodies were to be ingested through breastfeeding, they would probably be digested in the infant's gastrointestinal tract and not be absorbed. However, due to the potential for adverse effects that might be seen in a breastfed infant, the manufacturer recommends that women should not breastfeed while being treated with glofitamab and for at least 1 month after the last dose. Nevertheless, breastfeeding while using this drug should be based on the mother's clinical need for treatment. If used, the infant should be monitored for the most common reported adult side effects of musculoskeletal pain (leading to irritability), lethargy, rash, cytokine release syndrome, and various laboratory abnormalities (see PI).

Reference

1. Product Information. Columvi. Genentech, Inc; 2023.

GLUCAGON

Antidote/Diagnostic

PREGNANCY RECOMMENDATION: Limited Human Data—Animal Data Suggest Low Risk (Maternal Benefit May Outweigh Embryofetal Risk)

BREASTFEEDING RECOMMENDATION: Compatible

PREGNANCY SUMMARY

One report describing the use of glucagon in human pregnancy was located, which described the use of glucagon for severe hypoglycemia. Seven pregnant women received glucagon for severe hypoglycemia on 12 occasions during pregnancy, and no adverse effects were reported in the newborns at delivery. The gestational ages at which the drug was used were not provided. A second case report described the use of glucagon in treating a severe β-blocker overdose. A fetal demise occurred, but the drug was successful in reversing the severe β-blocker effects. Glucagon does not appear to cross the human placenta, so fetal exposure is not likely to occur. Animal data did not show any embryofetal toxicity in two species at doses greater than 10 times the RHD. Due to the indication for use of this drug, the mother's clinical need for treatment should outweigh any potential fetal risk that might occur from exposure, especially when intravenous (IV) glucose cannot be administered in a timely manner.

BREASTFEEDING SUMMARY

No reports describing the use of glucagon during human lactation have been located. The drug will not likely be found in breast milk, so infant exposure will probably not occur. Additionally, if any of the polypeptide were to be ingested through breastfeeding, it would probably be digested in the infant's gastrointestinal tract and not absorbed. Breastfeeding while using this drug should be based on the mother's clinical need for treatment versus any potential infant risks that might occur. If used, the infant should be monitored for the most common reported adult side effects of nausea, headache, and dizziness (all leading to irritability), vomiting, decreased blood pressure, paleness, diarrhea, and lethargy.

References

1. Prescribing Information. Glucagon. Fresenius Kabi USA, LLC; 2019.
2. Moore RS, Lumbers ER. Renal and metabolic effects of glucagon in the fetus. *J Dev Physiol*. 1992;17:47-49.
3. Johnston DI, Bloom SR, Greene KR, et al. Failure of the human placenta to transfer pancreatic glucagon. *Biol Neonate*. 1972;21:375-380.
4. Moore WMO, Ward BS, Gordon C. Human placental transfer of glucagon. *Clin Sci Mol Med*. 1974;46:125-129.
5. Spellacy WN, Buhi WC. Glucagon, insulin and glucose levels in maternal and umbilical cord plasma with studies of placental transfer. *Obstet Gynecol*. 1976;47:291-294.
6. Rayburn W, Piehl E, Sanfield J, et al. Reversing severe hypoglycemia during pregnancy with glucagon therapy. *Am J Perinatol*. 1987;4:259-261.
7. Tai YT, Lo CW, Chow WH, et al. Successful resuscitation and survival following massive overdose of metoprolol. *Br J Clin Pract*. 1990;44:746-747.
8. Bailey B. Are there teratogenic risks associated with antidotes used in the acute management of poisoned pregnant women? *Birth Defects Res A Clin Mol Teratol*. 2003;67:133-140.

GLUCARPIDASE

Antidote (Enzyme-Methotrexate Toxicity)

PREGNANCY RECOMMENDATION: No Human Data and No Relevant Animal Data (Maternal Benefit May Outweigh Embryofetal Risk)

BREASTFEEDING RECOMMENDATION: Probably Compatible

PREGNANCY SUMMARY

No reports describing the use of glucarpidase in human pregnancy have been located. Based on likely negligible placental transfer, fetal exposure would probably be clinically insignificant. However, the absence of human pregnancy experience prevents a complete assessment of the embryofetal risk. No animal reproduction studies have been conducted. The use of methotrexate in pregnancy is contraindicated (see Methotrexate). However, if the drug was used because a pregnant woman inadvertently received methotrexate, the risk-benefit ratio would favor glucarpidase.

BREASTFEEDING SUMMARY

No reports describing the use of glucarpidase during human lactation have been located. However, reports of its use during breastfeeding are unlikely because of its indication. The drug will likely not be found in breast milk. Additionally, if any enzyme were to be ingested through breastfeeding, it would probably be digested in the infant's gastrointestinal tract and not absorbed. If the clinical decision is to use this drug while breastfeeding, the infant should be monitored for the most common reported adult side effects of paresthesia, nausea, headache (all leading to irritability), flushing, vomiting, and hypotension.

Reference

1. Prescribing Information. Voraxaze. BTG International; 2020.

GLUCOSAMINE

Nutritional Supplement

PREGNANCY RECOMMENDATION: Limited Human Data—Animal Data Suggest Low Risk

BREASTFEEDING RECOMMENDATION: Probably Compatible

PREGNANCY SUMMARY

One report describing the use of glucosamine in 54 human pregnancies found no increased risk for major malformations or other adverse fetal effects. First-trimester exposure occurred in 34 cases. Some glucosamine will probably cross the placenta, so fetal exposure might occur. However, unbound glucosamine is concentrated in articular cartilage but is undetectable in plasma. Therefore, it appears that the amount of free drug at the maternal-fetal interface is likely limited. Nevertheless, this limited human pregnancy experience prevents a complete assessment of the embryofetal risk. Animal data did not show teratogenicity in two species. Using this supplement during pregnancy should be based on the pros and cons of the mother's clinical need for treatment versus any potential fetal risk that might occur from exposure.

BREASTFEEDING SUMMARY

No reports describing the use of glucosamine during human lactation have been located. This supplement may be found in breast milk, so infant exposure might occur. However, unbound glucosamine is undetectable in the plasma. Therefore, it appears that little, if any, of this supplement will be excreted into breast milk. *N*-acetylglucosamine is a derivative of glucosamine and is a normal component of human breast milk with levels that vary from about 600 mcg/mL to 1.5 mg/mL. In addition, levels of this normal compound appear to be higher in smokers when compared to nonsmokers.

References

1. Glucosamine. *The Review of Natural Products*. Wolters Kluwer Health; 2004.
2. Glucosamine hydrochloride. *Natural Medicines Comprehensive Database*. Therapeutic Research Faculty; 2003:626-628.
3. Glucosamine sulfate. *Natural Medicines Comprehensive Database*. Therapeutic Research Faculty; 2003:628-631.
4. Glucosamine. *PDR Health*. Accessed March 20, 2006. http://www.pdrhealth.com/drug_info/nmdrugprofiles/nutsupdrugs/glu_0122.shtml
5. Glucosamine. *Micromedex® Healthcare Series*. Accessed March 24, 2006. http://126.0.10.223/mdxcgi/display.exe?CTL=D:\Root\MMDX\MDX\MDXCGI\MEGAT
6. Didock KA, Jackson D, Robson JM. The action of some nucleotoxic substances in pregnancy. *Br J Pharmacol*. 1956;11:437-441. As cited in Schardein JL. *Chemically Induced Birth Defects*. 3rd ed. Marcel Dekker; 2000:699.
7. Sivojelezova A, Koren G, Einarson A. Glucosamine use in pregnancy: an evaluation of pregnancy outcome. *J Womens Health (Larchmt)*. 2007;16:345-348.
8. Stumpf JL, Lin SW. Effect of glucosamine on glucose control. *Ann Pharmacother*. 2006;40:694-698.

GLYBURIDE

Antidiabetic (Sulfonylurea)

PREGNANCY RECOMMENDATION: Limited Human Data—Animal Data Suggest Low Risk

BREASTFEEDING RECOMMENDATION: Probably Compatible

PREGNANCY SUMMARY

Numerous studies were located that describe the use of glyburide during human pregnancy. The rates of congenital anomalies with first-trimester exposure are higher than the expected rates for anomalies in the United States, but are usually lower than the rates when compared with no treatment or insulin therapy in diabetics. Therefore, the anomalies are likely related to glucose control in the first trimester. However, a recent meta-analysis found that glyburide was associated with higher rates of neonatal hypoglycemia and NICU admission duration when compared with insulin. Despite these findings, no difference has been shown in glycemic control when comparing glyburide and insulin. The drug crosses the placenta, so some fetal exposure will occur. Animal studies did not show any embryofetal toxicity in two species at doses greater than 10 times the RHD. ACOG and the ADA recommend that insulin be used for types 1 and 2 diabetes occurring during pregnancy and, if diet therapy alone is not successful, for gestational diabetes. Oral agents such as metformin and glyburide should not be used as first-line agents, as both cross the placenta. Other oral medications and injectable glucose-lowering medications lack safety data.

BREASTFEEDING SUMMARY

Three studies were located that have evaluated the use of glyburide during human lactation. In 11 patients, glyburide was not detected in breast milk in all cases (lower limit of detection was 5 ng/mL in 8 cases and 80 ng/mL in 3 cases). In one other case, the drug was detected in breast milk, but the patient had a genetic mutation that required high daily doses of glyburide. In this case, drug levels were also detected in the infant's blood. Breastfeeding while using this drug should be based on the mother's clinical need for treatment versus any potential infant risks that might occur. If used, the infant should be monitored for the most common reported adult side effects of nausea (leading to irritability), diarrhea, and signs of hypoglycemia such as sweating, poor feeding, tremors, lethargy, low tone, seizures, paleness, shortness of breath, and hypothermia.

References

1. ACOG Practice Bulletin No. 190: gestational diabetes mellitus. *Obstet Gynecol*. 2018;131:e49-e64.
2. American Diabetes Association Professional Practice Committee; 15. Management of diabetes in pregnancy: standards of care in diabetes—2024. *Diabetes Care*. 2024;47(suppl 1):S282-S294.
3. Prescribing Information. Glyburide. Cadila Pharmaceuticals Limited; 2022.
4. Shepard TH. *Catalog of Teratogenic Agents*. 8th ed. The Johns Hopkins University Press; 1995:202.
5. Sivan E, Feldman B, Dolitzki M, et al. Glyburide crosses the placenta in vivo in pregnant rats. *Diabetologia*. 1995;38:753-756.
6. Elliott BD, Langer O, Schenker S, et al. Insignificant transfer of glyburide occurs across the human placenta. *Am J Obstet Gynecol*. 1991;165:807-812.
7. Elliott BD, Bynum D, Langer O. Glyburide does not cross the diabetic placenta in significant amounts. Society of Perinatal Obstetricians Abstracts. *Am J Obstet Gynecol*. 1993;168:360.
8. Elliott BD, Bynum D, Langer O. Maternal hyperglycemia does not alter in-vitro placental transfer of the oral hypoglycemic agent glyburide. Society of Perinatal Obstetricians Abstracts. *Am J Obstet Gynecol*. 1993;168:360.
9. Elliott B, Langer O, Schenker S, et al. Glyburide is insignificantly transported to the fetal circulation by the human placenta in vitro (abstract). *Am J Obstet Gynecol*. 1991;164:247.
10. Elliott BD, Schenker S, Langer O, et al. Comparative placental transport of oral hypoglycemic agents in humans: a model of human placental drug transfer. *Am J Obstet Gynecol*. 1994;171:653-660.
11. Elliott BD, Crosby-Schmidt C, Langer O. Human placental glucose uptake and transport are not altered by pharmacologic levels of the oral hypoglycemic agent, glyburide. Society of Perinatal Obstetricians Abstracts. *Am J Obstet Gynecol*. 1994;170:321.
12. Koren G. Glyburide and fetal safety; transplacental pharmacokinetic considerations. *Reprod Toxicol*. 2001;15:227-229.
13. Kraemer J, Klein J, Lubetsky A, et al. Perfusion studies of glyburide transfer across the human placenta: implications for fetal safety. *Am J Obstet Gynecol*. 2006;195:270-274.
14. Piacquadio K, Hollingsworth DR, Murphy H. Effects of in-utero exposure to oral hypoglycaemic drugs. *Lancet*. 1991;338:866-869.
15. Coetzee EJ, Jackson WPU. Diabetes newly diagnosed during pregnancy. A 4-year study at Groote Schuur Hospital. *S Afr Med J*. 1979;56:467-475.
16. Coetzee EJ, Jackson WPU. Pregnancy in established non-insulin-dependent diabetics; a five-and-a-half year study at Groote Schuur Hospital. *S Afr Med J*. 1980;58:795-802.
17. Coetzee EJ, Jackson WPU. Oral hypoglycaemics in the first trimester and fetal outcome. *S Afr Med J*. 1984;65:635-637.
18. Coetzee EJ, Jackson WPU. The management of non-insulin-dependent diabetes during pregnancy. *Diabetes Res Clin Pract*. 1986;5:281-287.
19. Ravina A. Insulin-dependent diabetes of pregnancy treated with the combination of sulfonylurea and insulin. *Isr J Med Sci*. 1995;31:623-625.
20. Towner D, Kjos SL, Leung B, et al. Congenital malformations in pregnancies complicated by NIDDM. *Diabetes Care*. 1995;18:1446-1451.
21. Langer O, Conway DL, Berkus MD, et al. A comparison of glyburide and insulin in women with gestational diabetes mellitus. *N Engl J Med*. 2000;343:1134-1138.
22. Greene MF. Oral hypoglycemic drugs for gestational diabetes. *N Engl J Med*. 2000;343:1178-1179.
23. Velazquez MD, Bolnick J, Cloakey D, et al. The use of glyburide in the management of gestational diabetes. *Obstet Gynecol*. 2003;101(suppl):88S.
24. Kremer CJ, Duff P. Glyburide for the treatment of gestational diabetes. *Am J Obstet Gynecol*. 2004;190:1438-1439.
25. Jacobson GF, Ramos GA, Ching JV, et al. Comparison of glyburide and insulin for the management of gestational diabetes in a large managed care organization. *Am J Obstet Gynecol*. 2005;193:118-124.
26. Rochon M, Rand L, Roth L, et al. Glyburide for the management of gestational diabetes: risk factors predictive of failure and associated pregnancy outcomes. *Am J Obstet Gynecol*. 2006;195:1090-1094.
27. Kahn BF, Davies JK, Lynch AM, et al. Predictors of glyburide failure in the treatment of gestational diabetes. *Obstet Gynecol*. 2006;107:1303-1309.
28. Durnwald C, Landon MB. Glyburide: the new alternative for treating gestational diabetes? *Am J Obstet Gynecol*. 2005;193:1-2.
29. Feig DS, Briggs GG, Kraemer JM, et al. Transfer of glyburide and glipizide into breast milk. *Diabetes Care*. 2005;28:1851-1855.
30. Feig DS, Kraemer JM, Moskovitz DN, et al. The transfer of glyburide into breast milk. *Clin Pharmacol Ther*. 2004;75:P24.
31. Myngheer N, Allegaert K, Hattersley A, et al. Fetal macrosomia and neonatal hyperinsulinemic hypoglycemia associated with transplacental transfer of sulfonylurea in a mother with KCNJ11-related neonatal diabetes. *Diabetes Care*. 2014;37:3333-3335.
32. Wang X, Liu W, Chen H, Chen Q. Comparison of insulin, metformin, and glyburide on perinatal complications of gestational diabetes mellitus: a systematic review and meta-analysis. *Gynecol Obstet Invest*. 2021;86:218-220.
33. Bidhendi Yarandi R, Amiri M, Ramezani Tehrani F, Behboudi-Gandevani S. Effectiveness of antidiabetic agents for treatment of gestational diabetes: a methodological quality assessment of meta-analyses and network meta-analysis. *J Diabetes Investig*. 2021;12:2247-2258.
34. Yu DQ, Xu GX, Teng XY, et al. Glycemic control and neonatal outcomes in women with gestational diabetes mellitus treated using glyburide, metformin, or insulin: a pairwise and network meta-analysis. *BMC Endocr Disord*. 2021;21:199.
35. Li C, Gao C, Zhang X, et al. Comparison of the effectiveness and safety of insulin and oral hypoglycemic drugs in the treatment of gestational diabetes mellitus: a meta-analysis of 26 randomized controlled trials. *Gynecol Endocrinol*. 2022;38:303-309.

GLYCERIN

Gastrointestinal (Osmotic Laxative)

PREGNANCY RECOMMENDATION: Limited Human Data—No Relevant Animal Data

BREASTFEEDING RECOMMENDATION: Probably Compatible

PREGNANCY SUMMARY

One case report was located that described the oral use of glycerin in a pregnant patient at 22 weeks of gestation to treat elevated intracranial pressure. No adverse newborn effects were reported. Glycerin may cross the placenta, so some fetal exposure might occur. However, systemic absorption is thought to be negligible with rectal use. However, this limited human pregnancy experience prevents a complete assessment of the embryofetal risk. No animal reproduction studies have been conducted. Glycerin suppositories are generally considered acceptable for use during pregnancy.

BREASTFEEDING SUMMARY

No reports describing the use of glycerin during human lactation have been located. Glycerin with rectal use is likely minimally absorbed systemically, which should limit excretion into breast milk. Because of this, glycerin suppositories are generally considered acceptable for use during breastfeeding. If used while breastfeeding, the infant should be monitored for the most common reported side effects of gas and stomach cramps (leading to irritability) and diarrhea.

References

1. Prescribing Information. Glycerin. Rite Aid; 2023.
2. Yoshida M, Matsuda H, Furuya K. Successful prognosis of brain abscess during pregnancy. *J Reprod Infertil*. 2013;14:152-155.

GLYCOPYRROLATE

Autonomic (Anticholinergic)

PREGNANCY RECOMMENDATION: Limited Human Data—Animal Data Suggest Low Risk

BREASTFEEDING RECOMMENDATION: Probably Compatible

PREGNANCY SUMMARY

At least nine reports describing the use of glycopyrrolate in human pregnancy were located. The majority involved the use of the drug with cesarean section at delivery. The drug use in these cases did not appear to cause any adverse neonatal effects. A few first-trimester exposures have been described, but specific information on the presence of birth anomalies specific to glycopyrrolate was not provided. Because this drug is a quaternary ammonium compound that is fully ionized, transplacental passage should be limited. Low concentrations of glycopyrrolate have been found in umbilical cord blood and amniotic fluid after intramuscular (IM) administration. However, this limited human pregnancy experience prevents a complete assessment of the embryofetal risk. Animal data did not show embryofetal toxicity in two species at doses of 10 times or more than the MRHD. Using this drug during pregnancy should be based on the pros and cons of the mother's clinical need for treatment versus any potential fetal risk that might occur from exposure.

BREASTFEEDING SUMMARY

No reports describing the use of glycopyrrolate during human lactation have been located. The drug will probably be found in breast milk, so some infant exposure may occur. However, the poor oral bioavailability (only 3%) should greatly limit any infant systemic exposure. Breastfeeding while using this drug should be based on the mother's clinical need for treatment versus any potential infant risks that might occur. If used, the infant should be monitored for the most common reported adult side effects of drowsiness, flushing, vomiting, constipation, tachycardia, and urinary retention.

References

1. Prescribing Information. Glycopyrrolate. Fresenius Kabi USA, LLC; 2024.
2. Prescribing Information. Glycopyrrolate. Leading Pharma, LLC; 2022.
3. Heinonen OP, Slone D, Shapiro S. *Birth Defects and Drugs in Pregnancy*. Publishing Sciences Group; 1977:346-353.
4. Diaz DM, Diaz SF, Marx GF. Cardiovascular effects of glycopyrrolate and belladonna derivatives in obstetric patients. *Bull NY Acad Med*. 1980;56:245-248.
5. Abboud TK, Read J, Miller F, et al. Use of glycopyrrolate in the parturient: effect on the maternal and fetal heart and uterine activity. *Obstet Gynecol*. 1981;57:224-227.
6. Roper RE, Salem MG. Effects of glycopyrrolate and atropine combined with antacid on gastric acidity. *Br J Anaesth*. 1981;53:1277-1280.
7. Abboud T, Raya J, Sadri S, et al. Fetal and maternal cardiovascular effects of atropine and glycopyrrolate. *Anesth Analg*. 1983;62:426-430.
8. Ure D, James KS, McNeill M, et al. Glycopyrrolate reduces nausea during spinal anaesthesia for Caesarean section without affecting neonatal outcome. *Br J Anaesth*. 1999;82:277-279.
9. Chamchad D, Horrow JC, Nakhamchik L, et al. Prophylactic glycopyrrolate prevents bradycardia after spinal anesthesia for Cesarean section: a randomized, double-blind, placebo-controlled prospective trial with heart rate variability correlation. *J Clin Anesth*. 2011;23:361-366.
10. Wise MG, Ward SC, Townsend-Parchman W, et al. Case report of ECT during high-risk pregnancy. *Am J Psychiatry*. 1984;141:99-101.
11. Ngan Kee WD, See SW, Khaw KS, et al. Haemodynamic effects of glycopyrrolate pre-treatment before phenylephrine infusion during spinal anaesthesia for caesarean delivery. *Int J Obstet Anesth*. 2013;22:179-187.
12. Patel SD, Habib AS, Phillips S, et al. The effect of glycopyrrolate on the incidence of hypotension and vasopressor requirement during spinal anesthesia for cesarean delivery: a meta-analysis. *Anesth Analg*. 2018;126:552-558.
13. Grover S, Sikka P, Saini SS, et al. Use of modified bilateral electroconvulsive therapy during pregnancy: a case series. *Indian J Psychiatry*. 2017;59:487-492.

GOLIMUMAB

Immunologic (Monoclonal Antibody—Tumor Necrosis Factor-α Inhibitor)

PREGNANCY RECOMMENDATION: Limited Human Data—Animal Data Suggest Low Risk

BREASTFEEDING RECOMMENDATION: Probably Compatible

PREGNANCY SUMMARY

Three reports describing the use of golimumab with first-trimester exposure in about 151 human pregnancies found 32 (21%) spontaneous abortions, but many of these were also exposed to methotrexate. There were 3 (2.5%) major anomalies in 119 live births, with no pattern seen in the defects. Other retrospective analyses have described higher anomaly rates, but these were biased toward the reporting of poor outcomes. As an IgG antibody, it likely crosses the placenta (as shown in one case), especially during the second half of gestation, so some fetal exposure will occur. However, this limited human pregnancy experience prevents a complete assessment of the embryofetal risk. Animal data did not show any embryofetal toxicity in one species at doses of much greater than 10 times the RHD. The American College of Rheumatology guidelines conditionally recommend continuing tumor necrosis factor inhibitor therapy with golimumab prior to and during pregnancy. However, due to increased placental transfer in the third trimester, if the patient's disease is under good control, the medication may be discontinued in the third trimester.

BREASTFEEDING SUMMARY

Two reports describing the use of golimumab during human lactation found that the drug was not detected in one report and was almost undetectable in a second report. These levels are consistent with the knowledge that IgG antibodies can be found in human breast milk. However, they are not found in the neonatal circulation because IgG antibodies are likely to be digested in the infant's gastrointestinal tract and not be absorbed. The American College of Rheumatology guidelines and recommendations consider golimumab to be compatible with breastfeeding. If the clinical decision is to use this drug while breastfeeding, the infant should be monitored for the most common reported adult side effects of upper respiratory infection, viral infection, bronchitis, hypertension, rash, and various laboratory abnormalities (see PI).

References

1. Prescribing Information. Simponi Aria. Janssen Biotech; 2021.
2. Khanna D, McMahon M, Furst DE. Safety of tumor necrosis factor-α antagonists. *Drug Saf.* 2004;27:307-324.
3. Martin PL, Oneda S, Treacy G. Effects of an anti-TNF-α monoclonal antibody, administered throughout pregnancy and lactation, on the development of the macaque immune system. *Am J Reprod Immunol.* 2007;58:138-149.
4. Benoit L, Mir O, Berveiller P. Treating ulcerative colitis during pregnancy: evidence of materno-fetal transfer of golimumab. *J Crohns Colitis.* 2019;13:669-670.
5. Lau A, Clark M, Harrison DD, et al. THU0153 pregnancy outcomes in women exposed to the tumor necrosis factor inhibitor, golimumab. *Ann Rheum Dis.* 2014;73:232-233.
6. Weber-Schoendorfer C, Oppermann M, Wacker E, et al. Pregnancy outcome after TNF-α inhibitor therapy during the first trimester: a prospective multicenter cohort study. *Br J Clin Pharmacol.* 2015;80:727-729.
7. Esslinger S, Otero-Lobato M, Gabriel S, Clark M, Sheridan P, Geldhof A. P599 trimester exposure and pregnancy outcomes in women exposed to golimumab: results from the company pharmacovigilance database. *J Crohn's Colitis.* 2020;14:S500-S501.
8. Sammaritano LR, Bermas BL, Chakravarty EE, et al. 2020 American College of Rheumatology Guideline for the Management of Reproductive Health in Rheumatic and Musculoskeletal Diseases. *Arthritis Rheumatol.* 2020;72:529-556.
9. Matro R, Martin CF, Wolf D, et al. Exposure concentrations of infants breastfed by women receiving biologic therapies for inflammatory bowel diseases and effects of breastfeeding on infections and development. *Gastroenterology.* 2018;155:696-704.
10. Saito J, Yakuwa N, Hosokawa Y, et al. Establishment of a measurement system to evaluate breast milk transfer of biological agents using dry filter paper: a multi-institutional study. *Br J Clin Pharmacol.* 2004;90:146-157.

GOLODIRSEN

Genetic (Antisense Oligonucleotide—Duchenne Muscular Dystrophy)

PREGNANCY RECOMMENDATION: No Human Data and No Relevant Animal Data (Maternal Benefit May Outweigh Any Embryofetal Risk)

BREASTFEEDING RECOMMENDATION: Probably Compatible

PREGNANCY SUMMARY

No reports describing the use of golodirsen in human pregnancy have been located. Based on likely negligible placental transfer, fetal exposure would probably be clinically insignificant. However, the absence of human pregnancy experience prevents a complete assessment of the embryofetal risk. No animal studies have been conducted. DMD is primarily seen in males (X-linked recessive genetic disorder). Females with severe DMD who are of reproductive age are exceedingly rare.

(continued)

Using this drug during pregnancy should be based on the pros and cons of the mother's clinical need for treatment versus any potential fetal risk that might occur from exposure.

BREASTFEEDING SUMMARY

No reports describing the use of golodirsen during human lactation have been located. The drug will likely not be found in breast milk. Additionally, if any amount of the drug were to be ingested through breastfeeding, it would probably be digested in the infant's gastrointestinal tract and not absorbed. Breastfeeding while using this drug should be based on the mother's clinical need for treatment. If used, the infant should be monitored for the most common reported adult side effects of nausea, headache, and abdominal pain (all leading to irritability), fever, cough, and vomiting.

Reference

1. Prescribing Information. Vyondys 53. Sarepta Therapeutics; 2021.

G

GRANISETRON

Gastrointestinal (Antiemetic)

PREGNANCY RECOMMENDATION: Limited Human Data—Animal Data Suggest Low Risk

BREASTFEEDING RECOMMENDATION: Probably Compatible

PREGNANCY SUMMARY

In one study, 94 pregnancies were exposed to granisetron in the first trimester for treating nausea and vomiting of pregnancy, and 3 (3.2%) major anomalies were identified at delivery. No pattern to the anomalies was seen. Limited other reports were found describing the use of granisetron in nausea and vomiting of pregnancy, but newborn outcomes were not provided. The drug has also been used for prevention of nausea and vomiting during cesarean section. The drug will probably cross the placenta, so some fetal exposure will likely occur. However, this limited human pregnancy experience prevents a complete assessment of the embryofetal risk. Animal data did not show any embryofetal toxicity in two species at doses of more than 10 times the RHD. Using this drug during pregnancy should be based on the pros and cons of the mother's clinical need for treatment versus any potential fetal risk that might occur from exposure. Granisetron is associated with QT prolongation.

BREASTFEEDING SUMMARY

No reports describing the use of granisetron during human lactation have been located. The drug will probably be excreted into breast milk, so some infant exposure will likely occur. Breastfeeding while using this drug should be based on the mother's clinical need for treatment versus any potential infant risks that might occur. If used, the infant should be monitored for the most common reported adult side effects of headache and abdominal pain (both leading to irritability), weakness, diarrhea, and reflux. The IV product contains the preservative benzyl alcohol, which has been associated with serious and possibly fatal reactions in neonates, including "gasping syndrome" when consumed orally. However, benzyl alcohol is rapidly metabolized to benzoic acid in the maternal liver, which then binds to glycine and is excreted as hippuric acid. Therefore, exposure to a breastfeeding newborn is not likely to occur.

References

1. Prescribing Information. Granisetron. Breckenridge Pharmaceutical; 2019.
2. Nair B. Final report on the safety assessment of benzyl alcohol, benzoic acid, and sodium benzoate. *Int J Toxicol*. 2001;20(suppl 3):23-50.
3. Julius JM, Tindall A, Moise KJ, et al. Evaluation of the maternal-fetal transfer of granisetron in an ex vivo placenta perfusion model. *Reprod Toxicol*. 2014;49:43-47.
4. Fujii Y. Prevention of emetic episodes during cesarean delivery performed under regional anesthesia in parturients. *Curr Drug Saf*. 2007;2:25-32.
5. Merimsky O, Le Cesne A. Soft tissue and bone sarcomas in association with pregnancy. *Acta Oncol*. 1998;37:721-727.
6. Merimsky O, Le Chevalier T, Missenard G, et al. Management of cancer in pregnancy: a case of Ewing's sarcoma of the pelvis in the third trimester. *Ann Oncol*. 1999;10:345-350.
7. Aleyasin A, Saffarich E, Torkamandi H, et al. Comparison of efficacy of granisetron and promethazine in control of hyperemesis gravidarum. *J Obstet Gynaecol India*. 2016;66:409-414.
8. Caritis S, Zhao Y, Chen HJ, Venkataramanan R. Pharmacodynamics of transdermal granisetron in women with nausea and vomiting of pregnancy. *Am J Obstet Gynecol*. 2016;215:93.e1-e4.
9. Le TN, Adler MT, Ouillette H, et al. Observational case series evaluation of the granisetron transdermal patch system (Sancuso) for the management of nausea/vomiting of pregnancy. *Am J Perinatol*. 2017;34:851-855.
10. Shapira M, Avrahami I, Mazaki-Tovi S, Shai D, Zemet R, Barzilay E. The safety of early pregnancy exposure to granisetron. *Eur J Obstet Gynecol Reprod Biol*. 2020;245:35-38.

GRISEOFULVIN

Anti-Infective (Antifungal)

PREGNANCY RECOMMENDATION: Limited Human Data—Animal Data Suggest Risk

BREASTFEEDING RECOMMENDATION: Potential Toxicity

PREGNANCY SUMMARY

From two studies, griseofulvin was used in the first trimester of 71 pregnancies, and 3 (4.2%) major anomalies were found. No pattern to the anomalies was identified. In an earlier evaluation, there was a question of whether or not the drug could cause conjoined twins. However, several later reports involving several million deliveries have not confirmed this finding. Griseofulvin crosses the placenta, so fetal exposure will occur. However, this limited human pregnancy experience prevents a complete assessment of the embryofetal risk. Embryofetal toxicity with malformations was observed in two animal species at doses less than 10 times the MRHD. According to the manufacturer, griseofulvin is contraindicated in women who are or may become pregnant during treatment. It was previously considered pregnancy category X. The manufacturer also recommends that males should wait at least 6 months from the last dose before fathering a child. Nevertheless, using this drug during pregnancy should be based on the pros and cons of the mother's clinical need for treatment versus any potential fetal risk that might occur from exposure.

BREASTFEEDING SUMMARY

No reports describing the use of griseofulvin during human lactation have been located. The drug will probably be found in breastmilk, so some infant exposure will likely occur. However, due to the concern for tumorigenicity in animal studies, the manufacturer recommends that a decision be made whether to discontinue nursing or to discontinue the drug, considering the importance of the drug to the mother. Nevertheless, breastfeeding while using this drug should be based on the mother's clinical need for treatment versus any potential infant risks that might occur. If used, the infant should be monitored for the most common reported adult side effects of rash and itching.

References

1. Prescribing Information. Griseofulvin. Sigmapharm Laboratories; 2022.
2. Rubin A, Dvornik D. Placental transfer of griseofulvin. *Am J Obstet Gynecol*. 1965;92:882-883.
3. Pacifici GM. Placental transfer of antibiotics administered to the mother: a review. *Int J Clin Pharmacol Ther*. 2006;44:57-63.
4. Rosa FW, Hernandez C, Carlo WA. Griseofulvin teratology, including two thoracopagus conjoined twins. *Lancet*. 1987;1:171.
5. Metneki J, Czeizel A. Griseofulvin teratology. *Lancet*. 1987;1:1042.
6. Knudsen LB. No association between griseofulvin and conjoined twinning. *Lancet*. 1987;2:1097.
7. Moudgal VV, Sobel JD. Antifungal drugs in pregnancy: a review. *Expert Opin Drug Saf*. 2003;2:475-483.
8. Czeizel AE, Metneki J, Kazy Z, et al. A population-based case-control study of oral griseofulvin treatment during pregnancy. *Acta Obstet Gynecol*. 2004;83:827-831.

GUAIFENESIN

Respiratory (Mucolytic/Expectorant)

PREGNANCY RECOMMENDATION: Human Data Suggest Low Risk—No Relevant Animal Data

BREASTFEEDING RECOMMENDATION: Probably Compatible

PREGNANCY SUMMARY

Four reports describing the use of guaifenesin in the first trimester of human pregnancy were located. From 893 exposed pregnancies, there were 21 (2.5%) major birth anomalies identified. No pattern to the anomalies was seen. The drug will probably cross the placenta, so some fetal exposure will likely occur. However, this human pregnancy experience suggests that the drug is low risk. No animal reproduction studies have been located. Using this drug during pregnancy should be based on the pros and cons of the mother's clinical need for treatment versus any potential fetal risk that might occur from exposure.

BREASTFEEDING SUMMARY

No reports describing the use of guaifenesin during human lactation have been located. The drug will probably be found in breast milk, so some infant exposure will likely occur. Breastfeeding while using this drug should be based on the mother's clinical need for treatment versus any potential infant risks that might occur. If used, the infant should be monitored for the most common reported adult side effects of nausea (leading to irritability), vomiting, diarrhea, and constipation.

References

1. Prescribing Information. Guaifenesin. Major Pharmaceuticals; 2019.
2. Ward KE. Can Robitussin DM be used to treat cough during pregnancy? *Med Health R I*. 2005;88:99-100.
3. Werler MM, Mitchell AA, Hernandez-Diaz S, et al; National Birth Defects Prevention Study. Use of over-the-counter medications during pregnancy. *Am J Obstet Gynecol*. 2005;193:771-777.
4. Silva R, Lee JH, Tweed E. Is guaifenesin safe during pregnancy? *J Fam Pract*. 2007;56:669-670.
5. Heinonen OP, Slone D, Shapiro S. *Birth Defects and Drugs in Pregnancy*. Publishing Sciences Group; 1977.
6. Aselton P, Jick H, Milunsky A, et al. First-trimester drug use and congenital disorders. *Obstet Gynecol*. 1985;65:451-455.
7. Chasnoff IJ, Diggs G, Schnoll SH. Fetal alcohol effects and maternal cough syrup abuse. *Am J Dis Child*. 1981;135:968.

GUANFACINE

Antihypertensive/Mental Health

PRENANCY RECOMMENDATION: Limited Human Data—Animal Data Suggest Low Risk

BREASTFEEDING RECOMMENDATION: Probably Compatible

G

PREGNANCY SUMMARY

A case report of a patient who was participating in a clinical trial for the drug in treating hypertension, became pregnant during treatment. The drug was discontinued at approximately 8 weeks' gestation, and she later delivered a healthy newborn.

A second study reported the use of guanfacine for the treatment of hypertension secondary to preeclampsia in 30 women. The gestational ages of the women at the time of treatment were not specified, but they were beyond the first trimester. No drug-induced adverse effects were observed in any of the infants postdelivery, and all were developing normally on follow-up. The drug will likely cross the placenta, so fetal exposure will probably occur. However, the absence of human pregnancy experience prevents a complete assessment of the embryofetal risk. Animal data did not show embryofetal toxicity in two animal species at doses of less than 10 times the MRHD. Using this drug during pregnancy should be based on the pros and cons of the mother's clinical need for treatment versus any potential fetal risk that might occur from exposure.

BREASTFEEDING SUMMARY

No reports describing the use of guanfacine during human lactation have been located. The drug will probably be found in breast milk, so infant exposure will likely occur. Guanfacine reduces serum prolactin concentrations in some patients and, theoretically, could inhibit milk secretion. Breastfeeding while using this drug should be based on the mother's clinical need for treatment. If used, the infant should be monitored for the most common reported pediatric side effects of nausea (leading to irritability), hypotension, sleepiness, and fatigue (lethargy).

References

1. Prescribing Information. Guanfacine Hydrochloride. Amneal Pharmaceuticals; 2018.
2. Prescribing Information. Intuniv. Shire US Inc; 2019.
3. Karesoja M, Takkunen H. Guanfacine, a new centrally acting antihypertensive agent in long-term therapy. *Curr Ther Res*. 1981;29:60-65.
4. Philipp E. Guanfacine in the treatment of hypertension due to pre-eclamptic toxaemia in thirty women. *Br J Clin Pharmacol*. 1980;10(suppl 1):137S-140S.
5. Hauger-Klevene JH, Balossi EC, Scornavacchi JC. Effects of guanfacine on growth hormone, prolactin, renin, lipoproteins and glucose in essential hypertension. *Am J Cardiol*. 1986;57:27E-31E.

GUSELKUMAB

Immunologic (Monoclonal Antibody—Antipsoriatic)

PREGNANCY RECOMMENDATION: Limited Human Data—Animal Data Suggest Potential Risk

BREASTFEEDING RECOMMENDATION: Probably Compatible

PREGNANCY SUMMARY

There is a case report of a woman who conceived while on guselkumab, but the drug was discontinued at 4 weeks of gestation (2 weeks postconception). Her therapy changed to certolizumab, and this was continued up to delivery. The newborn was delivered at term and was healthy with no abnormalities reported. The VigiBase pharmacovigilance database reported 19 cases of pregnancy exposure to guselkumab, and no newborn abnormalities were reported. However, the gestational ages of exposure and duration of use were not supplied. As an IgG antibody, the drug likely crosses the placenta, so some fetal exposure will probably occur. Animal data did not show any embryofetal toxicity, but there was an increase in newborn deaths postdelivery (the significance of which was uncertain). Using this drug during pregnancy should be based on the pros and cons of the mother's clinical need for treatment versus any potential fetal risk that might occur from exposure. There is a pregnancy exposure registry that monitors pregnancy outcomes in women using this drug. Health care providers are encouraged to call the Tremfya Pregnancy Exposure Registry at 1-877-311-8972.

BREASTFEEDING SUMMARY

No reports describing the use of guselkumab during human lactation have been located. The drug is likely present in breast milk. However, it is known that IgG antibodies can be found in human breast milk, but are not found in the neonatal or infant circulation. Additionally, if any IgG antibodies were to be ingested through breastfeeding, they would probably be digested in the infant's gastrointestinal tract and not be absorbed. However, breastfeeding while using this drug should be based on the mother's clinical need for treatment. If used, the infant should be monitored for the most common reported adult side effects of headache and arthralgias (both leading to irritability), diarrhea, and various infections.

References

1. Product Information. Tremfya. Janssen Biotech, Inc; 2020.
2. AL-Khawaga S, Krishnankutty R, Sher G, et al. Treatment and molecular profiling of acrodermatitis continua of Hallopeau during pregnancy using targeted therapy. *JAAD Case Rep*. 2021;16:164-167.
3. Dernoncourt A, Liabeuf S, Bennis Y, et al. Fetal and neonatal adverse drug reactions associated with biologics taken during pregnancy by women with autoimmune diseases: insights from an analysis of the World Health Organization Pharmacovigilance database (VigiBase). *BioDrugs*. 2022;37:73-87.

G

H

HALCINONIDE

Corticosteroid (Topical)

PREGNANCY RECOMMENDATION: No Human Data and No Relevant Animal Data

BREASTFEEDING RECOMMENDATION: Probably Compatible

PREGNANCY SUMMARY

No reports describing the use of halcinonide in human pregnancy have been located. Some amount of the drug will probably cross the placenta, but fetal exposure is likely limited. However, the absence of human pregnancy experience prevents a complete assessment of the embryofetal risk. Animal reproduction studies have not been conducted. Using this drug during pregnancy should be based on the pros and cons of the mother's clinical need for treatment versus any potential fetal risk that might occur from exposure. Regarding topical steroids in general, the amount that is systemically absorbed depends on many factors, including the vehicle, occlusion, and skin integrity. Given the absence of human and animal data, an alternative agent might be considered during pregnancy (see Hydrocortisone).

BREASTFEEDING SUMMARY

No reports describing the use of halcinonide during human lactation have been located. The drug will probably be excreted into breast milk, but infant exposure is probably limited. As seen with other corticosteroids (see Hydrocortisone), trace amounts are excreted into breast milk. Breastfeeding while using this drug should be based on the mother's clinical need for treatment. Because of the topical use and lack of studies on absorption, adult systemic side effects were not reported. Regarding topical steroids in general, the amount that is systemically absorbed depends on many factors, including the vehicle, occlusion, and skin integrity. Halcinonide should not be applied to the breast or nipple, if possible, but if used in this area, it should be thoroughly wiped off prior to breastfeeding. Given the absence of human and animal data, an alternative agent might be considered during breastfeeding (see Hydrocortisone).

Reference

1. Prescribing Information. Halog. Mylan Pharmaceuticals; 2019.

HALOBETASOL

Corticosteroid (Topical)

PREGNANCY RECOMMENDATION: No Human Data—Animal Data Suggest Potential Risk

BREASTFEEDING RECOMMENDATION: Probably Compatible

PREGNANCY SUMMARY

No reports describing the use of halobetasol in human pregnancy have been located. Some amount of the drug will probably cross the placenta, but fetal exposure should be limited. However, the absence of human pregnancy experience prevents a complete assessment of the embryofetal risk. The drug was found to be teratogenic in one animal species at levels 3 times those seen with the human topical dose. Using this drug during pregnancy should be based on the pros and cons of the mother's clinical need for treatment versus any potential fetal risk that might occur from exposure. Regarding topical steroids in general, the amount that is systemically absorbed depends on many factors, including the vehicle, occlusion, and skin integrity.

BREASTFEEDING SUMMARY

No reports describing the use of halobetasol during human lactation have been located. The drug will probably be found in breast milk, but infant exposure should be limited. As seen with other corticosteroids (see Hydrocortisone), trace amounts are excreted into breast milk, but the amount that is absorbed depends on many factors, including the vehicle, occlusion, and skin integrity. Breastfeeding while using this drug should be based on the mother's clinical need for treatment. Because of the topical use and low plasma absorption, adult systemic side effects were not reported. Halobetasol should not be applied to the breast or nipple, if possible, but if used in this area, it should be thoroughly wiped off prior to breastfeeding.

Reference

1. Prescribing Information. Halobetasol. Sola Pharmaceuticals; 2019.

HALOPERIDOL

Mental Health (First-Generation Antipsychotic)

PREGNANCY RECOMMENDATION: Limited Human Data—Animal Data Suggest Risk

BREASTFEEDING RECOMMENDATION: Potential Toxicity

H

PREGNANCY SUMMARY

In combined data from the Michigan Medicaid Surveillance study recipients and the European Network of Teratology Information Services (ENTIS), a total of 192 pregnancies were exposed to haloperidol in the first trimester, and 6 (3.1%) anomalies were identified. Based on a few earlier case reports, there was a potential concern that haloperidol might increase the risk for limb defects. However, this has not been seen in these larger studies. Numerous other case reports were located that described the use of haloperidol in treating chorea gravidarum, bipolar illness, and other psychoses in the second and third trimesters, without any major complications noted, other than the potential for a withdrawal syndrome if high doses are used near delivery. The drug crosses the placenta, so fetal exposure will occur. Animal studies did show some embryofetal toxicity in two species at doses of less than 10 times the recommended human dose (RHD). Using this drug during pregnancy should be based on the pros and cons of the mother's clinical need for treatment versus any potential fetal risk that might occur from exposure. Haloperidol can increase prolactin levels in some patients, but this should not affect an established pregnancy. In addition, the drug can prolong the QT interval, usually with higher dosages.

BREASTFEEDING SUMMARY

Several studies have reported that haloperidol is excreted into breast milk. The reported levels ranged from undetectable to 32 ng/mL, all with varying amounts of daily dosing. Calculated relative infant doses (RIDs) are less than 10%. Most newborn breastfed infants exposed only to haloperidol do well. However, there are a few reports of neonatal sedation and decreased feeding with high doses or in combination with other antipsychotic medications. The manufacturer recommends that the drug not be used while breastfeeding. Nevertheless, breastfeeding while using this drug should be based on the mother's clinical need for treatment versus any potential infant risks that might occur. If used, the infant should be monitored for the most common reported adult side effects of nausea and dizziness (both leading to irritability), sedation, constipation, decreased appetite (monitor infant growth), tongue thrusting, and tremor. The drug can produce elevated prolactin levels, but this should not affect breastfeeding.

References

1. Product information. Haloperidol. Hikma Pharmaceuticals USA; 2019.
2. Tuchmann-Duplessis H, Mercier-Parot L. Influence of neuroleptics on prenatal development in mammals. In: Tuchmann-Duplessis H, Fanconi G, Burgio GR, eds. *Malformations, Tumors and Mental Defects, Pathogenetic Correlations*. Carlo Erba Foundation; 1971. As cited in Shepard TH. *Catalog of Teratogenic Agents*. 6th ed. The Johns Hopkins University Press; 1989:308-309.
3. Gill TS, Guram MS, Geber WF. Haloperidol teratogenicity in the fetal hamster. *Dev Pharmacol Ther*. 1982;4:1-5. As cited in Elia J, Katz IR, Simpson GM. Teratogenicity of psychotherapeutic medications. *Psychopharmacol Bull*. 1987;23:531-586.
4. Bignami G, Laviola G, Alleva E, et al. Developmental aspects of neurobehavioural toxicity. *Toxicol Lett*. 1992;64/65:231-237.
5. Newport DJ, Calamaras MR, DeVane CL, et al. Atypical antipsychotic administration during late pregnancy: placental passage and obstetrical outcomes. *Am J Psychiatry*. 2007;164:1214-1220.
6. Kuniyoshi M, Inanaga K. Haloperidol and biperiden plasma levels in a pregnant atypical psychotic woman and a neonate—a case report. *Kurume Med J*. 1985;32:199-202.
7. Dieulangard P, Coignet J, Vidal JC. Sur un cas d'ectro-phocomelie peut-etre d'origine medicamenteuse. *Bull Fed Gynecol Obstet*. 1966;18:85-87.
8. Kopelman AE, McCullar FW, Heggeness L. Limb malformations following maternal use of haloperidol. *JAMA*. 1975;231:62-64.
9. Diav-Citrin O, Shechtman S, Ornoy S, et al. Safety of haloperidol and penfluridol in pregnancy: a multicenter, prospective, controlled study. *J Clin Psychiatry*. 2005;66:317-322.
10. Van Waes A, Van de Velde E. Safety evaluation of haloperidol in the treatment of hyperemesis gravidarum. *J Clin Pharmacol*. 1969;9:224-227.
11. Hanson JW, Oakley GP. Haloperidol and limb deformity. *JAMA*. 1975;231:26.
12. Ayd FJ Jr. Haloperidol: fifteen years of clinical experience. *Dis Nerv Syst*. 1972;33:459-469.
13. Magnier P. On hyperemesis gravidarum; a therapeutical study of R 1625. *Gynecol Prat*. 1964;15:17-23.
14. Loke KH, Salleh R. Electroconvulsive therapy for the acutely psychotic pregnant patient: a review of 3 cases. *Med J Malaysia*. 1983;38:131-133.
15. Donaldson JO. Control of chorea gravidarum with haloperidol. *Obstet Gynecol*. 1982;59:381-382.
16. Nurnberg HG. Treatment of mania in the last six months of pregnancy. *Hosp Community Psychiatry*. 1980;31:122-126.
17. Sexon WR, Barak Y. Withdrawal emergent syndrome in an infant associated with maternal haloperidol therapy. *J Perinatol*. 1989;9:170-172.
18. Collins KO, Comer JB. Maternal haloperidol therapy associated with dyskinesia in a newborn. *Am J Health-Syst Pharm*. 2003;60:2253-2255.

19. Nishiwaki T, Tanaka K, Sekiya S. Acute lithium intoxication in pregnancy. *Int J Gynecol Obstet*. 1996;52:191-192.
20. Stewart RB, Karas B, Springer PK. Haloperidol excretion in human milk. *Am J Psychiatry*. 1980;137:849-850.
21. Whalley LJ, Blain PG, Prime JK. Haloperidol secreted in breast milk. *Br Med J*. 1981;282:1746-1747.
22. Ohkubo T, Shimoyama R, Sugawara K. Measurement of haloperidol in human breast milk by high-performance liquid chromatography. *J Pharm Sci*. 1992;81:947-949.
23. Yoshida K, Smith B, Craggs M, Kumar R. Neuroleptic drugs in breast milk: a study of pharmacokinetics and of possible adverse effects in breast-fed infants. *Psychol Med*. 1998;28:81-91.
24. Committee on Drugs, American Academy of Pediatrics. The transfer of drugs and other chemicals into human milk. *Pediatrics*. 2001;108:776-789.

HEMIN

Hematologic (Hematopoietic)

PREGNANCY RECOMMENDATION: Limited Human Data—No Relevant Animal Data

BREASTFEEDING RECOMMENDATION: Probably Compatible

H

PREGNANCY SUMMARY

A case report was located that describes a pregnancy where hemin was administered during the first trimester for an exacerbation of acute intermittent porphyria. A term delivery occurred, and no adverse fetal effects or anomalies were identified. It is not fully known if hemin treatment is indicated during pregnancy, but using this drug may shorten the duration of an acute intermittent porphyria attack and reduce its severity. Because it is a substance that is normally found in blood, it is not known if it will cross the placenta in any clinically significant amount. However, this limited human pregnancy experience prevents a complete assessment of the embryofetal risk. No animal reproduction studies have been conducted. Using this drug during pregnancy should be based on the pros and cons of the mother's clinical need for treatment versus any potential fetal risk that might occur from exposure. Although multiple steps have been taken to lessen the chance of blood-borne infections, because hemin is derived from human blood, a theoretical risk still exists for the transmission of infectious agents, such as viruses and the agents that can cause Creutzfeldt-Jakob disease. It is recommended that health care providers report any infections thought to be transmitted by this product to Recordati Rare Diseases at 1-888-575-8344.

BREASTFEEDING SUMMARY

No reports describing the use of hemin during human lactation have been located. Hemin is a substance that is normally found in blood, so it is doubtful if any clinically significant amount will be found in breast milk. However, even if small amounts were excreted, they would probably be digested in the infant's gastrointestinal tract. One study was found that examined the effect of hematin on bilirubin binding. In an in vitro experiment, hematin was added to bilirubin-enriched cord blood and was found to have a significant adverse effect on bilirubin binding. However, the high concentrations required were not physiologic, and therefore, were not thought to have clinical significance. Breastfeeding while using this drug should be based on the mother's clinical need for treatment. If used, the infant should be monitored for the most common reported adult side effects of headache (leading to irritability) and pyrexia.

References

1. Prescribing Information. Panhematin. Recordati Rare Diseases; 2020.
2. Wenger S, Meisinger V, Brücke T, Deecke L. Acute porphyric neuropathy during pregnancy—effect of haematin therapy. *Eur Neurol*. 1998;39:187-188.
3. Kanaan C, Veille JC, Lakin M. Pregnancy and acute intermittent porphyria. *Obstet Gynecol Surv*. 1989;44:244-249.
4. Kirk JJ, Ritter DA, Kenny JD. The effect of hematin on bilirubin binding in bilirubin-enriched neonatal cord serum. *Biol Neonate*. 1984;45:53-57.

HEPARIN

Hematologic (Anticoagulant)

PREGNANCY RECOMMENDATION: Human Data Suggest Compatible

BREASTFEEDING RECOMMENDATION: Compatible

PREGNANCY SUMMARY

In a Michigan Medicaid Surveillance study, 65 newborns had been exposed to heparin during the first trimester, and 7 (11%) major birth defects were observed (3 expected). However, no pattern to the anomalies was seen. A few other reports have not shown an elevated risk for congenital anomalies above the expected baseline. Because heparin does not cross the placenta, fetal complications or anomalies are likely related to the severe maternal disease necessitating anticoagulant therapy. Long-term use of heparin can lead to thrombocytopenia, and it is recommended that maternal platelet counts be obtained periodically. The drug has also been associated with osteopenia, but this should reverse when therapy is completed. Animal studies did show some embryofetal toxicity, but no teratogenicity, in two species at doses of about 10 times the maximum recommended human dose (MRHD). Using this drug during pregnancy should be based on the pros and cons of the mother's clinical need for treatment versus any potential fetal risk that might occur from exposure. Per the American College of Obstetricians and Gynecologists (ACOG), heparin is the preferred medication for treating deep vein thrombosis in pregnancy.

BREASTFEEDING SUMMARY

Heparin excretion into breast milk has not been specifically studied. However, low-molecular-weight heparins are not found in breast milk. Therefore, because the molecular weight (MW) of heparin chains is 3 times larger, heparin will not be found in breast milk. Furthermore, the drug is not absorbed from the gastrointestinal tract with oral administration. Therefore, the use of heparin while breastfeeding is considered compatible.

References

1. Hall JG, Pauli RM, Wilson KM. Maternal and fetal sequelae of anticoagulation during pregnancy. *Am J Med*. 1980;68:122-140.
2. Nageotte MP, Freeman RK, Garite TJ, Block RA. Anticoagulation in pregnancy. *Am J Obstet Gynecol*. 1981;141:472.
3. Flessa HC, Kapstrom AB, Glueck HI, et al. Placental transport of heparin. *Am J Obstet Gynecol*. 1965;93:570-573.
4. Russo R, Bortolotti U, Schivazappa L, Girolami A. Warfarin treatment during pregnancy: a clinical note. *Haemostasis*. 1979;8:96-98.
5. Moe N. Anticoagulant-therapy in the prevention of placental infarction and perinatal death. *Obstet Gynecol*. 1982;59:481-483.
6. Hellgren M, Nygards EB. Long-term therapy with subcutaneous heparin during pregnancy. *Gynecol Obstet Invest*. 1982;13:76-89.
7. Cohen AW, Gabbe SG, Mennuti MT. Adjusted-dose heparin therapy by continuous intravenous infusion for recurrent pulmonary embolism during pregnancy. *Am J Obstet Gynecol*. 1983;146:463-464.
8. Howell R, Fidler J, Letsky E. The risks of antenatal subcutaneous heparin prophylaxis: a controlled trial. *Br J Obstet Gynaecol*. 1983;90:1124-1128.
9. Vellenga E, van Imhoff GW, Aarnoudse JG. Effective prophylaxis with oral anticoagulants and low-dose heparin during pregnancy in an antithrombin III deficient woman. *Lancet*. 1983;2:224.
10. Bergqvist A, Bergqvist D, Hallbook T. Deep vein thrombosis during pregnancy. *Acta Obstet Gynecol Scand*. 1983;62:443-448.
11. Michiels JJ, Stibbe J, Vellenga E, van Vliet HHDM. Prophylaxis of thrombosis in antithrombin III-deficient women during pregnancy and delivery. *Eur J Obstet Gynecol Reprod Biol*. 1984;18:149-153.
12. Nelson DM, Stempel LE, Fabri PJ, Talbert M. Hickman catheter use in a pregnant patient requiring therapeutic heparin anticoagulation. *Am J Obstet Gynecol*. 1984;149:461-462.
13. Romero R, Duffy TP, Berkowitz RL, et al. Prolongation of a preterm pregnancy complicated by death of a single twin in utero and disseminated intravascular coagulation: effects of treatment with heparin. *N Engl J Med*. 1984;310:772-774.
14. Ginsberg JS, Kowalchuk G, Hirsh J, Brill-Edwards P, Burrows R. Heparin therapy during pregnancy: risks to the fetus and mother. *Arch Intern Med*. 1989;149:2233-2236.
15. Wise PH, Hall AJ. Heparin-induced osteopenia in pregnancy. *Br Med J*. 1980; 281:110-111.
16. Aarskog D, Aksnes L, Lehmann V. Low 1,25-dihydroxyvitamin D in heparin-induced osteopenia. *Lancet*. 1980;2:650-651.
17. Aarskog D, Aksnes L, Markestad T, et al. Heparin-induced inhibition of 1,25-dihydroxyvitamin D formation. *Am J Obstet Gynecol*. 1984;148:1141-1142.
18. De Swiet M, Dorrington Ward P, Fidler J, et al. Prolonged heparin therapy in pregnancy causes bone demineralization. *Br J Obstet Gynaecol*. 1983;90: 1129-1134.
19. Griffiths HT, Liu DTY. Severe heparin osteoporosis in pregnancy. *Postgrad Med J*.1984;60:424-425.

HEXACHLOROPHENE

Anti-Infective (Detergent Cleanser)

PREGNANCY RECOMMENDATION: Human Data Suggest Low Risk (Topical Skin/Excludes Mucous Membranes)

BREASTFEEDING RECOMMENDATION: Probably Compatible (With Normal Use)

PREGNANCY SUMMARY

A study from Sweden reported that the rate of major birth anomalies in 3,007 infants (with high maternal exposure to hexachlorophene) did not have a higher rate of major birth anomalies compared with 1,653 infants born from mothers with low hexachlorophene exposure. This study followed a report (also from Sweden) that hexachlorophene hand soap was teratogenic in humans, but it was later learned that the concerning study had several methodologic issues. No other studies have been located that describe an increase in risk for birth defects with first-trimester use of this topical hand scrub. Hexachlorophene crosses the placenta following topical use, so fetal exposure will occur. Therefore, this overall limited first-trimester human pregnancy experience prevents a complete assessment of the embryofetal risk. Animal studies did not show any embryofetal toxicity or malformations in one species with low oral doses. Because of fairly rapid skin absorption, hexachlorophene should not be used on mucous membranes or injured skin.

BREASTFEEDING SUMMARY

Hexachlorophene has been found in breast milk. In 11 breast milk samples, the levels were low, ranging from undetectable to a maximum of 9 ng/mL. The specific history of hexachlorophene use by the women was not available. The authors concluded that the low breast milk concentrations of hexachlorophene found in their study do not pose a risk to nursing infants.

However, excessive maternal skin washing and any newborn washing with hexachlorophene are not recommended.

References

1. Product Information. Phisohex. Sanofi-Aventis US, LLC; 2023.
2. Lockhart JD. How toxic is hexachlorophene? *Pediatrics*. 1972;50:220-235.
3. Gillespie WA, Corner BD, Burman D, Alder VG. Absorption of hexachlorophene from dusting powder on newborn infants' skin. *J Hyg (Cambridge)*. 1974;73:311-315.
4. Strickland DM, Leonard RG, Stavchansky S, et al. Vaginal absorption of hexachlorophene during labor. *Am J Obstet Gynecol*. 1983;147:769-772.
5. Curley A, Hawk RE, Kimbrough RD, et al. Dermal absorption of hexachlorophene in infants. *Lancet*. 1971;2:296-297.
6. Halling H. Suspected link between exposure to hexachlorophene and malformed infants. *Ann NY Acad Sci*. 1979;320:426-435.
7. Birth defects linked to hexachlorophene. *Sci News*. 1978;114:21.
8. Can hexachlorophene soap cause birth defects? *Med World News*. 1978; 19:20-24.
9. Check W. New study shows hexachlorophene is teratogenic in humans. *JAMA*.1978;240:513-514.
10. Hexachlorophene-birth defect link debated. *Hosp Infect Control*. 1978;5: 125-127.
11. Källen B. Hexachlorophene teratogenicity in humans disputed. *JAMA*. 1978;240:1585-1586.
12. Janerich DT. Environmental causes of birth defects: the hexachlorophene issue. *JAMA*. 1979;241:830-831.
13. Baltzar B, Ericson A, Källen B. Pregnancy outcome among women working in Swedish hospitals. *N Engl J Med*. 1979;300:627-628.
14. West RW, Wilson DJ, Schaffner W. Hexachlorophene concentrations in human milk. *Bull Environ Contam Toxicol*. 1975;13:167-169.

H

HOMATROPINE

Autonomic (Parasympatholytic/Anticholinergic)

PREGNANCY RECOMMENDATION: Limited Human Data—No Relevant Animal Data

BREASTFEEDING RECOMMENDATION: Probably Compatible

PREGNANCY SUMMARY

The Collaborative Perinatal Project reported 26 patients with first-trimester exposure to homatropine, and 1 (3.8%) newborn was identified with a malformation. Overall, there were 86 exposures to homatropine at any time during the pregnancy, with 3 (3.5%) malformations reported. No specific pattern was noted, and coexposures to other drugs occurred. Based on likely placental transfer, some fetal exposure will probably occur. Therefore, this limited human pregnancy experience prevents a complete assessment of the embryofetal risk. Animal reproduction studies have not been conducted. Parasympathetic blocking agents (see Atropine) can alter the appearance of the fetal heart monitor tracing by causing an elevation of the baseline rate and decreasing variability. Lastly, this drug is only available orally in the United States, combined with hydrocodone (as an antitussive agent—see Hydrocodone).

BREASTFEEDING SUMMARY

No reports describing the use of homatropine during human lactation have been located. The drug will probably be found in breast milk, so some infant exposure will likely occur. Breastfeeding while using this drug should be based on the mother's clinical need for treatment. If used, the infant should be monitored for the most common reported adult side effects of nausea, abdominal pain, and headache (all leading to irritability), diarrhea, lethargy, vomiting, constipation, dry mouth, tachycardia, and urinary retention. In addition, because this drug has anticholinergic effects, there is the possibility of interfering with breast milk production development in the early stages of breastfeeding and may decrease breast milk supply over time.

References

1. Prescribing Information. Hycodan. Endo Pharmaceuticals, Inc; 2018.
2. Heinonen OP, Slone D, Shapiro S. *Birth Defects and Drugs in Pregnancy*. Publishing Sciences Group; 1983:346-347,439.

HOMATROPINE OPHTHALMIC

Ophthalmic (Mydriatic/Anticholinergic)

PREGNANCY RECOMMENDATION: No Human Data and No Relevant Animal Data

BREASTFEEDING RECOMMENDATION: Probably Compatible

PREGNANCY SUMMARY

No reports describing the use of homatropine ophthalmic in human pregnancy have been located. The Collaborative Perinatal Project reported first-trimester exposure to oral homatropine in 26 patients, with 1 (3.8%) newborn identified who had a malformation. Overall, there were 86 exposures to homatropine at any time during the pregnancy, with 3 (3.5%)

malformations reported. No specific pattern to the anomalies was noted, and coexposures to other drugs occurred. Based on likely placental transfer, some fetal exposure might occur. However, systemic absorption is minimal with ophthalmic use, so exposure should be negligible. Therefore, this limited human pregnancy experience prevents a complete assessment of the embryofetal risk. Parasympathetic blocking agents (see Atropine) can alter the appearance of the fetal heart monitor tracing by causing an elevation of the baseline rate and decreasing variability. If used during pregnancy, consider placing pressure over the tear duct in the corner of the eye for at least 1 minute, and then remove any excess solution with absorbent tissue to decrease the amount of drug reaching the systemic circulation even further.

BREASTFEEDING SUMMARY

No reports describing the use of homatropine ophthalmic during human lactation have been located. The drug will probably be found in breast milk, but the overall amount should be negligible with ophthalmic use. Breastfeeding while using this drug should be based on the mother's clinical need for treatment. If used, the infant should be monitored for the most common reported adult side effects of nausea, abdominal pain, and headache (all leading to irritability), diarrhea, lethargy, vomiting, constipation, dry mouth, tachycardia, and urinary retention. In addition, because this drug has anticholinergic effects, there is the possibility of interfering with breast milk production development in the early stages of breastfeeding and decreasing breast milk supply over time (though this is unlikely with ophthalmic use). A method to reduce systemic absorption is described above in the Pregnancy Summary.

References

1. Prescribing Information. Homatropine. Altaire Pharmaceuticals, Inc; 2022.
2. Heinonen OP, Slone D, Shapiro S. *Birth Defects and Drugs in Pregnancy*. Publishing Sciences Group; 1983:346-347,439.

H

HYDRALAZINE

Antihypertensive (Vasodilator)

PREGNANCY RECOMMENDATION: Limited Human Data—Animal Data Suggest Low Risk (Maternal Benefit May Outweigh Embryofetal Risk With Severe Hypertension)

BREASTFEEDING RECOMMENDATION: Probably Compatible

PREGNANCY SUMMARY

A total of 50 first-trimester exposures to hydralazine were reported from the combined data of the Collaborative Perinatal Project and the Michigan Medicaid Surveillance study recipients. Only one (2%) major anomaly was identified. Many other studies have been published on the use of hydralazine in treating hypertension in pregnancy, with use primarily in the second and third trimesters. The drug crosses the placenta, so fetal exposure will occur. Therefore, this limited human pregnancy experience with first-trimester exposure prevents a complete assessment of the embryofetal risk. Animal studies did not show any embryofetal toxicity or teratogenicity in one species at doses of less than 10 times the RHD. Using this drug during pregnancy should be based on the pros and cons of the mother's clinical need for treatment versus any potential fetal risk that might occur from exposure. However, in cases of severe hypertension, maternal benefit probably outweighs any embryofetal risk. For treating hypertension in pregnancy, ACOG recommends nifedipine and labetalol as first-line agents.

BREASTFEEDING SUMMARY

Hydralazine was found to be excreted into breast milk at low concentrations. In one study, a level of about 130 ng/mL was reported. The calculated RID would be about 0.9%. No adverse effects were noted in the nursing infant from this small concentration. Serum levels in neonates exposed to hydralazine through breastfeeding are also low. Breastfeeding while using this drug should be based on the mother's clinical need for treatment versus any potential infant risks that might occur. If used, the infant should be monitored for the most common reported adult side effects of nausea, headache, and arthralgia (all leading to irritability), diarrhea, vomiting, tachycardia, hypotension, and rash.

References

1. Product information. Hydralazine Hydrochloride. Akorn; 2017.
2. De Swiet M. Antihypertensive drugs in pregnancy. *Br Med J*. 1985;291:365-366.
3. Liedholm H, Wahlin-Boll E, Ingemarsson I, Melander A. Transplacental passage and breast milk concentrations of hydralazine. *Eur J Clin Pharmacol*. 1982;21:417-419.
4. Widerlov E, Karlman I, Storsater J. Hydralazine-induced neonatal thrombocytopenia. *N Engl J Med*. 1980;303:1235.
5. Brazy JE, Grimm JK, Little VA. Neonatal manifestations of severe maternal hypertension occurring before the thirty-sixth week of pregnancy. *J Pediatr*. 1982;100:265-271.
6. Sibai BM, Anderson GD. Pregnancy outcome of intensive therapy in severe hypertension in first trimester. *Obstet Gynecol*. 1986;67:517-522.
7. Heinonen OP, Slone D, Shapiro S. *Birth Defects and Drugs in Pregnancy*. Publishing Sciences Group; 1977.
8. Bott-Kanner G, Schweitzer A, Schoenfeld A, et al. Treatment with propranolol and hydralazine throughout pregnancy in a hypertensive patient. *Isr J Med Sci*. 1978;14:466-468.
9. Pritchard JA, Pritchard SA. Standardized treatment of 154 consecutive cases of eclampsia. *Am J Obstet Gynecol*. 1975;123:543-552.
10. Chapman ER, Strozier WE, Magee RA. The clinical use of Apresoline in the toxemias of pregnancy. *Am J Obstet Gynecol*. 1954;68:1109-1117.

11. Johnson GT, Thompson RB. A clinical trial of intravenous Apresoline in the management of toxemia of late pregnancy. *J Obstet Gynecol.* 1958;65:360-366.
12. Kuzniar J, Skret A, Piela A, et al. Hemodynamic effects of intravenous hydralazine in pregnant women with severe hypertension. *Obstet Gynecol.* 1985;66:453-458.
13. Hogstedt S, Lindeberg S, Axelsson O, et al. A prospective controlled trial of metoprolol-hydralazine treatment in hypertension during pregnancy. *Acta Obstet Scand.* 1985;64:505-510.
14. Gallery EDM, Ross MR, Gyory AZ. Antihypertensive treatment in pregnancy: analysis of different responses to oxprenolol and methyldopa. *Br Med J.* 1985;291:563-566.
15. Horvath JS, Korda A, Child A, Henderson-Smart D, Phippard A, Duggin GG, Hall BM, Tiller DJ. Hypertension in pregnancy: a study of 142 women presenting before 32 weeks' gestation. *Med J Aust.* 1985;143:19-21.
16. Rosenfeld J, Bott-Kanner G, Boner G, et al. Treatment of hypertension during pregnancy with hydralazine monotherapy or with combined therapy with hydralazine and pindolol. *Eur J Obstet Gynecol Reprod Biol.* 1986;22:197-204.
17. Mabie WC, Gonzalez AR, Sibai BM, Amon E. A comparative trial of labetalol and hydralazine in the acute management of severe hypertension complicating pregnancy. *Obstet Gynecol.* 1987;70:328-333.
18. Owen J, Hauth JC. Polyarteritis nodosa in pregnancy: a case report and brief literature review. *Am J Obstet Gynecol.* 1989;160:606-607.
19. Rossouw HJ, Howarh G, Odendaal HJ. Ketanserin and hydralazine in hypertension in pregnancy—a randomised double-blind trial. *S Afr Med J.* 1995;86:525-528.
20. Henrich WL, Cronin R, Miller PD, Anderson RJ. Hypotensive sequelae of diazoxide and hydralazine therapy. *JAMA.* 1977;237:264-265.
21. Lodeiro JG, Feinstein SJ, Lodeiro SB. Fetal premature atrial contractions associated with hydralazine. *Am J Obstet Gynecol.* 1989;160:105-107.
22. Yemini M, Shoham (Schwartz) Z, Dgani R, et al. Lupus-like syndrome in a mother and newborn following administration of hydralazine: a case report. *Eur J Obstet Gynecol Reprod Biol.* 1989;30:193-197.
23. Magee LA, Cham C, Waterman EJ, et al. Hydralazine for treatment of severe hypertension in pregnancy: meta-analysis. *BMJ.* 2003;327:955-960.
24. Daily JW. Anticoagulant and cardiovascular drugs. In: Wilson JT, ed. *Drugs in Breast Milk.* ADIS Press; 1981:61-64.

HYDROCHLOROTHIAZIDE

Urinary (Diuretic)

SEE CHLOROTHIAZIDE

HYDROCODONE

Pain (Opioid)

PREGNANCY RECOMMENDATION: Human Data Suggest Low Risk (First Trimester)/Human Data Suggest Risk for Chronic Use

BREASTFEEDING RECOMMENDATION: Potential Toxicity

PREGNANCY SUMMARY

In combined data from the Michigan Medicaid Surveillance study and the Collaborative Perinatal Project, a total of 24 (7%) major fetal anomalies were identified in 344 first-trimester hydrocodone exposed pregnancies (14 expected). However, no specific pattern was seen, except that there were five cardiovascular defects noted (three expected). The National Birth Defects Prevention Study reported an overall rate of 2.6% for major birth anomalies in patients who filled any opioid prescription in the first trimester. This rate was significantly higher than the 2.0% rate in the unexposed control group, but falls within the expected rate of 2% to 4% for major birth defects in the United States. Though the exact number of cases was not supplied, 34.5% of the opioids reportedly used were hydrocodone. In the hydrocodone group, there was a higher rate for cardiovascular and neural tube defects (NTDs), as well as gastroschisis and cleft palate, compared with the control group. However, self-reported recall history can be flawed (in some cases, the interview occurred up to 3 years after the patient's first trimester); verification of actual drug use, the dosage, and exact timing of use during the first trimester cannot be confirmed; and, recall may be affected by whether or not a mother delivered a newborn with an anomaly. A few other large database studies have been conducted that were linked to pharmacy prescriptions filled for opioid drugs. Most showed no higher rate for major anomalies when compared with controls. None of these studies could be controlled for illicit opioid use. Lastly, several studies have identified smaller newborn head circumferences at birth in neonates exposed to opiates chronically throughout gestation. The clinical significance of this is unknown. The drug will probably cross the placenta, so fetal exposure will likely occur. Therefore, this limited human first-trimester hydrocodone exposure experience prevents a complete assessment of the embryofetal risk. Animal studies did show some embryofetal toxicity in one species at doses of less than 10 times the RHD and in another species at 10 times the RHD. However, no teratogenicity was seen at these doses. Hydrocodone is metabolized into six active metabolites, including hydromorphone (see Hydromorphone). The drug carries a boxed warning for a risk of misuse, addiction, life-threatening respiratory depression, neonatal opioid withdrawal syndrome, and, when combined with benzodiazepines and other central nervous system (CNS) depressants, profound sedation, coma, and death. The drug is a Schedule II controlled substance. In the United States, the drug is not available as a single agent, but is usually available with acetaminophen.

BREASTFEEDING SUMMARY

Hydrocodone has been found in the breast milk of numerous patients with levels that range from about 5 to 130 ng/mL. The calculated RIDs were all under 10%. Because hydromorphone is one of the active metabolites of hydrocodone, this drug was also assessed in 30 patients. It was undetectable in 18 cases (<1 ng/mL), and in the remaining 12 patients, the median drug level was only 1.9 ng/mL. However, there are a few reports of significant infant sedation with opioid use while breastfeeding. Therefore, it is recommended that use be limited to a few days, if possible. Breastfeeding while using this drug should be based on the mother's clinical need for treatment versus any potential infant risks that might occur. If used, the infant should be monitored for the most common reported adult side effects of nausea, headache, dizziness, pruritus, and abdominal pain (all leading to irritability), somnolence, lethargy, vomiting, constipation, and tremor.

References

1. Prescribing Information. Hydrocodone. Pernix Therapeutics, LLC; 2018.
2. Heinonen OP, Slone D, Shapiro S. *Birth Defects and Drugs in Pregnancy*. Publishing Sciences Group; 1983:287-288.
3. Broussard CS, Rasmussen SA, Reefhuis J, et al.; for the National Birth Defects Prevention Study. Maternal treatment with opioid analgesics and risk for birth defects. *Am J Obstet Gynecol*. 2011;204:314-317.
4. Bodley V, Powers D. Long-term treatment of a breastfeeding mother with fluconazole-resolved nipple pain caused by yeast: a case study. *J Hum Lact*. 1997;13:307-311.
5. Meyer D, Tobias JD. Adverse effects following the inadvertent administration of opioids to infants and children. *Clin Pediatr (Phil)*. 2005;44:499-503.
6. Anderson PO, Sauberan JB, Lane JR, Rossi SS. Hydrocodone excretion into breast milk: the first two reported cases. *Breastfeed Med*. 2007;2:10-14.
7. Sauberan JB, Anderson PO, Lane JR, et al. Breast milk hydrocodone and hydromorphone levels in mothers using hydrocodone for postpartum pain. *Obstet Gynecol*. 2011;117:611-617.

HYDROCORTISONE

Corticosteroid

PREGNANCY RECOMMENDATION: Human Data Suggest Potential Risk (First Trimester) (Maternal Benefit May Outweigh Embryofetal Risk With Some Disorders)

BREASTFEEDING RECOMMENDATION: Probably Compatible

PREGNANCY SUMMARY

The Collaborative Perinatal Project reported 55 patients with first-trimester exposure to hydrocortisone, and 3 (5.5%) newborns were identified who had malformations. However, no specific pattern was noted, and coexposures to other drugs were not described. In a second study that analyzed seventeen published series of any corticosteroid use in the first trimester, 16 (3.5%) neonates with anomalies were reported out of 457 births (no different than the expected rate). A third study reported 14 (4.6%) anomalies in 311 pregnancies with any corticosteroid use in the first trimester compared with 21 (2.7%) anomalies in 790 controls. This comparison was not significant, and no cases of cleft lip and/or palate occurred in the exposed group. Because cleft lip and palate were seen in animal studies at a higher-than-expected rate, several large population studies have been published evaluating for this risk. Overall, most of these studies report an increased risk of cleft lip and/or palate with first-trimester use of corticosteroids when compared to controls, but the rates for these two specific birth anomalies were well below 1%. Numerous case reports have been published describing cleft lip and/or palate along with other birth anomalies. However, because of the anomaly and drug exposure, the reporting of these cases can be biased. Most maternal hydrocortisone is extensively metabolized by placental 11β-hydroxysteroid dehydrogenase, converting it to cortisone (which is inactive). Therefore, only a limited amount of maternal hydrocortisone will cross the placenta. However, some fetal exposure can occur. Regardless, this limited human first-trimester pregnancy experience prevents a complete assessment of the embryofetal risk. Animal studies reported an increased risk for cleft lip and/or palate, along with some embryofetal toxicity in two species at doses less than 10 times the RHD. Because the benefits of corticosteroids in many clinical settings appear to outweigh any potential fetal risks, these agents should not be withheld if the mother's condition requires their use. Therefore, using this drug during pregnancy should be based on the pros and cons of the mother's clinical need for treatment versus any potential fetal risk that might occur from exposure.

BREASTFEEDING SUMMARY

Trace amounts of endogenous hydrocortisone are excreted into breast milk. The amount of the drug in breast milk varied from 0.2 to 32 ng/mL, with the highest mean concentrations (25.5 ng/mL) measured in colostrum. The concentration of hydrocortisone in colostrum averages about 7.5% of the maternal plasma level. No reports describing the excretion of exogenous hydrocortisone or cortisone into human breast milk have been located. It is unlikely, however, that these agents pose a risk to a nursing infant. Prednisone, a corticosteroid more potent than hydrocortisone, is excreted in trace amounts into breast milk and is considered compatible with breastfeeding (see Prednisone). Breastfeeding while using this drug should be based on the mother's clinical need for treatment versus any potential infant risks that might occur. If used, the infant should be monitored for the most common reported adult side effects of headaches and abdominal pain (both leading to irritability), weakness (lethargy), impaired wound healing, edema, increased sodium levels, low potassium, and hyperglycemia.

References

1. American Hospital Formulary Service. *Drug Information 1999*. American Society of Health-System Pharmacists; 1999:2637.
2. Fraser FC, Fainstat TD. Production of congenital defects in the offspring of pregnant mice treated with cortisone. Progress report. *Pediatrics*. 1951;8: 527-533.
3. Fraser FC, Kalter H, Walker BE, Fainstat TD. The experimental production of cleft palate with cortisone and other hormones. *J Cell Comp Physiol*. 1954;43(suppl 1):235-259.
4. Fraser FC, Walker BE, Trasler DG. Experimental production of congenital cleft palate: genetic and environmental factors. *Pediatrics*. 1957;19:782-787.
5. Kalter H, Fraser FC. Production of congenital defects in the offspring of pregnant mice treated with compound F. *Nature*. 1952;169:665.
6. Kalter H. Factors influencing the frequency of cortisone-induced cleft palate in mice. *J Exp Zool*. 1957;134:449-467.
7. Kalter H. Fetal growth restriction induced by cortisone 40 years ago. *Am J Obstet Gynecol*. 1998;179:835.
8. Pinsky L, DiGeorge AM. Cleft palate in the mouse: a teratogenic index of glucocorticoid potency. *Science*. 1965;147:402-403.
9. Rogoyski A, Trzcinska-Dabrowska Z. Corticosteroid-induced cataract and palatoschisis in the mouse fetus. *Am J Ophthalmol*. 1969;68:128-133.
10. DeCosta EJ, Abelman MA. Cortisone and pregnancy. An experimental and clinical study of the effects of cortisone on gestation. *Am J Obstet Gynecol*. 1952;64:746-767.
11. Fainstat T. Cortisone-induced congenital cleft palate in rabbits. *Endocrinology*. 1954;55:502-508.
12. Kotas RV, Mims LC, Hart LK. Reversible inhibition of lung cell number after glucocorticoid injection into fetal rabbits to enhance surfactant appearance. *Pediatrics*. 1974;53:358-361.
13. Van Geijn HP, Zuspan FP, Copeland SJ, Vorys AS, Zuspan MF, Scott GD. The effects of hydrocortisone on the development of the amine system in the fetal brain. *Am J Obstet Gynecol*. 1979;135:743-750.
14. Crocker JFS, Ogborn MR. Glucocorticoid teratogenesis in the developing nephron. *Teratology*. 1991;43:571-574.
15. Shepard TH. *Catalog of Teratogenic Agents*. 8th ed. The Johns Hopkins University Press; 1995.
16. Beitins IZ, Bayard F, Ances IG, Kowarski A, Migeon CJ. The metabolic clearance rate, blood production, interconversion and transplacental passage of cortisol and cortisone in pregnancy near term. *Pediatr Res*. 1973;7:509-519.
17. Pearson Murphy BE, Clark SJ, Donald IR, et al. Conversion of maternal cortisol to cortisone during placental transfer to the human fetus. *Am J Obstet Gynecol*. 1974;118:538-541.
18. Levitz M, Jansen V, Dancis J. The transfer and metabolism of corticosteroids in the perfused human placenta. *Am J Obstet Gynecol*. 1978;132:363-366.
19. Ballard PL, Liggins GC. Glucocorticoid activity in cord serum: comparison of hydrocortisone and betamethasone regimens. *J Pediatr*. 1982;101:468-470.
20. Heinonen OP, Slone D, Shapiro S. *Birth Defects and Drugs in Pregnancy*. Publishing Sciences Group; 1977.
21. Guilbeau JA Jr. Effects of cortisone on fetus. *Am J Obstet Gynecol*. 1953; 64:227.
22. Reisman LE, Matheny A. Corticosteroids in pregnancy. *Lancet*. 1968;1:592-593.
23. Khudr G, Olding L. Cyclopia. *Am J Dis Child*. 1973;125;120-122.
24. Malpas P. Foetal malformation and cortisone therapy. *Br Med J*. 1965;1:795.
25. Kraus AM. Congenital cataract and maternal steroid ingestion. *J Pediat Ophthalmol*. 1975;12:107-108.
26. Fraser FC, Sajoo A. Teratogenic potential of corticosteroids in humans. *Teratology*. 1995;51:45-46.
27. Harris JWS, Ross IP. Cortisone therapy in early pregnancy: relation to cleft palate. *Lancet*. 1956;1:1045-1047.
28. Doig RK, Coltman OM. Cleft palate following cortisone therapy in early pregnancy. *Lancet*. 1956;2:730.
29. Popert AJ. Pregnancy and adrenocortical hormones. Some aspects of the interaction in rheumatic diseases. *Br Med J*. 1962;1:967-972.
30. Bongiovanni AM, McPadden AJ. Steroids during pregnancy and possible fetal consequences. *Fertil Steril*. 1960;11:181-186.
31. Robert E, Vollset SE, Botto L, et al. Malformation surveillance and maternal drug exposure: the MADRE project. *Int J Risk Safety Med*. 1994;6:75-118.
32. Pradat P, Robert-Gnansia E, Di Tanna GL, et al; all contributors to the MADRE database. First trimester exposure to corticosteroids and oral clefts. *Birth Defects Res A Clin Mol Teratol*. 2003;67:968-970.
33. Rodriguez-Pinilla E, Martinez-Frias ML. Corticosteroids during pregnancy and oral clefts: a case-control study. *Teratology*. 1998;58:2-5.
34. Czeizel AE, Rockenbauer M. Population-based case-control study of teratogenic potential of corticosteroids. *Teratology*. 1997;56:335-340.
35. Carmichael SL, Shaw GM. Maternal corticosteroid use and risk of selected congenital anomalies. *Am J Med Genet*. 1999;86:242-244.
36. Mygind H, Thulstrup AM, Pedersen L, Larsen H. Risk of intrauterine growth restriction, malformations and other birth outcomes in children after topical use of corticosteroids in pregnancy. *Acta Obstet Gynecol Scand*. 2002;81: 234-239.
37. Gur C, Diav-Citrin O, Shechtman S, Arnon J, Ornoy A. Pregnancy outcome after first trimester exposure to corticosteroids: a prospective controlled study. *Reprod Toxicol*. 2004;18:93-101.
38. David M, Forest MG. Prenatal treatment of congenital adrenal hyperplasia resulting from 21-hydroxylase deficiency. *J Pediatr*. 1984;105:799-803.
39. Taeusch HW Jr. Glucocorticoid prophylaxis for respiratory distress syndrome: a review of potential toxicity. *J Pediatr*. 1975;87:617-623.
40. Dluholucky S, Babic J, Taufer I. Reduction of incidence and mortality of respiratory distress syndrome by administration of hydrocortisone to mother. *Arch Dis Child*. 1976;51:420-423.
41. Zuspan FP, Cordero L, Semchyshyn S. Effects of hydrocortisone on lecithin-sphingomyelin ratio. *Am J Obstet Gynecol*. 1977;128:571-574.
42. Morrison JC, Whybrew WD, Bucovaz ET, Schneider JM. Injection of corticosteroids into mother to prevent neonatal respiratory distress syndrome. *Am J Obstet Gynecol*. 1978;131:358-366.
43. Beck JC, Johnson JWC. Maternal administration of glucocorticoids. *Clin Obstet Gynecol*. 1980;23:93-113.
44. Semchyshyn S, Zuspan FP, Cordero L. Cardiovascular response and complications of glucocorticoid therapy in hypertensive pregnancies. *Am J Obstet Gynecol*. 1983;145:530-533.
45. Schmidt PL, Sims ME, Strassner HT, et al. Effect of antepartum glucocorticoid administration upon neonatal respiratory distress syndrome and perinatal infection. *Am J Obstet Gynecol*. 1984;148:178-186.
46. Iams JD, Barrows H. Management of preterm prematurely ruptured membranes: a retrospective comparison of observation versus use of steroids and timed delivery. *Am J Obstet Gynecol*. 1984;150:977-981.
47. Iams JD, Talbert ML, Barrows H, Sachs L. Management of preterm prematurely ruptured membranes: a prospective randomized comparison of observation versus use of steroids and timed delivery. *Am J Obstet Gynecol*. 1985;151:32-38.
48. Ward RM. Pharmacologic enhancement of fetal lung maturation. *Clin Perinatol*. 1994;21:523-542.
49. Wells CN. Treatment of hyperemesis gravidarum with cortisone. I. Fetal results. *Am J Obstet Gynecol*. 1953;66:598-601.
50. Taylor R. Successful management of hyperemesis gravidarum using steroid therapy. *QJM*. 1996;89:103-107.
51. Greenberg F. The potential teratogenicity of allergy and asthma treatment in pregnancy. *Immunol Aller Prac*. 1985;7:15-20.
52. D'Alonzo GE. The pregnant asthmatic patient. *Sem Perinatol*. 1990;14: 119-129.
53. Schatz M, Zeiger RS, Harden K, et al. The safety of asthma and allergy medications during pregnancy. *J Allergy Clin Immunol*. 1997;100:301-306.
54. Venkataraman MT, Shanies HM. Pregnancy and asthma. *J Asthma*. 1997;34: 265-271.
55. Schatz M, Zeiger RS. Asthma and allergy in pregnancy. *Clin Perinatol*. 1997; 24:407-432.
56. Report of the Working Group on Asthma and Pregnancy. *Management of asthma during pregnancy: National Institutes of Health*. NIH Publication No. 93-3279, 1993:18-19.
57. Rosner W, Beers PC, Awan T, Khan MS. Identification of corticosteroid-binding globulin in human milk: measurement with a filter disk assay. *J Clin Endocrinol Metab*. 1976;42:1064-1073.
58. Kulski JK, Hartmann PE. Changes in the concentration of cortisol in milk during different stages of human lactation. *Aust J Exp Biol Med Sci*. 1981;59: 769-778.

HYDROCORTISONE TOPICAL

Corticosteroid (Topical)

PREGNANCY RECOMMENDATION: Limited Human Data—Animal Data Suggest Potential Risk

BREASTFEEDING RECOMMENDATION: Probably Compatible

PREGNANCY SUMMARY

No reports describing the specific use of hydrocortisone topical cream in human pregnancy have been located. One report from a Danish prescription database and birth registry was located that described the use of topical corticosteroids during pregnancy. However, a breakdown of the individual types of topical steroids was not provided. There were 3 (1.8%) birth anomalies identified in 170 pregnancies with first-trimester exposure that was lower (but not significant) than the control group rate of 3.6% (332/9,263). For anytime use in pregnancy, no associations were found regarding low birth weight and preterm delivery. Stratification by corticosteroid strength (weak to very strong) did not change any of the results. In most clinical applications, in conjunction with extensive hydrocortisone conversion to inactive cortisone by placental 11β-hydroxysteroid dehydrogenase, only a limited amount of drug may cross the placenta, but some fetal exposure might occur. Therefore, this limited human pregnancy experience prevents a complete assessment of the embryofetal risk. Animal studies found some embryofetal toxicity with malformations in one species at doses of less than 10 times the RHD. Because the benefits of corticosteroids in many clinical settings appear to outweigh any potential fetal risks, these agents should not be withheld if the mother's condition requires their use. Therefore, using this drug during pregnancy should be based on the pros and cons of the mother's clinical need for treatment versus any potential fetal risk that might occur from exposure.

BREASTFEEDING SUMMARY

Trace amounts of endogenous hydrocortisone are excreted into breast milk. The amount of drug in breast milk varied from 0.2 to 32 ng/mL, with the highest concentrations being found in colostrum. The concentration of hydrocortisone in colostrum averages about 7.5% of the maternal plasma level. No reports describing the use of hydrocortisone cream during human lactation have been located. Prednisone, a corticosteroid more potent than hydrocortisone, is excreted in trace amounts into breast milk and is considered compatible with breastfeeding (see Prednisone). Therefore, it is unlikely that these agents pose any significant risk to a nursing infant. Breastfeeding while using this drug should be based on the mother's clinical need for treatment versus any potential infant risks that might occur. If used, the infant should be monitored for the most common reported adult side effects of headaches and abdominal pain (both leading to irritability), weakness (lethargy), impaired wound healing, edema, increased sodium levels, low potassium, and hyperglycemia.

References

1. Prescribing Information. Hydrocortisone Cream. Fougera Pharmaceuticals, Inc; 2019.
2. Beitins IZ, Bayard F, Ances IG, Kowarski A, Migeon CJ. The metabolic clearance rate, blood production, interconversion and transplacental passage of cortisol and cortisone in pregnancy near term. *Pediatr Res*. 1973;7:509-519.
3. Pearson Murphy BE, Clark SJ, Donald IR, et al. Conversion of maternal cortisol to cortisone during placental transfer to the human fetus. *Am J Obstet Gynecol*. 1974;118:538-541.
4. Mygind H, Thulstrup AM, Pedersen L, Larsen H. Risk of intrauterine growth restriction, malformations and other birth outcomes in children after topical use of corticosteroids in pregnancy. *Acta Obstet Gynecol Scand*. 2002;81:234-239.
5. Rosner W, Beers PC, Awan T, Khan MS. Identification of corticosteroid-binding globulin in human milk: measurement with a filter disk assay. *J Clin Endocrinol Metab*. 1976;42:1064-1073.
6. Kulski JK, Hartmann PE. Changes in the concentration of cortisol in milk during different stages of human lactation. *Aust J Exp Biol Med Sci*. 1981;59:769-778.

HYDROFLUMETHIAZIDE

Cardiovascular (Thiazide Diuretic)

PREGNANCY RECOMMENDATION: No Human Data and No Relevant Animal Data

BREASTFEEDING RECOMMENDATION: Potential Toxicity

PREGNANCY SUMMARY

The Collaborative Perinatal Project reported on one first-trimester exposure to hydroflumethiazide, but specific outcome data for this case were not supplied. There were 206 total first-trimester exposures to all thiazide diuretics, and 12 (5.8%) malformations were identified. However, no specific pattern was seen, and many of the patients were on other drugs at the

(continued)

time. Hydroflumethiazide will probably cross the placenta, so some fetal exposure will likely occur. Therefore, the absence of human pregnancy experience prevents a complete assessment of the embryofetal risk. Animal reproduction studies have not been performed. Using this drug during pregnancy should be based on the pros and cons of the mother's clinical need for treatment versus any potential fetal risk that might occur from exposure.

BREASTFEEDING SUMMARY

No reports describing the use of hydroflumethiazide in human lactation have been located. The drug will probably be excreted into breast milk, so some fetal exposure will likely occur. Breastfeeding while using this drug should be based on the mother's clinical need for treatment. If used, the infant should be monitored for the most common reported adult side effects of nausea, headache, and abdominal cramping (all leading to irritability), vomiting, diarrhea, jaundice, rash, and constipation.

References

1. Prescribing Information. Diucardin. Dipharma; 2018.
2. Heinonen OP, Slone D, Shapiro S. *Birth Defects and Drugs in Pregnancy*. Publishing Sciences Group; 1983:372.

H

HYDROMORPHONE

Pain (Opioid)

PREGNANCY RECOMMENDATION: Limited Human Data (First Trimester)/Human Data Suggest Risk for Chronic Use

BREASTFEEDING RECOMMENDATION: Potential Toxicity

PREGNANCY SUMMARY

The Collaborative Perinatal Project reported a total of 12 exposures to hydromorphone in the first trimester, and no major fetal malformations were identified. The National Birth Defects Prevention Study reported an overall rate of 2.6% for major birth anomalies in patients who filled any opioid prescription in the first trimester. This rate was significantly higher than the 2.0% rate in the unexposed control group, but falls within the expected rate of 2% to 4% for major birth defects in the United States. Separate numbers for hydromorphone were not provided. For the opioid exposed group, there was a higher rate for cardiovascular and NTDs, as well as gastroschisis, when compared with the control group. However, self-reported recall history can be flawed (in some cases, the interview occurred up to 3 years after the patient's first trimester); verification of actual drug use, the dosage, and exact timing of use during the first trimester cannot be confirmed; and, recall may be affected by whether or not a mother delivered a newborn with an anomaly. A few other large database studies have been conducted that were linked to pharmacy prescriptions filled for opioid drugs. Most showed no higher rate for major anomalies when compared with controls. None of these studies could be controlled for illicit opioid use. Lastly, several studies have identified smaller newborn head circumferences at birth in neonates exposed to opiates chronically throughout gestation. The clinical significance of this is unknown. The drug crosses the placenta, so fetal exposure will occur. Therefore, this limited human first-trimester exposure experience prevents a complete assessment of the embryofetal risk. Animal studies did show some embryofetal toxicity with malformations in one species at doses of less than 10 times the RHD. No embryofetal toxicity or malformations were seen in two other species at doses of less than and more than 10 times the RHD, despite maternal toxicity. The drug carries a boxed warning for a risk of misuse, addiction, life-threatening respiratory depression, neonatal opioid withdrawal syndrome, and, when combined with benzodiazepines and other CNS depressants, profound sedation, coma, and death. The drug is a Schedule II controlled substance.

BREASTFEEDING SUMMARY

Hydromorphone was found to be excreted into breast milk, but at low levels. The mean breast milk level from eight healthy lactating women was only 1 ng/mL. The RID was less than 1%. Because hydromorphone is one of the active metabolites of hydrocodone, this drug was also assessed in 30 patients taking hydrocodone postpartum. Hydromorphone was undetectable in 18 cases (<1 ng/mL), and in the remaining 12 patients, the median drug level was only 1.9 ng/mL. However, there are a few reports of significant infant sedation with opioid use while breastfeeding. Therefore, it is recommended that use be limited to a few days, if possible. Breastfeeding while using this drug should be based on the mother's clinical need for treatment versus any potential infant risks that might occur. If used, the infant should be monitored for the most common reported adult side effects of nausea, headache, dizziness, pruritus, and abdominal pain (all leading to irritability), somnolence, lethargy, vomiting, constipation, and tremor.

References

1. Bonica J. *Principles and Practice of Obstetric Analgesia and Anesthesia*. FA Davis; 1967:251.
2. Product information. Dilaudid. Fresenius Kabi USA; 2018.
3. Broussard CS, Rasmussen SA, Reefhuis J, et al.; for the National Birth Defects Prevention Study. Maternal treatment with opioid analgesics and risk for birth defects. *Am J Obstet Gynecol*. 2011;204:314-317.
4. Edwards JE, Rudy AC, Wermeling DP, et al. Hydromorphone transfer into breast milk after intranasal administration. *Pharmacotherapy*. 2003;23:153-158.
5. Sauberan JB, Anderson PO, Lane JR, et al. Breast milk hydrocodone and hydromorphone levels in mothers using hydrocodone for postpartum pain. *Obstet Gynecol*. 2011;117:611-617.

HYDROQUINONE

Dermatologic (Topical—Depigmentation)

PREGNANCY RECOMMENDATION: Limited Human Data—Animal Data Suggest Low Risk

BREASTFEEDING RECOMMENDATION: Probably Compatible

PREGNANCY SUMMARY

One study was located that described mostly first-trimester exposure to topical hydroquinone use in 64 pregnancies. No newborn complications or anomalies were reported. The drug will probably cross the placenta; however, due to the topical use of the drug, fetal exposure is likely to be small. Therefore, this limited human pregnancy experience prevents a complete assessment of the embryofetal risk. Animal studies have not been conducted with topical hydroquinone, and studies that involved oral doses were more than 10 times the RHD topically but were not found to be teratogenic. Using this drug during pregnancy should be based on the pros and cons of the mother's clinical need for treatment versus any potential fetal risk that might occur from exposure.

H

BREASTFEEDING SUMMARY

No reports describing the use of topical hydroquinone during human lactation have been located. The drug will probably be found in breast milk, but the levels should be low due to the topical use of the drug. Breastfeeding while using this drug should be based on the mother's clinical need for treatment. If used, the infant should be monitored for the most common reported adult side effects of nausea (leading to irritability), diarrhea, lethargy, and vomiting. Hydroquinone should not be applied to the breast or nipple, but if used in this area, it should be thoroughly wiped off prior to breastfeeding.

References

1. Prescribing Information. Hydroquinone. Sohm, Inc; 2023.
2. Bucks DAW, McMaster JR, Guy RH, Maibach HI. Percutaneous absorption of hydroquinone in humans: effect of 1-dodecylazacycloheptin-2-one (azone) and the 2-ethylhexyl ester of 4-(dimethylamino)benzoic acid (escalol 507). *J Toxicol Environ Health*. 1988;24:279-289.
3. Wester RC, Melendres J, Hui X, et al. Human in vivo and in vitro hydroquinone topical bioavailability, metabolism, and disposition. *J Toxicol Environ Health*. 1998;54:301-317.
4. Bolanca I, Bolanca Z, Kuna K, et al. Chloasma—the mask of pregnancy. *Coll Antropol*. 2008;32(suppl 2):139-141.
5. Mahe A, Perret JL, Ly F, et al. The cosmetic use of skin-lightening products during pregnancy in Dakar, Senegal: a common and potentially hazardous practice. *Trans R Soc Trop Med Hyg*. 2007;101:183-187.

HYDROXYCHLOROQUINE

Anti-Infective/Immunologic (Antimalarial—Antirheumatic)

PREGNANCY RECOMMENDATION: Human Data Suggest Low Risk—No Relevant Animal Data

BREASTFEEDING RECOMMENDATION: Probably Compatible

PREGNANCY SUMMARY

The rate of major birth anomalies from about 3,000 first trimester exposures (in pregnant women with lupus or rheumatoid arthritis) ranged from about 3.5% up to about 8.5%. These rates were either equal to or higher than those seen in patients without disease or drug exposure. However, no difference in anomaly rates were seen when compared with lupus and rheumatoid arthritis patients who were not exposed. No pattern to the defects were found. The drug will cross the placenta, so fetal exposure will occur. No animal reproduction studies have been conducted with hydroxychloroquine. Animal studies with chloroquine did not show any embryofetal toxicity or malformations in one species at doses of less than 10 times the RHD. No reports of retinal or ototoxicity after in utero exposure have been located. The US Centers for Disease Control and Prevention (CDC) has stated that hydroxychloroquine may be used during pregnancy for antimalarial prophylaxis since, in prophylactic doses, the agent is not harmful to the fetus. The use of higher doses for prolonged periods, such as those used for systemic lupus erythematosus (SLE), acute attacks of malaria, and rheumatoid arthritis, probably represents an increased fetal risk, but the magnitude of this increase is unknown. Moreover, stopping therapy when a pregnancy becomes known would not stop exposure to the embryo or fetus, because of the very long elimination half-life. Stopping the drug could increase the risk of a relapse of active disease. The drug can prolong the QT interval and has been associated with life-threatening cardiotoxicity, including cardiomyopathy.

BREASTFEEDING SUMMARY

Numerous reports have been published that have measured hydroxychloroquine in breast milk, reporting levels that ranged between 10 ng/mL and 4 mcg/mL. The calculated RIDs were all under 10% (one was 9.8%). However, breastfeeding during daily therapy with hydroxychloroquine should be undertaken cautiously, because the long elimination half-life increases the potential for accumulation of a toxic amount in the infant. The administration of once-weekly doses, such as those used for malaria prophylaxis, would markedly reduce the amount of drug available to a nursing infant and, consequently, produce a much lower risk of accumulation and toxicity. The amount of hydroxychloroquine in breast milk is insufficient to protect against malaria in the infant. Breastfeeding while using this drug should be based on the mother's clinical need for treatment versus any potential infant risks that might occur. If used, the infant should be monitored for the most common reported adult side effects of nausea and abdominal pain (both leading to irritability), diarrhea, and vomiting.

H

References

1. Prescribing Information. Plaquenil. Concordia Pharmaceuticals, 2021.
2. Nguyen NV, Svenungsson E, Dominicus A, et al. Hydroxychloroquine in lupus or rheumatoid arthritis pregnancy and risk of major congenital malformations: a population-based cohort study. Rheumatology. 2025;64:117-125.
3. Chambers CD, Johnson DL, Xu R, et al. Birth Outcomes in Women Who Have Taken Hydroxycholoroquine During Pregnancy: A Prospective Cohort Study. Arthritis Rheumatol 2022;74:711-724.
4. Andersson NW, Skov L, Andersen JT. Fetal safety of chloroquine and hydroxychloroquine use during pregnancy: a nationwide cohort study. Rheumatology. 2021;60:2317-26.
5. Huybrechts KF, Bateman BT, Zhu Y, et al. Hydroxychloroquine early in pregnancy and risk of birth defects. Am J Obstet Gynecol. 2021;224:290.e1-290.e22.
6. Parke AL, Rothfield NF. Antimalarial drugs in pregnancy—the North American experience. *Lupus*. 1996;5(suppl 1):567-569.
7. Parke A, West B. Hydroxychloroquine in pregnant patients with systemic lupus erythematosus. *J Rheumatol*. 1996;23:1715-1718.
8. Heinonen OP, Slone D, Shapiro S. *Birth Defects and Drugs in Pregnancy*. Publishing Sciences Group; 1977:299.
9. Ross JB, Garatsos S. Absence of chloroquine-induced ototoxicity in a fetus. *Arch Dermatol*.1974;109:573.
10. Suhonen R. Hydroxychloroquine administration in pregnancy. *Arch Dermatol*. 1983;119:185-186.
11. Nation RL, Hackett LP, Dusci LJ, Ilett KF. Excretion of hydroxychloroquine in human milk. *Br J Clin Pharmacol*. 1984;17:368-369.
12. Ostensen M, Brown ND, Chiang PK, Aarbakke J. Hydroxychloroquine in human breast milk. *Eur J Clin Pharmacol*. 1985;28:357.
13. Anderson PO. Drug use during breast-feeding. *Clin Pharm*. 1991;10:594-624.
14. Committee on Drugs, American Academy of Pediatrics. The transfer of drugs and other chemicals into human milk. *Pediatrics*. 2001;108:776-789.

HYDROXYUREA

Antineoplastic (Antimetabolite)

PREGNANCY RECOMMENDATION: Limited Human Data—Animal Data Suggest Risk

BREASTFEEDING RECOMMENDATION: Potential Toxicity

PREGNANCY SUMMARY

Numerous case reports were located that (combined) described 25 first-trimester exposures to hydroxyurea. Of these, there were four (16%) spontaneous abortions, and one (4%) was delivered at term with multiple anomalies (ambiguous genitalia, several hemivertebrae, and 11 ribs). These percentages are within the expected rates for the general population. Of the remaining 20 pregnancies, no fetal anomalies were identified. Three deliveries were preterm at 36 weeks, 32 weeks, and one at 26 weeks of gestation, a stillbirth (no identified anomalies) following an eclamptic seizure (unrelated to the medication). The remaining 17 were all healthy term newborns with no reported complications. An additional nine cases were found with hydroxyurea exposure in the second and third trimesters. Of these, one had an NTD, but exposure in this case occurred at about 13 to 14 weeks of gestation, and therefore, was not the cause of the NTD. Of the remaining eight pregnancies, one was electively terminated at about 20 weeks' gestation (no anomalies found in the abortus) and the other seven delivered healthy neonates with no anomalies or complications (though two were preterm at 30 and 31 weeks' gestation). The drug will probably cross the placenta, so some fetal exposure will likely occur. Therefore, this limited human pregnancy experience prevents a complete assessment of the embryofetal risk. Animal studies did show embryofetal toxicity with malformations in eight species at doses less than 10 times the RHD. Based on animal studies and the drug's mechanism of action, the manufacturer recommends that women with reproductive potential use effective contraception during treatment and for 6 months after the last dose. They also recommend that males with female partners of reproductive potential use effective contraception during treatment and for 1 year after the last dose. Nevertheless, using this drug during pregnancy should be based on the pros and cons of the mother's clinical need for treatment versus any potential fetal risk that might occur from exposure. There is a registry for women who are pregnant and have cancer. For more information, women and health care providers are encouraged to contact the Cancer and Pregnancy Registry at 1-877-635-4499.

BREASTFEEDING SUMMARY

Hydroxyurea is excreted into human breast milk with identified levels ranging from 0.51 to 19.24 mcg/mL. Depending on the maternal size, these higher values could exceed 10% for an RID. Another study showed that the highest breast milk levels for hydroxyurea occurred in the first 2 to 3 hours after a dose. The breast milk levels were about 84% of the maternal plasma levels. All breast milk levels were negative (undetected) at 24 hours, consistent with the drug's short elimination half-life. The manufacturer recommends not breastfeeding while being treated with this drug. Nevertheless, breastfeeding while using this drug should be based on the mother's clinical need for treatment versus any potential infant risks that might occur. If used, the infant should be monitored for the most common reported adult side effects of nausea and headache (both leading to irritability), pyrexia, infections, neutropenia, anemia, and thrombocytopenia. Breastfeeding more than 3 hours after a dose should decrease the amount of infant exposure.

References

1. Product information. Droxia. E.R. Squibb & Sons; 2019.
2. Shepard TH. *Catalog of Teratogenic Agents*. 7th ed. The Johns Hopkins University Press; 1992:206-207.
3. Platzek T, Schwabe R. Combined prenatal toxicity of 6-mercaptopurine riboside and hydroxyurea in mice. *Teratog Carcinog Mutagen*. 1999;19:223-232.
4. Doney KC, Kraemer KG, Shepard TH. Combination chemotherapy for acute myelocytic leukemia during pregnancy: three case reports. *Cancer Treat Rep*. 1979;63:369-371.
5. Patel M, Dukes IAF, Hull JC. Use of hydroxyurea in chronic myeloid leukemia during pregnancy: a case report. *Am J Obstet Gynecol*. 1991;165:565-566.
6. Tertian G, Tchernia G, Papiernik E, Elefant E. Hydroxyurea and pregnancy. *Am J Obstet Gynecol*. 1992;166:1868.
7. Zemlickis D, Lishner M, Degendorfer P, et al. Fetal outcome after in utero exposure to cancer chemotherapy. *Arch Intern Med*. 1992;152:573-576.
8. Delmer A, Rio B, Bauduer F, et al. Pregnancy during myelosuppressive treatment for chronic myelogenous leukaemia. *Br J Haematol*. 1992;82:783-784.
9. Jackson N, Shukri A, Ali K. Hydroxyurea treatment for chronic myeloid leukaemia during pregnancy. *Br J Haematol*. 1993;85:203-204.
10. Fitzgerald JM, McCann SR. The combination of hydroxyurea and leucapheresis in the treatment of chronic myeloid leukaemia in pregnancy. *Clin Lab Haematol*. 1993;15:63-65.
11. Szanto F, Kovacs L. Successful delivery following continuous cytostatic therapy of a leukemic pregnant woman. *Orv Hetil*.1994;134:527-529. (article in Hungarian). As cited in Diav-Citrin O, Hunnisett L, Sher GD, Koren G. Hydroxyurea use during pregnancy: a case report in sickle cell disease and review of the literature. *Am J Hematol*. 1999;60:148-150.
12. Martin J, Ramesh A, Devadasan L, et al. An uneventful pregnancy and delivery, in a case with chronic myeloid leukemia on imatinib. *Indian J Med Paediatr Oncol*. 2011;32:109-111.
13. Choudhary DR, Mishra P, Kumar R, et al. Pregnancy on imatinib: fatal outcome with meningocele. *Ann Oncol*. 2006;17:178-179.
14. Dolai TK, Bhargava R, Mahapatra M, Mishra P, Seth T, Pati HP, Saxena R. Is imatinib safe during pregnancy? *Leuk Res*. 2009;33:572-573.
15. Cinkotai KI, Wood P, Donnai P, Kendra J. Pregnancy after treatment with hydroxyurea in a patient with primary thrombocythaemia and a history of recurrent abortion. *J Clin Pathol*. 1994;47:769-770.
16. Fernandez H. Essential thrombocythemia and pregnancy. *J Gynecol Obstet Biol Reprod*. 1994;23:103-104. (article in French). As cited in Diav-Citrin O, Hunniset L, Sher GD, Koren G. Hydroxyurea use during pregnancy: a case report in sickle cell disease and review of the literature. *Am J Hematol*. 1999;60:148-150.
17. Dell'Isola A, De Rosa G, Catalano D. Essential thrombocythemia in pregnancy. A case report and general considerations. *Minerva Ginecol*. 1997;49:165-172. (article in Italian). As cited in Diav-Citrin O, Hunnisett L, Sher GD, Koren G. Hydroxyurea use during pregnancy: a case report in sickle cell disease and review of the literature. *Am J Hematol*. 1999;60:148-150.
18. Perez-Encinas M, Bello JL, Perez-Crespo S, et al. Familial myeloproliferative syndrome. *Am J Hematol*. 1994;46:225-229.
19. Beressi AH, Tefferi A, Silverstein MN, et al. Outcome analysis of 34 pregnancies in women with essential thrombocythemia. *Arch Intern Med*. 1995; 155:1217-1222.
20. Wright CA, Tefferi A. A single institutional experience with 43 pregnancies in essential thrombocythemia. *Eur J Haematol*. 2001;66:152-159.
21. Oskuie AE, Valizadeh N. Successful outcome of pregnancy in a case of essential thrombocytosis treated with hydroxyurea. *Indian J Cancer*. 2011;48: 268-269.
22. Charache S, Terrin ML, Moore RD, et al, The Investigators of the Multicenter Study of Hydroxyurea in Sickle Cell Anemia. Effect of hydroxyurea on the frequency of painful crises in sickle cell anemia. *N Engl J Med*. 1995;332:1317-1322.
23. Diav-Citrin O, Hunnisett L, Sher GD, Koren G. Hydroxyurea use during pregnancy: a case report in sickle cell disease and review of the literature. *Am J Hematol*. 1999;60:148-150.
24. Byrd DC, Pitts SR, Alexander CK. Hydroxyurea in two pregnant women with sickle cell anemia. *Pharmacotherapy*. 1999;19:1459-1462.
25. Ballas SK, McCarthy WF, Guo N, et al; The investigators of the Multicenter Study of Hydroxyurea in Sickle Cell Anemia. Exposure to hydroxyurea and pregnancy outcomes in patients with sickle cell anemia. *J Natl Med Assoc*. 2009;101:1046-1051.
26. Italia KY, Jijina FF, Chandrakala S, et al. Exposure to hydroxyurea during pregnancy in sickle-β thalassemia: a report of a case. *J Clin Pharmacol*. 2010;30:231-234.
27. Rustin GJS, Booth M, Dent J, et al. Pregnancy after cytotoxic chemotherapy for gestational trophoblastic tumours. *Br Med J*. 1984;288:103-106.
28. Woolas RP, Bower M, Newlands ES, et al. Influence of chemotherapy for gestational trophoblastic disease on subsequent pregnancy outcome. *Br J Obstet Gynaecol*. 1998;105:1032-1035.
29. Pajor A, Zimonyi I, Koos R, et al. Pregnancies and offspring in survivors of acute lymphoid leukemia and lymphoma. *Eur J Obstet Gynecol Reprod Biol*. 1991;40:1-5.
30. Pata O, Tok CE, Yazici G, et al. Polycythemia vera and pregnancy: a case report with the use of hydroxyurea in the first trimester. *Am J Perinatol*. 2004;21:135-137.
31. Saleh AJM, Alhejazi A, Ahmed SO, et al. Leukemia during pregnancy: long term follow up of 32 cases from a single institution. *Hematol Oncol Stem Cell Ther*. 2014;712:63-68.
32. Sylvester RK, Lobell M, Teresi ME, et al. Excretion of hydroxyurea into milk. *Cancer*. 1987;60:2177-2178.

HYDROXYZINE

Antihistamine (H_1 Receptor Antagonist)

PREGNANCY RECOMMENDATION: Human Data Suggest Low Risk

BREASTFEEDING RECOMMENDATION: Probably Compatible

PREGNANCY SUMMARY

In combined data from several studies, 55 (5.2%) anomalies were reported in 1,062 first-trimester exposures. Even though this is slightly higher than the expected rate for major anomalies in the United States, no pattern to the anomalies was seen. The drug will probably cross the placenta, so some fetal exposure will likely occur. Animal studies found embryofetal toxicity with malformations in two species, but at doses of more than 10 times the RHD. The manufacturer states that the drug is contraindicated for use in pregnancy. Nevertheless, using this drug during pregnancy should be based on the pros and cons of the mother's clinical need for treatment versus any potential fetal risk that might occur from exposure. ACOG lists hydroxyzine as a treatment option for anxiety during pregnancy.

BREASTFEEDING SUMMARY

No reports describing the use of hydroxyzine during human lactation have been located. The drug will probably be found in breast milk, so some infant exposure will likely occur. The manufacturer considers hydroxyzine to be contraindicated for use in nursing mothers. Nevertheless, breastfeeding while using this drug should be based on the mother's clinical need for treatment versus any potential infant risks that might occur. If used, the infant should be monitored for the most common reported adult side effects of nausea, headache, and dizziness (all leading to irritability), fatigue (lethargy), constipation, and somnolence.

References

1. Product information. Vistaril. Pfizer Laboratories Div Pfizer; 2019.
2. Product information. Atarax. Roerig; 2016.
3. King CTG, Howell J. Teratogenic effect of buclizine and hydroxyzine in the rat and chlorcyclizine in the mouse. *Am J Obstet Gynecol*. 1966;95:109-111.
4. Posner HS, Darr A. Fetal edema from benzhydrylpiperazines as a possible cause of oral-facial malformations in rats. *Toxicol Appl Pharmacol*. 1970;17:67-75.
5. Walker BE, Patterson A. Induction of cleft palate in mice by tranquilizers and barbiturates. *Teratology*. 1974;10:159-164.
6. Steffek AJ, King CTG, Wilk AL. Abortive effects and comparative metabolism of chlorcyclizine in various mammalian species. *Teratology*. 1968;1:399-406.
7. Erez S, Schifrin BS, Dirim O. Double-blind evaluation of hydroxyzine as an antiemetic in pregnancy. *J Reprod Med*. 1971;7:57-59.
8. Romero R, Olsen TG, Chervenak FA, Hobbins JC. Pruritic urticarial papules and plaques of pregnancy. A case report. *J Reprod Med*. 1983;28:615-619.
9. Heinonen OP, Slone D, Shapiro S. *Birth Defects and Drugs in Pregnancy*. Publishing Sciences Group; 1977.
10. Prenner BM. Neonatal withdrawal syndrome associated with hydroxyzine hydrochloride. *Am J Dis Child*. 1977;131:529-530.
11. Nageotte MP, Briggs GG, Towers CV, Asrat T. Droperidol and diphenhydramine in the management of hyperemesis gravidarum. *Am J Obstet Gynecol*. 1996;174:1801-1806.
12. Turcotte V, Ferreira E, Duperron L. Utilité du dropéridol et de la diphenhydramine dans l'hyperemesis gravidarum. *J Soc Obstet Gynaecol Can*. 2001; 23:133-139.
13. Einarson A, Bailey B, Jung G, et al. Prospective controlled study of hydroxyzine and cetirizine in pregnancy. *Ann Allergy Asthma Immunol*. 1997;78: 183-186.
14. Schatz M, Petitti D. Antihistamines and pregnancy. *Ann Allergy Asthma Immunol*. 1997;78:157-159.
15. Serreau R, Komiha M, Blanc F, et al. Neonatal seizures associated with maternal hydroxyzine in late pregnancy. *Reprod Toxicol*. 2005;20:573-574.
16. Zsigmond EK, Patterson RL. Double-blind evaluation of hydroxyzine hydrochloride in obstetric anesthesia. *Anesth Analg (Cleveland)*. 1967;46:275-280.
17. Amato G, Corsini D, Pelliccia E. Personal experience with a combination of Althesin and Atarax in caesarean section. *Minerva Anestesiol*. 1980;46: 671-674.
18. Petrie RH, Yeh S-Y, Murata Y, et al. The effects of drugs on fetal heart rate variability. *Am J Obstet Gynecol*. 1978;130:294-299.
19. Whaun JM, Smith GR, Sochor VA. Effect of prenatal drug administration on maternal and neonatal platelet aggregation and PF_4 release. *Haemostasis*. 1980;9:226-237.

HYOSCYAMINE

Autonomic (Parasympatholytic/Anticholinergic)

PREGNANCY RECOMMENDATION: Human Data Suggest Low Risk—No Relevant Animal Data

BREASTFEEDING RECOMMENDATION: Probably Compatible

PREGNANCY SUMMARY

In the combined data from the Michigan Medicaid US Food and Drug Administration (FDA) recipient study and the Collaborative Perinatal Project, a total of 603 first-trimester exposures to hyoscyamine were identified, and 26 (4.3%) infants with malformations were reported. No specific pattern was seen in the anomalies. Also from the Collaborative Perinatal Project, overall, there were 1,067 exposures to hyoscyamine at any time during the pregnancy, with 22 (2.1%) malformations reported. Again, no specific pattern was noted, and coexposures to other drugs occurred in both databases. Based on likely placental transfer, some fetal exposure will probably occur. Animal reproduction studies have not been performed. Using this drug during pregnancy should be based on the pros and cons of the mother's clinical need for treatment versus any potential fetal risk that might occur from exposure. Lastly, parasympathetic blocking agents can alter the appearance of the fetal heart monitor tracing by causing an elevation of the baseline rate and decreasing variability (see atropine).

BREASTFEEDING SUMMARY

No reports describing the use of hyoscyamine during human lactation have been located. The drug will probably be found in breast milk, so some infant exposure will likely occur. The manufacturer states that only traces of the drug are found in breast milk. Breastfeeding while using this drug should be based on the mother's clinical need for treatment. If used, the infant should be monitored for the most common reported adult side effects of nausea, abdominal pain, and headache (all leading to irritability), diarrhea, lethargy, vomiting, constipation, dry mouth, tachycardia, and urinary retention. In addition, because this drug has anticholinergic effects, there is a possibility of interfering with breast milk production development in the early stages of breastfeeding and may decrease breast milk supply over time.

References

1. Prescribing Information. Hyoscyamine. Wallace Pharmaceuticals, Inc; 2019.
2. Heinonen OP, Slone D, Shapiro S. *Birth Defects and Drugs in Pregnancy*. Publishing Sciences Group; 1983:346-347,350,354,439.

HYPERALIMENTATION

Nutrient (Total Parenteral Nutrition)

PREGNANCY RECOMMENDATION: Human Data Suggest Low Risk

BREASTFEEDING RECOMMENDATION: Probably Compatible

PREGNANCY SUMMARY

Numerous case reports and two literature reviews have described the use of hyperalimentation during pregnancy, including use in the first trimester. It is felt that the procedure is a relatively safe and effective method for reversing maternal malnutrition and promoting normal fetal growth and development. Because hyperalimentation products contain amino acids, lipids, and other nutrients normally found in the blood of humans, most, if not all, of these individual substances will cross the placenta (at their expected rate). Animal reproduction studies have not been performed. The use of total parenteral nutrition (TPN) does not pose a significant risk to the fetus or newborn, provided that normal procedures, as with nonpregnant patients, are followed to prevent maternal complications. Amino acid preparations pose a risk for vein damage or thrombosis, pulmonary embolism due to pulmonary vascular precipitates, and hyperglycemia (maternal glucose should be monitored). Lipid emulsions pose a risk for fat overload syndrome and hypertriglyceridemia. Both products pose risks for infections, hypersensitivity reactions, parenteral nutrition-associated liver disease, and aluminum toxicity. Therefore, using these products during pregnancy should be based on the pros and cons of the mother's clinical need for treatment versus any potential fetal risk that might occur from exposure.

BREASTFEEDING SUMMARY

Several case reports were located that described successful breastfeeding while receiving TPN. Overall, no complications were reported, and the infants did well. Breastfeeding while receiving these products should be based on the mother's clinical need for treatment versus any potential infant risks that might occur. If used, the infant should be monitored for growth.

References

1. Hew LR, Deitel M. Total parenteral nutrition in gynecology and obstetrics. *Obstet Gynecol.* 1980;55:464-468.
2. Tresadern JC, Falconer GF, Turnberg LA, Irving MH. Successful completed pregnancy in a patient maintained on home parenteral nutrition. *Br Med J.* 1983;286:602-603.
3. Tresadern JC, Falconer GF, Turnberg LA, Irving MH. Maintenance of pregnancy in a home parenteral nutrition patient. *J Parenter Enteral Nutr.* 1984;8:199-202.
4. Breen KJ, McDonald IA, Panelli D, Ihle B. Planned pregnancy in a patient who was receiving home parenteral nutrition. *Med J Aust.* 1987;146:215-217.
5. Levine MG, Esser D. Total parenteral nutrition for the treatment of severe hyperemesis gravidarum: maternal nutritional effects and fetal outcome. *Obstet Gynecol.* 1988;72:102-107.
6. Gineston JL, Capron JP, Delcenserie R, et al. Prolonged total parenteral nutrition in a pregnant woman with acute pancreatitis. *J Clin Gastroenterol.* 1984;6:249-252.
7. Lakoff KM, Feldman JD. Anorexia nervosa associated with pregnancy. *Obstet Gynecol.* 1972;39:699-701.
8. Lavin JP Jr, Gimmon Z, Miodovnik M, et al. Total parenteral nutrition in a pregnant insulin-requiring diabetic. *Obstet Gynecol.* 1982;59:660-664.
9. Weinberg RB, Sitrin MD, Adkins GM, Lin CC. Treatment of hyperlipidemic pancreatitis in pregnancy with total parenteral nutrition. *Gastroenterology.* 1982;83:1300-1305.
10. Di Costanzo J, Martin J, Cano N, et al. Total parenteral nutrition with fat emulsions during pregnancy—nutritional requirements: a case report. *JPEN.* 1982;6:534-538.
11. Young KR. Acute pancreatitis in pregnancy: two case reports. *Obstet Gynecol.* 1982;60:653-657.
12. Rivera-Alsina ME, Saldana LR, Stringer CA. Fetal growth sustained by parenteral nutrition in pregnancy. *Obstet Gynecol.* 1984;64:138-141.
13. Seifer DB, Silberman H, Catanzarite VA, et al. Total parenteral nutrition in obstetrics. *JAMA.* 1985;253:2073-2075.
14. Benny PS, Legge M, Aickin DR. The biochemical effects of maternal hyperalimentation during pregnancy. *NZ Med J.* 1978;88:283-285.
15. Cox KL, Byrne WJ, Ament ME. Home total parenteral nutrition during pregnancy: a case report. *JPEN.* 1981;5:246-249.
16. Gamberdella FR. Pancreatic carcinoma in pregnancy: a case report. *Am J Obstet Gynecol.* 1984;149:15-17.
17. Loludice TA, Chandrakaar C. Pregnancy and jejunoileal bypass: treatment complications with total parenteral nutrition. *South Med J.* 1980;73:256-258.
18. Main ANH, Shenkin A, Black WP, Russell RI. Intravenous feeding to sustain pregnancy in patient with Crohn's disease. *Br Med J.* 1981;283:1221-1222.
19. Webb GA. The use of hyperalimentation and chemotherapy in pregnancy: a case report. *Am J Obstet Gynecol.* 1980;137:263-266.
20. Stowell JC, Bottsford JE Jr, Rubel HR. Pancreatitis with pseudocyst and cholelithiasis in third trimester of pregnancy: management with total parenteral nutrition. *South Med J.* 1984;77:502-504.
21. Martin R, Trubow M, Bistrian BR, et al. Hyperalimentation during pregnancy: a case report. *JPEN.* 1985;9:212-215.
22. Herbert WNP, Seeds JW, Bowes WA, Sweeney CA. Fetal growth response to total parenteral nutrition in pregnancy: a case report. *J Reprod Med.* 1986;31:263-266.
23. Hatjis CG, Meis PJ. Total parenteral nutrition in pregnancy. *Obstet Gynecol.* 1985;66:585-589.
24. Adami GF, Friedman D, Cuneo S, et al. Intravenous nutritional support in pregnancy. Experience following biliopancreatic diversion. *Clin Nutr.* 1992;11:106-109.
25. Satin AJ, Twickler D, Gilstrap LC III. Esophageal achalasia in late pregnancy. *Obstet Gynecol.* 1992;79:812-814.
26. Teuscher AU, Sutherland DER, Robertson RP. Successful pregnancy after pancreatic islet autotransplantation. *Transplant Proc.* 1994;26:3520.
27. Lee RV, Rodgers BD, Young C, et al. Total parenteral nutrition during pregnancy. *Obstet Gynecol.* 1986;68:563-571.
28. Wolk RA, Rayburn WF. Parenteral nutrition in obstetric patients. *Nutr Clin Pract.* 1990;5:139-152.
29. Greenspoon JS, Masaki DI, Kurz CR. Cardiac tamponade in pregnancy during central hyperalimentation. *Obstet Gynecol.* 1989;73:465-466.
30. Jasnosz KM, Pickeral JJ, Graner S. Fat deposits in the placenta following maternal total parenteral nutrition with intravenous lipid emulsion. *Arch Pathol Lab Med.* 1995;119:555-557.

I

IBALIZUMAB

Antiviral (Antiretroviral/Monoclonal Antibody)

PREGNANCY RECOMMENDATION: No Human Data—Animal Data Suggest Potential Risk (Maternal Benefit May Outweigh Embryofetal Risk)

BREASTFEEDING RECOMMENDATION: *Contraindicated

PREGNANCY SUMMARY

No reports describing the use of ibalizumab in human pregnancy have been located. Immunoglobulin G (IgG) antibodies are known to cross the placenta, especially during the second half of gestation, so some fetal exposure will likely occur. The US Department of Health and Human Services AIDS Info guidelines (https://clinicalinfo.hiv.gov/en/guidelines/perinatal/) for the use of antiretroviral agents during pregnancy recommend that, in most cases, patients continue their regimen during pregnancy if it is tolerated, safe, and effective in suppressing viral replication. The guideline recommends that discussion and shared decision-making about the known and potential risks, as well as benefits to the mother and fetus, acknowledging limited data, should guide the selection of which antiretrovirals to use during pregnancy. Additionally, treatment initiation should not be delayed due to concerns about teratogenicity with first-trimester exposure. See the guideline for the most updated information. If indicated, ibalizumab should not be withheld in pregnancy since the expected benefit to the mother with HIV outweighs the unknown risk to the fetus. The guidelines note that ibalizumab is not recommended except in special circumstances. Additionally, based on animal studies, ibalizumab may cause reversible immunosuppression ($CD4^+$ T cell and B cell lymphocytopenia). The manufacturer recommends that infants exposed to ibalizumab undergo immune phenotyping of the peripheral blood, including $CD4^+$ T cell and B cell counts. Expert consultation is also recommended to provide guidance on the monitoring and management of exposed infants based on the degree of immunosuppression observed. Providers caring for pregnant patients with HIV and their infants can call the national Perinatal HIV/AIDS hotline (888-448-8765) for free clinical consultation. Additionally, there is a pregnancy exposure registry that monitors pregnancy outcomes in individuals exposed to antiretroviral medications during pregnancy. Health care providers are encouraged to register patients by calling the Antiretroviral Pregnancy Registry (APR) at 1-800-258-4263.

BREASTFEEDING SUMMARY

No reports describing the use of ibalizumab during human lactation have been located. It is known that IgG antibodies are excreted into breast milk but are not found in neonatal or infant circulation. Additionally, if any IgG antibodies were to be ingested through breastfeeding, they would probably be digested in the infant's gastrointestinal tract and not absorbed. The US Department of Health and Human Services AIDS Info guidelines state that using replacement of breast milk through formula or pasteurized donor human breast milk from a milk bank eliminates the risk of postnatal HIV transmission to the infant. Using antiretroviral therapy to achieve and maintain viral suppression during pregnancy and postpartum decreases the risk for infant transmission to less than 1% but not zero. *For patients not on therapy or those without viral load suppression during pregnancy (at a minimum of throughout the third trimester) and at delivery, replacement of breast milk is recommended. Patients on antiretroviral therapy who have a sustained undetectable viral load and who choose to breastfeed or use replacement of breast milk should be supported with this decision. If the clinical decision is to use this drug while breastfeeding, the infant should be monitored for the most common reported adult side effects of dizziness and nausea (both leading to irritability), diarrhea, and rash.

References

1. Prescribing Information. Trogarzo. Theratechnologies; 2023.
2. Panel on Treatment of HIV During Pregnancy and Prevention of Perinatal Transmission. Recommendations for the Use of Antiretroviral Drugs During Pregnancy and Interventions to Reduce Perinatal HIV Transmission in the United States. Department of Health and Human Services; 2024. Accessed March 4, 2024. https://clinicalinfo.hiv.gov/en/guidelines/perinatal

IBANDRONATE

Bone Health (Bisphosphonate)

PREGNANCY RECOMMENDATION: *Contraindicated

BREASTFEEDING RECOMMENDATION: *Contraindicated

PREGNANCY SUMMARY

One report describing the use of ibandronate in the third trimester of pregnancy resulted in a healthy infant with no malformations, anemia, or organ dysfunction detected. The drug will probably cross the placenta, so some fetal exposure can occur. However, this limited human pregnancy experience prevents a complete assessment of the embryofetal risk. Embryofetal toxicity was observed in one animal species at doses of less than 10 times the recommended human dose (RHD). *However, based on the drug's approval, it is for postmenopausal women, and therefore, would be contraindicated for use during pregnancy. Bisphosphonates are incorporated into the bone matrix and are gradually released over time. Moreover, animal data suggest that fetal bone has a greater uptake of bisphosphonates than that of maternal bone. Therefore, there is a potential risk of fetal harm, including hypocalcemia, skeletal, and other abnormalities.

BREASTFEEDING SUMMARY

No reports describing the use of ibandronate during human lactation have been located. The drug will probably appear in breast milk, so some infant exposure would likely occur. Although the oral bioavailability in infants differs from that of adults, the very low adult oral bioavailability (<1%) and the binding of ibandronate by the calcium in breast milk suggest that the amount absorbed by the infant would be clinically insignificant. *However, based on the drug's approval, it is for postmenopausal women, and therefore, would be contraindicated for use during breastfeeding. If used while breastfeeding, the infant should be monitored for the most common reported adult side effects of headache, pain in extremity, muscle pain, and back pain (all leading to irritability), reflux, and diarrhea.

References

1. Prescribing Information. Boniva Tablets. Roche Therapeutics, Inc; 2015.
2. Prescribing Information. Boniva Injection. Roche Therapeutics, Inc; 2015.
3. El-Safadi S, Wuesten O, Muenstedt K. Primary diagnosis of metastatic breast cancer in the third trimester of pregnancy: a case report and review of the literature. *J Obstet Gynaecol Res*. 2012;38:589-592.
4. Djokanovic N, Klieger-Grossmann C, Koren G. Does treatment with bisphosphonates endanger the human pregnancy? *J Obstet Gynaecol Can*. 2008; 30(12):1146-1148.
5. Levy S, Fayez I, Taguchi N, et al. Pregnancy outcome following in utero exposure to bisphosphonates. *Bone*. 2009;44:428-430.
6. Stathopoulos IP, Liakou CG, Katsalira A, et al. The use of bisphosphonates in women prior to or during pregnancy and lactation. *Hormones (Athens)*. 2011;10:280-291.
7. Green SB, Pappas AL. Effects of maternal bisphosphonate use on fetal and neonatal outcomes. *Am J Health Syst Pharm*. 2014;71:2029-2036.
8. Machairiotis N, Ntali G, Kouroutou P, Michala L. Clinical evidence of the effect of bisphosphonates on pregnancy and the infant. *Horm Mol Biol Clin Investig*. 2019;40.
9. Sokal A, Elefant E, Leturcq T, et al. Pregnancy and newborn outcomes after exposure to bisphosphonates: a case-control study. *Osteoporos Int*. 2019;30: 221-229.

IBREXAFUNGERP

Antifungal

PREGNANCY RECOMMENDATION: Limited Human Data—Animal Data Suggest Potential Risk

BREASTFEEDING RECOMMENDATION: Probably Compatible

PREGNANCY SUMMARY

Limited reports describing ibrexafungerp exposure during human pregnancy have been located. In the clinical trials, four pregnancy exposures were reported, of which one was electively terminated. The other three cases (unknown gestational ages of exposure) resulted in live births without any reported adverse effects or malformations. No other information about the pregnancies or infants is available. Based on likely placental transfer of some of the drug, fetal exposure will probably occur. Therefore, this limited human pregnancy experience prevents a complete assessment of the embryofetal risk. Embryofetal toxicity with malformations was observed in one animal species. Based on the animal studies, the manufacturer recommends that women with reproductive potential use effective contraception during treatment and for at least 4 days after the last dose. In women with reproductive potential using ibrexafungerp for reduction in the incidence of recurrent vulvovaginal candidiasis, the manufacturer also recommends that the patient use effective contraception throughout the 6-month treatment period and for 4 days after the last dose. Nevertheless, using this drug during pregnancy should be based on the pros and cons of the mother's clinical need for treatment versus any potential fetal risk that might occur from exposure. There is a pregnancy exposure registry that monitors pregnancy outcomes in women using this drug. Health care providers and women are encouraged to contact the Brexafemme Pregnancy Safety Study at 1-888-982-7299.

BREASTFEEDING SUMMARY

No reports describing the use of ibrexafungerp during human lactation have been located. The drug will likely be found in breast milk, so some infant exposure will probably occur. Breastfeeding while using this drug should be based on the mother's clinical need for treatment. If used, the infant should be monitored for the most common reported adult side effects of nausea, abdominal pain, and headache (all leading to irritability), diarrhea, vomiting, urinary tract infection, and lethargy.

References

1. Prescribing Information. Brexafemme. Scynexis; 2022.
2. Sobel R, Nyirjesy P, Ghannoum MA, et al. Efficacy and safety of oral ibrexafungerp for the treatment of acute vulvovaginal candidiasis: a global phase 3, randomised, placebo-controlled superiority study (VANISH 306). *BJOG*. 2022;129:412-420.
3. Nyirjesy P, Schwebke JR, Angulo DA, et al. Phase 2 randomized study of oral ibrexafungerp vs fluconazole in vulvovaginal candidiasis. *Clin Infect Dis*. 2022;74:2129-2135.
4. Schwebke JR, Sobel R, Gersten JK, et al. Ibrexafungerp versus placebo for vulvovaginal candidiasis treatment: a phase 3, randomized, controlled superiority trial (VANISH 303). *Clin Infect Dis*. 2022;74:1979-1985.

IBRITUMOMAB TIUXETAN

Antineoplastic (Monoclonal Antibody)

PREGNANCY RECOMMENDATION: *Contraindicated

BREASTFEEDING RECOMMENDATION: *Contraindicated

PREGNANCY SUMMARY

No reports describing the use of ibritumomab tiuxetan in human pregnancy have been located. IgG antibodies are known to cross the placenta, especially during the third trimester, so some fetal exposure will likely occur. However, the absence of human pregnancy experience prevents a complete assessment of the embryofetal risk. No animal reproduction studies have been conducted. *Because the tiuxetan agent is radioactive, the manufacturer recommends that women with reproductive potential who are taking ibritumomab tiuxetan use effective contraception during treatment and for at least 12 months after the last dose. They also recommend that males with female partners of reproductive potential use effective contraception during treatment and for at least 12 months after the last dose. There is a registry for women who are pregnant and have cancer. For more information, women and health care providers are encouraged to contact the Cancer and Pregnancy Registry at 1-877-635-4499.

BREASTFEEDING SUMMARY

No reports describing the use of ibritumomab tiuxetan during human lactation have been located. It is known that IgG antibodies are excreted into breast milk but are not found in neonatal or infant circulation. Additionally, if any IgG antibodies were to be ingested through breastfeeding, they would probably be digested in the infant's gastrointestinal tract and not absorbed. *However, because the tiuxetan agent is radioactive, the manufacturer recommends that women not breastfeed while being treated with this drug and for at least 6 months after the last dose. If the clinical decision is to use this drug while breastfeeding, the infant should be monitored for the most common reported adult side effects of nausea and abdominal pain (both leading to irritability), fatigue (lethargy), cough, diarrhea, fever, and various laboratory abnormalities (see Prescribing Information [PI]).

Reference

1. Prescribing Information. Zevalin. Acrotech Biopharma LLC; 2019.

IBRUTINIB

Antineoplastic (Tyrosine Kinase Inhibitor)

PREGNANCY RECOMMENDATION: No Human Data—Animal Data Suggest Risk

BREASTFEEDING RECOMMENDATION: Potential Toxicity

PREGNANCY SUMMARY

No reports describing the use of ibrutinib in human pregnancy have been located. The drug will probably cross the placenta, so some fetal exposure will likely occur. However, the absence of human pregnancy experience prevents a complete assessment of the embryofetal risk. Embryofetal toxicity was observed in two animal species at doses of less than 10 times the RHD. Based on these animal studies and the drug's mechanism of action, the manufacturer recommends that women with reproductive potential use effective contraception during treatment and for 1 month after the last dose. They also recommend that males with female partners of reproductive potential use effective contraception during treatment and for 1 month after the last dose. Nevertheless, using this drug during pregnancy should be based on the pros and cons of the mother's clinical need for treatment versus any potential fetal risk that might occur from exposure. There is a registry for women who are pregnant and have cancer. For more information, women and health care providers are encouraged to contact the Cancer and Pregnancy Registry at 1-877-635-4499.

BREASTFEEDING SUMMARY

No reports describing the use of ibrutinib during human lactation have been located. The drug will probably appear in breast milk, so some infant exposure will likely occur. However, due to a concern for potential serious adverse effects that might be seen in a breastfed infant, the manufacturer recommends that women not breastfeed while being treated with this drug and for at least 1 week after the last dose. Nevertheless, breastfeeding while using this drug should be based on the mother's clinical need for treatment versus any potential infant risks that might occur. If used, the infant should be monitored for the most common reported adult side effects of nausea, musculoskeletal pain, and abdominal pain (all leading to irritability), fatigue (lethargy), diarrhea, bruising, rash, fever, bleeding, and various laboratory abnormalities (see PI).

Reference

1. Prescribing Information. Imbruvica. Pharmacyclics LLC; 2024.

I

IBUPROFEN

Pain (Nonsteroidal Anti-Inflammatory Drug)

PREGNANCY RECOMMENDATION: Human Data Suggest Risk (Second and Third Trimesters)

BREASTFEEDING RECOMMENDATION: Probably Compatible

PREGNANCY SUMMARY

Numerous reports describing the use of ibuprofen in all trimesters of human pregnancy have been located. Many have suggested the possibility of producing major fetal anomalies, but overall, the studies have been contradictory, and no specific pattern to the anomalies has been described. The drug crosses the placenta, so fetal exposure will occur. Animal data did not show embryofetal toxicity in two species at doses of greater than 10 times the RHD. Nonsteroidal anti-inflammatory drugs (NSAIDs) can cause premature stricture or closure of the fetal ductus arteriosus when used in the latter portion of gestation. In some instances, this can produce pulmonary hypertension in the neonate. These drugs have also been reported to produce fetal renal dysfunction leading to oligohydramnios when used after 20 weeks' gestation. The US Food and Drug Administration (FDA) recommends that NSAIDs be avoided in women 20 weeks or later in pregnancy. If deemed necessary by a health care provider, the use of NSAIDs between 20 and 30 weeks should be limited to the lowest effective dose and shortest duration. If treatment extends beyond 48 hours, providers should consider an ultrasound to monitor amniotic fluid levels.

BREASTFEEDING SUMMARY

One report describing 21 infant outcomes of ibuprofen use during human lactation has been located. No adverse effects were reported. Very low amounts of ibuprofen are present in breast milk. Breastfeeding while using this drug should be based on the mother's clinical need for treatment versus any potential infant risks that might occur. If used, the infant should be monitored for the most common reported adult side effects of gastrointestinal distress (leading to irritability), diarrhea, and vomiting. Overall, short-term use of NSAIDs is probably compatible.

References

1. Levin DL. Effects of inhibition of prostaglandin synthesis on fetal development, oxygenation, and the fetal circulation. *Semin Perinatol*. 1980;4:35-44.
2. Van Marter LJ, Leviton A, Allred EN, et al. Persistent pulmonary hypertension of the newborn and smoking and aspirin and nonsteroidal antiinflammatory drug consumption during pregnancy. *Pediatrics*. 1996;97:658-663.
3. Alano MA, Ngougmna E, Ostrea EM Jr, Konduri GG. Analysis of nonsteroidal antiinflammatory drugs in meconium and its relation to persistent pulmonary hypertension of the newborn. *Pediatrics*. 2001;107:519-523.
4. Fuchs F. Prevention of prematurity. *Am J Obstet Gynecol*. 1976;126:809-820.
5. Powell JG, Cochrane RL. The effects of a number of non-steroidal anti-inflammatory compounds on parturition in the rat. *Prostaglandins*. 1982;23:469-488.
6. Matt DW, Borzelleca JF. Toxic effects on the female reproductive system during pregnancy, parturition, and lactation. In: Witorsch RJ, ed. *Reproductive Toxicology*. 2nd ed. Raven Press; 1995:175-193.
7. Dawood MY. Nonsteroidal antiinflammatory drugs and reproduction. *Am J Obstet Gynecol*. 1993;169:1255-1265.
8. Prescribing Information. RedPharm Drug, Inc; 2024.
9. Barry WS, Meinzinger MM, Howse CR. Ibuprofen overdose and exposure in utero: results from a postmarketing voluntary reporting system. *Am J Med*. 1984;77(1A):35-39.
10. Nielsen GL, Sorensen HT, Larsen H, Pedersen L. Risk of adverse birth outcome and miscarriage in pregnant users of non-steroidal anti-inflammatory drugs: population based observational study and case-control study. *Br Med J*. 2001;322:266-270.
11. Li DK, Liu L, Odouli R. Exposure to non-steroidal anti-inflammatory drugs during pregnancy and risk of miscarriage: population based cohort study. *Br Med J*. 2003;327:368-371.
12. Ericson A, Kallen BAJ. Nonsteroidal anti-inflammatory drugs in early pregnancy. *Reprod Toxicol*. 2001;15:371-375.
13. Kallen BAJ, Olausson PO. Maternal drug use in early pregnancy and infant cardiovascular defect. *Reprod Toxicol*. 2003;17:255-261.

14. Torfs CP, Katz EA, Bateson TF, et al. Maternal medications and environmental exposures as risk factors for gastroschisis. *Teratology*. 1996;54:84-92.
15. Ofori B, Oraichi D, Blais L, et al. Risk of congenital anomalies in pregnant users of non-steroidal anti-inflammatory drugs: a nested case-control study. *Birth Defects Res B Dev Reprod Toxicol*. 2006;77:268-279.
16. Cleves MA, Savell VH Jr, Raj S, et al.; the National Birth Defects Prevention Study. Maternal use of acetaminophen and nonsteroidal anti-inflammatory drugs (NSAIDs), and muscular ventricular septal defects. *Birth Defects Res A Clin Mol Teratol*. 2004;70:107-113.
17. Hickok DE, Hollenbach KA, Reilley SF, Nyberg DA. The association between decreased amniotic fluid volume and treatment with nonsteroidal anti-inflammatory agents for preterm labor. *Am J Obstet Gynecol*. 1989;160:1525-1531.
18. Wiggins DA, Elliott JP. Oligohydramnios in each sac of a triplet gestation caused by Motrin—fulfilling Kock's postulates. *Am J Obstet Gynecol*. 1990;162:460-461.
19. Hennessy MD, Livingston EC, Papagianos J, Killam AP. The incidence of ductal constriction and oligohydramnios during tocolytic therapy with ibuprofen (abstract). *Am J Obstet Gynecol*. 1992;166:324.
20. Glover DD, Amonkar M, Rybeck BF, Tracy TS. Prescription, over-the-counter, and herbal medicine use in a rural, obstetric population. *Am J Obstet Gynecol*. 2003;188:1039-1045.
21. Hernandez RK, Werler MM, Romitti P, et al.; National Birth Defects Prevention Study. Nonsteroidal antiinflammatory drug use among women and the risk of birth defects. *Am J Obstet Gynecol*. 2012;206:228.e1-228.e8.
22. Brandlistuen RE, Ystrom E, Nulman I, et al. Prenatal paracetamol exposure and child neurodevelopment: a sibling-controlled cohort study. *Int J Epidemiol*. 2013;42:1702-1713.
23. Townsend RJ, Benedetti T, Erickson S, et al. A study to evaluate the passage of ibuprofen into breast milk (abstract). *Drug Intell Clin Pharm*. 1982;16:482-483.
24. Townsend RJ, Benedetti TJ, Erickson S, et al. Excretion of ibuprofen into breast milk. *Am J Obstet Gynecol*. 1984;149:184-186.
25. Weibert RT, Townsend RJ, Kaiser DG, Naylor AJ. Lack of ibuprofen secretion into human milk. *Clin Pharm*. 1982;1:457-458.
26. Walter K, Dilger C. Ibuprofen in human milk. *Br J Clin Pharmacol*. 1997;44:209-213.
27. Ito S, Blajchman A, Stephenson M. Prospective follow-up of adverse reactions in breast-fed infants exposed to maternal medication. *Am J Obstet Gynecol*. 1993;168:1393-1399.
28. Leverrier-Penna S, Mitchell RT, Becker E, et al. Ibuprofen is deleterious for the development of first trimester human fetal ovary ex vivo. *Hum Reprod*. 2018;33:482-493.
29. U.S. Food and Drug Administration. FDA recommends avoiding use of NSAIDs in pregnancy at 20 weeks or later because they can result in low amniotic fluid. FDA Drug Safety Communication; Accessed September 12, 2024. https://www.fda.gov/drugs/drug-safety-and-availability/fda-recommends-avoiding-use-nsaids-pregnancy-20-weeks-or-later-because-they-can-result-low-amniotic

I

IBUTILIDE

Cardiovascular (Antiarrhythmic)

PREGNANCY RECOMMENDATION: Limited Human Data—Animal Data Suggest Potential Risk

BREASTFEEDING RECOMMENDATION: Probably Compatible

PREGNANCY SUMMARY

Two reports have described the successful use of ibutilide to convert three women to a sinus rhythm during the second half of pregnancy. All three pregnancies resulted in a healthy term delivery. No additional information was provided on the status of the newborns. Some amount of the drug will probably cross the placenta, so fetal exposure will likely occur. However, this limited human pregnancy experience prevents a complete assessment of the embryofetal risk. Embryofetal toxicity with malformations was observed in one animal species at doses of less than 10 times the RHD. Using this drug during pregnancy should be based on the pros and cons of the mother's clinical need for treatment versus any potential fetal risk that might occur from exposure. Ibutilide is associated with QT prolongation.

BREASTFEEDING SUMMARY

No reports describing the use of ibutilide during human lactation have been located. The drug will probably be excreted into breast milk, so some infant exposure will likely occur. However, its low oral bioavailability suggests that a nursing infant would absorb minimal amounts. However, due to the lack of data, the manufacturer recommends that women should not breastfeed during treatment with this drug. Nevertheless, breastfeeding while using this drug should be based on the mother's clinical need for treatment versus any potential infant risks that might occur. If used, the infant should be monitored for the most common reported adult side effects of nausea and headache (both leading to irritability) and tachycardia.

References

1. Prescribing Information. Corvert, Pharmacia & Upjohn Company LLC; 2023.
2. Marks TA, Terry RD. Developmental toxicity of ibutilide fumarate in rats (abstract). *Teratology*. 1995;49:406.
3. Marks TA, Terry RD. Developmental toxicity of ibutilide fumarate in rats after oral administration. *Teratology*. 1996;54:157-164.
4. Burkart TA, Kron J, Miles WM, et al. Successful termination of atrial flutter by ibutilide during pregnancy. *Pacing Clin Electrophysiol*. 2007;30:283-286.
5. Kockova R, Kocka V, Kiernan T, Fahy GJ. Ibutilide-induced cardioversion of atrial fibrillation during pregnancy. *J Cardiovasc Electrophysiol*. 2007;18:545-547.

ICATIBANT

Miscellaneous (Bradykinin B_2 Receptor Antagonist)

PREGNANCY RECOMMENDATION: Limited Human Data—Animal Data Suggest Risk

BREASTFEEDING RECOMMENDATION: Probably Compatible

PREGNANCY SUMMARY

Six reports describing the use of icatibant in 12 human pregnancies in all trimesters have been located. All infants were healthy at delivery, and all, except one, were delivered at term. A limited amount of the drug may cross the placenta, so some fetal exposure might occur. However, this limited human pregnancy experience prevents a complete assessment of the embryofetal risk. Embryofetal toxicity was observed in two animal species at doses less than 10 times the RHD. Using this drug during pregnancy should be based on the pros and cons of the mother's clinical need for treatment versus any potential fetal risk that might occur from exposure.

BREASTFEEDING SUMMARY

One report was located that described the use of icatibant as needed in treating hereditary angioedema attacks in a breastfeeding mother. Icatibant was used after the final breastfeeding before bedtime and resumed 6 hours or more after the last dose of icatibant. No adverse effects were reported. The drug may be excreted into breast milk, so some infant exposure might occur. Additionally, as a peptide, it will probably be digested in the infant's gastrointestinal tract and not absorbed. The manufacturer also states that systemic absorption of icatibant in infants is not expected. If the clinical decision is to use this drug while breastfeeding, the infant should be monitored for the most common reported adult side effects of fever, elevated transaminases, rash, and dizziness (leading to irritability).

References

1. Prescribing Information. Firazyr. Takeda Pharmaceuticals America, Inc; 2024.
2. Boufleur K, Delcaro L, Cordeiro DL, et al. Successful and safe use of icatibant for life-threatening angioedema attack during pregnancy in a patient with hereditary angioedema type 1. *J Allergy Clin Immunol*. 2014;133:AB36.
3. Zanichelli A, Mansi M, Periti G. Icatibant exposure during pregnancy in a patient with hereditary angioedema. *J Investig Allergol Clin Immunol*. 2015; 25:447-448.
4. Farkas H, Kojalmi KV, Veszeli N, et al. First report of icatibant treatment in a pregnant patient with hereditary angioedema. *J Obstet Gynaecol Res*. 2016;42:1026-1028.
5. Kaminsky LW, Kelbel T, Ansary F, Craig T. Multiple doses of icatibant used during pregnancy. *Allergy Rhinol*. 2017;8:178-181.
6. Hakl R, Kuklinek P, Krcmova I, et al. Treatment of hereditary angioedema attacks with icatibant and recombinant C1 inhibitor during pregnancy. *J Clin Immunol*. 2018;38:810-815.
7. Šimac DV, Štimac T, Novak S. Is icatibant safe for the treatment of hereditary angioedema during pregnancy? *Curr Allergy Asthma Rep*. 2022;22: 135-140.
8. Kondo Y, Yoshimura A, Azuma N. Successful management of hereditary angioedema with icatibant during the postpartum period. *J Cutan Immunol Allergy*. 2023;6:26-27.

IDARUBICIN

Antineoplastic (Anthracycline/Topoisomerase II Inhibitor)

PREGNANCY RECOMMENDATION: Limited Human Data—Animal Data Suggest Potential Risk

BREASTFEEDING RECOMMENDATION: Potential Toxicity

PREGNANCY SUMMARY

Eight reports describing the use of an idarubicin-containing regimen in 21 human pregnancies have been located. First-trimester exposure occurred in five pregnancies, where one patient died, there were three therapeutic abortions, and one spontaneous abortion. The exposure in the other 16 pregnancies (one set of twins) occurred in the second and third trimesters, resulting in 12 healthy infants, 4 fetal losses, and 1 infant who developed cardiomyopathy attributed to the chemotherapy (especially idarubicin). The drug probably will cross the placenta, so some fetal exposure will likely occur. However, this limited human pregnancy experience prevents a complete assessment of the embryofetal risk. Embryofetal toxicity (without maternal toxicity) was observed in one animal species at doses less than 10 times the RHD. Based on animal studies and the drug's mechanism of action, the manufacturer recommends that women with reproductive potential use effective contraception during treatment and for 6.5 months after the last dose. They also recommend that males with female partners of reproductive potential use effective contraception during treatment and for 3.5 months after the last dose. Nevertheless, using this drug during pregnancy should be based on the pros and cons of the mother's clinical need for treatment versus any potential fetal risk that might occur from exposure. There is a registry for women who are pregnant and have cancer. For more information, women and health care providers are encouraged to contact the Cancer and Pregnancy Registry at 1-877-635-4499.

BREASTFEEDING SUMMARY

No reports describing the use of idarubicin during human lactation have been located. The drug will probably be excreted into breast milk, so some infant exposure will likely occur. However, due to a concern for potential serious adverse effects that might be seen in a breastfed infant, the manufacturer recommends that women not breastfeed while being treated with this drug and for at least 2 weeks after the last dose. Nevertheless, breastfeeding while using this drug should be based on the mother's clinical need for treatment versus any potential infant risks that might occur. If used, the infant should be monitored for the most common reported adult side effects of nausea, headache, and abdominal pain (all leading to irritability), infections, hair loss, vomiting, diarrhea, bleeding, fever, and various laboratory abnormalities (see PI).

References

1. Prescribing Information. Idamycin PFS. Pharmacia and Upjohn; 2015.
2. Reynoso EE, Huerta F. Acute leukemia and pregnancy—fatal fetal outcome after exposure to idarubicin during the second trimester. *Acta Oncol*. 1994;33:703-716.
3. Claahsen HL, Semmekrot BA, van Dongen PWJ, Mattijssen V. Successful fetal outcome after exposure to idarubicin and cytosine-arabinoside during the second trimester of pregnancy—a case report. *Am J Perinatol*. 1998; 15:295-297.
4. Achtari C, Hohlfeld P. Cardiotoxic transplacental effect of idarubicin administered during the second trimester of pregnancy. *Am J Obstet Gynecol*. 2000;183:511-512.
5. Baumgartner AK, Oberhoffer R, Jacobs VR, et al. Reversible foetal cerebral ventriculomegaly and cardiomyopathy under chemotherapy for maternal AML. *Onkologie*. 2009;32:40-43.
6. Sanz MA, Montesinos P, Casale MF, et al. Maternal and fetal outcomes in pregnant women with acute promyelocytic leukemia. *Ann Hematol*. 2015; 94:1357-1361.
7. Maruyama S, Sato Y, Moriuchi K, et al. Fetal death following idarubicin treatment for acute promyelocytic leukemia in pregnancy-a case report. *Eur J Obstet Gynecol Reprod Biol*. 2017;218:140.
8. Dang CC, Guan YK, Lau NS, Chan SY. Two successful deliveries of healthy children by a young woman diagnosed and treated during induction and relapsed therapy for acute promyelocytic leukemia. *J Oncol Pharm Pract*. 2020;26:2034-2037.
9. Droc G, Stancioaica MC, Soare CG, et al. Acute promyelocytic leukemia and severe differentiation syndrome in pregnancy-a management challenge. *Life (Basel)*. 2023;13:1141.

I

IDARUCIZUMAB

Antidote (Monoclonal Antibody)

PREGNANCY RECOMMENDATION: No Human Data and No Relevant Animal Data

BREASTFEEDING RECOMMENDATION: Probably Compatible

PREGNANCY SUMMARY

No reports describing the use of idarucizumab in human pregnancy have been located. As a Fab-only portion of an immunoglobulin G (IgG) antibody, the drug will not likely cross the placenta, so fetal exposure should be negligible. However, the absence of human pregnancy experience prevents a complete assessment of the embryofetal risk. Animal reproduction studies have not been performed. Using this drug during pregnancy should be based on the pros and cons of the mother's clinical need for treatment versus any potential fetal risk that might occur from exposure.

BREASTFEEDING SUMMARY

No reports describing the use of idarucizumab during human lactation have been located. Limited amounts of the drug may be excreted into breast milk. However, it is known that IgG antibodies can be found in human breast milk but are not found in the neonatal or infant circulation. Additionally, if any IgG antibodies were to be ingested through breastfeeding, they would probably be digested in the infant's gastrointestinal tract and not be absorbed. Breastfeeding while using this drug should be based on the mother's clinical need for treatment. If used while breastfeeding, the infant should be monitored for the most common reported adult side effects of nausea and headache (both leading to irritability) and constipation.

Reference

1. Prescribing Information. Praxbind. Boehringer Ingelheim Pharmaceuticals, Inc; 2021.

IDELALISIB

Antineoplastic (Phosphatidylinositol 3-Kinase Inhibitor)

PREGNANCY RECOMMENDATION: No Human Data and No Relevant Animal Data

BREASTFEEDING RECOMMENDATION: Potential Toxicity

PREGNANCY SUMMARY

No reports describing the use of idelalisib in human pregnancy have been located. The drug will probably cross the placenta, so some fetal exposure will likely occur. However, the absence of human pregnancy experience prevents a complete assessment of the embryofetal risk. No relevant animal studies have been conducted. Based on animal studies and the drug's mechanism of action, the manufacturer recommends that women with reproductive potential use effective contraception during treatment and for 1 month after the last dose. They also recommend that males with female partners of reproductive potential use effective contraception during treatment and for 3 months after the last dose. Nevertheless, using this drug during pregnancy should be based on the pros and cons of the mother's clinical need for treatment versus any potential fetal risk that might occur from exposure. There is a registry for women who are pregnant and have cancer. For more information, women and health care providers are encouraged to contact the Cancer and Pregnancy Registry at 1-877-635-4499.

BREASTFEEDING SUMMARY

No reports describing the use of idelalisib during human lactation have been located. The drug will probably be found in breast milk, so some infant exposure will likely occur. However, due to a concern for potential serious adverse effects that might be seen in a breastfed infant, the manufacturer recommends that women not breastfeed while being treated with this drug and for at least 1 month after the last dose. Nevertheless, breastfeeding while using this drug should be based on the mother's clinical need for treatment versus any potential infant risks that might occur. If used, the infant should be monitored for the most common reported adult side effects of nausea (leading to irritability), diarrhea, fever, rash, lethargy, cough, and various laboratory abnormalities (see PI).

Reference

1. Prescribing Information. Zydelig. Gilead Sciences; 2016.

I

IDURSULFASE

Genetic (Enzyme)

PREGNANCY RECOMMENDATION: No Human Data—Animal Data Suggest Low Risk

BREASTFEEDING RECOMMENDATION: Probably Compatible

PREGNANCY SUMMARY

No reports describing the use of idursulfase in human pregnancy have been located. Placental transfer is likely to be clinically insignificant. However, the absence of human pregnancy experience prevents a complete assessment of the embryofetal risk. Animal data did not show any embryofetal toxicity in one animal species at doses of less than 10 times the RHD. Using this drug during pregnancy should be based on the pros and cons of the mother's clinical need for treatment versus any potential fetal risk that might occur from exposure.

BREASTFEEDING SUMMARY

No reports describing the use of idursulfase during human lactation have been located. The drug is not likely to be found in breast milk. If any amount of the drug were to be excreted, it would likely be clinically insignificant. Additionally, because idursulfase is an enzyme, if it were to be ingested through breastfeeding, it would probably be digested in the infant's gastrointestinal tract and not absorbed. If the clinical decision is to use this drug while breastfeeding, the infant should be monitored for the most common reported side effects in children of itching (leading to irritability), fever, rash, and vomiting.

Reference

1. Prescribing Information. Elaprase. Shire Human Genetic Therapies, Inc; 2021.

IFOSFAMIDE

Antineoplastic (Alkylating Agent)

PREGNANCY RECOMMENDATION: Limited Human Data—Animal Data Suggest Risk

BREASTFEEDING RECOMMENDATION: Potential Toxicity

PREGNANCY SUMMARY

Limited reports describing the use of ifosfamide in human pregnancy have been located. No first-trimester exposures were described. Overall, there were about 10 other cases with exposure usually in the late second trimester. Fetal growth

(*continued*)

restriction and neonatal anemia were reported, but these patients were also on other chemotherapeutic agents. In two cases, decreased amniotic fluid was seen, suggestive of fetal renal dysfunction. The drug will probably cross the placenta, so some fetal exposure will likely occur. However, the limited human pregnancy experience prevents a complete assessment of the embryofetal risk. Embryofetal toxicity with malformations was observed in three animal species at doses of less than 10 times the RHD. Based on these animal studies and the drug's mechanism of action, the manufacturer recommends that women with reproductive potential use effective contraception during treatment and for 6 months after the last dose. They also recommend that males with female partners of reproductive potential use effective contraception during treatment and for 6 months after the last dose. Nevertheless, using this drug during pregnancy should be based on the pros and cons of the mother's clinical need for treatment versus any potential fetal risk that might occur from exposure. There is a registry for women who are pregnant and have cancer. For more information, women and health care providers are encouraged to contact the Cancer and Pregnancy Registry at 1-877-635-4499.

BREASTFEEDING SUMMARY

No reports describing the use of ifosfamide during human lactation have been located. The drug is likely to be excreted into breast milk, so some infant exposure will probably occur. Due to a concern for potential serious adverse effects that might be seen in a breastfed infant, the manufacturer recommends that women not breastfeed while being treated with this drug. Nevertheless, breastfeeding while using this drug should be based on the mother's clinical need for treatment. If used, the infant should be monitored for the most common reported adult side effects of nausea (leading to irritability), vomiting, alopecia, leukopenia, anemia, and infections.

References

1. Prescribing Information. Ifosfamide. Hikma Pharmaceuticals USA, Inc; 2024.
2. Bus JS, Gibson JE. Teratogenicity and neonatal toxicity of ifosfamide in mice. *Proc Soc Exp Biol Med*. 1973;143:965-970.
3. Ypsilantis P, Papaioannou N, Psalla D, et al. Effects of single dose administration of ifosfamide on testes and semen characteristics in the rabbit. *Reprod Toxicol*. 2003;17:237-245.
4. Ypsilantis P, Papaioannou N, Psalla D, et al. Effects of subchronic ifosfamide-mesna treatment on testes and semen characteristics in the rabbit. *Reprod Toxicol*. 2003;17:699-708.
5. Pont J, Albrecht W. Fertility after chemotherapy for testicular germ cell cancer. *Fertil Steril*. 1997;68:1-5.
6. Longhi A, Macchiagodena M, Vitali G, Bacci G. Fertility in male patients treated with neoadjuvant chemotherapy for osteosarcoma. *J Pediatr Hematol Oncol*. 2003;25:292-296.
7. Chow EJ Stratton KL, Leisenring WM, Sklar CA, et al. Pregnancy after chemotherapy in male and female survivors of childhood cancer treated between 1970 and 1999: a report from the childhood cancer survivor study cohort. *Lancet Oncol*. 2016;17:567-576.
8. Fernandez H, Diallo A, Baume D, Papiernik E. Anhydramnios and cessation of fetal growth in a pregnant mother with polychemotherapy during the second trimester. *Prenat Diag*. 1989;9:681-682.
9. Merimsky O, Chevalier TL, Missenard G, et al. Management of cancer in pregnancy: a case of Ewing's sarcoma of the pelvis in the third trimester. *Ann Oncol*. 1999;10:345-350.
10. Nakajima W, Ishida A, Takahashi M, et al. Good outcome for infant of mother treated with chemotherapy for Ewing sarcoma at 25-30 weeks' gestation. *J Pediatr Hematol Oncol*. 2004;26:308-311.
11. Lam MSH. Treatment of Burkitt's lymphoma during pregnancy. *Ann Pharmacother*. 2006;40:2048-2052.
12. Mir O, Berrada N, Domont J, et al. Doxorubicin and ifosfamide for high-grade sarcoma during pregnancy. *Cancer Chemother Pharmacol*. 2012;69:357-367.
13. Miller D, Livingston JA, Park Y, et al. Pregnancy outcomes related to the treatment of sarcomas with anthracyclines and/or ifosfamide during pregnancy. *Cancer Med*. 2022;11:3471-3478.

ILOPERIDONE

Mental Health (Second-Generation Antipsychotic)

PREGNANCY RECOMMENDATION: No Human Data—Animal Data Suggest Low Risk

BREASTFEEDING RECOMMENDATION: Probably Compatible

PREGNANCY SUMMARY

No reports describing the use of iloperidone in human pregnancy have been located. The drug will probably cross the placenta, so some fetal exposure will likely occur. However, the absence of human pregnancy experience prevents a complete assessment of the embryofetal risk. Animal data did not show any embryofetal toxicity in two species at doses less than 10 times the RHD. The American College of Obstetricians and Gynecologists (ACOG) notes that second-generation antipsychotics are more often prescribed than first-generation antipsychotics due to fewer extrapyramidal side effects and better tolerability despite limited reproductive safety data. General principles for treatment in pregnancy include using the minimum effective dose and avoiding polypharmacy, if possible. While treatment in pregnancy poses an exposure risk, the risk is lower than the risk of symptom exacerbation and relapse. The manufacturer reports that neonates exposed to antipsychotic drugs, including iloperidone, during the third trimester, are at risk for extrapyramidal and/or withdrawal symptoms, such as agitation, hypertonia, hypotonia, tremor, somnolence, respiratory distress, and feeding intolerance. If continued during pregnancy, neonates should be monitored for extrapyramidal and/or withdrawal symptoms postdelivery. Some neonates recovered within hours or days without specific treatment, while others required prolonged hospitalization. There is a pregnancy exposure registry that monitors pregnancy outcomes in women using atypical antipsychotic drugs. Health care providers are encouraged to contact the National Pregnancy Registry for Atypical Antipsychotics at 1-866-961-2388. Iloperidone is also associated with QT prolongation.

BREASTFEEDING SUMMARY

No reports describing the use of iloperidone during human lactation have been located. The drug will probably appear in breast milk, so some infant exposure will likely occur. ACOG recommendations state that individuals with mental health conditions should not be discouraged from breastfeeding. If a woman is stable on a particular medication throughout pregnancy, the medication should not be changed postpartum. Breastfeeding while using this drug should be based on the mother's clinical need for treatment versus any potential infant risks that might occur. If used, the infant should be monitored for the most common reported adult side effects of dizziness (leading to irritability), fatigue (lethargy), somnolence, and tachycardia.

References

1. Prescribing Information. Fanapt. Vanda Pharmaceuticals; 2014.
2. American College of Obstetricians and Gynecologists. Use of psychiatric medications during pregnancy and lactation. ACOG Practice Bulletin. No. 92, April 2008. *Obstet Gynecol*. 2008;111:1001-1019.
3. Treatment and management of mental health conditions during pregnancy and postpartum: ACOG Clinical Practice Guideline No. 5. *Obstet Gynecol*. 2023;141:1262-1288.
4. Viguera AC, Vanderkruik R, Gaccione P, et al. Breastfeeding practices among women taking second-generation antipsychotics: findings from the National Pregnancy Registry for Atypical Antipsychotics. *Arch Womens Ment Health*. 2022;25:511-516.

I

ILOPROST

Cardiovascular (Vasodilator/Prostacyclin)

PREGNANCY RECOMMENDATION: Limited Human Data—Animal Data Suggest Potential Risk (Maternal Benefit May Outweigh Any Embryofetal Risk)

BREASTFEEDING RECOMMENDATION: Potential Toxicity

PREGNANCY SUMMARY

Six case reports and a retrospective observational study describing the use of iloprost in human pregnancy have been located. Pregnancy exposure to iloprost occurred in all trimesters. All 18 pregnancies resulted in live births with no adverse effects or congenital abnormalities. The drug will probably cross the placenta, so some fetal exposure will likely occur. However, the limited human pregnancy experience prevents a complete assessment of the embryofetal risk. Embryofetal toxicity with malformations was observed in one animal species at doses of less than 10 times the RHD. Due to the significant medical complications, including mortality of pregnant women with pulmonary arterial hypertension, ACOG advises against becoming pregnant. If the pregnancy occurs and is continued, despite limited evidence, prostacyclins, such as iloprost, are considered low risk for use in pregnancy.

BREASTFEEDING SUMMARY

No reports describing the use of iloprost during human lactation have been located. The drug will probably appear in breast milk, so some infant exposure will likely occur. Breastfeeding while using this drug should be based on the mother's clinical need for treatment versus any potential infant risks that might occur. If used, the infant should be monitored for the most common reported adult side effects of headache, nausea, back pain, and muscle cramps (all leading to irritability), cough, insomnia, hypotension, vomiting, increased alkaline phosphatase levels, and increased gamma-glutamyl transferase (GGT).

References

1. Prescribing Information. Ventavis. Actelion Pharmaceuticals US, Inc; 2022.
2. Prescribing Information. Aurlumyn. Eicos Sciences; 2024.
3. Elliot CA, Stewart P, Webster VJ, et al. The use of iloprost in early pregnancy in patients with pulmonary hypertension. *Eur Respir J*. 2005;26:168-173.
4. Cotrim C, Simoes O, Loureiro MJ, et al. Acute resynchronization with inhaled iloprost in a pregnant woman with idiopathic pulmonary artery hypertension. *Rev Port Cardiol*. 2006;25:529-533.
5. Streit M, Speich R, Fischler M, Ulrich S. Successful pregnancy in pulmonary arterial hypertension associated with systemic lupus erythematosus: a case report. *J Med Case Rep*. 2009;3:7255.
6. Terek D, Kayikcioglu M, Kultursay H, et al. Pulmonary arterial hypertension and pregnancy. *J Res Med Sci*. 2013;18:73-76.
7. Horng M, Mohammad I, Smith ZR, et al. Inhaled iloprost for chronic thromboembolic pulmonary hypertension (CTEPH) during pregnancy: a case report. *Pharmacotherapy*. 2016;36:e142-e147.
8. Mirdamadi A, Gharavi H, Behjati M. Role of meticulous observation: successful pregnancy in a 30-year-old woman with severe pulmonary hypertension. *Tanaffos*. 2016;15:187-190.
9. Kiely DG, Condliffe R, Webster V, et al. Improved survival in pregnancy and pulmonary hypertension using a multiprofessional approach. *BJOG*. 2009;117:565-574.
10. Moussa HN, Rajapreyar I. ACOG practice bulletin no. 212: pregnancy and heart disease. *Obstet Gynecol*. 2019;134(4):881-882.
11. Humbert M, Kovacs G, Hoeper MM, et al. 2022 ESC/ERS Guidelines for the diagnosis and treatment of pulmonary hypertension. *Eur Heart J*. 2022;43:3618-3731.

IMATINIB

Antineoplastic (Tyrosine Kinase Inhibitor)

PREGNANCY RECOMMENDATION: Limited Human Data—Animal Data Suggest Potential Risk

BREASTFEEDING RECOMMENDATION: Potential Toxicity

PREGNANCY SUMMARY

Numerous case reports and small series have reported the use of imatinib during human pregnancy. Where pregnancy outcome was known, of 49 first-trimester exposures, there were 7 (14%) spontaneous abortions, 42 normal infants without any identified birth anomalies, and 3 (7%) with congenital defects (one with a neural tube defect [NTD], one with pyloric stenosis, and one twin with multiple anomalies). Some amount of the drug may cross the placenta, so fetal exposure will probably occur. However, this limited human pregnancy experience prevents a complete assessment of the embryofetal risk. Embryofetal toxicity with malformations was observed in one animal species at doses of less than 10 times the RHD. Based on the animal studies and the drug's mechanism of action, the manufacturer recommends that women with reproductive potential use effective contraception during treatment and for 2 weeks after the last dose. Nevertheless, using this drug during pregnancy should be based on the pros and cons of the mother's clinical need for treatment versus any potential fetal risk that might occur from exposure. Because agents in this subclass inhibit angiogenesis, a critical component of embryonic and fetal development, avoiding the drug in pregnancy during organogenesis is the safest course. There is a registry for women who are pregnant and have cancer. For more information, women and health care providers are encouraged to contact the Cancer and Pregnancy Registry at 1-877-635-4499.

BREASTFEEDING SUMMARY

Four case reports describing the use of imatinib during human lactation have been located. No adverse effects were noted in the infants. However, due to a concern for potential serious adverse effects that might be seen in a breastfed infant, the manufacturer recommends that women not breastfeed while being treated with this drug and for at least 1 month after the last dose. Nevertheless, breastfeeding while using this drug should be based on the mother's clinical need for treatment versus any potential infant risks that might occur. If used, the infant should be monitored for the most common reported adult side effects of nausea, muscle cramps, musculoskeletal pain, and abdominal pain (all leading to irritability), peripheral edema, vomiting, diarrhea, rash, and fatigue (lethargy).

References

1. Prescribing Information. Gleevec. Novartis Pharmaceuticals; 2024.
2. Hensley ML, Ford JM. Imatinib treatment: specific issues related to safety, fertility, and pregnancy. *Semin Hematol*. 2003;40(2 suppl 2):21-25.
3. Heartin E, Walkinshaw S, Clark RE. Successful outcome of pregnancy in chronic myeloid leukaemia treated with imatinib. *Leuk Lymphoma*. 2004; 45:1307-1308.
4. Ali R, Ozkalemkas F, Ozcelik T, et al. Pregnancy under treatment of imatinib and successful labor in a patient with chronic myelogenous leukemia (CML). Outcome of discontinuation of imatinib therapy after achieving a molecular remission. *Leuk Res*. 2005;29:971-973.
5. AlKindi S, Dennison D, Pathare A. Imatinib in pregnancy. *Eur J Haematol*. 2005;74:535-537.
6. Prabhash K, Sastry PSRK, Biswas G, et al. Pregnancy outcome of two patients treated with imatinib. *Ann Oncol*. 2005;16:1983-1984.
7. Choudhary DR, Mishra P, Kumar R, et al. Pregnancy on imatinib: fatal outcome with meningocele. *Ann Oncol*. 2006;17:178-179.
8. Koh LP, Kanagalingam D. Pregnancies in patients with chronic myeloid leukemia in the era of imatinib. *Int J Hematol*. 2006;84:459-462.
9. Ault P, Kantarjian H, O'Brien S, et al. Pregnancy among patients with chronic myeloid leukemia treated with imatinib. *J Clin Oncol*. 2006;24:1204-1208.
10. Klamova J, Markova M, Moravcova J, et al. Response to treatment in women with chronic myeloid leukemia during pregnancy and after delivery. *Leuk Res*. 2009;33:1567-1569.
11. Dolai TK, Bhargava R, Mahapatra M, et al. Is imatinib safe during pregnancy? *Leuk Res*. 2009;33:572-573.
12. Martin J, Ramesh A, Devadasan L, et al. An uneventful pregnancy and delivery, in a case with chronic myeloid leukemia on imatinib. *Indian J Med Paediatr Oncol*. 2011;32:109-111.
13. Ali R, Ozkalemkas F, Kimya Y, et al. Imatinib use during pregnancy and breast feeding: a case report and review of the literature. *Arch Gynecol Obstet*. 2009;280:169-175.
14. Yadav U, Solanki SL, Yadav R. Chronic myeloid leukemia with pregnancy: successful management of pregnancy and delivery with hydroxyurea and imatinib continued till delivery. *J Cancer Res Ther*. 2013;9:484-486.
15. Iqbal J, Ali Z, Khan AUN, Aziz Z. Pregnancy outcomes in patients with chronic myeloid leukemia treated with imatinib mesylate: short report from a developing country. *Leuk Lymph*. 2014;55:2109-2113.
16. Jain N, Sharma D, Agrawal R, Jain A. A newborn with teratogenic effect of imatinib mesylate: a very rare case report. *Med Princ Pract*. 2015;24:291-293.
17. Gambacorti-Passerini CB, Tornaghi L, Marangon E, et al. Imatinib concentrations in human milk. *Blood*. 2007;109:1790.
18. Kronenberger R, Schleyer E, Bornhauser M, et al. Imatinib in breast milk. *Ann Hematol*. 2009;88:1265-1266.
19. Alizadeh H, Jaafar H, Kajtar B. Outcome of 3 pregnancies in a patient with chronic myeloid leukemia who received 3 types of tyrosine kinase inhibitors each in different pregnancy: follow-up of the case with a review of published reports. *Ann Saudi Med*. 2015;35:468-471.
20. Terao R, Nii M, Asai H, et al. Breastfeeding in a patient with chronic myeloid leukemia during tyrosine kinase inhibitor therapy. *J Oncol Pharm Pract*. 2020;27:756-760.
21. Jiang Q, Jiang B, Chen SS, et al. Pregnancy outcome among patients with chronic myelogenous leukemia treated with tyrosine kinase inhibitors. 2012;33:6-9.

IMETELSTAT

Hematologic (Oligonucleotide Human Telomerase Inhibitor)

PREGNANCY RECOMMENDATION: No Human Data—Animal Data Suggest Potential Risk (Maternal Benefit May Outweigh Any Embryofetal Risk)

BREASTFEEDING RECOMMENDATION: Probably Compatible

PREGNANCY SUMMARY

No reports describing the use of imetelstat in human pregnancy have been located. The drug will not likely cross the placenta in significant amounts, so fetal exposure should be negligible. However, the absence of human pregnancy experience prevents a complete assessment of the embryofetal risk. Animal reproduction studies did show some embryofetal toxicity in one species at doses of less than 10 times the RHD, but drug administration occurred 2 to 3 times a week rather than once a month (the frequency recommended for humans). It is not possible to determine the effect of this frequency difference. Using this drug during pregnancy should be based on the pros and cons of the mother's clinical need for treatment versus any potential fetal risk that might occur from exposure.

I

BREASTFEEDING SUMMARY

No reports describing the use of imetelstat during human lactation have been located. The drug will not likely be excreted into breast milk. In addition, because it is an oligonucleotide, if any drug were to be ingested through breastfeeding, it would probably be digested in the infant's gastrointestinal tract and not be absorbed. However, due to a concern for potential serious adverse effects that might be seen in a breastfed infant, the manufacturer recommends that women not breastfeed while being treated with this drug and for at least 1 week after the last dose. Nevertheless, breastfeeding while using this drug should be based on the mother's clinical need for treatment versus any potential infant risks that might occur. If used, the infant should be monitored for the most common reported adult side effects of headache, myalgia, and arthralgia (all leading to irritability), fatigue (lethargy), and various laboratory abnormalities (see PI).

Reference

1. Prescribing Information. Rytelo. Geron Corp; 2024.

IMIGLUCERASE

Genetic (Enzyme)

PREGNANCY RECOMMENDATION: Limited Human Data—No Relevant Animal Data

BREASTFEEDING RECOMMENDATION: Probably Compatible

PREGNANCY SUMMARY

Seven case reports describing the use of imiglucerase throughout pregnancy in seven human pregnancies have been located. No congenital abnormalities were reported. Successful pregnancy outcomes in patients treated with imiglucerase included six healthy live-born singletons and one set of healthy live-born twins. Placental transfer is likely to be clinically insignificant. However, this limited human pregnancy experience prevents a complete assessment of the embryofetal risk. No reproduction animal studies have been conducted. Pregnancy has been shown to exacerbate existing symptoms or result in new symptoms of Gaucher disease. Enzyme replacement therapy has also been shown to reduce the risk of spontaneous abortion and bleeding. Therefore, patients requiring treatment should continue imiglucerase during pregnancy, and for symptomatic patients, it can be started. There is also a pregnancy exposure registry that monitors pregnancy outcomes in women exposed to imiglucerase during pregnancy. Pregnant women exposed to imiglucerase and health care providers are encouraged to contact the Gaucher patient registry at 1-800-745-4447.

BREASTFEEDING SUMMARY

Four reports describing the use of imiglucerase during human lactation in five pregnancies have been located. Breastfeeding ranged from 9 to 12 months (when known), and four infants had noted normal development ranging from 13 to 36 months. Imiglucerase is a synthetic form of β-glucocerebrosidase that is a normal component of breast milk. Two reports have described the excretion of small amounts of imiglucerase in human breast milk, which resulted in lower β-glucocerebrosidase activity than that of normal mothers. However, if imiglucerase were to be ingested through breastfeeding, the enzyme would probably be digested in the infant's gastrointestinal tract and not absorbed. If the clinical decision is to use this drug while breastfeeding, the infant should be monitored for the most common reported adult side effects of nausea, headache, back pain, dizziness, and abdominal pain (all leading to irritability), fatigue (lethargy), rash, fever, and vomiting.

References

1. Prescribing Information. Cerezyme. Genzyme; 2022.
2. Mrsic M, Fumic K, Vrcic H, et al. Successful pregnancy on enzyme replacement therapy with Cerezyme. *Clin Ther*. 2007;29(suppl C):S84.
3. Zimran A, Morris E, Mengel E, et al. The female Gaucher patient: the impact of enzyme replacement therapy around key reproductive events (menstruation, pregnancy, and menopause). *Blood Cells Mol Dis*. 2009;43:264-288.
4. Granovsky-Grisaru S, Belmatoug N, vom Dahl S, et al. The management of pregnancy in Gaucher disease. *Eur J Obstet Gynecol Reprod Biol*. 2011; 156:3-8.
5. Sherer Y, Dulitzki M, Levy Y, et al. Successful pregnancy outcome in a patient with Gaucher's disease and antiphospholipid syndrome. *Ann Hematol*. 2002;81:161-163.
6. Malinova V, Poupetova H, Dvorakova L, Zeman J. Enzyme replacement therapy for Gaucher disease in twin pregnancy. *Int J Gynaecol Obstet*. 2009; 106:64-66.
7. Sekijima Y, Ohashi T, Ohira S, et al. Successful pregnancy and lactation outcome in a patient with Gaucher disease receiving enzyme replacement therapy, and the subsequent distribution and excretion of imiglucerase in human breast milk. *Clin Ther*. 2010;32:2048-2052.
8. Dornelles AD, Netto CBO, Vairo F, et al. Breastfeeding in Gaucher disease: is enzyme replacement therapy safe? *Clin Ther*. 2014;36:990-991.
9. Giannubilo SR, Pasculli A, Tidu E, Ciavattini A. Replacement therapy for Gaucher disease during pregnancy: a case report. *J Reprod Infertil*. 2015;16: 53-57.
10. Korkmazer E, Solak N, Tokgoz VY. Pregnancy and lactation in a patient with Gaucher disease receiving enzyme replacement therapy: case report. *Turk J Clin Obstet Gynecol*. 2015;25:224-226.

I

IMIPENEM-CILASTATIN

Antibacterial (Carbapenem)

PREGNANCY RECOMMENDATION: Limited Human Data—Animal Data Suggest Low Risk

BREASTFEEDING RECOMMENDATION: Probably Compatible

PREGNANCY SUMMARY

One report describing the use of imipenem-cilastatin in 100 human pregnancies for the treatment of preterm premature rupture of membranes (PPROM) has been located. The mean time from PPROM to delivery in the study and control groups was 11 and 6 days, respectively. No infants died within 1 year of birth in the study group compared with five infants in the controls. Imipenem-cilastatin crosses the placenta, so fetal exposure will occur. However, this limited human pregnancy experience (especially the first trimester) prevents a complete assessment of the embryofetal risk. Animal data did not show any embryofetal toxicity in two animal species at doses of less than 10 times the RHD. Using this drug during pregnancy should be based on the pros and cons of the mother's clinical need for treatment versus any potential fetal risk that might occur from exposure.

BREASTFEEDING SUMMARY

No reports describing the use of imipenem-cilastatin during human lactation have been located. Two reports have found small amounts of imipenem in breast milk. Cilastatin was undetectable in all samples of all women tested. Breastfeeding while using this drug should be based on the mother's clinical need for treatment versus any potential infant risks that might occur. If used, the infant should be monitored for the most common reported neonatal side effects of diarrhea, decreased urine output, oral thrush, rash, and increased heart rate.

References

1. Prescribing Information. Primaxin. Merck & Co; 2016.
2. Matsuda S, Suzuki M, Oh K, et al. Pharmacokinetic and clinical studies on imipenem/cilastatin sodium in the perinatal period. *Jpn J Antibiot*. 1988;11:1731-1741.
3. Hirabayashi K, Okada E. Pharmacokinetic and clinical studies of imipenem/cilastatin sodium in the perinatal period. *Jpn J Antibiot*. 1988;11:1797-1804.
4. Cho N, Fukunaga K, Kunii K, et al. Studies on imipenem/cilastatin sodium in the perinatal period. *Jpn J Antibiot*. 1988;11:1758-1773.
5. Heikkila A, Renkonen O-V, Erkkola R. Pharmacokinetics and transplacental passage of imipenem during pregnancy. *Antimicrob Agents Chemother*. 1992;36:2652-2655.
6. Ryo E, Ikeya M, Sugimoto M. Clinical study of the effectiveness of imipenem/cilastatin sodium as the antibiotics of first choice in the expectant management of patients with preterm premature rupture of membranes. *J Infect Chemother*. 2005;11:32-36.
7. Ito K, Izumi K, Takagi H, Tamaya T, Hayasaki M. Fundamental and clinical evaluation of imipenem/cilastatin sodium in the perinatal period. *Jpn J Antibiot*. 1988;41:1778-1785.

IMIPENEM, CILASTATIN, AND RELEBACTAM

Antibacterial

PREGNANCY RECOMMENDATION: Limited Human Data—Animal Data Suggest Potential Risk

BREASTFEEDING RECOMMENDATION: Probably Compatible

PREGNANCY SUMMARY

No human data specific to birth anomalies from exposure to imipenem, cilastatin, and relebactam have been located. It has been shown and/or is expected that all three drugs cross the human placenta, so fetal exposure will probably occur. Therefore, the absence of human pregnancy experience prevents a complete assessment of the embryofetal risk. Animal data did not show any embryofetal toxicity for imipenem and cilastatin, but was seen with relebactam. No adverse pregnancy outcomes were seen with imipenem and cilastatin when used in the late second and early third trimesters (see Imipenem-Cilastatin).

BREASTFEEDING SUMMARY

Small amounts of imipenem and cilastatin are excreted into human breast milk (see Imipenem-Cilastatin). Relebactam is also probably found in human breast milk. Breastfeeding while using this drug should be based on the mother's clinical need for treatment. If used, the infant should be monitored for the most common adult side effects of nausea and pruritus (both leading to irritability), diarrhea, vomiting, rash, and lethargy.

Reference

1. Prescribing Information. Recarbrio. Merck Sharp & Dohme, L; 2020.

IMIPRAMINE

Mantal Health (Antidepressant—Tricyclic)

PREGNANCY RECOMMENDATION: Limited Human Data—Animal Data Suggest Low Risk

BREASTFEEDING RECOMMENDATION: Probably compatible

PREGNANCY SUMMARY

Limited reports describing the use of imipramine in human pregnancy have been located. From two large databases, a total of 46 first-trimester exposures to imipramine were described. Of these, there were three (6.5%) with birth anomalies (one not described, one omphalocele, and one polydactyly). No pattern to the defects was identified. However, this limited human pregnancy experience prevents a complete assessment of the embryofetal risk. Animal data did not show any teratogenicity in three animal species at doses of less than 10 times the RHD. Neonatal withdrawal is a potential complication when the drug is used near birth. Imipramine and its active metabolite desimipramine cross the placenta. Using this drug during pregnancy should be based on the pros and cons of the mother's clinical need for treatment versus any potential fetal risk that might occur from exposure. There is a pregnancy exposure registry that monitors pregnancy outcomes in women using antidepressant drugs. Health care providers are encouraged to call the National Pregnancy Registry for Antidepressants at 1-844-405-6185.

BREASTFEEDING SUMMARY

Four reports describing the use of imipramine during human lactation have been located. No adverse effects were reported in 25 infants whose mothers were treated with imipramine while breastfeeding. Imipramine and its metabolite, desipramine, enter breast milk in low concentrations but are not detected in the serum of breastfed infants. Breastfeeding while using this drug should be based on the mother's clinical need for treatment versus any potential infant risks that might occur. If used, the infant should be monitored for the most common reported adult side effects of gastrointestinal disturbances (leading to irritability), insomnia, and sedation.

References

1. Prescribing Information. Imipramine Hydrochloride. Leading Pharma, LLC; 2022.
2. Shepard TH. *Catalog of Teratogenic Agents*. 6th ed. The Johns Hopkins University Press; 1989:345-346.
3. Sailee FR, Pollock BG. Clinical pharmacokinetics of imipramine and desipramine, *Clin Pharm*. 1990;18:346-364.
4. Shepard TH. *Catalog of Teratogenic Agents*. 13th ed. The Johns Hopkins University Press; 2010:1697.
5. McBride WG. Limb deformities associated with iminodibenzyl hydrochloride. *Med J Aust*. 1972;1:492.
6. Heinonen OP, Slone D, Shapiro S. *Birth Defects and Drugs in Pregnancy*. Publishing Sciences Group; 1977:336-337.
7. Kuenssberg EV, Knox JDE. Imipramine in pregnancy. *Br Med J*. 1972;2:29.
8. Barson AJ. Malformed infant. *Br Med J*. 1972;2:45.
9. Idanpaan-Heikkila J, Saxen L. Possible teratogenicity of imipramine/chloropyramine. *Lancet*. 1973;2:282-283.
10. Crombie DL, Pinsent R, Fleming D. Imipramine in pregnancy. *Br Med J*. 1972;1:745.
11. Sim M. Imipramine and pregnancy. *Br Med J*. 1972;2:45.
12. Scanlon FJ. Use of antidepressant drugs during the first trimester. *Med J Aust*. 1969;2:1077.
13. Rachelefsky GS, Flynt JW, Eggin AJ, Wilson MG. Possible teratogenicity of tricyclic antidepressants. *Lancet*. 1972;1:838.
14. Banister P, Dafoe C, Smith ESO, Miller J. Possible teratogenicity of tricyclic antidepressants. *Lancet*. 1972;1:838-839.
15. Jacobs D. Imipramine (Tofranil). *S Afr Med J*. 1972;46:1023.
16. Australian Drug Evaluation Committee. Tricyclic antidepressant and limb reduction deformities. *Med J Aust*. 1973;1:766-769.

17. Morrow AW. Imipramine and congenital abnormalities. *NZ Med J*. 1972; 75:228-229.
18. Wilson JG. Present status of drugs as teratogens in man. *Teratology*. 1973; 7:3-15.
19. McElhatton PR, Garbis HM, Elefant E, et al. The outcome of pregnancy in 689 women exposed to therapeutic doses of antidepressants. A collaborative study of the European Network of Teratology Information Services (ENTIS). *Reprod Toxicol*. 1996;10:285-294.
20. Hill RM. Will this drug harm the unborn infant? *South Med J*. 1977;67: 1476-1480.
21. Eggermont E. Withdrawal symptoms in neonate associated with maternal imipramine therapy. *Lancet*. 1973;2:680.
22. Shrand H. Agoraphobia and imipramine withdrawal? *Pediatrics*. 1982; 70:825.
23. Shearer WT, Schreiner RL, Marshall RE. Urinary retention in a neonate secondary to maternal ingestion of nortriptyline. *J Pediatr*. 1972;81:570-572.
24. Nulman I, Rovet J, Stewart DE, et al. Child development following exposure to tricyclic antidepressants or fluoxetine throughout fetal life: a prospective, controlled study. *Am J Psychiatry*. 2002;159:1889-1895.
25. Sovner R, Orsulak PJ. Excretion of imipramine and desipramine in human breast milk. *Am J Psychiatry*. 1979;136:451-452.
26. Erickson SH, Smith GH, Heidrich F. Tricyclics and breast-feeding. *Am J Psychiatry*. 1979;136:1483.
27. Yoshida K, Smith B, Craggs M, Kumar RC. Investigation of pharmacokinetics and of possible adverse effects in infants exposed to tricyclic antidepressants in breast-milk. *J Affect Disord*. 1997;43:225-237.
28. Douglas BH, Hume AS. Placental transfer of imipramine, a basic, lipid-soluble drug. *Am J Obstet Gynecol*. 1967;99(4):573-575.
29. Birnbaum CS, Cohen LS, Bailey JW, et al. Serum concentrations of antidepressants and benzodiazepines in nursing infants: a case series. *Pediatrics*. 1999;104:e11.
30. Misri S, Sivertz K. Tricyclic drugs in pregnancy and lactation: a preliminary report. *Int J Psychiatry Med*. 1991;21:157-171.
31. Uguz F, Aydin A, Ak M, et al. Low-dose imipramine for the treatment of panic disorder during postpartum period: a retrospective analysis of 6 cases. *J Clin Psychopharmacol*. 2016;36:292-293.

I

IMIQUIMOD

Dermatologic (Topical)

PREGNANCY RECOMMENDATION: Limited Human Data—Animal Data Suggest Low Risk

BREASTFEEDING RECOMMENDATION: Probably Compatible

PREGNANCY SUMMARY

Four reports describing the use of imiquimod during human pregnancy have been located. Twenty-six pregnant women described in these reports were exposed in all three trimesters. No adverse effects or congenital abnormalities were observed in any of the reports. The drug will probably cross the placenta, so some fetal exposure will likely occur if it reaches the placental interface. However, because systemic absorption with topical use produces low concentrations, the actual exposure is probably clinically insignificant. Nevertheless, this limited human pregnancy experience prevents a complete assessment of the embryofetal risk. Animal data did not show any embryofetal toxicity in two animal species at doses of less than 10 times the maximum recommended human dose (MRHD). Using this drug during pregnancy should be based on the pros and cons of the mother's clinical need for treatment versus any potential fetal risk that might occur from exposure.

BREASTFEEDING SUMMARY

No reports describing the use of imiquimod during human lactation have been located. The drug will probably be excreted into breast milk if it is present in the maternal circulation. However, the amount absorbed systemically with topical use is very low and probably is clinically insignificant. Direct application to the nipple or breast areas, where the infants' skin may come into direct contact, should be avoided. Breastfeeding while using this drug should be based on the mother's clinical need for treatment versus any potential infant risks that might occur. If used, the infant should be monitored for the most common reported adult side effects of headache, nausea, and itching (all leading to irritability), and fatigue (lethargy).

References

1. Prescribing Information. Imiquimod. Taro Pharmaceutical; 2021.
2. Manlove JM, Zaher FM, Tomai M, et al. Effect of imiquimod on cytokine induction in first trimester trophoblasts. *Infect Dis Obstet Gynecol*. 2000;8:105-111.
3. Maw RD. Treatment of external genital warts with 5% imiquimod cream during pregnancy: a case report. *BJOG*. 2004;111:1475.
4. Einarson A, Costei A, Kalra S, et al. The use of topical 5% imiquimod during pregnancy: a case series. *Reprod Toxicol*. 2006;21:1-2.
5. Audisio T, Roca FC, Piatti C. Topical imiquimod therapy for external anogenital warts in pregnant women. *Int J Gynaecol Obstet*. 2008;110:275-286.
6. Ciavattini A, Tsiroglou D, Vichi M, et al. Topical imiquimod 5% cream therapy for external anogenital warts in pregnant women: report of four cases and review of the literature. *J Matern Fetal Neonatal Med*. 2012;25:873-876.

IMMUNE GLOBULIN, HEPATITIS B (HBIG)

Immunologic (Antibody)

PREGNANCY RECOMMENDATION: Human Data Suggest Compatible

BREASTFEEDING RECOMMENDATION: Probably Compatible

PREGNANCY SUMMARY

Hepatitis B immune globulin (HBIG) use in pregnancy is well reported throughout the literature. Five meta-analyses of up to 37 randomized clinical trials have been located that have evaluated the benefit and harm of HBIG with or without hepatitis B vaccine during pregnancy for prevention of mother-to-child transmission of hepatitis B virus (HBV). While the benefit of antenatal HBIG administration to mothers with HBV on newborn outcomes is uncertain, no adverse risk to the fetus from the immune globulin has been reported. HBIG contains antibodies (IgG) to hepatitis B that passively diffuse across the placenta to the fetus, primarily in the second half of gestation. Diffusion is highest during the third trimester of pregnancy. ACOG recommends that pregnant health care workers with accidental and occupational exposure to hepatitis B should be managed the same way as those who are not pregnant, including the use of HBIG when indicated. It does not recommend the use of maternal HBIG to decrease the risk of neonatal infection. No known risk exists for the fetus from passive immunization of pregnant women with immune globulin preparations.

BREASTFEEDING SUMMARY

No reports describing the use of HBIG during human lactation have been located. It is known that IgG antibodies are excreted into breast milk but are not found in neonatal or infant circulation. Additionally, if any IgG antibodies were to be ingested through breastfeeding, they would probably be digested in the infant's gastrointestinal tract and not absorbed. HBIG is recommended along with hepatitis B vaccine in all infants postdelivery whose mothers are positive for hepatitis. Women with hepatitis B are encouraged to breastfeed their infants. If used while breastfeeding, the infant should be monitored for the most common reported systemic adult side effects of nausea, headache, and myalgia (all leading to irritability), vomiting, and malaise (lethargy).

References

1. Prescribing Information. Nabi-HB. ADMA Biologics; 2019.
2. Shi Z, Li X, Ma L, Yang Y. Hepatitis B immunoglobulin injection in pregnancy to interrupt hepatitis B virus mother-to-child transmission—a meta-analysis. *International Journal of Infectious Diseases*. 2010;14(7):e622-e634.
3. Jin H, Zhao Y, Tan Z, Zhang X, Zhao Y, Wang B, et al. Immunization interventions to interrupt hepatitis B virus mother-to-child transmission: a meta-analysis of randomized controlled trials. *BMC Pediatrics*. 2014;14(1):307.
4. Xu H, Zeng T, Liu J-Y, Lei Y, Zhong S, Sheng Y-J, et al. Measures to reduce mother-to-child transmission of hepatitis B virus in China: a meta-analysis. *Dig Dis Sci*. 2014;59(2):242-258.
5. Eke AC, Eleje GU, Eke UA, et al. Hepatitis B immunoglobulin during pregnancy for prevention of mother-to-child transmission of hepatitis B virus. *Cochrane Database Syst Rev*. 2017;2:2-3.
6. Chen Z, Zeng M, Liu D, et al. Antenatal administration of hepatitis B immunoglobulin and hepatitis B vaccine to prevent mother to child transmission in hepatitis B virus surface antigen positive pregnant women: a systematic review and meta-analysis. *Medicine*. 2020;99:e19886.
7. Viral hepatitis in pregnancy: ACOG Clinical Practice Guideline No. 6. *Obstet Gynecol*. 2023;142:745-759.
8. CDC. Guidelines for vaccinating pregnant women. Accessed April 5, 2024. https://www.cdc.gov/vaccines/pregnancy/hcp-toolkit/guidelines.html

IMMUNE GLOBULIN, INTRAVENOUS (IVIG)

Immunologic (Antibody)

PREGNANCY RECOMMENDATION: Human Data Suggest Compatible

BREASTFEEDING RECOMMENDATION: Probably Compatible

PREGNANCY SUMMARY

Several case reports and cohort studies describing the use of intravenous immune globulin (IVIG) to effectively treat diseases in pregnancy have been located. No embryofetal risk has been associated with IVIG. Exogenous immune globulin has been shown to cross the human placenta in the second half of gestation, but in greater amounts at 32 weeks' gestation and after. Placental transfer has also been shown to be a function of dose, duration of treatment, and possibly method of preparation. No relevant animal studies have been conducted. Using this drug during pregnancy should be based on the pros and cons of the mother's clinical need for treatment versus any potential fetal risk that might occur from exposure.

BREASTFEEDING SUMMARY

Several reports describing the use of IVIG during human lactation have been located. No serious adverse effects were reported in breastfed infants. Human IgG is excreted into breast milk during the first few days after birth. IgG levels in breast milk were normal to high after receiving IVIG therapy. If used while breastfeeding, the infant should be monitored for rash and the most common reported adult side effects of headache (leading to irritability), fatigue (lethargy), and fever.

References

1. Prescribing Information. Gammagard. Takeda Pharmaceuticals U.S.A., Inc; 2024.

2. Sidiropoulos D, Herrmann U Jr, Morell A, et al. Transplacental passage of intravenous immunoglobulin in the last trimester of pregnancy. *J Pediatr*. 1986;109:505-508.
3. Smith CIE, Hammarström SL. Intravenous immunoglobulin in pregnancy. *Obstet Gynecol*. 1985;66(suppl):39S-40S.
4. Sacher RA, King JC. Intravenous gamma-globulin in pregnancy: a review. *Obstet Gynecol Surv*. 1988;44:25-34.
5. Lynch L, Bussel JB, McFarland JG, et al. Antenatal treatment of alloimmune thrombocytopenia. *Obstet Gynecol*. 1992;80:67-71.
6. Wenstrom KD, Weiner CP, Williamson RA. Antenatal treatment of fetal alloimmune thrombocytopenia. *Obstet Gynecol*. 1992;80:433-435.
7. Scott JR, Branch DW, Kochenour NK, Ward K. Intravenous immunoglobulin treatment of pregnant patients with recurrent pregnancy loss caused by antiphospholipid antibodies and Rh immunization. *Am J Obstet Gynecol*. 1988;159:1055-1056.
8. Orvieto R, Achiron A, Ben-Rafael Z, Achiron R. Intravenous immunoglobulin treatment for recurrent abortions caused by antiphospholipid antibodies. *Fertil Steril*. 1991;56:1013-1020.
9. Kaaja R, Julkunen H, Ämmälä P, et al. Congenital heart block: successful prophylactic treatment with intravenous gamma globulin and corticosteroid therapy. *Am J Obstet Gynecol*. 1991;165:1333-1334.
10. Chitkara U, Bussel J, Alvarez M, et al. High-dose intravenous gamma globulin: does it have a role in the treatment of severe erythroblastosis fetalis? *Obstet Gynecol*. 1990;76:703-708.
11. Marzusch K, Tinneberg H, Mueller-Eckhardt G, et al. Is immunotherapy justified for recurrent spontaneous abortion? *Lancet*. 1992;339:1543.
12. Palmeria P, Costa-Carvalho BT, Arsianian C, et al. Transfer of antibodies across the placenta and in breast milk from mothers on intravenous immunoglobulin. *Pediatr Allergy Immunol*. 2009;20:528-535.
13. Achiron A, Kishner I, Doley M, et al. Effect of intravenous immunoglobulin treatment on pregnancy and post-partum-related relapses in multiple sclerosis. *J Neurol*. 2004;251:1133-1137.
14. Haas J. High dose IVIG in the postpartum period for prevention of exacerbation in MS. *Mult Scler*. 2000;6(suppl 2):S18-S20.
15. Saab W, Seshadri S, Huang C, et al. A systematic review of intravenous immunoglobulin G treatment in women with recurrent implantation failures and recurrent pregnancy losses. *Am J Reprod Immunol*. 2021;85:e13395.
16. Shi Y, Tan D, Hao B, et al. Efficacy of intravenous immunoglobulin in the treatment of recurrent spontaneous abortion: a systematic review and meta-analysis. *Am J Reprod Immunol*. 2022;88:e13615.

IMMUNE GLOBULIN, RABIES

Immunologic (Antibody)

PREGNANCY RECOMMENDATION: Limited Human Data—No Relevant Animal Data (Maternal Benefit May Outweigh Any Embryofetal Risk)

BREASTFEEDING RECOMMENDATION: Probably Compatible

PREGNANCY SUMMARY

Six reports and a prospective study describing the use of rabies immune globulin in about 231 human pregnancies have been located. No congenital abnormalities or increased risk for adverse effects were reported. While specific information is not available, human IgG antibodies are known to cross the placenta, especially during the third trimester, which suggests that some transfer will occur. However, this limited human pregnancy experience prevents a complete assessment of the embryofetal risk. No animal studies have been conducted. The Advisory Committee on Immunization Practices (ACIP) recommends that postexposure prophylaxis include passive immunization with human rabies immune globulin and rabies vaccine. Pregnancy is not a contraindication to postexposure prophylaxis. No known risk exists for the fetus from passive immunization of pregnant women with immune globulin preparations. Preexposure prophylaxis may be indicated during pregnancy if there is significant risk for rabies exposure.

BREASTFEEDING SUMMARY

No reports describing the use of rabies immune globulin during human lactation have been located. Maternal IgG antibodies are excreted into breast milk but are not found in the neonatal or infant circulation. Additionally, if any IgG antibodies were to be ingested through breastfeeding, they would probably be digested in the infant's gastrointestinal tract and not absorbed. If used while breastfeeding, the infant should be monitored for the most common reported systemic pediatric side effects of headache (leading to irritability), fever, fatigue (lethargy), and vomiting.

References

1. Prescribing Information. Kedrab. Kamada Ltd; 2021.
2. American College of Obstetricians and Gynecologists. ACOG Committee opinion. Immunization during pregnancy. *Obstet Gynecol*. 2003;101: 207-212.
3. Manning SE, Rupprecht CE, Fishbein D, et al. Human rabies prevention—United States, 2008: recommendations of the Advisory Committee on Immunization Practices. *MMWR Recomm Rep*. 2008;57:1-28.
4. Chutivongse S, Wilde H. Postexposure rabies vaccination during pregnancy: experience with 21 patients. *Vaccine*. 1989;7:546-548.
5. Chutivongse S, Wilde H, Benjavongkulchai M, et al. S. Postexposure rabies vaccination during pregnancy: effect on 202 women and their infants. *Clin Infect Dis*. 1995;20:818-820.
6. Sudarshan MK, Ananda Giri MS. Assessing the safety of post-exposure rabies immunization in pregnancy. *Hum Vaccin*. 2007;3:87-89.
7. Fayaz A, Simani S, Fallahian V, et al. Rabies antibody levels in pregnant women and their newborns after rabies post-exposure prophylaxis. *Iran J Reprod Med*. 2012;10:161-163.
8. Aguèmon CT, Tarantola A, Zoumènou E, et al. Rabies transmission risks during peripartum—two cases and a review of the literature. *Vaccine*. 2016; 34:1752-1757.
9. Windrim C, McGeer AJ, Murphy KE. Exposure to rabies during pregnancy. *CMAJ*. 2018;190:E1281-E1283.
10. Mondal PC, Char D, Mandal D, Das S. Rabies in a pregnant woman and delivery of a live fetus. *Int J Gynaecol Obstet*. 2014;125:171-172.
11. CDC. Guidelines for vaccinating pregnant women. Accessed April 5, 2024. https://www.cdc.gov/vaccines/pregnancy/hcp-toolkit/guidelines.html

IMMUNE GLOBULIN, TETANUS

Immunologic (Antibody)

PREGNANCY RECOMMENDATION: **No Human Data and No Relevant Animal Data (Maternal Benefit May Outweigh Embryofetal Risk)**

BREASTFEEDING RECOMMENDATION: **Probably Compatible**

PREGNANCY SUMMARY

No reports describing the use of tetanus immune globulin in human pregnancy have been located. While specific information is not available, human IgG antibodies are known to cross the placenta, especially during the third trimester, which suggests that some transfer will occur. However, the absence of human pregnancy experience prevents a complete assessment of the embryofetal risk. No animal studies have been conducted. ACOG recommends the use of tetanus immune globulin in pregnancy for postexposure prophylaxis. No known risk exists for the fetus from passive immunization of pregnant women with immune globulin preparations.

I

BREASTFEEDNG SUMMARY

No reports describing the use of tetanus immune globulin during human lactation have been located. Maternal IgG antibodies are excreted into breast milk but are not found in the neonatal or infant circulation. Additionally, if any IgG antibodies were to be ingested through breastfeeding, they would probably be digested in the infant's gastrointestinal tract and not absorbed. If used while breastfeeding, the infant should be monitored for the most common reported systemic side effects of slight temperature elevation.

References

1. Prescribing Information. HyperTET. Grifols Therapeutics LLC; 2022.
2. American College of Obstetricians and Gynecologists. Immunization during pregnancy. Technical Bulletin. No. 160, October 1991.
3. Guidelines for vaccinating pregnant women. Accessed April 5, 2024. https://www.cdc.gov/vaccines/pregnancy/hcp-toolkit/guidelines.html

IMMUNE GLOBULIN, VARICELLA-ZOSTER (VZIG)

Immunologic (Antibody)

PREGNANCY RECOMMENDATION: **Human Data Suggest Compatible**

BREASTFEEDING RECOMMENDATION: **Probably Compatible**

PREGNANCY SUMMARY

Seven reports describing the use of varicella-zoster immune globulin (VZIG) in human pregnancy have been located. No congenital abnormalities or adverse effects have been associated with VZIG use. IgG antibodies are known to cross the placenta, especially during the third trimester, which suggests that some transfer will occur. No animal studies have been conducted. ACOG and the US Centers for Disease Control and Prevention (CDC) recommend that pregnant women who are not immune to varicella-zoster virus and are exposed to someone with chickenpox should receive VZIG as soon as possible, ideally within 96 hours of exposure. The CDC also states that when VZIG cannot be given within the ideal window, it may still be given up to 10 days after exposure. No known risk exists for the fetus from passive immunization of pregnant women with immune globulin preparations.

BREASTFEEDING SUMMARY

No reports describing the use of VZIG during human lactation have been located. IgG antibodies are excreted into breast milk but are not found in neonatal or infant circulation. Additionally, if any IgG antibodies were to be ingested through breastfeeding, they would probably be digested in the infant's gastrointestinal tract and not absorbed. If used while breastfeeding, the infant should be monitored for the most common reported systemic side effect of headache (leading to irritability).

References

1. Prescribing Information. Varizig. Saol Therapeutics, Inc; 2021.
2. Enders G. Management of varicella-zoster contact and infection in pregnancy using a standardized varicella-zoster ELISA test. *Postgrad Med J*. 1985; 61(suppl 4):23-30.
3. McGregor JA, Mark S, Crawford GP, Levin MJ. Varicella zoster antibody testing in the care of pregnant women exposed to varicella. *Am J Obstet Gynecol*. 1987;157:281-284.
4. Koren G, Money D, Boucher M, et al. Serum concentrations, efficacy, and safety of a new, intravenously administered varicella zoster immune globulin in pregnant women. *J Clin Pharmacol*. 2002;42:267-274.

5. Centers for Disease Control and Prevention. Updated recommendations for use of VariZIG—United States, 2013. *MMWR*. 2013;62:574-576.
6. Cytomegalovirus, parvovirus B19, varicella zoster, and toxoplasmosis in pregnancy. Practice bulletin no. 151. American College of Obstetricians and Gynecologists. *Obstet Gynecol*. 2015;125:1510-1525.
7. Trotta M, Borchi B, Niccolai A, et al. Epidemiology, management and outcome of varicella in pregnancy: a 20-year experience at the Tuscany Reference Centre for Infectious Diseases in Pregnancy. *Infection*. 2018;46:693-699.
8. Levin MJ, Duchon JM, Swamy GK, Gershon AA. Varicella zoster immune globulin (VARIZIG) administration up to 10 days after varicella exposure in pregnant women, immunocompromised participants, and infants: varicella outcomes and safety results from a large, open-label, expanded-access program. *PLoS One*. 2019;14:e0217749.
9. Swamy GK, Dotters-Katz SK. Safety and varicella outcomes after varicella zoster immune globulin administration in pregnancy. *Am J Obstet Gynecol*. 2019;221:655-656.
10. Sile B, Brown KE, Gower C, et al. Effectiveness of oral acyclovir in preventing maternal chickenpox: a comparison with VZIG. *J Infect*. 2022;85:147-151.
11. CDC. Guidelines for vaccinating pregnant women. Accessed April 27, 2024. https://www.cdc.gov/vaccines/pregnancy/hcp-toolkit/guidelines.html

INCLISIRAN

Antilipemic (Small Interfering Ribonucleic Acid Agent)

PREGNANCY RECOMMENDATION: No Human Data—Animal Data Suggest Low Risk

BREASTFEEDING RECOMMENDATION: Probably Compatible

I

PREGNANCY SUMMARY

No reports describing the use of inclisiran in human pregnancy have been located. Inclisiran is not likely to cross the placenta, so any infant exposure will probably be clinically insignificant. However, the absence of human pregnancy experience prevents a complete assessment of the embryofetal risk. Animal data did not show any embryofetal toxicity. The manufacturer recommends discontinuing inclisiran when a pregnancy is discovered. Nevertheless, using this drug during pregnancy should be based on the pros and cons of the mother's clinical need for treatment versus any potential fetal risk that might occur from exposure.

BREASTFEEDING SUMMARY

No reports describing the use of inclisiran during human lactation have been located. In general, there is poor oral bioavailability with oligonucleotide-based products. Therefore, any drug levels that might be found in breast milk will probably be negligible. However, breastfeeding while using this drug should be based on the mother's clinical need for treatment. If used, the infant should be monitored for the most common reported adult side effects of arthralgia and extremity pain (both leading to irritability), urinary tract infection, diarrhea, and dyspnea.

Reference

1. Prescribing Information. Leqvio. Novartis Pharmaceuticals; 2021.

INDAPAMIDE

Antihypertensive/Cardiovascular (Diuretic)

PREGNANCY RECOMMENDATION: Limited Human Data—Animal Data Suggest Low Risk

BREASTFEEDING RECOMMENDATION: Probably Compatible

PREGNANCY SUMMARY

One report describing the use of indapamide during the first trimester in 46 human pregnancies was located. Three major birth defects were observed (two expected). No pattern to the anomalies was seen. The drug will probably cross the placenta, so some fetal exposure will likely occur. However, this limited human pregnancy experience prevents a complete assessment of the embryofetal risk. Animal data did not show any embryofetal toxicity in two species at doses of greater than 10 times the RHD. Using this drug during pregnancy should be based on the pros and cons of the mother's clinical need for treatment versus any potential fetal risk that might occur from exposure.

BREASTFEEDING SUMMARY

No reports describing the use of indapamide during human lactation have been located. The closely related thiazide diuretics have been used to suppress lactation (see Chlorothiazide). The drug will likely be found in breast milk, so some infant exposure will probably occur. If the clinical decision is to use this drug while breastfeeding, the infant should be monitored for the most common reported adult side effects of headache, pain, dizziness, and back pain (all leading to irritability), and infections.

References

1. Prescribing Information. Indapamide. Teva Pharmaceuticals; 2022.
2. Seki T, Fujitani M, Osumi S, et al. Reproductive studies of indapamide. *Yakuri Chiryo*. 1982;10:1325-1335, 1337-1353, 1355-1414. As cited in Shepard TH. *Catalog of Teratogenic Agents*. 6th ed. The Johns Hopkins University Press; 1989:347.

INDIGOTINDISULFONATE (INDIGO CARMINE)

Diagnostic (Urologic)

PREGNANCY RECOMMENDATION: Limited Human Data—No Relevant Animal Data

BREASTFEEDING RECOMMENDATION: Probably Compatible

PREGNANCY SUMMARY

No reports linking the use of indigotindisulfonate with congenital defects have been located. Use in the first trimester of pregnancy has not been located. Intra-amniotic injections have occurred after the first trimester without apparent effect on the fetus. The diagnostic agent will likely cross the placenta, so some fetal exposure will probably occur. Therefore, this limited human pregnancy experience prevents a complete assessment of the embryofetal risk. No animal reproduction studies have been conducted. Because of its known toxicities after IV administration, the dye should not be considered low risk for use in pregnancy.

BREASTFEEDING SUMMARY

No reports describing the use of indigotindisulfonate during human lactation have been located. The diagnostic agent will probably appear in breast milk, so some infant exposure will likely occur. However, the low oral availability suggests that if excretion into breast milk occurs, it is unlikely to be absorbed in a clinically significant amount. If used while breastfeeding, adverse effects on the breastfed infant are not expected.

References

1. Prescribing Information. Bludigo. Provepharm, Inc; 2022.
2. Elias S, Gerbie AB, Simpson JL, et al. Genetic amniocentesis in twin gestations. *Am J Obstet Gynecol*. 1980;138:169-174.
3. Horger EO III, Moody LO. Use of indigo carmine for twin amniocentesis and its effect on bilirubin analysis. *Am J Obstet Gynecol*. 1984;150:858-860.
4. Pijpers L, Jahoda MGJ, Vosters RPL, et al. Genetic amniocentesis in twin pregnancies. *Br J Obstet Gynaecol*. 1988;95:323-326.
5. Quintero RA, Morales WJ, Allen M, et al. Treatment of iatrogenic previable premature rupture of membranes with intra-amniotic injection of platelets and cryoprecipitate (amniopatch): preliminary experience. *Am J Obstet Gynecol*. 1999;181;744-749.
6. Fribourg S. Safety of intra-amniotic injection of indigo carmine. *Am J Obstet Gynecol*. 1981;140:350-351.
7. Van Der Pol JG, Wolf H, Boer K, et al. Jejunal atresia related to the use of methylene blue in genetic amniocentesis in twins. *Br J Obstet Gynaecol*. 1992;99:141-143.
8. McFadyen I. The dangers of intra-amniotic methylene blue. *Br J Obstet Gynaecol*. 1992;99:89-90.
9. Adekola H, Gill N, Sakr S, et al. Outcomes following intra-amniotic instillation with indigo carmine to diagnose prelabor rupture of membranes in singleton pregnancies: a single center experience. *J Matern Fetal Neonatal Med*. 2016;29:544-549.
10. Cragan JD, Martin ML, Khoury MJ, Fernhoff PM. Dye use during amniocentesis and birth defects. *Lancet*. 1993;341:1352.

INDOMETHACIN

Pain (Nonsteroidal Anti-Inflammatory Drug)

PREGNANCY RECOMMENDATION: Human Data Suggest Risk (Second and Third Trimesters)

BREASTFEEDING RECOMMENDATION: Probably Compatible (Short-Term Use)

PREGNANCY SUMMARY

The use of indomethacin in all trimesters of human pregnancy has been reported. Many have suggested the possibility of producing major fetal anomalies, but overall, the studies have been contradictory, and no specific pattern to the anomalies has been described. Indomethacin is often used to treat preterm labor. The drug crosses the placenta, so some fetal exposure will occur. Animal data did not show embryofetal toxicity in two species at less than 10 times the RHD. NSAIDs can cause premature stricture or closure of the fetal ductus arteriosus when used in the latter portion of gestation. In some instances, this can produce pulmonary hypertension in the neonate. These drugs have also been reported to produce fetal renal dysfunction leading to oligohydramnios when used after 20 weeks' gestation. The FDA recommends that NSAIDs be avoided in women 20 weeks or later in pregnancy. If deemed necessary by a health care provider, the use of NSAIDs between 20 and 30

(*continued*)

weeks should be limited to the lowest effective dose and shortest duration. If treatment extends beyond 48 hours, providers should consider an ultrasound to monitor amniotic fluid levels.

BREASTFEEDING SUMMARY

Two reports were located that described the use of indomethacin in eight infants whose mothers breastfed while receiving treatment. In one case report, an infant experienced a possible indomethacin-induced seizure on the day and the day after indomethacin was stopped. However, the causal link between the two events has been questioned. Indomethacin is excreted into human breast milk in low amounts. If used while breastfeeding, the infant should be monitored for the most common reported adult side effects of dizziness and gastrointestinal discomfort (both leading to irritability). Overall, short-term use of NSAIDs is probably compatible with breastfeeding, though indomethacin is one of the stronger products. Therefore, the use of a weaker agent (eg, ibuprofen) may be preferred.

I

References

1. Shepard TH. *Catalog of Teratogenic Agents*. 6th ed. The Johns Hopkins University Press; 1989:348-349.
2. Montenegro MA, Palomino H. Induction of cleft palate in mice by inhibitors of prostaglandin synthesis. *J Craniofac Genet Dev Biol*. 1990;10:83-94.
3. Moise KJ Jr, Ou C-N, Kirshon B, et al. Placental transfer of indomethacin in the human pregnancy. *Am J Obstet Gynecol*. 1990;162:549-554.
4. Nielsen GL, Sorensen HT, Larsen H, Pedersen L. Risk of adverse birth outcome and miscarriage in pregnant users of non-steroidal anti-inflammatory drugs: population based observational study and case-control study. *Br Med J*. 2001;322:266-270.
5. Ericson A, Kallen BAJ. Nonsteroidal anti-inflammatory drugs in early pregnancy. *Reprod Toxicol*. 2001;15:371-375.
6. Li DK, Liu L, Odouli R. Exposure to non-steroidal anti-inflammatory drugs during pregnancy and risk of miscarriage: population based cohort study. *Br Med J*. 2003;327:368-371.
7. Tassinari MS, Cook JC, Hurtt ME. NSAIDs and developmental toxicity. *Birth Defects Res B Dev Reprod Toxicol*. 2003;68:3-4.
8. Atad J, David A, Moise J, Abramovici H. Classification of threatened premature labor related to treatment with a prostaglandin inhibitor: indomethacin. *Biol Neonate*. 1980;37:291-296.
9. Gonzalez CHL, Jimenez PG, Pezzotti y R MA, Favela EL. Hipertension pulmonar persistente en el recien nacido por uso prenatal de inhibidores de las prostaglandinas (indometacina). Informe de un caso. *Ginecol Obstet Mex*. 1980;48:103-110.
10. Sureau C, Piovani P. Clinical study of indomethacin for prevention of prematurity. *Eur J Obstet Gynecol Reprod Biol*. 1983;46:400-402.
11. Van Kets H, Thiery M, Derom R, et al. Perinatal hazards of chronic antenatal tocolysis with indomethacin. *Prostaglandins*. 1979;18:893-907.
12. Van Kets H, Thiery M, Derom R, et al. Prostaglandin synthase inhibitors in preterm labor. *Lancet*. 1980;2:693.
13. Blake DA, Niebyl JR, White RD, et al. Treatment of premature labor with indomethacin. *Adv Prostaglandin Thromboxane Res*. 1980;8:1465-1467.
14. Grella P, Zanor P. Premature labor and indomethacin. *Prostaglandins*. 1978;16:1007-1017.
15. Karim SMM. On the use of blockers of prostaglandin synthesis in the control of labor. *Adv Prostaglandin Thromboxane Res*. 1978;4:301-306.
16. Katz Z, Lancet M, Yemini M, et al. Treatment of premature labor contractions with combined ritodrine and indomethacin. *Int J Gynaecol Obstet*. 1983;21:337-342.
17. Niebyl JR, Blake DA, White RD, et al. The inhibition of premature labor with indomethacin. *Am J Obstet Gynecol*. 1980;136:1014-1019.
18. Peteja J. Indometacyna w zapobieganiu porodom przedwczesnym. *Ginekol Pol*. 1980;51:347-353.
19. Reiss U, Atad J, Rubinstein I, Zuckerman H. The effect of indomethacin in labour at term. *Int J Gynaecol Obstet*. 1976;14:369-374.
20. Souka AR, Osman N, Sibaie F, Einen MA. Therapeutic value of indomethacin in threatened abortion. *Prostaglandins*. 1980;19:457-460.
21. Spearing G. Alcohol, indomethacin, and salbutamol. *Obstet Gynecol*. 1979;53:171-174.
22. Chimura T. The treatment of threatened premature labor by drugs. *Acta Obstet Gynaecol Jpn*. 1980;32:1620-1624.
23. Suzanne F, Fresne JJ, Portal B, Baudon J. Essai therapeutique de l'indometacine dans les menaces d'accouchement premature: a propos de 30 observations. *Therapie*. 1980;35:751-760.
24. Tinga DJ, Aranoudse JG. Post-partum pulmonary oedema associated with preventive therapy for premature labor. *Lancet*. 1979;1:1026.
25. Dudley DKL, Hardie MJ. Fetal and neonatal effects of indomethacin used as a tocolytic agent. *Am J Obstet Gynecol*. 1985;151:181-184.
26. Gamissans O, Canas E, Cararach V, et al. A study of indomethacin combined with ritodrine in threatened preterm labor. *Eur J Obstet Gynecol Reprod Biol*. 1978;8:123-128.
27. Wiqvist N, Lundstrom V, Green K. Premature labor and indomethacin. *Prostaglandins*. 1975;10:515-526.
28. Wiqvist N, Kjellmer I, Thiringer K, et al. Treatment of premature labor by prostaglandin synthetase inhibitors. *Acta Biol Med Germ*. 1978;37:923-930.
29. Zuckerman H, Reiss U, Rubinstein I. Inhibition of human premature labor by indomethacin. *Obstet Gynecol*. 1974;44:787-792.
30. Zuckerman H, Reiss U, Atad J, et al. The effect of indomethacin on plasma levels of prostaglandin F2α in women in labour. *Br J Obstet Gynaecol*. 1977;84:339-343.
31. Zuckerman H, Shalev E, Gilad G, Katzuni E. Further study of the inhibition of premature labor by indomethacin. Part I. *J Perinat Med*. 1984;12:19-23.
32. Zuckerman H, Shalev E, Gilad G, Katzuni E. Further study of the inhibition of premature labor by indomethacin. Part II. Double-blind study. *J Perinat Med*. 1984;12:25-29.
33. Niebyl JR. Prostaglandin synthetase inhibitors. *Semin Perinatol*. 1981;5:274-287.
34. Niebyl JR, Witter FR. Neonatal outcome after indomethacin treatment for preterm labor. *Am J Obstet Gynecol*. 1986;155:747-749.
35. Besinger RE, Niebyl JR, Keyes WG, Johnson TRB. Randomized comparative trial of indomethacin and ritodrine for the long-term treatment of preterm labor. *Am J Obstet Gynecol*. 1991;164:981-988.
36. Evans DJ, Kofinas AD, King K. Intraoperative amniocentesis and indomethacin treatment in the management of an immature pregnancy with completely dilated cervix. *Obstet Gynecol*. 1992;79:881-882.
37. Leonardi MR, Hankins GDV. What's new in tocolytics. *Clin Perinatol*. 1992;19:367-384.
38. Higby K, Xenakis EM-J, Pauerstein CJ. Do tocolytic agents stop preterm labor? A critical and comprehensive review of efficacy and safety. *Am J Obstet Gynecol*. 1993;168:1247-1259.
39. Morales WJ, Smith SG, Angel JL, et al. Efficacy and safety of indomethacin versus ritodrine in the management of preterm labor: a randomized study. *Obstet Gynecol*. 1989;74:567-572.
40. Morales WJ, Madhav H. Efficacy and safety of indomethacin compared with magnesium sulfate in the management of preterm labor: a randomized study. *Am J Obstet Gynecol*. 1993;169:97-102.
41. Levin DL. Effects of inhibition of prostaglandin synthesis on fetal development, oxygenation, and the fetal circulation. *Semin Perinatol*. 1980;4:35-44.
42. Csaba IF, Sulyok E, Ertl T. Relationship of maternal treatment with indomethacin to persistence of fetal circulation syndrome. *J Pediatr*. 1978;92:484.
43. Levin DL, Fixler DE, Morriss FC, Tyson J. Morphologic analysis of the pulmonary vascular bed in infants exposed in utero to prostaglandin synthetase inhibitors. *J Pediatr*. 1978;92:478-483.
44. Rubaltelli FF, Chiozza ML, Zanardo V, Cantarutti F. Effect on neonate of maternal treatment with indomethacin. *J Pediatr*. 1979;94:161.
45. Manchester D, Margolis HS, Sheldon RE. Possible association between maternal indomethacin therapy and primary pulmonary hypertension of the newborn. *Am J Obstet Gynecol*. 1976;126:467-469.
46. Goudie BM, Dossetor JFB. Effect on the fetus of indomethacin given to suppress labour. *Lancet*. 1979;2:1187-1188.
47. Mogilner BM, Ashkenazy M, Borenstein R, Lancet M. Hydrops fetalis caused by maternal indomethacin treatment. *Acta Obstet Gynecol Scand*. 1982;61:183-185.
48. Moise KJ Jr, Huhta JC, Sharif DS, et al. Indomethacin in the treatment of premature labor: effects on the fetal ductus arteriosus. *N Engl J Med*. 1988;319:327-331.

49. Van Den Veyver I, Moise K Jr, Ou C-N, Carpenter RJ Jr. The effect of gestational age and fetal indomethacin levels on the incidence of constriction of the fetal ductus arteriosus (abstract). *Am J Obstet Gynecol*. 1993;168:373.
50. Van Den Veyver IB, Moise KJ Jr, Ou C-N, Carpenter RJ Jr. The effect of gestational age and fetal indomethacin levels on the incidence of constriction of the fetal ductus arteriosus. *Obstet Gynecol*. 1993;82:500-503.
51. Moise KJ Jr. Effect of advancing gestational age on the frequency of fetal ductal constriction in association with maternal indomethacin use. *Am J Obstet Gynecol*. 1993;168:1350-1353.
52. Ovadia M. Effects of indomethacin on the fetus. *N Engl J Med*. 1988; 319:1484.
53. Moise KJ Jr, Huhta JC, Mari G. Effects of indomethacin on the fetus. *N Engl J Med*. 1988;319:1485.
54. Atad J, Lissak A, Rofe A, Abramovici H. Patent ductus arteriosus after prolonged treatment with indomethacin during pregnancy: case report. *Int J Gynaecol Obstet*. 1987;25:73-76.
55. Itskovitz J, Abramovici H, Brandes JM. Oligohydramnion, meconium and perinatal death concurrent with indomethacin treatment in human pregnancy. *J Reprod Med*. 1980;24:137-140.
56. Veersema D, de Jong PA, van Wijck JAM. Indomethacin and the fetal renal nonfunction syndrome. *Eur J Obstet Gynecol Reprod Biol*. 1983;16:113-121.
57. Cabrol D, Landesman R, Muller J, et al. Treatment of polyhydramnios with prostaglandin synthetase inhibitor (indomethacin). *Am J Obstet Gynecol*. 1987;157:422-426.
58. Kirshon B, Cotton DB. Polyhydramnios associated with a ring chromosome and low maternal serum α-fetoprotein levels managed with indomethacin. *Am J Obstet Gynecol*. 1988;158:1063-1064.
59. De Wit W, Van Mourik I, Wiesenhaan PF. Prolonged maternal indomethacin therapy associated with oligohydramnios: case reports. *Br J Obstet Gynecol*. 1988;95:303-305.
60. Goldenberg RL, Davis RO, Baker RC. Indomethacin-induced oligohydramnios. *Am J Obstet Gynecol*. 1989;160:1196-1197.
61. Hickok DE, Hollenbach KA, Reilley SF, Nyberg DA. The association between decreased amniotic fluid volume and treatment with nonsteroidal anti-inflammatory agents for preterm labor. *Am J Obstet Gynecol*. 1989;160:1525-1531.
62. Kirshon B, Moise KJ Jr, Wasserstrum N, et al. Influence of short-term indomethacin therapy on fetal urine output. *Obstet Gynecol*. 1988;72:51-53.
63. Demandt E, Legius E, Devlieger H, et al. Prenatal indomethacin toxicity in one member of monozygous twins; a case report. *Eur J Obstet Gynecol Reprod Biol*. 1990;35:267-269.
64. Eronen M, Pesonen E, Kurki T, et al. The effects of indomethacin and a β-sympathomimetic agent on the fetal ductus arteriosus during treatment of premature labor: a randomized double-blind study. *Am J Obstet Gynecol*. 1991;164:141-146.
65. Hallak M, Reiter AA, Ayres NA, Moise KJ Jr. Indomethacin for preterm labor: fetal toxicity in a dizygotic twin gestation. *Obstet Gynecol*. 1991;78:911-913.
66. Rosemond RL, Boehm FH, Moreau G, Karmo H. Tricuspid regurgitation: a method of monitoring patients treated with indomethacin (abstract). *Am J Obstet Gynecol*. 1992;166:336.
67. Bivins HA Jr, Newman RB, Fyfe DA, et al. Randomized comparative trial of indomethacin and terbutaline for the long term treatment of preterm labor (abstract). *Am J Obstet Gynecol*. 1993;168:375.
68. Norton M, Merril J, Kuller J, Clyman R. Neonatal complications after antenatal indomethacin for preterm labor (abstract). *Am J Obstet Gynecol*. 1993;168:303.
69. Norton ME, Merrill J, Cooper BAB, et al. Neonatal complications after the administration of indomethacin for preterm labor. *N Engl J Med*. 1993;329:1602-1607.
70. Carlan SJ, Stromquist C, Angel JL, et al. Cocaine and indomethacin: fetal anuria, neonatal edema, and gastrointestinal bleeding. *Obstet Gynecol*. 1991; 78:501-503.
71. Kirshon B, Mari G, Moise KJ Jr. Indomethacin therapy in the treatment of symptomatic polyhydramnios. *Obstet Gynecol*. 1990;75:202-205.
72. Mari G, Moise KJ Jr, Deter RL, et al. Doppler assessment of the renal blood flow velocity waveform during indomethacin therapy for preterm labor and polyhydramnios. *Obstet Gynecol*. 1990;75:199-201.
73. Mamopoulos M, Assimakopoulos E, Reece EA, et al. Maternal indomethacin therapy in the treatment of polyhydramnios. *Am J Obstet Gynecol*. 1990;162:1225-1229.
74. Kirshon B, Mari G, Moise KJ Jr, Wasserstrum N. Effect of indomethacin on the fetal ductus arteriosus during treatment of symptomatic polyhydramnios. *J Reprod Med*. 1990;35:529-532.
75. Smith LG Jr, Kirshon B, Cotton DB. Indomethacin treatment of polyhydramnios and subsequent infantile nephrogenic diabetes insipidus. *Am J Obstet Gynecol*. 1990;163:98-99.
76. Ash K, Harman CR, Gritter H. TRAP sequence—successful outcome with indomethacin treatment. *Obstet Gynecol*. 1990;76:960-962.
77. Malas HZ, Hamlett JD. Acute recurrent polyhydramnios—management with indomethacin. *Br J Obstet Gynaecol*. 1991;98:583-587.
78. Nordstrom L, Westgren M. Indomethacin treatment for polyhydramnios. Effective but potentially dangerous? *Acta Obstet Gynecol Scand*. 1992;71:239-241.
79. Dolkart LA, Eshwar KP, Reimers FT. Indomethacin therapy and chronic hemodialysis during pregnancy. A case report. *J Reprod Med*. 1992;37:181-183.
80. Buderus S, Thomas B, Fahnenstich H, Kowalewski S. Renal failure in two preterm infants: toxic effect of prenatal maternal indomethacin treatment? *Br J Obstet Gynaecol*. 1993;100:97-98.
81. Deeny M, Haxton MJ. Indomethacin use to control gross polyhydramnios complicating triplet pregnancy. *Br J Obstet Gynaecol*. 1993;100:281-282.
82. Murray HG, Stone PR, Strand L, Flower J. Fetal pleural effusion following maternal indomethacin therapy. *Br J Obstet Gynaecol*. 1993;100:277-282.
83. Moise KJ Jr. Indomethacin therapy in the treatment of symptomatic polyhydramnios. *Clin Obstet Gynecol*. 1991;34:310-318.
84. Schoenfeld A, Freedman S, Hod M, Ovadia Y. Antagonism of antihypertensive drug therapy in pregnancy by indomethacin? *Am J Obstet Gynecol*. 1989;161:1204-1205.
85. Mousavy SM. Indomethacin induces hypertensive crisis in preeclampsia irrespective of prior antihypertensive drug therapy. *Am J Obstet Gynecol*. 1991;165:1577.
86. Hansen PD. *Drug Interactions*. 5th ed. Lea & Febiger; 1985:36.
87. Vanhaesebrouck P, Thiery M, Leroy JG, et al. Oligohydramnios, renal insufficiency, and ileal perforation in preterm infants after intrauterine exposure to indomethacin. *J Pediatr*. 1988;113:738-743.
88. Di Battista C, Landizi L, Tamborino G. Focomelia ed agenesia del pene in neonato. *Minerva Pediatr*. 1975;27:675. As cited in Dukes MNG, ed. *Side Effects of Drugs Annual 1*. Excerpta Medica; 1977:89.
89. Van Marter LJ, Leviton A, Allred EN, et al. Persistent pulmonary hypertension of the newborn and smoking and aspirin and nonsteroidal antiinflammatory drug consumption during pregnancy. *Pediatrics*. 1996;97:658-663.
90. Matt DW, Borzelleca JF. Toxic effects on the female reproductive system during pregnancy, parturition, and lactation. In: Witorsch RJ, ed. *Reproductive Toxicology*. 2nd ed. Raven Press; 1995:175-193.
91. Dawood MY. Nonsteroidal antiinflammatory drugs and reproduction. *Am J Obstet Gynecol*. 1993;169:1255-1265.
92. Eeg-Olofsson O, Malmros I, Elwin CE, Steen B. Convulsions in a breast-fed infant after maternal indomethacin. *Lancet*. 1978;2:215.
93. Lebedevs TH, Wojnar-Horton RE, Yapp P, et al. Excretion of indomethacin in breast milk. *Br J Clin Pharmacol*. 1991;32:751-754.
94. Fairhead FW. Convulsions in a breast-fed infant after maternal indomethacin. *Lancet*. 1978;2:576.
95. Prescribing Information. Indomethacin. Chartwell RX, LLC; 2023.

INEBILIZUMAB

Central Nervous System (CD19-Directed Cytolytic—Monoclonal Antibody)

PREGNANCY RECOMMENDATION: No Human Data—Animal Data Suggest Potential Risk

BREASTFEEDING RECOMMENDATION: Probably Compatible

PREGNANCY SUMMARY

No reports describing the use of inebilizumab in human pregnancy have been located. As an IgG antibody, inebilizumab likely crosses the placenta. Therefore, the absence of human pregnancy experience prevents a complete assessment of embryofetal risk. Animal data did not show fetotoxic effects but did demonstrate a marked decrease in B cells and a persistent reduction in immune function. Due to these findings from animal studies, the manufacturer recommends that women with reproductive potential use effective contraception during treatment and for at least 6 months after the last dose. Nevertheless, using this drug during pregnancy should be based on the pros and cons of the mother's clinical need for treatment versus any potential fetal risk that might occur from exposure.

BREASTFEEDING SUMMARY

No reports describing the use of inebilizumab during human lactation have been located. The drug is likely present in breast milk. However, it is known that IgG antibodies can be found in human breast milk but are not found in neonatal or infant circulation. Additionally, if any IgG antibodies were to be ingested through breastfeeding, they would probably be digested in the infant's gastrointestinal tract and not be absorbed. Breastfeeding while using this drug should be based on the mother's clinical need for treatment versus any potential adverse infant effects, including B-cell depletion. If used, the infant should be monitored for the most common reported adult side effects of arthralgia (leading to irritability) and urinary tract infection.

I

Reference

1. Prescribing Information. Uplizna. Horizon Therapeutics USA, Inc; 2021.

INFIGRATINIB

Antineoplastic (Fibroblast Growth Factor Receptor Kinase Inhibitor)

PREGNANCY RECOMMENDATION: No Human Data—Animal Data Suggest Potential Risk

BREASTFEEDING RECOMMENDATION: Potential Toxicity

PREGNANCY SUMMARY

No reports describing the use of infigratinib in human pregnancy have been located. Infigratinib will likely cross the placenta, so some fetal exposure will probably occur. Therefore, the absence of human pregnancy experience prevents a complete assessment of embryofetal risk. Embryofetal toxicity with malformations was observed in animal studies. Based on the animal studies and the drug's mechanism of action, the manufacturer recommends that women with reproductive potential use effective contraception during treatment and for 1 month after the last dose. They also recommend that males with female partners of reproductive potential use effective contraception during treatment and for 1 month after the last dose. Nevertheless, using this drug during pregnancy should be based on the pros and cons of the mother's clinical need for treatment versus any potential fetal risk that might occur from exposure. There is a registry for women who are pregnant and have cancer. For more information, women and health care providers are encouraged to contact the Cancer and Pregnancy Registry at 1-877-635-4499.

BREASTFEEDING SUMMARY

No reports describing the use of infigratinib during human lactation have been located. The drug will likely be excreted into breast milk, so some infant exposure will probably occur. Due to the concern for potential serious adverse effects that might be seen in a breastfed infant, the manufacturer recommends that women not breastfeed while taking infigratinib or for 1 month after the last dose. Nevertheless, breastfeeding while using this drug should be based on the mother's clinical need for treatment. If used, the infant should be monitored for the most common reported adult side effects of nausea, abdominal pain, and arthralgia (all leading to irritability), diarrhea, lethargy, alopecia, vomiting, constipation, and decreased appetite (monitor growth) and various laboratory abnormalities (see PI).

Reference

1. Prescribing Information. Truseltiq. QED Therapeutics; 2021.

INFLIXIMAB

Gastrointestinal/Immunologic (Monoclonal Antibody—Tumor Necrosis Factor Inhibitor)

PREGNANCY RECOMMENDATION: Human Data and Animal Data Suggest Low Risk (Contraindicated If Combined With Methotrexate)

BREASTFEEDING RECOMMENDATION: Probably Compatible

PREGNANCY SUMMARY

Numerous reports have described the use of infliximab in human pregnancy. These reports included over 2,600 infliximab exposures in all trimesters. Of more than 1,500 first-trimester exposures, no significant adverse effects or increased rate of major malformations attributed to the drug were found. Infliximab has been shown to cross the placenta in late gestation, consistent with IgG antibodies. Animal data did not show any embryofetal toxicity in two species at doses or greater than 10 times the RHD. While the safety of tumor necrosis factor (TNF) inhibitors, such as infliximab, is emerging, ACOG considers them as low risk to continue or initiate during pregnancy. The American College of Rheumatology and British Society for Rheumatology also consider TNF-α inhibitors compatible for use in pregnancy.

I

BREASTFEEDING SUMMARY

Several reports describing the use of infliximab during human lactation have been found, and no adverse effects have been reported. Infliximab can be found in human breast milk of some women, but not all. However, if any IgG antibodies were to be ingested through breastfeeding, they would probably be digested in the infant's gastrointestinal tract and not absorbed. ACOG and the Society for Maternal-Fetal Medicine recommend that women not discontinue these medications during pregnancy or breastfeeding. Additionally, the American College of Rheumatology and British Society for Rheumatology consider TNF-α inhibitors to be compatible for use in breastfeeding. If used while breastfeeding, the infant should be monitored for the most common reported adult side effect of infection.

References

1. Gisbert JP. Safety of immunomodulators and biologics for the treatment of inflammatory bowel disease during pregnancy and breast-feeding. *Inflamm Bowel Dis*. 2010;16:881-895.
2. El Mourabet M, El-Hachem S, Harrison JR, Binion DG. Anti-TNF antibody therapy for inflammatory bowel disease during pregnancy: a clinical review. *Curr Drug Targets*. 2010;234-241.
3. Mahadevan U, Cucchiara S, Hyams JS, et al. The London position statement of the World Congress of Gastroenterology on biological therapy for IBD with the European Crohn's and Colitis Organization: pregnancy and pediatrics. *Am J Gastroenterol*. 2011;106:214-223.
4. Prescribing Information. Infliximab. Janssen Biotech, Inc; 2021.
5. Treacy G. Using an analogous monoclonal antibody to evaluate the reproductive and chronic toxicity potential for a humanized anti-TNFα monoclonal antibody. *Hum Exp Toxicol*. 2000;19:226-228.
6. Mahadevan U, Wolf DC, Dubinsky M, et al. Placental transfer of anti-tumor necrosis factor agents in pregnant patients with inflammatory bowel disease. *Clin Gastroenterol Hepatol*. 2013;11:286-292.
7. Srinivasan R. Infliximab treatment and pregnancy outcome in active Crohn's disease. *Am J Gastroenterol*. 2001;96:2274-2275.
8. Stein RB, Hanauer SB. Comparative tolerability of treatments for inflammatory bowel disease. *Drug Saf*. 2000;23:429-448.
9. Antoni CE, Furst D, Manger B, Lichtenstein GR, et al. Outcome of pregnancy in women receiving Remicade (infliximab) for the treatment of Crohn's disease or rheumatoid arthritis (abstract). *Arthritis Rheum*. 2001;44(suppl 9):S152.
10. Burt MJ, Frizelle FA, Barbezar GO. Pregnancy and exposure to infliximab (anti-tumor necrosis factor-alpha monoclonal antibody). *J Gastroenterol Hepatol*. 2003;18:465-466.
11. Chakravarty EF, Sanchez-Yamamoto D, Bush TM. The use of disease modifying antirheumatic drugs in women with rheumatoid arthritis of childbearing age: a survey of practice patterns and pregnancy outcomes. *J Rheumatol*. 2003;30:241-246.
12. Khanna D, McMahon M, Furst DE. Safety of tumour necrosis factor-α antagonists. *Drug Saf*. 2004;27:307-324.
13. Chambers CD, Johnson DL, Jones KL; The OTIS Collaborative Research Group. Pregnancy outcome in women exposed to anti-TNF-alpha medications: the OTIS Rheumatoid Arthritis in Pregnancy study (abstract). *Arthritis Rheum*. 2004;50:S479.
14. Chambers CD, Johnson DL, Jones KL. Safety of anti-TNF-α medications in pregnancy (abstract). *J Am Acad Dermatol*. 2005;52(suppl 1):P196.
15. Katz JA, Antoni C, Keenan GF, et al. Outcome of pregnancy in women receiving infliximab for the treatment of Crohn's disease and rheumatoid arthritis. *Am J Gastroenterol*. 2004;99:2385-2392.
16. Hyrich KL, Symmons DPM, Watson KD, Silman AJ. Pregnancy outcome in women who were exposed to anti-tumor necrosis factor agents: results from a national population register. *Arthritis Rheum*. 2006;54:2701-2702.
17. Vasiliauskas EA, Church JA, Silverman N, et al. Case report: evidence for transplacental transfer of maternally administered infliximab to the newborn. *Clin Gastroenterol Hepatol*. 2006;4:1255-1258.
18. Stengel JZ, Arnold HL. Is infliximab safe to use while breastfeeding? *World J Gastroenterol*. 2008;14:3085-3087.
19. Carter JD, Ladhani A, Ricca LR, et al. A safety assessment of tumor necrosis factor antagonists during pregnancy: a review of the Food and Drug Administration database. *J Rheumatol*. 2009;36:635-641.
20. Koren G, Inoue M. Do tumor necrosis factor inhibitors cause malformations in humans? *J Rheumatol*. 2009;36:465-466.
21. Berthelot JM, De Bandt M, Goupille P, et al.; on behalf of CRI (Club Rhumatismes et Inflammation). Exposition to anti-TNF drugs during pregnancy: outcome of 15 cases and review of the literature. *Joint Bone Spine*. 2009;76:28-34.
22. Kane S, Ford J, Cohen R, Wagner C. Absence of infliximab in infants and breast milk from nursing mothers receiving therapy for Crohn's disease before and after delivery. *J Clin Gastroenterol*. 2009;43:613-616.
23. Weber-Schoendorfer C, Oppermann M, Wacker E, et al. Pregnancy outcome after TNF-α inhibitor therapy during the first trimester: a prospective multicenter cohort study. *Br J Clin Pharmacol*. 2015;80:727-729.
24. Diav-Citrin O, Otcheretianski-Volodarsky A, Schechtman S, Ornoy A. Pregnancy outcome following gestational exposure to TNF-α-inhibitors: a prospective, comparative, observational study. *Reprod Toxicol*. 2014;43:78-84.
25. Gotestam Skorpen C, Hoeltzenbein M, Tincani A, et al. The EULAR points to consider for use of antirheumatic drugs before pregnancy, and during pregnancy and lactation. *Ann Rheum Dis*. 2016;75:795-810.
26. Immune modulating therapies in pregnancy and lactation. ACOG Committee Opinion No. 776. American College of Obstetricians and Gynecologists. *Obstet Gynecol*. 2019;133:e287-e295.
27. Russell MD, Dey M, Flint J, et al.; BSR Standards, Audit and Guidelines Working Group. British Society for Rheumatology guideline on prescribing drugs in pregnancy and breastfeeding: immunomodulatory anti-rheumatic drugs and corticosteroids. *Rheumatology (Oxford)*. 2023;62:e48-e88.

INOTERSEN

Miscellaneous (Antisense Oligonucleotide)

PREGNANCY RECOMMENDATION: No Human Data—Animal Data Suggest Low Risk

BREASTFEEDING RECOMMENDATION: Probably Compatible

PREGNANCY SUMMARY

No reports describing the use of inotersen in human pregnancy have been located. Placental transfer is unlikely to be clinically significant. However, the absence of human pregnancy experience prevents a complete assessment of the embryofetal risk. No embryofetal toxicity was observed in one animal species at doses of less than 10 times the RHD (despite being administered every other day for about 2 weeks). Standard dosing in humans is administration once per week. Using this drug during pregnancy should be based on the pros and cons of the mother's clinical need for treatment versus any potential fetal risk that might occur from exposure. There is a pregnancy exposure registry that monitors pregnancy outcomes in women exposed to inotersen during pregnancy. Health care providers are encouraged to register patients, and pregnant women are encouraged to register themselves by calling 1-877-465-7510. Due to the risk of serious bleeding caused by severe thrombopenia and glomerulonephritis, inotersen is only available through a restricted distribution program.

I

BREASTFEEDING SUMMARY

No reports describing the use of inotersen during human lactation have been located. The drug is not likely to be found in breast milk at clinically significant levels. In addition, because it is an oligonucleotide, if the drug were to be ingested through breastfeeding, it would probably be partially digested in the infant's gastrointestinal tract and not be absorbed. Breastfeeding while using this drug should be based on the mother's clinical need for treatment versus any potential infant risks that might occur. If used, the infant should be monitored for the most common reported adult side effects of nausea and headache (both leading to irritability), fatigue (lethargy), thrombocytopenia, and fever.

Reference

1. Prescribing Information. Tegsedi. Akcea Therapeutics; 2024.

INOTUZUMAB OZOGAMICIN

Antineoplastic (CD22-Directed—Monoclonal Antibody)

PREGNANCY RECOMMENDATION: No Human Data—Animal Data Suggest Potential Risk

BREASTFEEDING RECOMMENDATION: Potential Toxicity

PREGNANCY SUMMARY

No reports describing the use of inotuzumab ozogamicin in human pregnancy have been located. As an IgG antibody, the drug likely crosses the placenta, so some fetal exposure will probably occur. Ozogamicin is calicheamicin plus a linker agent. The potential effect of free calicheamicin is unknown. Therefore, the absence of human pregnancy experience prevents a complete assessment of the embryofetal risk. Animal data did show fetotoxic effects. Based on the drug's mechanism of action and animal studies, the manufacturer recommends that women with reproductive potential use effective contraception during treatment and for at least 8 months after the last dose. They also recommend that males with female partners of reproductive potential use effective contraception during treatment and for 5 months after the last dose. Nevertheless, using this drug during pregnancy should be based on the pros and cons of the mother's clinical need for treatment versus any potential fetal risk that might occur from exposure. The drug may also prolong the QT interval. There is a registry for women who are pregnant and have cancer. For more information, women and health care providers are encouraged to contact the Cancer and Pregnancy Registry at 1-877-635-4499.

BREASTFEEDING SUMMARY

No reports describing the use of inotuzumab ozogamicin during human lactation have been located. The drug is likely present in breast milk. However, it is known that IgG antibodies can be found in human breast milk but are not found in the neonatal or infant circulation. Additionally, if any IgG antibodies were to be ingested through breastfeeding, they would probably be digested in the infant's gastrointestinal tract and not be absorbed. Though plasma calicheamicin by itself in most cases is below quantitation, it is believed that a limited to negligible amount would be found in breast milk. However, the manufacturer recommends that women not breastfeed while being treated with this drug and for at least 2 months after the last dose. Nevertheless, breastfeeding while using this drug should be based on the mother's clinical need for treatment versus any potential adverse infant effects that might occur. If used, the infant should be monitored for the most common reported adult side effects of abdominal pain and nausea (both leading to irritability), pyrexia, lethargy, infections, and numerous laboratory abnormalities (see PI).

Reference

1. Prescribing Information. Besponsa. Wyeth Pharmaceuticals, Inc; 2017.

INSULIN, HUMAN

Antidiabetic

PREGNANCY RECOMMENDATION: Human Data Suggest Compatible

BREASTFEEDING RECOMMENDATION: Compatible

PREGNANCY SUMMARY

The use of insulin during pregnancy is well reported throughout the literature. Human insulin reportedly does not cross the placenta, so fetal exposure does not occur. ACOG and the American Diabetes Association (ADA) recommend the use of insulin as first-line pharmacologic therapy for the treatment of pregestational and gestational diabetes. Hypoglycemia may occur in patients treated with insulin. Glucose levels should be closely monitored, and insulin doses adjusted, as needed.

BREASTFEEDING SUMMARY

Insulin is naturally found in human breast milk. One report evaluated the excretion of exogenous insulin into human breast milk. While insulin is excreted into breast milk, most of it will probably be digested in the infant's gastrointestinal tract and not absorbed. ACOG and the ADA recommend breastfeeding for all mothers with diabetes. No adverse effects have been reported in breastfed infants whose mothers received human insulin.

References

1. Prescribing Information. Humulin R. Eli Lilly and Company; 2023.
2. Prescribing Information. Humulin N. Eli Lilly and Company; 2022.
3. Menon RK, Cohen RM, Sperling MA, et al. Transplacental passage of insulin in pregnant women with insulin-dependent diabetes mellitus. *N Engl J Med*. 1990;323:309-315.
4. Kimmerle R, Chantelau EA. Transplacental passage of insulin. *N Engl J Med*. 1991;324:198.
5. Weiss PA, Kainer F, Haas J. Cord blood insulin to assess the quality of treatment in diabetic pregnancies. *Early Hum Dev*. 1998;51:187-195.
6. Lindsay RS, Ziegler AG, Hamilton BA, et al. Scottish Multicentre Study of Diabetes in Pregnancy. Type 1 diabetes-related antibodies in the fetal circulation: prevalence and influence on cord insulin and birth weight in offspring of mothers with type 1 diabetes. *J Clin Endocrinol Metab*. 2004;89:3436-3439.
7. American College of Obstetricians and Gynecologists' Committee on Practice Bulletins—Obstetrics. Practice bulletin no. 190: gestational diabetes mellitus. *Obstet Gynecol*. 2018;131:e49-e64.
8. American College of Obstetricians and Gynecologists' Committee on Practice Bulletins—Obstetrics. ACOG practice bulletin no. 201: pregestational diabetes mellitus. *Obstet Gynecol*. 2018;132:e228-e248.
9. Yu DQ, Xu GX, Teng XY, et al. Glycemic control and neonatal outcomes in women with gestational diabetes mellitus treated using glyburide, metformin, or insulin: a pairwise and network meta-analysis. *BMC Endocr Disord*. 2021;21:199.
10. Bidhendi YR, Amiri M, Ramezani TF, Behboudi-Gandevani S. Effectiveness of antidiabetic agents for treatment of gestational diabetes: a methodological quality assessment of meta-analyses and network meta-analysis. *J Diabetes Investig*. 2021;12:2247-2258.
11. Musa OAH, Syed A, Mohamed AM, et al. Metformin is comparable to insulin for pharmacotherapy in gestational diabetes mellitus: a network meta-analysis evaluating 6046 women. *Pharmacol Res*. 2021;167:105546.
12. Wang X, Liu W, Chen H, Chen Q. Comparison of insulin, metformin, and glyburide on perinatal complications of gestational diabetes mellitus: a systematic review and meta-analysis. *Gynecol Obstet Invest*. 2021;86:218-230.
13. He K, Guo Q, Ge J, Li J, Li C, Jing Z. The efficacy and safety of metformin alone or as an add-on therapy to insulin in pregnancy with GDM or T2DM: a systematic review and meta-analysis of 21 randomized controlled trials. *J Clin Pharm Ther*. 2022;47(2):168-177.
14. Li C, Gao C, Zhang X, et al. Comparison of the effectiveness and safety of insulin and oral hypoglycemic drugs in the treatment of gestational diabetes mellitus: a meta-analysis of 26 randomized controlled trials. *Gynecol Endocrinol*. 2022;38:303-309.
15. Li F, Liu L, Hu Y, et al. Efficacy and safety of metformin compared to insulin in gestational diabetes: a systematic review and meta-analysis of Chinese randomized controlled trials. *Int J Clin Pharm*. 2022;44:1102-1113.
16. Sheng B, Ni J, Lv B, et al. Short-term neonatal outcomes in women with gestational diabetes treated using metformin versus insulin: a systematic review and meta-analysis of randomized controlled trials. *Acta Diabetol*. 2023;60:595-608.
17. Kattini R, Kelly L, Hummelen R. Systematic review of the use of metformin compared to insulin for the management of gestational diabetes: implications for low-resource settings. *Can J Rural Med*. 2023;28:59-65.
18. Fisher SA, Huang J, DuBord AY, et al. Continuous subcutaneous infusion versus multiple daily injections of insulin for pregestational diabetes in pregnancy: a systematic review and meta-analysis. *J Diabetes Sci Technol*. 2023;17:1337-1363.
19. Zhang L, Mai Y, Wang X, et al. Comparative study of the impact of metformin versus insulin on adverse pregnancy outcomes in women diagnosed with gestational diabetes mellitus: a meta-analysis. *Altern Ther Health Med*. 2024;30:460-465.
20. Wu R, Zhang Q, Li Z. A meta-analysis of metformin and insulin on maternal outcome and neonatal outcome in patients with gestational diabetes mellitus. *J Matern Fetal Neonatal Med*. 2024;37:2295809.
21. American Diabetes Association Professional Practice Committee. 15. Management of diabetes in pregnancy: standards of care in diabetes—2024. *Diabetes Care*. 2024;47(suppl 1):S282-S294.
22. Whitmore TJ, Trengove NJ, Graham DF, Hartmann PE. Analysis of insulin in human breast milk in mothers with type 1 and type 2 diabetes mellitus. *Int J Endocrinol*. 2012;2012:296368.

INSULIN ASPART

Antidiabetic (Rapid-Acting)

PREGNANCY RECOMMENDATION: Human Data Suggest Compatible

BREASTFEEDING RECOMMENDATION: Compatible

PREGNANCY SUMMARY

The use of insulin analogs during pregnancy is well reported throughout the literature. Insulin analogues, including insulin aspart, reportedly do not cross the placenta. ACOG and the ADA recommend the use of insulin as first-line pharmacologic therapy for the treatment of pregestational and gestational diabetes mellitus. Rapid-acting insulins, such as aspart, are considered acceptable insulins for use in pregnancy. Hypoglycemia may occur in patients treated with insulin. Glucose levels should be closely monitored, and insulin doses adjusted if necessary.

I

BREASTFEEDING SUMMARY

Insulin is naturally found in human breast milk. One report has evaluated the excretion of exogenous insulin, including aspart, into human breast milk. While insulin is excreted into breast milk, most of it will probably be digested in the infant's gastrointestinal tract and not absorbed. ACOG and the ADA recommend breastfeeding for all mothers with diabetes. No adverse effects have been reported in breastfed infants whose mothers received insulin aspart.

References

1. Prescribing Information. Novolog. Novo Nordisk; 2023.
2. Menon RK, Cohen RM, Sperling MA, et al. Transplacental passage of insulin in pregnant women with insulin-dependent diabetes mellitus. *N Engl J Med*. 1990;323:309-315.
3. Kimmerle R, Chantelau EA. Transplacental passage of insulin. *N Engl J Med*. 1991;324:198.
4. Weiss PA, Kainer F, Haas J. Cord blood insulin to assess the quality of treatment in diabetic pregnancies. *Early Hum Dev*. 1998;51:187-195.
5. Lindsay RS, Ziegler AG, Hamilton BA, et al.; Scottish Multicentre Study of Diabetes in Pregnancy. Type 1 diabetes-related antibodies in the fetal circulation: prevalence and influence on cord insulin and birth weight in offspring of mothers with type 1 diabetes. *J Clin Endocrinol Metab*. 2004;89:3436-3439.
6. Pettitt DJ, Ospina P, Howard C, et al. Efficacy, safety and lack of immunogenicity of insulin aspart compared with regular human insulin for women with gestational diabetes mellitus. *Diabet Med*. 2007;24:1129-1135.
7. Whitmore TJ, Trengove NJ, Graham DF, Hartmann PE. Analysis of insulin in human breast milk in mothers with type 1 and type 2 diabetes mellitus. *Int J Endocrinol*. 2012;2012:296368.
8. Ranasinghe PD, Maruthur NM, Nicholson WK, et al. Comparative effectiveness of continuous subcutaneous insulin infusion using insulin analogs and multiple daily injections in pregnant women with diabetes mellitus: a systematic review and meta-analysis. *J Womens Health (Larchmt)*. 2015;24:237-249.
9. Lv S, Wang J, Xu Y. Safety of insulin analogs during pregnancy: a meta-analysis. *Arch Gynecol Obstet*. 2015;292:749-756.
10. de Jong J, Garne E, Wender-Ozegowska E, et al. Insulin analogues in pregnancy and specific congenital anomalies: a literature review. *Diabetes Metab Res Rev*. 2016;32:366-375.
11. Nørgaard K, Sukumar N, Rafnsson SB, Saravanan P. Efficacy and safety of rapid-acting Insulin analogs in special populations with type 1 diabetes or gestational diabetes: systematic review and meta-analysis. *Diabetes Ther*. 2018;9:891-917.
12. American College of Obstetricians and Gynecologists' Committee on Practice Bulletins—Obstetrics. Practice bulletin no. 190: gestational diabetes mellitus. *Obstet Gynecol*. 2018;131:e49-e64.
13. American College of Obstetricians and Gynecologists' Committee on Practice Bulletins—Obstetrics. ACOG practice bulletin no. 201: pregestational diabetes mellitus. *Obstet Gynecol*. 2018;132:e228-e248.
14. American Diabetes Association Professional Practice Committee. 15. Management of diabetes in pregnancy: standards of care in diabetes—2024. *Diabetes Care*.2024;47(suppl 1):S282-S294.

INSULIN DEGLUDEC

Antidiabetic (Long-Acting)

PREGNANCY RECOMMENDATION: Limited Human Data but Probably Low Risk

BREASTFEEDING RECOMMENDATION: Probably Compatible

PREGNANCY SUMMARY

Four case reports or series and three studies describing the use of insulin degludec in 209 human pregnancies have been located. No adverse effects or congenital abnormalities related to this form of insulin were reported. When compared to other long-acting agents, maternal and neonatal outcomes were similar. Insulin analogues, including insulin degludec, reportedly do not cross the placenta. However, the limited human pregnancy experience prevents a complete assessment of the embryofetal risk. ACOG and the ADA recommend the use of insulin as first-line pharmacologic therapy for the treatment of pregestational and gestational diabetes. However, no mention of insulin degludec is found in these recommendations. Hypoglycemia may occur in patients treated with insulin. Glucose levels should be closely monitored, and insulin doses adjusted as needed. The elimination half-life of this form of insulin is 25 hours, so shorter-acting insulins might be preferred.

BREASTFEEDING SUMMARY

No reports describing the use of insulin degludec during human lactation have been located. Insulin is naturally found in breast milk. One report has evaluated the excretion of exogenous insulin into human breast milk. While insulin is excreted into breast milk, most of it will probably be digested in the infant's gastrointestinal tract and not absorbed. ACOG and the ADA recommend breastfeeding for all mothers with diabetes. No adverse effects have been reported in breastfed infants whose mothers received insulin degludec. The elimination half-life of this form of insulin is 25 hours, so shorter-acting insulins might be preferred.

References

1. Prescribing Information. Tresiba. Novo Nordisk; 2022.
2. Whitmore TJ, Trengove NJ, Graham DF, Hartmann PE. Analysis of insulin in human breast milk in mothers with type 1 and type 2 diabetes mellitus. *Int J Endocrinol*. 2012;2012:296368.
3. Milluzzo A, Tumminia A, Scalisi NM, et al. Insulin degludec in the first trimester of pregnancy: report of two cases. *J Diabetes Investig*. 2017;9:629-631.
4. Formoso G, Ginestra F, Di Dalmazi G, Consoli A. Empagliflozin, metformin and insulin degludec, during pregnancy: a case report. *Acta Diabetol*. 2018;55: 759-761.
5. Bonora BM, Avogaro A, Fadini GP. Exposure to insulin degludec during pregnancy: report of a small series and review of the literature. *J Endocrinol Invest*. 2019;42(3):345-349.
6. Keller MF, Vestgaard M, Damm P, et al. Treatment with the long-acting insulin analog degludec during pregnancy in women with type 1 diabetes: an observational study of 22 cases. *Diabetes Res Clin Pract*. 2019;152: 58-64.
7. Hiranput S, Ahmed SH, Macaulay D, Azmi S. Successful outcomes with Insulin degludec in pregnancy: a case series. *Diabetes Ther*. 2019;10:283-289.
8. Ringholm L, Do NC, Damm P, Mathiesen ER. Pregnancy outcomes in women with type 1 diabetes using insulin degludec. *Acta Diabetol*. 2022;59:721-727.
9. Mathiesen ER, Alibegovic AC, Corcoy R, et al.; EXPECT study group. Insulin degludec versus insulin detemir, both in combination with insulin aspart, in the treatment of pregnant women with type 1 diabetes (EXPECT): an open-label, multinational, randomised, controlled, non-inferiority trial. *Lancet Diabetes Endocrinol*. 2023;11:86-95.
10. American College of Obstetricians and Gynecologists' Committee on Practice Bulletins—Obstetrics. Practice bulletin no. 190: gestational diabetes mellitus. *Obstet Gynecol*. 2018;131:e49-e64.
11. American College of Obstetricians and Gynecologists' Committee on Practice Bulletins—Obstetrics. ACOG practice bulletin no. 201: pregestational diabetes mellitus. *Obstet Gynecol*. 2018;132:e228-e248.
12. American Diabetes Association Professional Practice Committee. 15. Management of diabetes in pregnancy: standards of care in diabetes—2024. *Diabetes Care*.2024;47(suppl 1):S282-S294.

INSULIN DETEMIR

Antidiabetic (Long-Acting)

PREGNANCY RECOMMENDATION: Human Data Suggest Compatible

BREASTFEEDING RECOMMENDATION: Compatible

PREGNANCY SUMMARY

Seven randomized control trials of about 1,251 pregnant women receiving insulin detemir and three recent systematic reviews and meta-analyses describing the use of insulin detemir in human pregnancy have been located. No adverse outcomes or congenital abnormalities related to insulin detemir were reported. When compared to NPH, insulin detemir may be associated with a greater gestational age at delivery and a lower incidence of hypoglycemic events. Insulin analogues, including insulin detemir, reportedly do not cross the placenta. ACOG and the ADA recommend the use of insulin as first-line pharmacologic therapy for the treatment of pregestational and gestational diabetes. Longer-acting agents, including insulin detemir, may be used to maintain euglycemia between meals and in the fasting state. The elimination half-life is about an hour longer than neutral protamine Hagedorn (NPH) insulin. Hypoglycemia may occur in patients treated with insulin. Glucose levels should be closely monitored, and insulin doses adjusted if necessary.

BREASTFEEDING SUMMARY

No reports describing the use of insulin detemir during human lactation have been located. Insulin is naturally found in breast milk. One report has evaluated the excretion of exogenous insulin into human breast milk. While insulin is excreted into breast milk, most of it will probably be digested in the infant's gastrointestinal tract and not absorbed. ACOG and the ADA recommend breastfeeding for all mothers with diabetes. No adverse effects have been reported in breastfed infants whose mothers received exogenous insulin, including insulin detemir.

References

1. Prescribing Information. Levemir. Novo Nordisk; 2022.
2. Whitmore TJ, Trengove NJ, Graham DF, Hartmann PE. Analysis of insulin in human breast milk in mothers with type 1 and type 2 diabetes mellitus. *Int J Endocrinol*. 2012;2012:296368.
3. Mathiesen ER, Hod M, Ivanisevic M, et al. Maternal efficacy and safety outcomes in a randomized, controlled trial comparing insulin detemir with

NPH insulin in 310 pregnant women with type 1 diabetes. *Diabetes Care*. 2012;35:2012-2017.
4. Hod M, Mathiesen ER, Jovanovič L, et al. A randomized trial comparing perinatal outcomes using insulin detemir or neutral protamine Hagedorn in type 1 diabetes. *J Matern Fetal Neonatal Med*. 2014;27:7-13.
5. Ji J, He Z, Yang Z, et al. Comparing the efficacy and safety of insulin detemir versus neutral protamine Hagedorn insulin in treatment of diabetes during pregnancy: a randomized, controlled study. *BMJ Open Diabetes Res Care*. 2020;8:e001155.
6. Herrera KM, Rosenn BM, Foroutan J, et al. Randomized controlled trial of insulin detemir versus NPH for the treatment of pregnant women with diabetes. *Am J Obstet Gynecol*. 2015;213:e1-e7.
7. Fishel Bartal M, Ward C, Blackwell SC, et al. Detemir vs neutral protamine Hagedorn insulin for diabetes mellitus in pregnancy: a comparative effectiveness, randomized controlled trial. *Am J Obstet Gynecol*. 2021;225:87.e1-87.e10.
8. Ji J, He Z, Yang Z, et al. Comparing the efficacy and safety of insulin detemir versus neutral protamine hagedorn insulin in treatment of diabetes during pregnancy: a randomized, controlled study. *BMJ Open Diabetes Res Care*. 2020;8:e001155.
9. Wang J, Ji X, Liu T, Zhao N. Maternal and neonatal outcomes with the use of long acting, compared to intermediate acting basal insulin (NPH) for managing diabetes during pregnancy: a systematic review and meta-analysis. *Diabetol Metab Syndr*. 2022;14:154.
10. Athanasiadou KI, Paschou SA, Stamatopoulos T, et al. Safety and efficacy of insulin detemir versus NPH in the treatment of diabetes during pregnancy: systematic review and meta-analysis of randomized controlled trials. *Diabetes Res Clin Pract*. 2022;190:110020.
11. Fatima K, Siddiqi AK, Shakil S, et al. Safety and efficacy of insulin detemir vs. insulin NPH in pregnant women with diabetes: a systematic review and meta-analysis. *Minerva Obstet Gynecol*. 2024;76:578.
12. Mathiesen ER, Alibegovic AC, Corcoy R, et al.; EXPECT Study Group. Insulin degludec versus insulin detemir, both in combination with insulin aspart, in the treatment of pregnant women with type 1 diabetes (EXPECT): an open-label, multinational, randomized, controlled, non-inferiority trial. *Lancet Diabetes Endocrinol*. 2023;11:86-95.
13. American College of Obstetricians and Gynecologists' Committee on Practice Bulletins—Obstetrics. Practice bulletin no. 190: gestational diabetes mellitus. *Obstet Gynecol*. 2018;131:e49-e64.
14. American College of Obstetricians and Gynecologists' Committee on Practice Bulletins—Obstetrics. ACOG practice bulletin no. 201: pregestational diabetes mellitus. *Obstet Gynecol*. 2018;132:e228-e248.
15. American Diabetes Association Professional Practice Committee. 15. Management of diabetes in pregnancy: standards of care in diabetes—2024. *Diabetes Care*. 2024;47(suppl 1):S282-S294.

INSULIN GLARGINE

Antidiabetic (Long-Acting)

PREGNANCY RECOMMENDATION: Human Data Suggest Compatible

BREASTFEEDING RECOMMENDATION: Compatible

PREGNANCY SUMMARY

Four meta-analyses that included at least 10 observational studies have evaluated the use of insulin glargine in pregnancy. Additionally, two literature reviews discussed the available evidence and recommendations on the use of insulin glargine in pregnancy. No adverse outcomes or congenital abnormalities related to insulin glargine were reported. When compared to NPH, insulin glargine has similar maternal and neonatal outcomes. Insulin analogues, including insulin glargine, reportedly do not cross the placenta. ACOG and the ADA recommend the use of insulin as first-line pharmacologic therapy for the treatment of pregestational and gestational diabetes. Longer-acting agents, including insulin glargine, may be used to maintain euglycemia between meals and in the fasting state. Hypoglycemia may occur in patients treated with insulin. Glucose levels should be closely monitored, and insulin doses adjusted as needed.

BREASTFEEDING SUMMARY

Insulin is naturally found in breast milk. One report has evaluated the excretion of exogenous insulin into human breast milk. While insulin is excreted into breast milk, most of it will probably be digested in the infant's gastrointestinal tract and not absorbed. ACOG and the ADA recommend breastfeeding for all mothers with diabetes. No adverse effects have been reported in breastfed infants whose mothers received exogenous insulin, including insulin glargine.

References

1. Prescribing Information. Lantus. Sanofi-Aventis; 2023.
2. Whitmore TJ, Trengove NJ, Graham DF, Hartmann PE. Analysis of insulin in human breast milk in mothers with type 1 and type 2 diabetes mellitus. *Int J Endocrinol*. 2012;2012:296368.
3. Pollex E, Moretti ME, Koren G, Feig DS. Safety of insulin glargine use in pregnancy: a systematic review and meta-analysis. *Ann Pharmacother*. 2011; 45:9-16.
4. Lepercq J, Lin J, Hall GC, et al. Meta-analysis of maternal and neonatal outcomes associated with the use of insulin glargine versus NPH insulin during pregnancy. *Obstet Gynecol Int*. 2012;2012:649070.
5. Lv S, Wang J, Xu Y. Safety of insulin analogs during pregnancy: a meta-analysis. *Arch Gynecol Obstet*. 2015;292:749-756.
6. de Jong J, Garne E, Wender-Ozegowska E, et al. Insulin analogues in pregnancy and specific congenital anomalies: a literature review. *Diabetes Metab Res Rev*. 2016;32:366-375.
7. Jethwani P, Saboo B, Jethwani L, Chawla R, Maheshwari A, Agarwal S, Jaggi S. Use of insulin glargine during pregnancy: a review. *Diabetes Metab Syndr*. 2021;15:379-384.
8. Wang J, Ji X, Liu T, Zhao N. Maternal and neonatal outcomes with the use of long acting, compared to intermediate acting basal insulin (NPH) for managing diabetes during pregnancy: a systematic review and meta-analysis. *Diabetol Metab Syndr*. 2022;14:154.
9. American College of Obstetricians and Gynecologists' Committee on Practice Bulletins—Obstetrics. Practice bulletin no. 190: gestational diabetes mellitus. *Obstet Gynecol*. 2018;131:e49-e64.
10. American College of Obstetricians and Gynecologists' Committee on Practice Bulletins—Obstetrics. ACOG practice bulletin no. 201: pregestational diabetes mellitus. *Obstet Gynecol*. 2018;132:e228-e248.
11. American Diabetes Association Professional Practice Committee. 15. Management of diabetes in pregnancy: standards of care in diabetes—2024. *Diabetes Care*.2024;47(suppl 1):S282-S294.

INSULIN GLULISINE

Antidiabetic (Rapid-Acting)

PREGNANCY RECOMMENDATION: No Human Data and No Relevant Animal Data

BREASTFEEDING RECOMMENDATION: Probably Compatible

PREGNANCY SUMMARY

No reports describing the use of insulin glulisine in human pregnancy have been located. Insulin analogues reportedly do not cross the placenta. However, the absence of human pregnancy experience prevents a complete assessment of the embryofetal risk. ACOG and the ADA recommend the use of insulin as first-line pharmacologic therapy for the treatment of pregestational and gestational diabetes mellitus. However, no mention of insulin glulisine is found in these recommendations. Hypoglycemia may occur in patients treated with insulin. Glucose levels should be closely monitored, and insulin doses adjusted as needed. The elimination half-life of this insulin is only about 40 minutes.

BREASTFEEDING SUMMARY

No reports describing the use of insulin glulisine during human lactation have been located. Insulin is naturally found in breast milk. One report has evaluated the excretion of exogenous insulin into human breast milk. While insulin is excreted into breast milk, most of it will probably be digested in the infant's gastrointestinal tract and not absorbed. ACOG and the ADA recommend breastfeeding for all mothers with diabetes. However, no mention of insulin glulisine is found in these recommendations. No adverse effects have been reported in breastfed infants whose mothers received exogenous insulin, including insulin glulisine. The elimination half-life of this insulin is only about 40 minutes.

References

1. Prescribing Information. Apidra. Sanofi-Aventis; 2020.
2. Whitmore TJ, Trengove NJ, Graham DF, Hartmann PE. Analysis of insulin in human breast milk in mothers with type 1 and type 2 diabetes mellitus. *Int J Endocrinol*. 2012;2012:296368.
3. American College of Obstetricians and Gynecologists' Committee on Practice Bulletins—Obstetrics. Practice bulletin no. 190: gestational diabetes mellitus. *Obstet Gynecol*. 2018;131:e49-e64.
4. American College of Obstetricians and Gynecologists' Committee on Practice Bulletins—Obstetrics. ACOG practice bulletin no. 201: pregestational diabetes mellitus. *Obstet Gynecol*. 2018;132:e228-e248.
5. American Diabetes Association Professional Practice Committee. 15. Management of diabetes in pregnancy: standards of care in diabetes—2024. *Diabetes Care*. 2024;47(suppl 1):S282-S294.

INSULIN LISPRO

Antidiabetic (Rapid-Acting)

PREGNANCY RECOMMENDATION: Human Data Suggest Compatible

BREASTFEEDING RECOMMENDATION: Compatible

PREGNANCY SUMMARY

The use of insulin analogs during pregnancy is well reported throughout the literature. Insulin analogues, including insulin lispro, reportedly do not cross the placenta. ACOG and the ADA recommend the use of insulin as first-line pharmacologic therapy for the treatment of pregestational and gestational diabetes. Rapid-acting insulins, such as lispro, are considered the preferred insulins in pregnancy. Hypoglycemia may occur in patients treated with insulin. Glucose levels should be closely monitored, and insulin doses adjusted as needed. The elimination half-life of this insulin is only about 60 minutes.

BREASTFEEDING SUMMARY

Insulin is naturally found in breast milk. One report has evaluated the excretion of exogenous insulin, including lispro, into human breast milk. While insulin is excreted into breast milk, most of it will probably be digested in the infant's gastrointestinal tract and not absorbed. ACOG and the ADA recommend breastfeeding for all mothers with diabetes. No adverse effects have been reported in breastfed infants whose mothers received exogenous insulin, including insulin lispro. The elimination half-life of this insulin is only about 60 minutes

References

1. Prescribing Information. Humalog. Eli Lilly and Company; 2023.
2. Rosenn B, Kosssenjans W, Eis A, Brockman D, Myatt L. Does lispro insulin cross the human placenta? *Am J Obstet Gynecol*. 2001;184:S69.
3. Boskovic R, Knie B, Feig DS, Portnoi G, Derewlany L, Koren G. Transfer of insulin lispro across the human placenta. *Diabetes Care*. 2003;26:1390-1394.
4. Holcberg G, Tsadkin-Tamir M, Sapir O, Wiznizer A, Segal D, Polachek H. Transfer of insulin lispro across the human placenta. *Eur J Obstet Gynecol Reprod Biol*. 2004;115:117-118.
5. Whitmore TJ, Trengove NJ, Graham DF, Hartmann PE. Analysis of insulin in human breast milk in mothers with type 1 and type 2 diabetes mellitus. *Int J Endocrinol*. 2012;2012:296368.

6. Ranasinghe PD, Maruthur NM, Nicholson WK, et al. Comparative effectiveness of continuous subcutaneous insulin infusion using insulin analogs and multiple daily injections in pregnant women with diabetes mellitus: a systematic review and meta-analysis. *J Womens Health (Larchmt)*. 2015;24:237-249.
7. Lv S, Wang J, Xu Y. Safety of insulin analogs during pregnancy: a meta-analysis. *Arch Gynecol Obstet*. 2015;292:749-756.
8. de Jong J, Garne E, Wender-Ozegowska E, et al. Insulin analogues in pregnancy and specific congenital anomalies: a literature review. *Diabetes Metab Res Rev*. 2016;32:366-375.
9. Nørgaard K, Sukumar N, Rafnsson SB, Saravanan P. Efficacy and safety of rapid-acting insulin analogs in special populations with type 1 diabetes or gestational diabetes: systematic review and meta-analysis. *Diabetes Ther*. 2018;9:891-917.
10. American College of Obstetricians and Gynecologists' Committee on Practice Bulletins—Obstetrics. Practice bulletin no. 190: gestational diabetes mellitus. *Obstet Gynecol*. 2018;131:e49-e64.
11. American College of Obstetricians and Gynecologists' Committee on Practice Bulletins—Obstetrics. ACOG practice bulletin no. 201: pregestational diabetes mellitus. *Obstet Gynecol*. 2018;132:e228-e248.
12. American Diabetes Association Professional Practice Committee. 15. Management of diabetes in pregnancy: standards of care in diabetes—2024. *Diabetes Care*. 2024;47(suppl 1):S282-S294.

INTERFERON BETA-1A

Immunologic (Immunomodulator)

PREGNANCY RECOMMENDATION: Human Data and Animal Data Suggest Low Risk

BREASTFEEDING RECOMMENDATION: Probably Compatible

I

PREGNANCY SUMMARY

At least 14 studies describing the use of interferon beta-1a for the treatment of multiple sclerosis in human pregnancy have been located. Three small early reports suggested that interferon beta-1a exposure during pregnancy was associated with low birth weight. However, larger studies did not support this finding. Additionally, studies have not found an increase in adverse pregnancy outcomes (including spontaneous abortion and congenital anomalies) with interferon beta-la exposure. Placental transfer, if it occurs, is unlikely to be clinically significant. Animal data did not show embryofetal toxicity in two species at doses less than 10 times the RHD. Using this drug during pregnancy should be based on the pros and cons of the mother's clinical need for treatment versus any potential fetal risk that might occur from exposure.

BREASTFEEDING SUMMARY

Five reports describing the use of interferon beta or interferon beta-1a during human lactation have been found. No adverse infant effects attributable to interferon exposure were reported. Minimal amounts of interferon beta-1a have been detected in breast milk. However, if excreted into breast milk, interferon beta will probably be digested in the infant's gastrointestinal tract and not be absorbed. If the clinical decision is to use this drug while breastfeeding, the infant should be monitored for the most common reported adult side effects of flu-like symptoms, myalgia, and abdominal pain (all leading to irritability), fever, weakness (lethargy), and various laboratory abnormalities (see PI).

References

1. Prescribing Information. Rebif. EMD Serono; 2023.
2. Prescribing Information. Avonex. Biogen; 2023.
3. Boskovic R, Wide R, Wolpin J, Bauer DJ, Koren G. The reproductive effects of beta interferon therapy in pregnancy: a longitudinal cohort. *Neurology*. 2005;65:807-811.
4. Weber-Schoendorfer C, Schaefer C. Multiple sclerosis, immunomodulators, and pregnancy outcome: a prospective observational study. *Mult Scler*. 2009;15:1037-1042.
5. Hellwig K, Haghikia A, Gold R. Parenthood and immunomodulation in patients with multiple sclerosis. *J Neurol*. 2010;257:580-583.
6. Amato MP, Portaccio E, Ghezzi A, et al. Pregnancy and fetal outcomes after interferon-beta exposure in multiple sclerosis. *Neurology*. 2010;75:1794-1802.
7. Hellwig K, Gold R. Glatiramer acetate and interferon-beta throughout gestation and postpartum in women with multiple sclerosis. *J Neurol*. 2011;258:502-503.
8. Hale TW, Siddiqui AA, Baker TE. Transfer of interferon beta-1a into human breastmilk. *Breastfeed Med*. 2012;7:123-125.
9. Hellwig K, Haghikia A, Rockhoff M, Gold R. Multiple sclerosis and pregnancy: experience from a nationwide database in Germany. *Ther Adv Neurol Disord*. 2012;5(5):247-253.
10. Fragoso YD, Adoni T, Alves-Leon SV, et al. Longterm effects of exposure to disease-modifying drugs in the offspring of mothers with multiple sclerosis: a retrospective chart review. *CNS Drugs*. 2013;27:955-961.
11. Thiel S, Langer-Gould A, Rockhoff M, et al. Interferon-beta exposure during first trimester is safe in women with multiple sclerosis-a prospective cohort study from the German Multiple Sclerosis and Pregnancy Registry. *Mult Scler*. 2016;22:801-809.
12. Burkill S, Vattulainen P, Geissbuehler Y, et al. The association between exposure to interferon-beta during pregnancy and birth measurements in offspring of women with multiple sclerosis. *PLoS ONE*. 2019;14:e0227120.
13. Hellwig K, Geissbuehler Y, Sabido M, et al. Pregnancy outcomes in interferon-beta-exposed patients with multiple sclerosis: results from the European Interferon-beta Pregnancy Registry. *J Neurol*. 2020;267:1715-1723.
14. Hakkarainen KM, Juuti R, Burkill S, et al. Pregnancy outcomes after exposure to interferon beta: a register-based cohort study among women with MS in Finland and Sweden. *Ther Adv Neurol Disord*. 2020;13:1756286420951072.
15. Ciplea AI, Langer-Gould A, Stahl A, et al. Safety of potential breast milk exposure to IFN-beta or glatiramer acetate: one-year infant outcomes. *Neurol Neuroimmunol Neuroinflamm*. 2020;7:e757.
16. Korjagina M, Hakkarainen KM, Burkill S, et al. Prevalence of adverse pregnancy outcomes after exposure to interferon beta prior to or during pregnancy in women with MS: stratification by maternal and newborn characteristics in a register based cohort study in Finland and Sweden. *Mult Scler Relat Disord*. 2021;48:102694.
17. Windfeld-Mathiasen J, Horwitz H, Andersen JB, et al. Interferon-beta exposure in-utero and the risk of infections in early childhood. *Mult Scler Relat Disord*. 2023;77:104867.
18. Klehmet J, Begus-Nahrmann Y, Taipale K, et al. Pregnancy outcomes in female multiple sclerosis patients exposed to intramuscular interferon beta-1a or peginterferon beta-1a reported in a German Patient Support Programme—results from the non-interventional post-authorization safety study PRIMA. *Ther Adv Neurol Disord*. 2023;16:17562864231214041.
19. Weinstock-Guttman B, Ross AP, Planton J, et al. Analysis of pregnancy outcomes following exposure to intramuscular interferon beta-1a: the AVONEX® pregnancy exposure registry. *Drugs Real World Outcomes*. 2023;10:503-511.

INTERFERON BETA-1B

Immunologic (Immunomodulator)

PREGNANCY RECOMMENDATION: Human Data Suggest Low Risk

BREASTFEEDING RECOMMENDATION: Probably Compatible

PREGNANCY SUMMARY

Five reports describing the use of interferon beta-1b during human lactation have been located. Two small early reports suggested that interferon beta-1b exposure during pregnancy was associated with low birth weight. However, larger studies did not support this finding. Additionally, studies have not found an increase in adverse pregnancy outcomes (including spontaneous abortion and congenital anomalies) with interferon beta-1b exposure. Placental transfer, if it occurs, is unlikely to be clinically significant. Using this drug during pregnancy should be based on the pros and cons of the mother's clinical need for treatment versus any potential fetal risk that might occur from exposure.

BREASTFEEDING SUMMARY

Only one case report describing the use of interferon beta-1b during human lactation was found. The infant was developing well with no abnormalities at 5 months of age. Minimal amounts of interferon beta-1a have been detected in breast milk. Therefore, interferon beta-1b will also probably be found in breast milk at low levels. However, if excreted into breast milk, it will probably be digested in the infant's gastrointestinal tract and not be absorbed. If the clinical decision is to use this drug while breastfeeding, the infant should be monitored for the most common reported adult side effects of flu-like symptoms, myalgia, and abdominal pain (all leading to irritability), fever, weakness (lethargy), poor sleeping, and various laboratory abnormalities (see PI).

References

1. Prescribing Information. Betaseron. Bayer Healthcare Pharmaceuticals; 2023.
2. Boskovic R, Wide R, Wolpin J, Bauer DJ, Koren G. The reproductive effects of beta interferon therapy in pregnancy: a longitudinal cohort. *Neurology*. 2005;65:807-811.
3. Weber-Schoendorfer C, Schaefer C. Multiple sclerosis, immunomodulators, and pregnancy outcome: a prospective observational study. *Mult Scler*. 2009;15:1037-1042.
4. Hale TW, Siddiqui AA, Baker TE. Transfer of interferon α-1a into human breastmilk. *Breastfeed Med*. 2012;7:123-125.
5. Fragoso YD, Adoni T, Alves-Leon SV, et al. Long-term effects of exposure to disease-modifying drugs in the offspring of mothers with multiple sclerosis: a retrospective chart review. *CNS Drugs*. 2013;27:955-961.
6. Coyle PK, Sinclair SM, Scheuerle AE, et al. Final results from the Betaseron (interferon β-1b) Pregnancy Registry: a prospective observational study of birth defects and pregnancy-related adverse events. *BMJ Open*. 2014;4:e004536.
7. Romero RS, Lünzmann C, Bugge JP. Pregnancy outcomes in patients exposed to interferon beta-1b. *J Neurol Neurosurg Psychiatry*. 2015;86:587-589.
8. Hellwig K, Duarte Caron F, Wicklein EM, et al. Pregnancy outcomes from the global pharmacovigilance database on interferon beta-1b exposure. *Ther Adv Neurol Disord*. 2020;13:1756286420910310.

INTERFERON GAMMA-1B

Immunologic (Immunomodulator)

PREGNANCY RECOMMENDATION: No Human Data and No Relevant Animal Data

BREASTFEEDING RECOMMENDATION: Probably Compatible

PREGNANCY SUMMARY

No reports describing the use of interferon gamma-1b in human pregnancy have been located. Placental transfer is likely to be clinically insignificant. However, the absence of human pregnancy experience prevents a complete assessment of the embryofetal risk. Embryofetal toxicity was observed in two animal species, but at doses greater than 10 times the RHD. Using this drug during pregnancy should be based on the pros and cons of the mother's clinical need for treatment versus any potential fetal risk that might occur from exposure.

BREASTFEEDING SUMMARY

No reports describing the use of interferon gamma-1b during human lactation have been located. The drug, if excreted into breast milk, is unlikely to be clinically significant. Additionally, if excreted into breast milk, it will probably be digested in the infant's gastrointestinal tract and not be absorbed. If the clinical decision is to use this drug while breastfeeding, the infant should be monitored for the most common reported adult side effects of headache (leading to irritability), rash, fever, fatigue (lethargy), and diarrhea.

References

1. Prescribing Information. Actimmune. Horizon Therapeutics USA; 2023.
2. Vassiliadis S, Athanassakis I. Type II interferon may be a potential hazardous therapeutic agent during pregnancy. *Br J Haematol*. 1992;82:782-783.

IODINE

Anti-Infective (Topical—Antiseptic)

PREGNANCY RECOMMENDATION: Limited Human Data—No Relevant Animal Data

BREASTFEEDING RECOMMENDATION: Potential Toxicity

I

PREGNANCY SUMMARY

At least eight reports describing the perinatal or prenatal exposure to iodine-based skin disinfectants have been located. Neonatal hypothyroidism has been reported with the use of iodine-based skin disinfectants. Iodine crosses the placenta. However, the limited human pregnancy experience prevents a complete assessment of the embryofetal risk. No animal reproduction studies have been located. Iodine is a natural element that is needed for producing thyroid hormones. It is found in eggs, dairy products, seafood, and iodized salt. Excess iodine can lead to thyroid damage. Using this drug during pregnancy should be based on the pros and cons of the mother's clinical need for treatment versus any potential fetal risk that might occur from exposure.

BREASTFEEDING SUMMARY

Four reports describing the use of iodine during human lactation have been located. Three case reports that involved the use of iodine for wound management resulted in abnormal infant thyroid function tests. Levothyroxine was started, and breastfeeding was discontinued. The infants' thyroid function tests then normalized. A study examined the neurodevelopmental outcomes of children whose breastfeeding mothers received iodine until 12 months postpartum. No evidence was found of delayed neurodevelopment. Iodine is a normal component of breast milk. Iodine is excreted into breast milk in concentrations depending on the maternal use and area applied. If used while breastfeeding, the infant should be monitored for the most common reported side effect of hypothyroidism.

References

1. Pyati SP, Ramamurthy RS, Krauss MT, et al. Absorption of iodine in the neonate following topical use of povidone iodine. *J Pediatr*. 1977;91:825-828.
2. Jackson HJ, Sutherland RM. Effect of povidone-iodine on neonatal thyroid function (Letter). *Lancet*. 1981;2:992.
3. Dela Cruz F, Brown DH, Leikin JB, et al. Iodine absorption after topical administration. *West J Med*. 1987;146:43-45.
4. l'Allemand D, Grüters AJ, Heidemann P, Schürnbrand. Iodine-induced alterations of thyroid function in newborn infants after prenatal and perinatal exposure to povidone iodine. *J Pediatr*. 1983;102:935-938.
5. L'Allemand D, Grüters A, Beyer P, Weber B. Iodine in contrast agents and skin disinfectants is the major cause for hypothyroidism in infants during intensive care. *Horm Res*. 1987;28:42-49.
6. Smerdely P, Boyages SC, Wu D, et al. Topical iodine-containing antiseptics and neonatal hypothyroidism in very-low-birthweight infants. *Lancet*. 1989;2:661-664.
7. Gordon CM, Rowitch DH, Mitchell ML, Kohane IS. Topical iodine and neonatal hypothyroidism. *Arch Pediatr Adoles Med*. 1995;149:1336-1339.
8. Brown RS, Bloomfield S, Bednarek FJ, et al. Routine skin cleansing with povidone-iodine is not a common cause of transient neonatal hypothyroidism in North America: a prospective controlled study. *Thyroid*. 1997;7:395-400.
9. Aitken J, Williams FLR. A systematic review of thyroid dysfunction in preterm neonates exposed to topical iodine. *Arch Dis Child*. 2014;99:F21-F28.
10. Williams FL, Watson J, Day C, et al. Thyroid dysfunction in preterm neonates exposed to iodine. *J Perinat Med*. 2017;45:135-143.
11. Fuse Y, Ogawa H, Tsukahara Y, et al. Iodine metabolism and thyroid function during the perinatal period: maternal-neonatal correlation and effects of topical povidone-iodine skin disinfectants. *Biol Trace Elem Res*. 2023;201:2685-2700.
12. Casteels K, Punt S, Bramswig J. Transient neonatal hypothyroidism during breastfeeding after post-natal maternal topical iodine treatment. *Eur J Pediatr*. 2000;159:716-717.
13. Smith VC, Svoren BM, Wolfsdorf JI. Hypothyroidism in a breast-fed preterm infant resulting from maternal topical iodine exposure. *J Pediatr*. 2006;149:566-567.
14. Kurtoğlu S, Akın L, Akın MA, et al. Iodine overload and severe hypothyroidism in two neonates. *J Clin Res Pediatr Endocrinol*. 2009;1:275-277.
15. Nazeri P, Tahmasebinejad Z, Pearce EN, et al. Does maternal iodine supplementation during the lactation have a positive impact on neurodevelopment of children? Three-year follow up of a randomized controlled trial. *Eur J Nutr*. 2021;60:4083-4091.
16. Mégier C, Dumery G, Luton D. Iodine and thyroid maternal and fetal metabolism during pregnancy. *Metabolites*. 2023;13(5):633.

IODIXANOL

Diagnostic (Radiologic—Iodinated Contrast Media)

PREGNANCY RECOMMENDATION: No Human Data—Animal Data Suggest Low Risk

BREASTFEEDING RECOMMENDATION: Probably Compatible

PREGNANCY SUMMARY

No reports describing the use of iodixanol in human pregnancy have been located. The drug is unlikely to cross the placenta in clinically significant amounts. However, iodinated contrast media have been shown to cross the human placenta and enter the fetus in measurable quantities. No documented cases of neonatal hypothyroidism from maternal intravascular water-soluble iodinated contrast agents have been reported. However, the absence of human pregnancy experience with iodixanol prevents a complete assessment of the embryofetal risk. Animal data did not show any embryofetal toxicity in two animal species at doses of less than 10 times the RHD. ACOG and the American College of Radiology do not recommend routine screening for pregnancy prior to iodinated contrast medium or withholding iodinated contrast in pregnant or potentially pregnant patients. Additionally, given the current available data and routine evaluation of newborns for congenital hypothyroidism by measurement of thyrotropin (TSH) at birth, no extra monitoring of the infant is felt to be necessary.

BREASTFEEDING SUMMARY

No reports describing the use of iodixanol during human lactation have been located. Less than 1% of a maternal dose of iodinated contrast medium is excreted into breast milk in the first 24 hours, and of that, less than 1% is absorbed from the infant's gastrointestinal tract. ACOG and the American College of Radiology feel it is low risk to continue breastfeeding after receiving iodinated contrast medium. If the mother is concerned about any potential effect to the infant, she can hold breastfeeding and be advised to pump and discard breast milk for up to 12 hours (five plus half-lives). While the likelihood of adverse effects is extremely low, infants should be monitored for the most common reported adult side effects of nausea and headache (both leading to irritability) and rash.

References

1. Prescribing Information. Visipaque. GE HealthCare, Inc; 2022.
2. Guidelines for Diagnostic Imaging During Pregnancy and Lactation. Committee Opinion No. 723. American College of Obstetricians and Gynecologists. *Obstet Gynecol*. 2017;133:e201-e206.
3. American College of Radiology. ACR Manual on Contrast Media. Accessed February 6, 2024. https://www.acr.org/-/media/ACR/Files/Clinical-Resources/Contrast_Media.pdf

IODOQUINOL

Dermatologic (Amebicide)

PREGNANCY RECOMMENDATION: **Limited Human Data—No Relevant Animal Data**

BREASTFEEDING RECOMMENDATION: **Probably Compatible**

PREGNANCY SUMMARY

Three reports describing the use of iodoquinol in 171 human pregnancies have been located. One case report of exposure in the second and third trimesters resulted in a dwarf with achondroplasia (an autosomal dominant disorder), while the second case report with exposure throughout pregnancy resulted in a normal term birth. The Collaborative Perinatal Project identified an additional 169 cases that had first-trimester exposure to iodoquinol. Nine infants were born with a congenital malformation, six (3.6%) of which were major anomalies. The drug will probably cross the placenta, so some fetal exposure will likely occur. However, iodoquinol is likely minimally absorbed systemically following topical administration, which should limit placental transfer. However, this limited human pregnancy experience prevents a complete assessment of the embryofetal risk. No animal reproduction studies have been conducted. Using this drug during pregnancy should be based on the pros and cons of the mother's clinical need for treatment versus any potential fetal risk that might occur from exposure.

BREASTFEEDING SUMMARY

No reports describing the use of topical iodoquinol during human lactation have been located. The drug probably will appear in breast milk if found in the maternal circulation. However, systemic absorption is likely to be minimal following topical administration, which should limit infant exposure. Breastfeeding while using this drug should be based on the mother's clinical need for treatment. Because of the topical use, adult systemic side effects were not reported. Iodoquinol should not be applied to the breast or nipple area, if possible, but if used in this area, it should be thoroughly wiped off prior to breastfeeding.

References

1. Prescribing Information. Hydrocortisone Iodoquinol. Syntenza Pharmaceuticals LLC; 2018.
2. Vedder JS, Griem S. Acrodermatitis enteropathica (Danbolt-Closs) in five siblings: efficacy of diodoquin in its management. *J Pediatr*. 1956;48:212-219.
3. Verburg DJ, Burd LI, Hoxtell EO, Merrill LK. Acrodermatitis enteropathica and pregnancy. *Obstet Gynecol*. 1974;44:233-237.
4. Heinonen OP, Slone D, Shapiro S. *Birth Defects and Drugs in Pregnancy*. Publishing Sciences Group; 1977.

IOFLUPANE IODINE 123

Diagnostic (Radiologic— Radioactive Iodinated Contrast Media)

PREGNANCY RECOMMENDATION: *Contraindicated

BREASTFEEDING RECOMMENDATION: *Contraindicated (Hold Breastfeeding)

PREGNANCY SUMMARY

No reports describing the use of ioflupane iodine 123 in human pregnancy have been located. Radioactive iodine products cross the placenta, so fetal exposure occurs. In humans, a dose of 185 MBq (the higher RHD) results in an absorbed radiation dose to the uterus of about 0.3 rads. Radiation doses of more than 15 rads have been associated with congenital anomalies but doses less than 5 rads generally have not. However, the absence of human pregnancy experience prevents a complete assessment of the embryofetal risk. No animal reproduction studies have been conducted. *Depending on the stage of fetal development, radioactive iodine products can permanently impair fetal thyroid function. The fetal thyroid does not start sequestering iodine until about 10 to 12 weeks' gestation. Therefore, use of ioflupane iodine 123 in a pregnant woman after 10 weeks gestation is not recommended, if possible.

I

BREASTFEEDING SUMMARY

No reports describing the use of ioflupane iodine 123 during human lactation have been located. Iodine 123 is present in breast milk, so infant exposure will occur. *The manufacturer recommends that breastfeeding should not be started before the diagnostic agent is administered, or if breastfeeding is already underway, it should be interrupted. Per the manufacturer, based on the physical half-life of iodine 123, nursing women should pump and discard breast milk for 6 days to minimize risks to a nursing infant. In contrast, the Advisory Committee on the Medical Uses of Isotopes recommends that nursing mothers discontinue breastfeeding for only 3 days (five half-lives) to achieve a maximum dose of 0.1 rad or less to a nursing infant. It is also advised for the mother to continue to pump during the interruption period. Breast milk that has been pumped during this period should either be discarded or stored in a refrigerator. If needed, the stored breast milk can be held for iodine 123 decay after the same length of the interruption period and then used to feed the infant.

References

1. Prescribing Information. DaTscan. GE Healthcare, Medi-Physics; 2022.
2. Djang DS, Janssen MJ, Bohnen N, et al. SNM practice guideline for dopamine transporter imaging with 123I-ioflupane SPECT 1.0. *J Nucl Med.* 2012;53:154-163.
3. Advisory Committee on the Medical Uses of Isotopes. Sub-Committee on Nursing Mother Guidelines for the Medical Administration of Radioactive Materials. Accessed March 22, 2024. https://www.nrc.gov/docs/ML1903/ML19038A498.pdf

IOHEXOL

Diagnostic (Radiologic—Iodinated Contrast Media)

PREGNANCY RECOMMENDATION: *Limited Human Data—Animal Data Suggest Low Risk

BREASTFEEDING RECOMMENDATION: Probably Compatible

PREGNANCY SUMMARY

One report evaluating thyroid function in 343 newborns whose mothers received IV iohexol during pregnancy was located. The concern was the potential adverse effects that iodide might have on the fetal thyroid gland. All newborns had a normal thyroxine (T_4) concentration at birth. Iohexol crosses the placenta and reaches the fetal tissues in small amounts. No documented cases of neonatal hypothyroidism from maternal intravascular water-soluble iodinated contrast agents have been reported. However, this limited human pregnancy experience prevents a complete assessment of the embryofetal risk. Animal data did not show any embryofetal toxicity in two species at doses of less than 10 times the RHD. ACOG and the American College of Radiology do not recommend routine screening for pregnancy prior to iodinated contrast medium use or withholding iodinated contrast in pregnant or potentially pregnant patients. *However, iohexol for hysterosalpingography is contraindicated during pregnancy or suspected pregnancy due to the risk to the fetus from an intrauterine procedure. Additionally, given the current available data and routine evaluation of newborns for congenital hypothyroidism by measurement of TSH at birth, no extra monitoring of the infant is felt to be necessary.

BREASTFEEDING SUMMARY

One report of four lactating women following iohexol use during lactation found low levels of the diagnostic agent in breast milk. The amount excreted over a 24-hour period was 0.5% of the maternal weight-adjusted dose. Furthermore, oral bioavailability of iohexol is only 1%, so if any amount of the diagnostic agent were to be in breast milk, the amount absorbed is likely to be clinically insignificant. ACOG and the American College of Radiology feel it is low risk to continue breastfeeding after receiving iodinated contrast medium. If the mother is concerned about any potential effect on the infant, she can hold breastfeeding and be advised to pump and discard breast milk, but five half-lives would be about 3 days. While the likelihood of adverse effects is extremely low, infants should be monitored for the most common reported adult side effects of nausea, headache, and pain (all leading to irritability), rash, and vomiting.

References

1. Prescribing Information. Omnipaque. GE Healthcare; 2022.
2. Bourrinet P, Dencausse A, Havard P, et al. Transplacental passage and milk excretion of iobitridol. *Invest Radiol*. 1995;30:156-158.
3. Bourjeily G, Chalhoub M, Phornphutkul C, et al. Neonatal thyroid function: effect of a single exposure to iodinated contrast medium in utero. *Radiology*. 2010;256:744-750.
4. Kochi MH, Kaloudis EV, Ahmed W, Moore WH. Effect of in utero exposure of iodinated intravenous contrast on neonatal thyroid function. *J Comput Assist Tomogr*. 2012;36:165-169.
5. Guidelines for Diagnostic Imaging During Pregnancy and Lactation. Committee Opinion No. 723. American College of Obstetricians and Gynecologists. *Obstet Gynecol*. 2017;133:e201
6. American College of Radiology. ACR Manual on Contrast Media. Accessed February 6, 2024. https://www.acr.org/-/media/ACR/Files/Clinical-Resources/Contrast_Media.pdf
7. Nielsen ST, Matheson I, Rasmussen JN, et al. Excretion of iohexol and metrizoate in human breast milk. *Acta Radiol*. 1987;28:523-526.

I

IOPAMIDOL

Diagnostic (Radiologic—Iodinated Contrast Media)

PREGNANCY RECOMMENDATION: Limited Human Data—Animal Data Suggest Low Risk

BREASTFEEDING RECOMMENDATION: Probably Compatible

PREGNANCY SUMMARY

Five case reports and a retrospective study describing the use of iopamidol in human pregnancies have been located. These reports include 31 pregnancies and 32 infants with exposure in the second or third trimesters. Four infants had TSH levels drawn that were found to be normal. Of the remaining infants, one infant was reported as healthy, another was born preterm, and 26 had no information regarding newborn outcomes. Iopamidol crosses the human placenta and reaches the fetal tissues. No documented cases of neonatal hypothyroidism from maternal intravascular water-soluble iodinated contrast agents have been reported. However, this limited human pregnancy experience prevents a complete assessment of the embryofetal risk. Animal data did not show embryofetal toxicity in two species at doses less than 10 times the RHD. ACOG and the American College of Radiology do not recommend routine screening for pregnancy prior to iodinated contrast medium use or withholding iodinated contrast in pregnant or potentially pregnant patients. Additionally, given the current available data and routine evaluation of newborns for congenital hypothyroidism by measurement of TSH at birth, no extra monitoring of the infant is felt to be necessary.

BREASTFEEDING SUMMARY

No reports describing the use of iopamidol during human lactation have been located. Due to its low lipid solubility and low absorption with oral use, the amount of iopamidol excreted into breast milk is thought to be negligible. ACOG and the American College of Radiology feel it is low risk to continue breastfeeding after receiving iodinated contrast medium. If the mother is concerned about any potential effect to the infant, she can hold breastfeeding and be advised to pump and discard breast milk for 12 hours (five elimination half-lives). While the likelihood of adverse effects is extremely low, infants should be monitored for the most common reported adult side effects of nausea, headache, and pain (all leading to irritability), rash, and vomiting.

References

1. Prescribing Information. Isovue. Bracco Diagnostics; 2023.
2. Fitzpatrick J, Speakman J, Kapfer SA, Holston AM. Transplacental passage of the non-ionic contrast agent iopamidol in twins. *Pediatr Radiol*. 2011;41:534-536.
3. Atwell TD, Lteif AN, Brown DL, et al. Neonatal thyroid function after administration of IV iodinated contrast agent to 21 pregnant patients. *AJR Am J Roentgenol*. 2008;191:268-271.
4. Ridge CA, McDermott S, Freyne BJ, et al. Pulmonary embolism in pregnancy: comparison of pulmonary CT angiography and lung scintigraphy. *Am J Roentgenol*. 2009;193:1223-1227.
5. McCaulley JA, Deering SH, Pates JA. Severe thrombocytopenia after contrast infusion in pregnancy. *Obstet Gynecol*. 2013;121:473-475.
6. Huang TK, Reese J, Weitkamp JH, Stancombe BB. Congenital radiocontrast agent in the neonatal gut. *J Pediatr*. 2014;164(5):1236.
7. Goto Y, Ebisu T, Mineura K. Ruptured intracranial aneurysm during pregnancy with false-negative computed tomography angiography findings: a case report. *Emerg Radiol*. 2015;22(3):343-346.
8. Guidelines for Diagnostic Imaging During Pregnancy and Lactation. Committee Opinion No. 723. American College of Obstetricians and Gynecologists. *Obstet Gynecol*. 2017;133:e201.
9. American College of Radiology. ACR Manual on Contrast Media. Accessed February 6, 2024. https://www.acr.org/-/media/ACR/Files/Clinical-Resources/Contrast_Media.pdf

IOTHALAMATE MEGLUMINE

Diagnostic (Radiologic—Iodinated Contrast Media)

PREGNANCY RECOMMENDATION: Limited Human Data—Animal Data Suggest Low Risk

BREASTFEEDING RECOMMENDATION: Probably Compatible

PREGNANCY SUMMARY

Two reports describing the use of iothalamate meglumine in 18 human pregnancies have been located. The diagnostic agent was used in all trimesters. No adverse effects related to iothalamate meglumine were reported. No documented cases of neonatal hypothyroidism from maternal intravascular water-soluble iodinated contrast agents have been reported. Iothalamate salts cross the placental barrier, so fetal exposure will occur. However, this limited human pregnancy experience prevents a complete assessment of the embryofetal risk. Animal data did not show any embryofetal toxicity in three species at doses less than 10 times the RHD. ACOG and the American College of Radiology do not recommend routine screening for pregnancy prior to iodinated contrast medium use or withholding iodinated contrast agents in pregnant or potentially pregnant patients. Additionally, given the current available data and routine evaluation of newborns for congenital hypothyroidism by measurement of TSH at birth, no extra monitoring of the infant is felt to be necessary.

BREASTFEEDING SUMMARY

No reports describing the use of iothalamate meglumine during human lactation have been located. Due to its low lipid solubility and low oral bioavailability, the amount excreted into human breast milk is thought to be minimal. However, due to a concern for potential serious adverse effects that might be seen in a breastfed infant, the manufacturer recommends that women not breastfeed while being treated with this agent. Nevertheless, ACOG and the American College of Radiology feel it is low risk to continue breastfeeding after receiving iodinated contrast medium. If the mother is concerned about any potential effect to the infant, she can hold breastfeeding and be advised to pump and discard breast milk for 8 hours (five half-lives). While the likelihood of adverse effects is low, infants should be monitored for the most common reported adult side effects of nausea and feeling of body warmth (both leading to irritability), facial flushing, and vomiting.

References

1. Prescribing Information. Conray. Liebel-Flarsheim Company LLC; 2017.
2. Dunnihoo DR, Harris RE. The diagnosis of monoamniotic twinning by amniography. *Am J Obstet Gynecol*. 1966;96:894-895.
3. Kierkegaard A. Incidence and diagnosis of deep vein thrombosis associated with pregnancy. *Acta Obstet Gynecol Scand*. 1983;62:239-243.
4. Guidelines for Diagnostic Imaging During Pregnancy and Lactation. Committee Opinion No. 723. American College of Obstetricians and Gynecologists. *Obstet Gynecol*. 2017;133:e201
5. American College of Radiology. ACR Manual on Contrast Media. Accessed February 6, 2024. https://www.acr.org/-/media/ACR/Files/Clinical-Resources/Contrast_Media.pdf

IPILIMUMAB

Antineoplastic (Monoclonal Antibody)

PREGNANCY RECOMMENDATION: Limited Human Data—Animal Data Suggest Potential Risk

BREASTFEEDING RECOMMENDATION: Probably Compatible

PREGNANCY SUMMARY

Four case reports describing the use of ipilimumab in 11 human pregnancies were located. Exposure was in the first and second trimesters (when known). No congenital anomalies were reported in three live births. (The other pregnancy outcomes were three no outcome data, two elective terminations, one ectopic, and two spontaneous losses). IgG antibodies are known to cross the placenta, especially during the third trimester, which suggests that some transfer will occur. However, this limited human pregnancy experience prevents a complete assessment of the embryofetal risk. Embryofetal toxicity with malformations was observed in one species at doses less than 10 times the RHD. Based on animal studies and the drug's mechanism of action, the manufacturer recommends that women with reproductive potential use effective contraception during treatment and for 3 months after the last dose. Nevertheless, using this drug during pregnancy should be based on the pros and cons of the mother's clinical need for treatment versus any potential fetal risk that might occur from exposure. There is a registry for women who are pregnant and have cancer. For more information, women and health care providers are encouraged to contact the Cancer and Pregnancy Registry at 1-877-635-4499.

BREASTFEEDING SUMMARY

One report evaluating the excretion of ipilimumab into human breast milk was located. The patient desired to breastfeed her infant, so she pumped throughout treatment and then began feeding her infant 3 weeks after cessation of ipilimumab. Ipilimumab was present in the breast milk samples during treatment, with peak levels 4 days after infusion. Detectable levels were present until 19 days after the infusion. However, if the IgG antibody were to be ingested through breastfeeding, it would probably be digested in the infant's gastrointestinal tract and not absorbed. Regardless, due to a concern for potential serious adverse effects that might be seen in a breastfed infant, the manufacturer recommends that women not breastfeed while being treated with this drug and for at least 3 months after the last dose. Nevertheless, breastfeeding while using this drug should be based on the mother's clinical need for treatment versus any potential infant risks that might occur. If used, the infant should be monitored for the most common reported adult side effects of pruritus (leading to irritability), fatigue (lethargy), diarrhea, and rash.

References

1. Prescribing Information. Yervoy. Bristol-Myers Squibb; 2011.
2. Ross E, Robinson SE, Amato C, et al. Therapeutic monoclonal antibodies in human breast milk: a case report. *Melanoma Res*. 2014;24:177-180.
3. Mehta A, Kim KB, Minor DR. Case report of a pregnancy during ipilimumab therapy. *J Glob Oncol*. 2018;4:1-3.
4. Burotto M, Gormaz JG, Samtani S, et al. Viable pregnancy in a patient with metastatic melanoma treated with double checkpoint immunotherapy. *Semin Oncol*. 2018;45:164-169.
5. Menzer C, Beedgen B, Rom J, et al. Immunotherapy with ipilimumab plus nivolumab in a stage IV melanoma patient during pregnancy. *Eur J Cancer*. 2018;104:239-242.
6. Zambrana F, Barbancho C, Huelves M, et al. Successful pregnancy and cancer outcomes with ipilimumab and nivolumab for metastatic renal cell carcinoma: case report and review of the literature. *J Immunother*. 2023;46:27-28.

I

IPRATROPIUM

Respiratory (Anticholinergic—Inhalation/Nasal Spray)

PREGNANCY RECOMMENDATION: Limited Human Data—Animal Data Suggest Low Risk

BREASTFEEDING RECOMMENDATION: Probably Compatible

PREGNANCY SUMMARY

A surveillance study describing the use of ipratropium in human pregnancy reported 37 first-trimester exposures with 1 (2.7%) malformation (renal obstruction). The drug will probably cross the placenta if found in the maternal circulation, but is unlikely to be clinically significant due to the low systemic absorption following oral inhalation and nasal administration. However, this limited human pregnancy experience prevents a complete assessment of the embryofetal risk. Animal data did not show any embryofetal toxicity in two species at doses greater than 10 times the MRHD. Using this drug during pregnancy should be based on the pros and cons of the mother's clinical need for treatment versus any potential fetal risk that might occur from exposure.

BREASTFEEDING SUMMARY

No reports describing the use of ipratropium during human lactation have been located. The drug will probably appear in breast milk. However, ipratropium is poorly absorbed systemically following oral inhalation and nasal administration, which should produce clinically insignificant amounts in breast milk. If the clinical decision is to use this drug while breastfeeding, the infant should be monitored for the most common reported adult side effects of nausea, headache, and pain (all leading to irritability) and upper respiratory infection.

References

1. Prescribing Information. Atrovent HFA. Boehringer Ingelheim Pharmaceuticals, Inc; 2023.
2. Prescribing Information. Ipratropium Bromide Inhalation Solution, 0.02%. Nephron Pharmaceuticals Corporation; 2017.
3. Prescribing Information. Ipratropium Bromide Nasal Solution, 0.03%. Boehringer Ingelheim Pharmaceuticals; 2014.
4. Gilchrist DM, Friedman JM, Werker D. Life-threatening status asthmaticus at 12.5 weeks' gestation. *Chest*. 1991;100:285-286.
5. Schardein JL. *Chemically Induced Birth Defects*. 2nd ed. Marcel Dekker; 1993:343.
6. Shepard TH. *Catalog of Teratogenic Agents*. 8th ed. The Johns Hopkins University Press; 1995:238.

IPTACOPAN

Hematologic (Complement Factor B Inhibitor)

PREGNANCY RECOMMENDATION: No Human Data—Animal Data Suggest Low Risk (Maternal Benefit May Outweigh Any Embryofetal Risk)

BREASTFEEDING RECOMMENDATION: Probably Compatible

PREGNANCY SUMMARY

No reports describing the use of iptacopan in human pregnancy have been located. The drug will likely cross the placenta, so some fetal exposure will probably occur. Therefore, the absence of human pregnancy experience prevents a complete assessment of the embryofetal risk. Animal studies did not show any embryofetal toxicity or malformations in two species at doses of less than 10 times the RHD. Using this drug during pregnancy should be based on the pros and cons of the mother's clinical need for treatment versus any potential fetal risk that might occur from exposure. The drug does carry a boxed warning for an increased risk of serious infections caused by encapsulated bacteria, including *Neisseria meningitidis*, *Streptococcus pneumoniae*, and *Haemophilus influenzae* type B. Pregnant patients with paroxysmal nocturnal hemoglobinuria and primary immunoglobulin A nephropathy have complicated pregnancies with a high rate of poor pregnancy outcomes. Therefore, maternal treatment might be needed despite any embryofetal risk.

BREASTFEEDING SUMMARY

No reports describing the use of iptacopan during human lactation have been located. The drug will likely be found in breast milk, so some infant exposure will probably occur. Due to a concern for potential serious adverse effects that might be seen in a breastfed infant, including infections with encapsulated bacteria (see boxed warning described above in the Pregnancy Summary), the manufacturer recommends that women not breastfeed while being treated with this drug and for at least 5 days after the last dose. However, breastfeeding while using this drug should be based on the mother's clinical need for treatment versus any potential infant risk that might occur. If used, the infant should be monitored for the most common reported adult side effects of headache, abdominal pain, and nausea (all leading to irritability), diarrhea, and rash. Patients with paroxysmal nocturnal hemoglobinuria and primary immunoglobulin A nephropathy have complicated medical histories with a high rate of complications. Therefore, maternal treatment might be needed despite any infant risk.

Reference

1. Prescribing Information. Fabhalta. Novartis Pharmaceuticals Corp; 2024.

IRBESARTAN

Antihypertensive (Angiotensin II Receptor Blocker)

PREGNANCY RECOMMENDATION: ***Contraindicated (Second and Third Trimesters)**

BREASTFEEDING RECOMMENDATION: **Potential Toxicity**

PREGNANCY SUMMARY

Three case reports describing the use of irbesartan in five human pregnancies with first- and second-trimester exposures were found. One pregnancy was terminated due to exencephaly detected at 13 weeks. Autopsy revealed a partial exencephaly and unilateral renal agenesis. Of the four remaining pregnancies, outcomes included a spontaneous loss due to a chromosomal abnormality in one and polydactyly in a second. The drug will probably cross the placenta, so some fetal exposure will likely occur. However, this limited human pregnancy experience prevents a complete assessment of the embryofetal risk. Embryofetal toxicity was observed in two species at doses of less than 10 times the RHD. Irbesartan is an angiotensin II receptor blocker with a similar mechanism of action as angiotensin-converting enzyme (ACE) inhibitors. That is, the former selectively blocks the binding of angiotensin II to angiotensin receptors, whereas the latter blocks the formation of angiotensin II itself. *The use of ACE inhibitors and ARBs during the second and third trimesters of pregnancy may cause severe fetal/neonatal renal toxicity. The fetal renal dysfunction produces oligohydramnios, leading to findings of Potter sequence with pulmonary hypoplasia and neonatal death. In some cases, this renal dysfunction is permanent, and in others, it is reversible. As a result, irbesartan carries a boxed warning regarding fetal toxicity due to direct effects on the renin-angiotensin system, which can cause injury and death to the developing fetus. The boxed warning recommends that irbesartan be discontinued as soon as possible once pregnancy is detected.

BREASTFEEDING SUMMARY

No reports describing the use of irbesartan during human lactation have been located. The drug will probably appear in breast milk, so some infant exposure will likely occur. However, due to a concern for potential serious adverse effects that might be seen in a breastfed infant, the manufacturer recommends that women not breastfeed while being treated with this drug. Nevertheless, breastfeeding while using this drug should be based on the mother's clinical need for treatment versus any potential infant risks that might occur. If used, the infant should be monitored for the most common reported adult side effects of dizziness (leading to irritability), hypotension, and hyperkalemia.

References

1. Prescribing Information. Irbesartan. Camber Pharmaceuticals, Inc; 2023.
2. Boix E, Zapater P, Pico A, Moreno O. Teratogenicity with angiotensin II receptor antagonists in pregnancy. *J Endocrinol Invest*. 2005;28:1029-1031.
3. Moel DI. Renal agenesis, unilateral. In: Buyse ML, ed. *Birth Defects Encyclopedia*. Blackwell Scientific Publications; 1990:1461.
4. Velazquez-Armenta EY, Han JY, Choi JS, et al. Angiotensin II receptor blockers in pregnancy: a case report and systematic review of the literature. *Hypertens Pregnancy*. 2007;26:51-66.
5. Gersak K, Cvijic M, Cerar LK. Angiotensin II receptor blockers in pregnancy: a report of 5 cases. *Reprod Toxicol*. 2009;28:109-112.
6. Polifka JE. Is there an embryopathy associated with first-trimester exposure to angiotensin-converting enzyme inhibitors and angiotensin receptor antagonists? A critical review of the evidence. *Birth Defects Res A*. 2012; 94:576-598.

IRINOTECAN

Antineoplastic (Topoisomerase I Inhibitor)

PREGNANCY RECOMMENDATION: Limited Human Data—Animal Data Suggest Risk

BREASTFEEDING RECOMMENDATION: Potential Toxicity

PREGNANCY SUMMARY

Three case reports describing the use of irinotecan (as part of a combination chemotherapy regimen) during human pregnancy were located. These reports include four pregnancies with exposure in the second and third trimesters. All pregnancies resulted in successful delivery of healthy infants. No congenital abnormalities were reported. All infants had normal development and growth at routine follow-up visits. Some amount of the drug will probably cross the placenta, so fetal exposure will likely occur. However, the limited human pregnancy experience prevents a complete assessment of the embryofetal risk. Embryofetal toxicity with malformations was observed in two species at doses of less than 10 times the RHD. Based on animal studies and the drug's mechanism of action, the manufacturer recommends that women with reproductive potential use effective contraception during treatment and for at least 6 and 7 months after the last conventional and liposomal dose, respectively. They also recommend that males with female partners of reproductive potential use effective contraception during treatment and for at least 3 and 4 months after the last conventional and liposomal dose, respectively. Nevertheless, using this drug during pregnancy should be based on the pros and cons of the mother's clinical need for treatment versus any potential fetal risk that might occur from exposure. There is a registry for women who are pregnant and have cancer. For more information, women and health care providers are encouraged to contact the Cancer and Pregnancy Registry at 1-877-635-4499.

BREASTFEEDING SUMMARY

One report evaluating the excretion of irinotecan into human breast milk was found. Irinotecan levels were detected on days 2 and 3, whereas the metabolite was detected up to the last day tested (day 7). The authors estimated a relative infant dose (RID) of about 8% for the infant. Due to a concern for potential serious adverse effects that might be seen in a breastfed infant, the manufacturer recommends that women not breastfeed while being treated with this drug and for at least 7 days and 1 month after the last conventional and liposomal dose, respectively. Nevertheless, breastfeeding while using this drug should be based on the mother's clinical need for treatment versus any potential infant risks that might occur. If used, the infant should be monitored for the most common reported adult side effects of nausea, headache, and abdominal pain (all leading to irritability), vomiting, diarrhea, constipation, anorexia (monitor infant growth), bone marrow suppression, hair loss, lethargy, and fever.

References

1. Prescribing Information. Camptosar. Pharmacia & Upjohn; 2022.
2. Prescribing Information. Onivyde. Ipsen Biopharmaceuticals, Inc; 2024.
3. Taylor J, Amanze A, Di Federico E, Verschraegen C. Irinotecan use during pregnancy. *Obstet Gynecol*. 2009;114:451-452.
4. Cirillo M, Musola M, Cassandrini PA, et al. Irinotecan during pregnancy in metastatic colon cancer. *Tumori*. 2012;98:e155-e157.
5. Nakagawa J, Terui K, Hosoi K, et al. Passage of irinotecan and its active metabolite, SN-38, into human milk. *J Clin Pharm Ther*. 2016;41:579-582.
6. Kozai L, Benavente K, Obeidat A, Acoba J. FOLFOXIRI in pregnant women with colorectal cancer: a case report and review of the literature. *Case Rep Oncol*. 2022;15:447-454.

ISATUXIMAB

Antineoplastic (Monoclonal Antibody)

PREGNANCY RECOMMENDATION: No Human Data—Animal Data Suggest Risk

BREASTFEEDING RECOMMENDATION: Probably Compatible

PREGNANCY SUMMARY

No reports describing the use of isatuximab in human pregnancy have been located. As an IgG antibody, it likely crosses the placenta, so some fetal exposure will occur. Animal models suggest fetal risk. *The combination use of isatuximab and pomalidomide in pregnancy is contraindicated as pomalidomide is a thalidomide analogue that can cause severe birth defects and death of the unborn child (see Pomalidomide). The manufacturer recommends that women with reproductive potential on isatuximab in combination with pomalidomide use effective contraception during treatment and for 5 months after the last dose. Regarding isatuximab with carfilzomib and dexamethasone, using this combination during pregnancy should be based on the pros and cons of the mother's clinical need for treatment versus any potential fetal risk that might occur from exposure (see Carfilzomib and Dexamethasone). There is a registry for women who are pregnant and have cancer. For more information, women and health care providers are encouraged to contact the Cancer and Pregnancy Registry at 1-877-635-4499.

BREASTFEEDING SUMMARY

Isatuximab is probably found in human breast milk, but IgG antibodies are not found in the neonatal or infant circulation. Additionally, if any IgG antibodies were to be ingested through breastfeeding, they would probably be digested in the infant's gastrointestinal tract and not be absorbed. However, due to the concern for potential serious adverse effects with the co-use of dexamethasone and pomalidomide, the manufacturer recommends that women not breastfeed while using isatuximab in combination with these agents (see Carfilzomib and Dexamethasone). However, if the clinical decision is to use this drug while breastfeeding, the infant should be monitored for the most common reported adult side effects of back pain (leading to irritability), upper respiratory tract infections, diarrhea, lethargy, and cough.

Reference

1. Prescribing Information. Sarclisa. Sanofi-Aventis U.S. LLC; 2020.

ISAVUCONAZONIUM

Antifungal (Azole)

PREGNANCY RECOMMENDATION: No Human Data—Animal Data Suggest Risk

BREASTFEEDING RECOMMENDATION: Potential Toxicity

PREGNANCY SUMMARY

No reports describing the use of isavuconazonium during human pregnancy have been located. Some amount of the drug may cross the placenta, so fetal exposure will probably occur. However, the absence of human pregnancy experience prevents a complete assessment of the embryofetal risk. Embryofetal toxicity with malformations was observed in two animal species at doses of less than 10 times the RHD. Based on animal studies and the drug's mechanism of action, the manufacturer recommends that women with reproductive potential use effective contraception during treatment and for 4 weeks after the last dose. Nevertheless, using this drug during pregnancy should be based on the pros and cons of the mother's clinical need for treatment versus any potential fetal risk that might occur from exposure.

BREASTFEEDING SUMMARY

No reports describing the use of isavuconazonium during human lactation have been located. The drug will probably be excreted into breast milk, so some infant exposure will likely occur. However, due to a concern for potential serious adverse effects that might be seen in a breastfed infant, the manufacturer recommends that women not breastfeed while being treated with this drug. Nevertheless, breastfeeding while using this drug should be based on the mother's clinical need for treatment versus any potential infant risks that might occur. If used, the infant should be monitored for the most common reported adult side effects of nausea, headache, itching, and abdominal pain (all leading to irritability), vomiting, diarrhea, elevated liver enzymes, and rash.

Reference

1. Prescribing Information. Cresemba. Astellas Pharma US; 2023.

ISOCARBOXAZID

Mental Health (Antidepressant/Monoamine Oxidase Inhibitor)

PREGNANCY RECOMMENDATION: No Human Data and No Relevant Animal Data

BREASTFEEDING RECOMMENDATION: Potential Toxicity

PREGNANCY SUMMARY

No reports describing the use of isocarboxazid in human pregnancy have been located. The drug will probably cross the placenta, so some fetal exposure will likely occur. Therefore, the absence of human pregnancy experience prevents a complete assessment of the embryofetal risk. No animal reproduction studies have been conducted. Using this drug during pregnancy should be based on the pros and cons of the mother's clinical need for treatment versus any potential fetal risk that might occur from exposure. There is a pregnancy exposure registry that monitors pregnancy outcomes in women using antidepressant drugs. Health care providers are encouraged to call the National Pregnancy Registry for Antidepressants at 1-844-405-6185.

BREASTFEEDING SUMMARY

No reports describing the use of isocarboxazid during human lactation have been located. The drug will probably appear in breast milk, so some infant exposure will likely occur. However, due to a lack of information, the manufacturer recommends that isocarboxazid should only be used in women who are breastfeeding, if clearly needed. If the clinical decision is to use this drug while breastfeeding, the infant should be monitored for the most common reported adult side effects of headache and dizziness (both leading to irritability) and difficulty sleeping.

References

1. Prescribing Information. Marplan. Validus Pharmaceuticals, LLC; 2020.
2. Sato T, Yamamoto S, Moroi K. The metabolism and placental transfer of isocarboxazid in pregnant rats. *Jpn J Pharmacol*. 1972;22:629-633.

I

ISOFLURANE

Anesthetic

PREGNANCY RECOMMENDATION: Limited Human Data—Animal Data Suggest Potential Risk

BREASTFEEDING RECOMMENDATION: Probably Compatible

PREGNANCY SUMMARY

No reports of isoflurane use in the first trimester of human gestation have been located. The drug has been used immediately prior to delivery for analgesia and anesthesia. This use does not appear to affect the newborn any differently from other general anesthetic agents. Isoflurane freely crosses the placenta to the fetus. However, this limited human pregnancy experience prevents a complete assessment of the embryofetal risk. Embryofetal toxicity was observed in one species, but a human dosing comparison was not provided. ACOG has described the use of isoflurane to maintain anesthesia until delivery as acceptable. Concentrations should be kept low due to the effect on uterine tone. Isoflurane is associated with QT prolongation.

BREASTFEEDING SUMMARY

Although isoflurane has been administered during labor and delivery, no reports of its effects on the infant (who begins nursing immediately after birth) have been described. The drug will probably appear in breast milk, so some infant exposure will likely occur. The risk to a nursing infant from exposure to isoflurane is probably very low. With an elimination half-life of only 10 minutes, the drug would be out of the maternal system within an hour of the last dose. Breastfeeding can likely be resumed as soon as the mother has recovered from anesthesia without any expected adverse infant effects.

References

1. Eger EI II. Desflurane animal and human pharmacology: aspects of kinetics, safety, and MAC. *Anesth Analg*. 1992;75:S3-S9.
2. Kennedy GL Jr, Smith SH, Keplinger ML, Calandra JG. Reproductive and teratologic studies with isoflurane. *Drug Chem Toxicol*. 1977-1978;1:75-88.
3. Mazze RI, Wilson AI, Rice SA, Baden JM. Fetal development in mice exposed to isoflurane. *Teratology*. 1985;32:339-345.
4. Mazze RI, Fujinaga M, Rice SA, et al. Reproductive and teratogenic effects of nitrous oxide, halothane, isoflurane, and enflurane in Sprague-Dawley rats. *Anesthesiology*. 1986;64:339-344.
5. Trevor AJ, Miller RD. General anesthetics. In: Katzung BG, ed. *Basic and Clinical Pharmacology*. 8th ed. McGraw-Hill; 2001:426.
6. O'Leary G, Bacon CL, Odumeru O, et al. Antiproliferative actions of inhalational anesthetics: comparisons to the valproate teratogen. *Int J Dev Neurosci*. 2000;18:39-45.
7. Palahniuk RJ, Shnider SM, Eger EI II. Pregnancy decreases the requirement for inhaled anesthetic agents. *Anesthesiology*. 1974;41:82-83.
8. Gin T, Chan MTV. Decrease minimum alveolar concentration of isoflurane in pregnant humans. *Anesthesiology*. 1994;81:829-832.
9. Friedman JM. Teratogen update: anesthetic agents. *Teratology*. 1988;37:69-77.
10. Kanto J. Risk-benefit assessment of anaesthetic agents in the puerperium. *Drug Saf*. 1991;6:285-301.
11. Dwyer R, Fee JPH, Moore J. Uptake of halothane and isoflurane by mother and baby during caesarean section. *Br J Anaesthesia*. 1995;74:379-383.
12. Merritt WT, Dickstein R, Beattie C, et al. Liver transplantation during pregnancy: anesthesia for two procedures in the same patient with successful outcome of pregnancy. *Transplant Proc*. 1991;23:1996-1997.
13. McLeod DD, Ramayya GP, Tunstall ME. Self-administered isoflurane in labour. A comparative study with Entonox. *Anaesthesia*. 1985;40:424-426.
14. Abboud TK, Gangolly J, Mosaad P, Crowell D. Isoflurane in obstetrics. *Anesth Analg*. 1989;68:388-391.
15. Wee MYK, Hasan MA, Thomas TA. Isoflurane in labour. *Anaesthesia*. 1993;48:369-372.
16. Ghaly RG, Flynn RJ, Moore J. Isoflurane as an alternative to halothane for caesarean section. *Anaesthesia*. 1988;43:5-7.
17. Abboud TK, Zhu J, Richardson M, et al. Intravenous propofol vs. thiamylal-isoflurane for caesarean section, comparative maternal and neonatal effects. *Acta Anaesthesiol Scand*. 1995;39:205-209.
18. Stuart JC, Kan AF, Rowbottom SJ, et al. Acid aspiration prophylaxis for emergency caesarean section. *Anaesthesia*. 1996;51:415-421.

19. Warren TM, Datta S, Ostheimer GW, et al. Comparison of the maternal and neonatal effects of halothane, enflurane, and isoflurane for cesarean section. *Anesth Analg*. 1983;62:516-520.
20. Munson ES, Embro WJ. Enflurane, isoflurane, and halothane and isolated human uterine muscle. *Anesthesiology*. 1977;46:11-14.
21. Abadir AR, Humayun SG, Calvello D, Gintautas J. Effects of isoflurane and oxytocin on gravid human uterus in vitro (abstract). *Anesth Analg*. 1987; 66:S1.
22. Sessler DI, Badgwell JM. Exposure of postoperative nurses to exhaled anesthetic gases. *Anesth Analg*. 1998;87:1083-1088.
23. Lee JJ, Rubin AP. Breastfeeding and anaesthesia. *Anaesthesia*. 1993;48: 616-625.
24. Spigset O. Anaesthetic agents and excretion in breast milk. *Acta Anaesthesiol Scand*. 1994;38:94-103.
25. Prescribing Information. Isofllurane. Piramal Critical Care, Inc; 2023.
26. Obstetric analgesia and anesthesia. ACOG practice bulletin no. 209. American College of Obstetricians and Gynecologists. *Obstet Gynecol*. 2019;133: e208-e225.

ISONIAZID

Antibacterial (Antitubercular Agent)

PREGNANCY RECOMMENDATION: Human Data Suggest Low Risk—Animal Data Suggest Risk (Maternal Benefit May Outweigh Embryofetal Risk)

BREASTFEEDING RECOMMENDATION: Probably Compatible

I

PREGNANCY SUMMARY

Several reports involving over 5,000 pregnancy exposures have been described in all trimesters. No increased risk for major birth anomalies has been found. The drug crosses the placenta, so fetal exposure will occur. Isoniazid was found to cause some embryofetal toxicity in two animal species, but a human dosing comparison was not supplied. Isoniazid is recommended as part of the initial treatment regimen used to treat active tuberculosis (TB). Hepatotoxicity may occur with isoniazid use in pregnancy. However, due to the poor maternal and fetal outcomes with untreated active TB, the benefits of treatment outweigh the potential risk from the medications. Therefore, monitoring for signs and symptoms of hepatitis is recommended. Treatment of latent TB can be delayed until 2 to 3 months postpartum to avoid unnecessary medication exposure. However, treatment is recommended in women who are at high risk of progression from latent to active TB, such as those who are a recent contact of someone with infectious TB.

BREASTFEEDING SUMMARY

Limited reports describing the use of isoniazid during human lactation have found no adverse effects. Both isoniazid and its metabolite are excreted in breast milk in low amounts. The amount of the drug in breast milk is below therapeutic levels. Breastfeeding should not be discouraged in women who are being treated with isoniazid. If used while breastfeeding, the infant should be monitored for the most common reported adult side effects of peripheral neuropathy (leading to irritability) and hepatotoxicity (jaundice). Pyridoxine administration is also recommended for all breastfeeding mothers taking isoniazid for the prevention of peripheral neuropathy.

References

1. Prescribing Information. Isoniazid. Eon Labs; 2018.
2. American Thoracic Society. Treatment of tuberculosis and tuberculosis infection in adults and children. *Am Rev Respir Dis*. 1986;134:355-363.
3. Medchill MT, Gillum M. Diagnosis and management of tuberculosis during pregnancy. *Obstet Gynecol Surv*. 1989;44:81-84.
4. Bromberg YM, Salzberger M, Bruderman I. Placental transmission of isonicotinic acid hydrazide. *Gynaecologia*. 1955;140:141-144.
5. Miceli JN, Olson WA, Cohen SN. Elimination kinetics of isoniazid in the newborn infant. *Dev Pharmacol Ther*. 1981;2:235-239.
6. Holdiness MR. Transplacental pharmacokinetics of the antituberculosis drugs. *Clin Pharmacokinet*. 1987;13:125-129.
7. Weinstein L, Dalton AC. Host determinants of response to antimicrobial agents. *N Engl J Med*. 1968;279:524-531.
8. Lowe CR. Congenital defects among children born to women under supervision or treatment for pulmonary tuberculosis. *Br J Prev Soc Med*. 1964;18: 14-16.
9. Heinonen OP, Slone D, Shapiro S. *Birth Defects and Drugs in Pregnancy*. Publishing Sciences Group; 1977.
10. Marynowski A, Sianozecka E. Comparison of the incidence of congenital malformations in neonates from healthy mothers and from patients treated because of tuberculosis. *Ginekol Pol*. 1972;43:713.
11. Jentgens H. Antituberkulose Chemotherapie und Schwangerschaftsabbruch. *Prax Klin Pneumol*. 1973;27:479.
12. Ludford J, Doster B, Woolpert SF. Effect of isoniazid on reproduction. *Am Rev Respir Dis*. 1973;108:1170-1174.
13. Scheinhorn DJ, Angelillo VA. Antituberculosis therapy in pregnancy: risks to the fetus. *West J Med*. 1977;127:195-198.
14. Good JT, Iseman MD, Davidson PT, et al. Tuberculosis in association with pregnancy. *Am J Obstet Gynecol*. 1981;140:492-498.
15. Kingdom JCP, Kennedy DH. Tuberculous meningitis in pregnancy. *Br J Obstet Gynaecol*. 1989;96:233-235.
16. Snider DE Jr, Layde PM, Johnson MW, Lyle MA. Treatment of tuberculosis during pregnancy. *Am Rev Respir Dis*. 1980;122:65-79.
17. Tuman KJ, Chilcote RR, Gerkow RI, Moohr JW. Mesothelioma in child with prenatal exposure to isoniazid. *Lancet*. 1980;2:362.
18. Hammond DC, Silidoff IJ, Robitzek EH. Isoniazid therapy in relation to later occurrence of cancer in adults and in infants. *Br Med J*. 1967;2:792-795.
19. Eggermont E, Logghe N, Van De Casseye W, et al. Haemorrhagic disease of the newborn in the offspring of rifampicin and isoniazid treated mothers. *Acta Paediatr Belg*. 1976;29:87-90.
20. Snider DE Jr, Powell KE. Should women taking antituberculosis drugs breast-feed? *Arch Intern Med*. 1984;144:589-590.
21. Berlin CM Jr, Lee C. Isoniazid and acetylisoniazid disposition in human milk, saliva and plasma. *Fed Proc*. 1979;38:426.
22. Vorherr H. Drugs excretion in breast milk. *Postgrad Med*. 1974;56:97-104.
23. Ricci G, Copaitich T. Modalita di eliminazione dell'isoniazide somministrata per via orale attraverso il latte di donna. *Rass Clin Ter*. 1954-1955;209:53-54.
24. Singh N, Golani A, Patel Z, Maitra A. Transfer of isoniazid from circulation to breast milk in lactating women on chronic therapy for tuberculosis. *Br J Clin Pharmacol*. 2008;65:418-422.
25. Miele K, Bamrah Morris S, Tepper NK. Tuberculosis in pregnancy. *Obstet Gynecol*. 2020;135:1444-1453.
26. Centers for Disease Control and Prevention (CDC). Treatment for TB During Pregnancy. Accessed October 2, 2024. https://www.cdc.gov/tb/topic/treatment/pregnancy.htm

ISOPROTERENOL

Autonomic (Sympathomimetic—β_1 and β_2 Agonist)

PREGNANCY RECOMMENDATION: Limited Human Data—No Relevant Animal Data

BREASTFEEDING RECOMMENDATION: Probably Compatible

PREGNANCY SUMMARY

Seven reports describing the use of isoproterenol in 113 human pregnancies have been located. One (3.2%) congenital anomaly was reported in 31 first-trimester exposures. The remaining uses were mostly at the time of delivery. The drug will probably cross the placenta, so some fetal exposure will likely occur. However, the limited human pregnancy experience prevents a complete assessment of the embryofetal risk. Animal reproduction studies found some embryofetal toxicity in one animal species, but not in two others. However, a human dosing comparison was not provided. The manufacturer reports that isoproterenol can inhibit contractions; therefore, it should be avoided during the second stage of labor, if possible. Regardless, in cases of shock, isoproterenol may improve maternal hypotension, but this could theoretically also result in uterine vasoconstriction and potential decreased uterine blood flow. However, studies have not shown any changes in the fetal heart rate with its use for maternal tachycardia. Using this drug during pregnancy should be based on the pros and cons of the mother's clinical need for treatment versus any potential fetal risk that might occur from exposure.

I

BREASTFEEDING SUMMARY

No reports describing the use of isoproterenol during human lactation have been located. The drug may appear in breast milk, but the very short half-life (minutes) would limit infant exposure. If the clinical decision is to use this drug while breastfeeding, the infant should be monitored for the most common reported adult side effect of tachycardia.

References

1. Prescribing Information. Isuprel. Bausch Health; 2022.
2. Heinonen OP, Slone D, Shapiro S. *Birth Defects and Drugs in Pregnancy*. Publishing Sciences Group; 1977.
3. Nishimura H, Tanimura T. *Clinical Aspects of the Teratogenicity of Drugs*. American Elsevier; 1976:231-232.
4. Shepard TH. *Catalog of Teratogenic Agents*. 3rd ed. The Johns Hopkins University Press; 1980:191.
5. DeSimone CA, Leighton BL, Norris MC, et al. The chronotropic effect of isoproterenol is reduced in term pregnant women. *Anesthesiology*. 1988;69:626-628.
6. Marcus MA, Vertommen JD, Van Aken H, et al. Hemodynamic effects of intravenous isoproterenol versus saline in the parturient. *Anesth Analg*. 1997;84:1113-1116.
7. Marcus MA, Vertommen JD, Van Aken H, et al. The effects of adding isoproterenol to 0.125% bupivacaine on the quality and duration of epidural analgesia in laboring parturients. *Anesth Analg*. 1998;86:749-752.
8. Sharif-Kazemi MB, Emkanjoo Z, Tavoosi A, et al. Electrical storm in Brugada syndrome during pregnancy. *Pacing Clin Electrophysiol*. 2011;34:e18-e21.
9. Burrows K, Fox J, Biblo LA, Roth JA. Pregnancy and short-coupled torsades de pointes. *Pacing Clin Electrophysiol*. 2013;36:e77-e79.
10. Mittadodla PS, Salen PN, Traub DM. Isoproterenol as an adjunct for treatment of idiopathic ventricular fibrillation storm in a pregnant woman. *Am J Emerg Med*. 2012;30:251.e3-251.e5.

ISOSORBIDE DINITRATE

Cardiovascular (Vasodilator/Antianginal)

PREGNANCY RECOMMENDATION: Limited Human Data—No Relevant Animal Data

BREASTFEEDING RECOMMENDATION: Probably Compatible

PREGNANCY SUMMARY

Numerous studies describing the use of isosorbide dinitrate in several hundred human pregnancies have been located. None of the analyses involved the first trimester of human pregnancy. All reports described the use of isosorbide dinitrate in cervical ripening, labor induction, and in treating hypertension in patients with preeclampsia. Overall, no higher rate of adverse effects related to the drug was seen when compared to other antihypertensive medications, including dinoprostone and misoprostol. The drug will probably cross the placenta, so some fetal exposure will likely occur. However, this limited human pregnancy experience, especially first-trimester use, prevents a complete assessment of the embryofetal risk. Embryofetal toxicity was observed in two animal species but at doses greater than 10 times the MRHD. Using this drug during pregnancy should be based on the pros and cons of the mother's clinical need for treatment versus any potential fetal risk that might occur from exposure.

BREASTFEEDING SUMMARY

No reports describing the use of isosorbide dinitrate during human lactation have been located. The drug will probably appear in breast milk, so some infant exposure will likely occur. If the clinical decision is to use this drug while breastfeeding, the infant should be monitored for the most common reported adult side effects of headache and lightheadedness (both leading to irritability).

References

1. Prescribing Information. Isosorbide Dinitrate. Par Pharmaceutical; 2021.
2. Thaler I, Amit A, Jakobi P, Itskovitz-Eldor J. The effect of isosorbide dinitrate on uterine artery and umbilical artery flow velocity waveforms at mid-pregnancy. *Obstet Gynecol*. 1996;88:838-843.
3. Nakatsuka M, Tada K, Kimura Y, et al. Clinical experience of long-term transdermal treatment with nitric oxide donor for women with preeclampsia. *Gynecol Obstet Invest*. 1999;47:13-19.
4. Martínez-Abundis E, González-Ortiz M, Hernández-Salazar F, Huerta-J-Lucas MT. Sublingual isosorbide dinitrate in the acute control of hypertension in patients with severe preeclampsia. *Gynecol Obstet Invest*. 2000;50:39-42.
5. Thaler I, Amit A, Kamil D, Itskovitz-Eldor J. The effect of isosorbide dinitrate on placental blood flow and maternal blood pressure in women with pregnancy induced hypertension. *Am J Hypertens*. 1999;12:341-347.
6. Romero-Gutierrez G, Gonzalez OEB, Ponce-Ponce de Leon A. Isosorbide and dinoprostone for induction of labor. *Ginecologia y Obstetricia de Mexico*. 2011;79:285-291.
7. Haghighi L, Homam H, Raoofi Z, Najmi Z. Intravaginal isosorbide dinitrate or misoprostol for cervical ripening prior to induction of labour: a randomized controlled trial. *J Obstet Gynaecol*. 2013;33:272-276.
8. Haghighi L, Moukhah S, Goshtasbi A. Comparing the effect of oral and vaginal isosorbide dinitrate in pre-induction cervical ripening in term pregnancy: a controlled clinical trial. *Advanced Biomedical Research*. 2015;4:129.
9. Ghosh A, Lattey KR, Kelly AJ. Nitric oxide donors for cervical ripening and induction of labour. *Cochrane Database Syst Rev*. 2016;12:CD006901.
10. Ghafarzadeh M, Shakarami A, Yari F. Prevention of preterm labor by isosorbide dinitrate and nitroglycerin patch. *Cardiovasc Hematol Disord Drug Targets*. 2023;23:130-135.

I

ISOSORBIDE MONONITRATE

Cardiovascular (Vasodilator/Antianginal)

PREGNANCY RECOMMENDATION: Limited Human Data—No Relevant Animal Data

BREASTFEEDING RECOMMENDATION: Probably Compatible

PREGNANCY SUMMARY

A number of reports have described the use of isosorbide mononitrate for cervical ripening at term. No adverse fetal effects were observed. None of the studies describes the use of the drug in the first trimester. Isosorbide mononitrate will probably cross the placenta, so some fetal exposure will likely occur. However, this limited human pregnancy experience prevents a complete assessment of the embryofetal risk. Embryofetal toxicity was observed in two animal species, but at doses of more than 10 times the RHD. Using this drug during pregnancy should be based on the pros and cons of the mother's clinical need for treatment versus any potential fetal risk that might occur from exposure.

BREASTFEEDING SUMMARY

No reports describing the use of isosorbide mononitrate during human lactation have been located. The drug will probably appear in breast milk, so some infant exposure will likely occur. If the clinical decision is to use this drug while breastfeeding, the infant should be monitored for the most common reported adult side effect of headache (leading to irritability).

References

1. Prescribing Information. Ismo. Reddy Pharmaceuticals; 2007.
2. Nicoll AE, MacKenzie F, Greer IA, Norman JE. Vaginal application of the nitric oxide donor isosorbide mononitrate for preinduction cervical ripening: a randomized controlled trial to determine effects on maternal and fetal hemodynamics. *Am J Obstet Gynecol*. 2001;184:958-964.
3. Chanrachakul B, Herabutya Y, Punyavachira P. Randomized trial of isosorbide mononitrate versus misoprostol for cervical ripening at term. *Int J Gynaecol Obstet*. 2002;78:139-145.
4. Ekerhovd E, Bullarbo M, Andersch B, Norstrom A. Vaginal administration of the nitric oxide donor isosorbide mononitrate for cervical ripening at term—a randomized controlled study. *Am J Obstet Gynecol*. 2003;189:1692-1697.
5. Wolfler MM, Facchinetti F, Venturini P, et al. Induction of labor at term using isosorbide mononitrate simultaneously with dinoprostone compared to dinoprostone treatment alone: a randomized, controlled trial. *Am J Obstet Gynecol*. 2006;195:1617-1622.
6. Osman I, MacKenzie F, Norrie J, et al. The "PRIM" study: a randomized comparison of prostaglandin E2 gel with the nitric oxide donor isosorbide mononitrate for cervical ripening before the induction of labor at term. *Am J Obstet Gynecol*. 2006;194:1012-1021.
7. Bullarbo M, Orrskog ME, Andersch B, et al. Outpatient vaginal administration of the nitric oxide donor isosorbide mononitrate for cervical ripening and labor induction postterm: a randomized controlled study. *Am J Obstet Gynecol*. 2007;196:50.e1-50.e5.
8. Rameez MF, Goonewardene IM. Nitric oxide donor isosorbide mononitrate for pre-induction cervical ripening at 41 weeks' gestation: a randomized controlled trial. *J Obstet Gynaecol Res*. 2007;33:452-456.
9. Habib SM, Emam SS, Saber AS. Outpatient cervical ripening with nitric oxide donor isosorbide mononitrate prior to induction of labor. *Int J Gynaecol Obstet*. 2008;101:57-61.
10. Bollapragada SS, MacKenzie F, Norrie JD, et al. Randomized placebo-controlled trial of outpatient (at home) cervical ripening with isosorbide mononitrate (IMN) prior to induction of labour-clinical trial with analyses of efficacy and acceptability. The IMOP study. *BJOG*. 2009;116;1185-1195.
11. Eddama O, Petrou S, Schroeder L, et al. The cost-effectiveness of outpatient (at home) cervical ripening with isosorbide mononitrate prior to induction of labour. *BJOG*. 2009;116:1196-1203.
12. Hatanaka AR, Moron AF, Auxiliadora de Aquino MM, et al. Interruption of a study of cervical ripening with isosorbide mononitrate due to adverse effects. *Clin Exp Obstet Gynecol*. 2012;39:175-180.

ISOTRETINOIN

Dermatologic (Retinoic Acid)

PREGNANCY RECOMMENDATION: Contraindicated

BREASTFEEDING RECOMMENDATION: Contraindicated

PREGNANCY SUMMARY

Isotretinoin is a known teratogen, primarily involving the fetal central nervous system. Of critical importance is the fact that a high percentage of the recipients of this drug are women with childbearing potential. Due to the high risk of life-threatening birth defects, the manufacturer recommends that women with reproductive potential who are taking isotretinoin be advised to use two effective forms of contraception at least one month prior to treatment, during treatment, and for at least 1 month after the last dose. Any suspected fetal exposure during or one month after isotretinoin therapy must immediately be reported to the FDA via the MedWatch number 1-800-FDA-1088 and the iPLEDGE Pregnancy Registry at 1-866-495-0654. Isotretinoin carries a boxed warning regarding life-threatening birth defects. Due to isotretinoin's teratogenicity and to minimize fetal exposure, it is approved for marketing only under a special restricted distribution or REMS program approved by the FDA called iPLEDGE.

I

BREASTFEEDING SUMMARY

No reports describing the use of isotretinoin during human lactation have been located. The drug will probably appear in breast milk, so some infant exposure will likely occur. In addition, the closely related retinoid, vitamin A, is excreted into breast milk, so the presence of isotretinoin should be expected. Due to a concern for potential serious adverse effects that might be seen in a breastfed infant, the manufacturer recommends that women not breastfeed while being treated with this drug. If the clinical decision is to use this drug while breastfeeding, the infant should be monitored for the most common reported adult side effects of headache, dizziness, nausea, stomach, bone and muscle problems (all leading to irritability), vomiting, seizures, and skin problems.

References

1. Prescribing Information. Claravis. Teva Pharmaceuticals USA, Inc; 2022.
2. Voorhees JJ, Orfanos CE. Oral retinoids. *Arch Dermatol*. 1981;117:418-421.
3. Kamm JJ. Toxicology, carcinogenicity, and teratogenicity of some orally administered retinoids. *J Am Acad Dermatol*. 1982;6:652-659.
4. Kubow S. Inhibition of isotretinoin teratogenicity by acetylsalicylic acid pretreatment in mice. *Teratology*. 1992;45:55-63.
5. Lammer EJ, Chen DT, Hoar RM, et al. Retinoic acid embryopathy. *N Engl J Med*. 1985;313:837-841.
6. Webster WS, Johnston MC, Lammer EJ, Sulik KK. Isotretinoin embryopathy and the cranial neural crest: an in vivo and in vitro study. *J Craniofac Genet Dev Biol*. 1986;6:211-222.
7. Dai WS, LaBraico JM, Stern RS. Epidemiology of isotretinoin exposure during pregnancy. *J Am Acad Dermatol*. 1992;26:599-606.
8. Benifla JL, Ville Y, Imbert MC, et al. Fetal tissue dosages of retinoids. Experimental study concerning a case of isotretinoin (Roaccutan) administration and pregnancy. *Fetal Diagn Ther*. 1995;10:189-191.
9. United Kingdom Teratology Information Service (UKTIS). Use of isotretinoin in pregnancy [Internet]; 2018. Accessed November 20, 2020. http://www.uktis.org./index.html
10. Choi EJ, Kim N, Kwak HS, et al. The rates of major malformations after gestational exposure to isotretinoin: a systematic review and meta-analysis. *Obstet Gynecol Sci*. 2021;64:364-373.

ISRADIPINE

Antihypertensive (Calcium Channel Blocker)

PREGNANCY RECOMMENDATION: Limited Human Data—Animal Data Suggest Low Risk

BREASTFEEDING RECOMMENDATION: Probably Compatible

PREGNANCY SUMMARY

Several studies have described the use of isradipine in pregnant women to treat hypertension or preeclampsia. No adverse fetal effects attributable to the drug were observed. No data were found on first-trimester exposure. Isradipine crosses the placenta, at least at term, so fetal exposure will occur. However, this limited human pregnancy experience prevents a complete assessment of the embryofetal risk. Animal data did not show any embryofetal toxicity in two species at doses less than 10 times the RHD in one and more than 10 times the RHD in the second. Using this drug during pregnancy should be based on the pros and cons of the mother's clinical need for treatment versus any potential fetal risk that might occur from exposure.

BREASTFEEDING SUMMARY

No reports describing the use of isradipine during human lactation have been located. The drug will probably appear in breast milk, so some infant exposure will likely occur. If the clinical decision is to use this drug while breastfeeding, the infant should be monitored for the most common reported adult side effects of nausea, headache, and dizziness (all leading to irritability), peripheral edema, tachycardia, lethargy, and flushing.

References

1. Prescribing Information. Isradipine. Teva Pharmaceuticals; 2023.
2. Lunell NO, Garoff L, Grunewald C, et al. Isradipine, a new calcium antagonist: effects on maternal and fetal hemodynamics. *J Cardiovasc Pharmacol.* 1991;18(suppl 3):S37-S40.
3. Lunell NO, Grunewald C, Nisell H. Effect of isradipine on responses to standardized physical stress tests in hypertension of pregnancy. *J Cardiovasc Pharmacol.* 1992;19(suppl 3):S99-S101.
4. Lunnell NO, Bondesson U, Grunewald C, et al. Transplacental passage of isradipine in the treatment of pregnancy-induced hypertension. *Am J Hypertens.* 1993;6:110S-111S.
5. Wide-Swensson DH, Ingemarsson I, Lunell NO, et al. Calcium channel blockade (isradipine) in treatment of hypertension in pregnancy: a randomized placebo-controlled study. *Am J Obstet Gynecol.* 1995;173:872-878.
6. Maharaj B, Khedun SM, Moodley J, et al. Intravenous isradipine in the management of severe hypertension in pregnant and nonpregnant patients. A pilot study. *Am J Hypertens.* 1994;7:61S-63S.
7. Fletcher H, Roberts G, Mullings A, Forrester T. An open trial comparing isradipine with hydralazine and methyldopa in the treatment of patients with severe pre-eclampsia. *J Obstet Gynaecol.* 2009;19:235-238.

ISTRADEFYLLINE

Central Nervous System (Anti-Parkinson—Adenosine Receptor Antagonist)

PREGNANCY RECOMMENDATION: No Human Data—Animal Data Suggest Risk

BREASTFEEDING RECOMMENDATION: Potential Toxicity

PREGNANCY SUMMARY

No reports describing the use of istradefylline in human pregnancy have been located. The drug will probably cross the placenta, so some fetal exposure will likely occur. However, the absence of human pregnancy experience prevents a complete assessment of the embryofetal risk. Embryofetal toxicity was observed in two animal species at doses less than 10 times the RHD. Based on these animal studies, the manufacturer recommends that women with reproductive potential use effective contraception during treatment. Nevertheless, using this drug during pregnancy should be based on the pros and cons of the mother's clinical need for treatment versus any potential fetal risk that might occur from exposure.

BREASTFEEDING SUMMARY

No reports describing the use of istradefylline during human lactation have been located. The drug will probably appear in breast milk, so some infant exposure will likely occur. Breastfeeding while using this drug should be based on the mother's clinical need for treatment versus any potential infant risks that might occur. If used, the infant should be monitored for the most common reported adult side effects of nausea, dizziness, and hallucinations (all leading to irritability), uncontrolled movements, constipation, and sleep difficulties.

Reference

1. Prescribing Information. Nourianz. Kyowa Kirin; 2023.

ITRACONAZOLE

Antifungal (Azole)

PREGNANCY RECOMMENDATION: Limited Human Data—Animal Data Suggest Potential Risk

BREASTFEEDING RECOMMENDATION: Probably Compatible

PREGNANCY SUMMARY

A few reports and a meta-analysis describing the use of itraconazole (and other antifungal agents) during the first trimester of human pregnancy have been located. No increased risk for congenital malformations or spontaneous abortion has been found in more than 100 exposures. Some amount of the drug may cross the placenta, so fetal exposure will likely occur. However, this limited human pregnancy experience still prevents a complete assessment of the embryofetal risk. Embryofetal toxicity was observed in two animal species at doses of about equal to the RHD, but maternal toxicity also occurred. Based on these animal studies, the manufacturer recommends that women with reproductive potential use effective contraception during treatment and for 2 months after the last dose. Nevertheless, using this drug during pregnancy should be based on the pros and cons of the mother's clinical need for treatment versus any potential fetal risk that might occur from exposure.

BREASTFEEDING SUMMARY

One report was found that described the use of itraconazole during human lactation. The drug was shown to be excreted into breast milk. It is estimated that the calculated RID was about 1.5% of the mother's weight-adjusted dose. If the clinical decision is to use this drug while breastfeeding, the infant should be monitored for the most common reported adult side effects of nausea and headache (both leading to irritability), rash, vomiting, and peripheral edema.

References

1. Prescribing Information. Sporanox. Janssen Pharmaceuticals, Inc; 2024.
2. Jick SS. Pregnancy outcomes after maternal exposure to fluconazole. *Pharmacotherapy*. 1999;19:221-222.
3. Bar-Oz B, Moretti ME, Bishai R, et al. Pregnancy outcome after in utero exposure to itraconazole: a prospective cohort study. *Am J Obstet Gynecol*. 2000;183:617-620.
4. De Santis M, Gianantonio ED, Cesari E, et al. First-trimester itraconazole exposure and pregnancy outcome: a prospective cohort study of women contacting teratology information services in Italy. *Drug Safety*. 2009;32: 239-244.
5. Mølgaard-Nielsen D, Pasternak B, Hviid A. Use of oral fluconazole during pregnancy and the risk of birth defects. *N Engl J Med*. 2013;369:830-839.
6. Mølgaard-Nielsen D, Svanström H, Melbye M, et al. Association between use of oral fluconazole during pregnancy and risk of spontaneous abortion and stillbirth. *JAMA*. 2016;315:58-67.
7. Liu D, Zhang C, Wu L, Zhang L, Zhang L. Fetal outcomes after maternal exposure to oral antifungal agents during pregnancy: a systematic review and meta-analysis. *Int J Gynaecol Obstet*. 2020;148:6-13.
8. McNamara PJ, Abbassi M. Neonatal exposure to drugs in breast milk. *Pharm Res*. 2004;21:555-566.

IVABRADINE

Cardiovascular (Heart Failure)

PREGNANCY RECOMMENDATION: Limited Human Data—Animal Data Suggest Risk

BREASTFEEDING RECOMMENDATION: Potential Toxicity

PREGNANCY SUMMARY

Three case reports and an observational study describing the use of ivabradine in human pregnancy have been located. These reports included 44 pregnancies with 41 exposures in the first trimester. After excluding elective terminations and spontaneous abortions, there were 2 (5.7%) major anomalies seen in 35 live births. Both were different; they both were exposed to other drugs, and one mother had diabetes (glucose control not provided). The drug will probably cross the placenta, so some fetal exposure will likely occur. However, this limited human pregnancy experience prevents a complete assessment of the embryofetal risk. Embryofetal toxicity with malformations was observed in one animal species, and embryotoxicity only in the second animal species at doses less than 10 times the RHD. Based on these animal studies, the manufacturer recommends that women with reproductive potential use effective contraception during treatment. The American College of Cardiology (ACC), the American Heart Association (AHA), the Heart Failure Society of America (HFSA), and the European Society of Cardiology (ESC) all consider ivabradine use as contraindicated for heart failure during pregnancy. They recommend discontinuing treatment prior to conception or when the woman is found to be pregnant, as other better-studied drugs are available. Nevertheless, using this drug during pregnancy should be based on the pros and cons of the mother's clinical need for treatment versus any potential fetal risk that might occur from exposure.

BREASTFEEDING SUMMARY

One case report describing the use of ivabradine during human lactation was located. The infant was only breastfed, and neither bradycardia nor cardiac dysfunction was observed. The drug will probably appear in breast milk, so some infant exposure will likely occur. However, due to a concern for potential serious adverse effects that might be seen in a breastfed infant, the manufacturer recommends that women not breastfeed while being treated with this drug. Additionally, the ESC guidelines consider ivabradine contraindicated for use during breastfeeding. Regardless, if the clinical decision is to use this drug while breastfeeding, the infant should be monitored for the most common reported adult side effects of vision changes (leading to irritability), bradycardia, hypotension, and atrial fibrillation.

References

1. Prescribing Information. Corlanor. Amgen; 2021.
2. Babic Z, Gabric ID, Pintaric H. Successful primary percutaneous coronary intervention in the first trimester of pregnancy. *Catheter Cardiovasc Interv*. 2011;77:522-525.
3. Sağ S, Çoşkun H, Baran İ, et al. Inappropriate sinus tachycardia-induced cardiomyopathy during pregnancy and successful treatment with ivabradine. *Anatol J Cardiol*. 2016;16:212-213.
4. Tonko JB, Douglas H, Wright MJ. Ivabradine-sensitive incessant atrial tachycardia during pregnancy: a case report. *Eur Heart J Case Rep*. 2021;5:ytab367.
5. Hoeltzenbein M, Lehmann ML, Beck E, et al. Ivabradine use in pregnant women-treatment indications and pregnancy outcome: an evaluation of the German Embryotox database. *Eur J Clin Pharmacol*. 2021;77:1029-1037.

6. Regitz-Zagrosek V, Roos-Hesselink JW, Bauersachs J, et al. 2018 ESC Guidelines for the management of cardiovascular diseases during pregnancy. *Eur Heart J*. 2018;39:3165-3241.
7. Heidenreich PA, Bozkurt B, Aguilar D, et al. 2022 AHA/ACC/HFSA guideline for the management of heart failure: a report of the American College of Cardiology/American Heart Association Joint Committee on Clinical Practice Guidelines. *J Am Coll Cardiol*. 2022;79:e263-e421.

IVACAFTOR

Genetic (Cystic Fibrosis—Transmembrane Conductance Regulator Potentiator)

PREGNANCY RECOMMENDATION: Limited Human Data—Animal Data Suggest Low Risk

BREASTFEEDING RECOMMENDATION: Potential Toxicity

PREGNANCY SUMMARY

Ten reports describing the use of ivacaftor alone or in combination throughout 13 pregnancies were located. Ivacaftor did not appear to be associated with congenital anomalies or significant adverse fetal effects in these few cases. The drug crosses the placenta, so some fetal exposure will occur. However, this limited human pregnancy experience prevents a complete assessment of the embryofetal risk. Animal data did not show any embryofetal toxicity in two species at doses less than 10 times the RHD in one and more than 10 times the RHD in the second. Using this drug during pregnancy should be based on the pros and cons of the mother's clinical need for treatment versus any potential fetal risk that might occur from exposure.

I

BREASTFEEDING SUMMARY

Nine reports describing the use of ivacaftor alone or in combination in 63 breastfeeding women have been located. No adverse effects were noted in 60 breastfed infants. However, three infants whose mothers took ivacaftor (in combination with other treatments) during pregnancy and while breastfeeding presented with bilateral cataracts. Cataracts were seen in one animal reproduction study. Cataracts have also been associated with cystic fibrosis. This potential risk needs further study. If the clinical decision is to use this drug while breastfeeding, the infant should be monitored for the most common reported adult side effects of nausea, headache, dizziness, oropharyngeal and abdominal pain (all leading to irritability), diarrhea, rash, and cataracts.

References

1. Prescribing Information. Kalydeco. Vertex Pharmaceuticals; 2023.
2. Jones GH, Walshaw MJ. Potential impact on fertility of new systemic therapies for cystic fibrosis. *Paediatr Respir Rev*. 2015;16(suppl 1):25-27.
3. Trimble A, McKinzie C, Terrell M, et al. Measured fetal and neonatal exposure to lumacaftor and ivacaftor during pregnancy and while breastfeeding. *J Cyst Fibros*. 2018;17:779-782.
4. Kaminski R, Nazareth D. A successful uncomplicated CF pregnancy while remaining on ivacaftor. *J Cyst Fibros*. 2016;15:133-134.
5. Collins B, Fortner C, Cotey A, et al. Drug exposure to infants born to mothers taking elexacaftor, tezacaftor, and ivacaftor. *J Cyst Fibros*. 2022;21:725-727.
6. Mainz JG, Michl RK, Beiersdorf N, et al. Successful pregnancy of a patient with cystic fibrosis genotype F508del/F508del and progressed pulmonary destruction on lumacaftor/ivacaftor. *Klin Padiatr*. 2019;231:271-273.
7. Ladores S, Bray LA, Brown J. Two unanticipated pregnancies while on cystic fibrosis gene-specific drug therapy. *J Patient Exp*. 2020;7:4-7.
8. Vekaria S, Popowicz N, White SW, Mulrennan S. To be or not to be on CFTR modulators during pregnancy: risks to be considered. *J Cyst Fibros*. 2020;19:e7-e8.
9. Fortner CN, Seguin JM, Kay DM. Normal pancreatic function and false-negative CF newborn screen in a child born to a mother taking CFTR modulator therapy during pregnancy. *J Cyst Fibros*. 2021;20:835-836.
10. Goodwin J, Quon BS, Wilcox PG. Experience to date with CFTR modulators during pregnancy and breastfeeding in the British Columbia Cystic Fibrosis clinic. *Respir Med Case Rep*. 2022;40:101778.26.
11. Balmpouzis Z, Faure van Rossum A, Baud D, et al. Successful pregnancy in a cystic fibrosis patient with a severe impairment of lung function receiving elexacaftor-tezacaftor-ivacaftor. *Respir Med Case Rep*. 2022;40:101776.27.
12. Chamagne M, Farabet C, Grenet D, Ayoubi JM. Comparison of two pregnancies with and without elexacaftor-tezacaftor-ivacaftor in a woman with cystic fibrosis. *Respir Med Res*. 2023;83:100953.
13. Nash EF, Middleton PG, Taylor-Cousar JL. Outcomes of pregnancy in women with cystic fibrosis (CF) taking CFTR modulators—an international survey. *J Cyst Fibros*. 2020;19:521-526.
14. Taylor-Cousar JL, Jain R. Maternal and fetal outcomes following elexacaftor-tezacaftor-ivacaftor use during pregnancy and lactation. *J Cyst Fibros*. 2021;20:402-406.
15. Szentpetery S, Foil K, Hendrix S, et al. A case report of CFTR modulator administration via carrier mother to treat meconium ileus in a F508del homozygous fetus. *J Cyst Fibros*. 2022;21:721-724.
16. Gómez-Montes E, Salcedo Lobato E, Galindo Izquierdo A, et al. Prenatal cystic fibrosis transmembrane conductance regulator modulator therapy: a promising way to change the impact of cystic fibrosis. *Fetal Diagn Ther*. 2023;50:136-142.
17. Ripani P, Mucci M, Pantano S, et al. Maternal, newborn and breast milk concentrations of elexacaftor/tezacaftor/ivacaftor in a F508del heterozygous woman with cystic fibrosis following successful pregnancy. *Front Med (Lausanne)*. 2023;10:1274303.
18. Jain R, Wolf A, Molad M, et al. Congenital bilateral cataracts in newborns exposed to elexacaftor-tezacaftor-ivacaftor in utero and while breast feeding. *J Cyst Fibros*. 2022;21:1074-1076.

IVERMECTIN

Anti-Infective (Anthelmintic—Avermectin)

PREGNANCY RECOMMENDATION: Limited Human Data—Animal Data Suggest Risk

BREASTFEEDING RECOMMENDATION: Potential Toxicity

PREGNANCY SUMMARY

Most ivermectin exposure during human pregnancy has occurred during mass drug administration campaigns, when a pregnant woman may be inadvertently exposed. No increased risk for congenital anomalies or adverse fetal effects has been attributed to ivermectin in more than 100 first-trimester exposures. Some amount of the drug may cross the placenta, so fetal exposure may occur. However, P-glycoprotein found in the placenta has been shown to prevent avermectins from penetrating the placenta. Therefore, fetal exposure may be negligible. However, this limited human pregnancy experience prevents a complete assessment of the embryofetal risk. Embryofetal toxicity with malformations was observed in three animal species at doses less than 10 times the RHD. Using this drug during pregnancy should be based on the pros and cons of the mother's clinical need for treatment versus any potential fetal risk that might occur from exposure.

BREASTFEEDING SUMMARY

Two reports evaluating the excretion of ivermectin into human breast milk have been located. Ivermectin was found in breast milk in low amounts after oral administration, but its effect on a nursing infant has not been reported. The amount of excretion into breast milk after topical administration should be much lower than oral administration. Avoid topical application to the areas where the infants' skin may come into direct contact. If the clinical decision is to use this drug while breastfeeding, the infant should be monitored for the most common reported adult side effects of itching (leading to irritability), rash, and fever.

References

1. Prescribing Information. Ivermectin. Edenbridge Pharmaceuticals LLC; 2023.
2. Lankas GR, Wise LD, Cartwright ME, et al. Placental P-glycoprotein deficiency enhances susceptibility to chemically induced birth defects in mice. *Reprod Toxicol.* 1998;12:457-463.
3. Brown KR. Changes in the use profile of Mectizan: 1987-1997. *Ann Trop Med Parasitol.* 1998;92(suppl 1):61-64.
4. Pacque M, Munoz B, Poetschke G, Foose J, Greene BM, Taylor HR. Pregnancy outcome after inadvertent ivermectin treatment during community-based distribution. *Lancet.* 1990;336:1486-1489.
5. Doumbo O, Soula G, Kodio B, Perrenoud M. Ivermectin and pregnancy in mass treatment in Mali. *Bull Soc Pathol Exot.* 1992;85:247-251.
6. Chippaux JP, Gardon-Wendel N, Gardon J, Ernould JC. Absence of any adverse effect of inadvertent ivermectin treatment during pregnancy. *Tran R Soc Trop Med Hyg.* 1993;87:318.
7. Gyapong J, Chinbuah M, Gyapong M. Inadvertent exposure of pregnant women to ivermectin and albendazole during mass drug administration for lymphatic filariasis. *Trop Med Int Health.* 2003;8:1093-1101.
8. Makene C, Malecela M, Kabali C, Charles E, Swai E, Lekashingo L. Inadvertent treatment of pregnant women in the Tanzanian mass drug administration program for the elimination of lymphatic filariasis. Paper presented at: *52nd Annual Meeting and Centennial Celebration—American Society of Tropical Medicine and Hygiene*; Philadelphia, USA; 2003.
9. Ndyomugyenyi R, Kabatereine N, Olsen A, Magnussen P. Efficacy of ivermectin and albendazole alone and in combination for treatment of soil-transmitted helminths in pregnancy and adverse events: a randomized open label controlled intervention trial in Masindi district, Western Uganda. *Am J Trop Med Hyg.* 2008;79:856-863.
10. Nicolas P, Maia MF, Bassat Q, et al. Safety of oral ivermectin during pregnancy: a systematic review and meta-analysis. *Lancet Glob Health.* 2020;8:e92-e100.
11. Ogbuokiri JE, Ozumba BC, Okonkwo PO. Ivermectin levels in human breastmilk. *Eur J Clin Pharmacol.* 1993;45:389-390.
12. Rodari P, Buonfrate D, Pomari E, et al. Ivermectin concentration in breastmilk of a woman with Strongyloides stercoralis and human T-lymphotropic virus-I co-infection. *Acta Trop.* 2020;202:105249.

IVOSIDENIB

Antineoplastic (Isocitrate Dehydrogenase Inhibitor)

PREGNANCY RECOMMENDATION: No Human Data—Animal Data Suggest Potential Risk

BREASTFEEDING RECOMMENDATION: Potential Toxicity

PREGNANCY SUMMARY

No reports describing the use of ivosidenib in human pregnancy have been located. Some amount of the drug may cross the placenta, so fetal exposure will likely occur. However, the absence of human pregnancy experience prevents a complete assessment of the embryofetal risk. Embryofetal toxicity without maternal toxicity was observed in one animal species at doses of less than 10 times the RHD. Using this drug during pregnancy should be based on the pros and cons of the mother's clinical need for treatment versus any potential fetal risk that might occur from exposure. Ivosidenib is associated with QT prolongation. Monitor QTc interval prior to and during ivosidenib treatment. There is a registry for women who are pregnant and have cancer. For more information, women and health care providers are encouraged to contact the Cancer and Pregnancy Registry at 1-877-635-4499.

BREASTFEEDING SUMMARY

No reports describing the use of ivosidenib during human lactation have been located. The drug may be excreted into breast milk, so some infant exposure will likely occur. However, due to a concern for potential serious adverse effects that might be seen in a breastfed infant, the manufacturer recommends that women not breastfeed while being treated with this drug and for at least 1 month after the last dose. Nevertheless, breastfeeding while using this drug should be based on the mother's clinical need for treatment versus any potential infant risks that might occur. If used, the infant should be monitored for the most common reported adult side effects of nausea and abdominal pain (both leading to irritability), fatigue (lethargy), diarrhea, cough, decreased appetite (monitor infant growth), vomiting, rash, and various laboratory abnormalities (see PI).

Reference

1. Prescribing Information. Tibsovo. Servier Pharmaceuticals LLC; 2023.

IXABEPILONE

Antineoplastic (Antimicrotubular)

PREGNANCY RECOMMENDATION: No Human Data—Animal Data Suggest Potential Risk

BREASTFEEDING RECOMMENDATION: Potential Toxicity

PREGNANCY SUMMARY

No reports describing the use of ixabepilone during human pregnancy have been located. The drug will probably cross the placenta, so some fetal exposure will likely occur. However, the absence of human pregnancy experience prevents a complete assessment of the embryofetal risk. Embryofetal toxicity was observed in two animal species at doses less than the RHD, but these doses also produced maternal toxicity. Based on these animal studies and the drug's mechanism of action, the manufacturer recommends that women with reproductive potential use effective contraception during treatment and for 7 months after the last dose. They also recommend that males with female partners of reproductive potential use effective contraception during treatment and for 4 months after the last dose. Nevertheless, using this drug during pregnancy should be based on the pros and cons of the mother's clinical need for treatment versus any potential fetal risk that might occur from exposure. There is a registry for women who are pregnant and have cancer. For more information, women and health care providers are encouraged to contact the Cancer and Pregnancy Registry at 1-877-635-4499.

BREASTFEEDING SUMMARY

No reports describing the use of ixabepilone during human lactation have been located. The drug will likely be excreted into breast milk, so some infant exposure will probably occur. Due to a concern for potential serious adverse effects that might be seen in a breastfed infant, the manufacturer recommends that women not breastfeed while being treated with this drug and for at least 2 weeks after the last dose. Nevertheless, breastfeeding while using this drug should be based on the mother's clinical need for treatment versus any potential infant risks that might occur. If used, the infant should be monitored for the most common reported adult side effects of nausea, neuropathy, myalgia, and arthralgia (all leading to irritability), fatigue (lethargy), alopecia, vomiting, diarrhea, and various laboratory abnormalities (see PI).

Reference

1. Prescribing Information. Ixempra. R-Pharm US Operating; 2023.

IXAZOMIB

Antineoplastic (Proteasome Inhibitor)

PREGNANCY RECOMMENDATION: *Contraindicated in the First Trimester—No Human Data and No Relevant Animal Data (Second and Third Trimesters)

BREASTFEEDING RECOMMENDATION: Potential Toxicity

PREGNANCY SUMMARY

No reports describing the use of ixazomib in human pregnancy have been located. The drug will probably cross the placenta, so some fetal exposure will likely occur. Therefore, the absence of human pregnancy experience prevents a complete assessment of the embryofetal risk. Embryofetal toxicity was observed in animal studies at doses that were also maternally toxic. Due to the findings from the animal studies and the drug's mechanism of action, the manufacturer recommends that women with reproductive potential use effective nonhormonal contraception during treatment and for at least 90 days after the last dose. They also recommend that males with female partners of reproductive potential use effective contraception during treatment and for at least 90 days after the last dose. *Additionally, ixazomib is administered in combination with lenalidomide (a thalidomide derivative), which can be a significant teratogen, and therefore is contraindicated, especially in the first trimester of pregnancy. There is a registry for women who are pregnant and have cancer. For more information, women and health care providers are encouraged to contact the Cancer and Pregnancy Registry at 1-877-635-4499.

BREASTFEEDING SUMMARY

No reports describing the use of ixazomib during human lactation have been located. The drug will probably be found in breast milk, so some infant exposure will likely occur. Due to the concern for potential serious adverse effects that might be seen in a breastfed infant, the manufacturer recommends that women not breastfeed while being treated with ixazomib and for at least 90 days after the last dose. Nevertheless, breastfeeding while using this drug should be based on the mother's clinical need for treatment. If used, the infant should be monitored for the most common reported adult side effects of nausea and peripheral neuropathy (both leading to irritability), vomiting, rash, diarrhea, peripheral edema, thrombocytopenia, and neutropenia.

Reference

1. Prescribing Information. Ninlaro. Takeda Pharmaceuticals America, Inc; 2022.

IXEKIZUMAB

Immunologic (Antipsoriatic—Monoclonal Antibody)

PREGNANCY RECOMMENDATION: Limited Human Data—Animal Data Suggest Low Risk

BREASTFEEDING RECOMMENDATION: Probably Compatible

PREGNANCY SUMMARY

Maternal exposure to ixekizumab during human pregnancy has been reported in clinical trials and postmarketing reports. Excluding those cases lost to follow-up, the spontaneous abortion rate in 70 pregnancies was 20% and 1 anomaly (2.6%) of 39 deliveries was identified. Seventeen pregnancies were terminated. The anomaly was an esophageal atresia with a tracheoesophageal fistula and hypospadias (genetics not reported). A retrospective comparative study of the EudraVigilance database identified 29 pregnant patients exposed (from 3 months before conception to term) to ixekizumab. However, the exact timing of the exposures was not noted. Of these 29 cases, 1 (3.4%) congenital malformation was reported that involved a neurologic genetic disorder. IgG antibodies are known to cross the placenta, especially during the third trimester, which suggests that some fetal exposure will probably occur. Therefore, this limited human pregnancy experience prevents a complete assessment of the embryofetal risk. Embryofetal toxicity was not observed in animal studies. Using this drug during pregnancy should be based on the pros and cons of the mother's clinical need for treatment versus any potential fetal risk that might occur from exposure. There is a pregnancy exposure registry that monitors pregnancy outcomes in women exposed to ixekizumab during pregnancy. Health care providers or patients are encouraged to contact the TALTZ Pregnancy Registry by calling 1-800-284-1695.

BREASTFEEDING SUMMARY

No reports describing the use of ixekizumab during human lactation have been located. It is known that IgG antibodies are excreted into breast milk but are not found in the neonatal or infant circulation. Additionally, if any IgG antibodies were to be ingested through breastfeeding, they would probably be digested in the infant's gastrointestinal tract and not be absorbed. If the clinical decision is to use this drug while breastfeeding, the infant should be monitored for the most common reported adult side effects of nausea (leading to irritability) and infections.

References

1. Prescribing Information. Talz. Eli Lilly and Company; 2022.
2. Egeberg A, Iversen L, Kimball AB, et al. Pregnancy outcomes in patients with psoriasis, psoriatic arthritis, or axial spondyloarthritis receiving ixekizumab. *Journal of Dermatological Treatment*. 2022;33:2503-2509.
3. Ghalandari N, Crijns HJMJ, Bergman JEH, et al. Reported congenital malformations after exposure to non-tumour necrosis factor inhibitor biologics: a retrospective comparative study in EudraVigilance. *Br J Clin Pharmacol*. 2022;88:5378-5388.

K

KETAMINE

Anesthetic (General)

PREGNANCY RECOMMENDATION: Limited Human Data—Animal Data Suggest Risk

BREASTFEEDING RECOMMENDATION: Probably Compatible

PREGNANCY SUMMARY

No reports describing the use of ketamine in the first trimester of human pregnancy have been located. The drug will probably cross the placenta, so some fetal exposure will likely occur. Therefore, the absence of human pregnancy experience prevents a complete assessment of the embryofetal risk. Numerous studies were located that report ketamine use as part of anesthesia for surgical delivery. In addition, several reports describe that the drug may have some oxytocic effects and can increase maternal blood pressure. It also may cause neonatal depression when used near delivery; however, this effect can be avoided with the use of lower maternal doses. Animal studies did show some embryofetal toxicity in two species at doses less than 10 times the recommended human dose (RHD). In a third species, no embryofetal toxicity was seen at doses less than 10 times the RHD. Using this drug during pregnancy should be based on the pros and cons of the mother's clinical need for treatment versus any potential fetal risk that might occur from exposure. Ketamine is a Schedule III controlled substance and has a risk potential for misuse and dependence. The drug is available on the street illicitly in tablet and powder form for use both orally and through snorting. Common street names for the drug are K, Special K, Vitamin K, and Super K.

BREASTFEEDING SUMMARY

Because ketamine is a general anesthetic agent, breastfeeding would not be possible during use of the drug. No reports have been located that have measured the amount of ketamine in breast milk. With the very short elimination half-life, the drug should be undetectable in the mother's plasma a few hours after treatment. Nursing after this time should not expose the infant to pharmacologically significant amounts of ketamine.

References

1. Friedman JM. Teratogen update: anesthetic agents. *Teratology*. 1988;37:69-77.
2. Prescribing Information. Ketamine. Civica; 2019.
3. Nishimura H, Tanimura T. *Clinical Aspects of the Teratogenicity of Drugs*. American Elsevier; 1976:178.
4. Schardein JL. *Chemically Induced Birth Defects*. 2nd ed. Marcel Dekker; 1993:148.
5. Onnis A, Grella P. *The Biochemical Effects of Drugs in Pregnancy*. Vol 1. Ellis Norwood; 1984:18-19.
6. El-Karum AHA, Benny R. Embryotoxic and teratogenic action of ketamine. *Ain Shams Med J*. 1976;27:459-463.
7. Nishijima M. Ketamine in obstetric anesthesia: special reference to placental transfer and its concentration in blood plasma. *Acta Obstet Gynaecol Jpn*. 1972;19:80-93. As cited in Anonymous. Operative obstetrics and anesthesia. *Obstet Gynecol Surv*. 1975;30:605-606.
8. Chodoff P, Stella JG. Use of CI-581 a phencyclidine derivative for obstetric anesthesia. *Anesth Analg*. 1966;45:527-530.
9. Bovill JG, Coppel DL, Dundee JW, Moore J. Current status of ketamine anaesthesia. *Lancet*. 1971;1:1285-1288.
10. Moore J, McNabb TG, Dundee JW. Preliminary report on ketamine in obstetrics. *Br J Anaesth*. 1971;43:779-782.
11. Little B, Chang T, Chucot L, et al. Study of ketamine as an obstetric anesthetic agent. *Am J Obstet Gynecol*. 1972;113:247-260.
12. McDonald JS, Mateo CV, Reed EC. Modified nitrous oxide or ketamine hydrochloride for cesarean section. *Anesth Analg*. 1972;51:975-983.
13. Peltz B, Sinclair DM. Induction agents for caesarean section. A comparison of thiopentone and ketamine. *Anaesthesia*. 1973;28:37-42.
14. Meer FM, Downing JW, Coleman AJ. An intravenous method of anaesthesia for caesarean section. Part II: ketamine. *Br J Anaesth*. 1973;45:191-196.
15. Galbert MW, Gardner AE. Ketamine for obstetrical anesthesia. *Anesth Analg*. 1973;52:926-930.
16. Corssen G. Ketamine in obstetric anesthesia. *Clin Obstet Gynecol*. 1974;17:249-258.
17. Janeczko GF, El-Etr AA, Younes S. Low-dose ketamine anesthesia for obstetrical delivery. *Anesth Analg*. 1974;53:828-831.
18. Akamatsu TJ, Bonica JJ, Rehmet R, et al. Experiences with the use of ketamine for parturition. I. Primary anesthetic for vaginal delivery. *Anesth Analg*. 1974;53:284-287.
19. Krantz ML. Ketamine in obstetrics: comparison with methoxyflurane. *Anesth Analg*. 1974;53:890-893.
20. Downing JW, Mahomedy MC, Jeal DE, Allen PJ. Anaesthesia for caesarean section with ketamine. *Anaesthesia*. 1976;31:883-892.
21. Galloon S. Ketamine for obstetric delivery. *Anesthesiology*. 1976;44:522-524.
22. Ellingson A, Haram K, Sagen N. Ketamine and diazepam as anaesthesia for forceps delivery. A comparative study. *Acta Anaesth Scand*. 1977;21:37-40.
23. Maduska AL, Hajghassemali M. Arterial blood gases in mothers and infants during ketamine anesthesia for vaginal delivery. *Anesth Analg*. 1978;57:121-123.
24. Dich-Nielsen J, Holasek J. Ketamine as induction agent for caesarean section. *Acta Anaesth Scand*. 1982;26:139-142.
25. White PF, Way WL, Trevor AJ. Ketamine—its pharmacology and therapeutic uses. *Anesthesiology*. 1982;56:119-136.
26. Hill CR, Schultetus RR, Dharamraj CM, et al. Wakefulness during cesarean section with thiopental, ketamine, or thiopental-ketamine combination (abstract). *Anesthesiology*. 1993;59:A419.
27. Schultetus RR, Paulus DA, Spohr GL. Haemodynamic effects of ketamine and thiopentone during anaesthetic induction for caesarean section. *Can Anaesth Soc J*. 1985;32:592-596.
28. Bernstein K, Gisselsson L, Jacobsson L, Ohrlander S. Influence of two different anaesthetic agents on the newborn and the correlation between foetal

oxygenation and induction-delivery time in elective caesarean section. *Acta Anaesthesiol Scand*. 1985;29:157-160.
29. Schultetus RR, Hill CR, Dharamraj CM, et al. Wakefulness during cesarean section after anesthetic induction with ketamine, thiopental, or ketamine and thiopental combined. *Anesth Analg*. 1986;65:723-728.
30. Reich DL, Silvay G. Ketamine: an update on the first twenty-five years of clinical experience. *Can J Anaesth*. 1989;36:186-197.
31. Baraka A, Louis F, Dalleh R. Maternal awareness and neonatal outcome after ketamine induction of anaesthesia for caesarean section. *Can J Anaesth*. 1990;37:641-644.
32. Rowbottom SJ, Gin T, Cheung LP. General anaesthesia for caesarean section in a patient with uncorrected complex cyanotic heart disease. *Anaesth Intensive Care*. 1994;22:74-78.
33. Krissel J, Dick WF, Leyser KH, et al. Thiopentone, thiopentone/ketamine, and ketamine for induction of anaesthesia in caesarean section. *Eur J Anaesthesiol*. 1994;11:115-122.
34. Conway JB, Posner M. Anaesthesia for caesarean section in a patient with Watson's syndrome. *Can J Anaesth*. 1994;41:1113-1116.
35. Maleck W. Ketamine and thiopentone in caesarean section. *Eur J Anaesthesiol*. 1995;12:533.
36. Marx GF, Hwang HS, Chandra P. Postpartum uterine pressures with different doses of ketamine. *Anesthesiology*. 1979;50:163-166.
37. Marx GF, Cabe CM, Kim YI, Eidelman AI. Neonatal blood pressures. *Anaesthesist*. 1976;25:318-322.
38. Oats JN, Vasey DP, Waldron BA. Effects of ketamine on the pregnant uterus. *Br J Anaesth*. 1979;51:1163-1166.
39. Galloon S. Ketamine and the pregnant uterus. *Can Anaesth Soc J*. 1973;20:141-145.
40. Hodgkinson R, Marx GF, Kim SS, Miclat NM. Neonatal neurobehavioral tests following vaginal delivery under ketamine, thiopental, and extradural anesthesia. *Anesth Analg*. 1977;56:548-553.
41. Hodgkinson R, Bhatt M, Kim SS, et al. Neonatal neurobehavioral tests following cesarean section under general and spinal anesthesia. *Am J Obstet Gynecol*. 1978;132:670-674.

KETOCONAZOLE

Anti-infective (Antifungal)

PREGNANCY RECOMMENDATION: Limited Human Data—No Relevant Animal Data

BREASTFEEDING RECOMMENDATION: Probably Compatible

PREGNANCY SUMMARY

In a surveillance study of Michigan Medicaid recipients, 20 newborns had been exposed to ketoconazole during the first trimester and no fetal anomalies were found. On the other hand, a case report described a normal karyotypic newborn with multiple fetal anomalies and hydrops. Ketoconazole was used in the first 7 weeks of gestation. Because the drug can impair cortisol synthesis, it has been used in treating Cushing syndrome. A few case reports described the use of the drug in the second half of pregnancy to aid in the treatment of Cushing syndrome. No reported complications related to the drug or newborn effects were noted. Some of the drug may likely cross the placenta, so some fetal exposure will probably occur. Therefore, this limited human pregnancy experience prevents a complete assessment of the embryofetal risk. Animal studies did show some embryofetal toxicity with malformations in one species at doses of 10 times the RHD, but this dose also caused maternal toxicity. Using this drug during pregnancy should be based on the pros and cons of the mother's clinical need for treatment versus any potential fetal risk that might occur from exposure. The drug can also prolong the QT interval.

BREASTFEEDING SUMMARY

Ketoconazole was found in breast milk in a single patient using 200 mg/d for 10 days. The maximum breast milk concentration was 220 ng/mL. The weight-adjusted overall relative infant dose (RID) was 0.4% with a maximum RID of about 1.4%. The manufacturer recommends that the drug not be used while breastfeeding. Nevertheless, breastfeeding while using this drug should be based on the mother's clinical need for treatment versus any potential infant risks that might occur. If used, the infant should be monitored for the most commonly reported adult side effects of nausea, headache, dizziness, and abdominal pain (all leading to irritability), diarrhea, vomiting, rash, and insomnia.

References

1. Prescribing Information. Ketoconazole tablet. Mylan Pharmaceuticals; 2018.
2. Prescribing Information. Ketoconazole cream. Northstar RX; 2019.
3. Lind J. Limb malformations in a case of hydrops fetalis with ketoconazole use during pregnancy (abstract). *Arch Gynecol*. 1985;237(suppl):398.
4. Minkoff HL. Care of pregnant women infected with human immunodeficiency virus. *JAMA*. 1987;258:2714-2717.
5. Hobbs ER. Coccidioidomycosis. *Dermatol Clin*. 1989;7:227-239.
6. Pont A, Williams PL, Loose DS, et al. Ketoconazole blocks adrenal steroid synthesis. *Ann Intern Med*. 1982;97:370-372.
7. Engelhardt D, Mann K, Hormann R, et al. Ketoconazole inhibits cortisol secretion of an adrenal adenoma in vivo and in vitro. *Klin Wochenschr*. 1983;61:373-375.
8. Divers MJ. Ketoconazole treatment of Cushing's syndrome in pregnancy. *Am J Obstet Gynecol*. 1990;163:1101.
9. Aron DC, Schnall AM, Sheeler LR. Cushing's syndrome and pregnancy. *Am J Obstet Gynecol*. 1990;162:244-252.
10. Amado JA, Pesquera C, Gonzalez EM, et al. Successful treatment with ketoconazole of Cushing's syndrome in pregnancy. *Postgrad Med J*. 1990;66:221-223.
11. Lim WH, Torpy DJ, Jeffries WS. The medical management of Cushing's syndrome during pregnancy. *Eur J Obstet Gynecol Reprod Biol*. 2013;168:1-6.
12. Costenaro F, Rodrigues TC, de Lima PB, et al. A successful case of Cushing's disease pregnancy treated with ketoconazole. *Gynecol Endocrinol*. 2015;31:176-178.
13. Zieleniewski W, Michalak R. A successful case of pregnancy in a woman with ACTH-independent Cushing's syndrome treated with ketoconazole and metyrapone. *Gynecol Endocrinol*. 2017;33:349-352.
14. Patel VM, Schwartz RA, Lambert WC. Topical antiviral and antifungal medications in pregnancy: a review of safety profiles. *J Eur Acad Dermatol Venereol*. 2017;31:1440-1446.
15. Moretti ME, Ito S, Koren G. Disposition of maternal ketoconazole in breast milk. *Am J Obstet Gynecol*. 1995;173:1625-1628.
16. American Academy of Pediatrics Committee on Drugs. The transfer of drugs and other chemicals into human milk. *Pediatrics*. 2001;108:776-789.

KETOCONAZOLE TOPICAL

Dermatologic (Topical Antifungal)

PREGNANCY RECOMMENDATION: No Human Data and No Relevant Animal Data

BREASTFEEDING RECOMMENDATION: Probably Compatible

PREGNANCY SUMMARY

No reports describing the use of ketoconazole topical in human pregnancy have been located. If any drug were to cross the placenta, the overall amount would be clinically insignificant. However, the absence of human pregnancy experience prevents a complete assessment of the embryofetal risk. In a surveillance study of Michigan Medicaid recipients, 20 newborns had been exposed to oral ketoconazole during the first trimester, and no fetal anomalies were found. Animal studies did show some embryofetal toxicity with malformations in one species at oral doses of 10 times the RHD, but this dose also caused maternal toxicity. Using this drug during pregnancy should be based on the pros and cons of the mother's clinical need for treatment versus any potential fetal risk that might occur from exposure.

BREASTFEEDING SUMMARY

Oral ketoconazole was found in breast milk in a single patient using 200 mg/d for 10 days. The maximum breast milk concentration was 220 ng/mL. The weight-adjusted overall RID was 0.4% with a maximum RID of about 1.4%. However, the lack of systemic absorption with other pK parameters suggests that if any drug were to be present, it would be clinically insignificant. Breastfeeding while using this drug should be based on the mother's clinical need for treatment versus any potential infant risks that might occur. Due to the lack of any measurable systemic absorption, clinical side effects were not evaluated.

K

Reference

1. Prescribing Information. Ketoconazole cream. Northstar RX; 2020.

KETOPROFEN

Pain (NSAID)

PREGNANCY RECOMMENDATION: Human Data Suggest Risk in the Third Trimester

BREASTFEEDING RECOMMENDATION: Probably Compatible

PREGNANCY SUMMARY

In a surveillance study of Michigan Medicaid recipients, 112 newborns had been exposed to ketoprofen during the first trimester, and only 3 (2.7%) were found to have major anomalies (5 expected). In a second study involving the Danish birth registry, 46 (4.2%) total congenital anomalies were seen in 1,106 pregnancies with probable nonsteroidal anti-inflammatory drug (NSAID) usage compared with 564 (3.3%) anomalies in 17,259 control pregnancies. This rate was not significantly different. Specific data on the type of NSAID were not provided. This study also did not show any increased risks for low birth weight or preterm delivery. There was a higher risk for spontaneous abortion, but the reported rates were only 1.4% in the NSAID group and 1.1% in the control group. The drug appears to cross the placenta, so some fetal exposure will occur. Animal studies did not show any embryofetal toxicity or teratogenicity in two species at doses of less than 10 times the RHD. However, NSAIDs can cause premature stricture or closure of the fetal ductus arteriosus when used in late gestation. In some instances, this can produce pulmonary hypertension in the neonate. These drugs have also been reported to produce fetal renal dysfunction leading to oligohydramnios when used after 20 weeks' gestation (see Indomethacin). Therefore, if possible, use between 20 and 30 weeks' gestation should be limited, and, if possible, no usage after 30 weeks' gestation. If used more than a few days continuously after 20 weeks' gestation, an ultrasound to evaluate amniotic fluid volume is suggested. The manufacturer states that the drug is contraindicated for use in labor and delivery.

BREASTFEEDING SUMMARY

No reports describing the use of ketoprofen while actively breastfeeding have been located. However, one study did evaluate breast milk for the presence of ketoprofen in 18 postpartum women. The mean and maximum ketoprofen milk concentrations were 57 and 91 ng/mL, respectively. The calculated maximum RID was 0.5%. The ketoprofen levels measured in this study are low, consistent with the very high plasma protein binding. The manufacturer recommends that the drug not be used while breastfeeding. Nevertheless, breastfeeding while using this drug should be based on the mother's clinical need for treatment versus any potential infant risks that might occur. If used, the infant should be monitored for the most commonly reported adult side effects of nausea, headache, and abdominal pain (all leading to irritability), diarrhea, vomiting, and rash.

References

1. Levin DL. Effects of inhibition of prostaglandin synthesis on fetal development, oxygenation, and the fetal circulation. *Semin Perinatol*. 1980;4:35-44.
2. Van Marter LJ, Leviton A, Allred EN, et al. Persistent pulmonary hypertension of the newborn and smoking and aspirin and nonsteroidal antiinflammatory drug consumption during pregnancy. *Pediatrics*. 1996;97:658-663.
3. Fuchs F. Prevention of prematurity. *Am J Obstet Gynecol*. 1976;126:809-820.
4. Powell JG, Cochrane RL. The effects of a number of non-steroidal anti-inflammatory compounds on parturition in the rat. *Prostaglandins*. 1982;23:469-488.
5. Matt DW, Borzelleca JF. Toxic effects on the female reproductive system during pregnancy, parturition, and lactation. In: Witorsch RJ, ed. *Reproductive Toxicology*. 2nd ed. Raven Press; 1995:175-193.
6. Dawood MY. Nonsteroidal antiinflammatory drugs and reproduction. *Am J Obstet Gynecol*. 1993;169:1255-1265.
7. Prescribing Information. Ketoprofen. Mylan Pharmaceuticals; 2018.
8. Shepard TH. *Catalog of Teratogenic Agents*. 6th ed. The Johns Hopkins University Press; 1989:364.
9. Lagrange F, Pehourcq F, Bannwarth B, et al. Passage of S-(+)- and R-(−)-ketoprofen across the human isolated perfused placenta. *Fundam Clin Pharmacol*. 1998;12:286-291.
10. Labat L, Llanas B, Demotes-Mainard F, et al. Accumulation of S-ketoprofen in neonates after maternal administration of the racemate. *Fundam Clin Pharmacol*. 1995;9:62. As cited in Lagrange F, Pehourcq F, Bannwarth B, et al. Passage of S-(+)- and R-(−)-ketoprofen across the human isolated perfused placenta. *Fundam Clin Pharmacol*. 1998;12:286-291.
11. Nielsen GL, Sorensen HT, Larsen H, Pedersen L. Risk of adverse birth outcome and miscarriage in pregnant users of non-steroidal anti-inflammatory drugs: population based observational study and case-control study. *Br Med J*. 2001;322:266-270.
12. Ericson A, Kallen BAJ. Nonsteroidal anti-inflammatory drugs in early pregnancy. *Reprod Toxicol*. 2001;15:371-375.
13. Li DK, Liu L, Odouli R. Exposure to non-steroidal anti-inflammatory drugs during pregnancy and risk of miscarriage: population based cohort study. *Br Med J*. 2003;327:368-371.
14. Tassinari MS, Cook JC, Hurtt ME. NSAIDs and developmental toxicity. *Birth Defects Res B Dev Reprod Toxicol*. 2003;68:3-4.
15. Grignaffini A, Soncini E, Ronzoni E, et al. Clinical practice evaluation of combination of atosiban, ritodrine and ketoprofen for inhibiting preterm labor. *Minerva Ginecol*. 2007;59:481-489.
16. Jacqz-Aigrain E, Serreau R, Boissinot C, et al. Excretion of ketoprofen and nalbuphine in human milk during treatment of maternal pain after delivery. *Ther Drug Monit*. 2007;29:815-818.
17. Soussan C, Gouraud A, Portolan G, et al. Drug-induced adverse reaction via breastfeeding: a descriptive study in the French Pharmacovigilance Database. *Eur J Clin Pharmacol*. 2014;70:1361-1366.

K

KETOROLAC

Pain (NSAID)

PREGNANCY RECOMMENDATION: Human Data Suggest Risk in the Third Trimester

BREASTFEEDING RECOMMENDATION: Probably Compatible

PREGNANCY SUMMARY

No specific study evaluating first trimester use of ketorolac for the risk of increasing congenital anomalies has been located. In a study involving the Danish birth registry, 46 (4.2%) total congenital anomalies were seen in 1,106 pregnancies with probable NSAID usage compared with 564 (3.3%) anomalies in 17,259 control pregnancies. This rate was not significantly different. Specific data on the type of NSAID were not provided. This study also did not show any increased risks for low birth weight or preterm delivery. There was a higher risk for spontaneous abortion but the reported rates were only 1.4% in the NSAID group and 1.1% in the control group. The drug will probably cross the placenta, so some fetal exposure will likely occur. Animal studies did not show any embryofetal toxicity or teratogenicity in two species at doses of less than 10 times the RHD. However, NSAIDs can cause premature stricture or closure of the fetal ductus arteriosus when used in late gestation. In some instances, this can produce pulmonary hypertension in the neonate. These drugs have also been reported to produce fetal renal dysfunction leading to oligohydramnios when used after 20 weeks' gestation (see Indomethacin). Therefore, if possible, use between 20 and 30 weeks' gestation should be limited, and, if possible, no usage after 30 weeks' gestation. If used more than a few days continuously after 20 weeks' gestation, an ultrasound to evaluate amniotic fluid volume is suggested. The manufacturer states that the drug is contraindicated for use in labor and delivery.

BREASTFEEDING SUMMARY

Ketorolac was found to be excreted into breast milk. Ten postpartum women were given oral ketorolac, and in four cases, breast milk concentrations were not detected (lower limit of detection 5 ng/mL). In the remaining six women, the levels ranged from 5.2 to 7.9 ng/mL (RID overall of less than 0.2%). Breastfeeding while using this drug should be based on the mother's clinical need for treatment versus any potential infant risks that might occur. If used, the infant should be monitored for the most commonly reported adult side effects of nausea, headache, and abdominal pain (all leading to irritability), diarrhea, hypertension, and rash.

References

1. Levin DL. Effects of inhibition of prostaglandin synthesis on fetal development, oxygenation, and the fetal circulation. *Semin Perinatol*. 1980;4:35-44.
2. Van Marter LJ, Leviton A, Allred EN, et al. Persistent pulmonary hypertension of the newborn and smoking and aspirin and nonsteroidal antiinflammatory drug consumption during pregnancy. *Pediatrics*. 1996;97:658-663.
3. Matt DW, Borzelleca JF. Toxic effects on the female reproductive system during pregnancy, parturition, and lactation. In: Witorsch RJ, ed. *Reproductive Toxicology*. 2nd ed. Raven Press; 1995:175-193.
4. Dawood MY. Nonsteroidal antiinflammatory drugs and reproduction. *Am J Obstet Gynecol*. 1993;169:1255-1265.
5. Prescribing Information. Ketorolac Tromethamine. West-Ward Pharmaceuticals; 2018.
6. Rauk PN, Laifer SA. Ketorolac blocks ritodrine-stimulated production of $PGF_{2\alpha}$ in pregnant sheep (abstract). *Am J Obstet Gynecol*. 1992;166:274.

7. Rauk PN, Laifer SA. The prostaglandin synthesis inhibitor ketorolac blocks ritodrine-stimulated production of prostaglandin $F_{2\alpha}$ in pregnant sheep. *Obstet Gynecol*. 1993;81:323-326.
8. Nielsen GL, Sorensen HT, Larsen H, Pedersen L. Risk of adverse birth outcome and miscarriage in pregnant users of non-steroidal anti-inflammatory drugs: population based observational study and case-control study. *Br Med J*. 2001;322:266-270.
9. Ericson A, Kallen BAJ. Nonsteroidal anti-inflammatory drugs in early pregnancy. *Reprod Toxicol*. 2001;15:371-375.
10. Li DK, Liu L, Odouli R. Exposure to non-steroidal anti-inflammatory drugs during pregnancy and risk of miscarriage: population based cohort study. *Br Med J*. 2003;327:368-371.
11. Tassinari MS, Cook JC, Hurtt ME. NSAIDs and developmental toxicity. *Birth Defects Res B Dev Reprod Toxicol*. 2003;68:3-4.
12. Walker JJ, Johnston J, Fairlie FM, et al. A comparative study of intramuscular ketorolac and pethidine in labour pain. *Eur J Obstet Gynecol Reprod Biol*. 1992;46:87-94.
13. Schorr SJ, Ascarelli MH, Rust OA, et al. Ketorolac is a safe and effective drug for acute tocolysis (abstract). *Am J Obstet Gynecol*. 1997;176:S7.
14. Schorr SJ, Ascarelli MH, Rust OA, et al. A comparative study of ketorolac (Toradol) and magnesium sulfate for arrest of preterm labor. *South Med J*. 1998;91:1028-1032.
15. Wischnik A, Manth SM, Lloyd J, et al. The excretion of ketorolac tromethamine into breast milk after multiple oral dosing. *Eur J Clin Pharmacol*. 1989;36:521-524.

KETOROLAC OPHTHALMIC

Ophthalmic (Topical NSAID)

PREGNANCY RECOMMENDATION: No Human Data—Animal Data Suggest Low Risk

BREASTFEEDING RECOMMENDATION: Probably Compatible

PREGNANCY SUMMARY

No reports describing the use of ketorolac ophthalmic in human pregnancy have been located. The drug may cross the placenta, but the amount is likely negligible and thus clinically insignificant. However, the absence of human pregnancy experience prevents a complete assessment of the embryofetal risk. Animal studies did not show any embryofetal toxicity or teratogenicity in two species at doses of more than 10 times the RHD. Based on the prostaglandin-inhibiting effect of NSAIDs and the potential for premature closure of the ductus arteriosus, the manufacturer recommends that the drug not be used in late pregnancy. Nevertheless, using this drug during pregnancy should be based on the pros and cons of the mother's clinical need for treatment versus any potential fetal risk that might occur from exposure. If used during pregnancy, consider placing pressure over the tear duct in the corner of the eye for at least 1 minute, and then remove any excess solution with absorbent tissue to decrease the amount of drug reaching the systemic circulation even further.

K

BREASTFEEDING SUMMARY

No reports describing the use of ketorolac ophthalmic during human lactation have been located. The drug may be found in breast milk, but the overall amount is likely to be clinically insignificant. One study did evaluate oral ketorolac levels in breast milk (lower limit of detection of 5 ng/mL) with dosing of 10 mg 4 times per day in 10 women. The drug was not detected in four patients, and in the remaining six, the levels ranged from 5.2 to 7.9 ng/mL (RID of less than 0.2%). Breastfeeding while using this drug should be based on the mother's clinical need for treatment versus any potential infant risks that might occur. Due to the minimal systemic absorption with topical ocular use, systemic side effects were not evaluated. A method to further decrease some systemic absorption with ophthalmic use is described in the Pregnancy Summary.

References

1. Prescribing Information. Ketorolac Tromethamine. Micro Labs; 2019.
2. Wischnik A, Manth SM, Lloyd J, et al. The excretion of ketorolac tromethamine into breast milk after multiple oral dosing. *Eur J Clin Pharmacol*. 1989;36:521-524.

KETOTIFEN

Antihistamine (H1 Receptor Antagonist/Mast Cell Stabilizer)

PREGNANCY RECOMMENDATION: Limited Human Data—Animal Data Suggest Low Risk

BREASTFEEDING RECOMMENDATION: Probably Compatible

PREGNANCY SUMMARY

One study did report the outcome of 40 human pregnancies exposed to oral ketotifen during pregnancy. Seven of these had exposure in the first trimester and continued it throughout the pregnancy. No fetal anomalies were identified. The drug will probably cross the placenta, so fetal exposure will likely occur. However, this limited human pregnancy experience prevents a complete assessment of the embryofetal risk. Animal studies did not show any embryofetal toxicity or teratogenicity in two species at doses of more than 10 times the RHD. Using this drug during pregnancy should be based on the pros and cons of the mother's clinical need for treatment versus any potential fetal risk that might occur from exposure.

BREASTFEEDING SUMMARY

No reports describing the use of ketotifen during human lactation have been located. The drug will probably be found in breast milk, so some infant exposure will likely occur. Breastfeeding while using this drug should be based on the mother's clinical need for treatment versus any potential infant risks that might occur. If used, the infant should be monitored for the most commonly reported adult side effects of rash, fatigue (lethargy), and somnolence.

References

1. Prescribing Information. Zaditen. Teve Canada Limited; 2020.
2. Maclay WP, Crowder D, Spiro S, Turner P. Postmarketing surveillance: practical experience with ketotifen. *BMJ*. 1984;288:911-914.

KETOTIFEN OPHTHALMIC AND DRUG-ELUTING CONTACT LENSES

Antihistamine (Topical H1 Receptor Antagonist/Mast Cell Stabilizer)

PREGNANCY RECOMMENDATION: No Human Data—Animal Data Suggest Low Risk

BREASTFEEDING RECOMMENDATION: Probably Compatible

PREGNANCY SUMMARY

No reports describing the use of ketotifen ophthalmic in human pregnancy have been located. One study did report the outcome of 40 human pregnancies exposed to oral ketotifen during pregnancy. Seven of these had exposure in the first trimester and continued it throughout the pregnancy. No fetal anomalies were identified. The drug may cross the placenta, but the amount is likely negligible and thus clinically insignificant. However, this limited human pregnancy experience prevents a complete assessment of the embryofetal risk. Animal studies did not show any embryofetal toxicity or teratogenicity in two species at doses of more than 10 times the RHD. Using this drug during pregnancy should be based on the pros and cons of the mother's clinical need for treatment versus any potential fetal risk that might occur from exposure. If used during pregnancy, consider placing pressure over the tear duct in the corner of the eye for at least 1 minute, and then remove any excess solution with absorbent tissue to decrease the amount of drug reaching the systemic circulation even further. The drug-eluting contact lenses contain a slightly lower amount of ketotifen when compared with the amount of drug applied to an individual eye with the ophthalmic drops. The manufacturer states that the drug is not absorbed systemically with use of the lenses (or is at least below the level of detection in the low picogram range). Therefore, overall findings would be consistent with the ocular drops.

BREASTFEEDING SUMMARY

No reports describing the use of ketotifen ophthalmic during human lactation have been located. The drug may be found in breast milk, but the overall amount is likely to be clinically insignificant. Breastfeeding while using this drug should be based on the mother's clinical need for treatment versus any potential infant risks that might occur. Due to the negligible systemic absorption with topical ocular use, systemic side effects were not evaluated. A method to further decrease some systemic absorption with ophthalmic use is described in the Pregnancy Summary. The drug-eluting contact lenses contain a slightly lower amount of ketotifen when compared with the amount of drug applied to an individual eye with the ophthalmic drops. The manufacturer states that the drug is not absorbed systemically with use of the lenses (or is at least below the level of detection in the low picogram range). Therefore, overall findings would be consistent with the ocular drops.

References

1. Prescribing Information. Ketotifen Ophthalmic. Alaway; 2020.
2. Prescribing Information. Acuvue Theravision. Johnson & Johnson Vision Care Inc; 2022.
3. Maclay WP, Crowder D, Spiro S, Turner P. Postmarketing surveillance: practical experience with ketotifen. *BMJ*. 1984;288:911-914.

L

LABETALOL

Antihypertensive (β-Blocker With α-Blocking Activity)

PREGNANCY RECOMMENDATION: Human Data Suggest Low Risk

BREASTFEEDING RECOMMENDATION: Probably Compatible

PREGNANCY SUMMARY

The use of labetalol in human pregnancy is well established. Available studies have found no significant evidence of an increased risk of congenital anomalies or adverse effects. The drug crosses the placenta, so fetal exposure occurs. The American College of Obstetricians and Gynecologists (ACOG) considers oral labetalol as one of the preferred agents for the maintenance treatment of hypertension during pregnancy. Intravenous (IV) labetalol is also recommended for treating severe hypertension in pregnancy. However, labetalol should be used with caution in women with asthma, preexisting myocardial disease, decompensated cardiac function, heart block, and bradycardia.

BREASTFEEDING SUMMARY

Limited reports describing the effects of labetalol during human lactation have been located. No adverse effects in breastfed infants have been reported. Labetalol is excreted into human breast milk in low amounts, so some infant exposure will occur. ACOG considers labetalol as one of the preferred treatments for hypertension during lactation. If used while breastfeeding, the infant should be monitored for bradycardia, hypotension, and the most common reported adult side effects of nausea and dizziness (both leading to irritability) and lethargy.

References

1. Michael CA. Use of labetalol in the treatment of severe hypertension during pregnancy. *Br J Clin Pharmacol*. 1979;8(suppl 2):211S-215S.
2. Riley AJ. Clinical pharmacology of labetalol in pregnancy. *J Cardiovasc Pharmacol*. 1981;3(suppl 1):S53-S59.
3. Andrejak M, Coevoet B, Fievet P, et al. Effect of labetalol on hypertension and the renin-angiotensin-aldosterone and adrenergic systems in pregnancy. In: Riley A, Symonds EM, eds. *The Investigation of Labetalol in the Management of Hypertension in Pregnancy*. Excerpta Medica; 1982:77-87.
4. Lunell NO, Hjemdahl P, Fredholm B, et al. Acute effects of labetalol on maternal metabolism and uteroplacental circulation in hypertension of pregnancy. In: Riley A, Symonds EM, eds. *The Investigation of Labetalol in the Management of Hypertension in Pregnancy*. Excerpta Medica; 1982:34-45.
5. Nylund L, Lunell NO, Lewander R, et al. Labetalol for the treatment of hypertension in pregnancy. *Acta Obstet Gynecol Scand*. 1984;118(suppl):71-73.
6. Lunell NO, Kulas J, Rane A. Transfer of labetalol into amniotic fluid and breast milk in lactating women. *Eur J Clin Pharmacol*. 1985;28:597-599.
7. Rubin PC. Drugs in pregnancy. In: Riley A, Symonds EM, eds. *The Investigation of Labetalol in the Management of Hypertension in Pregnancy*. Excerpta Medica; 1982:28-33.
8. Rubin PC, Butters L, Kelman AW, et al. Labetalol disposition and concentration-effect relationships during pregnancy. *Br J Clin Pharmacol*. 1983; 15:465-470.
9. Lamming GD, Broughton Pipkin F, Symonds EM. Comparison of the alpha and beta blocking drug, labetalol, and methyl dopa in the treatment of moderate and severe pregnancy-induced hypertension. *Clin Exp Hypertens*. 1980;2:865-895.
10. Lotgering FK, Derkx FMH, Wallenburg HCS. Primary hyperaldosteronism in pregnancy. *Am J Obstet Gynecol*. 1986;155:986-988.
11. Mabie WC, Gonzalez AR, Sibai BM, Amon E. A comparative trial of labetalol and hydralazine in the acute management of severe hypertension complicating pregnancy. *Obstet Gynecol*. 1987;70:328-333.
12. Plouin PF, Breart G, Maillard F, et al. Comparison of antihypertensive efficacy and perinatal safety of labetalol and methyldopa in the treatment of hypertension in pregnancy: a randomized controlled trial. *Br J Obstet Gynaecol*. 1988;95:868-876.
13. Pickles CJ, Symonds EM, Broughton Pipkin F. The fetal outcome in a randomized trial of labetalol versus placebo in pregnancy-induced hypertension. *Br J Obstet Gynaecol*. 1989;96:38-43.
14. Lardoux H, Gerard J, Blazquez G, et al. Hypertension in pregnancy: evaluation of two beta blockers atenolol and labetalol. *Eur Heart J*. 1983;4(suppl G):35-40.
15. Sibai BM, Gonzalez AR, Mabie WC, Moretti M. A comparison of labetalol plus hospitalization versus hospitalization alone in the management of preeclampsia remote from term. *Obstet Gynecol*. 1987;70:323-327.
16. Michael CA, Potter JM. A comparison of labetalol with other antihypertensive drugs in the treatment of hypertensive disease of pregnancy. In: Riley A, Symonds EM, eds. *The Investigation of Labetalol in the Management of Hypertension in Pregnancy*. Excerpta Medica; 1982:111-122.
17. Davey DA, Dommisse J, Garden A. Intravenous labetalol and intravenous dihydralazine in severe hypertension in pregnancy. In: Riley A, Symonds EM, eds. *The Investigation of Labetalol in the Management of Hypertension in Pregnancy*. Excerpta Medica; 1982:52-61.
18. MacPherson M, Broughton Pipkin F, Rutter N. The effect of maternal labetalol on the newborn infant. *Br J Obstet Gynaecol*. 1986;93:539-542.
19. Redman CWG. A controlled trial of the treatment of hypertension in pregnancy: labetalol compared with methyldopa. In: Riley A, Symonds EM, eds. *The Investigation of Labetalol in the Management of Hypertension in Pregnancy*. Excerpta Medica; 1982:101-110.
20. Walker JJ, Crooks A, Erwin L, Calder AA. Labetalol in pregnancy-induced hypertension: fetal and maternal effects. In: Riley A, Symonds EM, eds. *The Investigation of Labetalol in the Management of Hypertension of Pregnancy*. Excerpta Medica; 1982:148-160.
21. Thulesius O, Lunell NO, Ibrahim M, et al. The effect of labetalol on contractility of human myometrial preparations. *Acta Obstet Gynecol*. 1987;66: 237-240.
22. Lamming GD, Symonds EM. Use of labetalol and methyldopa in pregnancy-induced hypertension. *Br J Clin Pharmacol*. 1979;8(suppl 2): 217S-222S.
23. Jorge CS, Fernandes L, Cunha S. Labetalol in the hypertensive states of pregnancy. In: Riley A, Symonds EM, eds. *The Investigation of Labetalol in*

the Management of Hypertension of Pregnancy. Excerpta Medica; 1982: 124-130.
24. Lunell NO, Nylund L, Lewander R, Sarby B. Acute effect of an antihypertensive drug, labetalol, on uteroplacental blood flow. *Br J Obstet Gynaecol.* 1982;89:640-644.
25. Jouppila P, Kirkinen P, Koivula A, Ylikorkala O. Labetalol does not alter the placental and fetal blood flow or maternal prostanoids in pre-eclampsia. *Br J Obstet Gynaecol.* 1986;93:543-547.
26. Michael CA. The evaluation of labetalol in the treatment of hypertension complicating pregnancy. *Br J Clin Pharmacol.* 1982;13(suppl):127S-131S.
27. Symonds EM, Lamming GD, Jadoul F, Broughton Pipkin F. Clinical and biochemical aspects of the use of labetalol in the treatment of hypertension in pregnancy: comparison with methyldopa. In: Riley A, Symonds EM, eds. *The Investigation of Labetalol in the Management of Hypertension in Pregnancy.* Excerpta Medica; 1982:62-76.
28. Smith AM. Beta-blockers for pregnancy hypertension. *Lancet.* 1983;1: 708-709.
29. Walker JJ, Bonduelle M, Greer I, Calder AA. Antihypertensive therapy in pregnancy. *Lancet.* 1983;1:932-933.
30. Prescribing Information. Labetalol. Endo USA, Inc; 2024.
31. Frishman WH, Chesner M. Beta-adrenergic blockers in pregnancy. *Am Heart J.* 1988;115:147-152.
32. Magee LA, Elran E, Bull SB, Logan A, Koren G. Risks and benefits of β-receptor blockers for pregnancy hypertension: overview of the randomized trials. *Eur J Obstet Gynecol Reprod Biol.* 2000;88:15-26.
33. Leitz F, Bariletto S, Gural R, et al. Secretion of labetalol in breast milk of lactating women. *Fed Proc.* 1983;42:378.
34. Atkinson HC, Begg EJ, Darlow BA. Drugs in human milk. Clinical pharmacokinetic considerations. *Clin Pharmacokin.* 1988;14:217-240.
35. American College of Obstetricians and Gynecologists. ACOG practice bulletin no. 203: chronic hypertension in pregnancy. *Obstet Gynecol.* 2019;133: e26-e50.
36. Freppel R, Gaboriau L, Richardson M, et al. Beta-blockers and breastfeeding: a real-life prospective study. *Eur J Clin Pharmacol.* 2024;80:1937-1943.

LACTITOL

Gastrointestinal (Laxative)

PREGNANCY RECOMMENDATION: No Human Data—Animal Data Suggest Low Risk

BREASTFEEDING RECOMMENDATION: Probably Compatible

PREGNANCY SUMMARY

No reports describing the use of lactitol in human pregnancy have been located. Based on minimal systemic absorption, a negligible amount of lactitol may cross the placenta. However, the absence of human pregnancy experience prevents a complete assessment of any embryofetal risk. Animal data did not show any embryofetal toxicity in two species at doses of less than 10 times the recommended human dose (RHD). Using this drug during pregnancy should be based on the pros and cons of the mother's clinical need for treatment versus any potential fetal risk that might occur from exposure.

BREASTFEEDING SUMMARY

Minimal maternal systemic absorption of lactitol should limit infant exposure through breast milk. If lactitol is used while breastfeeding, the infant should be monitored for the most common reported adult side effects of abdominal distention (leading to irritability), flatulence, and diarrhea.

Reference

1. Prescribing Information. Lactitol. Braintree Laboratories, Inc; 2020.

LACTULOSE

Gastrointestinal (Laxative)

PREGNANCY RECOMMENDATION: No Human Data—Animal Data Suggest Low Risk

BREASTFEEDING RECOMMENDATION: Probably Compatible

PREGNANCY SUMMARY

No reports describing the use of lactulose during human pregnancy have been located. The drug is minimally absorbed systemically (<3%) following oral administration, which should greatly limit placental transfer. However, the absence of human pregnancy experience prevents a complete assessment of the embryofetal risk. Animal data did not show any embryofetal toxicity in three animal species at doses of less than 10 times the RHD. Using this drug during pregnancy should be based on the pros and cons of the mother's clinical need for treatment versus any potential fetal risk that might occur from exposure.

BREASTFEEDING SUMMARY

No reports describing the use of lactulose during human lactation have been located. The drug is minimally absorbed systemically (<3%) with oral use, which should significantly limit excretion into breast milk. If used while breastfeeding, the infant should be monitored for the most common reported adult side effects of gas, burping, and abdominal discomfort (leading to irritability).

Reference

1. Prescribing Information. Lactulose. VistaPharm, Inc; 2019.

LAMIVUDINE

Antiviral (HIV-1 and HBV)

PREGNANCY RECOMMENDATION: **Human Data Suggest Low Risk (Maternal Benefit May Outweigh Embryofetal Risk—for Both HIV and HBV)**

BREASTFEEDING RECOMMENDATION: ***Contraindicated (HIV)—Probably Compatible (HBV)**

PREGNANCY SUMMARY

In 2023, the updated US Department of Health and Human Services AIDS Info guidelines for the use of antiretroviral agents during pregnancy recommend that, in most cases, patients continue their regimen during pregnancy if it is tolerated, safe, and effective in suppressing viral replication. Additionally, treatment initiation should not be delayed due to concerns about teratogenicity with first-trimester exposure. See the guideline for the most updated information. If indicated, lamivudine should not be withheld in pregnancy since the expected benefit to the mother with HIV outweighs the unknown risk to the fetus. The same applies to the product used for treating hepatitis B. The data regarding first-trimester exposure to lamivudine is not associated with an increased risk of congenital anomalies or adverse infant outcomes. For HIV, there is a pregnancy exposure registry that monitors pregnancy outcomes in women exposed to antiretrovirals during pregnancy. Health care providers are encouraged to register patients by calling the Antiretroviral Pregnancy Registry (APR) at 1-800-258-4263.

BREASTFEEDING SUMMARY

In 2023, the updated US Department of Health and Human Services AIDS Info guidelines state that using replacement of breast milk through formula or pasteurized donor human breast milk from a milk bank eliminates the risk of postnatal HIV transmission to the infant. Using antiretroviral therapy to achieve and maintain viral suppression during pregnancy and postpartum decreases the risk for infant transmission to less than 1%, but not zero. *For patients not on therapy or those without viral load suppression during pregnancy (at a minimum of throughout the third trimester) and at delivery, replacement of breast milk is recommended. Patients on antiretroviral therapy who have a sustained undetectable viral load and who choose to breastfeed or use replacement of breast milk should be supported with this decision. Using lamivudine in treating hepatitis B virus (HBV) during lactation should be compatible. If used while breastfeeding, the infant should be monitored for the most common reported pediatric side effects of fever and cough.

References

1. Prescribing Information. Epivir. ViiV Healthcare Company; 2024.
2. Prescribing Information. Epivir HBV. GlaxoSmithKline LLC; 2021.
3. Moodley J, Moodley D, Pillay K, et al. Pharmacokinetics and antiretroviral activity of lamivudine alone or when coadministered with zidovudine in human immunodeficiency virus type 1-infected pregnant women and their offspring. *J Infect Dis*. 1998;178:1327-1333.
4. Benaboud S, Treluyer JM, Urien S, et al. Pregnancy-related effects on lamivudine pharmacokinetics in a population study with 228 women. *Antimicrob Agents Chemother*. 2012;56(2):776-782.
5. Antiretroviral Pregnancy Registry Steering Committee. Antiretroviral pregnancy registry interim report for 1 January 1989 through 31 July 2023. Registry Coordinating Center; 2023. Accessed January 26, 2024. https://www.apregistry.com/forms/interim_report.pdf
6. Sibiude J, Mandelbrot L, Blanche S, et al. Association between prenatal exposure to antiretroviral therapy and birth defects: an analysis of the French perinatal cohort study (ANRS CO1/CO11). *PLoS Med*. 2014;11:e1001635.
7. Vannappagari V, Koram N, Albano J, Tilson H, Gee C. Abacavir and lamivudine exposures during pregnancy and non-defect adverse pregnancy outcomes: data from the antiretroviral pregnancy registry. *J Acquir Immune Defic Syndr*. 2015;68:359-364.
8. Blanche S, Tardieu M, Rustin P, et al. Persistent mitochondrial dysfunction and perinatal exposure to antiretroviral nucleoside analogues. *Lancet*. 1999;354:1084-1089.
9. Panel on Treatment of HIV During Pregnancy and Prevention of Perinatal Transmission. Recommendations for the use of antiretroviral drugs during pregnancy and interventions to reduce perinatal HIV transmission in the United States. Recommendations for the use of antiretroviral drugs during pregnancy. Department of Health and Human Services. Accessed January 26, 2024. https://clinicalinfo.hiv.gov/en/guidelines/perinatal
10. Centers for Disease Control and Prevention. Hepatitis B and C infections. Accessed January 23, 2020. https://www.cdc.gov/breastfeeding-special-circumstances/hcp/illnesses-conditions/hepatitis-b-c.htmlange
11. Shapiro RL, Rossi S, Ogwu Moss M, et al. Therapeutic levels of lopinavir in late pregnancy and abacavir passage into breast milk in the Mma Bana study, Botswana. *Antiviral Ther*. 2013;18:585-590.
12. Mirochnick M, Thomas T, Capparelli E, et al. Antiretroviral concentrations in breast-feeding infants of mothers receiving highly active antiretroviral therapy. *Antimicrob Agents Chemother*. 2009;53:1170-1176.
13. Corbett AH, Kayira D, White NR, et al. Antiretroviral pharmacokinetics in mothers and breastfeeding infants from 6 to 24 weeks post partum: results of the BAN study. *Antivir Ther*. 2014;19:587-595.

14. Pirillo MF, Scarcella P, Andreotti M, et al. Hepatitis B virus mother-to-child transmission among HIV-infected women receiving lamivudine-containing antiretroviral regimens during pregnancy and breastfeeding. *J Viral Hepat*. 2015;22:289-296.
15. Ngoma MS, Hunter JA, Harper JA, et al. Cognitive and language outcomes in HIV-uninfected infants exposed to combined antiretroviral therapy in utero and through extended breast-feeding. *AIDS*. 2014;28(suppl 3):S323-S330.

LAMOTRIGINE

Central Nervous System (Antiseizure)

PREGNANCY RECOMMENDATION: Human Data Suggest Low Risk

BREASTFEEDING RECOMMENDATION: Potential Toxicity

PREGNANCY SUMMARY

Numerous studies, pregnancy registries, and meta-analyses describing the use of lamotrigine in several thousand human pregnancies have been located. Lamotrigine has not been associated with an increase in congenital malformations in more than 1,500 first-trimester exposures. One large study suggested a potential increase in risk (<1% increase) for oral clefts; however, this was not confirmed by other large evaluations. The drug crosses the placenta, so fetal exposure will occur. Embryofetal and maternal toxicity was observed in two animal species, one at doses less than 10 times the RHD and the other at more than 10 times the RHD. In a third species, no embryofetal or maternal toxicity occurred at doses of less than 10 times the RHD. Using this drug during pregnancy should be based on the pros and cons of the mother's clinical need for treatment versus any potential fetal risk that might occur from exposure. There is a pregnancy exposure registry that monitors pregnancy outcomes in women using antiseizure drugs. Health care providers are encouraged to call the North American Antiepileptic Drug Pregnancy Registry at 1-888-233-2334.

BREASTFEEDING SUMMARY

Several reports describing the use of lamotrigine during human lactation have been located. No adverse effects were observed in most infants. Occasional reports of varying issues have been reported in some infants, including rash, apnea, drowsiness, poor feeding, and withdrawal symptoms (that include loss of appetite, irritability, and tremors). Lamotrigine does not appear to affect infant growth and development. The drug is excreted into breast milk, with infant plasma levels reaching up to 50% of maternal levels. Breastfeeding while using this drug should be based on the mother's clinical need for treatment versus any potential infant risks that might occur. If used, the infant should be monitored for the most common reported adult side effects of rash, drowsiness, poor sucking, and poor weight gain.

References

1. Dichter MA, Brodie MJ. New antiepileptic drugs. *N Engl J Med*. 1996;334:1583-1590.
2. Morrell MJ. The new antiepileptic drugs and women: efficacy, reproductive health, pregnancy, and fetal outcome. *Epilepsia*. 1996;37(suppl 6):S34-S44.
3. Holmes LB, Wyszynski DF, Baldwin EJ, et al. Increased risk for non-syndromic cleft palate among infants exposed to lamotrigine during pregnancy (abstract). *Birth Defects Res A Clin Mol Teratol*. 2006;76:318.
4. Holmes LB, Hernandez-Diaz S. Newer anticonvulsants: lamotrigine, topiramate, and gabapentin. *Birth Defects Res A Clin Mol Teratol*. 2012;94:599-606.
5. The Lamotrigine Pregnancy Registry. Final report: 1 September 1992 through 31 March 2010. GlaxoSmithKline. 2010. https://pregnancyregistry.gsk.com/documents/lam_spring_2010_final_report.pdf
6. Prescribing Information. Lamictal. GlaxoSmithKline; 2023.
7. Betts T, Goodwin G, Withers RM, Yuen AWC. Human safety of lamotrigine. *Epilepsia*. 1991;32(suppl 2):S17-S21.
8. Rambeck B, Kurlemann G, Stodieck SRG, et al. Concentrations of lamotrigine in a mother on lamotrigine treatment and her newborn child. *Eur J Clin Pharmacol*. 1997;51:481-484.
9. Tomson T, Ohman I, Vitols S. Lamotrigine in pregnancy and lactation: a case report. *Epilepsia*. 1997;38:1039-1041.
10. Ohman I, Vitols S, Tomson T. Lamotrigine in pregnancy: pharmacokinetics during delivery, in the neonate, and during lactation. *Epilepsia*. 2000;41:709-713.
11. de Haan GJ, Edelbroek P, Segers J, et al. Gestation-induced changes in lamotrigine pharmacokinetics: a monotherapy study. *Neurology*. 2004;63:571-573.
12. Chambers CD, Kao KK, Felix RJ, et al. Pregnancy outcome in infants prenatally exposed to newer anticonvulsants (abstract). *Birth Defects Res A Clin Mol Teratol*. 2005;73:316.
13. Wilton LV, Pearce GL, Martin RM, Mackay FJ, Mann RD. The outcomes of pregnancy in women exposed to newly marketed drugs in general practice in England. *Br J Obstet Gynaecol*. 1998;105:882-889.
14. Holmes LB, Baldwin EJ, Smith CR, et al. Increased frequency of isolated cleft palate in infants exposed to lamotrigine during pregnancy. *Neurology*. 2008;70:2152-2158.
15. Dolk H, Jentink J, Loane M, Morris J, de Jong-van den Berg LTW. Does lamotrigine use in pregnancy increase orofacial cleft risk relative to other malformations? *Neurology*. 2008;71:714-722.
16. Meador KJ, Penovich P. What is the risk of orofacial clefts from lamotrigine exposure during pregnancy? *Neurology*. 2008;71:706-707.
17. Meador KJ, Baker GA, Browning N, et al; for the NEAD Study Group. Fetal antiepileptic drug exposure and cognitive outcomes at age 6 years (NEAD study): a prospective observational study. *Lancet Neurol*. 2013;12:244-252.
18. Nordmo E, Aronsen L, Wasland K, et al. Severe apnea in an infant exposed to lamotrigine in breast milk. *Ann Pharmacother*. 2009;43:1983-1987.
19. Gentile S. Prophylactic treatment of bipolar disorder in pregnancy and breastfeeding: focus on emerging mood stabilizers. *Bipolar Disord*. 2006;8:207-220.
20. Almgren M, Kallen B, Lavebratt C. Population-based study of antiepileptic drug exposure in utero—influence on head circumference in newborns. *Seizure*. 2009;18:672-675.
21. Pariente G, Leibson T, Shulman T, et al. Pregnancy outcomes following in utero exposure to lamotrigine: a systematic review and meta-analysis. *CNS Drugs*. 2017;31(6):439-450.
22. Dolk H, Wang H, Loane M, et al. Lamotrigine use in pregnancy and risk of orofacial cleft and other congenital anomalies. *Neurology*. 2016;86:1716-1725.
23. Tran TA, Leppik IE, Blesi K, et al. Lamotrigine clearance during pregnancy. *Neurology*. 2002;59:251-255.

24. Liporace J, Kao A, D'Abreu A. Concerns regarding lamotrigine and breast-feeding. *Epilepsy Behav*. 2004;5:102-105.
25. Gentile S. Lamotrigine in pregnancy and lactation. *Arch Womens Ment Health*. 2005;8:57-58.
26. Page-Sharp M, Kristensen JH, Hackett IP, et al. Transfer of lamotrigine into breast milk. *Ann Pharmacother*. 2006;40:1470-1471.
27. Newport DJ, Pennell PB, Calamaras MR, et al. Lamotrigine in breast milk and nursing infants: determination of exposure. *Pediatrics*. 2008;122:e223-e231.
28. Bar-Oz B, Nulman I, Koren G, Ito S. Anticonvulsants and breast feeding—a critical review. *Paediatr Drugs*. 2000;2:113-126.
29. Meador KJ, Baker GA, Browning N, et al; for the NEAD Study Group. Effects of breastfeeding in children of women taking antiepileptic drugs. *Neurology*. 2010;75:1954-1960.
30. Meador KJ, Baker GA, Browning N, et al; Neurodevelopmental Effects of Antiepileptic Drugs (NEAD) Study Group. Breastfeeding in children of women taking antiepileptic drugs: cognitive outcomes at age 6 years. *JAMA Pediatr*. 2014;168:729-736.

LANADELUMAB

Genetic/Cardiovascular (Kallikrein Inhibitor—Monoclonal Antibody)

PREGNANCY RECOMMENDATION: No Human Data—Animal Data Suggest Low Risk

BREASTFEEDING RECOMMENDATION: Probably Compatible

PREGNANCY SUMMARY

No reports describing the use of lanadelumab during human pregnancy have been located. Immunoglobulin G (IgG) antibodies are known to cross the placenta, especially during the third trimester, which suggests that some transfer will occur. However, the absence of human pregnancy experience prevents a complete assessment of the embryofetal risk. Animal data did not show any embryofetal toxicity in one animal species at doses of more than 10 times the RHD. Using this drug during pregnancy should be based on the pros and cons of the mother's clinical need for treatment versus any potential fetal risk that might occur from exposure.

L

BREASTFEEDING SUMMARY

No reports describing the use of lanadelumab during human lactation have been located. It is known that IgG antibodies can be found in human breast milk, but are not found in the neonatal or infant circulation. Additionally, if any IgG antibodies were to be ingested through breastfeeding, they would probably be digested in the infant's gastrointestinal tract and not be absorbed. Breastfeeding while using this drug should be based on the mother's clinical need for treatment. If used, the infant should be monitored for the most common reported adult side effects of headache and dizziness (leading to irritability), upper respiratory infection, rash, diarrhea, and weakness (lethargy).

Reference

1. Prescribing Information. Takhzyro. Takeda Pharmaceuticals; 2023.

LACOSAMIDE

Central Nervous System (Antiseizure)

PREGNANCY RECOMMENDATION: Limited Human Data—Animal Data Suggest Potential Risk

BREASTFEEDING RECOMMENDATION: Potential Toxicity

PREGNANCY SUMMARY

A few reports describing the use of lacosamide in 71 human pregnancies during all trimesters were located. No increased risk for congenital abnormalities was seen in those with first-trimester exposure. The drug crosses the placenta, so some fetal exposure will occur. However, this limited human pregnancy experience prevents a complete assessment of the embryofetal risk. Embryofetal toxicity was observed in one animal species but not the second species at doses less than 10 times the RHD. Maternal toxicity occurred in both species. Using this drug during pregnancy should be based on the pros and cons of the mother's clinical need for treatment versus any potential fetal risk that might occur from exposure. There is a pregnancy exposure registry that monitors pregnancy outcomes in women using antiseizure drugs. Health care providers are encouraged to call the North American Antiepileptic Drug Pregnancy Registry at 1-888-233-2334.

BREASTFEEDING SUMMARY

Seven reports describing the use of lacosamide during human lactation in eight women were located. The drug was excreted into breast milk, with a calculated relative infant dose (RID) of up to about 30% in one case. No adverse effects were reported in seven of the breastfed infants. Poor feeding and sleepiness were reported in one infant also exposed to levetiracetam. Nevertheless, breastfeeding while using this drug should be based on the mother's clinical need for treatment versus any potential infant risks that might occur. If used, the infant should be monitored for the most common reported adult side effects of poor feeding and sleepiness. Because of the high RID observed in one case, if used, close newborn monitoring is needed.

References

1. Prescribing Information. Vimpat. UCB; 2019.
2. Ylikotila P, Ketola R, Timonen S, et al. Early pregnancy cerebral venous thrombosis and status epilepticus treated with levetiracetam and lacosamide throughout pregnancy. *Reprod Toxicol*. 2015;57:204-206.
3. Zarubova J, Kremlackova V, Borecka K, Marusic P. Plasma and breast milk levels of lacosamide before, during, and post pregnancy. *Epilepsia*. 2016; 57:69.
4. Landmark CJ, Rektorli L, Burns ML, et al. Pharmacokinetic data on brivaracetam, lacosamide and perampanel during pregnancy and lactation. *Epileptic Disord*. 2021;23:426-431.
5. Lattanzi S, Cagnetti C, Foschi N, et al. Lacosamide during pregnancy and breastfeeding. *Neurol Neurochir Pol*. 2017;51:266-269.
6. Kohn E, Dinavitser N, Gandelman-Marton R, et al. Lacosamide levels in blood and breastmilk during pregnancy and lactation: a case report. *Reprod Toxicol*. 2020;97:10-26.
7. Monfort A, Jutras M, Martin B, et al. New data on the transfer of untested medication into breast milk. *Birth Defect Res*. 2021;113:829-831.
8. Hoeltzenbein M, Slimi S, Fietz AK, et al. Increasing use of newer antiseizure medication during pregnancy: an observational study with special focus on lacosamide. *Seizure*. 2023;107:107-113.
9. Cercos M, Seqat I, Facile A, et al. Lacosamide use during breastfeeding: a case report and a literature review. *Fundam Clin Pharmacol*. 2024;38:575-578.

LANREOTIDE

Endocrine (Somatostatin Analogue)

PREGNANCY RECOMMENDATION: Limited Human Data—Animal Data Suggest Risk

BREASTFEEDING RECOMMENDATION: Probably Compatible

PREGNANCY SUMMARY

Four case reports describing the use of lanreotide in five human pregnancies have been located. All pregnancies resulted in healthy newborns with no adverse effects or congenital anomalies. A limited amount of the drug may cross the placenta, so fetal exposure is possible. However, the limited human pregnancy experience prevents a complete assessment of the embryofetal risk. Embryofetal toxicity with malformations was observed in two animal species at doses less than 10 times the RHD. Using this drug during pregnancy should be based on the pros and cons of the mother's clinical need for treatment versus any potential fetal risk that might occur from exposure.

BREASTFEEDING SUMMARY

One case report describing the use of lanreotide during human lactation was located. The child had normal growth and development. Some amount of the drug may be excreted into breast milk, so infant exposure might occur. However, even if it is excreted into breast milk, the peptide will probably be digested in the infant's gastrointestinal tract and not be absorbed. Regardless, due to a concern for potential serious adverse effects that might be seen in a breastfed infant, the manufacturer recommends that women not breastfeed while being treated with this drug and for at least 6 months after the last dose. If the clinical decision is to use this drug while breastfeeding, the infant should be monitored for the most common reported adult side effects of nausea and abdominal pain (both leading to irritability) and diarrhea.

References

1. Prescribing Information. Lanreotide injection. Cipla USA, Inc; 2021.
2. de Menis E, Billeci D, Marton E, Gussoni G. Uneventful pregnancy in an acromegalic patient treatment with slow-release lanreotide: a case report. *J Clin Endocrinol Metab*. 1999;84:1489.
3. Ben Salem Hachmi L, Kammoun I, et al. Management of acromegaly in pregnant woman. *Ann Endocrinol (Paris)*. 2010;71:60-63.
4. Teltayev D, Akshulakov S, Ryskeldiev N, et al. Pregnancy in women after successful acromegaly treatment, including surgical removal of pituitary adenoma and postoperative therapy using lanreotide acetate. *Gynecol Endocrinol*. 2017;33(suppl 1):50-51.
5. Meoni G, Giommoni E, Petreni P, et al. Somatostatin analogs in pregnant patients with neuroendocrine tumor. *Anticancer Drugs*. 2020;31:1096-1098.
6. Popescu AD, Carsote M, Valea A, et al. Approach of acromegaly during pregnancy. *Diagnostics (Basel)*. 2022;12:2669.

LANSOPRAZOLE

Gastrointestinal (Proton Pump Inhibitor)

PREGNANCY RECOMMENDATION: Limited Human Data—Animal Data Suggest Low Risk

BREASTFEEDING RECOMMENDATION: Probably Compatible

PREGNANCY SUMMARY

Numerous reports and meta-analyses evaluating the use of proton pump inhibitors in pregnancy were located. Overall, as a group, there did not appear to be any increased risk for major congenital anomalies. From these, about 80 first-trimester exposures to lansoprazole were found. Three (3.7%) major anomalies were described, and all were different. The drug will probably cross the placenta, so some fetal exposure will likely occur. However, the limited human pregnancy experience with lansoprazole alone prevents a complete assessment of the embryofetal risk. Animal data did not show any embryofetal toxicity in two species at doses of more than 10 times the RHD. Using this drug during pregnancy should be based on the pros and cons of the mother's clinical need for treatment versus any potential fetal risk that might occur from exposure.

BREASTFEEDING SUMMARY

No reports describing the use of lansoprazole during human lactation have been located. The drug will probably appear in breast milk, so some infant exposure will likely occur. Breastfeeding while using this drug should be based on the mother's clinical need for treatment versus any potential infant risks that might occur. If used, the infant should be monitored for the most common reported adult side effects of nausea and abdominal pain (both leading to irritability), diarrhea, and constipation.

References

1. Prescribing Information. Lansoprazole. Teva Pharmaceuticals USA, Inc; 2022.
2. Schardein JL, Furuhashi T, Ooshima Y. Reproductive and developmental toxicity studies of lansoprazole (AG-1749) in rats and rabbits. *Yakuri to Rinsho*. 1990;18:S2773-S2783. As cited in Shepard TH. *Catalog of Teratogenic Agents*. 8th ed. Johns Hopkins University Press; 1995:245.
3. Schardein JL, Furuhashi T, Ooshima Y. Reproductive and developmental toxicity studies of lansoprazole (AG-1749) in rats and rabbits. *Jpn Pharmacol Ther*. 1990;18(suppl 10):119-129. As cited in Schardein JL. *Chemically Induced Birth Defects*. 2nd ed. Marcel Dekker; 1993:447.
4. Wilton LV, Pearce GL, Martin RM, et al. The outcomes of pregnancy in women exposed to newly marketed drugs in general practice in England. *Br J Obstet Gynaecol*. 1998;105:882-889.
5. Kallen B. Delivery outcome after the use of acid-suppressing drugs in early pregnancy with special reference to omeprazole. *Br J Obstet Gynaecol*. 1998;105:877-881.
6. Nielsen GL, Sorensen HT, Thulstrup AM, Tage-Jensen U, Olesen C, Ekbom A. The safety of proton pump inhibitors in pregnancy. *Aliment Pharmacol Ther*. 1999;13:1085-1089.
7. Nikfar S, Abdollahi M, Moretti ME, et al. Use of proton pump inhibitors during pregnancy and rates of major malformations: a meta-analysis. *Dig Dis Sci*. 2002;47:1526-1529.
8. Diav-Citrin O, Arnon J, Shechtman S, et al. The safety of proton pump inhibitors in pregnancy: a multicentre prospective controlled trial. *Aliment Pharmacol Ther*. 2005;21:269-275.
9. Mayer A, Sheiner E, Holcherg G. Zollinger Ellison syndrome, treated with lansoprazole, during pregnancy. *Arch Gynecol Obstet*. 2007;276:171-173.
10. Dehlink E, Yen E, Leichtner AM, et al. First evidence of a possible association between gastric acid suppression during pregnancy and childhood asthma: a population-based register study. *Clin Exp Allergy*. 2009;39:246-253.
11. Gill SK, O'Brien L, Einarson TR, Koren G. The safety of proton pump inhibitors (PPIs) in pregnancy: a meta-analysis. *Am J Gastroenterol*. 2009;104:1541-1545.
12. Pasternak B, Hviid A. Use of proton-pump inhibitors in early pregnancy and the risk of birth defects. *N Engl J Med*. 2010;363:2114-2123.
13. Mitchell AA. Proton-pump inhibitors and birth defects—some reassurance, but more needed. *N Engl J Med*. 2010;363:2161-2163.
14. Anderka M, Mitchell AA, Louik C, et al; the National Birth Defects Prevention Study. Medications used to treat nausea and vomiting of pregnancy and the risk of selected birth defects. *Birth Defects Res A Clin Mol Teratol*. 2012;94:22-30.
15. Erichsen R, Mikkelsen E, Pedersen L, Sorensen HT. Maternal use of proton pump inhibitors during early pregnancy and the prevalence of hypospadias in male offspring. *Am J Ther*. 2014;21(4):254-259.
16. Matok I, Levy A, Wiznitzer A, et al. The safety of fetal exposure to proton-pump inhibitors during pregnancy. *Dig Dis Sci*. 2012;57:699-705.
17. Broussard CN, Richter JE. Treating gastro-oesophageal reflux disease during pregnancy and lactation. What are the safest therapy options? *Drug Saf*. 1998;19:325-337.
18. Katz PO, Castell DO. Gastroesophageal reflux disease during pregnancy. *Gastroenterol Clin North Am*. 1998;27:153-167.
19. Ramakrishnan A, Katz PO. Pharmacologic management of gastroesophageal reflux disease. *Curr Treat Options Gastroenterol*. 2002;5:301-310.
20. Richter JE. Gastroesophageal reflux disease during pregnancy. *Gastroenterol Clin N Am*. 2003;32:235-261.
21. Richter JE. Review article: the management of heartburn in pregnancy. *Aliment Pharmacol Ther*. 2005;22:749-757.
22. Li CM, Zhernakova A, Engstrand L, Wijmenga C, Brusselaers N. Systematic review with meta-analysis: the risks of proton pump inhibitors during pregnancy. *Aliment Pharmacol Ther*. 2020;51:410-420.
23. Choi A, Noh Y, Jeong HE, et al. Association between proton pump inhibitor use during early pregnancy and risk of congenital malformations. *JAMA Netw Open*. 2023;6:e2250366.
24. Peron A, Ripoche E, Picot C, et al. Use of proton pump inhibitors during pregnancy: a systematic review and meta-analysis of congenital malformations. *Reprod Toxicol*. 2023;119:108419.
25. Nguyen PY, Armari E, Bradfield Z, et al. The effects of proton pump inhibitors during pregnancy on treatment of preeclampsia, and related outcomes: a systematic review and meta-analysis. *Am J Obstet Gynecol MFM*. 2024;6:101478.

LANTHANUM CARBONATE

Antidote (Phosphate Binder)

PREGNANCY RECOMMENDATION: No Human Data—Animal Data Suggest Low Risk

BREASTFEEDING RECOMMENDATION: Probably Compatible

PREGNANCY SUMMARY

No reports describing the use of lanthanum carbonate in human pregnancy have been located. The very low systemic absorption (<0.002%) following oral use suggests that negligible amounts will cross the placenta, and therefore, would likely be clinically insignificant. However, the absence of human pregnancy experience prevents a complete assessment of the embryofetal risk. Animal data did not show any embryofetal toxicity in two species at doses of less than 10 times the RHD. Using this drug during pregnancy should be based on the pros and cons of the mother's clinical need for treatment versus any potential fetal risk that might occur from exposure.

BREASTFEEDING SUMMARY

No reports describing the use of lanthanum carbonate during human lactation have been located. The very low systemic absorption (<0.002%) following oral use suggests that negligible amounts will be excreted into breast milk. Moreover, even if some amount of the drug were to be found in breast milk, it would likely bind with milk phosphate, resulting in a nonabsorbable complex. Breastfeeding while using this drug should be based on the mother's clinical need for treatment versus any potential infant risks that might occur. Due to the lack of absorption, systemic side effects were not evaluated.

Reference

1. Prescribing Information. Lanthanum carbonate. Teva Pharmaceuticals USA, Inc; 2023.

LAPATINIB

Antineoplastic (Tyrosine Kinase Inhibitor)

PREGNANCY RECOMMENDATION: **No Human Data—Animal Data Suggest Potential Risk**

BREASTFEEDING RECOMMENDATION: **Potential Toxicity**

PREGNANCY SUMMARY

Three reports describing the use of lapatinib in human pregnancy have been located. Two reports described 13 exposures while being treated during a clinical trial. Of these, six patients elected to continue the pregnancies, and no congenital defects were noted at delivery. The third study found an association with higher rates of oligohydramnios and neonatal kidney failure in women exposed to anti-ERBB2 agents as a group in pregnancy when compared to other anticancer agents. Additionally, an increased risk for intrauterine growth restriction was seen in the 18 women specifically exposed to lapatinib. Some amount of the drug may cross the placenta, so fetal exposure will likely occur. However, this limited human pregnancy experience prevents a complete assessment of the embryofetal risk. Embryofetal toxicity with malformations was observed in two animal species at doses less than 10 times the RHD, one of which was less than the RHD. Maternal toxicity also occurred in both species at these doses. Based on these animal studies and the drug's mechanism of action, the manufacturer recommends that women with reproductive potential use effective contraception during treatment and for 1 week after the last dose. They also recommend that males with female partners of reproductive potential use effective contraception during treatment and for 1 week after the last dose. Nevertheless, using this drug during pregnancy should be based on the pros and cons of the mother's clinical need for treatment versus any potential fetal risk that might occur from exposure. There is a registry for women who are pregnant and have cancer. For more information, women and health care providers are encouraged to contact the Cancer and Pregnancy Registry at 1-877-635-4499.

BREASTFEEDING SUMMARY

No reports describing the use of lapatinib during human lactation have been located. The drug will probably appear in breast milk, so some infant exposure will likely occur. However, due to a concern for potential serious adverse effects that might be seen in a breastfed infant, the manufacturer recommends that women not breastfeed while being treated with this drug and for at least 1 week after the last dose. Nevertheless, breastfeeding while using this drug should be based on the mother's clinical need for treatment versus any potential infant risks that might occur. If used, the infant should be monitored for the most common reported adult side effects of nausea (leading to irritability), diarrhea, vomiting, and rash.

References

1. Prescribing Information. Tykerb. Novartis. 2018.
2. Kelly H, Graham M, Humes E, et al. Delivery of a healthy baby after first-trimester maternal exposure to lapatinib. *Clin Breast Cancer*. 2006;7:339-341.
3. Lambertini M, Martel S, Campbell C, et al. Pregnancies during and after trastuzumab and/or lapatinib in patients with human epidermal growth factor receptor 2–positive early breast cancer: analysis from the NeoALTTO (BIG 1-06) and ALTTO (BIG 2-06) trials. *Cancer*. 2019;125:307-316.
4. Gougis P, Grandal B, Jochum F, et al. Treatments during pregnancy targeting ERBB2 and outcomes of pregnant individuals and newborns. *JAMA Netw Open*. 2023;6:e2339934.

LARONIDASE

Endocrine/Genetic (Enzyme)

PREGNANCY RECOMMENDATION: Limited Human Data—Animal Data Suggest Low Risk

BREASTFEEDING RECOMMENDATION: Probably Compatible

PREGNANCY SUMMARY

Two case reports and manufacturer data describing the use of laronidase in about 33 human pregnancies have been located. One (3%) major anomaly was described (Potter sequence). The remaining 32 had no congenital defects. Placental transfer is unlikely to be clinically significant, especially in the first trimester. However, this limited human pregnancy experience prevents a complete assessment of the embryofetal risk. Animal data did not show any embryofetal toxicity in one species at doses of less than 10 times the RHD. Using this drug during pregnancy should be based on the pros and cons of the mother's clinical need for treatment versus any potential fetal risk that might occur from exposure. Hypertension has been reported in up to 10% of patients treated with this drug during the clinical trials. If used, blood pressure should be monitored. There is a mucopolysaccharidosis (MPS) I Registry established for pregnant women that monitors pregnancy outcomes in women exposed to laronidase during pregnancy. For more information, health care providers or patients are encouraged to contact 1-800-745-4447.

BREASTFEEDING SUMMARY

One case report and manufacturer postmarketing data have found no adverse effects with the use of laronidase during human lactation. The drug will not likely be excreted into breast milk. In one report, the breast milk was negative for laronidase before and 60 minutes after the infusion at 1 and 3 months postpartum. Additionally, because it is a large protein, if any laronidase were to be ingested through breastfeeding, it would probably be digested in the infant's gastrointestinal tract and not be absorbed. If the clinical decision is to use this drug while breastfeeding, the infant should be monitored for the most common reported side effects in children and adults of tingling and numbness (both leading to irritability), rash, upper respiratory tract infection, and flushing.

References

1. Prescribing Information. Aldurazyme. Genzyme Corporation; 2023.
2. Anbu AT, Mercer J, Wraith JE. Effect of discontinuing of laronidase in a patient with mucopolysaccharidosis type 1. *J Inherit Metab Dis*. 2006;29:230-231.
3. Castorina M, Antuzzi D, Richards SM, et al. Successful pregnancy and breastfeeding in a woman with mucopolysaccharidosis type I while receiving laronidase enzyme replacement therapy. *Clin Exp Obstet Gynecol*. 2015; 42:108-113.

LAROTRECTINIB

Antineoplastic (Kinase Inhibitor)

PREGNANCY RECOMMENDATION: No Human Data—Animal Data Suggest Potential Risk

BREASTFEEDING RECOMMENDATION: Potential Toxicity

PREGNANCY SUMMARY

No reports describing the use of larotrectinib in human pregnancy have been located. The drug will probably cross the placenta, so some fetal exposure will likely occur. However, the absence of human pregnancy experience prevents a complete assessment of the embryofetal risk. Embryofetal toxicity was observed in one animal species at doses of less than 10 times the RHD and in a second species at doses of more than 10 times the RHD. Based on animal studies and the drug's mechanism of action, the manufacturer recommends that women with reproductive potential use effective contraception during treatment and for 1 week after the last dose. They also recommend that males with female partners of reproductive potential use effective contraception during treatment and for 1 week after the last dose. Nevertheless, using this drug during pregnancy should be based on the pros and cons of the mother's clinical need for treatment versus any potential fetal risk that might occur from exposure. There is a registry for women who are pregnant and have cancer. For more information, women and health care providers are encouraged to contact the Cancer and Pregnancy Registry at 1-877-635-4499.

BREASTFEEDING SUMMARY

No reports describing the use of larotrectinib during human lactation have been located. The drug will probably appear in breast milk, so some infant exposure will likely occur. However, due to a concern for potential serious adverse effects that might be seen in a breastfed infant, the manufacturer recommends that women not breastfeed while being treated with this drug and for at least 1 week after the last dose. Nevertheless, breastfeeding while using this drug should be based on the mother's clinical need for treatment versus any potential infant risks that might occur. If used, the infant should be monitored for the most common reported adult side effects of nausea, dizziness, and abdominal pain (all leading to irritability), lethargy, cough, diarrhea, fever, vomiting, and various laboratory abnormalities (see Prescribing Information [PI]).

Reference

1. Prescribing Information. Vitrakvi. Bayer HealthCare Pharmaceuticals, Inc; 2023.

LASMIDITAN

Central Nervous System (Antimigraine)

PREGNANCY RECOMMENDATION: No Human Data—Animal Data Suggest Potential Risk

BREASTFEEDING RECOMMENDATION: Potential Toxicity

PREGNANCY SUMMARY

No reports describing the use of lasmiditan in human pregnancy have been located. The drug will probably cross the placenta, so some fetal exposure will likely occur. However, the absence of human pregnancy experience prevents a complete assessment of the embryofetal risk. Embryofetal toxicity with malformations was observed in one animal species at doses equal to the RHD and in a second species at more than 10 times the RHD. Using this drug during pregnancy should be based on the pros and cons of the mother's clinical need for treatment versus any potential fetal risk that might occur from exposure. There is a pregnancy exposure registry that monitors pregnancy outcomes in women exposed to lasmiditan during pregnancy. For more information, health care providers or patients are encouraged to contact 1-833-464-4724.

BREASTFEEDING SUMMARY

No reports describing the use of lasmiditan during human lactation have been located. The drug will probably appear in breast milk, so some infant exposure will likely occur. Breastfeeding while using this drug should be based on the mother's clinical need for treatment. If used, the infant should be monitored for the most common reported adult side effects of tingling and dizziness (both leading to irritability), sleepiness, and fatigue.

Reference

1. Prescribing Information. Reyvow. Eli Lilly; 2022.

LATANOPROST OPHTHALMIC

Ophthalmic (Antiglaucoma—Topical Prostaglandin)

PREGNANCY RECOMMENDATION: Limited Human Data—Animal Data Suggest Potential Risk

BREASTFEEDING RECOMMENDATION: Probably Compatible

PREGNANCY SUMMARY

Ten cases with reported outcomes of latanoprost exposure in the first trimester of human pregnancy have been reported. One ended in a spontaneous abortion, and the other nine women delivered normal infants with no reported congenital defects. Prostaglandins can increase uterine tone and may lead to premature labor. However, there is no evidence that doses given to reduce elevated ophthalmic pressure would increase the risk for uterine contraction. The drug will probably cross the placenta, but the amount is expected to be clinically insignificant. However, this limited human pregnancy experience prevents a complete assessment of the embryofetal risk. Embryofetal toxicity with malformations was observed in one animal species and embryolethality in a second animal species at IV doses less than 10 times the maximum recommended human ophthalmic dose (MRHOD). But this would assume 100% systemic absorption with topical ocular use. Using this drug during pregnancy should be based on the pros and cons of the mother's clinical need for treatment versus any potential fetal risk that might occur from exposure. If used during pregnancy, consider placing pressure over the tear duct in the corner of the eye for at least 1 minute, and then remove any excess solution with absorbent tissue to decrease the amount of drug reaching the systemic circulation even further.

BREASTFEEDING SUMMARY

No reports describing the use of latanoprost during human lactation have been located. The drug may be found in breast milk, but the amount is likely to be clinically insignificant. If the clinical decision is to use this drug while breastfeeding, the infant should be monitored for the most common reported systemic adult side effects of abdominal cramps (leading to irritability) and tremors. A method to decrease some systemic absorption with ophthalmic use is described above in the Pregnancy Summary.

References

1. Prescribing Information. Xalatan. Pfizer; 2022.
2. Lipitz S, Grisaru D, Libshiz A, et al. Intra-amniotic prostaglandin F2 alpha for pregnancy termination in the second and early third trimesters of pregnancy. *J Reprod Med*. 1997;42:235-238.
3. Salamalekis E, Kassanos D, Hassiakos D, et al. Intra/extra-amniotic administration of prostaglandin F2a in fetal death, missed and therapeutic abortions. *Clin Exp Obstet Gynecol*. 1990;17:17-21.
4. De Santis M, Lucchese A, Carducci B, et al. Latanoprost exposure in pregnancy. *Am J Ophthalmol*. 2004;138:305-306.
5. Netland P. *Glaucoma Medical Therapy: Principles and Management*. Oxford University Press; 2008;31-155.

LATANOPROSTENE BUNOD

Ophthalmic (Prostaglandin Analogue—Topical)

PREGNANCY RECOMMENDATION: No Human Data—Animal Data Suggest Low Risk

BREASTFEEDING RECOMMENDATION: Probably Compatible

PREGNANCY SUMMARY

No reports describing the use of latanoprostene bunod in human pregnancy have been located. Though placental transfer is possible, fetal exposure is probably negligible because of insignificant absorption after ophthalmic use. However, the absence of human pregnancy experience prevents a complete assessment of the embryofetal risk. Animal data did not show any embryofetal toxicity despite the drug being administered IV. If used during pregnancy, consider placing pressure over the tear duct in the corner of the eye for at least 1 minute, and then remove any excess solution with absorbent tissue to decrease the amount of drug reaching the systemic circulation even further.

L

BREASTFEEDING SUMMARY

No reports describing the use of latanoprostene bunod in human lactation have been located. Because the drug has negligible absorption after ophthalmic use, any drug found in breast milk would not likely have a clinical effect. Breastfeeding while using this drug should be based on the mother's clinical need for treatment. A method to decrease some systemic absorption with ophthalmic use is described above in the Pregnancy Summary.

Reference

1. Prescribing Information. Vyzulta. Bausch and Lomb, Inc; 2019.

LAZERTINIB

Antineoplastic (Epidermal Growth Factor Receptor (EGFR) Kinase Inhibitor)

PREGNANCY RECOMMENDATION: No Human Data—Animal Data Suggest Risk

BREASTFEEDING RECOMMENDATION: Potential Toxicity

PREGNANCY SUMMARY

No reports describing the use of lazertinib in human pregnancy have been located. The drug will likely cross the placenta, so some fetal exposure will probably occur. Therefore, the absence of human pregnancy experience prevents a complete assessment of the embryofetal risk. Animal studies did show embryofetal toxicity with malformations in two species at doses of less than 10 times the RHD. Based on these animal studies and the drug's mechanism of action, the manufacturer recommends that women with reproductive potential use effective contraception during treatment and for 3 weeks after the last dose. They also recommend that males with female partners of reproductive potential use effective contraception during treatment and for 3 weeks after the last dose. Nevertheless, using this drug during pregnancy should be based on the pros and cons of the mother's clinical need for treatment versus any potential fetal risk that might occur from exposure. There is a registry for women who are pregnant and have cancer. For more information, women and health care providers are encouraged to contact the Cancer and Pregnancy Registry at 1-877-635-4499.

BREASTFEEDING SUMMARY

No reports describing the use of lazertinib during human lactation have been located. The drug will likely be found in breast milk, so some infant exposure will probably occur. Due to a concern for potential serious adverse effects that might be seen in a breastfed infant, the manufacturer recommends that women not breastfeed while being treated with this drug and for 3 weeks after the last dose. Nevertheless, breastfeeding while using this drug should be based on the mother's clinical need for treatment versus any potential infant risk that might occur. If used, the infant should be monitored for the most common reported adult side effects of nausea, pruritus, and musculoskeletal pain (all leading to irritability), fatigue (lethargy), rash, peripheral edema, constipation, decreased appetite (monitor infant growth), and various laboratory abnormalities (see PI).

Reference

1. Prescribing Information. Lazcluze. Janssen Biotech, Inc; 2024.

LEBRIKIZUMAB

Dermatologic/Immunologic (Monoclonal Antibody—Interleukin 13 Antagonist)

PREGNANCY RECOMMENDATION: No Human Data—Animal Data Suggest Low Risk

BREASTFEEDING RECOMMENDATION: Probably Compatible

PREGNANCY SUMMARY

No reports describing the use of lebrikizumab in human pregnancy have been located. As an IgG antibody, the drug will likely cross the placenta, so some fetal exposure will probably occur. However, the absence of human pregnancy experience prevents a complete assessment of the embryofetal risk. Animal reproduction studies did not show any embryofetal toxicity or malformations in one species at doses of more than 10 times the RHD. Using this drug during pregnancy should be based on the pros and cons of the mother's clinical need for treatment versus any potential fetal risk that might occur from exposure. The manufacturer states that because the drug interferes with the immune response, the administration of live vaccines should be delayed in newborns. There is a pregnancy exposure registry that monitors pregnancy outcomes in patients using this drug during gestation. Health care providers are encouraged to call Eli Lilly and Company at 800-545-5979.

BREASTFEEDING SUMMARY

No reports describing the use of lebrikizumab during human lactation have been located. It is known that IgG antibodies can be found in human breast milk, but are not found in the neonatal or infant circulation. Additionally, if any IgG antibodies were to be ingested through breastfeeding, they would probably be digested in the infant's gastrointestinal tract and not be absorbed. Breastfeeding while using this drug should be based on the mother's clinical need for treatment. If used, the infant should be monitored for the most common reported adult side effect of infections.

Reference

1. Prescribing Information. Ebglyss. Eli Lilly and Company; 2024.

LECANEMAB

Central Nervous System (Monoclonal Antibody—Alzheimer)

PREGNANCY RECOMMENDATION: No Human Data and No Relevant Animal Data

BREASTFEEDING RECOMMENDATION: Probably Compatible

PREGNANCY SUMMARY

No reports describing the use of lecanemab in human pregnancy have been located. As an IgG antibody, the drug will likely cross the placenta, so some fetal exposure will probably occur. However, the absence of human pregnancy experience prevents a complete assessment of the embryofetal risk. Animal reproduction studies have not been conducted. Using this drug during pregnancy should be based on the pros and cons of the mother's clinical need for treatment versus any potential fetal risk that might occur from exposure.

BREASTFEEDING SUMMARY

No reports describing the use of lecanemab during human lactation have been located. It is known that IgG antibodies can be found in human breast milk, but are not found in the neonatal or infant circulation. Additionally, if any IgG antibodies were to be ingested through breastfeeding, they would probably be digested in the infant's gastrointestinal tract and not be absorbed. Breastfeeding while using this drug should be based on the mother's clinical need for treatment. If used, the infant should be monitored for the most common reported adult side effects of headache (leading to irritability) and edema.

Reference

1. Prescribing Information. Leqembi. Eisai, Inc; 2023.

LEFAMULIN

Antibacterial

PREGNANCY RECOMMENDATION: No Human Data—Animal Data Suggest Risk

BREASTFEEDING RECOMMENDATION: Potential Toxicity

PREGNANCY SUMMARY

No reports describing the use of lefamulin in human pregnancy have been located. Some amount of the drug may cross the placenta, so fetal exposure will likely occur. However, the absence of human pregnancy experience prevents a complete assessment of the embryofetal risk. Embryofetal toxicity with malformations was observed in two animal species at doses of less than 10 times the RHD. Based on these animal studies, the manufacturer recommends that women with reproductive potential use effective contraception during treatment and for 2 days after the last dose. Nevertheless, using this drug during pregnancy should be based on the pros and cons of the mother's clinical need for treatment versus any potential fetal risk that might occur from exposure. Lefamulin is associated with QT prolongation. Monitor QTc interval prior to and during drug treatment.

BREASTFEEDING SUMMARY

No reports describing the use of lefamulin during human lactation have been located. The drug will probably appear in breast milk, so some infant exposure will likely occur. However, due to a concern for potential serious adverse effects that might be seen in a breastfed infant, the manufacturer recommends that women not breastfeed while being treated with this drug and for at least 2 days after the last dose. Nevertheless, breastfeeding while using this drug should be based on the mother's clinical need for treatment versus any potential infant risks that might occur. If used, the infant should be monitored for the most common reported adult side effects of nausea and headache (both leading to irritability), increased liver enzymes, hypokalemia, sleep abnormalities, vomiting, and diarrhea.

Reference

1. Prescribing Information. Xenleta. Nabriva Therapeutics US, Inc; 2019.

LEFLUNOMIDE

Immunologic (Antirheumatic)

PREGNANCY RECOMMENDATION: *Human Data Suggest Low Risk—Animal Data Suggest Risk

BREASTFEEDING RECOMMENDATION: Potential Toxicity

PREGNANCY SUMMARY

Numerous reports describing the use of leflunomide in human pregnancy have been located. Leflunomide exposure in over 750 periconceptual and first-trimester exposures identified a major malformation rate of about 3.6%, many of which underwent a washout procedure. In addition, no pattern to the congenital defects was seen. The drug will probably cross the placenta, so some fetal exposure will likely occur. However, this human pregnancy experience needs further study. Embryofetal toxicity with malformations was observed in two animal species at doses of less than 10 times the RHD. Based on these animal studies and the drug's mechanism of action, the manufacturer recommends that women with reproductive potential use effective contraception during treatment until teriflunomide (the active metabolite) concentrations are below 20 mcg/mL. *Because it may take up to 2 years to reach plasma levels below 20 mcg/mL of the active metabolite, the manufacturer has developed a drug elimination procedure in the event that a woman taking leflunomide becomes pregnant. It is also recommended that all women of childbearing potential undergo this accelerated elimination procedure after stopping leflunomide treatment. This is consistent with the American College of Rheumatology (ACR) guidelines that recommend leflunomide be discontinued 24 months prior to conception. A cholestyramine washout is also recommended if there are detectable levels prior to or once pregnancy is confirmed. There is a registry that monitors pregnancy outcomes in women exposed to leflunomide during pregnancy. For more information, health care providers or patients are encouraged to contact 1-877-311-8972. Leflunomide carries a boxed warning regarding embryofetal toxicity and hepatotoxicity.

BREASTFEEDING SUMMARY

No reports describing the use of leflunomide during human lactation have been located. The drug will probably appear in breast milk, so some infant exposure will likely occur. However, due to a concern for potential serious adverse effects that might be seen in a breastfed infant, the manufacturer recommends that women not breastfeed while being treated with this drug. A washout period (described above in the Pregnancy Summary) may be indicated. If the clinical decision is to use this drug while breastfeeding, the infant should be monitored for the most common reported adult side effects of nausea (leading to irritability), diarrhea, rash, reflux, and abnormal liver function tests.

References

1. Prescribing Information. Arava. Sanofi-Aventis Pharmaceuticals; 2022.
2. Chambers CD, Johnson DL, Macaraeg GR, Jones KL. Pregnancy outcome following early gestational exposure to leflunomide: the OTIS rheumatoid in pregnancy study (abstract). *Pharmacoepidemiol Drug Saf*. 2004;13: S126-S127.
3. Chakravarty EF, Sanchez-Yamamoto D, Bush TM. The use of disease modifying antirheumatic drugs in women with rheumatoid arthritis of childbearing age: a survey of practice patterns and pregnancy outcomes. *J Rheumatol*. 2003;30:241-246.
4. De Santis M, Straface G, Cavaliere A, et al. Paternal and maternal exposure to leflunomide: pregnancy and neonatal outcome. *Ann Rheum Dis*. 2005; 64:1096-1097.
5. Neville CE, McNally J. Maternal exposure to leflunomide associated with blindness and cerebral palsy. *Rheumatology*. 2007;46:1506.
6. Paulus W, Schloemp S, Sterzik K. The use of leflunomide in fertile patients with rheumatoid arthritis [abstract]. *Reprod Toxicol*. 2006;22:28.
7. Kraemer B, Abele H, Hahn M, et al. A successful pregnancy in a patient with Takayasu's arteritis. *Hypertens Pregnancy*. 2008;27:247-252.
8. Heine K, Poets CF. A pair of twins born after maternal exposure to leflunomide. *J Perinatol*. 2008;28:841-842.
9. Hajdyla-Banas I, Banas T, Rydz-Stryszowska I, et al. Pregnancy course and neonatal outcome after exposure to leflunomide–2 cases report and review of literature. *Przegl Lek*. 2009;66:1069-1071.
10. Sayarlioglu M, Sahin M, Cetin GY, Avan R, Cerit M. Maternal exposure to leflunomide and methotrexate in a patient with adult-onset Still's disease. *Rheumatology (Oxford)*. 2010;49:1787-1789.
11. Chambers CD, Johnson DL, Robinson LK, et al; The Organizations of Teratology Information Specialists Collaborative Research Group. Birth outcomes in women who have taken leflunomide during pregnancy. *Arthritis Rheum*. 2010;62:1494-1503.
12. Cassina M, Johnson DL, Robinson LK, et al; Organization of Teratology Information Specialists Collaborative Research Group. Pregnancy outcome in women exposed to leflunomide before or during pregnancy. *Arthritis Rheum*. 2012;64:2085-2094.
13. Karadag O, Kilic L, Erbil AA, et al. Pregnancy outcomes of rheumatic patients with pre/peri gestational leflunomide exposure. *Ann Rheum Dis*. 2013; 72:A896-A897.
14. Berard A, Zhao J, Shui I, Colilla S. Leflunomide use during pregnancy and the risk of adverse pregnancy outcomes. *Ann Rheum Dis*. 2018;77:500-509.
15. Pfaller B, Pupco A, Leibson T, et al. A critical review of the reproductive safety of leflunomide. *Clin Rheumatol*. 2020;39:607-612.
16. Henson LJ, Afsar S, Davenport L, et al. Pregnancy outcomes in patients treated with leflunomide, the parent compound of the multiple sclerosis drug teriflunomide. *Reprod Toxicol*. 2020;95:45-50.
17. Sammaritano LR, Bermas BL, Chakravarty EE, et al. 2020 American College of Rheumatology guideline for the management of reproductive health in rheumatic and musculoskeletal diseases. *Arthritis Care Res*. 2020;72: 461-488.
18. Alothman R, Yeung J, Waterman E, et al. Leflunomide exposure through second trimester of pregnancy: a case report. *Birth Defects Res*. 2023;115: 1566-1569.

LEMBOREXANT

Miscellaneous (Orexin Receptor Antagonist—Insomnia)

PREGNANCY RECOMMENDATION: No Human Data—Animal Data Suggest Low Risk

BREASTFEEDING RECOMMENDATION: Potential Toxicity

PREGNANCY SUMMARY

No reports describing the use of lemborexant in human pregnancy have been located. The drug will probably cross the placenta, so some fetal exposure will likely occur. Therefore, the absence of human pregnancy experience prevents a complete assessment of the embryofetal risk. Animal data did not show any embryofetal toxicity. Using this drug during pregnancy should be based on the pros and cons of the mother's clinical need for treatment versus any potential fetal risk that might occur from exposure. The drug is a controlled substance (Schedule IV) and has the risk for misuse, but does not appear to produce dependence. There have been reports of sleep paralysis (an inability to move or speak for up to several minutes during sleep-wake transitions), hallucinations, and complex sleep behaviors (sleep-walking, sleep-driving, and engaging in other activities while not fully awake) in some patients using this drug. There is a pregnancy exposure registry that monitors pregnancy outcomes in women using lemborexant. Health care providers are encouraged to call the Dayvigo Pregnancy Registry at 1-888-274-2378.

BREASTFEEDING SUMMARY

Lemborexant probably enters breast milk. Breastfeeding while using this drug should be based on the mother's clinical need for treatment. If used, the infant should be monitored for the most common reported adult side effect of sedation.

Reference

1. Prescribing Information. Dayvigo. Eisai, Inc; 2019.

LENACAPAVIR

Antiretroviral (Capsid Inhibitor)

PREGNANCY RECOMMENDATION: No Human Data—Animal Data Suggest Low Risk (Maternal Benefit May Outweigh Any Embryofetal Risk)

BREASTFEEDING RECOMMENDATION: *Contraindicated

PREGNANCY SUMMARY

No reports describing the use of lenacapavir in human pregnancy have been located. The drug will likely cross the placenta, so some fetal exposure will probably occur. Therefore, the absence of human pregnancy experience prevents a complete assessment of the embryofetal risk. Animal data did not show any embryofetal toxicity. Using this drug during pregnancy should be based on the pros and cons of the mother's clinical need for treatment versus any potential fetal risk that might occur from exposure. There is a pregnancy exposure registry that monitors pregnancy outcomes in women using this drug. Health care providers are encouraged to call the APR at 1-800-258-4263.

BREASTFEEDING SUMMARY

No reports describing the use of lenacapavir during human lactation have been located. A limited amount of the drug will likely be found in breast milk, so some infant exposure will probably occur. *However, the current Centers for Disease Control and Prevention recommendation is that mothers infected with HIV should not breastfeed their infants in order to reduce the risk of postnatal transmission of the virus to the neonate. In a clinical setting where a mother is not infected with HIV (or in cases where the HIV viral load is negative), the drug by itself is probably compatible. If the clinical decision is to use this drug while breastfeeding, the infant should be monitored for the most common reported adult side effect of nausea (leading to irritability).

Reference

1. Prescribing Information. Sunlenca. Gilead Sciences, Inc; 2022.

LENALIDOMIDE

Antineoplastic (Angiogenesis Inhibitor)

PREGNANCY RECOMMENDATION: *Contraindicated

BREASTFEEDING RECOMMENDATION: Potential Toxicity

PREGNANCY SUMMARY

No reports describing the use of lenalidomide in human pregnancy have been located. The drug will probably cross the placenta, so fetal exposure will likely occur. However, the absence of human pregnancy experience prevents a complete assessment of the embryofetal risk. Embryofetal toxicity with malformations was observed in one animal species at doses of less than 10 times the maximum recommended human dose (MRHD). *As a thalidomide analogue, lenalidomide is contraindicated for use in pregnancy due to thalidomide's known teratogenicity, which was also seen in female monkeys exposed to lenalidomide. Due to this embryofetal risk, lenalidomide is only available through the Lenalidomide REMS program. Patients must comply with the REMS program, which requires that females with reproductive potential who are taking lenalidomide must agree to abstain (continuously) from heterosexual intercourse or use two forms of effective contraception during treatment and for at least 4 weeks before and after therapy. They also recommend that males with female partners of reproductive potential use condoms during treatment and for at least 4 weeks before and after therapy. There is a pregnancy exposure registry that monitors pregnancy outcomes in women exposed to lenalidomide during pregnancy. For more information, health care providers or patients are encouraged to contact the MedWatch program at 1-800-FDA-1088 and the REMS call center at 1-888-423-5436. Lenalidomide carries a boxed warning regarding this embryofetal toxicity risk.

BREASTFEEDING SUMMARY

No reports describing the use of lenalidomide during human lactation have been located. The drug will probably appear in breast milk, so infant exposure will likely occur. Due to a concern for potential serious adverse effects that might be seen in a breastfed infant, the manufacturer recommends that women not breastfeed while being treated with this drug. However, if the clinical decision is to use this drug while breastfeeding, the infant should be monitored for the most common reported adult side effects of nausea, arthralgia, itching, and back pain (all leading to irritability), rash, diarrhea, constipation, fatigue (lethargy), fever, and peripheral swelling.

Reference

1. Prescribing Information. Revlimid. Bristol Myers Squibb; 2023.

LENIOLISIB

Antimetabolic (Kinase Inhibitor)

PREGNANCY RECOMMENDATION: **No Human Data—Animal Data Suggest Potential Risk**

BREASTFEEDING RECOMMENDATION: **Potential Toxicity**

PREGNANCY SUMMARY

No reports describing the use of leniolisib in human pregnancy have been located. The drug will likely cross the placenta, so some fetal exposure will probably occur. Therefore, the absence of human pregnancy experience prevents a complete assessment of the embryofetal risk. Animal data showed embryofetal toxicity at doses that also produced maternal toxicity. However, based on these animal studies, the manufacturer recommends that women with reproductive potential use effective contraception during treatment and for 1 week after the last dose. Nevertheless, using this drug during pregnancy should be based on the pros and cons of the mother's clinical need for treatment versus any potential fetal risk that might occur from exposure.

BREASTFEEDING SUMMARY

No reports describing the use of leniolisib during human lactation have been located. The drug will likely be excreted into breast milk, so some infant exposure will probably occur. Due to the concern for potential serious adverse effects that might be seen in a breastfed infant, the manufacturer recommends that women not breastfeed while being treated with this drug and for at least 1 week after the last dose. Nevertheless, breastfeeding while using this drug should be based on the mother's clinical need for treatment. If used, the infant should be monitored for the most common reported adult side effects of headache (leading to irritability), sinusitis, and atopic dermatitis (see PI).

Reference

1. Prescribing Information. Joenja. Pharming Technologies B.V.; 2023.

LENVATINIB

Antineoplastic (Kinase Inhibitor)

PREGNANCY RECOMMENDATION: **No Human Data—Animal Data Suggest Risk**

BREASTFEEDING RECOMMENDATION: **Potential Toxicity**

PREGNANCY SUMMARY

No reports describing the use of lenvatinib in human pregnancy have been located. Some amount of the drug may cross the placenta, so fetal exposure will likely occur. However, the absence of human pregnancy experience prevents a complete assessment of the embryofetal risk. Embryofetal toxicity with malformations was observed in two animal species at doses of less than 10 times the RHD. Based on animal studies and the drug's mechanism of action, the manufacturer recommends that women with reproductive potential use effective contraception during treatment and for 30 days after the last dose. Nevertheless, using this drug during pregnancy should be based on the pros and cons of the mother's clinical need for treatment versus any potential fetal risk that might occur from exposure. Hypertension has been reported in patients treated with this drug. If used, blood pressure should be monitored. There is a registry for women who are pregnant and have cancer. For more information, women and health care providers are encouraged to contact the Cancer and Pregnancy Registry at 1-877-635-4499.

BREASTFEEDING SUMMARY

No reports describing the use of lenvatinib during human lactation have been located. Some amount of the drug may be excreted into breast milk, so infant exposure will likely occur. However, due to the concern for potential serious adverse effects that might be seen in a breastfed infant, the manufacturer recommends that women not breastfeed while being treated with lenvatinib and for at least 1 week after the last dose. Nevertheless, breastfeeding while using this drug should be based on the mother's clinical need for treatment versus any potential infant risks that might occur. If used, the infant should be monitored for the most common reported adult side effects of nausea, headache, abdominal pain, joint pain, and muscle pain (all leading to irritability), high blood pressure, lethargy, diarrhea, decreased appetite (follow infant growth), flushing, and vomiting.

Reference

1. Prescribing Information. Lenvima. Eisai, Inc; 2023.

LETERMOVIR

Antiviral (Cytomegalovirus)

PREGNANCY RECOMMENDATION: No Human Data—Animal Data Suggest Low Risk

BREASTFEEDING RECOMMENDATION: Probably Compatible

PREGNANCY SUMMARY

No reports describing the use of letermovir in human pregnancy have been located. An ex vivo placental perfusion study demonstrated that the drug will cross the placenta (in small amounts). Therefore, some fetal exposure will probably occur. However, the absence of human pregnancy experience prevents a complete assessment of the embryofetal risk. In developed countries, congenital cytomegalovirus (CMV) is the most common nongenetic cause for fetal malformations. A study that analyzed trophoblastic tissue infected with CMV showed that letermovir inhibited CMV replication without damage to the trophoblastic cells. Therefore, this drug may be evaluated in the future as a potential prevention or treatment of CMV in pregnancy. In animal studies, at doses that did not produce maternal toxicity, embryofetal toxicity was not found. Using this drug during pregnancy should be based on the pros and cons of the mother's clinical need for treatment versus any potential fetal risk that might occur from exposure.

BREASTFEEDING SUMMARY

No reports describing the use of letermovir in human lactation have been located. Some amount of the drug is probably found in breast milk. Breastfeeding while using this drug should be based on the mother's clinical need for treatment. If used, the infant should be monitored for the most common reported adult side effects of abdominal pain, headache, and nausea (all leading to irritability), diarrhea, vomiting, peripheral edema, lethargy, and cough.

References

1. Prescribing Information. Prevymis. Merck Sharp & Dohme, LLC; 2022.
2. Bardon VF, Peytavin G, Le MP, et al. Placental transfer of letermovir & maribavir in the ex vivo human cotyledon perfusion model. New perspectives for in utero treatment of congenital cytomegalovirus infection. *PLoS One*. 2020:15:e0232140.
3. Hamilton ST, Marschall M, Rawlinson WD. Investigational antiviral therapy models for the prevention and treatment of congenital cytomegalovirus infection during pregnancy. *Antimicrob Agents Chemother*. 2021;65:e01627-20.

LETIBOTULINUMTOXINA

Toxins (Botulinum)

PREGNANCY RECOMMENDATION: No Human Data and No Relevant Animal Data

BREASTFEEDING RECOMMENDATION: Probably Compatible

PREGNANCY SUMMARY

No reports describing the use of letibotulinumtoxinA in human pregnancy have been located. An analysis of data regarding onabotulinumtoxinA from the Allergan Global Safety Database described a total of 195 prospective pregnancies resulting in 197 newborns. Most of these exposures occurred preconception or in the first trimester (before pregnancy was known). After eliminating 13 elective terminations, there were 32 (17.4%) spontaneous abortions and 152 live births. Of the live births, there was one major and two minor anomalies (2.0%). These rates fall within the expected range for spontaneous abortion and birth defects in the United States. Botulinum toxin type A has not been detected in the systemic circulation following intramuscular (IM) or intradermal administration. However, it has been found in breast milk (described below in Breastfeeding Summary), which suggests that some amount of the toxin may enter the maternal bloodstream in some cases and possibly cross the placenta . Regardless, based on the very low levels detected any amount present at the placental interface would likely lead to negligible amounts that cross the placenta. Animal reproduction studies with letibotulinumtoxinA did produce some embryofetal toxicity and malformations in one species at doses of less than 10 times the RHD, but injections occurred daily for 12 days (normal human administration is every 3 months) and maternal toxicity occurred. Using this drug during pregnancy should be based on the pros and cons of the mother's clinical need for treatment versus any potential fetal risk that might occur from exposure. In many instances, treatment of glabellar lines can be postponed until after pregnancy is completed.

BREASTFEEDING SUMMARY

No reports have been located that describe the use of letibotulinumtoxinA during human lactation. Two reports have been located that have evaluated breast milk for the presence of a different botulinum toxin type A in seven breastfeeding women. In two women, the toxin was not detected (lower limit of detection was 46 pg/mL for these two patients). In the other five women, the toxin was detected with a peak level of 747 pg/mL in one mother's breast milk and 422 pg/mL in a second mother's breast milk. The other three cases had peak levels all below 50 pg/mL. Using the highest peak level obtained, the infant would receive about 112 ng/kg/d. However, because these toxins are large proteins, if they were to be ingested through breastfeeding, they would probably be digested in the infant's gastrointestinal tract and not be absorbed. Therefore, breastfeeding while using this drug should be based on the mother's clinical need for treatment versus any potential infant risks that might occur. If used, the infant should be monitored for the most common reported adult side effect of headache (leading to irritability). In many instances, treatment of glabellar lines can be postponed until after breastfeeding is completed.

References

1. Prescribing Information. Letybo. Hugel; 2024.
2. Tsui JKC. Botulinum toxin as a therapeutic agent. *Pharmacol Ther*. 1996; 72:13-24.
3. Hart LG, Dixon RL, Long JP, Mackay B. Studies using clostridium botulinum toxin—type A. *Toxicol Appl Pharmacol*. 1965;7:84-89.
4. Brin MF, Kirby RS, Slavotinek A, et al. Pregnancy outcomes in patients exposed to onabotulinumtoxinA treatment: a cumulative 29-year safety update. *Neurology*. 2023;101:e103-e113.
5. Trivedi MK, Kroumpouzos G, Murase JE. A review of the safety of cosmetic procedures during pregnancy and lactation. *Int J Womens Dermatol*. 2017;3:6-10.

L

LETROZOLE

Antineoplastic (Aromatase Inhibitor)

PREGNANCY RECOMMENDATION: Limited Human Data—Animal Data Suggest Risk

BREASTFEEDING RECOMMENDATION: Potential Toxicity

PREGNANCY SUMMARY

No reports describing the use of letrozole in human pregnancy have been located. However, the manufacturer states that in postmarketing reports, letrozole use during pregnancy has resulted in spontaneous abortions and congenital birth defects (no further information supplied). The drug will probably cross the placenta, so some fetal exposure will likely occur. However, this limited human pregnancy experience prevents a complete assessment of the embryofetal risk. Embryofetal toxicity with malformations was observed in two animal species at doses of less than 10 times the RHD. Based on animal studies and the drug's mechanism of action, the manufacturer recommends that women with reproductive potential use effective contraception during treatment and for 3 weeks after the last dose. Nevertheless, using this drug during pregnancy should be based on the pros and cons of the mother's clinical need for treatment versus any potential fetal risk that might occur from exposure. There is a registry for women who are pregnant and have cancer. For more information, women and health care providers are encouraged to contact the Cancer and Pregnancy Registry at 1-877-635-4499.

BREASTFEEDING SUMMARY

No reports describing the use of letrozole during human lactation have been located. The drug will probably appear in breast milk, so some infant exposure will likely occur. However, due to a concern for potential serious adverse effects that might be seen in a breastfed infant, the manufacturer recommends that women not breastfeed while being treated with this drug and for at least 3 weeks after the last dose. Nevertheless, breastfeeding while using this drug should be based on the mother's clinical need for treatment versus any potential infant risks that might occur. If used, the infant should be monitored for the most common reported adult side effects of hot flashes, headache, bone, joint, and musculoskeletal pain (all leading to irritability), flushing, lethargy, peripheral edema, elevated cholesterol, and sweating.

References

1. Prescribing Information. Femara. Novartis Pharmaceuticals; 2020.
2. American College of Obstetricians and Gynecologists. Polycystic ovary syndrome. ACOG Practice Bulletin No. 194. *Obstet Gynecol*. 2018;131:e157-e171.
3. Mitwally MF, Biljan MM, Casper RF. Pregnancy outcome after the use of an aromatase inhibitor for ovarian stimulation. *Am J Obstet Gynecol*. 2005;192:381-386.
4. Thatcher SS, Jackson EM. Pregnancy outcome in infertile patients with polycystic ovary syndrome who were treated with metformin. *Fertil Steril*. 2006;85:1002-1009.
5. Tulandi T, Martin J, Al-Fadhli R, et al. Congenital malformations among 911 newborns conceived after infertility treatment with letrozole or clomiphene citrate. *Fertil Steril*. 2006;85:1761-1765.
6. Dickerson RD, Pinto AB, Putman JM, Lee-Messinger JR. Use of letrozole in polycystic ovary syndrome patients resistant to clomiphene (abstract). *Obstet Gynecol*. 2006;107(suppl):41S.
7. Forman R, Gill S, Moretti M, et al. Fetal safety of letrozole and clomiphene citrate for ovulation induction. *J Obstet Gynaecol Can*. 2007;29:668-671.
8. Badawy A, Shokeir T, Allam FA, Abdelhady H. Pregnancy outcome after ovulation induction with aromatase inhibitors or clomiphene citrate in unexplained infertility. *Acta Obstet Gynecol Scand*. 2009;88:187-191.
9. Hashim HA, Shokeir T, Badawy A. Letrozole versus combined metformin and clomiphene citrate for ovulation induction in clomiphene-resistant women with polycystic ovary syndrome: a randomized controlled trial. *Fertil Steril*. 2010;94:1405-1409.
10. Kamath MS, Aleyamma TK, Chandy A, George K. Aromatase inhibitors in women with clomiphene citrate resistance: a randomized, double-blind, placebo-controlled trial. *Fertil Steril*. 2010;94:2857-2859.
11. Badawy A, Elnashar A, Totongy M. Clomiphene citrate or aromatase inhibitors combined with gonadotropins for superovulation in women undergoing intrauterine inseminations: a prospective randomised trial. *J Obstet Gynaecol*. 2010;30:617-621.
12. Zeinalzadeh M, Basirat Z, Esmailpour M. Efficacy of letrozole in ovulation induction compared to that of clomiphene citrate in patients with polycystic ovarian syndrome. *J Reprod Med*. 2010;55:36-40.
13. Akar ME, Johnston-MacAnanny EB, Carrillo AJ, et al. The pregnancy outcome of retrieved excess eggs collected during selective follicular reduction from patients with three or more preovulatory follicles undergoing controlled ovarian stimulation and IUI. *Hum Reprod*. 2010;25:2931.
14. Wagman I, Levin I, Kapustiansky R, et al. Clomiphene citrate vs. letrozole for cryopreserved-thawed embryo transfer; a randomized, controlled trial. *J Reprod Med*. 2010;55:134-138.
15. Abdellah MS. Reproductive outcome after letrozole versus laparoscopic ovarian drilling for clomiphene-resistant polycystic ovary syndrome. *Int J Gynecol Obstet*. 2011;113:218-221.
16. Requena A, Herrero J, Landeras J, et al; Reproductive Endocrinology Interest Group of the Spanish Society of Fertility. Use of letrozole in assisted reproduction: a systematic review and meta-analysis. *Human Reprod Update*. 2008;14:571-582.
17. Elizur SE, Tulandi T. Drugs in infertility and fetal safety. *Fertil Steril*. 2008; 89:1595-1602.
18. Gill SK, Moretti M, Koren G. Is the use of letrozole to induce ovulation teratogenic? *Can Fam Physician*. 2008;54:353-354.
19. Eckmann KR, Kockler DR. Aromatase inhibitors for ovulation and pregnancy in polycystic ovary syndrome. *Ann Pharmacother*. 2009;43:1338-1346.
20. Polyzos NP, Tzioras S, Badawy AM, et al. Aromatase inhibitors for female infertility: a systematic review of the literature. *Reprod Biomed Online*. 2009; 19:456-471.
21. Pritts EA. Letrozole for ovulation induction and controlled ovarian hyperstimulation. *Curr Opin Obstet Gynecol*. 2010;22:289-294.
22. Franik S, Eltrop SM, Kremer JA, et al. Aromatase inhibitors (letrozole) for subfertile women with polycystic ovary syndrome. *Cochrane Database Syst Rev*. 2018;5:CD101287.
23. Pundir J, Achilli C, Bhide P, et al. Risk of foetal harm with letrozole use in fertility treatment: a systematic review and meta-analysis. *Hum Reprod Update*. 2021;27:474-485.
24. Baradwan S, Al-Shalhoub F, Alshahrani MS, et al. Effects of letrozole alone or in combination with gonadotropins on ovulation induction and clinical pregnancy in women with polycystic ovarian syndrome: a systematic review and meta-analysis of randomized controlled trials. *Hormones (Athens)*. 2024;23:497-508.

L

LEUCOVORIN CALCIUM

Antidote/Vitamin

PREGNANCY RECOMMENDATION: Limited Human Data—Likely Low Risk

BREASTFEEDING RECOMMENDATION: Compatible

PREGNANCY SUMMARY

No reports describing the use of leucovorin in human pregnancy have been located. Three reports describe the use of folinic acid (which is the same as leucovorin) in pregnancy. No increase in adverse effects was seen in 60 pregnant women who received a supplement of folinic acid during pregnancy. Some amount of the drug will probably cross the placenta, so fetal exposure will likely occur. Folic acid crosses the placenta. No animal reproduction studies have been conducted. Using this drug during pregnancy should be based on the pros and cons of the mother's clinical need for treatment versus any potential fetal risk that might occur from exposure.

BREASTFEEDING SUMMARY

No reports describing the use of leucovorin during human lactation have been located. Some amount of the drug may be excreted into breast milk, so infant exposure will likely occur. If the clinical decision is to use this drug while breastfeeding, the infant should be monitored for the most common reported adult side effect of urticaria (leading to irritability).

References

1. Prescribing Information. Leucovorin calcium. Fresenius Kabi USA, LLC; 2022.
2. Prescribing Information. Leucovorin calcium. Teva Pharmaceuticals USA, Inc; 2019.
3. Scott JM. Folinic acid in megaloblastic anaemia of pregnancy. *Br Med J*. 1957:2:270-272.
4. Chanarin I, Rothman D. Response to folic and folinic acid in megaloblastic anaemia in pregnancy. *J Obstet Gynaecol Br Commonw*. 1965;72:374-375.
5. Bumrungpert A, Pavadhgul P, Piromsawasdi T, Mozafari MR. Efficacy and safety of ferrous bisglycinate and folinic acid in the control of iron deficiency in pregnant women: a randomized, controlled trial. *Nutrients*. 2022;14:452.

LEUPROLIDE

Antineoplastic/Miscellaneous (Gonadotropin-Releasing Hormone Agonist)

PREGNANCY RECOMMENDATION: *Contraindicated

BREASTFEEDING RECOMMENDATION: *Contraindicated

PREGNANCY SUMMARY

No published reports describing the use of leuprolide in human pregnancy have been located. A limited amount of the drug may cross the placenta, so fetal exposure may occur. However, the absence of human pregnancy experience prevents a complete assessment of the embryofetal risk. Embryofetal toxicity with malformations was observed in one animal species at doses less than the RHD. *Nevertheless, the drug should not be used during pregnancy because of its approved uses (prostate cancer, endometriosis, uterine fibroids, and precocious puberty). The manufacturer recommends that women with reproductive potential use effective contraception during treatment. However, the drug is used off-label for infertility, so inadvertent pregnancy exposure may occur.

BREASTFEEDING SUMMARY

No reports describing the use of leuprolide during human lactation have been located. The drug may be excreted into breast milk, so some infant exposure may occur. *Nevertheless, the drug should not be used while breastfeeding because of its approved uses (prostate cancer, endometriosis, uterine fibroids, and precocious puberty). The manufacturer recommends that women should not breastfeed during treatment with this drug.

References

1. Prescribing Information. Lupron depot. AbbVie; 2023.
2. Chetkowski RJ, Kruse LR, Nass TE. Improved pregnancy outcome with the addition of leuprolide acetate to gonadotropins for in vitro fertilization. *Fertil Steril*. 1989;52:250-255.
3. Wilshire GB, Emmi AM, Gagliardi CC, Weiss G. Gonadotropin-releasing hormone agonist administration in early human pregnancy is associated with normal outcomes. *Fertil Steril*. 1993;60:980-983.

L

LEVALBUTEROL

Respiratory (β_2-Agonist)

PREGNANCY RECOMMENDATION: No Human Data—Animal Data Suggest Low Risk

BREASTFEEDING RECOMMENDATION: Probably Compatible

PREGNANCY SUMMARY

No reports describing the specific use of levalbuterol in human pregnancy have been located. The National Asthma Education and Prevention Program (NAEPP) expert panel reviewed 6 studies involving 1,599 women who had taken β_2-agonists during pregnancy. The panel concluded that these drugs, as a class, are considered low risk for use during pregnancy. Levalbuterol will probably cross the placenta, so fetal exposure will likely occur. However, the absence of human pregnancy experience with levalbuterol prevents a complete assessment of the embryofetal risk. Animal data did not show any embryofetal toxicity in two animal species at doses of more than 10 times the maximum recommended human daily inhalation dose (MRHDID). ACOG states that inhaled short-acting β_2-agonists are the rescue therapy of choice in treating asthma during pregnancy. While inhaled albuterol is the first choice for this use, other agents may be appropriate. Neonatal hyperglycemia may be seen when high doses of β-agonists are given within the last 48 hours prior to delivery. There is a pregnancy exposure registry that monitors pregnancy outcomes in women exposed to asthma medications during pregnancy. Health care providers or patients are encouraged to call 877-311-8972 for more information about patient enrollment in the Organization of Teratology Information Specialists (OTIS) study.

BREASTFEEDING SUMMARY

No reports describing the use of levalbuterol during human lactation have been located. The drug will probably appear in breast milk, so infant exposure will likely occur. If the clinical decision is to use this drug while breastfeeding, the infant should be monitored for the most common reported pediatric side effects of headache (leading to irritability), tachycardia, and fever.

References

1. Prescribing Information. Xopenex HFA. Oak Pharmaceuticals, Inc; 2018.
2. National Heart, Lung, and Blood Institute; National Asthma Education and Prevention Program Asthma and Pregnancy Working Group. NAEPP Expert Panel

Report. Managing asthma during pregnancy: recommendations for pharmacologic treatment-2004 update. *J Allergy Clin Immunol*. 2005;115:34-46.
3. American College of Obstetricians and Gynecologists. ACOG practice bulletin no. 90: asthma in pregnancy. *Obstet Gynecol*. 2008;111:457-464.
4. Global Initiative for Asthma. Global strategy for asthma management and prevention. Published 2023. Updated July 2023. Accessed January 29, 2024. https://ginasthma.org/wp-content/uploads/2023/07/GINA-2023-Full-report-23_07_06-WMS.pdf

LEVETIRACETAM

Central Nervous System (Antiseizure)

PREGNANCY RECOMMENDATION: Human Data Suggest Low Risk—Animal Data Suggest Risk

BREASTFEEDING RECOMMENDATION: Probably Compatible

PREGNANCY SUMMARY

Several reports and pregnancy registries describing the use of levetiracetam have been located. No significant evidence for an increased risk of congenital anomalies, spontaneous abortion, or neurodevelopmental abnormalities was seen in more than 1,000 exposures. The drug crosses the placenta, so fetal exposure will occur. Embryofetal toxicity was observed in two animal species at doses less than 10 times the RHD. Using this drug during pregnancy should be based on the pros and cons of the mother's clinical need for treatment versus any potential fetal risk that might occur from exposure. There is a pregnancy exposure registry that monitors pregnancy outcomes in women exposed to antiseizure drugs during pregnancy. For more information, health care providers or patients are encouraged to contact the Antiepileptic Drug Pregnancy Registry by calling 888-233-2334.

L

BREASTFEEDING SUMMARY

Several reports describing the use of levetiracetam during human lactation have been located. Maternal blood levels to breast milk levels are about equal. The drug has been found in the serum of some infants. In one case, the infant serum level was 13% of the maternal blood level. There are cases where the breast milk and infant serum levels were undetectable. Sedation and poor feeding were reported in some breastfed infants. Levetiracetam was found to be excreted into human breast milk, so infant exposure will occur. If the clinical decision is to use this drug while breastfeeding, the infant should be monitored for sedation and poor feeding along with the most common reported adult side effects of somnolence and irritability.

References

1. Prescribing Information. Levetiracetam ER. Westminster. Pharmaceuticals, LLC; 2024.
2. Dooley M, Plosker GL. Levetiracetam. A review of its adjunctive use in the management of partial onset seizures. *Drugs*. 2000;60:871-893.
3. Ten Berg K, Samren EB, van Oppen AC, et al. Levetiracetam use and pregnancy outcome. *Reprod Toxicol*. 2005;20:175-178.
4. The Lamotrigine Pregnancy Registry. Final report: 1 September 1992 through 31 March 2010. GlaxoSmithKline; 2010.
5. Ylikotila P, Ketola R, Timonen S, et al. Early pregnancy cerebral venous thrombosis and status epilepticus treated with levetiracetam and lacosamide throughout pregnancy. *Reprod Toxicol*. 2015;57:204-206.
6. Tomson T, Battino D, Bonizzoni E, et al. Antiepileptic drugs and intrauterine death. A prospective observational study from EURAP. *Neurology*. 2015; 85:580-588.
7. Chaudhry SA, Jong G, Koren G. The fetal safety of levetiracetam: a systematic review. *Reprod Toxicol*. 2014;46:40-45.
8. Johannessen SI, Helde G, Brodtkorb. Levetiracetam concentrations in serum and in breast milk at birth and during lactation. *Epilepsia*. 2005;46:775-777.
9. Tomson T, Palm R, Kallen K, et al. Pharmacokinetics of levetiracetam during pregnancy, delivery, in the neonatal period, and lactation. *Epilepsia*. 2007; 48:1111-1116.
10. Bromley RL, Calderbank R, Cheyne CP, et al. UK epilepsy and pregnancy register. *Neurology*. 2016;87:1943-1953.
11. Arkilo D, Hanna J, Dickens D, et al. Pregnancy and neurodevelopmental outcomes with in-utero antiepileptic agent exposure. A pilot study. *Eur J Paediatr Neurol*. 2015;19:37-40.
12. Shallcross R, Bromley RL, Cheyne CP, et al; Liverpool and Manchester Neurodevelopment Group; UK Epilepsy and Pregnancy Register. In utero exposure to levetiracetam vs valproate: development and language at 3 years of age. *Neurology*. 2014;82:213-221.
13. Kramer G, Hosli I, Glanzmann R, Holzgreve W. Levetiracetam accumulation in human breast milk [Abstract]. *Epilepsia*. 2002;43:105.
14. Nathalie P, Aurore G, Nathalie B, et al. Long-term follow-up of infants exposed to levetiracetam during breastfeeding: comparison to a control group [Abstract]. *Birth Defects Res A Clin Mol Teratol*. 2014;100:537-538.
15. Campbell E, Kennedy F, Russell A, et al. Malformation risks of antiepileptic drug monotherapies in pregnancy: updated results from the UK and Ireland epilepsy and pregnancy registers. *J Neurol Neurosurg Psychiatry*. 2014;85:1029-1034.
16. Tomson T, Battino D, Bonizzoni E, et al. Comparative risk of major congenital malformations with eight different antiepileptic drugs: a prospective cohort study of the EURAP registry. *Lancet Neurol*. 2018;17:530-538.
17. Holmes LB, Hernandez-Diaz S, Pennell B, et al. Latest study data—through 2023. North American Antiepileptic Drug Pregnancy Registry. Accessed May 19, 2022. https://www.aedpregnancyregistry.org/latest-data/
18. Weston J, Bromley R, Jackson CF, et al. Monotherapy treatment of epilepsy in pregnancy: congenital malformation outcomes in the child. *Cochrane Database Syst Rev*. 2016;11:CD010224.
19. Tomson T, Battino D, Bonizzoni E, et al. Comparative risk of major congenital malformations with eight different antiepileptic drugs: a prospective cohort study of the EURAP registry. *Lancet Neurol*. 2018;17:530-538.
20. Meador KJ, Cohen MJ, Loring DW, et al; Maternal Outcomes and Neurodevelopmental Effects of Antiepileptic Drugs Investigator Group. Two-year-old cognitive outcomes in children of pregnant women with epilepsy in the maternal outcomes and neurodevelopmental effects of antiepileptic drugs study. *JAMA Neurol*. 2021;78:927-936.

LEVOBUNOLOL OPHTHALMIC

Ophthalmic (β-Blocker, Nonselective—Antiglaucoma)

PREGNANCY RECOMMENDATION: No Human Data and No Relevant Animal Data

BREASTFEEDING RECOMMENDATION: Probably Compatible

PREGNANCY SUMMARY

No reports describing the use of levobunolol ophthalmic in human pregnancy have been located. While the amount of systemic absorption is not known, levobunolol is likely minimally absorbed systemically following topical ocular administration. This should significantly limit placental transfer. However, the absence of human pregnancy experience prevents a complete assessment of the embryofetal risk. Embryofetal toxicity was seen in two animal species, but at doses well above 100 times the RHD. Using this drug during pregnancy should be based on the pros and cons of the mother's clinical need for treatment versus any potential fetal risk that might occur from exposure. If used during pregnancy, consider placing pressure over the tear duct in the corner of the eye for at least 1 minute, and then remove any excess solution with absorbent tissue to decrease the amount of drug reaching the systemic circulation even further.

BREASTFEEDING SUMMARY

No reports describing the use of levobunolol during human lactation have been located. While the amount of systemic absorption is not known, levobunolol is likely minimally absorbed systemically following topical ocular administration. This should significantly limit excretion into breast milk. If the clinical decision is to use this drug while breastfeeding, the infant should be monitored for the most common reported adult side effects of decreased heart rate and blood pressure. A method to decrease some systemic absorption with ophthalmic use is described above in the Pregnancy Summary.

Reference

1. Prescribing Information. Levocetirizine dihydrochloride. A-S Medication Solutions; 2020.

L

LEVOCETIRIZINE

Antihistamine (Histamine H_1 Antagonist, Second Generation)

PREGNANCY RECOMMENDATION: No Human Data—Animal Data Suggest Low Risk

BREASTFEEDING RECOMMENDATION: Probably Compatible

PREGNANCY SUMMARY

No reports describing the use of levocetirizine in human pregnancy have been located. The drug will probably cross the placenta, so some infant exposure will likely occur. However, the absence of human pregnancy experience prevents a complete assessment of the embryofetal risk. Animal data did not show any embryofetal toxicity in two species at doses of more than 100 times the RHD. Using this drug during pregnancy should be based on the pros and cons of the mother's clinical need for treatment versus any potential fetal risk that might occur from exposure. ACOG and the American College of Allergy, Asthma and Immunology recommend that first-generation antihistamines (eg, chlorpheniramine or hydroxyzine) be considered first, if antihistamine therapy during pregnancy (especially in the first trimester) is required. The second-generation agents are considered acceptable alternatives if a first-generation antihistamine is not tolerated.

BREASTFEEDING SUMMARY

Two reports have evaluated the levels of levocetirizine in human breast milk. In over 200 lactating women, median breast milk levels were less than 15 ng/mL with calculated RIDs of about 2.7%. Many breast milk samples were undetectable (lower limit of quantification (LLQ) of 0.4 ng/mL). The peak level of all samples was about 70 ng/mL. Breastfeeding while using this drug should be based on the mother's clinical need for treatment versus any potential infant risks that might occur. If used, the infant should be monitored for the most common reported adult side effects of sedation and constipation.

References

1. Prescribing Information. Levocetirizine dihydrochloride. Apotex; 2019.
2. Mazzotta P, Loebstein R, Koren G. Treating allergic rhinitis in pregnancy. Safety considerations. *Drug Saf.* 1999;20:361-375.
3. Horak F, Stubner UP. Comparative tolerability of second-generation antihistamines. *Drug Saf.* 1999;20:385-401.
4. Joint committee of the American College of Obstetricians and Gynecologists (ACOG) and the American College of Allergy, Asthma and Immunology

(ACAAI). Position statement. The use of newer asthma and allergy medications during pregnancy. *Ann Allergy Asthma Immunol*. 2000;84:475-480.
5. Wegler C, Saleh A, Lindqvist A, et al. Simple and rapid quantification of cetirizine, venlafaxine, and O-desmethylvenlafaxine in human breast milk, and metformin in human milk and plasma with UHPLC-MS/MS. *J Chromatogr B Analyt Technol Biomed Life Sci*. 2022;1205:123340.
6. Nordeng H, Wegler C, Lindqvist A, et al. Transfer of cetirizine/levocetirizine into human breast milk and estimation of drug exposure to infants through breastfeeding: a human lactation study from the ConcePTION project. *Basic Clin Pharmacol Toxicol*. 2024;134:153-164.

LEVODOPA

Central Nervous System (Anti-Parkinson Agent)

PREGNANCY RECOMMENDATION: Limited Human Data—Animal Data Suggest Risk

BREASTFEEDING RECOMMENDATION: Potential Toxicity

PREGNANCY SUMMARY

Because Parkinson disease is relatively uncommon in women of childbearing age, limited case reports have been located that describe the use of levodopa, with or without carbidopa, in human pregnancy. No adverse outcomes associated with this drug have been observed in a small number of human pregnancies. Levodopa crosses the placenta, so fetal exposure will occur. However, this limited human pregnancy experience prevents a complete assessment of the embryofetal risk. Embryofetal toxicity with malformations was observed in two animal species at doses of less than 10 times the RHD. Using this drug during pregnancy should be based on the pros and cons of the mother's clinical need for treatment versus any potential fetal risk that might occur from exposure.

L

BREASTFEEDING SUMMARY

Two case reports describing the use of levodopa during human lactation found no infant adverse effects. In one patient, the calculated infant dose was less than 1% of the maternal dose. This showed that the drug is excreted into breast milk, so some infant exposure occurs. No adverse infant effects were seen in two cases with breast milk exposure. Levodopa inhibits prolactin release in humans and may suppress lactation. Breastfeeding while using this drug should be based on the mother's clinical need for treatment versus any potential infant risks that might occur. If used, the infant should be monitored for the most common reported adult side effects of nausea (leading to irritability), tremors, and abnormal movements.

References

1. Prescribing Information. Carbidopa and levodopa. Dr. Reddy's Laboratories, Inc; 2024.
2. Staples RE, Mattis PA. Teratology of l-dopa (abstract). *Teratology*. 1973; 8:238.
3. Cotzia GC, Miller ST, Tang LC, Papavila PS. Levodopa, fertility, and longevity. *Science*. 1977;196:549-550.
4. Kitchin KT, DiStefano V. l-Dopa and brown fat hemorrhage in the rat pup. *Toxicol Appl Pharmacol*. 1976;38:251-263.
5. Seybold VS, Miller JW, Lewis PR. Investigation of a dopaminergic mechanism for regulating oxytocin release. *J Pharmacol Exp Ther*. 1978;207:605-610.
6. Allain H, Bentue-Ferrer D, Milon D, et al. Pregnancy and parkinsonism. A case report without problem. *Clin Neuropharmacol*. 1989;12:217-219.
7. Merchant CA, Cohen G, Mytilineou C, et al. Human transplacental transfer of carbidopa/levodopa. *J Neural Transm Park Dis Dement Sect*. 1995;9: 239-242.
8. Cook DG, Klawans HL. Levodopa during pregnancy. *Clin Neuropharmacol*. 1985;8:93-95.
9. Golbe LI. Parkinson's disease and pregnancy. *Neurology*. 1987;37:1245-1249.
10. Ball MC, Sagar HJ. Levodopa in pregnancy. *Mov Disord*. 1995;10:115.
11. Nomoto M, Kaseda S, Iwata S, et al. Levodopa in pregnancy. *Mov Disord*. 1997;12:261.
12. Watanabe T, Matsubara S, Baba Y, et al. Successful management of pregnancy in a patient with Segawa disease: case report and literature review. *J Obstet Gynaecol Res*. 2009;35:562-564.
13. Hagell P, Odin P, Vinge E. Pregnancy in Parkinson' disease: a review of the literature and a case report. *Mov Disord*. 1998;13:34-38.
14. Kupsch A, Oertel WH. Selegiline, pregnancy, and Parkinson's disease. *Mov Disord*. 1998;13:175-194.
15. Thulin PC, Woodward WR, Carter JH, Nutt JG. Levodopa in human breast milk: clinical implications. *Neurology*. 1998;50:1920-1921.
16. von Graeventiz KS, Shulman LM, Revell SP. Levodopa in pregnancy. *Mov Disord*. 1996;11:115-116.
17. Bauherz G. Pregnancy and Parkinson's disease. A case report. *N Trends Clin Neuropharmacol*. 1994;8:142.
18. Lindh J. Short episode of seizures in a newborn of mother treated with levodopa/carbidopa/entacapone and bromocriptine. *Mov Disord*. 2007;22: 1515.
19. De Mari M, Zenzola A, Lamberti P. Antiparkinsonian treatment in pregnancy. *Mov Disord*. 2002;17:428-429.
20. Scott M, Chowdhury M. Pregnancy in Parkinson's disease: unique case report and review of the literature. *Mov Disord*. 2005;20:1078-1079.
21. Pujol-Amat P, Gamissans O, Calaf J, et al. Influence of l-dopa on serum prolactin, human chorionic somatomammotrophin (HCS) and human chorionic gonadotrophin (HCG) during the last trimester of pregnancy. In: Human Prolactin. Proceedings of the International Symposium on Human Prolactin, Brussels, June 12-14, 1973. American Elsevier;1973:316-320.
22. Datta DV, Maheshwari YK, Aggarwal ML. Levodopa in fulminant hepatic failure: preliminary report. *Am J Med Sci*. 1976;272:95-99.
23. Chajek T, Friedman G, Berry EM, Abramsky O. Treatment of acute hepatic encephalopathy with l-dopa. *Postgrad Med J*. 1977;53:262-265.
24. Kaulhausen H, Oney T, Feldmann R, Leyendecker G. Decrease of vascular angiotensin sensitivity by l-dopa during human pregnancy. *Am J Obstet Gynecol*. 1981;140:671-675.
25. Kaulhausen H, Oney T, Leyendecker G. Inhibition of the renin-aldosterone axis and of prolactin secretion during pregnancy by l-dopa. *Br J Obstet Gynaecol*. 1982;89:483-488.
26. Ayalon D, Peyser MR, Toaff R, et al. Effect of l-dopa on galactopoiesis and gonadotropin levels in the inappropriate lactation syndrome. *Obstet Gynecol*. 1974;44:159-170.
27. Zlotnik Y, Giladi N, Hilel A, et al. Levodopa-carbidopa intestinal gel (LCIG) infusion during pregnancy and delivery: first documented case. *Parkinsonism Relat Disord*. 2014;20:1317-1318.

LEVOFLOXACIN

Antibiotic (Fluoroquinolone)

PREGNANCY RECOMMENDATION: Limited Human Data—Animal Data Suggest Potential Risk

BREASTFEEDING RECOMMENDATION: Potential Toxicity

PREGNANCY SUMMARY

Two reports describing the use of levofloxacin in about 150 human pregnancies were located. Only one reported case of first-trimester levofloxacin exposure resulted in a major birth defect. Several studies on fluoroquinolones as a group have been analyzed, and no increase in major birth defects has been found. Early on, there was a question of fluoroquinolones causing bone abnormalities and arthropathy, but larger studies have not found this association. Levofloxacin crosses the human placenta, so fetal exposure occurs. However, this limited human pregnancy experience with levofloxacin prevents a complete assessment of the embryofetal risk. Embryofetal toxicity was observed in one animal species at doses of less than 10 times the RHD. Using this drug during pregnancy should be based on the pros and cons of the mother's clinical need for treatment versus any potential fetal risk that might occur from exposure.

BREASTFEEDING SUMMARY

One report describing the use of levofloxacin during human lactation was located. The drug was excreted into breast milk, producing a peak concentration of 8.2 mcg/mL. The estimated absolute infant dose was 1.23 mg/kg/d based on the highest breast milk level, producing a RID of 10% to 17%. Due to a concern for potential serious adverse effects that might be seen in a breastfed infant, the manufacturer recommends that women not breastfeed while being treated with this drug. If the clinical decision is to use this drug while breastfeeding, the infant should be monitored for possible effects on the gastrointestinal flora (diarrhea, thrush, or diaper rash) along with the most common reported adult side effects of nausea, dizziness, and headache (all leading to irritability), insomnia, and constipation.

References

1. Prescribing Information. Levofloxacin. Hospira, Inc; 2019.
2. Ozyuncu O, Nemutlu E, Katlan D, et al. Maternal and fetal blood levels of moxifloxacin, levofloxacin, cefepime and cefoperazone. *Int J Antimicrob Agents*. 2010;36:175-178.
3. Ozyuncu O, Beksac MS, Nemutlu E, et al. Maternal blood and amniotic fluid levels of moxifloxacin, levofloxacin and cefixime. *J Obstet Gynecol*. 2010;36:484-487.
4. Cahill JB Jr, Bailey EM, Chien S, Johnson GM. Levofloxacin secretion in breast milk: a case report. *Pharmacotherapy*. 2005;25:116-118.
5. Padberg S, Wacker E, Meister R, et al. Observational cohort study of pregnancy outcome after first-trimester exposure to fluoroquinolones. *Antimicrob Agents Chemother*. 2014;58:4392-4398.
6. Muanda FT, Sheehy O, Bérard A. Use of antibiotics during pregnancy and risk of spontaneous abortion. *CMAJ*. 2017;189:E625-E633.
7. Ziv A, Masarwa R, Perlman A, Ziv D, Matok I. Pregnancy outcomes following exposure to quinolone antibiotics—a systematic-review and meta-analysis. *Pharm Res*. 2018;35:109.
8. Yefet E, Schwartz N, Chazan B, Salim R, Romano S, Nachum Z. The safety of quinolones and fluoroquinolones in pregnancy: a meta-analysis. *BJOG*. 2018;125(9):1069-1076.
9. Acar S, Keskin-Arslan E, Erol-Coskun H, et al. Pregnancy outcomes following quinolone and fluoroquinolone exposure during pregnancy: a systematic review and meta-analysis. *Reprod Toxicol*. 2019;85:65-74.
10. Cahill JB Jr, Bailey EM, Chien S, Johnson GM. Levofloxacin secretion in breast milk: a case report. *Pharmacotherapy*. 2005;25:116-118.

LEVOFLOXACIN OPHTHALMIC

Ophthalmic/Antibiotic (Fluoroquinolone)

PREGNANCY RECOMMENDATION: No Human Data—Animal Data Suggest Low Risk

BREASTFEEDING RECOMMENDATION: Probably Compatible

PREGNANCY SUMMARY

No reports describing the use of levofloxacin ophthalmic solution during human pregnancy have been located. While the amount of systemic absorption is not known, levofloxacin is likely minimally absorbed systemically following ocular administration. This should significantly limit placental transfer. However, the absence of human pregnancy experience prevents a complete assessment of the embryofetal risk. Animal data did not show any embryofetal toxicity in one species at more than 10 times the maximum recommended human ophthalmic dose. Using this drug during pregnancy should be based on the pros and cons of the mother's clinical need for treatment versus any potential fetal risk that might occur from exposure. If used during pregnancy, consider placing pressure over the tear duct in the corner of the eye for at least 1 minute, and then remove any excess solution with absorbent tissue to decrease the amount of drug reaching the systemic circulation even further.

BREASTFEEDING SUMMARY

No reports describing the use of levofloxacin ophthalmic during human lactation have been located. While the amount of systemic absorption is not known, levofloxacin is likely minimally absorbed systemically following ocular administration. This should significantly limit excretion into breast milk. If used while breastfeeding, the infant should be monitored for the most common reported adult side effect of headache (leading to irritability). A method to decrease some systemic absorption with ophthalmic use is described above in the Pregnancy Summary.

Reference

1. Prescribing Information. Levofloxacin. Micro Labs Limited; 2019.

LEVOLEUCOVORIN

Antidote (Chemotherapy Rescue Agent)

PREGNANCY RECOMMENDATION: No Human Data and No Relevant Animal Data

BREASTFEEDING RECOMMENDATION: *Potential Toxicity

PREGNANCY SUMMARY

No reports describing the use of levoleucovorin in human pregnancy have been located. Some amount of drug may cross the placenta, so fetal exposure may occur. However, the absence of human pregnancy experience prevents a complete assessment of the embryofetal risk. No animal reproduction studies have been conducted. Levoleucovorin is administered after the use of methotrexate or fluorouracil, both drugs that may lead to embryofetal harm. (See Methotrexate and Fluorouracil for additional information.) However, using this drug during pregnancy should be based on the pros and cons of the mother's clinical need for treatment versus any potential fetal risk that might occur from exposure.

L

BREASTFEEDING SUMMARY

No reports describing the use of levoleucovorin during human lactation have been located. The drug may be excreted into breast milk, so some fetal exposure might occur. *Levoleucovorin is administered after the use of methotrexate or fluorouracil, both of which can be potentially toxic (See Methotrexate and Fluorouracil for additional information). However, if the clinical decision is to use this drug while breastfeeding, the infant should be monitored for the most common reported adult side effects of nausea (leading to irritability), vomiting, and mouth sores.

Reference

1. Prescribing Information. Levoleucovorin. Meitheal Pharmaceuticals; 2020.

LEVORPHANOL

Pain (Opioid)

PREGNANCY RECOMMENDATION: Limited Human Data—No Relevant Animal Data

BREASTFEEDING RECOMMENDATION: Potential Toxicity

PREGNANCY SUMMARY

One first-trimester exposure to levorphanol was reported in the Collaborative Perinatal Project, and no malformations were described at delivery. The drug will probably cross the placenta, so fetal exposure will likely occur. However, this limited human pregnancy experience with levorphanol prevents a complete assessment of the embryofetal risk. Embryofetal toxicity with malformations was observed in one animal species, but at doses of more than 10 times the RHD. Using this drug during pregnancy should be based on the pros and cons of the mother's clinical need for treatment versus any potential fetal risk that might occur from exposure. Levorphanol carries a boxed warning regarding life-threatening respiratory depression and neonatal opioid withdrawal syndrome. The drug is classified as a Schedule II controlled substance with a risk for tolerance, dependence, and misuse.

BREASTFEEDING SUMMARY

No reports describing the use of levorphanol during human lactation have been located. The drug will probably appear in breast milk, so some infant exposure will likely occur. Breastfeeding while using this drug should be based on the mother's clinical need for treatment versus any potential infant risks that might occur. If used, the infant should be monitored for the most common reported adult side effects of excess sedation and respiratory depression. Additionally, withdrawal symptoms can occur in breastfed infants when maternal opioid administration or breastfeeding is abruptly stopped.

Reference

1. Prescribing Information. Levorphanol tartrate. Mallinckrodt Pharmaceuticals; 2021
2. Heinonen OP, Slone D, Shapiro S. *Birth Defects and Drugs in Pregnancy*. Wright PSB; 1983:287.

LEVOTHYROXINE

Endocrine (Thyroid Hormone)

PREGNANCY RECOMMENDATION: Human Data Suggest Compatible

BREASTFEEDING RECOMMENDATION: Compatible

PREGNANCY SUMMARY

The use of levothyroxine in human pregnancy has been well reported in the literature. The drug has not been associated with any increased risk of congenital malformations or miscarriage. Levothyroxine (T_4) crosses the placenta in very small amounts throughout pregnancy (which are clinically insignificant in most instances). No animal reproduction studies have been conducted. ACOG and the American Thyroid Association recommend supplementing with levothyroxine during pregnancy to treat maternal hypothyroidism.

BREASTFEEDING SUMMARY

Several studies describing the use of levothyroxine during human lactation have been located. No reported adverse effects on infants have been described. Levothyroxine is excreted into human breast milk in low amounts. ACOG and the American Thyroid Association recommend using levothyroxine during lactation if the patient has hypothyroidism. If used while breastfeeding, adverse effects on the breastfed infant are not expected.

References

1. Thyroid disease in pregnancy: ACOG Practice Bulletin, Number 223. *Obstet Gynecol*. 2020;135(6):e261-e274.
2. Jafek BW, Small R, Lillian DL. Congenital radioactive-iodine induced stridor and hypothyroidism. *Arch Otolaryngol*. 1974;99:369-371.
3. Alexander EK, Pearce EN, Brent GA, et al. 2017 guidelines of the American thyroid association for the diagnosis and management of thyroid disease during pregnancy and the postpartum. *Thyroid*. 2017;27:315-389.
4. Prescribing Information. Synthroid. AbbVie, Inc; 2022.
5. Grumbach MM, Werner SC. Transfer of thyroid hormone across the human placenta at term. *J Clin Endocrinol Metab*. 1956;16:1392-1395.
6. Kearns JE, Hutson W. Tagged isomers and analogues of thyroxine (their transmission across the human placenta and other studies). *J Nucl Med*. 1963; 4:453-461.
7. Fisher DA, Lehman H, Lackey C. Placental transport of thyroxine. *J Clin Endocrinol Metab*. 1964;24:393-400.
8. Fisher DA, Klein AH. Thyroid development and disorders of thyroid function in the newborn. *N Engl J Med*. 1981;304:702-712.
9. Van Herle AJ, Young RT, Fisher DA, et al. Intrauterine treatment of a hypothyroid fetus. *J Clin Endocrinol Metab*. 1975;40:474-477.
10. Bachrach LK, Burrow GN. Maternal-fetal transfer of thyroxine. *N Engl J Med*. 1989;321:1549.
11. Vulsma T, Gons MH, de Vijlder JJM. Maternal-fetal transfer of thyroxine in congenital hypothyroidism due to a total organification defect or thyroid agenesis. *N Engl J Med*. 1989;321:13-16.
12. Burrow GN, Fisher DA, Larsen PR. Maternal and fetal thyroid function. *N Engl J Med*. 1994;331:1072-1078.
13. Larsen PR. Maternal thyroxine and congenital hypothyroidism. *N Engl J Med*. 1989;321:44-46.
14. Lightner ES, Fisher DA, Giles H, Woolfenden J. Intra-amniotic injection of thyroxine (T4) to a human fetus. *Am J Obstet Gynecol*. 1977;127:487-490.
15. Klein AH, Hobel CJ, Sack J, Fisher DA. Effect of intraamniotic fluid thyroxine injection on fetal serum and amniotic fluid iodothyronine concentrations. *J Clin Endocrinol Metab*. 1978;47:1034-1037.
16. Mashiach S, Barkai G, Sach J, et al. Enhancement of fetal lung maturity by intra-amniotic administration of thyroid hormone. *Am J Obstet Gynecol*. 1978;130:289-293.
17. Weiner S, Scharf JI, Bolognese RJ, Librizzi RJ. Antenatal diagnosis and treatment of fetal goiter. *J Reprod Med*. 1980;24:39-42.
18. Heinonen OP, Slone D, Shapiro S. *Birth Defects and Drugs in Pregnancy*. Publishing Sciences Group; 1977.
19. Potter JD. Hypothyroidism and reproductive failure. *Surg Gynecol Obstet*. 1980;150:251-255.
20. Pekonen F, Teramo K, Ikonen E, et al. Women on thyroid hormone therapy: pregnancy course, fetal outcome, and amniotic fluid thyroid hormone level. *Obstet Gynecol*. 1984;63:635-638.
21. Man EB, Shaver BA Jr, Cooke RE. Studies of children born to women with thyroid disease. *Am J Obstet Gynecol*. 1958;75:728-741.
22. Montoro M, Collea JV, Frasier SD, Mestman JH. Successful outcome of pregnancy in women with hypothyroidism. *Ann Intern Med*. 1981;94:31-34.
23. Haddow JE, Palomaki GE, Allan WC, et al. Maternal thyroid deficiency during pregnancy and subsequent neuropsychological development of the child. *N Engl J Med*. 1999;341:549-555.
24. Sack J, Amado O, Lunenfeld B. Thyroxine concentration in human milk. *J Clin Endocrinol Metab*. 1977;45:171-173.
25. Bode HH, Vanjonack WJ, Crawford JD. Mitigation of cretinism by breast-feeding. *Pediatrics*. 1978;62:13-16.
26. Hahn HB Jr, Spiekerman AM, Otto WR, Hossalla DE. Thyroid function tests in neonates fed human milk. *Am J Dis Child*. 1983;137:220-222.
27. Varma SK, Collins M, Row A, et al. Thyroxine, triiodothyronine, and reverse triiodothyronine concentrations in human milk. *J Pediatr*. 1978;93:803-806.
28. Abbassi V, Steinour TA. Successful diagnosis of congenital hypothyroidism in four breast-fed neonates. *J Pediatr*. 1980;97:259-261.
29. Letarte J, Guyda H, Dussault JH, Glorieux J. Lack of protective effect of breast-feeding in congenital hypothyroidism: report of 12 cases. *Pediatrics*. 1980;65:703-705.
30. Franklin R, O'Grady C, Carpenter L. Neonatal thyroid function: comparison between breast-fed and bottle-fed infants. *J Pediatr*. 1985;106:124-126.
31. Mizuta H, Amino N, Ichihara K, et al. Thyroid hormones in human milk and their influence on thyroid function of breast-fed babies. *Pediatr Res*. 1983;17:468-471.
32. Jansson L, Ivarsson S, Larsson I, Ekman R. Tri-iodothyronine and thyroxine in human milk. *Acta Paediatr Scand*. 1983;72:703-705.
33. Moller B, Bjorkhem I, Falk O, et al. Identification of thyroxine in human breast milk by gas chromatography-mass spectrometry. *J Clin Endocrinol Metab*. 1983;56:30-34.
34. Jiao XF, Zhang M, Chen J, et al. The impact of levothyroxine therapy on the pregnancy, neonatal and childhood outcomes of subclinical hypothyroidism during pregnancy: an updated systematic review, meta-analysis and trial sequential analysis. *Front Endocrinol (Lausanne)*. 2022;13:964084.

LIDOCAINE

Anesthetic (Local)/Cardiovascular (Antiarrhythmic)

PREGNANCY RECOMMENDATION: Limited Human Data—Animal Data Suggest Low Risk

BREASTFEEDING RECOMMENDATION: Probably Compatible

PREGNANCY SUMMARY

A few studies describing the use of lidocaine during human pregnancy were located. In the Collaborative Perinatal Project, there were 4 (1.4%) major malformations in 293 first-trimester exposures. Other studies describe its use near delivery. One case report described the use of lidocaine in resuscitating a patient at 18 weeks' gestation with a cardiac arrest associated with a ventricular arrhythmia. The resuscitation was successful, and she delivered at term a healthy newborn progressing normally at 17 months of age. The drug rapidly crosses the placenta, so fetal exposure will occur. However, this limited human pregnancy experience prevents a complete assessment of the embryofetal risk. Animal data did not show any embryofetal toxicity in one animal species at doses less than 10 times the RHD. Using this drug during pregnancy should be based on the pros and cons of the mother's clinical need for treatment versus any potential fetal risk that might occur from exposure. ACOG supports the use of lidocaine as a local anesthetic for obstetrical cases.

BREASTFEEDING SUMMARY

Two reports of lidocaine use during human lactation have been located, with no infant adverse effects. Small amounts of lidocaine are excreted into breast milk, so some infant exposure occurs. Breastfeeding while using this drug should be based on the mother's clinical need for treatment versus any potential infant risks that might occur. If used, adverse effects on the breastfed infant are not expected.

References

1. Prescribing Information. Lidocaine hydrochloride. Hospira, Inc; 2018.
2. Prescribing Information. Lidocaine hydrochloride. Pfizer; 2021.
3. Shnider SM, Way EL. The kinetics of transfer of lidocaine (Xylocaine) across the human placenta. *Anesthesiology*. 1968;29:944-950.
4. Shnider SM, Way EL. Plasma levels of lidocaine (Xylocaine) in mother and newborn following obstetrical conduction anesthesia: clinical applications. *Anesthesiology*. 1968;29:951-958.
5. Lurie AO, Weiss JB. Blood concentrations of mepivacaine and lidocaine in mother and baby after epidural anesthesia. *Am J Obstet Gynecol*. 1970;106: 850-856.
6. Petrie RH, Paul WL, Miller FC, et al. Placental transfer of lidocaine following paracervical block. *Am J Obstet Gynecol*. 1974;120:791-801.
7. Zador G, Lindmark G, Nilsson BA. Pudendal block in normal vaginal deliveries. Clinical efficacy, lidocaine concentrations in maternal and foetal blood, foetal and maternal acid-base values and influence on uterine activity. *Acta Obstet Gynecol Scand Suppl*. 1974;34:51-64.
8. Blankenbaker WL, DiFazio CA, Berry FA Jr. Lidocaine and its metabolites in the newborn. *Anesthesiology*. 1975;42:325-330.
9. Brown WU Jr, Bell GC, Lurie AO, et al. Newborn blood levels of lidocaine and mepivacaine in the first postnatal day following maternal epidural anesthesia. *Anesthesiology*. 1975;42:698-707.
10. Kuhnert BR, Knapp DR, Kuhnert PM, Prochaska AL. Maternal, fetal, and neonatal metabolism of lidocaine. *Clin Pharmacol Ther*. 1979;26: 213-220.
11. Abboud TK, Sarkis F, Blikian A, Varakian L. Lack of adverse neurobehavioral effects of lidocaine. *Anesthesiology*. 1982;57(suppl):A404.
12. Kileff M, James FM III, Dewan D, et al. Neonatal neurobehavioral responses after epidural anesthesia for cesarean section with lidocaine and bupivacaine. *Anesthesiology*. 1982;57(suppl):A403.
13. Abboud TK, David S, Costandi J, et al. Comparative maternal, fetal and neonatal effects of lidocaine versus lidocaine with epinephrine in the parturient. *Anesthesiology*. 1984;61(suppl):A405.
14. Philipson EH, Kuhnert BR, Syracuse CD. Maternal, fetal, and neonatal lidocaine levels following local perineal infiltration. *Am J Obstet Gynecol*. 1984;149:403-407.
15. Brown WU Jr, Bell GC, Alper MH. Acidosis, local anesthetics, and the newborn. *Obstet Gynecol*. 1976;48:27-30.
16. Scanlon JW, Brown WU Jr, Weiss JB, Alper MH. Neurobehavioral responses of newborn infants after maternal epidural anesthesia. *Anesthesiology*. 1974; 40:121-128.
17. Abboud TK, Williams V, Miller F, et al. Comparative fetal, maternal, and neonatal responses following epidural analgesia with bupivacaine, chloroprocaine, and lidocaine. *Anesthesiology*. 1981;55(suppl):A315.
18. Chestnut DH, Bates JN, Choi WW. Continuous infusion epidural analgesia with lidocaine: efficacy and influence during the second stage of labor. *Obstet Gynecol*. 1987;69:323-327.
19. Liston WA, Adjepon-Yamoah KK, Scott DB. Foetal and maternal lignocaine levels after paracervical block. *Br J Anaesth*. 1973;45:750-754.
20. Kim WY, Pomerance JJ, Miller AA. Lidocaine intoxication in a newborn following local anesthesia for episiotomy. *Pediatrics*. 1979;64:643-645.
21. Tamari I, Eldar M, Rabinowitz B, Neufeld HN. Medical treatment of cardiovascular disorders during pregnancy. *Am Heart J*. 1982;104:1357-1363.
22. Rotmensch HH, Elkayam U, Frishman W. Antiarrhythmic drug therapy during pregnancy. *Ann Intern Med*. 1983;98:487-497.
23. Stokes IM, Evans J, Stone M. Myocardial infarction and cardiac arrest in the second trimester followed by assisted vaginal delivery under epidural analgesia at 38 weeks gestation. Case report. *Br J Obstet Gynaecol*. 1984;91: 197-198.
24. Heinonen OP, Slone D, Shapiro S. *Birth Defects and Drugs in Pregnancy*. Publishing Sciences Group; 1977.
25. Zeisler JA, Gaarder TD, De Mesquita SA. Lidocaine excretion in breast milk. *Drug Intell Clin Pharm*. 1986;20:691-693.
26. American College of Obstetricians and Gynecologists' Committee on Practice Bulletins—Obstetrics. ACOG Practice Bulletin No. 209: obstetric analgesia and anesthesia. *Obstet Gynecol*. 2019;133:e208-e225.
27. Ortega D, Viviand X, Lorec AM, et al. Excretion of lidocaine and bupivacaine in breast milk following epidural anesthesia for cesarean delivery. *Acta Anaesthesiol Scand*. 1999;43:394-397.
28. Juanatey A, Ruíz M, Blanco L, et al. Results of peripheral nerve blocks in migraine patients during pregnancy and breastfeeding. *Cephalalgia*. 2016;36(1 suppl):24.

LIDOCAINE OPHTHALMIC

Ophthalmic (Anesthetic-Local)

PREGNANCY RECOMMENDATION: No Human Data—Animal Data Suggest Low Risk

BREASTFEEDING RECOMMENDATION: Probably Compatible

PREGNANCY SUMMARY

No reports describing the use of lidocaine ophthalmic in human pregnancy have been located. While the amount of systemic absorption is not known, lidocaine is likely minimally absorbed systemically following ocular administration; therefore, the amount of drug at the placental interface is likely to be negligible. However, the absence of human pregnancy experience prevents a complete assessment of the embryofetal risk. Animal data did not show any embryofetal toxicity in two animal species at doses of more than 10 times the RHD. Using this drug during pregnancy should be based on the pros and cons of the mother's clinical need for treatment versus any potential fetal risk that might occur from exposure. If used during pregnancy, consider placing pressure over the tear duct in the corner of the eye for at least 1 minute, and then remove any excess gel with absorbent tissue to decrease the amount of drug reaching the systemic circulation even further.

BREASTFEEDING SUMMARY

No reports describing the use of lidocaine ophthalmic during human lactation have been located. While the amount of systemic absorption is not known, lidocaine is likely minimally absorbed systemically following ocular administration, suggesting that the amount of drug excreted into breast milk is likely to be negligible. If the clinical decision is to use this drug while breastfeeding, the infant should be monitored for the most common systemic adult side effect of headache (leading to irritability). A method to decrease some systemic absorption with ophthalmic use is described above in the Pregnancy Summary.

Reference

1. Prescribing Information. Akten. Akorn; 2022.

LIFITEGRAST

Ophthalmic (Topical)

PREGNANCY RECOMMENDATION: No Human Data—Animal Data Suggest Low Risk

BREASTFEEDING RECOMMENDATION: Probably Compatible

PREGNANCY SUMMARY

No reports describing the use of lifitegrast in human pregnancy have been located. Fetal exposure is likely to be clinically insignificant. However, the absence of human pregnancy experience prevents a complete assessment of the embryofetal risk. Animal studies did not show any embryofetal toxicity despite being administered IV. Using this drug during pregnancy should be based on the pros and cons of the mother's clinical need for treatment. If used during pregnancy, consider placing pressure over the tear duct in the corner of the eye for at least 1 minute, and then remove any excess solution with absorbent tissue to decrease the amount of drug reaching the systemic circulation even further.

BREASTFEEDING SUMMARY

No reports describing the use of lifitegrast during human lactation have been located. The amount of drug found in breast milk is likely to be insignificant. Breastfeeding while using this drug should be based on the mother's clinical need for treatment. A method to decrease some systemic absorption with ophthalmic use is described above in the Pregnancy Summary.

Reference

1. Prescribing Information. Xiidra. Novartis Pharmaceuticals Corporation; 2020.

LINACLOTIDE

Gastrointestinal

PREGNANCY RECOMMENDATION: Human Data Suggest Low Risk—Animal Data Suggest Low Risk

BREASTFEEDING RECOMMENDATION: Probably Compatible

PREGNANCY SUMMARY

No reports describing the use of linaclotide in human pregnancy have been located. Based on the absence of quantifiable plasma concentrations of the drug and its active metabolite following oral administration, fetal exposure is likely negligible. However, the absence of human pregnancy experience prevents a complete assessment of the embryofetal risk. Animal data did not show any embryofetal toxicity in two species at doses much higher than the RHD. Using this drug during pregnancy should be based on the pros and cons of the mother's clinical need for treatment versus any potential fetal risk that might occur from exposure.

BREASTFEEDING SUMMARY

One report evaluating the levels of linaclotide and its active metabolite in seven lactating women found that all breast milk samples were below the LLQ at all time points tested. This is consistent with the absence of quantifiable systemic concentrations after oral administration. If used while breastfeeding, the infant should be monitored for the most common reported adult side effects of abdominal pain (leading to irritability), diarrhea, and abdominal distension. However, linaclotide carries a boxed warning regarding serious dehydration in pediatric patients less than 2 years of age.

L

References

1. Prescribing Information. Linzess. AbbVie and Ironwood Pharmaceuticals, Inc; 2023.
2. Crittenden N, McGeeney D, Assouline-Dayan Y, et al. Linaclotide is not detectable in breast milk of lactating women: an open-label, phase 1 study. *J Can Assoc Gastroenterol*. 2021;4(suppl 1):285-287.

LINAGLIPTIN

Antidiabetic (Dipeptidyl Peptidase-4 Inhibitor)

PREGNANCY RECOMMENDATION: No Human Data—Animal Data Suggest Low Risk

BREASTFEEDING RECOMMENDATION: Probably Compatible

PREGNANCY SUMMARY

No reports describing the use of linagliptin in human pregnancy have been located. The drug will probably cross the placenta, so some fetal exposure will likely occur. However, the absence of human pregnancy experience prevents a complete assessment of the embryofetal risk. Animal data did not show any embryofetal toxicity in two species at doses of more than 10 times the RHD. ACOG and the American Diabetes Association (ADA) recommend that insulin be used for types 1 and 2 diabetes occurring during pregnancy and, if diet therapy alone is not successful, for gestational diabetes. Oral agents such as metformin and glyburide should not be used as first-line agents, as both cross the placenta, and in general, other hypoglycemic agents do not provide adequate glycemic control.

BREASTFEEDING SUMMARY

No reports describing the use of linagliptin during human lactation have been located. The drug will probably appear in breast milk, so some infant exposure will likely occur. Breastfeeding while using this drug should be based on the mother's clinical need for treatment versus any potential infant risks that might occur. If used, the infant should be monitored for the most common reported adult side effects of hypoglycemia, jitteriness, excessive sleepiness, poor feeding, apnea, and paleness.

References

1. Prescribing Information. Tradjenta. Boehringer Ingelheim Pharmaceuticals and Eli Lilly; 2023.
2. ACOG Practice Bulletin No. 190: gestational diabetes mellitus. *Obstet Gynecol*. 2018;131:e49-e64.
3. American Diabetes Association Professional Practice Committee. Management of diabetes in pregnancy: standards of medical care in diabetes—2022. *Diabetes Care*. 2022;45(suppl_1):S232-S243.

LINCOMYCIN

Antibiotic (Lincosamide)

PREGNANCY RECOMMENDATION: Limited Human Data—Animal Data Suggest Low Risk

BREASTFEEDING RECOMMENDATION: Probably Compatible

PREGNANCY SUMMARY

Two reports describing the use of lincomycin in 647 human pregnancies have been located. One report from the manufacturer of 345 pregnancies exposed to lincomycin at various stages of pregnancy reported no adverse effects related to the drug. A second study of 302 women, also treated at various stages of pregnancy, observed no increase in malformations or delayed developmental defects when compared to the control group. However, exact numbers on first-trimester use are limited. Lincomycin crosses the placenta, achieving cord serum levels about 25% of the maternal serum level. Therefore, this limited human pregnancy experience still prevents a complete assessment of the embryofetal risk. Animal data did not show any embryofetal toxicity in one species at doses of less than 10 times the RHD. Using this drug during pregnancy should be based on the pros and cons of the mother's clinical need for treatment versus any potential fetal risk that might occur from exposure. Lincomycin carries a boxed warning regarding *Clostridium difficile* toxin–associated diarrhea.

BREASTFEEDING SUMMARY

Two reports involving nine women taking lincomycin during human lactation found that the drug is excreted into breast milk. Breast milk levels ranged from 20% to 90% of the maternal blood levels. A breast milk concentration of 2.5 mcg/mL was noted, resulting in a calculated RID of about 1.3%. However, due to a concern for potential serious adverse effects that might be seen in a breastfed infant, the manufacturer recommends that women not breastfeed while being treated with this drug. Nevertheless, breastfeeding while using this drug should be based on the mother's clinical need for treatment versus any potential infant risks that might occur. If used, the infant should be monitored for potential effects on the infant's gastrointestinal flora, such as diarrhea, thrush, diaper rash, or blood in the stool.

References

1. Prescribing Information. Lincomycin. XGEN Pharmaceuticals; 2022.
2. Medina A, Fiske N, Hjelt-Harvey I, et al. Absorption, diffusion, and excretion of a new antibiotic, lincomycin. *Antimicrob Agents Chemother*. 1963; 189-196.
3. Duignan NM, Andrews J, Williams JD. Pharmacological studies with lincomycin in late pregnancy. *Br Med J*. 1973;3:75-78.
4. Mickal A, Panzer JD. The safety of lincomycin in pregnancy. *Am J Obstet Gynecol*. 1975;121:1071-1074.
5. Wilson JT. Milk/plasma ratios and contraindicated drugs. In: Wilson JT, ed. *Drugs in Breast Milk*. ADIS Press; 1981:78-79.

LINEZOLID

Antibiotic (Oxazolidinone)

PREGNANCY RECOMMENDATION: Limited Human Data—Animal Data Suggest Low Risk

BREASTFEEDING RECOMMENDATION: Probably Compatible

PREGNANCY SUMMARY

Seven studies describing the use of linezolid in 31 pregnant women have been reported. Most cases were beyond the first trimester. No major malformations or adverse effects were reported in any of the cases. The drug will probably cross the placenta, so some fetal exposure will likely occur. However, this limited human pregnancy experience prevents a complete assessment of the embryofetal risk. Animal data did not show any embryofetal toxicity in two species at doses of less than 10 times the RHD. Using this drug during pregnancy should be based on the pros and cons of the mother's clinical need for treatment versus any potential fetal risk that might occur from exposure.

BREASTFEEDING SUMMARY

Three reports evaluating the levels of linezolid in lactating women found that the drug is excreted into breast milk. The calculated daily infant doses were about 2 mg/kg/d, which is well below the recommended infant dose of 30 mg/kg/d. However, when compared to the maternal dose, the RID was about 15%. Breastfeeding while using this drug should be based on the mother's clinical need for treatment versus any potential infant risks that might occur. If used, the infant should be monitored for the most common reported adult side effects of headache (leading to irritability), diarrhea, and vomiting.

References

1. Prescribing Information. Zyvox. Pharmacia & Upjohn; 2018.
2. Mercieri M, Di Rosa R, Pantosti A, et al. Critical pneumonia complicating early-stage pregnancy. *Anesth Analg*. 2010;110:852-854.
3. Jaspard M, Elefant-Amoura E, Melonio I, et al. Bedaquiline and linezolid for extensively drug-resistant tuberculosis in pregnant woman. *Emerg Infect Dis*. 2017;23:1731-1732.
4. Van Kampenhout E, Bolhuis MS, Alffenaar JC, et al. Pharmacokinetics of moxifloxacin and linezolid during and after pregnancy in a patient with multidrug-resistant tuberculosis. *Eur Respir J*. 2017;49:1601724.
5. Loveday M, Hughes J, Sunkari B, et al. Maternal and infant outcomes among pregnant women treated for multidrug/rifampicin-resistant tuberculosis in South Africa. *Clin Infect Dis*. 2021;72:1158-1168.
6. Acquah R, Mohr-Holland E, Daniels J, et al. Outcomes of children born to pregnant women with drug-resistant tuberculosis treated with novel drugs in Khayelitsha, South Africa: a report of five patients. *Pediatr Infect Dis J*. 2021;40:e191-e192.
7. Alene KA, Murray MB, van de Water BJ, et al. Treatment outcomes among pregnant patients with multidrug-resistant tuberculosis. *JAMA Netw Open*. 2022;5:e2216527.
8. Zhu Z, Zhang M, Li Y. Anti-tuberculosis drug-induced acute liver failure requiring transplantation in the second trimester of pregnancy: a case report. *BMC Pregnancy Childbirth*. 2021;21:592.
9. Sagirli O, Onal A, Toker S, Oztunc A. Determination of linezolid in human breast milk by high-performance liquid chromatography with ultraviolet detection. *J AOAC Int*. 2009;92:1658-1662.
10. Rowe HE, Felkins K, Cooper SD, Hale TW. Transfer of linezolid into breast milk. *J Hum Lact*. 2014;30:410-412.
11. Lim FH, Lovering AM, Currie A, et al. Linezolid and lactation: measurement of drug levels in breast milk and the nursing infant. *J Antimicrob Chemother*. 2017;72:2677-2678.
12. Navarro S, Keith K, Stafylis C, Konda K, Klausner JD. Safety of linezolid during pregnancy. *Sex Transm Dis*. 2023;50:e37-e40.

LIOTHYRONINE

Endocrine (Thyroid Agent)

PREGNANCY RECOMMENDATION: Human Data Suggest Low Risk—No Relevant Animal Data

BREASTFEEDING RECOMMENDATION: Probably Compatible

L

PREGNANCY SUMMARY

One report describing the use of liothyronine in 34 human pregnancies in the first trimester found no significant evidence of an increased risk of congenital anomalies or adverse effects. It appears that a small amount of triiodothyronine (T_3) will cross the human placenta following very high doses. However, the overall amount is clinically insignificant in most instances. No animal reproduction studies have been conducted. The use of liothyronine is not the preferred treatment in maternal hypothyroidism as it does not provide sufficient levels of T_4.

BREASTFEEDING SUMMARY

No reports describing the effects of liothyronine during human lactation have been located. Liothyronine is excreted into breast milk in low concentrations. If the clinical decision is to use this drug while breastfeeding, the infant should be monitored for the most common reported adult side effects of headache, heat intolerance, and chest pain (all leading to irritability), rapid or irregular heart rate, shortness of breath, insomnia, tremors, muscle weakness, weight loss, diarrhea, and skin rash.

References

1. Thyroid disease in pregnancy: ACOG practice bulletin, number 223. *Obstet Gynecol*. 2020;135(6):e261-e274.
2. Haddow JE, Palomaki GE, Allan WC, et al. Maternal thyroid deficiency during pregnancy and subsequent neuropsychological development of the child. *N Engl J Med*. 1999;341:549-555.
3. Alexander EK, Pearce EN, Brent GA, et al. 2017 guidelines of the American Thyroid Association for the diagnosis and management of thyroid disease during pregnancy and the postpartum. *Thyroid*. 2017;27:315-389.
4. Prescribing Information. Liothyronine sodium. AvKARE; 2024.
5. Grumbach MM, Werner SC. Transfer of thyroid hormone across the human placenta at term. *J Clin Endocrinol Metab*. 1956;16:1392-1395.
6. Kearns JE, Hutson W. Tagged isomers and analogues of thyroxine (their transmission across the human placenta and other studies). *J Nucl Med*. 1963;4:453-461.
7. Fisher DA, Lehman H, Lackey C. Placental transport of thyroxine. *J Clin Endocrinol Metab*. 1964;24:393-400.
8. Raiti S, Holzman GB, Scott RI, Blizzard RM. Evidence for the placental transfer of tri-iodothyronine in human beings. *N Engl J Med*. 1967;277:456-459.
9. Dussault J, Row VV, Lickrish G, Volpe R. Studies of serum triiodothyronine concentration in maternal and cord blood: transfer of triiodothyronine across the human placenta. *J Clin Endocrinol Metab*. 1969;29:595-606.
10. Burrow GN, Fisher DA, Larsen PR. Maternal and fetal thyroid function. *N Engl J Med*. 1994;331:1072-1078.
11. Heinonen OP, Slone D, Shapiro S. *Birth Defects and Drugs in Pregnancy*. Publishing Sciences Group; 1977:388-400.
12. Potter JD. Hypothyroidism and reproductive failure. *Surg Gynecol Obstet*. 1980;150:251-255.
13. Montoro M, Collea JV, Frasier SD, Mestman JH. Successful outcome of pregnancy in women with hypothyroidism. *Ann Intern Med*. 1981;94:31-34.
14. Bode HH, Vanjonack WJ, Crawford JD. Mitigation of cretinism by breast-feeding. *Pediatrics*. 1978;62:13-16.
15. Varma SK, Collins M, Row A, et al. Thyroxine, triiodothyronine, and reverse triiodothyronine concentrations in human milk. *J Pediatr*. 1978;93:803-806.
16. Hahn HB Jr, Spiekerman AM, Otto WR, Hossalla DE. Thyroid function tests in neonates fed human milk. *Am J Dis Child*. 1983;137:220-222.
17. Abbassi V, Steinour TA. Successful diagnosis of congenital hypothyroidism in four breast-fed neonates. *J Pediatr*. 1980;97:259-261.
18. Letarte J, Guyda H, Dussault JH, Glorieux J. Lack of protective effect of breast-feeding in congenital hypothyroidism: report of 12 cases. *Pediatrics*. 1980;65:703-705.
19. Franklin R, O'Grady C, Carpenter L. Neonatal thyroid function: comparison between breast-fed and bottle-fed infants. *J Pediatr*. 1985;106:124-126.
20. Mizuta H, Amino N, Ichihara K, et al. Thyroid hormones in human milk and influence on thyroid function of breast-fed babies. *Pediatr Res*. 1983;17:468-471.
21. Jansson L, Ivarsson S, Larsson I, Ekman R. Tri-iodothyronine and thyroxine in human milk. *Acta Paediatr Scand*. 1983;72:703-705.
22. Prescribing Information. Liothyronine sodium. XGen Pharmaceuticals DJB, Inc; 2023.

LIPID EMULSION

Nutrition/Nutritional Supplements

PREGNANCY RECOMMENDATION: Limited Human Data and No Relevant Animal Data

BREASTFEEDING RECOMMENDATION: Probably Compatible

PREGNANCY SUMMARY

Limited reports describing the use of lipid emulsion in human pregnancy have been located. The available studies have shown overall that lipid emulsion does not pose a significant risk to the fetus. However, if a pregnant woman needs hyperalimentation with lipids, her disease condition could lead to pregnancy complications. Some of the fats in the emulsion will probably cross the placenta. Regardless, this limited human pregnancy experience prevents a complete assessment of the embryofetal risk. No animal reproduction studies have been conducted. Using this product during pregnancy should be based on the pros and cons of the mother's clinical need for treatment versus any potential fetal risk that might occur from exposure.

BREASTFEEDING SUMMARY

Although there are no reports describing the use of lipid emulsion during lactation, there does not appear to be any risk to a nursing infant. If used while breastfeeding, adverse effects on the breastfed infant are not expected as the incidence of adult systemic reactions is less than 1%. However, the disease state of a mother that requires hyperalimentation with lipids postdelivery could lead to difficulties with breastfeeding.

References

1. Elphick MC, Filshie GM, Hull D. The passage of fat emulsion across the human placenta. *Br J Obstet Gynaecol*. 1978;85:610-618.
2. Hendrickse W, Stammers JP, Hull D. The transfer of free fatty acids across the human placenta. *Br J Obstet Gynaecol*. 1985;92:945-952.
3. Hew LR, Deitel M. Total parenteral nutrition in gynecology and obstetrics. *Obstet Gynecol*. 1980;55:464-468.
4. Tresadern JC, Falconer GF, Turnberg LA, Irving MH. Successful completed pregnancy in a patient maintained on home parenteral nutrition. *Br Med J*. 1983;286:602-603.
5. Tresadern JC, Falconer GF, Turnberg LA, Irving MH. Maintenance of pregnancy in a home parenteral nutrition patient. *JPEN*. 1984;8:199-202.
6. Seifer DB, Silberman H, Catanzarite VA, et al. Total parenteral nutrition in obstetrics. *JAMA*. 1985;253;2073-2075.
7. Lavin JP Jr, Gimmon Z, Miodovnik M, et al. Total parenteral nutrition in a pregnant insulin-requiring diabetic. *Obstet Gynecol*. 1982;59:660-664.
8. Rivera-Alsina ME, Saldana LR, Stringer CA. Fetal growth sustained by parenteral nutrition in pregnancy. *Obstet Gynecol*. 1984;64:138-141.
9. Di Costanzo J, Martin J, Cano N, et al. Total parenteral nutrition with fat emulsions during pregnancy—nutritional requirements: a case report. *JPEN*. 1982;6:534-538.
10. Young KR. Acute pancreatitis in pregnancy: two case reports. *Obstet Gynecol*. 1982;60:653-657.
11. Breen KJ, McDonald IA, Panelli D, Ihle B. Planned pregnancy in a patient who was receiving home parenteral nutrition. *Med J Aust*. 1987;146:215-217.
12. Levine MG, Esser D. Total parenteral nutrition for the treatment of severe hyperemesis gravidarum: maternal nutritional effects and fetal outcome. *Obstet Gynecol*. 1988;72:102-107.
13. Herbert WNP, Seeds JW, Bowes WA, Sweeney CA. Fetal growth response to total parenteral nutrition in pregnancy: a case report. *J Reprod Med*. 1986; 31:263-266.
14. Hatjis CG, Meis PJ. Total parenteral nutrition in pregnancy. *Obstet Gynecol*. 1985;66:585-589.
15. Heller L. Parenteral nutrition in obstetrics and gynecology. In: Greep JM, Soeters PB, Wesdorp RIC, Grant JP, eds. *Current Concepts in Parenteral Nutrition*. Martinus Nijhoff Medical Division; 1977:179-186.
16. Neri A. Fetal growth sustained by parenteral nutrition in pregnancy. *Obstet Gynecol*. 1986;67:753.
17. Saldana LR. Fetal growth sustained by parenteral nutrition in pregnancy (in reply). *Obstet Gynecol*. 1986;67:753.
18. Lee RV, Rodgers BD, Young C, et al. Total parenteral nutrition during pregnancy. *Obstet Gynecol*. 1986;68:563-571.
19. Neldam S, Hornnes PJ, Kuhl C. Effect of maternal triglyceride ingestion on fetal respiratory movements. *Obstet Gynecol*. 1982;59:640-642.
20. Greenspoon JS, Masaki DI, Kurz CR. Cardiac tamponade in pregnancy during central hyperalimentation. *Obstet Gynecol*. 1989;73:465-466.
21. Jasnosz KM, Pickeral JJ, Graner S. Fat deposits in the placenta following maternal total parenteral nutrition with intravenous lipid emulsion. *Arch Pathol Lab Med*. 1995;119:555-557.
22. Prescribing Information. Intralipid 20%. Fresenius Kabi AB; 2022.

LIRAGLUTIDE

Antidiabetic (Glucagon-Like Peptide 1 [GLP-1] Receptor Agonist)

PREGNANCY RECOMMENDATION: Limited Human Data—Animal Data Suggest Risk

BREASTFEEDING RECOMMENDATION: Probably Compatible

PREGNANCY SUMMARY

Two case reports describing the use of liraglutide in the first trimester in two human pregnancies resulted in healthy term infants with no identified anomalies. The drug does not appear to cross the human placenta. Therefore, any exposure is

(*continued*)

likely to be clinically insignificant. However, this limited human pregnancy experience prevents a complete assessment of the embryofetal risk. Embryofetal toxicity with malformations was observed in two animal species at doses less than 10 times the RHD. ACOG and the ADA recommend that insulin be used for types 1 and 2 diabetes occurring during pregnancy and, if diet therapy alone is not successful, for gestational diabetes. Oral agents such as metformin and glyburide should not be used as first-line agents, as both cross the placenta. Other oral medications, including liraglutide, need further safety data.

BREASTFEEDING SUMMARY

No reports describing the use of liraglutide during human lactation have been located. The drug is not likely to be excreted into breast milk. Additionally, if any were to be ingested through breastfeeding, the peptide would probably be digested in the infant's gastrointestinal tract and not absorbed. If used while breastfeeding, the infant should be monitored for the most common reported adult side effects of nausea (leading to irritability), diarrhea, reflux, vomiting, and decreased appetite (monitor infant growth).

References

1. Prescribing Information. Liraglutide. Teva Pharmaceuticals USA, Inc; 2024.
2. Greco D. Normal pregnancy outcome after first-trimester exposure to liraglutide in a woman with type 2 diabetes. *Diabetes Med*. 2015;32(10):e29-e30.
3. Ivanišević M, Herman M, Horvatiček M, Lovrenč ić Vuč ić M, Đelmiš J. Pregnancy outcome and liraglutide levels in serum and umbilical vein blood of a woman with type 2 diabetes. A case report. *Gynaecol Perinatol*. 2018;27(3-4):70-72.
4. Muller DRP, Stenvers DJ, Malekzadeh A, et al. Effects of GLP-1 agonists and SGLT2 inhibitors during pregnancy and lactation on offspring outcomes: a systematic review of the evidence. *Front Endocrinol (Lausanne)*. 2023;14:1215356.
5. Drummond RF, Seif KE, Reece EA. Glucagon-like peptide-1 receptor agonist use in pregnancy: a review. *Am J Obstet Gynecol*. 2025;232:17-33.
6. ACOG Practice Bulletin No. 190: gestational diabetes mellitus. *Obstet Gynecol*. 2018;131:e49-e64.
7. American Diabetes Association Professional Practice Committee. Management of diabetes in pregnancy: standards of care in diabetes—2024. *Diabetes Care*. 2024;47(suppl 1):S282-S294.

LISDEXAMFETAMINE

L

Mental Health (Central Nervous System Stimulant)

PREGNANCY RECOMMENDATION: Limited Human Data—Animal Data Suggest Low Risk

BREASTFEEDING RECOMMENDATION: Potential Toxicity

PREGNANCY SUMMARY

Two reports describing the use of lisdexamfetamine in pregnancy have been located. In one study, about 40 pregnant women were exposed to the drug in the first trimester, and no birth anomalies were described. The drug will probably cross the placenta, so fetal exposure will likely occur. However, the limited human pregnancy experience prevents a complete assessment of the embryofetal risk. Animal data did not show any embryofetal toxicity in two species at doses less than 10 times the RHD in one and more than 10 times the RHD in the second. Lisdexamfetamine is related to the amphetamine drug class. Amphetamines cause vasoconstriction and may produce hypertension and decrease placental perfusion. Infants exposed to amphetamines near term should be monitored for withdrawal symptoms, including feeding difficulties, irritability, agitation, and excessive drowsiness. Using this drug to curb eating is not recommended during pregnancy. There is a pregnancy exposure registry that monitors pregnancy outcomes in women exposed to attention-deficit/hyperactivity disorder (ADHD) medications during pregnancy. Health care providers are encouraged to register patients by calling the National Pregnancy Registry for Psychostimulants at 1-866-961-2388.

BREASTFEEDING SUMMARY

One report describing the use of lisdexamfetamine in 13 lactating women for ADHD has been located. At 18 months, five infants had experienced an adverse reaction possibly related to amphetamine in breast milk. However, all infants had normal Denver Developmental Scale and pediatric quality of life scores. The drug will probably appear in breast milk, so infant exposure will likely occur. Using this drug to curb eating is not recommended while breastfeeding. If the clinical decision is to use this drug while breastfeeding, the infant should be monitored for the most common reported adult side effects of nausea, dizziness, and abdominal pain (all leading to irritability), decreased appetite (monitor infant growth), diarrhea, insomnia, and vomiting.

References

1. Prescribing Information. Lisdexamfetamine. Apotex Corp; 2024.
2. Szpunar MJ, Freeman MP, Kobylski LA, et al. Risk of major malformations in infants after first-trimester exposure to stimulants: results from the Massachusetts General Hospital National Pregnancy Registry for psychiatric medications. *J Clin Psychopharmacol*. 2023;43:326-332.
3. Camacho X, Zoega H, Gomes T, et al. The association between psychostimulant use in pregnancy and adverse maternal and neonatal outcomes: results from a distributed analysis in two similar jurisdictions. *Int J Epidemiol*. 2023;52:190-202.
4. Benassayag Kaduri N, Hazan A, De-Haan T, et al. Amphetamine use for attention deficit hyperactive disorder during breastfeeding and children's neurodevelopmental outcomes: a pilot study. *Psychiatry Res*. 2024;339:116047

LISINOPRIL

Antihypertensive (Angiotensin-Converting Enzyme Inhibitor)

PREGNANCY RECOMMENDATION: Contraindicated (Second and Third Trimesters)

BREASTFEEDING RECOMMENDATION: Probably Compatible

PREGNANCY SUMMARY

Several reports describing the use of lisinopril in human pregnancy have been located. Regarding first-trimester exposure only, there were 2 (4.9%) major anomalies in 41 exposures, and both defects were different. Regarding angiotensin-converting enzyme (ACE) inhibitors in general, use during the second and third trimesters of pregnancy has been associated with fetal renal toxicity, as stated by the boxed warning for this drug. Numerous cases of severe oligohydramnios leading to findings of limb contractures, craniofacial deformation, and pulmonary hypoplasia with neonatal death have been reported. These fetal renal effects are often permanent, but if the drug is discontinued as soon as possible, they can be reversible in some cases. However, ACE inhibitors should not be used in the second and third trimesters, if at all possible. Regarding first-trimester exposure to ACE inhibitors in general, there was some concern about teratogenicity, especially cardiac and central nervous system. However, two large studies of more than 4,450 first-trimester exposures to ACE inhibitors did not find any increased risks for anomalies compared with other pregnant patients with hypertension on treatment with other antihypertensive agents or on no treatment at all. Therefore, the final summary determined that the use of ACE inhibitors in the first trimester did not increase the risk for fetal malformations compared with other pregnant women with hypertension. Lisinopril will cross the placenta, so fetal exposure will occur. However, this limited human pregnancy experience with lisinopril prevents a complete assessment of the embryofetal risk. Animal reproduction studies were not located for this drug. Women of reproductive age using lisinopril should be informed of these risks, so that they can closely monitor if pregnancy transpires. If a positive pregnancy test occurs, she and her health care providers can modify treatment (if possible) so that the drug is not used in the second or third trimesters. For treating hypertension in pregnancy, ACOG recommends nifedipine and labetalol as first-line agents.

L

BREASTFEEDING SUMMARY

No reports describing the use of lisinopril during human lactation have been located. No adverse effects of other ACE inhibitors in breast milk have been reported. The drug will probably appear in breast milk, so some infant exposure will likely occur. However, if lisinopril is similar to other ACE inhibitors, drug levels in breast milk should be low. Nevertheless, due to a concern for potential serious adverse effects that might be seen in a breastfed infant, the manufacturer recommends that women not breastfeed while being treated with this drug. Regardless, ACOG and the American Heart Association (AHA) consider ACE inhibitors low risk for use during breastfeeding. Breastfeeding while using this drug should be based on the mother's clinical need for treatment. If used, the infant should be monitored for the most common reported adult side effects of headache (leading to irritability) and cough.

References

1. Prescribing Information. Lisinopril. Camber Pharmaceuticals, Inc; 2024.
2. Rosa F, Bosco L. Infant renal failure with maternal ACE inhibition (abstract). *Am J Obstet Gynecol*. 1991;164:273.
3. Tomlinson AJ, Campbell J, Walker JJ, Morgan C. Malignant primary hypertension in pregnancy treated with lisinopril. *Ann Pharmacother*. 2000; 34:180-182.
4. Bhatt-Mehta V, Deluga KS. Chronic renal failure (CRF) in a neonate due to in-utero exposure to lisinopril. Presented at the 12th Annual Meeting of the American College of Clinical Pharmacy; August 20, 1991; Minneapolis, MN. Abstract No. 43.
5. Pryde PG, Nugent CE, Sedman AB, Barr M Jr. ACE inhibitor fetopathy (abstract). *Am J Obstet Gynecol*. 1992;166:348.
6. Lip GYH, Churchill D, Beevers M, et al. Angiotensin-converting-enzyme inhibitors in early pregnancy. *Lancet*. 1997;350:1446-1447.
7. Barr M Jr, Cohen MM Jr. ACE inhibitor fetopathy and hypocalvaria: the kidney-skull connection. *Teratology*. 1991;44:485-495.
8. Brent RL, Beckman DA. Angiotensin-converting enzyme inhibitors, an embryopathic class of drugs with unique properties: information for clinical teratology counselors. *Teratology*. 1991;43:543-546.
9. Cooper WO, Hernandez-Diaz S, Arbogast PG, et al. Major congenital malformations after first-trimester exposure to ACE inhibitors. *N Engl J Med*. 2006;354:2443-2451.
10. Friedman JM. ACE inhibitors and congenital anomalies. *N Engl J Med*. 2006; 354:2498-2500.
11. Scialli AR, Lione A. ACE inhibitors and major congenital malformations. *N Engl J Med*. 2006;355:1280.
12. Cooper WO, Ray WA. ACE inhibitors and major congenital malformations. Reply. *N Engl J Med*. 2006;355:1281.
13. Barr M Jr. Teratogen update: angiotensin-converting enzyme inhibitors. *Teratology*. 1994;50:399-409.
14. Shotan A, Widerhorn J, Hurst A, Elkayam U. Risks of angiotensin-converting enzyme inhibition during pregnancy: experimental and clinical evidence, potential mechanisms, and recommendations for use. *Am J Med*. 1994;96:451-456.
15. Robillard JE, Nakamura KT, Matherne GP, Jose PA. Renal hemodynamics and functional adjustments to postnatal life. *Semin Perinatol*. 1988;12:143-150.
16. Guignard J-P, Gouyon J-B. Adverse effects of drugs on the immature kidney. *Biol Neonate*. 1988;53:243-252.
17. Polifka JE. Is there an embryopathy associated with first-trimester exposure to angiotensin-converting enzyme inhibitors and angiotensin receptor antagonists? A critical review of the evidence. *Birth Defects Res A Clin Mol Teratol*. 2012;94:576-598.
18. Hoeltzenbein M, Tissen-Diabate T, Fietz AK, et al. Increased rate of birth defects after first trimester use of angiotensin converting enzyme inhibitors – treatment or hypertension related? An observational cohort study. *Pregnancy Hypertens*. 2018;13:65-71.
19. Al-Maawali A, Walfisch A, Koren G. Taking angiotensin-converting enzyme inhibitors during pregnancy: is it safe? *Can Fam Physician*. 2012;5849-5851.
20. ACOG Practice Bulletin No. 203: chronic hypertension in pregnancy. *Obstetrics & Gynecology*. 2019;133:e26-e50..
21. Heidenreich PA, Bozkurt B, Aguilar D, et al. 2022 AHA/ACC/HFSA guideline for the management of heart failure: a report of the American College of Cardiology/American Heart Association Joint Committee on Clinical Practice Guidelines. *Circulation*. 2022;145:e895-e1032.

LITHIUM

Mental Health (Antimanic Agent)

PREGNANCY RECOMMENDATION: Human Data Suggest Potential Risk

BREASTFEEDING RECOMMENDATION: Potential Toxicity

PREGNANCY SUMMARY

Numerous reports describing the use of lithium in human pregnancy have been located. Overall, the rate of birth anomalies with first-trimester exposure does not appear to be elevated above what would be expected in the general population. However, many publications (but not all) have shown an increased risk for cardiac defects, including a rare disorder of Ebstein anomaly (a tricuspid valve defect). There is a Lithium Baby Registry that was formed in Denmark in 1968. More than 20 newborns exposed in the first trimester (in >300 exposed infants) had cardiac defects, and of these, there were several Ebstein anomalies. This type of data collection is biased toward the reporting of abnormal outcomes, but the incidence of Ebstein anomaly is 1 in 200,000 births or less. Lithium crosses the placenta, so fetal exposure will occur. In addition, fetal cardiac organogenesis is primarily 2 to 4 weeks after conception or 4 to 6 weeks' gestation. ACOG recommends that mood stabilizers, including lithium, be continued due to a risk of recurrence or exacerbation of mood symptoms. However, due to the potential risk for cardiac anomalies, a fetal ultrasound is recommended in the second trimester. Lithium dosing should also be closely monitored to maintain a therapeutic response and minimize fetal exposure.

BREASTFEEDING SUMMARY

Several reports describing the use of lithium during human lactation have been located. Most reports found no toxicity or developmental problems in exposed infants. However, case studies of increased lithium levels and toxicity (decreased muscle tone, poor weight gain, cyanosis, and T-wave inversion) have also been reported. Lithium is excreted into breast milk, producing infant serum levels that are approximately 10% to 50% of the maternal serum concentration. Breastfeeding while using this drug should be based on the mother's clinical need for treatment versus any potential infant risks that might occur. If used, the infant should be monitored for the most common reported adult side effects of lithium toxicity such as muscle stiffness, hypothermia, cyanosis, and electrocardiogram (ECG) changes.

References

1. Committee on Drugs, American Academy of Pediatrics. Use of psychoactive medication during pregnancy and possible effects on the fetus and newborn. *Pediatrics*. 2000;105:880-887.
2. Jacobson SJ, Jones K, Johnson K, et al. Prospective multicentre study of pregnancy outcome after lithium exposure during first trimester. *Lancet*. 1992; 339:530-533.
3. Cohen LS, Friedman JM, Jefferson JW, et al. A reevaluation of risk of in utero exposure to lithium. *JAMA*. 1994;271:146-150.
4. Prescribing Information. Lithium carbonate. American Health Packaging; 2024.
5. Lexi-Comp, Inc. (Lexi-drugs). Lexi-Comp, Inc; 2020.
6. Elia J, Katz IR, Simpson GM. Teratogenicity of psychotherapeutic medications. *Psychopharmacol Bull*. 1987;23:531-586.
7. Weinstein MR, Goldfield M. Lithium carbonate treatment during pregnancy: report of a case. *Dis Nerv Syst*. 1969;30:828-832.
8. Mizrahi EM, Hobbs JF, Goldsmith DI. Nephrogenic diabetes insipidus in transplacental lithium intoxication. *J Pediatr*. 1979;94:493-495.
9. Mackay AVP, Loose R, Glen AIM. Labour on lithium. *Br Med J*. 1976;1:878.
10. Schou M, Amdisen A. Lithium and placenta. *Am J Obstet Gynecol*. 1975; 122:541.
11. Sykes PA, Quarrie J, Alexander FW. Lithium carbonate and breast-feeding. *Br Med J*. 1976;2:1299.
12. van Gent EM, Verhoeven WMA. Bipolar illness, lithium prophylaxis, and pregnancy. *Pharmacopsychiatry*. 1992;25:187-191.
13. Schou M, Amdisen A. Lithium in pregnancy. *Lancet*. 1970;1:1391.
14. Aoki FY, Ruedy J. Severe lithium intoxication: management without dialysis and report of a possible teratogenic effect of lithium. *Can Med Assoc J*. 1971; 105:847-848.
15. Goldfield M, Weinstein MR. Lithium in pregnancy: a review with recommendations. *Am J Psychiatry*. 1971;127:888-893.
16. Goldfield MD, Weinstein MR. Lithium carbonate in obstetrics: guidelines for clinical use. *Am J Obstet Gynecol*. 1973;116:15-22.
17. Schou M, Goldfield MD, Weinstein MR, Villeneuve A. Lithium and pregnancy. I. Report from the register of lithium babies. *Br Med J*. 1973;2:135-136.
18. Weinstein MR, Goldfield MD. Cardiovascular malformations with lithium use during pregnancy. *Am J Psychiatry*. 1975;132:529-531.
19. Weinstein MR. Recent advances in clinical psychopharmacology. I. Lithium carbonate. *Hosp Form*. 1977;12:759-762.
20. Linden S, Rich CL. The use of lithium during pregnancy and lactation. *J Clin Psychiatry*. 1983;44:358-361.
21. Pitts FN. Lithium and pregnancy (editorial). *J Clin Psychiatry*. 1983;44:357.
22. Nora JJ, Nora AH, Toews WH. Lithium, Ebstein's anomaly, and other congenital heart defects. *Lancet*. 1974;2:594-595.
23. Rane A, Tomson G, Bjarke B. Effects of maternal lithium therapy in a newborn infant. *J Pediatr*. 1978;93:296-297.
24. Arnon RG, Marin-Garcia J, Peeden JN. Tricuspid valve regurgitation and lithium carbonate toxicity in a newborn infant. *Am J Dis Child*. 1981;135: 941-943.
25. Allan LD, Desai G, Tynan MJ. Prenatal echocardiographic screening for Ebstein's anomaly for mothers on lithium therapy. *Lancet*. 1982;2:875-876.
26. Schou M. What happened later to the lithium babies? A follow-up study of children born without malformations. *Acta Psychiatr Scand*. 1976;54:193-197.
27. Warkany J. Teratogen update: lithium. *Teratology*. 1988;38:593-596.
28. Källén B. Comments on teratogen update: lithium. *Teratology*. 1988;38:597.
29. Eikmeier G. Fetal malformations under lithium treatment. *Eur Psychiatry*. 1996;11:376-377.
30. Moel DI. Renal agenesis, bilateral. In: Buyse ML, ed. *Birth Defects Encyclopedia*. Vol II. Center for Birth Defects Information Service; 1990:1460-1461.
31. Leonard A, Hantson Ph, Gerber GB. Mutagenicity, carcinogenicity and teratogenicity of lithium compounds. *Mutat Res*. 1995;339:131-137.
32. Woody JN, London WL, Wilbanks GD Jr. Lithium toxicity in a newborn. *Pediatrics*. 1971;47:94-96.
33. Tunnessen WW Jr, Hertz CG. Toxic effects of lithium in newborn infants: a commentary. *J Pediatr*. 1972;81:804-807.
34. Piton M, Barthe ML, Laloum D, et al. Acute lithium intoxication. Report of two cases: mother and her newborn. *Therapie*. 1973;28:1123-1144.
35. Wilbanks GD, Bressler B, Peete CH Jr, et al. Toxic effects of lithium carbonate in a mother and newborn infant. *JAMA*. 1970;213:865-867.
36. Morrell P, Sutherland GR, Buamah PK, et al. Lithium toxicity in a neonate. *Arch Dis Child*. 1983;58:539-541.
37. Krause S, Ebbesen F, Lange AP. Polyhydramnios with maternal lithium treatment. *Obstet Gynecol*. 1990;75:504-506.

38. Silverman JA, Winters RW, Strande C. Lithium carbonate therapy during pregnancy: apparent lack of effect upon the fetus. *Am J Obstet Gynecol*. 1971;109:934-936.
39. Strothers JK, Wilson DW, Royston N. Lithium toxicity in the newborn. *Br Med J*. 1973;3:233-234.
40. Karlsson K, Lindstedt G, Lundberg PA, Selstam U. Transplacental lithium poisoning: reversible inhibition of fetal thyroid. *Lancet*. 1975;1:1295.
41. Stevens D, Burman D, Midwinter A. Transplacental lithium poisoning. *Lancet*. 1974;2:595.
42. Wilson N, Forfar JC, Godman MJ. Atrial flutter in the newborn resulting from maternal lithium ingestion. *Arch Dis Child*. 1983;58:538-539.
43. Ang MS, Thorp JA, Parisi VM. Maternal lithium therapy and polyhydramnios. *Obstet Gynecol*. 1990;76:517-519.
44. Pinelli JM, Symington AJ, Cunningham KA, Paes BA. Case report and review of the perinatal implications of maternal lithium use. *Am J Obstet Gynecol*. 2002;187:245-249.
45. Nishiwaki T, Tanaka K, Sekiya S. Acute lithium intoxication in pregnancy. *Int J Gynecol Obstet*. 1996;52:191-192.
46. Frayne J, Nguyen T, Kohan R, et al. The comprehensive management of pregnant women with major mood disorders: a case study involving phenelzine, lithium, and quetiapine. *Arch Womens Ment Health*. 2014;17:73-75.
47. Mallinger AG, Hanin I, Stumpf RL, et al. Lithium treatment during pregnancy: a case study of erythrocyte choline content and lithium transport. *J Clin Psychiatry*. 1983;44:381-384.
48. Levin RM, Amsterdam JD, Winokur A, Wein AJ. Effects of psychotropic drugs on human sperm motility. *Fertil Steril*. 1981;36:503-506.
49. Moore JA; IEHR Expert Scientific Committee. An assessment of lithium using the IEHR evaluative process for assessing human developmental and reproductive toxicity of agents. *Reprod Toxicol*. 1995;9:175-210.
50. Schou M, Amdisen A, Steenstrup OR. Lithium and pregnancy. II. Hazards to women given lithium during pregnancy and delivery. *Br Med J*. 1973;2:137-138.
51. Diav-Citron O, Shechtman S, Tahover E, et al. Pregnancy outcome following in utero exposure to lithium: a prospective, comparative, observational study. *Am J Psychiatry*. 2014;171:785-794.
52. Patorno E, Huybrechts KF, Bateman BT, et al. Lithium use in pregnancy and the risk of cardiac malformations. *N Engl J Med*. 2017;376:2245-2254.
53. Fries H. Lithium in pregnancy. *Lancet*. 1970;1:1233.
54. Schou M, Amdisen A. Lithium and pregnancy. III. Lithium ingestion by children breast-fed by women on lithium treatment. *Br Med J*. 1973;2:138.
55. Kirksey A, Groziak SM. Maternal drug use: evaluation of risks to breast-fed infants. *World Rev Nutr Diet*. 1984;43:60-79.
56. Moretti ME, Koren G, Verjee Z, Ito S. Monitoring lithium in breast milk: an individualized approach for breast-feeding mothers. *Ther Drug Monit*. 2003;25:364-366.
57. Bogen DL, Sit D, Genovese A, Wisner KL. Three cases of lithium exposure and exclusive breastfeeding. *Arch Womens Ment Health*. 2012;15:69-72.
58. Fornaro M, Maritan E, Ferranti R, et al. Lithium exposure during pregnancy and the postpartum period: a systematic review and meta-analysis of safety and efficacy outcomes. *Am J Psychiatry*. 2020;177:76-92.
59. American College of Obstetricians and Gynecologists. Treatment and management of mental health conditions during pregnancy and postpartum: clinical practice guideline no. 5. *Obstet Gynecol*. 2023;141:1262-1288.

LOFEXIDINE

Antidote (α_2-Adrenergic Agonist)

PREGNANCY RECOMMENDATION: No Human Data—Animal Data Suggest Risk

BREASTFEEDING RECOMMENDATION: Potential Toxicity

PREGNANCY SUMMARY

No reports describing the use of lofexidine in human pregnancy have been located. The drug will probably cross the placenta, so some fetal exposure will likely occur. However, the absence of human pregnancy experience prevents a complete assessment of the embryofetal risk. Embryofetal toxicity with maternal toxicity was observed in one animal species and in one species without maternal toxicity at doses less than the RHD. Using this drug during pregnancy should be based on the pros and cons of the mother's clinical need for treatment versus any potential fetal risk that might occur from exposure.

BREASTFEEDING SUMMARY

No reports describing the use of lofexidine during human lactation have been located. The drug will probably appear in breast milk, so some infant exposure will likely occur. Breastfeeding while using this drug should be based on the mother's clinical need for treatment versus any potential infant risks that might occur. If used, the infant should be monitored for the most common reported adult side effects of dizziness and dry mouth (both leading to irritability), low blood pressure, decreased heart rate, and sedation.

Reference

1. Prescribing Information. Lucemyra. US WorldMeds; 2020.

LOMITAPIDE

Antilipemic

PREGNANCY RECOMMENDATION: No Human Data—Animal Data Suggest Risk

BREASTFEEDING RECOMMENDATION: Potential Toxicity

PREGNANCY SUMMARY

No reports describing the use of lomitapide in human pregnancy have been located. Some amount of the drug may cross the placenta, so fetal exposure will probably occur. However, the absence of human pregnancy experience prevents a complete assessment of the embryofetal risk. Embryofetal toxicity with malformations was observed in two animal species at doses of less than 10 times the RHD. Due to the findings from these animal studies, the manufacturer recommends that women with reproductive potential who are taking lomitapide be advised to use effective contraception during treatment and for at least 2 weeks after the last dose. Nevertheless, using this drug during pregnancy should be based on the pros and cons of the mother's clinical need for treatment versus any potential fetal risk that might occur from exposure. There is a pregnancy exposure registry that monitors pregnancy outcomes in women exposed to lomitapide during pregnancy. For more information, health care providers or patients are encouraged to call the Global Lomitapide Pregnancy Exposure Registry at 1-877-902-4099.

BREASTFEEDING SUMMARY

No reports describing the use of lomitapide during human lactation have been located. The drug may be excreted into breast milk, so some infant exposure will likely occur. Due to a concern for potential serious adverse effects that might be seen in a breastfed infant, the manufacturer recommends that women not breastfeed while being treated with this drug. Nevertheless, if the clinical decision is to use this drug while breastfeeding, the infant should be monitored for the most common reported adult side effects of nausea and abdominal pain (both leading to irritability), diarrhea, reflux, and vomiting.

Reference

1. Prescribing Information. Juxtapid. Amryt Pharmaceuticals; 2020.

L

LONAFARNIB

Genetic (Farnesyltransferase Inhibitor)

PREGNANCY RECOMMENDATION: No Human Data—Animal Data Suggest Potential Risk

BREASTFEEDING RECOMMENDATION: Potential Toxicity

PREGNANCY SUMMARY

No reports describing the use of lonafarnib in human pregnancy have been located. Some amount of the drug most likely crosses the placenta, but fetal exposure is probably small. However, the absence of human pregnancy experience prevents a complete assessment of the embryofetal risk. Animal data did show fetotoxic effects, and because of this, the manufacturer recommends that women with reproductive potential use effective contraception while being treated with lonafarnib. Nevertheless, using this drug during pregnancy should be based on the pros and cons of the mother's clinical need for treatment versus any potential fetal risk that might occur from exposure. If the drug is used during pregnancy, it can produce hypertension, and therefore, blood pressure should be monitored closely.

BREASTFEEDING SUMMARY

Lonafarnib probably enters breast milk, but the amount is most likely small. Breastfeeding while using this drug should be based on the mother's clinical need for treatment. If used, the infant should be monitored for the most common reported adult side effects of abdominal pain, musculoskeletal pain, and headache (all leading to irritability), vomiting, diarrhea, decreased appetite, lethargy, increased liver enzymes, hypertension, and weight loss.

Reference

1. Prescribing Information. Zokinvy. Eiger BioPharmaceuticals, Inc; 2020.

LONAPEGSOMATROPIN

Endocrine (Growth Hormone)

PREGNANCY RECOMMENDATION: No Human Data—Animal Data Suggest Low Risk

BREASTFEEDING RECOMMENDATION: Probably Compatible

PREGNANCY SUMMARY

No reports describing the use of lonapegsomatropin in human pregnancy have been located. Lonapegsomatropin and released somatropin are not likely to cross the placenta. However, because it consists of a protein, it is not known whether some fetal exposure could occur. Nevertheless, the absence of human pregnancy experience prevents a complete assessment of the embryofetal risk. Studies on somatropin by itself have not identified any embryofetal toxicity or increased risk for malformations (see Somatropin). Animal data did not show any embryofetal toxicity. Using this drug during pregnancy should be based on the pros and cons of the mother's clinical need for treatment versus any potential fetal risk that might occur from exposure. This medication can unmask previously undiagnosed glucose intolerance, diabetes, and hypothyroidism.

BREASTFEEDING SUMMARY

No reports describing the use of lonapegsomatropin during human lactation have been located. Lonapegsomatropin is unlikely to be excreted into breast milk, but because it is a protein, if the drug were to be ingested through breastfeeding, it would probably be digested in the infant's gastrointestinal tract and not be absorbed. Exogenous somatropin does not increase growth hormone concentrations in human breast milk. Breastfeeding while using this drug should be based on the mother's clinical need for treatment. If used, the infant should be monitored for the most common reported adult side effects of abdominal pain, arthralgia, and nausea (all leading to irritability), viral infections, pyrexia, cough, vomiting, and diarrhea.

Reference

1. Prescribing Information. Skytrofa. Ascendis Pharma Endocrinology; 2022.

LONCASTUXIMAB TESIRINE

Antineoplastic (Monoclonal Antibody Drug Conjugate)

PREGNANCY RECOMMENDATION: No Human Data and No Relevant Animal Data

BREASTFEEDING RECOMMENDATION: Potential Toxicity

PREGNANCY SUMMARY

No reports describing the use of loncastuximab tesirine in human pregnancy have been located. As an IgG antibody, loncastuximab tesirine is likely to cross the placenta, so some fetal exposure will probably occur. Therefore, the absence of human pregnancy experience prevents a complete assessment of the embryofetal risk. Animal reproduction studies have not been conducted. Because the alkylating agent component of loncastuximab is toxic to rapidly dividing cells, there is a potential for embryofetal toxicity and teratogenicity. Based on the drug's mechanism of action, the manufacturer recommends that women with reproductive potential use effective contraception during treatment and for 9 months after the last dose. They also recommend that males with female partners of reproductive potential use effective contraception during treatment and for 6 months after the last dose. Nevertheless, using this drug during pregnancy should be based on the pros and cons of the mother's clinical need for treatment versus any potential fetal risk that might occur from exposure. Elevated glucose levels have been reported in patients treated with this drug.

BREASTFEEDING SUMMARY

No reports describing the use of loncastuximab tesirine during human lactation have been located. It is known that IgG antibodies can be found in human breast milk, but are not found in the neonatal or infant circulation. Additionally, if any IgG antibodies were to be ingested through breastfeeding, they would probably be digested in the infant's gastrointestinal tract and not be absorbed. A limited amount of tesirine by itself might appear in breast milk, but the gastrointestinal absorption of this drug by the infant is unknown. Due to the potential for serious adverse effects that might be seen in a breastfed infant, the manufacturer recommends that women not breastfeed while being treated with loncastuximab tesirine and for at least 3 months after the last dose. Nevertheless, breastfeeding while using this drug should be based on the mother's clinical need for treatment. If used, the infant should be monitored for the most common reported adult side effects of nausea and musculoskeletal pain (both leading to irritability), rash, peripheral edema, and various laboratory abnormalities (see PI).

Reference

1. Prescribing Information. Zynlonta. ADC Therapeutics America; 2021.

LOPERAMIDE

Gastrointestinal (Antidiarrheal)

PREGNANCY RECOMMENDATION: Limited Human Data—Animal Data Suggest Low Risk

BREASTFEEDING RECOMMENDATION: Probably Compatible

PREGNANCY SUMMARY

Three studies have been identified that describe the use of loperamide during human pregnancy. Overall, over 800 exposures were identified, many in the first trimester. The overall rate of congenital anomalies in these cases was higher than expected, but no pattern to the anomalies has been found. In addition, the oral bioavailability of the drug is less than 1%. Therefore, these anomalies may be related to the disease state for which the drug is used. A minimal amount of the drug may cross the placenta, so fetal exposure is likely to be negligible. However, this limited first-trimester human pregnancy experience prevents a complete assessment of the embryofetal risk. Animal data did not show any embryofetal toxicity in two animal species at doses of more than 10 times the RHD. Using this drug during pregnancy should be based on the pros and cons of the mother's clinical need for treatment versus any potential fetal risk that might occur from exposure. Loperamide carries a boxed warning regarding torsades de pointes, cardiac arrest, and death.

BREASTFEEDING SUMMARY

No reports describing the effects of loperamide during human lactation have been located. The drug may appear in breast milk, but due to the very poor oral bioavailability, the overall amount is likely to be negligible. If the clinical decision is to use this drug while breastfeeding, the infant should be monitored for the most common reported adult side effects of nausea, dizziness, and abdominal cramps (all leading to irritability) and constipation.

L

References

1. Prescribing Information. Loperamide. RedPharm Drug, Inc; 2024.
2. Pubchem. Loperamide. Accessed June 30, 2017. https://pubchem.ncbi.nlm.nih.gov/compound/loperamide#section=Top
3. Einarson A, Mastroiacovo P, Arnon J, et al. A prospective controlled, multicentre study of loperamide in pregnancy. *Can J Gastroenterol*. 2000;14:185-187.
4. Kallen B, Nilsson E, Otterblad Olausson P. Maternal use of loperamide in early pregnancy and delivery outcome. *Acta Paediatr*. 2008;97:541-545.
5. Nikodem VC, Hofmeyr GJ. Secretion of the antidiarrhoeal agent loperamide oxide in breast milk. *Eur J Clin Pharmacol*. 1992;42:695-696.

LOPINAVIR

Antiretroviral (Protease Inhibitor)

PREGNANCY RECOMMENDATION: Human Data Suggest Low Risk (Maternal Benefit May Outweigh Any Embryofetal Risk)

BREASTFEEDING RECOMMENDATION: *Contraindicated

PREGNANCY SUMMARY

Numerous large studies have evaluated the use of lopinavir with use during the first trimester. In more than 7,000 exposures, the overall congenital defect rate was about 2.8%. The drug crosses the placenta, so fetal exposure will occur. Animal studies did show some embryofetal toxicity (in combination with ritonavir) in one species at doses of less than the RHD (along with maternal toxicity). This was not seen in a second animal species. In 2024, the updated US Department of Health and Human Services AIDS Info guidelines for the use of antiretroviral agents during pregnancy recommend that, in most cases, patients continue their regimen during pregnancy if it is tolerated, safe, and effective in suppressing viral replication. Additionally, treatment initiation should not be delayed due to concerns about teratogenicity with first-trimester exposure. See the guideline for the most updated information. The guidelines note that first-trimester exposure to lopinavir/ritonavir is not associated with an increased risk for congenital abnormalities. There is a pregnancy exposure registry that monitors pregnancy outcomes in women exposed to lopinavir during pregnancy. For more information, health care providers or patients are encouraged to contact the APR at 1-800-258-4263.

BREASTFEEDING SUMMARY

Two reports describing the effects of the combination product, lopinavir/ritonavir, during human lactation have been located. No adverse effects in breastfed infants were identified. Lopinavir is excreted into breast milk in low levels. In 2024, the updated US Department of Health and Human Services AIDS Info guidelines state that using replacement of breast milk through formula or pasteurized donor human breast milk from a milk bank eliminates the risk of postnatal HIV transmission to the infant. Using antiretroviral therapy to achieve and maintain viral suppression during pregnancy and postpartum decreases the risk for infant HIV transmission to less than 1% but not zero. *For patients not on therapy or those without viral load suppression during pregnancy (at a minimum of throughout the third trimester) and at delivery, replacement of breast milk is recommended. Patients on antiretroviral therapy who have a sustained undetectable viral load and who choose to breastfeed or use replacement of breast milk should be supported with their decision. If the clinical decision is to use this drug while breastfeeding, the infant should be monitored for the most common reported adult side effects of nausea (leading to irritability), diarrhea, and vomiting.

References

1. Prescribing Information. Kaletra. AbbVie; 2023.
2. Panel on Treatment of HIV During Pregnancy and Prevention of Perinatal Transmission. Recommendations for the use of antiretroviral drugs during pregnancy and interventions to reduce perinatal HIV transmission in the United States. Recommendations for the use of antiretroviral drugs during pregnancy. Department of Health and Human Services. Accessed October 16, 2024. https://clinicalinfo.hiv.gov/en/guidelines/perinatal
3. Antiretroviral Pregnancy Registry Steering Committee. Antiretroviral pregnancy registry interim report for 1 January 1989 through 31 July 2023. Registry Coordinating Center; 2023. Accessed January 31, 2024. https://www.apregistry.com/InterimReport.aspx
4. Gandhi M, Mwesigwa J, Aweeka F, et al. Prevention of Malaria and HIV disease in Tororo (PROMOTE) study. Hair and plasma data show that lopinavir, ritonavir, and efavirenz all transfer from mother to infant in utero, but only efavirenz transfers via breastfeeding. *J Acquir Immune Defic Syndr*. 2013;63:578-584.
5. Sibiude J, Mandelbrot L, Blanche S, et al. Association between prenatal exposure to antiretroviral therapy and birth defects: an analysis of the French perinatal cohort study (ANRS CO1/CO11). *PLoS Med*. 2014;11:e1001635.
6. Williams PL, Crain M, Yildirim C, et al. Congenital anomalies and in utero antiretroviral exposure in human immunodeficiency virus-exposed uninfected infants. *JAMA Pediatr*. 2015;169:45-55.
7. Tookey PA, Thorne C, van Wyk J, Norton M. Maternal and foetal outcomes among 4118 women with HIV infection treated with lopinavir/ritonavir during pregnancy: analysis of population-based surveillance data from the national study of HIV in pregnancy and childhood in the United Kingdom and Ireland. *BMC Infect Dis*. 2016;16:65.
8. Fowler MG, Qin M, Fiscus SA, et al. Benefits and risks of antiretroviral therapy for perinatal HIV prevention. *N Engl J Med*. 2016;375:1726-1737.
9. Favarato G, Townsend CL, Bailey H, et al. Protease inhibitors and preterm delivery: another piece in the puzzle. *AIDS*. 2018;32:243-252.
10. Cowdell I, Beck K, Portwood C, Sexton H, et al. Adverse perinatal outcomes associated with protease inhibitor-based antiretroviral therapy in pregnant women living with HIV: a systematic review and meta-analysis. *EClinicalMedicine*. 2022;46:101368.
11. Corbett AH, Kayira D, White NR, et al; the BAN Study Team. Antiretroviral pharmacokinetics in mothers and breastfeeding infants from 6 to 24 weeks postpartum: results of the BAN study. *Antivir Ther*. 2014;19:587-595.
12. Ngoma MS, Hunter JA, Harper JA, et al. Cognitive and language outcomes in HIV-uninfected infants exposed to combined antiretroviral therapy in utero and through extended breast-feeding. *AIDS*. 2014;28(suppl 3):S323-S330.
13. Cohan D, Natureeba P, Koss CA, et al. Efficacy and safety of lopinavir/ritonavir versus efavirenz-based antiretroviral therapy in HIV-infected pregnant Ugandan women. *AIDS*. 2015;29:183-191.
14. Oumar AA, Bagayoko-Maiga K, Bahachimi A, et al. Efavirenz and lopinavir levels in HIV-infected women and their nursing infants, in Mali. *J Pharmacol Exp Ther*. 2018;366:479-484.

L

LORATADINE

Antihistamine (Histamine H_1 Antagonist)

PREGNANCY RECOMMENDATION: Limited Human Data—Animal Data Suggest Low Risk

BREASTFEEDING RECOMMENDATION: Probably Compatible

PREGNANCY SUMMARY

Several reports describing the use of loratadine in human pregnancy have been located. Five (3.1%) major anomalies were identified in 161 first-trimester exposures. In two other large studies that evaluated drug use in a population of infants with birth defects compared with a group of infants with no congenital anomalies. The use of loratadine was no different in the groups. The drug and it's active metabolite will probably cross the placenta, so some fetal exposure will likely occur. However, this limited human pregnancy experience with first-trimester exposure still prevents a complete assessment of the embryofetal risk. Animal data did not show any embryofetal toxicity in two animal species at doses of more than 10 times the RHD. Using this drug during pregnancy should be based on the pros and cons of the mother's clinical need for treatment versus any potential fetal risk that might occur from exposure.

BREASTFEEDING SUMMARY

Two studies describing the effects of loratadine during human lactation have been located. An initial study suggested a risk for minor sedation in exposed infants. A follow-up study compared the results of this initial study to a control group of mothers who took a drug known to be safe in breastfeeding. No differences in adverse effects were found. Loratadine and its metabolite, desloratadine, are excreted into human breast milk in low amounts, so some infant exposure will occur. Several RIDs have been calculated and all were less than1%. If the clinical decision is to use this drug while breastfeeding, the infant should be monitored for the most common reported adult side effects of headache, dizziness, nausea, and abdominal pain (all leading to irritability) and vomiting.

References

1. Mazzotta P, Loebstein R, Koren G. Treating allergic rhinitis in pregnancy. Safety considerations. *Drug Saf*. 1999;20:361-375.
2. Horak F, Stubner UP. Comparative tolerability of second-generation antihistamines. *Drug Saf*. 1999;20:385-401.
3. Joint committee of the American College of Obstetricians and Gynecologists (ACOG) and the American College of Allergy, Asthma and Immunology (ACAAI). Position statement. The use of newer asthma and allergy medications during pregnancy. *Ann Allergy Asthma Immunol*. 2000;84:475-480.

4. Prescribing Information. Loratadine. Schering; 2001.
5. McIntyre BS, Vancutsem PM, Treinen KA, Morrissey RE. Effects of perinatal loratadine exposure on male rat reproductive organ development. *Reprod Toxicol*. 2003;17:691-697.
6. Wilton LV, Pearce GL, Martin RM, et al. The outcomes of pregnancy in women exposed to newly marketed drugs in general practice in England. *Br J Obstet Gynaecol*. 1998;105:882-889.
7. Kallen B. Use of antihistamine drugs in early pregnancy and delivery outcome. *J Matern Fetal Neonatal Med*. 2002;11:146-152.
8. Moretti ME, Caprara D, Coutinho CJ, et al. Fetal safety of loratadine use in the first trimester of pregnancy: a multicenter study. *J Allergy Clin Immunol*. 2003;111:479-483.
9. Werler M, McCloskey C, Edmonds LD, et al. Evaluation of an association between loratadine and hypospadias—United States, 1997-2001. *MMWR Morb Mortal Wkly Rep*. 2004;53:219-221.
10. Li Q, Mitchell AA, Werler MM, et al. Antihistamine use in early pregnancy and risk of birth defects. *J Allergy Clin Immunol Pract*. 2013;1:666-674.
11. Hilbert J, Radwanski E, Affrime MB, et al. Excretion of loratadine in human breast milk. *J Clin Pharmacol*. 1988;28:234-239.
12. Diav-Citrin O, Shechtman S, Aharonovich A, et al. Pregnancy outcome after gestational exposure to loratadine or antihistamines: a prospective controlled cohort study. *J Allergy Clin Immunol*. 2003;111:1239-1243.
13. Källén B, Olausson PO. Monitoring of maternal drug use and infant congenital malformations. Does loratadine cause hypospadias? *Int J Risk Safety Med*. 2001;14:115-119.
14. Källén B, Olausson PO. No increased risk of infant hypospadias after maternal use of loratadine in early pregnancy. *Int J Med Sci*. 2006;3:106-107.
15. Messinis IE, Souvatzoglou A, Fais N, et al. Histamine H1 receptor participation in the control of prolactin secretion in postpartum. *J Endocrinol Invest*. 1985;8:143-146.
16. Merlob P, Stahl B. Prospective follow-up of adverse reactions in breast-fed infants exposed to loratadine treatment (1999-2001). *BELTIS Newsl*. 2002;10:43-51.

LORAZEPAM

Central Nervous System (Antiseizure)/Mental Health (Benzodiazepine)

PREGNANCY RECOMMENDATION: Limited Human Data—Animal Data Suggest Potential Risk

BREASTFEEDING RECOMMENDATION: Potential Toxicity

L

PREGNANCY SUMMARY

Limited reports describing the use of lorazepam in human pregnancy have been located. A few cases with first-trimester use have not shown any malformations. When used close to delivery, sedation and neonatal withdrawal have been reported. The long-term effects of in utero exposure on neurobehavior, especially when the exposure occurs in the latter half of pregnancy, have not been studied. Lorazepam crosses the placenta, achieving cord levels similar to maternal serum concentrations, so fetal exposure will occur. However, the limited human pregnancy experience prevents a complete assessment of the embryofetal risk. Embryofetal toxicity with malformations was observed in one animal species without a relationship to the dose. ACOG recommends that benzodiazepines be avoided or prescribed sparingly in pregnancy. Exposure during pregnancy has been associated with neonatal sedation, decreased muscle tone, respiratory distress, neonatal intensive care unit (NICU) admission, and neonatal withdrawal. Using this drug during pregnancy for seizure control should be based on the pros and cons of the mother's clinical need for treatment versus any potential fetal risk that might occur from exposure.

BREASTFEEDING SUMMARY

Three reports describing the effects of lorazepam in 66 breastfeeding mothers have been located. No adverse effects related to the drug in breastfed infants were reported. Lorazepam is excreted into breast milk in low concentrations. The calculated RID in one study using mean drug levels was 2.6%. The studies overall concluded that the use of benzodiazepines was not a reason to avoid breastfeeding. If the clinical decision is to use this drug while breastfeeding, the infant should be monitored for the most common reported adult side effects of sedation and poor feeding.

References

1. Prescribing Information. Lorazepam injection. Hikma Pharmaceuticals USA, Inc; 2024.
2. Prescribing Information. Lorazepam tablet. Amneal Pharmaceuticals LLC; 2022.
3. De Groot G, Maes RAA, Defoort P, Thiery M. Placental transfer of lorazepam. *IRCS Med Sci*. 1975;3:290.
4. McBride RJ, Dundee JW, Moore J, et al. A study of the plasma concentrations of lorazepam in mother and neonate. *Br J Anaesth*. 1979;51:971-978.
5. Kanto J, Aaltonen L, Liukko P, Maenpaa K. Transfer of lorazepam and its conjugate across the human placenta. *Acta Pharmacol Toxicol (Copenh)*. 1980;47:130-134.
6. Kanto JH. Use of benzodiazepines during pregnancy, labour and lactation, with particular reference to pharmacokinetic considerations. *Drugs*. 1982;23:354-380.
7. Di Michele V, Ramenghi LA, Sabatino G. Clozapine and lorazepam administration in pregnancy. *Eur Psychiatry*. 1996;11:214.
8. Bonnot O, Vollset SE, Godet PF, Robert E. Maternal exposure to lorazepam and anal atresia in newborns? Results from a hypothesis generating study of benzodiazepines and malformations (abstract). *Teratology*. 1999;59:439-440.
9. McAuley DM, O'Neill MP, Moore J, Dundee JW. Lorazepam premedication for labour. *Br J Obstet Gynaecol*. 1982;89:149-154.
10. Whitelaw AGL, Cummings AJ, McFadyen IR. Effect of maternal lorazepam on the neonate. *Br Med J*. 1981;282:1106-1108.
11. Summerfield RJ, Nielsen MS. Excretion of lorazepam into breast milk. *Br J Anaesth*. 1985;57:1042-1043.
12. Johnstone M. Effect of maternal lorazepam on the neonate. *Br Med J*. 1981;282:1973-1974.
13. Johnstone MJ. The effect of lorazepam on neonatal feeding behaviour at term. *Pharmatherapeutica*. 1982;3:259-262.
14. Kelly LE, Poon S, Madadi P, Koren G. Neonatal benzodiazepines exposure during breastfeeding. *J Pediatr*. 2012;161:448-451.
15. Sinha SK, Thomas Kishore M, Thippeswamy H, et al. Adverse effects and short-term developmental outcomes of infants exposed to atypical antipsychotics during breastfeeding. *Indian J Psychiatry*. 2021;63:52-57.
16. American College of Obstetricians and Gynecologists. Treatment and management of mental health conditions during pregnancy and postpartum: ACOG clinical practice guideline no. 5. *Obstet Gynecol*. 2023;141:1262-1288.

LORLATINIB

Antineoplastic (Kinase Inhibitor)

PREGNANCY RECOMMENDATION: No Human Data—Animal Data Suggest Risk

BREASTFEEDING RECOMMENDATION: Potential Toxicity

PREGNANCY SUMMARY

No reports describing the use of lorlatinib in human pregnancy have been located. Some amount of the drug will probably cross the placenta, so some fetal exposure will likely occur. However, the absence of human pregnancy experience prevents a complete assessment of the embryofetal risk. Embryofetal toxicity with malformations was observed in two animal species at doses equal to or less than the RHD. Based on animal studies and the drug's mechanism of action, the manufacturer recommends that women with reproductive potential use effective nonhormonal contraception (because the drug may reduce the effectiveness of oral contraceptives) during treatment and for 6 months after the last dose. They also recommend that males with female partners of reproductive potential use effective contraception during treatment and for 3 months after the last dose. Using this drug during pregnancy should be based on the pros and cons of the mother's clinical need for treatment versus any potential fetal risk that might occur from exposure.

BREASTFEEDING SUMMARY

No reports describing the use of lorlatinib during human lactation have been located. The drug will probably appear in breast milk, so some infant exposure will likely occur. Due to a concern for potential serious adverse effects that might be seen in a breastfed infant, the manufacturer recommends that women not breastfeed while being treated with this drug and for at least 1 week after the last dose. Nevertheless, breastfeeding while using this drug should be based on the mother's clinical need for treatment versus any potential infant risks that might occur. If used, the infant should be monitored for the most common reported adult side effects of nausea, peripheral neuropathy, arthralgia, and abdominal pain (all leading to irritability), peripheral edema, fatigue (lethargy), diarrhea, and cough.

Reference

1. Prescribing Information. Lorbrena. Pfizer Laboratories; 2023.

L

LOSARTAN

Antihypertensive (Angiotensin II Receptor Blocker—ARB)

PREGNANCY RECOMMENDATION: *Contraindicated (Second and Third Trimesters)

BREASTFEEDING RECOMMENDATION: Probably Compatible

PREGNANCY SUMMARY

Limited reports describing the use of losartan in human pregnancy have been located. Regarding first-trimester exposure, there are only a few cases described, and no apparent increased risk for major anomalies has been seen. *Regarding angiotensin II receptor blocker (ARB) inhibitors in general, use during the second and third trimesters of pregnancy has been associated with fetal renal toxicity, as stated by the boxed warning for this drug. Many of these were using losartan. Numerous cases of severe oligohydramnios leading to findings of limb contractures, craniofacial deformation, and pulmonary hypoplasia with neonatal death have been reported. These fetal renal effects are often permanent, but if the drug is discontinued as soon as possible, they can be reversible in some cases. However, like ACE inhibitors, ARBs should also not be used in the second and third trimesters, if at all possible. Other studies looking at ARB exposures in the first trimester as a group have reported that the use of these drugs did not increase the risk for fetal malformations compared with other pregnant women with hypertension. The drug will probably cross the placenta, so some fetal exposure will likely occur. However, this limited human pregnancy experience with losartan prevents a complete assessment of the embryofetal risk. Animal reproduction studies did show some embryofetal toxicity in one species at doses of less than 10 times the RHD. Women of reproductive age using losartan should be informed of these risks, so that they can closely monitor if pregnancy transpires. If a positive pregnancy test occurs, she and her health care providers can modify treatment (if possible) so that the drug is not used in the second or third trimesters. For treating hypertension in pregnancy, ACOG recommends nifedipine and labetalol as first-line agents.

BREASTFEEDING SUMMARY

No reports describing the use of losartan during human lactation have been located. The drug will probably appear in breast milk, so some infant exposure will likely occur. If the clinical decision is to use this drug while breastfeeding, the infant should be monitored for the most common reported adult side effects of dizziness and back pain (both leading to irritability) and upper respiratory tract infection.

References

1. Prescribing Information. Losartan potassium. Granules Pharmaceuticals, Inc; 2023.
2. Spence SG, Allen HL, Cukierski MA, et al. Defining the susceptible period of developmental toxicity for the AT1-selective angiotensin II receptor antagonist losartan in rats. *Teratology*. 1995;51:367-382.
3. Spence SG, Cukierski MA, Manson JM, et al. Evaluation of the reproductive and developmental toxicity of the AT1-selective angiotensin II receptor antagonist losartan in rats. *Teratology*. 1995;51:383-397.
4. Mann RD, Mackay F, Pearce G, et al. Losartan: a study of pharmacovigilance data on 14,522 patients. *J Hum Hypertens*. 1999;13:551-557.
5. Saji H, Yamanaka M, Hagiwara A, Ijiri R. Losartan and fetal toxic effects. *Lancet*. 2001;357:363.
6. Lambot MA, Vermeylen D, Noel JC. Angiotensin-II-receptor inhibitors in pregnancy. *Lancet*. 2001;357:1619-1620.
7. Martinovic J, Benachi A, Laurent N, et al. Fetal toxic effects and angiotensin-II-receptor antagonists. *Lancet*. 2001;358:241-242.
8. Bakkum JN, Brost BC, Johansen KL, et al. In utero losartan withdrawal and subsequent development of fetal inferior vena cava thrombosis. *Obstet Gynecol*. 2006;108:739-740.
9. Bass JK, Faix RG. Gestational therapy with an angiotensin II receptor antagonist and transient renal failure in a premature infant. *Am J Perinatol*. 2006;23:313-318.
10. Alwan S, Polifka JE, Friedman JM. Addendum: sartan treatment during pregnancy. *Birth Defects Res A Clin Mol Teratol*. 2005;73:904-905.
11. Gersak K, Cvijic M, Cerar LK. Angiotensin II receptor blockers in pregnancy: a report of 5 cases. *Reprod Toxicol*. 2009;28:109-112.
12. Polifka JE. Is there an embryopathy associated with first-trimester exposure to angiotensin-converting enzyme inhibitors and angiotensin receptor antagonists? A critical review of the evidence. *Birth Defects Res A Clin Mol Teratol*. 2012;94:576-598.
13. Korkes HA, de Oliveira LG, Berlinck L, et al. Human fetal malformations associated with the use of an angiotensin II receptor antagonist: case report. *J Bras Nefrol*. 2014;36:410-413.

LOTEPREDNOL OPHTHALMIC

Ophthalmic/Corticosteroid (Topical)

PREGNANCY RECOMMENDATION: No Human Data—Animal Data Suggest Low Risk

BREASTFEEDING RECOMMENDATION: Probably Compatible

L

PREGNANCY SUMMARY

No reports describing the use of loteprednol ophthalmic in human pregnancy have been located. Based on the absence of quantifiable plasma concentrations following topical ocular use, fetal exposure is likely negligible. However, the absence of human pregnancy experience prevents a complete assessment of the embryofetal risk. Embryofetal toxicity was not observed in two animal species at doses of less than 10 times the RHD. Using this drug during pregnancy should be based on the pros and cons of the mother's clinical need for treatment versus any potential fetal risk that might occur from exposure. If used during pregnancy, consider placing pressure over the tear duct in the corner of the eye for at least 1 minute, and then remove any excess solution with absorbent tissue to decrease the amount of drug reaching the systemic circulation even further.

BREASTFEEDING SUMMARY

No reports describing the use of loteprednol ophthalmic during human lactation have been located. Excretion into breast milk is likely to be clinically insignificant due to minimal systemic absorption following topical ocular use. If the clinical decision is to use this drug while breastfeeding, the infant should be monitored for the most common reported adult nonocular side effect of headache (leading to irritability). A method to decrease some systemic absorption with ophthalmic use is described above in the Pregnancy Summary.

References

1. Prescribing Information. Alrex. Bausch & Lomb; 2022.
2. Prescribing Information. Lotemax. Bausch & Lomb; 2023.

LOTILANER OPHTHALMIC

Ophthalmic (Topical—GABA Chloride Channel Inhibitor)

PREGNANCY RECOMMENDATION: No Human Data—Animal Data Suggest Low Risk

BREASTFEEDING RECOMMENDATION: Probably Compatible

PREGNANCY SUMMARY

No reports describing the use of lotilaner ophthalmic in human pregnancy have been located. Though placental transfer is possible, fetal exposure is probably negligible because of minimal systemic absorption after ophthalmic use. However, the absence of human pregnancy experience prevents a complete assessment of the embryofetal risk. Animal data did not show any embryofetal toxicity despite being administered orally. Using this drug during pregnancy should be based on the pros and cons of the mother's clinical need for treatment versus any potential fetal risk that might occur from exposure. If used during pregnancy, consider placing pressure over the tear duct in the corner of the eye for at least 1 minute, and then remove any excess solution with absorbent tissue to decrease the amount of drug reaching the systemic circulation even further.

BREASTFEEDING SUMMARY

No reports describing the use of lotilaner ophthalmic in human lactation have been located. Because the drug has minimal systemic absorption after ophthalmic use, any drug found in breast milk would not likely have a clinical effect. Breastfeeding while using this drug should be based on the mother's clinical need for treatment. A method to decrease some systemic absorption with ophthalmic use is described above in the Pregnancy Summary.

Reference

1. Prescribing Information. Xdemvy. Tarus Pharmaceuticals, Inc; 2023.

LOVASTATIN

Antilipemic (HMG-CoA Reductase Inhibitor)

PREGNANCY RECOMMENDATION: *Contraindicated

BREASTFEEDING RECOMMENDATION: *Contraindicated

PREGNANCY SUMMARY

Several studies and case reports have described the use of lovastatin in human pregnancy. The rate of birth anomalies with first-trimester use of lovastatin in more than 100 pregnancies was slightly elevated at 5.6%. However, no pattern to the defects was seen. In addition, a few large reviews and meta-analyses of ARB use as a group have not found an increased risk for congenital birth anomalies with first-trimester use. Many of these analyses included patients using lovastatin. The drug will probably cross the placenta, so some fetal exposure will likely occur. However, this limited human pregnancy experience with lovastatin prevents a complete assessment of the embryofetal risk. Animal data did show some embryofetal toxicity in one species at doses of less than 10 times the RHD, but not in a second species. *In 2021, the US Food and Drug Administration (FDA) removed the long-standing contraindication to statin use in all women contemplating pregnancy or who are pregnant. The removal was requested because the benefits, which include prevention of serious or fatal events, may outweigh the potential risk in a small group of very high-risk pregnant patients. Despite this removal, the FDA continues to recommend most patients stop statin use once they learn they are pregnant.

BREASTFEEDING SUMMARY

No reports describing the use of lovastatin during human lactation have been located. The drug will probably appear in breast milk, so some infant exposure will likely occur. *In 2021, the FDA reaffirmed its warning that patients should not breastfeed when taking a statin because the medicine may pass into breast milk and pose a risk to the baby. If possible, statins should be temporarily held until breastfeeding ends. However, patients requiring ongoing statin treatment should not breastfeed and instead use infant formula or other alternatives.

References

1. Prescribing Information. Mevacor. Sanis Health; 2017.
2. Manson JM, Freyssinges C, Ducrocq MB, Stephenson WP. Postmarketing surveillance of lovastatin and simvastatin exposure during pregnancy. *Reprod Toxicol*. 1996;10:439-446.
3. Pollack PS, Shields KE, Burnett DM, et al. Pregnancy outcomes after maternal exposure to simvastatin and lovastatin. *Birth Defects Res A Clin Mol Teratol*. 2005;73:888-896.
4. Rosa F. Anti-cholesterol agent pregnancy exposure outcomes. Presented at: The 7th International Organization for Teratology Information Services; April 1994; Woods Hole, MA.
5. Ghidini A, Sicherer S, Willner J. Congenital abnormalities (VATER) in baby born to mother using lovastatin. *Lancet*. 1992;339:1416-1417.
6. Hayes A, Gilbert A, Lopez G, Miller WA. Mevacor—a new teratogen? *Am J Hum Genet*. 1995;57(4 suppl):A92.
7. Edison RJ, Muenke M. Central nervous system and limb anomalies in case reports of first-trimester statin exposure. *N Engl J Med*. 2004;350:1579-1582.
8. Lecarpentier E, Morel O, Foumier T, et al. Statins and pregnancy: between supposed risks and theoretical benefits. *Drugs*. 2012;72:773-788.
9. Godfrey LM, Erramouspe J, Cleveland KW. Teratogenic risk of statins in pregnancy. *Ann Pharmacother*. 2012;46:1419-1424.
10. Zarek J, Koren G. The fetal safety of statins: a systematic review and meta-analysis. *J Obstet Gynaecol Can*. 2014;36(6):506-509.
11. Karalis DG, Hill AN, Clifton S, Wild RA. The risks of statin use in pregnancy: a systematic review. *J Clin Lipidol*. 2016;10(5):1081-1090

12. Vahedian-Azimi A, Makvandi S, Banach M, et al. Fetal toxicity associated with statins: a systematic review and meta-analysis. *Atherosclerosis*. 2021; 327:59-67
13. Vahedian-Azimi A, Bianconi V, Makvandi S, et al. A systematic review and meta-analysis on the effects of statins on pregnancy outcomes. *Atherosclerosis*. 2021;336:1-11.
14. Karadas B, Uysal N, Erol H, et al. Pregnancy outcomes following maternal exposure to statins: a systematic review and meta-analysis. *Br J Clin Pharmacol*. 2022;88:3962-3976.
15. Hirsch A, Ternovsky N, Zwas DR, et al. The effect of statins exposure during pregnancy on congenital anomalies and spontaneous abortions: a systematic review and meta-analysis. *Front Pharmacol*. 2022;13:1003060.
16. U.S. Food and Drug Administration. FDA requests removal of strongest warning against using cholesterol-lowering statins during pregnancy; still advises most pregnant patients should stop taking statins. Accessed July 20, 2021. https://www.fda.gov/drugs/drug-safety-and-availability/fda-requests-removal-strongest-warning-against-using-cholesterol-lowering-statins-during-pregnancy
17. Wu T, Shi Y, Zhu B. Pregnancy-related adverse events associated with statins: a real-world pharmacovigilance study of the FDA Adverse Event Reporting System (FAERS). *Expert Opin Drug Saf*. 2023;1:1-9.

LOXAPINE

Mental Health (First-Generation Antipsychotic)

PREGNANCY RECOMMENDATION: Limited Human Data—Animal Data Suggest Potential Risk

BREASTFEEDING RECOMMENDATION: Potential Toxicity

PREGNANCY SUMMARY

Three pregnancies with first-trimester use of loxapine were reported by the manufacturer. One delivered an infant with an autosomal genetic disorder, one had multiple unspecified anomalies, and one infant was normal without any identified birth defects. The drug will probably cross the placenta, so some fetal exposure will likely occur a greater risk to the infant.

However, the limited human pregnancy experience prevents a complete assessment of the embryofetal risk. Embryofetal toxicity was observed in one animal species at doses of less than 10 times the RHD. ACOG notes that second-generation antipsychotics are more often prescribed than first-generation antipsychotics due to fewer extrapyramidal side effects and better tolerability despite limited reproductive safety data. General principles for treatment in pregnancy include using the minimum effective dose and avoiding polypharmacy, if possible. While treatment in pregnancy presents an exposure risk, this risk appears to be lower than the risks of disease symptom exacerbation and relapse. The manufacturer reports that neonates exposed to antipsychotic drugs, including loxapine, during the third trimester are at risk for extrapyramidal and/or withdrawal symptoms postdelivery, such as agitation, hypertonia, hypotonia, tremor, somnolence, respiratory distress, and feeding intolerance. If used near delivery, neonates should be monitored for these symptoms. Some neonates recovered within hours or days without specific treatment, while others required prolonged hospitalization.

BREASTFEEDING SUMMARY

No reports describing the use of loxapine during human lactation have been located. The drug will probably appear in breast milk, so some infant exposure will likely occur. ACOG recommendations state that individuals with mental health conditions should not be discouraged from breastfeeding. If a woman is stable on a particular medication throughout pregnancy, the medication should not be changed postpartum, as maternal exacerbation is probably a greater risk to the infant than the drug exposure from breastfeeding. If new medications are initiated during lactation, passage into breast milk and available safety data should be considered. If the clinical decision is to use this drug while breastfeeding, the infant should be monitored for the most common reported adult side effects of sleepiness and extrapyramidal symptoms that include irritability, hypertonia, hypotonia, tremor, somnolence, respiratory distress, and feeding intolerance.

References

1. Prescribing Information. Loxapine. Watson Pharma; 2017.
2. Prescribing Information. Adasuve. Alexa Pharmaceuticals; 2022.
3. Einarson A, Boskovic R. Use and safety of antipsychotic drugs during pregnancy. *J Psychiatr Pract*. 2009;15:183-192.
4. American College of Obstetricians and Gynecologists. Use of psychiatric medications during pregnancy and lactation. ACOG Practice Bulletin. No. 92, April 2008. *Obstet Gynecol*. 2008;111:1001-1019.
5. American College of Obstetricians and Gynecologists. Treatment and management of mental health conditions during pregnancy and postpartum: ACOG clinical practice guideline no. 5. *Obstet Gynecol*. 2023;141:1262-1288.

LUBIPROSTONE

Gastrointestinal

PREGNANCY RECOMMENDATION: Limited Human Data—Animal Data Suggest Low Risk

BREASTFEEDING RECOMMENDATION: Probably Compatible

PREGNANCY SUMMARY

The manufacturer reported four women in clinical trials who became pregnant while taking lubiprostone. Therapy was stopped when the pregnancies were detected. One was lost to follow-up, but the other three delivered healthy newborns with no identified birth anomalies. Based on the absence of quantifiable plasma concentrations of lubiprostone and the low concentrations of its active metabolite, transplacental fetal exposure is likely to be clinically insignificant. However, this limited human pregnancy experience prevents a complete assessment of the embryofetal risk. Animal data did not show any embryofetal toxicity in three species at doses of more than 10 times the RHD. Using this drug during pregnancy should be based on the pros and cons of the mother's clinical need for treatment versus any potential fetal risk that might occur from exposure.

BREASTFEEDING SUMMARY

No reports describing the use of lubiprostone during human lactation have been located. It is not known if lubiprostone or the metabolite M3 is excreted into human breast milk. However, based on the absence of quantifiable plasma concentrations of lubiprostone and the low concentrations of its active metabolite, excretion into breast milk is likely to be clinically insignificant. If the clinical decision is to use this drug while breastfeeding, the infant should be monitored for the most common reported adult side effects of nausea and headache (both leading to irritability) and diarrhea.

Reference

1. Prescribing Information. Amitiza. Takeda Pharmaceuticals America; 2018.

LULICONAZOLE

Dermatologic (Antifungal—Topical)

PREGNANCY RECOMMENDATION: **No Human Data—Animal Data Suggest Low Risk**

BREASTFEEDING RECOMMENDATION: **Probably Compatible**

PREGNANCY SUMMARY

No reports describing the use of luliconazole in human pregnancy have been located. Based on the low plasma concentrations following topical administration, fetal exposure is likely negligible. However, the absence of human pregnancy experience prevents a complete assessment of the embryofetal risk. Animal data did not show any embryofetal toxicity in two species at doses of less than 10 times the RHD in one species and in more than 10 times the RHD in a second species. Using this drug during pregnancy should be based on the pros and cons of the mother's clinical need for treatment versus any potential fetal risk that might occur from exposure.

BREASTFEEDING SUMMARY

No reports describing the use of luliconazole during human lactation have been located. Based on the low plasma concentrations following topical administration, excretion into breast milk is likely to be negligible. Breastfeeding while using this drug should be based on the mother's clinical need for treatment versus any potential infant risks that might occur. Due to the topical use of the drug, systemic side effects were not evaluated.

Reference

1. Prescribing Information. Luzu. Bausch Health US; 2020.

LUMASIRAN

Genetic (Double-Stranded Small Interfering Ribonucleic Acid—Primary Hyperoxaluria)

PREGNANCY RECOMMENDATION: **No Human Data—Animal Data Suggest Low Risk**

BREASTFEEDING RECOMMENDATION: **Probably Compatible**

PREGNANCY SUMMARY

No reports describing the use of lumasiran in human pregnancy have been located. Placental transfer is not likely to occur or is negligible at best. However, the absence of human pregnancy experience prevents a complete assessment of the

(continued)

embryofetal risk. Animal data did not show any embryofetal toxicity. Using this drug during pregnancy should be based on the pros and cons of the mother's clinical need for treatment versus any potential fetal risk that might occur from exposure.

BREASTFEEDING SUMMARY

Lumasiran excretion into breast milk is likely to be negligible. Breastfeeding while using this drug should be based on the mother's clinical need for treatment. If used, the infant should be monitored for the most common reported adult side effect of abdominal pain (leading to irritability).

Reference

1. Prescribing Information. Oxlumo. Alnylam Pharmaceuticals, Inc; 2020.

LUMATEPERONE

Mental Health (Antipsychotic)

PREGNANCY RECOMMENDATION: **No Human Data—Animal Data Suggest Low Risk**

BREASTFEEDING RECOMMENDATION: **Potential Toxicity**

PREGNANCY SUMMARY

No reports describing the use of lumateperone in human pregnancy have been located. The drug probably crosses the placenta, so some fetal exposure will likely occur. Therefore, the absence of human pregnancy experience prevents a complete assessment of the embryofetal risk. Animal studies did not show any embryofetal toxicity. Using this drug during pregnancy should be based on the pros and cons of the mother's clinical need for treatment versus any potential fetal risk that might occur from exposure. Neonates exposed to antipsychotic drugs during the third trimester are at risk for showing extrapyramidal and/or withdrawal symptoms (agitation, hypertonia, hypotonia, tremor, somnolence, and feeding disorders) postdelivery. There is a pregnancy exposure registry that monitors pregnancy outcomes in women exposed to atypical antipsychotic drugs. Health care providers are encouraged to call the National Pregnancy Registry for Atypical Antipsychotics by calling 1-866-961-2388.

L

BREASTFEEDING SUMMARY

Lumateperone probably enters breast milk. Breastfeeding with antipsychotic drugs in general can produce sedation, irritability, and extrapyramidal symptoms (tremors and abnormal muscle movements) in newborns. Because of these risks and the effects seen in animals (at higher doses), the manufacturer recommends that women not breastfeed their infants. However, breastfeeding while using this drug should be based on the overall clinical situation. If used, the infant should be monitored for the most common reported adult side effects of nausea (leading to irritability) and sedation or lethargy.

Reference

1. Prescribing Information. Caplyta. Intra-Cellular Therapies, Inc; 2020.

LURASIDONE

Mental Health (Second-Generation Antipsychotic)

PREGNANCY RECOMMENDATION: **Limited Human Data—Animal Data Suggest Low Risk**

BREASTFEEDING RECOMMENDATION: **Probably Compatible**

PREGNANCY SUMMARY

One study reported a congenital anomaly rate of 2.2% in more than 130 first-trimester exposures to lurasidone. No pattern to the defects was identified. The drug will probably cross the placenta, so some fetal exposure will likely occur. However, the limited human pregnancy experience prevents a complete assessment of the embryofetal risk. Animal data did not show any embryofetal toxicity in two species at doses of less than 10 times the RHD. ACOG states that second-generation antipsychotics are more often prescribed than first-generation antipsychotics due to fewer extrapyramidal side effects and better tolerability despite limited reproductive safety data. General principles for treatment in pregnancy include using the minimum effective dose and avoiding polypharmacy, if possible. While treatment in pregnancy presents an exposure risk, this risk is lower than the risks of symptom exacerbation and relapse. The manufacturer reports that neonates exposed to antipsychotic drugs, including lurasidone, during the third trimester are at risk for extrapyramidal and/or withdrawal symptoms postdelivery, such as agitation, hypertonia, hypotonia, tremor, somnolence, respiratory distress, and feeding intolerance. If used near delivery, neonates should be monitored for these symptoms. Some neonates recovered within hours or days without specific treatment, while others required prolonged hospitalization. There is a pregnancy exposure registry that monitors pregnancy outcomes in women using atypical antipsychotic drugs. Health care providers are encouraged to contact the National Pregnancy Registry for Atypical Antipsychotics at 1-866-961-2388.

BREASTFEEDING SUMMARY

One case report describing the use of lurasidone while exclusively breastfeeding resulted in very low levels along with normal growth and development. Using the highest breast milk level obtained (16 ng/mL), the calculated RID was about 0.4%. Additionally, a study of the National Pregnancy Registry for Psychiatric Medications found no adverse effects among infants exposed to second-generation antipsychotics through breastfeeding. ACOG recommendations state that individuals with mental health conditions should not be discouraged from breastfeeding. If a woman is stable on a particular medication throughout pregnancy, the medication should not be changed postpartum, as maternal exacerbation is greater than the exposure risk from breastfeeding. If new medications are initiated during lactation, passage into breast milk and available safety data should be considered. If the clinical decision is to use this drug while breastfeeding, the infant should be monitored for the most common reported pediatric side effects of nausea (leading to irritability), insomnia, and extrapyramidal symptoms that include agitation, hypertonia, hypotonia, tremor, somnolence, respiratory distress, and feeding intolerance.

References

1. Prescribing Information. Latuda. Sunovion; 2022.
2. Kernizan N, Forinash A, Yancey A, et al. Mood stabilizers for the treatment of bipolar disorder in pregnancy and impact on neonatal outcomes. *Bipolar Dis* 2024;26:779-84.
3. Cohen LS, Church TR, Freeman MP, et al. Reproductive safety of lurasidone and quetiapine: update from the national pregnancy registry for psychiatric medications. *J Womens Health (Larchmt)*. 2023;32:452-462.
4. American College of Obstetricians and Gynecologists. ACOG practice bulletin no. 92: use of psychiatric medications during pregnancy and lactation. *Obstet Gynecol*. 2008;111:1001-1019.
5. American College of Obstetricians and Gynecologists. Treatment and management of mental health conditions during pregnancy and postpartum: ACOG clinical practice guideline no. 5. *Obstet Gynecol*. 2023;141:1262-1288.
6. Keightley P, Schmidt Sotomayor N, O'Hara K, et al. Lurasidone in lactation: a case study with laboratory and clinical outcomes. *Aust N Z J Psychiatry*. 2020;54:1035-1036.
7. Viguera AC, Vanderkruik R, Gaccione P, et al. Breastfeeding practices among women taking second-generation antipsychotics: findings from the national pregnancy registry for atypical antipsychotics. *Arch Womens Ment Health*. 2022;25:511-516.

L

LURBINECTEDIN

Antineoplastic (Alkylating Agent)

PREGNANCY RECOMMENDATION: No Human Data—Animal Data Suggest Potential Risk

BREASTFEEDING RECOMMENDATION: Potential Toxicity

PREGNANCY SUMMARY

No reports describing the use of lurbinectedin in human pregnancy have been located. Some amount of the drug will probably cross the placenta, so fetal exposure will likely occur. However, the absence of human pregnancy experience prevents a complete assessment of the embryofetal risk. Embryofetal toxicity was observed in animal studies. Based on these animal studies and the drug's mechanism of action, the manufacturer recommends that women with reproductive potential use effective contraception during treatment and for 6 months after the last dose. They also recommend that males with female partners of reproductive potential use effective contraception during treatment and for 4 months after the last dose. Nevertheless, using this drug during pregnancy should be based on the pros and cons of the mother's clinical need for treatment versus any potential fetal risk that might occur from exposure.

BREASTFEEDING SUMMARY

No reports describing the use of lurbinectedin during human lactation have been located. The drug will probably enter breast milk in limited amounts, so some infant exposure is likely to occur. However, due to the concern for potential adverse effects in a breastfed infant, the manufacturer recommends that women not breastfeed while being treated with lurbinectedin and for at least 2 weeks after the last dose. Breastfeeding while using this drug should be based on the mother's clinical need for treatment. If used, the infant should be monitored for the most common reported adult side effects of nausea and musculoskeletal pain (both leading to irritability), lethargy, decreased appetite, constipation, diarrhea, vomiting, and cough.

Reference

1. Prescribing Information. Zepzelca. Jazz Pharmaceuticals, Inc; 2021.

LUSPATERCEPT

Hematologic (Fusion Protein With an IgG Fc Domain)

PREGNANCY RECOMMENDATION: No Human Data—Animal Data Suggest Potential Risk

BREASTFEEDING RECOMMENDATION: Probably Compatible

PREGNANCY SUMMARY

No reports describing the use of luspatercept during human pregnancy have been located. Because luspatercept contains the Fc domain of an IgG antibody, some amount of the drug will likely cross the placenta in the second half of gestation. Therefore, the absence of human pregnancy experience prevents a complete assessment of the embryofetal risk. Embryofetal toxicity was observed in one animal species at doses less than 10 times the MRHD. It also caused embryofetal toxicity in a second species, but at doses of more than 10 times the RHD. Based on animal studies and the drug's mechanism of action, the manufacturer recommends that women with reproductive potential use effective contraception during treatment and for 3 months after the last dose. Nevertheless, using this drug during pregnancy should be based on the pros and cons of the mother's clinical need for treatment versus any potential fetal risk that might occur from exposure.

BREASTFEEDING SUMMARY

No reports describing the use of luspatercept during human lactation have been located. Because it is a fusion protein with an IgG Fc domain, it might be excreted in small amounts into breast milk. Regardless, if any of this drug were to be ingested through breastfeeding, it would probably be digested in the infant's gastrointestinal tract and not be absorbed. Nevertheless, due to a concern for potential serious adverse effects that might be seen in a breastfed infant, the manufacturer recommends that women not breastfeed while being treated with this drug and for at least 3 months after the last dose. However, breastfeeding while using this drug should be based on the mother's clinical need for treatment versus any potential infant risks that might occur. If used, the infant should be monitored for the most common reported adult side effects of headache, musculoskeletal pain, arthralgia, dizziness/vertigo, nausea, and abdominal pain (all leading to irritability), dyspnea, fatigue (lethargy), diarrhea, cough, peripheral edema, and hypertension.

Reference

1. Prescribing Information. Reblozyl. Bristol Meyers Squibb; 2024.

LUSUTROMBOPAG

Hematologic (Thrombopoietin Receptor Agonist)

PREGNANCY RECOMMENDATION: No Human Data and No Relevant Animal Data

BREASTFEEDING RECOMMENDATION: Potential Toxicity

PREGNANCY SUMMARY

No reports describing the use of lusutrombopag in human pregnancy have been located. Some amount of the drug may cross the placenta, so fetal exposure will likely occur. However, the absence of human pregnancy experience prevents a complete assessment of the embryofetal risk. Embryofetal toxicity with malformations was observed in one animal species, but at doses of more than 10 times the RHD. Using this drug during pregnancy should be based on the pros and cons of the mother's clinical need for treatment versus any potential fetal risk that might occur from exposure.

BREASTFEEDING SUMMARY

No reports describing the use of lusutrombopag during human lactation have been located. Some amount of the drug may be excreted into breast milk, so infant exposure will likely occur. However, due to a concern for potential serious adverse effects that might be seen in a breastfed infant, the manufacturer recommends that women not breastfeed while being treated with this drug and for at least 4 weeks after the last dose. Nevertheless, breastfeeding while using this drug should be based on the mother's clinical need for treatment versus any potential infant risks that might occur. If used, the infant should be monitored for the most common reported adult side effect of headache (leading to irritability).

Reference

1. Prescribing Information. Mulpleta. Shionogi; 2018.

LUTETIUM LU 177

Antineoplastic/Radiopharmaceutical

PREGNANCY RECOMMENDATION: Contraindicated

BREASTFEEDING RECOMMENDATION: Contraindicated

PREGNANCY SUMMARY

No reports describing the use of lutetium Lu 177 in human pregnancy have been located. Placental transfer is likely to be clinically insignificant. However, the absence of human pregnancy experience prevents a complete assessment of the embryofetal risk. No animal reproduction studies have been conducted. However, all radiopharmaceutical agents have the potential to cause fetal harm depending on the stage of fetal development and magnitude of the radiation dose. Furthermore, based on the drug's mechanism of action, the manufacturer recommends that women with reproductive potential use effective contraception during treatment and for 7 months after the last dose. They also recommend that males with female partners of reproductive potential use effective contraception during treatment and for 4 months after the last dose.

BREASTFEEDING SUMMARY

No reports describing the use of lutetium Lu 177 during human lactation have been located. Excretion into breast milk should be limited. However, all radiopharmaceutical agents have the potential to cause harm depending on the magnitude of the radiation dose. Due to a concern for potential serious adverse effects that might be seen in a breastfed infant, the manufacturer recommends that women not breastfeed while being treated with this drug and for at least 2.5 months after the last dose.

Reference

1. Prescribing Information. Lutathera. Advanced Accelerator Applications USA, Inc; 2023.

L

LUTETIUM LU 177 VIPIVOTIDE TETRAXETAN

Radiopharmaceutical

PREGNANCY RECOMMENDATION: *Contraindicated

BREASTFEEDING RECOMMENDATION: *Contraindicated

PREGNANCY SUMMARY

No reports describing the use of lutetium Lu 177 vipivotide tetraxetan in human pregnancy have been located. Based on likely placental transfer, fetal exposure would probably occur. However, the absence of human pregnancy experience prevents a complete assessment of the embryofetal risk. No animal reproduction studies have been performed. *Regardless, given the drug's approved use indication, it should not be used in women. Based on the drug's mechanism of action, the manufacturer recommends that male patients with female partners of reproductive potential use effective contraception during treatment and for 14 weeks after the last dose.

BREASTFEEDING SUMMARY

No reports describing the use of lutetium Lu 177 vipivotide tetraxetan during human lactation have been located. A limited amount of the drug could be found in breast milk. *However, given the drug's approved use indication, it should not be used in women.

Reference

1. Prescribing Information. Pluvicto. Novartis AG; 2022.

M

MACIMORELIN

Endocrine/Metabolic (Human Growth Hormone Secretagogue Receptor Agonist)

PREGNANCY RECOMMENDATION: No Human Data and No Relevant Animal Data

BREASTFEEDING RECOMMENDATION: Probably Compatible

PREGNANCY SUMMARY

No reports describing the use of macimorelin in human pregnancy have been located. Though placental transfer is most likely small, some fetal exposure will probably occur. However, the absence of human pregnancy experience prevents a complete assessment of the embryofetal risk. Animal reproduction studies have not been performed. The drug was found to prolong the QT interval.

BREASTFEEDING SUMMARY

It is not known if macimorelin is excreted into human breast milk. Some amount of the drug is probably excreted into breast milk, but the total amount is likely minimal. Breastfeeding while using this drug should be based on the mother's clinical need for diagnosis. If used, the infant should be monitored for the most common reported adult side effects of nausea and headache (both leading to irritability), lethargy, and diarrhea. Most drugs in general are fully eliminated after about four to five half-lives. Therefore, a secondary option would be to pump and discard for 16 to 24 hours after the single drug dose is administered.

Reference

1. Prescribing Information. Macrilen. Novo Nordisk, Inc; 2021.

MACITENTAN

Cardiovascular (Endothelin Receptor Antagonist/Vasodilator)

PREGNANCY RECOMMENDATION: No Human Data—Animal Data Suggest Risk (Maternal Benefit May Outweigh Any Potential Fetal Risk—if Pregnancy Occurs)

BREASTFEEDING RECOMMENDATION: Potential Toxicity

PREGNANCY SUMMARY

One report describing the use of macitentan in human pregnancy did not report any outcomes. The drug will probably cross the placenta, so some fetal exposure will likely occur. Therefore, the absence of human pregnancy experience prevents a complete assessment of the embryofetal risk. Embryofetal toxicity with malformations was observed in two animal species at all doses tested. Based on animal studies and the drug's mechanism of action, the manufacturer recommends that women with reproductive potential use effective contraception during treatment and for 1 month after the last dose. Macitentan carries a boxed warning regarding embryofetal toxicity and is only available through a restricted program called the Macitentan-Containing Products Risk Evaluation and Mitigation Strategy (REMS). In this program, females of reproductive potential must have monthly negative pregnancy tests to continue the medication. However, pulmonary artery hypertension in pregnancy is extremely high risk, and if a pregnancy inadvertently occurs, using this drug during pregnancy should be based on the pros and cons of the mother's clinical need for treatment versus any potential fetal risk that might occur from exposure.

BREASTFEEDING SUMMARY

No reports describing the use of macitentan during human lactation have been located. The drug will probably be found in human breast milk, so some infant exposure will likely occur. However, due to a concern for potential serious adverse effects that might be seen in a breastfed infant, the manufacturer recommends that women not breastfeed while being treated with this drug. Nevertheless, if the clinical decision is to use this drug while breastfeeding, the infant should be monitored for the most common reported adult side effects of headache (leading to irritability), anemia, and various infections.

References

1. Prescribing Information. Opsumit. Actelion Pharmaceuticals US; 2024.
2. Amann U, Wentzell N, Kollhorst B, Haug U. Prescribing of endothelin receptor antagonists and riociguat in women of childbearing age in a large German claims database study. *Reprod Toxicol*. 2023;119:108415.

MAFENIDE

Antibacterial/Dermatologic

PREGNANCY RECOMMENDATION: No Human Data—Animal Data Suggest Low Risk

BREASTFEEDING RECOMMENDATION: Potential Toxicity

PREGNANCY SUMMARY

No reports describing the use of mafenide during human pregnancy have been located. Both the cream and the topical solution are absorbed into the systemic circulation. Therefore, the drug will probably cross the placenta, so some fetal exposure will likely occur. However, the absence of human pregnancy experience prevents a complete assessment of the embryofetal risk. Animal data did not show any embryofetal toxicity in one species. Using this drug during pregnancy should be based on the pros and cons of the mother's clinical need for treatment versus any potential fetal risk that might occur from exposure.

BREASTFEEDING SUMMARY

No reports describing the use of mafenide during human lactation have been located. The drug will probably appear in breast milk, so some infant exposure will likely occur. Mafenide and its active metabolite inhibit carbonic anhydrase, which has caused metabolic acidosis in some patients with prolonged treatment. Because the approved indications for this agent suggest long-term exposure, the manufacturer recommends that nursing be avoided. Nevertheless, breastfeeding while using this drug should be based on the mother's clinical need for treatment versus any potential infant risks that might occur.

References

1. Prescribing Information. Sulfamylon cream. Rising Pharma Holdings, Inc; 2023.
2. Prescribing Information. Mafenide acetate. Par Pharmaceuticals; 2017.

MAGNESIUM SULFATE

Central Nervous System (Antiseizure)/Miscellaneous (Electrolyte)

PREGNANCY RECOMMENDATION: Human Data Suggest Low Risk

BREASTFEEDING RECOMMENDATION: Compatible

PREGNANCY SUMMARY

The use of magnesium sulfate in pregnancy is well established. Available studies have found no evidence of a significantly increased risk for congenital anomalies. Magnesium crosses the placenta, so fetal exposure will occur. Animal reproduction studies have not been conducted. Infusions of the drug for greater than 5 to 7 days may be associated with hypocalcemia in the fetus. Magnesium toxicity in the newborn, including neuromuscular or respiratory depression, may also occur with continuous infusion. Newborns exposed to magnesium sulfate close to delivery should be closely observed for signs of toxicity during the first 24 to 48 hours after birth.

BREASTFEEDING SUMMARY

No reports describing the effects of magnesium sulfate during human lactation have been located. Magnesium is excreted into human breast milk. Concentrations of the element in breast milk were only slightly increased after intravenous (IV) magnesium treatment. Oral absorption of magnesium is very poor; therefore, maternal treatment is not expected to increase the infant's serum magnesium level or result in any adverse infant effects.

References

1. Prescribing Information. Magnesium sulfate. Amneal Pharmaceuticals LLC; 2024.
2. Dangman BC, Rosen TS. Magnesium levels in infants of mothers treated with $MgSO_4$ (abstract #262). *Pediatr Res*. 1977;11:415.
3. Cruikshank DP, Pitkin RM, Reynolds WA, Williams GA, Hargis GK. Effects of magnesium sulfate treatment on perinatal calcium metabolism. I. Maternal and fetal responses. *Am J Obstet Gynecol*. 1979;134:243-249.
4. Donovan EF, Tsang RC, Steichen JJ, Strub RJ, Chen IW, Chen M. Neonatal hypermagnesemia: effect on parathyroid hormone and calcium homeostasis. *J Pediatr*. 1980;96:305-310.

5. Stone SR, Pritchard JA. Effect of maternally administered magnesium sulfate on the neonate. *Obstet Gynecol*. 1970;35:574-577.
6. Pruett KM, Kirshon B, Cotton DB, Adam K, Doody KJ. The effects of magnesium sulfate therapy on Apgar scores. *Am J Obstet Gynecol*. 1988; 159:1047-1048.
7. Heinonen OP, Slone D, Shapiro S. *Birth Defects and Drugs in Pregnancy*. Publishing Sciences Group; 1977:440.
8. Martin RW, Gaddy DK, Martin JN Jr, Lucas JA, Wiser WL, Morrison JC. Tocolysis with oral magnesium. *Am J Obstet Gynecol*. 1987;156:433-434.
9. Spatling L, Spatling G. Magnesium supplementation in pregnancy: a double-blind study. *Br J Obstet Gynaecol*. 1988;95:120-125.
10. Sibai BM, Villar MA, Bray E. Magnesium supplementation during pregnancy: a double-blind randomized controlled clinical trial. *Am J Obstet Gynecol*. 1989;161:115-119.
11. Lipsitz PJ, English IC. Hypermagnesemia in the newborn infant. *Pediatrics*. 1967;40:856-862.
12. Lipsitz PJ. The clinical and biochemical effects of excess magnesium in the newborn. *Pediatrics*. 1971;47:501-509.
13. Savory J, Monif GRG. Serum calcium levels in cord sera of the progeny of mothers treated with magnesium sulfate for toxemia of pregnancy. *Am J Obstet Gynecol*. 1971;110:556-559.
14. Rasch DK, Huber PA, Richardson CJ, L'Hommedieu CS, Nelson TE, Reddi R. Neurobehavioral effects of neonatal hypermagnesemia. *J Pediatr*. 1982;100: 272-276.
15. Green KW, Key TC, Coen R, Resnik R. The effects of maternally administered magnesium sulfate on the neonate. *Am J Obstet Gynecol*. 1983;146:29-33.
16. Sibai BM, Lipshitz J, Anderson GD, Dilts PV Jr. Reassessment of intravenous $MgSO_4$ therapy in preeclampsia-eclampsia. *Obstet Gynecol* 1981;57: 199-202.
17. Hutchinson HT, Nichols MM, Kuhn CR, Vasicka A. Effects of magnesium sulfate on uterine contractility, intrauterine fetus, and infant. *Am J Obstet Gynecol*. 1964;88:747-758.
18. Lamm CI, Norton KI, Murphy RJC, et al. Congenital rickets associated with magnesium sulfate infusion for tocolysis. *J Pediatr*. 1988;113:1078-1082.
19. Wilkins IA, Goldberg JD, Phillips RN, et al. Long-term use of magnesium sulfate as a tocolytic agent. *Obstet Gynecol*. 1986;67:38S-40S.
20. Dudley D, Gagnon D, Varner M. Long-term tocolysis with intravenous magnesium sulfate. *Obstet Gynecol*. 1989;73:373-378.
21. Brady JP, Williams HC. Magnesium intoxication in a premature infant. *Pediatrics*. 1967;40:100-103.
22. Brazy JE, Grimm JK, Little VA. Neonatal manifestations of severe maternal hypertension occurring before the thirty-sixth week of pregnancy. *J Pediatr*. 1982;100:265-271.
23. Holcomb WL Jr, Shackelford GD, Petrie RH. Prolonged magnesium therapy affects fetal bone (abstract). *Am J Obstet Gynecol*. 1991;164:386.
24. Smith LG Jr, Schanler RJ, Burns P, Moise KJ Jr. Effect of magnesium sulfate therapy (MgSO4) on the bone mineral content of women and their newborns (abstract). *Am J Obstet Gynecol*. 1991;164:427.
25. Holcomb WL Jr, Shackelford GD, Petrie RH. Magnesium tocolysis and neonatal bone abnormalities: a controlled study. *Obstet Gynecol*. 1991;78: 611-614.
26. Smith LG Jr, Burns PA, Schanler RJ. Calcium homeostasis in pregnant women receiving long-term magnesium sulfate therapy for preterm labor. *Am J Obstet Gynecol*. 1992;167:45-51.
27. Cruikshank DP, Chan GM, Doerrfeld D. Alterations in vitamin D and calcium metabolism with magnesium sulfate treatment of preeclampsia. *Am J Obstet Gynecol*. 1993;168:1170-1177.
28. L'Hommedieu CS, Nicholas D, Armes DA, et al. Potentiation of magnesium sulfate-induced neuromuscular weakness by gentamicin, tobramycin, and amikacin. *J Pediatr*. 1983;102:629-631.
29. L'Hommedieu CS, Huber PA, Rasch DK. Potentiation of magnesium-induced neuromuscular weakness by gentamicin. *Crit Care Med*. 1983;11:55-56.
30. Waisman GD, Mayorga LM, Camera MI, et al. Magnesium plus nifedipine: potentiation of hypotensive effect in preeclampsia? *Am J Obstet Gynecol* 1988;159:308-309.
31. Snyder SW, Cardwell MS. Neuromuscular blockade with magnesium sulfate and nifedipine. *Am J Obstet Gynecol*. 1989;161:35-36.
32. Rodis JF, Vintzileos AM, Campbell WA, et al. Maternal hypothermia: an unusual complication of magnesium sulfate therapy. *Am J Obstet Gynecol*. 1987;156:435-436.
33. Doyle LW, Crowther CA, Middleton P, et al. Magnesium sulphate for women at risk of preterm birth for neuroprotection of the fetus. *Cochrane Database Syst Rev*. 2009;(1):CD004661.
34. American College of Obstetricians and Gynecologists. Magnesium sulfate before anticipated preterm birth for neuroprotection. Committee opinion no. 455. *Obstet Gynecol*. 2010;115:669-671.
35. Baldwin WF. Clinical study of senna administration to nursing mothers: assessment of effects on infant bowel habits. *CMAJ*. 1963;89:566-568.
36. Cruikshank DP, Varner MW, Pitkin RM. Breast milk magnesium and calcium concentrations following magnesium sulfate treatment. *Am J Obstet Gynecol*. 1982;143:685-688.
37. Haldeman W. Can magnesium sulfate therapy impact lactogenesis? *JHL*. 1993;9:249-252.
38. Riaz M, Porat R, Brodsky NL, Hurt H. The effects of maternal magnesium sulfate treatment on newborns: a prospective controlled study. *J Perinatol*. 1998;18:449-454.
39. Cordero L, Valentine CJ, Samuels P, et al. Breastfeeding in women with severe preeclampsia. *Breastfeed Med*. 2012;7:457-463.
40. Morris ME, LeRoy S, Sutton SC. Absorption of magnesium from orally administered magnesium sulfate in man. *J Toxicol Clin Toxicol*. 1987;25:371-382.

MANNITOL

Cardiovascular (Diuretic)

PREGNANCY RECOMMENDATION: Limited Human Data—Animal Data Suggest Low Risk

BREASTFEEDING RECOMMENDATION: Probably Compatible

PREGNANCY SUMMARY

Four reports describing the use of mannitol in human pregnancy were located. These reports include 36 pregnancies with exposure in all trimesters. No congenital abnormalities or adverse effects were reported. Mannitol crosses the placenta, so fetal exposure will occur. However, the limited human pregnancy experience prevents a complete assessment of the embryofetal risk. Animal data did not show any embryofetal toxicity in three species. Using this drug during pregnancy should be based on the pros and cons of the mother's clinical need for treatment versus any potential fetal risk that might occur from exposure.

BREASTFEEDING SUMMARY

No reports describing the use of mannitol during human lactation have been located. The drug will probably appear in human breast milk, so some infant exposure will likely occur. Breastfeeding while using this drug should be based on the mother's clinical need for treatment versus any potential infant risks that might occur. If used, the infant should be monitored for the most common reported adult side effects of dehydration and lethargy.

References

1. Prescribing Information. Mannitol. Fresenius Kabi USA, LLC; 2023.
2. Demir BC, Ozerkan K, Ozbek SE, et al. Comparison of magnesium sulfate and mannitol in treatment of eclamptic women with posterior reversible encephalopathy syndrome. *Arch Gynecol Obstet*. 2012;286:287-293.
3. Ebke M, Jurgens KU, Tomandl B, et al. Surgical treatment of space occupying edema and hemorrhage due to cerebral venous thrombosis during pregnancy. *Neurocrit Care*. 2011;15:166-169.
4. Kazemi P, Villar G, Flexman AM. Anesthetic management of neurosurgical procedures during pregnancy: a case series. *J Neurosurg Anesthesiol*. 2014;26:234-240.
5. Handlogten KS, Sharpe EE, Brost BC, et al. Dexmedetomidine and mannitol for awake craniotomy in a pregnant patient. *Anesth Analg*. 2015; 120:1099-1103.

MARALIXIBAT

Gastrointestinal (Ileal Bile Acid Transporter Inhibitor)

PREGNANCY RECOMMENDATION: No Human Data—Animal Data Suggest Low Risk

BREASTFEEDING RECOMMENDATION: Probably Compatible

PREGNANCY SUMMARY

No reports describing the use of maralixibat in human pregnancy have been located. The amount of the drug that might cross the placenta is probably negligible, so fetal exposure is likely to be clinically insignificant. However, the absence of human pregnancy experience prevents a complete assessment of the embryofetal risk. Animal data did not show any embryofetal toxicity. Using this drug during pregnancy should be based on the pros and cons of the mother's clinical need for treatment versus any potential fetal risk that might occur from exposure. Maralixibat can lead to fat-soluble vitamin deficiency. The manufacturer recommends checking levels at baseline, then periodically during treatment, and supplementing if a deficiency occurs.

BREASTFEEDING SUMMARY

No reports describing the use of maralixibat during human lactation have been located. If this drug were to appear in breast milk, the level would most likely be clinically insignificant. Breastfeeding while using this drug should be based on the mother's clinical need for treatment. If used, the infant should be monitored for the most common reported adult side effects of abdominal pain (leading to irritability), diarrhea, vomiting, fat-soluble vitamin deficiency, liver test abnormalities, and gastrointestinal bleeding.

Reference

1. Prescribing Information. Livmarli. Mirum Pharmaceuticals; 2021.

MARAVIROC

Antiretroviral (Cellular Chemokine Receptor Antagonist—HIV-1)

PREGNANCY RECOMMENDATION: Limited Human Data—Animal Data Suggest Low Risk (Maternal Benefit May Outweigh Embryofetal Risk)

BREASTFEEDING RECOMMENDATION: *Contraindicated

PREGNANCY SUMMARY

The Antiretroviral Pregnancy Registry (APR) report for the period ending January 2024 described 1 (3.1%) major birth anomaly in 32 live births with first-trimester exposure to a maraviroc-based regimen. The US Department of Health and Human Services AIDS Info guidelines for the use of antiretroviral agents during pregnancy recommend that, in most cases, patients continue their regimen during pregnancy if it is tolerated, safe, and effective in suppressing viral replication. Additionally, treatment initiation should not be delayed due to concerns about teratogenicity with first-trimester exposure. See the guideline for the most updated information. If indicated, maraviroc should not be withheld in pregnancy since the expected benefit to the mother with HIV outweighs the unknown risk to the fetus. Providers caring for pregnant patients with HIV and their infants can call the national Perinatal HIV/AIDS hotline (888-448-8765) for free clinical consultation. Additionally, there is a pregnancy exposure registry that monitors pregnancy outcomes in individuals exposed to antiretroviral medications during pregnancy. Health care providers are encouraged to register patients by calling APR at 1-800-258-4263.

BREASTFEEDING SUMMARY

One case report describing the use of maraviroc during human lactation was located. Normal clinical and laboratory assessment, development, and HIV testing were noted at all times tested. The drug will probably be found in human breast milk, so some infant exposure will likely occur. In 2023, the updated US Department of Health and Human Services AIDS Info guidelines state that using replacement of breast milk through formula or pasteurized donor human breast milk from a milk bank eliminates the risk of postnatal HIV transmission to the infant. Using antiretroviral therapy to achieve and maintain viral suppression during pregnancy and postpartum decreases the risk for infant transmission to less than 1% but not zero. *For patients not on therapy or those without viral load suppression during pregnancy (at a minimum of throughout the third trimester) and at delivery, replacement of breast milk is recommended. Patients on antiretroviral therapy with a sustained undetectable viral load who choose to breastfeed or use replacement of breast milk should be supported with this decision. If the clinical decision is to use this drug while breastfeeding, the infant should be monitored for the most common reported pediatric side effects of dizziness, nausea, and abdominal pain (all leading to irritability), diarrhea, and vomiting.

References

1. Prescribing Information. Selzentry. ViiV Healthcare; 2022.
2. Calcagno A, Trentini L, Marinaro L, et al. Transplacental passage of etravirine and maraviroc in a multidrug-experienced HIV-infected woman failing on darunavir-based HAART in late pregnancy. *J Antimicrob Chemother*. 2013;68:1938-1939.
3. Colbers A, Best B, Schalkwijk S, et al; for the PANNA network and the IMPAACT 1026 Study Team. Maraviroc pharmacokinetics in HIV-1-infected pregnant women. *Clin Inf Dis*. 2015;61:1582-1589.
4. Vinot C, Gavard L, Treluyer JM, et al. Placental transfer of maraviroc in an *ex vivo* human cotyledon perfusion model and influence of ABC transporter expression. *Antimicrob Agents Chemother*. 2013;57:1415-1420.
5. Antiretroviral Pregnancy Registry Steering Committee. Antiretroviral Pregnancy Registry interim report for 1 January 1989 through 31 January 2024. Registry Coordinating Center. 2024. Accessed July 3, 2024. https://www.pregistry.com.
6. Panel on Treatment of HIV During Pregnancy and Prevention of Perinatal Transmission. Recommendations for the use of antiretroviral drugs during pregnancy and interventions to reduce perinatal HIV transmission in the United States. Recommendations for the use of antiretroviral drugs during pregnancy. Department of Health and Human Services. 2024. Accessed July 3, 2024. https://clinicalinfo.hiv.gov/en/guidelines/perinatal
7. Feiterna-Sperling C, Krüger R, Amara A, et al. Pharmacokinetics of maraviroc in plasma and breastmilk in a treatment-experienced perinatally HIV-1-infected woman. *AIDS*. 2019;33:2443-2444.

MARGETUXIMAB

Antineoplastic (Monoclonal Antibody)

PREGNANCY RECOMMENDATION: No Human Data—Animal Data Suggest Potential Risk

BREASTFEEDING RECOMMENDATION: Probably Compatible

PREGNANCY SUMMARY

No reports describing the use of margetuximab in human pregnancy have been located. Because it is an antibody of the immunoglobulin G (IgG) class, it probably crosses the placenta. In postmarketing reports for HER2-directed antibody treatments overall, oligohydramnios and oligohydramnios sequence (pulmonary hypoplasia, skeletal abnormalities, and neonatal death) have been described. The drug may lead to a reduction in left ventricular ejection fraction, and cardiac function should be evaluated prior to and during treatment. Animal data showed similar fetotoxic effects. The manufacturer recommends effective contraception for women of childbearing age while receiving this treatment and for 4 months after the last dose. However, if the clinical decision is to use this drug during gestation for maternal benefit, it is recommended that the pregnancy be followed closely by an ultrasound for fetal growth and amniotic fluid volume.

BREASTFEEDING SUMMARY

Margetuximab probably enters breast milk. However, it is known that IgG antibodies found in human breast milk are not found in neonatal or infant circulation. Additionally, if any IgG antibodies were to be ingested through breastfeeding, they would probably be digested in the infant's gastrointestinal tract and not be absorbed. Breastfeeding while using this drug should be based on the mother's clinical need for treatment. If used, the infant should be monitored for the most common reported adult side effects of extremity pain, abdominal pain, back pain, and nausea (all leading to irritability), lethargy, pyrexia, cough, vomiting, diarrhea, constipation, and decreased appetite.

Reference

1. Prescribing Information. Margenza. MacroGenics, Inc; 2020.

MARIBAVIR

Antiviral (Cytomegalovirus)

PREGNANCY RECOMMENDATION: No Human Data—Animal Data Suggest Potential Risk

BREASTFEEDING RECOMMENDATION: Potential Toxicity

PREGNANCY SUMMARY

No reports describing the use of maribavir in human pregnancy have been located. Maribavir crossed the placenta in a human ex vivo placental transfer study at a rate of about 10%, so some fetal exposure will likely occur. However, the absence of human pregnancy experience prevents a complete assessment of embryofetal risk. Embryofetal toxicity was observed in animal studies. Using this drug during pregnancy should be based on the pros and cons of the mother's clinical need for treatment versus any potential fetal risk that might occur from exposure.

BREASTFEEDING SUMMARY

No reports describing the use of maribavir during human lactation have been located. The drug will probably be found in breast milk, so some infant exposure will likely occur. Breastfeeding while using this drug should be based on the mother's clinical need for treatment. If used, the infant should be monitored for the most common reported adult side effects of nausea (leading to irritability), diarrhea, vomiting, and lethargy.

References

1. Prescribing Information. Livtencity. Takeda Pharmaceuticals America; 2022.
2. Faure Bardon V, Peytavin G, Le MP, et al. Placental transfer of letermovir & maribavir in the *ex vivo* human cotyledon perfusion model. New perspectives for *in utero* treatment of congenital cytomegalovirus infection. *PLoS One*. 2020;15:e0232140.

MAVACAMTEN

Cardiovascular (Cardiac Myosin Inhibitor)

PREGNANCY RECOMMENDATION: No Human Data—Animal Data Suggest Risk

BREASTFEEDING RECOMMENDATION: Potential Toxicity

PREGNANCY SUMMARY

No reports describing the use of mavacamten in human pregnancy have been located. The drug is likely to cross the placenta, so some fetal exposure will probably occur. Therefore, the absence of human pregnancy experience prevents a complete assessment of the embryofetal risk. Embryofetal toxicity with malformations was observed in animal studies. Based on these animal studies, the manufacturer recommends that women with reproductive potential use effective contraception during treatment and for 4 months after the last dose. Nevertheless, using this drug during pregnancy should be based on the pros and cons of the mother's clinical need for treatment versus any potential fetal risk that might occur from exposure. There is a pregnancy safety study for this drug if taken during pregnancy or if a patient becomes pregnant within 4 months after the last dose. Health care providers are encouraged to contact Bristol-Myers Squibb at 1-800-721-5072.

BREASTFEEDING SUMMARY

No reports describing the use of mavacamten during human lactation have been located. The drug will likely be found in breast milk, so some infant exposure will probably occur. Breastfeeding while using this drug should be based on the mother's clinical need for treatment. If used, the infant should be monitored for the most common reported adult side effect of dizziness (leading to irritability).

Reference

1. Prescribing Information. Camzyos. Bristol-Myers Squibb; 2023.

MAVORIXAFOR

Hematologic (Hematopoietic Stem Cell Mobilizer)

PREGNANCY RECOMMENDATION: No Human Data—Animal Data Suggest Potential Risk

BREASTFEEDING RECOMMENDATION: Potential Toxicity

PREGNANCY SUMMARY

No reports describing the use of mavorixafor in human pregnancy have been located. The drug will probably cross the placenta, so some fetal exposure will likely occur. Therefore, the absence of human pregnancy experience prevents a complete

(continued)

assessment of the embryofetal risk. Animal reproduction or fertility studies have not been conducted with motixafortide. However, disruption of chemokine receptor type 4 (CXCR4) and chemokine receptor type 4 (SDF-1α) signaling did increase the risk for embryofetal lethality in mice. Based on animal studies and the drug's mechanism of action, the manufacturer recommends that women with reproductive potential use effective contraception during treatment and for 3 weeks after the last dose. Regardless, using this drug during pregnancy should be based on the pros and cons of the mother's clinical need for treatment versus any potential fetal risk that might occur from exposure. Mavorixafor has also been shown to prolong the QT interval.

BREASTFEEDING SUMMARY

No reports describing the use of mavorixafor during human lactation have been located. The drug will probably be excreted into breast milk, so some infant exposure will likely occur. Due to a concern for potential serious adverse effects that might be seen in a breastfed infant, the manufacturer recommends that women not breastfeed while being treated with this drug and for at least 3 weeks after the last dose. Nevertheless, breastfeeding while using this drug should be based on the mother's clinical need for treatment. If used, the infant should be monitored for the most common reported adult side effects of dizziness (leading to irritability), vomiting, rash, and epistaxis.

Reference

1. Prescribing Information. Xolremdi. X4 Pharmaceuticals, Inc; 2024.

MEBENDAZOLE

Anti-Infective (Anthelmintic)

PREGNANCY RECOMMENDATION: Human Data Suggest Low Risk

BREASTFEEDING RECOMMENDATION: Probably Compatible

PREGNANCY SUMMARY

Several reports describing the use of mebendazole in all trimesters of human pregnancy have been located. The rate of major congenital birth anomalies was only 2.4% in more than 1,500 first-trimester exposures. In addition, no pattern to the defects was seen. Mebendazole will probably cross the placenta, but the low systemic blood levels for the drug suggest that the amount is likely to be negligible. Embryofetal toxicity with malformations was observed in two animal species at doses less than the maximum recommended human dose (MRHD) but not in two other species at doses that were more than the MRHD. The World Health Organization (WHO) recommends preventative therapy with mebendazole after the first trimester in populations at risk for soil-transmitted helminth infections.

BREASTFEEDING SUMMARY

One case series describing the effects of mebendazole in 45 breastfeeding mothers reported no adverse effects in infants. Mebendazole has been detected in breast milk. Most samples have levels below the limit of quantification, but one peak value obtained was 6 ng/mL. The amount of drug absorbed through breast milk with these low concentrations suggests that any amount of the drug that might be in the infant's circulation would be clinically insignificant. The WHO considers mebendazole compatible with breastfeeding. If used while breastfeeding, the infant should be monitored for the most common reported adult side effects of nausea and abdominal pain (both leading to irritability), anorexia (monitor infant growth), diarrhea, flatulence, vomiting, and rash.

References

1. Prescribing Information. Emverm. Amneal Pharmaceuticals; 2021.
2. World Health Organization. Soil-transmitted helminth infections. Accessed February 19, 2025. http://www.who.int/news-room/fact-sheets/detail/soil-transmitted-helminth-infections
3. Beard TC, Rickard MD, Goodman HT. Medical treatment for hydatids. *Med J Aust*. 1978;1:633-635.
4. de Silva NR, Sirisena JLGJ, Gunasekera DPS, et al. Effect of mebendazole therapy during pregnancy on birth outcome. *Lancet*. 1999;353:1145-1149.
5. Diav-Citrin O, Shechtman S, Arnon J, et al. Pregnancy outcome after gestational exposure to mebendazole: a prospective controlled cohort study. *Am J Obstet Gynecol*. 2003;188:282-285.
6. Acs N, Bánhidy F, Puho E, Czeizel AE. Population-based case-control study of mebendazole in pregnant women for birth outcomes. *Congenit Anom (Kyoto)*. 2005;45:85-88.
7. Larocque R, Casapia M, Gotuzzo E, et al. A double-blind randomized controlled trial of antenatal mebendazole to reduce low birthweight in a hookworm-endemic area of Peru. *Trop Med Int Health*. 2006;11:1485-1495.
8. Gyorkos TW, Larocque R, Casapia M, Gotuzzo E. Lack of risk of adverse birth outcomes after deworming in pregnant women. *Pediatr Infect Dis J*. 2006;25:791-794.
9. Torp-Pedersen A, Jimenez-Solem E, Andersen JT, et al. Exposure to mebendazole and pyrvinium during pregnancy: a Danish nationwide cohort study. *Infect Dis Obstet Gynecol*. 2012;2012:769851.
10. Torp-Pedersen A, Jimenez-Solem E, Cejvanovic V, et al. Birth outcomes after exposure to mebendazole and pyrvinium during pregnancy—a Danish nationwide cohort study. *J Obstet Gynaecol*. 2016;36:1020-1025.
11. Rao TS. Does mebendazole inhibit lactation? *N Z Med J*. 1983;96:589-590.
12. Kurzel RB, Toot PJ, Lambert LV, Mihelcic AS. Mebendazole and postpartum lactation. *N Z Med J*. 1994;107:439.
13. Dayan AD. Albendazole, mebendazole, and praziquantel. Review of non-clinical toxicity and pharmacokinetics. *Acta Tropica*. 2003;86:141-159.
14. Gyorkos TW, St-Denis K. Systematic review of exposure to albendazole or mebendazole during pregnancy and effects on maternal and child outcomes, with particular reference to exposure in the first trimester. *Int J Parasitol*. 2019;49:541-554.
15. Karra N, Cohen R, Berlin M, et al. Safety of mebendazole use during lactation: a case series report. *Drugs R D* 2016;16:251-254.
16. Stoukides C. Can a mother safely breastfeed while on mebendazole (Vermox)? *J Hum Lact*. 1994;10:269.

MECHLORETHAMINE

Antineoplastic (Alkylating Agent)

PREGNANCY RECOMMENDATION: No Human Data and No Relevant Animal Data

BREASTFEEDING RECOMMENDATION: Probably Compatible

PREGNANCY SUMMARY

No reports describing the use of topical mechlorethamine in human pregnancy have been located. If the drug is found in the systemic circulation, it will probably cross the placenta. However, systemic concentrations were undetectable. Regardless, the absence of human pregnancy experience prevents a complete assessment of the embryofetal risk. Embryofetal toxicity with malformations was observed in two animal species, but the drug was administered subcutaneously (SC). Due to human systemic case reports, findings from animal studies, and the drug's mechanism of action, the manufacturer recommends that women with reproductive potential who are taking mechlorethamine be advised to use effective contraception during treatment. They also recommend that males with female partners of reproductive potential use effective contraception during treatment. Nevertheless, using this drug during pregnancy should be based on the pros and cons of the mother's clinical need for treatment versus any potential fetal risk that might occur from exposure. There is a registry for women who are pregnant and have cancer. For more information, women and health care providers are encouraged to contact the Cancer and Pregnancy Registry at 1-877-635-4499.

BREASTFEEDING SUMMARY

No reports describing the use of topical mechlorethamine during human lactation have been located. If the drug is found in the systemic circulation, it will probably be found in human breast milk. However, systemic concentrations were undetectable. Nevertheless, due to a concern for potential serious adverse effects that might be seen in a breastfed infant, the manufacturer recommends that women not breastfeed while being treated with this drug. Regardless, breastfeeding while using this drug should be based on the mother's clinical need for treatment. Because of the topical use, adult systemic side effects were not reported. Direct contact of the infant's skin and the treated areas should be avoided.

Reference

1. Prescribing Information. Valchlor. Helsinn Pharmaceuticals; 2024.

MECLIZINE

Antihistamine (Histamine H_1 Antagonist)

PREGNANCY RECOMMENDATION: Human Data Suggest Compatible

BREASTFEEDING RECOMMENDATION: Probably Compatible

PREGNANCY SUMMARY

Numerous case reports, letters, and studies describing the use of meclizine in human pregnancy have been located. Three large studies of over 17,000 meclizine exposures during the first trimester found no association with an increased risk of congenital malformations, and no pattern to the defects was identified. The drug will probably cross the placenta, so fetal exposure will likely occur. Embryofetal toxicity was observed in one animal species at doses less than 10 times the MRHD. Using this drug during pregnancy should be based on the pros and cons of the mother's clinical need for treatment versus any potential fetal risk that might occur from exposure.

BREASTFEEDING SUMMARY

No reports describing the use of meclizine during human lactation have been located. The drug will probably appear in breast milk, so infant exposure will likely occur. Breastfeeding while using this drug should be based on the mother's clinical need for treatment versus any potential infant risks that might occur. If used, the infant should be monitored for the most common reported adult side effects of dry mouth and headache (both leading to irritability), fatigue (lethargy), somnolence, and vomiting.

References

1. Prescribing Information. Antivert. Casper Pharma; 2019.
2. Heinonen OP, Slone D, Shapiro S. *Birth Defects and Drugs in Pregnancy*. Publishing Sciences Group; 1977.
3. Shapiro S, Kaufman DW, Rosenberg L, et al. Meclizine in pregnancy in relation to congenital malformations. *Br Med J*. 1978;1:483.

4. Nelson MM, Forfar JO. Associations between drugs administered during pregnancy and congenital abnormalities of the fetus. *Br Med J*. 1971;1:523-527.
5. Yerushalmy J, Milkovich L. Evaluation of the teratogenic effect of meclizine in man. *Am J Obstet Gynecol*. 1965;93:553-562.
6. Milkovich L, Van den Berg BJ. An evaluation of the teratogenicity of certain antinauseant drugs. *Am J Obstet Gynecol*. 1976;125:244-248.
7. Kallen B, Mottet I. Delivery outcome after the use of meclozine in early pregnancy. *Eur J Epidemiol*. 2003;18:665-669.
8. Pubchem. Meclizine. Accessed July 5, 2024. https://pubchem.ncbi.nlm.nih.gov/compound/meclizine

MECLOFENAMATE SODIUM

Pain (Nonsteroidal Anti-Inflammatory Drug)

PREGNANCY RECOMMENDATION: Human Data Suggest Risk (Second and Third Trimesters)

BREASTFEEDING RECOMMENDATION: Probably Compatible (Short-Term Use)

PREGNANCY SUMMARY

One report of 166 newborns exposed to meclofenamate sodium in the first trimester was located. No association with an increased risk of congenital anomalies was found. The drug will probably cross the placenta, so some fetal exposure will likely occur. However, this limited human pregnancy experience prevents a complete assessment of the embryofetal risk. Embryofetal toxicity was observed in one animal species. Nonsteroidal anti-inflammatory drugs (NSAIDs) can cause premature stricture or closure of the fetal ductus arteriosus when used in the latter portion of gestation. In some instances, this can produce pulmonary hypertension in the neonate. These drugs have also been reported to produce fetal renal dysfunction leading to oligohydramnios when used after 20 weeks' gestation. The US Food and Drug Administration (FDA) recommends that NSAIDs be avoided in women 20 weeks or later in pregnancy. If deemed necessary by a health care provider, the use of NSAIDs between 20 and 30 weeks should be limited to the lowest effective dose and shortest duration. If treatment extends beyond 48 hours, providers should consider an ultrasound to monitor amniotic fluid levels.

BREASTFEEDING SUMMARY

No reports describing the use of meclofenamate sodium during human lactation have been located. The drug will probably appear in breast milk, so some infant exposure will likely occur. Breastfeeding while using this drug should be based on the mother's clinical need for treatment versus any potential infant risks that might occur. If used, the infant should be monitored for the most common reported adult side effects of nausea and abdominal pain (both leading to irritability), diarrhea, and vomiting.

References

1. Prescribing Information. Meclofenamate sodium. Mylan Pharmaceuticals; 2024.
2. Schardein JL, Blatz AT, Woosley ET, Kaump DH. Reproduction studies on sodium meclofenamate in comparison to aspirin and phenylbutazone. *Toxicol Appl Pharmacol* 1969;15:46-55. As cited in Schardein JL. *Chemically Induced Birth Defects*. 2nd ed. Marcel Dekker, Inc; 1993:131.
3. Petrere JA, Humphrey RR, Anderson JA, et al. Studies on reproduction in rats with meclofenamate sodium, a nonsteroidal anti-inflammatory agent. *Fund Appl Toxicol* 1985;5:665-671. As cited in Shepard TH. *Catalog of Teratogenic Agents*. 7th ed. Johns Hopkins University Press; 1992:244-245.
4. U.S. Food and Drug Administration. FDA recommends avoiding use of NSAIDs in pregnancy at 20 weeks or later because they can result in low amniotic fluid. FDA Drug Safety Communication. Accessed September 12, 2024. https://www.fda.gov/drugs/drug-safety-and-availability/fda-recommends-avoiding-use-nsaids-pregnancy-20-weeks-or-later-because-they-can-result-low-amniotic

MEDROXYPROGESTERONE ACETATE

Reproductive (Progestin)

PREGNANCY RECOMMENDATION: *Contraindicated

BREASTFEEDING RECOMMENDATION: Probably Compatible

PREGNANCY SUMMARY

Several reports describing the use of medroxyprogesterone acetate in human pregnancy have been located. While medroxyprogesterone should not be used during pregnancy, available studies have found no significant evidence of an increased risk of congenital anomalies in women who have inadvertently been exposed early in gestation. Hypospadias, clitoral enlargement, and labial fusion have been reported with exposure in the first trimester. The drug will probably cross the placenta, so some fetal exposure will likely occur. Medroxyprogesterone acetate demonstrates dose-related teratogenicity and toxicity in animals. *Due to the approved use for this drug, the mother's clinical need for treatment is unlikely.

BREASTFEEDING SUMMARY

Several reports describing the effects of medroxyprogesterone acetate during human lactation were located. No adverse effects on the growth and development of breastfed infants have been reported. The drug is excreted into human breast milk but does not appear to adversely affect the composition, quality, or supply of breast milk. If the clinical decision is to use this drug while breastfeeding, the infant should be monitored for the most common reported adult side effects of headache, dizziness, and abdominal pain (all leading to irritability).

References

1. Prescribing Information. Medroxyprogesterone acetate. Hikma Pharmaceuticals USA Inc; 2025.
2. Prescribing Information. Medroxyprogesterone acetate. American Health Packaging; 2024.
3. Prescribing Information. Depo-SubQ provera. Pharmacia and Upjohn; 2024.
4. Andrew FD, Staples RE. Prenatal toxicity of medroxyprogesterone acetate in rabbits, rats, and mice. *Teratology*. 1977;15:25-32.
5. Kimmel GL, Hartwell BS, Andrew FD. A potential mechanism in medroxyprogesterone acetate teratogenesis. *Teratology*. 1979;19:171-176.
6. Briggs MH. Hypospadias, androgen biosynthesis, and synthetic progestogens during pregnancy. *Int J Fertil*. 1982;27:70-72.
7. Eibs HG, Spielmann H, Hagele M. Teratogenic effects of cyproterone acetate and medroxyprogesterone treatment during the pre-and postimplantation period of mouse embryos. I. *Teratology*. 1982;25:27-36.
8. Marks TA. Comments on two recent papers dealing with the teratogenicity of medroxyprogesterone acetate. *Teratology*. 1984;31:313-315.
9. Spielmann H. Reply to comments on two articles dealing with the teratogenicity of cyproterone acetate (CA) and medroxyprogesterone acetate (MPA). *Teratology*. 1985;32:319-320.
10. Prahalada S, Carroad E, Hendrickx AG. Embryotoxicity and maternal serum concentrations of medroxyprogesterone acetate (MPA) in baboons (Papio cynocephalus). *Contraception*. 1985;32:497-515.
11. Carbone JP, Figurska K, Buck S, Brent RL. Effect of gestational sex steroid exposure on limb development and endochondral ossification in the pregnant C57B1/6J mouse: I. Medroxyprogesterone acetate. *Teratology*. 1990;42:121-130.
12. Elovitz M, Wang Z. Medroxyprogesterone acetate, but not progesterone, protects against inflammation-induced parturition and intrauterine fetal demise. *Am J Obstet Gynecol*. 2004;190:693-701.
13. Burstein R, Wasserman HC. The effect of Provera on the fetus. *Obstet Gynecol*. 1964;23:931-934.
14. Eller JL, Morton JM. Bizarre deformities in offspring of user of lysergic acid diethylamide. *N Engl J Med*. 1970;283:395-397.
15. Harlap S, Prywes R, Davies AM. Birth defects and oestrogens and progesterones in pregnancy. *Lancet*. 1975;1:682-683.
16. Aarskog D. Maternal progestins as a possible cause of hypospadias. *N Engl J Med*. 1979;300:75-78.
17. Yovich J, Puzey A, De'Atta R, et al. In-vitro fertilisation pregnancy with early progestogen support. *Lancet*. 1982;2:378-379.
18. Barlow SM. Medroxyprogesterone in in-vitro fertilisation. *Lancet*. 1982; 2:1408.
19. Heinonen OP, Slone D, Shapiro S. *Birth Defects and Drugs in Pregnancy*. Publishing Sciences Group; 1977.
20. Heinonen OP, Slone D, Monson RR, et al. Cardiovascular birth defects and antenatal exposure to female sex hormones. *N Engl J Med*. 1977;296:67-70.
21. Wiseman RA, Dodds-Smith IC. Cardiovascular birth defects and antenatal exposure to female sex hormones: a reevaluation of some base data. *Teratology*. 1984;30:359-370.
22. Wilson JG, Brent RL. Are female sex hormones teratogenic? *Am J Obstet Gynecol*. 1981;141:567-580.
23. Dahlberg K. Some effects of depo-medroxyprogesterone acetate (DMPA): observations in the nursing infant and in the long-term user. *Int J Gynaecol Obstet*. 1982;20:43-48.
24. Yovich JL, Stanger JD, Grauaug AA, et al. Fetal abnormality (Goldenhar syndrome) occurring in one of triplet infants derived from in vitro fertilization with possible monozygotic twinning. *J In Vitro Fert Embryo Transf*. 1985;2:27-32.
25. Katz Z, Lancet M, Skornik J, et al. Teratogenicity of progestogens given during the first trimester of pregnancy. *Obstet Gynecol*. 1985;65:775-780.
26. Resseguie LJ, Hick JF, Bruen JA, et al. Congenital malformations among offspring exposed in utero to progestins, Olmsted County, Minnesota, 1936-1974. *Fertil Steril*. 1985;43:514-519.
27. Pardthaisong T, Gray RH, McDaniel EB, Chandacham A. Steroid contraceptive use and pregnancy outcome. *Teratology*. 1988;38:51-58.
28. Pardthaisong T, Gray RH. In utero exposure to steroid contraceptives and outcome of pregnancy. *Am J Epidemiol*. 1991;134:795-803.
29. Gray RH, Pardthaisong T. In utero exposure to steroid contraceptives and survival during infancy. *Am J Epidemiol*. 1991;134:804-811.
30. Hogue CJR. Invited commentary: the contraceptive technology tightrope. *Am J Epidemiol*. 1991;134:812-815.
31. Gray RH, Pardthaisong T. The author's response to Hogue. *Am J Epidemiol*. 1991;134:816-817.
32. Pardthaisong T, Yenchit C, Gray R. The long-term growth and development of children exposed to Depo-Provera during pregnancy and lactation. *Contraception*. 1992;45:313-324.
33. Yovich JL, Turner SR, Draper R. Medroxyprogesterone acetate therapy in early pregnancy has no apparent fetal effects. *Teratology*. 1988;38: 135-144.
34. Blickstein I, Katz Z. Possible relationship of bladder exstrophy and epispadias with progestins taken during early pregnancy. *Br J Urol*. 1991;68: 105-106.
35. Guiloff E, Ibarra-Polo A, Zanartu J, et al. Effect of contraception on lactation. *Am J Obstet Gynecol*. 1974;118:42-45.
36. Karim M, Ammar R, El Mahgoub S, et al. Injected progesterone and lactation. *Br Med J*. 1971;1:200-203.
37. Schwallie PC. The effect of depot-medroxyprogesterone acetate on the fetus and nursing infant: a review. *Contraception*. 1981;23:375-386.
38. Ratchanon S, Taneepanichskul S. Depot medroxyprogesterone acetate and basal serum prolactin levels in lactating women. *Obstet Gynecol*. 2000; 96:926-928.
39. Sapire KE, Dommisse J. Injectable contraception and lactation. *S Afr Med J*. 1995;85:1302-1303.
40. Virutamasen P, Leepipatpaiboon S, Kriengsinyot R, et al. Pharmacodynamic effects of depot-medroxyprogesterone acetate (DMPA) administered to lactating women on their male infants. *Contraception*. 1996;54:153-157.
41. Pardthaisong T, Yenchit C, Gray R. The long-term growth and development of children exposed to depo-provera during pregnancy or lactation. *Contraception*. 1992;45:313-324.
42. World Health Organization Task Force for Epidemiological Research on Reproductive Health; Special Programme of Research, Development and Research Training in Human Reproduction. Progestogen-only contraceptives during lactation: I. Infant growth. *Contraception*. 1994;50:35-53.
43. World Health Organization, Task Force for Epidemiological Research on Reproductive Health; Special Programme of Research, Development, and Research Training in Human Reproduction. Progestogen-only contraceptives during lactation: II. Infant development. *Contraception*. 1994;50:55-68.
44. Zacharias S, Aguilera E, Assenzo JR, et al. Effects of hormonal and nonhormonal contraceptives on lactation and incidence of pregnancy. *Contraception*. 1986;33:203-213.
45. Díaz S, Zepeda A, Maturana X, et al. Fertility regulation in nursing women IX. Contraceptive performance, duration of lactation, infant growth, and bleeding patterns during use of progesterone vaginal rings, progestin-only pills, Norplant® implants, and Copper T 380-A intrauterine devices. *Contraception*. 1997;56:223-232.
46. Jimenez J, Ochoa M, Soler MP, et al. Long-term follow-up of children breastfed by mothers receiving depot-medroxyprogesterone acetate. *Contraception*. 1984;30:523-533.
47. Brito MB, Ferriani RA, Quintana SM, et al. Safety of the etonogestrel-releasing implant during the immediate postpartum period: a pilot study. *Contraception*. 2009;80:519-526.
48. Singhal S, Sarda N, Gupta S, et al. Impact of injectable progestogen contraception in early puerperium on lactation and infant health. *J Clin Diagn Res*. 2014;8:69-72.

MEFENAMIC ACID

Pain (Nonsteroidal Anti-Inflammatory Drug)

PREGNANCY RECOMMENDATION: Human Data Suggest Risk (Second and Third Trimesters)

BREASTFEEDING RECOMMENDATION: Probably Compatible (Short-Term Use)

PREGNANCY SUMMARY

A randomized study and case report describing the use of mefenamic acid for the prevention of preterm delivery in human pregnancy were located. No adverse effects were observed in the 80 newborns exposed in utero to the drug when compared with controls. Conversely, the case report described an infant delivered at 34 weeks' gestation with marked cyanosis after in utero exposure to mefenamic acid. This finding was thought to be caused by premature closure of the ductus arteriosus. Mefenamic acid crosses the placenta, so fetal exposure will occur. However, this limited human pregnancy experience prevents a complete assessment of the embryofetal risk. Embryofetal and maternal toxicity were observed in two animal species at doses of less than 10 times the MRHD. NSAIDs can cause premature stricture or closure of the fetal ductus arteriosus when used in the latter portion of gestation. In some instances, this can produce pulmonary hypertension in the neonate. These drugs have also been reported to produce fetal renal dysfunction leading to oligohydramnios when used after 20 weeks' gestation. The FDA recommends that NSAIDs should be avoided in women 20 weeks or later in pregnancy. If deemed necessary by a health care provider, the use of NSAIDs between 20 and 30 weeks should be limited to the lowest effective dose and shortest duration. If treatment extends beyond 48 hours, providers should consider an ultrasound to monitor amniotic fluid levels.

BREASTFEEDING SUMMARY

One report describing the use of mefenamic acid in 10 postpartum women has been located. Small amounts of mefenamic acid are excreted into human breast milk and absorbed by the nursing infant. Breastfeeding while using this drug should be based on the mother's clinical need for treatment versus any potential infant risks that might occur. If used, the infant should be monitored for the most common reported adult side effects of nausea, headache, heartburn, abdominal pain, pruritus, and dizziness (all leading to irritability), constipation, diarrhea, flatulence, vomiting, rash, and tinnitus.

M

References

1. Prescribing Information. Mefenamic acid. Lupin Pharmaceuticals; 2024.
2. MacKenzie IZ, Graf AK, Mitchell MD. Prostaglandins in the fetal circulation following maternal ingestion of a prostaglandin synthetase inhibitor during mid-pregnancy. *Int J Gynaecol Obstet*. 1985;23:455-458.
3. Mital P, Garg S, Khuteta RP, et al. Mefenamic acid in prevention of premature labor. *J R Soc Health*. 1992;112:214-216.
4. Menahem S. Administration of prostaglandin inhibitors to the mother; the potential risk to the fetus and neonate with duct-dependent circulation. *Reprod Fertil Dev*. 1991;3:489-494.
5. Buchanan RA, Eaton CJ, Koeff ST, Kinkel AW. The breast milk excretion of mefenamic acid. *Curr Ther Res Clin Exp*. 1968;10:592-596.
6. U.S. Food and Drug Administration. FDA recommends avoiding use of NSAIDs in pregnancy at 20 weeks or later because they can result in low amniotic fluid. FDA Drug Safety Communication. Accessed September 12, 2024. https://www.fda.gov/drugs/drug-safety-and-availability/fda-recommends-avoiding-use-nsaids-pregnancy-20-weeks-or-later-because-they-can-result-low-amniotic

MEFLOQUINE

Anti-Infective (Antimalarial)

PREGNANCY RECOMMENDATION: Human Data Suggest Low Risk (Maternal Benefit May Outweigh Any Potential Embryofetal Risk)

BREASTFEEDING RECOMMENDATION: Probably Compatible

PREGNANCY SUMMARY

Several reports describing the use of mefloquine in human pregnancy have been located. Over 700 first-trimester and more than 2,000 second and third-trimester exposures have found no significant evidence of an increased risk of congenital anomalies or adverse effects. The drug crosses the placenta, so fetal exposure will occur. Embryofetal and maternal toxicity were observed in one animal species at doses less than 10 times the recommended human dose (RHD). The Centers for Disease Control and Prevention (CDC) recommends that pregnant women of all gestations diagnosed with uncomplicated malaria acquired in areas with chloroquine resistance may be treated with mefloquine. Mefloquine may also be used as an interim oral treatment for severe malaria if other oral options are not available.

BREASTFEEDING SUMMARY

No reports describing the effects of mefloquine during human lactation have been located. The drug is excreted into human breast milk in low amounts (about 4% of a 250 mg maternal dose). While these amounts are not thought to be harmful to a nursing infant, they are insufficient to provide adequate protection against malaria. The CDC considers mefloquine acceptable for use during breastfeeding. If the clinical decision is to use this drug while breastfeeding, the infant should be monitored for the most common reported adult side effects of dizziness (leading to irritability), vomiting, and irregular heart rate.

References

1. Prescribing Information. Mefloquine hydrochloride. Chartwell RX, LLC; 2024.
2. Tan K, Abanyie F. Travel-associated infections & diseases: Malaria. In: *Yellow Book*. Accessed October 2024 https://wwwnc.cdc.gov/travel/yellowbook/2024/infections-diseases/malaria
3. Nosten F, Karbwang J, White NJ, et al. Mefloquine antimalarial prophylaxis in pregnancy: dose finding and pharmacokinetic study. *Br J Clin Pharmacol*. 1990;30:79-85.
4. Centers for Disease Control. Recommendations for the prevention of malaria among travelers. *MMWR Recomm Rep*. 1990;39:1-10.
5. World Health Organization. Practical chemotherapy of malaria. *World Health Organ Tech Rep Ser*. 1990;805:1-141.
6. Subramanian D, Moise KJ Jr, White AC Jr. Imported malaria in pregnancy: report of four cases and review of management. *Clin Infect Dis*. 1992; 15:408-413.
7. World Health Organization. Severe and complicated malaria. *Trans R Soc Trop Med Hyg* 1990;84(suppl 2):1-65.
8. Nathwani D, Currie PF, Douglas JG, et al. *Plasmodium falciparum* malaria in pregnancy: a review. *Br J Obstet Gynaecol*. 1992;99:118-121.
9. Phillips RE, Looareesuwan S, White NJ, et al. Quinine pharmacokinetics and toxicity in pregnant and lactating women with falciparum malaria. *Br J Clin Pharmacol*. 1986;21:677-683.
10. White NJ, Warrell DA, Chanthavanich P, et al. Severe hypoglycemia and hyperinsulinemia in falciparum malaria. *N Engl J Med*. 1983;309:61-66.
11. Bradley D. Prophylaxis against malaria for travelers from the United Kingdom. *Br Med J*. 1993;306:1247-1252.
12. Barry M, Bia F. Pregnancy and travel. *JAMA*. 1989;261:728-731.
13. Lackritz EM, Lobel HO, Howell BJ, et al. Imported *Plasmodium falciparum* malaria in American travelers to Africa. *JAMA*. 1991;265:383-385.
14. Palmer KJ, Holliday SM, Brogden RN. Mefloquine. A review of its antimalarial activity, pharmacokinetic properties and therapeutic efficacy. *Drugs*. 1993;45:430-475.
15. Baker L, Van Schoor JD, Bartlett GA, Lombard JH. Malaria prophylaxis—the South African viewpoint. *S Afr Med J*. 1993;83:126-129.
16. Raccurt CP, Le Bras M, Ripert C, et al. Paludisme d'importation à Bordeaux: évaluation du risque d'infectation par Plasmodium falciparum en fonction de la destination. *Bull World Health Organ*. 1991;69:85-91.
17. Collignon P, Hehir J, Mitchell D. Successful treatment of falciparum malaria in pregnancy with mefloquine. *Lancet*. 1989;1:967.
18. Elefant E, Boyer M, Roux C. Presentation at the 4th International Conference of Teratogen Information Services; April 18-20, 1991; Chicago, IL (F Rosa, personal communication, 1993).
19. Briand V, Escolano S, Journot V, et al. Mefloquine versus sulfadoxine-pyrimethamine for intermittent preventive treatment in pregnancy: a joint analysis on efficacy and tolerability. *Am J Trop Med Hyg*. 2015;93:300-304.
20. PREGACT Study Group; Pekyi D, Ampromfi AA, et al. Four artemisinin-based treatments in African pregnant women with malaria. *N Engl J Med*. 2016;374:913-927.
21. Rupérez M, Gonzalez R, Mombo-Ngoma G, et al. Mortality, morbidity, and developmental outcomes in infants born to women who received either mefloquine or sulfadoxine-pyrimethamine as intermittent preventative treatment of malaria in pregnancy: a cohort study. *PLoS Med*. 2016;13:e1001964.
22. Edstein MD, Veenendaal JR, Hyslop R. Excretion of mefloquine in human breast milk. *Chemotherapy (Basel)*. 1988;34:165-169.

MELATONIN

Miscellaneous (Pineal Gland Hormone)

PREGNANCY RECOMMENDATION: Limited Human Data—Animal Data Suggest Potential Risk

BREASTFEEDING RECOMMENDATION: Probably Compatible

PREGNANCY SUMMARY

Limited reports describing the use of exogenous melatonin in human pregnancy have been located. Available studies have found no significant evidence of an increased risk of adverse effects. Melatonin rapidly crosses the placenta, so fetal exposure occurs. However, the limited human pregnancy experience prevents a complete assessment of the embryofetal risk. Embryofetal toxicity was observed in one animal species at doses less than 10 times the RHD. Using this drug during pregnancy should be based on the pros and cons of the mother's clinical need for treatment versus any potential fetal risk that might occur from exposure.

BREASTFEEDING SUMMARY

One case report describing the effects of exogenous melatonin during human lactation was located. An 18-month-old breastfed infant exposed to melatonin and valerian had experienced bleeding episodes since birth. Melatonin was stopped for 3 months, and the infant's platelet aggregation test returned to normal. The infant had no further bleeding episodes. Bleeding has not been reported in other studies, including those where melatonin was administered directly to infants. Endogenous melatonin is excreted into human breast milk. The estimated breast milk melatonin level is 35% of the maternal serum concentration. Exogenous melatonin increases the serum melatonin concentrations. Thus, an expected increase in breast milk is expected as well. If the clinical decision is to use this drug while breastfeeding, the infant should be monitored for the most common reported adult side effects of drowsiness and lethargy.

References

1. Melatonin. *Natural Medicines Comprehensive Database*. Therapeutic Research Faculty; 2003:910-915.
2. Davis FC. Melatonin: role in development. *J Biol Rhythms*. 1997;12: 498-508.

3. Kennaway DJ. Melatonin and development: physiology and pharmacology. *Semin Perinatal*. 2000;24:258-266.
4. Cavallo A. The pineal gland in human beings: relevance to pediatrics. *J Pediatr*. 1993;123:843-851.
5. Melatonin. In: Reynolds JEF, ed. *Martindale: The Extra Pharmacopoeia*. 34th ed. Royal Pharmaceutical Society of Great Britain; 2005:1710-1711.
6. Melatonin. *The Review of Natural Products*. Facts and Comparisons; 2004.
7. Orphan Drugs. *Melatonin: Drug Facts and Comparisons*. Facts and Comparisons; 2006:KU-14g.
8. Pepping J. Alternative therapies: melatonin. *Am J Health Syst Pharm*. 1999;56:2520, 2523-2524, 2527.
9. Colmenero MD, Diaz B, Miguel JL, et al. Melatonin administration during pregnancy retards sexual maturation of female offspring in the rat. *J Pineal Res*. 1991;11:23-27.
10. Price CJ, Marr MC, Myers CB, Jahnke GD. Developmental toxicity evaluation of melatonin in rats (abstract). *Teratology*. 1998;57:245.
11. Jahnke G, Marr M, Myers C, et al. Maternal and developmental toxicity evaluation of melatonin administered orally to pregnant Sprague-Dawley rats. *Toxicol Sci*. 1999;50:271-279.
12. Okatani Y, Wakatsuki A, Kaneda C. Melatonin increases activities of glutathione peroxidase and superoxide dismutase in fetal rat brain. *J Pineal Res*. 2000;28:89-96.
13. Pubchem. Melatonin. Accessed February 16, 2020. https://pubchem.ncbi.nlm.nih.gov/compound/Melatonin
14. Thomas L, Drew JE, Abramovich DR, Williams LM. The role of melatonin in the human fetus. *Int J Mol Med*. 1998;1:539-543.
15. Hobson SR, Gurusinghe S, Lim R, et al. Melatonin improves endothelial function in vitro and prolongs pregnancy in women with early-onset preeclampsia. *J Pineal Res*. 2018;65:e12508.
16. Freeman MP, Sosinsky AZ, Moustafa D, et al. Supplement use by women during pregnancy: data from the Massachusetts General Hospital National pregnancy registry for atypical antipsychotics. *Arch Womens Ment Health*. 2016;19:437-441.
17. Chung S, Yeh T, Wu CH. Trend and pattern of herb and supplement use among pregnant women in the United States: findings from the 2002, 2007, and 2012 US National Health Interview Surveys. *Am J Obstet Gynecol*. 2017;216:189-190.
18. Fang JH, Zhang SH, Yu XM, Yang Y. Effects of quercetin and melatonin in pregnant and gestational diabetic women. *Lat Am J Pharm*. 2016;35:1420-1425.
19. Hobson SR, Gurusinghe S, Lim R, et al. Melatonin improves endothelial function in vitro and prolongs pregnancy in women with early-onset preeclampsia. *J Pineal Res*. 2018;65:e12508.
20. Miller SL, Yawno T, Alers NO, et al. Antenatal antioxidant treatment with melatonin to decrease newborn neurodevelopmental deficits and brain injury caused by fetal growth restriction. *J Pineal Res*. 2014;56:283-294.
21. Okatani Y, Okamoto K, Hayashi K, et al. Maternal-fetal transfer of melatonin in pregnant women near term. *J Pineal Res*. 1998;25:129-134.
22. Vine T, Brown GM, Frey BN. Melatonin use during pregnancy and lactation: a scoping review of human studies. *Braz J Psychiatry*. 2022;44:342-348.
23. Cohen Engler A, Hadash A, Shehadeh N, et al. Breastfeeding may improve nocturnal sleep and reduce infantile colic: potential role of breast milk melatonin. *Eur J Pediatr*. 2012;171:729-723.
24. Iavarone S, Massoud M, Di Felice G, et al. Antiplatelet effect of melatonin through breastfeeding: a pediatric case report. *Children (Basel)*. 2023;10:1839.
25. Illnerova H, Buresova M, Presi J. Melatonin rhythm in human milk. *J Clin Endocrinol Metab*. 1993;77:838-841.
26. DeMuro RL, Nafziger AN, Blask DE, et al. The absolute bioavailability of oral melatonin. *J Clin Pharmacol*. 2000;40:781-784.
27. Fourtillan JB, Brisson AM, Gobin P, et al. Bioavailability of melatonin in humans after day-time administration of D(7) melatonin. *Biopharm Drug Dispos*. 2000;21:15-22.
28. Markantonis SL, Tsakalozou E, Paraskeva A, et al. Melatonin pharmacokinetics in premenopausal and postmenopausal healthy female volunteers. *J Clin Pharmacol*. 2008;48:240-245.

M

MELOXICAM

Pain (Nonsteroidal Anti-Inflammatory Drug)

PREGNANCY RECOMMENDATION: Human Data Suggest Risk (Second and Third Trimesters)

BREASTFEEDING RECOMMENDATION: Probably Compatible (Short-Term Use)

PREGNANCY SUMMARY

No reports describing the use of meloxicam in human pregnancy have been located. The drug will probably cross the placenta, so some fetal exposure will likely occur. However, the absence of human pregnancy experience prevents a complete assessment of the embryofetal risk. Embryofetal toxicity was observed in one animal species at doses less than 10 times the MRHD. NSAIDs can cause premature stricture or closure of the fetal ductus arteriosus when used in the latter portion of gestation. In some instances, this can produce pulmonary hypertension in the neonate. These drugs have also been reported to produce fetal renal dysfunction leading to oligohydramnios when used after 20 weeks' gestation. The FDA recommends that NSAIDs be avoided in women 20 weeks or later in pregnancy. If deemed necessary by a health care provider, the use of NSAIDs between 20 and 30 weeks should be limited to the lowest effective dose and shortest duration. If treatment extends beyond 48 hours, providers should consider an ultrasound to monitor amniotic fluid levels.

BREASTFEEDING SUMMARY

No reports describing the use of meloxicam during lactation have been located. The drug will probably appear in breast milk, so some infant exposure will likely occur. Breastfeeding while using this drug should be based on the mother's clinical need for treatment versus any potential infant risks that might occur. If used, the infant should be monitored for the most common reported adult side effects of nausea and abdominal discomfort (both leading to irritability) and diarrhea.

References

1. Prescribing Information. Meloxicam. ANI Pharmaceuticals, Inc; 2024.
2. Levin DL. Effects of inhibition of prostaglandin synthesis on fetal development, oxygenation, and the fetal circulation. *Semin Perinatol*. 1980;4:35-44.
3. U.S. Food and Drug Administration. FDA recommends avoiding use of NSAIDs in pregnancy at 20 weeks or later because they can result in low amniotic fluid. FDA Drug Safety Communication. Accessed September 12, 2024. https://www.fda.gov/drugs/drug-safety-and-availability/fda-recommends-avoiding-use-nsaids-pregnancy-20-weeks-or-later-because-they-can-result-low-amniotic

MELPHALAN

Antineoplastic (Alkylating Agent)

PREGNANCY RECOMMENDATION: No Human Data—Animal Data Suggest Potential Risk

BREASTFEEDING RECOMMENDATION: Potential Toxicity

PREGNANCY SUMMARY

No reports describing the use of melphalan during human pregnancy have been located. The drug will probably cross the placenta, so some fetal exposure will likely occur. However, the absence of human pregnancy experience prevents a complete assessment of the embryofetal risk. Embryofetal toxicity with malformations was observed in one animal species at doses of less than 10 times the MRHD. Based on animal studies and the drug's mechanism of action, the manufacturer recommends that women with reproductive potential use effective contraception during treatment and for 6 months after the last dose. They also recommend that males with female partners of reproductive potential use effective contraception during treatment and for 3 months after the last dose. Nevertheless, using this drug during pregnancy should be based on the pros and cons of the mother's clinical need for treatment versus any potential fetal risk that might occur from exposure. There is a registry for women who are pregnant and have cancer. For more information, women and health care providers are encouraged to contact the Cancer and Pregnancy Registry at 1-877-635-4499.

BREASTFEEDING SUMMARY

No reports describing the use of melphalan during human lactation have been located. The drug will probably appear in breast milk, so some infant exposure will likely occur. However, due to a concern for potential serious adverse effects that might be seen in a breastfed infant, the manufacturer recommends that women not breastfeed while being treated with this drug and for at least 1 week after the last dose. Nevertheless, breastfeeding while using this drug should be based on the mother's clinical need for treatment versus any potential infant risks that might occur. If used, the infant should be monitored for the most common reported adult side effects of nausea and abdominal pain (both leading to irritability), diarrhea, vomiting, and oral ulceration.

Reference

1. Prescribing Information. Melphalan. Apotex; 2023.

M

MEPERIDINE

Pain (Opioid)

PREGNANCY RECOMMENDATION: *Human Data Suggest Risk

BREASTFEEDING RECOMMENDATION: Probably Compatible (Short-Term Use)

PREGNANCY SUMMARY

Numerous reports describing the use of meperidine as an analgesic agent or adjunct to anesthesia during human pregnancy were located. From the Collaborative Perinatal Project, 8 (3.0%) major anomalies were found in 266 first-trimester exposures. Meperidine crosses the placenta, so fetal exposure will occur. However, the limited human pregnancy experience prevents a complete assessment of the embryofetal risk. Formal animal reproduction studies have not been conducted. The National Birth Defects Prevention Study found evidence that opioid use during organogenesis is associated with a low absolute risk of congenital birth defects. However, using opioids during pregnancy should be based on the pros and cons of the mother's clinical need for treatment versus any potential fetal risk that might occur from exposure. *Neonatal abstinence syndrome (NAS) or neonatal opioid withdrawal syndrome (NOWS) may occur with prolonged exposure to opioids. Neonatal opioid withdrawal symptoms include irritability, hyperactivity, abnormal sleep patterns, high-pitched cry, tremor, vomiting, diarrhea, and failure to gain weight. The onset, duration, and severity of withdrawal vary based on the opioid used, duration of use, timing and amount of last maternal use, and elimination of the drug by the newborn. Infants exposed to opioids near birth should be monitored for symptoms of NOWS. The American College of Obstetricians and Gynecologists (ACOG) does not recommend using meperidine during labor because of the prolonged half-life of its active metabolite and lack of reversal by naloxone.

BREASTFEEDING SUMMARY

Limited reports describing the use of meperidine during human lactation have been located. Infant sedation and reduced willingness to feed have been observed with maternal meperidine use during breastfeeding. The drug and its metabolite are excreted into breast milk. However, the amount that reaches the infant after IV or epidural use during labor or shortly thereafter is expected to be small. If the clinical decision is to use this drug while breastfeeding, the infant should be monitored for drowsiness, sedation, difficulty feeding, or limpness.

References

1. Prescribing Information. Meperidine. Hikma Pharmaceuticals USA Inc; 2024.
2. Lexi-Comp, Inc. (Lexi-Drugs). Lexi-Comp, Inc; 2024.
3. American College of Obstetricians and Gynecologists' Committee on Practice Bulletins—Obstetrics. ACOG practice bulletin no. 209: Obstetric analgesia and anesthesia. *Obstet Gynecol*. 2019;133:e208-e225.
4. Crawford JS, Rudofsky S. The placental transmission of pethidine. *Br J Anaesth*. 1965;37:929-933.
5. Szanto HH, Zervoudakis IA, Cederquist LL, Inturrise CE. Amniotic fluid transfer of meperidine from maternal plasma in early pregnancy. *Obstet Gynecol*. 1978;52:59-62.
6. Apgar V, Burns JJ, Brodie BB, Papper EM. The transmission of meperidine across the human placenta. *Am J Obstet Gynecol*. 1952;64:1368-1370.
7. Snider SM, Way EL, Lord MJ. Rate of appearance and disappearance of meperidine in fetal blood after administration of narcotic to the mother. *Anesthesiology*. 1966;27:227-228.
8. Freeborn SF, Calvert RT, Black P, et al. Saliva and blood pethidine concentrations in the mother and the newborn baby. *Br J Obstet Gynaecol*. 1980;87:966-969.
9. Morrison JC, Wiser WL, Rosser SI, et al. Metabolites of meperidine related to fetal depression. *Am J Obstet Gynecol*. 1973;115:1132-1137.
10. Belfries P, Boreus LO, Hartvig P, et al. Neonatal depression after obstetrical analgesia with pethidine. The role of the injection-delivery time interval and the plasma concentrations of pethidine and norpethidine. *Acta Obstet Gynecol Scand*. 1981;60:43-49.
11. Morrison JC, Whybrew WD, Rosser SI, et al. Metabolites of meperidine in the fetal and maternal serum. *Am J Obstet Gynecol*. 1976;126:997-1002.
12. Clark RB, Lattin DL. Metabolites of meperidine in serum. *Am J Obstet Gynecol*. 1978;130:113-115.
13. Morrison JC. Reply to Drs. Clark and Lattin. *Am J Obstet Gynecol*. 1978; 130:115-117.
14. Nissen E, Widstrom AM, Lilja G, et al. Effects of routinely given pethidine during labour on infants' developing breastfeeding behavior. Effects of dose-delivery time interval and various concentrations of pethidine/norpethidine in cord plasma. *Acta Paediatr*. 1997;86:201-208.
15. Borgstede AD, Rosen MG. Medication during labor correlated with behavior and EEG of the newborn. *Am J Dis Child*. 1968;115:21-24.
16. Hodgkinson R, Bhatt M, Wang CN. Double-blind comparison of the neurobehaviour of neonates following the administration of different doses of meperidine to the mother. *Can Anaesth Soc J*. 1978;25:405-411.
17. Cooper LV, Stephen GW, Aggett PJA. Elimination of pethidine and bupivacaine in the newborn. *Arch Dis Child*. 1977;52:638-641.
18. Kushner BR, Kuhnert PM, Prochaska AL, Sokol RJ. Meperidine disposition in mother, neonate and nonpregnant females. *Clin Pharmacol Ther*. 1980;27:486-491.
19. Betsey EM, Rosenblatt DB, Lieberman BA, et al. The influence of maternal analgesia on neonatal behaviour. I. Pethidine. *Br J Obstet Gynaecol*. 1981; 88:398-406.
20. Buck C, Gregg R, Stavraky K, et al. The effect of single prenatal and natal complications upon the development of children of mature birthweight. *Pediatrics*. 1969;43:942-955.
21. Buck C. Drugs in pregnancy. *Can Med Assoc J*. 1975;112:1285.
22. Heinonen O, Slone D, Shapiro S. *Birth Defects and Drugs in Pregnancy*. Publishing Sciences Group; 1977.
23. Broussard CS, Rasmussen SA, Reefhuis J, et al. The National Birth Defects Prevention Study. *Am J Obstet Gynecol*. 2011;204:314-317.
24. Vorherr H. Drug excretion in breast milk. *Postgrad Med*. 1974;56:97-104.
25. Peiker G, Muller B, Ihn W, Noschel H. Excretion of pethidine in mother's milk. *Zentralbl Gynaekol*. 1980;102:537-541.
26. Wittels B, Scott DT, Sinatra RS. Exogenous opioids in human breast milk and acute neonatal neurobehavior: a preliminary study. *Anesthesiol*. 1990; 73:864-869.
27. Wittels B, Glosten B, Faure AM, et al. Postcesarean analgesia with both epidural morphine and intravenous patient-controlled analgesia: neurobehavioral outcomes among nursing neonates. *Anesth Analg*. 1997;85:600-606.
28. Al-Tamimi Y, Ilett KF, Paech MJ, et al. Estimation of infant dose and exposure to pethidine and norpethidine via breast milk following patient-controlled epidural pethidine for analgesia post caesarean delivery. *Int J Obstet Anesth*. 2011;20:128-134.
29. Dejbakht M, Montaseri Z, Saem J, et al. Effect of maternal pethidine on breast feeding behavior of infants in cesarean section by spinal anesthesia: a randomized controlled trial. *Arch Iran Med*. 2021;24:591-598.
30. American College of Obstetricians and Gynecologists. Opioid use and opioid use disorder in pregnancy: committee opinion no. 711. *Obstet Gynecol*. 2017;130:e81-e94.

MEPOLIZUMAB

Respiratory (Monoclonal Antibody)

PREGNANCY RECOMMENDATION: Limited Human Data—Animal Data Suggest Low Risk

BREASTFEEDING RECOMMENDATION: Probably Compatible

PREGNANCY SUMMARY

Two reports were located that describe two women who became pregnant while on mepolizumab therapy for severe eosinophilic asthma. Both delivered healthy infants at term with no congenital abnormalities identified. As an IgG antibody, it likely crosses the placenta, especially during the second half of gestation, so some fetal exposure will probably occur. However, this limited human pregnancy experience prevents a complete assessment of the embryofetal risk. Animal data did not show any embryofetal toxicity in one species at doses less than 10 times the MRHD. Using this drug during pregnancy should be based on the pros and cons of the mother's clinical need for treatment versus any potential fetal risk that might occur from exposure.

BREASTFEEDING SUMMARY

No reports describing the use of mepolizumab during human lactation have been located. It is known that IgG antibodies are excreted into breast milk but are not found in the neonatal or infant circulation. Additionally, if any IgG antibodies were to be ingested through breastfeeding, they would probably be digested in the infant's gastrointestinal tract and not be absorbed. Breastfeeding while using this drug should be based on the mother's clinical need for treatment. If used, the infant should be monitored for the most common reported adult side effects of headache and back pain (both leading to irritability) and fatigue (lethargy).

References

1. Prescribing Information. Nucala. GlaxoSmithKline; 2023.
2. Ozden G, Pinar Deniz P. May mepolizumab used in asthma correct subfertility? *Ann Med*. 2021;53:456-458.
3. Vittorakis SK, Giannakopoulou G, Samitas K, Zervas E. Successful and safe treatment of severe steroid depended eosinophilic asthma with mepolizumab in a woman during pregnancy. *Respir Med Case Rep*. 2022; 41:101785.

MEPROBAMATE

Mental Health (Antianxiety)

PREGNANCY RECOMMENDATION: Limited Human Data—No Relevant Animal Data

BREASTFEEDING RECOMMENDATION: Potential Toxicity

PREGNANCY SUMMARY

Nine reports describing the use of meprobamate in human pregnancy have been located. These reports include exposure in all trimesters. From these studies, more than 450 first-trimester exposures were described with a major birth anomaly rate of about 3.0%. No pattern to the defects was seen. The drug crosses the placenta, so fetal exposure will occur. However, the limited human pregnancy experience still prevents a complete assessment of the embryofetal risk. No relevant animal reproduction studies have been conducted. The manufacturer recommends avoiding the drug in the first trimester because of the potential risk for congenital defects. Nevertheless, using this drug during pregnancy should be based on the pros and cons of the mother's clinical need for treatment versus any potential fetal risk that might occur from exposure.

M

BREASTFEEDING SUMMARY

One case report of a mother who partially breastfed her infant while taking carisoprodol (which is metabolized to meprobamate) noted no adverse effects in the infant. Normal growth and psychomotor development were observed at 6 months of age. Per the manufacturer, meprobamate is excreted into breast milk at concentrations 2 to 4 times that of maternal plasma. If the clinical decision is to use this drug while breastfeeding, the infant should be monitored for sedation, poor feeding, and poor weight gain.

References

1. Prescribing Information. Meprobamate. Alembic Pharmaceuticals; 2023.
2. Schardein JL. *Chemically Induced Birth Defects*. 3rd ed. Marcel Dekker; 2000:243.
3. Milkovich L, van den Berg BJ. Effects of prenatal meprobamate and chlordiazepoxide hydrochloride on human embryonic and fetal development. *N Engl J Med*. 1974;291:1268-1271.
4. Ringrose CAD. The hazard of neurotropic drugs in the fertile years. *CMAJ*. 1972;106:1058.
5. Bogdanoff B, Rorke LB, Yanoff M, Warren WS. Brain and eye abnormalities: possible sequelae to prenatal use of multiple drugs including LSD. *Am J Dis Child*. 1972;123:145-148.
6. Crombie DL, Pinsent RJ, Fleming DM, et al. Fetal effects of tranquilizers in pregnancy. *N Engl J Med*. 1975;293:198-199.
7. Heinonen OP, Slone D, Shapiro S. *Birth Defects and Drugs in Pregnancy*. Publishing Sciences Group; 1977:336-337.
8. Hartz SC, Heinonen OP, Shapiro S, et al. Antenatal exposure to meprobamate and chlordiazepoxide in relation to malformations, mental development, and childhood mortality. *N Engl J Med*. 1975;292:726-728.
9. Belafsky HA, Breslow S, Hirsch LM, et al. Meprobamate during pregnancy. *Obstet Gynecol*. 1969;34:378-386.
10. Czeizel AE, Mosonyi A. Monitoring of early human fetal development in women exposed to large doses of chemicals. *Environ Mol Mutagen*. 1997; 30:240-244.
11. Timmermann G, Acs N, Bánhidy F, Czeizel AE. A study of teratogenic and fetotoxic effects of large doses of meprobamate used for a suicide attempt by 42 pregnant women. *Toxicol Ind Health*. 2008;24:97-107.
12. Nordeng H, Zahlsen K, Spigset O. Transfer of carisoprodol to breast milk. *Ther Drug Monit*. 2001;23:298-300.
13. Bailey DN, Briggs JR. Carisoprodol: an unrecognized drug of abuse. *Am J Clin Pathol*. 2002;117:396-400.

MERCAPTOPURINE

Antineoplastic (Antimetabolite)

PREGNANCY RECOMMENDATION: Limited Human Data—Animal Data Suggest Risk

BREASTFEEDING RECOMMENDATION: Potential Toxicity

PREGNANCY SUMMARY

Several reports describing the use of mercaptopurine in human pregnancy have been located. Available studies have found no evidence of a significantly increased risk for congenital anomalies. Mercaptopurine is the active metabolite of azathioprine. Thiopurines have been associated with an increased risk for stillbirth and preterm birth, but this can also be related to the disease for which the drug is used. Mercaptopurine metabolites cross the placenta, but placental binding has been shown to limit their transfer. However, the limited human pregnancy experience prevents a complete assessment of the embryofetal risk. Embryofetal toxicity with malformations was observed in four animal species at doses less than the RHD. Based on animal studies and the drug's mechanism of action, the manufacturer recommends that women with reproductive potential use effective contraception during treatment and for 6 months after the last dose. They also recommend that males with female partners of reproductive potential use effective contraception during treatment and for 3 months after the last dose. Nevertheless, using this drug during pregnancy should be based on the pros and cons of the mother's clinical need for treatment versus any potential fetal risk that might occur from exposure. Thiopurines, including mercaptopurine, carry a special alert by the FDA telling providers that there is a rare risk of intrahepatic cholestasis of pregnancy with their use. There is also a registry for women who are pregnant and have cancer. For more information, women and health care providers are encouraged to contact the Cancer and Pregnancy Registry at 1-877-635-4499.

BREASTFEEDING SUMMARY

Three reports describing the use of mercaptopurine (or azathioprine) in 153 breastfeeding infants have been located. No significant infant adverse effects were attributed to mercaptopurine or azathioprine. Mercaptopurine is present in breast milk, so infant exposure will occur. However, one report found undetectable levels 4 hours after maternal ingestion. Regardless, due to a concern for potential serious adverse effects that might be seen in a breastfed infant, the manufacturer recommends that women not breastfeed while being treated with this drug and for at least 1 week after the last dose. Nevertheless, if the clinical decision is to use this drug while breastfeeding, the infant should be monitored for the most common reported adult side effects of nausea (leading to irritability), myelosuppression (producing anemia, leukopenia, and thrombocytopenia), anorexia (monitor infant growth), vomiting, diarrhea, lethargy, and rash.

M

References

1. Prescribing Information. Mercaptopurine. Hikma Pharmaceuticals; 2024.
2. Moloney WC. Management of leukemia in pregnancy. *Ann N Y Acad Sci*. 1964;114:857-867.
3. Nicholson HO. Cytotoxic drugs in pregnancy: review of reported cases. *J Obstet Gynaecol Br Commonw*. 1968;75:307-312.
4. Gililland J, Weinstein L. The effects of cancer chemotherapeutic agents on the developing fetus. *Obstet Gynecol Surv*. 1983;38:6-13.
5. Wegelius R. Successful pregnancy in acute leukaemia. *Lancet*. 1975;2:1301.
6. Nicholson HO. Leukaemia and pregnancy: a report of five cases and discussion of management. *J Obstet Gynaecol Br Commonw*. 1968;75:517-520.
7. Pizzuto J, Aviles A, Noriega L, et al. Treatment of acute leukemia during pregnancy: presentation of nine cases. *Cancer Treat Rep*. 1980;64:679-683.
8. Burnier AM. Discussion. In Plows CW. Acute myelomonocytic leukemia in pregnancy: report of a case. *Am J Obstet Gynecol*. 1982;143:41-43.
9. Dara P, Slater LM, Armentrout SA. Successful pregnancy during chemotherapy for acute leukemia. *Cancer*. 1981;47:845-846.
10. McConnell JF, Bhoola R. A neonatal complication of maternal leukemia treated with 6-mercaptopurine. *Postgrad Med J*. 1973;49:211-213.
11. Diamond J, Anderson MM, McCreadie SR. Transplacental transmission of busulfan (Myleran) in a mother with leukemia: production of fetal malformation and cytomegaly. *Pediatrics*. 1960;25:85-90.
12. Khurshid M, Saleem M. Acute leukaemia in pregnancy. *Lancet*. 1978;2:534-535.
13. Okun DB, Groncy PK, Sieger L, Tanaka KR. Acute leukemia in pregnancy: transient neonatal myelosuppression after combination chemotherapy in the mother. *Med Pediatr Oncol*. 1979;7:315-319.
14. Doney KC, Kraemer KG, Shepard TH. Combination chemotherapy for acute myelocytic leukemia during pregnancy: three case reports. *Cancer Treat Rep*. 1979;63:369-371.
15. Schleuning M, Clemm C. Chromosomal aberrations in a newborn whose mother received cytotoxic treatment during pregnancy. *N Engl J Med*. 1987;317:1666-1667.
16. Turchi JJ, Villasis C. Anthracyclines in the treatment of malignancy in pregnancy. *Cancer*. 1988;61:435-440.
17. Feliu J, Juarez S, Ordonez A, Garcia-Paredes ML, Gonzalez-Baron M, Montero JM. Acute leukemia and pregnancy. *Cancer*. 1988;61:580-584.
18. Haerr RW, Pratt AT. Multiagent chemotherapy for sarcoma diagnosed during pregnancy. *Cancer*. 1985;56:1028-1033.
19. Frenkel EP, Meyers MC. Acute leukemia and pregnancy. *Ann Intern Med*. 1960;53:656-671.
20. Loyd HO. Acute leukemia complicated by pregnancy. *JAMA*. 1961;178:1140-1143.
21. Lee RA, Johnson CE, Hanlon DG. Leukemia during pregnancy. *Am J Obstet Gynecol*. 1962;84:455-458.
22. Coopland AT, Friesen WJ, Galbraith PA. Acute leukemia in pregnancy. *Am J Obstet Gynecol*. 1969;105:1288-1289.
23. Seinen ML, de Boer NKH, van Hoorn ME, et al. Safe use of allopurinol and low-dose mercaptopurine therapy during pregnancy in an ulcerative colitis patient. *Inflamm Bowel Dis*. 2013;19(3):E37. doi:10.1002/ibd.22945
24. de Meij TGL, Jharap B, Kneepkens MF, et al; for the Dutch Initiative on Crohn and Colitis. Long-term follow-up of children exposed intrauterine to maternal thiopurine therapy during pregnancy in females with inflammatory bowel disease. *Aliment Pharmacol Ther*. 2013;38:38-43.
25. U.S. Food and Drug Administration. FDA alerts health care professionals of pregnancy problems associated with thiopurines. Accessed July 16, 2024. https://www.fda.gov/drugs/drug-safety-and-availability/fda-alerts-health-care-professionals-pregnancy-problems-associated-thiopurines
26. Flanagan E, Wright EK, Hardikar W, et al; PICCOLO Study Group. Maternal thiopurine metabolism during pregnancy in inflammatory bowel disease and clearance of thiopurine metabolites and outcomes in exposed neonates. *Aliment Pharmacol Ther*. 2021;53:810-820.
27. de Meij TG, Jharap B, Kneepkens CM, et al. Long-term follow-up of children exposed intrauterine to maternal thiopurine therapy during pregnancy in females with inflammatory bowel disease. *Aliment Pharmacol Ther*. 2013;38:38-43.
28. Matro R, Martin CF, Wolf D, et al. Exposure concentrations of infants breastfed by women receiving biologic therapies for inflammatory bowel diseases and effects of breastfeeding on infections and development. *Gastroenterology*. 2018;155:696-704.
29. Beswick L, Shukla D, Friedman AB, et al. National audit: assessing the use and safety of allopurinol thiopurine co-therapy in pregnant females with inflammatory bowel disease. *J Gastroenterol Hepatol*. 2016;31 (suppl 2):128-129.
30. Coulam CB, Moyer TP, Jiang NS, Zincke H. Breast-feeding after renal transplantation. *Transplant Proc*. 1982;14:605-609.
31. Ter Horst P, Smolders EJ, den Besten D. Mercaptopurine and metabolites in breast milk. *Breastfeed Med*. 2020;15:277-279.
32. Hutson JR, Lubetsky A, Walfisch A, et al. The transfer of 6-mercaptopurine in the dually perfused human placenta. *Reprod Toxicol*. 2011;32:349-353.
33. Meyer A, Drouin J, Weill A, et al. Comparative study of pregnancy outcomes in women with inflammatory bowel disease treated with thiopurines and/or anti-TNF: a French nationwide study 2010-2018. *Aliment Pharmacol Ther*. 2021;54:302-311.

MEROPENEM

Antibacterial (Carbapenem)

PREGNANCY RECOMMENDATION: Limited Human Data—Animal Data Suggest Low Risk

BREASTFEEDING RECOMMENDATION: Probably Compatible

PREGNANCY SUMMARY

Seven case reports describing the use of meropenem during the second and third trimesters in human pregnancies were located. Five infants had reported outcomes. One infant born to a mother with acrorenal syndrome also had deformities consistent with the same syndrome. No other congenital abnormalities were reported. Incomplete transplacental passage of meropenem was found in an ex vivo human placental perfusion model. Therefore, this limited human pregnancy experience prevents a complete assessment of the embryofetal risk. Animal data did not show any embryofetal toxicity in two species at doses of less than 10 times the MRHD. Using this drug during pregnancy should be based on the pros and cons of the mother's clinical need for treatment versus any potential fetal risk that might occur from exposure.

BREASTFEEDING SUMMARY

Two case reports describing the use of meropenem during human lactation have been located. No adverse infant effects were reported. The peak breast milk concentration was about 0.644 mcg/mL. The calculated relative infant dose (RID) was less than 1%. Breastfeeding while using this drug should be based on the mother's clinical need for treatment versus any potential infant risks that might occur. If used, the infant should be monitored for the most common reported adult side effects of nausea and headache (both leading to irritability), constipation, diarrhea, anemia, vomiting, and rash.

References

1. Prescribing Information. Meropenem. B. Braun Medical; 2024.
2. Hnat M, Bawdon RE. Transfer of meropenem in the ex vivo human placenta perfusion model. *Infect Dis Obstet Gynecol*. 2005;13:223-227.
3. Shea K, Hilburger E, Baroco A, Oldfield E. Successful treatment of vancomycin-resistant *Enterococcus faecium* pyelonephritis with daptomycin during pregnancy. *Ann Pharmacother*. 2008;42:722-725.
4. Yoshida M, Matsuda H, Furuya K. Successful prognosis of brain abscess during pregnancy. *J Reprod Infertil*. 2013;14:152-155.
5. Sauberan JB, Bradley JS, Blumer J, Stellwagen LM. Transmission of meropenem in breast milk. *Pediatr Infect Dis J*. 2012;31:832-834.
6. Festini F, Ciuti R, Repetto T, et al. Safety of breast-feeding during an IV tobramycin course for infants of CF women (abstract). *Pediatr Pulmonol Suppl*. 2004;27:288-289. As cited in Meropenem—National Library of Medicine LactMed database, November 6, 2013.
7. Brady A, Aglan A. Critical COVID-19 in a pregnant patient who presented in starvation ketoacidosis with a background history of acrorenal syndrome. *BMJ Case Rep*. 2021;14:e244117.
8. Tchirikov M, Ocker R, Seliger G, et al. Treatment of mid-trimester preterm premature rupture of membranes (PPROM) with multi-resistant bacteria-colonized anhydramnion with continuous amnioinfusion and meropenem: a case report and literature review. *Arch Gynecol Obstet*. 2022;306:585-592.
9. Zhang M, Jin H, Liu X. Septic shock induced by acute pyelonephritis resulting from kidney stones treated by double-J ureteral stents in a pregnant woman: a case report and literature review. *Am J Case Rep*. 2022;23:e936967.
10. Saif HS, Al-Ansari B, Raza G, Ghorabah M. Approach to the management of hypertriglyceridemia complicated with acute pancreatitis in pregnancy: a case report. *Cureus*. 2024;16:e56006.

MEROPENEM/VABORBACTAM

Antibacterial

PREGNANCY RECOMMENDATION: No Human Data—Animal Data Suggest Potential Risk

BREASTFEEDING RECOMMENDATION: Potential Toxicity

PREGNANCY SUMMARY

No human data specific to birth anomalies from exposure to the combination drug meropenem/vaborbactam have been located. Both drugs will probably cross the placenta, so some fetal exposure will likely occur. However, the absence of human pregnancy experience prevents a complete assessment of the embryofetal risk. Animal data did show embryofetal toxicity for vaborbactam.

BREASTFEEDING SUMMARY

No reports of the combination drug meropenem/vaborbactam in human lactation have been reported. Meropenem has been found in breast milk at low levels. Vaborbactam is also probably found in breast milk. Therefore, infant exposure will likely occur for both drugs. Breastfeeding while using this drug should be based on the mother's clinical need for treatment.

If used, the infant should be monitored for the most common reported adult side effects of nausea and headache (both leading to irritability), diarrhea, and pyrexia.

Reference

1. Prescribing Information. Vabomere. Melinta Therapeutics, LLC; 2021.

MESALAMINE

Gastrointestinal (5-Aminosalicyclic Acid Derivative)

PREGNANCY RECOMMENDATION: Limited Human Data—Animal Data Suggest Low Risk (Maternal Benefit May Outweigh Any Embryofetal Risk)

BREASTFEEDING RECOMMENDATION: Probably Compatible

PREGNANCY SUMMARY

A few reports describing the use of mesalamine in human pregnancy have been located. The rate of major birth anomalies in more than 200 first-trimester exposures was in the expected range. The drug crosses the placenta, so some fetal exposure will occur. However, this limited human pregnancy experience still prevents a complete assessment of the embryofetal risk. Animal data did not show any embryofetal toxicity in two species at doses of less than 10 times the RHD. Using this drug during pregnancy should be based on the pros and cons of the mother's clinical need for treatment versus any potential fetal risk that might occur from exposure. The maternal benefits of therapy with mesalamine appear to outweigh the potential unknown risks to the fetus.

BREASTFEEDING SUMMARY

Five reports describing the effects of mesalamine in 129 infants exposed during human lactation have been located. Two cases of diarrhea have been reported in infants exposed to mesalamine. The concentration of the drug in breast milk ranged from about 0.02 to 0.44 mcg/mL. The calculated RIDs were less than 1%. The breast milk concentrations for 5-aminosalicylic acid were much higher, but this metabolite is not clinically active. Breastfeeding while using this drug should be based on the mother's clinical need for treatment versus any potential infant risks that might occur. If used, the infant should be monitored for the most common reported pediatric side effects of dizziness, headache, and abdominal pain (all leading to irritability), diarrhea, rash, and cough.

References

1. Prescribing Information. Mesalamine. Teva Pharmaceuticals USA, Inc; 2024.
2. Prescribing Information. Meslamine enema. ANI Pharmaceuticals, Inc; 2024
3. Jarnerot G, Andersen S, Esbjorner E, Sandstrom B, Brodersen R. Albumin reserve for binding of bilirubin in maternal and cord serum under treatment with sulphasalazine. *Scand J Gastroenterol*. 1981;16:1049-1055.
4. Christensen LA, Rasmussen SN, Hansen SH, et al. Salazosulfapyridine and metabolites in fetal and maternal body fluids with special reference to 5-aminosalicylic acid. *Acta Obstet Gynecol Scand*. 1987;66:433-435.
5. Klotz U, Harings-Kaim A. Negligible excretion of 5-aminosalicylic acid in breast milk. *Lancet*. 1993;342:618-619.
6. Kamm MA, Senapati A. Drug management of ulcerative colitis. *Br Med J*. 1992;305:35-38.
7. Habal FM, Hui G, Greenberg GR. Oral 5-aminosalicylic acid for inflammatory bowel disease in pregnancy: safety and clinical course. *Gastroenterology*. 1993;105:1057-1060.
8. Colombel J-F, Brabant G, Gubler M-C, et al. Renal insufficiency in infant: side-effect of prenatal exposure to mesalazine? *Lancet*. 1994;344:620-621.
9. Marteau P, Devaux CB. Mesalazine during pregnancy. *Lancet*. 1994;344:1708-1709.
10. Bell CM, Habal FM. Safety of topical 5-aminosalicylic acid in pregnancy. *Am J Gastroenterol* 1997;92:2201-2202.
11. Diav-Citrin O, Park Y-H, Veerasuntharam G, et al. The safety of mesalamine in human pregnancy: a prospective controlled cohort study. *Gastroenterology*. 1998;114:23-28.
12. Moskovitz DN, Bodian C, Chapman ML, et al. The effect on the fetus of medications used to treat pregnant inflammatory bowel-disease patients. *Am J Gastroenterol*. 2004;99:656-661.
13. Rahimi R, Nikfar S, Rezaie A, Abdollahi M. Pregnancy outcome in women with inflammatory bowel disease following exposure to 5-aminosalicyclic acid drugs: a meta-analysis. *Reprod Toxicol*. 2008;25:271-275.
14. Seinen ML, de Boer NKH, van Hoorn ME, et al. Safe use of allopurinol and low-dose mercaptopurine therapy during pregnancy in an ulcerative colitis patient. *Inflamm Bowel Dis*. 2013;19:E37.
15. Jenss H, Weber P, Hartmann F. 5-Aminosalicylic acid and its metabolite in breast milk during lactation. *Am J Gastroenterol*. 1990;85:331.
16. Miller LG, Hopkinson JM, Motil KJ, et al. Disposition of olsalazine and metabolites in breast milk. *J Clin Pharmacol*. 1993;33:703-706.
17. Nelis GF. Diarrhoea due to 5-aminosalicylic acid in breast milk. *Lancet*. 1989;1:383.
18. Ito S, Blajchman A, Stephenson M, et al. Prospective follow-up of adverse reactions in breast-fed infants exposed to maternal medication. *Am J Obstet Gynecol*. 1993;168:1393-1399.
19. Moretti ME, Spiczynski Y, Hashemi G, et al. Prospective follow-up of infants exposed to 5-aminosalicylic acid containing drugs through maternal milk. *J Clin Pharmacol*. 1998;38:867.
20. Xu YL, Tan B, Ma LK, et al. Inflammatory bowel disease in pregnancy: A report of 7 cases and review of the literature. *Int J Clin Exp Med* 2017;10:5525-32.

MESNA

Antineoplastic (Cytoprotective)

PREGNANCY RECOMMENDATION: Limited Human Data—Animal Data Suggest Low Risk

BREASTFEEDING RECOMMENDATION: Potential Toxicity

PREGNANCY SUMMARY

Limited reports describing the use of mesna in human pregnancy have been located. In all the cases, mesna was combined with ifosfamide in the second and third trimesters (see Ifosfamide). No adverse fetal effects were described. The drug will probably cross the placenta, so some fetal exposure will likely occur. However, the limited human pregnancy experience prevents a complete assessment of the embryofetal risk. Animal data did not show any embryofetal toxicity in two species at doses of about 10 times the MRHD. Mesna is always combined with ifosfamide (which is used in the treatment of numerous malignancies). Based on animal studies and the drug's mechanism of action, the manufacturer recommends that women with reproductive potential use effective contraception during treatment when combined with ifosfamide and for 1 month after the last dose. They also recommend that males with female partners of reproductive potential use effective contraception during treatment when combined with ifosfamide and for 1 month after the last dose. Regardless, using this drug during pregnancy should be based on the pros and cons of the mother's clinical need for treatment versus any potential fetal risk that might occur from exposure.

BREASTFEEDING SUMMARY

No reports describing the use of mesna during human lactation have been located. The drug will probably appear in breast milk, so some infant exposure will likely occur. However, mesna is always combined with ifosfamide. Therefore, the manufacturer recommends that women not breastfeed while being treated with ifosfamide and for at least 1 month after the last dose. Nevertheless, breastfeeding while using this drug should be based on the mother's clinical need for treatment versus any potential infant risks that might occur from exposure. If the clinical decision is to use this drug, the infant should be monitored for the most common reported adult side effects of nausea, headache, and abdominal pain (all leading to irritability), vomiting, constipation, fatigue, anorexia (monitor infant growth), diarrhea, alopecia, somnolence, and various laboratory abnormalities (see Prescribing Information [PI]).

References

1. Prescribing Information. Mesna. Fresenius Kabi USA, LLC; 2024.
2. Prescribing Information. Ifosfamide. Hikma Pharmaceuticals USA Inc; 2020.
3. Komai Y, Itoh I, Iriyam K, et al. Reproduction study of mesna—teratogenicity study in rats by intravenous administration. *Kiso to Rinsho*. 1990;24: 6553-6594. As cited by Shepard TH. *Catalog of Teratogenic Agents*. 10th ed. The Johns Hopkins University Press; 2001:323.
4. Komai Y, Itoh I, Ishimura K, et al. Reproduction study of mesna—teratogenicity study in rabbits by intravenous administration. *Kiso to Rinsho*. 1990;24:6596-6602. As cited in Shepard TH. *Catalog of Teratogenic Agents*. 10th ed. The Johns Hopkins University Press; 2001:323.

METAXALONE

Pain (Skeletal Muscle Relaxant)

PREGNANCY RECOMMENDATION: No Human Data—Animal Data Suggest Low Risk

BREASTFEEDING RECOMMENDATION: Probably Compatible

PREGNANCY SUMMARY

No reports describing the use of metaxalone in human pregnancy have been located. The drug will probably cross the placenta, so fetal exposure will likely occur. However, the absence of human pregnancy experience prevents a complete assessment of the embryofetal risk. Animal data did not show embryofetal toxicity in one species at an unknown dose. Using this drug during pregnancy should be based on the pros and cons of the mother's clinical need for treatment versus any potential fetal risk that might occur from exposure.

BREASTFEEDING SUMMARY

No reports describing the use of metaxalone during human lactation have been located. The drug will probably appear in breast milk, so infant exposure will likely occur. If the clinical decision is to use this drug while breastfeeding, the infant should be monitored for the most common reported adult side effects of nausea, dizziness, headache, and gastrointestinal upset (all leading to irritability), drowsiness, and vomiting.

Reference

1. Prescribing Information. Metaxalone. Pfizer; 2024.

METFORMIN

Antidiabetic (Biguanide)

PREGNANCY RECOMMENDATION: Limited Human Data (First Trimester)—Animal Data Suggest Low Risk

BREASTFEEDING RECOMMENDATION: Probably Compatible

PREGNANCY SUMMARY

The use of metformin in human pregnancy has been well reported. Recent meta-analyses found that metformin resulted in a significant reduction in pregnancy weight gain and neonatal hypoglycemia, along with a significant reduction in the risk of preeclampsia, induction of labor, cesarean delivery, macrosomia, neonatal intensive care unit (NICU) admission, and large for gestational age when compared with insulin. Several thousand pregnancies have been recorded, but mainly with second- and third-trimester use. Therefore, the limited human pregnancy experience with first-trimester exposure prevents a complete assessment of the embryofetal risk. The drug crosses the placenta, so fetal exposure will occur. Animal data did not show any embryofetal toxicity in two species at greater than 10 times the MRHD. ACOG and the American Diabetes Association (ADA) recommend that, despite metformin's well-reported use in pregnancy, insulin should be used for types 1 and 2 diabetes occurring during pregnancy and, if diet therapy alone is not successful, for gestational diabetes. Oral agents such as metformin and glyburide should not be used as first-line agents, as both cross the placenta. Other oral medications and injectable glucose-lowering medications lack safety data.

BREASTFEEDING SUMMARY

Four reports describing the effects of metformin use in 75 breastfed infants were located. No adverse effects were reported in the nursing infants. Metformin is excreted into breast milk, producing mean peak concentrations that range from about 0.25 to 1.1 mcg/mL. The calculated RIDs were all less than about 1.5%. If the clinical decision is to use this drug while breastfeeding, the infant should be monitored for the most common reported adult side effects of nausea, headache, indigestion, and abdominal discomfort (all leading to irritability), diarrhea, vomiting, flatulence, and lethargy.

M

References

1. Prescribing Information. Metformin. Chartwell RX, LLC; 2022.
2. ACOG Practice Bulletin No. 190: Gestational Diabetes Mellitus. *Obstet Gynecol.* 2018 Feb;131:e49-e64.
3. American Diabetes Association Professional Practice Committee. Management of diabetes in pregnancy: standards of care in diabetes—2024. *Diabetes Care.* 2024;47(suppl 1):S282-S294.
4. Elliott B, Schuessling F, Langer O. The oral antihyperglycemic agent metformin does not affect glucose uptake and transport in the human diabetic placenta (abstract). *Am J Obstet Gynecol.* 1997;176:S182.
5. Elliott B, Langer O, Schuessling F. Human placental glucose uptake and transport are not altered by the oral antihyperglycemic agent metformin. *Am J Obstet Gynecol.* 1997;176:527-530.
6. Nanovskaya TN, Nekhayeva IA, Patrikeeva SL, et al. Transfer of metformin across the dually perfused human placenta lobule. *Am J Obstet Gynecol.* 2006;195:1081-1085.
7. Vanky E, Zahlsen K, Spigset O, Carlsen SM. Placental passage of metformin in women with polycystic ovary syndrome. *Fertil Steril.* 2005;83:1575-1578.
8. Yu DQ, Xu GX, Teng XY, et al. Glycemic control and neonatal outcomes in women with gestational diabetes mellitus treated using glyburide, metformin, or insulin: a pairwise and network meta-analysis. *BMC Endocr Disord.* 2021;21:199.
9. Bidhendi YR, Amiri M, Ramezani TF, Behboudi-Gandevani S. Effectiveness of antidiabetic agents for treatment of gestational diabetes: a methodological quality assessment of meta-analyses and network meta-analysis. *J Diabetes Investig.* 2021;12:2247-2258.
10. Musa OAH, Syed A, Mohamed AM, et al. Metformin is comparable to insulin for pharmacotherapy in gestational diabetes mellitus: a network meta-analysis evaluating 6046 women. *Pharmacol Res.* 2021;167:105546.
11. Wang X, Liu W, Chen H, Chen Q. Comparison of insulin, metformin, and glyburide on perinatal complications of gestational diabetes mellitus: a systematic review and meta-analysis. *Gynecol Obstet Invest.* 2021;86:218-230.
12. He K, Guo Q, Ge J, et al. The efficacy and safety of metformin alone or as an add-on therapy to insulin in pregnancy with GDM or T2DM: a systematic review and meta-analysis of 21 randomized controlled trials. *J Clin Pharm Ther.* 2022;47(2):168-177.
13. Li C, Gao C, Zhang X, et al. Comparison of the effectiveness and safety of insulin and oral hypoglycemic drugs in the treatment of gestational diabetes mellitus: a meta-analysis of 26 randomized controlled trials. *Gynecol Endocrinol.* 2022;38:303-309.
14. Li F, Liu L, Hu Y, et al. Efficacy and safety of metformin compared to insulin in gestational diabetes: a systematic review and meta-analysis of Chinese randomized controlled trials. *Int J Clin Pharm.* 2022;44:1102-1113.
15. Sheng B, Ni J, Lv B, et al. Short-term neonatal outcomes in women with gestational diabetes treated using metformin versus insulin: a systematic review and meta-analysis of randomized controlled trials. *Acta Diabetol.* 2023;60:595-608.
16. Kattini R, Kelly L, Hummelen R. Systematic review of the use of metformin compared to insulin for the management of gestational diabetes: implications for low-resource settings. *Can J Rural Med.* 2023;28:59-65.
17. Zhang L, Mai Y, Wang X, et al. Comparative study of the impact of metformin versus insulin on adverse pregnancy outcomes in women diagnosed with gestational diabetes mellitus: a meta-analysis. *Altern Ther Health Med.* 2024;30:460-465.
18. Wu R, Zhang Q, Li Z. A meta-analysis of metformin and insulin on maternal outcome and neonatal outcome in patients with gestational diabetes mellitus. *J Matern Fetal Neonatal Med.* 2024;37:2295809.
19. Hale TW, Kristensen JH, Hackett LP, et al. Transfer of metformin into human milk. *Diabetologia.* 2002;45:1509-1514.
20. Gardiner SJ, Kirkpatrick CMJ, Begg EJ, et al. Transfer of metformin into human milk. *Clin Pharmacol Ther.* 2003;73:71-77.
21. Briggs GG, Ambrose PJ, Nageotte MP, et al. Excretion of metformin into breast milk and the effect on nursing infants. *Obstet Gynecol.* 2005;105:1437-1441.
22. Glueck CJ, Salehi M, Sieve L, Wang P. Growth, motor, and social development in breast-and formula-fed infants of metformin treated women with polycystic ovary syndrome. *J Pediatr.* 2006;148:628-632.

METHADONE

Pain/Antidote (Opioid Agonist)

PREGNANCY RECOMMENDATION: Limited Human Data (First Trimester)/*Human Data Suggest Risk

BREASTFEEDING RECOMMENDATION: Potential Toxicity

PREGNANCY SUMMARY

The use of methadone in pregnancy for the treatment of opioid use disorder has been well reported in the literature. However, reports on first-trimester use are more limited. No evidence of a significantly increased risk of congenital anomalies has been seen, but numbers are small. Methadone does cross the placenta, so fetal exposure will occur. Animal reproductive studies were not located. Using opioid drugs because of substance use disorder during pregnancy can lead to numerous maternal, fetal, and neonatal complications. In addition, street drugs lack purity, and if used, IV can increase other risks of infections, sepsis, emboli, and even death. Thus, methadone maintenance programs can minimize these risks. *Nevertheless, NAS or NOWS may occur with prolonged exposure to opioids, including methadone. Neonatal opioid withdrawal symptoms include irritability, hyperactivity, abnormal sleep patterns, high-pitched cry, tremor, vomiting, diarrhea, and failure to gain weight. The onset, duration, and severity of withdrawal vary based on the opioid used, duration of use, timing and amount of last maternal use, and elimination of the drug by the newborn. Infants exposed to opioids should be monitored for symptoms of NOWS. ACOG recommends methadone for opioid maintenance therapy during pregnancy.

BREASTFEEDING SUMMARY

Numerous studies have been located that describe the use of methadone during human lactation. The drug has been found in human breast milk with concentrations that range from undetectable (lower limit of quantification [LLQ] 5 ng/mL) up to nearly 6 mcg/mL. Calculated RIDs were all less than 10% and most were less than 3%. Most infants receive an estimated dose of methadone ranging from 2% to 3% of the mother's weight-adjusted methadone dose, which is less than the dosage used for treating NAS. If the clinical decision is to use this drug while breastfeeding, the infant should be monitored for the most common reported adult side effects of increased sleepiness, difficulty breathing, and lethargy.

References

1. Prescribing Information. Methadone. Hikma Pharmaceuticals USA Inc; 2024.
2. American College of Obstetricians and Gynecologists. Committee opinion no. 711 summary: opioid use and opioid use disorder in pregnancy. *Obstet Gynecol*. 2017;130:e81-e94.
3. Zelson C, Lee SJ, Casalino M. Neonatal narcotic addiction. *N Engl J Med*. 1973;289:1216-1220.
4. Blinick G, Jerez E, Wallach RC. Methadone maintenance, pregnancy and progeny. *JAMA*. 1973;225:477-479.
5. Strauss ME, Andresko M, Stryker JC, et al. Methadone maintenance during pregnancy: pregnancy, birth and neonate characteristics. *Am J Obstet Gynecol*. 1974;120:895-900.
6. Newman RG, Bashkow S, Calko D. Results of 313 consecutive live births of infants delivered to patients in the New York City methadone maintenance program. *Am J Obstet Gynecol*. 1975;121:233-237.
7. Ostrea EM, Chavez CJ, Strauss ME. A study of factors that influence the severity of neonatal narcotic withdrawal. *J Pediatr*. 1976;88:642-645.
8. Kandall SR, Gartner LM. Delayed presentation of neonatal methadone withdrawal. *Pediatr Res*. 1973;7:320.
9. Parekh A, Mukherjee TK, Jhaveri R, et al. Intrauterine exposure to narcotics and cord blood prolactin concentrations. *Obstet Gynecol*. 1981;57:447-449.
10. Pierson PS, Howard P, Kleber HD. Sudden deaths in infants born to methadone-maintained addicts. *JAMA*. 1972;220:1733-1734.
11. Chavez CJ, Ostrea EM, Stryker JC, Smialek Z. Sudden infant death syndrome among infants of drug-dependent mothers. *J Pediatr*. 1979;95:407-409.
12. Zuspan FP, Gumpel JA, Mejia-Zelaya A, et al. Fetal stress from methadone withdrawal. *Am J Obstet Gynecol*. 1975;122:43-46.
13. Rementeria JL, Nunag NN. Narcotic withdrawal in pregnancy: stillbirth incidence with a case report. *Am J Obstet Gynecol*. 1973;116:1152-1156.
14. Burstein Y, Giardina PJV, Rausen AR, et al. Thrombocytosis and increased circulating platelet aggregates in newborn infants of polydrug users. *J Pediatr*. 1979;94:895-899.
15. Broussard CS, Rasmussen SA, Reefhuis J, et al; for the National Birth Defects Prevention Study. Maternal treatment with opioid analgesics and risk for birth defects. *Am J Obstet Gynecol*. 2011;204:314-317.
16. Cleary BJ, Donnelly JM, Strawbridge JD, et al. Methadone and perinatal outcomes: a retrospective cohort study. *Am J Obstet Gynecol*. 2011;204:139-141.
17. Margolis S, Martin L. Anophthalmia in an infant of parents using LSD. *Ann Ophthalmol*. 1980;12:1378-1381.
18. Nelson LB, Ehrlich S, Calhoun JH, et al. Occurrence of strabismus in infants born to drug-dependent women. *Am J Dis Child*. 1987;141:175-178.
19. Gill AC, Oei J, Lewis NL, et al. Strabismus in infants of opiate dependent mothers. *Acta Paediatr*. 2003;92:379-385.
20. Jones HE, Jansson LM, O'Grady KE, Kaltenbach K. The relationship between maternal methadone dose at delivery and neonatal outcome: methodological and design considerations. *Neurotoxicol Teratol*. 2013;39:110-115.
21. Jones HE, Kaltenback K, Heil SH, et al. Neonatal abstinence syndrome after methadone or buprenorphine exposure (MOTHER Study). *N Engl J Med*. 2010;363:2320-2331.
22. Kaltenbach K, O'Grady KE, Heil SH, et al. Prenatal exposure to methadone or buprenorphine: early childhood developmental outcomes. *Drug Alcohol Depend*. 2018;185:40-49.
23. Blinick G, Inturrisi CE, Jerez E, Wallach RC. Methadone assays in pregnant women and progeny. *Am J Obstet Gynecol*. 1975;121:617-621.
24. Smialek JE, Monforte JR, Aronow R, Spitz WU. Methadone deaths in children. A continuing problem. *JAMA*. 1977;238:2516-2517.
25. Anonymous. Methadone in breast milk. *Med Lett Drugs Ther*. 1979;21:52.
26. Geraghty B, Graham EA, Logan B, Weiss EL. Methadone levels in breast milk. *J Hum Lact*. 1997;13:227-230.
27. McCarthy JJ, Posey BL. Methadone levels in human milk. *J Hum Lact*. 2000;16:115-120.
28. Wojnar-Horton RE, Kristensen JH, Yapp P, et al. Methadone distribution and excretion into breast milk of clients in a methadone maintenance programme. *Br J Clin Pharmacol*. 1997;44:543-547.
29. de Castro A, Jones HE, Johnson RE, et al. Maternal methadone dose, placental methadone concentrations, and neonatal outcomes. *Clin Chem*. 2011;57:449-458.
30. Kaltenback K, Finnegan LP. Development and outcomes of children born to methadone maintained women: a review of longitudinal studies. *Neurobehav Toxicol Teratol*. 1984;6:271-275.

METHAMPHETAMINE

Central Stimulant

See Amphetamine.

METHAZOLAMIDE

Ophthalmic (Carbonic Anhydrase Inhibitor/Antiglaucoma)

PREGNANCY RECOMMENDATION: No Human Data and No Relevant Animal Data

BREASTFEEDING RECOMMENDATION: Probably Compatible

PREGNANCY SUMMARY

No reports describing the use of methazolamide in human pregnancy have been located. The drug will probably cross the placenta, so some fetal exposure will likely occur. However, the absence of human pregnancy experience prevents a complete assessment of the embryofetal risk. No relevant animal studies have been conducted. Using this drug during pregnancy should be based on the pros and cons of the mother's clinical need for treatment versus any potential fetal risk that might occur from exposure.

BREASTFEEDING SUMMARY

No reports describing the use of methazolamide during human lactation have been located. The drug will probably be found in human breast milk, so some infant exposure will likely occur. Breastfeeding while using this drug should be based on the mother's clinical need for treatment versus any potential infant risks that might occur. If used, the infant should be monitored for the most common reported adult side effects of nausea, paresthesias, and tinnitus (all leading to irritability), fatigue (lethargy), loss of appetite (monitor infant growth), vomiting, diarrhea, and drowsiness.

Reference

1. Prescribing Information. Methazolamide. ANI Pharmaceuticals, Inc; 2023.

METHENAMINE

Antibacterial (Urinary Agent)

PREGNANCY RECOMMENDATION: Limited Human Data—Animal Data Suggest Potential Risk

BREASTFEEDING RECOMMENDATION: Probably Compatible

PREGNANCY SUMMARY

Three reports describing the use of methenamine during human pregnancy were located. From 49 first-trimester exposures, 2 (4.1%) major birth anomalies were described, and both were different. In another study of 190 exposures with anytime use in pregnancy, no increased risk for birth defects was seen. The drug crosses the placenta, so fetal exposure will occur. However, this limited human pregnancy experience still prevents a complete assessment of the embryofetal risk. Embryofetal toxicity with malformations was observed in one animal species at doses less than 10 times the RHD, but not in a second species. Using this drug during pregnancy should be based on the pros and cons of the mother's clinical need for treatment versus any potential fetal risk that might occur from exposure.

BREASTFEEDING SUMMARY

One report describing the use of methenamine in four breastfeeding mothers was located. The drug was found to be excreted into breast milk, and no adverse effects on the nursing infant were reported. If the clinical decision is to use this drug while breastfeeding, the infant should be monitored for the most common reported adult side effects of nausea, pruritus, and dysuria (all leading to irritability), vomiting, and rash.

References

1. Prescribing Information. Methenamine Mandelate. Chartwell RX, LLC; 2023.
2. Prescribing Information. Methenamine Hippurate. Alvogen; 2024.
3. Lexi-Comp, Inc. (Lexi-Drugs). Lexi-Comp, Inc; 2024.
4. Allgen LG, Holmberg G, Persson B, Sorbo B. Biological fate of methenamine in man. *Acta Obstet Gynecol Scand*. 1979;58:287-293.
5. Gordon SF. Asymptomatic bacteriuria of pregnancy. *Clin Med*. 1972; 79:22-24.
6. Furness ET, McDonald PJ, Beasley NV. Urinary antiseptics in asymptomatic bacteriuria of pregnancy. *N Z Med J*. 1975;81:417-419.
7. Heinonen OP, Slone D, Shapiro S. *Birth Defects and Drugs in Pregnancy*. Publishing Sciences Group; 1977.
8. Sapeika N. The excretion of drugs in human milk—a review. *J Obstet Gynaecol Br Emp*. 1947;54:426-431.

METHIMAZOLE

Endocrine/Metabolic (Antithyroid)

PREGNANCY RECOMMENDATION: Human Data Suggest Risk (First Trimester)

BREASTFEEDING RECOMMENDATION: Probably Compatible

PREGNANCY SUMMARY

Numerous case reports and small series describing the use of methimazole in human pregnancy have been located. Studies suggest a higher rate of congenital abnormalities, including aplasia cutis congenita, craniofacial malformations, gastrointestinal malformations, and umbilical defects in infants exposed to methimazole in the first trimester. The drug crosses the placenta, so fetal exposure will occur. ACOG recommends that pregnant women with overt hyperthyroidism be treated with methimazole or propylthiouracil. If possible, methimazole should be avoided during the first trimester due to the possible association with the above-described birth defects. Therefore, starting with propylthiouracil early in pregnancy and then converting to methimazole is often followed. When methimazole is used later in pregnancy, it is recommended that treatment occur with the lowest possible dose to maintain free T_4 levels slightly above or in the high-normal range, regardless of thyrotropin (TSH) levels. Hypothyroidism may still occur in the newborn, so this needs to be monitored.

BREASTFEEDING SUMMARY

Limited reports describing the effects of methimazole during human lactation were located. No adverse effects in infants, including changes in thyroid function, have been reported. Methimazole is excreted into breast milk with concentrations that range from about 40 ng/mL up to about 110 ng/mL. Most calculated RIDs are low, with a peak value of about 5%. Breastfeeding while using this drug should be based on the mother's clinical need for treatment versus any potential infant risks that might occur. If used, the infant should be monitored for the most common reported adult side effects of nausea, headache, epigastric distress, pruritus, myalgia, and arthralgia (all leading to irritability), rash, and drowsiness. Infant thyroid levels should also be monitored.

References

1. Wilson LC, Kerr BA, Wilkinson R, et al. Choanal atresia and hypothelia following methimazole exposure in utero: a second report. *Am J Med Genet*. 1998;75:220-222.
2. Clementi M, Di Gianantonio E, Pelo E, et al. Methimazole embryopathy: delineation of the phenotype. *Am J Med Genet*. 1999;83:43-46.
3. Martin-Danavit T, Edery P, Plauchu H, et al. Ectodermal abnormalities associated with methimazole intrauterine exposure. *Am J Med Genet*. 2000; 94:338-340.
4. Momotani N, Noh J, Oyanagi H, et al. Antithyroid drug therapy for Graves' disease during pregnancy: optimal regimen for fetal thyroid status. *N Engl J Med*. 1986;315:24-28.
5. Lexi-Comp, Inc. (Lexi-Drugs). Lexi-Comp, Inc; 2018.
6. Mortimer RH, Cannell GR, Addison RS, et al. Methimazole and propylthiouracil equally cross the perfused human term placental lobule. *J Clin Endocrinol Metab*. 1997;82:3099-3102.
7. Marchant B, Brownlie EW, Hart DM, et al. The placental transfer of propylthiouracil, methimazole and carbimazole. *J Clin Endocrinol Metab*. 1977; 45:1187-1193.
8. Milham S Jr, Elledge W. Maternal methimazole and congenital defects in children. *Teratology*. 1972;5:125.
9. Mujtaba Q, Burrow GN. Treatment of hyperthyroidism in pregnancy with propylthiouracil and methimazole. *Obstet Gynecol*. 1975;46:282-286.
10. Milham S Jr. Scalp defects in infants of mothers treated for hyperthyroidism with methimazole or carbimazole during pregnancy. *Teratology*. 1985;32:321.
11. Kalb RE, Grossman ME. The association of aplasia cutis congenita with therapy of maternal thyroid disease. *Pediatr Dermatol*. 1986;3:327-330.
12. Farine D, Maidman J, Rubin S, Chao S. Elevated alpha-fetoprotein in pregnancy complicated by aplasia cutis after exposure to methimazole. *Obstet Gynecol*. 1988;71:996-997.
13. Van Dijke CP, Heydendael RJ, De Kleine MJ. Methimazole, carbimazole, and congenital skin defects. *Ann Intern Med*. 1987;106:60-61.
14. Sugrue D, Drury MI. Hyperthyroidism complicating pregnancy: results of treatment by antithyroid drugs in 77 pregnancies. *Br J Obstet Gynaecol*. 1980;87:970-975.
15. Heinonen OP, Slone D, Shapiro S. *Birth Defects and Drugs in Pregnancy*. Publishing Sciences Group; 1977:388-400.
16. McCarroll AM, Hutchinson M, McAuley R, Montgomery DAD. Long-term assessment of children exposed in utero to carbimazole. *Arch Dis Child*. 1976;51:532-536.
17. Hawe P, Francis HH. Pregnancy and thyrotoxicosis. *Br Med J*. 1962;2:817-822.
18. Herbst AL. Selenkow HA. Combined antithyroid-thyroid therapy of hyperthyroidism in pregnancy. *Obstet Gynecol*. 1963;21:543-550.
19. Reveno WS, Rosenbaum H. Observation on the use of antithyroid drugs. *Ann Intern Med*. 1964;60:982-989.
20. Herbst AL, Selenkow HA. Hyperthyroidism during pregnancy. *N Engl J Med*. 1965;273:627-633.
21. Talbert LM, Thomas CG Jr, Holt WA, Rankin P. Hyperthyroidism during pregnancy. *Obstet Gynecol*. 1970;36:779-785.
22. Refetoff S, Ochi Y, Selenkow HA, Rosenfield RL. Neonatal hypothyroidism and goiter in one infant of each of two sets of twins due to maternal therapy with antithyroid drugs. *J Pediatr*. 1974;85:240-244.
23. Mestman JH, Manning PR, Hodgman J. Hyperthyroidism and pregnancy. *Ann Intern Med*. 1974;134:434-439.
24. Ramsay I. Attempted prevention of neonatal thyrotoxicosis. *Br Med J*. 1976;2:1110.
25. Low L, Ratcliffe W, Alexander W. Intrauterine hypothyroidism due to antithyroid-drug therapy for thyrotoxicosis during pregnancy. *Lancet*. 1978; 2:370-371.
26. Robinson PL, O'Mullane NH, Alderman B. Prenatal treatment of fetal thyrotoxicosis. *Br Med J*. 1979;1:383-384.
27. Kock HCLV, Merkus JMWM. Graves' disease during pregnancy. *Eur J Obstet Gynecol Reprod Biol*. 1983;14:323-330.
28. Pekonen F, Teramo K, Makinen T, et al. Prenatal diagnosis and treatment of fetal thyrotoxicosis. *Am J Obstet Gynecol*. 1984;150:893-894.
29. Jeffcoate WJ, Bain C. Recurrent pregnancy-induced thyrotoxicosis presenting as hyperemesis gravidarum. Case report. *Br J Obstet Gynaecol*. 1985; 92:413-415.
30. Johnson IR, Filshie GM. Hodgkin's disease diagnosed in pregnancy: case report. *Br J Obstet Gynaecol*. 1977;84:791-792.
31. Ramsay I, Kaur S, Krassas G. Thyrotoxicosis in pregnancy: results of treatment by antithyroid drugs combined with T4. *Clin Endocrinol (Oxf)*. 1983; 18:73-85.
32. Momotani N, Ito K, Hamada N, et al. Maternal hyperthyroidism and congenital malformation in the offspring. *Clin Endocrinol (Oxf)*. 1984;20: 695-700.

33. Greenberg F. Choanal atresia and athelia: methimazole teratogenicity or a new syndrome? *Am J Med Genet*. 1987;28:931-934.
34. Ramirez A, Espinosa de los Monteros A, Parra A, De Leon B. Esophageal atresia and tracheoesophageal fistula in two infants born to hyperthyroid women receiving methimazole (Tapazole) during pregnancy. *Am J Med Genet*. 1992;44:200-202.
35. Eisenstein Z, Weiss M, Katz Y, Bank H. Intellectual capacity of subjects exposed to methimazole or propylthiouracil in utero. *Eur J Pediatr*. 1992; 151:558-559.
36. Mandel SJ, Brent GA, Larsen PR. Review of antithyroid drug use during pregnancy and report of a case of aplasia cutis. *Thyroid*. 1994;4:129-133.
37. Vogt T, Stolz W, Landthaler M. Aplasia cutis congenita after exposure to methimazole: a causal relationship? *Br J Dermatol*. 1995;133:994-996.
38. Hall BD. Methimazole as a teratogenic etiology of choanal atresia/ multiple congenital anomaly syndrome (abstract). *Am J Hum Genet*. 1997;61(suppl):A100. As cited in Clementi M, Di Gianantonio E, Pelo E, Mammi I, Basile RT, Tenconi R. Methimazole embryopathy: delineation of the phenotype. *Am J Med Genet*. 1999;83:43-46.
39. Johnsson E, Larsson G, Ljunggren M. Severe malformations in infant born to hyperthyroid woman on methimazole. *Lancet*. 1997;350:1520.
40. Hardisty CA, Munro DS. Serum long acting thyroid stimulator protector in pregnancy complicated by Graves' disease. *Br Med J*. 1983;286:934-935.
41. Cove DH, Johnston P. Fetal hyperthyroidism: experience of treatment in four siblings. *Lancet*. 1985;1:430-432.
42. Burrow GN. The management of thyrotoxicosis in pregnancy. *N Engl J Med*. 1985;313:562-565.
43. Wing D, Millar L, Koonings P, et al. A comparison of PTU versus Tapazole in the treatment of hyperthyroidism (abstract). *Am J Obstet Gynecol*. 1992;166:308.
44. Wing DA, Millar LK, Koonings PP, et al. A comparison of propylthiouracil versus methimazole in the treatment of hyperthyroidism in pregnancy. *Am J Obstet Gynecol*. 1994;170:90-95.
45. Di Gianantonio E, Schaefer C, Mastroiacovo PP, et al. Adverse effects of prenatal methimazole exposure. *Teratology*. 2001;64:262-266.
46. Seoud M, Nassar A, Usta I, et al. Gastrointestinal malformations in two infants born to women with hyperthyroidism untreated in the first trimester. *Am J Perinatol*. 2003;20:59-62.
47. Ferraris S, Valenzise M, Lerone M, et al. Malformations following methimazole exposure in utero: an open issue. *Birth Defects Res A Clin Mol Teratol*. 2003;67:989-992.
48. Burr WA. Thyroid disease. *Clin Obstet Gynecol*. 1981;8:341-351.
49. Martinez-Frias ML, Cereijo A, Rodriguez-Pinilla E, Urioste M. Methimazole in animal feed and congenital aplasia cutis. *Lancet*. 1992;339:742-743.
50. Anonymous. Transplacental passage of thyroid hormones. *N Engl J Med*. 1967;277:486-487.
51. Mestman JH. Hyperthyroidism in pregnancy. *Clin Obstet Gynecol*. 1997; 40:45-64.
52. Diav-Citrin O, Ornoy A. Teratogen update: antithyroid drugs—methimazole, carbimazole, and propylthiouracil. *Teratology*. 2002;65:38-44.
53. Valdez RM, Barbero PM, Liascovich RC, et al. Methimazole embryopathy: a contribution to defining the phenotype. *Reprod Toxicol*. 2007;23: 253-255.
54. Bachrach LK, Burrow GN. Aplasia cutis congenita and methimazole. *CMAJ*. 1984;130:1264.
55. Low LCK, Lang J, Alexander WD. Excretion of carbimazole and propylthiouracil in breast milk. *Lancet*. 1979;2:1011.
56. Tegler L, Lindstrom B. Antithyroid drugs in milk. *Lancet*. 1980;2:591.
57. Johansen K, Andersen AN, Kampmann JP, et al. Excretion of methimazole in human milk. *Eur J Clin Pharmacol*. 1982;23:339-341.
58. Rylance GW, Woods CG, Donnelly MC, et al. Carbimazole and breastfeeding. *Lancet*. 1987;1:928.
59. Alexander EK, Pearce EN, Brent GA, et al. 2017 Guidelines of the American Thyroid Association for the diagnosis and management of thyroid disease during pregnancy and the postpartum. *Thyroid*. 2017;27:315-389.
60. Lamberg BA, Ikonen E, Osterlund K, et al. Antithyroid treatment of maternal hyperthyroidism during lactation. *Clin Endocrinol*. 1984;21:81-87.
61. Azizi F. Effect of methimazole treatment of maternal thyrotoxicosis on thyroid function in breast-feeding infants. *J Pediatr*. 1996;128:855-858.
62. Azizi F, Khoshniat M, Bahrainian M, Hedayati M. Thyroid function and intellectual development of infants nursed by mothers taking methimazole. *J Clin Endocrinol Metab*. 2000;85:3233-3238.
63. Prescribing Information. Methimazole. Bionpharma Inc; 2024.
64. Thyroid disease in pregnancy: ACOG practice bulletin, number 223. *Obstet Gynecol*. 2020;135:e261-e274.
65. Yu W, Wu N, Li L, et al. Side effects of PTU and MMI in the treatment of hyperthyroidism: a systematic review and meta-analysis. *Endocr Pract*. 2020;26:207-217.
66. Morales DR, Fonkwen L, Nordeng HME. Antithyroid drug use during pregnancy and the risk of birth defects in offspring: systematic review and meta-analysis of observational studies with methodological considerations. *Br J Clin Pharmacol*. 2021;87:3890-3900.
67. Agrawal M, Lewis S, Premawardhana L, et al. Antithyroid drug therapy in pregnancy and risk of congenital anomalies: systematic review and meta-analysis. *Clin Endocrinol (Oxf)*. 2022;96:857-868.
68. Liu Y, Li Q, Xu Y, et al. Comparison of the safety between propylthiouracil and methimazole with hyperthyroidism in pregnancy: a systematic review and meta-analysis. *PLoS One*. 2023;18:e0286097
69. Bhagat M, Singh P, Sunkara SM, et al. Effects of methimazole vs propylthiouracil in newborns: a comparative review. *Cureus*. 2023;15:e41505.

M

METHOCARBAMOL

Central Nervous System (Skeletal Muscle Relaxant)

PREGNANCY RECOMMENDATION: Limited Human Data—No Relevant Animal Data

BREASTFEEDING RECOMMENDATION: Probably Compatible (Short-Term Use)

PREGNANCY SUMMARY

Limited reports describing the use of methocarbamol in human pregnancy have been located. From three studies, the Michigan Medicaid Surveillance study, the Collaborative Perinatal Project, and the manufacturer, there were 14 (3.6%) major congenital birth anomalies seen in 389 first-trimester exposures. No pattern to the defects was seen. The drug will probably cross the placenta, so some fetal exposure will likely occur. However, this limited human pregnancy experience prevents a complete assessment of the embryofetal risk. No animal reproduction studies have been conducted. Using this drug during pregnancy should be based on the pros and cons of the mother's clinical need for treatment versus any potential fetal risk that might occur from exposure.

BREASTFEEDING SUMMARY

No reports describing the use of methocarbamol during human lactation have been located. The drug will probably be found in breast milk, so some infant exposure will likely occur. Therefore, if the clinical decision is to use this drug while breastfeeding, the infant should be monitored for the most common reported adult side effects of nausea, vertigo, and headache (all leading to irritability), drowsiness, rash, and fever.

References

1. Prescribing Information. Methocarbamol tablets. XLCare Pharmaceuticals Inc; 2024.
2. Prescribing Information. Methocarbamol injection. Slate Run Pharmaceuticals, LLC; 2024.
3. Heinonen OP, Slone D, Shapiro S. *Birth Defects and Drugs in Pregnancy*. Publishing Sciences Group; 1977.
4. Hall JG, Reed SD. Teratogens associated with congenital contractures in humans and in animals. *Teratology*. 1982;25:173-191.
5. Barrow MV, Souder DE. Propoxyphene and congenital malformations. *JAMA*. 1971;217:1551-1552.

METHOHEXITAL SODIUM

Anesthetic

PREGNANCY RECOMMENDATION: Limited Human Data—*Animal Data Suggest Low Risk

BREASTFEEDING RECOMMENDATION: Probably Compatible

PREGNANCY SUMMARY

A few studies describing the use of methohexital sodium during human pregnancy were located. From the Collaborative Perinatal Project, there were 2 anomalies (1 major—2.4%) in 41 first-trimester exposures. Another study evaluated 2 doses of methohexital in 26 women undergoing an elective cesarean section. In the group that received the higher dose, more infants required assisted ventilation, took more time to establish regular respiration, and had lower Apgar scores. The drug can also cause dose-related fetal heart rate (FHR) slowing and newborn sedation. Methohexital crosses the placenta, so fetal exposure will occur. However, the limited human pregnancy experience prevents a complete assessment of the embryofetal risk. Animal data did not show embryofetal toxicity in two animal species at less than 10 times the RHD. *However, based on animal studies, the FDA issued a warning regarding that repeated or prolonged use (>3 hours) of general anesthetics and sedation medications during the third trimester may affect the developing brain. Therefore, using this drug during pregnancy should be based on the pros and cons of the mother's clinical need for treatment versus any potential fetal risk that might occur from exposure.

BREASTFEEDING SUMMARY

No reports describing the effects of methohexital sodium in infants during human lactation have been located. Methohexital is excreted into human breast milk, with the obtained peak value of about 0.4 mcg/mL. The highest calculated RID was about 3.5%. Breastfeeding while using this drug should be based on the mother's clinical need for treatment versus any potential infant risks that might occur. If used, the infant should be monitored for the most common reported adult side effects of nausea, headache, pruritus, and abdominal pain (all leading to irritability), tremors, lethargy, vomiting, erythema, and salivation. If there is any concern, the drug should only be used once with surgery. Therefore, holding breastfeeding for about 15 hours (5 half-lives) would greatly decrease any exposure.

References

1. Prescribing Information. Methohexital sodium. Heritage Pharmaceuticals Inc; 2024.
2. U.S. Food and Drug Administration. FDA drug safety communication: FDA review results in new warnings about using general anesthetics and sedation drugs in young children and pregnant women. Accessed January 17, 2025. https://www.fda.gov/Drugs/DrugSafety/ucm532356.htm
3. U.S. Food and Drug Administration. FDA drug safety communication: FDA approved label changes for use of general anesthetics and sedation drugs in young children. Accessed January 17, 2025. https://www.fda.gov/drugs/drug-safety-and-availability/fda-drug-safety-communication-fda-approves-label-changes-use-general-anesthetic-and-sedation-drugs
4. Lexi-Comp, Inc. (Lexi-Drugs). Lexi-Comp, Inc; 2025.
5. Varga VJ, Machay T, Paulin F, Balazs M, Fedak L. Changes in serum level of methohexital (Brietal) in mothers and newborns during cesarean section. *Zbl Gynakol*. 1983;105:297-299.
6. Herman NL, Li A-T, Johnson RF, et al. Transfer of methohexital across the perfused human placenta. *J Clin Anesth*. 2000;12:25-30.
7. Holdcroft A, Robinson MJ, Gordon H, Whitwam JG. Comparison of effect of two induction doses of methohexitone on infants delivered by elective caesarean section. *Br Med J*. 1974;2:472.
8. Downing JW. Effect of methohexitone on infants delivered by caesarean section. *Br Med J*. 1974;3:411.
9. Anderson EL, Reti IM. ECT in pregnancy: a review of the literature from 1941 to 2007. *Psychosom Med*. 2009;71:235-242.
10. De Asis SJ, Helgeson L, Ostroff R. The use of propofol to prevent fetal deceleration during electroconvulsive therapy treatment. *J ECT*. 2013; 29(4):e57-e58.
11. Borgatta L, Jenny RW, Gruss L, et al. Clinical significance of methohexital, meperidine, and diazepam in breast milk. *J Clin Pharmacol*. 1997;37: 186-192.

METHOTREXATE

Antineoplastic/Immunologic

PREGNANCY RECOMMENDATION: *Contraindicated

BREASTFEEDING RECOMMENDATION: Potential Toxicity

PREGNANCY SUMMARY

A number of reports describing the use of methotrexate in human pregnancy have been located. The use of methotrexate during organogenesis is associated with a spectrum of congenital defects collectively called methotrexate embryopathy or the fetal aminopterin-methotrexate syndrome. The critical period of exposure is 6 to 8 weeks postconception (8-10 weeks' gestation), and the critical dose is thought to be greater than or equal to 10 mg per week. Exposure in the second and third trimesters may be associated with fetal toxicity and death. The drug crosses the placenta, so fetal exposure will occur. Based on animal studies and the drug's mechanism of action, the manufacturer recommends that women with reproductive potential use effective contraception during treatment and for 1 month after the last dose. They also recommend that males with female partners of reproductive potential use effective contraception during treatment and for 1 month after the last dose. *Methotrexate is contraindicated in pregnant women for non-neoplastic diseases. However, using this drug for neoplastic diseases during pregnancy should be based on the pros and cons of the mother's clinical need for treatment versus any potential fetal risk that might occur from exposure. Pregnant women with neoplastic diseases should be advised of the potential risk to the fetus. The drug carries a boxed warning regarding embryofetal toxicity (including fetal death), hypersensitivity, and other severe reactions. There is a registry for women who are pregnant and have cancer. For more information, women and health care providers are encouraged to contact the Cancer and Pregnancy Registry at 1-877-635-4499.

BREASTFEEDING SUMMARY

Two reports describing the effects of methotrexate in four breastfed infants were located. No adverse effects were noted in the infants. Methotrexate was found to be excreted into human breast milk in low concentrations. However, due to a concern for potential serious adverse effects that might be seen in a breastfed infant, the manufacturer recommends that women not breastfeed while being treated with this drug and for at least 1 week after the last dose. Nevertheless, if the clinical decision is to use this drug while breastfeeding, the infant should be monitored for the most common reported pediatric side effects of nausea (leading to irritability), vomiting, diarrhea, elevated liver enzymes, leukopenia, and mouth sores.

References

1. Prescribing Information. Methotrexate sodium tablet. Hikma Pharmaceuticals USA Inc; 2024.
2. Prescribing Information. Methotrexate injection. Accord Healthcare, Inc; 2025.
3. Del Campo M, Kosaki K, Bennett FC, Jones KL. Developmental delay in fetal aminopterin/methotrexate syndrome. *Teratology*. 1999;60:10-12.
4. Nicholson HO. Cytotoxic drugs in pregnancy: review of reported cases. *J Obstet Gynaecol Br Commonw*. 1968;75:307-312.
5. Milunsky A, Graef JW, Gaynor MF. Methotrexate-induced congenital malformations. *J Pediatr*. 1968;72:790-795.
6. Powell HR, Ekert H. Methotrexate-induced congenital malformations. *Med J Aust*. 1971;2:1076-1077.
7. Pizzuto J, Aviles A, Noriega L, et al. Treatment of acute leukemia during pregnancy: presentation of nine cases. *Cancer Treat Rep*. 1980;64:679-683.
8. Dara P, Slater LM, Armentrout SA. Successful pregnancy during chemotherapy for acute leukemia. *Cancer*. 1981;47:845-846.
9. Warkany J. Teratogenicity of folic acid antagonists. *Cancer Bull*. 1981;33:76-77.
10. Burnier AM. Discussion. In Plows CW. Acute myelomonocytic leukemia in pregnancy: report of a case. *Am J Obstet Gynecol*. 1982;143:41-43.
11. Khurshid M, Saleem M. Acute leukaemia in pregnancy. *Lancet*. 1978;2:534-535.
12. Okun DB, Groncy PK, Sieger L, Tanaka KR. Acute leukemia in pregnancy: transient neonatal myelosuppression after combination chemotherapy in the mother. *Med Pediatr Oncol*. 1979;7:315-319.
13. Doney KC, Kraemer KG, Shepard TH. Combination chemotherapy for acute myelocytic leukemia during pregnancy: three case reports. *Cancer Treat Rep*. 1979;63:369-371.
14. Karp GI, von Oeyen P, Valone F, et al. Doxorubicin in pregnancy: possible transplacental passage. *Cancer Treat Rep*. 1983;67:773-777.
15. Feliu J, Juarez S, Ordonez A, et al. Acute leukemia and pregnancy. *Cancer*. 1988;61:580-584.
16. Turchi JJ, Villasis C. Anthracyclines in the treatment of malignancy in pregnancy. *Cancer*. 1988;61:435-440.
17. Schleuning M, Clemm C. Chromosomal aberrations in a newborn whose mother received cytotoxic treatment during pregnancy. *N Engl J Med*. 1987;317:1666-1667.
18. Frenkel EP, Meyers MC. Acute leukemia and pregnancy. *Ann Intern Med*. 1960;53:656-671.
19. Coopland AT, Friesen WJ, Galbraith PA. Acute leukemia in pregnancy. *Am J Obstet Gynecol*. 1969;105:1288-1289.
20. Kozlowski RD, Steinbrunner JV, MacKenzie AH, et al. Outcome of first-trimester exposure to low-dose methotrexate in eight patients with rheumatic disease. *Am J Med*. 1990;88:589-592.
21. Feldkamp M, Carey JC. Clinical teratology counseling and consultation case report: low dose methotrexate exposure in the early weeks of pregnancy. *Teratology*. 1993;47:533-539.
22. Gangadharan VP, Chitrathara K, Satishkumar K, et al. Successful management of choriocarcinoma with pregnancy. *Acta Oncol*. 1994;33:76-77.
23. Donnenfeld AE, Pastuszak A, Noah JS, et al. Methotrexate exposure prior to and during pregnancy. *Teratology*. 1994;49:79-81.
24. Buckley LM, Bullaboy CA, Leichtman L, Marquez M. Multiple congenital anomalies associated with weekly low-dose methotrexate treatment of the mother. *Arthritis Rheum*. 1997;40:971-973.
25. Bawle EV, Conard JV, Weiss L. Adult and two children with fetal methotrexate syndrome. *Teratology*. 1998;57:51-55.
26. Giacalone PL, Laffargue F, Benos P. Chemotherapy for breast carcinoma during pregnancy. *Cancer*. 1999;86:2266-2272.
27. Wheeler M, O'Meara P, Stanford M. Fetal methotrexate and misoprostol exposure: the past revisited. *Teratology*. 2002;66:73-76.
28. Nguyen C, Duhl AJ, Escallon CS, Blakemore KJ. Multiple anomalies in a fetus exposed to low-dose methotrexate in the first trimester. *Obstet Gynecol*. 2002;99:599-602.
29. Chapa JB, Hibbard JU, Weber EM, et al. Prenatal diagnosis of methotrexate embryopathy. *Obstet Gynecol*. 2003;101:1104-1107.
30. Chakravarty EF, Sanchez-Yamamoto D, Bush TM. The use of disease modifying antirheumatic drugs in women with rheumatoid arthritis of childbearing age: a survey of practice patterns and pregnancy outcomes. *J Rheumatol*. 2003;30:241-246.
31. Walden PAM, Bagshawe KD. Pregnancies after chemotherapy for gestational trophoblastic tumours. *Lancet*. 1979;2:1241.
32. Charache S, Condit PT, Humphreys SR. Studies on the folic acid vitamins. IV. The persistence of amethopterin in mammalian tissues. *Cancer*. 1960;13:236-240.
33. Barnes AB, Link DA. Childhood dermatomyositis and pregnancy. *Am J Obstet Gynecol*. 1983;146:335-336.
34. Sivanesaratnam V, Sen DK. Normal pregnancy after successful treatment of choriocarcinoma with cerebral metastases: a case report. *J Reprod Med*. 1988;33:402-403.
35. Dobbing J. Pregnancy and leukaemia. *Lancet*. 1977;1:1155.
36. Schilsky RL, Lewis BJ, Sherins RJ, Young RC. Gonadal dysfunction in patients receiving chemotherapy for cancer. *Ann Intern Med*. 1980;93:109-114.
37. Johns DG, Rutherford LD, Keighton PC, Vogel CL. Secretion of methotrexate into human milk. *Am J Obstet Gynecol*. 1972;112:978-980.

38. Tanaka T, Walsh W, Verjee Z, et al. Methotrexate use in a lactating woman with an ectopic pregnancy. *Birth Defects Res A Clin Mol Teratol*. 2009; 85:494.
39. Thorne JC, Nadarajah T, Moretti M, Ito S. Methotrexate use in a breastfeeding patient with rheumatoid arthritis. *J Rheumatol*. 2014;41:2332.
40. Delaney S, Colantonio D, Ito S. Methotrexate in breast milk. *Birth Defects Res*. 2017;109:711.
41. Baker T, Datta P, Rewers-Felkins K, Hale TW. High-dose methotrexate treatment in a breastfeeding mother with placenta accreta: a case report. *Breastfeed Med*. 2018;13:450-452.
42. Centre de Référence sur les Agents Tératogènes. Méthotrexate—Grossesse et allaitement. 2020.

METHOXSALEN

Miscellaneous (Photoactive Substance)

PREGNANCY RECOMMENDATION: Limited Human Data—No Relevant Animal Data

BREASTFEEDING RECOMMENDATION: Potential Toxicity

PREGNANCY SUMMARY

Three reports describing the use of methoxsalen in over 70 human pregnancies at the time of conception or during early pregnancy were located. No major birth anomalies were identified. The drug will probably cross the placenta, so some infant exposure will likely occur. However, the limited human pregnancy experience prevents a complete assessment of the embryofetal risk. No relevant animal reproduction studies have been conducted. Using this drug during pregnancy should be based on the pros and cons of the mother's clinical need for treatment versus any potential fetal risk that might occur from exposure.

BREASTFEEDING SUMMARY

No reports describing the use of methoxsalen during human lactation have been located. Because the drug acts as a photosensitizer, breastfeeding should probably be stopped and the breast milk discarded, for at least 12 hours (six half-lives), if possible. Breastfeeding while using this drug should be based on the mother's clinical need for treatment versus any potential infant risks that might occur. If used, the infant should be monitored for the most common reported adult side effects of nausea with the oral product and hypotension with the extracorporeal solution.

References

1. Prescribing Information. Methoxsalen. Strides Pharma Science Limited; 2019.
2. Prescribing Information. Uvadex. Therakos LLC; 2024.
3. Stern RS, Lange R; Members of the Photochemotherapy Follow-Up Study. Outcomes of pregnancies among women and partners of men with a history of exposure to methoxsalen photochemotherapy (PUVA) for the treatment of psoriasis. *Arch Dermatol*. 1991;127:347-350.
4. Gunnarskog JG, Källén AJB, Lindelöf BG, Sigurgeirsson B. Psoralen photochemotherapy (PUVA) and pregnancy. *Arch Dermatol*. 1993;129: 320-323.
5. Garbis H, Eléfant E, Bertolotti E, et al. Pregnancy outcome after periconceptional and first-trimester exposure to methoxsalen photochemotherapy. *Arch Dermatol*. 1995;131:492-493.

M

METHSCOPOLAMINE

Gastrointestinal/Autonomic (Anticholinergic)

PREGNANCY RECOMMENDATION: Limited Human Data—No Relevant Animal Data

BREASTFEEDING RECOMMENDATION: Probably Compatible

PREGNANCY SUMMARY

From the Group Health Cooperative of Puget Sound, there were 2 (3.3%) major anomalies in about 60 first-trimester exposures to methscopolamine. In the Collaborative Perinatal Project, there were no methscopolamine exposures. However, there were 2,323 exposures to parasympatholytic agents in the first trimester. Of these, there were 71 (3.1%) major anomalies. As a subgroup of these, there were 4 (1.0%) major anomalies in 388 scopolamine and other scopolamine derivatives with first-trimester exposure. The drug will probably cross the placenta, so some fetal exposure will likely occur. Therefore, this limited human pregnancy experience prevents a complete assessment of the embryofetal risk. No animal reproduction studies have been located. Using this drug during pregnancy should be based on the pros and cons of the mother's clinical need for treatment versus any potential fetal risk that might occur from exposure.

BREASTFEEDING SUMMARY

No reports describing the use of methscopolamine during human lactation have been located. The drug will probably be found in human breast milk, so some infant exposure will likely occur. If the clinical decision is to use this drug while breastfeeding, the infant should be monitored for the most common reported adult side effects of sedation, irritability, constipation, urinary retention, and dry mouth. Milk supply may decrease due to the anticholinergic effects.

References

1. Prescribing Information. Methscopolamine bromide. Breckenridge Pharmaceuticals, Inc; 2024.
2. Jick H, Holmes LB, Hunter JR, et al. First-trimester drug use and congenital disorders. *JAMA*. 1981;246:343-346.
3. Heinonen OP, Slone D, Shapiro S. *Birth Defects and Drugs in Pregnancy*. Publishing Sciences Group; 1977:346-353.

METHSUXIMIDE

Central Nervous System (Antiseizure)

PREGNANCY RECOMMENDATION: Limited Human Data—No Relevant Animal Data

BREASTFEEDING RECOMMENDATION: Probably Compatible

PREGNANCY SUMMARY

Two reports describing the use of methsuximide during the first trimester in five pregnancies have been located. No adverse fetal effects were reported. The drug will probably cross the placenta. However, the limited human pregnancy experience prevents a complete assessment of the embryofetal risk. No animal reproduction studies have been located. Using this drug during pregnancy should be based on the pros and cons of the mother's clinical need for treatment versus any potential fetal risk that might occur from exposure. There is a pregnancy exposure registry that monitors pregnancy outcomes in women using antiseizure drugs. Health care providers are encouraged to call the North American Antiepileptic Drug Pregnancy Registry at 1-888-233-2334.

BREASTFEEDING SUMMARY

No reports describing the use of methsuximide during human lactation have been located. The drug will probably be found in human breast milk, so some infant exposure will likely occur. If the clinical decision is to use this drug while breastfeeding, the infant should be monitored for the most common reported adult side effects of nausea, headache, dizziness, and abdominal pain (all leading to irritability), vomiting, diarrhea, constipation, and drowsiness.

References

1. Prescribing Information. Celontin. Parke-Davis Div of Pfizer; 2023.
2. Annegers JF, Elveback LR, Hauser WA, Kurland LT. Do anticonvulsants have a teratogenic effect? *Arch Neurol*. 1974;31:364-373.
3. Heinonen OP, Slone D, Shapiro S. *Birth Defects and Drugs in Pregnancy*. Publishing Sciences Group; 1977:358-359.
4. Fabro S, Brown NA. Teratogenic potential of anticonvulsants. *N Engl J Med*. 1979;300:1280-1281.
5. The National Institutes of Health. Anticonvulsants found to have teratogenic potential. *JAMA*. 1981;241:36.

METHYLDOPA

Antihypertensive (α_2-Adrenergic Agonist)

PREGNANCY RECOMMENDATION: Limited Human Data (First Trimester)/Human Data Suggest Low Risk (Second and Third Trimesters)—Animal Data Suggest Low Risk

BREASTFEEDING RECOMMENDATION: Probably Compatible

PREGNANCY SUMMARY

The use of methyldopa as an antihypertensive in pregnancy is well established. Available studies have not found any evidence of a significantly increased risk for adverse effects. However, first-trimester exposure is limited. The drug crosses the placenta, so fetal exposure will occur. Therefore, this limited first-trimester human pregnancy experience prevents a complete assessment of the embryofetal risk. Animal data did not show any embryofetal toxicity or malformations in three species, two with doses less than 10 times the MRHD and one with doses more than 10 times the MRHD. ACOG considers methyldopa as one of the common medications for the management of chronic hypertension in pregnancy. It is generally less favored because it may be less effective than other agents.

BREASTFEEDING SUMMARY

Four reports describing the effects of methyldopa during human lactation were located. No adverse effects in 15 breastfed infants were reported. Methyldopa is excreted into breast milk with levels of the drug ranging from about 0.1 to 1 mcg/mL. The maximum calculated RID was less than 2%. Breastfeeding while using this drug should be based on the mother's clinical need for treatment versus any potential infant risks that might occur. If used, the infant should be monitored for the most common reported adult side effects of headache (leading to irritability), sedation, and lethargy.

References

1. Prescribing Information. Methyldopa. Chartwell RX, LLC; 2024.
2. Jones HMR, Cummings AJ. A study of the transfer of alpha-methyldopa to the human foetus and newborn infant. *Br J Clin Pharmacol*. 1978;6:432-434.
3. Jones HMR, Cummings AJ, Setchell KDR, Lawson AM. Pharmacokinetics of methyldopa in neonates. *Br J Clin Pharmacol*. 1979;8:433-440.
4. Cummings AJ, Whitelaw AGL. A study of conjugation and drug elimination in the human neonate. *Br J Clin Pharmacol*. 1981;12:511-515.
5. Heinonen OP, Slone D, Shapiro S. *Birth Defects and Drugs in Pregnancy*. Publishing Sciences Group; 1977:372.
6. Myerscough PR. Infant growth and development after treatment of maternal hypertension. *Lancet*. 1980;1:883.
7. Moar VA, Jefferies MA, Mutch LMM, et al. Neonatal head circumference and the treatment of maternal hypertension. *Br J Obstet Gynaecol*. 1978;85:933-937.
8. Dunsted M, Moar VA, Redman CWG. Infant growth and development following treatment of maternal hypertension. *Lancet*. 1980;1:705.
9. Redman CWG, Beilin LJ, Bonnar J, Ounsted MK. Fetal outcome in trial of antihypertensive treatment in pregnancy. *Lancet*. 1976;2:753-756.
10. Hamilton M, Kopelman H. Treatment of severe hypertension with methyldopa. *Br Med J*. 1963;1:151-155.
11. Abramowsky CR, Vegas ME, Swinehart G, Gyves MT. Decidual vasculopathy of the placenta in lupus erythematosus. *N Engl J Med*. 1980;303:668-672.
12. Gallery EDM, Sounders DM, Hunyor SN, Gyory AZ. Randomised comparison of methyldopa and oxprenolol for treatment of hypertension in pregnancy. *Br Med J*. 1979;1:1591-1594.
13. Gyory AZ, Gallery ED, Hunyor SN. Effect of treatment of maternal hypertension with oxprenolol and α-methyldopa on plasma volume, placental and birth weights (abstract 1098). Presented at Eighth World Congress of Cardiology; 1978; Tokyo.
14. Arias F, Zamora J. Antihypertensive treatment and pregnancy outcome in patients with mild chronic hypertension. *Obstet Gynecol*. 1979;53:489-494.
15. Redman CWG, Beilin LJ, Bonnar J. A trial of hypotensive treatment in pregnancy. *Clin Sci Mol Med* 1975;49:3-4.
16. Tcherdakoff P, Milliez P. Traitement de l'hypertension arterielle par alpha-methyldopa au cours de la grossesse. In Proceedings Premier Symposium National, Hypertension Arterielle, Cannes; 1970:207-209.
17. Leather HM, Humphreys DM, Baker P, Chadd MA. A controlled trial of hypotensive agents in hypertension in pregnancy. *Lancet*. 1968;2:488-490.
18. Hamilton H. Some aspects of the long-term treatment of severe hypertension with methyldopa. *Postgrad Med J*. 1968;44:66-69.
19. Skacel K, Sklendvsky A, Gazarek F, et al. Therapeutic use of alpha-methyldopa in cases of late toxemia of pregnancy. *Cesk Gynekol*. 1967;32:78-80.
20. Kincaid-Smith P, Bullen M. Prolonged use of methyldopa in severe hypertension in pregnancy. *Br Med J*. 1966;1:274-276.
21. Whitelaw A. Maternal methyldopa treatment and neonatal blood pressure. *Br Med J*. 1981;283:471.
22. Molvi SN, Mir S, Rana VS, et al. Role of antihypertensive therapy in mild to moderate pregnancy-induced hypertension: a prospective randomized study comparing labetalol with alpha methyldopa. *Arch Gynecol Obstet*. 2012;285:1553-1562.
23. Ylikorkala O. Congenital anomalies and clomiphene. *Lancet*. 1975;2:1262-1263.
24. Hoeltzenbein M, Beck E, Fietz AK, et al. Pregnancy outcome after first trimester use of Methyldopa: a prospective cohort study. *Hypertension*. 2017;70:201-208.
25. Abalos E, Duley L, Steyn DW, Gialdini C. Antihypertensive drug therapy for mild to moderate hypertension during pregnancy. *Cochrane Database Syst Rev*. 2018;10:CD002252.
26. White WB, Andreoli JW, Cohn RD. Alpha-methyldopa disposition in mothers with hypertension and in their breast-fed infants. *Clin Pharmacol Ther*. 1985;37:387-390.
27. Hauser GJ, Almog S, Tirosh M, et al. Effect of alpha-methyldopa excreted in human milk on the breast-fed infant. *Helv Paediatr Acta*. 1985;40:83-86
28. Hoskins JA, Holliday SB. Determination of alpha-methyldopa and methyldopate in human breast milk and plasma by ion-exchange chromatography using electrochemical detection. *J Chromatogr*. 1982;230:162-167.
29. American College of Obstetricians and Gynecologists' Committee on Practice Bulletins—Obstetrics. ACOG practice bulletin no. 203: Chronic hypertension in pregnancy. *Obstet Gynecol*. 2019;133:e26-e50.

M

METHYLENE BLUE

Antidote (Oxidation-Reduction Agent)

PREGNANCY RECOMMENDATION: *Contraindicated

BREASTFEEDING RECOMMENDATION: Potential Toxicity

PREGNANCY SUMMARY

The Collaborative Perinatal Project reported no birth anomalies in nine first-trimester exposures to the drug. However, several studies have described the use of methylene blue in the second and third trimesters of pregnancy. In these cases, the agent was used in intra-amniotic instillation with amniocentesis in twins and also in diagnosing preterm premature rupture of the membranes. In these obstetrical uses, there were numerous reports of adverse effects that included hemolytic anemia, methemoglobinemia, prolonged skin staining, respiratory distress, and intestinal atresia. The drug will probably cross the placenta when found in the systemic circulation, so some fetal exposure may occur. However, the limited first-trimester human pregnancy experience prevents a complete assessment of the embryofetal risk. Animal studies did show some embryofetal toxicity in two species, but at doses of more than 10 times the RHD. *Because of the numerous adverse obstetrical outcomes reported with use of the drug in the second and third trimesters, using this drug during pregnancy should be avoided if at all possible.

BREASTFEEDING SUMMARY

No reports describing the use of methylene blue during human lactation have been located. The drug will probably appear in breast milk if found in the systemic circulation. Therefore, some infant exposure could occur. However, due to a concern for potential serious adverse effects that might be seen in a breastfed infant, the manufacturer recommends that women not breastfeed while being treated with this drug and for at least 8 days after treatment. If used while breastfeeding, the infant should be monitored for the most common reported adult side effects of nausea and headache (both leading to irritability), diarrhea, hypokalemia, hypomagnesemia, and myoclonus.

References

1. Prescribing Information. Methylene blue. Zydus Pharmaceuticals USA Inc; 2024.
2. Cragan JD. Teratogen update: methylene blue. *Teratology*. 1999;60:42-48.
3. Heinonen OP, Slone D, Shapiro S. *Birth Defects and Drugs in Pregnancy*. Publishing Sciences Group; 1977.
4. Plunkett GD. Neonatal complications. *Obstet Gynecol*. 1973;41:476-477.
5. Cowett RM, Hakanson DO, Kocon RW, Oh W. Untoward neonatal effect of intraamniotic administration of methylene blue. *Obstet Gynecol*. 1976; 48:74S-75S.
6. Kirsch IR, Cohen HJ. Heinz body hemolytic anemia from the use of methylene blue in neonates. *J Pediatr*. 1980;96:276-278.
7. Crooks J. Haemolytic jaundice in a neonate after intra-amniotic injection of methylene blue. *Arch Dis Child*. 1982;57:872-873.
8. McEnerney JK, McEnerney LN. Unfavorable neonatal outcome after intraamniotic injection of methylene blue. *Obstet Gynecol*. 1983;61:35S-36S.
9. Serota FT, Bernbaum JC, Schwartz E. The methylene-blue baby. *Lancet*. 1979;2:1142-1143.
10. Vincer MJ, Allen AC, Evans JR, et al. Methylene-blue-induced hemolytic anemia in a neonate. *CMAJ*. 1987;136:503-504.
11. Spahr RC, Salsburey DJ, Krissberg A, Prin W. Intraamniotic injection of methylene blue leading to methemoglobinemia in one of twins. *Int J Gynaecol Obstet*. 1980;17:477-478.
12. Poinsot J, Guillois B, Margis D, et al. Neonatal hemolytic anemia after intraamniotic injection of methylene blue. *Arch Fr Pediatr*. 1988;45:657-660.
13. Fish WH, Chazen EM. Toxic effects of methylene blue on the fetus. *Am J Dis Child*. 1992;146:1412-1413.
14. Troche BI. The methylene-blue baby. *N Engl J Med*. 1989;320:1756-1757.
15. Katz Z, Lancet M. Inadvertent intrauterine injection of methylene blue in early pregnancy. *N Engl J Med*. 1981;304:1427.
16. Nicolini U, Monni G. Intestinal obstruction in babies exposed in utero to methylene blue. *Lancet*. 1990;336:1258-1259.
17. Lancaster PAL, Pedisich EL, Fisher CC, Robertson RD. Intra-amniotic methylene blue and intestinal atresia in twins (abstract). *J Perinat Med*. 1992;20(suppl 1):262.
18. Van Der Pol JG, Wolf H, Boer K, et al. Jejunal atresia related to the use of methylene blue in genetic amniocentesis in twins. *Br J Obstet Gynaecol*. 1992;99:141-143.

METHYLERGONOVINE MALEATE

Miscellaneous (Ergot Derivative)

PREGNANCY RECOMMENDATION: *Contraindicated

BREASTFEEDING RECOMMENDATION: Probably Compatible

PREGNANCY SUMMARY

Limited reports describing the use of methylergonovine in human pregnancy have been located. No major birth anomalies were identified in five first-trimester exposures reported by the Collaborative Perinatal Project. The drug can cause sustained, uterine contractions that can result in FHR decelerations. The drug will probably cross the placenta, so fetal exposure will likely occur. However, the limited human pregnancy experience prevents a complete assessment of the embryofetal risk. Animal reproduction studies have not been located. *Methylergonovine is contraindicated during predelivery pregnancy because of its uterotonic effects. It is primarily used postpartum in the treatment of uterine atony.

BREASTFEEDING SUMMARY

One prospective case-control study was located that compared the outcome of 29 infants whose mothers had taken methylergonovine. No differences in health or development at 17 months postpartum were observed. Methylergonovine was found to be excreted into breast milk with levels that ranged from undetectable (LLQ <0.5 ng/mL) up to about 1.3 ng/mL. The highest calculated RID was about 5%. These levels came from a maternal dose of about 250 mcg. Some manufacturers recommend that women not breastfeed while using methylergonovine and for at least 12 hours after the last dose. However, if the clinical decision is to use this drug while breastfeeding, the infant should be monitored for the most common reported adult side effects of nausea and abdominal pain (both leading to irritability), vomiting, and hypertension (associated in several cases with headache and/or hypotension).

References

1. Prescribing Information. Methylergonovine maleate tablet. Teva Pharmaceuticals USA, Inc; 2024.
2. Prescribing Information. Methylergonovine maleate injection. Breckenridge Pharmaceutical, Inc; 2024.
3. Heinonen OP, Slone D, Shapiro S. *Birth Defects and Drugs in Pregnancy*. Publishing Sciences Group; 1977:357-365.
4. Wong R, Paul RH. Methergine-induced uterine tetany treated with epinephrine: case report. *Am J Obstet Gynecol*. 1979;134:602-603.
5. Moise KJ Jr, Carpenter RJ Jr. Methylergonovine-induced hypertonus in term pregnancy. A case report. *J Reprod Med*. 1988;33:771-773.
6. Erkkola R, Kanto J, Allonen H, et al. Excretion of methylergometrine (methylergonovine) into the human breast milk. *Int J Clin Pharmacol Biopharm*. 1978;16:579-580.
7. Allonen H, Juvakoski R, Kanto J, et al. Methylergometrine: comparison of plasma concentrations and clinical response of two brands. *Int J Clin Pharmacol Biopharm*. 1978;16:340-342.
8. Iwamura S, Kambegawa A. Determination of methylergometrine and dihydroergotoxine in biological fluids. *J Pharmacobiodyn*. 1981;4:275-281.
9. Vogel D, Burkhardt T, Rentsch K, et al. Misoprostol versus methylergometrine: pharmacokinetics in human milk. *Am J Obstet Gynecol*. 2004;191:2168-2173.

10. Nakamichi T, Yawata A, Hojo H, et al. Monitoring of methylergometrine in human breast milk by solid-phase extraction and high-performance liquid chromatography with fluorimetric detection. *Pharmazie*. 2012;67:482-484.

11. Gilad O, Merlob P, Stahl B, et al. Outcome of breastfed infants following post-partum methylergonovine treatment. *J Matern Fetal Neonatal Med*. 2017;30:1569-1573.

METHYLNALTREXONE

Gastrointestinal (Opioid Antagonist)

PREGNANCY RECOMMENDATION: No Human Data—Animal Data Suggest Low Risk

BREASTFEEDING RECOMMENDATION: *Potential Toxicity

PREGNANCY SUMMARY

No reports describing the use of methylnaltrexone in human pregnancy have been located. The drug will probably cross the placenta, so some fetal exposure will likely occur. However, the absence of human pregnancy experience prevents a complete assessment of the embryofetal risk. Animal data did not show any embryofetal toxicity in two species at doses of less than 10 times the MRHD. The use of methylnaltrexone may precipitate opioid withdrawal in pregnant women with chronic opioid use and in infants exposed to opioids near delivery. Using this drug during pregnancy should be based on the pros and cons of the mother's clinical need for treatment versus any potential fetal risk that might occur from exposure.

BREASTFEEDING SUMMARY

No reports describing the use of methylnaltrexone during human lactation have been located. The drug will probably be found in human breast milk, so some infant exposure will likely occur. Due to a concern for potential serious adverse effects that might be seen in a breastfed infant, the manufacturer recommends that women not breastfeed while being treated with this drug. *Nevertheless, if the clinical decision is to use this drug while breastfeeding, infants exposed to opioids during pregnancy or lactation should be monitored for signs of opioid withdrawal. Additionally, infants should also be monitored for the most common reported adult side effects of nausea, dizziness, and abdominal pain (all leading to irritability), flatulence, and diarrhea.

Reference

1. Prescribing Information. Relistor. Salix Pharmaceuticals, Inc; 2024.

M

METHYLPHENIDATE

Central Nervous System (Stimulant)

PREGNANCY RECOMMENDATION: Limited Human Data—Animal Data Suggest Potential Risk

BREASTFEEDING RECOMMENDATION: Potential Toxicity

PREGNANCY SUMMARY

Numerous reports describing the use of methylphenidate in human pregnancy have been located. Most exposures involved the misuse of the drug. Some suggested an elevated risk for birth anomalies and/or cardiac defects. However, in more than 3,000 cases, no consistent findings for cardiac defects were found. In addition, the prevalence of overall defects was higher in some studies, but the rate was not elevated above the expected rate for major birth defects in the general population. The drug will probably cross the placenta, so some fetal exposure will likely occur. Embryofetal toxicity was observed in one animal species at doses less than 10 times the MRHD. Using this drug during pregnancy should be based on the pros and cons of the mother's clinical need for treatment versus any potential fetal risk that might occur from exposure.

BREASTFEEDING SUMMARY

Five reports describing the effects of methylphenidate during human lactation found no adverse infant effects related to the drug. Methylphenidate was found to be excreted into human breast milk, but at levels that were less than 1% of the maternal weight-adjusted doses. Three infant blood levels were tested, and the drug was not detected (though the LLQ was only 1 mcg/mL). If the clinical decision is to use this drug while breastfeeding, the infant should be monitored for the most common reported adult side effects of agitation, insomnia, and anorexia (monitor infant growth).

References

1. Prescribing Information. Methylphenidate hydrochloride. Camber Pharmaceutical Inc; 2024.

2. Heinonen OP, Slone D, Shapiro S. *Birth Defects and Drugs in Pregnancy*. Publishing Sciences Group; 1977:346-347.

3. Smithells RW. Thalidomide and malformations in Liverpool. *Lancet*. 1962; 1:1270-1273.
4. Kopelman AE, McCullar FW, Heggeness L. Limb malformations following maternal use of haloperidol. *JAMA*. 1975;231:62-64.
5. Debooy VD, Seshia MMK, Tenenbein M, Casiro OG. Intravenous pentazocine and methylphenidate abuse during pregnancy. Maternal lifestyle and infant outcome. *Am J Dis Child*. 1993;147:1062-1065.
6. Cohen JM, Hernandez-Diaz S, Bateman BT, et al. Placental complications associated with psychostimulant use in pregnancy. *Obstet Gynecol*. 2017; 130(6):1192-1201.
7. Huybrechts KF, Broms G, Christensen LB, et al. Association between methylphenidate and amphetamine use in pregnancy and risk of congenital malformations. A cohort study from the international pregnancy safety study consortium. *JAMA Psychol*. 2018;75:167-175.
8. Noby U, Winbladh B, Kallen K. Perinatal outcomes after treatment with ADHD medication during pregnancy. *Pediatrics*. 2017;140:e20170747.
9. Diav-Citrin O, Schechtman S, Arnon J, et al. Methylphenidate in pregnancy: a multicenter, prospective comparative, observational study. *J Clin Psychiatry*. 2016;77:1176-1181.
10. Pottegard A, Hallas J, Andersen JT, et al. First-trimester exposure to methylphenidate: a population-based cohort study. *J Clin Psychol*. 2014;75:e88-e93.
11. Hackett LP, Kristensen JH, Hale TW, et al. Methylphenidate and breast-feeding. *Ann Pharmacother*. 2006;40:1890-1891.
12. Collin-Lévesque L, El-Ghaddaf Y, Genest M, et al. Infant exposure to methylphenidate and duloxetine during lactation. *Breastfeed Med*. 2018; 13:221-225.
13. Anderson PO, Pochop SL, Manoguerra AS. Adverse drug reactions in breastfed infants: less than imagined. *Clin Pediatr*. 2003;42:325-340.
14. Shah NS, Yates JD. Placental transfer and tissue distribution of dextroamphetamine in the mouse. *Arch Int Pharmacodyn Ther*. 1978;233:200-208.
15. Burchfield DJ, Lucas VW, Abrams RM, Miller RL, DeVane CL. Disposition and pharmacodynamics of methamphetamine in pregnant sheep. *JAMA*. 1991;265:1968-1973.
16. Dideriksen D, Pottegård A, Hallas J, Aagaard L, Damkier P. First trimester in utero exposure to methylphenidate. *Basic Clin Pharmacol Toxicol*. 2013; 112:73-76.
17. Bolea-Alamanac BM, Green A, Verma G, Maxwell P, Davies SJ. Methylphenidate use in pregnancy and lactation: a systematic review of evidence. *Br J Clin Pharmacol*. 2014;77(1):96-101.
18. Jiang HY, Zhang X, Jiang CM, Fu HB. Maternal and neonatal outcomes after exposure to ADHD medication during pregnancy: a systematic review and meta-analysis. *Pharmacoepidemiol Drug Saf*. 2019;28:288-295.
19. Koren G, Barer Y, Ornoy A. Fetal safety of methylphenidate—A scoping review and meta analysis. *Reprod Toxicol*. 2020;93:230-234.
20. di Giacomo E, Confalonieri V, Tofani F, Clerici M. Methylphenidate and atomoxetine in pregnancy and possible adverse fetal outcomes: a systematic review and meta-analysis. *JAMA Netw Open*. 2024;7(11):e2443648.
21. Hackett LP, Ilett KF, Kristensen JH, et al. Infant dose and safety of breastfeeding for dexamphetamine and methylphenidate in mothers with attention deficit hyperactivity disorder. *Ther Drug Monit*. 2005;27:220-221.
22. Bolea-Alamanac BM, Green A, Verma G, et al. Methylphenidate use in pregnancy and lactation: a systematic review of evidence. *Br J Clin Pharmacol*. 2014;77:96-101.
23. Collin-Lévesque L, El-Ghaddaf Y, Genest M, et al. Infant exposure to methylphenidate and duloxetine during lactation: a case report. *Breastfeed Med*. 2018;13:221-225.
24. Bello G, Poirier J, Sharkey KM. Successful lactation after resuming methylphenidate in a woman with narcolepsy. *J Clin Sleep Med*. 2022;18:1891-1894.
25. Spigset O, Brede WR, Zahlsen K. Excretion of methylphenidate in breast milk. *Am J Psychiatry*. 2007;164:348.

METHYLTESTOSTERONE

Androgenic Hormone

SEE TESTOSTERONE

M

METOCLOPRAMIDE

Gastrointestinal (Dopamine Antagonist)

PREGNANCY RECOMMENDATION: Human and Animal Data Suggest Low Risk

BREASTFEEDING RECOMMENDATION: Probably Compatible

PREGNANCY SUMMARY

Numerous reports describing the use of metoclopramide in all stages of human pregnancy have been located. Available studies analyzing the use of the drug in the first trimester in more than 4,000 pregnancies have not found a significant increased risk for congenital anomalies or adverse pregnancy/newborn effects. The drug crosses the placenta, so fetal exposure will occur. Animal studies did not show any embryofetal toxicity or teratogenicity in three species at doses of more than 10 times the RHD. ACOG considers metoclopramide as one of the agents for the adjunctive treatment of nausea and vomiting in pregnancy. However, the drug carries a boxed warning regarding an increased risk for tardive dyskinesia (especially with prolonged use); therefore, the manufacturer recommends use for only 12 weeks.

BREASTFEEDING SUMMARY

Several reports describing the effects of metoclopramide during human lactation were located. The drug was found to be excreted into human breast milk in low amounts. Breast milk concentrations produced daily doses of about 1 to 45 mcg/kg, which is much less than the maximum daily recommended infant dose of 500 mcg/kg or the 100 mcg/kg/d dosage for premature infants. The drug was detected in the plasma of one of five infants whose mothers were taking 30 mg daily. Mild adverse effects have been reported in only a few nursing infants. The drug can elevate prolactin levels, but this should not adversely affect breastfeeding. Metoclopramide has actually been used to help promote breast milk production in cases where breast milk supply is low. If the clinical decision is to use this drug while breastfeeding, the infant should be monitored for the most common reported adult side effects of dystonic reactions (involuntary muscle contractions), restlessness, drowsiness, and fatigue (lethargy).

References

1. Prescribing Information. Metoclopramide. Ipca Laboratories Limited; 2025.
2. Prescribing Information. Metoclopramide injection. Hospira, Inc; 2025.
3. Bylsma-Howell M, Riggs KW, McMorland GH, et al. Placental transport of metoclopramide: assessment of maternal and neonatal effects. *Can Anaesth Soc J*. 1983;30:487-492.
4. Arvela P, Jouppila R, Kauppila A, et al. Placental transfer and hormonal effects of metoclopramide. *Eur J Clin Pharmacol*. 1983;24:345-348.
5. Lyonnet R, Lucchini G. Metoclopramide in obstetrics. *J Med Chir Prat*. 1967;138:352-355.
6. Sidhu MS, Lean TH. The use of metoclopramide (Maxolon) in hyperemesis gravidarum. *Proc Obset Gynaecol Soc Singapore*. 1970;1:1-4.
7. Guikontes E, Spantideas A, Diakakis J. Ondansetron and hyperemesis gravidarum. *Lancet*. 1992;340:1223.
8. Martynshin MYA, Arkhengel'skii AE. Experience in treating early toxicoses of pregnancy with metoclopramide. *Akush Ginekol*. 1981;57:44-45.
9. Pinder RM, Brogden RN, Sawyer PR, et al. Metoclopramide: a review of its pharmacological properties and clinical use. *Drugs*. 1976;12:81-131.
10. Harrington RA, Hamilton CW, Brogden RN, et al. Metoclopramide: an update review of its pharmacological properties and clinical use. *Drugs*. 1983;25:451-494.
11. McGarry JM. A double-blind comparison of the anti-emetic effect during labour of metoclopramide and perphenazine. *Br J Anaesth*. 1971;43:613-615.
12. Howard FA, Sharp DS. Effect of metoclopramide on gastric emptying during labour. *Br Med J*. 1973;1:446-448.
13. Brock-Utne JG, Dow TGB, Welman S, et al. The effect of metoclopramide on the lower oesophageal sphincter in late pregnancy. *Anaesth Intensive Care*. 1978;6:26-29.
14. Hey VMF, Ostick DG. Metoclopramide and the gastrooesophageal sphincter. *Anaesthesia*. 1978;33:462-465.
15. Feeney JG. Heartburn in pregnancy. *Br Med J*. 1982;284:1138-1139.
16. Murphy DF, Nally B, Gardiner J, Unwin A. Effect of metoclopramide on gastric emptying before elective and emergency caesarean section. *Br J Anaesth*. 1984;56:1113-1116.
17. Vella L, Francis D, Houlton P, Reynolds F. Comparison of the antiemetics metoclopramide and promethazine in labour. *Br Med J*. 1985;290:1173-1175.
18. Messinis IE, Lolis DE, Dalkalitsis N, et al. Effect of metoclopramide on maternal and fetal prolactin secretion during labor. *Obstet Gynecol*. 1982; 60:686-688.
19. Bohnet HG, Kato K. Prolactin secretion during pregnancy and puerperium: response to metoclopramide and interactions with placental hormones. *Obstet Gynecol*. 1985;65:789-792.
20. Roti E, Robuschi G, Emanuele R, et al. Failure of metoclopramide to affect thyrotropin concentration in the term human fetus. *J Clin Endocrinol Metab*. 1983;56:1071-1075.
21. Milo R, Neuman M, Klein C, et al. Acute intermittent porphyria in pregnancy. *Obstet Gynecol*. 1989;73:450-452.
22. Nageotte MP, Briggs GG, Towers CV, Asrat T. Droperidol and diphenhydramine in the management of hyperemesis gravidarum. *Am J Obstet Gynecol*. 1996;174:1801-1806.
23. Turcotte V, Ferreira E, Duperron L. Utilité du dropéridol et de la diphenhydramine dans l'hyperemesis gravidarum. *J Soc Obstet Gynaecol Can*. 2001;23:133-139.
24. Sorensen HT, Nielsen GL, Christensen K, et al; the Euromap Study Group. Birth outcome following maternal use of metoclopramide. *Br J Clin Pharmacol*. 2000;49:264-268.
25. Berkovitch M, Elbirt D, Addis A, et al. Fetal effects of metoclopramide therapy for nausea and vomiting of pregnancy. *N Engl J Med*. 2000;343:445-446.
26. Eisenach JC, Dewan DM. Metoclopramide exaggerates stress-induced tachycardia in pregnant sheep. *Anesth Analg*. 1996;82:607-611.
27. Shenhav S, Gemer O, Sassoon E, Segal S. Acute intermittent porphyria precipitated by hyperemesis and metoclopramide treatment in pregnancy. *Acta Obstet Gynecol Scand*. 1997;76:484-485.
28. Matok I, Gorodischer R, Koren G, et al. The safety of metoclopramide use in the first trimester of pregnancy. *N Engl J Med*. 2009;360:2528-2535.
29. Pasternak B, Svanstrom H, Molgaard-Nielsen D, et al. Metoclopramide in pregnancy and risk of major congenital malformations and fetal death. *JAMA*. 2013;310:1601-1611.
30. Orr DA, Bill KM, Gillon KRW, et al. Effects of omeprazole, with and without metoclopramide, in elective obstetric anaesthesia. *Anaesthesia*. 1993; 48:114-119.
31. Stuart JC, Kan AF, Rowbottom SJ, et al. Acid aspiration prophylaxis for emergency caesarean section. *Anaesthesia*. 1996;51:415-421.
32. Robuschi G, Emanuele R, d'Amato L, et al. Failure of metoclopramide to release GH in pregnant women. *Horm Metab Res*. 1983;15:460-461.
33. Lewis PJ, Devenish C, Kahn C. Controlled trial of metoclopramide in the initiation of breast feeding. *Br J Clin Pharmacol*. 1980;9:217, 219.
34. Pelkonen O, Arvela P, Kauppila A, et al. Metoclopramide in breast milk and newborn (abstract). *Acta Physiol Scand*. 1982;(suppl 502):62.
35. Kauppila A, Arvela P, Koivisto M, et al. Metoclopramide and breast feeding: transfer into milk and the newborn. *Eur J Clin Pharmacol*. 1983;25: 819-823.
36. Sousa PLR. Metoclopramide and breast-feeding. *Br Med J*. 1975;1:512.
37. Guzman V, Toscano G, Canales ES, Zarate A. Improvement of defective lactation by using oral metoclopramide. *Acta Obstet Gynecol Scand*. 1979; 58:53-55.
38. Kauppila A, Kivinen S, Ylikorkala O. Metoclopramide increases prolactin release and milk secretion in puerperium without stimulating the secretion of thyrotropin and thyroid hormones. *J Clin Endocrinol Metab*. 1981; 52:436-439.
39. Kauppila A, Kivinen S, Ylikorkala O. A dose response relation between improved lactation and metoclopramide. *Lancet*. 1981;1:1175-1177.
40. de Gezelle H, Ooghe W, Thiery M, Dhont M. Metoclopramide and breast milk. *Eur J Obstet Gynecol Reprod Biol*. 1983;15:31-36.
41. Kauppila A, Anunti P, Kivinen S, et al. Metoclopramide and breast feeding: efficacy and anterior pituitary responses of the mother and the child. *Eur J Obstet Gynecol Reprod Biol*. 1985;19:19-22.
42. Gupta AP, Gupta PK. Metoclopramide as a lactogogue. *Clin Pediatr*. 1985; 24:269-272.
43. Ehrenkranz RA, Ackerman BA. Metoclopramide effect on faltering milk production by mothers of premature infants. *Pediatrics*. 1986;78:614-620.
44. Budd SC, Erdman SH, Long DM, et al. Improved lactation with metoclopramide. *Clin Pediatr*. 1993;32:53-57.
45. Toppare MF, Laleli Y, Senses DA, et al. Metoclopramide for breast milk production. *Nutr Res*. 1994;14:1019-1029.
46. Sankaran K, Yeboah E, Bingham WT, Ninan A. Use of metoclopramide in preterm infants. *Dev Pharmacol Ther*. 1982;5:114-119.
47. Lewis JH, Weingold AB; The Committee on FDA-Related Matters, American College of Gastroenterology. The use of gastrointestinal drugs during pregnancy and lactation. *Am J Gastroenterol*. 1985;80:912-923.
48. Ertl T, Sulyok E, Ezer E, et al. The influence of metoclopramide on the composition of human breast milk. *Acta Paediatr Hung*. 1991;31:415-422.
49. Bellouard M, Abe E, Etting I, et al. Metoclopramide intoxication through breast milk: relevance of blood and hair analyses. *Indian J Pediatr*. 2023; 90(3):314.
50. Sun L, Xi Y, Wen X, Zou W. Use of metoclopramide in the first trimester and risk of major congenital malformations: a systematic review and meta-analysis. *PLoS One*. 2021;16:e0257584.
51. Committee on Practice Bulletins-Obstetrics. ACOG practice bulletin no. 189: nausea and vomiting of pregnancy. *Obstet Gynecol*. 2018;131:e15-e30.

METOLAZONE

Cardiovascular (Diuretic, Thiazide-Related)

PREGNANCY RECOMMENDATION: No Human Data—Animal Data Suggest Low Risk

BREASTFEEDING RECOMMENDATION: Potential Toxicity

PREGNANCY SUMMARY

No reports describing the use of metolazone in human pregnancy have been located. It is structurally related to the thiazide diuretics. There is no evidence that thiazide diuretics are teratogenic. The drug crosses the placenta, so fetal exposure will likely occur. However, the absence of human pregnancy experience prevents a complete assessment of the embryofetal risk. Animal data did not show any embryofetal toxicity or teratogenicity in three species at doses of more than 10 times the MRHD based on weight. The use of diuretics in normal pregnancies is generally not recommended. Metolazone use in edema from pathologic causes in pregnancy may be considered. Nevertheless, using this drug during pregnancy should be based on the pros and cons of the mother's clinical need for treatment versus any potential fetal risk that might occur from exposure.

BREASTFEEDING SUMMARY

No reports describing the use of metolazone during human lactation have been located. The drug will probably be found in breast milk, so some infant exposure will likely occur. However, due to a concern for potential serious adverse effects that might be seen in a breastfed infant, the manufacturer recommends that women not breastfeed while being treated with this drug. Nevertheless, breastfeeding while using this drug should be based on the mother's clinical need for treatment versus any potential infant risks that might occur. If used, the infant should be monitored for the most common reported side effects of tachycardia, hypokalemia, and hyperbilirubinemia.

References

1. Prescribing Information. Metolazone. Ingenus Pharmaceuticals LLC; 2024.

METOPROLOL

Antihypertensive (β-Blocker)

PREGNANCY RECOMMENDATION: Human Data Suggest Potential Risk (Second and Third Trimesters)

BREASTFEEDING RECOMMENDATION: Probably Compatible

M

PREGNANCY SUMMARY

Several reports describing the use of metoprolol in human pregnancy have been located. Most publications involve the use of the drug in treating hypertension during pregnancy. From the Michigan Medicaid Surveillance study, there were 2 (3.8%) major anomalies in 52 first-trimester exposures. Inconsistent findings are reported for intrauterine growth restriction, preterm birth, and perinatal mortality with maternal use of metoprolol. The drug crosses the placenta, so some fetal exposure will occur. Embryofetal toxicity was observed in one animal species, but at doses greater than 10 times the RHD. Metoprolol has caused hyperglycemia in pregnant women treated during gestation. Additionally, persistent β-blockade has been observed in newborns exposed to other members of this class near delivery. Therefore, newborns exposed in utero to metoprolol should be closely observed during the first 24 to 48 hours after birth for bradycardia, neonatal hypoglycemia, and other β-blocker symptoms. Some β-blocker drugs may cause intrauterine growth restriction and reduced placental weight, especially those lacking intrinsic sympathomimetic activity. Metoprolol does not possess intrinsic sympathomimetic activity. Treatment beginning early in the second trimester results in the greatest newborn weight reductions, whereas treatment restricted to the third trimester primarily affects placental weight. Although growth restriction is a serious concern, the benefits of maternal therapy, in some cases, might outweigh the risks to the fetus and must be judged on a case-by-case basis.

BREASTFEEDING SUMMARY

Three reports describing the effects on infants of eight breastfeeding mothers taking metoprolol were located. No adverse effects in the breastfed infants were reported. The drug was found to be excreted into human breast milk with mean levels of about 0.23 mcg/mL. The calculated RIDs were about 0.5% to 2%. If the clinical decision is to use this drug while breastfeeding, the infant should be monitored for the most common reported adult side effects of hypotension, hypoglycemia, bradycardia, and respiratory depression.

References

1. Prescribing Information. Metoprolol succinate. Actavis Pharma, Inc; 2023.
2. Prescribing Information. Metoprolol tartrate. Baxter Healthcare Corporation; 2025.
3. Sandstrom B. Antihypertensive treatment with the adrenergic beta-receptor blocker metoprolol during pregnancy. *Gynecol Invest*. 1978;9:195-204.
4. Lundborg P, Agren G, Ervik M, Lindeberg S, Sandstrom B. Disposition of metoprolol in the newborn. *Br J Clin Pharmacol*. 1981;12:598-600.
5. Lindeberg S, Sandstrom B, Lundborg P, Regardh CG. Disposition of the adrenergic blocker metoprolol in the late-pregnant woman, the amniotic fluid, the cord blood and the neonate. *Acta Obstet Gynecol Scand*. 1984; 118(suppl):61-64.

6. Hogstedt S, Lindberg B, Rane A. Increased oral clearance of metoprolol in pregnancy. *Eur J Clin Pharmacol*. 1983;24:217-220.
7. Venuto R, Burstein P, Schneider R. Pheochromocytoma: antepartum diagnosis and management with tumor resection in the puerperium. *Am J Obstet Gynecol*. 1984;150:431-432.
8. Robson DJ, Jeeva Ray MV, Storey GAC, Holt DW. Use of amiodarone during pregnancy. *Postgrad Med J*. 1985;61:75-77.
9. Coen G, Cugini P, Gerlini G, et al. Successful treatment of long-lasting severe hypertension with captopril during a twin pregnancy. *Nephron*. 1985;40:498-500.
10. Gallery EDM. Hypertension in pregnant women. *Med J Aust*. 1985;143:23-7.
11. Hogstedt S, Lindeberg S, Axelsson O, et al. A prospective controlled trial of metoprolol-hydralazine treatment in hypertension during pregnancy. *Acta Obstet Gynecol Scand*. 1985;64:505-510.
12. Frishman WH, Chesner M. Beta-adrenergic blockers in pregnancy. *Am Heart J*. 1988;115:147-152.
13. Ryu RJ, Eyal S, Easterling TR, et al. Pharmacokinetics of metoprolol during pregnancy and lactation. *J Clin Pharmacol*. 2016;56:581-589.
14. Suonio S, Saarikoski S, Tahvanainen K, et al. Acute effects of dihydralazine mesylate, furosemide, and metoprolol on maternal hemodynamics in pregnancy-induced hypertension. *Am J Obstet Gynecol*. 1985;155:122-125.
15. Braverman AC, Bromley BS, Rutherford JD. New onset ventricular tachycardia during pregnancy. *Int J Cardiol*. 1991;33:409-412.
16. Brodsky M, Doria R, Allen B, Sato D, Thomas G, Sada M. New-onset ventricular tachycardia during pregnancy. *Am Heart J*. 1992;123:933-941.
17. Kaaja R, Hiilesmaa V, Holma K, Jarvenpaa A-L. Maternal antihypertensive therapy with beta-blockers associated with poor outcome in very-low birthweight infants. *Int J Gynecol Obstet*. 1992;38:195-199.
18. Bateman BT, Patorno E, Desai RJ, et al. Late pregnancy β blocker exposure and risks of neonatal hypoglycemia and bradycardia. *Pediatrics*. 2016;138:e20160731.
19. Sandstrom B, Regardh CG. Metoprolol excretion into breast milk. *Br J Clin Pharmacol*. 1980;9:518-519.
20. Liedholm H, Melander A, Bitzen PO, et al. Accumulation of atenolol and metoprolol in human breast milk. *Eur J Clin Pharmacol*. 1981;20:229-231.
21. Kulas J, Lunell NO, Rosing U, Steen B, Rane A. Atenolol and metoprolol. A comparison of their excretion into human breast milk. *Acta Obstet Scand*. 1984;118(suppl):65-69.
22. Ho TK, Moretti ME, Schaeffer JK, et al. Maternal beta-blocker usage and breast feeding in the neonate. *Pediatr Res*. 1999;45 (4, pt 2):67A.
23. Schimmel MS, Eidelman AI, Wilschanski MA, et al. Toxic effects of atenolol consumed during breast feeding. *J Pediatr*. 1989;114:476-478.
24. Freppel R, Gaboriau L, Richardson M, et al. Beta-blockers and breastfeeding: a real-life prospective study. *Eur J Clin Pharmacol*. 2024;80:1937-1943.

METRELEPTIN

Endocrine/Metabolic (Human Leptin Analogue)

PREGNANCY RECOMMENDATION: No Human Data—Animal Data Suggest Potential Risk

BREASTFEEDING RECOMMENDATION: Probably Compatible

PREGNANCY SUMMARY

No reports describing the use of metreleptin in human pregnancy have been located. Because it is a protein, it is not known whether some placental transfer might occur in the second half of gestation. Therefore, the absence of human pregnancy experience prevents a complete assessment of the embryofetal risk. Animal data did show some embryofetal toxicity along with maternal toxicity but at doses about equal to the RHD. Using this drug during pregnancy should be based on the pros and cons of the mother's clinical need for treatment versus any potential fetal risk that might occur from exposure. There is a pregnancy exposure registry that monitors pregnancy outcomes in women using this drug. Health care providers are encouraged to call the Metreleptin Pregnancy Exposure Registry at 1-855-669-2537. Metreleptin is only available through a restricted program called the MYALEPT REMS Program.

BREASTFEEDING SUMMARY

No reports describing the use of metreleptin during human lactation have been located, but endogenous leptin is found in human breast milk. Because it is a protein, if the drug were to be ingested through breastfeeding, it would probably be digested in the infant's gastrointestinal tract and not be absorbed. Breastfeeding while using this drug should be based on the mother's clinical need for treatment versus any potential infant risks that might occur. If used, the infant should be monitored for the most common reported adult side effects of headache and abdominal pain (both leading to irritability), hypoglycemia, and decreased appetite (monitor infant growth).

Reference

1. Prescribing Information. Myalept. Chiesi USA, Inc; 2024.

METRONIDAZOLE

Anti-Infective (Nitroimidazole)

PREGNANCY RECOMMENDATION: Human Data Suggest Low Risk

BREASTFEEDING RECOMMENDATION: Potential Toxicity

PREGNANCY SUMMARY

Numerous studies evaluating the use of metronidazole during human pregnancy have been located. Published studies that include more than 4,000 pregnant women have found no significant increased risk of congenital anomalies or adverse pregnancy effects. No consistent pattern to the defects has been described. However, because the use of metronidazole has been found to be carcinogenic in some animals, concern was raised about its use in pregnancy. However, available studies have not shown an increased risk of childhood cancer following metronidazole use in pregnancy. The drug crosses the placenta, so fetal exposure will occur. Animal studies did not show any embryofetal toxicity or teratogenicity in three species at doses of about equal to the RHD. The CDC guidelines recommend oral metronidazole treatment for trichomoniasis and oral or vaginal treatment for bacterial vaginosis during pregnancy at any gestation. For other indications, metronidazole can be used during pregnancy if there are no other alternatives with established safety profiles.

BREASTFEEDING SUMMARY

Four reports describing the effects of metronidazole during human lactation in 62 breastfed infants have been located. Metronidazole was found to be excreted into human breast milk with concentrations that vary with the maternal dosage. Mean breast milk levels were about 6 mcg/mL with a 600 mg dose, increasing up to about 60 mcg/mL with a 2-g dosage. The calculated RIDs ranged from about 5% up to 30%. Seven infants had average plasma levels of 1.6 mcg/mL for metronidazole and 1.4 mcg/mL for hydroxymetronidazole. These levels corresponded to 12.5% and 25.6% of the maternal metronidazole and hydroxymetronidazole blood concentrations. Due to the concern that metronidazole has been found to be tumorigenic in some animals, concern has been raised about its use in breastfeeding. The manufacturer recommends that women not breastfeed while being treated with this drug. Nevertheless, breastfeeding while using this drug should be based on the mother's clinical need for treatment versus any potential infant risks that might occur. Alternatively, the nursing mother may pump and discard the breast milk while being treated with metronidazole and for at least 24 hours after the last dose. If the clinical decision is to use this drug while breastfeeding, the infant should be monitored for the most common reported pediatric side effects of diarrhea, thrush, and diaper rash.

References

1. Prescribing Information. Metronidazole injection. Baxter Healthcare Corporation; 2024.
2. Prescribing Information. Metronidazole tablet. Alembic Pharmaceuticals; 2024.
3. Prescribing Information. Metronidazole vaginal gel, 0.75%. Encube Ethicals Private Limited; 2024.
4. Prescribing Information. Metronidazole topical gel, 0.75%. Encube Ethicals Private Limited; 2025.
5. Lexi-Comp, Inc. (Lexi-Drugs). Lexi-Comp, Inc; 2025.
6. Amon K, Amon I, Huller H. Maternal-fetal passage of metronidazole. In: Advances in Antimicrobial and Antineoplastic Chemotherapy. Proceedings of the VII International Congress of Chemotherapy; Prague; 1971:113-115.
7. Heisterberg L. Placental transfer of metronidazole in the first trimester of pregnancy. *J Perinat Med*. 1984;12:43-45.
8. Karhunen M. Placental transfer of metronidazole and tinidazole in early human pregnancy after a single infusion. *Br J Clin Pharmacol*. 1984;18: 254-257.
9. Amon I, Amon K, Franke G, Mohr C. Pharmacokinetics of metronidazole in pregnant women. *Chemotherapy*. 1981;27:73-79.
10. Visser AA, Hundt HKL. The pharmacokinetics of a single intravenous dose of metronidazole in pregnant patients. *J Antimicrob Chemother*. 1984;13:279-283.
11. Anonymous. Is Flagyl dangerous? *Med Lett Drugs Ther*. 1975;17:53-54.
12. Finegold SM. Metronidazole. *Ann Intern Med*. 1980;93:585-587.
13. Beard CM, Noller KL, O'Fallon WM, et al. Lack of evidence for cancer due to use of metronidazole. *N Engl J Med*. 1979;301:519-522.
14. Carvajal A, Sanchez A, Hurtarte G. Metronidazole during pregnancy. *Int J Gynecol Obstet*. 1995;48:323-324.
15. Thapa PB, Whitlock JA, Brockman Worrell KG, et al. Prenatal exposure to metronidazole and risk of childhood cancer. A retrospective cohort study of children younger than 5 years. *Cancer*. 1998;83:1461-1468.
16. Berbel-Tornero O, Lopez-Andreu JA, Ferris-Tortajada J. Prenatal exposure to metronidazole and risk of childhood cancer. A retrospective cohort study of children younger than 5 years. *Cancer*. 1999;85:2494-2495.
17. Gray MS. *Trichomonas vaginalis* in pregnancy: the results of metronidazole therapy on the mother and child. *J Obstet Gynaecol Br Commonw*. 1961;68:723-729.
18. Robinson SC, Johnston DW. Observations on vaginal trichomoniasis. II. Treatment with metronidazole. *Can Med Assoc J*. 1961;85:1094-1096.
19. Luthra R, Boyd JR. The treatment of trichomoniasis with metronidazole. *Am J Obstet Gynecol*. 1962;83:1288-1293.
20. Schram M, Kleinman H. Use of metronidazole in the treatment of trichomoniasis. *Am J Obstet Gynecol*. 1962;83:1284-1287.
21. Andrews MC, Andrews WC. Systemic treatment of trichomonas vaginitis. *South Med J*. 1963;56:1214-1218.
22. Zacharias LF, Salzer RB, Gunn JC, Dierksheide EB. Trichomoniasis and metronidazole. *Am J Obstet Gynecol*. 1963;86:748-752.
23. Kotcher E, Frick CA, Giesel LO Jr. The effect of metronidazole on vaginal microbiology and maternal and neonatal hematology. *Am J Obstet Gynecol*. 1964;88:184-189.
24. Scott-Gray M. Metronidazole in obstetric practice. *J Obstet Gynaecol Br Commonw*. 1964;71:82-85.
25. Perl G. Metronidazole treatment of trichomoniasis in pregnancy. *Obstet Gynecol*. 1965;25:273-276.
26. Peterson WF, Stauch JE, Ryder CD. Metronidazole in pregnancy. *Am J Obstet Gynecol*. 1966;94:343-349.
27. Robinson SC, Mirchandani G. Trichomonas vaginalis. V. Further observations on metronidazole (Flagyl) (including infant follow-up). *Am J Obstet Gynecol*. 1965;93:502-505.
28. Mitchell RW, Teare AJ. Amoebic liver abscess in pregnancy. Case reports. *Br J Obstet Gynaecol*. 1984;91:393-395.
29. Morgan I. Metronidazole treatment in pregnancy. *Int J Gynaecol Obstet*. 1978;15:501-502.
30. Sands RX. Pregnancy, trichomoniasis, and metronidazole. *Am J Obstet Gynecol*. 1966;94:350-353.
31. Berget A, Weber T. Metronidazole and pregnancy. *Ugeskr Laeger*. 1972; 134:2085-2089. As cited in Shepard TH. *Catalog of Teratogenic Agents*. 6th ed. Johns Hopkins University Press; 1989:426.
32. Heinonen OP, Slone D, Shapiro S. *Birth Defects and Drugs in Pregnancy*. Publishing Sciences Group; 1977:298, 299, 302.
33. Cantu JM, Garcia-Cruz D. Midline facial defect as a teratogenic effect of metronidazole. *Birth Defects*. 1982;18:85-88.
34. Greenberg F. Possible metronidazole teratogenicity and clefting. *Am J Med Genet*. 1985;22:825.
35. Rosa FW, Baum C, Shaw M. Pregnancy outcomes after first-trimester vaginitis drug therapy. *Obstet Gynecol*. 1987;69:751-755.
36. Piper JM, Mitchel EF, Ray WA. Prenatal use of metronidazole and birth defects: no association. *Obstet Gynecol*. 1993;82:348-352.
37. Burtin P, Taddio A, Ariburnu O, et al. Safety of metronidazole in pregnancy: a meta-analysis. *Am J Obstet Gynecol*. 1995;172:525-529.
38. Caro-Paton T, Carvajal A, Martin de Diego I, et al. Is metronidazole teratogenic? A meta-analysis. *Br J Clin Pharmacol*. 1997;44:179-182.

39. Czeizel AE, Rockenbauer M. A population based case-control teratologic study of oral metronidazole treatment during pregnancy. *Br J Obstet Gynaecol*. 1998;105:322-327.
40. Kazy Z, Puho E, Czeizel AE. The possible association between the combination of vaginal metronidazole and miconazole treatment and polysyndactyly population-based case-control teratologic study. *Reprod Toxicol*. 2005;20:89-94.
41. Sorensen HT, Larsen H, Jensen ES, et al; the Euromap Study Group. Safety of metronidazole during pregnancy: a cohort study of risk of congenital abnormalities, preterm delivery and low birth weight in 124 women. *J Antimicrob Chemother*. 1999;44:854-855.
42. Damjanov I. Metronidazole and alcohol in pregnancy. *JAMA*. 1986;256:472.
43. Diav-Citrin O, Shechtman S, Gotteiner T, et al. Pregnancy outcome after gestational exposure to metronidazole: a prospective controlled cohort study. *Teratology*. 2001;63:186-192.
44. McDonald HM, O'Loughlin JA, Vigneswaran R, et al. Bacterial vaginosis in pregnancy and efficacy of short-course oral metronidazole treatment: a randomized controlled trial. *Obstet Gynecol*. 1994;84:343-348.
45. Morales WJ, Schorr S, Albritton J. Effect of metronidazole in patients with history of preterm birth and bacterial vaginosis: a placebo control double blind study (abstract). *Am J Obstet Gynecol*. 1993;168:377.
46. Morales WJ, Schorr S, Albritton J. Effect of metronidazole in patients with preterm birth in preceding pregnancy and bacterial vaginosis: a placebo-controlled, double-blind study. *Am J Obstet Gynecol*. 1994;171:345-349.
47. Hauth J, Goldenberg R, Andrews W, et al. Efficacy of metronidazole plus erythromycin to decrease bacterial vaginosis and other markers of altered vaginal flora (abstract). *Am J Obstet Gynecol*. 1993;168:421.
48. Hauth JC, Goldenberg RL, Andrews WW, et al. Reduced incidence of preterm delivery with metronidazole and erythromycin in women with bacterial vaginosis. *N Engl J Med*. 1995;333:1732-1736.
49. McDonald HM, O'Loughlin JA, Vigneswaran R, et al. Impact of metronidazole therapy on preterm birth in women with bacterial vaginosis flora (*Gardnerella vaginalis*): a randomized, placebo controlled trial. *Br J Obstet Gynaecol*. 1997;104:1391-1397.
50. Svare J, Langhoff-Roos J, Andersen LF, et al. Ampicillin-metronidazole treatment in idiopathic preterm labour: a randomized controlled multicentre trial. *Br J Obstet Gynaecol*. 1997;104:892-897.
51. Klebanoff M, Carey JC; for the NICHD MFMU Network, Bethesda, MD. Metronidazole did not prevent preterm birth in asymptomatic women with bacterial vaginosis (abstract). *Am J Obstet Gynecol*. 1999;180:S2.
52. Hauth JC; for the NICHD MFMU Network, Bethesda, MD. Response of the three components of a vaginal Gram stain score to metronidazole treatment and in relation to preterm birth (abstract). *Am J Obstet Gynecol*. 2000;182:S56.
53. Carey J, Klebanoff MA, Hauth JC, et al; the National Institute of Child Health and Human Development Network of Maternal-Fetal Medicine Units. Metronidazole to prevent preterm delivery in pregnant women with asymptomatic bacterial vaginosis. *N Engl J Med*. 2000;342:534-540.
54. Carey JC, Klebanoff M; for the NICHD MFMU Network, Bethesda MD. Metronidazole treatment increased the risk of preterm birth in asymptomatic women with trichomonas (abstract). *Am J Obstet Gynecol*. 2000; 182:Ss13.
55. Klebanoff MA, Carey JC, Hauth JC, et al; the National Institute of Child Health and Human Development Network of Maternal-Fetal Medicine Units. Failure of metronidazole to prevent preterm delivery among pregnant women with asymptomatic *Trichomonas vaginalis* infection. *N Engl J Med*. 2001;345:487-493.
56. Erickson SH, Oppenheim GL, Smith GH. Metronidazole in breast milk. *Obstet Gynecol*. 1981;57:48-50.
57. Heisterberg L, Branebjerg PE. Blood and milk concentrations of metronidazole in mothers and infants. *J Perinat Med* 1983;11:114-120.
58. Moore B, Collier J. Drugs and breast-feeding. *Br Med J*. 1979;2:211.
59. Clements CJ. Metronidazole and breast feeding. *N Z Med J*. 1980;92:329.
60. Passmore CM, McElnay JC, Rainey EA, D'Arcy PF. Metronidazole excretion in human milk and its effect on the suckling neonate. *Br J Clin Pharmacol*. 1988;26:45-51.
61. Centers for Disease Control and Prevention. Sexually transmitted infections treatment guidelines, 2021: trichomoniasis. Accessed February 21, 2025. https://www.cdc.gov/std/treatment-guidelines/trichomoniasis.htm
62. Centers for Disease Control and Prevention. Sexually transmitted infections treatment guidelines, 2021: bacterial vaginosis. Accessed February 21, 2025. https://www.cdc.gov/std/treatment-guidelines/bv.htm
63. Ajiji P, Uzunali A, Ripoche E, et al. Investigating the efficacy and safety of metronidazole during pregnancy; A systematic review and meta-analysis. *Eur J Obstet Gynecol Reprod Biol X*. 2021 May 14;11:100128.
64. Jick H, Holmes LB, Hunter JR, et al. First-trimester drug use and congenital disorders. *JAMA*. 1981;246:343-346.
65. Aselton P, Jick H, Milunsky A, et al. First-trimester drug use and congenital disorders. *Obstet Gynecol*. 1985;65:451-455.

METYROSINE

Antihypertensive (Tyrosine Hydroxylase Inhibitor)

PREGNANCY RECOMMENDATION: Limited Human Data—No Relevant Animal Data

BREASTFEEDING RECOMMENDATION: Probably Compatible (Short-Term Use)

PREGNANCY SUMMARY

One case report describing the use of metyrosine in human pregnancy was located. The infant was exposed in the third trimester, and no adverse effects related to the drug were described. The drug will probably cross the placenta, so fetal exposure will likely occur. However, this limited human pregnancy experience prevents a complete assessment of the embryofetal risk. No animal reproduction studies were located. Using this drug during pregnancy should be based on the pros and cons of the mother's clinical need for treatment versus any potential fetal risk that might occur from exposure.

BREASTFEEDING SUMMARY

No reports describing the use of metyrosine during human lactation have been located. The drug will probably be excreted into human breast milk, so some infant exposure will likely occur. The effects of this exposure on a nursing infant are unknown. If the clinical decision is to use this drug while breastfeeding, the infant should be monitored for the most common reported adult side effects of sedation, extrapyramidal signs (e.g., drooling and tremor), and diarrhea.

References

1. Prescribing Information. Metyrosine. Amneal Pharmaceuticals NY LLC; 2023.
2. Devoe LD, O'Dell BE, Castillo RA, et al. Metastatic pheochromocytoma in pregnancy and fetal biophysical assessment after maternal administration of alpha-adrenergic, beta-adrenergic, and dopamine antagonists. *Obstet Gynecol*. 1986;68:15S-18S.

MEXILETINE

Cardiovascular (Antiarrhythmic)

PREGNANCY RECOMMENDATION: Limited Human Data—Animal Data Suggest Risk

BREASTFEEDING RECOMMENDATION: Potential Toxicity

PREGNANCY SUMMARY

Five case reports describing the use of mexiletine in human pregnancy were located. No congenital anomalies or adverse effects attributed to mexiletine were reported. The drug will probably cross the placenta, so fetal exposure will likely occur. However, the limited human pregnancy experience prevents a complete assessment of the embryofetal risk. Embryofetal toxicity was observed in three animal species at doses of less than 10 times the MRHD. Using this drug during pregnancy should be based on the pros and cons of the mother's clinical need for treatment versus any potential fetal risk that might occur from exposure.

BREASTFEEDING SUMMARY

Two reports describing the effects of mexiletine in three breastfeeding infants were located. No adverse effects attributable to mexiletine were described. The drug was found to be excreted into human breast milk. Breast milk concentrations ranged from about 0.6 mcg/mL up to about 1 mcg/mL. The calculated RID was less than 2%. The drug was not detected in the serum of one tested infant. Breastfeeding while using this drug should be based on the mother's clinical need for treatment versus any potential infant risks that might occur. If used, the infant should be monitored for the most common reported adult side effects of nausea, heartburn, dizziness, and nervousness (all leading to irritability), vomiting, and tremor.

M

References

1. Prescribing Information. Mexiletine. Chartwell RX, LLC; 2024.
2. Lownes HE, Ives TJ. Mexiletine use in pregnancy and lactation. *Am J Obstet Gynecol*. 1987;157:446-447.
3. Lewis AM, Patel L, Johnston A, Turner P. Mexiletine in human blood and breast milk. *Postgrad Med J*. 1981;57:546-547.
4. Timmis AD, Jackson G, Holt DW. Mexiletine for control of ventricular dysrhythmias in pregnancy. *Lancet*. 1980;2:647-648.
5. Gregg AR, Tomich PG. Mexiletine use in pregnancy. *J Perinatol*. 1988;8:33-35.
6. Ben-Ami M, Battino S, Rosenfeld T, et al. Aortic valve replacement during pregnancy—a case report and review of the literature. *Acta Obstet Gynecol Scand*. 1990;69:651-653.
7. Monfort A, Morin C, Jutras M, et al. Transfer of mexiletine into breast milk: a case report. *Breastfeed Med*. 2023;18:489-493.

MICAFUNGIN

Antifungal (Echinocandin)

PREGNANCY RECOMMENDATION: No Human Data—Animal Data Suggest Potential Risk (Maternal Benefit May Outweigh Any Embryofetal Risk)

BREASTFEEDING RECOMMENDATION: Potential Toxicity

PREGNANCY SUMMARY

No reports describing the use of micafungin in human pregnancy have been located. A limited amount of the drug might cross the placenta, so some fetal exposure may occur. However, the absence of human pregnancy experience prevents a complete assessment of the embryofetal risk. Embryofetal toxicity was observed in one animal species at doses of less than 10 times the MRHD. Using this drug during pregnancy should be based on the pros and cons of the mother's clinical need for treatment versus any potential fetal risk that might occur from exposure.

BREASTFEEDING SUMMARY

No reports describing the use of micafungin during human lactation have been located. The drug might be found in human breast milk, so some infant exposure may occur. Breastfeeding while using this drug should be based on the mother's clinical need for treatment versus any potential infant risks that might occur. If used, the infant should be monitored for the most common reported adult side effects of acidosis, anemia, decreased oxygen saturation, and hypokalemia.

Reference

1. Prescribing Information. Micafungin. Zydus Pharmaceuticals USA Inc; 2025.

MICONAZOLE

Anti-Infective (Antifungal)

PREGNANCY RECOMMENDATION: Human Data Suggest Low Risk

BREASTFEEDING RECOMMENDATION: Probably Compatible

PREGNANCY SUMMARY

Several reports describing the use of miconazole for the treatment of vulvovaginal candidiasis in human pregnancy were located. The major malformation rate in over 7,600 first-trimester exposures was about 4%, and no pattern to the defects was identified. In two other large studies involving over 29,400 pregnancies that resulted in infants with major birth anomalies compared with more than 135,900 controls, the use of metronidazole was 2.4% versus 2.2%, respectively. The drug will probably cross the placenta, so fetal exposure will likely occur. However, the systemic absorption of miconazole is minimal following vaginal administration, which should limit placental transfer even further. Animal data did not show any embryofetal toxicity in two animal species with IV doses of less than 10 times the RHD. The CDC recommends that only topical azole products be used for 7 days to treat vulvovaginal candidiasis during pregnancy, if possible.

BREASTFEEDING SUMMARY

No reports describing the use of miconazole during human lactation have been located. The drug will probably appear in breast milk, so some infant exposure may occur. However, the systemic absorption of miconazole is minimal following vaginal administration, which should limit excretion into breast milk even further. If the clinical decision is to use this drug while breastfeeding, the infant should be monitored for the most common reported adult side effects of nausea, headache, and abdominal pain (all leading to irritability), diarrhea, and vomiting.

References

1. Prescribing Information. Monistat. Insight Pharmaceuticals LLC; 2024.
2. Prescribing Information. Oravig. Galt Pharmaceuticals; 2021.
3. Culbertson C. Monistat: a new fungicide for treatment of vulvovaginal candidiasis. *Am J Obstet Gynecol*. 1974;120:973-976.
4. Wade A, ed. *Martindale: The Extra Pharmacopoeia*. 27th ed. Pharmaceutical Press; 1977:648.
5. Davis JE, Frudenfeld JH, Goddard JL. Comparative evaluation of monistat and mycostatin in the treatment of vulvovaginal candidiasis. *Obstet Gynecol*. 1974;44:403-406.
6. Wallenburg HCS, Wladimiroff JW. Recurrence of vulvovaginal candidosis during pregnancy. Comparison of miconazole vs nystatin treatment. *Obstet Gynecol*. 1976;48:491-494.
7. McNellis D, McLeod M, Lawson J, Pasquale SA. Treatment of vulvovaginal candidiasis in pregnancy: a comparative study. *Obstet Gynecol*. 1977;50:674-678.
8. Weisberg M. Treatment of vaginal candidiasis in pregnant women. *Clin Ther*. 1986;8:563-567.
9. Rosa FW, Baum C, Shaw M. Pregnancy outcomes after first-trimester vaginitis drug therapy. *Obstet Gynecol*. 1987;69:751-755.
10. Kragie L, Turner SD, Patten CJ, et al. Assessing pregnancy risks of azole antifungals using a high throughput aromatase inhibition assay. *Endocr Res*. 2002;28:129-140.
11. Workowski KA, Bachmann LH, Chan PA, et al. Sexually transmitted infections treatment guidelines, 2021. *MMWR Recomm Rep*. 2021;70:1-187.
12. Harada N. Genetic analysis of human placental aromatase deficiency. *JSteroid Biochem Mol Biol*. 1993;44:331-340.
13. Kazy Z, Puho E, Czeizel AE. The possible association between the combination of vaginal metronidazole and miconazole treatment and poly-syndactyly population-based case-control teratologic study. *Reprod Toxicol*. 2005;20:89-94.
14. Daneshmend TK. Systemic absorption of miconazole from the vagina. *J Antimicrob Chemother*. 1986;18:507-511.
15. Jick H, Holmes LB, Hunter JR, et al. First-trimester drug use and congenital disorders. *JAMA*. 1981;246:343-346.

M

MIDAZOLAM

Central Nervous System/Mental Health (Benzodiazepine)

PREGNANCY RECOMMENDATION: Limited Human Data—Animal Data Suggest Low Risk

BREASTFEEDING RECOMMENDATION: Probably Compatible

PREGNANCY SUMMARY

Limited reports describing the use of midazolam in human pregnancy have been located. No reports have been located that describe the use of midazolam in humans during the first or second trimesters. Use of the drug has primarily occurred in the third trimester at or near delivery. The use of midazolam late in pregnancy can result in newborn sedation and symptoms of withdrawal. However, patients should not be denied medically necessary surgery regardless of the trimester. Midazolam crosses the placenta, so fetal exposure will occur. Therefore, this limited human pregnancy experience, especially first-trimester exposure, prevents a complete assessment of the embryofetal risk. Animal data did not show any embryofetal toxicity in two species at doses of less than 10 times the RHD. Using this drug during pregnancy should be based on the pros and cons of the mother's clinical need for treatment versus any potential fetal risk that might occur from exposure. Infants

(*continued*)

exposed to midazolam late in pregnancy should be monitored for sedation (respiratory depression, lethargy, and hypotonia) and withdrawal symptoms (hyperreflexia, irritability, restlessness, tremors, inconsolable crying, and feeding difficulties). There is a pregnancy registry that monitors pregnancy outcomes in women exposed to psychiatric medications, including midazolam, during pregnancy. Health care providers are encouraged to register patients by calling the National Pregnancy Registry for Psychiatric Medications at 1-866-961-2388.

BREASTFEEDING SUMMARY

One report describing the sedative effects of midazolam in 19 breastfeeding infants was located. Sedation was not observed in any of the infants. Midazolam is excreted into breast milk with concentrations that range from undetectable (LLQ of 3 ng/mL) to about 10 ng/mL. Breastfeeding while using this drug should be based on the mother's clinical need for treatment versus any potential infant risks that might occur. If used, the infant should be monitored for the most common reported adult side effects of sedation, somnolence, lethargy, poor feeding, and decreased appetite (monitor infant growth). The manufacturer suggests that a breastfeeding mother may consider pumping and discarding breast milk for at least 4 to 8 hours after receiving midazolam for sedation or anesthesia to minimize drug exposure to a breastfed infant.

References

1. Prescribing Information. Midazolam injection. Belcher Pharmaceuticals, LLC; 2024.
2. Prescribing Information. Midazolam hydrochloride syrup. American Health Packaging; 2023.
3. U.S. Food and Drug Administration. FDA drug safety communication: FDA review results in new warnings about using general anesthetics and sedation drugs in young children and pregnant women. Accessed February 23, 2035. https://www.fda.gov/Drugs/DrugSafety/ucm532356.htm
4. Kanto J, Sjovall S, Erkkola R, et al. Placental transfer and maternal midazolam kinetics. *Clin Pharmacol Ther*. 1983;33:786-791.
5. Bach V, Carl P, Ravlo O, et al. A randomized comparison between midazolam and thiopental for elective cesarean section anesthesia. III. Placental transfer and elimination in neonates. *Anesth Analg*. 1989;68:238-242.
6. Wilson CM, Dundee JW, Moore J, et al. A comparison of plasma midazolam levels in non-pregnant and pregnant women at parturition. *Br J Clin Pharmacol*. 1985;20:256P-257P.
7. Bland BAR, Lawes EG, Duncan PW, et al. Comparison of midazolam and thiopental for rapid sequence anesthetic induction for elective cesarean section. *Anesth Analg*. 1987;66:1165-1168.
8. Crawford ME, Carl P, Bach V, et al. A randomized comparison between midazolam and thiopental for elective cesarean section anesthesia. I. Mothers. *Anesth Analg*. 1989;68:229-233.
9. Ravlo O, Carl P, Crawford ME, et al. A randomized comparison between midazolam and thiopental for elective cesarean section anesthesia: II. Neonates. *Anesth Analg*. 1989;68:234-237.
10. Matheson I, Lunde PKM, Bredesen JE. Midazolam and nitrazepam in the maternity ward: milk concentrations and clinical effects. *Br J Clin Pharmacol*. 1990;30:787-793.
11. Kelly LE, Poon S, Madadi P, Koren G. Neonatal benzodiazepines exposure during breastfeeding. *J Pediatr*. 2012;161:448-451.
12. Nitsun M, Szokol JW, Saleh HJ, et al. Pharmacokinetics of midazolam, propofol, and fentanyl transfer to human breast milk. *Clin Pharmacol Ther*. 2006;79:549-557.
13. Frölich MA, Burchfield DJ, Euliano TY, Caton D. A single dose of fentanyl and midazolam prior to cesarean section have no adverse neonatal effects. *Can J Anaesth*. 2006;53(1):79-85.
14. Olutoye OA, Baker BW, Belfort MA, Olutoye OO. Food and Drug Administration warning on anesthesia and brain development: implications for obstetric and fetal surgery. *Am J Obstet Gynecol*. 2018;218(1):98-102.
15. Senel AC, Mergan F. Premedication with midazolam prior to caesarean section has no neonatal adverse effects. *Braz J Anesthesiol*. 2014;64(1):16-21.

MIDODRINE

Cardiovascular (α-Adrenergic Agonist)

PREGNANCY RECOMMENDATION: Limited Human Data—Animal Data Suggest Potential Risk

BREASTFEEDING RECOMMENDATION: Potential Toxicity

PREGNANCY SUMMARY

One report was located that described the use of midodrine in human pregnancy. The drug was used throughout pregnancy, and the delivered infant did not have any identified birth anomalies. The drug will probably cross the placenta, so fetal exposure will likely occur. However, the limited human pregnancy experience prevents a complete assessment of the embryofetal risk. Embryofetal toxicity was observed in one animal species at doses of less than 10 times the MRHD. Using this drug during pregnancy should be based on the pros and cons of the mother's clinical need for treatment versus any potential fetal risk that might occur from exposure. Midodrine has been associated with marked increases in systolic blood pressure, which could produce obstetrical complications.

BREASTFEEDING SUMMARY

No reports describing the use of midodrine in human lactation have been located. The drug will probably be found in human breast milk, so infant exposure will likely occur. Because severe systolic hypertension is a potential adverse effect of this drug, the manufacturer states that women should probably not breastfeed while using this drug. Nevertheless, if the clinical decision is to use this drug while breastfeeding, the infant should be monitored for the most common reported adult side effects of paresthesia and pruritus (both leading to irritability), supine and sitting hypertension, urinary retention, and urinary frequency.

References

1. Prescribing Information. Midodrine. Apotex; 2024.
2. Glatter KA, Tuteja D, Chiamvimonvat N, et al. Pregnancy in postural orthostatic tachycardia syndrome. *Pacing Clin Electrophysiol*. 2005;28:591-593.

MIDOSTAURIN

Antineoplastic (Kinase Inhibitor)

PREGNANCY RECOMMENDATION: Limited Human Data—Animal Data Suggest Risk

BREASTFEEDING RECOMMENDATION: Potential Toxicity

PREGNANCY SUMMARY

There is a single case report of a woman who had exposure to midostaurin at conception and the first trimester and delivered at 34 weeks' gestation by scheduled cesarean. The child was reported to be healthy (except for being late-preterm) with no reported anomalies. Based on the likely placental transfer of midostaurin, some fetal exposure will probably occur. However, the limited human pregnancy experience prevents a complete assessment of the embryofetal risk. Animal studies did show embryofetal toxicity. Based on the animal studies and the drug's mechanism of action, the manufacturer recommends that women with reproductive potential use effective contraception during treatment and for 4 months after the last dose. They also recommend that males with female partners of reproductive potential use effective contraception during treatment and for 4 months after the last dose. Nevertheless, using this drug during pregnancy should be based on the pros and cons of the mother's clinical need for treatment versus any potential fetal risk that might occur from exposure.

BREASTFEEDING SUMMARY

No reports describing the use of midostaurin during human lactation have been located. Some amount of the drug probably enters breast milk, so infant exposure will likely occur. However, due to the drug's mechanism of action and the adverse effects seen in animal studies, the manufacturer recommends that women not breastfeed while being treated with midostaurin and for 4 months after the last dose. Nevertheless, breastfeeding while using this drug should be based on the mother's clinical need for treatment. If used, the infant should be monitored for the most common reported adult side effects of nausea, headache, abdominal pain, and musculoskeletal pain (all leading to irritability), diarrhea, vomiting, edema, pyrexia, fatigue, upper respiratory tract infection, and neutropenia.

References

1. Prescribing Information. Rydapt. Novartis Pharmaceuticals Corporation; 2017.
2. Ojha S, Ooi MG. Pregnancy exposure to midostaurin in the first trimester. *Ann Hematol*. 2020;99:355-356.

M

MIFEPRISTONE

Endocrine/Metabolic (Antiprogestin/Cortisol Receptor Blocker)

PREGNANCY RECOMMENDATION: Contraindicated

BREASTFEEDING RECOMMENDATION: Potential Toxicity

PREGNANCY SUMMARY

A large number of studies have investigated the use of mifepristone for the termination of pregnancy, either when given alone or in combination with a prostaglandin analogue. Data are too limited to determine whether the drug is a human teratogen. Mifepristone rapidly crosses the placenta. Embryofetal toxicity was observed in three animal species, with teratogenicity in one at doses less than the RHD. Because the incidence of successful abortion after mifepristone is high, but not total, women should be informed of the risk for embryotoxicity if their pregnancy continues after use of this drug. Due to its antiprogestin activity, the manufacturer recommends that women with reproductive potential use effective contraception during treatment and for 1 month after the last dose. Mifepristone for treating Cushing syndrome carries a boxed warning regarding an increased risk for pregnancy termination. When used for medical pregnancy termination, it carries a boxed warning regarding an increased risk for serious and sometimes fatal infections or bleeding. Regardless, the drug is contraindicated for use during pregnancy.

BREASTFEEDING SUMMARY

One report was located that describes the use of mifepristone during human lactation. The drug was found in human breast milk, so infant exposure will occur. The estimated RID was calculated to be about 1.5%. Due to a concern for potential serious adverse effects that might be seen in a breastfed infant, the manufacturer recommends that women not breastfeed while being treated with this drug and for at least 18 to 21 days after the last dose. If the clinical decision is to use this drug while breastfeeding, the infant should be monitored for the most common reported adult side effects of nausea, headache, and dizziness (all leading to irritability), weakness, fever, vomiting, and diarrhea.

References

1. Prescribing Information. Mifeprex. Danco Laboratories LLC; 2023.
2. Prescribing Information. Corcept Therapeutics Incorporated; 2024.
3. Smith SK, Kelly RW. The effect of the antiprogestins RU 486 and ZK 98734 on the synthesis and metabolism of prostaglandins F2α and E2 in separated cells from early human decidua. *J Clin Endocrinol Metab*. 1987;65:527-534.
4. Das C, Catt KJ. Antifertility actions of the progesterone antagonist RU 486 include direct inhibition of placental hormone secretion. *Lancet*. 1987; 2:599-601.
5. Anonymous. Mifepristone—contragestive agent or medical abortifacient? *Lancet*. 1987;2:1308-1310.
6. Hill NCW, Selinger M, Ferguson J, et al. The physiological and clinical effects of progesterone inhibition with mifepristone (RU 486) in the second trimester. *Br J Obstet Gynaecol*. 1990;97:487-492.
7. Baulieu EE. RU-486 as an antiprogesterone steroid. From receptor to contragestion and beyond. *JAMA*. 1989;262:1808-1814.
8. Guillebaud J. Medical termination of pregnancy. Combined with prostaglandin RU 486 is effective. *Br Med J*. 1990;301:352-354.
9. Brogden RN, Goa KL, Faulds D. Mifepristone. A review of its pharmacodynamic and pharmacokinetic properties, and therapeutic potential. *Drugs*. 1993;45:384-409.
10. Spitz IM, Bardin CW. Mifepristone (RU 486)—a modulator of progestin and glucocorticoid action. *N Engl J Med*. 1993;329:404-412.
11. Frydman R, Taylor S, Ulmann A. Transplacental passage of mifepristone. *Lancet*. 1985;2:1252.
12. Hill NCW, Selinger M, Ferguson J, MacKenzie IZ. The placental transfer of mifepristone (RU 486) during the second trimester and its influence upon maternal and fetal steroid concentrations. *Br J Obstet Gynaecol*. 1990; 97:406-411.
13. Hill NC, Selinger M, Ferguson J, MacKenzie IZ. Transplacental passage of mifepristone and its influence on maternal and fetal steroid concentrations in the second trimester of pregnancy. *Hum Reprod*. 1991;6(3):458-462.
14. Kovacs L, Sas M, Resch BA, et al. Termination of very early pregnancy by RU 486—an antiprogestational compound. *Contraception*. 1984;29:399-410.
15. Haspels AA. Interruption of early pregnancy by an anti-progestational compound, RU 486. *Eur J Obstet Gynecol Reprod Biol*. 1985;20:169-175.
16. Vervest HAM, Haspels AA. Preliminary results with the antiprogestational compound RU-486 (mifepristone) for interruption of early pregnancy. *Fertil Steril*. 1985;44:627-632.
17. Bygdeman M, Swahn ML. Progesterone receptor blockage. Effect on uterine contractility and early pregnancy. *Contraception*. 1985;32:45-51.
18. Couzinet B, Strat NL, Ulmann A, et al. Termination of early pregnancy by the progesterone antagonist RU 486 (mifepristone). *N Engl J Med*. 1986;315:1565-1570.
19. Shoupe D, Mishell DR Jr, Brenner PF, Spitz IM. Pregnancy termination with a high and medium dosage regimen of RU 486. *Contraception*. 1986; 33:455-461.
20. Mishell DR Jr, Shouupe D, Brenner PF, et al. Termination of early gestation with the anti-progestin steroid RU 486: medium versus low dose. *Contraception*. 1987;35:307-321.
21. Urquhart DR, Templeton AA. Mifepristone (RU 486) and second-trimester termination. *Lancet*. 1987;2:1405.
22. Birgerson L, Odlind V. Early pregnancy termination with antiprogestins: a comparative clinical study of RU 486 given in two dose regimens and epostane. *Fertil Steril*. 1987;48:565-570.
23. Cameron IT, Michie AF, Baird DT. Therapeutic abortion in early pregnancy with antiprogestogen RU486 alone or in combination with prostaglandin analogue (Gemeprost). *Contraception*. 1986;34:459-468.
24. Grimes DA, Mishell DR Jr, Shoupe D, Lacarra M. Early abortion with a single dose of the antiprogestin RU-486. *Am J Obstet Gynecol*. 1988; 158:1307-1312.
25. Cameron IT, Baird DT. Early pregnancy termination: a comparison between vacuum aspiration and medical abortion using prostaglandin (16,16 dimethyl-trans-Ä2-PGE1 methyl ester) or the antiprogestogen RU 486. *Br J Obstet Gynaecol*. 1988;95:271-276.
26. Maria B, Stampf F, Goepp A, Ulmann A. Termination of early pregnancy by a single dose of mifepristone (RU 486), a progesterone antagonist. *Eur J Obstet Gynecol Reprod Biol*. 1988;28:249-255.
27. Frydman R, Fernandez H, Pons JC, Ulmann A. Mifepristone (RU486) and therapeutic late pregnancy termination: a double-blind study of two different doses. *Hum Reprod*. 1988;3:803-806.
28. Ylikorkala O, Alfthan H, Kaariainen M, et al. Outpatient therapeutic abortion with mifepristone. *Obstet Gynecol*. 1989;74:653-657.
29. Gottlieb C, Bygdeman M. The use of antiprogestin (RU 486) for termination of second trimester pregnancy. *Acta Obstet Gynecol Scand*. 1991; 70:199-203.
30. Rodger MW, Baird DT. Induction of therapeutic abortion in early pregnancy with mifepristone in combination with prostaglandin pessary. *Lancet*. 1987;2:1415-1418.
31. Swahn ML, Bygdeman M. The effect of the antiprogestin RU 486 on uterine contractility and sensitivity to prostaglandin and oxytocin. *Br J Obstet Gynaecol*. 1988;95:126-134.
32. Hill NCW, Ferguson J, MacKenzie IZ. The efficacy of oral mifepristone (RU 38,486) with a prostaglandin E1 analog vaginal pessary for the termination of early pregnancy: complications and patient acceptability. *Am J Obstet Gynecol*. 1990;162:414-417.
33. Silvestre L, Dubois C, Renault M, et al. Voluntary interruption of pregnancy with mifepristone (RU 486) and a prostaglandin analogue. *N Engl J Med*. 1990;322:645-648.
34. UK Multicentre Trial. The efficacy and tolerance of mifepristone and prostaglandin in first trimester termination of pregnancy. *Br J Obstet Gynaecol*. 1990;97:480-486.
35. Norman JE, Thong KJ, Baird DT. Uterine contractility and induction of abortion in early pregnancy by misoprostol and mifepristone. *Lancet*. 1991;338:1233-1236.
36. Anonymous. Misoprostol and legal medical abortion. *Lancet*. 1991;338: 1241-1242.
37. World Health Organization. Pregnancy termination with mifepristone and gemeprost: a multicenter comparison between repeated doses and a single dose of mifepristone. *Fertil Steril*. 1991;56:32-40.
38. Norman JE, Thong KJ, Rodger MW, Baird DT. Medical abortion in women of less than or equal to 56 days amenorrhoea: a comparison between gemeprost (a PGE1 analogue) alone and mifepristone and gemeprost. *Br J Obstet Gynaecol*. 1992;99:601-606.
39. Ulmann A, Silvestre L, Chemama L, et al. Medical termination of early pregnancy with mifepristone (RU 486) followed by a prostaglandin analogue; study in 16,369 women. *Acta Obstet Gynecol Scand*. 1992;71:278-283.
40. Baird DT, Norman JE, Thong KJ, Glasier AF. Misoprostol, mifepristone, and abortion. *Lancet*. 1992;339:313.
41. Thong KJ, Baird DT. A study of gemeprost alone, dilapan or mifepristone in combination with gemeprost for the termination of second trimester pregnancy. *Contraception*. 1992;46:11-17.
42. Thong KJ, Baird DT. Induction of abortion with mifepristone and misoprostol in early pregnancy. *Br J Obstet Gynaecol*. 1992;99:1004-1007.
43. Heard M, Guillebaud J. Medical abortion. Safe, effective, and legal in Britain. *Br Med J*. 1992;304:195-196.
44. Peyron R, Aubeny E, Targosz V, et al. Early termination of pregnancy with mifepristone (RU 486) and the orally active prostaglandin misoprostol. *N Engl J Med*. 1993;328:1509-1513.
45. Cabrol D, Bouvier D'Yvoire M, Mermet E, Cedard L, Sureau C, Baulieu EE. Induction of labour with mifepristone after intrauterine fetal death. *Lancet*. 1985;2:1019.
46. Cabrol D, Dubois C, Cronje H, et al. Induction of labor with mifepristone (RU 486) in intrauterine fetal death. *Am J Obstet Gynecol*. 1990;163: 540-542.
47. Radestad A, Christensen NJ, Stromberg L. Induced cervical ripening with mifepristone in first trimester abortion. A double-blind randomized biomechanical study. *Contraception*. 1988;38:301-312.
48. Durlot F, Dubois C, Brunerie J, Frydman R. Efficacy of progesterone antagonist RU486 (mifepristone) for pre-operative cervical dilatation during first trimester abortion. *Hum Reprod*. 1988;3:583-584.
49. Lefebvre Y, Proulx L, Elie R, et al. The effects of RU-38486 on cervical ripening. Clinical studies. *Am J Obstet Gynecol*. 1990;162:61-65.
50. Johnson N, Bryce FC. Could antiprogesterones be used as alternative cervical ripening agents? *Am J Obstet Gynecol*. 1990;162:688-690.
51. World Health Organization. The use of mifepristone (RU 486) for cervical preparation in first trimester pregnancy termination by vacuum aspiration. *Br J Obstet Gynaecol*. 1990;97:260-266.
52. Cohn M, Stewart P. Pretreatment of the primigravid uterine cervix with mifepristone 30 h prior to termination of pregnancy: a double blind study. *Br J Obstet Gynaecol*. 1991;98:778-782.

53. Frydman R, Taylor S, Pons JC, et al. Obstetrical indications for mifepristone. *Adv Contracept*. 1986;2:269-270.
54. Li Y, Perezgrovas R, Gazal OS, et al. Antiprogesterone, RU 486, facilitates parturition in cattle. *Endocrinology*. 1991;129:765-770.
55. Wolf JP, Sinosich M, Anderson TL, et al. Progesterone antagonist (RU 486) for cervical dilation, labor induction, and delivery in monkeys: effectiveness in combination with oxytocin. *Am J Obstet Gynecol*. 1989;160:45-47.
56. Frydman R, Lelaidier C, Baton-Saint-Mleux C, et al. Labor induction in women at term with mifepristone (RU 486): a double-blind randomized, placebo-controlled study. *Obstet Gynecol*. 1992;80:972-975.
57. Levin JH, Lacarra M, d'Ablain G, et al. Mifepristone (RU 486) failure in an ovarian heterotopic pregnancy. *Am J Obstet Gynecol*. 1990;163:543-544.
58. Pansky M, Golan A, Bukovsky I, Caspi E. Nonsurgical management of tubal pregnancy. Necessity in view of the changing clinical appearance. *Am J Obstet Gynecol*. 1991;164:888-895.
59. Ulmann A. Uses of RU 486 for contragestion: an update. *Contraception*. 1987;36(suppl):27-31.
60. Nieman LK, Choate TM, Chrousos GP, et al. The progesterone antagonist RU 486. A potential new contraceptive agent. *N Engl J Med*. 1987;316:187-191.
61. Psychoyos A, Prapas I. Inhibition of egg development and implantation in rats after post-coital administration of the progesterone antagonist RU 486. *J Reprod Fertil*. 1987;80:487-491.
62. Baulieu EE, Ulmann A, Philibert D. Contragestion by antiprogestin RU 486: a review. *Arch Gynecol Obstet*. 1987;241:73-85.
63. Lahteenmaki P, Rapeli T, Kaariainen M, et al. Late postcoital treatment against pregnancy with antiprogesterone RU 486. *Fertil Steril*. 1988;50:36-38.
64. Dubois C, Ulmann A, Baulieu EE. Contragestion with late luteal administration of RU 486 (mifepristone). *Fertil Steril*. 1988;50:593-596.
65. Couzinet B, Le Strat N, Silvestre L, Schaison G. Late luteal administration of the antiprogesterone RU486 in normal women: effects on the menstrual cycle events and fertility control in a long-term study. *Fertil Steril*. 1990;54:1039-1044.
66. Swahn ML, Gemzell K, Bygdeman M. Contraception with mifepristone. *Lancet*. 1991;338:942-943.
67. Glasier A, Thong KJ, Dewar M, et al. Postcoital contraception with mifepristone. *Lancet*. 1991;337:1414-1415.
68. Batista MC, Bristow TL, Mathews J, et al. Daily administration of the progesterone antagonist RU 486 prevents implantation in the cycling guinea pig. *Am J Obstet Gynecol*. 1991;165:82-86.
69. Glasier A, Thong KJ, Dewar M, et al. Mifepristone (RU 486) compared with high-dose estrogen and progestogen for emergency postcoital contraception. *N Engl J Med*. 1992;327:1041-1044.
70. Grimes DA, Cook RJ. Mifepristone (RU 486)—an abortifacient to prevent abortion? *N Engl J Med*. 1992;327:1088-1089.
71. Hamel RP, Lysaught MT. Mifepristone (RU 486)—an abortifacient to prevent abortion? *N Engl J Med*. 1993;328:354.
72. Grimes DA, Cook RJ. Mifepristone (RU 486)—an abortifacient to prevent abortion? Reply. *N Engl J Med*. 1993;328:355.
73. Henrion R. RU 486 abortions. *Nature*. 1989;338:110.
74. Pons JC, Imbert MC, Elefant E, et al. Development after exposure to mifepristone in early pregnancy. *Lancet*. 1991;338:763.
75. Ulmann A, Rubin I, Barnard J. Development after in-utero exposure to mifepristone. *Lancet*. 1991;338:1270.
76. Pons JC, Papiernik E. Mifepristone teratogenicity. *Lancet*. 1991;338:1332-1333.
77. Lim BH, Lees DAR, Bjornsson S, et al. Normal development after exposure to mifepristone in early pregnancy. *Lancet*. 1990;336:257-258.
78. Saav I, Fiala C, Hamalainen JM, et al. Medical abortion in lactating women—low levels of mifepristone in breast milk. *Acta Obstet Gynecol Scand*. 2010;89:618-622.

MIGALASTAT

Genetic (Fabry Disease—Pharmacologic Chaperone)

PREGNANCY RECOMMENDATION: Limited Human Data—Animal Data Suggest Low Risk

BREASTFEEDING RECOMMENDATION: Probably Compatible

PREGNANCY SUMMARY

A total of four patients have been reported with exposure to migalastat during pregnancy. One patient used migalastat from conception up to 18 weeks' gestation when the drug was discontinued. The pregnancy was delivered at term, and no fetal abnormalities were noted. The other three patients were exposed during the clinical trials. One of these had 34 days of exposure during pregnancy and delivered a healthy baby at term. The timing of gestation for the exposure was not reported. No data are available on the other two cases. The drug probably crosses the placenta, so some fetal exposure will likely occur. Animal data did not show any embryofetal toxicity in two species at doses greater than 10 times the RHD. Using this drug during pregnancy should be based on the pros and cons of the mother's clinical need for treatment versus any potential fetal risk that might occur from exposure. Health care providers are encouraged to register patients or obtain additional information by contacting the Pregnancy Coordinating Center at 1-888-239-0758.

BREASTFEEDING SUMMARY

Migalastat probably enters breast milk, so infant exposure will likely occur. If the clinical decision is to use this drug while breastfeeding, the infant should be monitored for the most common reported adult side effects of headache, abdominal pain, back pain, and nausea (all leading to irritability), diarrhea, pyrexia, and cough. There is a study that collects data on this drug used during lactation in women with Fabry disease and potential effects on their neonates and infants up to 1 year of age. Health care providers are encouraged to register patients or obtain additional information by contacting the Pregnancy Coordinating Center at 1-888-239-0758.

References

1. Prescribing Information. Galafold. Amicus Therapeutics U.S., Inc; 2024.
2. Haninger-Vacariu N, El-Hadi S, Pauler U, et al. Pregnancy outcome after exposure to migalastat for Fabry disease: a clinical report. *Case Rep Obstet Gynecol*. 2019;1030259.

MIGLITOL

Antidiabetic (α-Glucosidase Inhibitor)

PREGNANCY RECOMMENDATION: No Human Data—Animal Data Suggest Potential Risk

BREASTFEEDING RECOMMENDATION: Probably Compatible

PREGNANCY SUMMARY

No reports describing the use of miglitol during human pregnancy have been located. The drug will probably cross the placenta, so fetal exposure will likely occur. However, the absence of human pregnancy experience prevents a complete assessment of the embryofetal risk. Animal data did not show any embryofetal toxicity in one species at doses of less than 10 times the MRHD. ACOG and the ADA recommend that insulin be used for types 1 and 2 diabetes occurring during pregnancy and, if diet therapy alone is not successful, for gestational diabetes. Oral medications, such a miglitol, lack safety data.

BREASTFEEDING SUMMARY

One study was located that described the use of miglitol during human lactation. The drug was found to be excreted into human breast milk in very small amounts, though some infant exposure will occur. The calculated RID was less than 1%. Breastfeeding while using this drug should be based on the mother's clinical need for treatment versus any potential infant risks that might occur. If used, the infant should be monitored for the most common reported adult side effects of abdominal pain (leading to irritability), diarrhea, and flatulence.

References

1. Prescribing Information. Miglitol. Westminster Pharmaceuticals, LLC; 2021.
2. American College of Obstetricians and Gynecologists. Pregestational diabetes mellitus. ACOG practice bulletin no. 201. *Obstet Gynecol.* 2018; 132:e228-e248.
3. American College of Obstetricians and Gynecologists. Gestational diabetes. ACOG practice bulletin no. 190. *Obstet Gynecol.* 2018;131:e49-e64.

MIGLUSTAT

Endocrine/Metabolic (Enzyme Inhibitor)

PREGNANCY RECOMMENDATION: No Human Data—Animal Data Suggest Potential Risk

BREASTFEEDING RECOMMENDATION: Potential Toxicity

PREGNANCY SUMMARY

No reports describing the use of miglustat in human pregnancy have been located. The drug will probably cross the placenta, so fetal exposure will likely occur. However, the absence of human pregnancy experience prevents a complete assessment of the embryofetal risk. Embryofetal toxicity was observed in one animal species at doses of less than 10 times the RHD. Using this drug during pregnancy should be based on the pros and cons of the mother's clinical need for treatment versus any potential fetal risk that might occur from exposure.

BREASTFEEDING SUMMARY

No reports describing the use miglustat during human lactation have been located. The drug will probably be found in human breast milk, so some infant exposure will likely occur. Breastfeeding while using this drug should be based on the mother's clinical need for treatment versus any potential infant risks that might occur. If used, the infant should be monitored for the most common reported adult side effects of nausea, headache, and abdominal pain (all leading to irritability), diarrhea, flatulence, tremor, weakness, and decreased appetite (monitor infant growth).

References

1. Prescribing Information. Miglustat. ANI Pharmaceuticals, Inc; 2024.
2. Hollak CE, Hughes D, van Schaik IN, et al. Miglustat (Zavesca) in type I Gaucher disease: 5-year results of a post-authorisation safety surveillance programme. *Pharmacoepidemiol Drug Saf.* 2009;18:770-777.

MILNACIPRAN

Mental Health (Serotonin/Norepinephrine Reuptake Inhibitor)

PREGNANCY RECOMMENDATION: No Human Data—Animal Data Suggest Potential Risk

BREASTFEEDING RECOMMENDATION: Potential Toxicity

PREGNANCY SUMMARY

No reports describing the use of milnacipran in human pregnancy have been located. The drug will probably cross the placenta, so some infant exposure will likely occur. However, the absence of human pregnancy experience prevents a complete assessment of the embryofetal risk. Embryofetal toxicity was observed in one animal species at doses less than the MRHD, but no embryofetal toxicity was seen in two other species at doses of less than 10 times the MRHD. Using this drug during pregnancy should be based on the pros and cons of the mother's clinical need for treatment versus any potential fetal risk that might occur from exposure. There is a pregnancy exposure registry that monitors pregnancy outcomes in women exposed to milnacipran during pregnancy. Physicians and patients are encouraged to enroll in the Savella Pregnancy Registry by calling 1-877-643-3010.

BREASTFEEDING SUMMARY

One report was located that described the use of milnacipran during human lactation in eight women. The drug was found to be excreted into human breast milk. The calculated RID with a daily milnacipran dose of 50 mg was 5%. Breastfeeding while using this drug should be based on the mother's clinical need for treatment versus any potential infant risks that might occur. If used, the infant should be monitored for the most common reported adult side effects of sedation, agitation, irritability, and poor feeding (monitor infant growth).

Reference

1. Prescribing Information. Savella. AbbVie; 2024.

MILRINONE

Cardiovascular (Inotrope/Phosphodiesterase 3 Enzyme Inhibitor)

PREGNANCY RECOMMENDATION: Limited Human Data—Animal Data Suggest Potential Risk (Maternal Benefit May Outweigh Any Potential Embryofetal Risk)

BREASTFEEDING RECOMMENDATION: Potential Toxicity

PREGNANCY SUMMARY

One case report describing the use of milrinone in human pregnancy was located. The patient had Eisenmenger syndrome with preeclampsia and was treated at 28 weeks' gestation. No adverse obstetrical or fetal effects related to the drug were described. The drug will probably cross the placenta, so some fetal exposure will likely occur. Therefore, the absence of human pregnancy experience prevents a complete assessment of the embryofetal risk. Embryofetal toxicity was observed in one animal species at doses of less than 10 times the MRHD based on weight. Due to the indication of this drug, the mother's clinical need for treatment may outweigh the potential fetal risk that might occur from exposure.

BREASTFEEDING SUMMARY

No reports describing the use of milrinone during human lactation have been located. The drug will probably be found in human breast milk, so some infant exposure may occur. The effect of this exposure on a nursing infant is unknown. If the clinical decision is to use this drug while breastfeeding, the infant should be monitored for the most common reported adult side effects of headache (leading to irritability), increased heart rate, and ventricular arrhythmias.

References

1. Prescribing Information. Milrinone. Hikma Pharmaceuticals USA Inc; 2025.
2. Atkinson BD, Fishburne JI Jr, Hales KA, et al. Placental transfer of milrinone in the nonhuman primate (baboon). *Am J Obstet Gynecol* 1996;174:895-896.
3. Deepak Chakravarthy CD, Thangaswamy CR, Balachander H. Perioperative management of an obstetric patient with Eisenmenger syndrome and pre-eclampsia using milrinone. *Ann Card Anaesth*. 2024;27:277-279.

MILTEFOSINE

Anti-Infective (Antileishmanial)

PREGNANCY RECOMMENDATION: No Human Data—Animal Data Suggest Risk

BREASTFEEDING RECOMMENDATION: Potential Toxicity

PREGNANCY SUMMARY

No reports describing the use of miltefosine in human pregnancy have been located. The drug will probably cross the placenta, so some fetal exposure will likely occur. Therefore, the absence of human pregnancy experience prevents a complete assessment of the embryofetal risk. Embryofetal toxicity with malformations was observed in two animal species at doses of less than 10 times the MRHD. Based on the animal studies, the manufacturer recommends that women with reproductive potential use effective contraception during treatment and for 5 months after the last dose. Nevertheless, using this drug during pregnancy should be based on the pros and cons of the mother's clinical need for treatment versus any potential fetal risk that might occur from exposure. There is a pregnancy exposure registry that monitors pregnancy outcomes in women using this drug. Health care providers are encouraged to call the IMPAVIDO Pregnancy Exposure Registry at 1-866-588-5405. Miltefosine carries a boxed warning regarding embryofetal toxicity.

BREASTFEEDING SUMMARY

No reports describing the use of miltefosine during human lactation have been located. The drug will probably be found in human breast milk, so some infant exposure will likely occur. However, due to a concern for potential serious adverse effects that might be seen in a breastfed infant, the manufacturer recommends that women not breastfeed while being treated with this drug and for at least 5 months after the last dose. Nevertheless, breastfeeding while using this drug should be based on the mother's clinical need for treatment. If used, the infant should be monitored for the most common reported adult side effects or nausea, headache, dizziness, pruritus, and abdominal pain (all leading to irritability), vomiting, diarrhea, decreased appetite (monitor infant growth), somnolence, elevated transaminases, and elevated creatinine.

Reference

1. Prescribing Information. Impavido. Profounda, Inc; 2024.

MINERAL OIL

Gastrointestinal (Laxative—Lubricant)

PREGNANCY RECOMMENDATION: Limited Human Data—No Relevant Animal Data

BREASTFEEDING RECOMMENDATION: Probably Compatible

M

PREGNANCY SUMMARY

No reports describing the use of mineral oil in human pregnancy have been located. While the bioavailability is not known, mineral oil is likely minimally absorbed systemically following oral or rectal administration. Therefore, placental transfer should be limited. However, the absence of human pregnancy experience prevents a complete assessment of the embryofetal risk. No animal reproduction studies have been located. Prolonged use of mineral oil may reduce the absorption of fat-soluble vitamins, including vitamin K, which could lead to hemorrhagic complications for the mother and baby. Using this drug during pregnancy should be based on the pros and cons of the mother's clinical need for treatment versus any potential fetal risk that might occur from exposure.

BREASTFEEDING SUMMARY

One report describing the use of mineral oil in 50 postpartum women was located. All infant stools were normal in consistency. While the bioavailability is not known, mineral oil is likely minimally absorbed systemically following oral or rectal administration. This should limit excretion into breast milk. If the clinical decision is to use this drug while breastfeeding, the infant should be monitored for the most common reported adult side effects of nausea and abdominal cramps (both leading to irritability), vomiting, and diarrhea. Mineral oil may reduce the absorption of fat-soluble vitamins, so caution should be used with repeated use.

Reference

1. Baldwin WF. Clinical study of senna administration to nursing mothers: assessment of effects on infant bowel habits. *Can Med Assoc J.* 1963; 89:566-568.

MINOCYCLINE

Antibacterial (Tetracycline)

PREGNANCY RECOMMENDATION: Human Data Suggest Risk (Second and Third Trimesters) —Animal Data Suggest Potential Risk

BREASTFEEDING RECOMMENDATION: *Potential Toxicity

PREGNANCY SUMMARY

No reports describing the use of minocycline in human pregnancy have been located. The drug crosses the placenta, so fetal exposure will likely occur. However, the absence of human pregnancy experience prevents a complete assessment of the embryofetal risk. Embryofetal toxicity was observed in two animal species, but dosing was not supplied. Tetracycline drugs may cause permanent tooth discoloration and can produce bone stippling. Therefore, the drug should not be used in the second and third trimesters, if possible. Using this drug during pregnancy should be based on the pros and cons of the mother's clinical need for treatment versus any potential fetal risk that might occur from exposure.

BREASTFEEDING SUMMARY

No reports describing the effects of minocycline during human lactation have been located. Minocycline was found to be excreted into human breast milk, so infant exposure will occur. *Because it is a tetracycline, it is not recommended for use in children 8 years of age or younger due to the risk for permanent tooth discoloration and adverse effects on bone growth. Therefore, the manufacturer recommends that women not breastfeed while being treated with this drug. If the clinical decision is to use this drug while breastfeeding, the infant should be monitored for adverse effects on gastrointestinal flora, such as diarrhea, thrush, and diaper rash.

References

1. Prescribing Information. Minocycline. Actavis Pharma, Inc; 2024.
2. Prescribing Information. Amzeeq. Journey Medical Corporation; 2023.
3. Mizuno S, Taketa M, Sano S, et al. Minocycline. *Jpn J Antibiot*. 1969; 22:473-479.

MINOXIDIL

Cardiovascular (Antihypertensive/Vasodilator)

PREGNANCY RECOMMENDATION: *Contraindicated

BREASTFEEDING RECOMMENDATION: Potential Toxicity

PREGNANCY SUMMARY

Three case reports describing the use of oral minoxidil in four human pregnancies have been located. Two of four infants exposed to the drug had hypertrichosis, which has been reported in children and adults who have used this drug. Multiple congenital malformations were observed in a third neonate, and heart defects in the fourth. In addition, multiple anomalies were reported in two fetuses after topical minoxidil application. Although the doses applied in these two cases were not specified, only small amounts of the topical drug are absorbed into the systemic circulation. Minoxidil will probably cross the placenta, so fetal exposure will likely occur. However, this limited human pregnancy experience prevents a complete assessment of the embryofetal risk. Embryofetal toxicity was observed in two animal species at doses of less than 10 times the MRHD. *Even if these malformations are not related to the drug exposure, the potential toxicity of minoxidil is severe enough to preclude its use in pregnancy, if possible. If a patient's blood pressure is only controlled by this drug, then use might be indicated.

BREASTFEEDING SUMMARY

Two case reports describing the effects of minoxidil in two breastfeeding infants have been located. One preterm infant developed facial hypertrichosis while the mother was using 5% minoxidil topically twice a day. Minoxidil was discontinued, and the excess hair was lost by 6 months of age. No adverse effects were reported in the second-term infant whose mother was taking oral minoxidil throughout her pregnancy and postpartum. The drug was found in breast milk with concentrations that ranged from about 0.3 to about 42 ng/mL. The calculated RID was about 4.5%. If the clinical decision is to use this drug while breastfeeding, the infant should be monitored for the most common reported adult side effects of nausea (leading to irritability), hypertrichosis, peripheral edema, vomiting, and electrocardiogram (ECG) changes.

References

1. Prescribing Information. Minoxidil. Actavis Pharma, Inc; 2024.
2. Prescribing Information. Rogaine. Kenvue Brands LLC; 2024.
3. Carlson RG, Feenstra ES. Toxicologic studies with the hypotensive agent minoxidil. *Toxicol Appl Pharmacol*. 1977;39:1-11.
4. Valdivieso A, Valdes G, Spiro TE, Westerman RL. Minoxidil in breast milk. *Ann Intern Med*. 1985;102:135.
5. Kaler SG, Patrinos ME, Lambert GH, et al. Hypertrichosis and congenital anomalies associated with maternal use of minoxidil. *Pediatrics*. 1987; 79:434-436.
6. Rosa FW, Idanpaan-Heikkila J, Asanti R. Fetal minoxidil exposure. *Pediatrics*. 1987;80:120.
7. Rojansky N, Fasouliotis SJ, Ariel H, Nadjari M. Extreme caudal agenesis. Possible drug-related etiology? *J Reprod Med*. 2002;47:241-245.
8. Smorlesi C, Caldarella A, Caramelli L, et al. Topically applied minoxidil may cause fetal malformation: a case report. *Birth Defects Res A Clin Mol Teratol*. 2003;67:997-1001.
9. Trüeb RM, Caballero-Uribe N. Minoxidil-induced hypertrichosis in a breastfed infant. *J Eur Acad Dermatol Venereol*. 2022;36:e224-e225

MIRABEGRON

Urinary (β_3-Agonist)

PREGNANCY RECOMMENDATION: No Human Data and No Relevant Animal Data

BREASTFEEDING RECOMMENDATION: Potential Toxicity

PREGNANCY SUMMARY

No reports describing the use of mirabegron in human pregnancy have been located. The drug will probably cross the placenta, so some fetal exposure will likely occur. However, the absence of human pregnancy experience prevents a complete assessment of the embryofetal risk. Embryofetal toxicity was seen in two animal species, but at doses of well above 10 times the MRHD. Using this drug during pregnancy should be based on the pros and cons of the mother's clinical need for treatment versus any potential fetal risk that might occur from exposure.

BREASTFEEDING SUMMARY

No reports describing the use of mirabegron during human lactation have been located. The drug will probably be found in human breast milk, so some infant exposure will likely occur. The effect of this exposure on a nursing infant is unknown. If the clinical decision is to use this drug while breastfeeding, the infant should be monitored for the most common reported adult side effects of headache (leading to irritability), hypertension, nasopharyngitis, and urinary tract infections.

Reference

1. Prescribing Information. Mirabegron. Zydus Lifesciences Limited; 2024.

MIRIKIZUMAB

Gastrointestinal (Monoclonal Antibody—Ulcerative Colitis)

PREGNANCY RECOMMENDATION: No Human Data—Animal Data Suggest Low Risk

BREASTFEEDING RECOMMENDATION: Probably Compatible

PREGNANCY SUMMARY

No reports describing the use of mirikizumab in human pregnancy have been located. As an IgG antibody, it likely crosses the placenta, especially during the second half of pregnancy, so some fetal exposure will probably occur. Therefore, the absence of human pregnancy experience prevents a complete assessment of the embryofetal risk. Animal reproduction studies did not show any embryofetal toxicity or malformations in one species at doses of more than 10 times the MRHD. Using this drug during pregnancy should be based on the pros and cons of the mother's clinical need for treatment versus any potential fetal risk that might occur from exposure. There is a pregnancy exposure registry that monitors pregnancy outcomes in women using this drug. Health care providers are encouraged to call the Omvoh Pregnancy Exposure Registry with Eli Lilly and Company at 1-800-545-5979.

BREASTFEEDING SUMMARY

No reports describing the use of mirikizumab during human lactation have been located. It is known that IgG antibodies can be found in human breast milk but are not found in the neonatal or infant circulation. Additionally, if any IgG antibodies were to be ingested through breastfeeding, they would probably be digested in the infant's gastrointestinal tract and not be absorbed. Nevertheless, breastfeeding while using this drug should be based on the mother's clinical need for treatment. If used, the infant should be monitored for the most common reported adult side effects of nausea and arthralgia (both leading to irritability), rash, and infections.

Reference

1. Prescribing Information. Omvoh. Eli Lilly and Company; 2023.

MIRTAZAPINE

Mental Health (Antidepressant)

PREGNANCY RECOMMENDATION: Human Data Suggest Low Risk (First Trimester)/*Human Data Suggest Risk (Third Trimester)

BREASTFEEDING RECOMMENDATION: Probably Compatible

PREGNANCY SUMMARY

Numerous reports describing the use of mirtazapine in over 2,000 human pregnancies have been located. These available studies have found no evidence of significant adverse effects. Most studies did not find an increased risk of congenital malformations or spontaneous abortion; however, some data were conflicting. *Neonatal withdrawal symptoms have been associated with mirtazapine exposure late in pregnancy. The drug will probably cross the placenta, so some fetal exposure will likely occur. Animal data did show some embryofetal toxicity in one species, but not a second species, at doses of more than 10 times the MRHD. Using this drug during pregnancy should be based on the pros and cons of the mother's clinical need for treatment versus any potential fetal risk that might occur from exposure. Infants exposed to mirtazapine late in pregnancy should be monitored for symptoms of withdrawal that include irritability, hyperactivity, abnormal sleep patterns, high-pitched cry, tremor, vomiting, diarrhea, and failure to gain weight. There is a pregnancy exposure registry that monitors pregnancy outcomes in women using antidepressant drugs. Health care providers are encouraged to call the National Pregnancy Registry for Antidepressants at 1-844-405-6185.

BREASTFEEDING SUMMARY

Seven reports describing the effects of mirtazapine during human lactation in 63 women were located, and no consistent infant adverse effects were noted. However, breastfeeding was associated with a lower risk of newborn withdrawal. The drug was found to be excreted into human breast milk with concentrations that range from undetectable (<1 ng/mL) up to about 35 ng/mL. Calculated RIDs were about 2% for the drug and active metabolite combined. A few infant blood samples have been analyzed for the drug, and most were undetectable. The highest infant level was 10 ng/mL, which would be considered therapeutic. If the clinical decision is to use this drug while breastfeeding, the infant should be monitored for the most common reported adult side effects of dizziness (leading to irritability), sleepiness, and increased appetite.

References

1. Prescribing Information. Mirtazapine. Apotex Corp; 2024.
2. Mirtazapine. In: Sweetman SC, ed. *Martindale: The Complete Drug Reference*. 34th ed. Pharmaceutical Press; 2005:307-308.
3. Kesim M, Yaris F. Mirtazapine use in two pregnant women: is it safe? *Teratology*. 2002;66:204.
4. Biswas PN, Wilton LV, Shakir SAW. The pharmacovigilance of mirtazapine: results of a prescription event monitoring study on 13554 patients in England. *J Psychopharmacol*. 2003;17:121-126.
5. Rohde A, Dembinski J, Dorn C. Mirtazapine (Remergil) for treatment resistant hyperemesis gravidarum: rescue of a twin pregnancy. *Arch Gynecol Obstet*. 2003;268:219-221.
6. Guclu S, Gol M, Dogan E, Saygili U. Mirtazapine use in resistant hyperemesis gravidarum: report of three cases and review of the literature. *Arch Gynecol Obstet*. 2005;272:298-300.
7. Yaris F, Kadioglu M, Kesim M, et al. Newer antidepressants in pregnancy: prospective outcome of a case series. *Reprod Toxicol*. 2004;19:235-238.
8. Djulus J, Koren G, Einarson TR, et al. Exposure to mirtazapine during pregnancy: a prospective, comparative study of birth outcomes. *J Clin Psychiatry*. 2006;67:1280-1284.
9. Einarson A, Choi J, Einarson TR, Koren G. Incidence of major malformations in infants following antidepressant exposure in pregnancy: results of a large prospective cohort study. *Can J Psychiatry*. 2009;54:242-246.
10. Winterfeld U, Klinger G, Panchaud A, et al. Pregnancy outcome following maternal exposure to mirtazapine. *J Clin Psychopharmacol*. 2015;35:250-259.
11. Omay O, Einarson A. Is mirtazapine an effective treatment for nausea and vomiting of pregnancy? A case series. *J Clin Pyschopharmacol*. 2017;37:260-261.
12. Tonn P, Reuter SC, Hiemke C, Dahmen N. High mirtazapine plasma levels in infant after breast feeding. Case report and review of the literature. *J Clin Psychopharmacol*. 2009;29:191-192.
13. Aichhorn W, Whitworth AB, Weiss U, Stuppaeck C. Mirtazapine and breastfeeding. *Am J Psychiatry*. 2004;161:2325.
14. Kristensen JH, Ilett KF, Rampono J, et al. Transfer of the antidepressant mirtazapine into breast milk. *Br J Clin Pharmacol*. 2007;63:322-327.
15. Klier CM, Mossaheb N, Lee A, Zernig G. Mirtazapine and breastfeeding: maternal and infant plasma levels. *Am J Psychiatry*. 2007;164:348-349.
16. Smit M, Wennink H, Heres M, et al. Mirtazapine in pregnancy and lactation: data from a case series. *J Clin Psychopharmacol*. 2015;35:163-167.
17. Uguz F. Short-term safety of paroxetine plus low-dose mirtazapine during lactation. *Breastfeed Med*. 2019;14:131-132.
18. Güngör BB, Öztürk N, Atar AÖ, Aydın N. Comparison of the groups treated with mirtazapine and selective serotonine reuptake inhibitors with respect to birth outcomes and severity of psychiatric disorder. *Psychiatry Clin Psychopharmacol*. 2019;29:822-831.
19. Ostenfeld A, Petersen TS, Pedersen LH, et al. Mirtazapine exposure in pregnancy and fetal safety: a nationwide cohort study. *Acta Psychiatr Scand*. 2022;145(6):557-567.
20. Ostenfeld A, Lyngholm S, Christensen SE, et al. Mirtazapine in pregnancy and lactation: a systematic review of adverse outcomes. *Acta Psychiatr Scand*. 2025;151:6-32.

MIRVETUXIMAB SORAVTANSINE

Antineoplastic (Antifolate Receptor Alpha Monoclonal Antibody/Microtubule Inhibitor)

PREGNANCY RECOMMENDATION: No Human Data and No Relevant Animal Data

BREASTFEEDING RECOMMENDATION: Potential Toxicity

PREGNANCY SUMMARY

No reports describing the use of mirvetuximab soravtansine in human pregnancy have been located. As an IgG antibody, mirvetuximab will likely cross the placenta, so some fetal exposure will probably occur. In addition, some fetal exposure will

(*continued*)

probably occur for the microtubule inhibitor (DM4) as well. Therefore, the absence of human pregnancy experience prevents a complete assessment of the embryofetal risk. No reproduction animal studies have been conducted. Based on the drug's mechanism of action, the manufacturer recommends that women with reproductive potential use effective contraception during treatment and for 7 months after the last dose. Nevertheless, using this drug during pregnancy should be based on the pros and cons of the mother's clinical need for treatment versus any potential fetal risk that might occur from exposure. Women who are pregnant and have cancer are encouraged to contact the Cancer and Pregnancy Registry at 877-635-4499.

BREASTFEEDING SUMMARY

No reports describing the use of mirvetuximab soravtansine during human lactation have been located. It is known that IgG antibodies can be found in human breast milk but are not found in the neonatal or infant circulation. Additionally, if any IgG antibodies were to be ingested through breastfeeding, they would probably be digested in the infant's gastrointestinal tract and not be absorbed. Regardless, the microtubule inhibitor (DM4) will also probably be excreted into breast milk, so some infant exposure to this drug will also likely occur. Therefore, due to the concern for potential serious adverse effects that might be seen in a breastfed infant, the manufacturer recommends that women not breastfeed while being treated with this drug and for at least 1 month after the last dose. Nevertheless, breastfeeding while using this drug should be based on the mother's clinical need for treatment. If used, the infant should be monitored for the most common reported adult side effects of nausea (leading to irritability), lethargy, diarrhea, constipation, dry eye, and various laboratory abnormalities (see PI).

Reference

1. Prescribing Information. Elahere. ImmunoGen, Inc; 2022.

MISOPROSTOL

Gastrointestinal (Prostaglandin)

PREGNANCY RECOMMENDATION: *Contraindicated (First Trimester)

BREASTFEEDING RECOMMENDATION: Probably Compatible

M

PREGNANCY SUMMARY

Numerous reports describing the use of misoprostol in human pregnancy were located. Many of these involve its use for cervical ripening in term pregnancies and as a potential abortifacient in early pregnancy for attempted legal and illegal (depending on the country) pregnancy termination. The amount of drug used in these clinical cases is often much higher than would be administered for the drug's approved use. *If the attempted abortion fails, these studies showed an increased risk for various anomalies related to vascular disruption. Use during the second and third trimesters has demonstrated the utility of misoprostol for labor induction and cervical ripening. However, uterine rupture has been reported with misoprostol use to induce labor (especially in patients with a prior uterine incision). The drug crosses the placenta, so fetal exposure will occur. Due to the adverse effects seen in pregnant women with early pregnancy exposure, the manufacturer recommends that women with reproductive potential use effective contraception during treatment. *Misoprostol carries a boxed warning regarding its administration to pregnant women, including risks for birth defects, abortion, premature birth, and uterine rupture. It also includes the warning that misoprostol should not be used to decrease the risk of NSAID-induced ulcers in women of childbearing age unless the patient is at high risk for complications related to gastric ulcers or developing gastric ulceration. However, ACOG considers low-dose (eg, 25 mcg) intravaginal misoprostol to be effective for inducing labor in pregnant women who have unfavorable cervices near delivery.

BREASTFEEDING SUMMARY

A few reports were located that describe the use of misoprostol during human lactation. Following 200 and 600 mcg doses, peak breast milk levels were about 5 and 21 pg/mL, respectively. Calculated RIDs were all less than 1%. No reports describing infant effects from misoprostol use during breastfeeding have been located. Endogenous prostaglandin E_1 normally appears in colostrum and breast milk. The effect of this small additional exposure on a nursing infant is unknown. If used while breastfeeding, the infant should be monitored for the most common reported adult side effects of abdominal pain (leading to irritability) and diarrhea.

References

1. Prescribing Information. Misoprostol. AvPAK; 2024.
2. Clemens GR, Hilbish KG, Hartnagel RE Jr, et al. Developmental toxicity including teratogenicity of E1 prostaglandins in rabbits. *Toxicologist*. 1997;36:260. As cited in Gonzalez CH, Marques-Dias MJ, Kim CA, et al. Congenital abnormalities in Brazilian children associated with misoprostol misuse in first trimester of pregnancy. *Lancet*. 1998;351:1624-1627.
3. Lewis JH. Summary of the 29th meeting of the Gastrointestinal Drugs Advisory Committee, Food and Drug Administration—June 10, 1985. *Am J Gastroenterol*. 1985;80:743-745.
4. Anonymous. Misoprostol and legal medical abortion. *Lancet*. 1991;338:1241-1242.
5. Baird DT, Norman JE, Thong KJ, Glasier AF. Misoprostol, mifepristone, and abortion. *Lancet*. 1992;339:313.

6. Norman JE, Thong KJ, Baird DT. Uterine contractility and induction of abortion in early pregnancy by misoprostol and mifepristone. *Lancet*. 1991; 338:1233-1236.
7. Peyron R, Aubeny E, Targosz V, et al. Early termination of pregnancy with mifepristone (RU 486) and the orally active prostaglandin misoprostol. *N Engl J Med*. 1993;328:1509-1513.
8. Schonhofer PS. Brazil: misuse of misoprostol as an abortifacient may induce malformations. *Lancet*. 1991;337:1534-1535.
9. Fonseca W, Alencar AJC, Mota FSB, Coelho HLL. Misoprostol and congenital malformations. *Lancet*. 1991;338:56.
10. Fonseca W, Alencar AJC, Pereira RMM, Misago C. Congenital malformation of the scalp and cranium after failed first trimester abortion attempt with misoprostol. *Clin Dysmorphol*. 1993;2:76-80.
11. Costa SH, Vessey MP. Misoprostol and illegal abortion in Rio de Janeiro, Brazil. *Lancet*. 1993;341:1258-1261.
12. Coêlho HLL, Teixeira AC, Santos AP, et al. Misoprostol and illegal abortion in Fortaleza, Brazil. *Lancet*. 1993;341:1261-1263.
13. Schuler L, Ashton PW, Sanseverino MT. Teratogenicity of misoprostol. *Lancet*. 1992;339:437.
14. Gonzalez CH, Vargas FR, Perez ABA, et al. Limb deficiency with or without Möbius sequence in seven Brazilian children associated with misoprostol use in the first trimester of pregnancy. *Am J Med Genet*. 1993;47:59-64.
15. Brent RL. Congenital malformation case reports: the editor's and reviewer's dilemma. *Am J Med Genet*. 1993;47:872-874.
16. Shepard TH. Möbius syndrome after misoprostol: a possible teratogenic mechanism. *Lancet*. 1995;346:780.
17. Shepard TH, Lemire RJ. Möbius syndrome: a possible teratogenic mechanism (abstract). *Teratology*. 1996;53:86.
18. Pastuszak AL, Schuler L, Speck-Martins CE, et al. Use of misoprostol during pregnancy and Möbius' syndrome in infants. *N Engl J Med*. 1998;338: 1881-1885.
19. Pastuszak AL, Schuler L, Coelho KA, et al. Misoprostol use during pregnancy is associated with an increased risk for Möbius sequence (abstract). *Teratology*. 1997;55:36.
20. Genest DR, Richardson A, Rosenblatt M, Holmes L. Limb defects and omphalocele in a 17 week fetus following first trimester misoprostol exposure (abstract). *Teratology*. 1994;49:418.
21. Castilla EE, Orioli IM. Teratogenicity of misoprostol: data from the Latin-American Collaborative Study of Congenital Malformations (ECLAMC). *Am J Med Genet*. 1994;51:161-162.
22. Orioli IM, Castilla EE. Epidemiological assessment of misoprostol teratogenicity. *Br J Obstet Gynaecol*. 2000;107:519-523.
23. Hall JG. Arthrogryposis associated with unsuccessful attempts at termination of pregnancy. *Am J Med Genet*. 1996;63:293-300.
24. Vargas FR, Brunoni D, Gonzalez C, et al. Investigation of the teratogenic potential of misoprostol (abstract). *Teratology*. 1997;55:104.
25. Hofmeyr GJ, Milos D, Nikodem VC, de Jager M. Limb reduction anomaly after failed misoprostol abortion. *S Afr Med J*. 1998;88:566-567.
26. Gonzalez CH, Marques-Dias MJ, Kim CA, et al. Congenital abnormalities in Brazilian children associated with misoprostol misuse in first trimester of pregnancy. *Lancet*. 1998;351:1624-1627.
27. Schuler L, Pastuszak A, Sanseverino MT, et al. Pregnancy outcome after abortion attempt with misoprostol (abstract). *Teratology*. 1997;55:36.
28. Schuler L, Pastuszak A, Sanseverino MTV, et al. Pregnancy outcome after exposure to misoprostol in Brazil: a prospective, controlled study. *Reprod Toxicol*. 1999;13:147-151.
29. Coelho KEFA, Sarmento MVF, Veiga CM, et al. Misoprostol embryotoxicity: clinical evaluation of fifteen patients with arthrogryposis. *Am J Med Genet*. 2000;95:297-301.
30. Vargas FR, Schuler-Faccini L, Brunoni D, et al. Prenatal exposure to misoprostol and vascular disruption defects: a case-control study. *Am J Med Genet*. 2000;95:302-306.
31. Bond GR, Zee AV. Overdosage of misoprostol in pregnancy. *Am J Obstet Gynecol*. 1994;171:561-562.
32. de Silva Dal Pizzol T, Knop FP, Mengu SS. Prenatal exposure to misoprostol and congenital anomalies: systematic review and meta-analysis. *Reprod Toxicol*. 2006;22:666-671.
33. Mariani-Neto C, Leao EJ, Barreto EMCP, et al. Use of misoprostol for labor induction in stillbirth. *Rev Paul Med*. 1987;105:325-328.
34. Bugalho A, Bique C, Machungo F, Faúndes A. Induction of labor with intravaginal misoprostol in intrauterine fetal death. *Am J Obstet Gynecol*. 1994;171:538-541.
35. Jain JK, Mishell DR Jr. A comparison of intravaginal misoprostol with prostaglandin E2 for termination of second-trimester pregnancy. *N Engl J Med*. 1994;331:290-293.
36. Bugalho A, Bique C, Almeida L, Bergström S. Pregnancy interruption by vaginal misoprostol. *Gynecol Obstet Invest*. 1993;36:226-229.
37. Bugalho A, Bique C, Almeida L, Faúndes A. The effectiveness of intravaginal misoprostol (Cytotec) in inducing abortion after eleven weeks of pregnancy. *Stud Fam Plann*. 1993;24:319-323.
38. Margulies M, Perez GC, Voto LS. Misoprostol to induce labour. *Lancet*. 1992;339:64.
39. Sanchez-Ramos L, Kaunitz AM, Del Valle GO, et al. Labor induction with the prostaglandin E1 methyl analogue misoprostol versus oxytocin: a randomized trial. *Obstet Gynecol*. 1993;81:332-336.
40. Fletcher HM, Mitchell S, Frederick J, Brown D. Intravaginal misoprostol as a cervical ripening agent. *Br J Obstet Gynaecol*. 1993;100:641-644.
41. Sanchez-Ramos L, Chen A, Briones D, et al. Premature rupture of membranes at term: induction of labor with intravaginal misoprostol tablets (PGE1) or intravenous oxytocin (abstract). *Am J Obstet Gynecol*. 1994;170:380.
42. Fletcher H, Mitchell S, Frederick J, et al. Intravaginal misoprostol versus dinoprostone as cervical ripening and labor-inducing agents. *Obstet Gynecol*. 1994;83:244-247.
43. Sanchez-Ramos L, Kaunitz A. Intravaginal misoprostol versus dinoprostone as cervical ripening and labor-inducing agents. *Obstet Gynecol*. 1994; 83:799-800.
44. Fletcher H. Intravaginal misoprostol versus dinoprostone as cervical ripening and labor-inducing agents (reply). *Obstet Gynecol*. 1994;83:800-801.
45. American College of Obstetricians and Gynecologists Committee on Obstetric Practice. Induction of labor with misoprostol. Committee opinion no. 228. 1999.
46. American College of Obstetricians and Gynecologists Committee on Obstetric Practice. Response to Searle's drug warning on misoprostol. Committee opinion no. 248. 2000.
47. Fonseca W, Misago C, Kanji N. Misoprostol plus mifepristone. *Lancet*. 1991;338:1594.
48. Abdel-Aleem H, Villar J, Gulmezoglu M, et al. The pharmacokinetics of the prostaglandin E1 analogue misoprostol in plasma and colostrum after postpartum oral administration. *Eur J Obstet Gynecol*. 2003;108:25-28.
49. Vogel D, Burkhardt T, Rentsch K, et al. Misoprostol versus methylergometrine: pharmacokinetics in human milk. *Am J Obstet Gynecol*. 2004; 191:2168-2173.
50. Shimizu T, Yamashiro Y, Yabuta K. Prostaglandins E1, E2, and F2 alpha in human milk and plasma. *Biol Neonate*. 1992;61:222-225.
51. de Oliveira Filgueira GC, de Fátima Pinto Rodrigues G, Benzi JRL, et al. Determination of misoprostol acid in plasma samples by UPLC-MS/MS with application in a maternal-fetal pharmacokinetic study following a low misoprostol dose vaginally to induce labor. *J Pharm Biomed Anal*. 2021; 202:114138.
52. Yin J, Li Y, Chen Y, et al. Intracervical Foley catheter plus intravaginal misoprostol compared to intravaginal misoprostol-only for cervical ripening: a systematic review and meta-analysis. *Eur J Obstet Gynecol Reprod Biol*. 2023;281:76-84.
53. Taliento C, Manservigi M, Tormen M, et al. Safety of misoprostol vs dinoprostone for induction of labor: a systematic review and meta-analysis. *Eur J Obstet Gynecol Reprod Biol*. 2023;289:108-128.
54. Yenuberi H, Mathews J, George A, et al. The efficacy and safety of 25 μg or 50 μg oral misoprostol versus 25 μg vaginal misoprostol given at 4- or 6-hourly intervals for induction of labour in women at or beyond term with live singleton pregnancies: a systematic review and meta-analysis. *Int J Gynaecol Obstet*. 2024;164(2):482-498.
55. Vilchez G, Meislin R, Lin L, et al. Outpatient cervical ripening and labor induction with low-dose vaginal misoprostol reduces the interval to delivery: a systematic review and network meta-analysis. *Am J Obstet Gynecol*. 2024;230(3S):S716-S728.e61.
56. Jingran G, Yan D, Xiaoying Y. Risk of teratogenicity in continued pregnancy after gestational exposure to mifepristone and/or misoprostol: a systematic review and meta-analysis. *Arch Gynecol Obstet*. 2024;310:1331-1342.
57. Ramadan M, Bashour G, Eldokmery E, et al. The efficacy and safety of oral and vaginal misoprostol versus dinoprostone on women experiencing labor: a systematic review and updated meta-analysis of 53 randomized controlled trials. *Medicine (Baltimore)*. 2024;103:e39861.

MITAPIVAT

Hematologic (Pyruvate Kinase Activator)

PREGNANCY RECOMMENDATION: No Human Data—Animal Data Suggest Low Risk

BREASTFEEDING RECOMMENDATION: Probably Compatible

PREGNANCY SUMMARY

No reports describing the use of mitapivat in human pregnancy have been located. A limited amount of the drug may cross the placenta. Therefore, the absence of human pregnancy experience prevents a complete assessment of the embryofetal risk. Animal data did not show any embryofetal toxic effects. Using this drug during pregnancy should be based on the pros and cons of the mother's clinical need for treatment versus any potential fetal risk that might occur from exposure. Untreated pyruvate kinase (PK) deficiency during pregnancy increases the risk for spontaneous abortion, acute hemolysis, severe anemia requiring frequent transfusion, and preterm labor. In addition, an increased risk for hypertension and preeclampsia has been observed.

BREASTFEEDING SUMMARY

No reports describing the use of mitapivat during human lactation have been located. A limited amount of the drug may be found in breast milk, so some infant exposure might occur. Breastfeeding while using this drug should be based on the mother's clinical need for treatment. If used, the infant should be monitored for the most common reported adult side effects of back pain and arthralgia (both leading to irritability), decreased levels of estrone and estradiol (males), and increased urate levels.

Reference

1. Prescribing Information. Pyrukynd. Agios Pharmaceuticals, Inc; 2022.

M

MITOMYCIN

Antineoplastic (Antibiotic)

PREGNANCY RECOMMENDATION: No Human Data—Animal Data Suggest Risk

BREASTFEEDING RECOMMENDATION: Potential Toxicity (Hold Breastfeeding)

PREGNANCY SUMMARY

No reports describing the use of mitomycin in human pregnancy have been located. The drug will probably cross the placenta, so some fetal exposure will likely occur. However, the absence of human pregnancy experience prevents a complete assessment of the embryofetal risk. Embryofetal toxicity with malformations was observed in three animal species. Using this drug during pregnancy should be based on the pros and cons of the mother's clinical need for treatment versus any potential fetal risk that might occur from exposure. There is a registry for women who are pregnant and have cancer. For more information, women and health care providers are encouraged to contact the Cancer and Pregnancy Registry at 1-877-635-4499.

BREASTFEEDING SUMMARY

No reports describing the use of mitomycin during human lactation have been located. The drug will probably be found in human breast milk, so some infant exposure will likely occur. However, due to a concern for potential serious adverse effects that might be seen in a breastfed infant, the manufacturer recommends that women not breastfeed while being treated with this drug. Nevertheless, breastfeeding while using this drug should be based on the mother's clinical need for treatment versus any potential infant risks that might occur. Because the drug is given as a single dose at 6- to 8-week intervals, pumping and dumping for a few hours after a dose should decrease some exposure to a nursing infant. If used, the infant should be monitored for the most common reported adult side effects of nausea (leading to irritability), bone marrow suppression, anorexia (monitor infant growth), vomiting, and fever.

References

1. Prescribing Information. Mitomycin. Accord Healthcare; 2019.
2. Shepard TH, Lemire RJ. *Catalog of Teratogenic Agents*. 12th ed. The Johns Hopkins University Press; 2007:297.
3. Schardein JL. *Chemically Induced Birth Defects*. 3rd ed. Marcel Dekker; 2000:567, 574.

MITOMYCIN OPHTHALMIC

Ophthalmic (Antiglaucoma—Topical)

PREGNANCY RECOMMENDATION: No Human Data—No Relevant Animal Data

BREASTFEEDING RECOMMENDATION: Probably Compatible

PREGNANCY SUMMARY

No reports describing the use of mitomycin ophthalmic in human pregnancy have been located. The drug will probably cross the placenta if found in the maternal circulation. However, while the amount of systemic absorption is not known, mitomycin is likely minimally absorbed systemically following ophthalmic administration. However, the absence of human pregnancy experience prevents a complete assessment of the embryofetal risk. No animal reproduction studies have been conducted using mitomycin ophthalmic. Using this drug during pregnancy should be based on the pros and cons of the mother's clinical need for treatment versus any potential fetal risk that might occur from exposure. If used during pregnancy, consider placing pressure over the tear duct in the corner of the eye for at least 1 minute, and then remove any excess solution with absorbent tissue to decrease the amount of drug reaching the systemic circulation even further.

BREASTFEEDING SUMMARY

No reports describing the use of mitomycin ophthalmic during human lactation have been located. The drug will probably appear in breast milk if found in the maternal circulation. However, mitomycin is likely minimally absorbed systemically following topical ocular administration, which should limit infant exposure. Regardless, due to a concern for potential serious adverse effects that might be seen in a breastfed infant, the manufacturer recommends that women not breastfeed while being treated with this drug and for at least 1 week after the last dose. Because of the ophthalmic usage, systemic adverse reactions were not analyzed. A method to decrease some systemic absorption with ophthalmic use is described above in the Pregnancy Summary.

Reference

1. Prescribing Information. Mitosol. Mobius Therapeutics; 2024.

M

MITOXANTRONE

Antineoplastic (Anthracenedione)

PREGNANCY RECOMMENDATION: Limited Human Data—Animal Data Suggest Risk

BREASTFEEDING RECOMMENDATION: Potential Toxicity

PREGNANCY SUMMARY

Six reports describing the use of mitoxantrone in seven human pregnancies have been located. Six of the seven exposures occurred in the second trimester and included combination use with other chemotherapeutic agents. The remaining exposure to mitoxantrone (along with odansetron) occurred in the first trimester prior to the detection of a pregnancy at 10 weeks' gestation. At delivery, the neonate was found to have Pierre Robin sequence (which is a genetic disorder, most often caused by a new mutation). One exposed infant was delivered stillborn, and another experienced cardiomyopathy, which were both attributed to idarubicin. The drug will probably cross the placenta, so some fetal exposure will likely occur. However, the limited human pregnancy experience prevents a complete assessment of the embryofetal risk. Embryofetal toxicity was observed in two animal species at doses less than the RHD. Using this drug during pregnancy should be based on the pros and cons of the mother's clinical need for treatment versus any potential fetal risk that might occur from exposure.

BREASTFEEDING SUMMARY

One case report describing the effects of mitoxantrone in a breastfeeding infant was located. The infant had no reported adverse effects. The drug was found in breast milk and was still present 28 days after the last dose. However, due to a concern for potential serious adverse effects that might be seen in a breastfed infant, the manufacturer recommends that women not breastfeed while being treated with this drug. Nevertheless, if the clinical decision is to use this drug while breastfeeding, the infant should be monitored for the most common reported adult side effects of nausea (leading to irritability), alopecia, upper respiratory tract infection, urinary tract infection, diarrhea, and various laboratory abnormalities (see PI).

References

1. Prescribing Information. Mitoxantrone. Hospira; 2025.

2. Reynoso EE, Huerta F. Acute leukemia and pregnancy—fatal fetal outcome after exposure to idarubicin during the second trimester. *Acta Oncologica*. 1994;33:703-716.
3. Azuno Y, Kaku K, Fujita N, et al. Mitoxantrone and etoposide in breast milk. *Am J Hematol*. 1995;48:131-132.
4. Giacalone PL, Laffargue F, Benos P. Chemotherapy for breast carcinoma during pregnancy. *Cancer*. 1999;86:2266-2272.
5. Baumgartner AK, Oberhoffer R, Jacobs VR, et al. Reversible foetal cerebral ventriculomegaly and cardiomyopathy under chemotherapy for maternal AML. *Onkologie*. 2009;32:40-43.
6. Hellwig K, Schimrigk S, Chan A, et al. A newborn with Pierre Robin sequence after preconceptional mitoxantrone exposure of a female with multiple sclerosis. *J Neurol Sci*. 2011;307:164-165.
7. Karagiannis P, Alsdorf W, Tallarek AC, et al. Treatment of refractory acute myeloid leukaemia during pregnancy with venetoclax, high-dose cytarabine and mitoxantrone. *Br J Haematol*. 2021;192:e60-e63.

MOBOCERTINIB

Antineoplastic (Kinase Inhibitor)

PREGNANCY RECOMMENDATION: No Human Data and No Relevant Animal Data

BREASTFEEDING RECOMMENDATION: Potential Toxicity

PREGNANCY SUMMARY

No reports describing the use of mobocertinib in human pregnancy have been located. The drug and its active metabolites are likely to cross the placenta, so some fetal exposure will probably occur. Therefore, the absence of human pregnancy experience prevents a complete assessment of the embryofetal risk. Animal data showed embryofetal toxicity, but maternal toxicity was also seen. Based on animal studies and the drug's mechanism of action, the manufacturer recommends that women with reproductive potential use effective contraception during treatment and for 1 month after the last dose. They also recommend that males with female partners of reproductive potential use effective contraception during treatment and for 1 week after the last dose. Nevertheless, using this drug during pregnancy should be based on the pros and cons of the mother's clinical need for treatment versus any potential fetal risk that might occur from exposure. Mobocertinib can also prolong the QT interval, and there is a risk for torsades de pointes (an uncommon, distinct form of ventricular tachycardia that can lead to sudden death).

M

BREASTFEEDING SUMMARY

No reports describing the use of mobocertinib during human lactation have been located. The drug and its metabolites will likely be excreted into breast milk, so some infant exposure will probably occur. Due to the concern for potential serious adverse effects that might be seen in a breastfed infant, the manufacturer recommends that women not breastfeed while being treated with this drug and for at least 1 week after the last dose. Nevertheless, breastfeeding while using this drug should be based on the mother's clinical need for treatment. If used, the infant should be monitored for the most common reported adult side effects of nausea and musculoskeletal pain (both leading to irritability), diarrhea, lethargy, vomiting, decreased appetite, rash, and various laboratory abnormalities (see PI).

Reference

1. Prescribing Information. Exkivity. Takeda Pharmaceuticals America; 2021.

MODAFINIL

Central Nervous System (Stimulant)

PREGNANCY RECOMMENDATION: Limited Human Data—Animal Data Suggest Risk

BREASTFEEDING RECOMMENDATION: Potential Toxicity

PREGNANCY SUMMARY

Limited reports describing the use of modafinil in human pregnancy have been located. Available studies have found conflicting evidence of an increased risk of congenital anomalies. Some studies have reported a congenital malformation prevalence rate of up to 13%, while other studies found prevalence rates as low as 2%. With combined data, the overall rate is slightly higher than would be expected at about 5.5% in more than 450 first-trimester exposures. No pattern to the defects was identified. Modafinil will probably cross the placenta, so some fetal exposure will likely occur. However, this limited human pregnancy experience needs more study to better determine the embryofetal risk. Embryofetal toxicity was observed in two animal species at doses of less than or about equal to the RHD. Using this drug during pregnancy should be based on the pros and cons of the mother's clinical need for treatment versus any potential fetal risk that might occur from exposure.

BREASTFEEDING SUMMARY

Two reports describing the use of modafinil in seven breastfed infants found no adverse effects. The drug was found in human breast milk in low amounts. Breastfeeding while using this drug should be based on the mother's clinical need for treatment versus any potential infant risks that might occur. If used, the infant should be monitored for the most common reported adult side effects of nausea, headache, dizziness, dyspepsia, and back pain (all leading to irritability), rhinitis, and diarrhea.

References

1. Prescribing Information. Modafinil. Apotex Corp; 2024.
2. Williams SF, Alvarez JR, Pedro HF, Apuzzio JJ. Glutaric aciduria type II and narcolepsy in pregnancy. *Obstet Gynecol*. 2008;111:522-524.
3. Haervig KB, Mortensen LH, Hansen AV, Strandberg-Larsen K. Use of ADHD medication during pregnancy from 1999 to 2010: a Danish register-based study. *Pharmacoepidemiol Drug Saf*. 2014;23:526-533.
4. Damkier P, Broe A. First-trimester pregnancy exposure to modafinil and risk of congenital malformations. *JAMA*. 2020;323:374-376.
5. Leggett C, Ritchie U, Costi L, et al. Infant exposure to armodafinil through human milk following maternal use of modafinil. *J Hum Lact*. 2022;39:218-222.
6. Calvo-Ferrandiz E, Peraita-Adrados R. Narcolepsy with cataplexy and pregnancy: a case-control study. *J Sleep Res*. 2018;27:268-267.
7. Damkier P, Broe A. First-trimester pregnancy exposure to modafinil and risk of congenital malformations. *JAMA*. 2020;323:374-376.
8. Cesta CE, Engeland A, Karlsson P, et al. Incidence of malformations after early pregnancy exposure to modafinil in Sweden and Norway. *JAMA*. 2020;324:895-897.
9. Kaplan S, Braverman DL, Frishman I, Bartov N. Pregnancy and fetal outcomes following exposure to modafinil and armodafinil during pregnancy. *JAMA Intern Med*. 2021;181:275-277.
10. Onken M, Lohse L, Coulm B, et al. Effects of maternal modafinil treatment on fetal development and neonatal growth parameters—a multicenter case series of the European Network of Teratology Information Services (ENTIS). *Acta Psychiatr Scand*. 2024;150:372-384.
11. Aurora S, Aurora N, Datta P, et al. Evaluating transfer of modafinil into human milk during lactation: a case report. *J Clin Sleep Med*. 2018;14:2087-2089.
12. Anderson PO. Armodafinil in milk. *J Hum Lact*. 2023;39:223.

MOEXIPRIL

Antihypertensive (Angiotensin-Converting Enzyme Inhibitor)

PREGNANCY RECOMMENDATION: *Contraindicated (Second and Third Trimesters)

BREASTFEEDING RECOMMENDATION: Potential Toxicity

PREGNANCY SUMMARY

No reports specifically describing the use of moexipril in human pregnancy have been located. A few large studies have reported a risk for congenital anomalies with first-trimester exposure to angiotensin-converting enzyme (ACE) inhibitors as a class of drugs. These publications reported overall malformation rates of about 5% to 6%, which is higher than the expected rate of 2% to 4%. However, most of these studies also reported similar fetal anomaly rates in pregnant patients with hypertension not on treatment. The impression was that these findings might be related to the disease and not the drug. Likewise, some of these studies also reported an increase in risk for cardiac defects, but again, it was not certain as to whether this elevated risk was related to the drug or the disease. Furthermore, no pattern to the anomalies has been identified. Moexipril probably crosses the placenta, so some fetal exposure will likely occur. Therefore, the absence of first-trimester human pregnancy experience for this drug prevents a complete assessment of the embryofetal risk. Animal studies did not show any embryofetal toxicity in two species at doses of more than 10 times the MRHD in one species and less than 10 times the MRHD in the second species. *Regarding the use of ACE inhibitors in the second half of pregnancy, numerous case reports and reviews have reported that these drugs can, in some cases, produce severe fetal renal dysfunction. This can lead to anomalies related to longstanding oligohydramnios and fetal/neonatal death. There are cases, however, where the process reverses itself when the drug is discontinued. These findings are similar to those seen with angiotensin receptor blockers (ARBs). The drug actually carries a boxed warning for these risks. Women of reproductive age using moexipril should be informed of these risks, so they can be closely monitored if pregnancy transpires. If a positive pregnancy test occurs, she and her health care providers can modify treatment (if possible) so that the drug is not used in the second or third trimesters. For treating hypertension in pregnancy, ACOG recommends nifedipine and labetalol as first-line agents.

BREASTFEEDING SUMMARY

No reports describing the use of moexipril in human lactation have been located. The drug will probably be found in human breast milk, so some infant exposure will likely occur. The manufacturer recommends caution in using this drug while breastfeeding. Nevertheless, breastfeeding while using moexipril should be based on the mother's clinical need for treatment versus any potential infant risks that might occur. If used, the infant should be monitored for the most common reported adult side effects of headache, nausea, myalgia, and dizziness (all leading to irritability), cough, rash, hypotension, diarrhea, and fatigue (lethargy). ACOG and the American Heart Association (AHA) consider ACE inhibitors compatible for use during breastfeeding.

References

1. Prescribing Information. Moexipril. Glenmark Pharmaceuticals Inc; 2024.
2. Cooper WO, Hernandez-Diaz S, Arbogast PG, et al. Major congenital malformations after first-trimester exposure to ACE inhibitors. *N Engl J Med*. 2006;354:2443-2451.
3. Friedman JM. ACE inhibitors and congenital anomalies. *N Engl J Med*. 2006;354:2498-2500.
4. Scialli AR, Lione A. ACE inhibitors and major congenital malformations. *N Engl J Med*. 2006;355:1280.
5. Cooper WO, Ray WA. Reply—ACE inhibitors and major congenital malformations. *N Engl J Med*. 2006;355:1281.
6. Barr M Jr. Teratogen update: angiotensin-converting enzyme inhibitors. *Teratology*. 1994;50:399-409.
7. Shotan A, Widerhorn J, Hurst A, Elkayam U. Risks of angiotensin-converting enzyme inhibition during pregnancy: experimental and clinical evidence, potential mechanisms, and recommendations for use. *Am J Med*. 1994;96:451-456.
8. Robillard JE, Nakamura KT, Matherne GP, Jose PA. Renal hemodynamics and functional adjustments to postnatal life. *Semin Perinatol*. 1988;12:143-150.
9. Guignard J-P, Gouyon J-B. Adverse effects of drugs on the immature kidney. *Biol Neonate*. 1988;53:243-252.
10. Brent RL, Beckman DA. Angiotensin-converting enzyme inhibitors, an embryopathic class of drugs with unique properties: information for clinical teratology counselors. *Teratology*. 1991;43:543-546.
11. Polifka JE. Is there an embryopathy associated with first-trimester exposure to angiotensin-converting enzyme inhibitors and angiotensin receptor antagonists? A critical review of the evidence. *Birth Defects Res A Clin Mol Teratol*. 2012;94:576-598.
12. Hoeltzenbein M, Tissen-Diabate T, Fietz AK, et al. Increased rate of birth defects after first trimester use of angiotensin converting enzyme inhibitors—treatment or hypertension related? An observational cohort study. *Pregnancy Hypertens*. 2018;13:65-71.
13. American College of Obstetricians and Gynecologists' Committee on Practice Bulletins—Obstetrics. ACOG practice bulletin no. 203: chronic hypertension in pregnancy. *Obstet Gynecol*. 2019;133:e26-e50.
14. Heidenreich PA, Bozkurt B, Aguilar D, et al. 2022 AHA/ACC/HFSA guideline for the management of heart failure: a report of the American College of Cardiology/American Heart Association Joint Committee on Clinical Practice Guidelines. *Circulation*. 2022;145:e895-e1032.

MOGAMULIZUMAB

Antineoplastic (Monoclonal Antibody)

PREGNANCY RECOMMENDATION: No Human Data—Animal Data Suggest Low Risk

BREASTFEEDING RECOMMENDATION: Probably Compatible

M

PREGNANCY SUMMARY

No reports describing the use of mogamulizumab in human pregnancy have been located. As an IgG antibody, it likely crosses the placenta, especially during the second half of gestation, so some fetal exposure will probably occur. Therefore, the absence of human pregnancy experience prevents a complete assessment of the embryofetal risk. Animal data did not show any embryofetal toxicity in one species at doses of greater than 10 times the RHD. However, based on the drug's mechanism of action, the manufacturer recommends that women with reproductive potential use effective contraception during treatment and for 3 months after the last dose. Nevertheless, using this drug during pregnancy should be based on the pros and cons of the mother's clinical need for treatment versus any potential fetal risk that might occur from exposure.

BREASTFEEDING SUMMARY

No reports describing the use of mogamulizumab during human lactation have been found. It is known that IgG antibodies can be found in human breast milk but are not found in the neonatal or infant circulation. Additionally, if any IgG antibodies were to be ingested through breastfeeding, they would probably be digested in the infant's gastrointestinal tract and not be absorbed. If the clinical decision is to use this drug while breastfeeding, the infant should be monitored for the most common reported adult side effects of musculoskeletal pain (leading to irritability), rash, fatigue (lethargy), diarrhea, and upper respiratory tract infection.

Reference

1. Prescribing Information. Poteligeo. Kyowa Kirin; 2025.

MOMELOTINIB

Antineoplastic (Janus Kinase Inhibitor)

PREGNANCY RECOMMENDATION: No Human Data—Animal Data Suggest Risk

BREASTFEEDING RECOMMENDATION: Potential Toxicity

PREGNANCY SUMMARY

No reports describing the use of momelotinib in human pregnancy have been located. The drug will likely cross the placenta, so some fetal exposure will probably occur. Therefore, the absence of human pregnancy experience prevents a complete assessment of the embryofetal risk. Animal studies did show embryofetal toxicity with malformations in two species at doses of less than the RHD. Based on these animal studies and the drug's mechanism of action, the manufacturer recommends that women with reproductive potential use effective contraception during treatment and for 1 week after the last dose. Nevertheless, using this drug during pregnancy should be based on the pros and cons of the mother's clinical need for treatment versus any potential fetal risk that might occur from exposure. There is a registry for women who are pregnant and have cancer. For more information, women and health care providers are encouraged to contact the Cancer and Pregnancy Registry at 1-877-635-4499.

BREASTFEEDING SUMMARY

No reports describing the use of momelotinib during human lactation have been located. The drug will likely be found in breast milk, so some infant exposure will probably occur. Due to a concern for potential serious adverse effects that might be seen in a breastfed infant, the manufacturer recommends that women not breastfeed while being treated with this drug and for 2 weeks after the last dose. Nevertheless, breastfeeding while using this drug should be based on the mother's clinical need for treatment versus any potential infant risk that might occur. If used, the infant should be monitored for the most common reported adult side effects of nausea, dizziness, headache, and abdominal pain (all leading to irritability), fatigue (lethargy), rash, fever, diarrhea, and various laboratory abnormalities (See PI).

Reference

1. Prescribing Information. Ojjaara. GlaxoSmithKline; 2023.

MOMETASONE

Corticosteroid

PREGNANCY RECOMMENDATION: Limited Human Data—Animal Data Suggest Risk

BREASTFEEDING RECOMMENDATION: Probably Compatible

PREGNANCY SUMMARY

One study describing the use of intranasal mometasone in more than 1,100 pregnancies reported no association with an increased risk for congenital anomalies. The drug will probably cross the placenta, but the very low systemic bioavailability suggests that the amount should be clinically insignificant. Embryofetal toxicity with malformations was observed in three animal species at doses less than 10 times the MRHD. ACOG recommends that, while budesonide is considered the inhaled corticosteroid of choice during pregnancy, women who are well controlled by other inhaled corticosteroids prior to pregnancy should continue using those agents. Use of occlusive dressings with topical use can increase the amount of systemic absorption. Topical use of corticosteroids during pregnancy should be limited to the least potent effective dose, shortest duration, and the smallest area of skin possible while avoiding areas with high absorption, such as the eyelids, skin folds, and vulva.

BREASTFEEDING SUMMARY

No reports describing the use of mometasone during human lactation have been located. The National Asthma Education and Prevention Program expert panel considers inhaled corticosteroids compatible with breastfeeding. If the drug were to be found in the maternal circulation, it would likely be found in human breast milk. However, the very low systemic concentrations obtained after use of the inhaled, intranasal, and topical formulations suggest that any excreted amount would likely be clinically insignificant. Topical use of corticosteroids while breastfeeding should be limited to the least potent effective dose and the smallest area of skin possible, avoiding the areas where the infant's skin may come into direct contact. Direct application to the nipple or areola should be avoided. If needed, lower-potency, water-miscible cream or gel products should be used and applied after breastfeeding, then wiped off prior to the next feeding.

References

1. Prescribing Information. Asmanex Twisthaler. Organon & Co; 2021.
2. Prescribing Information. Nasonex. L. Perrigo Company; 2024.
3. Prescribing Information. Mometasone furoate. Cosette Pharmaceuticals Inc; 2023.
4. National Heart, Lung, and Blood Institute; National Asthma Education and Prevention Program Asthma and Pregnancy Working Group. NAEPP expert panel report. Managing asthma during pregnancy: recommendations for pharmacologic treatment-2004 update. *J Allergy Clin Immunol*. 2005; 115:34-46.
5. Asthma in pregnancy. ACOG practice bulletin no. 90. American College of Obstetricians and Gynecologists. *Obstet Gynecol*. 2008;111:457-464.
6. Alhussien AH, Alhedaithy RA, Alsaleh SA. Safety of intranasal corticosteroid sprays during pregnancy: an updated review. *Eur Arch Otorhinolaryngol*. 2018;275:325-333.

MONTELUKAST

Respiratory (Leukotriene Receptor Antagonist)

PREGNANCY RECOMMENDATION: Human Data and Animal Data Suggest Low Risk

BREASTFEEDING RECOMMENDATION: Probably Compatible

PREGNANCY SUMMARY

Numerous studies were located that describe the use of montelukast in human pregnancy. From a total of more than 1,250 first-trimester exposures, the prevalence rate of major malformations was 2.9%, and no pattern to the defects was seen. In addition, a recent 2024 review and meta-analysis also reported no significant increase in major birth defects with early pregnancy usage of montelukast. The drug will probably cross the placenta, so some fetal exposure will likely occur. Animal data did not show any embryofetal toxicity in two species at doses of more than 10 times the MRHD. While ACOG considers long-acting β-agonists as the preferred add-on controller therapy for asthma in pregnancy, leukotriene receptor antagonists, such as montelukast, may be used as alternative add-on therapies.

BREASTFEEDING SUMMARY

One report of seven lactating women was located that described the use of montelukast during human lactation. The drug was found in human breast milk with a peak concentration of about 10 ng/mL and a mean concentration of about 5.3 ng/mL. The calculated RID was less than 1%. Breastfeeding while using this drug should be based on the mother's clinical need for treatment versus any potential infant risks that might occur. If used, the infant should be monitored for the most common reported adult side effects of headache and abdominal pain (both leading to irritability), fever, cough, diarrhea, and various infections.

M

References

1. Prescribing Information. Montelukast. XLCare Pharmaceuticals; 2023.
2. American College of Obstetricians and Gynecologists. Asthma in pregnancy: ACOG practice bulletin no. 90. *Obstet Gynecol*. 2008;111:457-464.
3. Bakhireva LN, Jones KL, Schatz M, et al; the Organization of Teratology Information Specialists Collaborative Research Group. Safety of leukotriene receptor antagonists in pregnancy. *J Allergy Clin Immunol*. 2007;119:618-625.
4. Sarkar M, Koren G, Kalra S, et al. Montelukast use during pregnancy: a multicentre, prospective, comparative study of infant outcomes. *Eur J Clin Pharmacol*. 2009;65:1259-1264.
5. Cavero-Carbonell C, Vinkel-Hansen A, Rabanque-Hernandez MJ, et al. Fetal exposure to montelukast and congenital anomalies: a population based study in Denmark. *Birth Defects Res*. 2017;109:452-459.
6. Datta P, Rewers-Felkins K, Baker T, Hale TW. Transfer of montelukast into human milk during lactation. *Breastfeed Med*. 2017;12:54-57.
7. Hatakeyama S, Goto M, Yamamoto A, et al. The safety of pranlukast and montelukast during the first trimester of pregnancy: a prospective, two-centered cohort study in Japan. *Congenit Anom (Kyoto)*. 2022;62:161-168.
8. Fareed A, Siblini D, Vaid R, et al. Montelukast use in pregnancy: a systematic review and meta-analysis of maternal and fetal outcomes in asthma treatment. *Congenit Anom (Kyoto)*. 2024;64:220-227.

MORPHINE

Pain (Opioid Agonist)

PREGNANCY RECOMMENDATION: *Human Data Suggest Risk

BREASTFEEDING RECOMMENDATION: Probably Compatible

PREGNANCY SUMMARY

The Collaborative Perinatal Project reported 70 first-trimester exposures to morphine, with 2 (2.9%) major anomalies identified. Similar to other opioid analgesics, the use of morphine late in pregnancy has the potential to cause respiratory depression and withdrawal symptoms in the newborn. The use of opioids, including morphine, during pregnancy should be based on the pros and cons of the mother's clinical need for treatment versus any potential fetal risk that might occur from exposure. *NAS or NOWS may occur with prolonged exposure to opioids. The onset, duration, and severity of withdrawal vary based on the opioid used, duration of use, timing and amount of last maternal use, and elimination of the drug by the newborn. Infants exposed to opioids should be monitored for symptoms of NOWS postdelivery.

BREASTFEEDING SUMMARY

Limited reports describing the use of morphine during human lactation have been located. The drug is excreted into human breast milk, so infant exposure will occur. However, the amount that reaches the infant after IV or epidural use during labor or shortly thereafter is expected to be small and likely not cause any adverse effects in the infant. Breastfeeding while using this drug should be based on the mother's clinical need for treatment versus any potential infant risks that might occur. If used, the infant should be monitored for the most common reported adult side effects of drowsiness, sedation, difficulty feeding, and lethargy.

References

1. Prescribing Information. Morphine sulfate. Amneal Pharmaceuticals of New York LLC; 2024.
2. Perlstein MA. Congenital morphinism. A rare cause of convulsions in the newborn. *JAMA*. 1947;135:633.
3. Fisher DE, Paton JB. The effect of maternal anesthetic and analgesic drugs on the fetus and newborn. *Clin Obstet Gynaecol*. 1974;17:275-287.
4. Bonica JJ. *Principles and Practice of Obstetric Analgesia and Anesthesia*. FA Davis; 1967:247.
5. McMullin GP, Mobarak AN. Congenital narcotic addiction. *Arch Dis Child*. 1970;45:140-141.
6. Cobrinik RW, Hodd RT Jr, Chusid E. The effect of maternal narcotic addiction on the newborn infant. *Pediatrics*. 1959;24:288-304.
7. Gilbert G, Dixon AB. Observations on demerol as an obstetric analgesic. *Am J Obstet Gynecol*. 1943;45:320-326.
8. Way WL, Costley EC, Way EL. Respiratory sensitivity of the newborn infant to meperidine and morphine. *Clin Pharmacol Ther*. 1965;6:454-461.
9. Nybell-Lindahl G, Carlsson C, Ingemarsson I, et al. Maternal and fetal concentrations of morphine after epidural administration during labor. *Am J Obstet Gynecol*. 1981;139:20-21.
10. Baraka A, Noueihid R, Hajj S. Intrathecal injection of morphine for obstetric analgesia. *Anesthesiology*. 1981;54:136-140.
11. Bonnardot JP, Maillet M, Colau JC, et al. Maternal and fetal concentration of morphine after intrathecal administration during labour. *Br J Anaesth*. 1982;54:487-489.
12. Brizgys RV, Shnider SM. Hyperbaric intrathecal morphine analgesia during labor in a patient with Wolff-Parkinson-White syndrome. *Obstet Gynecol*. 1984;64:44S-46S.
13. Heinonen OP, Slone D, Shapiro S. *Birth Defects and Drugs in Pregnancy*. Publishing Sciences Group; 1977.
14. Broussard CS, Rasmussen SA, Reefhuis J, et al. The National Birth Defects Prevention Study. *Am J Obstet Gynecol*. 2011;204:314-317.
15. Terwilliger WG, Hatcher RA. The elimination of morphine and quinine in human milk. *Surg Gynecol Obstet*. 1934;58:823-826.
16. Kwit NT, Hatcher RA. Excretion of drugs in milk. *Am J Dis Child*. 1935; 49:900-904.
17. Anonymous. Drugs in breast milk. *Med Lett Drugs Ther*. 1979;21:21-24.
18. Robieux I, Koren G, Vandenbergh H, Schneiderman J. Morphine excretion in breast milk and resultant exposure of a nursing infant. *J Toxicol Clin Toxicol*. 1990;28:365-370.
19. American College of Obstetricians and Gynecologists. Opioid use and opioid use disorder in pregnancy: committee opinion no. 711. *Obstet Gynecol*. 2017;130:e81-e94.
20. American College of Obstetricians and Gynecologists. Obstetric analgesia and anesthesia: ACOG practice bulletin no. 209. *Obstet Gynecol*. 2019;133: e208-e225.
21. Kopecky EA, Simone C, Knie B, Koren G. Transfer of morphine across the human placenta and its interaction with naloxone. *Life Sci*. 1999; 65:2359-2371.

MOSUNETUZUMAB

Antineoplastic (Anti-CD3 and Anti-CD20—Monoclonal Antibody)

PREGNANCY RECOMMENDATION: No Human Data and No Relevant Animal Data

BREASTFEEDING RECOMMENDATION: Probably Compatible

PREGNANCY SUMMARY

No reports describing the use of mosunetuzumab in human pregnancy have been located. As an IgG antibody, the drug will likely cross the placenta, so some fetal exposure will probably occur. Therefore, the absence of human pregnancy experience prevents a complete assessment of embryofetal risk. No animal studies have been conducted. Theoretically, pregnancy maintenance may be compromised due to T-cell activation and cytokine release caused by mosunetuzumab. Additionally, B-cell depletion has been observed in nonpregnant animals, so use during pregnancy may result in B-cell lymphocytopenia in exposed infants. Based on the drug's mechanism of action, the manufacturer recommends that women with reproductive potential use effective contraception during treatment and for 3 months after the last dose. Nevertheless, using this drug during pregnancy should be based on the pros and cons of the mother's clinical need for treatment versus any potential fetal risk that might occur from exposure. Women who are pregnant and have cancer are encouraged to contact the Cancer and Pregnancy Registry at 877-635-4499.

BREASTFEEDING SUMMARY

No reports describing the use of mosunetuzumab during human lactation have been located. It is known that IgG antibodies can be found in human breast milk, but are not found in the neonatal or infant circulation. Additionally, if any IgG antibodies were to be ingested through breastfeeding, they would probably be digested in the infant's gastrointestinal tract and not be absorbed. Based on the drug's mechanism of action, the manufacturer recommends that women not breastfeed while using mosunetuzumab and for 3 months after the last dose. Nevertheless, breastfeeding while using this drug should be based on the mother's clinical need for treatment. If used, the infant should be monitored for the most common reported adult side effects of headache (leading to irritability), cytokine release syndrome, lethargy, rash, pyrexia, and various laboratory abnormalities (see PI).

Reference

1. Prescribing Information. Lunsumio. Genentech, Inc; 2022.

MOTIXAFORTIDE

Hematologic (Hematopoietic Stem Cell Mobilizer)

PREGNANCY RECOMMENDATION: No Human Data—Animal Data Suggest Potential Risk

BREASTFEEDING RECOMMENDATION: Probably Compatible

PREGNANCY SUMMARY

No reports describing the use of motixafortide in human pregnancy have been located. The drug is not likely to cross the placenta; however, because it consists of a protein, it is not known whether some fetal exposure could occur in the second half of gestation. Nevertheless, the absence of human pregnancy experience prevents a complete assessment of the embryofetal risk. Animal reproduction or fertility studies have not been conducted with motixafortide. However, disruption of CXCR4 and SDF-1α signaling did increase the risk for embryofetal lethality in mice. Based on animal studies and the drug's mechanism of action, the manufacturer recommends that women with reproductive potential use effective contraception during treatment and for 8 days after the last dose. Regardless, using this drug during pregnancy should be based on the pros and cons of the mother's clinical need for treatment versus any potential fetal risk that might occur from exposure.

BREASTFEEDING SUMMARY

No reports describing the use of motixafortide during human lactation have been located. The drug will probably not be excreted into breast milk in clinically significant amounts. In addition, because it is a peptide, if the drug were to be ingested through breastfeeding, it would probably be digested in the infant's gastrointestinal tract and not be absorbed. However, due to a concern for potential serious adverse effects that might be seen in a breastfed infant, the manufacturer recommends that women not breastfeed while being treated with this drug and for at least 8 days after the last dose. Nevertheless, breastfeeding while using this drug should be based on the mother's clinical need for treatment. If used, the infant should be monitored for the most common reported adult side effects of pruritus and back pain (both leading to irritability) and flushing.

M

Reference

1. Prescribing Information. Aphexda. BioLineRx; 2023.

MOXETUMOMAB PASUDOTOX

Antineoplastic (Monoclonal Antibody)

PREGNANCY RECOMMENDATION: No Human Data and No Relevant Animal Data

BREASTFEEDING RECOMMENDATION: Potential Toxicity

PREGNANCY SUMMARY

No reports describing the use of moxetumomab pasudotox in human pregnancy have been located. Because it is an antibody, it probably crosses the placenta, so some fetal exposure will likely occur. However, the absence of human pregnancy experience prevents a complete assessment of the embryofetal risk. Animal reproduction studies were not performed. The drug has the potential to cause capillary leak syndrome and hemolytic uremic syndrome. Because of the mechanism of action, the manufacturer recommends that females of reproductive potential use effective contraception during treatment with moxetumomab pasudotox and for at least 30 days after the last dose. Nevertheless, using this drug during pregnancy should be based on the pros and cons of the mother's clinical need for treatment versus any fetal risk that might occur from exposure.

BREASTFEEDING SUMMARY

Moxetumomab pasudotox probably enters human breast milk. However, it is known that antibodies can be found in breast milk but are not found in the neonatal or infant circulation. Furthermore, because the immunoglobulin and the endotoxin are both proteins, if ingested through breastfeeding, they most likely would be digested in the infant's gastrointestinal tract and not be absorbed. Regardless, the manufacturer recommends that women not breastfeed their infants if treated with this drug. Nevertheless, breastfeeding while using moxetumomab pasudotox should be based on the mother's clinical need for treatment. If used, the infant should be monitored for the most common reported adult side effects of nausea and headache (both leading to irritability), edema, lethargy, pyrexia, constipation, and diarrhea.

Reference

1. Prescribing Information. Lumoxiti. AstraZeneca Pharmaceuticals LP; 2018.

MOXIDECTIN

Anti-Infective (Anthelmintic)

PREGNANCY RECOMMENDATION: No Human Data—Animal Data Suggest Low Risk

BREASTFEEDING RECOMMENDATION: Probably Compatible

PREGNANCY SUMMARY

No reports describing the use of moxidectin in human pregnancy have been located. Some amount of the drug will probably cross the placenta, so fetal exposure will likely occur. However, the absence of human pregnancy experience prevents a complete assessment of the embryofetal risk. Animal data did not show any embryofetal toxicity. Using this drug during pregnancy should be based on the pros and cons of the mother's clinical need for treatment versus any potential fetal risk that might occur from exposure. A serious and possibly even fatal encephalopathy can occur in patients coinfected with Loa loa who are treated with moxidectin.

BREASTFEEDING SUMMARY

Moxidectin was evaluated in the breast milk of 12 lactating women over a period of 28 days. The total mean amount of drug found in the breast milk was 56 ng (if an infant consumed all the breast milk during that time period). The overall RID was about 9% of the maternal dose. Breastfeeding while using this drug should be based on the mother's clinical need for treatment. If used, the infant should be monitored for the most common reported adult side effects of pruritus, musculoskeletal pain, headache, and abdominal pain (all leading to irritability), hypotension, pyrexia, cough, diarrhea, and peripheral swelling.

References

1. Prescribing Information. Moxidectin. Medicines Development for Global Health; 2018.
2. Korth-Bradley JM, Parks V, Chalon S, et al. Excretion of moxidectin into breast milk and pharmacokinetics in healthy lactating women. *Antimicrob Agents Chemother*. 2011;55(11):5200-5204.

M

MOXIFLOXACIN

Antibacterial (Fluoroquinolone)

PREGNANCY RECOMMENDATION: *Limited Human Data—Animal Data Suggest Potential Risk

BREASTFEEDING RECOMMENDATION: Potential Toxicity

PREGNANCY SUMMARY

Four reports describing the use of moxifloxacin in human pregnancy have been located. According to reports, the drug was not found to have an increased risk of major congenital anomalies when compared with controls. *However, three studies found a higher rate of major congenital anomalies with first-trimester use when compared with other fluoroquinolones. No specific pattern to the defects was seen except for one. The FDA Adverse Event Reporting System demonstrated a signal that indicated a potential increase in multiple congenital cardiac abnormalities. Moxifloxacin crosses the placenta, so fetal exposure will occur. Therefore, this limited human pregnancy experience still prevents a complete assessment of the embryofetal risk. Embryofetal and maternal toxicity were observed in two animal species at doses less than 10 times the MRHD. Using this drug during pregnancy should be based on the pros and cons of the mother's clinical need for treatment versus any potential fetal risk that might occur from exposure. Regardless, alternate fluoroquinolone drugs might be considered for early pregnancy use until further analysis of this specific drug occurs. Moxifloxacin is associated with QT prolongation. Monitor QTc interval prior to and during treatment.

BREASTFEEDING SUMMARY

No reports describing the use of moxifloxacin in human lactation have been located. The drug will probably be found in human breast milk, so some infant exposure will likely occur. The effect of this exposure on a nursing infant is unknown. Breastfeeding while using this drug should be based on the mother's clinical need for treatment versus any potential infant risks that might occur. If used, the infant should be monitored for the most common reported adult side effects of nausea, headache, and dizziness (all leading to irritability), and diarrhea.

References

1. Prescribing Information. Moxifloxacin Hydrochloride. Teva Pharmaceuticals; 2024.
2. Prescribing Information. Moxifloxacin Hydrochloride Injection. Mylan Institutional LLC; 2024.
3. Ozyuncu O, Nemutlu E, Katlan D, et al. Maternal and fetal blood levels of moxifloxacin, levofloxacin, cefepime and cefoperazone. *Int J Antimicrob Agents*. 2010;36:175-178.
4. Ozyuncu O, Beksac MS, Nemutlu E, et al. Maternal blood and amniotic fluid levels of moxifloxacin, levofloxacin and cefixime. *J Obstet Gynecol*. 2010;36:484-487.
5. Padberg S, Wacker E, Meiser R, et al. Observational cohort study of pregnancy outcome after first-trimester exposure to fluoroquinolones. *Antimicrob Agents Chemother*. 2014;58:4392-4398.
6. Muanda FT, Sheehy O, Berard A. Use of antibiotics during pregnancy and the risk of major congenital malformations: a population based cohort study. *Br J Clin Pharmacol*. 2017;83:2557-2571.
7. Cuff RD, Carter E, Taam R, et al. Effect of antibiotic treatment of amniotic fluid sludge. *Am J Obstet Gynecol MFM*. 2020;2:100073.
8. Xiang DC, Xie WL, Cheng GY, et al J. Pregnancy related adverse events and congenital disorders associated with fluoroquinolones: a real-world pharmacovigilance study of the FDA adverse event reporting system (FAERS). *Heliyon*. 2024;10:e37547.

MOXIFLOXACIN OPHTHALMIC

Antibacterial/Ophthalmic (Fluoroquinolone)

PREGNANCY RECOMMENDATION: No Human Data—Animal Data Suggest Low Risk

BREASTFEEDING RECOMMENDATION: Probably Compatible

PREGNANCY SUMMARY

No reports describing the use of moxifloxacin ophthalmic in human pregnancy have been located. The drug will probably cross the placenta, so some fetal exposure will likely occur. Therefore, the absence of human pregnancy experience prevents a complete assessment of the embryofetal risk. Animal data did not show any embryofetal toxicity in two species at doses of more than 10 times the recommended human ophthalmic dose (RHOD). Using this drug during pregnancy should be based on the pros and cons of the mother's clinical need for treatment versus any potential fetal risk that might occur from exposure. If used during pregnancy, consider placing pressure over the tear duct in the corner of the eye for at least 1 minute, and then remove any excess solution with absorbent tissue to decrease the amount of drug reaching the systemic circulation even further.

M

BREASTFEEDING SUMMARY

No reports describing the use of moxifloxacin ophthalmic during human lactation have been located. The drug will probably be found in human breast milk if found in the maternal circulation, but the low systemic concentrations seen with ocular use suggest that the amount is likely to be clinically insignificant. Breastfeeding while using this drug should be based on the mother's clinical need for treatment versus any potential infant risks that might occur. A method to decrease some systemic absorption with ophthalmic use is described above in the Pregnancy Summary.

Reference

1. Prescribing Information. Moxifloxacin Hydrochloride Solution/Drops. Somerset Therapeutics, LLC; 2024.

MUPIROCIN

Antibacterial (Topical)

PREGNANCY RECOMMENDATION: No Human Data—Animal Data Suggest Low Risk

BREASTFEEDING RECOMMENDATION: Probably Compatible

PREGNANCY SUMMARY

No reports describing the use of mupirocin in human pregnancy have been located. The drug will probably cross the placenta, so some fetal exposure will likely occur. Therefore, the absence of human pregnancy experience prevents a complete assessment of the embryofetal risk. Animal data did not show any embryofetal toxicity in two species at doses of more than 10 times the human topical dose. Using this drug during pregnancy should be based on the pros and cons of the mother's clinical need for treatment versus any potential fetal risk that might occur from exposure.

BREASTFEEDING SUMMARY

One report describing the use of topical mupirocin cream by a breastfeeding mother reported no infant adverse effects. The drug may be found in human breast milk, but the minimal systemic absorption following topical administration should limit excretion. Breastfeeding while using this drug should be based on the mother's clinical need for treatment versus any potential infant risks that might occur. Because of the topical use, adult systemic side effects were not reported. Mupirocin should not be applied to the breast or nipple area, if possible, but if used in this area, it should be thoroughly wiped off prior to breastfeeding.

References

1. Prescribing Information. Mupirocin. NuCare Pharmaceuticals, Inc; 2024.
2. Kaplan YC, Keskin-Arslan E, Acar S, et al. Teicoplanin use during breastfeeding. *Breastfeed Med* 2017;12:124

MYCOPHENOLATE MOFETIL

Immunologic (Immunosuppressive)

PREGNANCY RECOMMENDATION: Human Data Suggest Risk

BREASTFEEDING RECOMMENDATION: Potential Toxicity

PREGNANCY SUMMARY

Numerous studies have been located that describe the use of mycophenolate mofetil (MMF) during human pregnancy. Most involve case reports that have resulted in numerous fetal anomalies. In large analyses, the rate of major congenital malformations is elevated from the expected baseline rate in the 6% to 8% range. However, when smaller studies are combined, the risk may be higher. Overall, there may be an MMF fetopathy that involves cleft lip and palate, external ear defects (including absent ear canals), distal limb or digit defects, and esophageal, renal, and cardiac abnormalities. The FDA reported this in 2007 and changed the pregnancy rating for this drug at that time from category C to D. Additionally, the risk of first-trimester loss with use of this drug has been reported to be as high as 45%. It is not fully known if the active moiety of MMF, mycophenolic acid (MPA), crosses the placenta, but based on pK parameters, it likely does, so fetal exposure probably occurs. Animal studies also showed embryofetal toxicity in two species at doses of less than the RHD. Due to this spectrum of reported congenital malformations, the manufacturer recommends that women with reproductive potential use effective contraception during treatment and for 6 weeks after the last dose. They also recommend that males with female partners of reproductive potential use effective contraception during treatment and for at least 90 days after the last dose. There is a pregnancy exposure registry that monitors pregnancy outcomes in women exposed to mycophenolate during pregnancy and those who become pregnant within 6 weeks of discontinuing MMF treatment. To report a pregnancy or obtain information about the registry, health care providers should call 1-800-617-8191. Mycophenolate carries a boxed warning regarding embryofetal toxicity.

BREASTFEEDING SUMMARY

Four reports describing the use of a MMF during human lactation have been located. No adverse infant outcomes were reported in two case series that included 12 infants. The drug will probably be found in human breast milk, so some infant exposure will likely occur. Breastfeeding while using this drug should be based on the mother's clinical need for treatment versus any potential infant risks that might occur. If used, the infant should be monitored for the most common reported adult side effects of diarrhea, leukopenia, infection, vomiting, and certain types of opportunistic infections.

References

1. Prescribing Information. Mycophenolate Mofetil. Lupin Pharmaceuticals, Inc; 2023.
2. Prescribing Information. Mycophenolate Mofetil, Meitheal Pharmaceuticals; 2023.
3. Pisoni CN, D'Cruz DP. The safety of mycophenolate mofetil in pregnancy. *Expert Opin Drug Saf.* 2008;7:219-222.
4. Casele HL, Laifer SA. Pregnancy after liver transplantation. *Semin Perinatol.* 1998;22:149-155.
5. Pergola PE, Kancharla A, Riley DJ. Kidney transplantation during the first trimester of pregnancy: immunosuppression with mycophenolate mofetil, tacrolimus, and prednisone. *Transplantation.* 2001;71:994-997.
6. Le Ray C, Coulomb A, Elefant E, et al. Mycophenolate mofetil in pregnancy after renal transplantation: a case of major fetal malformations. *Obstet Gynecol.* 2004;103:1091-1094.
7. Gutierrez MJ, Acebedo-Ribo M, Garcia-Donaire JA, et al. Pregnancy in renal transplant recipients. *Transplant Proc.* 2005;37:3721-3722.
8. Armenti VT, Radomski JS, Moritz MJ, et al. Report from the National Transplantation Pregnancy Registry (NTPR): outcomes of pregnancy after transplantation. *Clin Transpl.* 2005:69-83.
9. Sifontis NM, Coscia LA, Constantinescu S, et al. Pregnancy outcomes in solid organ transplant recipients with exposure to mycophenolate mofetil or sirolimus. *Transplantation.* 2006;82:1698-1702.
10. Naqvi R, Nor H, Ambaries S, et al. Outcome of pregnancy in renal allograft recipients: SIUT experience. *Transplant Proc.* 2006;38:2001-2002.
11. Tjeertes IFA, Bastiaans DET, van Ganzewinkel CJLM, Zegers SHJ. Neonatal anemia and hydrops fetalis after maternal mycophenolate mofetil use. *J Perinatal.* 2007;27:62-64.
12. El Sebaaly Z, Charpentier B, Snanoudj R. Fetal malformations associated with mycophenolate mofetil for lupus nephritis. *Nephrol Dial Transplant.* 2007;22:2722.
13. Schoner K, Steinhard J, Figiel J, Rehder H. Severe facial clefts in acrofacial dysostosis. *Obstet Gynecol.* 2008;111:483-486.

M

14. Velinov M, Zellers N. The fetal mycophenolate mofetil syndrome. *Clin Dysmorphol*. 2008;17:77-78.
15. Ghafari A, Sanadgol H. Pregnancy after renal transplantation: ten-year single-center experience. *Transplant Proc*. 2008;40:251-252.
16. Perez-Aytes A, Ledo A, Boso V, et al. In utero exposure to mycophenolate mofetil: a characteristic phenotype? *Am J Med Genet A*. 2008;146A:1-7.
17. King RW, Baca MJ, Armenti VT, Kaplan B. Pregnancy outcomes related to mycophenolate exposure in female kidney transplant recipients. *Am J Transplant*. 2017;17:151-160.
18. Constantinescu S, Pai A, Coscia LA, et al. Breast-feeding after transplantation. *Best Pract Res Clin Obstet Gynaecol*. 2014;28:1163-1173.
19. Punnoose LR, Coscia LA, Armenti DP, et al. Pregnancy outcomes in heart transplant recipients. *J Heart Lung Transplant*. 2020;39:473-480.
20. Mohamed-Ahmed O, Nelson-Piercy C, Bramham K, et al. Pregnancy outcomes in liver and cardiothoracic transplant recipients: a UK national cohort study. *PLoS One*. 2014;9:e89151.
21. Boyle S, Sung-Him Mew T, Lust K, et al. Pregnancy following heart transplantation: a single centre case series and review of the literature. *Heart Lung Circ*. 2021;30:144-153.

N

NABUMETONE

Pain (Nonsteroidal Anti-Inflammatory Drug)

PREGNANCY RECOMMENDATION: Human Data Suggest Risk (Second and Third Trimesters)

BREASTFEEDING RECOMMENDATION: Potential Toxicity

PREGNANCY SUMMARY

One report describing the use of nabumetone in human pregnancy has been located. The report assessed the risk of preterm birth in 130,815 pregnancies exposed to nonsteroidal anti-inflammatory drugs (NSAIDs), 947 of which received nabumetone. Overall, NSAIDs were associated with an increased risk for premature birth, including nabumetone. The drug will probably cross the placenta, so some fetal exposure will likely occur. Therefore, this limited first-trimester human pregnancy experience prevents a complete assessment of the embryofetal risk. Embryofetal toxicity was observed in one animal species at doses of about equal to the maximum recommended human dose (MRHD). NSAIDs can cause premature stricture or closure of the fetal ductus arteriosus when used in the latter portion of gestation. In some instances, this can produce persistent pulmonary hypertension in the neonate. These drugs have also been reported to produce fetal renal dysfunction leading to oligohydramnios when used after 20 weeks' gestation. The US Food and Drug Administration (FDA) recommends that NSAIDs be avoided in women 20 weeks or later in pregnancy. If deemed necessary by a health care provider, the use of NSAIDs between 20 and 30 weeks should be limited to the lowest effective dose and shortest duration. If treatment extends beyond 48 hours, providers should consider an ultrasound to monitor amniotic fluid levels.

BREASTFEEDING SUMMARY

No reports describing the use of nabumetone during human lactation have been located. The drug will probably appear in breast milk, so some infant exposure will likely occur. Breastfeeding while using this drug should be based on the mother's clinical need for treatment versus any potential infant risks that might occur. If used, the infant should be monitored for the most common reported adult side effects of nausea, upset stomach, and abdominal pain (all leading to irritability).

References

1. Levin DL. Effects of inhibition of prostaglandin synthesis on fetal development, oxygenation, and the fetal circulation. *Semin Perinatol*. 1980;4:35-44.
2. Van Marter LJ, Leviton A, Allred EN, et al. Persistent pulmonary hypertension of the newborn and smoking and aspirin and nonsteroidal antiinflammatory drug consumption during pregnancy. *Pediatrics*. 1996;97:658-663.
3. Matt DW, Borzelleca JF. Toxic effects on the female reproductive system during pregnancy, parturition, and lactation. In: Witorsch RJ, ed. *Reproductive Toxicology*. 2nd ed. Raven Press; 1995:175-193.
4. Dawood MY. Nonsteroidal antiinflammatory drugs and reproduction. *Am J Obstet Gynecol*. 1993;169:1255-1265.
5. Prescribing Information. Nabumetone. LGM Pharma Solutions LLC; 2024.
6. Toshiyaki F, Kadoh Y, Fujimoto Y, et al. Toxicity study of nabumetone (iii)—teratological studies. *Kiso to Rinsho*. 1988;22:2975-2985. As cited in Shepard TH. *Catalog of Teratogenic Agents*. 7th ed. The Johns Hopkins University Press; 1992:275-276.
7. Quantin C, Yamdjieu Ngadeu C, Cottenet J, et al. Early exposure of pregnant women to non-steroidal anti-inflammatory drugs delivered outside hospitals and preterm birth risk: nationwide cohort study. *BJOG*. 2021;128: 1575-1584.
8. U.S. Food and Drug Administration. FDA recommends avoiding use of NSAIDs in pregnancy at 20 weeks or later because they can result in low amniotic fluid. FDA Drug Safety Communication. Accessed September 12, 2024. https://www.fda.gov/drugs/drug-safety-and-availability/fda-recommends-avoiding-use-nsaids-pregnancy-20-weeks-or-later-because-they-can-result-low-amniotic

NADOLOL

Antihypertensive (β-Blocker)

PREGNANCY RECOMMENDATION: Limited Human Data—Animal Data Suggest Potential Risk

BREASTFEEDING RECOMMENDATION: Potential Toxicity

PREGNANCY SUMMARY

Four case reports and a study describing the use of nadolol in all trimesters of human pregnancy have been located. No congenital abnormalities were reported. Of the four case reports, two of the infants were born healthy at term, while the remaining two infants experienced a decreased heart rate, hypoglycemia, and growth restriction. The cause of some or all of the effects may have been β-blockade. However, a more recent study of 27 nadolol exposures in pregnancy did not observe an increased rate of intrauterine growth restriction. Nadolol crosses the placenta, so fetal exposure will occur. Therefore, this limited human pregnancy experience prevents a complete assessment of the embryofetal risk. Embryofetal toxicity was observed in one animal species at doses less than 10 times the MRHD. Using this drug during pregnancy should be based on the pros and cons of the mother's clinical need for treatment versus any potential fetal risk that might occur from exposure.

BREASTFEEDING SUMMARY

A few reports describing the use of nadolol during human lactation were located. In 12 lactating women ingesting 80 mg once daily, mean steady-state levels of nadolol were approximately 357 ng/mL. The calculated relative infant doses (RIDs) ranged from 2% to 7%. Hypoglycemia was not observed, and only one case of bradycardia was reported. Breastfeeding while using this drug should be based on the mother's clinical need for treatment versus any potential infant risks that might occur. If used, the infant should be monitored for the most common reported adult side effects of β-blockade, including bradycardia and lethargy due to hypoglycemia.

References

1. Prescribing Information. Nadolol. Alembic Pharmaceuticals Inc; 2024.
2. Saegusa T, Suzuki T, Narama I. Reproduction studies of nadolol a new β-adrenergic blocking agent. *Yakuri Chiryo.* 1983;11:5119-5138. As cited in Shepard TH, Lemire RJ. *Catalog of Teratogenic Agents.* 12th ed. The Johns Hopkins University Press; 2007:304.
3. Fox RE, Marx C, Stark AR. Neonatal effects of maternal nadolol therapy. *Am J Obstet Gynecol.* 1985;152:1045-1046.
4. Solomon CG, Thiet M, Moore F Jr, Seely EW. Primary hyperaldosteronism in pregnancy. A case report. *J Reprod Med.* 1996;41:255-258.
5. Kambire Y, Konate L, Millogo GRC, et al. Right ventricular outflow tract tachycardia worsened during pregnancy. *Pan African Med J.* 2015;20:1-5.
6. King-Mallory R, Barker S, McGrogan K, Franks AM. Nadolol in pregnancy: a medical student's reflection on her pregnancy. *Marshall J Med.* 2018;4:16.
7. Hammond BH, El Assaad I, Herber JM, et al. Contemporary maternal and fetal outcomes in the treatment of LQTS during pregnancy: is nadolol bad for the fetus? *Heart Rhythm.* 2022;19:1516-1521.
8. Devlin RG, Duchin KL, Fleiss PM. Nadolol in human serum and breast milk. *Br J Clin Pharmacol.* 1981;12:393-396.

N

NAFCILLIN

Antibacterial (Penicillin)

PREGNANCY RECOMMENDATION: No Human Data—Animal Data Suggest Low Risk

BREASTFEEDING RECOMMENDATION: Probably Compatible

PREGNANCY SUMMARY

No reports describing the use of nafcillin in human pregnancy have been located. However, penicillins in general are considered low risk in pregnancy. The drug will probably cross the placenta, so some fetal exposure will likely occur. However, the absence of human pregnancy experience prevents a complete assessment of the embryofetal risk. Animal data did not show embryofetal toxicity in two species at doses of less than 10 times the recommended human dose (RHD). Using this drug during pregnancy should be based on the pros and cons of the mother's clinical need for treatment versus any potential fetal risk that might occur from exposure.

BREASTFEEDING SUMMARY

No reports describing the use of nafcillin during human lactation have been located. The drug will probably appear in breast milk, so some infant exposure will likely occur. Penicillins are generally considered compatible with breastfeeding. Breastfeeding while using this drug should be based on the mother's clinical need for treatment versus any potential infant risks that might occur. If used, the infant should be monitored for the most common reported adult side effects of rash, vomiting, and changes in gastrointestinal flora, including diarrhea and thrush.

Reference

1. Prescribing Information. Nafcillin. Eugia Pharma Specialties Limited; 2024.

NAFTIFINE

Anti-Infective (Antifungal - Topical)

PREGNANCY RECOMMENDATION: No Human Data—Animal Data Suggest Low Risk

BREASTFEEDING RECOMMENDATION: Probably Compatible

PREGNANCY SUMMARY

No reports describing the use of naftifine in human pregnancy have been located. The drug will probably cross the placenta, so some fetal exposure may occur. However, the low systemic bioavailability (6%) suggests that any exposure is likely to be minimal. Regardless, the absence of human pregnancy experience prevents a complete assessment of the embryofetal risk. Animal data did not show any embryofetal toxicity in two species at doses of less than 10 times the MRHD. Using this drug during pregnancy should be based on the pros and cons of the mother's clinical need for treatment versus any potential fetal risk that might occur from exposure.

BREASTFEEDING SUMMARY

No reports describing the use of naftifine during human lactation have been located. The drug will probably be excreted into breast milk, so some infant exposure will likely occur. However, the low systemic bioavailability (6%) suggests that exposure should be minimal. Breastfeeding while using this drug should be based on the mother's clinical need for treatment versus any potential infant risks that might occur. Because of the topical use of the drug, adult systemic side effects were not reported. Naftifine should not be applied to the breast or nipple, if possible, but if used in this area, it should be thoroughly wiped off prior to breastfeeding.

Reference

1. Prescribing Information. Naftin. Sebela Pharmaceuticals Inc; 2020.

N

NALBUPHINE

Pain (Opioid Agonist/Antagonist)

PREGNANCY RECOMMENDATION: Limited Human Data—Animal Data Suggest Potential Risk

BREASTFEEDING RECOMMENDATION: Probably Compatible

PREGNANCY SUMMARY

Nalbuphine is used for pain management during labor. However, there are limited reports of nalbuphine use earlier in pregnancy. Available studies have not reported any congenital anomalies. Fetal bradycardia and sinusoidal-like fetal heart rate (FHR) patterns have been reported with use of this drug during labor. The FHR pattern should be monitored closely. The drug crosses the placenta, so some fetal exposure will occur. Therefore, this limited early human pregnancy experience prevents a complete assessment of the embryofetal risk. Embryofetal toxicity was observed in one animal species at doses less than 10 times the MRHD. Using this drug during pregnancy should be based on the pros and cons of the mother's clinical need for treatment versus any potential fetal risk that might occur from exposure.

BREASTFEEDING SUMMARY

No reports describing the use of nalbuphine during human lactation have been located. The manufacturer states that small amounts (<1% of the mother's dose) are excreted into human breast milk, and these amounts are clinically insignificant. Breastfeeding while using this drug should be based on the mother's clinical need for treatment versus any potential infant risks that might occur. If used, the infant should be monitored for the most common reported adult side effects of sedation and respiratory depression.

References

1. Miller RR. Evaluation of nalbuphine hydrochloride. *Am J Hosp Pharm.* 1980;37:942-949.
2. Prescribing Information. Nalbuphine hydrochloride. Hospira; 2024.
3. Guillonneau M, Jacqz-Aigrain E, De Grepy A, Zeggout H. Perinatal adverse effects of nalbuphine given during parturition. *Lancet.* 1990;335:1588.
4. Sgro C, Escousse A, Tennenbaum D, Gouyon JB. Perinatal adverse effects of nalbuphine given during labour. *Lancet.* 1990;336:1070.
5. Wilson CM, McClean E, Moore J, Dundee JW. A double-blind comparison of intramuscular pethidine and nalbuphine in labour. *Anaesthesia.* 1986;41:1207-1213.
6. Frank M, McAteer EJ, Cattermole R, Loughnan B, Stafford LB, Hitchcock AM. Nalbuphine for obstetric analgesia. *Anaesthesia.* 1987;42:697-703.
7. Wilson SJ, Errick JK, Balkon J. Pharmacokinetics of nalbuphine during parturition. *Am J Obstet Gynecol.* 1986;155:340-344.
8. Nicolle E, Devillier P, Delanoy B, Durand C, Bessard G. Therapeutic monitoring of nalbuphine: transplacental transfer and estimated pharmacokinetics in the neonate. *Eur J Clin Pharmacol.* 1996;49:485-489.
9. Feinstein SJ, Lodeiro JG, Vintzileos AM, Campbell WA, Montgomery JT, Nochimson DJ. Sinusoidal fetal heart rate pattern after administration

of nalbuphine hydrochloride: a case report. *Am J Obstet Gynecol*. 1986; 154:159-160.

10. Podlas J, Breland BD. Patient-controlled analgesia with nalbuphine during labor. *Obstet Gynecol*. 1987;70:202-204.
11. Dan U, Rabinovici Y, Barkai G, Modan M, Etchin A, Mashiach S. Intravenous pethidine and nalbuphine during labor: a prospective double-blind comparative study. *Gynecol Obstet Invest*. 1991;32:39-43.
12. Jacqz-Aigrain E, Serreau R, Boissinot C, et al. Excretion of ketoprofen and nalbuphine in human milk during treatment of maternal pain after delivery. *Ther Drug Monit*. 2007;29:815-818.

NALDEMEDINE

Antidote (Opioid Antagonist)

PREGNANCY RECOMMENDATION: No Human Data—Animal Data Suggest Low Risk

BREASTFEEDING RECOMMENDATION: Probably Compatible

PREGNANCY SUMMARY

No reports describing the use of naldemedine in human pregnancy have been located. A limited amount of the drug probably crosses the placenta, so some fetal exposure will likely occur. However, the absence of human pregnancy experience prevents a complete assessment of the embryofetal risk. Animal studies did not demonstrate any embryofetal toxicity. When using opioid antagonists in patients with opioid use disorder, there is a theoretical concern that a precipitated withdrawal could occur.

BREASTFEEDING SUMMARY

No reports describing the use of naldemedine in human lactation have been located. A limited amount of the drug is probably found in breast milk. Because of the theoretical concern for precipitating neonatal opioid withdrawal in a breastfed infant delivered of a patient with opioid use disorder, the manufacturer recommends that women consider not using this drug while breastfeeding. However, breastfeeding while using this drug should be based on the mother's clinical need for treatment. If used, the infant should be monitored for the most common reported adult side effects of abdominal pain and nausea (both leading to irritability) and diarrhea.

Reference

1. Prescribing Information. Symproic. Shionogi Group; 2017.

N

NALOXEGOL

Gastrointestinal (Opioid Antagonist)

PREGNANCY RECOMMENDATION: No Human Data—Animal Data Suggest Low Risk

BREASTFEEDING RECOMMENDATION: Probably Compatible

PREGNANCY SUMMARY

No reports describing the use of naloxegol in human pregnancy have been located. The drug may cross the placenta, so some fetal exposure will likely occur. If it does reach the fetus, and the drug is chronically used during the pregnancy, then there is a possibility of fetal opioid withdrawal postdelivery. However, the absence of human pregnancy experience prevents a complete assessment of the embryofetal risk. Animal data did not show any embryofetal toxicity in two species at doses greater than 10 times the MRHD. Using this drug during pregnancy should be based on the pros and cons of the mother's clinical need for treatment versus any potential fetal risk that might occur from exposure.

BREASTFEEDING SUMMARY

No reports describing the use of naloxegol during human lactation have been located. The drug may be excreted into breast milk, so some infant exposure might occur. Due to a concern for potential serious adverse effects, including opioid withdrawal that may be seen in breastfed infants, the manufacturer recommends that women not breastfeed during treatment with this drug. Nevertheless, breastfeeding while using this drug should be based on the mother's clinical need for treatment versus any potential infant risks that might occur. If used, the infant should be monitored for the most common reported adult side effects of nausea, headache, and abdominal pain (all leading to irritability), diarrhea, flatulence, and vomiting.

Reference

1. Prescribing Information. Movantik. AstraZeneca Pharmaceuticals; 2023.

NALOXONE

Antidote (Opioid Antagonist)

PREGNANCY RECOMMENDATION: Limited Human Data—Animal Data Suggest Low Risk

BREASTFEEDING RECOMMENDATION: Probably Compatible

PREGNANCY SUMMARY

Limited reports describing the use of naloxone in human pregnancy have been located. Available studies have not found any significant evidence of an increased risk of congenital anomalies or adverse effects. However, most studies involve use after the first trimester. Naloxone crosses the placenta, so fetal exposure will occur. However, the limited human pregnancy experience prevents a complete assessment of the embryofetal risk. Animal data did not show any embryofetal toxicity in two species at doses of less than 10 times the RHD. Using this drug during pregnancy should be based on the pros and cons of the mother's clinical need for treatment versus any potential fetal risk that might occur from exposure. The American College of Obstetricians and Gynecologists (ACOG) recommends the use of small doses of naloxone for opioid-induced pruritus. It also states that despite the possibility of induced fetal withdrawal, naloxone should not be withheld in the case of maternal opioid overdose.

BREASTFEEDING SUMMARY

One report describing the use of naloxone in combination with buprenorphine during human lactation was located. In four patients, naloxone was found in breast milk in small amounts but was not detected in the plasma of breastfed infants. This is consistent with its low oral bioavailability of 2% or less. Breastfeeding while using this drug should be based on the mother's clinical need for treatment versus any potential infant risks that might occur. If used while breastfeeding, the infant should be monitored for symptoms of withdrawal in opioid using mothers.

References

1. Prescribing Information. Naloxone. Dr. Reddy's Laboratories, Inc; 2024.
2. Prescribing Information. Buprenorphine and Naloxone. Akorn Operating Company LLC; 2023.
3. Clark RB. Transplacental reversal of meperidine depression in the fetus by naloxone. *J Arkansas Med Soc*. 1971;68:128-130.
4. Clark RB, Beard AG, Greifenstein FE, Barclay DL. Naloxone in the parturient and her infant. *South Med J*. 1976;69:570-575.
5. Hodgkinson R, Bhatt M, Grewal G, Marx GF. Neonatal neurobehavior in the first 48 hours of life: effect of the administration of meperidine with and without naloxone in the mother. *Pediatrics*. 1978;62:294-298.
6. Brookshire GL, Shnider SM, Abboud TK, et al. Effects of naloxone on the mother and neonate after intrathecal morphine for labor analgesia. *Anesthesiology*. 1983;59:A417.
7. Evans JM, Hogg MIJ, Rosen M. Reversal of narcotic depression in the neonate by naloxone. *Br Med J*. 1976;2:1098-1100.
8. Wiener PC, Hogg MIJ, Rosen M. Effects of naloxone on pethidine-induced neonatal depression. II. Intramuscular naloxone. *Br Med J*. 1977;2:229-231.
9. Wiener PC, Hogg MIJ, Rosen M. Effects of naloxone on pethidine-induced neonatal depression. I. Intravenous naloxone. *Br Med J*. 1977;2:228-229.
10. Gerhardt T, Bancalari E, Cohen H, Rocha LF. Use of naloxone to reverse narcotic respiratory depression in the newborn infant. *J Pediatr*. 1977;90:1009-1012.
11. Bonta BW, Gagliardi JV, Williams V, Warshaw JB. Naloxone reversal of mild neurobehavioral depression in normal newborn infants after routine obstetric analgesia. *J Pediatr*. 1979;94:102-105.
12. Welles B, Belfrage P, de Chateau P. Effects of naloxone on newborn infant behavior after maternal analgesia with pethidine during labor. *Acta Obstet Gynecol Scand*. 1984;63:617-619.
13. Goodlin RC. Naloxone and its possible relationship to fetal endorphin levels and fetal distress. *Am J Obstet Gynecol*. 1981;139:16-19.
14. Arduini D, Rizzo G, Dell'Acqua S, Mancuso S, Romanini C. Effect of naloxone on fetal behavior near term. *Am J Obstet Gynecol*. 1987;156:474-478.
15. Jumah NA, Edwards C, Balfour-Boehm J, et al. Observational study of the safety of buprenorphine+naloxone in pregnancy in a rural and remote population. *BMJ Open*. 2016;6:e01174.
16. Jansson LM, McConnell K, Velez M, Spencer N, Gomonit M, Swortwood MJ. Buprenorphine-naloxone maintenance and lactation. *J Hum Lact*. 2024;40:113-119.
17. American College of Obstetricians and Gynecologists. ACOG practice bulletin no. 209: obstetric analgesia and anesthesia. *Obstet Gynecol*. 2019;133:e208-e225.
18. American College of Obstetricians and Gynecologists. Opioid use and opioid use disorder in pregnancy: committee opinion no. 711. *Obstet Gynecol*. 2017;130:e81-e94.

NALTREXONE

Antidote (Opioid Antagonist)

PREGNANCY RECOMMENDATION: Limited Human Data—Animal Data Suggest Potential Risk

BREASTFEEDING RECOMMENDATION: Probably Compatible

PREGNANCY SUMMARY

Numerous reports were located that describe the use of naltrexone during human pregnancy. From one study, there were 22 first-trimester exposures, and no fetal anomalies were identified. Several small reports and series have shown that the

(continued)

drug can be safely used during pregnancy. When used up to delivery, the rate of neonatal abstinence syndrome is lower when compared with methadone or buprenorphine. One of the primary concerns is overdose if the patient discontinues the drug and relapses to opioid drugs. The drug crosses the placenta, so fetal exposure will occur. Therefore, this limited early human pregnancy experience prevents a complete assessment of the embryofetal risk. Animal data did show show some embryo-fetal toxicity in one species at doses of less than 10 times the MRHD. Using this drug during pregnancy should be based on the pros and cons of the mother's clinical need for treatment versus any potential fetal risk that might occur from exposure.

BREASTFEEDING SUMMARY

One study was located that described the use of naltrexone during human pregnancy. The drug and its active metabolite were found in breast milk with mean breast milk concentrations of 1.6 ng/mL and 46 ng/mL, respectively. Using the mean combined drug levels, the calculated RID was about 1%. The infant was reported to be achieving expected milestones and had no identified adverse effects. Although this report is reassuring, additional data are warranted, and use during lactation should be evaluated on a case-by-case basis. Breastfeeding while using this drug should be based on the mother's clinical need for treatment versus any potential infant risks that might occur. If used, the infant should be monitored for the most common reported adult side effects of headache, abdominal cramps, and nausea (all leading to irritability), vomiting, and fatigue (lethargy).

References

1. Prescribing Information. Naltrexone. Accord Healthcare; 2019.
2. Prescribing Information. Vivitrol. Alkermes; 2015.
3. American College of Obstetricians and Gynecologists. Opioid use and opioid use disorder in pregnancy: committee opinion no. 711. *Obstet Gynecol*. 2017;130:e81-e94.
4. Christian MS. Reproductive toxicity and teratology evaluations of naltrexone. *J Clin Psychiatry*. 1984;45:7-10.
5. Zagon IS, Hurst WJ, McLaughlin PJ. Transplacental transfer of naltrexone in rats. *Life Sci*. 1997;61:1261-1267.
6. Keshet GI, Weinstock M. Maternal naltrexone prevents morphological and behavioral alterations induced in rats by prenatal stress. *Pharmacol Biochem Behav*. 1995;50:413-419.
7. McLaughlin PJ, Tobias SW, Lang CM, Zagon IS. Chronic exposure to the opioid antagonist naltrexone during pregnancy: maternal and offspring effects. *Physiol Behav*. 1997;62:501-508.
8. Harry GJ, Rosecrans JA. Behavioral effects of perinatal naltrexone exposure: a preliminary investigation. *Pharmacol Biochem Behav*. 1979;11(suppl):19-22.
9. Zagon IS, Tobias SW, Hytrek SD, McLaughlin PJ. Opioid receptor blockade throughout prenatal life confers long-term insensitivity to morphine and alters μ opioid receptors. *Pharmacol Biochem Behav*. 1998;59:201-207.
10. Caba M, Poindron P, Krehbiel D, Levy F, Romeyer A, Venier G. Naltrexone delays the onset of maternal behavior in primiparous parturient ewes. *Pharmacol Biochem Behav*. 1995;52:743-748.
11. Cohen E, Keshet G, Shavit Y, Weinstock M. Prenatal naltrexone facilitates male sexual behavior in the rat. *Pharmacol Biochem Behav*. 1996;54:183-188.
12. McLaughlin PJ, Tobias SW, Lang CM, Zagon IS. Opioid receptor blockade during prenatal life modifies postnatal behavioral development. *Pharmacol Biochem Behav*. 1997;58:1075-1082.
13. Zagon IS, Hurst WJ, McLaughlin PJ. Naltrexone is not detected in preweaning rats following transplacental exposure: implications for growth modulation. *Life Sci*. 1998;62:221-228.
14. Wildt L, Leyendecker G, Sir-Petermann T, Waibel-Treber S. Treatment with naltrexone in hypothalamic ovarian failure: induction of ovulation and pregnancy. *Hum Reprod*. 1993;8:350-358.
15. Kelty E, Hulse G. A retrospective cohort study of obstetric outcomes in opioid-dependent women treated with implant naltrexone, oral methadone, or sublingual buprenorphine, and non-dependent controls. *Drugs*. 2017;77:1199-1210.
16. Kelty E, Hulse G. A retrospective cohort study of birth outcomes in neonates exposed to naltrexone in utero: a comparison with methadone-, buprenorphine- and non-opioid-exposed neonates. *Drugs*. 2017;77:1211-1219.
17. Kelty E, Hulse G. A retrospective cohort study of the health of children prenatally exposed to methadone, buprenorphine or naltrexone compared with non-exposed control children. *Am J Addict*. 2017;26:845-851.
18. Wildt L, Sir-Petermann T, Leyendecker G, Waibel-Treber S, Rabenbauer B. Opiate antagonist treatment of ovarian failure. *Hum Reprod*. 1993;8(suppl 2):168-174.
19. Couzinet B, Young J, Brailly S, Chanson P, Schaison G. Even after priming with ovarian steroids or pulsatile gonadotropin-releasing hormone administration, naltrexone is unable to induce ovulation in women with functional hypothalamic amenorrhea. *J Clin Endocrinol Metab*. 1995;80:2102-2107.
20. Chan CF, Page-Sharp M, Kristensen JH, O'Neil G, Ilett KF. Transfer of naltrexone and its metabolite 6,β-naltrexol into human milk. *J Hum Lact*. 2004; 20:322-326.
21. Towers CV, Katz E, Weitz B, Visconti K. Use of naltrexone in treating opioid use disorder in pregnancy. *Am J Obstet Gynecol*. 2020;222(1):83.e1-83.e8.
22. Atluru S, Bruehlman AK, Vaughn P, Schauberger CW, Smid MC. Naltrexone compared with buprenorphine or methadone in pregnancy: a systematic review. *Obstet Gynecol*. 2024;143(3):403-410.
23. Hulse G, O'Neil G. Using naltrexone implants in the management of the pregnant heroin user. *Aust N Z J Obstet Gynaecol*. 2002;42:569-573.
24. Wachman EM, Saia K, Miller M, et al. Naltrexone treatment for pregnant women with opioid use disorder compared with matched buprenorphine control subjects. *Clin Ther*. 2019;41:1681-1689.

NAPHAZOLINE OPHTHALMIC

Ophthalmic (Vasoconstrictor)

PREGNANCY RECOMMENDATION: Limited Human Data—No Relevant Animal Data

BREASTFEEDING RECOMMENDATION: Probably Compatible

PREGNANCY SUMMARY

No reports describing the use of naphazoline ophthalmic solution during human pregnancy were located. Two cases of fetal constriction of the ductus arteriosus were reported after overuse of nasal naphazoline, which is not available in the United States. The Collaborative Perinatal Project (CPP) reported the use of the nasal spray in 20 pregnancies in the first trimester, and no congenital anomalies were identified. While the drug will likely cross the placenta, because of the ocular use, it is doubtful that the amount would be clinically significant. However, this limited human pregnancy experience prevents a complete assessment of the embryofetal risk. Animal reproduction studies have not been conducted. Using this drug during pregnancy should be based on the pros and cons of the mother's clinical need for treatment versus any potential fetal risk that might occur from exposure. If used during pregnancy, consider placing pressure over the tear duct in the corner of the eye for at least 1 minute, and then remove any excess solution with absorbent tissue to decrease the amount of drug reaching the systemic circulation even further.

BREASTFEEDING SUMMARY

No reports describing the use of naphazoline ophthalmic during human lactation have been located. The drug may be found in breast milk; however, naphazoline is likely minimally absorbed systemically following ophthalmic administration, which should significantly limit excretion into breast milk. If the clinical decision is to use this drug while breastfeeding, a method to decrease some systemic absorption with ophthalmic use is described above in the Pregnancy Summary. Additionally, the infant should be monitored for the most common reported adult side effects of nausea, headache, and dizziness (all leading to irritability), sweating, drowsiness, elevated blood pressure, and hyperglycemia.

References

1. Prescribing Information. Naphazoline Hydrochloride Ophthalmic Solution. Akorn, Inc; 2016.
2. Lopes LM, Carrilho MC, Francisco RPV, Lopes MAB, Krebs VLJ, Zugaib M. Fetal ductus arteriosus constriction and closure: analysis of the causes and perinatal outcome related to 45 consecutive cases. *J Matern Fetal Neonatal Med*. 2016;29:638-645.

NAPROXEN

Pain (Nonsteroidal Anti-Inflammatory Drug)

PREGNANCY RECOMMENDATION: Human Data Suggest Risk (Second and Third Trimesters)

BREASTFEEDING RECOMMENDATION: Probably Compatible

PREGNANCY SUMMARY

Numerous reports describing the use of naproxen in human pregnancy were located. From the Michigan Medicaid Surveillance study, a total of 70 (4.8%) birth anomalies were described in 1,448 first-trimester exposures. Though the rate was slightly increased, no pattern to the defects was identified. This has been reported in a few smaller studies. In addition, some studies have suggested an increased risk for cardiac anomalies and cleft lip and palate, but again, these findings have not been consistently found. Data from other evaluations analyzing NSAIDs as a group have also not found any increased risk or pattern to the defects. Naproxen crosses the placenta, so some fetal exposure will occur. NSAIDs can cause premature stricture or closure of the fetal ductus arteriosus when used in the latter portion of gestation. In some instances, this can produce persistent pulmonary hypertension in the neonate. These drugs have also been reported to produce fetal renal dysfunction leading to oligohydramnios when used after 20 weeks' gestation. The FDA recommends that NSAIDs be avoided in women 20 weeks or later in pregnancy. If deemed necessary by a health care provider, the use of NSAIDs between 20 and 30 weeks should be limited to the lowest effective dose and shortest duration. If treatment extends beyond 48 hours, providers should consider an ultrasound to monitor amniotic fluid levels.

BREASTFEEDING SUMMARY

Two reports describing the use of naproxen in 21 breastfeeding women were located. Naproxen was found in human breast milk, with a peak concentration of 1.25 mcg/mL following a 500 mg daily dose and 2.37 mcg/mL with a 750 mg daily dose. Calculated RIDs were about 2.6% and 3.3%. One infant was reported to have experienced a prolonged bleeding time, thrombocytopenia, and acute anemia, possibly due to naproxen. Breastfeeding while using this drug should be based on the mother's clinical need for treatment versus any potential infant risks that might occur. If used, the infant should be monitored for the most common reported adult side effects of stomach upset, abdominal pain, nausea, and headache (all leading to irritability), rash, bruising, and edema.

References

1. Prescribing Information. Anaprox DS. Canton Laboratories; 2021.
2. Nielsen GL, Sorensen HT, Larsen H, Pedersen L. Risk of adverse birth outcome and miscarriage in pregnant users of non-steroidal anti-inflammatory drugs: population based observational study and case-control study. *Br Med J*. 2001;322:266-270.
3. Anonymous. PG-synthetase inhibitors in obstetrics and after. *Lancet*. 1980;2:185-186.
4. Matt DW, Borzelleca JF. Toxic effects on the female reproductive system during pregnancy, parturition, and lactation. In: Witorsch RJ, ed. *Reproductive Toxicology*. 2nd ed. Raven Press; 1995:175-193.
5. Dawood MY. Nonsteroidal antiinflammatory drugs and reproduction. *Am J Obstet Gynecol*. 1993;169:1255-1265.
6. Glover DD, Amonkar M, Rybeck BF, Tracy TS. Prescription, over-the-counter, and herbal medicine use in a rural, obstetric population. *Am J Obstet Gynecol*. 2003;188:1039-1045.
7. Fuchs F. Prevention of prematurity. *Am J Obstet Gynecol*. 1976;126:809-820.

8. Montenegro MA, Palomino H. Induction of cleft palate in mice by inhibitors of prostaglandin synthesis. *J Craniofac Genet Del Biol*. 1990;10:83-94.
9. Siu SSN, Yeung JHK, Lau TK. An in-vivo study on placental transfer of naproxen in early human pregnancy. *Hum Reprod*. 2002;17:1056-1059.
10. Wilkinson AR. Naproxen levels in preterm infants after maternal treatment. *Lancet*. 1980;2:591-592.
11. Ericson A, Kallen BAJ. Nonsteroidal anti-inflammatory drugs in early pregnancy. *Reprod Toxicol*. 2001;15:371-375.
12. Li DK, Liu L, Odouli R. Exposure to non-steroidal anti-inflammatory drugs during pregnancy and risk of miscarriage: population based cohort study. *Br Med J*. 2003;327:368-371.
13. Tassinari MS, Cook JC, Hurtt ME. NSAIDs and developmental toxicity. *Birth Defects Res B Dev Reprod Toxicol*. 2003;68:3-4.
14. Kallen B. Maternal drug use and infant cleft lip/palate with special reference to corticoids. *Cleft Palate Craniofac J*. 2003;40:624-628.
15. Kallen BAJ, Olausson PO. Maternal drug use in early pregnancy and infant cardiovascular defect. *Reprod Toxicol*. 2003;17:255-261.
16. Kajantie E, Somer M. Bilateral cleft lip and palate, hypertelorism and hypoplastic toes. *Clin Dysmorphol*. 2004;13:195-196.
17. Ofori B, Oraichi D, Blais L, Rey E, Bérard A. Risk of congenital anomalies in pregnant users of non-steroidal anti-inflammatory drugs: a nested case-control study. *Birth Defects Res B Dev Reprod Toxicol*. 2006;77:268-279.
18. Levin DL. Effects of inhibition of prostaglandin synthesis on fetal development, oxygenation, and the fetal circulation. *Semin Perinatol*. 1980;4:35-44.
19. Rudolph AM. The effects of nonsteroidal antiinflammatory compounds on fetal circulation and pulmonary function. *Obstet Gynecol*. 1981;58(suppl):63s-67s.
20. Van Marter LJ, Leviton A, Allred EN, et al. Persistent pulmonary hypertension of the newborn and smoking and aspirin and nonsteroidal antiinflammatory drug consumption during pregnancy. *Pediatrics*. 1996;97:658-663.
21. Wilkinson AR, Aynsley-Green A, Mitchell MD. Persistent pulmonary hypertension and abnormal prostaglandin E levels in preterm infants after maternal treatment with naproxen. *Arch Dis Child*. 1979;54:942-945.
22. Alano MA, Ngougmna E, Ostrea EM Jr, Konduri GG. Analysis of nonsteroidal antiinflammatory drugs in meconium and its relation to persistent pulmonary hypertension of the newborn. *Pediatrics*. 2001;107:519-523.
23. Gerris J, Jonckheer M, Sacre-Smits L. Acute hyperthyroidism during pregnancy: a case report and critical analysis. *Eur J Obstet Gynecol Reprod Biol*. 1981;12:271-280.
24. Wiqvist N, Kjellmer I, Thiringer K, et al. Treatment of premature labor by prostaglandin synthetase inhibitors. *Acta Biol Med Germ*. 1978;37:923-930.
25. Talati AJ, Salim MA, Korones SB. Persistent pulmonary hypertension after maternal naproxen ingestion in a term newborn: a case report. *Am J Perinatol*. 2000;17:69-71.
26. Hernandez RK, Werler MM, Romitti P, Sun L, Anderka M; National Birth Defects Prevention Study. Nonsteroidal antiinflammatory drug use among women and the risk of birth defects. *Am J Obstet Gynecol*. 2012;206:228.e1-228.e8.
27. Nezvalova-Henriksen K, Spigset O, Nordeng H. Effects of ibuprofen, diclofenac, naproxen, and piroxicam on the course of pregnancy and pregnancy outcome: a prospective cohort study. *BJOG*. 2013;120:948-959.
28. Jamali F, Tam YK, Stevens RD. Naproxen excretion in breast milk and its uptake by suckling infant (abstract). *Drug Intell Clin Pharm*. 1982;16:475.
29. Jamali F, Stevens DRS. Naproxen excretion in milk and its uptake by the infant. *Drug Intell Clin Pharm*. 1983;17:910-911.
30. Fidalgo I, Correa R, Gómez Carrasco JA, Martínez Quiroga F. Acute anemia, rectorrhagia and hematuria caused by ingestion of naproxen. *An Esp Pediatr*. 1989;30:317-319.
31. Ito S, Blajchman A, Stephenson M, Eliopoulos C, Koren G. Prospective follow-up of adverse reactions in breast-fed infants exposed to maternal medication. *Am J Obstet Gynecol*. 1993;168:1393-1399.
32. U.S. Food and Drug Administration. FDA recommends avoiding use of NSAIDs in pregnancy at 20 weeks or later because they can result in low amniotic fluid. FDA Drug Safety Communication. Accessed September 12, 2024. https://www.fda.gov/drugs/drug-safety-and-availability/fda-recommends-avoiding-use-nsaids-pregnancy-20-weeks-or-later-because-they-can-result-low-amniotic

NARATRIPTAN

Central Nervous System (Antimigraine)

PREGNANCY RECOMMENDATION: Limited Human Data—Animal Data Suggest Potential Risk

BREASTFEEDING RECOMMENDATION: Potential Toxicity

PREGNANCY SUMMARY

Four reports describing the use of naratriptan in 323 human pregnancies have been located. Exposure has occurred in all trimesters. No association with major congenital anomalies has been found in those with first-trimester exposure. The drug will probably cross the placenta, so some fetal exposure will likely occur. However, this limited human pregnancy experience prevents a complete assessment of the embryofetal risk. Embryofetal toxicity was observed in one animal species at doses of less than 10 times the MRHD. ACOG suggests the cautious use of triptans, preferably sumatriptan, as second-line therapy for patients uncontrolled by acetaminophen alone or a combination therapy with caffeine or metoclopramide with diphenhydramine. It is also recommended that triptans not be used in pregnant patients with cardiac disease or hypertension due to their possible vasoconstrictive effects. Using this drug during pregnancy should be based on the pros and cons of the mother's clinical need for treatment versus any potential fetal risk that might occur from exposure.

BREASTFEEDING SUMMARY

One report evaluating the transfer of triptans, including naratriptan, into breast milk has been located. Naratriptan is present in breast milk. The estimated RID was 5%, which was the highest among the triptans tested. Despite low infant exposure, ACOG suggests avoiding breastfeeding for 24 hours after the use of triptans (except sumatriptan). Breastfeeding while using this drug should be based on the mother's clinical need for treatment versus any potential infant risks that might occur. If used, the infant should be monitored for the most common reported adult side effects of nausea, paresthesia, and dizziness (all leading to irritability), drowsiness, and lethargy.

References

1. Prescribing Information. Naratriptan. Bionpharma Inc; 2023.
2. Cunnington M, Ephross S, Churchill P. The safety of sumatriptan and naratriptan in pregnancy: what have we learned? *Headache*. 2009;49:1414-1422.
3. Nezvalova-Henriksen K, Spigset O, Nordeng H. Triptan exposure during pregnancy and the risk of major congenital malformations and adverse pregnancy outcomes: results from the Norwegian Mother and Child Cohort Study. *Headache*. 2010;50:563-575.

4. Ephross SA, Sinclair SM. Final results from the 16-year sumatriptan, naratriptan, and treximet pregnancy registry. *Headache*. 2014;54:1158-1172.
5. Yusuf A, Chia V, Xue F, Mikol DD, Bollinger L, Cangialose C. Use of existing electronic health care databases to evaluate medication safety in pregnancy: triptan exposure in pregnancy as a case study. *Pharmacoepidemiol Drug Saf*. 2018;27:1309-1315.
6. Amundsen S, Nordeng H, Fuskevåg OM, Nordmo E, Sager G, Spigset O. Transfer of triptans into human breast milk and estimation of infant drug exposure through breastfeeding. *Basic Clin Pharmacol Toxicol*. 2021;128:795-804.
7. Headaches in pregnancy and postpartum: ACOG clinical practice guideline no. 3. *Obstet Gynecol*. 2022;139:944-972.

NATALIZUMAB

Immunologic (Monoclonal Antibody—Immunomodulator)

PREGNANCY RECOMMENDATION: Limited Human Data—Animal Data Suggest Risk

BREASTFEEDING RECOMMENDATION: Probably Compatible

PREGNANCY SUMMARY

Several case reports and series describing the use of natalizumab in all trimesters of human pregnancy have been located. The major birth anomaly rate was less than 3% in more than 200 first-trimester exposures. Anemia and thrombocytopenia have been reported in a few infants exposed to natalizumab during pregnancy. As an immunoglobulin G (IgG) antibody, it likely crosses the placenta, especially during the second half of gestation, so some fetal exposure will probably occur. However, this limited human pregnancy experience prevents a complete assessment of the embryofetal risk. Embryofetal toxicity was observed in two animal species at doses less than 10 times the RHD. Using this drug during pregnancy should be based on the pros and cons of the mother's clinical need for treatment versus any potential fetal risk that might occur from exposure.

BREASTFEEDING SUMMARY

Two reports describing the effects of natalizumab in 25 breastfeeding mothers. In eight women who received natalizumab or another biologic while breastfeeding, no difference in infant growth, development, or infection rate was observed when compared to no treatment. In a second study, no adverse effects in breastfed infants related to natalizumab were reported in the four infants only exposed during breastfeeding. Natalizumab has been detected in the breast milk of some but not all women. However, as an IgG antibody, natalizumab will probably be digested in the infant's gastrointestinal tract and not absorbed. Breastfeeding while using this drug should be based on the mother's clinical need for treatment versus any potential infant risks that might occur. If used, the infant should be monitored for the most common reported adult side effects of nausea and headache (both leading to irritability), upper respiratory tract infections, and fatigue (lethargy).

References

1. Prescribing Information. Tysabri. Biogen Inc; 2023.
2. Mahadevan U, Cucchiara S, Hyams JS, et al. The London position statement of the World Congress of Gastroenterology on biological therapy for IBD with the European Crohn's and Colitis Organization: pregnancy and pediatrics. *Am J Gastroenterol*. 2011;106:214-223.
3. Hellwig K, Haghikia A, Gold R. Pregnancy and natalizumab: results of an observational study in 35 accidental pregnancies during natalizumab treatment. *Mult Scler*. 2011;17:958-963.
4. Hoevenaren IA, de Vries LC, Rijnders RJP, Lotgering FK. Delivery of healthy babies after natalizumab use for multiple sclerosis: a report of two cases. *Acta Neurol Scand*. 2011;123:430-433.
5. Bayas A, Penzien J, Hellwig K. Accidental natalizumab administration in pregnancy in multiple sclerosis. *Acta Neurol Scand*. 2012;126:e5-e6. doi:10.1111/j.1600-0404.2011.01636.x
6. Schneider H, Weber CE, Hellwig K, Schroten H, Tenenbaum T. Natalizumab treatment during pregnancy—effects on the neonatal immune system. *Acta Neurol Scand*. 2013;127:e1-e4. doi:10.1111/ane.12004
7. Haghikia A, Langer-Gould A, Rellensmann G, et al. Natalizumab use during the third trimester of pregnancy. *JAMA Neurol*. 2014;71:891-895.
8. Friend S, Richman S, Bloomgren G, Cristiano LM, Wenten M. Evaluation of pregnancy outcomes from the Tysabri (natalizumab) pregnancy exposure registry: a global, observational, follow-up study. *BMC Neurol*. 2016;16:150.
9. Ebrahimi N, Herbstritt S, Gold R, Amezcua L, Koren G, Hellwig K. Pregnancy and fetal outcomes following natalizumab exposure in pregnancy. A prospective, controlled observational study. *Mult Scler J*. 2015;21:198-205.
10. Baker TE, Cooper SD, Kessler MD, Hale TW. Transfer of natalizumab into breast milk in a mother with multiple sclerosis. *J Human Lact*. 2015;31:233-236.
11. Matro R, Martin CF, Wolf D, Shah SA, Mahadevan U. Exposure concentrations of infants breastfed by women receiving biologic therapies for inflammatory bowel diseases and effects of breastfeeding on infections and development. *Gastroenterology*. 2018;156:696-704.
12. Friend S, Richman S, Bloomgren G, Cristiano LM, Wenten M. Evaluation of pregnancy outcomes from the Tysabri® (natalizumab) pregnancy exposure registry: a global, observational, follow-up study. *BMC Neurol*. 2016;16:150.
13. Portaccio E, Annovazzi P, Ghezzi A, et al. Pregnancy decision-making in women with multiple sclerosis treated with natalizumab: I: fetal risks. *Neurology*. 2018;90:e823-e831.
14. Ebrahimi N, Herbstritt S, Gold R, Amezcua L, Koren G, Hellwig K. Pregnancy and fetal outcomes following natalizumab exposure in pregnancy. A prospective, controlled observational study. *Mult Scler J*. 2014;21:198-205.
15. Haghikia A, Langer-Gould A, Rellensmann G, et al. Natalizumab use during the third trimester of pregnancy. *JAMA Neurol*. 2014;71:891-895.
16. Kümpfel T, Thiel S, Meinl I, et al. Long-term exposure to natalizumab during pregnancy—a prospective case series from the German Multiple Sclerosis and Pregnancy Registry. Poster presented at: 7th Joint ECTRIMS-ACTIRMS Meeting; October 25-27, 2017; Paris, France.
17. Landi D, Bovis F, Grimaldi A, et al. Exposure to natalizumab throughout pregnancy: effectiveness and safety in an Italian cohort of women with multiple sclerosis. *J Neurol Neurosurg Psychiatry*. 2022.
18. Ciplea AI, Langer-Gould A, de Vries A, et al. Monoclonal antibody treatment during pregnancy and/or lactation in women with MS or neuromyelitis optica spectrum disorder. *Neurol Neuroimmunol Neuroinflamm*. 2020;7:e723.

NATAMYCIN OPHTHALMIC

Ophthalmic (Antifungal - Topical)

PREGNANCY RECOMMENDATION: No Human Data and No Relevant Animal Data

BREASTFEEDING RECOMMENDATION: Probably Compatible

PREGNANCY SUMMARY

No reports describing the use of natamycin ophthalmic suspension in human pregnancy have been located. Systemic concentrations are not expected with ocular use. However, the absence of human pregnancy experience prevents a complete assessment of the embryofetal risk. Animal reproduction studies have not been conducted. Using this drug during pregnancy should be based on the pros and cons of the mother's clinical need for treatment versus any potential fetal risk that might occur from exposure. If used during pregnancy, consider placing pressure over the tear duct in the corner of the eye for at least 1 minute, and then remove any excess solution with absorbent tissue to decrease the amount of drug reaching the systemic circulation even further.

BREASTFEEDING SUMMARY

No reports describing the use of natamycin ophthalmic during human lactation have been located. The drug may be found in breast milk, but systemic concentrations are not expected with ocular use. Therefore, any amount is likely to be clinically insignificant. Breastfeeding while using this drug should be based on the mother's clinical need for treatment versus any potential infant risks that might occur. Because of the ophthalmic use, systemic side effects were not assessed. No systemic side effects are expected. If the clinical decision is to use this drug while breastfeeding, a method to decrease some systemic absorption with ophthalmic use is described above in the Pregnancy Summary.

Reference

1. Prescribing Information. Natacyn. Eyevance Pharmaceuticals, LLC; 2020.

N

NATEGLINIDE

Antidiabetic (Meglitinide)

PREGNANCY RECOMMENDATION: Limited Human Data—Animal Data Suggest Low Risk

BREASTFEEDING RECOMMENDATION: Probably Compatible

PREGNANCY SUMMARY

One report describing the use of nateglinide in the first 24 weeks of pregnancy resulted in a healthy infant. The drug will probably cross the placenta, so some fetal exposure will likely occur. However, this limited human pregnancy experience prevents a complete assessment of the embryofetal risk. Animal data did not show any embryofetal toxicity in two species, one at doses of less than 10 times the MRHD and one at doses of more than 10 times the MRHD. ACOG and the American Diabetes Association (ADA) recommend that insulin be used for types 1 and 2 diabetes occurring during pregnancy and, if diet therapy alone is not successful, for gestational diabetes. Oral agents such as metformin and glyburide should not be used as first-line agents, if possible, as both cross the placenta, and in general, may not provide adequate glycemic control. Other oral medications and injectable glucose-lowering medications lack safety data.

BREASTFEEDING SUMMARY

No reports describing the use of nateglinide during human lactation have been located. The drug will probably appear in breast milk, so some infant exposure will likely occur. Breastfeeding while using this drug should be based on the mother's clinical need for treatment versus any potential infant risks that might occur. If used, the infant should be monitored for the most common reported adult side effects of dizziness, arthropathy, and back pain (all leading to irritability), hypoglycemia (producing drowsiness, lethargy, paleness, sweating, and tremors), upper respiratory tract infection, and diarrhea.

References

1. Prescribing Information. Nateglinide. Activas Pharma, Inc; 2023.
2. Teelucksingh S, Youssef JE, Sohan K, Ramsewak S. Prolonged inadvertent pravastatin use in pregnancy. *Reprod Toxicol.* 2004;18:299-300.
3. ACOG practice bulletin no. 190: gestational diabetes mellitus. *Obstet Gynecol.* 2018;131:e49-e64.
4. American Diabetes Association Professional Practice Committee. Management of diabetes in pregnancy: standards of care in diabetes—2024. *Diabetes Care.* 2024;47(suppl 1):S282-S294.

NAXITAMAB

Antineoplastic (Monoclonal Antibody)

PREGNANCY RECOMMENDATION: No Human Data and No Relevant Animal Data

BREASTFEEDING RECOMMENDATION: Probably Compatible

PREGNANCY SUMMARY

No reports describing the use of naxitamab in human or animal pregnancies have been located. Because it is an antibody of the IgG class, it probably crosses the placenta. Therefore, the absence of human pregnancy experience prevents a complete assessment of the embryofetal risk. Naxitamab may cause serious infusion-related reactions, including cardiac arrest, anaphylaxis, hypotension, and bronchospasm. It may also lead to severe neurotoxicity, including severe neuropathic pain, transverse myelitis, and reversible posterior leukoencephalopathy syndrome. Hypertension was also reported in up to 44% of patients treated with this drug in clinical trials. The manufacturer recommends effective contraception for women of childbearing age while receiving this treatment and for 2 months after the last dose.

BREASTFEEDING SUMMARY

Naxitamab probably enters breast milk. However, if used while breastfeeding, newborn effects would be expected to be negligible due to probable digestion of the antibody in the infant's gastrointestinal tract. However, based on mechanism of action and the significant risk for serious adult side effects, the manufacturer recommends that women not breastfeed while being treated with this drug and for up to 2 months after the last dose.

Reference

1. Prescribing Information. Danyelza. Y-mAbs Therapeutics, Inc; 2020.

NEBIVOLOL

Antihypertensive (β-Blocker)

PREGNANCY RECOMMENDATION: Limited Human Data—Animal Data Suggest Potential Risk

BREASTFEEDING RECOMMENDATION: Probably Compatible

PREGNANCY SUMMARY

Two reports describing the use of nebivolol in 58 human pregnancies have been located. In one study, 57 pregnant women received nebivolol for treating hypertension in pregnancy, and no adverse effects related to the drug were reported. In addition, the drug was found to produce good blood pressure control. The second study was a case report of a fetus exposed to the drug at delivery that had hypoglycemia, jaundice, mild thrombocytopenia, with prolonged prothrombin time. The infant's condition gradually improved and was in good clinical condition with normal clinical and laboratory parameters at discharge. The drug will probably cross the placenta, so some fetal exposure will likely occur. Therefore, the absence of the first-trimester human pregnancy experience prevents a complete assessment of the embryofetal risk. Embryofetal toxicity was observed in one animal species at doses less than 10 times the MRHD, but not in a second species at doses of about 10 times the MRHD. Using this drug during pregnancy should be based on the pros and cons of the mother's clinical need for treatment versus any potential fetal risk that might occur from exposure. Neonates of women who are treated with β-blockers during the third trimester may be at increased risk for hypotension, bradycardia, hypoglycemia, and respiratory depression. If used during the third trimester of pregnancy, newborns should be observed for these effects.

BREASTFEEDING SUMMARY

No reports describing the use of nebivolol during human lactation have been located. The drug will probably be found in breast milk, so some infant exposure will likely occur. Breastfeeding while using this drug should be based on the mother's clinical need for treatment versus any potential infant risks that might occur. If used, the infant should be monitored for the most common reported adult side effects of headache (leading to irritability), fatigue (lethargy), hypotension, bradycardia, and hypoglycemia.

References

1. Prescribing Information. Bystolic. Allergan USA; 2023.
2. Sullo MG, Perri D, Sibilio M, et al. Hypoglycemia, polycythemia and hyponatremia in a newborn exposed to nebivolol during pregnancy. *J Pharmacol Pharmacother*. 2015;6:45-48.
3. Humenna IY, Heryak SN, Dobryanska VY. Rational control of arterial pressure during labor in women with arterial hypertension. *Ginekol Pol*. 2019;90:206-211.

N

NECITUMUMAB

Antineoplastic (Monoclonal Antibody—EGFR Inhibitor)

PREGNANCY RECOMMENDATION: No Human Data—Animal Data Suggest Risk

BREASTFEEDING RECOMMENDATION: Probably Compatible

PREGNANCY SUMMARY

No reports describing the use of necitumumab in human pregnancy have been located. As an IgG antibody, necitumumab likely crosses the placenta, so some fetal exposure will probably occur. Therefore, the absence of human pregnancy experience prevents a complete assessment of the embryofetal risk. Embryofetal toxicity was observed in animal studies with disruption of the epidermal growth factor receptor (EGFR). Due to these findings in animal studies and the drug's mechanism of action, the manufacturer recommends that women with reproductive potential use effective contraception during treatment and for at least 3 months after the last dose. Nevertheless, using this drug during pregnancy should be based on the pros and cons of the mother's clinical need for treatment versus any potential fetal risk that might occur from exposure.

BREASTFEEDING SUMMARY

No reports describing the use of necitumumab during human lactation have been located. A limited amount of the drug will probably be excreted into breast milk. However, it is known that IgG antibodies can be found in human breast milk but are not found in the neonatal or infant circulation. Additionally, if any IgG antibodies were to be ingested through breastfeeding, they would probably be digested in the infant's gastrointestinal tract and not be absorbed. However, due to the concern for potential serious adverse effects that might be seen in a breastfed infant, the manufacturer recommends that women should not breastfeed during treatment with this drug and for 3 months after the final dose. Nevertheless, breastfeeding while using this drug should be based on the mother's clinical need for treatment. If used, the infant should be monitored for the most common reported adult side effects of nausea (leading to irritability), rash, and hypomagnesemia.

Reference

1. Prescribing Information. Portrazza. Eli Lilly and Company; 2015.

NEDOSIRAN

Renal/Genetic (Double-Stranded Small Interfering RNA)

PREGNANCY RECOMMENDATION: No Human Data—Animal Data Suggest Potential Risk

BREASTFEEDING RECOMMENDATION: Probably Compatible

PREGNANCY SUMMARY

No reports describing the use of nedosiran in human pregnancy have been located. The drug will not likely cross the placenta in significant amounts, so fetal exposure should be minimal. However, the absence of human pregnancy experience prevents a complete assessment of the embryofetal risk. Animal reproduction studies did show some embryofetal toxicity in one species at doses of about equal to MRHD, but maternal toxicity also occurred. No embryofetal toxicity was seen in a second species at doses of more than 10 times the MRHD. Using this drug during pregnancy should be based on the pros and cons of the mother's clinical need for treatment versus any potential fetal risk that might occur from exposure.

BREASTFEEDING SUMMARY

No reports describing the use of nedosiran during human lactation have been located. The drug might be found in breast milk, but any levels are likely to be clinically insignificant. In addition, because it is a small nucleotide, if any amount of the drug were to be ingested through breastfeeding, it would probably be somewhat digested in the infant's gastrointestinal tract and not be absorbed. Breastfeeding while using this drug should be based on the mother's clinical need for treatment versus any potential infant risks that might occur. If used, the infant should be monitored for the most common reported adult side effects of rash and flushing.

Reference

1. Prescribing Information. Rivfloza Novo Nordisk, Inc; 2023.

NEFAZODONE

Mental Health (Antidepressant)

PREGNANCY RECOMMENDATION: Limited Human Data—Animal Data Suggest Potential Risk

BREASTFEEDING RECOMMENDATION: Potential Toxicity

PREGNANCY SUMMARY

Two prospective studies and a meta-analysis that involved the use of nefazodone in human pregnancy were located. Of 147 pregnancies exposed in the first trimester to either nefazodone or trazodone, only 2 (0.7%) major anomalies were identified. Two other studies analyzed a large number of antidepressant medications for the risk of birth defects when used during the first trimester, and in both, the rate was not increased above the 2% to 4% expected rate. Nefazodone was used in both studies. The drug will probably cross the placenta, so some fetal exposure will likely occur. Therefore, this limited human pregnancy experience with nefazodone prevents a complete assessment of the embryofetal risk. Embryofetal toxicity was observed in one animal species at doses less than 10 times the MRHD, but not in a second species with doses of less than 10 times the MRHD. Using this drug during pregnancy should be based on the pros and cons of the mother's clinical need for treatment versus any potential fetal risk that might occur from exposure. There is a pregnancy exposure registry that monitors pregnancy outcomes in women using antidepressant drugs. Health care providers are encouraged to call the National Pregnancy Registry for Antidepressants at 1-844-405-6185.

BREASTFEEDING SUMMARY

A few reports describing the use of nefazodone during human lactation were located. Breast milk levels ranged from less than 50 ng/mL up to about 690 ng/mL. The highest possible calculated RID was about 7%, with most less than 3%. No abnormal development difficulties were observed in the two nursing infants. Breastfeeding while using this drug should be based on the mother's clinical need for treatment versus any potential infant risks that might occur. If used, the infant should be monitored for the most common reported adult side effects of nausea and dizziness (both leading to irritability).

References

1. Prescribing Information. Nefazodone. Teva Pharmaceuticals USA, Inc; 2021.
2. Einarson A, Bonari L, Voyer-Lavigne S, et al. A multicentre prospective controlled study to determine the safety of trazodone and nefazodone use during pregnancy. *Can J Psychiatry*. 2003;48:106-109.
3. Einarson TR, Einarson A. Newer antidepressants in pregnancy and rates of major malformations: a meta-analysis of prospective comparative studies. *Pharmacoepidemiol Drug Saf*. 2005;14:823-827.
4. Einarson A, Choi J, Einarson TR, Koren G. Incidence of major malformations in infants following antidepressant exposure in pregnancy: results of a large prospective cohort study. *Can J Psychiatry*. 2009;54:242-246.
5. Dodd S, Buist A, Burrows GD, et al. Determination of nefazodone and its pharmacologically active metabolites in human blood plasma and breast milk by high-performance liquid chromatography. *J Chromatogr B Biomed Sci Appl*. 1999;730:249-255.
6. Dodd S, Maguire KP, Burrows GD, Norman TR. Nefazodone in the breast milk of nursing mothers: a report of two patients. *J Clin Psychopharmacol*. 2000;20:717-718.
7. Yapp P, Ilett KF, Kristensen JH, Hackett LP, Paech MJ, Rampono J. Drowsiness and poor feeding in a breast-fed infant: association with nefazodone and its metabolites. *Ann Pharmacother*. 2000;34:1269-1272.

N

NELARABINE

Antineoplastic (Antimetabolite)

PREGNANCY RECOMMENDATION: No Human Data—Animal Data Suggest Potential Risk

BREASTFEEDING RECOMMENDATION: Potential Toxicity

PREGNANCY SUMMARY

No reports describing the use of nelarabine in human pregnancy have been located. The drug will probably cross the placenta, so some fetal exposure will likely occur. Therefore, the absence of human pregnancy experience prevents a complete assessment of the embryofetal risk. Embryofetal toxicity with malformations was observed in one animal species at doses less than the RHD. Based on animal studies and the drug's mechanism of action, the manufacturer recommends that women with reproductive potential use effective contraception during treatment. They also recommend that males with female partners of reproductive potential use effective contraception during treatment and for 3 months after the last dose. Nevertheless, using this drug during pregnancy should be based on the pros and cons of the mother's clinical need for treatment versus any potential fetal risk that might occur from exposure. There is a registry for women who are pregnant and have cancer. For more information, women and health care providers are encouraged to contact the Cancer and Pregnancy Registry at 1-877-635-4499.

BREASTFEEDING SUMMARY

No reports describing the use of nelarabine during lactation have been located. The drug will probably appear in breast milk, so some infant exposure will likely occur. Due to a concern for potential serious adverse effects that might be seen in a breastfed infant, the manufacturer recommends that women not breastfeed while being treated with this drug. Nevertheless, breastfeeding while using this drug should be based on the mother's clinical need for treatment versus any potential infant risks that might occur. If used, the infant should be monitored for the most common reported adult side effects of headache and peripheral neuropathy (both leading to irritability), and various laboratory abnormalities (see Prescribing Information [PI]).

Reference

1. Prescribing Information. Nelarabine. Amneal Pharmaceuticals LLC; 2023.

NELFINAVIR

Antiretroviral (Protease Inhibitor)

PREGNANCY RECOMMENDATION: *Contraindicated

BREASTFEEDING RECOMMENDATION: *Contraindicated

PREGNANCY SUMMARY

From the January 2024 interim report of the Antiretroviral Pregnancy Registry (APR), there were 47 (3.9%) birth anomalies in 1,216 first-trimester exposures. In 2024, the updated US Department of Health and Human Services AIDS Info guidelines for the use of antiretroviral agents during pregnancy recommend that, in most cases, patients continue their regimen during pregnancy if it is tolerated, safe, and effective in suppressing viral replication. The guideline recommends that the discussion and shared decision-making process about the known and potential risks, as well as benefits to the mother and fetus, should guide the selection of which antiretrovirals to use during pregnancy. Additionally, treatment initiation should not be delayed due to concerns about teratogenicity with first-trimester exposure. See the guideline for the most updated information. management. *The guidelines note that nelfinavir should not be used during pregnancy due to inferior virologic efficacy. There is a pregnancy exposure registry that monitors pregnancy outcomes in patients using antiretroviral medicines during pregnancy. Health care providers are encouraged to call the APR at 1-800-258-4263.

N

BREASTFEEDING SUMMARY

A few studies were located that describe the use of nelfinavir during human lactation. The drug was found in human breast milk, so some infant exposure will occur. In 2023, the updated US Department of Health and Human Services AIDS Info guidelines state that using replacement of breast milk through formula or pasteurized donor human breast milk from a milk bank eliminates the risk of postnatal HIV transmission to the infant. Using antiretroviral therapy to achieve and maintain viral suppression during pregnancy and postpartum decreases the risk for infant transmission to less than 1% but not zero. *For patients not on therapy or those without viral load suppression during pregnancy (at a minimum throughout the third trimester) and at delivery, replacement of breast milk is recommended. Patients on antiretroviral therapy who have a sustained undetectable viral load and who choose to breastfeed or use replacement of breast milk should be supported with this decision. If the clinical decision is to use this drug while breastfeeding, the infant should be monitored for the most common reported pediatric side effects of irritability, rash, diarrhea, hepatotoxicity, and hyperbilirubinemia.

References

1. Prescribing Information. Viracept. Agouron; 2023.
2. Covington DL, Conner SD, Doi PA, et al. Risk of birth defects associated with nelfinavir exposure during pregnancy. *Obstet Gynecol*. 2004;103:1181-1189.
3. Antiretroviral Pregnancy Registry Steering Committee. Antiretroviral Pregnancy Registry interim report for 1 January 1989 through 31 January 2024. Registry Coordinating Center; 2023. Accessed October 28, 2024. https://www.apregistry.com/forms/interim_report.pdf
4. McGowan JP, Crane M, Wiznia AA, Blum S. Combination antiretroviral therapy in human immunodeficiency virus-infected pregnant women. *Obstet Gynecol*. 1999;94:641-646.
5. Centers for Disease Control and Prevention. Public Health Service Task Force recommendations for the use of antiretroviral drugs in pregnant women infected with HIV-1 for maternal health and for reducing perinatal HIV-1 transmission in the United States. *MMWR Recomm Rep*. 1998;47(RR-2):1-30.
6. Fassett M, Kramer F, Stek A. Treatment with protease inhibitors in pregnancy is not associated with an increased incidence of gestational diabetes (abstract). *Am J Obstet Gynecol*. 2000;182:S97.
7. Stek A, Kramer F, Fassett M, Khoury M. The safety and efficacy of protease inhibitor therapy for HIV infection during pregnancy (abstract). *Am J Obstet Gynecol*. 1999;180:S7.
8. Morris AB, Cu-Uvin S, Harwell JI, et al. Multicenter review of protease inhibitors in 89 pregnancies. *J Acquir Immune Defic Syndr*. 2000;25:306-311.
9. Carpenter CCJ, Fischi MA, Hammer SM, et al. Antiretroviral therapy for HIV infection in 1996. *JAMA*. 1996;276:146-154.
10. Minkoff H, Augenbraun M. Antiretroviral therapy for pregnant women. *Am J Obstet Gynecol*. 1997;176:478-489.
11. Minkoff H. Human immunodeficiency virus infection in pregnancy. *Obstet Gynecol*. 2003;101:797-810.
12. Panel on Treatment of HIV During Pregnancy and Prevention of Perinatal Transmission. Recommendations for the use of antiretroviral drugs during pregnancy and interventions to reduce perinatal HIV transmission in the United States. Department of Health and Human Services. Accessed January 31, 2024. https://clinicalinfo.hiv.gov/en/guidelines/perinatal
13. Brown ZA, Watts DH. Antiviral therapy in pregnancy. *Clin Obstet Gynecol*. 1990;33:276-289.

14. De Martino M, Tovo P-A, Pezzotti P, et al. HIV-1 transmission through breast-milk: appraisal of risk according to duration of feeding. *AIDS*. 1992;6: 991-997.
15. Van de Perre P. Postnatal transmission of human immunodeficiency virus type 1: the breast-feeding dilemma. *Am J Obstet Gynecol*. 1995;173:483-487.
16. Else LJ, Taylor S, Back DJ, Khoo SH. Pharmacokinetics of antiretroviral drugs in anatomical sanctuary sites: the fetal compartment (placenta and amniotic fluid). *Antivir Ther*. 2011;16:1139-1147.
17. Benaboud S, Ekouevi DK, Urien S, et al. Population pharmacokinetics of nevirapine in HIV-1-infected pregnant women and their neonates. *Antimicrob Agents Chemother*. 2011;55:331-337.
18. Palombi L, Pirillo MF, Andreotti M, et al. Antiretroviral prophylaxis for breastfeeding transmission in Malawi: drug concentrations, virological efficacy and safety. *Antivir Ther*. 2012;17:1511-1519.
19. Shapiro RL, Rossi S, Ogwu A, et al. Therapeutic levels of lopinavir in late pregnancy and abacavir passage into breast milk in the Mma Bana Study, Botswana. *Antivir Ther*. 2013;18:585-590.
20. Minniear TD, Zeh C, Polle N, et al. Rash, hepatotoxicity and hyperbilirubinemia among Kenyan infants born to HIV-infected women receiving triple-antiretroviral drugs for the prevention of mother-to-child HIV transmission. *Pediatr Infect Dis J*. 2012;31:1155-1157.

NEMOLIZUMAB

Immunologic/Dermatologic (Interleukin 31 Receptor Antagonist)

PREGNANCY RECOMMENDATION: No Human Data—Animal Data Suggest Low Risk

BREASTFEEDING RECOMMENDATION: Probably Compatible

PREGNANCY SUMMARY

No reports describing the use of nemolizumab in human pregnancy have been located. As an IgG antibody, it likely crosses the placenta, especially during the second half of pregnancy, so some fetal exposure will probably occur. Therefore, the absence of human pregnancy experience prevents a complete assessment of the embryofetal risk. Animal studies did not show any embryofetal toxicity in one species at doses of more than 10 times the MRHD. Using this drug during pregnancy should be based on the pros and cons of the mother's clinical need for treatment versus any potential fetal risk that might occur from exposure.

BREASTFEEDING SUMMARY

No reports describing the use of nemolizumab during human lactation have been located. It is known that IgG antibodies can be found in human breast milk but are not found in the neonatal or infant circulation. Additionally, if any IgG antibodies were to be ingested through breastfeeding, they would probably be digested in the infant's gastrointestinal tract and not be absorbed. Breastfeeding while using this drug should be based on the mother's clinical need for treatment versus any potential infant risks that might occur. If used, the infant should be monitored for the most common reported adult side effects of headache, arthralgia, and myalgia (all leading to irritability) and rash.

Reference

1. Prescribing Information. Nemluvio. Galderma Laboratories, L.P.; 2024.

NEOMYCIN

Antibiotic (Aminoglycoside)

PREGNANCY RECOMMENDATION: Limited Human Data—No Relevant Animal Data

BREASTFEEDING RECOMMENDATION: Probably Compatible

PREGNANCY SUMMARY

From the Collaborative Perinatal Project (CPP), no birth defects were seen in 30 cases of first-trimester exposure to neomycin. From a second study of more than 61,000 pregnancies (a major birth defect group was compared with a no-anomaly control group), the use of neomycin was no different between the groups. The drug will probably cross the placenta if found in the systemic circulation. However, oral bioavailability (<3%) and systemic absorption from the skin, eye, and ear are minimal. So, any fetal exposure will likely be clinically insignificant. However, the limited human pregnancy experience prevents a complete assessment of the embryofetal risk. Animal reproduction studies have not been conducted. Using this drug during pregnancy should be based on the pros and cons of the mother's clinical need for treatment versus any potential fetal risk that might occur from exposure.

N

BREASTFEEDING SUMMARY

No reports describing the use of neomycin during human lactation have been located. The very limited systemic bioavailability of oral neomycin (<3%) and minimal absorption from topical, ophthalmic, and otic use suggest that any amounts of neomycin in breast milk are likely to be clinically insignificant. If topical neomycin is applied to the breast or nipple, it should be thoroughly wiped off prior to breastfeeding. Additionally, only water-miscible cream or gel products are recommended for application to the breast. If the clinical decision is to use this drug while breastfeeding, the infant should be monitored for alterations in the gastrointestinal flora, including diarrhea, thrush, and diaper rash, along with the additional most common adult side effects of nausea (leading to irritability) and vomiting.

References

1. Prescribing Information. Neomycin sulfate. Chartwell RX, LLC; 2023.
2. Heinonen OP, Slone D, Shapiro S. *Birth Defects and Drugs in Pregnancy*. Publishing Sciences Group; 1977:297-301.
3. Czeizel AE, Rockenbauer M, Olsen J, Sorensen HT. A teratological study of aminoglycoside antibiotic treatment during pregnancy. *Scand J Infect Dis*. 2000;32:309-313.

NEOSTIGMINE

Antidote (Acetylcholinesterase Inhibitor)

PREGNANCY RECOMMENDATION: Limited Human Data—Animal Data Suggest Low Risk

BREASTFEEDING RECOMMENDATION: Probably Compatible

PREGNANCY SUMMARY

Several reports describing the use of neostigmine to reverse muscle relaxation during general anesthesia for cesarean section have been located. A few case reports and data from the CPP described first-trimester exposure in about 24 cases, with one major anomaly reported. It is thought that neostigmine crosses the placenta, so fetal exposure probably occurs (though this has not been confirmed). However, this limited human pregnancy experience prevents a complete assessment of the embryofetal risk. Animal data did not show any embryofetal toxicity in two species at doses of less than the MRHD. Using this drug during pregnancy should be based on the pros and cons of the mother's clinical need for treatment versus any potential fetal risk that might occur from exposure.

N

BREASTFEEDING SUMMARY

A few studies describing the use of neostigmine during human lactation were located. In several lactating women, the drug was not detected in breast milk. This is consistent with the lack of any significant systemic absorption with oral, topical, ophthalmic, and otic use. If the clinical decision is to use this drug while breastfeeding, the infant should be monitored for the most common reported adult side effects of nausea and abdominal cramps (both leading to irritability), bradycardia, and vomiting.

References

1. Prescribing Information. Neostigmine. Amneal Pharmaceuticals; 2024.
2. Clark RB, Brown MA, Lattin DL. Neostigmine, atropine, and glycopyrrolate: does neostigmine cross the placenta? *Anesthesiology*. 1996;84:450-452.
3. Heinonen OP, Slone D, Shapiro S. *Birth Defects and Drugs in Pregnancy*. Publishing Sciences Group; 1977:345-356.
4. Brunclik V, Hauser GA. Short-term therapy in secondary amenorrhea. *Ther Umsch*. 1973;30:496-502.
5. McNall PG, Jafarnia MR. Management of myasthenia gravis in the obstetrical patient. *Am J Obstet Gynecol*. 1965;92:518-525.
6. Foldes FF, McNall PG. Myasthenia gravis: a guide for anesthesiologists. *Anesthesiology*. 1962;23:837-872.
7. Chambers DC, Hall JE, Boyce J. Myasthenia gravis and pregnancy. *Obstet Gynecol*. 1967;29:597-603.
8. Hay DM. Myasthenia gravis and pregnancy. *J Obstet Gynaecol Br Commonw*. 1969;76:323-329.
9. Blackhall MI, Buckley GA, Roberts DV, Roberts JB, Thomas BH, Wilson A. Drug-induced neonatal myasthenia. *J Obstet Gynaecol Br Commonw*. 1969;76:157-162.
10. Eden RD, Gall SA. Myasthenia gravis and pregnancy: a reappraisal of thymectomy. *Obstet Gynecol*. 1983;62:328-333.
11. Plauche WC. Myasthenia gravis in pregnancy: an update. *Am J Obstet Gynecol*. 1979;135:691-697.
12. Fraser D, Turner JWA. Myasthenia gravis and pregnancy. *Proc R Soc Med*. 1963;56:379-381.
13. Lefvert AK, Osterman PO. Newborn infants to myasthenic mothers: a clinical study and an investigation of acetylcholine receptor antibodies in 17 children. *Neurology*. 1983;33:133-138.
14. Wilson JT. Pharmacokinetics of drug excretion. In: Wilson JT, ed. *Drugs in Breast Milk*. ADIS Press; 1981:17.
15. Habib AS, Gan TJ. Use of neostigmine in the management of acute postoperative pain and labour pain: a review. *CNS Drugs*. 2006;20(10):821-839.

NEPAFENAC OPHTHALMIC

Ophthalmic (Nonsteroidal Anti-Inflammatory Drug)

PREGNANCY RECOMMENDATION: No Human Data—Animal Data Suggest Low Risk

BREASTFEEDING RECOMMENDATION: Probably Compatible

PREGNANCY SUMMARY

No reports describing the use of the nepafenac ophthalmic in human pregnancy have been located. The drug and its active metabolite will probably cross the placenta. However, the amount of systemic absorption is low, which should limit placental transfer. Therefore, the amount is likely to be clinically insignificant. Nevertheless, the absence of human pregnancy experience prevents a complete assessment of the embryofetal risk. Animal data did not show any embryofetal toxicity in two species at doses of more than 10 times the Maximum recommended human ophthalmic dose (MRHOD). Using this drug during pregnancy should be based on the pros and cons of the mother's clinical need for treatment versus any potential fetal risk that might occur from exposure. If used during pregnancy, consider placing pressure over the tear duct in the corner of the eye for at least 1 minute, and then remove any excess solution with absorbent tissue to decrease the amount of drug reaching the systemic circulation even further.

BREASTFEEDING SUMMARY

No reports describing the use of nepafenac ophthalmic during human lactation have been located. The drug, if found in the systemic circulation, will probably be excreted into breast milk. However, systemic absorption is low with ophthalmic use. Therefore, the amount is likely to be clinically insignificant. Breastfeeding while using this drug should be based on the mother's clinical need for treatment versus any potential infant risks that might occur. If the clinical decision is to use this drug while breastfeeding, a method to decrease some systemic absorption with ophthalmic use is described above in the Pregnancy Summary. Due to low systemic absorption, systemic side effects are not expected.

Reference

1. Prescribing Information. Nevanac. Novartis Pharmaceuticals; 2020.

NERATINIB

Antineoplastic (Kinase Inhibitor)

PREGNANCY RECOMMENDATION: No Human Data—Animal Data Suggest Potential Risk

BREASTFEEDING RECOMMENDATION: Potential Toxicity

PREGNANCY SUMMARY

No reports describing the use of neratinib in human pregnancy have been located. Some amount of the drug will probably cross the placenta, so fetal exposure will likely occur. However, the absence of human pregnancy experience prevents a complete assessment of the embryofetal risk. Animal studies showed embryofetal toxicity and teratogenicity. Based on animal studies and the drug's mechanism of action, the manufacturer recommends that women with reproductive potential use effective contraception during treatment and for 1 month after the last dose. They also recommend that males with female partners of reproductive potential use effective contraception during treatment and for 3 months after the last dose. However, using this drug during pregnancy should be based on the pros and cons of the mother's clinical need for treatment versus any potential fetal risk that might occur from exposure.

BREASTFEEDING SUMMARY

No reports describing the use of neratinib during human lactation have been located. Some amount of the drug probably enters breast milk, so infant exposure will likely occur. However, due to the concern for potential serious adverse effects in a breastfed infant, the manufacturer recommends that women not breastfeed while being treated with neratinib and for at least 1 month after the last dose. Nevertheless, breastfeeding while using this drug should be based on the mother's clinical need for treatment. If used, the infant should be monitored for the most common reported adult side effects of nausea and abdominal pain (both leading to irritability), decreased appetite, diarrhea, vomiting, rash, lethargy, and urinary tract infection.

Reference

1. Prescribing Information. Nerlynx. Puma Biotechnology, Inc; 2017.

NETARSUDIL OPHTHALMIC

Ophthalmic (Rho Kinase Inhibitor—Topical)

PREGNANCY RECOMMENDATION: No Human Data—Animal Data Suggest Low Risk

BREASTFEEDING RECOMMENDATION: Probably Compatible

N

PREGNANCY SUMMARY

No reports describing the use of netarsudil ophthalmic in human pregnancy have been located. Though placental transfer is possible, fetal exposure is probably negligible because of insignificant absorption after ophthalmic use. However, the absence of human pregnancy experience prevents a complete assessment of the embryofetal risk. Animal data did not show any embryofetal toxicity despite being administered intravenously (IV). If used during pregnancy, consider placing pressure over the tear duct in the corner of the eye for at least 1 minute, and then remove any excess solution with absorbent tissue to decrease the amount of drug reaching the systemic circulation even further.

BREASTFEEDING SUMMARY

No reports describing the use of netarsudil ophthalmic in human lactation have been located. Because the drug has negligible absorption after ophthalmic use, any amount of the drug found in breast milk would not likely have a clinical effect. Breastfeeding while using this drug should be based on the mother's clinical need for treatment. A method to decrease some systemic absorption with ophthalmic use is described above in the Pregnancy Summary.

Reference

1. Prescribing Information. Rhopressa. Aerie Pharmaceuticals Inc; 2019.

NETUPITANT (FOSNETUPITANT)/PALONOSETRON

Gastrointestinal (Antiemetic)

PREGNANCY RECOMMENDATION: No Human Data—Animal Data Suggest Potential Risk

BREASTFEEDING RECOMMENDATION: Potential Toxicity

PREGNANCY SUMMARY

No reports describing the use of netupitant/fosnetupitant and palonosetron in human pregnancy have been located. All three drugs most likely cross the placenta to some extent, so fetal exposure will likely occur (though probably negligible for fosnetupitant). However, the absence of human pregnancy experience prevents a complete assessment of the embryofetal risk for these agents. Animal studies did not show embryofetal toxicity for palonosetron (see Palonosetron), but embryofetal toxicity was seen for netupitant/fosnetupitant. The overall fetal effect of this combination drug is not fully known. Both the oral and IV administrations are used in conjunction with dexamethasone (see Dexamethasone). Using this drug during pregnancy should be based on the pros and cons of the mother's clinical need for treatment versus any potential fetal risk that might occur from exposure.

BREASTFEEDING SUMMARY

Netupitant and palonosetron are probably excreted into human breast milk, so infant exposure will likely occur. Fosnetupitant is rapidly converted to netupitant. Both the oral and IV forms of these drugs are used in conjunction with dexamethasone (see Dexamethasone). Breastfeeding while using netupitant/fosnetupitant and palonosetron should be based on the mother's clinical need for treatment. If used, the infant should be monitored for the most common reported adult side effects of headache and dyspepsia (both leading to irritability), lethargy, constipation, and erythema.

Reference

1. Prescribing Information. Akynzeo. Helsinn Birex Pharmaceuticals; 2018.

N

NEVIRAPINE

Antiretroviral (Reverse Transcriptase Inhibitor)

PREGNANCY RECOMMENDATION: Human Data Suggest Low Risk (Maternal Benefit May Outweigh Any Embryofetal Risk)

BREASTFEEDING RECOMMENDATION: *Contraindicated

PREGNANCY SUMMARY

From the January 2024 interim report of APR, there were 36 (3.1%) birth anomalies in 1,180 first-trimester exposures. No pattern to the defects was seen. In 2024, the updated US Department of Health and Human Services AIDS Info guidelines for the use of antiretroviral agents during pregnancy recommend that, in most cases, patients continue their regimen during pregnancy if it is tolerated, safe, and effective in suppressing viral replication. The guidelines recommend that discussion and shared decision-making process about the known and potential risks as well as benefits to the mother and fetus should guide the selection of which antiretrovirals to use during pregnancy. The guidelines note that first-trimester exposure to nevirapine is not associated with an increased risk of congenital abnormalities. Additionally, treatment initiation should not be delayed due to concerns about teratogenicity with first-trimester exposure. See the guidelines for the most updated information. management. There is a pregnancy exposure registry that monitors pregnancy outcomes in patients using antiretroviral medicines during pregnancy. Health care providers are encouraged to call the APR at 1-800-258-4263.

BREASTFEEDING SUMMARY

A few studies were located that describe the use of nevirapine during human lactation. The manufacturer reports, based on five publications, that nevirapine is excreted into breast milk with a median breast milk to maternal plasma ratio of 59% to 88%. Therefore, some infant exposure will occur. In 2023, the updated US Department of Health and Human Services AIDS Info guidelines state that using replacement of breast milk through formula or pasteurized donor human breast milk from a milk bank eliminates the risk of postnatal HIV transmission to the infant. Using antiretroviral therapy to achieve and maintain viral suppression during pregnancy and postpartum decreases the risk for infant transmission to less than 1% but not zero. *For patients not on therapy or those without viral load suppression during pregnancy (at a minimum of throughout the third trimester) and at delivery, replacement of breast milk is recommended. Patients on antiretroviral therapy who have a sustained undetectable viral load and who choose to breastfeed or use replacement of breast milk should be supported with this decision. If the clinical decision is to use this drug while breastfeeding, the infant should be monitored for the most common reported pediatric side effects of rash and hyperbilirubinemia.

References

1. Prescribing Information. Nevirapine. Camber Pharmaceuticals; 2022.
2. Mirochnick M, Fenton T, Gagnier P, et al; for the Pediatric AIDS Clinical Trials Group Protocol 250 team. Pharmacokinetics of nevirapine in human immunodeficiency virus type 1-infected pregnant women and their neonates. *J Infect Dis*. 1998;178:368-374.
3. Musoke P, Guay LA, Bagenda D, et al. A phase I/II study of the safety and pharmacokinetics of nevirapine in HIV-1-infected pregnant Ugandan women and their neonates (HIVNET 006). *AIDS*. 1999;13:479-486.
4. Antiretroviral Pregnancy Registry Steering Committee. Antiretroviral Pregnancy Registry interim report for 1 January 1989 through 31 January 2024. Registry Coordinating Center; 2023. Accessed October 29, 2024. https://www.apregistry.com/forms/interim_report.pdf
5. Richardson MP, Osrin D, Donaghy S, et al. Spinal malformations in the fetuses of HIV infected women receiving combination antiretroviral therapy and co-trimoxazole. *Eur J Obstet Gynecol Reprod Biol*. 2000;93:215-217.
6. McGowan JP, Crane M, Wiznia AA, Blum S. Combination antiretroviral therapy in human immunodeficiency virus-infected pregnant women. *Obstet Gynecol*. 1999;94:641-646.
7. Guay LA, Musoke P, Fleming T, et al. Intrapartum and neonatal single-dose nevirapine compared with zidovudine for prevention of mother-to-child transmission of HIV-1 in Kampala, Uganda: HIVNET 012 randomised trial. *Lancet*. 1999;354:795-802.
8. Marseille E, Kahn JG, Mmiro F, et al. Cost effectiveness of single-dose nevirapine regimen for mothers and babies to decrease vertical HIV-1 transmission in sub-Saharan Africa. *Lancet*. 1999;354:803-809.
9. Taylor GP, Lyall EGH, Back D, et al. Pharmacological implications of lengthened in-utero exposure to nevirapine. *Lancet*. 2000;355:2134-2135.
10. Mofenson LM, McIntyre JA. Advances and research directions in the prevention of mother-to-child HIV-1 transmission. *Lancet*. 2000;355:2237-2244.
11. Panel on Treatment of HIV During Pregnancy and Prevention of Perinatal Transmission. Recommendations for the use of antiretroviral drugs during pregnancy and interventions to reduce perinatal HIV transmission in the United States. Department of Health and Human Services. Accessed October 29, 2024. https://clinicalinfo.hiv.gov/en/guidelines/perinatal

N

NIACIN

Vitamin/Antilipemic

PREGNANCY RECOMMENDATION: Human Data Suggest Compatible (Recommended Usage)

BREASTFEEDING RECOMMENDATION: Compatible (Recommended Usage)/*Potential Toxicity (Extra Usage)

PREGNANCY SUMMARY

Two reports describing the use of niacin supplementation in human pregnancy have been located. Adverse effects were not reported. Niacin (also known as Vitamin B_3) crosses the placenta. No animal studies have been conducted. Niacin helps support immunity and normal cholesterol balance and can lower low-density lipoprotein (LDL) cholesterol levels. The recommended daily allowance (RDA) for niacin during pregnancy is about 18 mg. If the diet of the pregnant woman adequately supplies this amount, extra supplementation is not needed. Maternal supplementation with niacin is primarily recommended for those patients with inadequate nutritional intake. This vitamin is not stored and ingesting too much from diet is not really possible. However, it is not known if using large amounts of supplemental niacin can be harmful.

BREASTFEEDING SUMMARY

No reports describing the effects of niacin during human lactation have been located. Niacin is actively excreted into breast milk. The RDA for niacin during lactation is 17 mg. If the diet of the lactating woman adequately supplies this amount, extra supplementation is not needed. Maternal supplementation with niacin is primarily recommended for those patients with inadequate nutritional intake. *However, if the mother is receiving extra niacin for its lipid-altering effects, the manufacturer recommends that a decision should be made whether to discontinue nursing or to discontinue the supplementation, considering the importance of the vitamin to the mother.

References

1. Prescribing Information. Niacin. Emerald Therapeutics, LLC; 2021.
2. Hart BF, McConnell WT. Vitamin B factors in toxic psychosis of pregnancy and the puerperium. *Am J Obstet Gynecol*. 1943;46:283.
3. Deodhar AD, Rajalakshmi R, Ramakrishnan CV. Studies on human lactation. Part III. Effect of dietary vitamin supplementation on vitamin contents of breast milk. *Acta Paediatr Scand*. 1964;53:42-48.
4. Ford JE, Zechalko A, Murphy J, Brooke OG. Comparison of the B vitamin composition of milk from mothers of preterm and term babies. *Arch Dis Child*. 1983;58:367-372.
5. Husebye ESN, Riedel B, Bjørke-Monsen AL, et al. Vitamin B status and association with antiseizure medication in pregnant women with epilepsy. *Epilepsia*. 2021;62:2968-2980.
6. Institute of Medicine (US) Standing Committee on the Scientific Evaluation of Dietary Reference Intakes and Its Panel on Folate, Other B Vitamins, and Choline. *Dietary Reference Intakes for Thiamin, Riboflavin, Niacin, Vitamin B_6, Folate, Vitamin B_{12}, Pantothenic Acid, Biotin, and Choline*. National Academies Press (US); 1998.

NIACINAMIDE

Vitamin

PREGNANCY RECOMMENDATION: Human Data Suggest Compatible (Recommended Usage)

BREASTFEEDING RECOMMENDATION: Compatible (Recommended Usage)

PREGNANCY SUMMARY

No reports describing the use of niacinamide supplementation in human pregnancy have been located. Niacinamide (an analogue of niacin, vitamin B_3) crosses the placenta. No animal studies have been conducted. Niacinamide is beneficial for skin, joints, glucose control, and immunity. It is not involved in supporting cholesterol balance. Like niacin, it is also not stored in the body. The RDA for niacinamide during lactation is 18 mg. If the diet of the pregnant woman adequately supplies this amount, supplementation with niacinamide is not needed. Maternal supplementation is primarily recommended for those patients with inadequate nutritional intake.

N

BREASTFEEDING SUMMARY

No reports describing the effects of niacinamide during human lactation have been located. Niacinamide, an analogue of niacin, is actively excreted into breast milk. Reports on the amount of niacinamide excreted in human breast milk have not been located. The RDA for niacinamide during lactation is 17 mg. If the diet of the lactating woman adequately supplies this amount, supplementation with extra niacinamide is not needed. Maternal supplementation with niacinamide is primarily recommended for those patients with inadequate nutritional intake.

References

1. American Hospital Formulary Service. *Drug Information 1997*. American Society of Health-System Pharmacists; 1997:2811-2813.
2. Hobson W. A dietary and clinical survey of pregnant women with particular reference to toxaemia of pregnancy. *J Hyg (Lond)*. 1948;46:198-216.
3. Hill EP, Longo LD. Dynamics of maternal-fetal nutrient transfer. *Fed Proc*. 1980;39:239-244.
4. Kaminetzky HA, Baker H, Frank O, Langer A. The effects of intravenously administered water-soluble vitamins during labor in normovitaminemic and hypovitaminemic gravidas on maternal and neonatal blood vitamin levels at delivery. *Am J Obstet Gynecol*. 1974;120:697-703.
5. Baker H, Frank O, Thomson AD, et al. Vitamin profile of 174 mothers and newborns at parturition. *Am J Clin Nutr*. 1975;28:59-65.
6. Baker H, Frank O, Deangelis B, Feingold S, Kaminetzky HA. Role of placenta in maternal-fetal vitamin transfer in humans. *Am J Obstet Gynecol*. 1981;141:792-796.
7. Baker H, Thind IS, Frank O, DeAngelis B, Caterini H, Louria DB. Vitamin levels in low-birth-weight newborn infants and their mothers. *Am J Obstet Gynecol*. 1977;129:521-524.
8. Wertz AW, Lojkin ME, Bouchard BS, Derby MB. Tryptophan-niacin relationships in pregnancy. *Am J Nutr*. 1958;64:339-353.
9. Deodhar AD, Rajalakshmi R, Ramakrishnan CV. Studies on human lactation. Part III. Effect of dietary vitamin supplementation on vitamin contents of breast milk. *Acta Paediatr Scand*. 1964;53:42-48.
10. Ford JE, Zechalko A, Murphy J, Brooke OG. Comparison of the B vitamin composition of milk from mothers of preterm and term babies. *Arch Dis Child*. 1983;58:367-372.
11. Institute of Medicine (US) Standing Committee on the Scientific Evaluation of Dietary Reference Intakes and Its Panel on Folate, Other B Vitamins, and Choline. *Dietary Reference Intakes for Thiamin, Riboflavin, Niacin, Vitamin B_6, Folate, Vitamin B_{12}, Pantothenic Acid, Biotin, and Choline*. National Academies Press (US); 1998.

NICARDIPINE

Antihypertensive (Calcium Channel Blocker)

PREGNANCY RECOMMENDATION: Limited Human Data—Animal Data Suggest Low Risk (Oral)/ Potential Toxicity (IV Use)

BREASTFEEDING RECOMMENDATION: Probably Compatible (Oral Use)/Potential Toxicity (IV Use)

PREGNANCY SUMMARY

Limited reports describing the use of nicardipine in human pregnancy have been located. Available studies have found no significant evidence of an increased risk of congenital anomalies or significant adverse effects with first-trimester exposure. The drug has primarily been used in the second and third trimesters to treat hypertension. Nicardipine crosses the human placenta in low amounts, so some fetal exposure will occur. However, this limited first-trimester human pregnancy experience prevents a complete assessment of the embryofetal risk. No embryofetal toxicity or teratogenicity was seen in two animal species with oral doses less than 10 times the RHD in one species and more than 10 times the RHD in the second species. However, embryofetal toxicity was seen with IV doses at about equal to the RHD. Using this drug during pregnancy should be based on the pros and cons of the mother's clinical need for treatment versus any potential fetal risk that might occur from exposure.

BREASTFEEDING SUMMARY

A few studies were located that describe the use of nicardipine during human lactation. Breast milk levels ranged from undetectable to about 20 ng/mL. The calculated RIDs were all less than 1%. Breastfeeding while using this drug should be based on the mother's clinical need for treatment versus any potential infant risks that might occur. If used, the infant should be monitored for the most common reported adult side effects of nausea and headache (both leading to irritability), hypotension, tachycardia, and vomiting.

References

1. Prescribing Information. Nicardipine Hydrochloride. Epic Pharma, LLC; 2023.
2. Prescribing Information. Nicardipine Hydrochloride. Armas Pharmaceuticals Inc; 2024.
3. Matsumura H, Takagi K, Seki H, et al. Placental transfer of intravenous nicardipine and disposition into breast milk during the control of hypertension in women with pre-eclampsia. *Hypertens Pregnancy.* 2014;33:93-101.
4. Bartels PA, Hanff LM, Mathot RAA, Steegers EAP, Vulto AG, Visser W. Nicardipine in pre-eclamptic patients: placental transfer and disposition in breast milk. *BJOG*. 2007;114:230-233.
5. Cornette J, Buijs AB, Duvekot JJ, et al. Hemodynamic effects of intravenous nicardipine in severely pre-eclamptic women with a hypertensive crisis. *Ultrasound Obstet Gynecol*. 2016;47:89-95.
6. Jannet D, Abankwa A, Guyard B, Carbonne B, Marpeau L, Milliez J. Nicardipine versus salbutamol in the treatment of premature labor. A prospective randomized study. *Eur J Obstet Gynaecol Reprod Med*. 1997;73:11-16.
7. Ross EL, Ross BS, Dickerson GA, et al. Oral nicardipine versus intravenous magnesium sulfate for the treatment of preterm labor (abstract). *Am J Obstet Gynecol*. 1998;178:S181.
8. Larmon JE, Ross BS, May WL, Dickerson GA, Fischer RG, Morrison JC. Oral nicardipine versus intravenous magnesium sulfate for the treatment of preterm labor. *Am J Obstet Gynecol*. 1999;181:1432-1437.
9. Melis M, Cupelli A, Sottosanti L, et al. Off-label use of nicardipine as tocolytic and acute pulmonary oedema: a post-marketing analysis of adverse drug reaction reports in EudraVigilance. *Pharmacoepidemiol Drug Saf*. 2015;24:1220-1224.
10. Walker JJ, Mathers A, Bjornsson S, Cameron AD, Fairlie FM. The effect of acute and chronic antihypertensive therapy on maternal and fetoplacental Doppler velocimetry. *Eur J Obstet Gynecol Reprod Biol*. 1992;43:193-199.
11. Carbonne B, Jannet D, Touboul C, Khelifati Y, Milliez J. Nicardipine treatment of hypertension during pregnancy. *Obstet Gynecol*. 1993;81:908-914.
12. Jannet D, Carbonne B, Sebban E, Milliez J. Nicardipine versus metoprolol in the treatment of hypertension during pregnancy: a randomized comparative trial. *Obstet Gynecol*. 1994;84:354-359.
13. Jarreau PH, Le Beller C, Guillonneau M, Jacqz-Aigrain E. Excretion of nicardipine in human milk. *Pediat Perinat Drug Ther*. 2000;4:28-30.

N

NICOTINE REPLACEMENT THERAPY

Central Nervous System (Smoking Cessation Aid)

PREGNANCY RECOMMENDATION: Limited Human Data—Animal Data Suggest Risk

BREASTFEEDING RECOMMENDATION: Probably Compatible

PREGNANCY SUMMARY

The use of nicotine replacement therapy (NRT) during pregnancy is reported throughout the literature. Since 2020, at least five meta-analyses or systematic reviews have evaluated the outcomes of NRT in pregnancy. Available studies have not found significant evidence of an increased risk of congenital anomalies or a statistically significant difference in smoking cessation. While most studies found no adverse effects on fetal or neonatal outcomes, the evidence is poor and inconsistent. Nicotine crosses the placenta, so fetal exposure will occur. However, the inconsistent human pregnancy experience prevents a complete assessment of the embryofetal risk. The US Preventive Services Task Force (USPSTF) and ACOG have concluded that the current evidence is insufficient to assess the balance of benefits and harms of pharmacotherapy interventions for tobacco cessation in pregnant persons. ACOG also recommends that NRT should be considered only after a detailed discussion with the patient of the known risks of continued smoking, the possible risks of NRT, and the need for close supervision.

BREASTFEEDING SUMMARY

One report describing the use of nicotine patches found that nicotine and its metabolite cotinine are excreted into breast milk at much lower levels than those found with cigarette smoking. The American Academy of Pediatrics (AAP) states that NRT may be used while breastfeeding. Short-acting agents (gum or lozenges) are preferred over patches. If used while breastfeeding, the infant should be monitored for nausea (leading to irritability), vomiting, diarrhea, and tachycardia.

References

1. Prescribing Information. Nicotrol inhaler. Pharmacia and Upjohn Company; 2024.
2. Shepard TH. *Catalog of Teratogenic Agents*. 10th ed. The Johns Hopkins University Press; 2001:361-362.
3. Schardein JL. *Chemically Induced Birth Defects*. 3rd ed. Marcel Dekker; 2000:981-982.
4. Ilett KF, Hale TW, Page-Sharp M, Kristensen JH, Kohan R, Hackett LP. Use of nicotine patches in breast-feeding mothers: transfer of nicotine and cotinine into human milk. *Clin Pharmacol Ther*. 2003;74:516-524.
5. American College of Obstetricians and Gynecologist. Tobacco and nicotine cessation during pregnancy: ACOG Committee Opinion No. 807. *Obstet Gynecol*. 2020;135:e221-e229.
6. Claire R, Chamberlain C, Davey MA, et al. Pharmacological interventions for promoting smoking cessation during pregnancy. *Cochrane Database Syst Rev*. 2020;3(3):CD010078.
7. Blanc J, Tosello B, Ekblad MO, Berlin I, Netter A. Nicotine replacement therapy during pregnancy and child health outcomes: a systematic review. *Int J Environ Res Public Health*. 2021;18(8):4004.
8. Taylor L, Claire R, Campbell K, et al. Fetal safety of nicotine replacement therapy in pregnancy: systematic review and meta-analysis. *Addiction*. 2021;116(2):239-277.
9. Patnode CD, Henderson JT, Coppola EL, Melnikow J, Durbin S, Thomas RG. Interventions for tobacco cessation in adults, including pregnant persons: updated evidence report and systematic review for the US Preventive Services Task Force. *JAMA*. 2021;325(3):280-298.
10. Morales-Suárez-Varela M, Puig BM, Kaerlev L, Peraita-Costa I, Perales-Marín A. Safety of nicotine replacement therapy during pregnancy: a narrative review. *Int J Environ Res Public Health*. 2022;20(1):250.
11. Sachs HC; Committee on Drugs. The transfer of drugs and therapeutics into human breast milk: an update on selected topics. *Pediatrics*. 2013;132(3):e796-809.
12. Meek JY, Noble L; Section on Breastfeeding. Policy statement: breastfeeding and the use of human milk. *Pediatrics*. 2022;150(1):e2022057988.

NIFEDIPINE

Antihypertensive (Calcium Channel Blocker)

PREGNANCY RECOMMENDATION: Human Data Suggest Low Risk

BREASTFEEDING RECOMMENDATION: Probably Compatible

PREGNANCY SUMMARY

The use of nifedipine for tocolysis, hypertension, and hypertensive emergency in pregnancy is well reported in the literature. Available studies have found no significant evidence of an increased risk of congenital anomalies, though the number of first-trimester exposures are small. Overall, nifedipine is considered low risk for use in pregnancy. Nifedipine crosses the placenta, so fetal exposure will occur. Animal studies did show some embryofetal toxicity in one species at doses of about 5 times the MRHD, but most studies involved doses of more than 10 times the MRHD. Though further studies would be helpful regarding first-trimester use, ACOG considers oral nifedipine as a first-line agent for the treatment of hypertension during pregnancy and for postpartum hypertension. Nifedipine extended-release is also recommended for chronic maintenance treatment in pregnancy.

N

BREASTFEEDING SUMMARY

Nine reports describing the use of nifedipine in Raynaud phenomenon of the nipple in breastfeeding mothers have been located. No adverse effects in breastfed infants have been reported. Nifedipine is excreted into breast milk in low amounts, so infant exposure will occur. Breastfeeding while using this drug should be based on the mother's clinical need for treatment versus any potential infant risks that might occur. If used, the infant should be monitored for the most common reported adult side effects of nausea, dizziness, and headache (all leading to irritability), constipation, fatigue, flushing, and edema.

References

1. Prescribing Information. Nifedipine extended-release. Chartwell RX, LLC; 2024.
2. Lindow SW, Davies N, Davey DA, Smith JA. The effect of sublingual nifedipine on uteroplacental blood flow in hypertensive pregnancy. *Br J Obstet Gynaecol*. 1988;95:1276-1281.
3. Walters BNJ, Redman CWG. Treatment of severe pregnancy-associated hypertension with the calcium antagonist nifedipine. *Br J Obstet Gynaecol*. 1984;91:330-336.
4. Constantine G, Beevers DG, Reynolds AL, Luesley DM. Nifedipine as a second line antihypertensive drug in pregnancy. *Br J Obstet Gynaecol*. 1987;94:1136-1142.
5. Bird LM, Anderson NC Jr, Chandler ML, Young RC. The effects of aminophylline and nifedipine on contractility of isolated pregnant human myometrium. *Am J Obstet Gynecol*. 1987;157:171-177.
6. Ulmsten U, Andersson K-E, Wingerup L. Treatment of premature labor with the calcium antagonist nifedipine. *Arch Gynecol*. 1980;229:1-5.
7. Kaul AF, Osathanondh R, Safon LE, et al. The management of preterm labor with the calcium channel-blocking agent nifedipine combined with the beta-mimetic terbutaline. *Drug Intell Clin Pharm*. 1985;19:369-371.
8. Read MD, Wellby DE. The use of a calcium antagonist (nifedipine) to suppress preterm labour. *Br J Obstet Gynaecol*. 1986;93:933-937.
9. Snyder SW, Cardwell MS. Neuromuscular blockade with magnesium sulfate and nifedipine. *Am J Obstet Gynecol*. 1989;161:35-36.
10. Waisman GD, Mayorga LM, Camera MI, Vignolo CA, Martinotti A. Magnesium plus nifedipine: potentiation of hypotensive effect in preeclampsia? *Am J Obstet Gynecol*. 1988;159:308-309.
11. Magee LA, Schick B, Donnenfeld AE, et al. The safety of calcium channel blockers in human pregnancy: a prospective, multicenter cohort study. *Am J Obstet Gynecol*. 1996;174:823-828.
12. Weber-Schoendorfer C, Hannemann D, Meister R, et al. The safety of calcium channel blockers during pregnancy: a prospective, multicenter, observational study. *Reprod Toxicol*. 2008;26:24-30.
13. Ehrenkranz RA, Ackerman BA, Hulse JD. Nifedipine transfer into human milk. *J Pediatr*. 1989;114:478-480.
14. Prevost RR, Akl SA, Whybrew WD, Sibai BM. Oral nifedipine pharmacokinetics in pregnancy-induced hypertension. *Pharmacotherapy*. 1992;12(3):174-177.
15. American College of Obstetricians and Gynecologists. Chronic hypertension in pregnancy: ACOG practice bulletin no. 203. *Obstet Gynecol*. 2019;133:e26-e50.

16. American College of Obstetricians and Gynecologists. Practice bulletin no. 171: management of preterm labor. *Obstet Gynecol*. 2016;128:e155-e164.
17. Anderson PO. Drug treatment of Raynaud's phenomenon of the nipple. *Breastfeed Med*. 2020;15:686-688.
18. Penny WJ, Lewis MJ. Nifedipine is excreted in human milk. *Eur J Clin Pharmacol*. 1989;36:427-428.
19. Manninen AK, Juhakoski A. Nifedipine concentrations in maternal and umbilical serum, amniotic fluid, breast milk and urine of mothers and offspring. *Int J Clin Pharmacol Res*. 1991;11:231-236.
20. Taddio A, Oskamp M, Ito S, et al. Is nifedipine use during labour and breastfeeding safe for the neonate? *Clin Investig Med*. 1996;19:S11.
21. Malfará BN, Benzi JRI, de Oliveira Filgueira GC, et al. ABCG2 c.421C>A polymorphism alters nifedipine transport to breast milk in hypertensive breastfeeding women. *Reprod Toxicol*. 2019;85:1-5.
22. Lawlor-Smith LS, Lawlor-Smith CL. Raynaud's phenomenon of the nipple: a preventable cause of breastfeeding failure? *Med J Aust*. 1996;166:448.
23. Garrison CP. Nipple vasospasm, Raynaud's syndrome, and nifedipine. *J Hum Lact*. 2002;18:382-385.
24. Anderson JE, Held N, Wright K. Raynaud's phenomenon of the nipple: a treatable cause of painful breastfeeding. *Pediatrics*. 2004;113:e360-e364.
25. Page SM, McKenna DS. Vasospasm of the nipple presenting as painful lactation. *Obstet Gynecol*. 2006;108(3 part 2):806-808.
26. O'Sullivan S, Keith MP. Raynaud phenomenon of the nipple: a rare finding in rheumatology clinic. *J Clin Rheumatol*. 2011;17:371-372.
27. Wu M, Chason R, Wong M. Raynaud's phenomenon of the nipple. *Obstet Gynecol*. 2012;119(2 pt 2):447-449.
28. Barrett ME, Heller MM, Fullerton Stone H, Murase JE. Raynaud phenomenon of the nipple in breastfeeding mothers: an underdiagnosed cause of nipple pain. *JAMA Dermatol*. 2013;149:300-306.

NIFURTIMOX

Anti-Infective (Antiprotozoal)

PREGNANCY RECOMMENDATION: Limited Human Data—Animal Data Suggest Potential Risk

BREASTFEEDING RECOMMENDATION: Probably Compatible

PREGNANCY SUMMARY

No human data specific to birth anomalies from exposure to nifurtimox have been reported. The drug will probably cross the placenta. Animal data did show fetotoxic effects in one species at doses below the MRHD. However, the absence of human pregnancy experience prevents a complete assessment of the embryofetal risk. From a clinical standpoint, most patients (including newborns) are asymptomatic when infected with Chagas disease in the early stages. However, long-term effects from chronic disease over time can be significant. The World Health Organization considers Chagas disease a "neglected tropical disease." The risk of perinatal transmission of Chagas disease during gestation is estimated to be about 5%. While the benefits of treating an asymptomatic mother during pregnancy are not clear, identifying and treating an infected newborn could be crucial. Decisions to treat during pregnancy should be based on full informed consent with pros and cons. There is a pregnancy safety study for this drug if administered during pregnancy, if a patient becomes pregnant while being treated, or if a patient is pregnant within 6 months of the last dose. Health care providers are encouraged to call 1-888-842-2937. Because of the potential adverse fetal effects seen in animal studies, the manufacturer recommends that women with reproductive potential use effective contraception during treatment with nifurtimox and for 6 months after the last dose. They also recommend that males with female partners of reproductive potential use condoms during treatment and for 3 months after the final dose. Nitrofurantoin is a similar nitrofuran analogue used primarily in treating urinary tract infections (see Nitrofurantoin).

BREASTFEEDING SUMMARY

A study of 10 lactating women found that nifurtimox was excreted into human breast milk but at low levels (<15% of the recommended daily dose for pediatric patients with Chagas disease). None of the neonates demonstrated any adverse effects during and after study treatment. In a separate study, the presence of Trypanosoma cruzi was not found in the breast milk of 21 lactating women. The presence of Trypanosoma cruzi in breast milk is possible with cracked/bleeding nipples; however, Chagas disease is not a reason to avoid breastfeeding. If nifurtimox is used while breastfeeding, the infant should be monitored for the most common reported side effects of vomiting, decreased appetite, rash, pyrexia, and irritability.

References

1. Prescribing Information. Lampit. Bayer Healthcare Pharmaceuticals Inc; 2020.
2. Schnid C, Kuemmerle A, Blum J, et al. In-hospital safety in field conditions of nifurtimox eflornithine combination therapy (NECT) for T. b. gambiense sleeping sickness. *PLoS Negl Trop Dis*. 2012;6(11):e1920.
3. Livingston EG, Duggal R, Dotters-Katz S. Screening for Chagas disease during pregnancy in the United States—a literature review. *Trop Med Infect Dis*. 2021;6(4):202-215.
4. Moroni S, Marson ME, Moscatelli G, et al. Negligible exposure to nifurtimox through breast milk during maternal treatment for Chagas Disease. *PLoS Negl Trop Dis*. 2019;13(8):e0007647.
5. Garcia-Bournissen F, Moroni S, Marson ME, et al. Limited infant exposure to benznidazole through breast milk during maternal treatment for Chagas disease. *Arch Dis Child*. 2015;100(1):90-94.
6. Bittencourt AL, Sadigursky M, Da Silva AA, et al. Evaluation of Chagas disease transmission through breast-feeding. *Mem Inst Oswaldo Cruz*. 1988;83(1):37-39.
7. Campos R, Pinto PL, Moreira AA, et al. Experimental study on the transmission of Chagas disease by milk. *Rev Hosp Clin Fac Med Sao Paulo*. 1988;43:146-147.
8. Ferreira CS, Martinho PC, Amato Neto V, Cruz RR. Pasteurization of human milk to prevent transmission of Chagas disease. *Rev Inst Med Trop Sao Paula*. 2001;43:161-162.

NILOTINIB

Antineoplastic (Tyrosine Kinase Inhibitor)

PREGNANCY RECOMMENDATION: Limited Human Data—Animal Data Suggest Risk

BREASTFEEDING RECOMMENDATION: Potential Toxicity

PREGNANCY SUMMARY

Ten reports describing the use of nilotinib in at least 60 human pregnancies have been located. In most cases, nilotinib exposure occurred in the first trimester and was discontinued when pregnancy was discovered. The majority of these cases resulted in healthy deliveries. Two miscarriages, one omphalocele, and a case of intrauterine death of one twin with congenital transposition of great vessels have been reported. Nilotinib has limited placental transfer, but some fetal exposure will occur. However, this limited human pregnancy experience prevents a complete assessment of the embryofetal risk. Embryofetal toxicity was observed in two animal species at doses less than 10 times the RHD. Based on animal studies and the drug's mechanism of action, the manufacturer recommends that women with reproductive potential use effective contraception during treatment and for 2 weeks after the last dose. However, current recommendations suggest that it may be advisable to stop tyrosine kinase inhibitor therapy at the first detection of pregnancy, but if needed, nilotinib may be considered after 16 weeks' gestation. Additionally, there is a registry for women who are pregnant and have cancer. For more information, women and health care providers are encouraged to contact the Cancer and Pregnancy Registry at 1-877-635-4499. Nilotinib carries a boxed warning regarding QT prolongation and risk for sudden death.

BREASTFEEDING SUMMARY

One report describing the case of a mother who received nilotinib for 9 months while breastfeeding has been located. No adverse effects were reported in the infant. Nilotinib was found in every sample with a peak value of 129 ng/mL. The calculated RID was less than 1%. However, due to a concern for potential serious adverse effects that might be seen in a breastfed infant, the manufacturer recommends that women not breastfeed while being treated with this drug and for at least 2 weeks after the last dose. Nevertheless, breastfeeding while using this drug should be based on the mother's clinical need for treatment versus any potential infant risks that might occur. If used, the infant should be monitored for the most common reported adult side effects of nausea, headache, pruritus, and arthralgia (all leading to irritability), rash, fatigue (lethargy), vomiting, diarrhea, cough, constipation, fever, night sweats, and various laboratory abnormalities (see PI).

N

References

1. Prescribing Information. Tasigna. Novartis Pharmaceuticals; 2024.
2. Conchon M, Sanabani SS, Bendit I, Maria Santos F, Serpa M, Dorliac-Llacer PE. Two successful pregnancies in a woman with chronic myeloid leukemia exposed to nilotinib during the first trimester of her second pregnancy: case study. *J Hematol Oncol*. 2009;2:42.
3. Hadiji Mseddi S, Kallel F, Amouri H, Affes H, Mdhaffar M, Elloumi M. Delivery of two normal twins exposed to imatinib and nilotinib during the first trimester of pregnancy in a woman with chronic myeloid leukemia. *J Hematol Malig*. 2012;2:838.
4. Sweany SJ. TKIs and the treatment of CML in pregnant women. *HemOnc Today*. October 25, 2011. https://www.healio.com/hematology-oncology/leukemia/news/print/hemonc-today/%7Bff202790-727e-43aa-9d19-d403b622c670%7D/tkis-and-the-treatment-of-cml-in-pregnant-women
5. Arnall J, Muluneh B. Loss of pregnancy in a patient with chronic myeloid leukemia during treatment with nilotinib. *J Hematol Oncol Pharm*. 2016;6:22-27.
6. Abruzzese E, Trawinska MM, Perrotti AP, De Fabritiis P. Tyrosine kinase inhibitors and pregnancy. *Mediterr J Hematol Infect Dis*. 2014;6:e2014028.
7. Alizadeh H, Jaafar H, Kajtár B. Outcome of 3 pregnancies in a patient with chronic myeloid leukemia who received 3 types of tyrosine kinase inhibitors each in different pregnancy: follow-up of the case with a review of published reports. *Ann Saudi Med*. 2015;35:468.
8. Chelysheva E, Turkina A, Polushkina E, et al. Placental transfer of tyrosine kinase inhibitors used for chronic myeloid leukemia treatment. *Leuk Lymphoma*. 2018;59:733-738.
9. Dou X, Qin Y, Huang X, Jiang Q. Planned pregnancy in female patients with chronic myeloid leukemia receiving tyrosine kinase inhibitor therapy. *Oncologist*. 2019;24(11):e1141-e1147.
10. Abruzzese E, Mauro M, Apperley J, Chelysheva E. Tyrosine kinase inhibitors and pregnancy in chronic myeloid leukemia: opinion, evidence, and recommendations. *Ther Adv Hematol*. 2020;11:2040620720966120.
11. Abruzzese E, Aureli S, Bondanini F, et al. Chronic myeloid leukemia and pregnancy: when dreams meet reality. State of the art, management and outcome of 41 cases, nilotinib placental transfer. *J Clin Med*. 2022;11:180.
12. Chethan R, Malik PS, Sahoo RK, et al. Fertility and pregnancy in chronic myeloid leukemia: real-world experience from an Indian tertiary care institution. *Ann Hematol*. 2023;10:2087-2096.
13. Abruzzese E, Trawinska MM, De Fabritiis P, Bernardi S. SOHO state of the art updates and next questions: chronic myeloid leukemia and pregnancy: "Per Aspera Ad Astra". *Clin Lymphoma Myeloma Leuk*. 2024;24:214-223.
14. Chelysheva E, Aleshin S, Polushkina E, et al. Breastfeeding in patients with chronic myeloid leukaemia: case series with measurements of drug concentrations in maternal milk and review of literature. *Mediterr J Hematol Infect Dis*. 2018;10:e2018027.

NIMODIPINE

Central Nervous System (Calcium Channel Blocker)

PREGNANCY RECOMMENDATION: Limited Human Data—Animal Data Suggest Risk

BREASTFEEDING RECOMMENDATION: Probably Compatible

PREGNANCY SUMMARY

Four small reports and a large randomized controlled trial (RCT) were located that describe the use of nimodipine in more than 850 pregnant women. Nearly all of the pregnancies were in the late second and third trimester in treating preeclampsia compared with other drugs, such as magnesium sulfate. No differences were observed in neonatal outcomes between groups, but magnesium was more effective than nimodipine for the prevention of seizures in women with severe preeclampsia. A few first-trimester exposures were found, but the numbers are too small to identify any risks. Nimodipine crosses the placenta, so some fetal exposure will occur. However, this limited human pregnancy experience prevents a complete assessment of the embryofetal risk. Embryofetal toxicity was observed in two animal species at doses less than 10 times the RHD. Using this drug during pregnancy should be based on the pros and cons of the mother's clinical need for treatment versus any potential fetal risk that might occur from exposure.

BREASTFEEDING SUMMARY

Two reports were located that describe the use of nimodipine during human lactation. Nimodipine was found to be excreted into breast milk with levels ranging from about 0.4 ng/mL up to about 16 ng/mL. Calculated RIDs were less than 1%. Breastfeeding while using this drug should be based on the mother's clinical need for treatment versus any potential infant risks that might occur. If used, the infant should be monitored for the most common reported adult side effects of headache (leading to irritability) and hypotension.

References

1. Prescribing Information. Nimodipine. Heritage Pharmaceuticals Inc; 2024.
2. Belfort M, Saade G, Cruz A, et al. Nimodipine as an alternative to magnesium sulfate in the management of severe preeclampsia: maternal and fetal effects (abstract). *Am J Obstet Gynecol*. 1994;170:412.
3. Belfort MA, Saade GR, Moise KJ Jr, et al. Nimodipine in the management of preeclampsia: maternal and fetal effects. *Am J Obstet Gynecol*. 1994; 171:417-424.
4. Magee LA, Schick B, Donnenfeld AE, et al. The safety of calcium channel blockers in human pregnancy: a prospective, multicenter cohort study. *Am J Obstet Gynecol*. 1996;174:823-828.
5. Horn EH, Filshie M, Kerslake RW, Jaspan T, Worthington BS, Rubin PC. Widespread cerebral ischaemia treated with nimodipine in a patient with eclampsia. *Br Med J*. 1990;301:794.
6. Belfort MA, Carpenter RJ Jr, Kirshon B, et al. The use of nimodipine in a patient with eclampsia: color flow Doppler demonstration of retinal artery relaxation. *Am J Obstet Gynecol*. 1993;169:204-206.
7. Anthony J, Mantel G, Johanson R, Dommisse J. The haemodynamic and respiratory effects of intravenous nimodipine used in the treatment of eclampsia. *Br J Obstet Gynaecol*. 1996;103:518-522.
8. Belfort M, Anthony J, Saade GR, Allen JC; the Nimodipine Study Group. Interim report of the nimodipine vs. magnesium sulfate for seizure prophylaxis in severe preeclampsia study: an international, randomized, controlled trial (abstract). *Am J Obstet Gynecol*. 1998;178:S7.
9. Belfort MA, Saade GR, Yared M, et al. Change in estimated cerebral perfusion pressure after treatment with nimodipine or magnesium sulfate in patients with preeclampsia. *Am J Obstet Gynecol*. 1999;181:402-407.
10. Carcas AJ, Abad-Santos F, de Rosendo JM, Frias J. Nimodipine transfer into human breast milk and cerebrospinal fluid. *Ann Pharmacother*. 1996;30:148-150.
11. Tonks AM. Nimodipine levels in breast milk. *Aust N Z J Surg*. 1995;65: 693-694.
12. Hollenberg NK. A comparison of magnesium sulfate and nimodipine for the prevention of eclampsia. *Curr Hypertens Rep*. 2003;5(4):288-289.
13. Belfort MA, Anthony J, Saade GR, Allen JC Jr; Nimodipine Study Group. A comparison of magnesium sulfate and nimodipine for the prevention of eclampsia. *N Engl J Med*. 2003;348:304-311.

N

NINTEDANIB

Respiratory (Tyrosine Kinase Inhibitor)

PREGNANCY RECOMMENDATION: No Human Data—Animal Data Suggest Risk

BREASTFEEDING RECOMMENDATION: Potential Toxicity

PREGNANCY SUMMARY

No reports describing the use of nintedanib in human pregnancy have been located. Some amount of the drug may cross the placenta, so fetal exposure will likely occur. However, the absence of human pregnancy experience prevents a complete assessment of the embryofetal risk. Embryofetal toxicity with malformations was observed in two animal species at doses less than 10 times the MRHD. Based on animal studies and the drug's mechanism of action, the manufacturer recommends that women with reproductive potential use effective contraception during treatment and for 3 months after the last dose. Nevertheless, using this drug during pregnancy should be based on the pros and cons of the mother's clinical need for treatment versus any potential fetal risk that might occur from exposure.

BREASTFEEDING SUMMARY

No reports describing the use of nintedanib during human lactation have been located. The drug will probably be found in breast milk, so some infant exposure will likely occur. Due to a concern for potential serious adverse effects that might be seen in a breastfed infant, the manufacturer recommends that women not breastfeed while being treated with this drug. Nevertheless, breastfeeding while using this drug should be based on the mother's clinical need for treatment versus any potential infant risks that might occur. If used, the infant should be monitored for the most common reported adult side effects of nausea, headache, and abdominal pain (all leading to irritability), diarrhea, vomiting, liver enzyme elevation, decreased appetite (monitor infant growth), and hypertension.

Reference

1. Prescribing Information. Ofev. Boehringer Ingelheim Pharmaceuticals, Inc; 2022.

NIRAPARIB

Antineoplastic (Poly [ADP-Ribose] Polymerase Inhibitor)

PREGNANCY RECOMMENDATION: No Human Data and No Relevant Animal Data

BREASTFEEDING RECOMMENDATION: Potential Toxicity

PREGNANCY SUMMARY

No reports describing the use of niraparib in human pregnancy have been located. Some amount of the drug will probably cross the placenta, so fetal exposure will likely occur. However, the absence of human pregnancy experience prevents a complete assessment of the embryofetal risk. Animal reproductive studies have not been performed. Based on the drug's mechanism of action, the manufacturer recommends that women with reproductive potential use effective contraception during treatment and for 6 months after the last dose. However, using this drug during pregnancy should be based on the pros and cons of the mother's clinical need for treatment versus any potential fetal risk that might occur from exposure.

BREASTFEEDING SUMMARY

No reports describing the use of niraparib during human lactation have been located. Some amount of the drug probably enters breast milk, so infant exposure will likely occur. However, due to the concern for potential serious adverse effects in a breastfed infant, the manufacturer recommends that women not breastfeed while being treated with niraparib and for at least 1 month after the last dose. Nevertheless, breastfeeding while using this drug should be based on the mother's clinical need for treatment. If used, the infant should be monitored for the most common reported adult side effects of nausea, headache, abdominal pain, and musculoskeletal pain (all leading to irritability), diarrhea, vomiting, rash, lethargy, cough, constipation, decreased appetite, and various laboratory abnormalities (see PI).

Reference

1. Prescribing Information. Zejula. GlaxoSmithKline; 2020.

N

NIROGACESTAT

Miscellaneous (Gamma Secretase Inhibitor)

PREGNANCY RECOMMENDATION: No Human Data—Animal Data Suggest Potential Risk

BREASTFEEDING RECOMMENDATION: Potential Toxicity

PREGNANCY SUMMARY

No reports describing the use of nirogacestat in human pregnancy have been located. The drug will probably cross the placenta, so some fetal exposure will likely occur. However, the absence of human pregnancy experience prevents a complete assessment of the embryofetal risk. Animal reproduction studies did show some embryofetal toxicity in one species at doses of less than the RHD. Using this drug during pregnancy should be based on the pros and cons of the mother's clinical need for treatment versus any potential fetal risk that might occur from exposure.

BREASTFEEDING SUMMARY

No reports describing the use of nirogacestat during human lactation have been located. The drug will probably be found in breast milk, so some infant exposure will likely occur. Due to a concern for potential serious adverse effects that might be seen in a breastfed infant, the manufacturer recommends that women not breastfeed while being treated with this drug and for at least 1 week after the last dose. Nevertheless, breastfeeding while using this drug should be based on the mother's clinical need for treatment versus any potential infant risks that might occur. If used, the infant should be monitored for the most common reported adult side effects of nausea, headache, and abdominal pain (all leading to irritability), diarrhea, cough, rash, and fatigue (lethargy).

Reference

1. Prescribing Information. Ogsiveo. Spring Works Therapeutics, Inc; 2023.

NIRSEVIMAB

Antiviral (Monoclonal Antibody—Respiratory Syncytial Virus (RSV))

PREGNANCY RECOMMENDATION: *Contraindicated

BREASTFEEDING RECOMMENDATION: *Contraindicated

PREGNANCY SUMMARY

No reports describing the use of nirsevimab in human pregnancy have been located. As an IgG antibody, it would likely cross the placenta, especially during the second half of pregnancy, so some fetal exposure could occur. *However, this drug is not indicated for use in women with reproductive potential. Animal reproduction studies have not been performed.

BREASTFEEDING SUMMARY

No reports describing the use of nirsevimab during human lactation have been located. It is known that IgG antibodies can be found in human breast milk but are not found in the neonatal or infant circulation. Additionally, if any IgG antibodies were to be ingested through breastfeeding, they would probably be digested in the infant's gastrointestinal tract and not be absorbed. *However, this drug is not indicated for use in women with reproductive potential.

Reference

1. Prescribing Information. Beyfortus. Sanofi Pasteur, Inc; 2023.

NISOLDIPINE

Antihypertensive (Calcium Channel Blocker)

PREGNANCY RECOMMENDATION: No Human Data—Animal Data Suggest Risk

BREASTFEEDING RECOMMENDATION: Probably Compatible

PREGNANCY SUMMARY

No reports describing the use of nisoldipine in human pregnancy have been located. The drug will probably cross the placenta, so some fetal exposure will likely occur. However, the absence of human pregnancy experience prevents a complete assessment of the embryofetal risk. Embryofetal and maternal toxicity were observed in two animal species at doses less than or equal to 10 times the MRHD. Using this drug during pregnancy should be based on the pros and cons of the mother's clinical need for treatment versus any potential fetal risk that might occur from exposure. Other calcium channel blockers have been extensively used in human pregnancy as antihypertensives and tocolytics without evidence of major congenital defects or fetal toxicity.

BREASTFEEDING SUMMARY

No reports describing the use of nisoldipine in human lactation have been reported. The drug will probably be found in breast milk, so infant exposure will likely occur. Breastfeeding while using this drug should be based on the mother's clinical need for treatment versus any potential infant risks that might occur. If used, the infant should be monitored for the most common reported adult side effects of headache (leading to irritability) and peripheral edema.

Reference

1. Prescribing Information. Sular. Mylan Pharmaceuticals Inc; 2022.

NITAZOXANIDE

Anti-Infective (Antiprotozoal)

PREGNANCY RECOMMENDATION: Limited Human Data—Animal Data Suggest Low Risk

BREASTFEEDING RECOMMENDATION: Probably Compatible

N

PREGNANCY SUMMARY

One report was located describing the use of nitazoxanide in 51 COVID-19 pregnancies (in combination with levofloxacin and clarithromycin during the second and third trimesters). No adverse effects attributed to nitazoxanide were reported. Nitazoxanide is a prodrug. The prodrug active metabolites, tizoxanide and tizoxanide glucuronide, will probably cross the placenta, so some fetal exposure might occur. However, due to the absence of quantifiable plasma concentrations of nitazoxanide and the lack of metabolite accumulation, fetal exposure is likely minimal. Regardless, this limited first-trimester human pregnancy experience prevents a complete assessment of the embryofetal risk. Animal data did not show any embryofetal toxicity in two species at doses less than 10 times the MRHD. Using this drug during pregnancy should be based on the pros and cons of the mother's clinical need for treatment versus any potential fetal risk that might occur from exposure.

BREASTFEEDING SUMMARY

One report of a lactating mother found low levels of the main nitazoxanide metabolite (tizoxanide) in human breast milk. The peak concentration was 1.4 ng/mL, producing a calculated RID well below 1%. Breastfeeding while using this drug should be based on the mother's clinical need for treatment versus any potential infant risks that might occur. If used, the infant should be monitored for the most common reported adult side effects of nausea, headache, and abdominal pain (all leading to irritability) and abnormal urine color.

References

1. Prescribing Information. Alinia. Rising Pharmaceuticals Inc; 2022.
2. Hadad GM, Abdel Salam, RA, Emara S. Validated and optimized high-performance liquid chromatographic determination of tizoxanide, the main active metabolite of nitazoxanide in human urine, plasma and breast milk. *J Chromatogr Sci*. 2012;50:509-515.
3. Enríquez López KY, Meneses Calderón J, de la Cruz Ávila L, et al. Evolution of COVID-19 pregnancies treated with nitazoxanide in a third-level hospital. *Cureus*. 2021;13:e15002.

NITROFURANTOIN

Anti-Infective (Urinary Germicide)

PREGNANCY RECOMMENDATION: Human Data Suggest Low Risk (First Trimester)

BREASTFEEDING RECOMMENDATION: *Potential Toxicity

N

PREGNANCY SUMMARY

Many reports describing the use of nitrofurantoin in human pregnancy have been located. No increased risk for major congenital anomalies was found in a 2015 meta-analysis of over 91,000 nitrofurantoin first-trimester exposures compared with more than 1.5 million unexposed controls. A few other institutional studies of several thousand exposures have also found no increased risk. There appears to be a small risk of hemolytic anemia in newborns exposed in utero to nitrofurantoin close to delivery. Nitrofurantoin crosses the placenta, so fetal exposure will occur. Animal data did not show any embryofetal toxicity in two animal species at doses less than 10 times the RHD. ACOG considers nitrofurantoin as a reasonable option in the first trimester if no alternatives are available. It also considers nitrofurantoin as a first-line treatment for a urinary tract infection in the second and third trimesters. However, the use of nitrofurantoin should be avoided in patients with glucose-6-phosphate dehydrogenase (G6PD) deficiency.

BREASTFEEDING SUMMARY

A few studies have evaluated the use of nitrofurantoin during human lactation. In a few cases, the drug was not detected in breast milk. In others, the drug was identified with levels ranging from about 0.3 mcg/mL up to 1.3 mcg/mL. The highest calculated RID was about 6%. *Due to the concern for hemolytic anemia in infants less than 1 month of age or those with G6PD deficiency, the manufacturer recommends that a decision be made whether to discontinue nursing or to discontinue the drug, considering the importance of the drug to the mother. Adverse effects in older infants without G6PD are unlikely. If the clinical decision is to use this drug while breastfeeding, the infant should be monitored for the most common reported adult side effects of nausea and headache (both leading to irritability) and diarrhea.

References

1. Prescribing Information. Nitrofurantoin. Micro Labs Limited; 2023.
2. Perry JE, Leblanc AL. Transfer of nitrofurantoin across the human placenta. *Tex Rep Biol Med*. 1967;25:265-269.
3. Hailey FJ, Fort H, Williams JC, Hammers B. Foetal safety of nitrofurantoin macrocrystals therapy during pregnancy: a retrospective analysis. *J Int Med Res*. 1983;11:364-369.
4. Lenke RR, VanDorsten JP, Schifrin BS. Pyelonephritis in pregnancy: a prospective randomized trial to prevent recurrent disease evaluating suppressive therapy with nitrofurantoin and close surveillance. *Am J Obstet Gynecol*. 1983;146:953-957.
5. Ben David S, Einarson T, Ben David Y, Nulman I, Pastuszak A, Koren G. The safety of nitrofurantoin during the first trimester of pregnancy: meta-analysis. *Fundam Clin Pharmacol*. 1995;9:503-507.
6. Kallen BAJ, Olausson PO. Maternal drug use in early pregnancy and infant cardiovascular defect. *Reprod Toxicol*. 2003;17:255-261.
7. Crider KS, Cleves MA, Reefhuis J, Berry RJ, Hobbs CA, Hu DJ. Antibacterial medication use during pregnancy and risk of birth defects. *Arch Pediatr Adolesc Med*. 2009;163:978-985.

8. Nordeng H, Lupattelli A, Romoren M, Koren G. Neonatal outcomes after gestational exposure to nitrofurantoin. *Obstet Gynecol*. 2013;121:306-313.
9. Muanda FT, Sheehy O, Berard A. Use of antibiotics during pregnancy and the risk of major congenital malformations: a population based cohort study. *Br J Clin Pharmacol*. 2017;83:2557-2571.
10. Gait JE. Hemolytic reactions to nitrofurantoin in patients with glucose-6-phosphate dehydrogenase deficiency: theory and practice. *DICP Ann Pharmacother*. 1990;24:1210-1213.
11. Bruel H, Guillemant V, Saladin-Thiron C, Chabrolle JP, Lahary A, Poinsot J. Hemolytic anemia in a newborn after maternal treatment with nitrofurantoin at the end of pregnancy. *Arch Pediatr*. 2000;7:745-747.
12. Hosbach RE, Foster RB. Absence of nitrofurantoin from human milk. *JAMA*. 1967;202:1057.
13. Varsano I, Fischl J, Shochet SB. The excretion of orally ingested nitrofurantoin in human milk. *J Pediatr*. 1973;82:886-887.
14. Gerk PM, Kuhn RJ, Desai NS, McNamara PJ. Active transport of nitrofurantoin into human milk. *Pharmacotherapy*. 2001;21:669-675.
15. Ito S, Blajchman A, Stephenson M, Eliopoulos C, Koren G. Prospective follow-up of adverse reactions in breast-fed infants exposed to maternal medication. *Am J Obstet Gynecol*. 1993;168:1393-1399.
16. Goldberg O, Koren G, Landau D, Lunenfeld E, Matok I, Levy A. Exposure to nitrofurantoin during the first trimester of pregnancy and the risk for major malformations. *J Clin Pharmacol*. 2013;53(9):991-995.
17. Goldberg O, Moretti M, Levy A, Koren G. Exposure to nitrofurantoin during early pregnancy and congenital malformations: a systematic review and meta-analysis. *J Obstet Gynaecol Can*. 2015;37(2):150-156.
18. Urinary Tract Infections in Pregnant Individuals. Clinical Consensus No. 4. American College of Obstetricians and Gynecologists. *Obstet Gynecol*. 2023; 142:435-445.

NITROGLYCERIN

Cardiovascular (Vasodilator/Antianginal Agent)

PREGNANCY RECOMMENDATION: Limited Human Data—Animal Data Suggest Low Risk (Maternal Benefit May Outweigh Any Embryofetal Risk—Cardiac Issues)

BREASTFEEDING RECOMMENDATION: Probably Compatible

PREGNANCY SUMMARY

Nitroglycerin has been used to control hypertension, treat angina, promote uterine relaxation in obstetrical procedures (eg, version or breech delivery), and as a tocolytic agent in pregnancy. Available studies have found no significant adverse obstetrical or fetal/neonatal effects. Minimal data exist regarding the use of the drug in the first trimester. Nitroglycerin crosses the placenta, so fetal exposure will occur. However, this limited human pregnancy experience prevents a complete assessment of the embryofetal risk. Animal data did not show any embryofetal toxicity in two species at doses of more than 10 times the RHD. Using this drug during pregnancy should be based on the pros and cons of the mother's clinical need for treatment versus any potential fetal risk that might occur from exposure.

BREASTFEEDING SUMMARY

One report describing the use of topical nitroglycerin for anal fissures in 40 breastfeeding mothers has been located. No infant adverse events were reported. The drug will probably be found in breast milk, so some fetal exposure is possible. However, with the very short elimination half-life, the overall amount is likely to be minimal. Nitroglycerin should not be applied to the nipple while breastfeeding. If the clinical decision is to use this drug while breastfeeding, the infant should be monitored for the most common reported adult side effects of headache, dizziness, and paresthesia (all leading to irritability).

References

1. Prescribing Information. Nitroglycerin tablet. Advagen Pharma Ltd; 2023.
2. Snyder SW, Wheeler AS, James FM III. The use of nitroglycerin to control severe hypertension of pregnancy during cesarean section. *Anesthesiology*. 1979;51:563-564.
3. Hood DD, Dewan DM, James FM III, Floyd HM, Bogard TD. The use of nitroglycerin in preventing the hypertensive response to tracheal intubation in severe preeclamptics. *Anesthesiology*. 1983;59:A423.
4. Diro M, Beydown SN, Jaramillo B, O'Sullivan MJ, Kieval J. Successful pregnancy in a woman with a left ventricular cardiac aneurysm: a case report. *J Reprod Med*. 1983;28:559-563.
5. Oketani Y, Mitsuzono T, Ichikawa K, et al. Toxicological studies on nitroglycerin (NK-843). 6. Teratological studies in rabbits. *Oyo Yakuri*. 1981;22:633-638. As cited in Schardein JL. *Chemically Induced Birth Defects*. 2nd ed. Marcel Dekker; 1993:91.
6. Oketani Y, Mitsuzono T, Ichikawa K, et al. Toxicological studies on nitroglycerin (NK-843). 8. Teratological study in rats. *Oyo Yakuri*. 1981;22:737-751. As cited in Schardein JL. *Chemically Induced Birth Defects*. 2nd ed. Marcel Dekker; 1993:91.
7. Sato K, Taniguchi H, Ohtsuka T, et al. Reproductive studies of nitroglycerin applied dermally to pregnant rats and rabbits. *Clin Report*. 1984;18: 3511-3586. As cited in Shepard TH. *Catalog of Teratogenic Agents*. 7th ed. The Johns Hopkins University Press; 1992:285.
8. Wheeler AS, James FM III, Meis PJ, et al. Effects of nitroglycerin and nitroprusside on the uterine vasculature of gravid ewes. *Anesthesiology*. 1980;52:390-394.
9. Bootstaylor B, Roman C, Heymann MA, Parer JT. Fetal cardiorespiratory effects of nitroglycerin in the near term pregnant sheep (abstract). *Am J Obstet Gynecol*. 1994;170:281.
10. Heinonen OP, Slone D, Shapiro S. *Birth Defects and Drugs in Pregnancy*. Publishing Sciences Group; 1977:371-373.
11. Cotton DB, Jones MM, Longmire S, Dorman KF, Tessem J, Joyce TH III. Role of intravenous nitroglycerin in the treatment of severe pregnancy-induced hypertension complicated by pulmonary edema. *Am J Obstet Gynecol*. 1986;154:91-93.
12. Cotton DB, Longmire S, Jones MM, Dorman KF, Tessem J, Joyce TH III. Cardiovascular alterations in severe pregnancy-induced hypertension: effects of intravenous nitroglycerin coupled with blood volume expansion. *Am J Obstet Gynecol*. 1986;154:1053-1059.
13. Facchinetti F, Neri I, Volpe A. Glyceryl trinitrate lowers blood pressure in patients with gestational hypertension (abstract). *Am J Obstet Gynecol*. 1996; 174:455.
14. Grunewald C, Kublickas M, Carlstrom K, et al. Effects of nitroglycerin on the uterine and umbilical circulation in severe preeclampsia. *Obstet Gynecol*. 1995;86:600-604.
15. Longmire S, Leduc L, Jones MM, Hawkins JL, Joyce TH III, Cotton DB. The hemodynamic effects of intubation during nitroglycerin infusion in severe preeclampsia. *Am J Obstet Gynecol*. 1991;164:551-556.
16. Ottman EH, Gall SA. Myocardial infarction in the third trimester of pregnancy secondary to an aortic valve thrombus. *Obstet Gynecol*. 1993;81:804-805.

17. Sheikh AU, Harper MA. Myocardial infarction during pregnancy: management and outcome of two pregnancies. *Am J Obstet Gynecol*. 1993; 169:279-284.
18. Sanchez-Ramos L, Chami YG, Bass TA, Delvalle GO, Adair CD. Myocardial infarction during pregnancy: management with transluminal coronary angioplasty and metallic intracoronary stents. *Am J Obstet Gynecol*. 1994;171:1392-1393.
19. Roblin SH, Hew EM, Bernstein A. Uterine relaxation can be life saving. *Can J Anaesth*. 1991;38:939-940.
20. Mayer DC, Weeks SK. Antepartum uterine relaxation with nitroglycerin at caesarean delivery. *Can J Anaesth*. 1992;39:166-169.
21. Belfort MA. Intravenous nitroglycerin as a tocolytic agent for intrapartum external cephalic version. *S Afr Med J*. 1993;83:656.
22. Abouleish AE, Corn SB. Intravenous nitroglycerin for intrapartum external version of the second twin. *Anesth Analg*. 1994;78:808-809.
23. Greenspoon JS, Kovacic A. Breech extraction facilitated by glyceryl trinitrate sublingual spray. *Lancet*. 1991;338:124-125.
24. Rosen DJD, Velez J, Greenspoon JS. Total breech extraction of the second twin with uterine relaxation induced by nitroglycerin sublingual spray. *Israel J Obstet Gynecol*. 1994;5:18-21.
25. Dufour P, Vinatier D, Vanderstichele S, et al. Intravenous nitroglycerin for intrapartum internal podalic version of the second non-vertex twin. *Eur J Obstet Gynecol Reprod Biol*. 1996;70:29-32.
26. Lees C, Campbell S, Jauniaux E, et al. Arrest of preterm labour and prolongation of gestation with glyceryl trinitrate, a nitric oxide donor. *Lancet*. 1994;343:1325-1326.
27. Lees C, Campbell S, Martin J, et al. Glyceryl trinitrate in management of preterm labour. Authors' reply. *Lancet*. 1994;344:553-554.
28. Mercier FJ, Dounas M, Bouaziz H, Lhuissier C, Benhamou D. Intravenous nitroglycerin to relieve intrapartum fetal distress related to uterine hyperactivity: a prospective observational study. *Anesth Analg*. 1997;84:1117-1120.
29. Trapani A Jr, Gonçalves LF, Tranpani TF, Franco MJ, Galluzzo RN, Pires MMS. Comparison between transdermal nitroglycerin and sildenafil citrate in intrauterine growth restriction: effects on uterine, umbilical and fetal middle cerebral artery pulsatility indices. *Ultrasound Obstet Gynecol*. 2016;48:61-65.
30. Isquick S, Henry D, Nakagawa S, et al. The association between nitroglycerin use and adverse outcomes in women undergoing cesarean delivery in the second stage of labor. *J Matern Fetal Neonat Med*. 2017;30:1297-1301.
31. Peng ATC, Gorman RS, Shulman SM, DeMarchis E, Nyunt K, Blancato LS. Intravenous nitroglycerin for uterine relaxation in the postpartum patient with retained placenta. *Anesthesiology*. 1989;71:172-173.
32. DeSimone CA, Norris MC, Leighton BL. Intravenous nitroglycerin aids manual extraction of a retained placenta. *Anesthesiology*. 1990;73:787.
33. Altabef KM, Spencer JT, Zinberg S. Intravenous nitroglycerin for uterine relaxation of an inverted uterus. *Am J Obstet Gynecol*. 1992;166:1237-1238.
34. Dayan SS, Schwalbe SS. The use of small-dose intravenous nitroglycerin in a case of uterine inversion. *Anesth Anal*. 1996;82:1091-1093.
35. Taylor I, Kennedy D. Safety of topical glyceryl trinitrate in the treatment of anal fissure in breastfeeding women. *Birth Defects Res Part A*. 2008;82:411; Abstract.
36. Prescribing Information. Nitroglycerin injection. American Regent, Inc; 2021.
37. David M, Walka MM, Schmid B, Sinha P, Veit S, Lichtenegger W. Nitroglycerin application during cesarean delivery: plasma levels, fetal/maternal ratio of nitroglycerin, and effects in newborns. *Am J Obstet Gynecol*. 2000;182:955-961.
38. Bustard MA, Ryan G, Seaward G, Saleniak M-E, Smith GN. Human maternal and fetal plasma glyceryl trinitrate concentrations. *Am J Obstet Gynecol*. 2003; 189:1777-1778.
39. O'Sullivan S, Keith MP. Raynaud phenomenon of the nipple: a rare finding in rheumatology clinic. *J Clin Rheumatol*. 2011;17:371-372.
40. Prescribing Information. Nitroglycerin ointment. Cosette Pharmaceuticals, Inc; 2023.

NITROPRUSSIDE

Antihypertensive (Vasodilator)

PREGNANCY RECOMMENDATION: Limited Human Data—Animal Data Suggest Potential Risk (Maternal Benefit May Outweigh Any Embryofetal Risk—Some Cases)

BREASTFEEDING RECOMMENDATION: Potential Toxicity

N

PREGNANCY SUMMARY

Limited reports have described the use of nitroprusside in pregnancy to produce deliberate hypotension during aneurysm surgery or to treat severe hypertension. However, first-trimester use is lacking. One case of transient fetal bradycardia has been reported. Prolonged nitroprusside use may lead to possible cyanide exposure and toxicity. The drug will probably cross the placenta, so fetal exposure will likely occur. However, this limited human pregnancy experience prevents a complete assessment of the embryofetal risk. Fetal demise was observed in one animal species with higher doses. Using this drug during pregnancy should be based on the pros and cons of the mother's clinical need for treatment versus any potential fetal risk that might occur from exposure. In many clinical situations, use of this drug may outweigh any embryofetal risk.

BREASTFEEDING SUMMARY

No reports describing the use of nitroprusside during human lactation have been located. The drug will probably be found in breast milk, so some fetal exposure is possible. However, with the very short elimination half-life, the overall amount is likely to be minimal. However, the toxic metabolite, thiocyanide, is excreted into breast milk in concentrations ranging from 16% to 82%. Thiocyanide may also inhibit the transport of iodide into breast milk. Therefore, its use while breastfeeding should be limited, as would be expected for most of the approved uses. If the clinical decision is to use this drug while breastfeeding, the infant should be monitored for the most common reported adult side effects of hypotension and cyanide toxicity.

References

1. Donchin Y, Amirav B, Sahar A, Yarkoni S. Sodium nitroprusside for aneurysm surgery in pregnancy. *Br J Anaesth*. 1978;50:849-851.
2. Paull J. Clinical report of the use of sodium nitroprusside in severe pre-eclampsia. *Anesth Intensive Care*. 1975;3:72.
3. Rigg D, McDonogh A. Use of sodium nitroprusside for deliberate hypotension during pregnancy. *Br J Anaesth*. 1981;53:985-987.
4. Willoughby JS. Case reports: sodium nitroprusside, pregnancy and multiple intracranial aneurysms. *Anaesth Intensive Care*. 1984;12:358-360.
5. Stempel JE, O'Grady JP, Morton MJ, Johnson KA. Use of sodium nitroprusside in complications of gestational hypertension. *Obstet Gynecol*. 1982;60:533-538.
6. Shoemaker CT, Meyers M. Sodium nitroprusside for control of severe hypertensive disease of pregnancy: a case report and discussion of potential toxicity. *Am J Obstet Gynecol*. 1984;149:171-173.
7. Willoughby JS. Review article: sodium nitroprusside, pregnancy and multiple intracranial aneurysms. *Anaesth Intensive Care*. 1984;12:351-357.

8. de Swiet M. Antihypertensive drugs in pregnancy. *Br Med J*. 1985;291: 365-366.
9. Prescribing Information. Sodium nitroprusside. Slate Run Pharmaceuticals, LLC; 2024.
10. Lewis PE, Cefalo RC, Naulty JS, Rodkey RL. Placental transfer and fetal toxicity of sodium nitroprusside. *Gynecol Invest*. 1977;8:46.
11. Naulty J, Cefalo RC, Lewis PE. Fetal toxicity of nitroprusside in the pregnant ewe. *Am J Obstet Gynecol*. 1981;139(6):708-711.
12. Dorea JG. Maternal thiocyanate and thyroid status during breast-feeding. *J Am Coll Nutr*. 2004;23:97-101.
13. Funderburk CF, Van Middlesworth L. Effect of lactation and perchlorate on thiocyanate metabolism. *Am J Physiol*. 1967;213:1371-1377.
14. Meberg A, Sande H, Foss OP, Stenwig JT. Smoking during pregnancy—effects on the fetus and on thiocyanate levels in mother and baby. *Acta Paediatr Scand*. 1979;68:547-552.
15. Dasgupta PK, Kirk AB, Dyke JV, Ohira, S-I. Intake of iodine and perchlorate and excretion in human milk. *Environ Sci Technol*. 2008;42:8115-8121.

NITROUS OXIDE

Anesthetic (Inhalation)

PREGNANCY RECOMMENDATION: Limited Human Data—No Relevant Animal Data

BREASTFEEDING RECOMMENDATION: Probably Compatible

PREGNANCY SUMMARY

Numerous reports describing the use of nitrous oxide during human pregnancy were located. Of about 100 first-trimester exposures, the risk for major congenital malformations was not increased from the expected baseline risk, and no pattern to the anomalies was seen. Many other studies have evaluated the drug for use as an analgesic during labor or as part of the induction process for anesthesia. Again, no adverse fetal effects were identified. Lastly, occupational exposure to nitrous oxide can occur in dental offices and other outpatient surgery centers. There were some studies that indicated that this might increase the risk for spontaneous abortion, but this finding has not been seen in several other large studies. Due to the concern for occupational exposure, nitrous oxide levels must be measured every 6 months and maintained at less than 25 parts per million for nitrous oxide to be compliant with Occupational Safety and Health Administration standards. Nitrous oxide rapidly crosses the placenta, so some fetal exposure can occur. However, the short elimination half-life should limit the amount of exposure. However, this limited early human pregnancy experience prevents a complete assessment of the embryofetal risk. Animal reproduction data suggest risk, but the exposures to the gas were usually much higher and longer than the exposures that occur in humans. ACOG states that nitrous oxide may be used in the management of labor pain. While the analgesia provided by nitrous oxide is less effective than epidural analgesia, benefits include improved patient mobility, lack of required monitoring, patient control of effect, and quick termination of effect. Additionally, nitrous oxide may be safely used with other forms of analgesia.

BREASTFEEDING SUMMARY

No reports describing the use of nitrous oxide during human lactation have been located. The drug may be found in breast milk, but the very short elimination half-life suggests that the overall amount is likely to be minimal. Breastfeeding while using this drug should be based on the mother's clinical need for treatment versus any potential infant risks that might occur. If used, the infant should be monitored for the most common reported adult side effects of nausea and dizziness (leading to irritability), vomiting, and drowsiness.

References

1. Cohen EN, Paulson WJ, Wall J, Elert B. Thiopental, curare, and nitrous oxide anesthesia for cesarean section with studies on placental transmission. *Surg Gynecol Obstet*. 1953;97:456-462.
2. Marx GF, Joshi CW, Orkin LR. Placental transmission of nitrous oxide. *Anesthesiology*. 1970;32:429-432.
3. Heinonen OP, Sloan D, Shapiro S. *Birth Defects and Drugs in Pregnancy*. Publishing Sciences Group; 1977:358-360.
4. Cohen EN, Brown BW, Wu ML, et al. Occupational disease in dentistry and chronic exposure to trace anesthetic gases. *J Am Dent Assoc*. 1980; 101:21-31.
5. Heidam LZ. Spontaneous abortions among dental assistants, factory workers, painters, and gardening workers: a follow up study. *J Epidemiol Comm Health*. 1984;38:149-155.
6. Rowland AS, Baird DD, Shore DL, Weinberg CR, Savitz DA, Wilcox AJ. Nitrous oxide and spontaneous abortion in female dental assistants. *Am J Epidemiol*. 1995;141:531-538.
7. Axelsson G, Ahlborg G Jr, Bodin L. Shift work, nitrous oxide exposure, and spontaneous abortion among Swedish midwives. *Occup Environ Med*. 1996;53:374-378.
8. Crawford JS, Lewis M. Nitrous oxide in early human pregnancy. *Anaesthesia*. 1986;41:900-905.
9. Hale TW. Anesthetic medications in breastfeeding mothers. *J Hum Lact*. 1999;15:185-194.
10. Boivin JF. Risk of spontaneous abortion in women occupationally exposed to anaesthetic gases: a meta-analysis. *Occup Environ Med*. 1997;54:541-548.
11. Dutch Health Council. Nitrous oxide: evaluation of the effects on reproduction, recommendation for classification. 2000. https://www.gezondheidsraad.nl/binaries/gezondheidsraad/documenten/adviezen/2000/05/03/lachgas/advies-lachgas.pdf
12. Menon JML, van Luijk J, Swinkels J, et al. A health-based recommended occupational exposure limit for nitrous oxide using experimental animal data based on a systematic review and dose-response analysis. *Environ Res*. 2021;201:111575.
13. Rooks JP. Safety and risks of nitrous oxide labor analgesia: a review. *J Midwifery Womens Health*. 2011;56:557-565.
14. Rosen MA. Nitrous oxide for relief of labor pain: a systematic review. *Am J Obstet Gynecol*. 2002;186(5 suppl Nature):S110-S126.
15. Likis FE, Andrews JC, Collins MR, et al. Nitrous oxide for the management of labor pain: a systematic review. *Anesth Analg*. 2014;118:153-167.
16. American College of Obstetricians and Gynecologists. ACOG practice bulletin no. 209: obstetric analgesia and anesthesia. *Obstet Gynecol*. 2019;133: e208-e225.

N

17. Starosta A, Lundsberg L, Culhane J, Partridge C, Grechukhina O, Son M. Association between intrapartum nitrous oxide for labor analgesia and short-term neonatal outcomes. *Obstet Gynecol*. 2024;143:677-682.
18. National Institute for Occupational Safety and Health. 1977. *Criteria for a Recommended Standard: Occupational Exposure to Waste Anesthetic Gases and Vapors* [DHEW (NIOSH) Publication No. 77-140]. U.S. Department of Health, Education, and Welfare. Public Health Service. Center for Disease Control. National Institute for Occupational Safety and Health.

NIVOLUMAB

Antineoplastic (Programmed Death Receptor-1 Inhibitor—Monoclonal Antibody)

PREGNANCY RECOMMENDATION: Limited Human Data—Animal Data Suggest Potential Risk

BREASTFEEDING RECOMMENDATION: Probably Compatible

PREGNANCY SUMMARY

Seven case reports describing the use of nivolumab in pregnancy have been located. These reports included seven pregnancies and nine infants with exposure reported in all trimesters. No congenital abnormalities were reported. Human IgG antibodies are known to cross the placenta, especially during the second and third trimesters, which suggests that some transfer will occur. However, this limited human pregnancy experience prevents a complete assessment of the embryofetal risk. Embryofetal toxicity and premature infant death were observed in one animal species at doses less than 10 times the RHD. Based on animal studies and the drug's mechanism of action, the manufacturer recommends that women with reproductive potential use effective contraception during treatment and for 5 months after the last dose. Nevertheless, using this drug during pregnancy should be based on the pros and cons of the mother's clinical need for treatment versus any potential fetal risk that might occur from exposure. There is a registry for women who are pregnant and have cancer. For more information, women and health care providers are encouraged to contact the Cancer and Pregnancy Registry at 1-877-635-4499.

BREASTFEEDING SUMMARY

One case report was located that described the excretion and accumulation of nivolumab in human breast milk. The cumulative RID was 9.8%. However, if IgG antibodies were to be ingested through breastfeeding, they would probably be digested in the infant's gastrointestinal tract and not be absorbed. Regardless, due to a concern for potential serious adverse effects that might be seen in a breastfed infant, the manufacturer recommends that women not breastfeed while being treated with this drug and for at least 5 months after the last dose. Nevertheless, breastfeeding while using this drug should be based on the mother's clinical need for treatment versus any potential infant risks that might occur. If used, the infant should be monitored for the most common reported adult side effects of pruritus, nausea, headache, abdominal, back, and musculoskeletal pain (all leading to irritability), fatigue (lethargy), rash, diarrhea, cough, constipation, decreased appetite (monitor infant growth), upper respiratory infection, hypothyroidism, and urinary tract infection.

References

1. Prescribing Information. Opdivo. Bristol-Myers Squibb Company; 2024.
2. Menzer C, Beedgen B, Rom J, et al. Immunotherapy with ipilimumab plus nivolumab in a stage IV melanoma patient during pregnancy. *Eur J Cancer*. 2018;104:239-242.
3. Xu W, Moor RJ, Walpole ET, Atkinson VG. Pregnancy with successful foetal and maternal outcome in a melanoma patient treated with nivolumab in the first trimester: case report and review of the literature. *Melanoma Res*. 2019;29(3):333-337.
4. Bucheit AD, Hardy JT, Szender JB, Glitza Oliva IC. Conception and viable twin pregnancy in a patient with metastatic melanoma while treated with CTLA-4 and PD-1 checkpoint inhibition. *Melanoma Res*. 2020;30(4):423-425.
5. Haiduk J, Ziemer M. Pregnancy in a patient with metastatic uveal melanoma treated with nivolumab. *J Dtsch Dermatol Ges*. 2021;19(5):762-765.
6. Hutson JR, Eastabrook G, Garcia-Bournissen F. Pregnancy outcome after early exposure to nivolumab, a PD-1 checkpoint inhibitor for relapsed Hodgkin's lymphoma. *Clin Toxicol (Phila)*. 2022;60(4):535-536.
7. Gambichler T, Susok L. Uncomplicated pregnancy and delivery under ongoing nivolumab therapy for metastatic melanoma. *Melanoma Res*. 2022;32(2):131-132.
8. Zambrana F, Barbancho C, Huelves M, et al. Successful pregnancy and cancer outcomes with ipilimumab and nivolumab for metastatic renal cell carcinoma: case report and review of the literature. *J Immunother*. 2023;46(1):27-28.
9. de Jong K, Damoiseaux D, Pluim D, et al. High accumulation of nivolumab in human breast milk: a case report. *Biomed Pharmacother*. 2023;166:115354.

NIZATIDINE

Gastrointestinal (Histamine H_2 Antagonist)

PREGNANCY RECOMMENDATION: Limited Human Data—Animal Data Suggest Low Risk

BREASTFEEDING RECOMMENDATION: Probably Compatible

PREGNANCY SUMMARY

A few studies were located that describe the use of nizatidine in human pregnancy. Of the few numbers with first-trimester exposure, no increase in major birth anomalies was seen. A few larger studies that have analyzed histamine H_2 blockers as a group (>3,500 cases) have not identified an increased risk for major congenital defects. The drug will probably cross the placenta, so some fetal exposure will occur. However, the limited human pregnancy experience with nizatidine, specifically, prevents a complete assessment of the embryofetal risk. Animal data did not show any embryofetal toxicity in two species at doses more than 10 times the RHD. Using this drug during pregnancy should be based on the pros and cons of the mother's clinical need for treatment versus any potential fetal risk that might occur from exposure.

BREASTFEEDING SUMMARY

One report was located that described the use of nizatidine during human lactation. Small amounts of the drug were found in the breast milk of three lactating women; however, the total amount was less than 1% of the maternal dose. Breastfeeding while using this drug should be based on the mother's clinical need for treatment versus any potential infant risks that might occur. If used, the infant should be monitored for the most common reported adult side effects of nausea, headache, and abdominal pain (all leading to irritability), diarrhea, and rhinitis.

References

1. Prescribing Information. Nizatidine. Actavis Pharma, Inc; 2022.
2. Morton DM. Pharmacology and toxicology of nizatidine. *Scand J Gastroenterol*. 1987;22(suppl 136):1-8.
3. Dicke JM, Johnson RF, Henderson GI, Kuehl TJ, Schenker S. A comparative evaluation of the transport of H2-receptor antagonists by the human and baboon placenta. *Am J Med Sci*. 1988;295:198-206.
4. Magee LA, Inocencion G, Kamboj L, Rosetti F, Koren G. Safety of first trimester exposure to histamine H2 blockers. A prospective cohort study. *Dig Dis Sci*. 1996;41:1145-1149.
5. Kallen B. Delivery outcome after the use of acid-suppressing drugs in early pregnancy with special reference to omeprazole. *Br J Obstet Gynaecol*. 1998;105:877-881.
6. Dehlink E, Yen E, Leichtner AM, Hait EJ, Fiebiger E. First evidence of a possible association between gastric acid suppression during pregnancy and childhood asthma: a population-based register study. *Clin Exp Allergy*. 2009, 39:246-253.
7. Garbis H, Elefant E, Diav-Citrin O, et al. Pregnancy outcome after exposure to ranitidine and other H2-blockers—a collaborative study of the European Network of Teratology Information Services. *Reprod Toxicol*. 2005;19: 453-458.
8. Gill SK, O'Brien L, Koren G. The safety of histamine 2 (H2) blockers in pregnancy: a meta-analysis. *Dig Dis Sci*. 2009;54:1835-1838.
9. Broussard CN, Richter JE. Treating gasto-oesophageal reflux disease during pregnancy and lactation. What are the safest therapy options? *Drug Saf*. 1998;19:325-337.
10. Katz PO, Castell DO. Gastroesophageal reflux disease during pregnancy. *Gastroenterol Clin N Am*. 1998;27:153-167.
11. Ramakrishnan A, Katz PO. Pharmacologic management of gastroesophageal reflux disease. *Curr Treat Options Gastroenterol*. 2002;5:301-310.
12. Richter JE. Gastroesophageal reflux disease during pregnancy. *Gastroenterol Clin N Am*. 2003;32:235-261.
13. Richter JE. Review article: the management of heartburn in pregnancy. *Aliment Pharmacol Ther*. 2005;22:749-757.
14. Matok I, Gorodischer R, Koren G, et al. The safety of H2-blockers use during pregnancy. *J Clin Pharmacol*. 2010;50:81-87.
15. Obermeyer BD, Bergstrom RF, Callaghan JT, Knadler MP, Golichowski A, Rubin A. Secretion of nizatidine into human breast milk after single and multiple doses. *Clin Pharmacol Ther*. 1990;47:724-730.

NOGAPENDEKIN ALFA INBAKICEPT

Antineoplastic (Interleukin 15 Receptor Antagonist—Intravesical Use)

PREGNANCY RECOMMENDATION: No Human Data and No Relevant Animal Data

BREASTFEEDING RECOMMENDATION: Probably Compatible

PREGNANCY SUMMARY

No reports describing the use of nogapendekin alfa inbakicept in human pregnancy have been located. The drug will probably not cross the placenta in amounts that would have any clinical significance. However, the absence of human pregnancy experience prevents a complete assessment of the embryofetal risk. No animal reproduction or fertility studies have been conducted. Using this drug during pregnancy should be based on the pros and cons of the mother's clinical need for treatment versus any potential fetal risk that might occur from exposure. There is a registry for women who are pregnant and have cancer. For more information, women and health care providers are encouraged to contact the Cancer and Pregnancy Registry at 1-877-635-4499.

BREASTFEEDING SUMMARY

No reports describing the use of nogapendekin alfa inbakicept during human lactation have been located. The drug will probably not be excreted into breast milk. In addition, due to a lack of measurable systemic absorption following intravesical use, any amounts that might be present in breast milk would likely be clinically insignificant. Breastfeeding while using this drug should be based on the mother's clinical need for treatment. If used, the infant should be monitored for the most common reported adult side effects of musculoskeletal pain and chills (both leading to irritability) and fever.

Reference

1. Prescribing Information. Anktiva. Altor BioScience LLC; 2024.

NONOXYNOL-9

Reproductive (Spermicide)

PREGNANCY RECOMMENDATION: *Contraindicated

BREASTFEEDING RECOMMENDATION: Probably Compatible

PREGNANCY SUMMARY

Several studies have been located that describe human pregnancy exposure to nonoxynol-9. Initially, there was a study that suggested concerns for an increased risk of birth anomalies when early pregnancy was exposed to this drug. However, several follow-up studies have not found this risk. One study reported 17 (2.2%) major birth defects in 763 first-trimester exposures. In the CPP, there were 7 (2.0%) birth anomalies in 342 first-trimester exposures. In addition, no pattern to the defects was seen in either of these publications. In addition, some early studies suggest an increased risk for spontaneous abortion, but the observed rates have not been higher than the expected population rates. Therefore, the available evidence indicates that the use of vaginal spermicides, either before or during early pregnancy, does not pose a risk of congenital malformations or adverse pregnancy/fetal effects. If the drug is found in the systemic circulation, then some of it will probably cross the placenta. So, some fetal exposure might occur. Embryofetal toxicity was observed in one animal species. *While nonoxynol-9 does not pose a risk either before or early in pregnancy, its routine use is contraindicated because there is no benefit for its use in pregnancy.

BREASTFEEDING SUMMARY

One report describing the use of nonoxynol-9 in breastfeeding mothers found no observable adverse effects. It is not known if nonoxynol-9 is excreted into breast milk. If used while breastfeeding, adverse effects on the breastfed infant are not expected.

N

References

1. Jick H, Walker AM, Rothman KJ, et al. Vaginal spermicides and congenital disorders. *JAMA*. 1981;245:1329-1332.
2. Jick H, Walker AM, Rothman KJ. The relation between vaginal spermicides and congenital disorders. Reply. *JAMA*. 1987;258:2066.
3. Anonymous. Data do not support association between spermicides, birth defects. *FDA Drug Bull*. 1986;16:21.
4. Mills JL. Reporting provocative results: can we publish "hot" papers without getting burned? *JAMA*. 1987;258:3428-3429.
5. Holmes LB. Vaginal spermicides and congenital disorders: the validity of a study—in reply. *JAMA*. 1986;256:3096.
6. Chvapil M, Eskelson CD, Stiffel V, Owen JA, Droegemueller W. Studies on nonoxynol-9. II. Intravaginal absorption, distribution, metabolism and excretion in rats and rabbits. *Contraception*. 1980;22:325-339.
7. Smith ESO, Dafoe CS, Miller JR, Banister P. An epidemiological study of congenital reduction deformities of the limbs. *Br J Prev Soc Med*. 1977;31:39-41.
8. Rothman KJ. Spermicide use and Down's syndrome. *Am J Public Health*. 1982;72:399-401.
9. Polednak AP, Janerich DT, Glebatis DM. Birth weight and birth defects in relation to maternal spermicide use. *Teratology*. 1982;26:27-38.
10. Huggins G, Vessey M, Flavel R, Yeates D, McPherson K. Vaginal spermicides and outcome of pregnancy: findings in a large cohort study. *Contraception*. 1982;25:219-230.
11. Oakley GP Jr. Spermicides and birth defects. *JAMA*. 1982;247:2405.
12. Cordero JF, Layde PM. Vaginal spermicides, chromosomal abnormalities and limb reduction defects. *Fam Plann Perspect*. 1983;15:16-18.
13. Bracken MB. Spermicidal contraceptives and poor reproductive outcomes: the epidemiologic evidence against an association. *Am J Obstet Gynecol*. 1985;151:552-556.
14. Watkins RN. Vaginal spermicides and congenital disorders: the validity of a study. *JAMA*. 1986;256:3095.
15. Jick H, Walker A, Rothman KJ. Vaginal spermicides and congenital disorders: the validity of a study. Reply. *JAMA*. 1986;256:3095-3096.
16. Bracken MB, Vita K. Frequency of non-hormonal contraception around conception and association with congenital malformations in offspring. *Am J Epidemiol*. 1983;117:281-291.
17. Mills JL, Harley EE, Reed GF, Berendes HW. Are spermicides teratogenic? *JAMA*. 1982;248:2148-2151.
18. Mills JL, Reed GF, Nugent RP, Harley EE, Berendes HW. Are there adverse effects of periconceptional spermicide use? *Fertil Steril*. 1985;43:442-446.
19. Harlap S, Shiono PH, Ramcharan S. Congenital abnormalities in the offspring of women who used oral and other contraceptives around the time of conception. *Int J Fertil*. 1985;30:39-47.
20. Shapiro S, Slone D, Heinonen OP, et al. Birth defects and vaginal spermicides. *JAMA*. 1982;247:2381-2384.
21. Linn S, Schoenbaum SC, Monson RR, Rosner B, Stubblefield PG, Ryan KJ. Lack of association between contraceptive usage and congenital malformations in offspring. *Am J Obstet Gynecol*. 1983;147:923-928.
22. Louik C, Mitchell AA, Werler MM, Hanson JW, Shapiro S. Maternal exposure to spermicides in relation to certain birth defects. *N Engl J Med*. 1987;317:474-478.
23. Warburton D, Neugut RH, Lustenberger A, Nicholas AG, Kline J. Lack of association between spermicide use and trisomy. *N Engl J Med*. 1987;317:478-482.
24. Bracken MB. Vaginal spermicides and congenital disorders: study reassessed, not retracted. *JAMA*. 1987;257:2919.
25. Jick H, Shiota K, Shepard TH, et al. Vaginal spermicides and miscarriage seen primarily in the emergency room. *Teratog Carcinog Mutagen*. 1982;2:205-210.
26. Scholl TO, Sobel E, Tanfer K, Soefer EF, Saidman B. Effects of vaginal spermicides on pregnancy outcome. *Fam Plann Perspect*. 1983;15:244, 249-250.
27. Warburton D, Stein Z, Kline J, Strobino B. Environmental influences on rates of chromosome anomalies in spontaneous abortions (abstract). *Am J Hum Genet*. 1980;32:92A.
28. Strobino B, Kline J, Lai A, Stein Z, Susser M, Warburton D. Vaginal spermicides and spontaneous abortion of known karyotype. *Am J Epidemiol*. 1986;123:431-443.
29. Strobino B, Kline J, Stein Z, et al. Exposure to contraceptive creams, jellies and douches and their effect on the zygote (abstract). *Am J Epidemiol*. 1980;112:434.
30. Harlap S, Shiono PH, Ramcharan S. Spontaneous foetal losses in women using different contraceptives around the time of conception. *Int J Epidemiol*. 1980;9:49-56.
31. Porter JB, Hunter-Mitchell J, Jick H, Walker AM. Drugs and stillbirth. *Am J Public Health*. 1986;76:1428-1431.
32. Einarson TR, Koren G, Mattice D, Schechter-Tsafriri O. Maternal spermicide use and adverse reproductive outcome: a meta-analysis. *Am J Obstet Gynecol*. 1990;162:655-660.

33. Gallaway MS, Waller DK, Canfield MA, Scheuerle A; National Birth Defects Prevention Study. The association between use of spermicides or male condoms and major structural birth defects. *Contraception*. 2009;80:422-429.
34. Tryphonas L, Buttar HS. Effects of the spermicide nonoxynol-9 on the pregnant uterus and the conceptus of rat. *Toxicology*. 1986;39:177-186.
35. Peralta O, Díaz S, Juez G, et al. Fertility regulation in nursing women: V. Long-term influence of a low-dose combined oral contraceptive initiated at day 90 postpartum on lactation and infant growth. *Contraception*. 1983;27:27-38.

NOREPINEPHRINE

Autonomic (Sympathomimetic/Adrenergic)

PREGNANCY RECOMMENDATION: Limited Human Data—Animal Data Suggest Risk (Maternal Benefit May Outweigh Any Embryofetal Risk)

BREASTFEEDING RECOMMENDATION: Potential Toxicity

PREGNANCY SUMMARY

Limited reports have been located that describe the use of norepinephrine to maintain blood pressure with regional anesthesia at the time of cesarean delivery. Available studies have found no significant evidence of an increased risk of adverse fetal effects. First-trimester exposure studies have not been found. Despite the lack of evidence in septic shock, norepinephrine is considered to be a reasonable first-line vasopressor in pregnancy. The drug crosses the placenta, so fetal exposure can occur. However, the very short elimination half-life would suggest that exposure might be minimal. Regardless, this limited human pregnancy experience, especially with first-trimester use and in the setting of shock, prevents a complete assessment of the embryofetal risk. Embryofetal toxicity was observed in two animal species at doses less than or equal to 10 times the RHD. Using this drug during pregnancy should be based on the pros and cons of the mother's clinical need for treatment versus any potential fetal risk that might occur from exposure. Nevertheless, the maternal clinical need may outweigh any potential unknown fetal risk.

BREASTFEEDING SUMMARY

No reports describing the use of norepinephrine during human lactation have been located. The drug will probably be found in breast milk, so some infant exposure will likely occur. But the elimination half-life is so short that the amounts may be negligible. Breastfeeding while using this drug should be based on the mother's clinical need for treatment versus any potential infant risks that might occur. If used, the infant should be monitored for the most common reported adult side effects of anxiety and headache (both leading to irritability), bradycardia, and respiratory difficulty.

References

1. Prescribing Information. Norepinephrine bitartrate. Caplin Steriles Limited; 2024.
2. Fujinaga M, Maze M, Hoffman BB, Baden JM. Activation of α-1 adrenergic receptors modulates the control of left/right sidedness in rat embryos. *Dev Biol*. 1992;150:419-421. As cited in Shepard TH. *Catalog of Teratogenic Agents*. 9th ed. The Johns Hopkins University Press; 1998:340.
3. Pitel M, Lerman S. Studies on the fetal rat lens. Effects of intrauterine adrenaline and noradrenalin. *Invest Ophthalmol*. 1962;1:406-412. As cited in Shepard TH. *Catalog of Teratogenic Agents*. 9th ed. The Johns Hopkins University Press; 1998:340.
4. Gatling RR. The effect of sympathomimetic agents on the chick embryo. *Am J Pathol*. 1962;40:113-127.
5. Hirsch KS, Fritz HI. A comparison of mescaline with epinephrine and norepinephrine in the hamster. *Teratology*. 1974;9:A19-A20. As cited in Schardein TH. *Chemically Induced Birth Defects*. 3rd ed. Marcel Dekker; 2000:360, 364.
6. Stevens AD, Lumbers ER. Effects of intravenous infusions of noradrenaline into the pregnant ewe on uterine blood flow, fetal renal function, and lung liquid flow. *Can J Physiol. Pharmacol*. 1995;73:202-208.
7. Morgan CD, Sandler M, Panigel M. Placental transfer of catecholamines in vitro and in vivo. *Am J Obstet Gynecol*. 1972;112:1068-1075.
8. Evans L, Rhodes A, Alhazzani W, et al. Surviving sepsis campaign: international guidelines for management of sepsis and septic shock 2021. *Intensive Care Med*. 2021;47:1181-1247.
9. Ahmed S, Ahmad E, Fatima E, et al. Efficacy and safety of norepinephrine versus phenylephrine for post-spinal hypotension in preeclamptic patients: a systematic review and meta-analysis. *Eur J Obstet Gynecol Reprod Biol*. 2024;303:91-98.
10. Society for Maternal-Fetal Medicine (SMFM); Shields AD, Plante LA, Pacheco LD, Louis JM; SMFM Publications Committee. Society for Maternal-Fetal Medicine Consult Series #67: maternal sepsis. *Am J Obstet Gynecol*. 2023;229:B2-B19.

NORETHINDRONE

Reproductive (Progestin)

PREGNANCY RECOMMENDATION: *Contraindicated

BREASTFEEDING RECOMMENDATION: Probably Compatible

N

PREGNANCY SUMMARY

A few reports have been located that describe norethindrone exposure in early pregnancy. From the CPP and Michigan Medicaid Surveillance study, there were 26 (7.0%) major birth anomalies in 370 first-trimester exposures to norethindrone. However, after evaluating all the confounding variables, no pattern to the defects was seen. Additionally from the CPP, there were 35 (4.0%) major birth anomalies in 866 first-trimester exposures to progestins as a group. Masculinization of a female fetus and possibly hypospadias in a male fetus may be risk factors for exposure to this drug in early pregnancy. The drug will likely cross the placenta, so some fetal exposure will probably occur. No animal reproduction studies have been conducted. However, this limited human pregnancy experience prevents a complete assessment of the embryofetal risk. *Regardless, there is no indication for the use of norethindrone in pregnancy. The drug should be discontinued if a pregnancy is confirmed.

BREASTFEEDING SUMMARY

Several reports describing the effects of norethindrone during human lactation have been located. Breast milk supply, composition, infant growth, and neurodevelopment were not impacted by norethindrone use during lactation. Norethindrone was found to be excreted into breast milk in small amounts (about one-tenth maternal serum concentrations). The Centers for Disease Control and Prevention (CDC) states that progestin-only pills, such as norethindrone, may be restarted immediately postpartum in breastfeeding patients. Adverse effects are rarely reported in infants.

References

1. Hagler S, Schultz A, Hankin H, Kunstadter RN. Fetal effects of steroid therapy during pregnancy. *Am J Dis Child*. 1963;106:586-590.
2. Jacobson BD. Hazards of norethindrone therapy during pregnancy. *Am J Obstet Gynecol*. 1962;84:962-968.
3. Wilson JG, Brent RL. Are female sex hormones teratogenic? *Am J Obstet Gynecol*. 1981;141:567-580.
4. Bongiovanni AM, McFadden AJ. Steroids during pregnancy and possible fetal consequences. *Fertil Steril*. 1960;11:181-184.
5. Prescribing Information. Camila. Dr. Reddy's Laboratories Inc; 2024.
6. Heinonen OP, Slone D, Shapiro S. *Birth Defects and Drugs in Pregnancy*. Publishing Sciences Group; 1977.
7. Heinonen OP, Slone D, Monson RR, Hook EB, Shapiro S. Cardiovascular birth defects and antenatal exposure to female sex hormones. *N Engl J Med*. 1977;296:67-70.
8. Wiseman RA, Dodds-Smith IC. Cardiovascular birth defects and antenatal exposure to female sex hormones: a reevaluation of some base data. *Teratology*. 1984;30:359-370.
9. Dillon S. Congenital malformations and hormones in pregnancy. *Br Med J*. 1976;2:1446.
10. Carmichael SL, Shaw GM, Laurent C, Croughan MS, Olney RS, Lammer EJ. Maternal progestin intake and risk of hypospadias. *Arch Pediatr Adoles Med*. 2005;159:957-962.
11. Curtis KM, Tepper NK, Jatlaoui TC, et al. U.S. medical eligibility criteria for contraceptive use, 2016. *MMWR Recomm Rep*. 2016;65:1-103.
12. Faculty of Family Planning and Reproductive Health Care Clinical Effectiveness Unit. FFPRHC guidance (July 2004) contraceptive choices for breastfeeding women. *J Fam Plann Reprod Health Care*. 2004;30:181-189.
13. Phillips SJ, Tepper NK, Kapp N, Nanda K, Temmerman M, Curtis KM. Progestogen-only contraceptive use among breastfeeding women: a systematic review. *Contraception*. 2016;94:226-252.
14. Lopez LM, Grey TW, Stuebe AM, Chen M, Truitt ST, Gallo MF. Combined hormonal versus nonhormonal versus progestin-only contraception in lactation. *Cochrane Database Syst Rev*. 2015;3:CD003988.
15. World Health Organization Task Force for Epidemiological Research on Reproductive Health. Progestin-only contraceptives during lactation: I. Infant growth. *Contraception*. 1994;50:35-53.
16. World Health Organization Task Force for Epidemiological Research on Reproductive Health. Progestin-only contraceptives during lactation: II. Infant development. *Contraception*. 1994;50:54-68.
17. Saxena BN, Shrimanker K, Grudzinaskas JG. Levels of contraceptive steroids in breast milk and plasma of lactating women. *Contraception*. 1977;16:605-613.
18. Prescribing Information. Norethindrone Acetate. Amneal Pharmaceuticals LLC; 2024.
19. Charlton BM, Mølgaard-Nielsen D, Svanström H, Wohlfahrt J, Pasternak B, Melbye M. Maternal use of oral contraceptives and risk of birth defects in Denmark: prospective, nationwide cohort study. *BMJ*. 2016;352:h6712.
20. Curtis KM, Nguyen AT, Tepper NK, et al. U.S. selected practice recommendations for contraceptive use, 2024. *MMWR Recomm Rep*. 2024;73(No. RR-3):1-77.

NORTRIPTYLINE

Mental Health (Antidepressant—Tricyclic)

PREGNANCY RECOMMENDATION: Limited Human Data—No Relevant Animal Data

BREASTFEEDING RECOMMENDATION: Probably Compatible

PREGNANCY SUMMARY

From a few small series, there were no birth anomalies seen in seven cases of first-trimester exposure to nortriptyline. One infant exposed to nortriptyline during pregnancy experienced urinary retention. Nortriptyline and its active metabolite cross the human placenta, so fetal exposure will occur. However, this limited human pregnancy experience prevents a complete assessment of the embryofetal risk. No conclusive animal reproductive studies have been conducted with nortriptyline. Using this drug during pregnancy should be based on the pros and cons of the mother's clinical need for treatment versus any potential fetal risk that might occur from exposure. There is a pregnancy exposure registry that monitors pregnancy outcomes in women using antidepressant drugs. Health care providers are encouraged to call the National Pregnancy Registry for Antidepressants at 1-844-405-6185.

BREASTFEEDING SUMMARY

Several reports describing the effects of nortriptyline during human lactation have been located. The drug was found in human breast milk with levels ranging from about 50 to 410 ng/mL. The calculated breast milk to plasma ratios ranged from about 70% to more than double. However, the drug was not detected in the infant's serum, and only small amounts of the metabolite were detected. Breastfeeding while using this drug should be based on the mother's clinical need for treatment versus any potential infant risks that might occur. If used, the infant should be monitored for the most common reported adult side effects of dry mouth (leading to irritability), drowsiness, poor feeding (monitor infant growth), constipation, and urinary retention.

References

1. Yonkers KA, Wisner KL, Stewart DE, et al. The management of depression during pregnancy: a report from the American Psychiatric Association and the American College of Obstetricians and Gynecologists. *Obstet Gynecol*. 2009;114:703-713.
2. Prescribing Information. Nortriptyline Hydrochloride. Dr. Reddy's Laboratories; 2023.
3. Lexi-Comp, Inc. (Lexi-Drugs). Lexi-Comp, Inc; 2018.
4. Loughhead AM, Stowe ZN, Newport DJ, Ritchie JC, DeVane CL, Owens MJ. Placental passage of tricyclic antidepressants. *Biol Psychiatry*. 2006;59:287-290.
5. Bourke GM. Antidepressant teratogenicity? *Lancet*. 1974;1:98.
6. McBride WG. Limb deformities associated with iminobenzyl hydrochloride. *Med J Aust*. 1972;1:492.
7. Australian Drug Evaluation Committee. Tricyclic antidepressants and limb reduction deformities. *Med J Aust*. 1973;1:768-769.
8. Shearer WT, Schreiner RL, Marshall RE. Urinary retention in a neonate secondary to maternal ingestion of nortriptyline. *J Pediatr*. 1972;81:570-572.
9. McElhatton PR, Garbis HM, Elefant E, et al. The outcome of pregnancy in 689 women exposed to therapeutic doses of antidepressants. A collaborative study of the European Network of Teratology Information Services (ENTIS). *Reprod Toxicol*. 1996;10:285-294.
10. Nulman I, Rovet J, Stewart DE, et al. Child development following exposure to tricyclic antidepressants or fluoxetine throughout fetal life: a prospective, controlled study. *Am J Psychiatry*. 2002;159:1889-1895.
11. Bader TF, Newman K. Amitriptyline in human breast milk and the nursing infant's serum. *Am J Psychiatry*. 1980;137:855-856.
12. Erickson SH, Smith GH, Heidrich F. Tricyclics and breast feeding. *Am J Psychiatry*. 1979;136:1483.
13. Brixen-Rasmussen L, Halgrener J, Jorgensen A. Amitriptyline and nortriptyline excretion in human breast milk. *Psychopharmacology (Berlin)*. 1982; 76:94-95.
14. Matheson I, Skjaeraasen J. Milk concentrations of flupenthixol, nortriptyline and zuclopenthixol and between-breast differences in two patients. *Eur J Clin Pharmacol*. 1988;35:217-220.
15. Wisner KL, Perel JM. Serum nortriptyline levels in nursing mothers and their infants. *Am J Psychiatry*. 1991;148:1234-1236.
16. Wisner KL, Perel JM, Findling RL. Antidepressant treatment during breastfeeding. *Am J Psychiatry*. 1996;153:1132-1137.
17. Breyer-Pfaff U, Nill K, Entenmann A, Gaertner HJ. Secretion of amitriptyline and metabolites into breast milk. *Am J Psychiatry*. 1995;152:812-813.
18. Misri S, Sivertz K. Tricyclic drugs in pregnancy and lactation: a preliminary report. *Int J Psychiatry Med*. 1991;21:157-171.
19. Altshuler LL, Burt VK, McMullen M, Hendrick V. Breastfeeding and sertraline: a 24-hour analysis. *J Clin Psychiatry*. 1995;56:243-245.

NUSINERSEN

Central Nervous System (Survival Motor Neuron-2 Antisense Oligonucleotide)

PREGNANCY RECOMMENDATION: Limited Human Data—Animal Data Suggest Low Risk

BREASTFEEDING RECOMMENDATION: Probably Compatible

PREGNANCY SUMMARY

One case report describes a woman with type 3 spinal muscular atrophy (SMA) who unintentionally became pregnant during nusinersen treatment. She was found to have a twin gestation with one lost early in the first trimester. The surviving twin was delivered at term and followed up to 1 year of age. No anomalies or adverse consequences were reported. Biodistribution studies indicate that nusinersen does not cross the placenta. However, this limited human pregnancy experience prevents a complete assessment of the embryofetal risk. Animal studies did not show any embryo-fetal toxicity in one species at doses of less than 10 times the MRHD. Using this drug during pregnancy should be based on the pros and cons of the mother's clinical need for treatment versus any potential fetal risk that might occur from exposure.

BREASTFEEDING SUMMARY

No reports describing the use of nusinersen during human lactation have been located. The drug is unlikely to be found in breast milk. Breastfeeding while using this drug should be based on the mother's clinical need for treatment. If used, the infant should be monitored for the most common reported side effects of headache and back pain (both leading to irritability), constipation, vomiting, and pyrexia.

References

1. Prescribing Information. Spinraza. Biogen; 2020.
2. European Medicine Agency. Spinraza. Accessed March 19, 2023. https://www.ema.europa.eu/en/documents/assessment-report/spinraza-epar-public-assessment-report_en.pdf
3. Schön M, Domingues S, de Carvalho M, Santos MO. Nusinersen treatment in a type 3 spinal muscular atrophy patient during early pregnancy. *Neurol Sci*. 2023;44:1803-1804.

NYSTATIN

Anti-Infective (Antifungal)

PREGNANCY RECOMMENDATION: Human Data Suggest Low Risk—No Relevant Animal Data

BREASTFEEDING RECOMMENDATION: Probably Compatible

PREGNANCY SUMMARY

From two large databases, the CPP and the Michigan Medicaid Surveillance study, a total of 25 (4.0%) major birth anomalies were found in 631 first-trimester exposures. No pattern to the defects was identified. In a third study of more than 50,000 pregnancies (a major birth defect group was compared with a no-anomaly control group), the use of nystatin was no different between the groups. The drug will probably cross the placenta if found in the systemic circulation. However, oral bioavailability and systemic absorption from the skin are less than 1%. So, any fetal exposure will likely be clinically insignificant. Animal reproduction studies have not been conducted. Using this drug during pregnancy should be based on the pros and cons of the mother's clinical need for treatment versus any potential fetal risk that might occur from exposure.

BREASTFEEDING SUMMARY

No reports describing the use of nystatin during human lactation have been located. The drug may be excreted into breast milk if found in the systemic circulation. However, oral bioavailability and systemic absorption from the skin are less than 1%. So, any infant exposure will likely be clinically insignificant. Breastfeeding while using this drug should be based on the mother's clinical need for treatment versus any potential infant risks that might occur. Systemic side effects are not expected.

N

References

1. Prescribing Information. Nystatin cream. Crown Laboratories; 2021.
2. Prescribing Information. Nystatin tablet. Heritage Pharmaceuticals Inc; 2024.
3. Heinonen OP, Slone D, Shapiro S. *Birth Defects and Drugs in Pregnancy*. Publishing Sciences Group; 1977.
4. Culbertson C. Monistat: a new fungicide for treatment of vulvovaginal candidiasis. *Am J Obstet Gynecol*. 1974;120:973-976.
5. David JE, Frudenfeld JH, Goddard JL. Comparative evaluation of Monistat and Mycostatin in the treatment of vulvovaginal candidiasis. *Obstet Gynecol*. 1974;44:403-406.
6. Wallenburg HCS, Wladimiroff JW. Recurrence of vulvovaginal candidosis during pregnancy. Comparison of miconazole vs nystatin treatment. *Obstet Gynecol*. 1976;48:491-494.
7. Rosa FW, Baum C, Shaw M. Pregnancy outcomes after first-trimester vaginitis drug therapy. *Obstet Gynecol*. 1987;69:751-755.
8. Czeizel AE, Kazy Z, Puhó E. A population-based case-control teratological study of oral nystatin treatment during pregnancy. *Scand J Infect Dis*. 2003;35:830-835.

O

OBETICHOLIC ACID

Gastrointestinal

PREGNANCY RECOMMENDATION: No Human Data—Animal Data Suggest Low Risk

BREASTFEEDING RECOMMENDATION: Probably Compatible

PREGNANCY SUMMARY

No reports describing the use of obeticholic acid in human pregnancy have been located. The drug will probably cross the placenta, so some fetal exposure will likely occur. Therefore, the absence of human pregnancy experience prevents a complete assessment of the embryofetal risk. Animal studies did not show any embryofetal toxicity. Using this drug during pregnancy should be based on the pros and cons of the mother's clinical need for treatment versus any potential fetal risk that might occur from exposure.

BREASTFEEDING SUMMARY

No reports describing the use of obeticholic acid during human lactation have been located. Some amount of the drug will probably appear in breast milk, so infant exposure will likely occur. The manufacturer recommends that the developmental and health benefits of breastfeeding should be considered along with the mother's clinical need for treatment. If used, the infant should be monitored for the most common reported adult side effects of pruritus, arthralgia, and abdominal pain (all leading to irritability), rash, constipation, and lethargy.

Reference

1. Prescribing Information. Ocaliva. Intercept Pharmaceuticals, Inc; 2022.

OBILTOXAXIMAB

Antidote (Monoclonal Antibody—Anthrax)

PREGNANCY RECOMMENDATION: No Human Data—Animal Data Suggest Low Risk

BREASTFEEDING RECOMMENDATION: Probably Compatible

PREGNANCY SUMMARY

No reports describing the use of obiltoxaximab in human pregnancy have been located. Immunoglobulin G (IgG) antibodies are known to cross the placenta, especially during the third trimester, so some transfer will occur. Therefore, the absence of human pregnancy experience prevents a complete assessment of the embryofetal risk. Animal studies did not show any embryofetal toxicity. Anthrax infection during pregnancy is associated with a high risk of maternal, fetal, and neonatal deaths, especially without treatment. Using this drug during pregnancy should be based on the pros and cons of the mother's clinical need for treatment versus any potential fetal risk that might occur from exposure.

BREASTFEEDING SUMMARY

No reports describing the use of obiltoxaximab during human lactation have been located. It is known that IgG antibodies are excreted into breast milk but are not found in the neonatal or infant circulation. Additionally, if any IgG antibodies were to be ingested through breastfeeding, they would probably be digested in the infant's gastrointestinal tract and not be absorbed. Breastfeeding while using this drug should be based on the mother's clinical need for treatment. If used, the infant should be monitored for the most common reported adult side effects of headache, pruritus, and extremity pain (all leading to irritability), upper respiratory tract infection, cough, and rash.

References

1. Prescribing Information. Anthim. Elusys Therapeutics, Inc; 2019.
2. Meaney-Delman D, Zotti ME, Rasmussen SA, et al. Anthrax cases in pregnant and postpartum women: a systematic review. *Obstet Gynecol*. 2012;120:1439-1449.

OBINUTUZUMAB

Antineoplastic (Anti-CD20 Antigen—Monoclonal Antibody)

PREGNANCY RECOMMENDATION: No Human Data—Animal Data Suggest Risk

BREASTFEEDING RECOMMENDATION: Probably Compatible

PREGNANCY SUMMARY

No reports describing the use of obinutuzumab in human pregnancy have been located. As an IgG antibody, it likely crosses the placenta, especially during the second half of gestation, so some fetal exposure will probably occur. Therefore, the absence of human pregnancy experience prevents a complete assessment of the embryofetal risk. Obinutuzumab was not found to cause any embryofetal toxicity or teratogenicity in one animal species at doses of less than 10 times the recommended human dose (RHD). However, newborn B-cell levels were nearly completely depleted. B-cell concentrations returned to normal at about 6 months of age. Therefore, based on these animal studies and the drug's effect on neonatal B-cell concentrations, the manufacturer recommends that women with reproductive potential use effective contraception during treatment and for 6 months after the last dose. The manufacturer also recommends not administering newborn live vaccines until B-cell concentrations return to normal. Nevertheless, using this drug during pregnancy should be based on the pros and cons of the mother's clinical need for treatment versus any potential fetal risk that might occur from exposure. There is a registry for women who are pregnant and have cancer. For more information, women and health care providers are encouraged to contact the Cancer and Pregnancy Registry at 1-877-635-4499.

BREASTFEEDING SUMMARY

No reports describing the use of obinutuzumab during human lactation have been located. It is known that IgG antibodies can be found in human breast milk but are not found in the neonatal or infant circulation. Additionally, if any IgG antibodies were to be ingested through breastfeeding, they would probably be digested in the infant's gastrointestinal tract and not be absorbed. However, due to a concern for potential serious adverse effects that might be seen in a breastfed infant, the manufacturer recommends that women not breastfeed while being treated with this drug and for at least 6 months after the last dose. Nevertheless, breastfeeding while using this drug should be based on the mother's clinical need for treatment versus any potential infant risks that might occur. If used, the infant should be monitored for the most common reported adult side effects of musculoskeletal pain (leading to irritability), B-cell depletion, neutropenia, constipation, pyrexia, fatigue (lethargy), and cough.

Reference

1. Prescribing Information. Gazyva. Genentech; 2022.

OCRELIZUMAB

Central Nervous System (Multiple Sclerosis—Monoclonal Antibody)

PREGNANCY RECOMMENDATION: Limited Human Data—Animal Data Suggest Potential Risk

BREASTFEEDING RECOMMENDATION: Probably Compatible

PREGNANCY SUMMARY

There have been several reports regarding the use of ocrelizumab in human pregnancy. The data come from the German Multiple Sclerosis and Pregnancy Registry; the Clinical Trials and Post-Marketing Data as of March 2019, the Canadian Roche Patient Support Program; and a multiple sclerosis clinic in Western Australia. From these publications, there were 98 live births with probable exposure to the drug in the first trimester, and four anomalies were reported (4.1%). One anomaly was polydactyly in a family with a history of polydactyly. The other three were cardiac defects of a ventricular septal defect, an atrial septal defect with pulmonary stenosis, and a "hole in the heart." From the overall Roche Safety Data as of March 2021, 427 live births with 7 (1.6%) major anomalies were reported. However, some of the patients from the 98 cases discussed above are part of this database, and gestational age and the amount of exposure to the drug were not supplied. As an IgG antibody, it likely crosses the placenta, so some fetal exposure will probably occur. However, the limited human pregnancy experience prevents a complete assessment of the embryofetal risk. The drug can decrease peripheral B-lymphocyte counts. Blood levels of B cells in newborns were reported in two cases, and both pregnancies received an ocrelizumab infusion at about 19 weeks' gestation. One neonate had a normal B-cell count at delivery, and in the other, the count was reduced (but normalized by 2 months of age). Animal studies did show embryofetal toxicity. The manufacturer recommends that women with reproductive potential on ocrelizumab use effective contraception during treatment and for 6 months after the last dose. Nevertheless, using this drug during pregnancy should be based on the pros and cons of the mother's clinical need for treatment versus any potential fetal risk that might occur from exposure. There is a pregnancy exposure registry that monitors pregnancy outcomes in women using this drug. Health care providers are encouraged to call the Ocrevus Pregnancy Exposure Registry at 1-833-872-4370. Because three of the four anomalies (reported in the 98 cases mentioned earlier) were cardiac, this may need further evaluation in future studies.

BREASTFEEDING SUMMARY

A few reports describing the use of ocrelizumab during human lactation have been located. A total of 13 patients reportedly breastfed with exposure to ocrelizumab, and 7 had no adverse effects. The outcomes of breastfeeding in the other six were not supplied. Some amount of the drug is probably found in human breast milk. However, it is known that IgG antibodies can be found in breast milk but not in the neonatal or infant circulation. Additionally, if any IgG antibodies were to be ingested through breastfeeding, they would probably be digested in the infant's gastrointestinal tract and not be absorbed. Breastfeeding while using this drug should be based on the mother's clinical need for treatment. If used, the infant should be monitored for the most common reported adult side effects of respiratory tract infections, skin infections, and cough.

References

1. Prescribing Information. Ocrevus. Genentech, Inc (Roche Group); 2021.
2. Oreja-Guevara C, Wray S, Buffels R, et al. Pregnancy outcome in patients treated with ocrelizumab. *J Neurol Sci*. 2019;405:311-312.
3. Ciplea AI, Langer-Gould A, de Vries A, et al. Monoclonal antibody treatment during pregnancy and/or lactation in women with MS or neuromyelitis optica spectrum disorder. *Neurol Neuroimmunol Neuroinflamm*. 2020;7:e723(1-8).
4. Rolfes M, Rutatangwa A, Waubant E, Krysko KM. Ocrelizumab exposure in the second trimester of pregnancy without-B-cell depletion. *Mult Scler Relat Disord*. 2020;45:102398(1-4).
5. Kumpfel T, Thiel S, Meinl I, et al. Anti-CD20 therapies and pregnancy in neuroimmunologic disorders: a cohort study from Germany. *Neurol Neuroimmunol Neuroinflamm*. 2021;8:e913(1-11).
6. Chey SY, Kermode AG. Pregnancy outcome following exposure to ocrelizumab in multiple sclerosis. *Mult Scler J Exp Transl Clin*. 2022;8:20552173221085737(1-7).
7. Gitman V, Stavropoulos A, Saenz V, et al. Pregnancy outcomes of women with multiple sclerosis treated with ocrelizumab in Canada: a descriptive analysis of real-world data. *Mult Scler Relat Disord*. 2022;62:103792(1-8).

OCTREOTIDE

Endocrine/Metabolic (Somatostatin Analogue)

PREGNANCY RECOMMENDATION: Limited Human Data—Animal Data Suggest Low Risk

BREASTFEEDING RECOMMENDATION: Probably Compatible

O

PREGNANCY SUMMARY

Numerous case reports and series were located that describe the use of octreotide during human pregnancy. A total of 19 first-trimester exposures were found, and no major birth defects were described in the infants at delivery. The drug has been shown to cross the placenta, so fetal exposure will occur. Therefore, this limited human pregnancy experience prevents a complete assessment of the embryofetal risk. Animal studies did not show any embryofetal toxicity or teratogenicity in two species at doses of less than 10 times the maximum recommended human dose (MRHD) in one and more than 10 times the MRHD in the second. Using this drug during pregnancy should be based on the pros and cons of the mother's clinical need for treatment versus any potential fetal risk that might occur from exposure. In the clinical trials, the drug was shown to prolong the QT interval, and about 15% of patients had hyperglycemia.

BREASTFEEDING SUMMARY

A few reports were located that described the use of octreotide during human lactation. In one case, colostrum levels were low at 4.6 ng/mL. A calculated relative infant dose (RID) would be less than 2%. A few other infants were exposed to the drug through lactation, and no adverse effects were described. However, because it is an octapeptide, if the drug were to be ingested through breastfeeding, it would probably be digested in the infant's gastrointestinal tract and not be absorbed. This is consistent with the drug's poor oral bioavailability. Breastfeeding while using this drug should be based on the mother's clinical need for treatment versus any potential infant risks that might occur. If used, the infant should be monitored for the most common reported adult side effects of headache, nausea, dizziness, abdominal pain, and back pain (all leading to irritability), diarrhea, flatulence, and fatigue (lethargy).

References

1. Prescribing Information. Octreotide acetate. Wockhardt Limited; 2012.
2. Caron P, Gerbeau C, Pradayrol L. Maternal-fetal transfer of octreotide. *N Engl J Med*. 1995;333:601-602.
3. Caron P, Gerbeau C, Pradayrol L, et al. Successful pregnancy in an infertile woman with a thyrotropin-secreting macroadenoma treated with somatostatin analog (octreotide). *J Clin Endocrinol Metab*. 1996;81:1164-1168.
4. Landolt AM, Schmid J, Karlsson ERC, Boerlin V. Successful pregnancy in a previously infertile woman treated with SMS-201-995 for acromegaly. *N Engl J Med*. 1989;320:621-622.
5. Montini M, Pagani G, Gianola D, et al. Acromegaly and primary amenorrhea: ovulation and pregnancy induced by SMS 201-995 and bromocriptine. *J Endocrinol Invest*. 1990;13:193.

6. Takeuchi K, Funakoshi T, Oomori S, Maruo T. Successful pregnancy in an acromegalic woman treated with octreotide. *Obstet Gynecol*. 1999; 93:848.
7. Mozas J, Ocon E, Lopez de la Torre M, et al. Successful pregnancy in a woman with acromegaly treated with somatostatin analog (octreotide) prior to surgical resection. *Int J Gynecol Obstet*. 1999;65:71-73.
8. Neal JM. Successful pregnancy in a woman with acromegaly treated with octreotide. *Endocr Pract*. 2000;6:148-150.
9. Fassnacht M, Capeller B, Arit W, et al. Octreotide LAR treatment throughout pregnancy in an acromegalic woman. *Clin Endocrinol*. 2001;55:411-415.
10. Boulanger C, Vezzosi D, Bennet A, et al. Normal pregnancy in a woman with nesidioblastosis treated with somatostatin analog octreotide. *J Endocrinol Invest*. 2004;27:465-470.
11. Takano T, Saito J, Soyama A, et al. Normal delivery following an uneventful pregnancy in a Japanese acromegalic patient after discontinuation of octreotide long acting release formulation at an early phase of pregnancy. *Endocr J*. 2006;53:209-212.
12. Maffei P, Tamagno G, Nardelli GB, et al. Effects of octreotide exposure during pregnancy in acromegaly. *Clin Endocrinol (Oxf)*. 2010;72:668-677.
13. Naccache DD, Zaina A, Shen-Or Z, et al. Uneventful octreotide LAR therapy throughout three pregnancies, with favorable delivery and anthropometric measures for each newborn: a case report. *J Med Case Rep*. 2011;5:386.
14. Dias M, Boguszewski C, Gadelha M, et al. Acromegaly and pregnancy: a prospective study. *Eur J Endocrinol*. 2014;170:301-310.
15. Colao A, Merola B, Ferone D, Lombardi G. Acromegaly. *J Clin Endocrinol Metab*. 1997;82:2777-2781.

ODEVIXIBAT

Gastrointestinal (Ileal Bile Acid Transporter Inhibitor)

PREGNANCY RECOMMENDATION: No Human Data—Animal Data Suggest Potential Risk

BREASTFEEDING RECOMMENDATION: Probably Compatible

PREGNANCY SUMMARY

No reports describing the use of odevixibat in human pregnancy have been located. Clinically significant amounts of the drug are not likely to cross the placenta. However, the absence of human pregnancy experience prevents a complete assessment of embryofetal risk. Embryofetal toxicity with malformations (mainly cardiac) was observed in one animal species. Using this drug during pregnancy should be based on the pros and cons of the mother's clinical need for treatment versus any potential fetal risk that might occur from exposure. Odevixibat may reduce the absorption of fat-soluble vitamins. Therefore, the manufacturer recommends monitoring levels and increasing intake if a deficiency occurs.

BREASTFEEDING SUMMARY

No reports describing the use of odevixibat during human lactation have been located. Infant exposure to this drug through breast milk should be negligible. Breastfeeding while using this drug should be based on the mother's clinical need for treatment. If used, the infant should be monitored for the most common reported adult side effects of abdominal pain (leading to irritability), liver test abnormalities, diarrhea, vomiting, and fat-soluble vitamin deficiency. Because odevixibat may reduce the absorption of fat-soluble vitamins, the manufacturer recommends monitoring levels for deficiency.

Reference

1. Prescribing Information. Bylvay. Albireo Pharma; 2022.

OFATUMUMAB

Central Nervous System (Multiple Sclerosis—Monoclonal Antibody)

PREGNANCY RECOMMENDATION: Limited Human Data—Animal Data Suggest Potential Risk

BREASTFEEDING RECOMMENDATION: Probably Compatible

PREGNANCY SUMMARY

One report describing the use of ofatumumab in human pregnancy was located. A patient was inadvertently treated with the drug throughout gestation up to delivery. The infant did well with no identified birth anomalies. In addition, maternal B-cell levels were significantly low, but the newborn's B-cell concentrations were normal. As an IgG antibody, it likely crosses the placenta, especially during the second half of gestation, so some fetal exposure will probably occur. Therefore, this limited human pregnancy experience prevents a complete assessment of the embryofetal risk. Animal studies did not show any embryofetal toxicity or teratogenicity at doses well above the RHD. However, newborn B-cell levels were low, though again at doses well above 10 times the RHD. Based on these animal studies and the drug's potential effect on neonatal B-cell concentrations, the manufacturer recommends that women with reproductive potential use effective contraception during treatment and for 6 months after the last dose. The manufacturer also recommends not administering newborn live vaccines until B-cell concentrations return to normal. Nevertheless, using this drug during pregnancy should be based on the pros and cons of the mother's clinical need for treatment versus any potential fetal risk that might occur from exposure.

BREASTFEEDING SUMMARY

One report was located that described the use of ofatumumab during human lactation. A total of 12 mothers with multiple sclerosis were being treated with the drug. About 30% of the samples had undetectable levels (Lower Limit of Quantification (LLQ) of 1.5 ng/mL). Detectable concentrations ranged from 1.5 ng/mL up to about 56 ng/mL. All calculated RIDs were less than 1%. Infant B-cell levels were normal in the five that were tested, and in eight, live vaccines were administered, and no adverse reactions occurred. Lastly, no adverse effects were identified in infants. These findings are consistent with what would be expected in an IgG antibody. Breast milk levels are positive, but in low concentrations. Though infant blood concentrations for the drug were not evaluated, they would likely be clinically insignificant due to the IgG antibodies mostly being digested in the infant's gastrointestinal tract and not absorbed. Breastfeeding while using this drug should be based on the mother's clinical need for treatment versus any potential infant risks that might occur. If used, the infant should be monitored for the most common reported adult side effects of headache (leading to irritability) and upper respiratory tract infections.

References

1. Prescribing Information. Kesimpta. Novartis Pharmaceuticals Corp.; 2020.
2. Hefner S, Casaccia TL, Hofstaetter E, et al. Impact of continuous ofatumumab exposure during pregnancy in multiple sclerosis. *Neurol Clin Pract*. 2025;15:e200410.
3. Witt L, Dost-Kovalsky K, Friedmann N, et al. Ofatumumab-exposed breastfeeding in multiple sclerosis. *Mult Scler*. 2025;31:13524585241307165.

OFLOXACIN

Antibacterial (Fluoroquinolone)

PREGNANCY RECOMMENDATION: Limited Human Data—Animal Data Suggest Potential Risk

BREASTFEEDING RECOMMENDATION: Potential Toxicity

PREGNANCY SUMMARY

Several studies were located that describe the use of ofloxacin during human pregnancy. From 3 studies, 5 (2.5%) major birth anomalies were found in about 200 first-trimester exposures. In a few other larger studies analyzing the use of fluoroquinolones as a group, again, no overall increased risk for major birth anomalies was seen. The number of ofloxacin exposures in these studies was small. No pattern to the defects has been identified. The drug appears to cross the placenta, so some fetal exposure will occur. Therefore, this limited human pregnancy experience with ofloxacin prevents a complete assessment of the embryofetal risk. Animal data did show some embryofetal toxicity but no teratogenicity in two species at doses of less than 10 times the MRHD in one but more than 10 times the MRHD in the second. The drug carries a boxed warning for an increased risk of tendonitis and tendon rupture. Using this drug during pregnancy should be based on the pros and cons of the mother's clinical need for treatment versus any potential fetal risk that might occur from exposure. If possible, fluoroquinolones should be reserved for those cases where alternative treatment options are limited.

O

BREASTFEEDING SUMMARY

One study was located that described the use of ofloxacin during human lactation. The drug was found in the breast milk of 10 lactating women with a peak concentration of 2.41 mcg/mL. The calculated RID was about 3.2%. No infant drug levels have been analyzed. Breastfeeding while using this drug should be based on the mother's clinical need for treatment versus any potential infant risks that might occur. If used, the infant should be monitored for the most common reported adult side effects of dizziness, abdominal pain, and blurred vision (all leading to irritability), diarrhea, rash, insomnia, and cough.

References

1. Norrby SR, Lietman PS. Safety and tolerability of fluoroquinolones. *Drugs*. 1993;45(suppl 3):59-64.
2. Schaefer C, Amoura-Elefant E, Vial T, et al. Pregnancy outcome after prenatal quinolone exposure: evaluation of a case registry of the European Network of Teratology Information Services (ENTIS). *Eur J Obstet Gynecol Reprod Biol*. 1996;69:83-89.
3. U.S. Food and Drug Administration. FDA approves safety labeling changes for fluoroquinolones. Accessed May 24, 2016. http://www.fda.gov/Drugs/DrugSafety/InformationbyDrugClass/ucm500325.htm
4. Takayama S, Watanabe T, Akiyama Y, et al. Reproductive toxicity of ofloxacin. *Arzneim Forsch*. 1986;36:1244-1248. As cited in Shepard TH. Catalog of Teratogenic Agents. 7th ed. The Johns Hopkins University Press; 1992:296.
5. Prescribing Information. Ofloxacin. Dr. Reddy's Laboratories; 2018.
6. Giamarellou H, Kolokythas E, Petrikkos G, et al. Pharmacokinetics of three newer quinolones in pregnant and lactating women. *Am J Med*. 1989;87(suppl 5A):49S-51S.
7. Polachek H, Holcberg G, Sapir G, et al. Transfer of ciprofloxacin, ofloxacin and levofloxacin across the perfused human placenta in vitro. *Eur J Obstet Gynecol Reprod Biol*. 2005;122:61-65.
8. Loebstein R, Addis A, Ho E, et al. Pregnancy outcome following gestational exposure to fluoroquinolones: a multicenter prospective controlled study. *Antimicrob Agents Chemother*. 1998;42:1336-1339.
9. Padberg S, Wacker E, Meiser R, et al. Observational cohort study of pregnancy outcome after first-trimester exposure to fluoroquinolones. *Antimicrob Agents Chemother*. 2014;58:4392-4398.
10. Muanda FT, Sheehy O, Berard A. Use of antibiotics during pregnancy and the risk of major congenital malformations: a population based cohort study. *Br J Clin Pharmacol*. 2017;83:2557-2571.
11. Shin YJ, Choi JS, Chung JH, et al. Pregnancy outcomes in women reporting exposure to ofloxacin in early pregnancy. *J Obstet Gynaecol*. 2018;38:807-812.
12. American Academy of Pediatrics Committee on Drugs. The transfer of drugs and other chemicals into human milk. *Pediatrics*. 2001;108:776-789.

OFLOXACIN OPHTHALMIC

Ophthalmic/Antibacterial (Topical—Fluoroquinolone)

PREGNANCY RECOMMENDATION: No Human Data and No Relevant Animal Data

BREASTFEEDING RECOMMENDATION: Probably Compatible

PREGNANCY SUMMARY

No reports describing the use of ofloxacin ophthalmic in human pregnancy have been located. The drug will probably cross the placenta, so some fetal exposure will likely occur. However, systemic absorption is minimal with ocular use. Therefore, the absence of human pregnancy experience prevents a complete assessment of the embryofetal risk. Animal studies did show embryofetal toxicity, but at doses well above 10 times the Maximum Recommended Human Ophthalmic Dose (MRHOD). Using this drug during pregnancy should be based on the pros and cons of the mother's clinical need for treatment versus any potential fetal risk that might occur from exposure. If used during pregnancy, consider placing pressure over the tear duct in the corner of the eye for at least 1 minute, and then remove any excess solution with absorbent tissue to decrease the amount of drug reaching the systemic circulation even further.

BREASTFEEDING SUMMARY

No reports describing the use of ofloxacin ophthalmic during human lactation have been located. The drug will probably be found in human breast milk, but with the very low systemic levels seen with ocular use, the amount is likely to be clinically insignificant. Regardless, due to a concern for potential serious adverse effects that might be seen in a breastfed infant, the manufacturer recommends that women not breastfeed while being treated with this drug. Nevertheless, breastfeeding while using this drug should be based on the mother's clinical need for treatment versus any potential infant risks that might occur. Due to the ocular use, systemic side effects were not evaluated. A method to reduce the amount entering the systemic circulation is described above in the Pregnancy Summary.

Reference

1. Prescribing Information. Ofloxacin ophthalmic. Altaire Pharmaceuticals; 2020.

OLANZAPINE

Mental Health (Atypical Antipsychotic)

PREGNANCY RECOMMENDATION: Human Data Suggest Low Risk (First Trimester) / Human Data Suggest Possible Risk (Third Trimester) (Maternal Benefit May Outweigh Any Embryofetal Risk)

BREASTFEEDING RECOMMENDATION: Potential Toxicity

PREGNANCY SUMMARY

Numerous studies were located that describe the use of olanzapine during human pregnancy. From several case reports and small series, a total of 4 (2.6%) major birth anomalies were found in 137 first-trimester exposures. A recent systematic review reported 38 (3.5%) major defects in 1,090 early pregnancy exposures. No pattern to the defects was seen. The drug crosses the placenta, so fetal exposure will occur. Animal studies did show some embryofetal toxicity in one species at doses of about 9 times the MRHD. There is a risk of extrapyramidal and/or withdrawal symptoms in the newborn if the drug is used in the third trimester. Regardless, olanzapine is indicated for severe debilitating mental disease, and the benefits to the mother appear to outweigh any potential embryofetal risks. Therefore, using this drug during pregnancy should be based on the pros and cons of the mother's clinical need for treatment versus any potential fetal risk that might occur from exposure. The risk for hyperglycemia was also found to be increased during the clinical trials. There is a pregnancy exposure registry that monitors pregnancy outcomes in women using atypical antipsychotic drugs. Health care providers are encouraged to contact the National Pregnancy Registry for Atypical Antipsychotics at 1-866-961-2388.

BREASTFEEDING SUMMARY

Numerous studies were located that describe the use of olanzapine during human lactation. Breast milk from 21 lactating women was analyzed in mothers using this medication. Breast milk levels ranged from undetectable (LLQ of 1 ng/mL) up to a peak of 35 ng/mL (in a patient on 20 mg/d). The calculated RIDs were mostly less than 1% with the highest reported at 4%. A total of 13 infants had their blood analyzed for the drug when exposed through nursing. Of these, 12 had undetectable values (LLQ ranging from 1-5 ng/mL). In the remaining infant, concentrations ranged from 0.02 to 11 ng/mL. Overall, no adverse effects were reported other than sedation in the infant. The drug has also been shown to increase prolactin levels in some patients, but this should not adversely affect breastfeeding. However, due to a concern for potential serious adverse effects that might be seen in a breastfed infant, the manufacturer recommends that women not breastfeed while being treated with this drug. Nevertheless, breastfeeding while using this drug should be based on the mother's clinical need for treatment versus any potential infant risks that might occur. If used, the infant should be monitored for the most common reported adult side effects of dizziness (leading to irritability), constipation, somnolence, and tremors.

References

1. Altshuler LL, Cohen L, Szuba MP, et al. Pharmacologic management of psychiatric illness during pregnancy: dilemmas and guidelines. *Am J Psychiatry*. 1996;153:592-606.
2. Prescribing Information. Olanzapine. Dr. Reddy's Laboratories; 2019.
3. Schenker S, Yang Y, Mattiuz E, et al. Olanzapine transfer by human placenta. *Clin Exp Pharmacol Physiol*. 1999;26:691-697.
4. Newport DJ, Calamaras MR, DeVane CL, et al. Atypical antipsychotic administration during late pregnancy: placental passage and obstetrical outcomes. *Am J Psychiatry*. 2007;164:1214-1220.
5. Goldstein DJ, Corbin LA, Fung MC. Olanzapine-exposed pregnancies and lactation: early experience. *J Clin Psychopharmacol*. 2000;20:399-403.
6. Ernst CL, Goldberg JF. The reproductive safety profile of mood stabilizers, atypical antipsychotics, and broad-spectrum psychotropics. *J Clin Psychiatry*. 2002;63(suppl 4):42-55.
7. Littrell KH, Johnson CG, Peabody CD, Hilligoss N. Antipsychotics during pregnancy. *Am J Psychiatry*. 2000;157:1342.
8. Kirchheiner J, Berghofer A, Bolk-Weischedel D. Healthy outcome under olanzapine treatment in a pregnant woman. *Pharmacopsychiatry*. 2000;33:78-80.
9. Malek-Ahmadi P. Olanzapine in pregnancy. *Ann Pharmacother*. 2001;35:1294-1295.
10. Biwsas PN, Wilton LV, Pearce GL, et al. The pharmacovigilance of olanzapine: results of a post-marketing surveillance study on 8858 patients in England. *J Psychopharmacol*. 2001;15:265-271.
11. Lim LM. Olanzapine and pregnancy. *Aust N Z J Psychiatry*. 2001;35:856-857.
12. Dickson RA, Dawson DT. Olanzapine and pregnancy. *Can J Psychiatry*. 1998;43:196-197.
13. Mendhekar DN, War L, Sharma JB, Jiloha RC. Olanzapine and pregnancy. *Pharmacopsychiatry*. 2002;35:122-123.
14. McKenna K, Koren G, Tetelbaum M, et al. Pregnancy outcome of women using atypical antipsychotic drugs: a prospective comparative study. *J Clin Psychiatry*. 2005;66:444-449.
15. Gentile S. Prophylactic treatment of bipolar disorder in pregnancy and breastfeeding: focus on emerging mood stabilizers. *Bipolar Disord*. 2006;8:207-220.
16. Vigod SN, Gomes T, Wilton AS, et al. Antipsychotic drug use in pregnancy: high dimensional, propensity matched, population based cohort study. *Br Med J*. 2015;350:h2298.
17. Ennis ZN, Damkier P. Pregnancy exposure to olanzapine, quetiapine, risperidone, aripiprazole and risk of congenital malformations: a systematic review. *Basic Clin Pharmacol Toxicol*. 2015;116:315-320.
18. Croke S, Buist A, Hackett LP, et al. Olanzapine excretion in human breast milk: estimation of infant exposure. *Int J Neuropsychopharmacol*. 2002;5:243-247.
19. Gardiner SJ, Kristensen JH, Begg EJ, et al. Transfer of olanzapine into breast milk, calculation of infant drug dose, and effect on breast-fed infants. *Am J Psychiatry*. 2003;160:1428-1431.
20. Ambresin G, Berney P, Schulz P, Bryois C. Olanzapine excretion into breast milk: a case report. *J Clin Psychopharmacol*. 2004;24:93-95.
21. Aydin B, Nayir T. Olanzapine and quetiapine use during breastfeeding. *J Clin Psychopharmacol*. 2015;35:206-207.
22. Uguz F. Second-generation antipsychotics during the lactation period. *J Clin Psychopharmacol*. 2016;36:244-252.
23. American Academy of Pediatrics Committee on Drugs. The transfer of drugs and other chemicals into human milk. *Pediatrics*. 2001;108:776-789.

OLANZAPINE/SAMIDORPHAN

Mental Health (Antipsychotic and Opioid Antagonist)

PREGNANCY RECOMMENDATION: No Human Data—Animal Data Suggest Low Risk

BREASTFEEDING RECOMMENDATION: Potential Toxicity

O

PREGNANCY SUMMARY

No reports describing the use of olanzapine/samidorphan in human pregnancy have been located. Olanzapine and samidorphan are both likely to cross the placenta, so some fetal exposure will probably occur. From a retrospective cohort study of a Medicaid database, 9,258 women exposed to antipsychotic drugs during pregnancy did not show an overall increase in birth anomalies. See Olanzapine for further information on human exposure. However, the absence of human pregnancy experience for samidorphan prevents a complete assessment of the embryofetal risk. Animal data for samidorphan did not show any embryofetal toxicity. Uncontrolled bipolar disorder and schizophrenia have risks to pregnant women. Therefore, using this drug during pregnancy should be based on the pros and cons of the mother's clinical need for treatment versus any potential fetal risk that might occur from exposure. Samidorphan can also precipitate a severe opioid withdrawal if administered to a patient dependent on opioid drugs. Elevated glucose levels have also been reported in patients treated with this combination drug. If used during pregnancy, glucose levels should be monitored. There is a pregnancy exposure registry that monitors pregnancy outcomes in women using this drug. Health care providers are encouraged to call the National Pregnancy Registry for Atypical Antipsychotics at 1-866-961-2388.

BREASTFEEDING SUMMARY

No reports describing the use of olanzapine/samidorphan during human lactation have been located. Olanzapine is known to cross into breast milk (see Olanzapine). Samidorphan is likely present in breast milk, so infant exposure to this drug will also probably occur. Breastfeeding while using this drug should be based on the mother's clinical need for treatment. If used, the infant should be monitored for the most common reported adult side effects of nausea (leading to irritability), somnolence, constipation, and tremor. Additionally, because of olanzapine, the manufacturer recommends monitoring infants exposed to this drug through breastfeeding for the development of extrapyramidal symptoms (tremors and abnormal muscle movements).

Reference

1. Prescribing Information. Lybalvi. Alkermes; 2021.

OLAPARIB

Antineoplastic (Poly [ADP-Ribose] Polymerase Enzyme Inhibitor)

PREGNANCY RECOMMENDATION: No Human Data—Animal Data Suggest Potential Risk

BREASTFEEDING RECOMMENDATION: Potential Toxicity

PREGNANCY SUMMARY

No reports describing the use of olaparib during human pregnancy have been located. The drug will probably cross the placenta, so some fetal exposure will likely occur. Therefore, the absence of human pregnancy experience prevents a complete assessment of the embryofetal risk. Embryofetal toxicity and teratogenicity were seen in one animal species at doses of less than the MRHD. Based on animal studies and the drug's mechanism of action, the manufacturer recommends that women with reproductive potential use effective contraception during treatment and for 6 months after the last dose. They also recommend that males with female partners of reproductive potential use effective contraception during treatment and for 3 months after the last dose. Nevertheless, using this drug during pregnancy should be based on the pros and cons of the mother's clinical need for treatment versus any potential fetal risk that might occur from exposure. There is a registry for women who are pregnant and have cancer. For more information, women and health care providers are encouraged to contact the Cancer and Pregnancy Registry at 1-877-635-4499.

BREASTFEEDING SUMMARY

No reports describing the use of olaparib during human lactation have been located. The drug will probably be found in human breast milk, so some infant exposure will likely occur. Due to a concern for potential serious adverse effects that might be seen in a breastfed infant, the manufacturer recommends that women not breastfeed while being treated with this drug and for at least 1 month after the last dose. Nevertheless, breastfeeding while using this drug should be based on the mother's clinical need for treatment versus any potential infant risks that might occur. If used, the infant should be monitored for the most common reported adult side effects of nausea, headache, arthralgia, myalgia, back pain, and abdominal pain (all leading to irritability), diarrhea, fatigue (lethargy), vomiting, decreased appetite (monitor infant growth), rash, and cough.

Reference

1. Prescribing Information. Lynparza. AstraZeneca Pharmaceuticals; 2018.

O

OLICERIDINE

Analgesic (Opioid)

PREGNANCY RECOMMENDATION: No Human Data—Animal Data Suggest Low Risk

BREASTFEEDING RECOMMENDATION: Potential Toxicity

PREGNANCY SUMMARY

No reports describing the use of oliceridine in human pregnancy have been located. The drug probably crosses the placenta. Animal data did not show any embryofetal toxicity. However, the absence of human pregnancy experience prevents a complete assessment of the embryofetal risk. Because oliceridine is an opioid drug, there is a potential for addiction, serious life-threatening respiratory depression, profound sedation if used with other central nervous system (CNS) depressants, and a risk for neonatal opioid withdrawal syndrome (if used during pregnancy). If used during labor, neonatal depression can occur immediately postbirth. Oliceridine is a Schedule II controlled substance. Regarding strength, 1 mg of oliceridine is about 5 morphine milligram equivalents. Though it is recommended that the cumulative daily dose should not exceed 27 mg, daily cumulative doses greater than 27 mg may lead to prolongation of the QT interval.

BREASTFEEDING SUMMARY

Oliceridine probably enters breast milk. Because oliceridine is an opioid drug, there is a potential for profound sedation and serious life-threatening respiratory depression. Breastfeeding while using this drug should be based on the mother's clinical need for treatment. If used, the infant should be monitored for the most common reported adult side effects of nausea and pruritus (both leading to irritability), sedation, vomiting, and constipation.

Reference

1. Prescribing Information. Olinvyk. Trevena, Inc; 2020.

OLIPUDASE ALFA

Genetic (Lysosomal β-Glucuronidase Enzyme)

PREGNANCY RECOMMENDATION: No Human Data—*Animal Data Suggest Potential Risk

BREASTFEEDING RECOMMENDATION: Probably Compatible

PREGNANCY SUMMARY

No reports describing the use of olipudase alfa in human pregnancy have been located. The drug most likely does not cross the placenta; therefore, fetal exposure is probably nonexistent or extremely limited. However, the absence of human pregnancy experience prevents a complete assessment of the embryofetal risk. Animal studies did show embryofetal toxicity, with a potential concern for a rare CNS anomaly of exencephaly. *Therefore, use in the first trimester might be a concern. Based on animal studies, the manufacturer recommends that women with reproductive potential use effective contraception during treatment and for 2 weeks after the last dose. However, using this drug during the second and third trimesters of pregnancy should be based on the pros and cons of the mother's clinical need for treatment versus any potential fetal risk that might occur from exposure.

BREASTFEEDING SUMMARY

No reports describing the use of olipudase alfa during human lactation have been located. The drug most likely will not appear in breast milk. Furthermore, because it is an enzyme, if any drug were to be present in breast milk, it would most likely be digested in the infant's gastrointestinal tract and not be absorbed. Breastfeeding while using this drug should be based on the mother's clinical need for treatment. If used, the infant should be monitored for the most common reported adult side effects of headache, abdominal pain, nausea, arthralgias, and pruritus (all leading to irritability), diarrhea, rash, pyrexia, cough, and vomiting.

References

1. Prescribing Information. Xenpozyme. Genzyme Corporation; 2022.
2. Ross MM, Piorczynski TB, Harvey J, et al. Ceramide: a novel inducer for neural tube defects. *Dev Dyn*. 2019;248:979-996.

OLMESARTAN MEDOXOMIL

Antihypertensive (Angiotensin II Receptor Blocker—ARB)

PREGNANCY RECOMMENDATION: Human Data Suggest Risk (Second and Third Trimesters)

BREASTFEEDING RECOMMENDATION: Potential Toxicity

PREGNANCY SUMMARY

Two reports describing the use of olmesartan during the second and third trimesters in human pregnancy were located. Both resulted in oligohydramnios and anuria that resolved postdelivery in one case. Olmesartan probably crosses the placenta based on these two cases, so fetal exposure will occur. However, this limited first-trimester human pregnancy experience prevents a complete assessment of embryofetal risk. Decreased fetal renal function leading to anuria and oligohydramnios is commonly known as a major risk in the use of angiotensin II receptor blockers (ARBs) and angiotensin-converting enzyme (ACE) inhibitors, and this can lead to fetal lung hypoplasia, skeletal malformations, and death in some cases. However, it is not universally fatal, as seen in one of the cases described above. Therefore, use in the second and third trimesters should be avoided if at all possible. The drug carries a boxed warning regarding these fetal risks and to discontinue olmesartan as soon as possible when pregnancy is detected. If a mother has no appropriate alternative therapy, the manufacturer recommends educating the patient about the potential fetal risks. If used, serial ultrasounds to monitor amniotic fluid volume should be performed. Embryofetal toxicity or malformations were seen in two species at doses of less than 10 times the MRHD. Some embryofetal toxicity was seen in one animal species at doses that were about equal to the MRHD based on body surface area (BSA). Uncontrolled maternal hypertension is associated with an increased risk for preeclampsia, gestational diabetes, placental abruption, preterm delivery, intrauterine growth restriction, and intrauterine death.

BREASTFEEDING SUMMARY

No reports describing the use of olmesartan during human lactation have been located. The drug will probably be found in human breast milk, so some infant exposure will likely occur. Due to a concern for potential serious adverse effects that might be seen in a breastfed infant, the manufacturer recommends that women not breastfeed while being treated with this drug. Nevertheless, breastfeeding while using this drug should be based on the mother's clinical need for treatment versus any potential infant risks that might occur. If used, the infant should be monitored for the most common reported adult side effect of dizziness (leading to irritability).

References

1. Prescribing Information. Olmesartan medoxomil. Macleods Pharmaceuticals; 2019.
2. Sinelli MT, Cattarelli D, Cortinovis S, et al. Severe neonatal renal failure after maternal use of angiotensin II type 1 receptor antagonists. *Pediatr Med Chir*. 2008;30:306-308.
3. Polifka JE. Is there an embryopathy associated with first-trimester exposure to angiotensin-converting enzyme inhibitors and angiotensin receptor antagonists? A critical review of the evidence. *Birth Defects Res A Clin Mol Teratol*. 2012;94:576-598.
4. Perez-Iranzo A, Ferreres AN, Bou AJ. Maternal olmesartan exposure causing neonatal failure. *BMJ Case Rep*. 2017:bcr2016218921.

OLODATEROL

Respiratory (Bronchodilator—Long-Acting β_2-Adrenergic Agonist)

PREGNANCY RECOMMENDATION: No Human Data—Animal Data Suggest Low Risk

BREASTFEEDING RECOMMENDATION: Probably Compatible

PREGNANCY SUMMARY

No reports describing the use of olodaterol in human pregnancy have been located. Some amount of the drug will probably cross the placenta, so fetal exposure will likely occur. However, overall concentrations may be low due to inhalation use. Therefore, the absence of human pregnancy experience prevents a complete assessment of the embryofetal risk. Animal studies did not show any embryofetal toxicity or teratogenicity in two species with doses well above the Maximum Recommended Human Daily Inhalation Dose (MRHDID). Using this drug during pregnancy should be based on the pros and cons of the mother's clinical need for treatment versus any potential fetal risk that might occur from exposure.

BREASTFEEDING SUMMARY

No reports describing the use of olodaterol during human lactation have been located. The drug will probably be found in human breast milk, but overall levels may be low, with only 30% of the drug absorbed systemically with inhalation use. However, less than 1% of the drug is absorbed systemically with oral use. Therefore, any exposure to a breastfeeding infant is likely to be clinically insignificant. Breastfeeding while using this drug should be based on the mother's clinical need for treatment versus any potential infant risks that might occur.

Reference

1. Prescribing Information. Striverdi respimat. Boehringer Ingelheim Pharmaceuticals; 2020.

OLOPATADINE OPHTHALMIC

Ophthalmic/Antihistamine (Mast Cell Stabilizer—Topical)

PREGNANCY RECOMMENDATION: No Human Data and No Relevant Animal Data

BREASTFEEDING RECOMMENDATION: Probably Compatible

PREGNANCY SUMMARY

No reports describing the use of olopatadine ophthalmic in human pregnancy have been located. The drug will probably cross the placenta; however, because of the topical ocular use producing very low blood levels following systemic absorption, fetal exposure is probably clinically insignificant. However, the absence of human pregnancy experience prevents a complete assessment of the embryofetal risk. Embryofetal toxicity was seen in two animal species, but at doses well above 10 times the MRHOD. Using this agent during pregnancy should be based on the pros and cons of the mother's clinical need for treatment and to assess treatment options versus any potential fetal risk that might occur from exposure. If used during pregnancy, consider placing pressure over the tear duct in the corner of the eye for at least 1 minute, and then remove any excess solution with absorbent tissue to decrease the amount of drug reaching the systemic circulation even further.

BREASTFEEDING SUMMARY

No reports describing the use of olopatadine ophthalmic during human lactation have been located. The drug will probably be excreted into human breast milk. However, the amount of drug absorbed systemically is very low, suggesting that the levels would be clinically insignificant. Breastfeeding while using this drug should be based on the mother's clinical need for treatment versus any potential infant risks that might occur. If used, the infant should be monitored for the most common reported adult side effects of nausea, headache, and back pain (all leading to irritability) and cough. A method to decrease some systemic absorption with ophthalmic use is described above in the Pregnancy Summary.

References

1. Prescribing Information. Pataday. Alcon Laboratories; 2018.
2. Prescribing Information. Patanol. Alcon Laboratories; 2018.

OLSALAZINE

Gastrointestinal (5-Aminosalicylic Acid—Inflammatory Bowel Disease)

PREGNANCY RECOMMENDATION: Limited Human Data—Animal Data Suggest Potential Risk

BREASTFEEDING RECOMMENDATION: Probably Compatible

PREGNANCY SUMMARY

A 2008 meta-analysis studied the risk of adverse pregnancy outcomes in women with inflammatory bowel disease following exposure to 5-aminosalicylic acid (5-ASA) drugs (olsalazine, balsalazide, mesalazine, and sulfasalazine). In 7 studies, 1,158 received no medications, and 642 received 5-ASA drugs. There was no significant increase in birth defects, stillbirths, spontaneous abortion, preterm delivery, or low birth weight between the groups. The drug will probably cross the placenta, but levels will probably be clinically insignificant. However, this limited human pregnancy experience prevents a complete assessment of the embryofetal risk. Animal data did show some embryofetal toxicity in one species at doses of less than 10 times the RHD. Using this drug during pregnancy should be based on the pros and cons of the mother's clinical need for treatment versus any potential fetal risk that might occur from exposure.

BREASTFEEDING SUMMARY

The breast milk of two women was evaluated while using olsalazine during breastfeeding. The active metabolite, 5-ASA, and the inactive metabolite *N*-acetyl-5-aminosalicylic acid (*N*-ac-5-ASA) were analyzed. In both cases, 5-ASA was not detected (LLQ of 170 ng/mL in one and 20 ng/mL in the second). However, the inactive metabolite, *N*-ac-5-ASA, was detected with breast milk levels of 0.17 to 0.264 mcg/mL in one case and 1.2 to 3.8 mcg/mL in the second case. The calculated RIDs for the inactive metabolite were 0.6% and 2.6%. Therefore, the RIDs for the active metabolite are much less than this. In addition, the oral bioavailability is only 2.4%, so if any of the drug were to be ingested through breastfeeding, the amount would likely be clinically insignificant. Breastfeeding while using this drug should be based on the mother's clinical need for treatment versus any potential infant risks that might occur. If used, the infant should be monitored for the most common reported adult side effects of nausea and abdominal cramps (both leading to irritability), rash, and diarrhea.

References

1. Prescribing Information. Dipentum. MEDA Pharmaceuticals; 2019.
2. Rahimi R, Nikfar S, Rezaie A, Abdollahi M. Pregnancy outcome in women with inflammatory bowel disease following exposure to 5-aminosalicyclic acid drugs: a meta-analysis. *Reprod Toxicol*. 2008;25:271-275.
3. Miller LG, Hopkinson JM, Motil KJ, et al. Disposition of olsalazine and metabolites in breast milk. *J Clin Pharmacol*. 1993;33:703-706.
4. Ambrosius Christensen L, Rasmussen SN, Hansen SH, et al. Salazosulfapyridine and metabolites in fetal and maternal body fluids with special reference to 5-aminosalicylic acid. *Acta Obstet Gynecol Scand*. 1987;66:433-435.

O

OLUTASIDENIB

Antineoplastic (Mutated Isocitrate Dehydrogenase-1 Inhibitor)

PREGNANCY RECOMMENDATION: No Human Data—Animal Data Suggest Potential Risk

BREASTFEEDING RECOMMENDATION: Potential Toxicity

PREGNANCY SUMMARY

No reports describing the use of olutasidenib in human pregnancy have been located. Some amount of the drug will probably cross the placenta, so fetal exposure will likely occur. However, the absence of human pregnancy experience prevents a complete assessment of the embryofetal risk. Animal studies did show embryofetal toxicity in one species at doses of less than 10 times the RHD. Using this drug during pregnancy should be based on the pros and cons of the mother's clinical need for treatment versus any potential fetal risk that might occur from exposure.

BREASTFEEDING SUMMARY

No reports describing the use of olutasidenib during human lactation have been located. Some amount of the drug probably enters breast milk, so infant exposure will likely occur. However, due to the concern for potential serious adverse effects that might be seen in a breastfed infant, the manufacturer recommends that women not breastfeed while being treated with olutasidenib and for 2 weeks after the last dose. Nevertheless, breastfeeding while using this drug should be based on the mother's clinical need for treatment. If used, the infant should be monitored for the most common reported adult side effects of nausea and arthralgia (both leading to irritability), lethargy, constipation, dyspnea, pyrexia, rash, diarrhea, and several laboratory abnormalities (see Prescribing Information [PI]).

Reference

1. Prescribing Information. Reslidhea. Forma Therapeutics, Inc; 2022.

OMADACYCLINE

Antibacterial (Tetracycline Derivative)

PREGNANCY RECOMMENDATION: Contraindicated (Second and Third Trimesters)

BREASTFEEDING RECOMMENDATION: Potential Toxicity

PREGNANCY SUMMARY

No reports describing the use of omadacycline in human pregnancy have been located. The drug will probably cross the placenta, so some fetal exposure will likely occur. Therefore, the absence of human pregnancy experience prevents a complete assessment of the embryofetal risk. Animal data did show embryofetal toxicity. Numerous studies on tetracycline drugs have shown a risk for tooth discoloration, tooth enamel hypoplasia, and inhibition of bone growth when used in the second and third trimesters of pregnancy (see Tetracycline). Therefore, the manufacturer recommends that women of reproductive potential use effective contraception while using omadacycline.

BREASTFEEDING SUMMARY

It is not known if omadacycline is excreted into human breast milk. The drug will probably be found in breast milk, so some infant exposure will likely occur. Tooth discoloration, tooth enamel hypoplasia, and inhibition of bone growth are theoretically possible in an infant if the drug is used during breastfeeding, but the expected maternal treatment time should be short-term. The manufacturer recommends that a woman not breastfeed during treatment and for 4 days after the last dose. Nevertheless, breastfeeding while using this drug should be based on the mother's clinical need for treatment. If used, the infant should be monitored for the most common reported adult side effects of nausea and headache (both leading to irritability), vomiting, and diarrhea.

Reference

1. Prescribing Information. Nuzyra. Paratek Pharmaceuticals, Inc; 2018.

OMALIZUMAB

Respiratory (Monoclonal Antibody)

PREGNANCY RECOMMENDATION: Limited Human Data—Animal Data Suggest Low Risk

BREASTFEEDING RECOMMENDATION: Probably Compatible

PREGNANCY SUMMARY

Several studies were located that describe the use of omalizumab during human pregnancy. From 3 of these studies, 5 (2.8%) major anomalies were described in about 180 pregnancies with first-trimester exposure. No pattern to the defects was seen. As an IgG antibody, it likely crosses the placenta, especially during the second half of pregnancy, so some fetal exposure will probably occur. However, this limited human pregnancy experience prevents a complete assessment of the embryofetal risk. Animal studies did not show any embryofetal toxicity or teratogenicity in one species at doses of about 10 times the MRHD. Using this drug during pregnancy should be based on the pros and cons of the mother's clinical need for treatment versus any potential fetal risk that might occur from exposure.

BREASTFEEDING SUMMARY

Several publications regarding the use of omalizumab during human lactation were located. In one study, breast milk concentrations were evaluated in one mother who was treated with the drug during pregnancy. Breast milk samples were taken about 85 to 86 days after the last dose (~3.5 half-lives). One sample was positive at 8 ng/mL, while the remaining samples were negative (LLQ of 2 ng/mL). It is known that IgG antibodies can be found in human breast milk but are not found in the neonatal or infant circulation. However, if any IgG antibodies were to be ingested through breastfeeding, they would probably be digested in the infant's gastrointestinal tract and not be absorbed. Several other studies have reported no adverse infant effects when exposed to the drug through breastfeeding. Breastfeeding while using this drug should be based on the mother's clinical need for treatment versus any potential infant risks that might occur. If used, the infant should be monitored for the most common reported adult side effects of headache, arthralgia, dizziness, itching, abdominal pain, and nausea (all leading to irritability), fatigue (lethargy), fever, and cough.

References

1. Prescribing Information. Xolair. Genentech; 2018.
2. Namazy J, Cabana MD, Scheuerle AE, et al. The Xolair pregnancy registry (EXPECT): the safety of omalizumab use during pregnancy. *J Allergy Clin Immunol*. 2015;135:407-412.
3. Cuervo-Pardo L, Barcena-Blanch M, Radojicic C. Omalizumab use during pregnancy for CIU: a tertiary care experience. *Eur Ann Allergy Clin Immunol*. 2016;48:145-146.
4. Saito J, Yakuwa N, Sandaiji N, et al. Omalizumab concentrations in pregnancy and lactation: a case study. *J Allergy Clin Immunol Pract*. 2020;8:3603-3604.

OMAVELOXOLONE

Central Nervous System/Genetic (Friedreich Ataxia)

PREGNANCY RECOMMENDATION: No Human Data—Animal Data Suggest Risk

BREASTFEEDING RECOMMENDATION: Potential Toxicity

PREGNANCY SUMMARY

No reports describing the use of omaveloxolone in human pregnancy have been located. The drug will likely cross the placenta, so some fetal exposure will probably occur. Therefore, the absence of human pregnancy experience prevents a complete assessment of the embryofetal risk. Animal data showed embryofetal toxicity. The drug may decrease the efficacy of hormonal contraceptives. Therefore, the manufacturer recommends that women use alternate or additional contraceptive methods while being treated with this drug and for 1 month after the last dose. Nevertheless, using omaveloxolone during pregnancy should be based on the pros and cons of the mother's clinical need for treatment versus any potential fetal risk that might occur from exposure.

BREASTFEEDING SUMMARY

No reports describing the use of omaveloxolone during human lactation have been located. The drug will likely be excreted into breast milk, so some infant exposure will probably occur. Breastfeeding while using this drug should be based on the mother's clinical need for treatment. If used, the infant should be monitored for the most common reported adult side effects of headache, nausea, abdominal pain, and musculoskeletal pain (all leading to irritability), diarrhea, lethargy, and elevated liver function tests.

Reference

1. Prescribing Information. Skyclarys. Reata Pharmaceuticals, Inc; 2023.

OMEGA-3 FATTY ACIDS

Antilipemic/Nutrition/Nutritional Supplements

PREGNANCY RECOMMENDATION: Compatible

BREASTFEEDING RECOMMENDATION: Compatible

PREGNANCY SUMMARY

Numerous reports, including several meta-analyses describing the use of ω-3 fatty acids in pregnancy, have been located. Although research is still evolving regarding the effects of long-chain polyunsaturated fatty acids (LC-PUFAs) during pregnancy, human studies show that an increased intake of docosahexaenoic acid (DHA) and eicosapentaenoic acid (EPA) has

(continued)

been associated with the prevention of preterm birth. While most studies of higher maternal fish consumption during pregnancy have been associated with improvement in infant neurodevelopment, this association has not been confirmed in randomized trials of ω-3 fatty acid intervention (food, supplements). Supplementation during pregnancy has also shown a possible reduction in allergic outcomes. ω-3 Fatty acids, including EPA and DHA, are actively transported across the placenta. Experts recommend an average intake of 250 mg/d or more of DHA plus EPA and an additional 100 to 200 mg/d or more of DHA. Pregnant women with low DHA intake or blood levels at the beginning of pregnancy should have an average intake of 600 to 1,000 mg/d of DHA plus EPA or DHA alone, preferably beginning in the second trimester but no later than 20 weeks' gestation and continuing until birth or about 37 weeks' gestation.

BREASTFEEDING SUMMARY

Numerous reports, including several meta-analyses describing the use and effects of ω-3 fatty acids during human lactation, have been located. The potential benefits of ω-3 LC-PUFA use during lactation include improved language ability, improved vision and attention, reduced oxidative stress, greater ponderal index, and reduced insulin resistance in infants. No beneficial effects on childhood allergic diseases or the reduction of bronchopulmonary dysplasia were observed. No adverse effects in breastfed infants have been reported. DHA and EPA are present in breast milk. Supplementation with ω-3 fatty acids resulted in increased levels in breast milk. It is recommended that breastfeeding women consume at least 250 mg of DHA per day.

References

1. Benatti P, Peluso G, Nicolai R, Calvani M. Polyunsaturated fatty acids: biochemical, nutritional and epigenetic properties. *J Am Coll Nutr*. 2004; 23:281-302.
2. Otten JJ, Hellway JP, Meyers LD, eds. *Dietary Intakes IOM and Food and Nutrition Board*. National Academies Press; 2006:122-139.
3. Greenberg JA, Bell SJ, Ausdal WV. Omega-3 fatty acid supplementation during pregnancy. *Rev Obstet Gynecol*. 2008;1:162-169.
4. Coletta JM, Bell SJ, Roman AS. Omega-3 fatty acids and pregnancy. *Rev Obstet Gynecol*. 2010;3:163-171.
5. Koletzko B, Lien E, Agostoni C, et al.; World Association of Perinatal Medicine Dietary Guidelines Working Group. The roles of long-chain polyunsaturated fatty acids in pregnancy, lactation and infancy: review of current knowledge and consensus recommendations. *J Perinat Med*. 2008;36:5-14.
6. Makrides M, Gibson RA. Long-chain polyunsaturated fatty acid requirements during pregnancy and lactation. *Am J Clin Nutr*. 2000;71(suppl 1): 307S-311S.
7. Koletzko B, Rodriguez-Palmero M, Demmelmair H, et al. Physiological aspects of human milk lipids. *Early Hum Dev*. 2001;65(suppl):S3-S18.
8. Middleton P, Gomersall JC, Gould JF, et al. Omega-3 fatty acid addition during pregnancy. *Cochrane Database Syst Rev*. 2018;11(11):CD003402.
9. von Schacky C. Omega-3 fatty acids in pregnancy—the case for a target Omega-3 index. *Nutrients*. 2020;12(4):898.
10. Cetin I, Carlson SE, Burden C, et al.; Clinical Practice Guideline on behalf of Asia Pacific Health Association (Pediatric-Neonatology Branch), Child Health Foundation (Stiftung Kindergesundheit), European Academy of Paediatrics, European Board & College of Obstetrics and Gynaecology, European Foundation for the Care of Newborn Infants, European Society for Paediatric Research, and International Society for Developmental Origins of Health and Disease. Omega-3 fatty acid supply in pregnancy for risk reduction of preterm and early preterm birth. *Am J Obstet Gynecol MFM*. 2024;6:101251.
11. Vahdaninia M, Mackenzie H, Dean T, Helps S. ω-3 LCPUFA supplementation during pregnancy and risk of allergic outcomes or sensitization in offspring: a systematic review and meta-analysis. *Ann Allergy Asthma Immunol*. 2019; 122:302-313.e2.
12. Serra R, Peñailillo R, Monteiro LJ, et al. Supplementation of omega 3 during pregnancy and the risk of preterm birth: a systematic review and meta-analysis. *Nutrients*. 2021;13:1704.
13. Best KP, Gibson RA, Makrides M. ISSFAL statement number 7—Omega-3 fatty acids during pregnancy to reduce preterm birth. *Prostaglandins Leukot Essent Fatty Acids*. 2022;186:102495.
14. Delgado-Noguera MF, Calvache JA, Bonfill Cosp, X, et al. Supplementation with long chain polyunsaturated fatty acids (LCPUFA) to breastfeeding mothers for improving child growth and development. *Cochrane Database Syst Rev*. 2015;7:CD007901.
15. Lehner A, Staub K, Aldakak L, et al. Impact of omega-3 fatty acid DHA and EPA supplementation in pregnant or breast-feeding women on cognitive performance of children: systematic review and meta-analysis. *Nutr Rev*. 2021;79:585-598.
16. Quin C, Erland BM, Loeppky JL, et al. Omega-3 polyunsaturated fatty acid supplementation during the pre and post-natal period: a meta-analysis and systematic review of randomized and semi-randomized controlled trials. *J Nutr Intermediary Metab*. 2016;5:34-54.
17. Nevins JEH, Donovan SM, Snetselaar L, et al. Omega-3 fatty acid dietary supplements consumed during pregnancy and lactation and child neurodevelopment: a systematic review. *J Nutr*. 2021;151:3483-3494.
18. Liu Y, Zhong L, Sun Z, et al. N-3 fatty acid supplementation in mothers and infants for childhood psychomotor and cognitive development: an updated systematic review and meta-analysis. *Matern Child Nutr*. 2024;21:e13767.
19. Klemens CM, Berman DR, Mozurkewich EL. The effect of perinatal omega-3 fatty acid supplementation on inflammatory markers and allergic diseases: a systematic review. *BJOG*. 2011;118:916-925.
20. Gunaratne AW, Makrides M, Collins CT. Maternal prenatal and/or postnatal n-3 long chain polyunsaturated fatty acids (LCPUFA) supplementation for preventing allergies in early childhood. *Cochrane Database Syst Rev*. 2015;7:CD010085.
21. Lauritzen L, Eriksen SE, Hjorth MF, et al. Maternal fish oil supplementation during lactation is associated with reduced height at 13 years of age and higher blood pressure in boys only. *Br J Nutr*. 2016;116:2082-2090.

OMEPRAZOLE

Gastrointestinal (Proton Pump Inhibitor)

PREGNANCY RECOMMENDATION: Human Data Suggest Low Risk

BREASTFEEDING RECOMMENDATION: Probably Compatible (Short-Term Use)

PREGNANCY SUMMARY

Numerous studies have been located that describe the use of omeprazole during human pregnancy. The rate of major congenital anomalies from more than 2,800 first-trimester exposures was only 2.6%, and no pattern to the defects was identified. In addition, several studies have analyzed proton pump inhibitor use with first-trimester exposure in several thousand cases, and again, no increased risk for major birth defects has been seen. Lastly, a few reviews and meta-analyses have not shown any increased risk for omeprazole use during pregnancy. Though a few studies have suggested a higher rate of cardiac anomalies, clefts, or hypospadias, these have not been consistently found. The drug crosses the placenta, so fetal exposure will occur. Animal studies did show some embryofetal toxicity, but no teratogenicity, in two species at doses of about 5 times the MRHD. Using this drug during pregnancy should be based on the pros and cons of the mother's clinical need for treatment versus any potential fetal risk that might occur from exposure.

BREASTFEEDING SUMMARY

A few studies regarding the use of omeprazole during human lactation were located. In one woman, the drug was found in human breast milk with a peak level of about 20 ng/mL, producing a calculated RID of about 1%. In a few other studies, no consistent adverse effects were reported in infants upon use during breastfeeding. The drug has been shown to increase prolactin levels, but this should not adversely affect breastfeeding. However, due to a concern for potential serious adverse effects that might be seen in a breastfed infant, the manufacturer recommends that women not breastfeed while being treated with this drug. Nevertheless, breastfeeding while using this drug should be based on the mother's clinical need for treatment versus any potential infant risks that might occur. If used, the infant should be monitored for the most common reported adult side effects of nausea, headache, and abdominal pain (all leading to irritability), diarrhea, vomiting, and flatulence.

References

1. Prescribing Information. Prilosec. AstraZeneca; 2019.
2. Moore J, Flynn RJ, Sampaio M, et al. Effect of single-dose omeprazole on intragastric acidity and volume during obstetric anaesthesia. *Anaesthesia*. 1989;44:559-562.
3. Tsirigotis M, Yazdani N, Craft I. Potential effects of omeprazole in pregnancy. *Hum Reprod*. 1995;10:2177-2178.
4. Harper MA, McVeigh JE, Thompson W, et al. Successful pregnancy in association with Zollinger-Ellison syndrome. *Am J Obstet Gynecol*. 1995;173:863-864.
5. Kallen B. Delivery outcome after the use of acid-suppressing drugs in early pregnancy with special reference to omeprazole. *Br J Obstet Gynaecol*. 1998;105:877-881.
6. Kallen BAJ. Use of omeprazole during pregnancy—no hazard demonstrated in 955 infants exposed during pregnancy. *Eur J Obstet Gynecol Reprod Biol*. 2001;98:63-68.
7. Lalkin A, Loebstein R, Addis A, et al. The safety of omeprazole during pregnancy: a multicenter prospective controlled study. *Am J Obstet Gynecol*. 1998;179:727-730.
8. Wilton LV, Pearce GL, Martin RM, et al. The outcomes of pregnancy in women exposed to newly marketed drugs in general practice in England. *Br J Obstet Gynaecol*. 1998;105:882-889.
9. Brunner G, Meyer H, Athmann C. Omeprazole for peptic ulcer disease in pregnancy. *Digestion*. 1998;59:651-654.
10. Nielsen GL, Sorensen HT, Thulstrup AM, et al. The safety of proton pump inhibitors in pregnancy. *Aliment Pharmacol Ther*. 1999;13:1085-1089.
11. Ruigomez A, Rodriguez LAG, Cattaruzzi C, et al. Use of cimetidine, omeprazole, and ranitidine in pregnant women and pregnancy outcomes. *Am J Epidemiol*. 1999;150:476-481.
12. Marshall JK, Thomson ABR, Armstrong D. Omeprazole for refractory gastroesophageal reflux disease during pregnancy and lactation. *Can J Gastroenterol*. 1998;12:225-227.
13. Nikfar S, Abdollahi M, Moretti ME, et al. Use of proton pump inhibitors during pregnancy and rates of major malformations: a meta-analysis. *Dig Dis Sci*. 2002;47:1526-1529.
14. Diav-Citrin O, Arnon J, Shechtman S, et al. The safety of proton pump inhibitors in pregnancy: a multicentre prospective controlled trial. *Aliment Pharmacol Ther*. 2005;21:269-275.
15. Dehlink E, Yen E, Leichtner AM, et al. First evidence of a possible association between gastric acid suppression during pregnancy and childhood asthma: a population-based register study. *Clin Exp Allergy*. 2009;39:246-253.
16. Yau G, Kan AF, Gin T, Oh TE. A comparison of omeprazole and ranitidine for prophylaxis against aspiration pneumonitis in emergency caesarean section. *Anaesthesia*. 1992;47:101-104.
17. Orr DA, Bill KM, Gillon KRW, et al. Effects of omeprazole, with and without metoclopramide, in elective obstetric anaesthesia. *Anaesthesia*. 1993;48:114-119.
18. Rocke DA, Rout CC, Gouws E. Intravenous administration of the proton pump inhibitor omeprazole reduces the risk of acid aspiration at emergency cesarean section. *Anesth Analg*. 1994;78:1093-1098.
19. Gin T. Intravenous omeprazole before emergency cesarean section. *Anesth Analg*. 1995;80:848.
20. Rocke DA, Rout CC. Intravenous omeprazole before emergency cesarean section. *Anesth Analg*. 1995;80:848-849.
21. Stuart JC, Kan AF, Rowbottom SJ, Gin T. Acid aspiration prophylaxis for emergency caesarean section. *Anaesthesia*. 1996;51:415-421.
22. Gill SK, O'Brien L, Einarson TR, Koren G. The safety of proton pump inhibitors (PPIs) in pregnancy: a meta-analysis. *Am J Gastroenterol*. 2009;104:1541-1545.
23. Pasternak B, Hviid A. Use of proton-pump inhibitors in early pregnancy and the risk of birth defects. *N Engl J Med*. 2010;363:2114-2123.
24. Mitchell AA. Proton-pump inhibitors and birth defects—some reassurance, but more needed. *N Engl J Med*. 2010;363:2161-2163.
25. Anderka M, Mitchell AA, Louik C, et al.; the National Birth Defects Prevention Study. Medications used to treat nausea and vomiting of pregnancy and the risk of selected birth defects. *Birth Defects Res A Clin Mol Teratol*. 2012;94:22-30.
26. Erichsen R, Mikkelsen E, Pedersen L, Sorensen HT. Maternal use of proton pump inhibitors during early pregnancy and the prevalence of hypospadias in male offspring. *Am J Ther*. 2014;21(4):254-259.
27. Matok I, Levy A, Wiznitzer A, et al. The safety of fetal exposure to proton-pump inhibitors during pregnancy. *Dig Dis Sci*. 2012;57:699-705.
28. Broussard CN, Richter JE. Treating gastro-oesophageal reflux disease during pregnancy and lactation: what are the safest therapy options? *Drug Saf*. 1998;19:325-337.
29. Katz PO, Castell DO. Gastroesophageal reflux disease during pregnancy. *Gastroenterol Clin N Am*. 1998;27:153-167.
30. Ramakrishnan A, Katz PO. Pharmacologic management of gastroesophageal reflux disease. *Curr Treat Options Gastroenterol*. 2002;5:301-310.
31. Richter JE. Gastroesophageal reflux disease during pregnancy. *Gastroenterol Clin N Am*. 2003;32:235-261.
32. Richter JE. Review article: the management of heartburn in pregnancy. *Aliment Pharmacol Ther*. 2005;22:749-757.
33. Ito S. Drug therapy for breast-feeding women. *N Engl J Med*. 2000;343:118-126.
34. Lawrence RA, Lawrence RM. *Breastfeeding: A Guide for the Medical Profession*. 5th ed. St. Mosby; 1999:360.

OMIDENEPAG ISOPROPYL OPHTHALMIC

Ophthalmic (Antiglaucoma; Prostaglandin E_2 Receptor Agonist)

PREGNANCY RECOMMENDATION: No Human Data and No Relevant Animal Data

BREASTFEEDING RECOMMENDATION: Probably Compatible

PREGNANCY SUMMARY

No reports describing the use of omidenepag isopropyl ophthalmic in human pregnancy have been located. Based on likely minimal to no placental transfer, fetal exposure is probably negligible. However, the absence of human pregnancy experience prevents a complete assessment of the embryofetal risk. Embryofetal toxicity was observed in one animal species, but with subcutaneous doses at about 24 times the MRHOD. Using this drug during pregnancy should be based on the pros and cons of the mother's clinical need for treatment versus any potential fetal risk that might occur from exposure. If used during pregnancy, consider placing pressure over the tear duct in the corner of the eye for at least 1 minute, and then remove any excess solution with absorbent tissue to decrease the amount of drug reaching the systemic circulation even further.

BREASTFEEDING SUMMARY

No reports describing the use of omidenepag isopropyl ophthalmic during human lactation have been located. A negligible amount of the drug may be found in breast milk due to low systemic absorption after ocular use. However, if present, it most likely would be clinically insignificant. If the clinical decision is to use this drug while breastfeeding, the infant should be monitored for the most common reported adult systemic side effect of headache (leading to irritability). A method to reduce the amount entering the systemic circulation is described above in the Pregnancy Summary.

Reference

1. Prescribing Information. Omlonti. Santen, Inc; 2022.

ONDANSETRON

Gastrointestinal (Antiemetic)

PREGNANCY RECOMMENDATION: Human Data Suggest Potential Risk (First Trimester)

BREASTFEEDING RECOMMENDATION: Probably Compatible

O

PREGNANCY SUMMARY

Two large national studies, one from Denmark and the other from Sweden, regarding first-trimester use of ondansetron, found a significant increase in cardiac anomalies (but not cleft lip/palate) when compared with controls. However, another very large Medicaid study found a higher rate of cleft lip/palate (but not cardiac) when compared with controls. These overall risks are small, at possibly 3 to 5 more cases in 10,000 pregnancies, but are significant because of the total number of cases analyzed. The overall rate of major birth anomalies in these studies is about 2.5% to 3%, which falls within the expected rate for birth defects in the United States. In another study, there were 6 (3.4%) major birth defects (7 expected) in 176 first-trimester exposures, but three were hypospadias. An increased risk of hypospadias has not been seen in other evaluations. The drug crosses the placenta, so fetal exposure will occur. The only US Food and Drug Administration (FDA)-approved drug for nausea and vomiting in pregnancy is doxylamine-pyridoxine. This combination product does not cause birth defects and is not associated with harm in pregnancy (see Doxylamine). Consequently, the American College of Obstetricians and Gynecologists (ACOG) recommends doxylamine-pyridoxine as the treatment of choice for nausea and vomiting in pregnancy. Using this drug during pregnancy should be based on the pros and cons of the mother's clinical need for treatment versus any potential fetal risk that might occur from exposure. The drug has also been shown to prolong the QT interval.

BREASTFEEDING SUMMARY

One report was located that analyzed the use of ondansetron during human lactation. Maternal blood and breast milk were evaluated in 78 lactating women. Median peak breast milk levels were about 20 ng/mL with a calculated RID of about 3.5%. Breastfeeding while using this drug should be based on the mother's clinical need for treatment versus any potential infant risks that might occur. If used, the infant should be monitored for the most common reported adult side effects of headache (leading to irritability), fatigue (lethargy), constipation, and diarrhea.

References

1. Andersen JT, Jimenez-Solem E, Andersen NL, Poulsen HE. Ondansetron use in early pregnancy and the risk of congenital malformations—a registry based nationwide control study: International Society of Pharmaco-Epidemiology (abstract). *Pharmacoepidemiol Drug Saf*. 2013;22(suppl 1):13-14.
2. Koren G. Scary science: ondansetron safety in pregnancy—two opposing results from the same Danish registry. *Ther Drug Monit*. 2014;36:1-2.

3. Danielsson B, Wikner BN, Kallen B. Use of ondansetron during pregnancy and congenital malformations in the infant. *Reprod Toxicol*. 2014;50:134-137.
4. Huybrechts KF, Hernandez-Diaz S, Straub L, et al. Association of maternal first-trimester ondansetron use with cardiac malformations and oral clefts in offspring. *JAMA*. 2018;320:2429-2437.
5. American College of Obstetricians and Gynecologists. Nausea and vomiting of pregnancy: ACOG practice bulletin No. 189. *Obstet Gynecol*. 2018;131:e15-e30.
6. Prescribing Information. Ondansetron. Natco Pharma; 2018.
7. Siu SSN, Chan MTV, Lau TK. Placental transfer of ondansetron during early human pregnancy. *Clin Pharmacokinet*. 2006;45:419-423.
8. Guikontes E, Spantideas A, Diakakis J. Ondansetron and hyperemesis gravidarum. *Lancet*. 1992;340:1223.
9. World MJ. Ondansetron and hyperemesis gravidarum. *Lancet*. 1993;341:185.
10. Sullivan CA, Johnson CA, Roach H, et al. A prospective, randomized, double-blind comparison of the serotonin antagonist ondansetron to a standardized regimen of promethazine for hyperemesis gravidarum: a preliminary investigation (abstract). *Am J Obstet Gynecol*. 1995;172:299.
11. Sullivan CA, Johnson CA, Roach H, et al. A pilot study of intravenous ondansetron for hyperemesis gravidarum. *Am J Obstet Gynecol*. 1996;174:1565-1568.
12. Tincello DG, Johnstone MJ. Treatment of hyperemesis gravidarum with the 5-HT3 antagonist ondansetron (Zofran). *Postgrad Med J*. 1996;72:688-689.
13. Einarson A, Maltepe C, Navioz Y, et al. The safety of ondansetron for nausea and vomiting of pregnancy: a prospective comparative study. *Br J Obstet Gynaecol*. 2004;111:940-943.
14. Anderka M, Mitchell AA, Louik C, et al.; the National Birth Defects Prevention Study. Medications use to treat nausea and vomiting of pregnancy and the risk of selected birth defects. *Birth Defects Res (Part A)*. 2012;94:22-30.
15. Pasternak B, Svanstrom H, Hviid A. Ondansetron in pregnancy and risk of adverse fetal outcomes. *NEJM*. 2013;368:814-823.
16. Oliveira LG, Capp SM, You WB, et al. Ondansetron compared with doxylamine and pyridoxine for treatment of nausea in pregnancy: a randomized controlled trial. *Obstet Gynecol*. 2014;124:735-742.
17. Koren G, Maltepe C, Madjunkova S. Ondansetron compared with doxylamine and pyridoxine for treatment of nausea in pregnancy: a randomized controlled trial (letter). *Obstet Gynecol*. 2015;125:490.
18. Cunningham K. Ondansetron compared with doxylamine and pyridoxine for treatment of nausea in pregnancy: a randomized controlled trial (letter). *Obstet Gynecol*. 2015;125:490-491.
19. Oliveira L, Capp S. Ondansetron compared with doxylamine and pyridoxine for treatment of nausea in pregnancy: a randomized controlled trial (in reply). *Obstet Gynecol*. 2015;125:491.
20. Carstairs SD. Ondansetron use in pregnancy and birth defects: a systematic review. *Obstet Gynecol*. 2016;127:878-883.
21. Huybrechts KF, Hernandez-Diaz S, Straub L, et al. Intravenous ondansetron in pregnancy and risk of congenital malformations. *JAMA*. 2020;323:372-374.

OPICAPONE

Central Nervous System (Parkinson Treatment)

PREGNANCY RECOMMENDATION: No Human Data—Animal Data Suggest Potential Risk

BREASTFEEDING RECOMMENDATION: Potential Toxicity

PREGNANCY SUMMARY

No reports describing the use of opicapone in human pregnancy have been located. The drug will probably cross the placenta, so fetal exposure will likely occur. Therefore, the absence of human pregnancy experience prevents a complete assessment of embryofetal risk. Animal studies did show embryofetal toxicity in one species. Using this drug during pregnancy should be based on the pros and cons of the mother's clinical need for treatment versus any potential fetal risk that might occur from exposure.

BREASTFEEDING SUMMARY

No reports describing the use of opicapone during human lactation have been located. The drug will probably enter breast milk, so infant exposure will likely occur. Breastfeeding while using this drug should be based on the mother's clinical need for treatment. If used, the infant should be monitored for the most common reported adult side effects of involuntary movements, constipation, and decreased weight.

Reference

1. Prescribing Information. Ogentys. Neurocrine Biosciences, Inc; 2020.

ORAL CONTRACEPTIVES

Reproductive (Estrogenic/Progestogenic Hormones)

PREGNANCY RECOMMENDATION: *Contraindicated

BREASTFEEDING RECOMMENDATION: Probably Compatible

PREGNANCY SUMMARY

Limited reports describing the use of oral contraceptives in human pregnancy have been located. Available studies have found no significant evidence of an increased risk of congenital anomalies with inadvertent use during early pregnancy. Early reports suggested an association with the use of sex hormones late in pregnancy and masculinization of female fetuses; however, a meta-analysis of 14 studies including 65,567 women did not confirm this association. The various estrogens and progestins found in oral contraceptives cross the placenta, so some fetal exposure will occur. *However, oral contraceptives are contraindicated in pregnancy because there are usually no benefits from their use.

BREASTFEEDING SUMMARY

Limited reports describing the effects of oral contraceptives in 53 breastfeeding infants have been located. Four cases of breast enlargement that disappeared after stopping breastfeeding or contraception have been reported. Inconsistent data exists regarding the impact of combined oral contraceptive use on breastfeeding duration and success. Small amounts of estrogens and progestins are transferred to the infant through breast milk. Due to the risk of thromboembolism, the Centers for Disease Control and Prevention (CDC) recommends that combined oral contraceptives should not be used until at least 21 (preferably 30) days postpartum. However, if there are additional risk factors for Venous Thromboembolism (VTE), combined oral contraceptives should not be used until at least 42 days postpartum. Progestin-only contraception can be initiated at any time after delivery. The CDC Medical Eligibility Criteria for Contraceptive Use provides evidence-based clinical practice guidance for health care providers regarding the use of specific contraceptive methods, including oral contraceptives, by persons who have certain characteristics or medical conditions. An updated 2024 summary chart can be found at https://www.cdc.gov/contraception/media/pdfs/2024/07/us-mec-summary-chart-color-508.pdf.

References

1. Ambani LM, Joshi NJ, Vaidya RA, Devi PK. Are hormonal contraceptives teratogenic? *Fertil Steril*. 1977;28:791-797.
2. Wilson JG, Brent RL. Are female sex hormones teratogenic? *Am J Obstet Gynecol*. 1981;141:567-580.
3. Corcoran R, Entwistle GC. VACTERL congenital malformations and the male fetus. *Lancet*. 1975;2:981-982.
4. Nora JJ, Nora AH. Can the pill cause birth defects? *N Engl J Med*. 1974; 294:731-732.
5. Kasan PN, Andrews J. Oral contraceptives and congenital abnormalities. *Br J Obstet Gynaecol*. 1980;87:545-551.
6. Kullander S, Kallen B. A prospective study of drugs and pregnancy. *Acta Obstet Gynecol Scand*. 1976;55:221-224.
7. Oakley GP, Flynt JW. Hormonal pregnancy test and congenital malformations. *Lancet*. 1973;2:256-257.
8. Savolainen E, Saksela E, Saxen L. Teratogenic hazards of oral contraceptives analyzed in a national malformation register. *Am J Obstet Gynecol*. 1981;140:521-524.
9. Frost O. Tracheo-oesophageal fistula associated with hormonal contraception during pregnancy. *Br Med J*. 1976;3:978.
10. Redline RW, Abramowsky CR. Transposition of the great vessels in an infant exposed to massive doses of oral contraceptives. *Am J Obstet Gynecol*. 1981;141:468-469.
11. Farb HF, Thomason J, Carandang FS, et al. Anencephaly twins and HLA-B27. *J Reprod Med*. 1980;25:166-169.
12. Department of Medical and Public Affairs. *Population Reports*. George Washington University Medical Center; 1975;2:A29-A51.
13. Bongiovanni AM, DiGeorge AM, Grumbach MM. Masculinization of the female infant associated with estrogenic therapy alone during gestation: four cases. *J Clin Endocrinol Metab*. 1959;19:1004-1011.
14. Hagler S, Schultz A, Hankin H, Kunstadter RH. Fetal effects of steroid therapy during pregnancy. *Am J Dis Child*. 1963;106:586-590.
15. Bongiovanni AM, McFadden AJ. Steroids during pregnancy and possible fetal consequences. *Fertil Steril*. 1960;11:181-184.
16. Bracken MB, Srisuphan W. Oral contraception as a risk factor for preeclampsia. *Am J Obstet Gynecol*. 1982;142:191-196.
17. Harlap S, Eldor J. Births following oral contraceptive failures. *Obstet Gynecol*. 1980;55:447-452.
18. Matanoski GM, Wilson PD, Rubin JD, et al. Maternal hormone therapy and congenital heart disease. *Teratology*. 1980;21:225-239.
19. Rothman KJ, Fyler DC, Goldblatt A, Kreidberg MB. Exogenous hormones and other drug exposures of children with congenital heart disease. *Am J Epidemiol*. 1979;109:433-439.
20. Raman-Wilms L, Tseng AL, Wighardt S, et al. Fetal genital effects of first-trimester sex hormone exposure: a meta-analysis. *Obstet Gynecol*. 1995;85(1):141-149.
21. Miller GH, Hughes LR. Lactation and genital involution effects of a new low-dose oral contraceptive on breast-feeding mothers and their infants. *Obstet Gynecol*. 1970;35:44-50.
22. Kora SJ. Effect of oral contraceptives on lactation. *Fertil Steril*. 1969;20:419-423.
23. Guiloff E, Ibarra-Polo A, Zanartu J, et al. Effect of contraception on lactation. *Am J Obstet Gynecol*. 1974;118:42-45.
24. Lonnerdal B, Forsum E, Hambraeus L. Effect of oral contraceptives on consumption and volume of breast milk. *Am J Clin Nutr*. 1980;33:816-824.
25. American Academy of Pediatrics Committee on Drugs. Breast-feeding and contraception. *Pediatrics*. 1981;68:138-140.
26. Nilsson S, Nygren KC, Johansson EDB. d-Norgestrel concentrations in maternal plasma, milk, and child plasma during administration of oral contraceptives to nursing women. *Am J Obstet Gynecol*. 1977;129:178-183.
27. Van der Molen HJ, Hart PG, Wijmenga HG. Studies with 4-14C-lynestrol in normal and lactating women. *Acta Endocrinol*. 1969;61:255-274.
28. Farley KE, Huber LRB, Warren-Findlow J, Ersek JL. The association between contraceptive use at the time of conception and hypertensive disorders during pregnancy: a retrospective cohort study of prams participants. *Matern Child Health J*. 2014;18:1779-1785.
29. Chen XK, Wen SW, Sun LM, et al. Recent oral contraceptive use and adverse birth outcomes. *Eur J Obstet Gynecol Reprod Biol*. 2009;144:40-43.
30. Waller DK, Gallaway MS, Taylor LG, et al.; National Birth Defects Prevention Study. Use of oral contraceptives in pregnancy and major structural birth defects in offspring. *Epidemiology*. 2010;21:232-239.
31. Jensen E, Daniels J, Stürmer T et al. Hormonal contraceptive use before and after conception in relation to preterm birth and small for gestational age: an observational cohort study. *BJOG*. 2015;122:1349-1361.
32. Charlton BM, Mølgaard-Nielsen D, Svanström H, et al. Maternal use of oral contraceptives and risk of birth defects in Denmark: prospective, nationwide cohort study. *BMJ*. 2016;352:h6712.
33. Schreuder A, Mokadem I, Smeets NJL, et al. Associations of periconceptional oral contraceptive use with pregnancy complications and adverse birth outcomes. *Int J Epidemiol*. 2023;52:1388-1399.
34. Prescribing Information. Necon. Dr. Reddy's Laboratories, Inc; 2024.
35. Curtis EM. Oral-contraceptive feminization of a normal male infant. *Obstet Gynecol*. 1964;23:295-296.
36. Marriq P, Oddo G. Gynecomastia in the newborn induced by maternal milk? An unusual complication of oral contraceptives. *Nouv Presse Med*. 1974;3:2579.
37. Madhavapeddi R, Ramachandran P. Side effects of oral contraceptive use in lactating women—enlargement of breast in a breast-fed child. *Contraception*. 1985;32:437-443.
38. Mandel H, Berant M. Oral contraceptives and breastfeeding: haematological effects on the infant. *Arch Dis Child*. 1985;60:971-972.
39. Lopez LM, Grey TW, Stuebe AM, et al. Combined hormonal versus nonhormonal versus progestin-only contraception in lactation. *Cochrane Database Syst Rev*. 2015;2015:CD003988.
40. Tepper NK, Phillips SJ, Kapp N, et al. Combined hormonal contraceptive use among breastfeeding women: an updated systematic review. *Contraception*. 2016;94:262-274.
41. Bahamondes L, Bahamondes MV, Modesto W, et al. Effect of hormonal contraceptives during breastfeeding on infant's milk ingestion and growth. *Fertil Steril*. 2013;100:445-450.
42. Nguyen AT, Curtis KM, Tepper NK, et al. U.S. medical eligibility criteria for contraceptive use, 2024. *MMWR Recomm Rep*. 2024;73(No. RR-4):1-126.

ORITAVANCIN

Antibacterial (Lipoglycopeptide)

PREGNANCY RECOMMENDATION: No Human Data—Animal Data Suggest Low Risk

BREASTFEEDING RECOMMENDATION: Probably Compatible

PREGNANCY SUMMARY

No reports describing the use of oritavancin in human pregnancy have been located. The drug may cross the placenta, so some fetal exposure might occur. However, the absence of human pregnancy experience prevents a complete assessment of the embryofetal risk. No embryofetal toxicity or teratogenicity was seen in two animal species. Using this drug during pregnancy should be based on the pros and cons of the mother's clinical need for treatment versus any potential fetal risk that might occur from exposure.

BREASTFEEDING SUMMARY

No reports describing the use of oritavancin during human lactation have been located. The drug is not likely to be found in human breast milk in clinically significant amounts. In addition, because the oral bioavailability is less than 1%, if found in human breast milk, it is unlikely to cause any adverse effects in a nursing infant. Breastfeeding while using this drug should be based on the mother's clinical need for treatment versus any potential infant risks that might occur. If used, the infant should be monitored for the most common reported adult side effects of headache and nausea (both leading to irritability), vomiting, and diarrhea.

Reference

1. Prescribing Information. Orbactiv. The Melinta Therapeutics; 2021.

ORLISTAT

Gastrointestinal (Lipase Inhibitor)

PREGNANCY RECOMMENDATION: Limited Human Data—Animal Data Suggest Potential Risk

BREASTFEEDING RECOMMENDATION: Probably Compatible

PREGNANCY SUMMARY

Two studies were located that described the use of orlistat during human pregnancy. In one large series, the rate of major birth anomalies was not increased when compared with controls in 248 early pregnancy exposures. A case report was also found that described the use of the drug at conception and into the first trimester. The patient was on seven other drugs, but the infant was delivered at term with no identified birth defects. The drug may cross the placenta, but with the very low systemic absorption with oral use, the amount is likely to be clinically insignificant. However, this limited human pregnancy experience prevents a complete assessment of the embryofetal risk. Orlistat could cause a deficiency of fat-soluble vitamins (A, D, E, and K) if a multiple vitamin supplement is not taken. Using this drug during pregnancy should be based on the pros and cons of the mother's clinical need for treatment versus any potential fetal risk that might occur from exposure; however, use of weight loss medications during pregnancy is not recommended.

BREASTFEEDING SUMMARY

No reports describing the use of orlistat during human lactation have been located. If found in the systemic circulation, the drug will probably be excreted into human breast milk. However, systemic absorption is negligible. In addition, if the drug were to be ingested through breast milk, the amount absorbed systemically in the infant would also be negligible and thus clinically insignificant. Breastfeeding while using this drug should be based on the mother's clinical need for treatment versus any potential infant risks that might occur. If used, the infant should be monitored for the most common reported adult side effects of flatulence, fecal urgency, oily stool, and diarrhea.

References

1. Prescribing Information. Xenical. Genentech; 2016.
2. Kalyoncu NI, Yaris F, Kadioglu M, et al. Pregnancy outcome following exposure to orlistat, ramipril, glimepiride in a woman with metabolic syndrome. *Saudi Med J*. 2005;26:497-499.
3. Kallen BA. Antiobesity drugs in early pregnancy and congenital malformations in the offspring. *Obes Res Clin Pract*. 2014;8:e571-e576.

ORPHENADRINE

Pain (Skeletal Muscle Relaxant)

PREGNANCY RECOMMENDATION: Limited Human Data - No Relevant Animal Data

BREASTFEEDING RECOMMENDATION: Probably Compatible (Recommended Dosages)

PREGNANCY SUMMARY

From the Michigan Medicaid Surveillance and Collaborative Perinatal Project (CPP), there were 414 first-trimester exposures with 11 (2.7%) major birth defects observed (16 expected), and no pattern to the defects was seen. The drug will probably cross the placenta, so some fetal exposure will likely occur. No animal reproduction or fertility studies have been conducted. Using this drug during pregnancy should be based on the pros and cons of the mother's clinical need for treatment versus any potential fetal risk that might occur from exposure. Though some individuals have chronically misused orphenadrine for euphoric effects, it is not a controlled substance.

BREASTFEEDING SUMMARY

No reports describing the use of orphenadrine during human lactation have been located. The drug will probably be found in human breast milk, so some infant exposure will likely occur. Because it has some anticholinergic properties, it could result in decreased breast milk production. Breastfeeding while using this drug should be based on the mother's clinical need for treatment versus any potential infant risks that might occur. If used, the infant should be monitored for the most common reported adult side effects of nausea, headache, blurred vision, dizziness, and pruritus (all leading to irritability), weakness (lethargy), vomiting, constipation, and tremor.

Reference

1. Prescribing Information. Orphenadrine citrate. Eon Labs; 2019.

OSELTAMIVIR

Antiviral (Influenza)

PREGNANCY RECOMMENDATION: Human Data Suggest Low Risk (Maternal Benefit May Outweigh Any Potential Fetal Risk)

BREASTFEEDING RECOMMENDATION: Probably Compatible

PREGNANCY SUMMARY

Several studies have been identified that describe the use of oseltamivir during human pregnancy. Two (1.3%) major anomalies were described in more than 150 first-trimester exposures. In two other very large analyses of more than 6,000 oseltamivir exposures (all trimesters), the rate of congenital anomalies was not increased. It appears that the drug and active metabolite cross the placenta, but in low amounts, using ex vivo placental perfusion studies. Animal studies did not show any embryofetal toxicity or malformations in two species at doses of less than 10 times the RHD in one and more than 10 times the RHD in the second. Using this drug during pregnancy should be based on the pros and cons of the mother's clinical need for treatment versus any potential fetal risk that might occur from exposure. Because influenza infection in pregnancy is a high-risk condition, the maternal benefit probably outweighs any unknown fetal risk.

BREASTFEEDING SUMMARY

Three studies were located that describe the use of oseltamivir during human lactation. From a total of 14 lactating women, the drug and active metabolite, oseltamivir carboxylate, were found in breast milk with concentrations that ranged from less than 10 ng/mL up to about 70 ng/mL for oseltamivir and up to about 40 ng/mL for the metabolite. The calculated RIDs were all less than 1%. The FDA states that the drug can be administered to newborns aged 2 weeks or older. Breastfeeding while using this drug should be based on the mother's clinical need for treatment versus any potential infant risks that might occur. If used, the infant should be monitored for the most common reported adult side effects of nausea and abdominal pain (both leading to irritability), vomiting, and diarrhea.

References

1. Rasmussen SA, Jamieson DJ, MacFarlane K, et al.; Pandemic Influenza Pregnancy Working Group. Pandemic influenza and pregnant women: summary of a meeting of experts. *Am J Public Health*. 2009;99(suppl 2):S248-S254.
2. Prescribing Information. Oseltamivir. Amneal Pharmaceuticals; 2019.
3. Centers for Disease Control and Prevention (CDC). Novel influenza A (H1N1) virus infections in three pregnant women—United States, April-May 2009. *MMWR Morb Mortal Wkly Rep*. 2009;58(18):497-500.
4. Worley KC, Roberts SW, Bawdon RE. The metabolism and transplacental transfer of oseltamivir in the ex vivo human model. *Inf Dis Obstet Gynecol*. 2008;2008:Article ID 927574.
5. Huang H, Wang J, Li Q, et al. Transplacental transfer of oseltamivir phosphate and its metabolite oseltamivir carboxylate using the ex vivo human placenta perfusion model in Chinese Hans population. *J Matern Fetal Neonatal Med*. 2017;30:1288-1292.
6. Ward P, Small I, Smith J, et al. Oseltamivir (Tamiflu) and its potential for use in the event of an influenza pandemic. *J Antimicrob Chemother*. 2005;55(suppl S1):i5-i21.
7. Tanaka T, Nakajima K, Murashima A, et al. Safety of neuraminidase inhibitors against novel influenza A (H1N1) in pregnant and breastfeeding women. *CMAJ*. 2009;181:55-58.
8. Greer LG, Sheffield JS, Rogers VL, et al. Maternal and neonatal outcomes after antepartum treatment of influenza with antiviral medications. *Obstet Gynecol*. 2010;115:711-716.
9. Graner S, Svensson T, Beau AB, et al. Neuraminidase inhibitor during pregnancy and risk of adverse neonatal outcomes and congenital malformations: population based European register study. *Br Med J*. 2017;356:j629.

10. Ehrenstein V, Kristensen NR, Monz BU, et al. Oseltamivir in pregnancy and birth outcomes. *BMC Inf Dis*. 2018;18:519-529.
11. Wentges-van Holthe N, van Eijkeren M, van der Laan JW. Oseltamivir and breastfeeding. *Int J Infect Dis*. 2008;12:451.
12. Greer LG, Leff RD, Rogers VL, et al. Pharmacokinetics of oseltamivir in breast milk and maternal plasma. *Am J Obstet Gynecol*. 2011;204:524.e1-524.e4.
13. CDC. What should pregnant women should know about H1N1 (formerly called swine flu) virus. Accessed June 8, 2009. http://www.cdc.gov/h1n1flu/guidance/pregnant.htm

OSILODROSTAT

Endocrine/Metabolic (Cortisol Synthesis Inhibitor)

PREGNANCY RECOMMENDATION: No Human Data—Animal Data Suggest Low Risk

BREASTFEEDING RECOMMENDATION: Potential Toxicity

PREGNANCY SUMMARY

No reports describing the use of osilodrostat in human pregnancy have been located. The drug probably crosses the placenta. Osilodrostat did not cause any embryofetal toxicity at doses that did not cause maternal toxicity in animal studies. However, the absence of human pregnancy experience prevents a complete assessment of the embryofetal risk. Active Cushing syndrome during pregnancy has been associated with increased risks of maternal and fetal morbidity and mortality. Maternal and fetal benefits of treating Cushing disease may outweigh the risk of using osilodrostat during pregnancy. Osilodrostat is associated with QT prolongation. Monitor QTc interval prior to and during osilodrostat treatment.

BREASTFEEDING SUMMARY

No reports describing the use of osilodrostat during human lactation have been located. The drug is probably excreted into breast milk. Due to the concern for potential adverse effects, such as adrenal insufficiency, the manufacturer recommends that women withhold breastfeeding while being treated with osilodrostat and for one week after the last dose. However, breastfeeding while using this drug should be based on the mother's clinical need for treatment. If used, the infant should be monitored for the most common reported adult side effects of nausea and headache (both leading to irritability), lethargy, and edema. In addition, the infant should be monitored for adrenal insufficiency.

Reference

1. Prescribing Information. Isturisa. Recordati Rare Diseases, Inc; 2020.

O

OSIMERTINIB

Antineoplastic (Kinase Inhibitor)

PREGNANCY RECOMMENDATION: No Human Data—Animal Data Suggest Potential Risk

BREASTFEEDING RECOMMENDATION: Potential Toxicity

PREGNANCY SUMMARY

No reports describing the use of osimertinib in human pregnancy have been located. Some of the drug will probably cross the placenta, so fetal exposure will likely occur. Therefore, the absence of human pregnancy experience prevents a complete assessment of the embryofetal risk. Embryofetal toxicity was observed in animal studies. Due to the findings from the animal studies and the drug's mechanism of action, the manufacturer recommends that women with reproductive potential use effective contraception during treatment and for at least 6 weeks after the last dose. They also recommend that males with female partners of reproductive potential use effective contraception during treatment and for at least 4 months after the last dose. Nevertheless, using this drug during pregnancy should be based on the pros and cons of the mother's clinical need for treatment versus any potential fetal risk that might occur from exposure. In the clinical trials, 2.4% of patients developed cardiomyopathy, with an ejection fraction dropping below 50%. It is recommended that patients obtain a baseline echocardiogram prior to drug initiation.

BREASTFEEDING SUMMARY

No reports describing the use of osimertinib during human lactation have been located. Some amount of the drug will probably be found in breast milk, so infant exposure will likely occur. However, due to the concern for potential serious adverse effects that might be seen in a breastfed infant, the manufacturer recommends that women not breastfeed while being treated with osimertinib and for at least 2 weeks after the last dose. Nevertheless, breastfeeding while using this drug should be based on the mother's clinical need for treatment. If used, the infant should be monitored for the most common reported adult side effects of diarrhea and rash.

Reference

1. Prescribing Information. Tagrisso. AstraZeneca Pharmaceuticals LP; 2022.

OSPEMIFENE

Miscellaneous (Selective Estrogen Receptor Modulator)

PREGNANCY RECOMMENDATION: *Contraindicated

BREASTFEEDING RECOMMENDATION: *Contraindicated

PREGNANCY SUMMARY

No reports describing the use of ospemifene in human pregnancy have been located. The drug would probably cross the placenta in limited amounts. However, the absence of human pregnancy experience prevents a complete assessment of the embryofetal risk. Animal data did not show any embryofetal toxicity. The manufacturer states that ospemifene is contraindicated in women who are or may become pregnant. *Furthermore, the approved drug indication is for use during menopause.

BREASTFEEDING SUMMARY

No reports describing the use of ospemifene during human lactation have been located. The drug will probably be excreted into breast milk in limited amounts. *The manufacturer recommends that women should not breastfeed during treatment with this drug; however, the approved drug indication is for use during menopause.

Reference

1. Prescribing Information. Osphena. Duchesnay, Inc; 2019.

OTESECONAZOLE

Anti-Infective (Antifungal—Azole)

PREGNANCY RECOMMENDATION: No Human Data—Animal Data Suggest Risk

BREASTFEEDING RECOMMENDATION: Potential Toxicity

PREGNANCY SUMMARY

No reports describing the use of oteseconazole in human pregnancy have been located. The drug will likely cross the placenta, so some fetal exposure could occur. Therefore, the absence of human pregnancy experience prevents a complete assessment of the embryofetal risk. The manufacturer recommends that women of child bearing age should not use this drug. Embryofetal toxicity with malformations was observed in animal studies.

BREASTFEEDING SUMMARY

No reports describing the use of oteseconazole during human lactation have been located. The drug will likely be found in breast milk, so some infant exposure could occur. The manufacturer recommends that women should not breastfeed during treatment with this drug.

Reference

1. Prescribing Information. Vivjoa. Mycovia Pharmaceuticals; 2022.

OXACILLIN

Antibacterial (Penicillin)

PREGNANCY RECOMMENDATION: Limited Human Data—Animal Data Suggest Low Risk

BREASTFEEDING RECOMMENDATION: Probably Compatible

PREGNANCY SUMMARY

The Collaborative Perinatal Project (CPP) reported on 3,546 first-trimester exposures to penicillin derivatives. There were 88 (2.5%) major congenital anomalies identified, and no pattern to the defects was seen. The CPP data collection was from 1959 through 1965. Oxacillin was approved for use in 1962 and was probably used by some of the patients in this drug group. Despite the small numbers of oxacillin exposure, another study involving a large number of pregnancies resulting in birth anomalies was compared with a large number of pregnancies with no birth defects identified. The use of oxacillin was 0.02% in both groups. The drug crosses the placenta, so some fetal exposure will occur. However, the limited human pregnancy experience, specifically with oxacillin, prevents a complete assessment of the embryofetal risk. Animal studies did not show any embryofetal toxicity or malformations in three species at doses of more than 10 times the RHD. Using this drug during pregnancy should be based on the pros and cons of the mother's clinical need for treatment versus any potential fetal risk that might occur from exposure. It should not be used in treating infections susceptible to penicillin G.

BREASTFEEDING SUMMARY

Several studies have been located that describe the use of oxacillin during human lactation. From 6 studies, about 53 women had their breast milk analyzed. The drug was found in most samples at low levels. The drug concentration in breast milk ranged from about 0.18 mcg/mL up to 0.7 mcg/mL. The highest calculated RID was about 1.5%, with most being less than 1%. The drug was found in the urine of 10 infants exposed through breastfeeding. No adverse effects have been reported in nursing infants exposed to the drug, but there is a risk of a modification of bowel flora. Breastfeeding while using this drug should be based on the mother's clinical need for treatment versus any potential infant risks that might occur. If used, the infant should be monitored for the most common reported adult side effects of nausea, itching, and abdominal pain (all leading to irritability), diarrhea, fever, and rash.

References

1. Prescribing Information. Oxacillin. AuroMedics Pharma; 2019.
2. Heinonen OP, Slone D, Shapiro S. *Birth Defects and Drugs in Pregnancy*. Publishing Sciences Group; 1977.
3. Czeizel AE, Rockenbauer M, Sorensen HT, Olsen J. Teratogenic evaluation of oxacillin. *Scand J Infect Dis*. 1999;31:311-312.

OXALIPLATIN

Antineoplastic (Platinum Based)

PREGNANCY RECOMMENDATION: Limited Human Data—Animal Data Suggest Potential Risk

BREASTFEEDING RECOMMENDATION: Potential Toxicity

PREGNANCY SUMMARY

A few case reports and a small series described the use of oxaliplatin in six patients. Treatment was started in the second and third trimesters, and none of the infants had any major birth anomalies. There was one 33-week intrauterine fetal demise (no anatomical defects). The drug will probably cross the placenta, so some fetal exposure will likely occur. Therefore, this limited human pregnancy experience prevents a complete assessment of the embryofetal risk. Animal studies did show some embryofetal toxicity in one species at doses of less than the RHD, but the dosing frequency was daily for 5 to 6 days rather than once every 2 weeks (which is the recommended dosing cycle for humans). The effect of this increased dosing frequency is not known. Based on animal studies and the drug's mechanism of action, the manufacturer recommends that women with reproductive potential use effective contraception during treatment and for 9 months after the last dose. They also recommend that males with female partners of reproductive potential use effective contraception during treatment and for 6 months after the last dose. Nevertheless, using this drug during pregnancy should be based on the pros and cons of the mother's clinical need for treatment versus any potential fetal risk that might occur from exposure. The drug was also found to prolong the QT interval and produce ventricular arrhythmias during the clinical trials. There is a registry for women who are pregnant and have cancer. For more information, women and health care providers are encouraged to contact the Cancer and Pregnancy Registry at 1-877-635-4499.

BREASTFEEDING SUMMARY

One study was located that described the use of oxaliplatin during human lactation. Breast milk was analyzed for platinum at about 34 and 65 days after treatment. Levels were 7.8 and 10.3 ng/mL. The effect on an infant with these levels is not fully known. Due to a concern for potential serious adverse effects that might be seen in a breastfed infant, the manufacturer recommends that women not breastfeed while being treated with this drug and for at least 3 months after the last dose. Nevertheless, breastfeeding while using this drug should be based on the mother's clinical need for treatment versus any potential infant risks that might occur. If used, the infant should be monitored for the most common reported adult side effects of nausea and peripheral neuropathy (both leading to irritability), diarrhea, fatigue (lethargy), vomiting, and various laboratory abnormalities (see PI).

References

1. Prescribing Information. Oxaliplatin. Sanofi-Aventis U.S., LLC.; 2020.
2. Gensheimer M, Jones CA, Graves CR, Merchant NB, Lockhart AC. Administration of oxaliplatin to a pregnant woman with rectal cancer. *Cancer Chemother Pharmacol*. 2009;63:371-373.
3. Kanate AS, Auber ML, Higa GM. Priorities and uncertainties of administering chemotherapy in a pregnant woman with newly diagnosed colorectal cancer. *J Oncol Pharm Pract*. 2009;15:5-8.
4. Robson DE, Lewin J, Cheng AW, et al. Synchronous colorectal liver metastases in pregnancy and post-partum. *ANZ J Surg*. 2017;87:800-804.
5. Makoshi Z, Perrott C, Al-Khatani K, Al-Mohaisen F. Chemotherapeutic treatment of colorectal cancer in pregnancy: case report. *J Med Case Reports*. 2015;9:140.
6. Krutsch K, Adams K, Shinwari M, Baucom RB. Persistence of oxaliplatin transfer into human milk: a case report. *Breastfeed Med*. 2023;18:395-399.

OXAPROZIN

Pain (Nonsteroidal Anti-Inflammatory Drug)

PREGNANCY RECOMMENDATION: Human Data Suggest Risk (Second and Third Trimesters)

BREASTFEEDING RECOMMENDATION: Potential Toxicity

PREGNANCY SUMMARY

No reports describing the use of oxaprozin in human pregnancy have been located. The drug will probably cross the placenta, so some fetal exposure will likely occur. Therefore, the absence of human pregnancy experience prevents a complete assessment of the embryofetal risk. Animal data did not show any embryofetal toxicity or teratogenicity in two species at doses of about equal to the MRHD based on BSA. However, some embryofetal toxicity and teratogenicity were seen in a third species at doses of less than the MRHD based on BSA. Data from other evaluations analyzing nonsteroidal anti-inflammatory drugs (NSAIDs) as a group have not found any increased risk or pattern to the defects. NSAIDs can cause premature stricture or closure of the fetal ductus arteriosus when used in the latter portion of gestation. In some instances, this can produce persistent pulmonary hypertension in the neonate. These drugs have also been reported to produce fetal renal dysfunction leading to oligohydramnios when used after 20 weeks' gestation. The FDA recommends that NSAIDs be avoided in women 20 weeks or later in pregnancy. If deemed necessary by a health care provider, the use of NSAIDs between 20 and 30 weeks should be limited to the lowest effective dose and shortest duration. If treatment extends beyond 48 hours, providers should consider an ultrasound to monitor amniotic fluid levels.

O

BREASTFEEDING SUMMARY

No reports describing the use of oxaprozin during human lactation have been located. The MW and long elimination half-life suggest that the drug will cross, but the high plasma protein binding may limit some excretion. Breastfeeding while using this drug should be based on the mother's clinical need for treatment versus any potential infant risks that might occur. If used, the infant should be monitored for the most common reported adult side effects of nausea and dyspepsia (both leading to irritability), constipation, and rash. Because of the long elimination half-life (approximately 48 hours) and the unknown amount of oxaprozin that is excreted into breast milk, choosing a different NSAID with better *pK* parameters might be suggested.

References

1. Levin DL. Effects of inhibition of prostaglandin synthesis on fetal development, oxygenation, and the fetal circulation. *Semin Perinatol*. 1980;4:35-44.
2. Van Marter LJ, Leviton A, Allred EN, et al. Persistent pulmonary hypertension of the newborn and smoking and aspirin and nonsteroidal antiinflammatory drug consumption during pregnancy. *Pediatrics*. 1996;97:658-663.
3. Matt DW, Borzelleca JF. Toxic effects on the female reproductive system during pregnancy, parturition, and lactation. In: Witorsch RJ, ed. *Reproductive Toxicology*. 2nd ed. Raven Press; 1995:175-193.
4. Dawood MY. Nonsteroidal antiinflammatory drugs and reproduction. *Am J Obstet Gynecol*. 1993;169:1255-1265.
5. Prescribing Information. Oxaprozin. Amneal Pharmaceuticals; 2019.
6. Yamada T, Nishiyama T, Sasajima M, Nakane S. Reproduction studies of oxaprozin in the rat and rabbit. *Iyakuhin Kenkyu*. 1984;15:207-292. As cited in Shepard TH. Catalog of Teratogenic Agents. 7th ed. The Johns Hopkins University Press; 1992:299-300.
7. Yamada T, Norariya T, Sasajima M, Nakane S. Reproduction studies of oxaprozin. II. Teratology study in rats. *Iyakuhin Kenkyu*. 1984;15:225-249. As cited in Schardein JL. Chemically Induced Birth Defects. 2nd ed. Marcel Dekker; 1993:132-133.
8. Yamada T, Uchida H, Sasajima M, Nakane S. Reproduction studies of oxaprozin. III. Teratogenicity study in rabbits. *Iyakuhin Kenkyu*. 1984;15:250-264. As cited in Schardein JL. Chemically Induced Birth Defects. 2nd ed. Marcel Dekker; 1993:132-133.
9. Yamada T, Inoue T, Hara M, et al. Reproductive studies of oxaprozin and studies on the fetal ductus arteriosus. *Clin Report*. 1984;18:514-525, 528-536. As cited in Shepard TH. Catalog of Teratogenic Agents. 7th ed. The Johns Hopkins University Press; 1992:299-300.
10. Nielsen GL, Sorensen HT, Larsen H, Pedersen L. Risk of adverse birth outcome and miscarriage in pregnant users of non-steroidal anti-inflammatory drugs: population based observational study and case-control study. *Br Med J*. 2001;322:266-270.
11. Ericson A, Kallen BAJ. Nonsteroidal anti-inflammatory drugs in early pregnancy. *Reprod Toxicol*. 2001;15:371-375.
12. Li DK, Liu L, Odouli R. Exposure to non-steroidal anti-inflammatory drugs during pregnancy and risk of miscarriage: population based cohort study. *Br Med J*. 2003;327:368-371.
13. Tassinari MS, Cook JC, Hurtt ME. NSAIDs and developmental toxicity. *Birth Defects Res (Part B)*. 2003;68:3-4.
14. Anderson PO. Medication use while breast feeding a neonate. *Neonatal Pharmacol Q*. 1993;2:3-14.

OXAZEPAM

Central Nervous System (Benzodiazepine)

PREGNANCY RECOMMENDATION: Human Data Suggest Risk (Third Trimester)

BREASTFEEDING RECOMMENDATION: Potential Toxicity

PREGNANCY SUMMARY

Only a few case reports have been located that describe the use of oxazepam in human pregnancy. A few larger studies have analyzed the use of benzodiazepine drugs as a group, and no increased risk for birth defects was identified. However, the use of oxazepam in these evaluations was minimal. The drug has been shown to cross the placenta, so fetal exposure will occur. Embryofetal toxicity was not observed in three animal species at doses of less than 10 times the RHD based on weight. Using this drug during pregnancy should be based on the pros and cons of the mother's clinical need for treatment versus any potential fetal risk that might occur from exposure. Health care providers are encouraged to register women who are pregnant and have taken oxazepam at any time during pregnancy by contacting the National Pregnancy Registry for Psychiatry Medications at 866-961-2388. The drug carries a boxed warning for a risk from concomitant use with opioid drugs of misuse and addiction, with dependence and withdrawal reactions. An abrupt discontinuation of benzodiazepine drugs can produce seizures. Due to the adverse event profile and addictive potential, ACOG recommends avoiding benzodiazepines or using them sparingly as an anxiety treatment. If prescribed, ACOG recommends using the lowest effective dose and states that doses can be tapered down by 25% to 50% per week. Neonatal sedation, decreased muscle tone, respiratory compromise, and neonatal intensive care unit (NICU) admission have been associated with benzodiazepine use near delivery.

BREASTFEEDING SUMMARY

A few case reports were located that describe the use of oxazepam during human lactation. The drug was found in human breast milk in three cases, with drug concentrations that ranged from about 11 to 30 ng/mL. Calculated RIDs were 1% or less. Several studies have described infant sedation, irritability, and lethargy in a few infants when exposed to benzodiazepine drugs during nursing. Breastfeeding while using this drug should be based on the mother's clinical need for treatment versus any potential infant risks that might occur. If used, the infant should be monitored for the most common reported adult side effects of headache, nausea, blurred vision, and dizziness (all leading to irritability), drowsiness, lethargy, sedation, rash, and tremor.

References

1. Prescribing Information. Oxazepam. Actavis Pharma; 2016.
2. Kangas L, Erkkola R, Kanto J, Eronen M. Transfer of free and conjugated oxazepam across the human placenta. *Eur J Clin Pharmacol*. 1980;17:301-304.
3. Kanto J, Erkkola R, Sellman R. Perinatal metabolism of diazepam. *Br Med J*. 1974;1:641-642.
4. Mandelli M, Morselli PL, Nordio S, et al. Placental transfer of diazepam and its disposition in the newborn. *Clin Pharmacol Ther*. 1975;17:564-572.
5. Kanto JH. Use of benzodiazepines during pregnancy, labour and lactation, with particular reference to pharmacokinetic considerations. *Drugs*. 1982;23:354-380.
6. Gillberg C. "Floppy infant syndrome" and maternal diazepam. *Lancet*. 1977;2:612-613.
7. Drury KAD, Spalding E, Donaldson D, Rutherford D. Floppy-infant syndrome: is oxazepam the answer? *Lancet*. 1977;2:1126-1127.
8. Laegreid L, Olegard R, Walstrom J, Conradi N. Teratogenic effects of benzodiazepine use during pregnancy. *J Pediatr*. 1989;114:126-131.
9. Wretlind M. Excretion of oxazepam in breast milk. *Eur J Clin Pharmacol*. 1987;33:209-210.
10. Kelly LE, Poon S, Madadi P, Koren G. Neonatal benzodiazepine exposure during pregnancy. *J Pediatr*. 2012;161:448-451.
11. Patrick MJ, Tilstone WJ, Reavey P. Diazepam and breast-feeding. *Br Med J*. 1972;1:542-543.

O

OXCARBAZEPINE

Central Nervous System (Antiseizure)

PREGNANCY RECOMMENDATION: Limited Human Data—Animal Data Suggest Risk

BREASTFEEDING RECOMMENDATION: Potential Toxicity

PREGNANCY SUMMARY

Several small studies have been found that describe the use of oxcarbazepine during human pregnancy. A total of 3 (5.7%) major birth defects were described in 53 first-trimester exposures (2 expected). All three anomalies were different. The drug crosses the placenta, so fetal exposure will occur. Therefore, the human data are too limited to assess the risk to the embryo or fetus. In addition, the effect of oxcarbazepine on folic acid levels or metabolism is unknown. Animal studies did show

(continued)

some embryofetal toxicity with malformations in two species at doses of about equal to the MRHD. Nevertheless, using this drug during pregnancy (especially if the patient has good seizure control with this agent) should be based on the pros and cons of the mother's clinical need for treatment versus any potential fetal risk that might occur from exposure. There is a pregnancy exposure registry that monitors pregnancy outcomes in women using antiseizure drugs. Health care providers are encouraged to call the North American Antiepileptic Drug Pregnancy Registry at 1-888-233-2334.

BREASTFEEDING SUMMARY

A few studies were located that describe the use of oxcarbazepine during human lactation. Breast milk levels have been found to be about 50% to 70% maternal serum concentrations. From three lactating women, breast milk levels for oxcarbazepine ranged from about 0.19 to 7.8 mcg/mL, and for the maximum human dose (MHD) were 2.9 to 10.4 mcg/mL. A few calculated RIDs were more than 20%. However, blood levels were analyzed in about 10 infants. Concentrations ranged from undetectable (LLQ of 0.1 mcg/mL) up to about 0.2 mcg/mL or 2% up to 15% of the maternal blood levels. Several studies have reported no adverse effects in most infants exposed to the drug from breastfeeding, but a few have had irritability, tremors, and increased muscle tone reported. Due to a concern for potential serious adverse effects that might be seen in a breastfed infant, the manufacturer recommends that women not breastfeed while being treated with this drug. Nevertheless, breastfeeding while using this drug should be based on the mother's clinical need for treatment versus any potential infant risks that might occur. If used, the infant should be monitored for the most common reported adult side effects of nausea, arthralgias, dizziness, and abdominal pain (all leading to irritability), sedation, diarrhea, rash, anorexia (monitor infant growth), and constipation.

O

References

1. Morrell MJ. The new antiepileptic drugs and women: efficacy, reproductive health, pregnancy, and fetal outcome. *Epilepsia*. 1996;37(suppl 6):S34-S44.
2. Pienimaki P, Lampela E, Hakkola J, et al. Pharmacokinetics of oxcarbazepine and carbamazepine in human placenta. *Epilepsia*. 1997;38:309-316.
3. Grant SM, Faulds D. Oxcarbazepine: a review of its pharmacology and therapeutic potential in epilepsy, trigeminal neuralgia and affective disorders. *Drugs*. 1992;43:873-888.
4. Prescribing Information. Oxcarbazepine. Taro Pharmaceuticals; 2014.
5. Bennett GD, Amore BM, Finnell RH, et al. Teratogenicity of carbamazepine-10, 11-epoxide and oxcarbazepine in the SWV mouse. *J Pharmacol Exp Ther*. 1996;279:1237-1242.
6. Bulau P, Paar WD, von Unruh GE. Pharmacokinetics of oxcarbazepine and 10-hydroxy-carbazepine in the newborn child of an oxcarbazepine-treated mother. *Eur J Clin Pharmacol*. 1988;34:311-313.
7. Ohman I, Tomson T. Pharmacokinetics of oxcarbazepine in neonatal period and during lactation (Abstract E700). *Epilepsia*. 2009;50(suppl 4):2-262.
8. Andermann E. Pregnancy and oxcarbazepine. *Epilepsia*. 1994;35 (suppl 3):S26.
9. The Lamotrigine Pregnancy Registry. Final Report. 1 September 1992 through 31 March 2010. GlaxoSmithKline; July 2010.
10. Gentile S. Prophylactic treatment of bipolar disorder in pregnancy and breastfeeding: focus on emerging mood stabilizers. *Bipolar Disord*. 2006;8:207-220.
11. Veroniki AA, Rios P, Cogo E, et al. Comparative safety of antiepileptic drugs for neurological development in children exposed during pregnancy and breast feeding: a systematic review and network meta-analysis. *BMJ Open*. 2017;7:e017248.
12. Chen CY, Li X, Ma LY, et al. In utero oxcarbazepine exposure and neonatal abstinence syndrome: case report and brief review of the literature. *Pharmacotherapy*. 2017;37:e71-e75.
13. Tomson T, Battino D, Bonizzoni E, et al.; EURAP Study Group. Antiepileptic drugs and intrauterine death: a prospective observational study from EURAP. *Neurology*. 2015;85:580-588.
14. Lutz UC, Wiatr G, Gaertner HJ, Bartels M. Oxcarbazepine treatment during breast-feeding: a case report. *J Clin Psychopharmacol*. 2007;27:730-732.
15. Gentile S. Oxcarbazepine in pregnancy and lactation. *Clin Drug Investig*. 2003;23:687.
16. Bar-Oz B, Nulman I, Koren G, Ito S. Anticonvulsants and breast feeding—a critical review. *Paediatr Drugs*. 2000;2:113-126.

OXICONAZOLE

Anti-Infective (Antifungal—Topical)

PREGNANCY RECOMMENDATION: No Human Data—Animal Data Suggest Low Risk

BREASTFEEDING RECOMMENDATION: Probably Compatible

PREGNANCY SUMMARY

No reports describing the use of oxiconazole in human pregnancy have been located. The drug may cross the placenta, but the low systemic absorption with topical use suggests that the amount would be clinically insignificant. However, the absence of human pregnancy experience prevents a complete assessment of the embryofetal risk. Animal data did not show any embryofetal toxicity in three species with oral doses of more than 10 times the RHD based on BSA. Using this drug during pregnancy should be based on the pros and cons of the mother's clinical need for treatment versus any potential fetal risk that might occur from exposure.

BREASTFEEDING SUMMARY

No reports describing the use of oxiconazole during human lactation have been located. The drug may be found in human breast milk, but the low systemic absorption from topical use suggests that the amount is probably clinically insignificant. However, the manufacturer states that the drug is found in breast milk, but no further data were supplied. Breastfeeding while using this drug should be based on the mother's clinical need for treatment versus any potential infant risks that might occur. Due to the topical use of the drug, no systemic side effects were evaluated.

Reference

1. Prescribing Information. Oxiconazole nitrate cream. E. Fougera and Co a Division of Fougera Pharmaceuticals; 2019.

OXYBUTYNIN

Urinary (Antispasmodic)

PREGNANCY RECOMMENDATION: Limited Human Data—Animal Data Suggest Low Risk

BREASTFEEDING RECOMMENDATION: Probably Compatible (Short-Term Use)

PREGNANCY SUMMARY

A large analysis of drugs used for overactive bladder disorder compared 479 patients who filled a prescription during pregnancy (around 400 of these used oxybutynin) with those that did not. The rate of birth anomalies was no different between the groups. There was also a case report describing a woman with paraplegia who had used baclofen, oxybutynin, and trimethoprim throughout an uneventful pregnancy. At delivery, the infant was described as healthy with no identified birth defects. The drug will probably cross the placenta, so some fetal exposure will likely occur. Therefore, this limited human pregnancy experience prevents a complete assessment of the embryofetal risk. Animal studies did not show any embryofetal toxicity or teratogenicity in four species at doses of more than 10 times the MRHD based on body weight. Using this drug during pregnancy should be based on the pros and cons of the mother's clinical need for treatment versus any potential fetal risk that might occur from exposure.

BREASTFEEDING SUMMARY

No reports describing the use of oxybutynin during human lactation have been located. The drug will probably be found in human breast milk, so some infant exposure will likely occur. Because of the drug's anticholinergic properties, it has the potential to decrease breast milk supply. Breastfeeding while using this drug should be based on the mother's clinical need for treatment versus any potential infant risks that might occur. If used, the infant should be monitored for the most common reported adult side effects of headache, dizziness, and dry mouth (all leading to irritability), constipation, and somnolence.

References

1. Prescribing Information. Oxybutynin. Eywa Pharma; 2019.
2. Welk B, McClure JA, McArthur E, Leong Y. The association of adverse pregnancy outcomes with overactive bladder anticholinergics. *Urogynecology*. 2025;31:849-56.
3. Ratnayaka BDM, Dhaliwal H, Watkin S. Neonatal convulsions after withdrawal of baclofen. *Br Med J*. 2001;323:85.

OXYCODONE

Pain (Opioid Agonist)

PREGNANCY RECOMMENDATION: Human Data Suggest Risk (Prolonged Use)

BREASTFEEDING RECOMMENDATION: Potential Toxicity

PREGNANCY SUMMARY

Numerous studies have been located that describe the use of oxycodone during human pregnancy. The rate of major anomalies was about 4.5% in more than 350 first-trimester exposures, but no pattern to the defects was identified. Many papers discuss the risk for newborn dependence leading to a high rate of neonatal opioid withdrawal syndrome. The National Birth Defects Prevention study reported data of higher rates of opioid use in newborns with specific birth defects compared with newborns that did not have these defects. However, the two groups have many different risk factors. There are several studies regarding opioid use in general that have shown a decrease in head circumference at birth with prolonged use in pregnancy compared with controls. The significance of this is not known. The drug crosses the placenta, so fetal exposure will occur. Animal studies did not show any embryofetal toxicity in two species at doses of less than 10 times the RHD. Oxycodone is a Schedule II controlled substance with an overall morphine milligram equivalence of about 1.5. Using this drug during pregnancy should be based on the pros and cons of the mother's clinical need for treatment versus any potential

(*continued*)

fetal risk that might occur from exposure. The drug carries a boxed warning for an increased risk of addiction and misuse; life-threatening respiratory depression; neonatal opioid withdrawal syndrome, cytochrome P450 3A4 inhibitor interaction; and concomitant use with benzodiazepines or other CNS depressants.

BREASTFEEDING SUMMARY

Numerous studies have evaluated the use of oxycodone in human lactation. From a total of about 175 women, numerous samples have been analyzed. Drug levels in breast milk ranged from undetectable (LLQ of 1-5 ng/mL) up to a peak of about 230 ng/mL. Most calculated RIDs were 1% or less, but a few were at 8% to 9%. Approximately 66 infants have had blood levels analyzed. In 41 infants, 40 had negative blood levels (LLQ of 2 ng/mL). The one positive test was a concentration of 7.4 ng/mL. In another 25 cases, again, most samples were negative (LLQ of 0.1 ng/mL). The positive blood levels ranged from 0.2 to 0.4 ng/mL. Several reports were located that describe newborn sedation, lethargy, and apnea that required intubation in some instances in breastfeeding infants exposed to the drug. Breastfeeding while using this drug should be based on the mother's clinical need for treatment versus any potential infant risks that might occur. If used, the infant should be monitored for the most common reported adult side effects of nausea, pruritus, and dizziness (all leading to irritability), constipation, vomiting, lethargy, and somnolence. If the clinical decision is to use this drug, short-term pain treatment is recommended, if at all possible.

References

1. Prescribing Information. Oxycontin. Purdue Pharma; 2019.
2. Heinonen OP, Slone D, Shapiro S. *Birth Defects and Drugs in Pregnancy*. Publishing Sciences Group; 1977:287.
3. Schick B, Hom M, Tolosa J, et al. Preliminary analysis of first trimester exposure to oxycodone and hydrocodone (abstract): presented at the Ninth International Conference of the Organization of Teratology Information Services, Salt Lake City, Utah, May 2-4, 1996. *Reprod Toxicol*. 1996; 10:162.
4. Rampono J, Kristensen JH, Ilett KF, et al. Quetiapine and breast feeding. *Ann Pharmacother*. 2007;41:711-714.
5. Weintraub SJ, Naulty JS. Acute abstinence syndrome after epidural injection of butorphanol. *Anesth Analg*. 1985;64:452-453.
6. Rao R, Desai NS. OxyContin and neonatal abstinence syndrome. *J Perinatol*. 2002;22:324-325.
7. Broussard CS, Rasmussen SA, Reefhuis J, et al.; for the National Birth Defects Prevention Study. Maternal treatment with opioid analgesics and risk for birth defects. *Am J Obstet Gynecol*. 2011;204:314-317.
8. Marx CM, Pucino F, Carlson JD, et al. Oxycodone excretion in human milk in the puerperium (abstract). *Drug Intell Clin Pharm*. 1986;20:474.
9. Lam J, Kelly L, Ciszkowski C, et al. Central nervous system depression of neonates breastfed by mothers receiving oxycodone for postpartum analgesia. *J Pediatr*. 2012;160:33-37.

OXYMETAZOLINE CREAM

Dermatologic (Topical—α-Adrenergic Agonist)

PREGNANCY RECOMMENDATION: No Human Data—Animal Data Suggest Low Risk

BREASTFEEDING RECOMMENDATION: Probably Compatible

O

PREGNANCY SUMMARY

There were two patients in the Collaborative Perinatal Project (CPP) that had first-trimester exposure to oral oxymetazoline, and no birth anomalies were identified. No studies were located that describe the use of oxymetazoline cream in human pregnancy. The drug may cross the placenta, but the low systemic levels seen with topical skin use suggest that the amount would be clinically insignificant. Therefore, the absence of human pregnancy experience prevents a complete assessment of the embryofetal risk. Animal studies did not show any embryofetal toxicity in two species at doses of less than 10 times the MRHD in one species and more than 10 times the MRHD in the second. Using this drug during pregnancy should be based on the pros and cons of the mother's clinical need for treatment versus any potential fetal risk that might occur from exposure.

BREASTFEEDING SUMMARY

No reports describing the use of oxymetazoline cream during human lactation have been located. The drug may be found in human breast milk, but the low systemic levels seen with topical skin use suggest that the amount would be clinically insignificant. Breastfeeding while using this drug should be based on the mother's clinical need for treatment versus any potential infant risks that might occur. If used, the infant should be monitored for the most common reported adult side effects of nausea, headache, dizziness, blurred vision (all leading to irritability), elevated heart rate, and tremors.

References

1. Prescribing Information. Rhofade. Allergan; 2019.
2. Heinonen OP, Slone D, Shapiro S. *Birth Defects and Drugs in Pregnancy*. Wright PSB; 1983:346.

OXYMETAZOLINE NASAL SPRAY

Respiratory (α-Adrenergic Agonist)

PREGNANCY RECOMMENDATION: Limited Human Data—Animal Data Suggest Low Risk

BREASTFEEDING RECOMMENDATION: Probably Compatible

PREGNANCY SUMMARY

There were two patients in the Collaborative Perinatal Project (CPP) that had first-trimester exposure to oral oxymetazoline, and no birth anomalies were identified. Two studies described possible effects on the fetal heart rate (FHR). In one case, the mother used six treatments in each nostril in about a 16-hour period (instead of two doses in a 24-hour period). There was a nonreactive FHR tracing with decelerations that resolved about 6 hours after the last dose. However, in a second study, 12 women used the nasal spray as directed, and no FHR changes or other abnormalities occurred. The drug may cross the placenta, but the low systemic levels seen with nasal spray use suggest that the amount would be clinically insignificant. Therefore, this limited human pregnancy experience prevents a complete assessment of the embryofetal risk. Animal studies did not show any embryofetal toxicity in two species at doses of less than 10 times the MRHD in one and more than 10 times the MRHD in the second. Using this drug during pregnancy should be based on the pros and cons of the mother's clinical need for treatment versus any potential fetal risk that might occur from exposure.

BREASTFEEDING SUMMARY

No reports describing the use of oxymetazoline nasal spray during human lactation have been located. The drug may be found in human breast milk, but the low systemic levels seen with nasal spray use suggest that the amount would be clinically insignificant. Breastfeeding while using this drug should be based on the mother's clinical need for treatment versus any potential infant risks that might occur. If used, the infant should be monitored for the most common reported adult side effects of nausea, headache, dizziness, blurred vision (all leading to irritability), elevated heart rate, and tremors.

References

1. Prescribing Information. Rhofade. Allergan; 2019.
2. Heinonen OP, Slone D, Shapiro S. *Birth Defects and Drugs in Pregnancy*. Wright PSB; 1983:346.
3. Baxi LV, Gindoff PR, Pregenzer GJ, Parras MK. Fetal heart rate changes following maternal administration of a nasal decongestant. *Am J Obstet Gynecol*. 1985;153:799-800.
4. Rayburn WF, Anderson JC, Smith CV, et al. Uterine and fetal doppler flow changes from a single dose of a long-acting intranasal decongestant. *Obstet Gynecol*. 1990;76:180-182.

O

OXYMETAZOLINE OPHTHALMIC

Ophthalmic (Topical—α-Adrenergic Agonist)

PREGNANCY RECOMMENDATION: No Human Data—Animal Data Suggest Low Risk

BREASTFEEDING RECOMMENDATION: Probably Compatible

PREGNANCY SUMMARY

There were two patients in the CPP that had first-trimester exposure to oral oxymetazoline, and no birth anomalies were identified. No studies were located that describe the use of oxymetazoline ophthalmic in human pregnancy. The drug may cross the placenta, but the low systemic levels seen with ocular use suggest that the amount would be clinically insignificant. Therefore, the absence of human pregnancy experience prevents a complete assessment of the embryofetal risk. Animal studies did not show any embryofetal toxicity in two species at doses of less than 10 times the MRHOD in one and more than 10 times the MRHOD in the second. Using this drug during pregnancy should be based on the pros and cons of the mother's clinical need for treatment versus any potential fetal risk that might occur from exposure If used during pregnancy, consider placing pressure over the tear duct in the corner of the eye for at least 1 minute, and then remove any excess solution with absorbent tissue to decrease the amount of drug reaching the systemic circulation even further.

BREASTFEEDING SUMMARY

No reports describing the use of oxymetazoline ophthalmic during human lactation have been located. The drug may be found in human breast milk, but the low systemic levels seen with ocular use suggest that the amount would be clinically insignificant. Breastfeeding while using this drug should be based on the mother's clinical need for treatment versus any potential infant risks that might occur. Due to the ocular use of the drug, systemic side effects were not evaluated. A method to decrease some systemic absorption with ophthalmic use is described above in the Pregnancy Summary.

References

1. Prescribing Information. Upneeq. RVI Pharmaceuticals, Inc; 2020.
2. Heinonen OP, Slone D, Shapiro S. *Birth Defects and Drugs in Pregnancy*. Wright PSB; 1983:346.

OXYMORPHONE

Pain (Opioid Agonist)

PREGNANCY RECOMMENDATION: Human Data Suggest Risk (Prolonged Use)

BREASTFEEDING RECOMMENDATION: Potential Toxicity

PREGNANCY SUMMARY

Studies analyzing the use of oxymorphone in the first trimester are lacking. The drug has been used during labor and has caused neonatal respiratory depression to the same degree as other narcotic analgesics. Although oxymorphone was not included in a National Birth Defects Prevention study, the use of other opioid agonists during organogenesis was associated with a low absolute risk of congenital birth defects. The drug will probably cross the placenta, so some fetal exposure will likely occur. Therefore, the absence of the first-trimester human pregnancy experience prevents a complete assessment of the embryofetal risk. Animal studies did show some embryofetal toxicity in one species at doses of less than 10 times the RHD. The use of any opioid agonist during labor or close to delivery may cause neonatal respiratory depression. Use for prolonged periods or in high doses at term has the potential to cause neonatal abstinence syndrome or respiratory depression in the newborn. There are several studies regarding opioid use in general that have shown a decrease in head circumference at birth with prolonged use in pregnancy compared with controls. The significance of this is not known. Oxymorphone is a Schedule II controlled substance with an overall morphine milligram equivalence of about 3. Using this drug during pregnancy should be based on the pros and cons of the mother's clinical need for treatment versus any potential fetal risk that might occur from exposure. The drug carries a boxed warning for an increased risk of addiction and misuse; life-threatening respiratory depression; and interaction with alcohol.

BREASTFEEDING SUMMARY

No reports describing the use of oxymorphone during human lactation have been located. The drug will probably be excreted into breast milk, so some infant exposure will likely occur. Breastfeeding while using this drug should be based on the mother's clinical need for treatment versus any potential infant risks that might occur. If used, the infant should be monitored for the most common reported adult side effects of nausea, pruritus, dizziness, and abdominal pain (all leading to irritability), constipation, vomiting, lethargy, sedation, and somnolence. If the clinical decision is to use this drug, short-term pain treatment is recommended, if at all possible.

References

1. Prescribing Information. Oxymorphone. Aurolife Pharma; 2019.
2. Simeckova M, Shaw W, Pool E, Nichols EE. Numorphan in labor—a preliminary report. *Obstet Gynecol*. 1960;16:119-123.
3. Sentnor MH, Solomons E, Kohl SG. An evaluation of oxymorphone in labor. *Am J Obstet Gynecol*. 1962;84:956-961.
4. Eames GM, Pool KRS. Clinical trial of oxymorphone in labor. *Br Med J*. 1964;2:353-355.
5. Ransom S. Oxymorphone as an obstetric analgesic—a clinical trial. *Anesthesia*. 1966;21:464-471.

OZANIMOD

Immunologic

PREGNANCY RECOMMENDATION: Limited Human Data—Animal Data Suggest Low Risk

BREASTFEEDING RECOMMENDATION: Probably Compatible

PREGNANCY SUMMARY

Limited reports describing the use of ozanimod in human pregnancy have been located. The drug will probably cross the placenta, so fetal exposure will likely occur. Animal studies did not show embryofetal toxicity. Pregnancy data from the clinical development program reported on 60 pregnancies in women exposed to the drug in the first trimester. The spontaneous abortion rate was about 23%, and the fetal anomaly rate was 3.3% (1 anomaly in 30 births, a duplex kidney). However, due to the findings from animal studies with higher doses and its mechanism of action, the manufacturer recommends that women with reproductive potential who are taking ozanimod use effective contraception during treatment and for at least 3 months after the last dose. Women with multiple sclerosis who become pregnant during treatment with ozanimod should talk to their health care provider about registering with the ZEPOSIA Pregnancy Registry. The patient or health care provider can enroll the patient in this registry by calling 1-877-301-9314.

BREASTFEEDING SUMMARY

No reports describing the use of ozanimod during human lactation have been located. The drug will probably be excreted into breast milk, so infant exposure will likely occur. Breastfeeding while using this drug should be based on the mother's clinical need for treatment. If used, the infant should be monitored for the most common reported adult side effects of nausea, headache, abdominal pain, back pain, and arthralgias (all leading to irritability), upper respiratory tract infections, urinary tract infections, and pyrexia.

References

1. Prescribing Information. Zeposia. Celgene Corporation; 2021.
2. Dubinsky MC, Mahadevan U, Charles L, et al. Pregnancy outcomes in the ozanimod clinical development program in relapsing multiple sclerosis, ulcerative colitis, and Crohn's disease, DOP53. *J Crohn's Colitis*. 2021;15(suppl 1): S088-S089.

OZENOXACIN

Antibacterial (Topical Skin—Quinolone)

PREGNANCY RECOMMENDATION: No Human Data—Animal Data Suggest Low Risk

BREASTFEEDING RECOMMENDATION: Probably Compatible

PREGNANCY SUMMARY

No reports describing the use of ozenoxacin in human pregnancy have been located. Though placental transfer is possible, fetal exposure is probably negligible because of insignificant absorption after topical use. However, the absence of human pregnancy experience prevents a complete assessment of the embryofetal risk. Animal data did not show any embryofetal toxicity. The majority of patients with impetigo are 5 years of age and under. However, skin infections with *Staphylococcus aureus* and *Streptococcus pyogenes* organisms are theoretically possible at any age.

BREASTFEEDING SUMMARY

No reports describing the use of ozenoxacin in human lactation have been located. Because the drug has negligible absorption after topical use, any drug found in breast milk would not likely have any clinical effect. Breastfeeding while using this drug should be based on the mother's clinical need for treatment. Because the drug is used topically with insignificant plasma absorption, adverse systemic adult reactions were not reported. The drug should not be used on or around the nipple.

Reference

1. Prescribing Information. Xepi. Medimetriks Pharmaceuticals, Inc; 2017.

O

P

PACLITAXEL

Antineoplastic (Antimicrotubular)

PREGNANCY RECOMMENDATION: Limited Human Data—Animal Data Suggest Potential Risk

BREASTFEEDING RECOMMENDATION: Potential Toxicity

PREGNANCY SUMMARY

Several case reports describing the use of paclitaxel in human pregnancy have been located. The human pregnancy experience is limited to use in the second and third trimesters. No fetal or newborn toxicity has been reported following this use. Paclitaxel crosses the placenta in ex vivo placental perfusion studies, so fetal exposure will probably occur. Embryofetal and maternal toxicity were observed in one animal species at doses of less than the maximum recommended human dose (MRHD). However, this limited first-trimester human pregnancy experience prevents a complete assessment of embryofetal risk. Based on animal studies and the drug's mechanism of action, the manufacturer recommends that women with reproductive potential use effective contraception during treatment. However, using this drug during pregnancy should be based on the pros and cons of the mother's clinical need for treatment versus any potential fetal risk that might occur from exposure. There is a registry for women who are pregnant and have cancer. For more information, women and health care providers are encouraged to contact the Cancer and Pregnancy Registry at 1-877-635-4499.

BREASTFEEDING SUMMARY

Paclitaxel has been shown to be excreted into human breast milk. A lactating mother using the drug for cancer treatment had breast milk samples tested. The peak concentration was about 0.97 mcg/mL with a calculated relative infant dose (RID) of about 16%. Due to a concern for potential serious adverse effects that might be seen in a breastfed infant, the manufacturer recommends that women not breastfeed while being treated with this drug. Nevertheless, if the clinical decision is to use this drug while breastfeeding, the infant should be monitored for the most common reported adult side effects of peripheral neuropathy, myalgia/arthralgia, nausea, and mucositis (all leading to irritability), vomiting, diarrhea, hypersensitivity reactions, and various laboratory abnormalities (see Prescribing Information [PI]).

References

1. Prescribing Information. Paclitaxel. Alembic Pharmaceuticals Inc; 2024.
2. Nekhayeva IA, Nanovskaya TN, Hankins GDV, Ahmed MS. Role of human placental efflux transporter P-glycoprotein in the transfer of buprenorphine, levo-α-acetylmethadol, and paclitaxel. *Am J Perinatol*. 2006;23:423-430.
3. Seiden MV, Spitzer TR, McAfee S, Fuller AF. Successful pregnancy after high-dose cyclophosphamide, carboplatinum, and taxol with peripheral blood stem cell transplant in a young woman with ovarian cancer. *Gynecol Oncol*. 2001;83:412-414.
4. Sood AK, Shahin MS, Sorosky JI. Paclitaxel and platinum chemotherapy for ovarian carcinoma during pregnancy. *Gynecol Oncol*. 2001;83:599-600.
5. Méndez LE, Mueller A, Salom E, González-Quintero VH. Paclitaxel and carboplatin chemotherapy administered during pregnancy for advanced epithelial ovarian cancer. *Obstet Gynecol*. 2003;102:1200-1202.
6. Gadducci A, Cosio S, Fanucchi A, et al. Chemotherapy with epirubicin and paclitaxel for breast cancer during pregnancy: case report and review of the literature. *Anticancer Res*. 2003;23:5225-5229.
7. Adolph A, Le T, Khan K, Biem S. Recurrent metastatic fallopian tube carcinoma in pregnancy. *Gynecol Oncol*. 2001;81:110-112.
8. Gonzalez-Angulo AM, Walters RS, Carpenter RJ Jr, et al. Paclitaxel chemotherapy in a pregnant patient with bilateral breast cancer. *Clin Breast Cancer*. 2004;5:317-319.
9. Morris PG, King F, Kennedy MJ. Cytotoxic chemotherapy for pregnancy-associated breast cancer: a single institution case series. *J Oncol Pharm Practice*. 2009;15:241-247.
10. Palaia I, Pernice M, Graziano M, et al. Neoadjuvant chemotherapy plus radical surgery in locally advanced cervical cancer during pregnancy: a case report. *Am J Obstet Gynecol*. 2007;197:e5-e6.
11. Modares Giliani M, Karimi Zarchi M, Behtash N, et al. Preservation of pregnancy in a patient with advanced ovarian cancer at 20 weeks of gestation: case report and literature review. *Int J Gynecol Cancer*. 2007;17:1140-1143.
12. Hubalek M, Smekal-Schindelwig C, Zeimet AG, et al. Chemotherapeutic treatment of a pregnant patient with ovarian dysgerminoma. *Arch Gynecol Obstet*. 2007;276:179-183.
13. Doi D, Boh Y, Konishi H, et al. Combined chemotherapy with paclitaxel and carboplatin for mucinous cystadenocarcinoma of the ovary during pregnancy. *Arch Gynecol Obstet*. 2009;280:633-636.
14. Garcia-Gonzalez J, Cueva J, Lamus MJ, et al. Paclitaxel and cisplatin in the treatment of metastatic non-small-cell lung cancer during pregnancy. *Clin Transl Oncol*. 2008;10:375-376.
15. Azim HA Jr, Scarfone G, Peccatori FA. Carboplatin and weekly paclitaxel for the treatment of non-small cell lung cancer (NSCLC) during pregnancy. *J Thorac Oncol*. 2009;4:559-560.
16. Griffin SJ, Milla M, Baker TE, et al. Transfer of carboplatin and paclitaxel into breast milk. *J Hum Lact*. 2012;28:457-459.
17. Leslie KK. Chemotherapy and pregnancy. *Clin Obstet Gynecol*. 2002;45:153-164.

PACRITINIB

Antineoplastic (Janus Kinase Inhibitor)

PREGNANCY RECOMMENDATION: No Human Data—Animal Data Suggest Potential Risk

BREASTFEEDING RECOMMENDATION: Potential Toxicity

PREGNANCY SUMMARY

No reports describing the use of pacritinib in human pregnancy have been located. Some amount of the drug will probably cross the placenta, so fetal exposure will likely occur. However, the absence of human pregnancy experience prevents a complete assessment of the embryofetal risk. Animal studies did show embryofetal toxicity, but maternal toxicity also occurred. Using this drug during pregnancy should be based on the pros and cons of the mother's clinical need for treatment versus any potential fetal risk that might occur from exposure. The drug can also prolong the cardiac QT interval.

BREASTFEEDING SUMMARY

No reports describing the use of pacritinib during human lactation have been located. Some amount of the drug probably enters breast milk, so infant exposure will likely occur. However, due to the concern for potential serious adverse effects seen in adults, the manufacturer recommends that women not breastfeed while being treated with pacritinib and for 2 weeks after the last dose. Nevertheless, breastfeeding while using this drug should be based on the mother's clinical need for treatment. If used, the infant should be monitored for the most common reported adult side effects of nausea (leading to irritability), diarrhea, edema, anemia, and thrombocytopenia.

Reference

1. Prescribing Information. Vonjo. CTI BioPharm Corporation; 2022.

PAFOLACIANINE

Diagnostic (Imaging Agent)

PREGNANCY RECOMMENDATION: No Human Data—Animal Data Suggest Low Risk

BREASTFEEDING RECOMMENDATION: Probably Compatible

PREGNANCY SUMMARY

No reports describing the use of pafolacianine in human pregnancy have been located. This diagnostic agent will likely have limited placental transfer, so fetal exposure is probably minimal. However, the absence of human pregnancy experience prevents a complete assessment of the embryofetal risk. Animal data did not show any embryofetal toxicity. Regardless, the manufacturer states that based on the drug's mechanism of action, it may cause fetal harm if administered during pregnancy. They recommend that the patient have a negative pregnancy test prior to administration. Nevertheless, using this agent during pregnancy should be based on the pros and cons of the mother's clinical need for treatment versus any potential fetal risk that might occur from exposure. In addition, patients need to discontinue any intake of folic acid supplementation for about 48 hours prior to the single administration, but this would only have a theoretical concern at the very early stages of gestation.

BREASTFEEDING SUMMARY

No reports describing the use of pafolacianine during human lactation have been located. Pafolacianine may have limited transfer into breast milk, so infant exposure is likely minimal. Breastfeeding while using this diagnostic agent should be based on the mother's clinical need for treatment. If used, the infant should be monitored for the most common reported adult side effects of nausea, abdominal pain, and pruritus (all leading to irritability) and vomiting.

Reference

1. Prescribing Information. Cytalux. Grand River Aseptic Manufacturing; 2021.

PALBOCICLIB

Antineoplastic (Cyclin-Dependent Kinase Inhibitor)

PREGNANCY RECOMMENDATION: No Human Data—Animal Data Suggest Risk

BREASTFEEDING RECOMMENDATION: Potential Toxicity

PREGNANCY SUMMARY

No reports describing the use of palbociclib in human pregnancy have been located. The drug will probably cross the placenta, so some fetal exposure will likely occur. Therefore, the absence of human pregnancy experience prevents a complete assessment of the embryofetal risk. Embryofetal and maternal toxicity were observed in two animal species at doses of less than 10 times the recommended human dose (RHD). Based on animal studies and the drug's mechanism of action, the manufacturer recommends that women with reproductive potential use effective contraception during treatment and for 3 weeks after the last dose. They also recommend that males with female partners of reproductive potential use effective contraception during treatment and for 3 months after the last dose. Regardless, using this drug during pregnancy should be based on the pros and cons of the mother's clinical need for treatment versus any potential fetal risk that might occur from exposure. There is a registry for women who are pregnant and have cancer. For more information, women and health care providers are encouraged to contact the Cancer and Pregnancy Registry at 1-877-635-4499.

BREASTFEEDING SUMMARY

No reports describing the use of palbociclib during human lactation have been located. The drug will likely be excreted into breast milk, so some infant exposure will probably occur. However, because palbociclib is used with letrozole or fulvestrant, these agents also may be excreted into breast milk. Due to a concern for potential serious adverse effects that might be seen in a breastfed infant, the manufacturer recommends that women not breastfeed while being treated with this drug and for at least 3 weeks after the last dose. Nevertheless, if the clinical decision is to use this drug while breastfeeding, the infant should be monitored for the most common reported adult side effects of nausea and stomatitis (both leading to irritability), infections, fatigue (lethargy), alopecia, diarrhea, rash, vomiting, decreased appetite (monitor infant growth), pyrexia, and various laboratory abnormalities (see PI).

Reference

1. Prescribing Information. Ibrance. Pfizer Laboratories Div Pfizer Inc; 2024.

PALIFERMIN

Miscellaneous (Keratinocyte Growth Factor)

PREGNANCY RECOMMENDATION: No Human Data—Animal Data Suggest Potential Risk (Maternal Benefit May Outweigh Any Potential Fetal Risk)

BREASTFEEDING RECOMMENDATION: Probably Compatible

P

PREGNANCY SUMMARY

No reports describing the use of palifermin in human pregnancy have been located. The drug will probably cross the placenta, so some fetal exposure will likely occur. Therefore, the absence of human pregnancy experience prevents a complete assessment of the embryofetal risk. Embryofetal and maternal toxicity were observed in two animal species at doses of less than 10 times the RHD. The use of this agent by a pregnant patient implies that she is also probably receiving or has received chemotherapy that is toxic to the bone marrow and oral mucosa. The addition of palifermin to decrease maternal oral mucosal toxicity and allow a more rapid return to normal intake of food and fluids would appear to be an overall embryofetal benefit. Therefore, the maternal benefit may outweigh any unknown fetal risk. There is a registry for women who are pregnant and have cancer. For more information, women and health care providers are encouraged to contact the Cancer and Pregnancy Registry at 1-877-635-4499.

BREASTFEEDING SUMMARY

No reports describing the use of palifermin during human lactation have been located. The drug is not likely to be excreted into human breast milk in clinically significant amounts. In addition, because it is a protein of 140 amino acids, if the drug were to be ingested through breastfeeding, it would probably be digested in the infant's gastrointestinal tract and not be absorbed. The use of this agent by a postpartum woman implies that she is also probably receiving or has received chemotherapy that could have its own toxic effects on a breastfeeding infant. However, due to a concern for potential serious adverse effects that might be seen in a breastfed infant, the manufacturer recommends that women not breastfeed while being treated with this drug and for at least 2 weeks after the last dose. Nevertheless, if the clinical decision is to use this drug while breastfeeding, the infant should be monitored for the most common reported adult side effects of pruritus (leading to irritability), rash, fever, elevated serum amylase levels, erythema, and peripheral edema.

Reference

1. Prescribing Information. Kepivance. Swedish Orphan Biovitrum AB (publ); 2023.

PALIPERIDONE

Mental Health (Atypical Antipsychotic)

PREGNANCY RECOMMENDATION: Human Data Suggest Risk (Third Trimester)—Animal Data Suggest Low Risk

BREASTFEEDING RECOMMENDATION: Probably Compatible

PREGNANCY SUMMARY

Several reports were located that describe the use of atypical antipsychotics in human pregnancy, including two case reports of use with paliperidone. In the two case reports, both patients used the depot formulation and delivered full-term infants. One infant had talipes equinovarus, and the other had no anomalies. A large retrospective cohort study using a Medicaid database ($n = 9{,}258$) did not show a higher risk of birth defects in the women exposed to antipsychotics during pregnancy. The drug crosses the placenta, so fetal exposure will occur. However, the limited human pregnancy experience prevents a complete assessment of embryofetal risk. Animal data did not show any embryofetal toxicity in two species at doses of less than 10 times the MRHD. However, antipsychotic exposure in the third trimester has been associated with fetal/neonatal adverse reactions of extrapyramidal and/or withdrawal symptoms, including agitation, hypertonia, hypotonia, tremor, somnolence, respiratory distress, and feeding disorders. Duration varies from hours to days, with some infants requiring prolonged hospitalization. Using this drug during pregnancy should be based on the pros and cons of the mother's clinical need for treatment versus any potential fetal risk that might occur from exposure. The American College of Obstetricians and Gynecologists (ACOG) guidelines from 2023 state that the risks of uncontrolled bipolar disorder and schizophrenia in pregnancy include preterm delivery, fetal growth restriction, adverse neurodevelopmental outcomes, and postpartum psychosis risk. There is a pregnancy exposure registry that monitors pregnancy outcomes in women using atypical antipsychotic drugs. Health care providers are encouraged to contact the National Pregnancy Registry for Atypical Antipsychotics at 1-866-961-2388. Paliperidone can prolong the QTc interval. Although elevated glucose levels have been reported with atypical antipsychotic use during pregnancy, ACOG recommends checking for gestational diabetes using the standard recommendations.

BREASTFEEDING SUMMARY

Paliperidone has been shown to be excreted into human breast milk. There are three reports of mothers breastfeeding while taking risperidone and having paliperidone levels measured as well (see Risperidone). In summary, patients taking 1.5 to 6 mg/d of risperidone had RIDs for risperidone and paliperidone that were less than 1% up to about 3.5%, respectively. Paliperidone breast milk levels were higher than risperidone breast milk levels. All the infants were doing well at 2- to 12-month follow-ups. Although the combined amounts of risperidone and paliperidone measured in breast milk appear to be too low to cause extrapyramidal effects, concern was expressed for other potential adverse effects, such as neuroleptic malignant syndrome and effects on cognitive development. Breastfeeding while using this drug should be based on the mother's clinical need for treatment versus any potential infant risks that might occur. If used, the infant should be monitored for the most common reported adult side effects of excess sedation, failure to thrive, jitteriness, and extrapyramidal symptoms (tremors and abnormal muscle movements).

References

1. Prescribing Information. Paliperidone. Ajanta Pharma USA Inc; 2024.
2. Prescribing Information. Invega Trinza. Janssen Pharmaceuticals Inc; 2025.
3. Prescribing Information. Invega Hafyera. Janssen Pharmaceuticals Inc; 2024.
4. Prescribing Information. Invega Sustenna. Janssen Pharmaceuticals Inc; 2024.
5. American College of Obstetricians and Gynecologists. Treatment and management of mental health conditions during pregnancy and postpartum: ACOG clinical practice guideline No. 5. *Obstet Gynecol*. 2023;141:1262-1288.
6. Binns R, O'Halloran SJ, Teoh S, et al. Placental transfer of paliperidone during treatment with depot formulation. *J Clin Psychopharmacol*. 2017; 37:474-475.
7. Özdemir AK, Pak SC, Canan F, et al. Paliperidone palmitate use in pregnancy in a woman with schizophrenia. *Arch Womens Ment Health*. 2015; 18:739-740.
8. Viguera AC, McElheny SA, Caplin PS, et al. Risk of poor neonatal adaption syndrome among infants exposed to second-generation atypical antipsychotics compared to antidepressants. *J Clin Psychiatry*. 2023;84:22m14492.
9. Viguera A, Freeman MP, Goez-Mogollon L, et al. Reproduction safety of second generation antipsychotics: updated data from the Massachusetts General Hospital National Pregnancy Registry for atypical antipsychotics. *J Clin Psychiatry*. 2021;82:20m13745.
10. Huybrechts KF, Straub L, Karlsson P, et al. Association of in utero antipsychotic medication exposure with risk of congenital malformations in Nordic countries and the US. *JAMA Psychiatry*. 2023;80:156-166.
11. Wang Z, Chan AYL, Coghill D, et al. Association between prenatal exposure to antipsychotics and attention-deficit/hyperactivity disorder, autism spectrum disorder, preterm birth, and small for gestational age. *JAMA Intern Med*. 2021;181:1332-1340.
12. Westin AA, Brekke M, Molden E, et al. Treatment with antipsychotics in pregnancy: changes in drug disposition. *Clin Pharmacol Ther*. 2018; 103:477-484.
13. Park Y, Hernandez-Diaz S, Bateman BT, et al. Continuation of atypical antipsychotic medication during early pregnancy and the risk of gestational diabetes. *Am J Psychiatry*. 2018;175:564-574.
14. Kulkarni J, Gurvich C, Gilbert H, et al. The use of first and second generation antipsychotic drugs and the potential to develop gestational diabetes mellitus among perinatal patients with psychosis. *Schizophr Res*. 2023;254:22-26.
15. Heinonen E, Forsberg L, Norby U, et al. Antipsychotic use during pregnancy and risk for gestational diabetes: a national register-based cohort study in Sweden. *CNS Drugs*. 2022;36:529-539.
16. Hill RC, McIvor RJ, Wojnar-Horton RE, et al. Risperidone distribution and excretion into human milk: case report and estimated infant exposure during breast-feeding. *J Clin Psychopharmacol*. 2000;20:285-286.
17. Ilett KF, Hackett LP, Kristensen JH, et al. Transfer of risperidone and 9-hydroxyrisperidone into human milk. *Ann Pharmacother*. 2004;38: 273-276.
18. Aichhorn W, Stuppaeck C, Whitworth AB. Risperidone and breast-feeding. *J Psychopharmacol*. 2005;19:211-213.

PALIVIZUMAB

Anti-Infective (Monoclonal Antibody)

PREGNANCY RECOMMENDATION: No Human Data—No Relevant Animal Data

BREASTFEEDING RECOMMENDATION: Probably Compatible

PREGNANCY SUMMARY

No reports describing the use of palivizumab in human pregnancy have been located. As an immunoglobulin G (IgG) antibody, it likely crosses the placenta, especially during the second half of gestation, so some fetal exposure will probably occur. However, such reports are unlikely because the drug is currently only indicated for pediatric use. Nevertheless, the absence of human pregnancy experience prevents a complete assessment of embryofetal risk. No animal reproduction studies have been conducted. Using this drug during pregnancy should be based on the pros and cons of the mother's clinical need for treatment versus any potential fetal risk that might occur from exposure.

BREASTFEEDING SUMMARY

No reports describing the use of palivizumab during human lactation have been located, and this medication is not currently indicated for use in adults. However, it is known that IgG antibodies can be found in human breast milk but are not found in the neonatal or infant circulation. Additionally, if any IgG antibodies were to be ingested through breastfeeding, they would probably be digested in the infant's gastrointestinal tract and not be absorbed. If the clinical decision is to use this drug while breastfeeding, the infant should be monitored for the most common reported adult side effects of fever and rash.

Reference

1. Prescribing Information. Synagis. Swedish Orphan Biovitrum AB (publ); 2021.

PALONOSETRON

Gastrointestinal (5-HT_3 Receptor Antagonist—Antiemetic)

PREGNANCY RECOMMENDATION: Limited Human Data—Animal Data Suggest Low Risk

BREASTFEEDING RECOMMENDATION: Probably Compatible

P

PREGNANCY SUMMARY

One report describing the use of palonosetron in human pregnancy was located. A 2024 randomized, double-blind trial evaluated intravenous (IV) palonosetron (n = 27) and ondansetron (n = 27) on phenylephrine requirements during spinal anesthesia for patients undergoing cesarean delivery. No difference was observed in total phenylephrine dose, blood pressure, heart rate, Apgar scores, and postoperative nausea/vomiting at 2 and 24 hours postspinal anesthesia. The drug will probably cross the placenta, so some fetal exposure will likely occur. Therefore, the absence of the human first-trimester pregnancy experience prevents a complete assessment of the embryofetal risk. Animal data did not show any embryofetal toxicity in one species at doses of more than 10 times the RHD. Using this drug during pregnancy should be based on the pros and cons of the mother's clinical need for treatment versus any potential fetal risk that might occur from exposure. This medication can also prolong the QT interval.

BREASTFEEDING SUMMARY

No reports describing the use of palonosetron during human lactation have been located. The drug will likely be excreted into human breast milk, so some infant exposure will probably occur. However, due to a concern for potential serious adverse effects that might be seen in a breastfed infant, the manufacturer recommends that women not breastfeed while being treated with this drug. Nevertheless, because the use of palonosetron is normally for short periods, the risk of toxicity in a nursing infant appears remote. If the clinical decision is to use this drug while breastfeeding, the infant should be monitored for the most common reported adult side effects of headache (leading to irritability) and constipation.

References

1. Prescribing Information. Palonosetron Hydrochloride. Cipla USA Inc; 2022.
2. Kim MK, Kim I, Kang H, et al. Effect of intravenous palonosetron on hypotension induced by spinal anesthesia for cesarean section: a randomized controlled trial. *PLoS One*. 2024;19:e0305913.

PAMIDRONATE

Bone Health (Bisphosphonate)

PREGNANCY RECOMMENDATION: Limited Human Data—Animal Data Suggest Potential Risk

BREASTFEEDING RECOMMENDATION: Probably Compatible

PREGNANCY SUMMARY

Nine reports describing the use of pamidronate in 21 human pregnancies have been located. In two of the cases, pamidronate was given during the second trimester. Hypocalcemia was noted in one newborn but not the other. The amount of drug retained in bone and eventually released back into the systemic circulation is directly related to the dose and duration of treatment. Because pamidronate probably crosses the placenta, continuous fetal exposure most likely occurred throughout gestation in six cases. Therefore, these embryos were exposed during organogenesis to the low plasma concentrations resulting from the slow release of pamidronate from bone, not to the much higher concentrations obtained in the first few days after an IV dose. No major birth anomalies directly related to the drug were identified. However, the limited human pregnancy experience prevents a complete assessment of embryofetal risk. Embryofetal and maternal toxicity were observed in two animal species at doses of less than 10 times the MRHD. The manufacturer states that the use of pamidronate is not recommended in women who may become pregnant or during pregnancy. However, based solely on the limited human pregnancy experience, inadvertent exposure does not appear to represent a major risk to the embryo or fetus. However, infants should be monitored for hypocalcemia during the first few days after birth. Using this drug during pregnancy should be based on the pros and cons of the mother's clinical need for treatment versus any potential fetal risk that might occur from exposure.

BREASTFEEDING SUMMARY

Although the pK parameters suggest that pamidronate will be excreted into human breast milk, one study was unable to detect the drug in breast milk. In addition, the oral bioavailability of pamidronate is very low, at about 2% in the fasting state. Moreover, the drug is highly bound by calcium, and this should further limit absorption from breast milk. Based on these data, breastfeeding appears to be compatible with pamidronate therapy. If there is any concern, withholding nursing for 12 to 24 hours can further ensure that the infant is exposed to little or no drug. Breastfeeding while using this drug should be based on the mother's clinical need for treatment versus any potential infant risks that might occur. If used, the infant should be monitored for the most common reported adult side effects of nausea, dyspepsia, abdominal pain, arthralgia, myalgia, and skeletal pain (all leading to irritability), fatigue (lethargy), anorexia (monitor infant growth), vomiting, constipation, diarrhea, insomnia, cough, and various laboratory abnormalities (see PI).

References

1. Prescribing Information. Pamidronate. Mylan Institutional LLC; 2023.
2. Graepel P, Bentley P, Fritz H, et al. Reproduction toxicity studies with pamidronate. *Arzneimittelforschung*. 1992;42:654-667.
3. Dunlop DJ, Soukop M, McEwan HP. Antenatal administration of aminopropylidene diphosphate. *Ann Rheum Dis*. 1990;49:955.
4. Illidge TM, Hussey M, Godden CW. Malignant hypercalcaemia in pregnancy and antenatal administration of intravenous pamidronate. *Clin Oncol (R Coll Radiol)*. 1996;8:257-258.
5. Munns CFJ, Rauch F, Ward L, Glorieux FH. Maternal and fetal outcome after long-term pamidronate treatment before conception: a report of two cases. *J Bone Miner Res*. 2004;19:1742-1745.
6. Fleischnick EA, Kasser JR. Foot, talipes equinovarus (TEV). In: Buyse ML, ed. *Birth Defects Encyclopedia*. Vol 1. Blackwell Scientific Publications/Center for Birth Defects Information Services; 1990:744-746.
7. Culbert EC, Schfirin BS. Malignant hypercalcemia in pregnancy. Effect of pamidronate on uterine contractions. *Obstet Gynecol*. 2006;108:789-791.
8. Chan B, Zacharin M. Maternal and infant outcome after pamidronate treatment of polyostotic fibrous dysplasia and osteogenesis imperfecta before conception: a report of four cases. *J Clin Endocrinol Metab*. 2006; 91:217-220.
9. Cabar ER, Nomura RMY, Zugaib M. Maternal and fetal outcome of pamidronate treatment before conception: a case report. *Clin Exp Rheumatol*. 2007;25:344-345.
10. Djokanovic N, Klieger-Grossmann C, Koren G. Does treatment with bisphosphonates endanger the human pregnancy? *J Obstet Gynaecol Can*. 2008;30:1146-1148.
11. Mastaglia SR, Watman NP, Oliveri B. Intravenous bisphosphonate treatment and pregnancy: its effects on mother and infant bone health. *Osteoporos Int*. 2010;21:1959-1962.
12. Siminoski K, Fitzgerald AA, Flesch G, Gross MS. Intravenous pamidronate for treatment of reflex sympathetic dystrophy during breast feeding. *J Bone Miner Res*. 2000;15:2052-2055.

PANITUMUMAB

Antineoplastic (Monoclonal Antibody—Epidermal Growth Factor Receptor Inhibitor)

PREGNANCY RECOMMENDATION: No Human Data—Animal Data Suggest Potential Risk

BREASTFEEDING RECOMMENDATION: Probably Compatible

PREGNANCY SUMMARY

No reports describing the use of panitumumab in human pregnancy have been located. As an IgG antibody, it likely crosses the placenta, especially during the second half of gestation, so some fetal exposure will probably occur. Therefore, the absence of human pregnancy experience prevents a complete assessment of the embryofetal risk. Embryofetal toxicity was observed in one animal species at doses of less than 10 times the RHD. Based on animal studies and the drug's mechanism of action, the manufacturer recommends that women with reproductive potential use effective contraception during treatment and for 2 months after the last dose. Nevertheless, using this drug during pregnancy should be based on the pros and cons of the mother's clinical need for treatment versus any potential fetal risk that might occur from exposure. There is a registry for women who are pregnant and have cancer. For more information, women and health care providers are encouraged to contact the Cancer and Pregnancy Registry at 1-877-635-4499.

BREASTFEEDING SUMMARY

No reports describing the use of panitumumab during human lactation have been located. It is known that IgG antibodies can be found in human breast milk but are not found in the neonatal or infant circulation. Additionally, if any IgG antibodies were to be ingested through breastfeeding, they would probably be digested in the infant's gastrointestinal tract and not be absorbed. However, due to a concern for potential serious adverse effects that might be seen in a breastfed infant, the manufacturer recommends that women not breastfeed while being treated with this drug and for at least 2 months after the last dose. Nevertheless, if the clinical decision is to use this drug while breastfeeding, the infant should be monitored for the most common reported adult side effects of nausea (leading to irritability), rash, fatigue (lethargy), and diarrhea.

Reference

1. Prescribing Information. Vectibix. Amgen Inc; 2025.

PANTOPRAZOLE

Gastrointestinal (Proton Pump Inhibitor)

PREGNANCY RECOMMENDATION: Limited Human Data—Animal Data Suggest Low Risk

BREASTFEEDING RECOMMENDATION: Probably Compatible

PREGNANCY SUMMARY

Several reports describing the use of proton pump inhibitors (PPIs), including pantoprazole, in human pregnancy have been located. PPIs do not appear to increase the risk for major malformations. One study evaluated specific agents and did not find an increased risk with pantoprazole. Other publications did not find an increased risk for future allergic rhinitis, atopic dermatitis, or food allergy, but there are conflicting reports regarding the risk for childhood asthma. However, it is difficult to fully evaluate these findings because specific rates were not consistently provided for comparison to the expected background risks for these various events. In addition, all of these factors can be influenced by numerous confounding variables. A meta-analysis of PPIs in pregnancy compared 1,530 exposed patients with 133,410 not exposed and found no increased risk for major congenital malformations, spontaneous abortion, or preterm birth. The drug will probably cross the placenta, so some fetal exposure will likely occur. Therefore, the absence of human pregnancy experience prevents a complete assessment of the embryofetal risk. Animal studies did not show any embryofetal toxicity in two species at doses of more than 10 times the MRHD. Using this drug during pregnancy should be based on the pros and cons of the mother's clinical need for treatment versus any potential fetal risk that might occur from exposure.

BREASTFEEDING SUMMARY

Small amounts of pantoprazole were found to be excreted into human breast milk. A partially nursing mother was given a single 40-mg enteric-coated pantoprazole tablet. Several breast milk samples were obtained. The drug was detected only in the 2-hour sample at 36 ng/mL and the 4-hour sample at 24 ng/mL. The calculated RID was less than 1%. Breastfeeding while using this drug should be based on the mother's clinical need for treatment versus any potential infant risks that might occur. If used, the infant should be monitored for the most common reported adult side effects of headache, nausea, arthralgia, abdominal pain, and dizziness (all leading to irritability), diarrhea, vomiting, and flatulence.

References

1. Prescribing Information. Pantoprazole sodium delayed-release. Lifestar Pharma LLC; 2024.
2. Diav-Citrin O, Arnon J, Shechtman S, et al. The safety of proton pump inhibitors in pregnancy: a multicentre prospective controlled trial. *Aliment Pharmacol Ther*. 2005;21:269-275.

3. Peron A, Ripoche E, Picot C, et al. Use of proton pump inhibitors during pregnancy: a systematic review and meta-analysis of congenital malformations. *Reprod Toxicol*. 2023;119:108419.
4. Li CM, Zhernakova A, Engstrand L, et al. Systematic review with meta-analysis: the risks of proton pump inhibitors during pregnancy. *Aliment Pharmacol Ther*. 2020;51:410-420.
5. Choi A, Noh Y, Jeong HE, et al. Association between proton pump inhibitor use during early pregnancy and risk of congenital malformations. *JAMA Netw Open*. 2023;6:e2250366.
6. Noh Y, Jeong HE, Choi A, et al. Prenatal and infant exposure to acid-suppressive medication and risk of allergic diseases in children. *JAMA Pediatr*. 2023;177:267-277.
7. Lai T, Wu M, Liu J, et al. Acid-suppressive drug use during pregnancy and the risk of childhood asthma: a meta-analysis. *Pediatrics*. 2018;141:e20170889.
8. Choi A, Noh Y, Yon DK, Shin JY. Maternal proton pump inhibitor use during pregnancy and risk of low birth weight in offspring in Korea, 2008-2019. *JAMA Netw Open*. 2023;6:e237962.
9. Choi A, Noh Y, Park SH, et al. Exploration of proton pump inhibitors use during pregnancy and preeclampsia. *JAMA Netw Open*. 2023;4:e2124339.
10. Plante L, Ferron GM, Unruh M, Mayer PR. Excretion of pantoprazole in human breast milk. *J Reprod Med*. 2004;49:825-827.
11. Bor S, Karacaoglu S, Ergun P, et al. The levels of pantoprazole in human breast milk and plasma: two compartment model (Abstract). *Neurogastroenterol Motil*. 2017;29:79-80.

PANTOTHENIC ACID (VITAMIN B$_5$)

Vitamin (Water-Soluble Vitamin)

PREGNANCY RECOMMENDATION: Compatible

BREASTFEEDING RECOMMENDATION: Compatible

PREGNANCY SUMMARY

Pantothenic acid is found in many prenatal vitamins and has a recommended daily intake of 6 mg in the United States. This vitamin crosses the placenta. Because it is water soluble, the vitamin is not stored in the human body. Using this vitamin during pregnancy is recommended at the daily recommended allowance.

BREASTFEEDING SUMMARY

Pantothenic acid is normally excreted in human breast milk with concentrations directly proportional to intake. With a dietary intake of 8 to 15 mg/d, mean breast milk concentrations average about 1.9 to 2.4 mcg/mL. Breast milk levels in mothers who delivered preterm averaged higher amounts, at about 3.9 mcg/mL. For the term group, levels at 2 and 12 weeks postpartum were about 2.6 mcg/mL. The recommended daily allowance (RDA) for pantothenic acid in breastfeeding is 7 mg.

References

1. National Institutes of Health. Pantothenic acid: fact sheet for health professionals. Office of Dietary Supplements. Accessed February 5, 2025. https://ods.od.nih.gov/factsheets/PantothenicAcid-HealthProfessional/
2. National Library of Medicine. Pantothenic acid. PubChem. Accessed February 5, 2025. https://pubchem.ncbi.nlm.nih.gov/compound/Pantothenic-Acid
3. Baker H, Frank O, Thomson AD, et al. Vitamin profile of 174 mothers and newborns at parturition. *Am J Clin Nutr*. 1975;28:59-65.
4. Baker H, Frank O, Deangelis B, et al. Role of placenta in maternal-fetal vitamin transfer in humans. *Am J Obstet Gynecol*. 1981;141:792-796.
5. Hill EP, Longo LD. Dynamics of maternal-fetal nutrient transfer. *Fed Proc*. 1980;39:239-244.
6. Kaminetsky HA, Baker H, Frank O, Langer A. The effects of intravenously administered water-soluble vitamins during labor in normovitaminemic and hypovitaminemic gravidas on maternal and neonatal blood vitamin levels at delivery. *Am J Obstet Gynecol*. 1974;120:697-703.
7. Cohenour SH, Calloway DH. Blood, urine, and dietary pantothenic acid levels of pregnant teenagers. *Am J Clin Nutr*. 1972;25:512-517.
8. Baker H, Thind IS, Frank O, et al. Vitamin levels in low-birth-weight newborn infants and their mothers. *Am J Obstet Gynecol*. 1977;129:521-524.
9. Deodhar AD, Rajalakshmi R, Ramakrishnan CV. Studies on human lactation. Part III. Effect of dietary vitamin supplementation on vitamin contents of breast milk. *Acta Paediatr Scand*. 1964;53:42-48.
10. Song WO, Chan GM, Wyse BW, Hansen RG. Effect of pantothenic acid status on the content of the vitamin in human milk. *Am J Clin Nutr*. 1984;40:317-324.
11. Ford JE, Zechalko A, Murphy J, Brooke OG. Comparison of the B vitamin composition of milk from mothers of preterm and term babies. *Arch Dis Child*. 1983;58:367-372.

PARATHYROID HORMONE

Endocrine (Hormone)

PREGNANCY RECOMMENDATION: No Human Data—Animal Data Suggest Potential Risk

BREASTFEEDING RECOMMENDATION: Probably Compatible

PREGNANCY SUMMARY

No reports describing the use of parathyroid hormone in human pregnancy have been located. If placental transfer occurs, it is likely to be clinically insignificant. However, the absence of human pregnancy experience prevents a complete assessment

(continued)

of the embryofetal risk. Embryofetal toxicity was observed in animal studies. Due to a concern for osteosarcoma seen in animal studies, parathyroid hormone is only available through the NATPARA Risk Evaluation and Mitigation Strategy (REMS) Program. Additionally, in September of 2019, the manufacturer recalled all doses of NATPARA, and later, in October 2022, decided to discontinue manufacturing this drug at the end of 2024. Hypocalcemia in pregnant women may result in spontaneous abortion, premature labor, and possibly preeclampsia. Using this drug during pregnancy should be based on the pros and cons of the mother's clinical need for treatment versus any potential fetal risk that might occur from exposure.

BREASTFEEDING SUMMARY

No reports describing the use of parathyroid hormone during human lactation have been located. If excretion into breast milk occurs, it is likely to be clinically insignificant. Furthermore, the drug is a peptide, so if it were to be ingested through breastfeeding, it probably would be digested in the infant's gastrointestinal tract and not be absorbed. Breastfeeding while using this drug should be based on the mother's clinical need for treatment. If used, the infant should be monitored for the most common reported adult side effects of nausea, headache, arthralgia, and extremity pain (all leading to irritability), vomiting, diarrhea, and abnormal calcium levels.

Reference

1. Prescribing Information. Natpara. Shire-NPS Pharmaceuticals, Inc; 2020.

PARICALCITOL

Vitamin (Vitamin D Analogue)

PREGNANCY RECOMMENDATION: No Human Data—Animal Data Suggest Risk

BREASTFEEDING RECOMMENDATION: Potential Toxicity

PREGNANCY SUMMARY

No reports describing the use of paricalcitol in human pregnancy have been located. The drug will probably cross the placenta, so some fetal exposure will likely occur. Therefore, the absence of human pregnancy experience prevents a complete assessment of the embryofetal risk. Embryofetal and maternal toxicity were observed in two animal species at doses of less than 10 times the RHD. Using this drug during pregnancy should be based on the pros and cons of the mother's clinical need for treatment versus any potential fetal risk that might occur from exposure.

P

BREASTFEEDING SUMMARY

No reports describing the use of paricalcitol during human lactation have been located. The drug will likely be excreted into breast milk, so some infant exposure will probably occur. However, due to a concern for potential serious adverse effects, including hypercalcemia, that might be seen in a breastfed infant, the manufacturer recommends that women not breastfeed while being treated with this drug. Nevertheless, if the clinical decision is to use this drug while breastfeeding, the infant should be monitored for the most common reported adult side effects of dizziness and nausea (both leading to irritability), diarrhea, vomiting, hypertension, rash, flushing, hypersensitivity, and peripheral edema.

References

1. Prescribing Information. Paricalcitol capsule. Bionpharma Inc; 2023.
2. Prescribing Information. Paricalcitol injection. Amneal Pharmaceuticals LLC; 2014.

PAROMOMYCIN

Anti-Infective (Amebicide)

PREGNANCY RECOMMENDATION: Human Data Suggest Low Risk—No Relevant Animal Data

BREASTFEEDING RECOMMENDATION: Probably Compatible

PREGNANCY SUMMARY

Two reports describing the use of paromomycin in human pregnancy have been located. In one report, two women, one at 13 weeks and the other at 23 weeks, were treated for a symptomatic intestinal infection caused by *Giardia lamblia*. Both delivered normal female infants at term. In the other report, topical paromomycin plus methylbenzethonium chloride with/without sodium stibogluconate injections were utilized in five women with cutaneous leishmaniasis. There were no cases of teratogenicity or vertical transmission. Given the nearly absent absorption after oral administration, paromomycin is not expected to reach the fetus after oral administration. However, the limited human pregnancy experience prevents a complete assessment of embryofetal risk. No animal reproductive studies have been conducted. Using this drug during pregnancy should be based on the pros and cons of the mother's clinical need for treatment versus any potential fetal risk that might occur from exposure.

BREASTFEEDING SUMMARY

Paromomycin excretion in human breast milk is not expected, as the drug is not absorbed into the systemic circulation after oral dosing.

References

1. Prescribing Information. Humatin. Waylis Therapeutics LLC; 2023.
2. Kreutner AK, Del Bene VE, Amstey MS. Giardiasis in pregnancy. *Am J Obstet Gynecol*. 1981;140:895-901.
3. D'Alauro F, Lee RV, Pao-In K, Khairallah M. Intestinal parasites and pregnancy. *Obstet Gynecol*. 1985;66:639-643.
4. Bitton Y, Diav-Citron O. Cutaneous leishmaniasis: case series on pregnancy outcome. *Open Forum Infect Dis*. 2020;7:ofaa479.

PAROXETINE

Mental Health (Selective Serotonin Reuptake Inhibitor)

PREGNANCY RECOMMENDATION: Human Data Suggest Risk (Third Trimester)

BREASTFEEDING RECOMMENDATION: Probably Compatible

PREGNANCY SUMMARY

There are numerous publications describing the use of paroxetine in human pregnancy. In 2023, ACOG stated that selective serotonin reuptake inhibitors (SSRIs) do not appear to increase the risk for overall congenital malformations, cardiovascular malformations, growth restriction, preterm delivery, gestational diabetes, preeclampsia, or neurodevelopmental delays of speech-language, scholastic disorders, or motor disorders. However, its use near delivery is associated with an increased risk for poor neonatal adaptation syndrome. The manufacturer recommends advising the patient of the potential hazard to the fetus if the patient becomes pregnant while taking paroxetine. The drug crosses the placenta, so fetal exposure will occur. Embryofetal toxicity was observed in one animal species at doses of less than 10 times the MRHD. In a second species, no embryofetal toxicity was seen with doses of less than 10 times the MRHD. Using this drug during pregnancy should be based on the pros and cons of the mother's clinical need for treatment versus any potential fetal risk that might occur from exposure. There is a pregnancy exposure registry that monitors pregnancy outcomes in women using antidepressant drugs. Health care providers are encouraged to call the National Pregnancy Registry for Antidepressants at 1-844-405-6185. Paroxetine can prolong the QTc interval and should be used with caution in patients with risk factors for QTc prolongation. ACOG states that uncontrolled and undertreated depression is associated with a risk for limited engagement in medical care and self-care, substance use disorder, preterm birth, low birth weight, preeclampsia, postpartum depression, impaired infant attachment (which carries long-term infant developmental effects), disrupted relationships with partner, and suicide. Additionally, untreated and undertreated mental health disorders should be considered an exposure. Pregnancy and lactation alone should not be a reason to withhold or discontinue mental health medications.

BREASTFEEDING SUMMARY

Several studies were located that describe the use of paroxetine during human lactation. The drug has been found in nearly all breast milk samples, but in low concentrations. The mean RID has been calculated as about 0.3% up to about 1.4%. Most of the publications did not report any adverse infant events. Other studies have reported possible sleepiness, constipation, and irritability. In 18 exposed infants, only one had paroxetine detected in the plasma. A separate cohort study found that infants exposed to antidepressants during the third trimester of pregnancy had significantly lower rates of poor neonatal adaptation syndrome if they were breastfed either exclusively or mixed with formula compared to those that were formula-fed only. Regardless, due to a concern for potential serious adverse effects that might be seen in a breastfed infant, the manufacturer recommends that women not breastfeed while being treated with this drug. Nevertheless, if the clinical decision is to use this drug while breastfeeding, the infant should be monitored for the most common reported adult side effects of headache, nausea, dry mouth, and dizziness (all leading to irritability), fatigue (lethargy), constipation, decreased appetite (monitor infant growth), insomnia, somnolence, and tremor.

References

1. Prescribing Information. Paroxetine hydrochloride hemihydrate tablet. Mylan Pharmaceuticals Inc; 2024.
2. Product Information. Paroxetine. Padagis US LLC; 2023.
3. American College of Obstetricians and Gynecologists. Treatment and management of mental health conditions during pregnancy and postpartum. Clinical practice guideline No. 5. *Obstet Gynecol*. 2023;141:1262-1288.
4. Hendrick V, Stowe ZN, Altshuler LL, et al. Placental passage of antidepressant medications. *Am J Psychiatry*. 2003;160:993-996.
5. Huybrechts KF, Palmsten K, Avorn J, et al. Antidepressant use in pregnancy and the risk of cardiac defects. *N Engl J Med*. 2014;370:2397-2407.
6. Gao SY, Wu QJ, Sun C, et al. Selective serotonin reuptake inhibitor use during early pregnancy and congenital malformations: a systematic review and meta-analysis of cohort studies of more than 9 million births. *BMC Med*. 2018;16:205.
7. Wang XY, Ying XH, Jiang HY. Antidepressant use during pregnancy and the risk for gestational diabetes: a systematic review and meta-analysis. *J Matern Fetal Neonatal Med*. 2023;36:2162817.
8. Kievet N, Hoppenbrouwers C, Dolman KM, et al. Risk factors for poor neonatal adaption after exposure to antidepressants in utero. *Acta Paediatr*. 2015;104:384-391.
9. Masarwa R, Bar-Oz B, Gorelik E, et al. Prenatal exposure to selective serotonin reuptake inhibitors and serotonin norepinephrine reuptake inhibitors and risk for persistent pulmonary hypertension of the newborn: a systematic review, meta-analysis, and network meta-analysis. *Am J Obstet Gynecol*. 2019;220:57.e1-57.e13.
10. Spigset O, Carleborg L, Norstrom A, Sandlund M. Paroxetine level in breast milk. *J Clin Psychiatry*. 1996;57:39.
11. Ohman R, Hagg S, Carleborg L, Spigset O. Excretion of paroxetine into breast milk. *J Clin Psychiatry*. 1999;60:519-523.
12. Begg EJ, Duffull SB, Saunders DA, et al. Paroxetine in human milk. *Br J Clin Pharmacol*. 1999;48:142-147.
13. Stowe ZN, Cohen LS, Hostetter A, et al. Paroxetine in human breast milk and nursing infants. *Am J Psychiatry*. 2000;157:185-189.
14. Misri S, Kim J, Riggs KW, Kostaras X. Paroxetine levels in postpartum depressed women, breast milk, and infant serum. *J Clin Psychiatry*. 2000; 61:828-832.
15. Costei AM, Kozer E, Ho T, et al. Perinatal outcome following third trimester exposure to paroxetine. *Arch Pediatr Adolesc Med*. 2002;156:1129-1132.
16. Berle JO, Steen VM, Aamo TO, et al. Breastfeeding during maternal antidepressant treatment with serotonin reuptake inhibitors: infant exposure, clinical symptoms, and cytochrome P450 genotypes. *J Clin Psychiatry*. 2004; 65:1228-1234.

PASIREOTIDE

Endocrine/Metabolic (Somatostatin Analogue)

PREGNANCY RECOMMENDATION: No Human Data—Animal Data Suggest Potential Risk

BREASTFEEDING RECOMMENDATION: Probably Compatible

PREGNANCY SUMMARY

No reports describing the use of pasireotide in human pregnancy have been located. The drug is not likely to cross the placenta in significant amounts. However, because it is a small peptide of six amino acids, it is not known whether some fetal exposure could occur, especially in the second half of gestation. Nevertheless, the absence of human pregnancy experience prevents a complete assessment of the embryofetal risk. Embryofetal toxicity was observed in two animal species at doses of less than the MRHD, and one had maternal toxicity at all doses tested. However, the absence of human pregnancy experience prevents a complete assessment of embryofetal risk. Using this drug during pregnancy should be based on the pros and cons of the mother's clinical need for treatment versus any potential fetal risk that might occur from exposure. Hypertension was reported in up to 10% of patients treated with this drug in clinical trials, and it can also prolong the QT interval. Elevated glucose levels have also been reported in up to 40% of patients treated with this drug.

P

BREASTFEEDING SUMMARY

No reports describing the use of pasireotide during human lactation have been located. The drug might be excreted into human breast milk, but concentrations should be low. However, if any pasireotide were to be ingested through breastfeeding, this peptide would probably be digested in the infant's gastrointestinal tract and not absorbed. Breastfeeding while using this drug should be based on the mother's clinical need for treatment versus any potential infant risks that might occur. If used, the infant should be monitored for the most common reported adult side effects of nausea, headache, and abdominal pain (all leading to irritability), diarrhea, hyperglycemia, cholelithiasis, and fatigue (lethargy).

Reference

1. Prescribing Information. Signifor. Recordati Rare Diseases Inc; 2024.

PATIROMER

Antidote (Potassium Binder)

PREGNANCY RECOMMENDATION: No Human Data—Animal Data Suggest Low Risk

BREASTFEEDING RECOMMENDATION: Probably Compatible

PREGNANCY SUMMARY

No reports describing the use of patiromer in human pregnancy have been located. Patiromer is not systemically absorbed following oral administration; therefore, it should not cross the placenta or result in fetal risk. However, the absence of human pregnancy experience prevents a complete assessment of the embryofetal risk. Radioactivity studies showed that the drug was limited to the gastrointestinal tract, with no detectable level in any other tissues or organs. There is an increased risk of patiromer binding to other oral drugs that could reduce their absorption and overall effectiveness. Therefore, it is recommended that the use of other drugs be delayed by at least 6 hours after using patiromer.

BREASTFEEDING SUMMARY

No reports describing the use of patiromer during human lactation have been located. Patiromer is not absorbed systemically; therefore, it is not expected to appear in breast milk.

Reference

1. Prescribing Information. Veltassa. Vifor Pharma, Inc; 2023.

PATISIRAN

Immunologic (Small Interfering Ribonucleic Acid—Amyloidosis)

PREGNANCY RECOMMENDATION: No Human Data—Animal Data Suggest Low Risk

BREASTFEEDING RECOMMENDATION: Probably Compatible

PREGNANCY SUMMARY

No reports describing the use of patisiran in human pregnancy have been located. Placental transfer and embryofetal exposure are likely to be negligible. However, the absence of human pregnancy experience prevents a complete assessment of the embryofetal risk. Animal data did not show any embryofetal toxicity. Using this drug during pregnancy should be based on the pros and cons of the mother's clinical need for treatment versus any potential fetal risk that might occur from exposure. Patisiran can decrease vitamin A levels. Therefore, if used during pregnancy, it is imperative that patients use prenatal vitamins with the recommended amount of vitamin A. Excess vitamin A can be teratogenic; therefore, excess vitamin A intake beyond what is recommended for pregnancy is not indicated.

BREASTFEEDING SUMMARY

Patisiran excretion into human breast milk is likely to be negligible. Breastfeeding while using this drug should be based on the mother's clinical need for treatment. If used, the infant should be monitored for the most common reported adult side effect of upper respiratory tract infections.

Reference

1. Prescribing Information. Onpattro. Alnylam Pharmaceuticals, Inc; 2018.

PAZOPANIB

Antineoplastic (Kinase Inhibitor)

PREGNANCY RECOMMENDATION: No Human Data—Animal Data Suggest Risk

BREASTFEEDING RECOMMENDATION: Potential Toxicity

PREGNANCY SUMMARY

No reports describing the use of pazopanib in human pregnancy have been located. The drug will probably cross the placenta, so some fetal exposure will likely occur. Therefore, the absence of human pregnancy experience prevents a complete assessment of the embryofetal risk. Embryofetal toxicity with malformations was observed in two animal species at doses of less than the MRHD, one that also had maternal toxicity. Based on animal studies and the drug's mechanism of action, the manufacturer recommends that women with reproductive potential use effective contraception during treatment and for 2 weeks after the last dose. They also recommend that males with female partners of reproductive potential use effective

(*continued*)

contraception during treatment and for 2 weeks after the last dose. Nevertheless, using this drug during pregnancy should be based on the pros and cons of the mother's clinical need for treatment versus any potential fetal risk that might occur from exposure. There is a registry for women who are pregnant and have cancer. For more information, women and health care providers are encouraged to contact the Cancer and Pregnancy Registry at 1-877-635-4499. Hypertension was reported in up to 40% of patients treated with this drug in clinical trials. Pazopanib can also prolong the QT interval.

BREASTFEEDING SUMMARY

No reports describing the use of pazopanib during human lactation have been located. The drug will likely be excreted into human breast milk, so some infant exposure will likely occur. However, due to a concern for potential serious adverse effects that might be seen in a breastfed infant, the manufacturer recommends that women not breastfeed while being treated with this drug and for at least 2 weeks after the last dose. Nevertheless, if the clinical decision is to use this drug while breastfeeding, the infant should be monitored for the most common reported adult side effects of nausea, musculoskeletal pain, and headache (all leading to irritability), hypertension, hair color changes (depigmentation), decreased appetite (monitor infant growth), vomiting, fatigue (lethargy), diarrhea, and dyspnea.

Reference

1. Prescribing Information. Pazopanib. Novugen Pharma (USA) LLC; 2024.

PEGCETACOPLAN

Immunologic (Complement C3 Inhibitor)

PREGNANCY RECOMMENDATION: **No Human Data—Animal Data Suggest Potential Risk**

BREASTFEEDING RECOMMENDATION: **Probably Compatible**

PREGNANCY SUMMARY

No reports describing the use of pegcetacoplan in human pregnancy have been located. The drug is not likely to cross the placenta; however, because it consists of proteins, it is not known whether some fetal exposure could occur. Therefore, the absence of human pregnancy experience prevents a complete assessment of the embryofetal risk. Embryofetal toxicity was observed in animal studies. Because of the potential for embryofetal harm, the manufacturer recommends that women with reproductive potential use effective contraception during treatment and for at least 40 days after the last dose. Nevertheless, using this drug during pregnancy should be based on the pros and cons of the mother's clinical need for treatment versus any potential fetal risk that might occur from exposure. During pregnancy, paroxysmal nocturnal hemoglobin has been associated with thrombotic events, infections, bleeding, increased maternal mortality, spontaneous abortion, stillbirth, and premature delivery.

P

BREASTFEEDING SUMMARY

No reports describing the use of pegcetacoplan during human lactation have been located. It is unlikely that the drug will be excreted into breast milk. However, because the active portion of the drug is two peptides, if these peptides were to be ingested through breastfeeding, they would probably be digested in the infant's gastrointestinal tract and not be absorbed. Regardless, due to the potential for serious adverse effects that might be seen in a breastfed infant, the manufacturer recommends that women not breastfeed while taking pegcetacoplan and for 40 days after the last dose. Nevertheless, breastfeeding while using this drug should be based on the mother's clinical need for treatment. If used, the infant should be monitored for the most common reported adult side effects of abdominal pain (leading to irritability), infections, lethargy, and diarrhea.

Reference

1. Prescribing Information. Empaveli. Apellis Pharmaceuticals; 2021.

PEGFILGRASTIM

Hematologic (Leukocyte Growth Factor)

PREGNANCY RECOMMENDATION: **No Human Data—Animal Data Suggest Potential Risk**

BREASTFEEDING RECOMMENDATION: **Probably Compatible**

PREGNANCY SUMMARY

No reports describing the use of pegfilgrastim in human pregnancy have been located. Pegfilgrastim is a covalent conjugate of mono-methoxypolyethylene glycol and filgrastim, which is a 175-amino acid protein. Filgrastim reaches the fetus late in gestation in amounts sufficient to produce a biologic effect (see Filgrastim). The molecular weight (MW) of pegfilgrastim is twice that of filgrastim because of the polyethylene glycol portion. The addition of this non-amino acid moiety may prevent the transfer of pegfilgrastim in amounts sufficient to produce a biologic effect in the fetus. However, the absence of human pregnancy experience prevents a complete assessment of embryofetal risk. Animal data did show some embryofetal toxicity in one species at doses of less than 10 times the MRHD, but not in a second species at doses of 10 times the MRHD. Using this drug during pregnancy should be based on the pros and cons of the mother's clinical need for treatment versus any potential fetal risk that might occur from exposure. Filgrastim has been used in pregnancy without apparent fetal harm. Therefore, until human data are available, filgrastim might be preferred over pegfilgrastim in pregnancy. There is a registry for women who are pregnant and have cancer. For more information, women and health care providers are encouraged to contact the Cancer and Pregnancy Registry at 1-877-635-4499.

BREASTFEEDING SUMMARY

No reports describing the use of pegfilgrastim during human lactation have been located. Pegfilgrastim is composed of mono-methoxypolyethylene glycol and filgrastim that are chemically bound together. This produces a compound with a high MW, suggesting that excretion into breast milk is likely to be clinically insignificant. However, if it were to be found in human breast milk, the filgrastim portion would probably be digested in the infant's gastrointestinal tract and not be absorbed. Breastfeeding while using this drug should be based on the mother's clinical need for treatment versus any potential infant risks that might occur. If used, the infant should be monitored for the most common reported adult side effects of bone pain and extremity pain (both leading to irritability).

Reference

1. Prescribing Information. Fulphila. Biocon Biologics Inc; 2023.

PEGINTERFERON BETA-1A

Immunologic (Interferon)

PREGNANCY RECOMMENDATION: Limited Human Data—Animal Data Suggest Potential Risk

BREASTFEEDING RECOMMENDATION: Probably Compatible

PREGNANCY SUMMARY

One report describing the use of peginterferon beta-1a in human pregnancy was located. The study retrospectively evaluated pregnancy outcomes in patients with relapsing-remitting multiple sclerosis treated with interferon products before or during pregnancy. There were 426 women with 542 pregnancies included in the analysis. Of the total 424 live births, malformations were observed in 2.8%. Peginterferon beta-1a exposure occurred in 233 pregnancies (excluding elective terminations). In this exposed group, there were 37 (15.9%) spontaneous abortions, and there were 3 (1.5%) congenital anomalies in the 196 live births. Because it is a glycosylated protein, the drug may cross the placenta in the third trimester. However, the overall amount should be clinically insignificant. Nevertheless, the limited human pregnancy experience prevents a complete assessment of embryofetal risk. No animal reproduction studies have been located. However, peginterferon beta-1a showed abortifacient activity in pregnant monkeys after three to five doses (dosage not provided). Therefore, using this drug during pregnancy should be based on the pros and cons of the mother's clinical need for treatment versus any potential fetal risk that might occur from exposure.

BREASTFEEDING SUMMARY

Two reports describing the use of peginterferon beta-1a during human lactation have been located. In one publication, 72 and 66 women breastfed while using peginterferon beta-1a and intramuscular (IM) administration of interferon beta-1a, respectively. No adverse infant effects were reported in the peginterferon beta-1a group. The drug may be excreted into human breast milk, but the overall amount should be negligible. However, even if some amount of the drug were to be found in breast milk, because it is a protein, it would probably be digested in the infant's gastrointestinal tract and not be absorbed. Breastfeeding while using this drug should be based on the mother's clinical need for treatment versus any potential infant risks that might occur. If used, the infant should be monitored for the most common reported adult side effects of headache, myalgia, and arthralgia (all leading to irritability), fatigue (lethargy), and pyrexia.

References

1. Prescribing Information. Plegridy. Biogen Inc; 2023.

P

2. Klehmet J, Begus-Nahrmann Y, Taipale K, et al. Pregnancy outcomes in female multiple sclerosis patients exposed to intramuscular interferon beta-1a or peginterferon beta-1a reported in a German patient support programme—results from the non-interventional post-authorization safety study PRIMA. *Ther Adv Neurol Disord*. 2023;16:1-14.
3. Klehmet J, Begus-Nahrmann Y, Taipale K, et al. Impact of interferon beta exposure on birth outcome and child development-results from the post-authorisation safety study PRIMA. *Mult Scler Relat Disord*. 2023; 77:104844.

PEGLOTICASE

Endocrine/Metabolic (Antigout)

PREGNANCY RECOMMENDATION: No Human Data and No Relevant Animal Data

BREASTFEEDING RECOMMENDATION: Probably Compatible

PREGNANCY SUMMARY

No reports describing the use of pegloticase in human pregnancy have been located. The drug is not likely to cross the placenta in clinically significant amounts. However, the absence of human pregnancy experience prevents a complete assessment of embryofetal risk. Animal data did show embryofetal toxicity in two species, but at doses well above 10 times the MRHD. Using this drug during pregnancy should be based on the pros and cons of the mother's clinical need for treatment versus any potential fetal risk that might occur from exposure.

BREASTFEEDING SUMMARY

No reports describing the use of pegloticase during human lactation have been located. The drug is not likely to be excreted into human breast milk in clinically significant amounts. However, because it is a protein, if the drug were to be ingested through breastfeeding, it would probably be digested in the infant's gastrointestinal tract and not be absorbed. Regardless, the manufacturer recommends that pegloticase should not be used during breastfeeding unless the clear benefit to the mother can overcome the unknown risk to the newborn/infant. Nevertheless, if the clinical decision is to use this drug while breastfeeding, the infant should be monitored for the most common reported adult side effects of nausea and chest pain (both leading to irritability), ecchymosis, constipation, flushing, rash, and vomiting.

References

1. Prescribing Information. Krystexxa. Horizon Therapeutics USA Inc; 2022.
2. Sundy JS, Ganson NJ, Kelly SJ, et al. Pharmacokinetics and pharmacodynamics of intravenous PEGylated recombinant mammalian urate oxidase in patients with refractory gout. *Arthritis Rheum*. 2007;56:1021-1028.
3. Yue CS, Huang W, Alton M, et al. Population pharmacokinetic and pharmacodynamic analysis of pegloticase in subjects with hyperuricemia and treatment-failure gout. *J Clin Pharmacol*. 2008;48:708-718.

PEGULICIANINE

Miscellaneous (Optical Imaging Agent)

PREGNANCY RECOMMENDATION: No Human Data and No Relevant Animal Data

BREASTFEEDING RECOMMENDATION: Probably Compatible

PREGNANCY SUMMARY

No reports describing the use of pegulicianine in human pregnancy have been located. Though placental transfer may be possible, fetal exposure should be minimal. However, the absence of human pregnancy experience prevents a complete assessment of the embryofetal risk. Animal reproduction and fertility studies have not been conducted. Using this product during pregnancy should be based on the pros and cons of the mother's clinical need for treatment versus any potential fetal risk that might occur from exposure.

BREASTFEEDING SUMMARY

It is not known if pegulicianine is excreted into human breast milk. Negligible amounts of the drug should be found in breast milk. However, until further studies are performed, breast milk excretion is not known. Breastfeeding while using this drug should be based on the mother's clinical need for treatment versus any potential infant risks that might occur. If used, the infant should be monitored for the most common reported adult systemic side effects of pruritus (leading to irritability), blue-green discoloration of urine, rash, flushing, and wheezing.

Reference

1. Prescribing Information. Lumisight. Lumicell; 2024.

PEGUNIGALSIDASE ALFA

Genetic/Central Nervous System (Enzyme—Fabry Disease)

PREGNANCY RECOMMENDATION: No Human Data—Animal Data Suggest Low Risk

BREASTFEEDING RECOMMENDATION: Probably Compatible

PREGNANCY SUMMARY

No reports describing the use of pegunigalsidase alfa in human pregnancy have been located. The drug is not likely to cross the placenta; however, because it consists of a protein, it is not known whether some fetal exposure could occur. Therefore, the absence of human pregnancy experience prevents a complete assessment of the embryofetal risk. Animal studies did not show any embryofetal toxicity at doses that did not produce maternal toxicity. There is a pregnancy safety study for exposure to pegunigalsidase alfa during pregnancy. Health care providers are encouraged to call 1-888-661-9260.

BREASTFEEDING SUMMARY

No reports describing the use of pegunigalsidase alfa during human lactation have been located. The drug most likely will not appear in breast milk. Furthermore, because it is an enzyme, if any drug were to be present in breast milk, it would most likely be digested in the infant's gastrointestinal tract and not be absorbed. Breastfeeding while using this drug should be based on the mother's clinical need for treatment. If used, the infant should be monitored for the most common reported adult side effects of headache, nausea, back pain, and extremity pain (all leading to irritability), lethargy, diarrhea, and nasopharyngitis.

Reference

1. Prescribing Information. Elfabrio. Chiesi Farmaceutici S.p.A; 2023.

PEGVALIASE

Genetic (Phenylalanine-Metabolizing Enzyme—PKU)

PREGNANCY RECOMMENDATION: Limited Human Data—Animal Data Suggest Low Risk

BREASTFEEDING RECOMMENDATION: Probably Compatible

PREGNANCY SUMMARY

A case report of a patient with phenylketonuria (PKU) who used pegvaliase throughout the pregnancy delivered at term with no anomalies identified. The newborn had a normal head circumference and was discharged with the mother in good condition. The patient elected not to breastfeed. The pegvaliase level at birth was not evaluated. In a designated clinic for using pegvaliase in patients with PKU, three pregnancies were reported in two women, and all were spontaneously lost in the first trimester. Transplacental passage of this drug should be minimal, and therefore, fetal exposure during pregnancy should be negligible. Conversely, uncontrolled PKU during pregnancy (blood phenylalanine levels above 600-900 mcmol/L) can lead to birth anomalies of microcephaly and heart defects with a risk for future developmental delays. The goal of managing pregnant patients with PKU is to keep the phenylalanine level at 120 to 360 mcmol/L (and some medical opinions describe even tighter parameters). No embryofetal toxicity was found in relevant animal studies. There is a Palynziq pregnancy surveillance program for women who are exposed to this drug during pregnancy or who become pregnant within 1 month following the last dose that monitors pregnancy outcomes. Health care providers are encouraged to call 1-866-906-6100.

BREASTFEEDING SUMMARY

Two case reports of pegvaliase use during lactation have been reported in the same patient. Four breast milk samples were tested (one in the patient's first pregnancy after she discontinued breastfeeding, and three samples in her second pregnancy while breastfeeding her child). All four samples were negative for pegvaliase. This is consistent with what would be expected based on the MW of the drug. Furthermore, the enzyme portion of the drug, if excreted into breast milk, should be digested in the infant's gastrointestinal tract and not be absorbed. However, the use of pegvaliase while breastfeeding theoretically might result in low phenylalanine levels in breast milk. Phenylalanine levels were tested in the three samples from the patient's second pregnancy, discussed above. Overall, the phenylalanine levels were lower when compared to three control breast milk samples but not significantly different. However, only three samples were tested. Breastfeeding while using this drug should be based on the mother's clinical need for treatment. If used, the infant should be monitored for the most common reported adult side effects of arthralgias, headache, abdominal pain, oropharyngeal pain, pruritus, and nausea (all leading to irritability), vomiting, cough, diarrhea, and lethargy. In addition, phenylalanine levels should periodically be monitored in the infant.

References

1. Prescribing Information. Palynziq. BioMarin Pharmaceutical, Inc; 2018.
2. Boyer M, Skaar J, Sowa M, et al. Continuation of pegvaliase treatment during pregnancy: a case report. *Mol Genet Metab Rep*. 2021;26:100713.
3. Lah M, McPheron M. Palynziq clinic: one year and 43 patients later. *Mol Genet Metab*. 2021;133:250-256.
4. Rouse B, Azen C, Koch R, et al. Maternal phenylketonuria collaborative study (MPKUCS) offspring: facial anomalies, malformations, and early neurological sequela. *Am J Med Genet*. 1997;69:89-95.
5. Yano S, Moseley K, Bottiglieri T, et al. Maternal phenylketonuria international collaborative study revisited: evaluation of maternal nutritional risk factors besides phenylalanine for fetal congenital heart defects. *J Inherit Metab Dis*. 2014;37:39-42.
6. Rohr F, Kritzer A, Harding CO, et al. Discontinuation of pegvaliase therapy during maternal PKU pregnancy and postnatal breastfeeding: a case report. *Mol Genet Metab Rep*. 2020;22:100555.
7. Rohr F, Wessel A, Harding CO, et al. Restitution of pegvaliase therapy during lactation. *Mol Genet Metab Rep*. 2022;33:100938.

PEGVISOMANT

Endocrine/Metabolic (Growth Hormone Receptor Antagonist)

PREGNANCY RECOMMENDATION: Limited Human Data—Animal Data Suggest Potential Risk

BREASTFEEDING RECOMMENDATION: Probably Compatible

PREGNANCY SUMMARY

Two reports describing the use of pegvisomant in human pregnancy have been located. Both were exposed at conception, and one continued the drug through to delivery. No fetal malformations were described. The drug is not likely to cross the placenta in clinically significant amounts. However, because it consists of a protein, it is not known whether some fetal exposure could occur in the second half of gestation. Nevertheless, the absence of human pregnancy experience prevents a complete assessment of the embryofetal risk. Embryofetal toxicity was observed in one animal species at doses of less than 10 times the MRHD. Using this drug during pregnancy should be based on the pros and cons of the mother's clinical need for treatment versus any potential fetal risk that might occur from exposure.

BREASTFEEDING SUMMARY

One report was located that described the use of pegvisomant during human lactation. The mother was receiving 25 mg/d of the protein, and breast milk concentrations were undetectable (LLQ 50 ng/mL). The timing of the sample relative to the last dose or the time after birth was not reported. Regardless, even if some amount of the drug were to be excreted into breast milk, it would most likely be digested in the infant's gastrointestinal tract and not be absorbed. Breastfeeding while using this drug should be based on the mother's clinical need for treatment versus any potential infant risks that might occur. If used, the infant should be monitored for the most common reported adult side effects of nausea and joint pain (both leading to irritability), infection, diarrhea, abnormal liver function tests, and fatigue (lethargy).

References

1. Prescribing Information. Somavert. Pharmacia & Upjohn Company LLC; 2023.
2. Qureshi A, Kalu E, Ramanathan G, et al. IVF/ICSI in a woman with active acromegaly: successful outcome following treatment with pegvisomant. *J Assist Reprod Genet*. 2006;23:439-442.
3. Brian SR, Bidlingmaier M, Wajnrajch MP, et al. Treatment of acromegaly with pegvisomant during pregnancy: maternal and fetal effects. *J Clin Endocrinol Metab*. 2007;92:3374-3377.
4. Biermasz NR, Romijn JA, Pereira AM, Roelfsema F. Current pharmacotherapy for acromegaly: a review. *Expert Opin Pharmacother*. 2005;6:2393-2405.

PEMBROLIZUMAB

Antineoplastic (Monoclonal Antibody—Programmed Death Receptor Blocking Antibody)

PREGNANCY RECOMMENDATION: Limited Human Data—No Relevant Animal Data

BREASTFEEDING RECOMMENDATION: Potential Toxicity

PREGNANCY SUMMARY

Two case reports describing the use of pembrolizumab in human pregnancy were located. One exposure was at conception, and no adverse pregnancy or fetal effects were described. The other exposure started at 16 weeks' gestation with a last dose at 34 weeks' gestation. No fetal malformations or adverse effects were seen until 4 months of age, when the infant was hospitalized for severe immune-related gastroenterocolitis that was thought to be due to pembrolizumab exposure in utero. However, at that time, more than six half-lives had occurred from the last dose, so pembrolizumab should no longer be in the infant's system. The drug crosses the placenta. Infant blood concentrations about 7 days postdelivery were between 35 and 42 mcg/mL. However, the limited human pregnancy experience prevents a complete assessment of embryofetal risk. Animal reproduction studies have not been located. The programmed death receptor 1 (PD-1)/PD ligand 1 (PD-L1) pathway preserves pregnancy by maintaining maternal immune tolerance to the fetus. However, in PD-1 knockout mice, immune-mediated disorders have occurred, but no malformations. Based on the drug's mechanism of action, the manufacturer recommends that women with reproductive potential use effective contraception during treatment and for 4 months after the last dose. Nevertheless, using this drug during pregnancy should be based on the pros and cons of the mother's clinical need for treatment versus any potential fetal risk that might occur from exposure. There is a registry for women who are pregnant and have cancer. For more information, women and health care providers are encouraged to contact the Cancer and Pregnancy Registry at 1-877-635-4499.

BREASTFEEDING SUMMARY

No reports describing the use of pembrolizumab during human lactation have been located. It is known that IgG antibodies can be found in human breast milk but are not found in the neonatal or infant circulation. Additionally, if any IgG antibodies were to be ingested through breastfeeding, they would probably be digested in the infant's gastrointestinal tract and not be absorbed. However, due to a concern for potential serious adverse effects that might be seen in a breastfed infant, the manufacturer recommends that women not breastfeed while being treated with this drug and for at least 4 months after the last dose. Nevertheless, if the clinical decision is to use this drug while breastfeeding, the infant should be monitored for the most common reported adult side effects of musculoskeletal pain, abdominal pain, pruritus, and nausea (all leading to irritability), fatigue (lethargy), diarrhea, pyrexia, cough, decreased appetite (monitor infant growth), constipation, and decreased thyroid hormone levels.

References

1. Prescribing Information. Keytruda. Merck Sharp & Dohme LLC; 2024.
2. Baarslag MA, Heimovaara JH, Borgers JSW, et al. Severe immune-related enteritis after in utero exposure to pembrolizumab. *N Engl J Med*. 2023; 389:790-796.
3. Polnaszek B, Mullen M, Bligard K, et al. Term pregnancy after complete response of placental site trophoblastic tumor to immunotherapy. *Obstet Gynecol*. 2021;138:115-118.

PEMETREXED

Antineoplastic (Folate Analogue Metabolic Inhibitor)

PREGNANCY RECOMMENDATION: No Human Data—Animal Data Suggest Potential Risk

BREASTFEEDING RECOMMENDATION: Potential Toxicity

P

PREGNANCY SUMMARY

No reports describing the use of pemetrexed in human pregnancy have been located. The drug will probably cross the placenta, so some fetal exposure will likely occur. Therefore, the absence of human pregnancy experience prevents a complete assessment of the embryofetal risk. Embryofetal toxicity was observed in one animal species (only one species tested) at doses less than the RHD. Based on animal studies and the drug's mechanism of action, the manufacturer recommends that women with reproductive potential use effective contraception during treatment and for 6 months after the last dose. They also recommend that males with female partners of reproductive potential use effective contraception during treatment and for 3 months after the last dose. Nevertheless, using this drug during pregnancy should be based on the pros and cons of the mother's clinical need for treatment versus any potential fetal risk that might occur from exposure. There is a registry for women who are pregnant and have cancer. For more information, women and health care providers are encouraged to contact the Cancer and Pregnancy Registry at 1-877-635-4499. Hypertension was reported in up to 11% of patients treated with this drug in clinical trials.

BREASTFEEDING SUMMARY

No reports describing the use of pemetrexed during human lactation have been located. The drug will likely be excreted into breast milk, so some infant exposure will probably occur. However, due to a concern for potential serious adverse effects that might be seen in a breastfed infant, the manufacturer recommends that women not breastfeed while being treated with this drug and for at least 1 week after the last dose. Nevertheless, breastfeeding while using this drug should be based on the mother's clinical need for treatment versus any potential infant risks that might occur. If used, the infant should be monitored for the most common reported adult side effects of nausea (leading to irritability), fatigue (lethargy), and anorexia (monitor infant growth).

References

1. Prescribing Information. Pemetrexed dipotassium. Avyxa Pharma LLC; 2024.
2. Prescribing Information. Pemetrexed disodium. Dr. Reddy's Laboratories Inc; 2022.

PEMIGATINIB

Antineoplastic (Kinase Inhibitor)

PREGNANCY RECOMMENDATION: No Human Data—Animal Data Suggest Potential Risk

BREASTFEEDING RECOMMENDATION: Potential Toxicity

PREGNANCY SUMMARY

No reports describing the use of pemigatinib in human pregnancy have been located. The drug will probably cross the placenta, so some fetal exposure will likely occur. Therefore, the absence of human pregnancy experience prevents a complete assessment of the embryofetal risk. Animal studies showed embryofetal toxicity. Based on these animal studies and the drug's mechanism of action, the manufacturer recommends that women with reproductive potential use effective contraception during treatment and for 1 week after the last dose. They also recommend that males with female partners of reproductive potential use effective contraception during treatment and for 1 week after the last dose. Nevertheless, using this drug during pregnancy should be based on the pros and cons of the mother's clinical need for treatment versus any potential fetal risk that might occur from exposure.

BREASTFEEDING SUMMARY

No reports describing the use of pemigatinib during human lactation have been located. The drug will probably be excreted into breast milk, so some infant exposure will likely occur. However, due to the concern for potential serious adverse effects in a breastfed infant, the manufacturer recommends that women not breastfeed while being treated with this drug and for at least 1 week after the last dose. Nevertheless, if the clinical decision is to use this drug while breastfeeding, the infant should be monitored for the most common reported adult side effects of abdominal pain, back pain, arthralgias, and nausea (all leading to irritability), vomiting, diarrhea, constipation, lethargy, decreased appetite, alopecia, and dry skin.

Reference

1. Prescribing Information. Pemazyre. Incyte Corporation; 2021.

PENCICLOVIR

Antiviral (Herpes Simplex Virus Types 1 and 2)

PREGNANCY RECOMMENDATION: Limited Human Data—No Relevant Animal Data

BREASTFEEDING RECOMMENDATION: Probably Compatible

P

PREGNANCY SUMMARY

One report describing the use of penciclovir in human pregnancy was located. First-trimester exposure to penciclovir topical cream (n = 118) was not associated with a significant risk for congenital malformations (4.2% vs 2.4%, respectively) when compared to unexposed controls. Penciclovir cream is not systemically absorbed in clinically significant amounts after topical administration, so any amount at the placental interface is likely to be negligible. However, this limited human pregnancy experience prevents a complete assessment of embryofetal risk. No animal reproduction studies have been conducted. Using this drug during pregnancy should be based on the pros and cons of the mother's clinical need for treatment versus any potential fetal risk that might occur from exposure.

BREASTFEEDING SUMMARY

No reports describing the use of penciclovir during human lactation have been located. Since the topical cream is not systemically absorbed at levels that could be detected, breastfeeding is not expected to result in any clinically significant exposure to the infant. Breastfeeding while using this drug should be based on the mother's clinical need for treatment versus any potential infant risks that might occur. Due to the topical use of the drug, systemic side effects were not evaluated.

Reference

1. Prescribing Information. Penciclovir. Padagis Israel Pharmaceuticals Ltd; 2024.

PENICILLAMINE

Chelating Agent

PREGNANCY RECOMMENDATION: *Limited Human Data—Animal Data Suggest Potential Risk

BREASTFEEDING RECOMMENDATION: Probably Compatible

PREGNANCY SUMMARY

Several reports describing the use of penicillamine in human pregnancy have been located. Over 100 mothers were treated for rheumatoid arthritis, cystinuria, or Wilson disease. Most of the pregnancies resulted in healthy newborns who developed normally. *However, the manufacturer reported that characteristics for congenital cutis laxa and other associated malformations have been reported after penicillamine pregnancy exposure. The drug crosses the placenta, so some fetal exposure will occur. However, the limited human pregnancy experience prevents a complete assessment of embryofetal risk. Embryofetal toxicity was observed in one animal species at doses of less than 10 times the MRHD. Using this drug during pregnancy should be based on the pros and cons of the mother's clinical need for treatment versus any potential fetal risk that might occur from exposure. *Congenital cutis laxa is a rare genetic disorder that produces an inelastic property to the skin, resulting in looseness and sagginess. It has been reported as autosomal recessive and X-linked recessive. There is also an autosomal dominant form that is often a new mutation. At least five of these cases were reported in studies, mostly from the 1970s. Other, more recent, larger evaluations on the use of penicillamine in pregnancy have not found this disorder. The manufacturer recommends that penicillamine should only be used in women of childbearing potential when the expected benefits outweigh the possible hazards. In Wilson disease, continuing penicillamine during pregnancy can protect the mother against relapse, and discontinuation can have deleterious effects on the mother, some of which are fatal. The manufacturer recommends limiting the dose to 750 mg daily during pregnancy, if possible.

BREASTFEEDING SUMMARY

A few studies were located that describe the use of penicillamine during human lactation. In eleven lactating women being treated with the drug for Wilson disease, no breast milk samples had detectable drug concentrations. Overall, no adverse effects in infants were reported. However, due to a concern for potential serious adverse effects that might be seen in a breastfed infant, the manufacturer recommends that women not breastfeed while being treated with this drug. Nevertheless, breastfeeding while using this drug should be based on the mother's clinical need for treatment versus any potential infant risks that might occur. If used, the infant should be monitored for the most common reported adult side effects of epigastric pain and nausea (leading to irritability), anorexia (monitor infant growth), vomiting, and diarrhea.

References

1. Prescribing Information. Penicillamine. Ani Pharmaceuticals Inc; 2024.
2. Crawhall JC, Scowen EF, Thompson CJ, Watts RWE. Dissolution of cystine stones during d-penicillamine treatment of a pregnant patient with cystinuria. *Br Med J*. 1967;2:216-218.
3. Marecek Z, Graf M. Pregnancy in penicillamine-treated patients with Wilson's disease. *N Engl J Med*. 1976;295:841-842.
4. Endres W. D-penicillamine in pregnancy—to ban or not to ban? *Klin Wochenschr*. 1981;59:535-537.
5. Mjolnerod OK, Rasmussen K, Dommerud SA, Gjeruldsen ST. Congenital connective-tissue defect probably due to d-penicillamine treatment in pregnancy. *Lancet*. 1971;1:673–675.
6. Laver M, Fairley KF. D-penicillamine treatment in pregnancy. *Lancet*. 1971; 1:1019-1020.
7. Scheinberg IH, Sternlieb I. Pregnancy in penicillamine-treated patients with Wilson's disease. *N Engl J Med*. 1975;293:1300-1303.
8. Solomon L, Abrams G, Dinner M, Berman L. Neonatal abnormalities associated with d-penicillamine treatment during pregnancy. *N Engl J Med*. 1977;296:54-55.
9. Walshe JM. Pregnancy in Wilson's disease. *Q J Med*. 1977;46:73-83.
10. Lyle WH. Penicillamine in pregnancy. *Lancet*. 1978;1:606-607.
11. Linares A, Zarranz JJ, Rodriguez-Alarcon J, Diaz-Perez JL. Reversible cutis laxa due to maternal d-penicillamine treatment. *Lancet*. 1979;2:43.
12. Harpey JP, Jaudon MC, Clavel JP, et al. Cutis laxa and low serum zinc after antenatal exposure to penicillamine. *Lancet*. 1983;2:858.
13. Beck RB, Rosenbaum KN, Byers PH, Holbrook KA, Perry LW. Ultrastructural findings in the fetal penicillamine syndrome (abstract). Paper presented at: The 13th Annual Birth Defects Conference; June 1980; March of Dimes and University of California, San Diego.
14. Gal P, Ravenel SD. Contractures and hydrocephalus with penicillamine and maternal hypotension. *J Clin Dysmorphol*. 1984;2:9-12.
15. Gregory MC, Mansell MA. Pregnancy and cystinuria. *Lancet*. 1983;2:1158-1160.
16. Dupont P, Irion O, Béguin F. Pregnancy in a patient with treated Wilson's disease: a case report. *Am J Obstet Gynecol*. 1990;163:1527-1528.
17. Hartard C, Kunze K. Pregnancy in a patient with Wilson's disease treated with D-penicillamine and zinc sulfate. *Eur Neurol*. 1994;34:337-340.
18. Berghella V, Steele D, Spector T, et al. Successful pregnancy in a neurologically impaired woman with Wilson's disease. *Am J Obstet Gynecol*. 1997; 176:712-714.
19. Martinez-Frias ML, Rodriguez-Pinilla E, Bermejo E, Blanco M. Prenatal exposure to penicillamine and oral clefts: case report. *Am J Med Genet*. 1998;76:274-275.
20. Sternlieb I. Wilson's disease and pregnancy. *Hepatology*. 2000;31:531-532.
21. Nunns D, Hawthorne B, Goulding P, Maresh M. Wilson's disease in pregnancy. *Eur J Obstet Gynecol Reprod Biol*. 1995;62:141-143.
22. Oga M, Matsui N, Anai T, et al. Copper disposition of the fetus and placenta in a patient with untreated Wilson's disease. *Am J Obstet Gynecol*. 1993;169:196-198.
23. Demir K, Soyer OM, Karaca C, Besisk F, Kaymakoglu S, Besisik F. The course of pregnancy in Wilson's disease—one center, 20 years' experience (Abstract). *Gastroenterology*. 2014;146:S1009.
24. Dathe K, Beck E, Schaefer C. Pregnancy outcome after chelation therapy in Wilson disease. Evaluation of the German Embryotox Database. *Reprod Toxicol*. 2016;65:39-45.
25. European Association for the Study of the Liver. EASL clinical practice guidelines: Wilson's disease. *J Hepatol*. 2012;56:671-685.

P

PENICILLIN G/PENICILLIN G BENZATHINE/PENICILLIN V

Antibiotic (Penicillins)

PREGNANCY RECOMMENDATION: Human Data Suggest Compatible

BREASTFEEDING RECOMMENDATION: Probably Compatible

PREGNANCY SUMMARY

There are several reports describing the use of basic penicillins in human pregnancy. There are several formulations that include penicillin G (parenteral, aqueous), penicillin G benzathine (IM, suspension), and penicillin V (oral). Penicillin G is used routinely for maternal infections during pregnancy (commonly group G *Streptococcus* prophylaxis). The Collaborative Perinatal Project reported 88 (2.5%) major anomalies in 3,546 first-trimester exposures to basic penicillin derivatives. No pattern to the defects was seen. For penicillin V, two large databases, the Michigan Medicaid Surveillance study and the Group Health Cooperative of Puget Sound, reported 210 (4.0%) major birth anomalies (210 expected) in 5,243 first-trimester exposures. Again, no pattern to the defects was identified. These penicillins rapidly cross the placenta, with cord blood and maternal blood concentrations about equal. Animal data did not show any increased risk for embryofetal toxicity in three species. Using these drugs during pregnancy should be based on the pros and cons of the mother's clinical need for treatment versus any potential fetal risk that might occur from exposure.

BREASTFEEDING SUMMARY

These penicillins are excreted into human breast milk, so infant exposure will occur. Breast milk to maternal plasma ratios following IM benzathine doses appear to be lower than those obtained with IV or oral use. The oral and IV forms can be used in newborns and infants. Overall, no adverse infant effects have been reported, though there is a risk for modification of bowel flora. Breastfeeding while using this drug should be based on the mother's clinical need for treatment versus any potential infant risks that might occur. If used, the infant should be monitored for the most common reported adult side effects of nausea, headache, and myalgia (all leading to irritability), rash, and diarrhea.

P

References

1. Penicillin V potassium. Penicillin G potassium. Athenix Pharmaceutical Division LLC; 2025.
2. Penicillin V potassium. Lentocilin. Laboratorios Atral SA; 2024.
3. Penicillin V potassium. Aurobindo Pharm Limited; 2022.
4. Herrel W, Nichols D, Heilman D. Penicillin: its usefulness, limitations, diffusion and detection, with analysis of 150 cases in which it was employed. *JAMA*. 1944;125:1003-1011.
5. Woltz J, Zintel H. The transmission of penicillin to amniotic fluid and fetal blood in the human. *Am J Obstet Gynecol*. 1945;50:338-340.
6. Hutter A, Parks J. The transmission of penicillin through the placenta. A preliminary report. *Am J Obstet Gynecol*. 1945;49:663-665.
7. Woltz J, Wiley M. The transmission of penicillin to the previable fetus. *JAMA*. 1946;131:969-970.
8. Wasz-Hockert O, Nummi S, Vuopala S, Jarvinen P. Transplacental passage of azidocillin, ampicillin and penicillin G during early and late pregnancy. *Acta Paediatr Scand (Suppl)*. 1970;206:109-110.
9. Lentz J, Ingraham N Jr, Beerman H, Stokes J. Penicillin in the prevention and treatment of congenital syphilis. *JAMA*. 1944;126:408-413.
10. Leavitt H. Clinical action of penicillin on the uterus. *J Vener Dis Inf*. 1945;26:150-153.
11. McLachlan A, Brown D. The effects of penicillin administration on menstrual and other sexual functions. *Br J Vener Dis*. 1947;23:1-10.
12. Mazingarbe A. Le pencilline possede-t-elle une action abortive? *Gynecol Obstet*. 1946;45:487.
13. Perin L, Sissmann R, Detre F, Chertier A. La pencilline a-t-elle une action abortive? *Bull Soc Fr Dermatol*. 1950;57:534-538.
14. Kosim H. Intrauterine fetal death as a result of anaphylactic reaction to penicillin in a pregnant woman. *Dapim Refuiim*. 1959;18:136-137.
15. Nathan L, Bawdon RE, Sidawi JE, Stettler RW, McIntire DM, Wendel GD Jr. Penicillin levels following the administration of benzathine penicillin G in pregnancy. *Obstet Gynecol*. 1993;82:338-342.
16. Carter M, Wilson F. Antibiotics and congenital malformations. *Lancet*. 1963;1:1267-1268.
17. Carter M, Wilson F. Antibiotics in early pregnancy and congenital malformations. *Dev Med Child Neurol*. 1965;7:353-359.
18. Khudr G, Olding L. Cyclopia. *Am J Dis Child*. 1973;125:120-122.
19. Ravid R, Toaff R. On the possible teratogenicity of antibiotic drugs administered during pregnancy—a prospective study. In: Klingberg M, Abramovici A, Chemki J, eds. *Drugs and Fetal Development*. Plenum Press; 1972:505-510.
20. Heinonen OP, Slone D, Shapiro S. *Birth Defects and Drugs in Pregnancy*. Publishing Sciences Group; 1977.
21. Greene H, Burkhart B, Hobby G. Excretion of penicillin in human milk following parturition. *Am J Obstet Gynecol*. 1946;51:732-733.
22. Matheson I, Samseth M, Loberg R, Faegri A, Prentice A. Milk transfer of phenoxymethylpenicillin during puerperal mastitis. *Br J Clin Pharmacol*. 1988;25:33-40.

PENTAMIDINE

Anti-Infective (Antiprotozoal)

PREGNANCY RECOMMENDATION: Limited Human Data—Animal Data Suggest Potential Risk

BREASTFEEDING RECOMMENDATION: Potential Toxicity (Parenteral)/Probably Compatible (Aerosolized)

PREGNANCY SUMMARY

There are a few case reports describing the use of aerosolized and IV pentamidine in human pregnancy. No adverse fetal or obstetrical effects were noted. Of the two with first-trimester use, no major birth anomalies were described. The drug will probably cross the placenta, so some fetal exposure will likely occur. Therefore, this limited human pregnancy experience prevents a complete assessment of the embryofetal risk. Embryofetal toxicity was observed in one animal species at doses about equal to the MRHD. The manufacturer states that pentamidine can cause fetal harm when administered to a pregnant woman and should only be administered if clearly needed. However, the Guidelines for the Prevention and Treatment of Opportunistic Infections in Adults and Adolescents, along with HIV guidelines, recommend that trimethoprim-sulfamethoxazole be used for prophylaxis. Aerosolized pentamidine or oral atovaquone are alternative regimens for use in the first trimester for prophylaxis against *Pneumocystis jiroveci* in persons infected with HIV, and IV pentamidine is an alternative regimen to treat this infection during pregnancy. Nevertheless, the maternal benefit in many instances appears to outweigh any unknown embryofetal risk. Using this drug during pregnancy should be based on the pros and cons of the mother's clinical need for treatment versus any potential fetal risk that might occur from exposure.

BREASTFEEDING SUMMARY

No reports describing the use of pentamidine during human lactation have been located. Because systemic concentrations achieved with aerosolized pentamidine are very low, breast milk levels of the drug after administration are probably clinically insignificant. For the IV/IM use, the drug will likely be excreted into breast milk, so some infant exposure will probably occur. Due to a concern for potential serious adverse effects that might be seen in a breastfed infant, the manufacturer recommends that women not breastfeed while being treated with this drug. Nevertheless, breastfeeding while using this drug should be based on the mother's clinical need for treatment versus any potential infant risks that might occur. If used, the infant should be monitored for the most common reported adult side effects of nausea (leading to irritability), hypotension, anorexia (monitor infant growth), and various laboratory abnormalities (see PI).

References

1. Prescribing Information. Pentamidine isethionate (inhalant). Seton Pharmaceuticals; 2024.
2. Prescribing Information. Pentamidine isethionate (injection). Heritage Pharmaceuticals Inc d/b/a Avet Pharmaceuticals Inc; 2023.
3. Panel on Guidelines for the Prevention and Treatment of Opportunistic Infections in Adults and Adolescents with HIV. Guidelines for the prevention and treatment of opportunistic infections in adults and adolescents with HIV: Pneumocystis pneumonia. National Institutes of Health, Centers for Disease Control and Prevention, HIV Medicine Association, and Infectious Diseases Society of America. Updated September 16, 2024. Accessed February 11, 2025. https://clinicalinfo.hiv.gov/en/guidelines/adult-and-adolescent-opportunistic-infection
4. Fortunato SJ, Bawdon RE. Determination of pentamidine transfer in the in vitro perfused human cotyledon with high-performance liquid chromatography. *Am J Obstet Gynecol*. 1989;160:759-761.
5. Schwebke K, Fletcher CV, Acosta EP, Henry K. Pentamidine concentrations in a mother with AIDS and in her neonate. *Clin Infect Dis*. 1995;20:1569-1570.
6. Conover B, Goldsmith JC, Buehler BA, et al. Aerosolized pentamidine and pregnancy. *Ann Intern Med*. 1988;109:927.
7. Ito S, Koren G. Estimation of fetal risk from aerosolized pentamidine in pregnant healthcare workers. *Chest*. 1994;106:1460-1462.
8. Nana D, Tannenbaum I, Landesman S, et al. Pentamidine prophylaxis in pregnancy (abstract). *Am J Obstet Gynecol*. 1992;166:387.
9. Sperling RS, Stratton P, O'Sullivan MJ, et al. A survey of zidovudine use in pregnant women with human immunodeficiency virus infection. *N Engl J Med*. 1992;326:857-861.
10. Stratton P, Mofenson LM, Willoughby AD. Human immunodeficiency virus infection in pregnant women under care at AIDS clinical trials centers in the United States. *Obstet Gynecol*. 1992;79:364-368.
11. Gates HS Jr, Barker CD. Pneumocystis carinii pneumonia in pregnancy. A case report. *J Reprod Med*. 1993;38:483-486.
12. McGrane J, Bedford T, Kelly S. Successful pregnancy and delivery after concomitant temozolomide and radiotherapy treatment of glioblastoma multiforme. *Clin Oncol (R Coll Radiol)*. 2012;24:311.
13. Harstad TW, Little BB, Bawdon RE, et al. Embryofetal effects of pentamidine isethionate administered to pregnant Sprague-Dawley rats. *Am J Obstet Gynecol*. 1990;163:912-916.

PENTAZOCINE AND NALOXONE

Pain (Partial Opioid Agonist and Opioid Antagonist)

PREGNANCY RECOMMENDATION: Human Data Suggest Potential Risk

BREASTFEEDING RECOMMENDATION: Probably Compatible (Short-Term Use)

PREGNANCY SUMMARY

There are a few reports describing the use of pentazocine in human pregnancy. Pentazocine is a partial opioid agonist. Naloxone is an opioid antagonist but has no pharmacologic activity when administered orally. Naloxone is added as a deterrent for misuse. The Collaborative Perinatal Project reported 47 (3%) major congenital birth anomalies in 1,564 first-trimester exposures. No pattern to the defects was seen. In contrast, the National Birth Defects Prevention Study found evidence

(continued)

that opioid use during organogenesis is associated with a low absolute risk of congenital birth defects. Pentazocine rapidly crosses the placenta, resulting in cord blood levels that are 40% to 70% maternal serum concentrations. Embryofetal toxicity with malformations was observed in one animal species, but not in the second, at doses of less than the MRHD. However, the limited human pregnancy experience, specifically with pentazocine, prevents a complete assessment of embryofetal risk. Using opioid drugs during pregnancy should be based on the pros and cons of the mother's clinical need for treatment versus any potential fetal risk that might occur from exposure. Neonatal abstinence syndrome (NAS) or neonatal opioid withdrawal syndrome (NOWS) may occur with prolonged exposure to opioids. Neonatal opioid withdrawal symptoms include irritability, hyperactivity and abnormal sleep patterns, high-pitched cry, tremor, vomiting, diarrhea, and failure to gain weight. The onset, duration, and severity of withdrawal vary based on the opioid used, duration of use, timing and amount of last maternal use, and elimination of the drug by the newborn. Infants exposed to opioids near birth should be monitored for symptoms of NOWS. The drug carries a boxed warning for addiction and misuse, along with life-threatening respiratory depression, and risks with concomitant benzodiazepine use or other central nervous system (CNS) depressants. It also states that there is an increased risk for NOWS.

BREASTFEEDING SUMMARY

Pentazocine is excreted into human breast milk, so some infant exposure will occur. Breastfeeding while using this drug should be based on the mother's clinical need for treatment versus any potential infant risks that might occur. If used, the infant should be monitored for the most common reported adult side effects of drowsiness, sedation, difficulty feeding, respiratory depression, and lethargy. Additionally, withdrawal symptoms can occur in breastfed infants when maternal administration of an opioid analgesic is stopped or when breastfeeding is stopped.

References

1. Prescribing Information. Pentazocine and naloxone. Actavis Pharma Inc; 2023.
2. Beckett AH, Taylor JF. Blood concentrations of pethidine and pentazocine in mother and infant at time of birth. *J Pharm Pharmacol*. 1967;19(suppl):50S-52S.
3. Goetz RL, Bain RV. Neonatal withdrawal symptoms associated with maternal use of pentazocine. *J Pediatr*. 1974;84:887-888.
4. Scanlon JW. Pentazocine and neonatal withdrawal symptoms. *J Pediatr*. 1974;85:735-736.
5. Kopelman AE. Fetal addiction to pentazocine. *Pediatrics*. 1975;55:888-889.
6. Reeds TO. Withdrawal symptoms in a neonate associated with maternal pentazocine abuse. *J Pediatr*. 1975;87:324.
7. Preis O, Choi SJ, Rudolph N. Pentazocine withdrawal syndrome in the newborn infant. *Am J Obstet Gynecol*. 1977;127:205-206.
8. Filler WW, Filler NW. Effect of a potent non-narcotic analgesic agent (pentazocine) on uterine contractility and fetal heart rate. *Obstet Gynecol*. 1966;28:224-232.
9. Freedman H, Tafeen CH, Harris H. Parenteral Win 20,228 as analgesic in labor. *NY State J Med*. 1967;67:2849-2851.
10. Duncan SLB, Ginsburg J, Morris NF. Comparison of pentazocine and pethidine in normal labor. *Am J Obstet Gynecol*. 1969;105:197-202.
11. Moore J, Carson RM, Hunter RJ. A comparison of the effects of pentazocine and pethidine administered during labor. *J Obstet Gynaecol Br Commonw*. 1970;77:830-836.
12. Mowat J, Garrey MM. Comparison of pentazocine and pethidine in labour. *Br Med J*. 1970;2:757-759.
13. Levy DL. Obstetric analgesia. Pentazocine and meperidine in normal primiparous labor. *Obstet Gynecol*. 1971;38:907-911.
14. Moore J, Ball HG. A sequential study of intravenous analgesic treatment during labour. *Br J Anaesth*. 1974;46:365-372.
15. Refstad SO, Lindbaek E. Ventilatory depression of the newborn of women receiving pethidine or pentazocine. *Br J Anaesth*. 1980;52:265-270.
16. Dunn DW, Reynolds J. Neonatal withdrawal symptoms associated with "T's and Blue's" (pentazocine and tripelennamine). *Am J Dis Child*. 1982; 136:644-645.
17. Pastorek JG, Plauche WC, Faro S. Acute bacterial endocarditis in pregnancy: a report of three cases. *J Reprod Med*. 1983;28:611-614.
18. Chasnoff IJ, Hatcher R, Burns WJ, Schnoll SH. Pentazocine and tripelennamine ("T's and blue's"): effects on the fetus and neonate. *Dev Pharmacol Ther*. 1983;6:162-169.
19. Chasnoff IJ, Burns KA, Burns WJ, Schnoll SH. Prenatal drug exposure: effects on neonatal and infant growth and development. *Neurobehavior Toxicol Teratol*. 1986;8:357-362.
20. Von Almen WF II, Miller JM Jr. "Ts and blues" in pregnancy. *J Reprod Med*. 1986;31:236-239.
21. Debooy VD, Seshia MMK, Tenenbein M, Casiiro OG. Intravenous pentazocine and methylphenidate abuse during pregnancy. Maternal lifestyle and infant outcome. *Am J Dis Child*. 1993;147:1062-1065.
22. Broussard CS, Rasmussen SA, Reefhuis J, et al; National Birth Defects Prevention Study. Maternal treatment with opioid analgesics and risk for birth defects. *Am J Obstet Gynecol*. 2011;204:314-317.

P

PENTOBARBITAL

Central Nervous System (Barbiturate—Sedative/Hypnotic)

PREGNANCY RECOMMENDATION: Limited Human Data—No Relevant Animal Data

BREASTFEEDING RECOMMENDATION: Potential Toxicity

PREGNANCY SUMMARY

Data from the Collaborative Perinatal Project and Group Health Cooperative of Puget Sound reported 4 (1.2%) major birth anomalies in 332 first-trimester exposures. No pattern to the defects was seen. Long-term barbiturate exposure in utero may produce fetal dependence and result in acute withdrawal syndrome of seizures and hyperirritability presenting in the newborn following delivery. This neonatal response can occur shortly after birth or have a delayed onset of up to 14 days postdelivery. If barbiturates are used during labor and delivery, resuscitation equipment should be available. The drug crosses the placenta with cord blood levels about equal to maternal concentration levels. However, the limited human pregnancy experience still prevents a complete assessment of embryofetal risk. Using this drug during pregnancy should be based on the pros and cons of the mother's clinical need for treatment versus any potential fetal risk that might occur from exposure.

BREASTFEEDING SUMMARY

Pentobarbital has been shown to be excreted into human breast milk. Breast milk levels of 0.17 mcg/mL have been detected 19 hours after a daily dose of 100 mg. Any effect on the nursing infant is not known. The manufacturer states that caution should be exercised when a barbiturate is administered to a nursing woman. Therefore, if the clinical decision is to use this drug while breastfeeding, the infant should be monitored for the most common reported adult side effects of sedation and somnolence.

References

1. Prescribing Information. Pentobarbital. Akorn; 2024.
2. National Library of Medicine. Pentobarbital. PubChem. Accessed February 12, 2025. https://pubchem.ncbi.nlm.nih.gov/compound/Pentobarbital
3. U.S. Food and Drug Administration. FDA drug safety communication: FDA review results in new warnings about using general anesthetics and sedation drugs in young children and pregnant women. Accessed February 12, 2025. https://www.fda.gov/Drugs/DrugSafety/ucm532356.htm
4. Heinonen OP, Slone D, Shapiro S. *Birth Defects and Drugs in Pregnancy*. Publishing Sciences Group; 1977:336-337.
5. Wilson JT, Brown RD, Cherek DR, et al. Drug excretion in human breast milk: principles, pharmacokinetics and projected consequences. *Clin Pharmacokinet*. 1980;5:1-66.
6. Jick H, Holmes LB, Hunter JR, et al. First-trimester drug use and congenital disorders. *JAMA*. 1981;246:343-346.

PENTOSAN

Urinary (Analgesic)

PREGNANCY RECOMMENDATION: Limited Human Data—Animal Data Suggest Low Risk

BREASTFEEDING RECOMMENDATION: Probably Compatible

PREGNANCY SUMMARY

One report describing the use of pentosan in human pregnancy was located. The study evaluated whether the drug crosses the placenta in early pregnancy. The analysis involved whether fetal blood demonstrated anticoagulant effects seen in the mothers. No changes in fetal coagulation were seen. Therefore, it was felt that transplacental passage did not occur. This would be consistent with the drug's MW. However, the limited human pregnancy experience prevents a complete assessment of embryofetal risk. Animal data did not show any embryofetal toxicity when tested at doses of less than the RHD. Using this drug during pregnancy should be based on the pros and cons of the mother's clinical need for treatment versus any potential fetal risk that might occur from exposure.

P

BREASTFEEDING SUMMARY

No reports describing the use of pentosan during human lactation have been located. The drug will not likely be excreted into breast milk. In addition, oral absorption is only about 3%. Thus, the risk to a nursing infant from the drug is probably negligible. Breastfeeding while using this drug should be based on the mother's clinical need for treatment versus any potential infant risks that might occur. If used, the infant should be monitored for the most common reported adult side effects of nausea, headache, dyspepsia, abdominal pain, and dizziness (all leading to irritability), alopecia, diarrhea, rash, and abnormal liver function tests.

References

1. Product Information. Elmiron. Janssen Pharmaceuticals Inc; 2024.
2. Forestier F, Fischer AM, Daffos F, et al. Absence of transplacental passage of pentosan polysulfate during mid trimester of pregnancy. *Thromb Haemost*. 1986;56:247-249.

PENTOSTATIN

Antineoplastic (Antimetabolite)

PREGNANCY RECOMMENDATION: No Human Data—Animal Data Suggest Potential Risk

BREASTFEEDING RECOMMENDATION: Potential Toxicity

PREGNANCY SUMMARY

No reports describing the use of pentostatin in human pregnancy have been located. The drug will probably cross the placenta, so some fetal exposure will likely occur. Therefore, the absence of human pregnancy experience prevents a complete assessment of the embryofetal risk. Embryofetal toxicity with malformations was observed in one animal species at doses of less than the RHD based on weight. No embryofetal toxicity was seen in two other species, one at doses of less than the RHD and the other at doses of more than 10 times the RHD. Using this drug during pregnancy should be based on the pros and cons of the mother's clinical need for treatment versus any potential fetal risk that might occur from exposure. There is a registry for women who are pregnant and have cancer. For more information, women and health care providers are encouraged to contact the Cancer and Pregnancy Registry at 1-877-635-4499. Use with fludarabine phosphate is not recommended.

BREASTFEEDING SUMMARY

No reports describing the use of pentostatin during human lactation have been located. The drug will likely be excreted into breast milk, so some infant exposure will probably occur. However, due to a concern for potential serious adverse effects that might be seen in a breastfed infant, the manufacturer recommends that women not breastfeed while being treated with this drug. Nevertheless, breastfeeding while using this drug should be based on the mother's clinical need for treatment versus any potential infant risks that might occur. If used, the infant should be monitored for the most common reported adult side effects of nausea, myalgia, headache, pruritus, and abdominal pain (all leading to irritability), fever, rash, vomiting, fatigue (lethargy), cough, diarrhea, and anorexia (monitor infant growth).

Reference

1. Prescribing Information. Nipent. Hospira Inc; 2024.

PENTOXIFYLLINE

Cardiovascular (Blood Viscosity Reducing Agent)

PREGNANCY RECOMMENDATION: Limited Human Data Suggest Potential Risk—Animal Data Suggest Potential Risk

BREASTFEEDING RECOMMENDATION: Potential Toxicity

PREGNANCY SUMMARY

Three reports describing the use of pentoxifylline during human pregnancy were located. Regarding first-trimester use, 5 (14.7%) major anomalies were identified in 34 exposures (2 were cardiac, 1 was a neural tube defect (NTD), and 2 were other anomalies). Though this rate is higher than the expected rate for the general population, the numbers are too small to make any conclusions. The other two studies evaluated the drug in patients with preterm labor and in pregnancies with intrauterine growth restriction (IUGR). Pentoxifylline and its metabolite (M1) cross the placenta with fetal levels about equal to maternal concentrations. However, the limited human pregnancy experience prevents a complete assessment of embryofetal risk. Embryofetal toxicity was observed in one animal species at doses of less than 10 times the MRHD but not in the second species. Using this drug during pregnancy should be based on the pros and cons of the mother's clinical need for treatment versus any potential fetal risk that might occur from exposure.

BREASTFEEDING SUMMARY

Pentoxifylline has been found to be excreted into human breast milk. Five healthy women who had been breastfeeding for at least 6 weeks were given a single 400-mg sustained-release tablet. The mean breast milk to plasma ratio of pentoxifylline was about 87%. The mean breast milk concentration of pentoxifylline at 2 hours was about 74 ng/mL and at 4 hours was about 36 ng/mL. The calculated RID was less than 1%. Pentoxifylline and its metabolites are stable in breast milk for 3 weeks when stored at −15 °C. The effects of this exposure on a nursing infant are unknown. However, due to a concern for potential serious adverse effects that might be seen in a breastfed infant, the manufacturer recommends that women not breastfeed while being treated with this drug. Nevertheless, breastfeeding while using this drug should be based on the mother's clinical need for treatment versus any potential infant risks that might occur. If used, the infant should be monitored for the most common reported adult side effects of dyspepsia, nausea, dizziness, and headache (all leading to irritability) and flatulence.

References

1. Prescribing Information. Pentoxifylline. Ani Pharmaceuticals Inc; 2024.
2. Broekhuizen M, de Vries R, Smits MAW, et al. Pentoxifylline as a therapeutic option for pre-eclampsia: a study on its placental effects. *Br J Pharmacol.* 2022;179:5074-5088.
3. Lauterbach R, Rytlewski K, Pawlik D, et al. Effect of pentoxifylline, administered in preterm labour, on the foetal-placental circulation and neonatal outcome: a randomized, prospective pilot study. *Basic Clin Pharmacol Toxicol.* 2012;110:342-346.

4. Asadi N, Roozmeh S, Vafaei H, et al. Effectiveness of pentoxifylline in severe early-onset fetal growth restriction: a randomized double-blinded clinical trial. *Taiw J Obstet Gynecol*. 2022;61:612-619.
5. Shen MR, Chiang PH, Yang RC, et al. Pentoxifylline stimulates human sperm motility both in vitro and after oral therapy. *Br J Clin Pharmacol*. 1991;31:711-714.
6. Witter FR, Smith RV. The excretion of pentoxifylline and its metabolites into human breast milk. *Am J Obstet Gynecol*. 1985;151:1094-1097.
7. Bauza MT, Smith RV, Knutson DE, Witter FR. Gas chromatographic determination of pentoxifylline and its major metabolites in human breast milk. *J Chromatogr*. 1984;310:61-69.

PERAMIVIR

Antiviral (Influenza Virus Neuraminidase Inhibitor)

PREGNANCY RECOMMENDATION: Limited Human Data—Animal Data Suggest Risk (Maternal Benefit May Outweigh Any Potential Embryofetal Risk)

BREASTFEEDING RECOMMENDATION: Potential Toxicity

PREGNANCY SUMMARY

Four case reports describing the use of peramivir in five human pregnancies were located. In three exposures at unknown gestational ages, three healthy infants were born. In the other two cases, one was a first-trimester loss and the other an intrauterine fetal demise (IUFD) (probably related to maternal disease state). No influenza was detected in any of the fetal tissue during autopsy in the IUFD case. Peramivir will probably cross the placenta, so some fetal exposure will likely occur. Therefore, this limited human pregnancy experience prevents a complete assessment of the embryofetal risk. Embryofetal toxicity was observed in one animal species receiving continuous IV infusion at doses less than the RHD. With single injection exposures at 8 times the RHD, one animal species had embryofetal toxicity and a second species did not. Using this drug during pregnancy should be based on the pros and cons of the mother's clinical need for treatment versus any potential fetal risk that might occur from exposure.

BREASTFEEDING SUMMARY

No reports describing the use of peramivir during human lactation have been located. The drug will likely be excreted into breast milk, so some infant exposure will probably occur. Breastfeeding while using this drug should be based on the mother's clinical need for treatment versus any potential infant risks that might occur. If used, the infant should be monitored for the most common reported adult side effect of diarrhea.

References

1. Prescribing Information. Rapivab. BioCryst Pharmaceuticals Inc; 2024.
2. Hernandez JE, Adiga R, Armstrong R, et al; eIND Peramivir Investigators. Clinical experience in adults and children treated with intravenous peramivir for 2009 influenza A (H1N1) under an emergency IND program in the United States. *Clin Infect Dis*. 2011;52:695-706.
3. Jain S, Fry AM. Peramivir: another tool for influenza treatment? *Clin Infect Dis*. 2011;52:707-709.
4. Sorbello A, Jones C, Carter W, et al. Emergency use authorization for intravenous peramivir: evaluation of safety in the treatment of hospitalized patients infected with 2009 H1N1 influenza A virus. *Clin Infect Dis*. 2012; 55:1-7.
5. Wang J, Xu H, Mu C, et al. A study on mother-to-fetus/infant transmission of influenza A (H7N9) virus: two case reports and a review of the literature. *Clin Respir J*. 2018;12:2539-2545.

P

PERAMPANEL

Central Nervous System (Antiseizure)

PREGNANCY RECOMMENDATION: Limited Human Data—Animal Data Suggest Potential Risk

BREASTFEEDING RECOMMENDATION: Potential Toxicity

PREGNANCY SUMMARY

A small number of case reports describing the use of perampanel during human pregnancy have been located. No major birth anomalies were reported in the few that had first-trimester exposure. The drug will probably cross the placenta, so some fetal exposure will likely occur. Therefore, the absence of human pregnancy experience prevents a complete assessment of the embryofetal risk. Embryofetal toxicity was observed in one species at doses of about equal to the RHD but not in the second species at doses of less than 10 times the RHD. Using this drug during pregnancy should be based on the pros and cons of the mother's clinical need for treatment versus any potential fetal risk that might occur from exposure. There is a pregnancy exposure registry that monitors pregnancy outcomes in women using antiseizure drugs. Health care providers are encouraged to call the North American Antiepileptic Drug Pregnancy Registry at 1-888-233-2334.

BREASTFEEDING SUMMARY

Two studies were located that describe the use of perampanel in three lactating women. The drug was not detected in one case (lower limit of quantification [LLQ] of 10 ng/mL). In the other two cases, the highest breast milk concentration was 108 ng/mL in a mother on 8 mg daily and 60 ng/mL in a mother on 4 mg daily. The calculated RIDs were both about 15%. In both cases, infant blood was also analyzed. The drug concentrations in the first case (8 mg daily) were about 80 ng/mL in breast milk on day 1, which increased to 171 ng/mL by day 5, with a return to 80 ng/mL during week 5. In the second case (4 mg daily), infant serum levels were 160 ng/mL on day 4. (In these early samplings, based on the long elimination half-life, transplacental transfer could contribute to these concentrations if the drug crosses the placenta.) However, the infant's drug level obtained in the first case on week 5 should only be related to breastfeeding. Breastfeeding while using this drug should be based on the mother's clinical need for treatment versus any potential infant risks that might occur. If used, the infant should be monitored for the most common reported adult side effects of dizziness, irritability, nausea, headache, and abdominal pain (all leading to irritability), somnolence, fatigue (lethargy), and vomiting.

References

1. Prescribing Information. Fycompa. Catalyst Pharmaceuticals Inc; 2023.
2. Alicino AM, Falcicchio G, Boero G, et al. Perampanel during pregnancy: description of four cases. *Epilepsy Behav Rep*. 2021;16:100490.
3. Johannessen Landmark C, Rekcori L, Burns ML, et al. Pharmacokinetics data on brivaracetam, lacosamide, and perampanel during pregnancy and lactation. Epileptic Disorders. 2021;23:426-31.
4. Yamamoto Y, Akita N, Nogimoto H, et al. Changes in perampanel pharmacokinetics and cytochrome P450 3A4 activity before, during, and after pregnancy. *Therap Drug Monit*. 2024;46:548-551.
5. Kacirova I, Urinovska R, Grundmann M. Therapeutic monitoring of lacosamide, perampanel, and zonisamide during breastfeeding. *Epilepsy Res*. 2024;199:107264.

PERFLUOROHEXYLOCTANE OPHTHALMIC

Ophthalmic (Semi-Fluorinated Alkane Solution—Topical)

PREGNANCY RECOMMENDATION: **No Human Data—Animal Data Suggest Low Risk**

BREASTFEEDING RECOMMENDATION: **Probably Compatible**

PREGNANCY SUMMARY

No reports describing the use of perfluorohexyloctane in human pregnancy have been located. Though placental transfer is possible, fetal exposure is probably negligible because of minimal to no systemic absorption after ophthalmic use. However, the absence of human pregnancy experience prevents a complete assessment of the embryofetal risk. Animal data did not show any embryofetal toxicity despite being administered orally. Using this drug during pregnancy should be based on the pros and cons of the mother's clinical need for treatment versus any potential fetal risk that might occur from exposure.

P

BREASTFEEDING SUMMARY

No reports describing the use of perfluorohexyloctane in human lactation have been located. Because the drug has minimal to no systemic absorption after ophthalmic use, any drug found in breast milk would not likely have a clinical effect. Breastfeeding while using this drug should be based on the mother's clinical need for treatment.

References

1. Prescribing Information. Miebo. Bausch & Lomb, Inc; 2023.
2. Tauber J, Wirta, D, Sall K, et al. A randomized clinical trial study (SEECASE) to assess efficacy, safety, and tolerability of NOV03 for treatment of dry eye disease. *Cornea*. 2021;40:1132-1140.

PERINDOPRIL

Antihypertensive (Angiotensin-Converting Enzyme Inhibitor)

PREGNANCY RECOMMENDATION: ***Contraindicated (Second and Third Trimesters)**

BREASTFEEDING RECOMMENDATION: **Probably Compatible**

PREGNANCY SUMMARY

No reports specifically describing the use of perindopril in human pregnancy have been located. A few large studies have reported a risk for congenital anomalies with first-trimester exposure to angiotensin-converting enzyme (ACE) inhibitors as a class of drugs. These publications reported overall malformation rates of about 5% to 6%, which is higher than the expected rate of 2% to 4%. However, most of these studies also reported similar fetal anomaly rates in pregnant patients with hypertension not on treatment. The impression was that these findings might be related to the disease and not the drug. Likewise, some of these studies also reported an increase in risk for cardiac defects, but again, it was not certain as to whether this elevated risk was related to the drug or the disease. Furthermore, no pattern to the anomalies has been identified. Perindopril probably crosses the placenta, so some fetal exposure will likely occur. Therefore, the absence of first-trimester human pregnancy experience for this drug prevents a complete assessment of the embryofetal risk. No animal reproduction studies have been located. *Regarding the use of ACE inhibitors in the second half of pregnancy, numerous case reports and reviews have reported that these drugs can, in some cases, produce severe fetal renal dysfunction. This can lead to anomalies related to longstanding oligohydramnios and fetal/neonatal death. There are cases, however, where the process reverses itself when the drug is discontinued. These findings are similar to those seen with angiotensin receptor blockers (ARBs). The drug actually carries a boxed warning for these risks. Women of reproductive age using perindopril should be informed of these risks, so they can be closely monitored if pregnancy transpires. If a positive pregnancy test occurs, she and her health care providers can modify treatment (if possible) so that the drug is not used in the second or third trimesters. For treating hypertension in pregnancy, ACOG recommends nifedipine and labetalol as first-line agents.

BREASTFEEDING SUMMARY

Perindopril and its active metabolite, perindoprilat, are both excreted into human breast milk. One report described the use of the prodrug during human lactation. A lactating woman taking perindopril 10 mg twice daily for 2 weeks had breast milk samples obtained only once after dosing. Perindopril and perindoprilat breast milk levels at 9 hours postdose were about 1 ng/mL and 23 ng/mL, respectively. The calculated RID was about 1.3%. The effects on a nursing infant from this exposure are unknown. The manufacturer recommends caution in using this drug while breastfeeding. Nevertheless, breastfeeding while using perindopril should be based on the mother's clinical need for treatment versus any potential infant risks that might occur. If used, the infant should be monitored for the most common reported adult side effects of headache, dizziness, and back pain (all leading to irritability), cough, rash, and hypotension. ACOG and the American Heart Association (AHA) consider ACE inhibitors safe for use during breastfeeding.

References

1. Prescribing Information. Perindopril erbumine. Aurobindo Pharma Limited; 2024.
2. Cooper WO, Hernandez-Diaz S, Arbogast PG, et al. Major congenital malformations after first-trimester exposure to ACE inhibitors. *N Engl J Med*. 2006;354:2443-2451.
3. Friedman JM. ACE inhibitors and congenital anomalies. *N Engl J Med*. 2006;354:2498-500.
4. Scialli AR, Lione A. ACE inhibitors and major congenital malformations. *N Engl J Med*. 2006;355:1280.
5. Cooper WO, Ray WA. Reply—ACE inhibitors and major congenital malformations. *N Engl J Med*. 2006;355:1281.
6. Barr M Jr. Teratogen update: angiotensin-converting enzyme inhibitors. *Teratology*. 1994;50:399-409.
7. Shotan A, Widerhorn J, Hurst A, Elkayam U. Risks of angiotensin-converting enzyme inhibition during pregnancy: experimental and clinical evidence, potential mechanisms, and recommendations for use. *Am J Med*. 1994; 96:451-456.
8. Robillard JE, Nakamura KT, Matherne GP, Jose PA. Renal hemodynamics and functional adjustments to postnatal life. *Semin Perinatol*. 1988;12: 143-150.
9. Guignard J-P, Gouyon J-B. Adverse effects of drugs on the immature kidney. *Biol Neonate*. 1988;53:243-252.
10. Brent RL, Beckman DA. Angiotensin-converting enzyme inhibitors, an embryopathic class of drugs with unique properties: information for clinical teratology counselors. *Teratology*. 1991;43:543-546.
11. Lwin EMP, Gerber C, Song Y, et al. A new LC-MS/MS bioanalytical method for perindopril and perindoprilat in human plasma and milk. *Anal Bioanal Chem*. 2017;409:6141-6148.

PERMETHRIN

Anti-Infective (Topical—Pediculicide/Scabicide)

PREGNANCY RECOMMENDATION: Limited Human Data—Animal Data Suggest Low Risk

BREASTFEEDING RECOMMENDATION: Probably Compatible

PREGNANCY SUMMARY

Three reports describing the use of permethrin in over 100 human pregnancies have been located. It is not known how many of these were first-trimester exposures, but no reported increased risk for fetal malformations or adverse pregnancy outcomes was described. If the drug is found in the maternal circulation, it will likely cross the placenta. However, with very low systemic absorption following topical use, the amount is likely to be negligible. Nevertheless, this limited human pregnancy experience prevents a complete assessment of embryofetal risk. Using this drug during pregnancy should be based on the pros and cons of the mother's clinical need for treatment versus any potential fetal risk that might occur from exposure. The Centers for Disease Control and Prevention (CDC) 2021 sexually transmitted infection guidelines recommend permethrin 5% cream as the preferred treatment for scabies and pubic lice during pregnancy.

BREASTFEEDING SUMMARY

No reports describing the use of permethrin during human lactation have been located. If the drug is found in the maternal circulation, it will likely be found in human breast milk. However, with very low systemic absorption following topical use, the amount is likely to be negligible. If the clinical decision is to use this drug while breastfeeding, the infant should be monitored for the most common reported adult side effects of headache, dizziness, abdominal pain, and nausea (all leading to irritability), vomiting, fever, and diarrhea. The CDC 2021 sexually transmitted infection guidelines recommend permethrin 5% cream as the preferred treatment for scabies during lactation.

References

1. Prescribing Information. Elimite. Aurobindo Pharma Limited; 2024.
2. Centers for Disease Control and Prevention. 2015 Guidelines for treatment of sexually transmitted diseases. *MMWR Recomm Rep*. 2021;70:1-187.
3. Judge MR, Kobza-Black A. Crusted scabies in pregnancy. *Br J Dermatol*. 1995;132:116-119.
4. Kennedy D, Hurst V, Konradsdottir E, Einarson A. Pregnancy outcome following exposure to permethrin and use of teratogen information. *Am J Perinatol*. 2005;22:87-90.
5. Garayar Cantero M, Garabito Solovera E, Aguado Garcia A, et al. Use of permethrin in the treatment of rosacea fulminans during pregnancy: one case report. *Dermat Ther*. 2020;33:e13436.

PERPHENAZINE

Mental Health (First-Generation Antipsychotic/Typical Antipsychotic)

PREGNANCY RECOMMENDATION: **Limited Human Data (First Trimester)/Human Data Suggest Risk (Third Trimester)—No Relevant Animal Data**

BREASTFEEDING RECOMMENDATION: **Potential Toxicity**

PREGNANCY SUMMARY

A few reports describing the use of perphenazine in human pregnancy were located. The Collaborative Perinatal Project and Michigan Medicaid Surveillance study reported a total of 7 (3.4%) major malformations in 203 first-trimester exposures. Use of the drug near the end of gestation has resulted in newborns described as having extrapyramidal and/or withdrawal symptoms (agitation, hypertonia, hypotonia, tremor, somnolence, respiratory distress, and feeding disorders) in the exposed infants. Perphenazine will probably cross the placenta, so some fetal exposure will likely occur. Therefore, this limited human pregnancy experience still prevents a complete assessment of the embryofetal risk. Perphenazine is likely to cross the placenta. No animal reproduction studies have been located. Using this drug during pregnancy should be based on the pros and cons of the mother's clinical need for treatment versus any potential fetal risk that might occur from exposure. Perphenazine can prolong the QT interval.

P

BREASTFEEDING SUMMARY

Perphenazine has been shown to be excreted into human breast milk. A 50-kg lactating woman was taking 24 mg of perphenazine daily for postpartum psychosis. The mean breast milk concentration for the drug was 3.2 ng/mL. This dropped to 2.1 ng/mL when the daily dose was dropped to 16 mg. The calculated RIDs were both less than 1%. The mother continued to breastfeed for an additional 3.5 months, and no adverse infant effects were noted. As an antipsychotic, perphenazine can increase prolactin levels, but this should not adversely affect breastfeeding. Breastfeeding while using this drug should be based on the mother's clinical need for treatment versus any potential infant risks that might occur. If used, the infant should be monitored for the most common reported adult side effects of headache and nausea (both leading to irritability), extrapyramidal symptoms, sedation, somnolence, flushing, rash, and various laboratory abnormalities (see PI).

References

1. Prescribing Information. Perphenazine. Chartwell Rx LLC; 2024.
2. Moya F, Thorndike V. Passage of drugs across the placenta. *Am J Obstet Gynecol*. 1962;84:1778-1798.
3. Slone D, Siskind V, Heinonen OP, et al. Antenatal exposure to the phenothiazines in relation to congenital malformations, perinatal mortality rate, birth weight, and intelligence quotient score. *Am J Obstet Gynecol*. 1977;128:486-488.
4. Wertelecki W, Purvis-Smith SG, Blackburn WR. Amitriptyline/perphenazine maternal overdose and birth defects (abstract). *Teratology*. 1980;21:74A.
5. Handal M, Matheson I, Bechensteen AG, Lindemann R. Antipsychotic agents and pregnant women. A case report. *Tidsskr Nor Laegeforen*. 1995;115:2539-2540.
6. McGarry JM. A double-blind comparison of the anti-emetic effect during labour of metoclopramide and perphenazine. *Br J Anaesth*. 1971;43:613-615.
7. Einarson A, Boskovic R. Use and safety of antipsychotic drugs during pregnancy. *J Psychiatr Pract*. 2009;15:183-192.
8. Olesen OV, Bartels U, Poulsen JH. Perphenazine in breast milk and serum. *Am J Psychiatry*. 1990;147:1378-1379.

PERTUZUMAB

Antineoplastic (Anti-HER2; Monoclonal Antibody)

PREGNANCY RECOMMENDATION: **Limited Human Data—Animal Data Suggest Potential Risk**

BREASTFEEDING RECOMMENDATION: **Probably Compatible**

PREGNANCY SUMMARY

Two reports describing the use of pertuzumab in human pregnancy have been located. In a case report, a patient received pertuzumab and trastuzumab maintenance therapy, and a pregnancy was discovered at 20 weeks of gestation. Oligohydramnios and right renal agenesis were observed during an ultrasound. The pregnancy was terminated at 27 weeks due to anhydramnios and IUGR. Upon autopsy evaluation, macroscopic and microscopic right adrenal gland hyperplasia was found. No urinary system abnormalities were noted. A 2023 case-control study of anti-ErBB2 inhibitors included 55 pertuzumab exposures. Pertuzumab exposure was associated with a significantly higher risk for congenital respiratory tract malformations and oligohydramnios. As an IgG antibody, it likely crosses the placenta, especially during the second half of gestation, so some fetal exposure will probably occur. Therefore, this limited human pregnancy experience prevents a complete assessment of the embryofetal risk. Embryofetal toxicity was observed in one animal species at doses of less than 10 times the RHD. Based on animal studies and the drug's mechanism of action, the manufacturer recommends that women with reproductive potential use effective contraception during treatment and for 7 months after the last dose. The manufacturer further recommends monitoring for oligohydramnios in women exposed to pertuzumab in combination with trastuzumab during pregnancy or within 7 months prior to conception. If oligohydramnios occurs, perform fetal testing that is appropriate for gestational age. There is a pregnancy pharmacovigilance program for pertuzumab. If a patient is exposed to the drug during pregnancy or within 7 months following the last dose in combination with trastuzumab, health care providers should report the exposure to Genentech at 888-835-2555. There is also a registry for women who are pregnant and have cancer. For more information, women and health care providers are encouraged to contact the Cancer and Pregnancy Registry at 1-877-635-4499. The drug carries a boxed warning for left ventricular dysfunction and embryofetal toxicity.

BREASTFEEDING SUMMARY

No reports describing the use of pertuzumab during human lactation have been located. It is known that IgG antibodies can be found in human breast milk but are not found in the neonatal or infant circulation. Additionally, if any IgG antibodies were to be ingested through breastfeeding, they would probably be digested in the infant's gastrointestinal tract and not be absorbed. Breastfeeding while using this drug should be based on the mother's clinical need for treatment versus any potential infant risks that might occur. If used, the infant should be monitored for the most common reported adult side effects of nausea, peripheral neuropathy, headache, and myalgia (all leading to irritability), diarrhea, alopecia, fatigue (lethargy), rash, vomiting, constipation, and various laboratory abnormalities (see PI).

References

1. Prescribing Information. Perjeta. Genentech Inc; 2021.
2. Yildirim N, Bahceci A. Use of pertuzumab and trastuzumab during pregnancy. *Anti-Cancer Drugs*. 2018;29:810-813.
3. Gougis P, Grandal B, Jochum F, et al. Treatment during pregnancy targeting ERBB2 and outcomes of pregnant individuals and newborns. *JAMA Netw Open*. 2023;6:e2339934.

P

PEXIDARTINIB

Antineoplastic (Tyrosine Kinase Inhibitor)

PREGNANCY RECOMMENDATION: **No Human Data—Animal Data Suggest Risk**

BREASTFEEDING RECOMMENDATION: **Potential Toxicity**

PREGNANCY SUMMARY

No reports describing the use of pexidartinib in human pregnancy have been located. The drug will probably cross the placenta, so some fetal exposure will likely occur. Therefore, the absence of human pregnancy experience prevents a complete assessment of the embryofetal risk. Embryofetal toxicity with malformations was observed in two animal species at doses of less than 10 times the RHD. Based on animal studies and the drug's mechanism of action, the manufacturer recommends that women with reproductive potential use effective contraception during treatment and for 1 month after the last dose. They also recommend that males with female partners of reproductive potential use effective contraception during treatment and for 1 week after the last dose. Nevertheless, using this drug during pregnancy should be based on the pros and cons of the mother's clinical need for treatment versus any potential fetal risk that might occur from exposure. There is a registry for women who are pregnant and have cancer. For more information, women and health care providers are encouraged to contact the Cancer and Pregnancy Registry at 1-877-635-4499.

BREASTFEEDING SUMMARY

No reports describing the use of pexidartinib during human lactation have been located. The drug will likely be excreted into human breast milk, so some infant exposure will probably occur. However, due to a concern for potential serious adverse effects that might be seen in a breastfed infant, the manufacturer recommends that women not breastfeed while being treated with this drug and for at least 1 week after the last dose. Nevertheless, breastfeeding while using this drug should be based on the mother's clinical need for treatment versus any potential infant risks that might occur. If used, the infant should be monitored for the most common reported adult side effects of hair color changes, fatigue (lethargy), peripheral edema, rash, and various laboratory abnormalities (see PI).

Reference

1. Prescribing Information. Turalio. Daiichi Sankyo Inc; 2025.

PHENAZOPYRIDINE

Urinary (Analgesic)

PREGNANCY RECOMMENDATION: Human Data Suggest Low Risk

BREASTFEEDING RECOMMENDATION: Potential Toxicity

PREGNANCY SUMMARY

From the Collaborative Perinatal Project, Michigan Medicaid Surveillance study, and the Group Health Cooperative of Puget Sound, a total of 29 (2.8%) major anomalies were described with more than 1,000 first-trimester exposures to phenazopyridine. No pattern to the defects was seen. The drug has been reported to cross the placenta, so some fetal exposure will occur. Animal studies did not show any embryofetal toxicity in one species at doses of less than 10 times the MRHD. Using this drug during pregnancy should be based on the pros and cons of the mother's clinical need for treatment versus any potential fetal risk that might occur from exposure.

BREASTFEEDING SUMMARY

No reports describing the use of phenazopyridine during human lactation have been located. The drug will likely be excreted into breast milk, so some infant exposure will probably occur. However, phenazopyridine can cause methemoglobinemia, sulfhemoglobinemia, and hemolytic anemia in some patients so the manufacturer states that it should not be used during breastfeeding, especially with an infant under 1 month of age or with glucose-6-phosphate dehydrogenase (G6PD) deficiency. However, if the clinical decision is to use this drug while breastfeeding, the infant should be monitored for the most common reported adult side effects of headache, pruritus, and occasional gastrointestinal disturbance (all leading to irritability) and rash.

References

1. Prescribing Information. Phenazopyridine hydrochloride. Amneal Pharmaceuticals LLC; 2024.
2. Heinonen OP, Slone D, Shapiro S. *Birth Defects and Drugs in Pregnancy*. Publishing Sciences Group; 1977.
3. Lee M, Bozzo P, Einarson A, Koren G. Urinary tract infections in pregnancy. *Can Fam Physician*. 2008;54:853-854.
4. Aselton P, Jick H, Milunsky A, Hunter JR, Stergachis A. First-trimester drug use and congenital disorders. *Obstet Gynecol*. 1985;65:451-455.

PHENDIMETRAZINE

Autonomic (Sympathomimetic/Anorexiant)

PREGNANCY RECOMMENDATION: *Contraindicated

BREASTFEEDING RECOMMENDATION: *Contraindicated

PREGNANCY SUMMARY

No reports describing the use of phendimetrazine in human pregnancy have been located. The drug will probably cross the placenta, so some fetal exposure will likely occur. Therefore, the absence of human pregnancy experience prevents a complete assessment of the embryofetal risk. Animal reproduction studies have not been located. *However, it is doubtful if any real benefit is derived from the use of this drug for weight control during human pregnancy. Therefore, its use during gestation, especially during the first trimester, should be considered contraindicated. Using this drug during pregnancy should be based on the pros and cons of the mother's clinical need for treatment versus any potential fetal risk that might occur from exposure. Hypertension was reported in patients treated with this drug during the clinical trials.

BREASTFEEDING SUMMARY

No reports describing the use of phendimetrazine during human lactation have been located. The drug will likely be excreted into breast milk, so infant exposure will probably occur. *Because CNS stimulation and other adverse reactions may occur in a nursing infant exposed to this drug in breast milk, phendimetrazine should be considered contraindicated during breastfeeding. The manufacturer recommends that phendimetrazine should not be taken by women who are breastfeeding unless, in the opinion of the physician, the potential benefits outweigh the possible hazards. If the clinical decision is to use this drug while breastfeeding, the infant should be monitored for the most common reported adult side effects of agitation, dizziness, headache, nausea, and stomach pain (all leading to irritability), tachycardia, elevated blood pressure, ischemic events, insomnia, tremor, sweating, diarrhea, constipation, and urinary frequency.

Reference

1. Prescribing Information. Phendimetrazine tartrate. Elite Laboratories Inc; 2019.

PHENELZINE

Mental Health (Antidepressant—MAO Inhibitor)

PREGNANCY RECOMMENDATION: **Limited Human Data—No Relevant Animal Data**

BREASTFEEDING RECOMMENDATION: **Potential Toxicity**

PREGNANCY SUMMARY

Four reports describing the use of phenelzine in six human pregnancies have been located. All of the exposures were at conception and throughout the first trimester. The outcome of three was reported as normal with no identified fetal anomalies. The drug will probably cross the placenta, so some fetal exposure will likely occur. Therefore, this limited human pregnancy experience prevents a complete assessment of the embryofetal risk. No animal reproduction studies have been located. Using this drug during pregnancy should be based on the pros and cons of the mother's clinical need for treatment versus any potential fetal risk that might occur from exposure. There is a pregnancy exposure registry that monitors pregnancy outcomes in women using antidepressant drugs. Health care providers are encouraged to call the National Pregnancy Registry for Antidepressants at 1-844-405-6185. ACOG states that uncontrolled and undertreated depression is associated with a risk for limited engagement in medical care and self-care, substance use, preterm birth, low birth weight, preeclampsia, postpartum depression, impaired infant attachment (which carries long-term developmental effects), disrupted relationships with partner, and suicide. Additionally, untreated and undertreated mental health disorders should be considered as an exposure. Pregnancy and lactation alone should not be a reason to withhold or discontinue mental health medications.

BREASTFEEDING SUMMARY

No reports describing the use of phenelzine during human lactation have been located. The drug will likely be excreted into breast milk, so some infant exposure will probably occur. Breastfeeding while using this drug should be based on the mother's clinical need for treatment versus any potential infant risks that might occur. If used, the infant should be monitored for the most common reported adult side effects of dizziness, gastrointestinal disturbances, and headache (all leading to irritability), drowsiness, sleep disturbances, fatigue (lethargy), tremors, hyperreflexia, constipation, peripheral edema, and elevated serum transaminases.

References

1. Prescribing Information. Phenelzine. Greenstone LLC; 2020.
2. American College of Obstetricians and Gynecologists. Treatment and management of mental health conditions during pregnancy and postpartum. Clinical practice guideline No. 5. *Obstet Gynecol*. 2023;141:1262-1288.
3. Heinonen OP, Slone D, Shapiro S. *Birth Defects and Drugs in Pregnancy*. Publishing Sciences Group; 1977:336-337.
4. Pavy TJG, Kliffer AP, Douglas MJ. Anaesthetic management of labour and delivery in a woman taking long-term MAOI. *Can J Anaesth*. 1995; 42:618-620.
5. Gracious BL, Wisner KL. Phenelzine use throughout pregnancy and the puerperium: case report, review of the literature, and management recommendations. *Depress Anxiety*. 1997;6:124-128.
6. Frayne J, Nguyen T, Kohan R, et al. The comprehensive management of pregnant women with major mood disorders: a case study involving phenelzine, lithium, and quetiapine. *Arch Womens Ment Health*. 2014;17:73-75.

PHENIRAMINE OPHTHALMIC

Ophthalmic (Topical—Antihistamine)

PREGNANCY RECOMMENDATION: **Human Data Suggest Low Risk**

BREASTFEEDING RECOMMENDATION: **Probably Compatible**

PREGNANCY SUMMARY

One report describing the use of pheniramine in pregnancy was located. Pheniramine is only available combined with naphazoline as an ophthalmic preparation. The Collaborative Perinatal Project reported 28 (3.4%) major anomalies in 831 first-trimester exposures. No pattern to the defects was seen. If found in the maternal circulation, this drug will probably cross the placenta. However, the amount of drug that is systemically absorbed with ocular use is low and likely to be negligible. Animal reproduction studies have not been conducted. Using this drug during pregnancy should be based on the pros and cons of the mother's clinical need for treatment versus any potential fetal risk that might occur from exposure. If used during pregnancy, consider placing pressure over the tear duct in the corner of the eye for at least 1 minute, and then remove any excess solution with absorbent tissue to decrease the amount of drug reaching the systemic circulation even further.

BREASTFEEDING SUMMARY

No reports describing the use of pheniramine during human lactation have been located. The drug will likely be excreted into breast milk, so some infant exposure will probably occur. Breastfeeding while using this drug should be based on the mother's clinical need for treatment versus any potential infant risks that might occur. Due to the ophthalmic use of the drug, systemic side effects were not evaluated. A method to decrease some systemic absorption with ophthalmic use is described above in the Pregnancy Summary.

References

1. Prescribing Information. Eye allergy relief. CVS Pharmacy; 2020.
2. National Library of Medicine. Pheniramine. PubChem. Accessed February 16, 2025. https://pubchem.ncbi.nlm.nih.gov/compound/Pheniramine

PHENOBARBITAL

Central Nervous System (Antiseizure—Barbiturate)

PREGNANCY RECOMMENDATION: Human Data Suggest Potential Risk (First and Third Trimester)

BREASTFEEDING RECOMMENDATION: Potential Toxicity

PREGNANCY SUMMARY

Numerous studies have been located that describe the use of phenobarbital in human pregnancy. In combined data from several sources (including the Collaborative Perinatal Project, Michigan Medicaid Surveillance study, and others), the rate of major birth anomalies was about 3.8% in 1,850 first-trimester exposures. No specific pattern to the anomalies was identified. However, the American Academy of Neurology, American Epilepsy Society, and the Society for Maternal Fetal Medicine published joint guidelines in 2024 for epilepsy during pregnancy. They reported that phenobarbital has a slight but significantly increased risk for cardiac malformations and cleft lip/palate. Some small series suggest an increased risk of subtle birth defects associated with fetal hydantoin syndrome, but this has not been consistently seen. In addition, adverse effects on neurobehavioral development, head circumference, and intelligence have been reported. However, it is difficult to determine if this is related to the drug, use in conjunction with other medications, the disease, or a combination of all of these. Barbiturates can be addictive with long-term use, and neonatal withdrawal, including seizures, can occur when used near delivery. Regardless, uncontrolled seizures have a greater risk for poor pregnancy outcomes. The drug crosses the placenta, so fetal exposure will occur. No animal reproduction studies have been located. Using this drug during pregnancy should be based on the pros and cons of the mother's clinical need for treatment versus any potential fetal risk that might occur from exposure. There is a pregnancy exposure registry that monitors pregnancy outcomes in women using antiseizure drugs. Health care providers are encouraged to call the North American Antiepileptic Drug Pregnancy Registry at 1-888-233-2334.

BREASTFEEDING SUMMARY

Phenobarbital has been shown to be excreted into human breast milk. In two reports, the breast milk to maternal plasma ratio averaged about 50%. The amount of phenobarbital ingested by the nursing infant has been estimated to reach 2 to 4 mg/d. With normal maternal drug usage, this would result in an RID of less than about 3%. Reports have described infant withdrawal and seizures when the drug is abruptly stopped during nursing. Because of the long elimination half-life, accumulation may occur in the infant. Breastfeeding while using this drug should be based on the mother's clinical need for treatment versus any potential infant risks that might occur. If used, the infant should be monitored for the most common reported adult side effects of nausea, dizziness, headache, and dyspepsia (all leading to irritability), sedation, apnea, and rash.

References

1. Prescribing Information. Phenobarbital tablet. Chartwell Rx LLC; 2024.
2. Prescribing Information. Phenobarbital sodium injection. BPI Labs LLC; 2025.
3. Pack AM, Oskoui M, Williams S, et al. Teratogenesis, perinatal, and neurodevelopmental outcomes after in utero exposure to antiseizure medication. *Neurology*. 2024;102:e209279.
4. Tomson T, Battino D, Bromley R, et al. Management of epilepsy in pregnancy: a report from the International League Against Epilepsy task force on women and pregnancy. *Epileptic Disord*. 2019;21:497-517.

P

5. De Carolis MP, Romagnoli C, Frezza S, et al. Placental transfer of phenobarbital: what is new? *Dev Pharmacol Ther*. 1992;19:19-26.
6. Janz D, Fuchs V. Are anti-epileptic drugs harmful when given during pregnancy? *Ger Med Monogr*. 1964;9:20-23.
7. Hill RB. Teratogenesis and anti-epileptic drugs. *N Engl J Med*. 1973; 289:1089-1090.
8. Bodendorfer TW. Fetal effects of anticonvulsant drugs and seizure disorders. *Drug Intell Clin Pharm*. 1978;12:14-21.
9. Nakane Y, Okoma T, Takahashi R, et al. Multi-institutional study of the teratogenicity and fetal toxicity of anti-epileptic drugs: a report of a collaborative study group in Japan. *Epilepsia*. 1980;21:633-680.
10. Andermann E, Dansky L, Andermann F, et al. Minor congenital malformations and dermatoglyphic alterations in the offspring of epileptic women; a clinical investigation of the teratogenic effects of anticonvulsant medication. In: *Epilepsy, Pregnancy and the Child*. Proceedings of a Workshop in Berlin, September 1980; New York, NY: Raven Press; 1981.
11. Dansky L, Andermann E, Andermann F. Major congenital malformations in the offspring of epileptic patients. In: *Epilepsy, Pregnancy and the Child*. Proceedings of a Workshop in Berlin, September 1980New York, NY: Raven Press; 1981.
12. Van der Pol MC, Hadders-Algra M, Huisjes HJ, Touwen BCL. Antiepileptic medication in pregnancy: late effects on the children's central nervous system development. *Am J Obstet Gynecol*. 1991;164:121-128.
13. Hanson JW, Buehler BA. Fetal hydantoin syndrome: current status. *J Pediatr*. 1982;101:816-818.
14. Canger R, Battino D, Canevini MP, et al. Malformations in offspring of women with epilepsy: a prospective study. *Epilepsia*. 1999;40:1231-1236.
15. Holmes LB, Harvey EA, Coull BA, et al. The teratogenicity of anticonvulsant drugs. *N Engl J Med*. 2001;344:1132-1138.
16. Janz D. Antiepileptic drugs and pregnancy: altered utilization patterns and teratogenesis. *Epilepsia*. 1982;23(suppl 1):S53-S63.
17. Heinonen OP, Slone D, Shapiro S. *Birth Defects and Drugs in Pregnancy*. Publishing Sciences Group; 1977.
18. Hernandez-Diaz S, Werler MM, Walker AM, Mitchell AA. Folic acid antagonists during pregnancy and the risk of birth defects. *N Engl J Med*. 2000;343:1608-1614.
19. Rafla NM, Meehan FP. Thanatophoric dwarfism; drugs and antenatal diagnosis; a case report. *Eur J Obstet Gynecol Reprod Biol*. 1990;38:161-165.
20. Arpino C, Brescianini S, Robert E, et al. Teratogenic effects of antiepileptic drugs: use of an international database on malformations and drug exposure (MADRE). *Epilepsia*. 2000;41:1436-1443.
21. The Lamotrigine Pregnancy Registry. Final report. 1 September 1992 through 31 March 2010. GlaxoSmithKline; 2010.
22. Weston J, Bromley R, Jackson CF, et al. Monotherapy treatment of epilepsy in pregnancy: congenital malformation outcomes in the child. *Cochrane Database Syst Rev*. 2016;11:CD101224.
23. Desmond MM, Schwanecke RP, Wilson GS, et al. Maternal barbiturate utilization and neonatal withdrawal symptomatology. *J Pediatr*. 1972;80: 190-197.
24. Pritchard JA, Scott DE, Whalley PJ. Maternal folate deficiency and pregnancy wastage. IV. Effects of folic acid supplements, anticonvulsants, and oral contraceptives. *Am J Obstet Gynecol*. 1971;109:341-346.
25. Hiilesmaa VK, Teramo K, Granstrom ML, Bardy AH. Serum folate concentrations during pregnancy in women with epilepsy: relation to antiepileptic drug concentrations, number of seizures, and fetal outcome. *Br Med J*. 1983; 287:577-579.
26. Biale Y, Lewenthal H. Effect of folic acid supplementation on congenital malformations due to anticonvulsive drugs. *Eur J Obstet Reprod Biol*. 1984;18:211-216.
27. Morales WJ. Antenatal therapy to minimize neonatal intraventricular hemorrhage. *Clin Obstet Gynecol*. 1991;34:328-335.
28. Gaily E, Kantola-Sorsa E, Granstrom ML. Intelligence of children of epileptic mothers. *J Pediatr*. 1988;113:677-684.
29. Reinisch JM, Sanders SA, Mortensen EL, Rubin DB. In utero exposure to phenobarbital and intelligence deficits in adult men. *JAMA*. 1995;274:1518-1525.
30. Dessens AB, Cohen-Kettenis PT, Mellenbergh GJ, et al. Association of prenatal phenobarbital and phenytoin exposure with small head size at birth and with learning problems. *Acta Paediatr*. 2000;89:533-541.
31. Koch S, Jager-Roman E, Losche G, et al. Antiepileptic drug treatment in pregnancy: drug side effects in the neonate and neurological outcome. *Acta Paediatr*. 1996;84:739-746.
32. Shankaran S, Woldt E, Nelson J, et al. Antenatal phenobarbital therapy and neonatal outcome II: neurodevelopmental outcome at 36 months. *Pediatrics*. 1996;97:649-652.
33. Thorpe JA, Yeast JD, Cohen GR, et al. Does in-utero phenobarbital lower IQ: follow up of the intracranial hemorrhage prevention trial (abstract). *Am J Obstet Gynecol*. 1997;176:S117.
34. Thorp JA, O'Connor M, Jones AMH, et al. Does perinatal phenobarbital exposure affect developmental outcome at age 2? *Am J Perinatol*. 1999; 16:51-60.
35. Gopinath N, Muneer AK, Unnikrishnan S, et al. Children (10-12 years age) of women with epilepsy have lower intelligence, attention and memory: observations from a prospective cohort case control study. *Epilepsy Res*. 2015;117:58-62.
36. Tyson RM, Shrader EA, Perlman HN. Drugs transmitted through breast-milk. II. Barbiturates. *J Pediatr*. 1938;13:86-90.
37. Kaneko S, Sata T, Suzuki K. The levels of anticonvulsants in breast milk. *Br J Clin Pharmacol*. 1979;7:624-627.
38. Nau H, Kuhnz W, Egger HJ, et al. Anticonvulsants during pregnancy and lactation: transplacental, maternal and neonatal pharmacokinetics. *Clin Pharmacokinet*. 1982;7:508-543.
39. Horning MG, Stillwell WG, Nowlin J, et al. Identification and quantification of drugs and drug metabolites in human breast milk using GC-MS-COM methods. *Mod Probl Paediatr*. 1975;15:73-79.
40. Reith H, Schafer H. Antiepileptic drugs during pregnancy and the lactation period. Pharmacokinetic data. *Dtsch Med Wochenschr*. 1979;104:818-823.
41. Knott C, Reynolds F, Clayden G. Infantile spasms on weaning from breast milk containing anticonvulsants. *Lancet*. 1987;2:272-273.

P

PHENOXYBENZAMINE

Antihypertensive (α-Adrenergic Blocking Agent)

PREGNANCY RECOMMENDATION: Limited Human Data—No Relevant Animal Data (Maternal Benefit May Outweigh Any Embryofetal Risk)

BREASTFEEDING RECOMMENDATION: Potential Toxicity

PREGNANCY SUMMARY

A few reports describing the use of phenoxybenzamine in human pregnancy were located, but none of these reported use in the first trimester. No adverse fetal effects related to this drug treatment were identified when used in the second and third trimesters. The drug will probably cross the placenta, so some fetal exposure will likely occur. Therefore, the absence of human pregnancy experience prevents a complete assessment of the embryofetal risk. Animal reproduction studies have not been conducted. Using this drug during pregnancy should be based on the pros and cons of the mother's clinical need for treatment versus any potential fetal risk that might occur from exposure. Phenoxybenzamine is used to reduce maternal and fetal mortality that may occur with pheochromocytoma, especially after 24 weeks' gestation when surgical intervention is associated with high rates of these outcomes.

BREASTFEEDING SUMMARY

No reports describing the use of phenoxybenzamine during human lactation have been located. The drug will likely be excreted into breast milk, so some infant exposure will probably occur. However, due to a concern for potential serious adverse effects that might be seen in a breastfed infant, the manufacturer recommends that women not breastfeed while being treated with this drug. Nevertheless, if the clinical decision is to use this drug while breastfeeding, the infant should be monitored for the most common reported adult side effects of gastrointestinal irritation (leading to irritability), hypotension, tachycardia, nasal congestion, miosis, drowsiness, and fatigue (lethargy).

References

1. Prescribing Information. Phenoxybenzamine. Amneal Pharmaceuticals NY LLC; 2024.
2. Santeiro ML, Stromquist C, Wyble L. Phenoxybenzamine placental transfer during the third trimester. *Ann Pharmacother*. 1996;30:1249-1251.
3. Maughan GB, Shabanah EH, Toth A. Experiments with pharmacologic sympatholysis in the gravid. *Am J Obstet Gynecol*. 1967;97:764-776.
4. Wansbrough H, Nakanishi H, Wood C. The effect of adrenergic receptor blocking drugs on the human uterus. *J Obstet Gynaecol Br Commonw*. 1968;75:189-198.
5. Combs CA, Easterling TR, Schmucker BC, Benedetti TJ. Hemodynamic observations during paroxysmal hypertension in a pregnancy with pheochromocytoma. *Obstet Gynecol*. 1989;74:439-441.
6. Brown RB, Borowsky M. Further observations on intestinal lesions associated with pheochromocytomas. A case of malignant pheochromocytoma in pregnancy. *Ann Surg*. 1960;151:683-692.
7. Lawee D. Pheochromocytoma associated with pregnancy. *Can Med Assoc J*. 1970;103:1185-1187.
8. Simanis J, Amerson JR, Hendee AE, Anton AH. Unresectable pheochromocytoma in pregnancy. Pharmacology and biochemistry. *Am J Med*. 1972;53:381-385.
9. Brenner WE, Yen SSC, Dingfelder JR, Anton AH. Pheochromocytoma: serial studies during pregnancy. *Am J Obstet Gynecol*. 1972;113:779-788.
10. Smith AM. Phaeochromocytoma and pregnancy. *J Obstet Gynaecol Br Commonw*. 1973;80:848-851.
11. Griffith MI, Felts JH, James FM, et al. Successful control of pheochromocytoma in pregnancy. *JAMA*. 1974;229:437-439.
12. Awitti-Sunga SA, Ursell W. Phaeochromocytoma in pregnancy. Case report. *Br J Obstet Gynaecol*. 1975;82:426-428.
13. Coombes GB. Phaeochromocytoma presenting in pregnancy. *Proc R Soc Med*. 1976;69:224-225.
14. Leak D, Carroll JJ, Robinson DC, Ashworth EJ. Management of pheochromocytoma during pregnancy. *Can Med Assoc J*. 1977;116:371-375.
15. Burgess GE III. Alpha blockade and surgical intervention of pheochromocytoma in pregnancy. *Obstet Gynecol*. 1979;53:266-270.
16. Modlin IM, Farndon JR, Shepherd A, et al. Phaeochromocytomas in 72 patients: clinical and diagnostic features, treatment and long term results. *Br J Surg*. 1979;66:456-465.
17. Fudge TL, McKinnon WMP, Geary WL. Current surgical management of pheochromocytoma during pregnancy. *Arch Surg*. 1980;115:1224-1225.
18. Coetzee A, Hartwig N, Erasmus FR. Feochromositoom tydens swangerskap. Die narkosehantering van 'n pasient. *S Afr Med J*. 1981;59:861-862.
19. Stonham J, Wakefield C. Phaeochromocytoma in pregnancy: caesarean section under epidural analgesia. *Anaesthesia*. 1983;38:654-658.
20. Stenstrom G, Swolin K. Pheochromocytoma in pregnancy. Experience of treatment with phenoxybenzamine in three patients. *Acta Obstet Gynecol Scand*. 1985;64:357-361.
21. Bakri YN, Ingemansson SE, Ali A, Parikh S. Pheochromocytoma and pregnancy: report of three cases. *Acta Obstet Gynecol Scand*. 1992;71:301-304.
22. Miller C, Bernet V, Elkas JC, et al. Conservative management of extra-adrenal pheochromocytoma during pregnancy. *Obstet Gynecol*. 2005;105:1185-1188.
23. Lyons CW, Colmorgen GHC. Medical management of pheochromocytoma in pregnancy. *Obstet Gynecol*. 1988;72:450-451.
24. Schenker JG, Chowers I. Pheochromocytoma and pregnancy. Review of 89 cases. *Obstet Gynecol Surv*. 1971;26:739-747.

PHENTERMINE

Autonomic (Sympathomimetic/Anorexiant)

PREGNANCY RECOMMENDATION: *Contraindicated

BREASTFEEDING RECOMMENDATION: *Contraindicated

PREGNANCY SUMMARY

A few reports were located that describe the use of phentermine alone or in combination with fenfluramine in more than 200 human pregnancies. No higher rate of major anomalies was seen in about 100 cases with first-trimester exposure when compared with controls. The remainder of exposures came from older studies where the drug was used in the third trimester in treating obesity prior to delivery. The drug will probably cross the placenta, so some fetal exposure will likely occur. Therefore, this limited human pregnancy experience prevents a complete assessment of the embryofetal risk. Animal reproduction studies have not been located. *However, it is doubtful if any real benefit is derived from the use of this drug for weight control during human pregnancy. Therefore, its use during gestation, especially during the first trimester, should be considered contraindicated. Using this drug during pregnancy should be based on the pros and cons of the mother's clinical need for treatment versus any potential fetal risk that might occur from exposure. Hypertension was reported in patients treated with this drug during the clinical trials.

BREASTFEEDING SUMMARY

No reports describing the use of phentermine during human lactation have been located. The drug will likely be excreted into breast milk, so infant exposure will probably occur. *Because CNS stimulation and other adverse reactions may occur in a nursing infant exposed to this drug in breast milk, phentermine should be considered contraindicated during breastfeeding. The manufacturer recommends that phentermine should not be taken by women who are breastfeeding unless, in the opinion of the physician, the potential benefits outweigh the possible hazards. If the clinical decision is to use this drug while breastfeeding, the infant should be monitored for the most common reported adult side effects of agitation, dizziness, headache, nausea, and stomach pain (all leading to irritability), tachycardia, elevated blood pressure, ischemic events, insomnia, tremor, sweating, diarrhea, constipation, and urinary frequency.

References

1. Prescribing Information. Phentermine hydrochloride. Precision Dose Inc; 2023.
2. Sands RX. Obesity and pregnancy. Weight control with a resinate. *Am J Obstet Gynecol.* 1962;83:1617-1621.
3. Jones KL, Johnson KA, Dick LM, et al. Pregnancy outcomes after first trimester exposure to phentermine/fenfluramine. *Teratology.* 2002;65: 125-130.
4. D'Adesky N, Ghosh S. Phentermine use during first and second trimesters associated with fetal stroke. *Cureus.* 2019;11:e6170.

PHENTOLAMINE

Antihypertensive (α-Adrenergic Blocker)

PREGNANCY RECOMMENDATION: Limited Human Data—No Relevant Animal Data (Maternal Benefit May Outweigh Embryofetal Risk)

BREASTFEEDING RECOMMENDATION: Potential Toxicity (Hold Breastfeeding)

PREGNANCY SUMMARY

A few reports describing the use of phentolamine in human pregnancy have been located. A healthy newborn with no identified anomalies was delivered to one patient with first-trimester exposure. The rest of the drug administrations involved the diagnosis of or short-term treatment of pheochromocytoma. No adverse effects on the fetus or newborn attributable to phentolamine from this use were described. The drug is likely to cross the placenta, so some fetal exposure will probably occur. Therefore, this limited human pregnancy experience prevents a complete assessment of embryofetal risk. Embryofetal toxicity was observed in two animal species, but at doses of more than 10 times the RHD. Using this drug during pregnancy should be based on the pros and cons of the mother's clinical need for treatment versus any potential fetal risk that might occur from exposure. Hypotension can often occur in patients treated with this drug.

BREASTFEEDING SUMMARY

No reports describing the use of phentolamine during human lactation have been located. The drug will likely be excreted into breast milk, so some infant exposure will probably occur. However, due to a concern for potential serious adverse effects that might be seen in a breastfed infant, the manufacturer recommends that women not breastfeed while being treated with this drug. Nevertheless, breastfeeding while using this drug should be based on the mother's clinical need for treatment versus any potential infant risks that might occur. If used, the infant should be monitored for the most common reported adult side effects of nausea and dizziness (both leading to irritability), acute and prolonged hypotensive episodes, tachycardia, cardiac arrhythmias, weakness, flushing, vomiting, and diarrhea. Another option would be to hold breastfeeding for about 1.5 to 2 hours (five to six half-lives) if short-term usage is needed.

References

1. Prescribing Information. Phentolamine mesylate. Hikma Pharmaceuticals USA Inc; 2024.
2. Maughan GB, Shabanah EH, Toth A. Experiments with pharmacologic sympatholysis in the gravid. *Am J Obstet Gynecol.* 1967;97:764-776.
3. Wansbrough H, Nakanishi H, Wood C. The effect of adrenergic receptor blocking drugs on the human uterus. *J Obstet Gynaecol Br Commonw.* 1968;75:189-198.
4. Althabe O Jr, Schwarcz RL Jr, Sala NL, Fisch L. Effect of phentolamine methanesulfonate upon uterine contractility induced by l-norepinephrine in pregnancy. *Am J Obstet Gynecol.* 1968;101:1083-1088.
5. Jenssen H. Inhibition of oxytocin-induced uterine activity in midpregnancy by combined adrenergic α-blockade and β-stimulation. *Acta Obstet Gynecol Scand.* 1971;50:135-139.
6. Anton AH, Brenner WE, Yen SS, Dingfelder JR. Pheochromocytoma: studies during pregnancy, premature delivery and surgery. Paper presented at: 5th International Congress on Pharmacology; July 23-28, 1972; San Francisco, CA, Abstract No. 43, p. 8.
7. Simanis J, Amerson JR, Hendee AE, Anton AH. Unresectable pheochromocytoma in pregnancy. Pharmacology and biochemistry. *Am J Med.* 1972; 53:381-385.
8. Brenner WE, Yen SSC, Dingfelder JR, Anton AH. Pheochromocytoma: serial studies during pregnancy. *Am J Obstet Gynecol.* 1972;113:779-788.
9. Burgess GE III. Alpha blockade and surgical intervention of pheochromocytoma in pregnancy. *Obstet Gynecol.* 1979;53:266-270.
10. Schenker JG, Chowers I. Pheochromocytoma and pregnancy. Review of 89 cases. *Obstet Gynecol Surv.* 1971;26:739-747.
11. Hendee AE, Martin RD, Waters WC III. Hypertension in pregnancy: toxemia or pheochromocytoma? *Am J Obstet Gynecol.* 1969;105:64-72.
12. Smith AM. Phaeochromocytoma and pregnancy. *J Obstet Gynaecol Br Commonw.* 1973;80:848-851.
13. Heinonen OP, Slone D, Shapiro S. *Birth Defects and Drugs in Pregnancy.* Wright PSB; 1983:372-373.

PHENYLEPHRINE

Respiratory/Cardiovascular/Gastrointestinal (α_1-Agonist)

PREGNANCY RECOMMENDATION: Human Data Suggest Low Risk (Malformations)/Potential Risk (Blood Pressure)

BREASTFEEDING RECOMMENDATION: Probably Compatible (Short-Term Use)

P

PREGNANCY SUMMARY

Several reports describing the use of phenylephrine in human pregnancy have been located. It is approved for several routes of administration. From the Collaborative Perinatal Project and the Group Health Cooperative of Puget Sound databases (using worst-case possibility when needed), there were 46 (2.8%) major congenital anomalies seen in 1,650 first-trimester exposures. No pattern to the defects was seen. The oral and nasal spray products are for nasal and sinus congestion, whereas the IV product is for treating hypotension related to anesthesia (primarily used in the second or third trimesters). Lastly, the rectal form is for treating hemorrhoids. The drug will probably cross the placenta, so some fetal exposure will likely occur. Embryofetal toxicity was seen in two animal species at doses of less than 10 times the RHD. Using this drug during pregnancy should be based on the pros and cons of the mother's clinical need for treatment versus any potential fetal risk that might occur from exposure. Hypertension is not common in patients treated with this drug, especially those with chronic hypertension, hyperthyroidism, and cardiovascular disease.

BREASTFEEDING SUMMARY

No reports describing the use of phenylephrine during human lactation have been located. The drug will likely be excreted into breast milk, so some infant exposure will probably occur. Another systemic α-agonist, pseudoephedrine, resulted in decreased breast milk supply when used during lactation (see Pseudoephedrine). Therefore, this may occur with phenylephrine. Breastfeeding while using this drug should be based on the mother's clinical need for treatment versus any potential infant risks that might occur. If used, the infant should be monitored for the most common reported adult side effects of nausea and headache (both leading to irritability) and vomiting.

References

1. Prescribing Information. Phenylephrine hydrochloride (injection). Amneal Pharmaceuticals LLC; 2023.
2. Prescribing Information. McKesson Phenylephrine HCl (tablet). McKesson Medical-Surgical; 2024.
3. Food and Drug Administration. FDA News release. Accessed February 22, 2025. https://www.fda.gov/news-events/press-announcements/fda-proposes-ending-use-oral-phenylephrine-otc-monograph-nasal-decongestant-active-ingredient-after
4. Product Information. 4 Way fast acting (spray). Haleon US Holdings LLC; 2024.
5. Medscape. Phenylephrine nasal (OTC). Accessed February 22, 2025. https://reference.medscape.com/drug/neosynephrine-phenylephrine-nasal-343410#0
6. Product Information. Avedana hemorrhoidal pain relief. Unipack LLC; 2024.
7. Smith NT, Corbascio AN. The use and misuse of pressor agents. *Anesthesiology*. 1970;33:58-101.
8. Minzter BH, Johnson RF, Paschall RL, et al. The diverse effects of vasopressors on the fetoplacental circulation of the dual perfused placenta. *Anesth Analg*. 2010;110:857-862.
9. Heinonen OP, Slone D, Shapiro S. *Birth Defects and Drugs in Pregnancy*. Publishing Sciences Group; 1977.
10. Eguchi K, Yonezawa M, Hagegawa T, et al. Fetal activity determination and neosynephrine test for evaluation of fetal well-being in high risk pregnancies. *Nihon Sanka Fujinka Gakkai Zasshi*. 1980;32:663-668.
11. Yau WP, Mitchell AA, Lin KJ, et al. Use of decongestants during pregnancy and the risk of birth defects. *Am J Epidemiol*. 2013;178:198-208.
12. Dyer FA, Emmanuel A, Adams SC, et al. A randomized comparison of bolus phenylephrine and ephedrine for the management of spinal hypotension in patients with severe preeclampsia and fetal compromise. *Int J Obstet Anesth*. 2018;33:23-31.
13. Xu C, Liu S, Huang Y, et al. Phenylephrine vs ephedrine in cesarean delivery under spinal anesthesia: a systematic literature review and meta-analysis. *Int J Surg*. 2018;60:48-59.
14. Tan H, Chen Y, Jiang Y, et al. Determination of ED90s of phenylephrine and norepinephrine infusion for prevention of spinal anesthesia-induced hypotension in patients with preeclampsia during cesarean delivery. *Drug Des Devel Ther*. 2024;18:2813-2821.
15. Pan ZB, Sheng ZM, Zhu M, et al. Randomized double-blinded comparison of intermittent boluses phenylephrine and norepinephrine for the treatment of postspinal hypotension in patients with severe pre-eclampsia during cesarean section. *Drug Des Devel Ther*. 2024;18:639-650.

P

PHENYLEPHRINE OPHTHALMIC

Ophthalmic (α_1-Adrenergic Agonist)

PREGNANCY RECOMMENDATION: No Human Data—No Relevant Animal Data

BREASTFEEDING RECOMMENDATION: Probably Compatible

PREGNANCY SUMMARY

No reports describing the use of phenylephrine ophthalmic in human pregnancy have been located. The amount of the medication absorbed systemically has not been analyzed; however, systemic adverse effects have been reported to the manufacturer. These include cardiac effects, an increase in blood pressure, syncope, tachycardia, and arrhythmia. Therefore, the drug will probably cross the placenta, so some fetal exposure will likely occur. However, the absence of human pregnancy experience prevents a complete assessment of the embryofetal risk. No animal reproduction studies have been conducted. Using this drug during pregnancy should be based on the pros and cons of the mother's clinical need for treatment versus any potential fetal risk that might occur from exposure. If used during pregnancy, consider placing pressure over the tear duct in the corner of the eye for at least 1 minute, and then remove any excess solution with absorbent tissue to decrease the amount of drug reaching the systemic circulation even further. Hypertension is not common in patients treated with this drug, especially those with chronic hypertension, hyperthyroidism, and cardiovascular disease.

BREASTFEEDING SUMMARY

No reports describing the use of phenylephrine ophthalmic during human lactation have been located. The drug will likely be excreted into breast milk, so some infant exposure will probably occur. Although the amount of drug that might be in the maternal circulation after ophthalmic use is unknown, it has produced systemic side effects. If the clinical decision is to use this drug while breastfeeding, the infant should be monitored for the most common reported adult side effects of an increase in blood pressure, tachycardia, and arrhythmias. A method to decrease some systemic absorption with ophthalmic use is described above in the Pregnancy Summary.

Reference

1. Prescribing Information. Phenylephrine hydrochloride. Alcon Laboratories Inc; 2024.

PHENYTOIN

Central Nervous System (Antiseizure—Hydantoin)

PREGNANCY RECOMMENDATION: Human Data Suggest Potential Risk (First Trimester) (Maternal Benefit May Outweigh Embryofetal Risk)

BREASTFEEDING RECOMMENDATION: Potential Toxicity

PREGNANCY SUMMARY

Numerous studies have been located that describe the use of phenytoin during human pregnancy. From several sources, including the Collaborative Perinatal Project, Michigan Medicaid Surveillance study, and others, the malformation rate in about 550 first-trimester exposures was 4.2%. In these analyses, no specific pattern to the defects was seen. However, numerous reports exist that describe a pattern of defects (some of which are minor) that has been labeled fetal hydantoin syndrome (FHS). FHS includes hypoplastic or absent nails, distal phalange abnormalities, craniofacial anomalies with a flat nasal bridge and hypertelorism, abnormal or low-set ears, low hairline, and others. Data are mixed on neurocognitive outcomes, childhood intelligence, and newborn head circumference. The drug crosses the placenta, so some fetal exposure will occur. Embryofetal toxicity with malformations was observed in three animal species at doses of less than 10 times the MRHD based on body weight. Regardless, the risk to the mother and fetus is also high if the drug is not used to control seizures. The risk/benefit ratio, in this case, favors continued use of the drug during pregnancy. During pregnancy, uncontrolled epilepsy is associated with IUGR and preterm delivery, as well as an increased risk for hypoxia. There is a pregnancy exposure registry that monitors pregnancy outcomes in women using antiseizure drugs. Health care providers are encouraged to call the North American Antiepileptic Drug Pregnancy Registry at 1-888-233-2334. Elevated glucose levels have been reported in patients treated with this drug. In addition, phenytoin has also been shown to decrease vitamin K levels.

BREASTFEEDING SUMMARY

Phenytoin has been shown to be excreted into human breast milk. Breast milk to maternal plasma levels average about 40%. Reviewers have concluded that little risk to a nursing infant was present if maternal drug levels were kept in the therapeutic range. Most evaluations do not report any adverse infant effects when using this drug while breastfeeding. Overall, no adverse effects have been seen in childhood intelligence quotient (IQ) in children who had been breastfed while their mothers were taking phenytoin. Breastfeeding while using this drug should be based on the mother's clinical need for treatment versus any potential infant risks that might occur. If used, the infant should be monitored for the most common reported adult side effects of nystagmus and somnolence.

References

1. Prescribing Information. Dilantin. Parke-Davis Div of Pfizer Inc; 2022.
2. Prescribing Information. Phenytoin sodium. Acella Pharmaceuticals LLC; 2024.
3. Prescribing Information. Phenytoin (suspension). Greenstone LLC; 2022.
4. Tomson T, Battino D, Bromley R, et al. Management of epilepsy in pregnancy: a report from the International League Against Epilepsy task force on women and pregnancy. *Epileptic Disord*. 2019;21:497-517.
5. Hill RB. Teratogenesis and antiepileptic drugs. *N Engl J Med*. 1973;289:1089-1090.
6. Janz D. The teratogenic risk of antiepileptic drugs. *Epilepsia*. 1975;16:159-169.
7. Bodendorfer TW. Fetal effects of anticonvulsant drugs and seizure disorders. *Drug Intell Clin Pharm*. 1978;12:14-21.
8. Nakane Y, Okuma T, Takahashi R, et al. Multi-institutional study of the teratogenicity and fetal toxicity of antiepileptic drugs: a report of a collaborative study group in Japan. *Epilepsia*. 1980;21:663-680.
9. Andermann E, Dansky L, Andermann F, et al. Minor congenital malformations and dermatoglyphic alterations in the offspring of epileptic women: a clinical investigation of the teratogenic effects of anticonvulsant medication. In: *Epilepsy, Pregnancy and the Child*. Proceedings of a Workshop in Berlin, September 1980. Raven Press; 1981.
10. Dansky L, Andermann E, Andermann F. Major congenital malformations in the offspring of epileptic patients. In: *Epilepsy, Pregnancy and the Child*. Proceedings of a Workshop in Berlin, September 1980. Raven Press; 1981.
11. Hanson JW, Buehler BA. Fetal hydantoin syndrome: current status. *J Pediatr*. 1982;101:816-818.
12. Canger R, Battino D, Canevini MP, et al. Malformations in offspring of women with epilepsy: a prospective study. *Epilepsia*. 1999;40:1231-1236.
13. Holmes LB, Harvey EA, Coull BA, et al. The teratogenicity of anticonvulsant drugs. *N Engl J Med*. 2001;344:1132-1138.
14. Buehler BA, Delimont D, Van Waes M, Finnell RH. Prenatal prediction of risk of the fetal hydantoin syndrome. *N Engl J Med*. 1990;322:1567-1572.
15. Tiboni GM, Iammarrone E, Giampietro F, et al. Teratological interaction between the bis-triazole antifungal agent fluconazole and the anticonvulsant drug phenytoin. *Teratology*. 1999;59:81-87.
16. Meadow SR. Anticonvulsant drugs and congenital abnormalities. *Lancet*. 1968;2:1296.
17. Loughnan PM, Gold H, Vance JC. Phenytoin teratogenicity in man. *Lancet*. 1973;1:70-72.

18. Hill RM, Horning MG, Horning EC. Antiepileptic drugs and fetal well-being. In: Boreus L, ed. *Fetal Pharmacology*. Raven Press; 1973:375-379.
19. Janz D. Antiepileptic drugs and pregnancy: altered utilization patterns and teratogenesis. *Epilepsia*. 1982;23(suppl 1):S53-S63.
20. Allen RW Jr, Ogden B, Bentley FL, Jung AL. Fetal hydantoin syndrome, neuroblastoma, and hemorrhagic disease in a neonate. *JAMA*. 1980;244:1464-1465.
21. Ramilo J, Harris VJ. Neuroblastoma in a child with the hydantoin and fetal alcohol syndrome. The radiographic features. *Br J Radiol*. 1979;52:993-995.
22. Pendergrass TW, Hanson JW. Fetal hydantoin syndrome and neuroblastoma. *Lancet*. 1976;2:150.
23. Sherman S, Roizen N. Fetal hydantoin syndrome and neuroblastoma. *Lancet*. 1976;2:517.
24. Ehrenbard LT, Chaganti RSK. Cancer in the fetal hydantoin syndrome. *Lancet*. 1981;2:97.
25. Seeler RA, Israel JN, Royal JE, et al. Ganglioneuroblastoma and fetal hydantoin-alcohol syndromes. *Pediatrics*. 1979;63:524-527.
26. Jimenez JF, Seibert RW, Char F, et al. Melanotic neuroectodermal tumor of infancy and fetal hydantoin syndrome. *Am J Pediatr Hematol Oncol*. 1981;3:9-15.
27. Taylor WF, Myers M, Taylor WR. Extrarenal Wilms' tumour in an infant exposed to intrauterine phenytoin. *Lancet*. 1980;2:481-482.
28. Blattner WA, Hanson DE, Young EC, Fraumeni JF. Malignant mesenchymoma and birth defects. *JAMA*. 1977;238:334-335.
29. Kousseff BG. Subcutaneous vascular abnormalities in fetal hydantoin syndrome. *Birth Defects*. 1982;18:51-54.
30. Lipson A. Bale P. Ependymoblastoma associated with prenatal exposure to diphenylhydantoin and methylphenobarbitone. *Cancer*. 1985;55:1859-1862.
31. Corcoran R, Rizk MW. VACTERL congenital malformation and phenytoin therapy? *Lancet*. 1976;2:960.
32. Pinto W Jr, Gardner LI, Rosenbaum P. Abnormal genitalia as a presenting sign in two male infants with hydantoin embryopathy syndrome. *Am J Dis Child*. 1977;131:452-455.
33. Hoyt CS, Billson FA. Maternal anticonvulsants and optic nerve hypoplasia. *Br J Ophthalmol*. 1978;62:3-6.
34. Wilson RS, Smead W, Char F. Diphenylhydantoin teratogenicity: ocular manifestations and related deformities. *J Pediatr Ophthalmol Strabismus*. 1970;15:137-140.
35. Dabee V, Hart AG, Hurley RM. Teratogenic effects of diphenylhydantoin. *Can Med Assoc J*. 1975;112:75-77.
36. Anderson RC. Cardiac defects in children of mothers receiving anticonvulsant therapy during pregnancy. *J Pediatr*. 1976;89:318-319.
37. Hill RM, Verniaud WM, Horning MG, et al. Infants exposed in utero to antiepileptic drugs. A prospective study. *Am J Dis Child*. 1974;127:645-653.
38. Stankler L, Campbell AGM. Neonatal acne vulgaris: a possible feature of the fetal hydantoin syndrome. *Br J Dermatol*. 1980;103:453-455.
39. Ringrose CAD. The hazard of neurotropic drugs in the fertile years. *Can Med Assoc J*. 1972;106:1058.
40. Pettifor JM, Benson R. Congenital malformations associated with the administration of oral anticoagulants during pregnancy. *J Pediatr*. 1975;86:459-461.
41. Biale Y, Lewenthal H, Aderet NB. Congenital malformations due to anticonvulsant drugs and congenital abnormalities. *Obstet Gynecol*. 1975;45:439-442.
42. Aase JM. Anticonvulsant drugs and congenital abnormalities. *Am J Dis Child*. 1974;127:758.
43. Lewin PK. Phenytoin associated congenital defects with Y-chromosome variant. *Lancet*. 1973;1:559.
44. Yang TS, Chi CC, Tsai CJ, Chang MJ. Diphenylhydantoin teratogenicity in man. *Obstet Gynecol*. 1978;52:682-684.
45. Mallow DW, Herrick MK, Gathman G. Fetal exposure to anticonvulsant drugs. *Arch Pathol Lab Med*. 1980;104:215-218.
46. Hirschberger M, Kleinberg F. Maternal phenytoin ingestion and congenital abnormalities: report of a case. *Am J Dis Child*. 1975;129:984.
47. Hanson JW, Myrianthopoulos NC, Sedgwick Harvey MA, Smith DW. Risks to the offspring of women treated with hydantoin anticonvulsants, with emphasis on the fetal hydantoin syndrome. *J Pediatr*. 1976;89:662-668.
48. Shakir RA, Johnson RH, Lambie DG, et al. Comparison of sodium valproate and phenytoin as single drug treatment in epilepsy. *Epilepsia*. 1981;22:27-33.
49. Michalodimitrakis M, Parchas S, Coutselinis A. Fetal hydantoin syndrome: congenital malformation of the urinary tract—a case report. *Clin Toxicol*. 1981;18:1095-1097.
50. Phelan MC, Pellock JM, Nance WE. Discordant expression of fetal hydantoin syndrome in heteropaternal dizygotic twins. *N Engl J Med*. 1982;307:99-101.
51. Kousseff BG, Root ER. Expanding phenotype of fetal hydantoin syndrome. *Pediatrics*. 1982;70:328-329.
52. Wilker R, Nathenson G. Combined fetal alcohol and hydantoin syndromes. *Clin Pediatr*. 1982;21:331-334.
53. Kogutt MS. Fetal hydantoin syndrome. *South Med J*. 1984;77:657-658.
54. Krauss CM, Holmes LB, VanLang QN, Keith DA. Four siblings with similar malformations after exposure to phenytoin and primidone. *J Pediatr*. 1984;105:750-755.
55. Pearl KN, Dickens S, Latham P. Functional palatal incompetence in the fetal anticonvulsant syndrome. *Arch Dis Child*. 1984;59:989-990.
56. Trice JE, Ambler M. Multiple cerebral defects in an infant exposed in utero to anticonvulsants. *Arch Pathol Lab Med*. 1985;109:521-523.
57. D'Souza SW, Robertson IG, Donnai D, Mawer G. Fetal phenytoin exposure, hypoplastic nails, and jitteriness. *Arch Dis Child*. 1990;65:320-324.
58. Kotzot D, Weigl J, Huk W, Rott HD. Hydantoin syndrome with holoprosencephaly: a possible rare teratogenic effect. *Teratology*. 1993;48:15-19.
59. Shaw GM, Wasserman CR, O'Malley CD, et al. Orofacial clefts and maternal anticonvulsant use. *Reprod Toxicol*. 1995;9:97-98.
60. Sabry MA, Farag TI. Hand anomalies in fetal-hydantoin syndrome: from nail/phalangeal hypoplasia to unilateral acheiria. *Am J Med Genet*. 1996;62:410-412.
61. Holmes LB, Harvey EA. Holoprosencephaly and the teratogenicity of anticonvulsants. *Teratology*. 1994;49:82.
62. Rafla NM, Meehan FP. Thanatophoric dwarfism; drugs and antenatal diagnosis: a case report. *Eur J Obstet Gynecol Reprod Biol*. 1990;38:161-165.
63. Arpino C, Brescianini S, Robert E, et al. Teratogenic effects of antiepileptic drugs: use of an international database on malformations and drug exposure (MADRE). *Epilepsia*. 2000;41:1436-1443.
64. The Lamotrigine Pregnancy Registry. Final report. 1 September 1992 through 31 March 2010. GlaxoSmithKline; 2010.
65. Al-Shammri S, Guberman A, Hsu E. Neuroblastoma and fetal exposure to phenytoin in a child without dysmorphic features. *Can J Neurol Sci*. 1992;19:243-245.
66. Koren G, Demitrakoudis D, Weksberg R, et al. Neuroblastoma after prenatal exposure to phenytoin: cause and effect? *Teratology*. 1989;40:157-162.
67. Lawrence A. Antiepileptic drugs and the foetus. *Br Med J*. 1963;2:1267.
68. Kohler HG. Haemorrhage in newborn of epileptic mothers. *Lancet*. 1966;1:267.
69. Douglas H. Haemorrhage in the newborn. *Lancet*. 1966;1:816-817.
70. Monnet P, Rosenberg D, Bovier-Lapierre M. Thérapeutique anticomitiale administrée pendant la grossesse et maladie hémorragique du nouveau-né. Remarques critiques à propos de trois observations personnelles. *Rev Fr Gynecol Obstet*. 1968;63(12):695-702. As cited in Bleyer WA, Skinner AL. Fetal neonatal hemorrhage after maternal anticonvulsant therapy. *JAMA*. 1976;235:626-627.
71. Davis PP. Coagulation defect due to anticonvulsant drug treatment in pregnancy. *Lancet*. 1970;1:413.
72. Evans AR, Forrester RM, Discombe C. Neonatal haemorrhage following maternal anticonvulsant therapy. *Lancet*. 1970;1:517-518.
73. Stevensom MM, Bilbert EF. Anticonvulsants and hemorrhagic diseases of the newborn infant. *J Pediatr*. 1970;77:516.
74. Speidel BD, Meadow SR. Maternal epilepsy and abnormalities of the foetus and newborn. *Lancet*. 1972;2:839-840.
75. Truog WE, Feusner JH, Baker DL. Association of hemorrhagic disease and the syndrome of persistent fetal circulation with the fetal hydantoin syndrome. *J Pediatr*. 1980;96:112-114.
76. Solomon GE, Hilgartner MW, Kutt H. Coagulation defects caused by diphenylhydantoin. *Neurology*. 1972;22:1165-1171.
77. Griffiths AD. Neonatal haemorrhage associated with maternal anticonvulsant therapy. *Lancet*. 1981;2:1296-1297.
78. Page TE, Hoyme HE, Markarian M, Jones KL. Neonatal hemorrhage secondary to thrombocytopenia: an occasional effect of prenatal hydantoin exposure. *Birth Defects*. 1982;18:47-50.
79. Srinivasan G, Seeler RA, Tiruvury A, Pildes RS. Maternal anticonvulsant therapy and hemorrhagic disease of the newborn. *Obstet Gynecol*. 1982;59:250-252.
80. Payne NR, Hasegawa DK. Vitamin K deficiency in newborns: a case report in α-1-antitrypsin deficiency and a review of factors predisposing to hemorrhage. *Pediatrics*. 1984;73:712-716.
81. Lane PA, Hathaway WE. Vitamin K in infancy. *J Pediatr*. 1985;106:351-359.
82. Howe AM, Lipson AH, Sheffield LJ, et al. Prenatal exposure to phenytoin, facial development, and a possible role for vitamin K. *Am J Med Genet*. 1995;58:238-244.
83. Felding I, Rane A. Congenital liver damage after treatment of mother with valproic acid and phenytoin? *Acta Paediatr Scand*. 1984;73:565-568.

84. Biale Y, Lewenthal H. Effect of folic acid supplementation on congenital malformations due to anticonvulsive drugs. *Eur J Obstet Reprod Biol*. 1984; 18:211-216.
85. Pritchard JA, Scott DE, Whalley PJ. Maternal folate deficiency and pregnancy wastage. IV. Effects of folic acid supplements, anticonvulsants, and oral contraceptives. *Am J Obstet Gynecol*. 1971;109:341-346.
86. Hiilesmaa VK, Teramo K, Granstrom ML, Bardy AH. Serum folate concentrations during pregnancy in women with epilepsy: relation to antiepileptic drug concentrations, number of seizures, and fetal outcome. *Br Med J*. 1983;287:577-579.
87. Hernandez-Diaz S, Werler MM, Walker AM, Mitchell AA. Folic acid antagonists during pregnancy and the risk of birth defects. *N Engl J Med*. 2000;343:1608-1614.
88. Nau H, Kuhnz W, Egger HJ, Rating D, Helge H. Anticonvulsants during pregnancy and lactation: transplacental, maternal and neonatal pharmacokinetics. *Clin Pharmacokinet*. 1982;7:508-543.
89. Chen SS, Perucca E, Lee JN, Richens A. Serum protein binding and free concentrations of phenytoin and phenobarbitone in pregnancy. *Br J Clin Pharmacol*. 1982;13:547-552.
90. Van der Kligh E, Schobben F, Bree TB. Clinical pharmacokinetics of antiepileptic drugs. *Drug Intell Clin Pharm*. 1980;14:674-685.
91. Dansky L, Andermann E, Sherwin AL, Andermann F. Plasma levels of phenytoin during pregnancy and the puerperium. In: *Epilepsy, Pregnancy and the Child*. Proceedings of a Workshop held in Berlin, September 1980. Raven Press; 1981.
92. Dansky L, Andermann E, Andermann F, et al. Maternal epilepsy and congenital malformation: correlation with maternal plasma anticonvulsant levels during pregnancy. In: *Epilepsy, Pregnancy and the Child*. Proceedings of a Workshop held in Berlin, September 1980. Raven Press; 1981.
93. Hiilesmaa VK. Evaluation of placental function in women on antiepileptic drugs. *J Perinat Med*. 1983;11:187-192.
94. Carriero R, Andermann E, Chen MF, et al. Thyroid function in epileptic mothers and their infants at birth. *Am J Obstet Gynecol*. 1985;151:641-644.
95. Markestad T, Ulstein M, Strandjord RE, et al. Anticonvulsant drug therapy in human pregnancy: effects on serum concentrations of vitamin D metabolites in maternal and cord blood. *Am J Obstet Gynecol*. 1984; 150:254-258.
96. Tamari I, Eldar M, Rabinowitz B, Neufeld HN. Medical treatment of cardiovascular disorders during pregnancy. *Am Heart J*. 1982;104:1357-1363.
97. Rotmensch HH, Elkayam U, Frishman W. Antiarrhythmic drug therapy during pregnancy. *Ann Intern Med*. 1983;98:487-497.
98. Rotmensch HH, Rotmensch S, Elkayam U. Management of cardiac arrhythmias during pregnancy: current concepts. *Drugs*. 1987;33:623-633.
99. Ryan G, Lange IR, Naugler MA. Clinical experience with phenytoin prophylaxis in severe preeclampsia. *Am J Obstet Gynecol*. 1989;161:1297-1304.
100. Almgren M, Kallen B, Lavebratt C. Population-based study of antiepileptic drug exposure *in utero*—influence on head circumference in newborns. *Seizure*. 2009;18:672-675.
101. Weston J, Bromley R, Jackson CF, et al. Monotherapy treatment of epilepsy in pregnancy: congenital malformation outcomes in the child. *Cochrane Database Syst Rev*. 2016;11(11):CD101224.
102. Gaily E, Kantola-Sorsa E, Granstrom M-L. Intelligence of children of epileptic mothers. *J Pediatr*. 1988;113:677-684.
103. Scolnik D, Nulman I, Rovet J, et al. Neurodevelopment of children exposed in utero to phenytoin and carbamazepine monotherapy. *JAMA*. 1994;271:767-770.
104. Jeret JS. Neurodevelopment after in utero exposure to phenytoin and carbamazepine. *JAMA*. 1994;272:850.
105. Loring DW, Meador KJ, Thompson WO. Neurodevelopment of children exposed in utero to phenytoin and carbamazepine. *JAMA*. 1994;272: 850-851.
106. Koren G. Neurodevelopment of children exposed in utero to phenytoin and carbamazepine. *JAMA*. 1994;272:851.
107. Meador KJ, Baker GA, Browning N, et al; NEAD Study Group. Fetal antiepileptic drug exposure and cognitive outcomes at age 6 years (NEAD study): a prospective observational study. *Lancet Neurol*. 2013;12:244-252.
108. Koch S, Jager-Roman E, Losche G, et al. Antiepileptic drug treatment in pregnancy: drug side effects in the neonate and neurological outcome. *Acta Paediatr*. 1996;84:739-746.
109. Dessens AB, Cohen-Kettenis PT, Mellenbergh GJ, et al. Association of prenatal phenobarbital and phenytoin exposure with small head size at birth and with learning problems. *Acta Paediatr*. 2000;89:533-541.
110. Gopinath N, Muneer AK, Unnikrishnan S, et al. Children (10-12 years age) of women with epilepsy have lower intelligence, attention and memory: observations from a prospective cohort case control study. *Epilepsy Res*. 2015;117:58-62.
111. Horning MG, Stillwell WG, Nowling J, et al. Identification and quantification of drugs and drug metabolites in human breast milk using GC-MS-COM methods. *Mod Probl Pediatr*. 1975;15:73-79.
112. Svensmark O, Schiller PJ. 5-5-Diphenylhydantoin (Dilantin) blood level after oral or intravenous dosage in man. *Acta Pharmacol Toxicol*. 1960; 16:331-346.
113. Kok THHG, Taitz LS, Bennett MJ, Holt DW. Drowsiness due to clemastine transmitted in breast milk. *Lancet*. 1982;1:914-915.
114. Steen B, Rane A, Lonnerholm G, et al. Phenytoin excretion in human breast milk and plasma levels in nursed infants. *Ther Drug Monit*. 1982; 4:331-334.
115. Finch E, Lorber J. Methaemoglobinaemia in the newborn: probably due to phenytoin excreted in human milk. *J Obstet Gynaecol Br Emp*. 1954;61:833.
116. Meador KJ, Baker GA, Browning N, et al; NEAD Study Group. Effects of breastfeeding in children of women taking antiepileptic drugs. *Neurology*. 2010;75:1954-1960.
117. Meador KJ, Baker GA, Browning N, et al. Breastfeeding in children of women taking antiepileptic drugs: cognitive outcomes at age 6 years. *JAMA Pediatr*. 2014;168:729-736.

P

PHYSOSTIGMINE

Neurologic/Immunologic/Antidote (Acetylcholinesterase Inhibitor)

PREGNANCY RECOMMENDATION: Limited Human Data—No Relevant Animal Data

BREASTFEEDING RECOMMENDATION: Probably Compatible

PREGNANCY SUMMARY

A few reports describing the use of physostigmine in human pregnancy were located. The drug has been used to treat 15 women at term to reverse scopolamine-induced twilight sleep. It has also been used to treat some pregnant women with myasthenia gravis. No adverse effects related to the drug were described. No first-trimester exposures were identified. Physostigmine will probably cross the placenta, so some fetal exposure will likely occur. Therefore, this limited human pregnancy experience prevents a complete assessment of the embryofetal risk. No animal reproduction studies have been located. Using this drug during pregnancy should be based on the pros and cons of the mother's clinical need for treatment versus any potential fetal risk that might occur from exposure.

BREASTFEEDING SUMMARY

No reports describing the use of physostigmine during human lactation have been located. The drug will likely be excreted into breast milk, so some infant exposure will probably occur. Breastfeeding while using this drug should be based on the mother's clinical need for treatment versus any potential infant risks that might occur. If used, the infant should be monitored for the most common reported adult side effects of nausea (leading to irritability), vomiting, and excess salivation.

References

1. Prescribing Information. Physostigmine salicylate. HF Acquisition Co LLC DBA HealthFirst; 2023.
2. Smiller BG, Bartholomew EG, Sivak BJ, et al. Physostigmine reversal of scopolamine delirium in obstetric patients. *Am J Obstet Gynecol*. 1973; 116:326-329.
3. McNall PG, Jafarnia MR. Management of myasthenia gravis in the obstetrical patient. *Am J Obstet Gynecol*. 1965;92:518-525.
4. Blackhall MI, Buckley GA, Roberts DV, et al. Drug-induced neonatal myasthenia. *J Obstet Gynaecol Br Commonw*. 1969;76:157-162.
5. Plauche WC. Myasthenia gravis in pregnancy: an update. *Am J Obstet Gynecol*. 1979;135:691-697.

PHYTONADIONE

Vitamin (Fat-Soluble Vitamin K)

PREGNANCY RECOMMENDATION: Human Data Suggest Compatible

BREASTFEEDING RECOMMENDATION: Compatible

PREGNANCY SUMMARY

Several reports describing the use of phytonadione in human pregnancy have been located. Phytonadione (Vitamin K_1) is the treatment of choice for maternal hypoprothrombinemia (clotting factor II deficiency) and for the prevention of hemorrhagic disease of the newborn. Maternal supplementation is not needed except for patients deemed at risk for vitamin K deficiency. This vitamin crosses the placenta, so some fetal exposure will occur. However, the limited human pregnancy experience prevents a complete assessment of embryofetal risk. No animal reproduction studies have been conducted. Using this vitamin supplement during pregnancy should be based on the pros and cons of the mother's clinical need for treatment versus any potential fetal risk that might occur from exposure. Vitamin K deficiency, producing clotting factor II deficiency during pregnancy, may increase the risk for bleeding diatheses and hemorrhagic events at delivery. Additionally, subclinical maternal vitamin K deficiency during pregnancy has been implicated in rare cases of fetal intracranial hemorrhage. Some phytonadione injectable emulsion formulations contain benzyl alcohol, which has been associated with gasping syndrome in neonates. If injectable phytonadione is used during pregnancy, consider using a benzyl alcohol–free formulation. Vitamin K is a normal endogenous vitamin; however, it is fat soluble, so it can be stored over time, similar to other fat-soluble vitamins.

BREASTFEEDING SUMMARY

Phytonadione is present in human breast milk. The natural vitamin K content of breast milk is too low to protect the newborn from vitamin K deficiency, which can increase the risk for hemorrhagic disease in the newborn. The administration of vitamin K to the mother to increase breast milk concentrations may be possible but needs further study. Nevertheless, it is recommended that all newborns receive a parenteral prophylactic vitamin K injection shortly after delivery. Newborns of mothers using anticonvulsants or oral anticoagulants may require larger or repeated doses. In 20 lactating women, colostrum and mature breast milk concentrations for vitamin K were 2.3 and 2.1 ng/mL, respectively (less than half that found in cow's milk). Administration of a single 20-mg oral dose of phytonadione to one mother produced a concentration of 140 ng/mL at 12 hours. Concentrations at 48 hours were still about double normal values.

References

1. Prescribing Information. Phytonadione (tablet). Agnitio Inc; 2024.
2. Prescribing Information. Phytonadione (injection). Cipla USA Inc; 2024.
3. Shearer MJ, Rahim S, Barkhan P, Stimmler L. Plasma vitamin K_1 in mothers and their newborn babies. *Lancet*. 1982;2:460-463.
4. Kazzi NJ, Ilagan NB, Liang K-C, et al. Placental transfer of vitamin K_1 in preterm pregnancy. *Obstet Gynecol*. 1990;75:334-337.
5. Lane PA, Hathaway WE. Vitamin K in infancy. *J Pediatr*. 1985;106:351-359.
6. Payne NR, Hasegawa DK. Vitamin K deficiency in newborns: a case report in α-1-antitrypsin deficiency and a review of factors predisposing to hemorrhage. *Pediatrics*. 1984;73:712-716.
7. Wynn RM. The obstetric significance of factors affecting the metabolism of bilirubin, with particular reference to the role of vitamin K. *Obstet Gynecol Surv*. 1963;18:333-354.
8. Finkel MJ. Vitamin K_1 and the vitamin K analogues. *J Clin Pharmacol Ther*. 1961;2:795-814.
9. Blood Study Group of Gynecologists. Effect of vitamins K_2 and K_1 on the bleeding volume during parturition and the blood coagulation disturbance of newborns by a double blind controlled study. *Igaku no Ayumi*. 1971; 76:818. As cited in Nishimura H, Tanimura T. *Clinical Aspects of the Teratogenicity of Drugs*. American Elsevier; 1976:253.

10. Larsen JF, Jacobsen B, Holm HH, et al. Intrauterine injection of vitamin K before delivery during anticoagulant therapy of the mother. *Acta Obstet Gynecol Scand*. 1978;57:227-230.
11. American Academy of Pediatrics Committee on Nutrition. Vitamin K compounds and the water-soluble analogues. *Pediatrics*. 1961;28:501-507.
12. Haroon Y, Shearer MJ, Rahim S, et al. The content of phylloquinone (vitamin K_1) in human milk, cows' milk and infant formula foods determined by high-performance liquid chromatography. *J Nutr*. 1982;112:1105-1117.
13. Dyggve HV, Dam H, Sondergaard E. Influence on the prothrombin time of breast-fed newborn babies of one single dose of vitamin K_1 or synkavit given to the mother within 2 hours after birth. *Acta Obstet Gynecol Scand*. 1956;35:440-444.
14. American Academy of Pediatrics Committee on Nutrition. Vitamin and mineral supplement needs in normal children in the United States. *Pediatrics*. 1980;66:1015-1021.
15. Motohara K, Matsukura M, Matsuda I, et al. Severe vitamin K deficiency in breast-fed infants. *J Pediatr*. 1984;105:943-945.

PIFLUFOLASTAT F 18

Diagnostic (Prostate)

PREGNANCY RECOMMENDATION: Contraindicated

BREASTFEEDING RECOMMENDATION: Contraindicated

PREGNANCY SUMMARY

No reports describing the use of piflufolastat F 18 in human pregnancy have been located. The drug will probably cross the placenta. Animal studies have not been conducted. However, this radioactive diagnostic agent is not indicated for use in females. All radioactive agents have the potential to cause fetal harm based on the stage of fetal development and radiation dose.

BREASTFEEDING SUMMARY

Piflufolastat F 18 is probably excreted into human breast milk; however, this radioactive diagnostic agent is not indicated for use in females.

Reference

1. Prescribing Information. Pylarify. Progenics Pharmaceuticals; 2021.

PILOCARPINE

Autonomic (Cholinergic Agonist)

PREGNANCY RECOMMENDATION: No Human Data—Animal Data Suggest Potential Risk

BREASTFEEDING RECOMMENDATION: Potential Toxicity

PREGNANCY SUMMARY

No reports describing the use of pilocarpine in human pregnancy have been located. The drug will probably cross the placenta, so some fetal exposure will likely occur. Therefore, the absence of human pregnancy experience prevents a complete assessment of the embryofetal risk. Embryofetal toxicity was observed in one animal species at doses of less than 10 times the MRHD. Using this drug during pregnancy should be based on the pros and cons of the mother's clinical need for treatment versus any potential fetal risk that might occur from exposure.

BREASTFEEDING SUMMARY

No reports describing the use of pilocarpine during human lactation have been located. The drug will likely be excreted into breast milk, so some infant exposure will probably occur. However, due to a concern for potential serious adverse effects that might be seen in a breastfed infant, the manufacturer recommends that women not breastfeed while being treated with this drug. Nevertheless, breastfeeding while using this drug should be based on the mother's clinical need for treatment versus any potential infant risks that might occur. If used, the infant should be monitored for the most common reported adult side effects of nausea, dizziness, and headache (all leading to irritability), sweating, rhinitis, flushing, weakness, and increased urinary frequency.

Reference

1. Prescribing Information. Pilocarpine hydrochloride (tablet). Padagis US LLC; 2023.

P

PILOCARPINE OPHTHALMIC

Ophthalmic/Autonomic (Topical—Cholinergic Agonist)

PREGNANCY RECOMMENDATION: Limited Human Data—No Relevant Animal Data

BREASTFEEDING RECOMMENDATION: Probably Compatible

PREGNANCY SUMMARY

One report describing the use of pilocarpine ophthalmic in human pregnancy has been located. A woman with glaucoma was treated throughout gestation with topical pilocarpine (two drops twice daily), timolol (two drops each eye), and oral acetazolamide. At delivery, no adverse effects related to the drug were seen, and no fetal anomalies were identified. The drug will probably cross the placenta, so some fetal exposure will likely occur. However, the low concentrations in maternal plasma suggest that this exposure will likely be clinically insignificant. Nevertheless, this limited human pregnancy experience prevents a complete assessment of the embryofetal risk. No animal reproduction studies have been conducted. Using this drug during pregnancy should be based on the pros and cons of the mother's clinical need for treatment versus any potential fetal risk that might occur from exposure. If used during pregnancy, consider placing pressure over the tear duct in the corner of the eye for at least 1 minute, and then remove any excess solution with absorbent tissue to decrease the amount of drug reaching the systemic circulation even further.

BREASTFEEDING SUMMARY

No reports describing the use of pilocarpine ophthalmic during human lactation have been located. The drug will likely be excreted into breast milk. However, the low concentrations in maternal plasma suggest that this exposure will likely be clinically insignificant. Breastfeeding while using this drug should be based on the mother's clinical need for treatment versus any potential infant risks that might occur. If used, the infant should be monitored for the most common reported adult side effect of headache (leading to irritability). A method to decrease some systemic absorption with ophthalmic use is described above in the Pregnancy Summary.

References

1. Product Information. Pilocarpine hydrochloride. Somerset Therapeutics LLC; 2023.
2. Merlob P, Litwin A, Mor N. Possible association between acetazolamide administration during pregnancy and metabolic disorders in the newborn. *Eur J Obstet Gynecol Reprod Biol*. 1990;35:85-88.

PIMAVANSERIN

Mental Health (Antipsychotic)

PREGNANCY RECOMMENDATION: No Human Data—Animal Data Suggest Low Risk

BREASTFEEDING RECOMMENDATION: Probably Compatible

PREGNANCY SUMMARY

No reports describing the use of pimavanserin in human pregnancy have been located. A limited amount of the drug will probably cross the placenta, so some fetal exposure will likely occur. Therefore, the absence of human pregnancy experience prevents a complete assessment of the embryofetal risk. Animal data did not show any embryofetal toxicity. The drug may prolong the cardiac QT interval. Using this drug during pregnancy should be based on the pros and cons of the mother's clinical need for treatment versus any potential fetal risk that might occur from exposure.

BREASTFEEDING SUMMARY

No reports describing the use of pimavanserin during human lactation have been located. A limited amount of the drug will probably appear in breast milk, so the same infant exposure may occur. The manufacturer recommends that the developmental and health benefits of breastfeeding should be considered along with the mother's clinical need for treatment. If the clinical decision is to use this drug while breastfeeding, the infant should be monitored for the most common reported adult side effect of peripheral edema.

Reference

1. Prescribing Information. Nuplazid. Acadia Pharmaceuticals Inc; 2020.

PIMECROLIMUS

Immunologic/Dermatologic (Topical Calcineurin Inhibitor)

PREGNANCY RECOMMENDATION: No Human Data—No Relevant Animal Data

BREASTFEEDING RECOMMENDATION: Probably Compatible

PREGNANCY SUMMARY

No reports describing the use of pimecrolimus in human pregnancy have been located. Although pimecrolimus has the potential to cross the placenta, the low systemic absorption after topical application suggests that any amount would likely be clinically insignificant. However, the absence of human pregnancy experience prevents a complete assessment of embryofetal risk. Embryofetal toxicity was observed in two animal species, but with oral doses at more than 10 times the MRHD. Using this drug during pregnancy should be based on the pros and cons of the mother's clinical need for treatment versus any potential fetal risk that might occur from exposure. Pimecrolimus carries a boxed warning that the long-term safety of topical calcineurin inhibitors has not been established.

BREASTFEEDING SUMMARY

No reports describing the use of pimecrolimus during human lactation have been located. The drug has the potential to be excreted into human breast milk, but the low systemic absorption after topical application suggests that any amount would likely be clinically insignificant. However, due to a concern for potential serious adverse effects that might be seen in a breastfed infant, the manufacturer recommends that women not breastfeed while being treated with this drug. Nevertheless, breastfeeding while using this drug should be based on the mother's clinical need for treatment versus any potential infant risks that might occur. If used, the infant should be monitored for the most common reported adult side effects of headache (leading to irritability), cough, fever, and infections.

References

1. Prescribing Information. Pimecrolimus. Oceanside Pharmaceuticals; 2020.
2. Scott G, Osborne SA, Greig G, et al. Pharmacokinetics of pimecrolimus, a novel nonsteroid anti-inflammatory drug, after single and multiple oral administration. *Clin Pharmacokinet*. 2003;42:1305-1314.

PIMOZIDE

Mental Health (First-Generation Antipsychotic, Typical Antipsychotic)

PREGNANCY RECOMMENDATION: Limited Human Data—Animal Data Suggest Potential Risk

BREASTFEEDING RECOMMENDATION: Potential Toxicity

PREGNANCY SUMMARY

Two case reports describing the use of pimozide in human pregnancy were located. In both women, the drug was used to treat Tourette syndrome. Exposure occurred at conception and through most of the pregnancy. At delivery, no birth anomalies or adverse infant effects were described. The drug will probably cross the placenta, so some fetal exposure will likely occur. Therefore, the limited human pregnancy experience prevents a complete assessment of the embryofetal risk. Embryofetal toxicity was observed in two animal species at doses of less than 10 times the MRHD (with maternal toxicity in one). Using this drug during pregnancy should be based on the pros and cons of the mother's clinical need for treatment versus any potential fetal risk that might occur from exposure. The manufacturer notes that neonates exposed to antipsychotic drugs during the third trimester are at risk for extrapyramidal and/or withdrawal symptoms postdelivery. Symptoms include agitation, hypertonia, hypotonia, tremor, somnolence, respiratory distress, and feeding disorders. These complications vary in severity and have been self-limited in some cases; whereas in other cases, neonates have required neonatal intensive care unit (NICU) support and prolonged hospitalization. Pimozide has also been shown to prolong the QT interval.

BREASTFEEDING SUMMARY

No reports describing the use of pimozide during human lactation have been located. The drug will likely be excreted into human breast milk, so some infant exposure will probably occur. However, due to a concern for potential serious adverse effects that might be seen in a breastfed infant, the manufacturer recommends that women not breastfeed while being treated with this drug. Nevertheless, breastfeeding while using this drug should be based on the mother's clinical need for treatment versus any potential infant risks that might occur. If used, the infant should be monitored for the most common reported adult side effects of extrapyramidal reactions, sedation, and constipation.

References

1. Prescribing Information. Pimozide. Endo USA Inc; 2017.
2. National Library of Medicine. Pimozide. PubChem. Accessed February 23, 2025. https://pubchem.ncbi.nlm.nih.gov/compound/Pimozide
3. Bjarnason NH, Rode L, Dalhoff K. Fetal exposure to pimozide: a case report. *J Reprod Med*. 2006;51:443-444.
4. Prowler ML, Kim DR. Perinatal akathisia: implications for pharmacokinetic changes during pregnancy. *Am J Psychiatry*. 2009;166:1296-1297.

PINDOLOL

Antihypertensive (Nonselective β-Blocker)

PREGNANCY RECOMMENDATION: Limited Human Data—Animal Data Suggest Low Risk

BREASTFEEDING RECOMMENDATION: Potential Toxicity

PREGNANCY SUMMARY

Several reports describing the use of pindolol in human pregnancy have been located. No first-trimester exposures have been found. All of the publications describe the use of the drug in treating hypertension in the second half of gestation. The drug crosses the placenta, so some fetal exposure will occur. However, this limited human first-trimester pregnancy experience prevents a complete assessment of the embryofetal risk. Animal data did not show any embryofetal toxicity in one species at doses of more than 10 times the RHD. Some β-blockers may cause IUGR and reduced placental weight, especially those lacking intrinsic sympathomimetic activity (ISA). Pindolol possesses ISA. However, IUGR and reduced placental weight may potentially occur with all β-blocker drugs. Using this drug during pregnancy should be based on the pros and cons of the mother's clinical need for treatment versus any potential fetal risk that might occur from exposure. ACOG states that uncontrolled chronic hypertension has maternal risks of superimposed preeclampsia, placental abruption, postpartum hemorrhage, gestational diabetes, cerebrovascular accidents, pulmonary edema, renal insufficiency, myocardial infarction, and mortality, along with fetal risks of stillbirth or perinatal death, growth restriction, preterm birth, and congenital malformations. ACOG recommends labetalol or nifedipine as first-line agents in treating hypertension in pregnancy.

BREASTFEEDING SUMMARY

Pindolol has been shown to be excreted into human breast milk. One report evaluated breast milk concentrations of pindolol after delivery. Levels were higher in breast milk than the concentrations found in the maternal circulation for both the R- (1.9 vs 1.1 ng/mL, respectively) and S- (3.1 vs 1.4 ng/mL, respectively) enantiomers. However, therapeutic blood levels for pindolol in adults range from 10 to 30 ng/mL. Because β-blockade has been observed in nursing infants exposed to other β-blockers (see Atenolol), infants should be closely observed for bradycardia and other symptoms of β-blockade. Breastfeeding while using this drug should be based on the mother's clinical need for treatment versus any potential infant risks that might occur. If used, the infant should be monitored for the most common reported adult side effects of dizziness, muscle pain, and joint pain (all leading to irritability), fatigue (lethargy), peripheral edema, and insomnia.

References

1. Prescribing Information. Pindolol. ANI Pharmaceuticals Inc; 2023.
2. American College of Obstetricians and Gynecologists. Chronic hypertension in pregnancy. Practice bulletin No. 203. *Obstet Gynecol*. 2019;133:e26-e50.
3. Grunstein S, Ellenbogen A, Anderman S, et al. Transfer of pindolol across the placenta in hypertensive pregnant women. *Curr Ther Res*. 1985;37:587-591.
4. Goncalves PVB, Cavalli RC, da Cunha SP, Lanchote VL. Determination of pindolol enantiomers in amniotic fluid and breast milk by high-performance liquid chromatography: applications to pharmacokinetics in pregnant and lactating women. *J Chromatogr B Analyt Technol Biomed Life Sci*. 2007;852:640-645.
5. Lunell NO, Nylund L, Lewander R, et al. Uteroplacental blood flow in pregnancy hypertension after the administration of a beta-adrenoceptor blocker, pindolol. *Gynecol Obstet Invest*. 1984;18:269-274.
6. Meizner I, Paran E, Katz M, et al. Flow velocity analysis of umbilical and uterine artery flow in pre-eclampsia treated with propranolol or pindolol. *J Clin Ultrasound*. 1992;20:115-119.
7. Dubois D, Petitcolas J, Temperville B, et al. Treatment of hypertension in pregnancy with β-adrenoceptor antagonists. *Br J Clin Pharmacol*. 1982;13(suppl):375S-378S.
8. Sukerman-Voldman E. Pindolol therapy in pregnant hypertensive patients. *Br J Clin Pharmacol*. 1982;13(suppl):379S.
9. Ingemarsson I, Liedholm H, Montan S, et al. Fetal heart rate during treatment of maternal hypertension with beta-adrenergic antagonists. *Acta Obstet Gynecol Scand*. 1984;118(suppl):95-97.
10. Tuimala R, Hartikainen-Sorri A-L. Randomized comparison of atenolol and pindolol for treatment of hypertension in pregnancy. *Curr Ther Res*. 1988;44:579-584.
11. Rosenfeld J, Bott-Kanner G, Boner G, et al. Treatment of hypertension during pregnancy with hydralazine monotherapy or with combined therapy with hydralazine and pindolol. *Eur J Obstet Gynecol Reprod Biol*. 1986;22:197-204.
12. Montan S, Ingemarsson I, Marsal K, Sjoberg N-O. Randomized controlled trial of atenolol and pindolol in human pregnancy: effects on fetal haemodynamics. *Br Med J*. 1992;304:946-949.
13. Schoenfeld A, Freedman S, Hod M, Ovadia Y. Antagonism of antihypertensive drug therapy in pregnancy by indomethacin? *Am J Obstet Gynecol*. 1989;161:1204-1205.

PIOGLITAZONE

Antidiabetic (Thiazolidinedione)

PREGNANCY RECOMMENDATION: No Human Data—Animal Data Suggest Potential Risk

BREASTFEEDING RECOMMENDATION: Potential Toxicity

PREGNANCY SUMMARY

No reports describing the use of pioglitazone in human pregnancy have been located. The drug and active metabolites will probably cross the placenta, so some fetal exposure will likely occur. Therefore, the absence of human pregnancy experience prevents a complete assessment of the embryofetal risk. Embryofetal toxicity was observed in one animal species at doses of less than 10 times the MRHD. Using this drug during pregnancy should be based on the pros and cons of the mother's clinical need for treatment versus any potential fetal risk that might occur from exposure. Uncontrolled diabetes is associated with an increased risk for preeclampsia, spontaneous abortion, preterm delivery, IUFD, delivery complications, major congenital malformations, macrosomia-related morbidity, and maternal diabetic ketoacidosis. ACOG recommends that insulin be used for types 1 and 2 diabetes occurring during pregnancy and, if diet therapy alone is not successful, for gestational diabetes. If a woman becomes pregnant while taking pioglitazone, changing the therapy to insulin should be considered. Insulin does not cross the placenta, which eliminates the additional concern that the drug therapy could adversely affect the fetus.

BREASTFEEDING SUMMARY

No reports describing the use of pioglitazone during human lactation have been located. The drug and its active metabolites will likely be excreted into human breast milk, so some infant exposure will probably occur. Breastfeeding while using this drug should be based on the mother's clinical need for treatment versus any potential infant risks that might occur. If used, the infant should be monitored for the most common reported adult side effects of headache and myalgia (both leading to irritability) and infections.

References

1. Prescribing Information. Pioglitazone Hydrochloride. Aurobindo Pharma Limited; 2024.
2. American College of Obstetricians and Gynecologists. ACOG practice bulletin No. 201: pregestational diabetes mellitus. *Obstet Gynecol*. 2018; 132:e228-e248.
3. American College of Obstetricians and Gynecologists. ACOG practice bulletin No. 190: gestational diabetes. *Obstet Gynecol*. 2018;131:e49-e64.

PIPERACILLIN/TAZOBACTAM

Antibiotic (Penicillin/β-Lactam Inhibitor)

PREGNANCY RECOMMENDATION: Limited Human Data—Animal Data Suggest Potential Risk

BREASTFEEDING RECOMMENDATION: Probably Compatible

PREGNANCY SUMMARY

A few studies describing the use of piperacillin/tazobactam during human pregnancy have been located. Essentially, every study has described the use after the first trimester. No adverse fetal effects have been described. This drug combination has been shown to cross the placenta, so some fetal exposure will occur. Though human data for the penicillin class of drugs has been shown to be low risk for use in pregnancy, the absence of first-trimester human pregnancy experience with piperacillin/tazobactam prevents a complete assessment of the embryofetal risk. Embryofetal toxicity was observed in one animal species at doses of less than 10 times the MRHD but not in a second species. Using this drug during pregnancy should be based on the pros and cons of the mother's clinical need for treatment versus any potential fetal risk that might occur from exposure.

BREASTFEEDING SUMMARY

Piperacillin is excreted into breast milk. No reports describing the use of tazobactam during human lactation have been located. The drug will likely be excreted into human breast milk, so some infant exposure will probably occur. Breastfeeding while using this drug should be based on the mother's clinical need for treatment versus any potential infant risks that might occur. If used, the infant should be monitored for the most common reported adult side effects of nausea and headache (both leading to irritability), diarrhea, constipation, and insomnia.

References

1. Prescribing Information. Piperacillin sodium and tazobactam sodium. Xellia Pharmaceuticals USA LLC; 2022.

2. Brown CEL, Christmas JT, Bawdon RE. Placental transfer of cefazolin and piperacillin in pregnancies remote from term complicated by Rh isoimmunization. *Am J Obstet Gynecol*. 1990;163:938-943.
3. Heikkilä A, Erkkola R. Pharmacokinetics of piperacillin during pregnancy. *J Antimicrob Chemother*. 1991;28:419-423.
4. Bourget P, Sertin A, Lesne-Hulin A, et al. Influence of pregnancy on the pharmacokinetic behaviour and the transplacental transfer of the piperacillin-tazobactam combination. *Eur J Obstet Gynecol Reprod Biol*. 1998;76:21-27.
5. Lockwood CJ, Costigan K, Ghidini A, et al. Double-blind, placebo-controlled trial of piperacillin sodium in preterm membrane rupture (abstract). *Am J Obstet Gynecol*. 1993;168:378.

PIRFENIDONE

Respiratory (Pyridine)

PREGNANCY RECOMMENDATION: No Human Data—Animal Data Suggest Potential Risk

BREASTFEEDING RECOMMENDATION: Potential Toxicity

PREGNANCY SUMMARY

No reports describing the use of pirfenidone in human pregnancy have been located. The drug will probably cross the placenta, so some fetal exposure will likely occur. Therefore, the absence of human pregnancy experience prevents a complete assessment of the embryofetal risk. Embryofetal toxicity was observed in one animal species at doses of less than 10 times the MRHD but not in a second species. Using this drug during pregnancy should be based on the pros and cons of the mother's clinical need for treatment versus any potential fetal risk that might occur from exposure.

BREASTFEEDING SUMMARY

No reports describing the use of pirfenidone during human lactation have been located. The drug will likely be excreted into human breast milk, so some infant exposure will probably occur. Breastfeeding while using this drug should be based on the mother's clinical need for treatment versus any potential infant risks that might occur. If used, the infant should be monitored for the most common reported adult side effects of nausea, abdominal pain, headache, dyspepsia, dizziness, and arthralgia (all leading to irritability), diarrhea, fatigue (lethargy), decreased appetite (monitor infant growth), vomiting, infections, and insomnia.

Reference

1. Prescribing Information. Pirfenidone. Amneal Pharmaceuticals; 2023.

PIROXICAM

Pain (Nonsteroidal Anti-Inflammatory Drug)

PREGNANCY RECOMMENDATION: Human Data Suggest Potential Risk (Second and Third Trimesters)

BREASTFEEDING RECOMMENDATION: Probably Compatible

PREGNANCY SUMMARY

A few studies were located that described the use of piroxicam in the first trimester. Of 161 pregnancies with first-trimester exposure, there were 6 (3.7%) major anomalies identified. No pattern to the defects was seen. However, many studies described a risk of premature closure of the ductus arteriosus when used in the third trimester. This can lead to pulmonary hypertension in the newborn and other neonatal complications. Use in the second half of gestation has also been associated with a decrease in fetal urine production, leading to oligohydramnios. The drug will probably cross the placenta, so some fetal exposure will likely occur. Therefore, this limited human pregnancy experience prevents a complete assessment of the embryofetal risk. Animal studies did show some embryofetal toxicity in one species at doses of less than 10 times the RHD. However, no embryofetal toxicity was seen in a second species at doses of 10 times the RHD. Using this drug during pregnancy should be based on the pros and cons of the mother's clinical need for treatment versus any potential fetal risk that might occur from exposure. If possible, avoid use in the third trimester or limit use to a minimal number of doses.

BREASTFEEDING SUMMARY

Two studies were located that described the use of piroxicam during human lactation. In two lactating women, the drug's breast milk concentrations were from 50 ng/mL with 20 mg/d maternal use up to 220 ng/mL with 40 mg/d maternal use. Breast milk levels were about 1% maternal levels. Calculated RIDs were from about 6% up to about 9%. However infant serum was evaluated in one case, and the drug was not detected (LLQ of 10 ng/mL). Breastfeeding while using this drug should be based on the mother's clinical need for treatment versus any potential infant risks that might occur. If used, the infant should be monitored for the most common reported adult side effects of nausea, headache, abdominal pain, and dizziness (all leading to irritability), constipation, diarrhea, peripheral edema, and rash.

References

1. Prescribing Information. Piroxicam. Greenstone LLC; 2025.
2. Food and Drug Administration. Nonsteroidal anti-inflammatory drugs (NSAIDs): drug safety communication—avoid use of NSAIDs in pregnancy at 20 weeks or later. Accessed October 8, 2024. https://www.fda.gov/safety/medical-product-safety-information/nonsteroidal-anti-inflammatory-drugs-nsaids-drug-safety-communication-avoid-use-nsaids-pregnancy-20
3. Kumbasar S, Gul O, Sik A. Evaluation of the effect of indomethacin and piroxicam administration before embryo transfer on pregnancy rate. *J Obstet Gynaecol Res*. 2017;43:536-542.
4. Chen X, Yang Y, Chen L, et al. Pregnancy outcomes and birth defects in offspring following non-steroidal anti-inflammatory drugs exposure during pregnancy: a systematic review and meta-analysis. *Reprod Tox*. 2024;125:108561.
5. Ying XH, Bao DN, Jiang HY, Shi YD. Maternal non-steroidal anti-inflammatory drug exposure during pregnancy and risk of miscarriage: a systematic review and meta-analysis. *Eur J Clin Pharmacol*. 2022;78:171-180.
6. Ostensen M. Piroxicam in human breast milk. *Eur J Clin Pharmacol*. 1983;25:829-830.
7. Ostensen M, Husby G. Antirheumatic drug treatment during pregnancy and lactation. *Scand J Rheumatol*. 1985;14:1-7.

PIRTOBRUTINIB

Antineoplastic (Kinase Inhibitor)

PREGNANCY RECOMMENDATION: No Human Data—Animal Data Suggest Potential Risk

BREASTFEEDING RECOMMENDATION: Potential Toxicity

PREGNANCY SUMMARY

No reports describing the use of pirtobrutinib in human pregnancy have been located. The drug will likely cross the placenta, so some fetal exposure will probably occur. Therefore, the absence of human pregnancy experience prevents a complete assessment of the embryofetal risk. Animal data showed embryofetal toxicity. Based on these animal studies, the manufacturer recommends that women with reproductive potential use effective contraception during treatment and for 1 week after the last dose. Nevertheless, using this drug during pregnancy should be based on the pros and cons of the mother's clinical need for treatment versus any potential fetal risk that might occur from exposure.

BREASTFEEDING SUMMARY

No reports describing the use of pirtobrutinib during human lactation have been located. The drug will likely be excreted into breast milk, so some infant exposure will probably occur. Due to the concern for potential serious adverse effects that might be seen in a breastfed infant, the manufacturer recommends that women not breastfeed while being treated with this drug and for at least 1 week after the last dose. Nevertheless, breastfeeding while using this drug should be based on the mother's clinical need for treatment. If used, the infant should be monitored for the most common reported adult side effects of musculoskeletal pain (leading to irritability), diarrhea, lethargy, edema, bruising, and various laboratory abnormalities (see PI).

Reference

1. Prescribing Information. Jaypirca. Lilly USA, LLC; 2023.

PITAVASTATIN

Antilipemic (Statin—HMG-CoA Inhibitor)

PREGNANCY RECOMMENDATION: No Human Data—Animal Data Suggest Potential Risk

BREASTFEEDING RECOMMENDATION: Potential Toxicity

PREGNANCY SUMMARY

No reports describing the use of pitavastatin in human pregnancy have been located. A systematic review and meta-analysis evaluated pregnancy outcomes with first-trimester exposure to statins (n = 1,655) as a group compared with unexposed controls (n = 974,159). No significant difference was observed for major malformations, IUFD, or preterm delivery. The manufacturer reported that a Medicaid cohort linkage evaluated outcomes in 1,152 women taking statins (as a group) prior to pregnancy, then discontinuing at some point during the first trimester, compared with 886,996 unexposed pregnancies. After adjusting for confounders, statin exposure was not associated with an increased risk for congenital malformations. The drug will probably cross the placenta, so some fetal exposure will likely occur. Therefore, the absence of human pregnancy experience specifically with pitavastatin prevents a complete assessment of the embryofetal risk. Embryofetal and maternal

(*continued*)

toxicity were observed in two animal species but at doses of about equal to the MRHD in one and less than 10 times the MRHD in the second. The drug will probably cross the placenta, so some fetal exposure will likely occur. Therefore, the absence of human pregnancy experience prevents a complete assessment of the embryofetal risk. Cholesterol and other products of cholesterol biosynthesis are essential components for fetal development. Moreover, maternal cholesterol levels increase during pregnancy. Hyperlipidemia treatment is not generally necessary during pregnancy. Atherosclerosis is a chronic process, and stopping lipid-lowering therapy during pregnancy should have little impact on the outcome of these disorders. Therefore, the manufacturer recommends discontinuing this drug when a pregnancy is recognized. Nevertheless, using this drug during pregnancy should be based on the pros and cons of the mother's clinical need for treatment versus any potential fetal risk that might occur from exposure.

BREASTFEEDING SUMMARY

No reports describing the use of pitavastatin during human lactation have been located. The drug will likely be excreted into human breast milk, so some infant exposure will probably occur. Other statins are known to be excreted into breast milk (see Fluvastatin and Pravastatin). However, due to a concern for potential serious adverse effects that might be seen in a breastfed infant, the manufacturer recommends that women not breastfeed while being treated with this drug. Nevertheless, breastfeeding while using this drug should be based on the mother's clinical need for treatment versus any potential infant risks that might occur. If used, the infant should be monitored for the most common reported adult side effects of myalgia, back pain, and extremity pain (all leading to irritability), constipation, and diarrhea.

References

1. Prescribing Information. Pitavastatin. Camber Pharmaceuticals Inc; 2024.
2. Karadas B, Uysal N, Erol H, et al. Pregnancy outcomes following maternal exposure to statins: a systematic review and meta-analysis. *Br J Pharmacol.* 2022;88:3962-3976.

PITOLISANT

Central Nervous System (Histamine H_3 Receptor Antagonist/Inverse Agonist)

PREGNANCY RECOMMENDATION: Limited Human Data—Animal Data Suggest Low Risk

BREASTFEEDING RECOMMENDATION: Potential Toxicity

PREGNANCY SUMMARY

The manufacturer reports that exposures of pitolisant during human pregnancy are available from cases that occurred in the clinical trials and postmarketing reports. They stated that no increased risk for major malformations, spontaneous abortion, or adverse fetal or maternal outcomes was seen, but no additional data were provided. The drug will probably cross the placenta, so some fetal exposure will likely occur. Therefore, this limited human pregnancy experience prevents a complete assessment of the embryofetal risk. No embryofetal toxicity was seen in two species at doses of less than 10 times the MRHD. Using this drug during pregnancy should be based on the pros and cons of the mother's clinical need for treatment versus any potential fetal risk that might occur from exposure. There is a pregnancy exposure registry that monitors pregnancy outcomes in women using this drug. Health care providers are encouraged to call the Pitolisant Pregnancy Exposure Registry at 1-800-833-7460. Pitolisant can prolong the QT interval. The drug may reduce the effectiveness of hormonal contraceptives, and patients should be advised to use an alternative nonhormonal contraceptive method during treatment and for at least 21 days after the last dose.

BREASTFEEDING SUMMARY

Pitolisant has been shown to be excreted into human breast milk. In a study of eight lactating women administered a single dose of 35.6 mg, the drug was found in breast milk with a mean concentration of about 47.5 ng/mL (mean maternal serum concentration was about 61.4 ng/mL). The calculated RID was about 13%. Breastfeeding while using this drug should be based on the mother's clinical need for treatment versus any potential infant risks that might occur. If used, the infant should be monitored for the most common reported adult side effects of nausea and anxiety (both leading to irritability), and insomnia.

Reference

1. Prescribing Information. Wakix. Harmony Biosciences LLC; 2024.

PLAZOMICIN

Antibacterial (Aminoglycoside)

PREGNANCY RECOMMENDATION: No Human Data—Animal Data Suggest Low Risk

BREASTFEEDING RECOMMENDATION: Potential Toxicity

PREGNANCY SUMMARY

No human data specific to embryofetal toxicity from exposure to plazomicin have been reported. Some amount of the drug will probably cross the placenta, so fetal exposure will likely occur. However, the absence of human pregnancy experience prevents a complete assessment of the embryofetal risk. Animal data did not show any embryofetal toxicity. Studies on streptomycin have reported total, irreversible, bilateral, congenital deafness (see Streptomycin); however, the overall incidence of fetal ototoxicity is low with careful dosage calculations and limited time exposure. Therefore, using this drug during pregnancy should be based on the pros and cons of the mother's clinical need for treatment versus any potential fetal risk that might occur from exposure.

BREASTFEEDING SUMMARY

Plazomicin will probably be found in human breast milk, so some infant exposure will likely occur. Breastfeeding while using this drug should be based on the mother's clinical need for treatment. If used, the infant should be monitored for the most common reported adult side effects of headache and nausea (both leading to irritability), diarrhea, and vomiting.

Reference

1. Prescribing Information. Zemdri. Cipla USA, Inc; 2020.

PLECANATIDE

Gastrointestinal (Laxative)

PREGNANCY RECOMMENDATION: No Human Data—Animal Data Suggest Low Risk

BREASTFEEDING RECOMMENDATION: Probably Compatible

PREGNANCY SUMMARY

No reports describing the use of plecanatide in human pregnancy have been located. The drug most likely does not cross the placenta; therefore, fetal exposure is probably nonexistent or extremely limited. However, the absence of human pregnancy experience prevents a complete assessment of the embryofetal risk. Animal studies did not show any embryofetal toxicity. The drug is contraindicated in patients under the age of 6 and should be avoided in patients between the ages of 6 and 18.

BREASTFEEDING SUMMARY

No reports describing the use of plecanatide during human lactation have been located. The drug most likely will not appear in breast milk. Furthermore, because it is a peptide molecule, if any drug were to be present in breast milk, it would most likely be digested in the infant's gastrointestinal tract and not be absorbed. Breastfeeding while using this drug should be based on the mother's clinical need for treatment. If used, the infant should be monitored for the most common reported adult side effect of diarrhea.

Reference

1. Prescribing Information. Trulance. Synergy Pharmaceuticals Inc; 2017.

PLERIXAFOR

Hematologic (Hematopoietic Stem Cell Mobilizer)

PREGNANCY RECOMMENDATION: No Human Data—Animal Data Suggest Potential Risk

BREASTFEEDING RECOMMENDATION: Potential Toxicity

PREGNANCY SUMMARY

No reports describing the use of plerixafor in human pregnancy have been located. The drug will probably cross the placenta, so some fetal exposure will likely occur. Therefore, the absence of human pregnancy experience prevents a complete assessment of the embryofetal risk. Embryofetal toxicity with malformations was observed in one animal species at doses of about 10 times the MRHD. Based on animal studies and the drug's mechanism of action, the manufacturer recommends that women with reproductive potential use effective contraception during treatment and for 1 week after the last dose. They also recommend that males with female partners of reproductive potential use effective contraception during treatment and for 1 week after the last dose. Nevertheless, using this drug during pregnancy should be based on the pros and cons of the mother's clinical need for treatment versus any potential fetal risk that might occur from exposure.

BREASTFEEDING SUMMARY

No reports describing the use of plerixafor during human lactation have been located. The drug will likely be excreted into human breast milk, so some infant exposure will probably occur. However, due to a concern for potential serious adverse effects that might be seen in a breastfed infant, the manufacturer recommends that women not breastfeed while being treated with this drug and for at least 1 week after the last dose. Nevertheless, breastfeeding while using this drug should be based on the mother's clinical need for treatment versus any potential infant risks that might occur. If used, the infant should be monitored for the most common reported adult side effects of headache, arthralgia, and dizziness (all leading to irritability), diarrhea, fatigue (lethargy), and vomiting.

Reference

1. Prescribing Information. Plerixafor. Amneal Pharmaceuticals LLC; 2024.

PODOFILOX

Dermatologic (Topical—Keratolytic)

PREGNANCY RECOMMENDATION: *Contraindicated

BREASTFEEDING RECOMMENDATION: Probably Compatible

PREGNANCY SUMMARY

No reports describing the use of podofilox in human pregnancy have been located. If found in the maternal circulation, the drug will probably cross the placenta, so some fetal exposure could occur. However, the low systemic levels seen with the maximum daily topical application suggest that the amount would likely be clinically insignificant. Regardless, the absence of human pregnancy experience prevents a complete assessment of the embryofetal risk. Animal data did not show embryofetal toxicity in one species at doses of less than 10 times the MRHD. Using this drug during pregnancy should be based on the pros and cons of the mother's clinical need for treatment versus any potential fetal risk that might occur from exposure. *Nevertheless, the CDC recommends that podofilox, podophyllin, and sinecatechins be avoided during pregnancy.

BREASTFEEDING SUMMARY

No reports describing the use of podofilox during human lactation have been located. The drug might be excreted into human breast milk, but the low systemic absorption after topical application using the maximum recommended daily treatment suggests that the amount would likely be clinically insignificant. However, due to a concern for potential serious adverse effects that might be seen in a breastfed infant, the manufacturer recommends that women not breastfeed while being treated with this drug. Nevertheless, breastfeeding while using this drug should be based on the mother's clinical need for treatment versus any potential infant risks that might occur. Due to the topical use of the drug, systemic side effects were not evaluated.

References

1. Prescribing Information. Podofilox. Padagis US LLC; 2023.
2. Centers for Disease Control and Prevention. 2015 guidelines for treatment of sexually transmitted diseases. *MMWR Recomm Rep*. 2021;64:1-140.

PODOPHYLLUM

Dermatologic (Keratolytic)

PREGNANCY RECOMMENDATION: *Contraindicated

BREASTFEEDING RECOMMENDATION: Potential Toxicity

PREGNANCY SUMMARY

A few reports describing the use of podophyllum in human pregnancy were located. From about 15 oral exposures to the drug, 1 newborn with multiple congenital anomalies was described. Three other cases have been reported with the use of the topical drug in the second and third trimesters. In one of these, the topical application was 7.5 mL, or about 1.88 g—approximately 4 times the MRHD for topical application. An IUFD occurred 2 days later, but it is not possible to determine if this occurred due to the excessive topical application or some other obstetrical issue. If found in the maternal circulation, the drug may cross the placenta in minimal amounts. However, the low systemic levels seen with the maximum daily topical application suggest that any amount would likely be clinically insignificant. Regardless, the limited human pregnancy experience prevents a complete assessment of the embryofetal risk. No animal reproduction studies have been located. Using this drug during pregnancy should be based on the pros and cons of the mother's clinical need for treatment versus any potential fetal risk that might occur from exposure. *Nevertheless, the CDC recommends that podofilox, podophyllin, and sinecatechins be avoided during pregnancy.

BREASTFEEDING SUMMARY

No reports describing the use of podophyllum during human lactation have been located. The drug might be excreted into human breast milk, but the low systemic absorption after topical application using the maximum recommended daily treatment suggests that the amount would likely be clinically insignificant. Breastfeeding while using this drug should be based on the mother's clinical need for treatment versus any potential infant risks that might occur. If used, the infant should be monitored for the most common reported adult side effects of abdominal pain, nausea, agitation, and headache (all leading to irritability), diarrhea, tachycardia, vomiting, and lethargy.

References

1. Rosenstein G, Rosenstein H, Freeman M, Weston N. Podophyllum—a dangerous laxative. *Pediatrics*. 1976;57:419-421.
2. National Library of Medicine. Podophyllin. PubChem. Accessed February 27, 2025. https://pubchem.ncbi.nlm.nih.gov/compound/Podophyllin
3. Center for Disease Control and Prevention. 2015 guidelines for treatment of sexually transmitted diseases. *MMWR Recomm Rep*. 2021;64:1-140.
4. Cullis JE. Congenital deformities and herbal "slimming tablets." *Lancet*. 1962;2:511-512.
5. Balucani M, Zellers DD. Podophyllum resin poisoning with complete recovery. *JAMA*. 1964;189:639-640.
6. Chamberlain MJ, Reynolds AL, Yeoman WB. Toxic effect of podophyllum application in pregnancy. *Br Med J*. 1972;3:391-392.
7. Karol MD, Conner CS, Watanabe AS, Murphrey KJ. Podophyllum: suspected teratogenicity from topical application. *Clin Toxicol*. 1980;16:283-286.
8. Fraser FC. Letter to the editor. *Mod Med Canada*. 1981;36:1508.
9. Heinonen OP, Slone D, Shapiro S. *Birth Defects and Drugs in Pregnancy*. Publishing Sciences Group; 1977:385.

POLATUZUMAB VEDOTIN

Antineoplastic (CD79b-Directed Antibody Drug Conjugate—Monoclonal Antibody)

PREGNANCY RECOMMENDATION: No Human Data—Animal Data Suggest Potential Risk

BREASTFEEDING RECOMMENDATION: Potential Toxicity

PREGNANCY SUMMARY

No reports describing the use of polatuzumab vedotin in human pregnancy have been located. As an IgG antibody, it likely crosses the placenta, especially during the second half of gestation, so some fetal exposure will probably occur. However, the absence of human pregnancy experience prevents a complete assessment of the embryofetal risk. No animal reproduction studies have been conducted with polatuzumab. However, the antimitotic agent , monomethyl auristatin E (mmAE), did show some embryofetal toxicity with malformations in one animal species at doses of less than the RHD. Based on animal studies and the drug's mechanism of action, the manufacturer recommends that women with reproductive potential use effective contraception during treatment and for 3 months after the last dose. They also recommend that males with female partners of reproductive potential use effective contraception during treatment and for 5 months after the last dose. Nevertheless, using this drug during pregnancy should be based on the pros and cons of the mother's clinical need for treatment versus any potential fetal risk that might occur from exposure. There is a registry for women who are pregnant and have cancer. For more information, women and health care providers are encouraged to contact the Cancer and Pregnancy Registry at 1-877-635-4499.

BREASTFEEDING SUMMARY

No reports describing the use of polatuzumab vedotin during human lactation have been located. It is known that IgG antibodies can be found in human breast milk but are not found in the neonatal or infant circulation. Additionally, if any IgG antibodies were to be ingested through breastfeeding, they would probably be digested in the infant's gastrointestinal tract and not be absorbed. However, MMAE will also likely be found in human breast milk, and this antimitotic drug could cause some infant toxicity. Therefore, due to a concern for potential serious adverse effects that might be seen in a breastfed infant, the manufacturer recommends that women not breastfeed while being treated with this drug and for at least 2 months after the last dose. Nevertheless, breastfeeding while using this drug should be based on the mother's clinical need for treatment versus any potential infant risks that might occur. If used, the infant should be monitored for the most common reported adult side effects of nausea and peripheral neuropathy (both leading to irritability), diarrhea, constipation, alopecia, fatigue (lethargy), decreased appetite (monitor infant growth), and infections.

Reference

1. Prescribing Information. Polivy. Genentech Inc; 2023.

POLIDOCANOL

Cardiovascular (Sclerosing Agent)

PREGNANCY RECOMMENDATION: Limited Human Data—Animal Data Suggest Low Risk

BREASTFEEDING RECOMMENDATION: Probably Compatible

PREGNANCY SUMMARY

There are two published reports describing the use of polidocanol in human pregnancy. In both cases, the drug was used after the first trimester, and no apparent treatment-related adverse effects were noted. Additionally, the manufacturer reports no malformations, spontaneous abortions, or adverse maternal or fetal outcomes with exposure in a few case reports. The drug will probably cross the placenta, so some fetal exposure will likely occur. However, there is low systemic absorption seen in some patients treated for spider or reticular veins. Regardless, this limited human pregnancy experience prevents a complete assessment of the embryofetal risk. Polidocanol was not found to cause any embryofetal toxicity in two animal species at doses of about 10 times (or more) the RHD based on weight. In addition, the manufacturer noted that these studies were conducted in a manner to achieve systemic exposure, while the intended clinical use is local exposure at the injection site with minimal to no systemic exposure. Using this drug during pregnancy should be based on the pros and cons of the mother's clinical need for treatment versus any potential fetal risk that might occur from exposure.

BREASTFEEDING SUMMARY

No reports describing the use of polidocanol during human lactation have been located. The drug will likely be excreted into human breast milk if found in the maternal circulation. However, there is low systemic absorption seen in some patients treated for spider or reticular veins. The manufacturer recommends that the lactating woman may consider interrupting breastfeeding and pumping and discarding the breast milk for up to 8 hours (about five half-lives) after drug administration in order to minimize exposure to the breastfed infant. Nevertheless, breastfeeding while using this drug should be based on the mother's clinical need for treatment versus any potential infant risks that might occur. Systemic side effects have not been evaluated.

References

1. Prescribing Information. Asclera. Methapharm Inc; 2023.
2. Potzi R, Ferenci P, Gangl A. Endoscopic sclerotherapy of esophageal varices during pregnancy—a case report. *Z Gastroenterol*. 1991;29:246-247.
3. Bermudez C, Perez-Wulff J, Arcadipane M, et al. Percutaneous fetal sclerotherapy for congenital cystic adenomatoid malformation of the lung. *Fetal Diagn Ther*. 2008;24:237-240.

POLYETHYLENE GYLCOL-3350

Gastrointestinal (Osmotic Laxative)

PREGNANCY RECOMMENDATION: Human Data Suggest Low Risk

BREASTFEEDING RECOMMENDATION: Probably Compatible

PREGNANCY SUMMARY

Although the published human pregnancy experience is limited, polyethylene glycol (PEG)-3350 is likely compatible in pregnancy because less than 1% of the drug is absorbed systemically. In addition, PEG-3350 is not likely to cross the placenta. However, the limited human pregnancy experience prevents a complete assessment of embryofetal risk. No animal reproduction studies have been conducted. Using this drug during pregnancy should be based on the pros and cons of the mother's clinical need for treatment versus any potential fetal risk that might occur from exposure.

BREASTFEEDING SUMMARY

No reports describing the use of PEG-3350 during human lactation have been located. The drug is not likely to be excreted into breast milk due to its poor systemic absorption with maternal oral use (<1%). Breastfeeding while using this drug should be based on the mother's clinical need for treatment versus any potential infant risks that might occur. Systemic side effects have not been evaluated.

References

1. Prescribing Information. Miralax orange flavor. Bayer Healthcare LLC; 2024.

2. Kothari S, Afshar Y, Friedman LS, Ahn J. AGA clinical practice update on pregnancy-related gastrointestinal and liver disease: expert review. *Gastroenterol*. 2024;167:1033-45.
3. Neri I, Blasi I, Castro P, et al. Polyethylene glycol electrolyte solution (Isocolan) for constipation during pregnancy: an observational open-label study. *J Midwifery Women's Health*. 2004;49:355-358.
4. Van Ameyde KJ, Tenenbein M. Whole bowel irrigation during pregnancy. *Am J Obstet Gynecol*. 1989;160:646-647.
5. Raj VI, Hassan A, Hanafiah N, et al. Polyethylene glycol compared to lactulose for constipation in pregnancy: a randomized controlled trial. *Int J Gynecol Obstet*. 2024;166:828-836.

POLYMYXIN B

Antibiotic (Basic Polypeptide Antibiotic)

PREGNANCY RECOMMENDATION: Limited Human Data—No Relevant Animal Data

BREASTFEEDING RECOMMENDATION: Probably Compatible

PREGNANCY SUMMARY

Two reports describing the use of polymyxin B in human pregnancy have been located. Of seven first-trimester exposures (IV or IM), no major birth anomalies occurred. In another small study, the use of polymyxin B in a group of infants with birth anomalies was no higher when compared with a group of infants that did not have any birth defects. The drug will probably cross the placenta with IV or IM use in limited amounts, so some fetal exposure may occur. Systemic absorption with ophthalmic use is negligible. However, this limited human pregnancy experience prevents a complete assessment of the embryofetal risk. No animal reproduction studies have been conducted. Using this drug during pregnancy should be based on the pros and cons of the mother's clinical need for treatment versus any potential fetal risk that might occur from exposure. There is a boxed warning regarding IM, IV, and intrathecal use, in that it should only be administered to hospitalized patients in order to provide constant physician supervision.

BREASTFEEDING SUMMARY

No reports describing the use of polymyxin B during human lactation have been located. The drug will probably be found in human breast milk in small amounts, so some infant exposure will likely occur. However, polymyxin B is poorly absorbed from the gastrointestinal tract. Therefore, the overall infant exposure risk is probably clinically insignificant. If the clinical decision is to use this drug while breastfeeding, the infant should be monitored for the most common reported adult side effects for the injectable product of dizziness (leading to irritability), drowsiness, apnea, facial flushing, and various laboratory abnormalities (see PI).

References

1. Prescribing Information. Polymyxin B. Eugia US LLC; 2023.
2. Biolmol. Polymyxin B (sulfate). Accessed February 27, 2025. https://www.biomol.com/products/chemicals/antibiotics/polymyxin-b-sulfate-cay14157-500
3. Heinonen OP, Slone D, Shapiro S. *Birth Defects and Drugs in Pregnancy*. Publishing Sciences Group; 1977:297.
4. Kazy Z, Puho E, Czeizel AE. Parenteral polymyxin B treatment during pregnancy. *Reprod Toxicol*. 2005;20:181-182.

POMALIDOMIDE

Antineoplastic (Thalidomide Analogue)

PREGNANCY RECOMMENDATION: *Contraindicated

BREASTFEEDING RECOMMENDATION: Potential Toxicity

PREGNANCY SUMMARY

No reports describing the use of pomalidomide in human pregnancy have been located. The drug will probably cross the placenta. However, the absence of human pregnancy experience prevents a complete assessment of the embryofetal risk. Embryofetal toxicity with malformations was observed in animal studies. Thalidomide is a known significant teratogen that can cause severe birth defects and embryofetal toxicity, and pomalidomide is a thalidomide analogue. The manufacturer states that women with reproductive potential must use two forms of contraception or continuously abstain from heterosexual sex during treatment and for at least 4 weeks after the last dose. They also state that males with female partners of

(*continued*)

reproductive potential must use a condom during sexual contact while taking pomalidomide and for at least 4 weeks after the last dose, regardless of a successful vasectomy. Women with any suspected fetal exposure to pomalidomide should contact the US Food and Drug Administration (FDA) via the MedWatch program at 1-800-332-1088. There is also a pregnancy exposure registry that monitors pregnancy outcomes in women using this drug. Health care providers are encouraged to call 1-888-423-5436. *There could be clinical cases where a pregnant woman in the second half of her pregnancy might be a candidate for using this, who might consider treatment following an in-depth discussion of the pros and cons and risks and benefits.

BREASTFEEDING SUMMARY

No reports describing the use of pomalidomide during human lactation have been located. The drug will probably be found in breast milk, so infant exposure will likely occur. Breastfeeding while using this drug should be based on the mother's clinical need for treatment. If used, the infant should be monitored for the most common reported adult side effects of nausea and back pain (both leading to irritability), fatigue, rash, constipation, diarrhea, and various laboratory abnormalities (see PI).

Reference

1. Prescribing Information. Pomalyst. Bristol-Meyers Squibb Company; 2022.

PONATINIB

Antineoplastic (Tyrosine Kinase Inhibitor)

PREGNANCY RECOMMENDATION: No Human Data—Animal Data Suggest Potential Risk

BREASTFEEDING RECOMMENDATION: Potential Toxicity

PREGNANCY SUMMARY

No reports describing the use of ponatinib in human pregnancy have been located. The drug will probably cross the placenta, so some fetal exposure will likely occur. Therefore, the absence of human pregnancy experience prevents a complete assessment of the embryofetal risk. Embryofetal toxicity was observed in one animal species at doses of less than 10 times the MRHD. Based on animal studies and the drug's mechanism of action, the manufacturer recommends that women with reproductive potential use effective contraception during treatment and for 3 weeks after the last dose. Nevertheless, using this drug during pregnancy should be based on the pros and cons of the mother's clinical need for treatment versus any potential fetal risk that might occur from exposure. Hypertension was reported in up to 35% of patients treated with this drug in clinical trials.

BREASTFEEDING SUMMARY

No reports describing the use of ponatinib during human lactation have been located. The drug will likely be excreted into human breast milk, so some infant exposure will probably occur. However, due to a concern for potential serious adverse effects that might be seen in a breastfed infant, the manufacturer recommends that women not breastfeed while being treated with this drug and for at least 1 week after the last dose. Nevertheless, breastfeeding while using this drug should be based on the mother's clinical need for treatment versus any potential infant risks that might occur. If used, the infant should be monitored for the most common reported adult side effects of arthralgia, abdominal pain, headache, and nausea (all leading to irritability), rash, constipation, hypertension, fatigue (lethargy), peripheral edema, pyrexia, and various laboratory abnormalities (see PI).

Reference

1. Prescribing Information. Iclusig. Takeda Pharmaceuticals America Inc; 2024.

PONESIMOD

Immunologic (Sphingosine 1-Phosphate Receptor Modulator)

PREGNANCY RECOMMENDATION: No Human Data—Animal Data Suggest Risk

BREASTFEEDING RECOMMENDATION: Potential Toxicity

PREGNANCY SUMMARY

No reports describing the use of ponesimod in human pregnancy have been located. Ponesimod is likely to cross the placenta, so fetal exposure will probably occur. Therefore, the absence of human pregnancy experience prevents a complete assessment of the embryofetal risk. Embryofetal toxicity with malformations was observed in animal studies. Based on the animal studies, the manufacturer recommends that women with reproductive potential use effective contraception during treatment and for 1 week after the last dose. Nevertheless, using this drug during pregnancy should be based on the pros and cons of the mother's clinical need for treatment versus any potential fetal risk that might occur from exposure. Hypertension was reported in 10% of patients treated with this drug in clinical trials.

BREASTFEEDING SUMMARY

No reports describing the use of ponesimod during human lactation have been located. It is likely that some amount of the drug will be excreted into breast milk, so infant exposure will probably occur. Breastfeeding while using this drug should be based on the mother's clinical need for treatment. If used, the infant should be monitored for the most common reported adult side effects of upper respiratory tract infection, hepatic transaminase elevation, and hypertension.

Reference

1. Product Information. Ponvory. Janssen Pharmaceuticals; 2022.

PORFIMER

Antineoplastic (Photoactivated Radical Generator)

PREGNANCY RECOMMENDATION: No Human Data—Animal Data Suggest Potential Risk

BREASTFEEDING RECOMMENDATION: Potential Toxicity

PREGNANCY SUMMARY

No reports describing the use of porfimer in human pregnancy have been located. The drug may cross the placenta, so some fetal exposure might occur, but the total amount may be negligible. Therefore, the absence of human pregnancy experience prevents a complete assessment of the embryofetal risk. Embryofetal toxicity was seen in two animal species at doses of less than the RHD, but maternal toxicity also occurred. Based on animal studies and the drug's mechanism of action, the manufacturer recommends that women with reproductive potential use effective contraception during treatment and for 5 months after the last dose. They also recommend that males with female partners of reproductive potential use effective contraception during treatment and for 5 months after the last dose. Nevertheless, using this drug during pregnancy should be based on the pros and cons of the mother's clinical need for treatment versus any potential fetal risk that might occur from exposure. There is a registry for women who are pregnant and have cancer. For more information, women and health care providers are encouraged to contact the Cancer and Pregnancy Registry at 1-877-635-4499.

BREASTFEEDING SUMMARY

No reports describing the use of porfimer during human lactation have been located. The drug may be excreted into human breast milk, so some infant exposure might occur. However, the total amount may be negligible. Nevertheless, due to a concern for potential serious adverse effects that might be seen in a breastfed infant, the manufacturer recommends that women not breastfeed while being treated with this drug and for at least 5 months after the last dose. Regardless, breastfeeding while using this drug should be based on the mother's clinical need for treatment versus any potential infant risks that might occur. If used, the infant should be monitored for the most common reported adult side effects of nausea, chest pain, and abdominal pain (all leading to irritability), pleural effusion, pyrexia, constipation, anemia, dyspnea, photosensitivity reactions, cough, esophageal obstruction, and vomiting.

Reference

1. Prescribing Information. Photofrin. Pinnacle Biologics Inc; 2019.

POSACONAZOLE

Anti-Infective (Triazole Antifungal)

PREGNANCY RECOMMENDATION: No Human Data—Animal Data Suggest Potential Risk

BREASTFEEDING RECOMMENDATION: Potential Toxicity

P

PREGNANCY SUMMARY

No reports describing the use of posaconazole in human pregnancy have been located. The drug will probably cross the placenta, so some fetal exposure will likely occur. Therefore, the absence of human pregnancy experience prevents a complete assessment of the embryofetal risk. Embryofetal toxicity was observed in two animal species at doses of less than 10 times the MRHD, but maternal toxicity was seen in one. Using this drug during pregnancy should be based on the pros and cons of the mother's clinical need for treatment versus any potential fetal risk that might occur from exposure. Hypertension was reported in up to 20% of patients treated with this drug in the clinical trials. Posaconazole can also prolong the QT interval.

BREASTFEEDING SUMMARY

No reports describing the use of posaconazole during human lactation have been located. The drug will likely be excreted into human breast milk, so some infant exposure will probably occur. Breastfeeding while using this drug should be based on the mother's clinical need for treatment versus any potential infant risks that might occur. If used, the infant should be monitored for the most common reported adult side effects of nausea and headache (leading to irritability), diarrhea, fever, vomiting, coughing, and hypokalemia.

References

1. Prescribing Information. Posaconazole (tablet). Chartwell Rx LLC; 2022.
2. Prescribing Information. Posaconazole (injection). Endo USA Inc; 2022.

POTASSIUM CHLORIDE/GLUCONATE

Nutrition (Electrolyte)

PREGNANCY RECOMMENDATION: Compatible

BREASTFEEDING RECOMMENDATION: Compatible

PREGNANCY SUMMARY

The Michigan Medicaid Surveillance study reported 1 (2.9%) major fetal anomaly in 35 first-trimester exposures to potassium salts. Potassium crosses the placenta to the fetal circulation. Treating a patient with potassium chloride or potassium gluconate is for the purpose of correcting hypokalemia. High or low potassium levels can be detrimental to maternal and fetal cardiac function. No animal reproduction studies have been conducted. Using this product during pregnancy should be based on the pros and cons of the mother's clinical need for treatment versus any potential fetal risk that might occur from exposure.

P

BREASTFEEDING SUMMARY

Breast milk is naturally high in potassium, with levels that are 3 to 4 times those in plasma. Because potassium freely passes into and out of breast milk, the use of potassium chloride by a lactating woman with normal plasma potassium levels would have no adverse effect on a nursing infant. However, if the woman has hyperkalemia, this could result in higher breast milk potassium concentrations. In this case, nursing infants should be observed for gastrointestinal complaints commonly observed in adults with oral potassium, and plasma potassium concentrations should be monitored.

References

1. Prescribing Information. Potassium chloride (capsule). Lupin Limited; 2024.
2. National Library of Medicine. Potassium chloride. PubChem. Accessed March 1, 2025. https://pubchem.ncbi.nlm.nih.gov/compound/Potassium-Chloride
3. National Library of Medicine. Potassium gluconate. PubChem. Accessed March 1, 2025. https://pubchem.ncbi.nlm.nih.gov/compound/Potassium-gluconate-monohydrate
4. Zhao Y, Pasanen M, Rysa J. Placental ion channels: potential target of chemical exposure. *Biol Reprod*. 2023;108:41-51.
5. Lawrence RA, Lawrence RM. Biochemistry of human milk. In: *Breastfeeding. A Guide for the Medical Profession*. 5th ed. Mosby; 1999:127-129.

POTASSIUM CITRATE

Urinary (Urinary Alkalinizer)

PREGNANCY RECOMMENDATION: Limited Human Data—No Relevant Animal Data

BREASTFEEDING RECOMMENDATION: Probably Compatible

PREGNANCY SUMMARY

Two case reports describing the use of potassium citrate in human pregnancy have been located. Both involved the treatment of renal tubular acidosis after the first trimester. Potassium crosses the placenta. However, the limited human pregnancy experience prevents a complete assessment of the embryofetal risk. No animal reproduction studies have been conducted. Using this drug during pregnancy should be based on the pros and cons of the mother's clinical need for treatment versus any potential fetal risk that might occur from exposure.

BREASTFEEDING SUMMARY

One report describing the use of potassium citrate during human lactation was located. A patient with renal tubular acidosis, being treated with potassium citrate, breastfed her infant postdelivery with no reported complications. Breast milk is naturally high in potassium, with levels that are 3 to 4 times those in plasma. Because potassium freely passes into and out of breast milk, the use of potassium chloride by a lactating woman with normal plasma potassium levels would have no adverse effect on a nursing infant. However, if the woman has hyperkalemia, this could result in higher breast milk potassium concentrations. In this case, nursing infants should be observed for gastrointestinal complaints commonly observed in adults with oral potassium, and plasma potassium concentrations should be monitored.

References

1. Prescribing Information. Potassium citrate extended release. Strides Pharma Inc; 2023.
2. National Library of Medicine. Potassium citrate. Pubchem. Accessed March 1, 2025. https://pubchem.ncbi.nlm.nih.gov/compound/Potassium-Citrate
3. Zhao Y, Pasanen M, Rysa J. Placental ion channels: potential target of chemical exposure. *Biol Reprod*. 2023;108:41-51.
4. Yuvaraj A, Ghosh S, Shanmugasundaram L, Abraham G. Sjogren's with distal renal tubular acidosis complicating pregnancy. *J Obstet Gynaecol*. 2018;38:429-431.
5. Mellin GW. Drugs in the first trimester of pregnancy and the fetal life of Homo sapiens. *Am J Obstet Gynecol*. 1964;90:1169-1180.
6. Lawrence RA, Lawrence RM. Biochemistry of human milk. In: *Breastfeeding. A Guide for the Medical Profession*. 5th ed. Mosby; 1999:127.

POTASSIUM IODIDE

Antidote/Respiratory (Antidote—Expectorant)

PREGNANCY RECOMMENDATION: Limited Human Data—No Relevant Animal Data (Matenal Benefit May Outweigh Embryofetal Risk [Nuclear Radiation Emergency])

BREASTFEEDING RECOMMENDATION: Potential Toxicity

P

PREGNANCY SUMMARY

The Collaborative Perinatal Project reported 3 (5.4%) major anomalies (2 expected) with potassium iodide use in 56 first-trimester exposures. No pattern to the defects was seen. Potassium and iodide both cross the placenta. No animal reproduction studies have been conducted. Using this drug during pregnancy should be based on the pros and cons of the mother's clinical need for treatment versus any potential fetal risk that might occur from exposure. When used for prolonged periods or close to term, iodide may cause fetal/neonatal hypothyroidism and goiter. Therefore, the manufacturer of the expectorant recommends that the drug not be used if possible. Short-term use in preparation for maternal thyroid surgery probably represents a negligible risk. (See Potassium Chloride for effects of potassium.)

BREASTFEEDING SUMMARY

Iodide is excreted into and concentrated in breast milk. However, the concentration in breast milk depends on maternal levels. The adequate intake (recommended dietary allowance) for iodine is 110 mcg for infants 0 to 6 months old and 130 mcg for infants 7 to 12 months old. Breastfeeding while using this drug should be based on the mother's clinical need for treatment versus any potential infant risks that might occur. The manufacturer notes that the use of potassium iodide by nursing mothers may cause rash and thyroid suppression. Regarding the treatment of a nuclear radiation emergency, the benefit of treating the mother may outweigh any potential infant risk.

References

1. Prescribing Information. Potassium iodide. Mission Pharmacal Company; 2023.
2. Prescribing Information. SSKI. Avondale Pharmaceuticals LLC; 2024.
3. National Library of Medicine. Potassium iodide. PubChem. Accessed March 1, 2025. https://pubchem.ncbi.nlm.nih.gov/compound/Potassium-Iodide
4. National Library of Medicine. Iodine. Accessed March 1, 2025. https://ods.od.nih.gov/factsheets/Iodine-HealthProfessional/
5. Wolff J. Iodide goiter and the pharmacologic effects of excess iodide. *Am J Med*. 1969;47:101-124.

6. Herbst AL, Selenkow HA. Hyperthyroidism during pregnancy. *N Engl J Med.* 1965;273:627-633.
7. Selenkow HA, Herbst AL. Hyperthyroidism during pregnancy. *N Engl J Med.* 1966;274:165-166.
8. Mehta PS, Mehta SJ, Vorherr H. Congenital iodide goiter and hypothyroidism: a review. *Obstet Gynecol Surv.* 1983;38:237-247.
9. Postellon DC, Aronow R. Iodine in mother's milk. *JAMA.* 1982;247:463.
10. Casteels K, Punt S, Bramswig J. Transient neonatal hypothyroidism during breastfeeding after post-natal maternal topical iodine treatment. *Eur J Pediatr.* 2000;159:716-717.
11. Gushurst CA, Mueller JA, Green JA, Sedor F. Breast milk iodide: reassessment in the 1980s. *Pediatrics.* 1984;73:354-357.

POVIDONE IODINE

Anti-Infective (Topical)

PREGNANCY RECOMMENDATION: Limited Human Data—No Relevant Animal Data

BREASTFEEDING RECOMMENDATION: Potential Toxicity

PREGNANCY SUMMARY

The Collaborative Perinatal Project reported no major anomalies in six first-trimester exposures to povidone iodine. Four other studies have shown a potential hazard resulting from the use of topical povidone iodine during human pregnancy. In each case, significant absorption of iodine occurred in the mother and fetus following topical, vaginal, or perineal use before delivery. Transient hypothyroidism was demonstrated in some newborns. Iodide, the negative ion of iodine, readily crosses the placenta to the fetus. However, the limited human pregnancy experience prevents a complete assessment of embryofetal risk. No animal reproduction studies have been conducted. Using this drug during pregnancy should be based on the pros and cons of the mother's clinical need for treatment versus any potential fetal risk that might occur from exposure.

BREASTFEEDING SUMMARY

A few case reports have described excess iodine levels in breastfeeding infants of mothers using topical povidone iodine. Infant hypothyroidism has also been reported. Abnormal neonatal thyroid tests have even been identified when this topical agent was used just prior to delivery. Iodide is excreted into and concentrated in breast milk. However, the concentration in breast milk depends on maternal levels. Breastfeeding while using this drug should be based on the mother's clinical need for treatment versus any potential infant risks that might occur.

P

References

1. National Library of Medicine. Povidone iodine. PubChem. Accessed March 1, 2025. https://pubchem.ncbi.nlm.nih.gov/compound/410087
2. Wolff J. Iodide goiter and the pharmacologic effects of excess iodide. *Am J Med.* 1969;47:101-124.
3. Herbst AL, Selenkow HA. Hyperthyroidism during pregnancy. *N Engl J Med.* 1965;273:627-633.
4. Selenkow HA, Herbst AL. Hyperthyroidism during pregnancy. *N Engl J Med.* 1966;274:165-166.
5. Mehta PS, Mehta SJ, Vorherr H. Congenital iodide goiter and hypothyroidism: a review. *Obstet Gynecol Surv.* 1983;38:237-247.
6. l'Allemand D, Gruters A, Heidemann P, Schurnbrand P. Iodine-induced alterations of thyroid function in newborn infants after prenatal and perinatal exposure to povidone iodine. *J Pediatr.* 1983;102:935-938.
7. Bachrach LK, Burrow GN, Gare DJ. Maternal-fetal absorption of povidone-iodine. *J Pediatr.* 1984;104:158-159.
8. Jacobson JM, Hankins GV, Young RL, Hauth JC. Changes in thyroid function and serum iodine levels after prepartum use of a povidone-iodine vaginal lubricant. *J Reprod Med.* 1984;29:98-100.
9. Danziger Y, Pertzelan A, Mimouni M. Transient congenital hypothyroidism after topical iodine in pregnancy and lactation. *Arch Dis Child.* 1987;62:295-296.
10. National Library of Medicine. Iodine. Accessed March 1, 2025. https://ods.od.nih.gov/factsheets/Iodine-HealthProfessional/
11. Postellon DC, Aronow R. Iodine in mother's milk. *JAMA.* 1982;247:463.
12. Casteels K, Punt S, Bramswig J. Transient neonatal hypothyroidism during breastfeeding after post-natal maternal topical iodine treatment. *Eur J Pediatr.* 2000;159:716-717.
13. Chanoine JP, Boulvain M, Bourdoux P, et al. Increased recall rate at screening for congenital hypothyroidism in breast fed infants born to iodine overloaded mothers. *Arch Dis Child.* 1988;63:1207-1210.
14. Heinonen OP, Slone D, Shapiro S. *Birth Defects and Drugs in Pregnancy.* Wright PSB; 1983:300.

POVIDONE IODINE OPHTHALMIC

Ophthalmic (Anti-Infective)

PREGNANCY RECOMMENDATION: No Human Data—No Relevant Animal Data

BREASTFEEDING RECOMMENDATION: Probably Compatible

PREGNANCY SUMMARY

No reports describing the use of povidone iodine ophthalmic in human pregnancy have been located. The amount of systemic absorption following ocular use is unknown. Iodine readily crosses the human placenta. Therefore, this limited human pregnancy experience prevents a complete assessment of embryofetal risk. No animal reproduction studies have been conducted. Using this drug during pregnancy should be based on the pros and cons of the mother's clinical need for treatment versus any potential fetal risk that might occur from exposure. Prolonged exposure to iodine may cause hypothyroidism and goiter in the fetus and newborn, but short-term topical use (<10 days) most likely does not carry this risk. If used during pregnancy, consider placing pressure over the tear duct in the corner of the eye for at least 1 minute, and then remove any excess solution with absorbent tissue to decrease the amount of drug reaching the systemic circulation even further.

BREASTFEEDING SUMMARY

No reports describing the use of povidone iodine ophthalmic during human lactation have been located. Iodide, the negative ion of iodine, is concentrated in breast milk, but the amount of iodine in the systemic circulation after ocular use is unknown. Short-term use is probably low risk. However, due to a concern for potential serious adverse effects that might be seen in a breastfed infant, the manufacturer recommends that women not breastfeed while being treated with this drug. Nevertheless, breastfeeding while using this drug should be based on the mother's clinical need for treatment versus any potential infant risks that might occur. A method to decrease some systemic absorption with ophthalmic use is described above in the Pregnancy Summary.

References

1. Prescribing Information. Betadine. Alcon Laboratories; 2022.
2. National Library of Medicine. Povidone iodine. PubChem. Accessed March 1, 2025. https://pubchem.ncbi.nlm.nih.gov/compound/410087

POZELIMAB

Gastrointestinal (Monoclonal Antibody—Complement Protein 5 Inhibitor)

PREGNANCY RECOMMENDATION: No Human Data—Animal Data Suggest Low Risk

BREASTFEEDING RECOMMENDATION: Probably Compatible

PREGNANCY SUMMARY

No reports describing the use of pozelimab in human pregnancy have been located. As an IgG antibody, it likely crosses the placenta, especially during the second half of pregnancy, so some fetal exposure will probably occur. Therefore, the absence of human pregnancy experience prevents a complete assessment of the embryofetal risk. Animal reproduction studies did not show any embryofetal toxicity or malformations in one species at doses of less than 10 times the MRHD. Using this drug during pregnancy should be based on the pros and cons of the mother's clinical need for treatment versus any potential fetal risk that might occur from exposure.

BREASTFEEDING SUMMARY

No reports describing the use of pozelimab during human lactation have been located. It is known that IgG antibodies can be found in human breast milk but are not found in the neonatal or infant circulation. Additionally, if any IgG antibodies were to be ingested through breastfeeding, they would probably be digested in the infant's gastrointestinal tract and not be absorbed. Breastfeeding while using this drug should be based on the mother's clinical need for treatment. If used, the infant should be monitored for the most common reported adult side effects of upper respiratory infections, rash, alopecia, and fractures.

Reference

1. Prescribing Information. Veopoz. Regeneron; 2023.

PRABOTULINUM TOXIN TYPE A

Central Nervous System (Neuromuscular Blocker/Toxin)

PREGNANCY RECOMMENDATION: No Human Data—Animal Data Suggest Low Risk

BREASTFEEDING RECOMMENDATION: Probably Compatible

P

PREGNANCY SUMMARY

No reports describing the use of prabotulinum toxin type A in human pregnancy have been located. Because it most likely will not cross the placenta, fetal exposure is expected to be nonexistent. However, if the administration is done incorrectly, systemic exposure is possible. Therefore, the absence of human pregnancy experience prevents a complete assessment of the embryofetal risk. Animal data did not show any embryofetal toxicity. Using this drug during pregnancy should be based on the pros and cons of the mother's clinical need for treatment versus any potential fetal risk that might occur from exposure. However, based on drug indication, use during pregnancy is not recommended.

BREASTFEEDING SUMMARY

No reports describing the use of prabotulinum toxin type A during human lactation have been located. The lack of systemic absorption should limit infant exposure. However, if any toxin were to be ingested through breastfeeding, because it is a polypeptide, it would probably be digested in the infant's gastrointestinal tract and not be absorbed. Breastfeeding while using this drug should be based on the mother's clinical need for treatment. If used, the infant should be monitored for the most common reported adult side effect of headache (leading to irritability).

Reference

1. Prescribing Information. Jeuveau. Evolus Inc; 2023.

PRALATREXATE

Antineoplastic (Antimetabolite—Folate Analogue Metabolic Inhibitor)

PREGNANCY RECOMMENDATION: **No Human Data—Animal Data Suggest Risk**

BREASTFEEDING RECOMMENDATION: **Potential Toxicity**

PREGNANCY SUMMARY

No reports describing the use of pralatrexate in human pregnancy have been located. The drug will probably cross the placenta, so some fetal exposure will likely occur. Therefore, the absence of human pregnancy experience prevents a complete assessment of the embryofetal risk. Embryofetal toxicity was observed in two animal species at doses of about equal to the RHD. Based on animal studies and the drug's mechanism of action, the manufacturer recommends that women with reproductive potential use effective contraception during treatment and for 6 months after the last dose. They also recommend that males with female partners of reproductive potential use effective contraception during treatment and for 3 months after the last dose. Nevertheless, using this drug during pregnancy should be based on the pros and cons of the mother's clinical need for treatment versus any potential fetal risk that might occur from exposure. There is a registry for women who are pregnant and have cancer. For more information, women and health care providers are encouraged to contact the Cancer and Pregnancy Registry at 1-877-635-4499.

BREASTFEEDING SUMMARY

No reports describing the use of pralatrexate during human lactation have been located. The drug will likely be excreted into human breast milk, so some infant exposure will probably occur. However, due to a concern for potential serious adverse effects that might be seen in a breastfed infant, the manufacturer recommends that women not breastfeed while being treated with this drug and for at least 1 week after the last dose. Nevertheless, breastfeeding while using this drug should be based on the mother's clinical need for treatment versus any potential infant risks that might occur. If used, the infant should be monitored for the most common reported adult side effects of nausea (leading to irritability), fatigue (lethargy), and thrombocytopenia.

Reference

1. Prescribing Information. Pralatrexate. Fresenius Kabi USA LLC; 2022.

PRALIDOXIME

Antidote (Cholinesterase Reactivator)

PREGNANCY RECOMMENDATION: **Limited Human Data—No Relevant Animal Data (Maternal Benefit May Outweigh Any Potential Embryofetal Risk)**

BREASTFEEDING RECOMMENDATION: **Potential Toxicity (Hold Breastfeeding)**

PREGNANCY SUMMARY

Two reports describing the use of pralidoxime in three human pregnancies have been located. Exposures occurred during the second and third trimesters in treating organophosphate poisoning. Three healthy infants were born. The drug will probably cross the placenta, so some fetal exposure will likely occur. Therefore, the absence of human pregnancy experience prevents a complete assessment of the embryofetal risk. Animal reproduction studies have not been conducted. Using this drug during pregnancy should be based on the pros and cons of the mother's clinical need for treatment versus any potential fetal risk that might occur from exposure. Given the indication for use, the maternal benefit clearly outweighs any concern regarding embryofetal toxicity.

BREASTFEEDING SUMMARY

No reports describing the use of pralidoxime during human lactation have been located. The drug will likely be excreted into human breast milk, so some infant exposure will probably occur. The emergency nature of pralidoxime use suggests that nursing is unlikely when it might be indicated. However, the maternal benefit is clear, and breastfeeding can be held for about 6 to 7 hours (about five half-lives) after a dose is administered. If the clinical decision is to use this drug while breastfeeding, the infant should be monitored for the most common reported adult side effects of dizziness, headache, nausea, and blurred vision (all leading to irritability), tachycardia, increased blood pressure, hyperventilation, and lethargy.

References

1. Prescribing Information. Protopam chloride. Baxter Healthcare Corporation; 2018.
2. Karalliedde L, Senanayake N, Ariaratnam A. Acute organophosphorus insecticide poisoning during pregnancy. *Hum Toxicol*. 1988;7:363-364.
3. Kamha AA, Al Omary IYM, Zalabany HA, et al. Organophosphate poisoning in pregnancy: a case report. *Basic Clin Pharmacol Toxicol*. 2005;96:397-398.

PRALSETINIB

Antineoplastic (Tyrosine Kinase Inhibitor)

PREGNANCY RECOMMENDATION: No Human Data—Animal Data Suggest Potential Risk

BREASTFEEDING RECOMMENDATION: Potential Toxicity

PREGNANCY SUMMARY

No reports describing the use of pralsetinib in human pregnancy have been located. The drug most likely crosses the placenta in small amounts. Therefore, the absence of human pregnancy experience prevents a complete assessment of the embryofetal risk. Animal data did show fetotoxic effects, and because of this, the manufacturer recommends that women with reproductive potential use effective nonhormonal contraception while being treated with pralsetinib and for 2 weeks following the last dose. They also advise that males with female partners of reproductive potential also use effective contraception during treatment and for 1 week after the final dose. Because the drug can produce hypertension, if the clinical decision is to use this drug during pregnancy, blood pressure should be monitored closely.

BREASTFEEDING SUMMARY

Pralsetinib probably enters breast milk, but the amount is most likely small. Because of potential serious adverse reactions seen in adults treated with pralsetinib, the manufacturer recommends that women not breastfeed during treatment or for 1 week after the final dose. However, breastfeeding while taking this drug should be based on the mother's clinical need for treatment. If used, the infant should be monitored for the most common reported adult side effects of musculoskeletal pain and headache (both leading to irritability), lethargy, diarrhea, constipation, decreased appetite, pyrexia, hypertension, rash, cough, and pneumonia.

Reference

1. Prescribing Information. Gavreto. Genentech, Inc; 2020.

PRAMIPEXOLE

Central Nervous System (Anti-Parkinson—Dopamine Agonist)

PREGNANCY RECOMMENDATION: Limited Human Data—Animal Data Suggest Potential Risk

BREASTFEEDING RECOMMENDATION: Potential Toxicity

P

PREGNANCY SUMMARY

Three reports describing the use of pramipexole in about 13 human pregnancies in the first trimester have been located. No major malformations were described. The drug will probably cross the placenta, so some fetal exposure will likely occur. Therefore, this limited human pregnancy experience prevents a complete assessment of the embryofetal risk. Embryofetal toxicity was observed in one animal species at doses of about equal to the RHD, whereas no embryofetal toxicity was seen in a second animal species at doses well above 10 times the RHD. Using this drug during pregnancy should be based on the pros and cons of the mother's clinical need for treatment versus any potential fetal risk that might occur from exposure.

BREASTFEEDING SUMMARY

No reports describing the use of pramipexole during human lactation have been located. The drug will likely be excreted into human breast milk, so some infant exposure will probably occur. Because pramipexole inhibits prolactin secretion, it may inhibit lactation. Breastfeeding while using this drug should be based on the mother's clinical need for treatment versus any potential infant risks that might occur. If used, the infant should be monitored for the most common reported adult side effects of nausea and dizziness (both leading to irritability), somnolence, lethargy, insomnia, and constipation.

References

1. Prescribing Information. Pramipexole dihydrochloride. Alembic Pharmaceuticals Inc; 2023.
2. Mucchiut M, Belgrado E, Cutuli D, et al. Pramipexole-treated Parkinson's disease during pregnancy. *Mov Disord*. 2004;19:1114-1115.
3. Lamichhane D, Narayanan NS, Gonzalez-Alegre P. Two cases of pregnancy in Parkinson's disease. *Parkinsonism Relat Disorder*. 2014;20:239-240.
4. Tufekcioglu Z, Hanagasi H, Yalcin Cakmakli G, et al. Use of anti-Parkinson medication during pregnancy: a case series. *J Neurol*. 2018;265:1922-1929.

PRAMLINTIDE

Endocrine/Metabolic (Antidiabetic, Amylin Analogue)

PREGNANCY RECOMMENDATION: No Human Data—Animal Data Suggest Potential Risk

BREASTFEEDING RECOMMENDATION: Probably Compatible

PREGNANCY SUMMARY

No reports describing the use of pramlintide in human pregnancy have been located. With ex vivo placental perfusion studies, a minimal amount of the drug was found to cross the term placenta. However, the absence of human pregnancy experience prevents a complete assessment of embryofetal risk. Embryofetal toxicity with malformations was observed in one animal species at doses of about 10 times the RHD. In a second species, no embryofetal toxicity was seen at doses of less than 10 times the RHD, despite maternal toxicity. Using this drug during pregnancy should be based on the pros and cons of the mother's clinical need for treatment versus any potential fetal risk that might occur from exposure. This drug carries a boxed warning for an increased risk of severe hypoglycemia. Uncontrolled diabetes is associated with an increased risk for preeclampsia, spontaneous abortion, preterm delivery, IUFD, delivery complications, major malformations, and macrosomia-related morbidity. It is also a risk for maternal diabetic ketoacidosis. To lower this risk, ACOG recommends that insulin be used for types 1 and 2 diabetes occurring during pregnancy and, if diet therapy alone is not successful, for gestational diabetes. Insulin does not cross the placenta, which eliminates the additional concern that the drug therapy could adversely affect the fetus.

P

BREASTFEEDING SUMMARY

No reports describing the use of pramlintide during human lactation have been located. The drug may be found in human breast milk, but the amount is likely to be minimal. Furthermore, because it is a polypeptide of 37 amino acids, if the drug were to be ingested through breastfeeding, it would probably be digested in the infant's gastrointestinal tract and not be absorbed. Breastfeeding while using this drug should be based on the mother's clinical need for treatment versus any potential infant risks that might occur. If used, the infant should be monitored for the most common reported adult side effects of nausea and headache (both leading to irritability), vomiting, and anorexia (monitor infant growth).

References

1. Prescribing Information. Symlinpen. AstraZeneca; 2019.
2. American College of Obstetricians and Gynecologists. ACOG practice bulletin No. 201: pregestational diabetes mellitus. *Obstet Gynecol*. 2018;132:e228-e248.
3. American College of Obstetricians and Gynecologists. ACOG practice bulletin No. 190: gestational diabetes. *Obstet Gynecol*. 2018;131:e49-e64.
4. Hiles RA, Bawdon RE, Petrella EM. *Ex vivo* human placental transfer of the peptides pramlintide and exenatide (synthetic exendin-4). *Hum Exp Toxicol*. 2003;22:623-628.

PRAMOXINE

Pain (Topical—Local Anesthetic)

PREGNANCY RECOMMENDATION: Human Data Suggest Low Risk

BREASTFEEDING RECOMMENDATION: Probably Compatible

PREGNANCY SUMMARY

One report describing the use of pramoxine in human pregnancy was located. The study reported the use of pramoxine combined with hydrocortisone for the treatment of hemorrhoids in the third trimester of 204 women. Compared with controls, no adverse fetal or maternal effects were described. If found in the maternal circulation, the drug will probably cross the placenta. However, with minimal systemic absorption, the overall exposure would likely be clinically insignificant. However, the absence of human pregnancy experience prevents a complete assessment of the embryofetal risk. No animal reproduction studies have been located. Using this drug during pregnancy should be based on the pros and cons of the mother's clinical need for treatment versus any potential fetal risk that might occur from exposure.

BREASTFEEDING SUMMARY

No reports describing the use of pramoxine during human lactation have been located. If found in the maternal circulation, the drug will probably be excreted into human breast milk. However, with minimal systemic absorption, the overall exposure would likely be clinically insignificant. Therefore, the risk to a nursing infant is probably negligible. Breastfeeding while using this drug should be based on the mother's clinical need for treatment versus any potential infant risks that might occur. Due to the topical use of the drug, systemic side effects were not evaluated.

References

1. Prescribing Information. Anti itch soothing 1 pramoxine hydrochloride. The Honey Pot Company LLC; 2024.
2. National Library of Medicine. Pramoxine. PubChem. Accessed March 2, 2025. https://pubchem.ncbi.nlm.nih.gov/compound/Pramoxine
3. Lewis JH, Weingold AB; The Committee on FDA-Related Matters, American College of Gastroenterology. The use of gastrointestinal drugs during pregnancy and lactation. *Am J Gastroenterol*. 1985;80:912-923.
4. Ebrahimi N, Vohra S, Gedeon C, et al. The fetal safety of hydrocortisone-pramoxine (Proctofoam-HC) for the treatment of hemorrhoids in late pregnancy. *J Obstet Gynaecol Can*. 2011;33:153-158.

PRASUGREL

Cardiovascular ($P2Y_{12}$ Platelet Inhibitor, Antiplatelet)

PREGNANCY RECOMMENDATION: Limited Human Data—No Relevant Animal Data

BREASTFEEDING RECOMMENDATION: Probably Compatible

P

PREGNANCY SUMMARY

One report describing the use of prasugrel in human pregnancy was located. The patient used prasugrel and low-dose aspirin throughout pregnancy starting near the end of the first trimester/early second trimester. At delivery, no congenital anomalies or adverse neonatal effects were described. The prodrug prasugrel is not detected in plasma. However, the active metabolite will likely cross the placenta, so some fetal exposure will probably occur. Therefore, this limited human pregnancy experience prevents a complete assessment of embryofetal risk. Animal data did show some embryofetal toxicity in two species, but at doses of more than 10 times the MRHD. Using this drug during pregnancy should be based on the pros and cons of the mother's clinical need for treatment versus any potential fetal risk that might occur from exposure. If a woman's condition requires prasugrel combined with low-dose aspirin, the benefits will probably outweigh the unknown fetal risks, and the drug should not be withheld because of pregnancy. The drug carries a boxed warning for an increased risk of bleeding.

BREASTFEEDING SUMMARY

No reports describing the use of prasugrel during human lactation have been located. The prodrug prasugrel is not detected in plasma. However, the active metabolite will likely be excreted into breast milk, so some infant exposure will probably occur. Breastfeeding while using this drug should be based on the mother's clinical need for treatment versus any potential infant risks that might occur. If used, the infant should be monitored for the most common reported adult side effects of bleeding (that can be life-threatening in some cases). If a woman's condition requires prasugrel combined with low-dose aspirin, the benefits will probably outweigh any unknown infant risks, and the drug should not be withheld because of breastfeeding.

References

1. Prescribing Information. Prasugrel. Lupin Pharmaceuticals Inc; 2023.
2. Tello-Montoliu A, Seecheram NA, Angiolillo DJ. Successful pregnancy and delivery on prasugrel treatment: considerations for the use of dual antiplatelet therapy during pregnancy in clinical practice. *J Thromb Thrombolysis*. 2013;36:348-351.

PRAVASTATIN

Antilipemic (Statin—HMG-CoA Inhibitor)

PREGNANCY RECOMMENDATION: Limited Human Data—Animal Data Suggest Potential Risk

BREASTFEEDING RECOMMENDATION: Potential Toxicity

PREGNANCY SUMMARY

Publications specific to pravastatin regarding first-trimester exposure are limited. A systematic review and meta-analysis evaluated pregnancy outcomes with first-trimester exposure to statins (n = 1,655) as a group compared with unexposed controls (n = 974,159). No significant difference was observed for major malformations, IUFD, or preterm delivery. The manufacturer reported that a Medicaid cohort linkage evaluated outcomes in 1,152 women taking statins (as a group) prior to pregnancy, then discontinuing at some point during the first trimester, compared with 886,996 unexposed pregnancies. After adjusting for confounders, statin exposure was not associated with an increased risk for congenital malformations. Pravastatin was used in these two studies, but outcome data specifically related to this drug were not supplied. Based on ex vivo placental perfusion studies, pravastatin crosses the placenta, so some fetal exposure will occur. However, this limited human pregnancy experience, specifically with pravastatin, prevents a complete assessment of the embryofetal risk. Embryofetal toxicity was observed in one animal species at doses of about 10 times the MRHD but was not seen in a second species at the same exposure. Cholesterol and other products of cholesterol biosynthesis are essential components for fetal development. Moreover, maternal cholesterol levels increase during pregnancy. Hyperlipidemia treatment is not generally necessary during pregnancy. Atherosclerosis is a chronic process, and stopping lipid-lowering therapy during pregnancy should have little impact on the outcome of these disorders. Therefore, the manufacturer recommends discontinuing this drug when a pregnancy is recognized. Nevertheless, using this drug during pregnancy should be based on the pros and cons of the mother's clinical need for treatment versus any potential fetal risk that might occur from exposure.

P

BREASTFEEDING SUMMARY

Pravastatin has been shown to be excreted into human breast milk. One report has described the use of pravastatin during lactation in 11 women. The women, who were not breastfeeding, were given pravastatin 20 mg twice daily. Breast milk samples were obtained at various times after the fifth dose. Peak breast milk levels averaged 3.9 ng/mL. Using the peak level, the calculated RID was about 1.4% of the mother's weight-adjusted dose. However, due to a concern for potential serious adverse effects that might be seen in a breastfed infant, the manufacturer recommends that women not breastfeed while being treated with this drug. Nevertheless, breastfeeding while using this drug should be based on the mother's clinical need for treatment versus any potential infant risks that might occur. If used, the infant should be monitored for the most common reported adult side effects of musculoskeletal pain, nausea, and headache (all leading to irritability), diarrhea, vomiting, and upper respiratory tract infection.

References

1. Prescribing Information. Pravastatin sodium. Accord Healthcare Inc; 2022.
2. Zarek J, DeGorter MK, Lubetsky A, et al. The transfer of pravastatin in the dually perfused human placenta. *Placenta*. 2013;34:719-721.
3. Nanovskaya TN, Patrikeeva SL, Paul J, et al. Transplacental transfer and distribution of pravastatin. *Am J Obstet Gynecol*. 2013;209:373.e1-e5.
4. Balan A, Szaingurten-Solodkin I, Swissa SS, et al. The effects of pravastatin on the normal human placenta: lesson from ex-vivo models. *PLoS One*. 2017; 12:e0172174.
5. Teelucksingh S, Youssef JE, Sohan K, Ramsewak S. Prolonged inadvertent pravastatin use in pregnancy. *Reprod Toxicol*. 2004;18:299-300.
6. McElhatton P. Preliminary data on exposure to statins during pregnancy (abstract). *Reprod Toxicol*. 2005;20:471-472.
7. Taguchi N, Rubin ET, Hosokawa A, et al. Prenatal exposure to HMG-CoA reductase inhibitors: effects on fetal and neonatal outcomes. *Reprod Toxicol*. 2008;26:175-177.
8. Brownfoot FC, Tong S, Hannan NJ, et al. Effects of pravastatin on human placenta, endothelium, and women with severe preeclampsia. *Hypertension*. 2015;66:687-697.
9. Costantine MM, Cleary K, Hebert MF, et al; Eunice Kennedy Shriver National Institute of Child Health and Human Development Obstetric-Fetal Pharmacology Research Units Network. Safety and pharmacokinetics of pravastatin used for the prevention of preeclampsia in high-risk pregnant women: a pilot randomized controlled trial. *Am J Obstet Gynecol*. 2016;214:720.e1-e17.
10. Dobert M, Varouxaki AN, Mu AC, et al. Pravastatin versus placebo in pregnancies at high risk of term preeclampsia. *Circulation*. 2021;144:670-679.
11. Jurisic A, Jurisic Z, Lefkou E, et al. Pravastatin and L-arginine combination improves umbilical artery blood flow and neonatal outcomes in dichorionic twin pregnancies through an nitric-oxide dependent vasorelaxant effect. *Vascul Pharmacol*. 2018;110:64-70.
12. Otten LA, van der Ven K, Kuhr M, et al. Pravastatin for prevention of HELLP syndrome. A case report. *Medicine*. 2017;96:e8229.
13. Karadas B, Uysal N, Erol H, et al. Pregnancy outcomes following maternal exposure to statins: a systematic review and meta-analysis. *Br J Pharmacol*. 2022;88:3962-3976.
14. Pan H, Fleiss P, Moore L, et al. Excretion of pravastatin, an HMG CoA reductase inhibitor, in breast milk of lactating women. *J Clin Pharmacol*. 1988;28:942 (abstract).

PRAZIQUANTEL

Anti-Infective (Anthelmintic)

PREGNANCY RECOMMENDATION: Limited Human Data—Animal Data Suggest Low Risk

BREASTFEEDING RECOMMENDATION: Probably Compatible

PREGNANCY SUMMARY

A few reports were located that describe the use of praziquantel during human pregnancy. Praziquantel was not associated with any fetal or maternal harm compared with placebo when used in the second and third trimesters in more than 1,000 cases. One case report described use at about 8 weeks' gestation, and no birth anomalies were described at delivery. The drug will probably cross the placenta, so some fetal exposure will likely occur. Therefore, this limited first-trimester human pregnancy experience prevents a complete assessment of the embryofetal risk. Animal data did not show any embryofetal toxicity in two species at doses of about equal to or less than the RHD. Using this drug during pregnancy should be based on the pros and cons of the mother's clinical need for treatment versus any potential fetal risk that might occur from exposure. The World Health Organization (WHO) recommends that all praziquantel-based mass drug administration programs include pregnant and breastfeeding women.

BREASTFEEDING SUMMARY

No reports describing the use of praziquantel during human lactation have been located. The drug will likely be excreted into human breast milk, so some infant exposure will probably occur. Breastfeeding while using this drug should be based on the mother's clinical need for treatment versus any potential infant risks that might occur. If used, the infant should be monitored for the most common reported adult side effects of headache, dizziness, nausea, and abdominal discomfort (all leading to irritability), lethargy, pyrexia, and rash.

References

1. Prescribing Information. Praziquantel. Endo USA Inc; 2024.
2. National Library of Medicine. Pubchem. Praziquantel. Accessed March 2, 2025. https://pubchem.ncbi.nlm.nih.gov/compound/Praziquantel
3. Montero R, Ostrosky P. Genotoxic activity of praziquantel. *Mutat Res*. 1997;387:123-139.
4. Friedman JF, Olveda RM, Mirochnick MH, et al. Praziquantel for the treatment of schistosomiasis during human pregnancy. *Bull World Health Organ*. 2018;96:59-65.
5. Paparone PW, Menghetti RA. Case report: neurocysticercosis in pregnancy. *N J Med*. 1996;93:91-94.
6. Ndibazza J, Muhangi L, Akishule D, et al. Effects of deworming during pregnancy on maternal and perinatal outcomes in Entebbe, Uganda: a randomized controlled trial. *Clin Infect Dis*. 2010;50:531-540.
7. Olveda RM, Acosta LP, Tallo V, et al. A randomized double blind placebo controlled trial assessing the efficacy and safety of praziquantel for the treatment of human schistosomiasis during pregnancy. *Lancet Infect Dis*. 2016;16:199-208.
8. Namara B, Nash S, Lule S, et al. Effects of treating helminths during pregnancy and early childhood on risk of allergy-related outcomes: follow-up of a randomized controlled trial. *Pediatr Allergy Immunol*. 2017;28:784-792.

PRAZOSIN

Cardiovascular (Antihypertensive—α_1-Adrenergic Blocker)

PREGNANCY RECOMMENDATION: Limited Human Data—Animal Data Suggest Low Risk

BREASTFEEDING RECOMMENDATION: Probably Compatible

PREGNANCY SUMMARY

Several reports describing the use of prazosin in human pregnancy have been located. In nearly every study, prazosin was used to treat hypertension in the second or third trimesters, including hypertension associated with pheochromocytoma. No adverse effects related to the drug beyond what was expected were described. One case report of first-trimester administration through to delivery (along with minoxidil and metoprolol) did not produce any major birth anomalies, except for hypertrichosis (related to the minoxidil exposure). The drug crosses the placenta (cord blood levels about 10%-25% maternal serum concentrations), so fetal exposure will occur. Therefore, the limited first-trimester human pregnancy experience prevents a complete assessment of the embryofetal risk. Animal data did not show any embryofetal toxicity at doses of more than 10 times the MRHD. Using this drug during pregnancy should be based on the pros and cons of the mother's clinical need for treatment versus any potential fetal risk that might occur from exposure.

BREASTFEEDING SUMMARY

Prazosin was found to be excreted in small amounts into human breast milk. The manufacturer recommends exercising caution when prazosin is administered to a nursing woman. Breastfeeding while using this drug should be based on the mother's clinical need for treatment versus any potential infant risks that might occur. If used, the infant should be monitored for the most common reported adult side effects of dizziness, headache, and nausea (all leading to irritability), drowsiness, lethargy, and tachycardia.

References

1. Prescribing Information. Prazosin. Lannett Company Inc; 2023.
2. Bourget P, Fernandez H, Edouard D, et al. Disposition of a new rate-controlled formulation of prazosin in the treatment of hypertension during pregnancy: transplacental passage of prazosin. *Eur J Drug Metab Pharmacokinet*. 1995;20:233-241.
3. Lubbe WF, Hodge JV. Combined alpha- and beta-adrenoceptor antagonism with prazosin and oxprenolol in control of severe hypertension in pregnancy. *NZ Med J*. 1981;94:169-172.
4. Lubbe WF. More on beta-blockers in pregnancy. *N Engl J Med*. 1982;307:753.
5. Rosa FW, Idanpaan-Heikkila J, Asanti R. Fetal minoxidil exposure. *Pediatrics*. 1987;80:120.
6. Venuto R, Burstein P, Schneider R. Pheochromocytoma: antepartum diagnosis and management with tumor resection in the puerperium. *Am J Obstet Gynecol*. 1984;150:431-432.
7. Devoe LD, O'Dell BE, Castillo RA, et al. Metastatic pheochromocytoma in pregnancy and fetal biophysical assessment after maternal administration of alpha-adrenergic, beta-adrenergic, and dopamine antagonists. *Obstet Gynecol*. 1986;68:15S-18S.
8. Hall DR, Odendaal HJ, Steyn DW, Smith M. Nifedipine or prazosin as a second agent to control early severe hypertension in pregnancy: a randomised controlled trial. *Br J Obstet Gynaecol*. 2000;107:759-765.
9. Zitoun N, Campbell MK, Matsui D, Garcia-Bournissen F. Prospective evaluation of pregnancy outcomes after gestational exposure to prazosin. *Br J Clin Pharmacol*. 2023;89:3324-3329.

PREDNISOLONE OPTHALMIC

Ophthalmic (Topical—Corticosteroid)

PREGNANCY RECOMMENDATION: No Human Data—Animal Data Suggest Potential Risk

BREASTFEEDING RECOMMENDATION: Probably Compatible

PREGNANCY SUMMARY

No reports describing the use of prednisolone ophthalmic in human pregnancy have been located. If found in the maternal circulation, the drug will likely cross the placenta. However, with the low systemic bioavailability (≤2%) with ocular use, the amount would probably be clinically insignificant. Higher doses or prolonged use could produce higher systemic levels. Therefore, the absence of human pregnancy experience prevents a complete assessment of embryofetal risk. Embryofetal toxicity with malformations were observed in one animal species at doses of about equal to the maximum recommended human ophthalmic dose (MRHOD). Using this drug during pregnancy should be based on the pros and cons of the mother's clinical need for treatment versus any potential fetal risk that might occur from exposure. If used during pregnancy, consider placing pressure over the tear duct in the corner of the eye for at least 1 minute, and then remove any excess solution with absorbent tissue to decrease the amount of drug reaching the systemic circulation even further.

P

BREASTFEEDING SUMMARY

No reports describing the use of prednisolone ophthalmic during human lactation have been located. If found in the maternal circulation, the drug will likely be excreted into human breast milk. However, with the low systemic bioavailability (≤2%) with ocular use, the amount would probably be clinically insignificant. Breastfeeding while using this drug should be based on the mother's clinical need for treatment versus any potential infant risks that might occur. Due to the ophthalmic use, systemic side effects were not evaluated. A method to decrease some systemic absorption with ophthalmic use is described above in the Pregnancy Summary.

References

1. Prescribing Information. Pred Forte. Allergan Inc; 2024.
2. National Library of Medicine. Prednisolone. PubChem. Accessed March 2, 2025. https://pubchem.ncbi.nlm.nih.gov/compound/Prednisolone

PREDNISONE/PREDNISOLONE

Corticosteroids

PREGNANCY RECOMMENDATION: Human Data Suggest Potential Risk (First Trimester)

BREASTFEEDING RECOMMENDATION: Probably Compatible

PREGNANCY SUMMARY

Numerous studies have been located that describe the use of prednisone and prednisolone during human pregnancy. Prednisone is metabolized to prednisolone. In combined data from the Collaborative Perinatal Project, the Michigan Medicaid Surveillance study, and others, the congenital malformation rate was about 4.7% in about 550 first-trimester exposures. However, no pattern to the defects was identified. It has not been determined if this slight increase in risk is related to the medication use, the diseases for which they are used, or a combination of both. Both drugs cross the placenta, so some fetal exposure will occur. Regardless, further human study needs to occur to better assess any embryofetal risk. No animal reproduction studies were located. Using this drug during pregnancy should be based on the pros and cons of the mother's clinical need for treatment versus any potential fetal risk that might occur from exposure. Hypertension was reported in patients treated with this drug in the clinical trials. In addition, elevated glucose levels have been reported, so glucose levels should be monitored.

BREASTFEEDING SUMMARY

Prednisone and prednisolone have been shown to be excreted into human breast milk. In one study, the combined breast milk levels for both drugs were about 30 ng/mL, producing an RID of less than 1%. A few other analyses produced calculated RIDs of less than 1%. Breastfeeding while using this drug should be based on the mother's clinical need for treatment versus any potential infant risks that might occur. If used, the infant should be monitored for the most common reported adult side effects of dizziness and headache (both leading to irritability), infections, hypertension, peripheral edema, fatigue (lethargy), hypoglycemia, and various other laboratory abnormalities (see PI).

References

1. Prescribing Information. Prednisone. Jubilant Cadista Pharmaceuticals Inc; 2018.
2. Kraus AM. Congenital cataract and maternal steroid injection. *J Pediatr Ophthalmol*. 1975;12:107-108.
3. Durie BGM, Giles HR. Successful treatment of acute leukemia during pregnancy: combination therapy in the third trimester. *Arch Intern Med*. 1977;137:90-91.
4. Nolan GH, Sweet RL, Laros RK, Roure CA. Renal cadaver transplantation followed by successful pregnancies. *Obstet Gynecol*. 1974;43:732-739.
5. Grossman JH III, Littner MR. Severe sarcoidosis in pregnancy. *Obstet Gynecol*. 1977;50(suppl):81s-84s.
6. Cutting HO, Collier TM. Acute lymphocytic leukemia during pregnancy: report of a case. *Obstet Gynecol*. 1964;24:941-945.
7. Hanson GC, Ghosh S. Systemic lupus erythematosus and pregnancy. *Br Med J*. 1965;2:1227-1228.
8. Warrell DW, Taylor R. Outcome for the foetus of mothers receiving prednisolone during pregnancy. *Lancet*. 1968;1:117-118.
9. Walsh SD, Clark FR. Pregnancy in patients on long-term corticosteroid therapy. *Scott Med J*. 1967;12:302-306.
10. Zulman JI, Talal N, Hoffman GS, Epstein WV. Problems associated with the management of pregnancies in patients with systemic lupus erythematosus. *J Rheumatol*. 1980;7:37-49.
11. Hartikainen-Sorri AL, Kaila J. Systemic lupus erythematosus and habitual abortion: case report. *Br J Obstet Gynaecol*. 1980;87:729-731.
12. Minchinton RM, Dodd NJ, O'Brien H, et al. Autoimmune thrombocytopenia in pregnancy. *Br J Haematol*. 1980;44:451-459.
13. Tozman ECS, Urowitz MB, Gladman DD. Systemic lupus erythematosus and pregnancy. *J Rheumatol*. 1980;7:624-632.
14. Karpatkin M, Porges RF, Karpatkin S. Platelet counts in infants of women with autoimmune thrombocytopenia: effect of steroid administration to the mother. *N Engl J Med*. 1981;305:936-939.
15. Pratt WR. Allergic diseases in pregnancy and breast feeding. *Ann Allergy*. 1981;47:355-360.
16. Carmichael SL, Shaw GM. Maternal corticosteroid use and risk of selected congenital anomalies. *Am J Med Genet*. 1999;86:242-244.
17. Park-Wyllie L, Mazzotta P, Pastuszak A, et al. Birth defects after maternal exposure to corticosteroids: prospective cohort study and meta-analysis of epidemiological studies. *Teratology*. 2000;62:385-382.
18. Cote CJ, Meuwissen HJ, Pickering RJ. Effects on the neonate of prednisone and azathioprine administered to the mother during pregnancy. *J Pediatr*. 1974;85:324-328.
19. Cederqvist LL, Merkatz IR, Litwin SD. Fetal immunoglobulin synthesis following maternal immunosuppression. *Am J Obstet Gynecol*. 1977;129:687-690.
20. Tallent MB, Simmons RL, Najarian JS. Birth defects in child of male recipient of kidney transplant. *JAMA*. 1970;211:1854-1855.
21. Jensen MK. Chromosome studies in patients treated with azathioprine and amethopterin. *Acta Med Scand*. 1967;182:445-455.
22. Mancini RE, Larieri JC, Muller F, et al. Effect of prednisolone upon normal and pathologic human spermatogenesis. *Fertil Steril*. 1966;17:500-513.
23. Szabo I, Csaba I, Novak P, Drozgyik I. Single-dose glucocorticoid for prevention of respiratory-distress syndrome. *Lancet*. 1977;2:243.
24. Szabo I, Csaba I, Bodis J, et al. Effect of glucocorticoid on fetal lecithin and sphingomyelin concentrations. *Lancet*. 1980;1:320.
25. Katz FH, Duncan BR. Entry of prednisone into human milk. *N Engl J Med*. 1975;293:1154.
26. McKenzie SA, Selley JA, Agnew JE. Secretion of prednisone into breast milk. *Arch Dis Child*. 1975;50:894-896.
27. Ost L, Wettrell G, Bjorkhem I, Rane A. Prednisolone excretion in human milk. *J Pediatr*. 1985;106:1008-1011.
28. Greenberger PA, Odeh YK, Frederiksen MC, Atkinson AJ Jr. Pharmacokinetics of prednisolone transfer to breast milk. *Clin Pharmacol Ther*. 1993;53:324-328.

PREGABALIN

Central Nervous System (Antiseizure)

PREGNANCY RECOMMENDATION: Human Data Suggest Low Risk

BREASTFEEDING RECOMMENDATION: Potential Toxicity

PREGNANCY SUMMARY

Numerous studies have been located that describe the use of pregabalin in human pregnancy. Including a database (with more than 2,700 first-trimester exposures) reported by the manufacturer, combined with several other publications, more than 3,600 first-trimester uses have been recorded. No increased risk for major congenital anomalies was seen. In addition, no pattern to the defects was identified. However, important study limitations include uncertainty of whether a woman filled a prescription and took the medication, along with an inability to adequately control for the underlying disease and other potential confounders. The drug will probably cross the placenta, so some fetal exposure will likely occur. No embryofetal toxicity was observed in one animal species at doses of more than 10 times the MRHD. In a second species, no embryofetal toxicity was seen at doses of less than 10 times the MRHD but was seen at higher doses that were still less than 10 times the MRHD. Using this drug during pregnancy should be based on the pros and cons of the mother's clinical need for treatment versus any potential fetal risk that might occur from exposure. When used for partial seizures, there is a pregnancy exposure registry that monitors pregnancy outcomes. Health care providers are encouraged to call the North American Antiepileptic Drug Pregnancy Registry at 1-888-233-2334.

BREASTFEEDING SUMMARY

Pregabalin has been shown to be excreted into human breast milk. The manufacturer reports that breast milk levels are about 76% of maternal plasma levels. Mean breast milk levels are about 2 mcg/mL, with mean peak concentrations of about 4.6 mcg/mL. Calculated RIDs are about 7%. However, due to a concern for potential serious adverse effects that might be seen in a breastfed infant, the manufacturer recommends that women not breastfeed while being treated with this drug. Nevertheless, if the clinical decision is to use this drug while breastfeeding, the infant should be monitored for the most common reported adult side effects of dizziness, blurred vision, and dry mouth (all leading to irritability), somnolence, and peripheral edema.

References

1. Prescribing Information. *Pregabalin*. Actavis Pharma Inc; 2024.
2. Patorno E, Bateman BT, Huybrechts KF, et al. Pregabalin use early in pregnancy and the risk of major congenital malformations. *Neurology*. 2017; 88:2020-2025.
3. Winterfeld U, Merlob P, Baud D, et al. Pregnancy outcome following maternal exposure to pregabalin may call for concern. *Neurology*. 2016;86: 2251-2257.
4. Veiby G, Daltveit AK, Engelsen BA, Gilhus NE. Fetal growth restriction and birth defects with newer and older antiepileptic drugs during pregnancy. *J Neurol*. 2014;261:579-588.
5. Ohman I, De Flon O, Tomson T. Pregabalin kinetics in the neonatal period, and during lactation. *Epilepsia*. 2011;52(suppl 6):249
6. Lockwood PA, Pauer L, Scavone JM, Aet al. The Pharmacokinetics of Pregabalin in Breast Milk, Plasma, and Urine of Healthy Postpartum Women. J Hum Lact. 2016;32:NP1-NP8.
7. El Kenany S, El Tahan MR. Effect of preoperative pregabalin on post-caesarean delivery analgesia: a dose-response study. Int J Obstet Anesth. 2016;26:24-31.

P

PRETOMANID

Anti-Infective (Antituberculosis)

PREGNANCY RECOMMENDATION: No Human Data—Animal Data Suggest Potential Risk

BREASTFEEDING RECOMMENDATION: Potential Toxicity

PREGNANCY SUMMARY

No reports describing the use of pretomanid in human pregnancy have been located. The drug will probably cross the placenta, so some fetal exposure will likely occur. Therefore, the absence of human pregnancy experience prevents a complete assessment of the embryofetal risk. Embryofetal toxicity was observed in one animal species at doses of less than 10 times the MRHD but not in a second species. Using this drug during pregnancy should be based on the pros and cons of the mother's clinical need for treatment versus any potential fetal risk that might occur from exposure. Pretomanid can prolong the QT interval. Active tuberculosis in pregnancy is associated with adverse maternal and neonatal outcomes, including maternal anemia, preterm birth, low birth weight, and increased perinatal infant mortality.

BREASTFEEDING SUMMARY

No reports describing the use of pretomanid during human lactation have been located. The drug will likely be excreted into human breast milk, so some infant exposure will probably occur. If the clinical decision is to use this drug while breastfeeding, the infant should be monitored for the most common reported adult side effects of nausea, headache, musculoskeletal pain, pruritus, abdominal pain, and peripheral neuropathy (all leading to irritability), vomiting, rash, decreased appetite (monitor infant growth), and various laboratory abnormalities (see PI).

Reference

1. Prescribing Information. Pretomanid. Viatris Specialty LLC; 2024.

PRIMAQUINE

Anti-Infective (Antimalarial)

PREGNANCY RECOMMENDATION: No Human Data and No Relevant Animal Data

PREGNANCY SUMMARY

No reports describing the use of primaquine during human pregnancy have been located. The drug will probably cross the placenta, so some fetal exposure will likely occur. Therefore, the absence of human pregnancy experience prevents a complete assessment of the embryofetal risk. No animal reproduction studies have been conducted. However, based on the risk of producing hemolytic anemia in the fetus/newborn, the manufacturer recommends that women with reproductive potential use effective contraception during treatment and until completion of an ongoing ovulatory cycle (up to next menses) after stopping treatment. They also recommend that males with female partners of reproductive potential use a condom during treatment and for 3 months after the last dose. Nevertheless, using this drug during pregnancy should be based on the pros and cons of the mother's clinical need for treatment versus any potential fetal risk that might occur from exposure. Primaquine can prolong the QT interval. The drug may also cause hemolytic anemia in patients with G6PD deficiency. The CDC states that pregnant patients with malaria are 3 times more likely to develop severe disease compared to nonpregnant patients in the same geographic area. Malaria during pregnancy increases the risk for spontaneous abortion, preterm delivery, low birth weight, congenital infection, and perinatal death.

BREASTFEEDING SUMMARY

One report describing the use of primaquine during human lactation has been located. The study included 21 breastfeeding women with a history of *Plasmodium vivax* infection. The drug was not initiated until the infant was at least 28 days old, and neither the mother nor the infant had G6PD deficiency. Mothers received primaquine 0.5 mg base per kilogram daily for 14 days. No adverse events were reported for any of the mothers or infants. Peak maternal plasma levels of about 139 ng/mL were obtained. Peak breast milk levels of about 44 ng/mL occurred. Calculated RIDs were 1.8% or less. The CDC states that the mother and the infant should be tested for G6PD deficiency before the drug is used during breastfeeding. However, due to a concern for potential serious adverse effects that might be seen in a breastfed infant, the manufacturer recommends that women not breastfeed while being treated with this drug. Nevertheless, if the clinical decision is to use this drug while breastfeeding, the infant should be monitored for the most common reported adult side effects of nausea, epigastric distress, abdominal cramps, dizziness, and pruritus (all leading to irritability), vomiting, cardiac arrhythmia, rash, and various laboratory abnormalities (see PI).

References

1. Prescribing Information. Primaquine. Bayshore Pharmaceuticals LLC; 2024.
2. National Library of Medicine. Primaquine. PubChem. Accessed March 2, 2025. https://pubchem.ncbi.nlm.nih.gov/compound/Primaquine
3. Center for Disease Control and Prevention. Alternatives for pregnant women. Accessed March 2, 2025. https://www.cdc.gov/malaria/hcp/clinical-guidance/pregnant-women.html

PRIMIDONE

Central Nervous System (Antiseizure)

PREGNANCY RECOMMENDATION: Limited Human Data—No Relevant Animal Data

BREASTFEEDING RECOMMENDATION: Potential Toxicity

PREGNANCY SUMMARY

Several reports describing the use of primidone in human pregnancy have been located. In combined data from 3 studies, there were 3 (3.8%) major birth anomalies in 80 first-trimester pregnancy exposures. A Cochrane Review of 110 first-trimester monotherapy exposures to primidone did not show an increased risk for birth defects compared with controls. One of primidone's active metabolites is phenobarbital (see Phenobarbital). It is not known if primidone crosses the placenta, but phenobarbital does. Therefore, primidone will also probably cross the placenta, so some fetal exposure will likely occur. However, this limited first-trimester human pregnancy experience prevents a complete assessment of the embryofetal risk. No animal reproduction studies specifically for primidone have been located. Using this drug during pregnancy should be based on the pros and cons of the mother's clinical need for treatment versus any potential fetal risk that might occur from exposure. There is a pregnancy exposure registry that monitors pregnancy outcomes in women using antiseizure drugs. Health care providers are encouraged to call the North American Antiepileptic Drug Pregnancy Registry at 1-888-233-2334.

BREASTFEEDING SUMMARY

Primidone has been shown to be excreted into human breast milk. Mean breast milk levels are about 2.3 mcg/mL, with most calculated RIDs less than 10%. However, because primidone undergoes limited conversion to phenobarbital, breast milk concentrations of phenobarbital may also occur. The breast milk to maternal plasma ratio is about 80%. No reports linking adverse effects to the nursing infant have been located; however, patients who breastfeed should be instructed to watch for potential sedative effects in the infant. Due to a concern for potential serious adverse effects that might be seen in a breastfed infant, the manufacturer recommends that women not breastfeed while being treated with this drug. Nevertheless, breastfeeding while using this drug should be based on the mother's clinical need for treatment versus any potential infant risks that might occur. If used, the infant should be monitored for the most common reported adult side effects of nausea (leading to irritability), anorexia (monitor infant growth), vomiting, fatigue (lethargy), drowsiness, and rash.

P

References

1. Prescribing Information. Primidone. Advangen Pharma Limited; 2023.
2. Nakane Y, Okuma T, Takahashi R, et al. Multi-institutional study on the teratogenicity and fetal toxicity of antiepileptic drugs: a report of a collaborative study group in Japan. *Epilepsia*. 1980;21:663-680.
3. Lowe CR. Congenital malformations among infants born to epileptic women. *Lancet*. 1973;1:9-10.
4. Lander CM, Edwards BE, Eadie MJ, Tyrer JH. Plasma anticonvulsants concentrations during pregnancy. *Neurology*. 1977;27:128-131.
5. Speidel BD, Meadow SR. Maternal epilepsy and abnormalities of the fetus and newborn. *Lancet*. 1972;2:839-843.
6. McMullin GP. Teratogenic effects of anticonvulsants. *Br Med J*. 1971;4:430.
7. Fedrick J. Epilepsy and pregnancy: a report from the Oxford Record Linkage Study. *Br Med J*. 1973;2:442-448.
8. Biale Y, Lewenthal H, Aderet NB. Congenital malformations due to anticonvulsant drugs. *Obstet Gynecol*. 1975;45:439-442.
9. Thomas P, Buchanan N. Teratogenic effect of anticonvulsants. *J Pediatr*. 1981;99:163.
10. Myhree SA, Williams R. Teratogenic effects associated with maternal primidone therapy. *J Pediatr*. 1981;99:160-162.
11. Rudd NL, Freedom RM. A possible primidone embryopathy. *J Pediatr*. 1979; 94:835-837.
12. Heinonen OP, Slone D, Shapiro S. *Birth Defects and Drugs in Pregnancy*. Publishing Sciences Group; 1977:358.
13. Kutlay B, Bayramoglu S, Kutlar AI, Yesildaglar N. An acardiac acephalic monster following in-utero anti-epileptic drug exposure. *Eur J Obstet Gynecology Reprod Med*. 1996;65:245-248.
14. Hernandez-Diaz S, Werler MM, Walker AM, Mitchell AA. Folic acid antagonists during pregnancy and the risk of birth defects. *N Engl J Med*. 2000;343:1608-1614.
15. Canger R, Battino D, Canevini MP, et al. Malformations in offspring of women with epilepsy: a prospective study. *Epilepsia*. 1999;40:1231-1236.
16. The Lamotrigine Pregnancy Registry. Final report. 1 September 1992 through 31 March 2010. GlaxoSmithKline; 2010.
17. Martinez G, Snyder RD. Transplacental passage of primidone. *Neurology*. 1973;23:381-383.
18. Kohler HG. Haemorrhage in the newborn of epileptic mothers. *Lancet*. 1966;1:267.
19. Bleyer WA, Skinner AL. Fatal neonatal hemorrhage after maternal anticonvulsant therapy. *JAMA*. 1976;235:826-827.
20. Mountain KR, Hirsh J, Gallus AS. Neonatal coagulation defect due to anticonvulsant drug treatment in pregnancy. *Lancet*. 1970;1:265-268.
21. Evans AR, Forrester RM, Discombe C. Neonatal hemorrhage following maternal anticonvulsant therapy. *Lancet*. 1970;1:517-518.
22. Margolin DO, Kantor NM. Hemorrhagic disease of the newborn: an unusual case related to maternal ingestion of antiepileptic drug. *Clin Pediatr (Phila)*. 1972;11:59-60.
23. Weston J, Bromley R, Jackson CF, et al. Monotherapy treatment of epilepsy in pregnancy: congenital malformation outcomes in the child. *Cochrane Database Syst Rev*. 2016;11(11):CD101224.
24. Kaneko S, Sato T, Suzuki K. The levels of anticonvulsants in breast milk. *Br J Clin Pharmacol*. 1979;7:624-627.

PROBENECID

Endocrine/Metabolic (Antigout)

PREGNANCY RECOMMENDATION: Limited Human Data—No Relevant Animal Data

BREASTFEEDING RECOMMENDATION: Probably Compatible

PREGNANCY SUMMARY

A few reports describing the use of probenecid in human pregnancy have been located. From the Michigan Medicaid Surveillance study, 11 (3.2%) major birth anomalies in 339 first-trimester exposures were reported. No pattern to the defects was seen. The drug crosses the placenta, so some fetal exposure will occur. However, this limited human pregnancy experience prevents a complete assessment of the embryofetal risk. No animal reproduction studies have been located. Using this drug during pregnancy should be based on the pros and cons of the mother's clinical need for treatment versus any potential fetal risk that might occur from exposure.

BREASTFEEDING SUMMARY

Probenecid has been shown to be excreted into human breast milk. Mean breast milk concentration for the drug in a mother using 500 mg, 4 times per day, was about 0.964 mcg/mL. The calculated RID was less than 1%. Breastfeeding while using this drug should be based on the mother's clinical need for treatment versus any potential infant risks that might occur. If used, the infant should be monitored for the most common reported adult side effects of headache, dizziness, nausea, sore gums, pruritus, and costovertebral pain (all leading to irritability), vomiting, anorexia (monitor infant growth), urinary frequency, rash, flushing, and various laboratory abnormalities (see PI).

References

1. Prescribing Information. Probenecid. Actavis Pharma Inc; 2024.
2. Beidleman B. Treatment of chronic hypoparathyroidism with probenecid. *Metabolism*. 1958;7:690-698.
3. Lee FI, Loeffler FE. Gout and pregnancy. *J Obstet Gynaecol Br Commonw*. 1962;69:299.
4. Batt RE, Cirksena WJ, Lebhertz TB. Gout and salt-wasting renal disease during pregnancy. Diagnosis, management and follow-up. *JAMA*. 1963;186:835-838.
5. Hayashi TT. The effect of benemid on uric acid excretion in normal pregnancy and in pre-eclampsia. *Am J Obstet Gynecol*. 1957;73:17-22.
6. Czaczkes WJ, Ullmann TD, Sadowsky E. Plasma uric acid levels, uric acid excretion, and response to probenecid in toxemia of pregnancy. *J Lab Clin Med*. 1958;51:224-229.
7. Harris RE, Gilstrap LC III, Pretty A. Single-dose antimicrobial therapy for asymptomatic bacteriuria during pregnancy. *Obstet Gynecol*. 1982;59:546-549.
8. Cavenee MR, Farris JR, Spalding TR, Barnes DL, Castaneda YS, Wendel GD Jr. Treatment of gonorrhea in pregnancy. *Obstet Gynecol*. 1993;81:33-38.
9. Ilett KF, Hackett LP, Ingle B, Bretz PJ. Transfer of probenecid and cephalexin into breast milk. *Ann Pharmacother*. 2006;40:986-989.

PROCAINAMIDE

Cardiovascular (Antiarrhythmic)

PREGNANCY RECOMMENDATION: Limited Human Data—No Relevant Animal Data

BREASTFEEDING RECOMMENDATION: Potential Toxicity

PREGNANCY SUMMARY

Several case reports describing the use of procainamide during human pregnancy were found. Most of the pregnant patients were treated for ventricular arrhythmias or fetal arrhythmias. First-trimester exposure cases were not located. Though numbers are small, the limited human pregnancy data did not show any adverse maternal or fetal effects. The drug crosses the placenta with cord blood levels about equal to maternal serum concentrations. Therefore, some fetal exposure will occur. However, this limited human pregnancy experience prevents a complete assessment of the embryofetal risk. Animal reproduction studies have not been located. Using this drug during pregnancy should be based on the pros and cons of the mother's clinical need for treatment versus any potential fetal risk that might occur from exposure. The drug carries a boxed warning for the development of a positive anti-nuclear antibody (ANA) test, with or without symptoms of a lupus-like syndrome with prolonged administration. If a positive ANA titer develops, the benefits versus risks of continued procainamide therapy should be discussed. The drug can also prolong the QT interval.

BREASTFEEDING SUMMARY

One case report was located that described the use of procainamide during human lactation. The drug and its active metabolite, *N*-acetyl-procainamide, were found to have breast milk concentrations that were higher than maternal serum levels. The maternal procainamide dose was 500 mg, 4 times daily. Mean serum procainamide and *N*-acetyl-procainamide concentrations were 1.1 and 1.6 mcg/mL, respectively, while mean breast milk levels were 5.4 and 3.5 mcg/mL, respectively. The mean breast milk to maternal serum ratios for the drug and its metabolite were about 4.3 (range 1.0-7.3) and 3.8 (range 1.0-6.2), respectively. The calculated RID was less than 3%. However, due to a concern for potential serious adverse effects that might be seen in a breastfed infant, the manufacturer recommends that women not breastfeed while being treated with this drug. Nevertheless, breastfeeding while using this drug should be based on the mother's clinical need for treatment versus any potential infant risks that might occur. If used, the infant should be monitored for the most common reported adult side effects of pruritus, nausea, abdominal pain, and dizziness (all leading to irritability), flushing, rash, anorexia (monitor infant growth), lethargy, vomiting, diarrhea, and various laboratory abnormalities (see PI).

References

1. Prescribing Information. Procainamide hydrochloride. Nexus Pharmaceuticals LLC; 2024.
2. Allen NM, Page RL. Procainamide administration during pregnancy. *Clin Pharm*. 1993;12:58-60.
3. Rotmensch HH, Elkayam U, Frishman W. Antiarrhythmic drug therapy during pregnancy. *Ann Intern Med*. 1983;98:487-497.
4. Mendelson CL. Disorders of the heartbeat during pregnancy. *Am J Obstet Gynecol*. 1956;72:1268-1301.
5. Tamari I, Eldar M, Rabinowitz B, Neufeld HN. Medical treatment of cardiovascular disorders during pregnancy. *Am Heart J*. 1982;104:1357-1363.
6. Dumesic DA, Silverman NH, Tobias S, Golbus MS. Transplacental cardioversion of fetal supraventricular tachycardia with procainamide. *N Engl J Med*. 1982;307:1128-1131.
7. Weiner CP, Thompson MIB. Direct treatment of fetal supraventricular tachycardia after failed transplacental therapy. *Am J Obstet Gynecol*. 1988;158:570-573.
8. Little BB, Gilstrap LC III. Cardiovascular drugs during pregnancy. *Clin Obstet Gynecol*. 1989;32:13-20.
9. Kanzaki T, Murakami M, Kobayashi H, et al. Hemodynamic changes during cardioversion in utero: a case report of supraventricular tachycardia and atrial flutter. *Fetal Diagn Ther*. 1993;8:37-44.
10. Hallak M, Neerhof MG, Perry R, et al. Fetal supraventricular tachycardia and hydrops fetalis: combined intensive, direct, and transplacental therapy. *Obstet Gynecol*. 1991;78:523-525.
11. Pittard WB III, Glazier H. Procainamide excretion in human milk. *J Pediatr*. 1983;102:631-633.

PROCARBAZINE

Antineoplastic (Alkylating Agent)

PREGNANCY RECOMMENDATION: Limited Human Data—Animal Data Suggest Potential Risk

BREASTFEEDING RECOMMENDATION: Potential Toxicity

PREGNANCY SUMMARY

A few case reports were located that describe the use of procarbazine in human pregnancy. Several of these had major malformations, but the defects were all different. The drug and two active metabolites will probably cross the placenta, so some fetal exposure will likely occur. However, the limited human pregnancy experience prevents a complete assessment of the embryofetal risk. Embryofetal toxicity was observed in one animal species at doses of less than 10 times the MRHD. Using this drug during pregnancy should be based on the pros and cons of the mother's clinical need for treatment versus any potential fetal risk that might occur from exposure. There is a registry for women who are pregnant and have cancer. For more information, women and health care providers are encouraged to contact the Cancer and Pregnancy Registry at 1-877-635-4499.

P

BREASTFEEDING SUMMARY

No reports describing the use of procarbazine during human lactation have been located. The drug and two active metabolites will likely be excreted into breast milk, so some infant exposure will probably occur. However, due to the concern for tumorigenicity shown for procarbazine in animal studies, the manufacturer recommends that women not breastfeed while being treated with this drug. Nevertheless, breastfeeding while using this drug should be based on the mother's clinical need for treatment versus any potential infant risks that might occur. If used, the infant should be monitored for the most common reported adult side effects of nausea (leading to irritability), vomiting, and various laboratory abnormalities (see PI).

References

1. Prescribing Information. Matulane. Leadiant Biosciences; 2024.
2. Wells JH, Marshall JR, Carbone PP. Procarbazine therapy for Hodgkin's disease in early pregnancy. *JAMA*. 1968;205:935-937.
3. Garrett MJ. Teratogenic effects of combination chemotherapy. *Ann Intern Med*. 1974;80:667.
4. Mennuti MT, Shepard TH, Mellman WJ. Fetal renal malformation following treatment of Hodgkin's disease during pregnancy. *Obstet Gynecol*. 1975;46:194-196.
5. Thomas PRM, Peckham MJ. The investigation and management of Hodgkin's disease in the pregnant patient. *Cancer*. 1976;38:1443-1451.
6. Daly H, McCann SR, Hanratty TD, Temperley IJ. Successful pregnancy during combination chemotherapy for Hodgkin's disease. *Acta Haematol (Basel)*. 1980;64:154-156.
7. Daw EG. Procarbazine in pregnancy. *Lancet*. 1970;2:984.
8. Johnson IR, Filshie GM. Hodgkin's disease diagnosed in pregnancy: case report. *Br J Obstet Gynaecol*. 1977;84:791-792.
9. Jones RT, Weinerman ER. MOPP (nitrogen mustard, vincristine, procarbazine, and prednisone) given during pregnancy. *Obstet Gynecol*. 1979;54:477-478.
10. Dobbing J. Pregnancy and leukaemia. *Lancet*. 1977;1:1155.
11. Nicholson HO. Cytotoxic drugs in pregnancy: review of reported cases. *J Obstet Gynecol Br Commonw*. 1968;75:307-312.
12. Lee IP, Dixon RL. Mutagenicity, carcinogenicity and teratogenicity of procarbazine. *Mutat Res*. 1978;55:1-14.
13. Sherins RJ, DeVita VT Jr. Effect of drug treatment for lymphoma on male reproductive capacity: studies of men in remission after therapy. *Ann Intern Med*. 1973;79:216-220.
14. Sherins RJ, Olweny CLM, Ziegler JL. Gynecomastia and gonadal dysfunction in adolescent boys treated with combination chemotherapy for Hodgkin's disease. *N Engl J Med*. 1978;299:12-16.
15. Johnson SA, Goldman JM, Hawkins DF. Pregnancy after chemotherapy for Hodgkin's disease. *Lancet*. 1979;2:93.
16. Card RT, Holmes IH, Sugarman RG, et al. Successful pregnancy after high dose chemotherapy and marrow transplantation for treatment of aplastic anemia. *Exp Hematol*. 1980;8:57-60.
17. Schilsky RL, Sherins RJ, Hubbard SM, et al. Long-term follow-up of ovarian function in women treated with MOPP chemotherapy for Hodgkin's disease. *Am J Med*. 1981;71:552-556.
18. Shalet SM, Vaughan Williams CA, Whitehead E. Pregnancy after chemotherapy induced ovarian failure. *Br Med J*. 1985;290:898.

19. Whitehead E, Shalet SM, Blackledge G, et al. The effect of combination chemotherapy on ovarian function in women treated for Hodgkin's disease. *Cancer*. 1983;52:988-993.
20. Andrieu JM, Ochoa-Molina ME. Menstrual cycle, pregnancies and offspring before and after MOPP therapy for Hodgkin's disease. *Cancer*. 1983;52:435-438.
21. Schapira DV, Chudley AE. Successful pregnancy following continuous treatment with combination chemotherapy before conception and throughout pregnancy. *Cancer*. 1984;54:800-803.
22. Chow EJ, Stratton KL, Leisenring WM, et al. Pregnancy after chemotherapy in male and female survivors of childhood cancer treated between 1970 and 1999: a report from the Childhood Cancer Survivor Study cohort. *Lancet Oncol*. 2016;17:567-576.
23. Levine JM, Whitton JA, Ginsberg JP, et al. Non-surgical premature menopause and reproductive implications in survivors of childhood cancer: a report from the childhood cancer survivor study. *Cancer*. 2018;124:1044-1052.
24. Weibull CE, Johansson ALV, Eloranta S, et al. Contemporarily treated patients with Hodgkin lymphoma have childbearing potential in line with matched comparators. *J Clin Oncol*. 2018;36:2718-2725.

PROCHLORPERAZINE

Gastrointestinal/Mental Health (Phenothiazine—Antiemetic/Antipsychotic)

PREGNANCY RECOMMENDATION: Human Data Suggest Low Risk (First Trimester) Potential Risk (Third Trimester)

BREASTFEEDING RECOMMENDATION: Potential Toxicity

PREGNANCY SUMMARY

From the Collaborative Perinatal Project and the Michigan Medicaid Surveillance study, there were 58 (3.7%) major birth anomalies (63 expected) in 1,581 first-trimester exposures. No pattern to the defects was seen. The drug crosses the placenta, so some fetal exposure will occur. Animal reproduction studies have not been located. Prochlorperazine crosses the placenta. The manufacturer reports several instances of extrapyramidal symptoms and/or withdrawal symptoms seen in newborns that were exposed to the drug in late pregnancy or at delivery. Reported symptoms include agitation, hypotonia, hypertonia, tremor, somnolence, respiratory distress, and feeding disorders. Using this drug during pregnancy should be based on the pros and cons of the mother's clinical need for treatment versus any potential fetal risk that might occur from exposure. In the 2018 ACOG nausea and vomiting practice bulletin, prochlorperazine is a second-line option for use in pregnancy.

BREASTFEEDING SUMMARY

No reports describing the use of prochlorperazine during human lactation have been located. Because other phenothiazines are found in human breast milk, prochlorperazine should also be expected to be excreted into breast milk. The drug can increase prolactin levels, but this should not adversely affect breastfeeding. Breastfeeding while using this drug should be based on the mother's clinical need for treatment versus any potential infant risks that might occur. If used, the infant should be monitored for the most common reported adult side effects of dizziness and blurred vision (leading to irritability), sedation, rash, and hypotension.

References

1. Prescribing Information. Prochlorperazine (tablet). Ajanta Pharma USA Inc; 2024.
2. Prescribing Information. Prochlorperazine (injection). Amneal Pharmaceuticals LLC; 2023.
3. Prescribing Information. Prochlorperazine (suppository). Cosette Pharmaceuticals Inc; 2023.
4. National Library of Medicine. Prochlorperazine. In: *StatPearls* [Internet]. StatPearls Publishing. Accessed March 3, 2025. https://www.ncbi.nlm.nih.gov/books/NBK537083/
5. American College of Obstetricians and Gynecologists. Nausea and vomiting in pregnancy. ACOG practice bulletin No. 189. *Obstet Gynecol*. 2018;131:e15-e30.
6. Moya F, Thorndike V. Passage of drugs across the placenta. *Am J Obstet Gynecol*. 1962;84:1778-1798.
7. Reider RO, Rosenthal D, Wender P, Blumenthal H. The offspring of schizophrenics. Fetal and neonatal deaths. *Arch Gen Psychiatry*. 1975;32:200-211.
8. Milkovich L, Van den Berg BJ. An evaluation of the teratogenicity of certain antinauseant drugs. *Am J Obstet Gynecol*. 1976;125:244-248.
9. Slone D, Siskind V, Heinonen OP, et al. Antenatal exposure to the phenothiazines in relation to congenital malformations, perinatal mortality rate, birth weight, and intelligence quotient score. *Am J Obstet Gynecol*. 1977;128:486-488.
10. Platt JE, Friedhoff AJ, Broman SH, et al. Effects of prenatal exposure to neuroleptic drugs on children's growth. *Neuropsychopharmacology*. 1988;1:205-212.
11. Ho CK, Kaufman RL, McAlister WH. Congenital malformations. Cleft palate, congenital heart disease, absent tibiae, and polydactyly. *Am J Dis Child*. 1975;129:714-716.
12. Farag RA, Ananth J. Thanatophoric dwarfism associated with prochlorperazine administration. *NY State J Med*. 1978;78:279-282.
13. Freeman R. Limb deformities: possible association with drugs. *Med J Aust*. 1972;1:606-607.
14. Rafla N. Limb deformities associated with prochlorperazine. *Am J Obstet Gynecol*. 1987;156:1557.
15. Hall G. A case of phocomelia of the upper limbs. *Med J Aust*. 1983;1:449-450.
16. Mellin GW. Report of prochlorperazine during pregnancy from the fetal life study bank (abstract). *Teratology*. 1975;11:28A.
17. Reis M, Kallen B. Maternal use of antipsychotics in early pregnancy and delivery outcome. *J Clin Psychopharmacol*. 2008;28:279-288.
18. Molitch M. Medication-induced hyperprolactinemia. *Mayo Clin Proc*. 2005;80:1050-1057.

PROGUANIL/ATOVAQUONE

Anti-Infective (Antiprotozoal)

SEE ATOVAQUONE/PROGUANIL

PROMETHAZINE

Gastrointestinal/Antihistamine (Phenothiazine—Antiemetic)

PREGNANCY RECOMMENDATION: Human Data Suggest Low Risk (First Trimester)

BREASTFEEDING RECOMMENDATION: Probably Compatible (Short-Term Use)

PREGNANCY SUMMARY

Several reports describing the use of promethazine in human pregnancy have been located. From four large studies, including the Collaborative Perinatal Project, Michigan Medicaid Surveillance study, and the Group Health Cooperative of Puget Sound, there were 54 (3.5%) major birth anomalies (62 expected) in 1,539 first-trimester exposures. No pattern to the defects was seen. The drug crosses the placenta, so some fetal exposure will occur. Animal reproduction studies showed some embryofetal toxicity in one species at doses of less than 10 times the MRHD. A few reports describe some excess neonatal sedation with use near delivery, but these effects were short-term and not to the extent as seen with other phenothiazine drugs. Using this drug during pregnancy should be based on the pros and cons of the mother's clinical need for treatment versus any potential fetal risk that might occur from exposure. In the 2018 ACOG nausea and vomiting practice bulletin, promethazine is a second-line option for use in pregnancy.

BREASTFEEDING SUMMARY

No reports describing the use of promethazine during human lactation have been located. The drug will likely be excreted into breast milk, so some infant exposure will probably occur. However, due to a concern for potential serious adverse effects (primarily sedation) that might be seen in a breastfed infant, the manufacturer recommends that women not breastfeed while being treated with this drug. Nevertheless, breastfeeding while using this drug should be based on the mother's clinical need for treatment versus any potential infant risks that might occur. If used, the infant should be monitored for the most common reported adult side effects of nausea and dry mouth (leading to irritability), sedation, rash, vomiting, jaundice, nasal stuffiness, apnea, and various laboratory abnormalities (see PI). Though not described, the antihistamine effect could decrease prolactin levels.

P

References

1. Prescribing Information. Promethazine hydrochloride (tablet). Ameal Pharmaceuticals LLC; 2024.
2. Prescribing Information. Promethazine hydrochloride (suppository). Camber Pharmaceuticals Inc; 2022.
3. Prescribing Information. Promethazine hydrochloride (injection). Hikma Pharmaceuticals USA Inc; 2024.
4. American College of Obstetricians and Gynecologists. Nausea and vomiting in pregnancy. ACOG practice bulletin No. 189. *Obstet Gynecol*. 2018; 131:e15-e30.
5. Moya F, Thorndike V. The effects of drugs used in labor on the fetus and newborn. *Clin Pharmacol Ther*. 1963;4:628-653.
6. Heinonen OP, Slone D, Shapiro S. *Birth Defects and Drugs in Pregnancy*. Publishing Sciences Group; 1977.
7. Wheatley D. Drugs and the embryo. *Br Med J*. 1964;1:630.
8. Nelson MM, Forfar JO. Association between drugs administered during pregnancy and congenital abnormalities of the fetus. *Br Med J*. 1971;1:523-527.
9. Powe CE, Kiem IM, Fromhagen C, Cavanagh D. Propiomazine hydrochloride in obstetrical analgesia. *JAMA*. 1962;181:290-294.
10. Potts CR, Ullery JC. Maternal and fetal effects of obstetric analgesia. *Am J Obstet Gynecol*. 1961;81:1253-1259.
11. Carroll JJ, Moir RS. Use of promethazine (Phenergan) hydrochloride in obstetrics. *JAMA*. 1958;168:2218-2224.
12. Riffel HD, Nochimson DJ, Paul RH, Hon EH. Effects of meperidine and promethazine during labor. *Obstet Gynecol*. 1973;42:738-745.
13. Borgstedt AD, Rosen MG. Medication during labor correlated with behavior and EEG of the newborn. *Am J Dis Child*. 1968;115:21-24.
14. Zakut H, Mannor SM, Serr DM. Effect of promethazine on uterine contractions. *Harefuah* 1970;78:61-62. As cited in Anonymous. References and reviews. *JAMA*. 1970;211:1572.
15. Corby DG, Shulman I. The effects of antenatal drug administration on aggregation of platelets of newborn infants. *J Pediatr*. 1971;79:307-313.
16. Vella L, Francis D, Houlton P, Reynolds F. Comparison of the antiemetics metoclopramide and promethazine in labour. *Br Med J*. 1985;290:1173-1175.
17. Hall PF. Use of promethazine (Phenergan) in labour. *Can Med Assoc J*. 1987;136:690-691.
18. Montminy M, Teres D. Shock after phenothiazine administration in a pregnant patient with a pheochromocytoma: a case report and literature review. *J Reprod Med*. 1983;28:159-162.
19. Whaun JM, Smith GR, Sochor VA. Effect of prenatal drug administration on maternal and neonatal platelet aggregation and PF_4 release. *Haemostasis*. 1980;9:226-237.
20. Bierme S, Bierme R. Antihistamines in hydrops foetalis. *Lancet*. 1967;1:574.
21. Gusdon JP Jr. The treatment of erythroblastosis with promethazine hydrochloride. *J Reprod Med*. 1981;26:454-458.
22. Charles AG, Blumenthal LS. Promethazine hydrochloride therapy in severely Rh-sensitized pregnancies. *Obstet Gynecol*. 1982;60:627-630.
23. Bowman JM. Antenatal suppression of Rh alloimmunization. *Clin Obstet Gynecol*. 1991;34:296-303.
24. Dyson JL, Kohler HC. Anencephaly and ovulation stimulation. *Lancet*. 1973;1:1256-1257.
25. Aselton P, Jick H, Milunsky A, et al. First-trimester drug use and congenital disorders. *Obstet Gynecol*. 1985;65:451-455.

PROPAFENONE

Cardiovascular (Class 1C Antiarrhythmic)

PREGNANCY RECOMMENDATION: Limited Human Data—Animal Data Suggest Potential Risk

BREASTFEEDING RECOMMENDATION: Potential Toxicity

PREGNANCY SUMMARY

A few reports were located that describe the use of propafenone in human pregnancy. In all of the cases, the drug was started in the second or third trimester. No adverse effects were observed in the mother or fetus/newborn related to the drug. Propafenone and the active metabolite, 5-OH-propafenone, were both shown to cross the placenta, so fetal exposure will occur. However, the limited human pregnancy experience prevents a complete assessment of embryofetal risk. Embryofetal toxicity was observed in two animal species at doses of about equal to or less than 10 times the MRHD. Maternal toxicity also occurred in one of these species. Using this drug during pregnancy should be based on the pros and cons of the mother's clinical need for treatment versus any potential fetal risk that might occur from exposure. Propafenone can prolong the QT interval. The incidence of ventricular tachycardia is increased and may be more symptomatic during pregnancy. Ventricular arrhythmias most often occur in pregnant patients with underlying cardiomyopathy, congenital heart disease, valvular heart disease, or mitral valve prolapse. Breakthrough arrhythmias may also occur during pregnancy, as therapeutic treatment levels may be difficult to maintain due to the increased volume of distribution and increased drug metabolism inherent in the pregnant state.

BREASTFEEDING SUMMARY

Propafenone and 5-OH-propafenone are excreted into human breast milk. A woman took propafenone 300 mg, 3 times a day during the latter part of pregnancy and during breastfeeding. Three days postpartum, trough breast milk concentrations of propafenone and its active metabolite were 32 ng/mL and 47 ng/mL, respectively. The maternal plasma levels were 219 ng/mL and 86 ng/mL, respectively. The calculated RID was less than 1%. In a second patient, a single 150 mg oral dose of propafenone was administered. The drug was detected in breast milk and again the calculated RID was also less than 1%. Breastfeeding while using this drug should be based on the mother's clinical need for treatment versus any potential infant risks that might occur. If used, the infant should be monitored for the most common reported adult side effects of nausea, dizziness, and headache (all leading to irritability), vomiting, constipation, fatigue (lethargy), and ventricular conduction delay.

References

1. Prescribing Information. Propafenone HCl. Actavis Pharma Inc; 2019.
2. Libardoni M, Piovan D, Busato E, Padrini R. Transfer of propafenone and 5-OH-propafenone to foetal plasma and maternal milk. *Br J Clin Pharmacol.* 1991;32:527-528.
3. Brunozzi LT, Meniconi L, Chiocchi P, et al. Propafenone in the treatment of chronic ventricular arrhythmias in a pregnant patient. *Br J Clin Pharmacol.* 1988;26:489-490.
4. Santinelli V, De Paola M, Turco P, et al. Wolff-Parkinson-White at risk and propafenone. *J Am Coll Cardiol.* 1988;11:1138.
5. Gembruch U, Manz M, Bald R, et al. Repeated intravascular treatment with amiodarone in a fetus with refractory supraventricular tachycardia and hydrops fetalis. *Am Heart J.* 1989;118:1335-1338.
6. Capucci A, Boriani G. Propafenone in the treatment of cardiac arrhythmias. A risk-benefit appraisal. *Drug Saf.* 1995;12:55-72.
7. Wakaumi M, Tsuruoka S, Sakamoto K, et al. Pilsicainide in breast milk from a mother: comparison with disopyramide and propafenone. *Br J Clin Pharmacol.* 2005;59:120-122.

P

PROPARACAINE OPHTHALMIC

Ophthalmic (Topical—Anesthetic)

PREGNANCY RECOMMENDATION: No Human Data and No Relevant Animal Data

BREASTFEEDING RECOMMENDATION: Probably Compatible

PREGNANCY SUMMARY

No reports describing the use of proparacaine ophthalmic in human pregnancy have been located. If found in the maternal circulation, the drug will probably cross the placenta. However, with recommended use, the amount is likely to be clinically insignificant. However, the absence of human pregnancy experience prevents a complete assessment of the embryofetal risk. No animal reproduction studies have been located. Using this drug during pregnancy should be based on the pros and cons of the mother's clinical need for treatment versus any potential fetal risk that might occur from exposure. If used during pregnancy, consider placing pressure over the tear duct in the corner of the eye for at least 1 minute, and then remove any excess solution with absorbent tissue to decrease the amount of drug reaching the systemic circulation even further.

BREASTFEEDING SUMMARY

No reports describing the use of proparacaine ophthalmic during human lactation have been located. If found in the maternal circulation, the drug will probably be excreted into human breast milk. However, with recommended use, the amount is likely to be clinically insignificant. Breastfeeding while using this drug should be based on the mother's clinical need for treatment versus any potential infant risks that might occur. Due to the ophthalmic use, systemic side effects were not evaluated. A method to decrease some systemic absorption with ophthalmic use is described above in the Pregnancy Summary.

Reference

1. Prescribing Information. Proparacaine hydrochloride. Sandoz Inc; 2022.

PROPOFOL

Anesthetic (General)

PREGNANCY RECOMMENDATION: Limited Human Data—Animal Data Suggest Risk

BREASTFEEDING RECOMMENDATION: Probably Compatible

PREGNANCY SUMMARY

A few studies were located that describe the use of propofol in human pregnancy. All of the cases involved use at the time of delivery. Most of the studies analyzed neonatal neurobehavior and adaptation postdelivery, and no consistent adverse effects were identified. The drug was found to cross the placenta with cord blood levels about 70% of the maternal concentrations. However, the limited human pregnancy experience prevents a complete assessment of embryofetal risk. Embryofetal toxicity was observed in two animal species at doses of about equal to the RHD. Maternal toxicity occurred in one of these, as well as, a third species in which no embryofetal toxicity was seen. Using this drug during pregnancy should be based on the pros and cons of the mother's clinical need for treatment versus any potential fetal risk that might occur from exposure.

BREASTFEEDING SUMMARY

Propofol has been shown to be excreted into human breast milk, but at variable concentrations. No consistent adverse maternal or fetal/neonatal effects have been reported. Breast milk levels varied based on dosage and time from drug administration to breast milk sampling but ranged from about 48 ng/mL up to about 740 ng/mL. Using the peak values, the highest calculated RID would be about 5%. Breastfeeding while using this drug should be based on the mother's clinical need for treatment versus any potential infant risks that might occur. If used, the infant should be monitored for the most common reported adult side effects of pruritus (leading to irritability), bradycardia, tachycardia, hypotension, hypertension, apnea, and rash.

References

1. Prescribing Information. Propofol injectable emulsion. Dr. Reddy's Laboratories Inc; 2022.
2. Costantino P, Emanuelli M, Muratori F, Sebastiani M. Propofol versus thiopentone as induction agents in cesarean section. *Minerva Anestesiol*. 1990;56:865-870.
3. Food and Drug Administration. FDA drug safety communication: FDA review results in new warnings about using general anesthetics and sedation drugs in young children and pregnant women. Accessed March 3, 2025. https://www.fda.gov/drugs/drug-safety-and-availability/fda-drug-safety-communication-fda-review-results-new-warnings-about-using-general-anesthetics-and
4. Gin T, Gregory MA, Chan K, et al. Pharmacokinetics of propofol in women undergoing elective caesarean section. *Br J Anaesth*. 1990;64:148-153.
5. Dailland P, Lirzin JD, Cockshott ID, et al. Placental transfer and neonatal effects of propofol administered during cesarean section (abstract). *Anesthesiology.* 1987;67:A454.
6. Dailland P, Cockshott ID, Lirzin JD, et al. Intravenous propofol during cesarean section: placental transfer, concentrations in breast milk, and neonatal effects. A preliminary study. *Anesthesiology*. 1989;71:827-834.
7. Moore J, Bill KM, Flynn RJ, et al. A comparison between propofol and thiopentone as induction agents in obstetric anaesthesia. *Anaesthesia*. 1989;44:753-757.
8. Dailland P, Jacquinot P, Lirzin JD, et al. Neonatal effects of propofol administered to the mother in anesthesia in cesarean section. *Can Anesthesiol*. 1989;37:429-433.
9. Dailland P, Jacquinot P, Lirzin JD, et al. Comparative study of propofol with thiopental for general anesthesia in cesarean section. *Ann Fr Anesth Reanim*. 1989;8(suppl):R65.
10. Valtonen M, Kanto J, Rosenberg P. Comparison of propofol and thiopentone for induction of anaesthesia for elective caesarean section. *Anaesthesia*. 1989;44:758-762.
11. Gin T, Gregory MA. Propofol for caesarean section. *Anaesthesia*. 1990; 45:165.
12. Pagnoni B, Casalino S, Monzani R, et al. Placental transfer of propofol in elective cesarean section. *Minerva Anestesiol*. 1990;56:877-879.
13. Maglione F, Guarini MC, Montanari A, et al. Determination of propofol blood levels in mothers and newborns in anesthesia for cesarean section. *Minerva Anestesiol*. 1990;56:881-883.
14. Gin T, Gregory MA, Chan K, Oh TE. Maternal and fetal levels of propofol at caesarean section. *Anaesth Intensive Care*. 1990;18:180-184.
15. Gin T, Yau G, Chan K, et al. Disposition of propofol infusions for caesarean section. *Can J Anaesth*. 1991;38:31-36.
16. Celleno D, Capogna G, Tomassetti M, et al. Neurobehavioural effects of propofol on the neonate following elective caesarean section. *Br J Anaesth*. 1989;62:649-654.
17. Gin T, Yau G, Gregory MA. Propofol during cesarean section. *Anesthesiology*. 1990;73:789.
18. Gin T, Yau G, Chan K, et al. Recovery from propofol infusion anaesthesia for caesarean section. *Neurosci Lett (Suppl)*. 1990;37:S44.
19. Gregory MA, Gin T, Yau G, et al. Propofol infusion anaesthesia for caesarean section. *Can J Anaesth*. 1990;37:514-520.
20. Gin T, Gregory MA, Oh TE. The haemodynamic effects of propofol and thiopentone for induction of caesarean section. *Anaesth Intensive Care*. 1990;18:175-179.

21. Yau G, Gin T, Ewart MC, et al. Propofol for induction and maintenance of anaesthesia at caesarean section. *Anaesthesia*. 1991;46:20-23.
22. Costantino P, Emanuelli M, Muratori F, Sebastiani M. Propofol versus thiopentone as induction agents in cesarean section. *Minerva Anestesiol*. 1990;56:865-870.
23. Alberico FP. Propofol in anesthesia induction for cesarean section. *Minerva Anestesiol*. 1990;56:871.
24. Zhong L, Luo F, Zhao W, et al. Propofol exposure during late stages of pregnancy impairs learning and memory in rat offspring via the BDNF-TrkB signaling pathway. *J Cell Mol Med*. 2016;20:1920-1931.

PROPRANOLOL

Antihypertensive (Nonselective β-Blocker)

PREGNANCY RECOMMENDATION: Human Data Suggest Potential Risk (Second and Third Trimesters)

BREASTFEEDING RECOMMENDATION: Potential Toxicity

PREGNANCY SUMMARY

Numerous reports have been located that describe the use of propranolol during human pregnancy. From the Michigan Medicaid Surveillance study, 11 (4%) major birth anomalies (11 expected) were identified in 274 first-trimester exposures. No pattern to the defects was seen. Some β-blockers, including propranolol, may cause IUGR and reduced placental weight. However, IUGR and reduced placental weight are commonly seen in pregnancies complicated by hypertension. Although IUGR is a serious concern, the benefits of maternal therapy with β-blockers, in some cases, might outweigh the risks to the fetus and must be judged on a case-by-case basis. The drug crosses the placenta, so some fetal exposure will occur. Nevertheless, this limited first-trimester human pregnancy experience prevents a complete assessment of the embryofetal risk. Embryofetal toxicity was observed in one animal species at doses of about equal to the MRHD, but embryofetal toxicity was not seen in a second species at doses of less than 10 times the MRHD. Use of β-blocking agents near delivery can result in persistent β-blockade in the newborn producing hypotension and decreased heart rate. Thus, newborns exposed to propranolol in utero should be closely observed during the first 24 to 48 hours after birth. Using this drug during pregnancy should be based on the pros and cons of the mother's clinical need for treatment versus any potential fetal risk that might occur from exposure. ACOG states that uncontrolled chronic hypertension has maternal risks of preeclampsia, placental abruption, postpartum hemorrhage, cerebrovascular accidents, pulmonary edema, renal insufficiency, myocardial infarction, and mortality and fetal risks of stillbirth or perinatal death, growth restriction, and preterm birth. Labetalol and nifedipine are considered first-line medications in treating hypertension in pregnancy. Propranolol is not a preferred agent in pregnancy.

BREASTFEEDING SUMMARY

Propranolol has been shown to be excreted into human breast milk. Peak breast milk concentrations ranged from 4 to 64 ng/mL at about 2 to 3 hours after a dose. Calculated RIDs were less than 1%. Although adverse effects, such as respiratory depression, bradycardia, and hypoglycemia, have not been reported in nursing infants exposed to propranolol, close observation for symptoms of β-blockade should occur. Breastfeeding while using this drug should be based on the mother's clinical need for treatment versus any potential infant risks that might occur. If used, the infant should be monitored for the most common reported adult side effects of dizziness, blurred vision, and abdominal pain (all leading to irritability), fatigue (lethargy), decreased heart rate, hypoglycemia, diarrhea, vomiting, constipation, rash, and decreased appetite (monitor infant growth). ACOG states that labetalol and propranolol are preferred agents in lactation due to higher protein binding.

References

1. Prescribing Information. Propranolol hydrochloride (tablet). Amneal Pharmaceuticals NY LLC; 2023.
2. Prescribing Information. Propranolol hydrochloride (injection). Hikma Pharmaceuticals USA Inc; 2022.
3. American College of Obstetricians and Gynecologists. Chronic hypertension in pregnancy. Practice bulletin No. 203. *Obstet Gynecol*. 2019;133:e26-e50.
4. American College of Obstetricians and Gynecologists. Gestational hypertension and preeclampsia. Practice bulletin No. 202. *Obstet Gynecol*. 2019; 133:e1-25.
5. Langer A, Hung CT, McA'Nulty JA, et al. Adrenergic blockade: a new approach to hyperthyroidism during pregnancy. *Obstet Gynecol*. 1974;44:181-186.
6. Habib A, McCarthy JS. Effects on the neonate of propranolol administered during pregnancy. *J Pediatr*. 1977;91:808-811.
7. Levitan AA, Manion JC. Propranolol therapy during pregnancy and lactation. *Am J Cardiol*. 1973;32:247.
8. Cottrill CM, McAllister RG Jr, et al. Propranolol therapy during pregnancy, labor, and delivery: evidence for transplacental drug transfer and impaired neonatal drug disposition. *J Pediatr*. 1977;91:812-814.
9. Teuscher A, Boss E, Imhof P, Erb E, Stocker FP, Weber JW. Effect of propranolol on fetal tachycardia in diabetic pregnancy. *Am J Cardiol*. 1978;42:304-307.
10. Taylor EA, Turner P. Anti-hypertensive therapy with propranolol during pregnancy and lactation. *Postgrad Med J*. 1981;57:427-430.
11. Smith MT, Livingstone I, Eadie MJ, et al. Metabolism of propranolol in the human maternal-placental-foetal unit. *Eur J Clin Pharmacol*. 1983;24:727-732.
12. Erkkola R, Lammintausta R, Liukko P, Anttila M. Transfer of propranolol and sotalol across the human placenta. *Acta Obstet Gynecol Scand*. 1982; 61:31-34.
13. Datta S, Kitzmiller JL, Ostheimer GW, Schoenbaum SC. Propranolol and parturition. *Obstet Gynecol*. 1978;51:577-581.
14. Mitrani A, Oettinger M, Abinader EG, et al. Use of propranolol in dysfunctional labour. *Br J Obstet Gynaecol*. 1975;82:651-655.
15. Amy JJ, Karim SMM. Intrauterine administration of L-noradrenaline and propranolol during the second trimester of pregnancy. *J Obstet Gynaecol Br Commonw*. 1974;81:75-83.
16. Barden TP, Stander RW. Myometrial and cardiovascular effects of an adrenergic blocking drug in human pregnancy. *Am J Obstet Gynecol*. 1968; 101:91-99.
17. Wansbrough H, Nakanishi H, Wood C. The effect of adrenergic receptor blocking drugs on the human fetus. *J Obstet Gynaecol Br Commonw*. 1968;75:189-198.
18. Fylling P. Dexamethasone or propranolol blockade of induced increase in plasma progesterone in early human pregnancy. *Acta Endocrinol (Copenh)*. 1973;72:569-572.

19. Smith MT, Livingstone I, Eadie MJ, et al. Chronic propranolol administration during pregnancy: maternal pharmacokinetics. *Eur J Clin Pharmacol*. 1983;25:481-490.
20. Jackson GL. Treatment of hyperthyroidism in pregnancy. *Pa Med*. 1973; 76:56-57.
21. Bullock JL, Harris RE, Young R. Treatment of thyrotoxicosis during pregnancy with propranolol. *Am J Obstet Gynecol*. 1975;121:242-245.
22. Lightner ES, Allen HD, Loughlin G. Neonatal hyperthyroidism and heart failure: a different approach. *Am J Dis Child*. 1977;131:68-70.
23. Pruyn SC, Phelan JP, Buchanan GC. Long-term propranolol therapy in pregnancy: maternal and fetal outcome. *Am J Obstet Gynecol*. 1979;135:485-489.
24. Turner GM, Oakley CM, Dixon HG. Management of pregnancy complicated by hypertrophic obstructive cardiomyopathy. *Br Med J*. 1968;4:281-284.
25. Schroeder JS, Harrison DC. Repeated cardioversion during pregnancy. *Am J Cardiol*. 1971;27:445-446.
26. Reed RL, Cheney CB, Fearon RE, Hook R, Hehre FW. Propranolol therapy throughout pregnancy: a case report. *Anesth Analg (Cleve)*. 1974;53:214-218.
27. Fiddler GI. Propranolol and pregnancy. *Lancet*. 1974;2:722-723.
28. Bauer JH, Pape B, Zajicek J, Groshong T. Propranolol in human plasma and breast milk. *Am J Cardiol*. 1979;43:860-862.
29. Gladstone GR, Hordof A, Gersony WM. Propranolol administration during pregnancy: effects on the fetus. *J Pediatr*. 1975;86:962-964.
30. Tcherdakoff PH, Colliard M, Berrard E, et al. Propranolol in hypertension during pregnancy. *Br Med J*. 1978;2:670.
31. Eliahou HE, Silverberg DS, Reisin E, Romen I, Mashiach S, Serr DM. Propranolol for the treatment of hypertension in pregnancy. *Br J Obstet Gynaecol*. 1978;85:431-436.
32. Bott-Kanner G, Schweitzer A, Schoenfeld A, Joel-Cohen J, Rosenfeld JB. Treatment with propranolol and hydralazine throughout pregnancy in a hypertensive patient: a case report. *Isr J Med Sci*. 1978;14:466-468.
33. Bott-Kanner G, Reisner SH, Rosenfeld JB. Propranolol and hydralazine in the management of essential hypertension in pregnancy. *Br Obstet Gynaecol*. 1980;87:110-114.
34. O'Connor PC, Jick H, Hunter JR, Stergachis A, Madsen S. Propranolol and pregnancy outcome. *Lancet*. 1981;2:1168.
35. Caldroney RD. Beta-blockers in pregnancy. *N Engl J Med*. 1982;306:810.
36. Goodlin RC. Beta blocker in pregnancy-induced hypertension. *Am J Obstet Gynecol*. 1982;143:237.
37. Livingstone I, Craswell PW, Bevan EB, et al. Propranolol in pregnancy: three year prospective study. *Clin Exp Hypertens (B)*. 1983;2:341-350.
38. Duminy PC, Burger PD. Fetal abnormality associated with the use of captopril during pregnancy. *S Afr Med J*. 1981;60:805.
39. Tunstall ME. The effect of propranolol on the onset of breathing at birth. *Br J Anaesth*. 1969;41:792.
40. Lieberman BA, Stirrat GM, Cohen SL, et al. The possible adverse effect of propranolol on the fetus in pregnancies complicated by severe hypertension. *Br J Obstet Gynaecol*. 1978;85:678-683.
41. Rubin PC. Beta-blockers in pregnancy. *N Engl J Med*. 1981;305:1323-1326.
42. Redmond GP. Propranolol and fetal growth restriction. *Semin Perinatol*. 1982;6:142-147.
43. Jensen OH. Fetal heart rate response to a controlled sound stimulus after propranolol administration to the mother. *Acta Obstet Gynecol Scand*. 1984;63:199-202.
44. Margulis E, Binder D, Cohen AW. The effect of propranolol on the nonstress test. *Am J Obstet Gynecol*. 1984;148:340-341.
45. Karlberg B, Lundberg O, Aberg H. Excretion of propranolol in human breast milk. *Acta Pharmacol Toxicol (Copenh)*. 1974;34:222-224.

PROPYLTHIOURACIL

Endocrine/Metabolic (Antithyroid)

PREGNANCY RECOMMENDATION: Limited Human Data (Maternal Benefit Outweighs Any Embryofetal Risk)

BREASTFEEDING RECOMMENDATION: Probably Compatible

P

PREGNANCY SUMMARY

Numerous reports have been located that describe the use of propylthiouracil (PTU) in human pregnancy. In combined data from the Collaborative Perinatal Project, Michigan Medicaid Surveillance study, the Swedish nationwide register, and other studies, the rate of major birth anomalies was about 3.4% in more than 350 first-trimester exposures. The drug crosses the placenta with fetal concentrations about double maternal levels, so some fetal exposure will occur. No animal reproduction studies have been conducted. PTU is routinely used in pregnancy for the treatment of hyperthyroidism. The maternal benefit will usually outweigh the potential embryofetal risk. Nevertheless, there are cases of liver injury, including liver failure and death, in women treated with PTU during pregnancy. The drug carries a boxed warning for these risks. Because PTU may be safer for use in early pregnancy, the manufacturer, ACOG, and the American Thyroid Association recommend that if antithyroid medications are needed in pregnancy, PTU is the drug of choice in the first trimester, then switch patients to methimazole to decrease the risk for maternal liver injury.

BREASTFEEDING SUMMARY

PTU has been shown to be excreted into human breast milk. The manufacturer reported nine women who received 400 mg PTU. The breast milk concentration at 90 minutes was 0.7 mcg/mL. The calculated RID was about 1.8%. Breastfeeding while using this drug should be based on the mother's clinical need for treatment versus any potential infant risks that might occur. If used, the infant should be monitored for the most common reported adult side effects of dizziness, itching, arthralgia, nausea, abdominal pain, and headache (all leading to irritability), drowsiness, and rash.

References

1. Product Information. Propylthiouracil. Chartwell Rx LLC; 2023.
2. National Library of Medicine. Propylthiouracil. PubChem. Accessed March 3, 2025. https://pubchem.ncbi.nlm.nih.gov/compound/Propylthiouracil
3. Alexander EK, Pearce EN, Brent GA, et al. 2017 guidelines of the American Thyroid Association for the diagnosis and management of thyroid disease during pregnancy and the postpartum. *Thyroid*. 2017;27: 315-389.
4. Astwood EB, VanderLaan WP. Treatment of hyperthyroidism with propylthiouracil. *Ann Intern Med*. 1946;25:813-821.
5. Bain L. Propylthiouracil in pregnancy: report of a case. *South Med J*. 1947; 40:1020-1021.
6. Lahey FH, Bartels EC. The use of thiouracil, thiobarbital and propylthiouracil in patients with hyperthyroidism. *Ann Surg*. 1947;125:572-581.

7. Reveno WS. Propylthiouracil in the treatment of toxic goiter. *J Clin Endocrinol Metab*. 1948;8:866-874.
8. Eisenberg L. Thyrotoxicosis complicating pregnancy. *NY State J Med*. 1950; 50:1618-1619.
9. Astwood EB. The use of antithyroid drugs during pregnancy. *J Clin Endocrinol Metab*. 1951;11:1045-1056.
10. Aaron HH, Schneierson SJ, Siegel E. Goiter in newborn infant due to mother's ingestion of propylthiouracil. *JAMA*. 1955;159:848-850.
11. Waldinger C, Wermer OS, Sobel EH. Thyroid function in infant with congenital goiter resulting from exposure to propylthiouracil. *J Am Med Wom Assoc*. 1955;10:196-197.
12. Bongiovanni AM, Eberlein WR, Thomas PZ, Anderson WB. Sporadic goiter of the newborn. *J Clin Endocrinol Met*. 1956;16:146-152.
13. Krementz ET, Hooper RG, Kempson RL. The effect on the rabbit fetus of the maternal administration of propylthiouracil. *Surgery*. 1957:41:619-631.
14. Branch LK, Tuthill SW. Goiters in twins resulting from propylthiouracil given during pregnancy. *Ann Intern Med*. 1957;46:145-148.
15. Man EB, Shaver BA Jr, Cooke RE. Studies of children born to women with thyroid disease. *Am J Obstet Gynecol*. 1958;75:728-741.
16. Becker WF, Sudduth PG. Hyperthyroidism and pregnancy. *Ann Surg*. 1959; 149:867-874.
17. Greenman GW, Gabrielson MO, Howard-Flanders J, Wessel MA. Thyroid dysfunction in pregnancy. *N Engl J Med*. 1962;267:426-431.
18. Herbst AL, Selenkow HA. Combined antithyroid-thyroid therapy of hyperthyroidism in pregnancy. *Obstet Gynecol*. 1963;21:543-550.
19. Reveno WS, Rosenbaum H. Observations on the use of antithyroid drugs. *Ann Intern Med*. 1964;60:982-989.
20. Herbst AL, Selenkow HA. Hyperthyroidism during pregnancy. *N Engl J Med*. 1965;273:627-633.
21. Burrow GN. Neonatal goiter after maternal propylthiouracil therapy. *J Clin Endocrinol Metab*. 1965;25:403-408.
22. Burrow GN, Bartsocas C, Klatskin EH, Grunt JA. Children exposed in utero to propylthiouracil. *Am J Dis Child*. 1968;116:161-165.
23. Talbert LM, Thomas CG Jr, Holt WA, Rankin P. Hyperthyroidism during pregnancy. *Obstet Gynecol*. 1970;36:779-785.
24. Hollingsworth DR, Austin E. Thyroxine derivatives in amniotic fluid. *J Pediatr*. 1971;79:923-929.
25. Ayromlooi J. Congenital goiter due to maternal ingestion of iodides. *Obstet Gynecol*. 1972;39:818-822.
26. Worley RJ, Crosby WM. Hyperthyroidism during pregnancy. *Am J Obstet Gynecol*. 1974;119:150-155.
27. Refetoff S, Ochi Y, Selenkow HA, Rosenfield RL. Neonatal hypothyroidism and goiter in one infant of each of two sets of twins due to maternal therapy with antithyroid drugs. *J Pediatr*. 1974;85:240-244.
28. Mestman JH, Manning PR, Hodgman J. Hyperthyroidism and pregnancy. *Arch Intern Med*. 1974;134:434-439.
29. Goluboff LG, Sisson JC, Hamburger JI. Hyperthyroidism associated with pregnancy. *Obstet Gynecol*. 1974;44:107-116.
30. Mujtaba Q, Burrow GN. Treatment of hyperthyroidism in pregnancy with propylthiouracil and methimazole. *Obstet Gynecol*. 1975;46:282-286.
31. Serup J, Petersen S. Hyperthyroidism during pregnancy treated with propylthiouracil. *Acta Obstet Gynecol Scand*. 1977;56:463-466.
32. Petersen S, Serup J. Case report: neonatal thyrotoxicosis. *Acta Paediatr Scand*. 1977;66:639-642.
33. Serup J. Maternal propylthiouracil to manage fetal hyperthyroidism. *Lancet*. 1978;2:896.
34. Wallace EZ, Gandhi VS. Triiodothyronine thyrotoxicosis in pregnancy. *Am J Obstet Gynecol*. 1978;130:106-107.
35. Weiner S, Scharf JI, Bolognese RJ, Librizzi RJ. Antenatal diagnosis and treatment of a fetal goiter. *J Reprod Med*. 1980;24:39-42.
36. Sugrue D, Drury MI. Hyperthyroidism complicating pregnancy: results of treatment by antithyroid drugs in 77 pregnancies. *Br J Obstet Gynaecol*. 1980;87:970-975.
37. Cheron RG, Kaplan MM, Larsen PR, et al. Neonatal thyroid function after propylthiouracil therapy for maternal Graves' disease. *N Engl J Med*. 1981; 304:525-528.
38. Check JH, Rezvani I, Goodner D, Hopper B. Prenatal treatment of thyrotoxicosis to prevent intrauterine growth retardation. *Obstet Gynecol*. 1982; 60:122-124.
39. Kock HCLV, Merkus JMWM. Graves' disease during pregnancy. *Eur J Obstet Gynecol Reprod Biol*. 1983;14:323-330.
40. Hollingsworth DR, Austin E. Observations following I^{131} for Graves disease during first trimester of pregnancy. *South Med J*. 1969;62:1555-1556.
41. Burrow GN. The management of thyrotoxicosis in pregnancy. *N Engl J Med*. 1985;313:562-565.
42. Momotani N, Noh J, Oyanagi H, et al. Antithyroid drug therapy for Graves' disease during pregnancy. Optimal regiment for fetal thyroid status. *N Engl J Med*. 1986;315:24-28.
43. Marchant B, Brownlie EW, Hart DM, et al. The placental transfer of propylthiouracil, methimazole and carbimazole. *J Clin Endocrinol Metab*. 1977;45:1187-1193.
44. Gardner DF, Cruikshank DP, Hays PM, Cooper DS. Pharmacology of propylthiouracil (PTU) in pregnant hyperthyroid women: correlation of maternal PTU concentrations with cord serum thyroid function tests. *J Clin Endocrinol Metab*. 1986;62:217-220.
45. Ramsay I, Kaur S, Krassas G. Thyrotoxicosis in pregnancy: results of treatment by antithyroid drugs combined with T4. *Clin Endocrinol (Oxf)*. 1983;18:73-85.
46. Burr WA. Thyroid disease. *Clin Obstet Gynecol*. 1981;8:341-351.
47. Burrow GN. Hyperthyroidism during pregnancy. *N Engl J Med*. 1978;298: 150-153.
48. Burrow GN. Maternal-fetal considerations in hyperthyroidism. *Clin Endocrinol Metab*. 1978;7:115-125.
49. Burrow GN, Klatskin EH, Genel M. Intellectual development in children whose mothers received propylthiouracil during pregnancy. *Yale J Biol Med*. 1978;51:151-156.
50. Momotani N, Ito K, Hamada N, et al. Maternal hyperthyroidism and congenital malformations in the offspring. *Clin Endocrinol (Oxf)*. 1984;20:695-700.
51. Heinonen OP, Slone D, Shapiro S. *Birth Defects and Drugs in Pregnancy*. Publishing Sciences Group; 1977:388-400.
52. Wing D, Millar L, Koonings P, et al. A comparison of PTU versus Tapazole in the treatment of hyperthyroidism (abstract). *Am J Obstet Gynecol*. 1992;166:308.
53. Wing DA, Millar LK, Koonings PP, Montoro MN, Mestman JH. A comparison of propylthiouracil versus methimazole in the treatment of hyperthyroidism in pregnancy. *Am J Obstet Gynecol*. 1994;170:90-95.
54. Diav-Citrin O, Ornoy A. Teratogen update: antithyroid drugs—methimazole, carbimazole, and propylthiouracil. *Teratology*. 2002;65:38-44.
55. Anonymous. Transplacental passage of thyroid hormones. *N Engl J Med*. 1967;277:486-487.
56. Low LCK, Lang J, Alexander WD. Excretion of carbimazole and propylthiouracil in breast milk. *Lancet*. 1979;2:1011.
57. Bartnik CM, Maheshwari RN, Subramanian RM. Beating the odds: a full-term delivery after liver transplantation of a pregnant hyperthyroid patient at 19 weeks' gestation for propylthiouracil-induced acute liver failure. *Transplant Proc*. 2018;50:3995-3999.
58. Andersen SL, Lonn S, Vestergaard P, et al. Birth defects after use of antithyroid drugs in early pregnancy: a Swedish nationwide study. *Eur J Endocrinol*. 2017;177:369-378.
59. Kampmann JP, Johansen K, Hansen JM, Helweg J. Propylthiouracil in human milk. *Lancet*. 1980;1:736-738.
60. Lee A, Moretti ME, Collantes A, et al. Choice of breastfeeding and physicians' advice: a cohort study of women receiving propylthiouracil. *Pediatrics*. 2000;106:27-30.

P

PROTAMINE

Antidote/Hematologic (Antiheparin)

PREGNANCY RECOMMENDATION: No Human Data and No Relevant Animal Data (Maternal Benefit Will Probably Outweigh Any Embryofetal Risk)

BREASTFEEDING RECOMMENDATION: Probably Compatible

PREGNANCY SUMMARY

No reports describing the use of protamine in human pregnancy have been located. The drug will not likely cross the placenta in clinically significant amounts. However, the absence of human pregnancy experience prevents a complete assessment of the embryofetal risk. No animal reproduction studies have been conducted. Using this drug during pregnancy should be based on the pros and cons of the mother's clinical need for treatment versus any potential fetal risk that might occur from exposure. Nevertheless, since this medication would be used to reverse heparin toxicity, maternal benefit would likely outweigh any potential fetal risk.

BREASTFEEDING SUMMARY

No reports describing the use of protamine during human lactation have been located. Such reports are unlikely due to its approved indication. The drug is not likely to be found in human breast milk in clinically significant amounts. However, if protamine were to be excreted into breast milk and ingested through breastfeeding, because it is a protein, it would probably be digested in the infant's gastrointestinal tract and not absorbed. If the clinical decision is to use this drug while breastfeeding, the infant should be monitored for the most common reported adult side effects of nausea (leading to irritability), hypotension, bradycardia, flushing, dyspnea, and vomiting.

References

1. Product Information. Protamine sulfate. Fresenius Kabi USA LLC; 2024.
2. Haddadin AS, Faraday N. Hemostasis, coagulopathy, and tamponade. Accessed March 3, 2025. https://www.sciencedirect.com/topics/medicine-and-dentistry/protamine#:~:text=Protamine%20is%20polypeptide%20composed%20primarily,and%20is%20highly%20positively%20charged

PROTRIPTYLINE

Mental Health (Tricyclic Antidepressant)

PREGNANCY RECOMMENDATION: No Human Data and No Relevant Animal Data

BREASTFEEDING RECOMMENDATION: Potential Toxicity

PREGNANCY SUMMARY

No reports describing the use of protriptyline in human pregnancy have been located. The drug will probably cross the placenta, so some fetal exposure will likely occur. Therefore, the absence of human pregnancy experience prevents a complete assessment of the embryofetal risk. No animal reproduction studies have been conducted. Using this drug during pregnancy should be based on the pros and cons of the mother's clinical need for treatment versus any potential fetal risk that might occur from exposure. Other agents in this class have been associated with poor neonatal adaptation syndrome when used near delivery (see Amitriptyline). There is a pregnancy exposure registry that monitors pregnancy outcomes in women using antidepressant drugs. Health care providers are encouraged to call the National Pregnancy Registry for Antidepressants at 1-844-405-6185.

P

BREASTFEEDING SUMMARY

No reports describing the use of protriptyline during human lactation have been located. The drug will likely be excreted into human breast milk, so some infant exposure will probably occur. Breastfeeding while using this drug should be based on the mother's clinical need for treatment versus any potential infant risks that might occur. If used, the infant should be monitored for the most common reported adult side effects of irritability, tachycardia, and hypotension.

References

1. Prescribing Information. Protriptyline hydrochloride. Epic Pharma LLC; 2023.
2. American College of Obstetricians and Gynecologists. Treatment and management of mental health conditions during pregnancy and postpartum. Clinical practice guideline No. 5. *Obstet Gynecol.* 2023;141:1262-1288.

PRUCALOPRIDE

Gastrointestinal (Laxative)

PREGNANCY RECOMMENDATION: No Human Data—Animal Data Suggest Low Risk

BREASTFEEDING RECOMMENDATION: Probably Compatible

PREGNANCY SUMMARY

No reports describing the use of prucalopride in human pregnancy have been located. The drug will probably cross the placenta, so some fetal exposure will likely occur. Therefore, the absence of human pregnancy experience prevents a complete assessment of the embryofetal risk. Animal data did not show any embryofetal toxicity. Constipation is common during pregnancy, but other treatment options with greater experience may be available.

BREASTFEEDING SUMMARY

The manufacturer reports an open-label study of eight healthy lactating women who provided breast milk samples during the weaning stage. The breast milk to plasma ratio was 2.65:1, and the average amount passed to the infant was estimated to be about 1.74 mcg/kg/d (which is about 6% the maternal dose). If the clinical decision is to use this drug while breastfeeding, the infant should be monitored for the most common reported adult side effects of headache, abdominal pain, and nausea (all leading to irritability), diarrhea, vomiting, and lethargy.

Reference

1. Prescribing Information. Motegrity. Shire US, Inc; 2018.

PSEUDOEPHEDRINE

Respiratory (α-/β-Agonist—Decongestant—Sympathomimetic)

PREGNANCY RECOMMENDATION: *Human Data Suggest Low Risk

BREASTFEEDING RECOMMENDATION: Probably Compatible

PREGNANCY SUMMARY

Numerous reports were located that describe the use of pseudoephedrine in human pregnancy. From the Michigan Medicaid Surveillance study, the Group Health Cooperative of Puget Sound, the Slone Epidemiology Center Birth Defects study and the Collaborative Perinatal Project, a total of 101 (2.7%) major birth anomalies were described in 3,792 pregnancies with first-trimester exposure. No pattern to the defects was identified. *However, from two other large studies that analyzed drug exposure in pregnancies that delivered infants with gastroschisis, the use of pseudoephedrine in the first trimester was increased when compared with infants that had other birth anomalies. Confirmation of these findings is needed. The drug will probably cross the placenta, so some fetal exposure will likely occur. No animal reproduction studies have been conducted. Using this drug during pregnancy should be based on the pros and cons of the mother's clinical need for treatment versus any potential fetal risk that might occur from exposure. Hypertension was reported in patients treated with this drug. Elevated glucose levels have also been reported in patients treated with this drug. Therefore, if used during pregnancy, glucose levels and blood pressure should be monitored.

BREASTFEEDING SUMMARY

Pseudoephedrine has been shown to be excreted into human breast milk. A total of 11 lactating women have been evaluated. Pseudoephedrine milk levels were found to be higher in breast milk than the maternal serum concentrations, with a breast milk to maternal serum ratio that ranges from 2.6 to 3.9 times higher. Calculated RIDs for these patients ranged from less than 1% up to 4.3%. Breastfeeding while using this drug should be based on the mother's clinical need for treatment versus any potential infant risks that might occur. If used, the infant should be monitored for the most common reported adult side effects of headache, dyspepsia, nausea, and dry mouth (all leading to irritability), hypertension, tachycardia, palpitations, urinary retention, and sleep disturbances.

References

1. Prescribing Information. Good neighbor pharmacy nasal decongestant. Amerisource Bergen; 2024.
2. National Library of Medicine. Pseudoephedrine. PubChem. Accessed March 3, 2025. https://pubchem.ncbi.nlm.nih.gov/compound/Pseudoephedrine
3. Heinonen OP, Slone D, Shapiro S. *Birth Defects and Drugs in Pregnancy*. Publishing Sciences Group; 1977.
4. Werler MM, Mitchell AA, Shapiro S. First trimester maternal medication use in relation to gastroschisis. *Teratology*. 1992;45:361-367.
5. Werler MM, Sheehan JE, Mitchell AA. Maternal medication use and risks of gastroschisis and small intestinal atresia. *Am J Epidemiol*. 2002;155:26-31.
6. Werler MM. Teratogen update: pseudoephedrine. *Birth Defects Res A Clin Mol Teratol*. 2005;73:328.
7. Kallen BAJ, Olausson PO. Use of oral decongestants during pregnancy and delivery outcome. *Am J Obstet Gynecol*. 2006;194:480-485.
8. Chasnoff IJ, Diggs G. Fetal alcohol effects and maternal cough syrup abuse. *Am J Dis Child*. 1981;135:968.
9. Hernandez RK, Mitchell AA, Werler MM. Decongestant use during pregnancy and its association with preterm delivery. *Birth Defects Res A Clin Mol Teratol*. 2010;88:715-721.
10. Yau WP, Mitchell AA, Lin KJ, et al. Use of decongestants during pregnancy and the risk of birth defects. *Am J Epidemiol*. 2013;178:198-208.
11. Findlay JWA, Butz RF, Sailstad JM, et al. Pseudoephedrine and triprolidine in plasma and breast milk of nursing mothers. *Br J Clin Pharmacol*. 1984;18:901-906.
12. Aljazaf K, Hale TW, Hett KF, et al. Pseudoephedrine: effects on milk production in women and estimation of infant exposure via breastmilk. *Br J Clin Pharmacol*. 2003;56:18-24.
13. Jick H, Holmes LB, Hunter JR, et al. First-trimester drug use and congenital disorders. *JAMA*. 1981;246:343-346.
14. Aselton P, Jick H, Milunsky A, et al. First-trimester drug use and congenital disorders. *Obstet Gynecol*. 1985;65:451-455.

P

PYRANTEL PAMOATE

Anti-Infective (Anthelmintic)

PREGNANCY RECOMMENDATION: No Human Data and No Relevant Animal Data (Maternal Benefit May Outweigh Embryofetal Risk)

BREASTFEEDING RECOMMENDATION: Probably Compatible

PREGNANCY SUMMARY

No reports describing the use of pyrantel pamoate in human pregnancy have been located. The drug will probably cross the placenta, so some fetal exposure will likely occur. Therefore, the absence of human pregnancy experience prevents a complete assessment of the embryofetal risk. No animal reproduction studies have been conducted. Using this drug during pregnancy should be based on the pros and cons of the mother's clinical need for treatment versus any potential fetal risk that might occur from exposure. In mass drug administration campaigns, the WHO states that the benefits of treatment in the second and third trimesters of pregnancy probably outweigh any potential fetal risks. In pregnant patients with a soil-transmitted helminth infection, it is recommended to balance the benefits of treatment with the risks of disease progression.

BREASTFEEDING SUMMARY

No reports describing the use of pyrantel pamoate during human lactation have been located. If found in the maternal circulation, the drug will likely be excreted into breast milk. However, with low oral absorption, the amount of exposure to the nursing infant is probably limited (but this needs further study). Breastfeeding while using this drug should be based on the mother's clinical need for treatment versus any potential infant risks that might occur. If used, the infant should be monitored for the most common reported adult side effects of abdominal pain, dizziness, and headache (all leading to irritability), vomiting, diarrhea, rash, decreased appetite (monitor infant growth), lethargy, and sedation. The WHO states that pyrantel pamoate is compatible with breastfeeding.

References

1. National Library of Medicine. Pyrantel pamoate. PubChem. Accessed March 3, 2025. https://pubchem.ncbi.nlm.nih.gov/compound/Pyrantel-Pamoate
2. Centers for Disease Control and Prevention. Parasites—enterobiasis (also known as pinworm infection). Accessed March 3, 2025. https://www.cdc.gov/pinworm/hcp/clinical-overview/index.html

PYRAZINAMIDE

Anti-Infective (Antituberculosis)

PREGNANCY RECOMMENDATION: Limited Human Data—No Relevant Animal Data

BREASTFEEDING RECOMMENDATION: Probably Compatible

PREGNANCY SUMMARY

A few case reports and small series were located that describe the use of pyrazinamide in human pregnancy. A total of about 13 cases were reported, with a few that had first-trimester exposure. No fetal malformations were identified in these cases, and overall, no adverse maternal or fetal effects were seen. The drug and its active metabolite will probably cross the placenta, so some fetal exposure will likely occur. Therefore, the absence of human pregnancy experience prevents a complete assessment of the embryofetal risk. No animal reproduction studies have been conducted. Using this drug during pregnancy should be based on the pros and cons of the mother's clinical need for treatment versus any potential fetal risk that might occur from exposure. Untreated tuberculosis has more risk to the pregnant woman and her fetus than the risk of medications. The CDC recommends starting treatment when there is a moderate to high probability of active tuberculosis; however, pyrazinamide is not listed as a recommended treatment due to unknown fetal effects. The American Thoracic Society/CDC/and Infectious Disease Society of America—Tuberculosis Guidelines recommend evaluating pyrazinamide use in pregnancy on a case-by-case basis.

BREASTFEEDING SUMMARY

Pyrazinamide has been shown to be excreted into human breast milk. A lactating woman was given an oral 1-g dose of pyrazinamide. The peak breast milk concentration was 1.5 mcg/mL, which occurred at 3 hours postadministration. The peak maternal plasma concentration was 42 mcg/mL, producing a breast milk to maternal plasma concentration of about 4%. The calculated RID was about 1.6%. Breastfeeding while using this drug should be based on the mother's clinical need for treatment versus any potential infant risks that might occur. If used, the infant should be monitored for the most common reported adult side effects of nausea and arthralgia (both leading to irritability), fever, loss of appetite (monitor infant growth), vomiting, rash, and thrombocytopenia.

References

1. Prescribing Information. Pyrazinamide. Marlex Pharmaceuticals Inc; 2024.
2. The Center for Disease Control and Prevention. Tuberculosis. Treatment for TB during pregnancy. Accessed January 1, 2026. https://www.cdc.gov/tb/hcp/clinical-care/pregnancy.html.
3. Nahid P, Dorman SE, Alipanah N, et al. Official American Thoracic Society/Centers for Disease Control and Prevention/Infectious Diseases Society of America Clinical Practice Guidelines: treatment of drug-susceptible tuberculosis. *Clin Inf Dis*. 2016;63:e147-e195.
4. Bothamley G, Elston W. Pregnancy does not mean that patients with tuberculosis must stop treatment. *BMJ*. 1991;318:1286.
5. Margono F, Mroueh J, Garely A, et al. Resurgence of active tuberculosis among pregnant women. *Obstet Gynecol*. 1994;83:911-914.
6. Hamadeh MA, Glassroth J. Tuberculosis and pregnancy. *Chest*. 1992;101:1114-1120.
7. Jana N, Vasishta K, Saha SC, Ghosh K. Obstetrical outcomes among women with extrapulmonary tuberculosis. *N Engl J Med*. 1999;341:645-649.
8. Klaus-Dieter KLL, Qarah S. Multidrug-resistant tuberculosis in pregnancy—case report and review of the literature. *Chest*. 2003;123:953-956.
9. Keskin N, Yilmaz S. Pregnancy and tuberculosis: to assess tuberculosis cases in pregnancy in a developing region retrospectively and two case reports. *Arch Gynecol Obstet*. 2008;278:451-455.
10. Holdiness MR. Antituberculosis drugs and breast-feeding. *Arch Intern Med*. 1984;144:1888.

PYRETHRINS WITH PIPERONYL BUTOXIDE

Anti-Infective (Topical—Antiparasitic/Pediculicide)

PREGNANCY RECOMMENDATION: No Human Data and No Relevant Animal Data

BREASTFEEDING RECOMMENDATION: Probably Compatible

PREGNANCY SUMMARY

No reports describing the use of pyrethrins with piperonyl butoxide in human pregnancy have been located. If found in the maternal circulation, both drugs will probably cross the placenta. However, systemic absorption with topical use is only about 2% from the skin and about 8% from the scalp. Therefore, the overall amount of fetal exposure is likely to be minimal. Nevertheless, the absence of human pregnancy experience prevents a complete assessment of the embryofetal risk. No animal reproduction studies have been conducted. Using this drug during pregnancy should be based on the pros and cons of the mother's clinical need for treatment versus any potential fetal risk that might occur from exposure. The CDC 2021 sexually transmitted infection guidelines state that pyrethrin with piperonyl butoxide cream and permethrin 1% are the recommended regimens for pubic lice during pregnancy.

BREASTFEEDING SUMMARY

No reports describing the use of pyrethrin and piperonyl butoxide during human lactation have been located. If found in the maternal circulation, both drugs will probably cross the placenta. However, systemic absorption with topical use is only about 2% from the skin and about 8% from the scalp. Therefore, the overall amount of the drug that may be found in human breast milk is likely to be minimal. Pyrethrin is absorbed orally, but piperonyl butoxide is poorly absorbed orally. However, overall exposure to a nursing infant for both drugs is likely to be negligible. Breastfeeding while using this drug should be based on the mother's clinical need for treatment versus any potential infant risks that might occur. Due to the topical use of the drug, systemic side effects were not evaluated.

References

1. Prescribing Information. Liceout. Bob Barker Company Inc; 2024.
2. Agency for Toxic Substances and Disease Registry. Public health statement for pyrethrins and pyrethroids. Accessed March 4, 2025. https://wwwn.cdc.gov/TSP/PHS/PHS.aspx?phsid=785&toxid=153
3. National Library of Medicine. Pyrethrum extract. PubChem. Accessed March 4, 2025. https://pubchem.ncbi.nlm.nih.gov/compound/pyrethrum%20extract
4. National Library of Medicine. Piperonyl butoxide. PubChem. Accessed March 4, 2025. https://pubchem.ncbi.nlm.nih.gov/compound/Piperonyl-Butoxide
5. Wester RC, Bucks DA, Maibach HI. Human in vivo percutaneous absorption of pyrethrin and piperonyl butoxide. *Food Chem Toxicol*. 1994;32:51-53.
6. Centers for Disease Control and Prevention. 2015 Guidelines for treatment of sexually transmitted diseases. *MMWR Recomm Rep*. 2021;70:1-187.

PYRIDOSTIGMINE

Central Nervous System (Cholinesterase Inhibitor)

PREGNANCY RECOMMENDATION: Limited Human Data—No Relevant Animal Data (Maternal Treatment May Outweigh Risks in Some Cases)

BREASTFEEDING RECOMMENDATION: Probably Compatible

PREGNANCY SUMMARY

Several case reports and small series have been located that describe the use of pyridostigmine in human pregnancy. No major birth anomalies were noted in more than 20 cases, except one. The drug will cross the placenta, so some fetal exposure will occur. However, this limited human pregnancy experience prevents a complete assessment of the embryofetal risk. No animal reproduction studies have been located. Oral pyridostigmine is the first-line treatment for myasthenia gravis during pregnancy. Fetal and neonatal myasthenia gravis have been reported and are caused by transplacental passage of antiacetylcholine receptor IgG antibodies. The inhibited fetal skeletal muscle movement and development can result in a lack of fetal breathing and swallowing, leading to pulmonary hypoplasia and polyhydramnios. Arthrogryposis multiplex can also occur. Additionally, patients are at an increased risk for exacerbations and preterm delivery. Using this drug during pregnancy should be based on the pros and cons of the mother's clinical need for treatment versus any potential fetal risk that might occur from exposure. Nevertheless, maternal treatment in some cases may outweigh any potential fetal risks because this can lower both maternal and fetal morbidity.

BREASTFEEDING SUMMARY

Pyridostigmine has been shown to be excreted into human breast milk in two lactating women. Breast milk concentrations were about 2 and 25 ng/mL with maternal doses of 120 to 300 mg/d. Breast milk to maternal serum levels ranged from 40% to 110%. Calculated RIDs were well below 1%. The infant's blood level in one case was undetectable (LLQ of 1 ng/mL). Breastfeeding while using this drug should be based on the mother's clinical need for treatment versus any potential infant risks that might occur. If used, the infant should be monitored for the most common reported adult side effects of nausea, abdominal cramps, and muscle cramps (all leading to irritability), vomiting, diarrhea, increased salivation, increased bronchial secretions, miosis, and weakness.

References

1. Prescribing Information. Pyridostigmine bromide (tablet). Amneal Pharmaceuticals of New York LLC; 2024.
2. Product Information. Pyridostigmine bromide (injection). Sandoz Inc; 2022.
3. Lefvert AK, Osterman PO. Newborn infants to myasthenic mothers: a clinical study and an investigation of acetylcholine receptor antibodies in 17 children. *Neurology*. 1983;33:133-138.
4. Plauche WC. Myasthenia gravis in pregnancy: an update. *Am J Obstet Gynecol*. 1979;135:691-697.
5. Braga AC, Pinto C, Santos E, Braga J. Myasthenia gravis in pregnancy: experience of a Portuguese center. *Muscle Nerve*. 2016;54:715-720.
6. Niesen CE, Shah NS. Pyridostigmine-induced microcephaly. *Neurology*. 2000;54:1873-1874.
7. Sharon I. Myasthenia gravis and pregnancy. Medscape. Updated May 8, 2024. Accessed March 4, 2025. https://emedicine.medscape.com/article/261815-overview?form=fpf
8. Foldes FF, McNall PG. Myasthenia gravis: a guide for anesthesiologists. *Anesthesiology*. 1962;23:837-872.
9. McNall PG, Jafarnia MR. Management of myasthenia gravis in the obstetric patient. *Am J Obstet Gynecol*. 1965;92:518-525.
10. Plauche WC. Myasthenia gravis in pregnancy. *Am J Obstet Gynecol*. 1964;88:404-409.
11. Chambers DC, Hall JE, Boyce J. Myasthenia gravis and pregnancy. *Obstet Gynecol*. 1967;29:597-603.
12. Hay DM. Myasthenia gravis and pregnancy. *J Obstet Gynaecol Br Commonw*. 1969;76:323-329.
13. Heinonen OP, Slone D, Shapiro S. *Birth Defects and Drugs in Pregnancy*. Publishing Sciences Group; 1977:345-356.
14. Blackhall MI, Buckley GA, Roberts DV, et al. Drug-induced neonatal myasthenia. *J Obstet Gynaecol Br Commonw*. 1969;76:157-162.
15. Rolbin SH, Levinson G, Shnider SM, Wright RG. Anesthetic considerations for myasthenia gravis and pregnancy. *Anesth Analg (Cleve)*. 1978;57:441-447.
16. Plauche WC. Myasthenia gravis in pregnancy: an update. *Am J Obstet Gynecol*. 1979;135:691-697.
17. Eden RD, Gall SA. Myasthenia gravis and pregnancy: a reappraisal of thymectomy. *Obstet Gynecol*. 1983;62:328-333.
18. Cohen BA, London RS, Goldstein PJ. Myasthenia gravis and preeclampsia. *Obstet Gynecol*. 1976;48(suppl):35S-37S.
19. Catanzarite VA, McHargue AM, Sandberg EC, Dyson DC. Respiratory arrest during therapy for premature labor in a patient with myasthenia gravis. *Obstet Gynecol*. 1984;64:819-822.
20. Hardell LI, Lindstrom B, Lonnerholm G, Osterman PO. Pyridostigmine in human breast milk. *Br J Clin Pharmacol*. 1982;14:565-567.
21. Carr SR, Gilchrist JM, Abuelo DN, Clark D. Treatment of antenatal myasthenia gravis. *Obstet Gynecol*. 1991;78:485-489.
22. Niesen CE, Shah NS. Pyridostigmine-induced microcephaly. *Neurology*. 2000;54:1873-1874.
23. Gilchrist JM. Muscle disease in the pregnant woman. *Adv Neurol*. 1994;64:193-208.

P

PYRILAMINE

Antihistamine (First Generation H_1-Antihistamine)

PREGNANCY RECOMMENDATION: Limited Human Data—No Relevant Animal Data

BREASTFEEDING RECOMMENDATION: Probably Compatible

PREGNANCY SUMMARY

One report was located that described the use of pyrilamine in human pregnancy. The Collaborative Perinatal Project described 5 (4.1%) major anomalies in 121 first-trimester exposures. No pattern to the defects was seen. The drug will probably cross the placenta, so some fetal exposure will likely occur. Therefore, this limited human pregnancy experience prevents a complete assessment of the embryofetal risk. No animal reproduction studies have been conducted. Using this drug during pregnancy should be based on the pros and cons of the mother's clinical need for treatment versus any potential fetal risk that might occur from exposure.

BREASTFEEDING SUMMARY

No reports describing the use of pyrilamine during human lactation have been located. The drug will likely be excreted into breast milk, so some infant exposure will probably occur. Because it is an antihistamine, there is always a possibility that it could decrease prolactin levels, which could then affect breast milk supply. Breastfeeding while using this drug should be based on the mother's clinical need for treatment versus any potential infant risks that might occur. If used, the infant should be monitored for the most common reported adult side effects of dizziness, blurred vision, epigastric discomfort, and dry mouth (all leading to irritability), constipation, sleep disorder, sedation, rash, and tachycardia.

References

1. National Library of Medicine. Pyrilamine. PubChem. Accessed March 4, 2025. https://pubchem.ncbi.nlm.nih.gov/compound/Pyrilamine
2. Heinonen OP, Slone D, Shapiro S. *Birth Defects and Drugs in Pregnancy*. Publishing Sciences Group; 1977.

PYRIMETHAMINE

Anti-Infective (Folic Acid Antagonist—Antiparasitic)

PREGNANCY RECOMMENDATION: Limited Human Data—Animal Data Suggest Risk

BREASTFEEDING RECOMMENDATION: Potential Toxicity

PREGNANCY SUMMARY

Numerous case reports and small series have been located that describe the use of pyrimethamine in human pregnancy. Of the few cases with first-trimester exposure, the overall risk for major congenital birth anomalies does not appear to be increased. For use in other trimesters, there does not appear to be any increased risk for adverse maternal or fetal effects. Although some folic acid antagonists are human teratogens (see Methotrexate), this does not seem to occur with pyrimethamine. With an ex vivo placental perfusion study, the drug was found to cross the placenta with fetal levels about 30% of maternal concentrations. Therefore, fetal exposure appears to occur. Embryofetal toxicity with malformations was observed in two animal species at doses of less than 10 times the RHD. Using this drug during pregnancy should be based on the pros and cons of the mother's clinical need for treatment versus any potential fetal risk that might occur from exposure.

BREASTFEEDING SUMMARY

Pyrimethamine has been shown to be excreted into human breast milk. Mothers treated with 25 to 75 mg orally produced peak concentrations of 3.1 to 3.3 mcg/mL at 6 hours. The drug was detectable up to 48 hours after a dose. Malaria parasites were completely eliminated in infants up to 6 months of age who were entirely breastfed. In another study, three women were treated with a combination tablet containing 100 mg of dapsone and 12.5 mg of pyrimethamine at 2 to 5 days postpartum. Blood and breast milk samples were collected up to 227 hours after the dose. The breast milk to plasma ratio was about 55%. The calculated RID ranged from about 17% to 46% of the maternal doses during a 9-day period. Due to a concern for potential serious adverse effects that might be seen in a breastfed infant, the manufacturer recommends that women not breastfeed while being treated with this drug. Nevertheless, if the clinical decision is to use this drug while breastfeeding, the infant should be monitored for the most common reported adult side effects of nausea and pruritus (leading to irritability), rash, flushing, anorexia (monitor infant growth), vomiting, and various laboratory abnormalities (see PI). The WHO and American Academy of Pediatrics state that pyrimethamine is compatible with breastfeeding; however, exercise caution when it is used in combination with other medications.

References

1. Prescribing Information. Pyrimethamine. Alvogen Inc; 2021.
2. Centers for Disease Control and Prevention. Clinical care of toxoplasmosis. Accessed March 4, 2025. https://www.cdc.gov/toxoplasmosis/hcp/clinical-care/index.html
3. Peytavin G, Leng JJ, Forestier F, et al. Placental transfer of pyrimethamine studied in an ex vivo placental perfusion model. *Biol Neonate*. 2000; 78:83-85.
4. Anonymous. Prevention of malaria in pregnancy and early childhood. *Br Med J (Clin Res Ed)*. 1984;289:1296-1297.
5. Spracklen FHN. Malaria 1984. Part I. Malaria prophylaxis. *S Afr Med J*. 1984;65:1037-1041.
6. Spracklen FHN, Monteagudo FSE. Therapeutic protocol no. 3. Malaria prophylaxis. *S Afr Med J*. 1986;70:316.
7. Brown GV. Chemoprophylaxis of malaria. *Med J Aust*. 1986;144:696-702.
8. Cook GC. Prevention and treatment of malaria. *Lancet*. 1988;1:32-37.
9. Barry M, Bia F. Pregnancy and travel. *JAMA*. 1989;261:728-731.
10. Stekette RW, Wirima JJ, Slutsker L, et al. The problem of malaria and malaria control in pregnancy in sub-Saharan Africa. *Am J Trop Med Hyg*. 1996;55:2-7.
11. Harpey J-P, Darbois Y, Lefebvre G. Teratogenicity of pyrimethamine. *Lancet*. 1983;2:399.

12. Main EK, Main DM, Krogstad DJ. Treatment of chloroquine-resistant malaria during pregnancy. *JAMA*. 1983;249:3207-3209.
13. Smithells RW, Sheppard S. Teratogenicity of debendox and pyrimethamine. *Lancet*. 1983;2:623-624.
14. Luzzi GA, Peto TEA. Adverse effects of antimalarials. An update. *Drug Saf*. 1993;8:295-311.
15. Anonymous. Pyrimethamine combinations in pregnancy. *Lancet*. 1983;2: 1005-1007.
16. Morley D, Woodland M, Cuthbertson WFJ. Controlled trial of pyrimethamine in pregnant women in an African village. *Br Med J*. 1964;1:667-668.
17. Gilles HM, Lawson JB, Sibelas M, et al. Malaria, anaemia and pregnancy. *Ann Trop Med Parasitol*. 1969;63:245-263.
18. Heinonen OP, Slone D, Shapiro S. *Birth Defects and Drugs in Pregnancy*. Wright PSB; 1983:299.
19. Bruce-Chwatt LJ. Malaria and pregnancy. *Br Med J*. 1983;286:1457-1458.
20. Anonymous. Malaria in pregnancy. *Lancet*. 1983;2:84-85.
21. Strang A, Lachman E, Pitsoe SB, et al. Malaria in pregnancy with fatal complications. Case report. *Br J Obstet Gynaecol*. 1984;91:399-403.
22. Nahlen BL, Akintunde A, Alakija T, et al. Lack of efficacy of pyrimethamine prophylaxis in pregnant Nigerian women. *Lancet*. 1989;2:830-834.
23. Keuter M, van Eijk A, Hoogstrate M, et al. Comparison of chloroquine, pyrimethamine and sulfadoxine, and chlorproguanil and dapsone as treatment for falciparum malaria in pregnant and non-pregnant women, Kakamega district, Kenya. *Br Med J*. 1990;301:466-470.
24. Greenwood AM, Armstrong JRM, Byass P, et al. Malaria chemoprophylaxis, birth weight and child survival. *Trans Roy Soc Trop Med Hyg*. 1992; 86:483-485.
25. Greenwood AM, Menendez C, Todd J, Greenwood BM. The distribution of birth weights in Gambian women who received malaria chemoprophylaxis during their first pregnancy and in control women. *Trans Roy Soc Trop Med Hyg*. 1994;88:311-312.
26. Schultz LJ, Steketee RW, Macheso A, et al. The efficacy of antimalarial regimens containing sulfadoxine-pyrimethamine and/or chloroquine in preventing peripheral and placental *Plasmodium falciparum* infection among pregnant women in Malawi. *Am J Trop Med Hyg*. 1994;51:515-522.
27. Menendez C, Todd J, Alonso PL, et al. Malaria chemoprophylaxis, infection of the placenta and birth weight in Gambian primigravidae. *J Trop Med Hyg*. 1994;97:244-248.
28. Sowunmi A, Akindele JA, Omitowoju GO, et al. Intramuscular sulfadoxine-pyrimethamine in uncomplicated chloroquine-resistant falciparum malaria during pregnancy. *Trans Roy Soc Trop Med Hyg*. 1993;87:472.
29. Clyde DF, Shute GT, Press J. Transfer of pyrimethamine in human milk. *J Trop Med Hyg*. 1956;59:277-284.
30. Edstein MD, Veerendaal JR, Newman K, Hyslop R. Excretion of chloroquine, dapsone and pyrimethamine in human milk. *Br J Clin Pharmacol*. 1986; 22:733-735.

Q

QUAZEPAM

Mental Health (Benzodiazepine)

PREGNANCY RECOMMENDATION: Limited Human Data—No Relevant Animal Data

BREASTFEEDING RECOMMENDATION: Potential Toxicity

PREGNANCY SUMMARY

No reports describing the use of quazepam in human pregnancy have been located. The data for the risk of malformations with benzodiazepines have been mixed. Although early studies with other benzodiazepines found an association with malformations, a systematic review and meta-analysis of eight publications and data from the Massachusetts General Pregnancy Registry for Psychiatric Medications did not find an increased risk for malformations with first-trimester benzodiazepine use. Another systematic review and meta-analysis has been published on the benzodiazepine class of drugs, suggesting an increased risk for potential adverse pregnancy and delivery outcomes (spontaneous abortion, preterm birth, small for gestational age, low birth weight, low 5-minute Apgar score, and neonatal intensive care unit [NICU] admission). However, it is difficult to fully evaluate these findings because specific rates were not provided for comparison to the expected background risks for these various events. In addition, all of these factors can be influenced by numerous confounding variables. Attention-deficit/hyperactivity disorder (ADHD) risk was significantly increased with first- and second-trimester exposure but not third-trimester exposure or when compared to unexposed controls and sibling controls. No difference in autism spectrum disorder risk between benzodiazepine use in any trimester compared to unexposed controls or sibling controls was seen. Quazepam is likely to cross the placenta, so fetal exposure will probably occur. Animal studies showed embryofetal toxicity with malformations in one species (but not a second species) at doses of more than 10 times the recommended human dose (RHD). However, this limited human pregnancy experience prevents a complete assessment of the embryofetal risk. Using this drug during pregnancy should be based on the pros and cons of the mother's clinical need for treatment versus any potential fetal risk that might occur from exposure. Due to the adverse event profile and addictive potential, the American College of Obstetricians and Gynecologists (ACOG) recommends avoiding (or using sparingly) the use of benzodiazepines as anxiety treatment. If prescribed, ACOG recommends using the lowest effective dose and states that doses can be tapered down by 25% to 50% per week. Withdrawal symptoms and seizures can occur with abrupt cessation. Neonatal sedation, decreased muscle tone, respiratory compromise, and NICU admission have been associated with benzodiazepine use in pregnancy, especially near delivery.

BREASTFEEDING SUMMARY

Quazepam and metabolites are excreted into human breast milk. From four healthy, lactating volunteers, who agreed not to breastfeed their infants, mean cumulative amounts were 11.6 mcg (range 2.4-32.8 mcg) quazepam, 4.0 mcg (range 1.3-10.0 mcg) 2-oxoquazepam, and 1.0 mcg (range 0.4-1.6 mcg) *N*-desalky-2-oxoquazepam (following a single 15 mg dose). These amounts represented 0.08%, 0.02%, and 0.09% the administered dose, respectively. Breast milk concentrations of quazepam and 2-oxoquazepam were always higher than those in the maternal plasma, with milk:plasma ratios of 4.18 and 2.02, respectively. Because of the lipophilic properties of quazepam, these ratios are much higher than those observed with diazepam (see Diazepam). The investigators estimated that following a multiple-dose regimen, only 28.7 mcg/d of the three compounds combined would be excreted into breast milk, representing 0.19% of the daily dose. Although these amounts are small, the effects, if any, on a nursing infant's central nervous system function are unknown. The manufacturer recommends that the developmental and health benefits of breastfeeding should be considered along with the mother's clinical need for quazepam and any potential adverse effects on the breastfed infant or from the underlying maternal condition. Because infants exposed to benzodiazepine drugs through breast milk have experienced adverse effects of sedation, poor feeding, and poor weight gain, exposed infants should be monitored for these effects, along with the most common reported adult side effects of headache, dizziness, dry mouth, and dyspepsia (all leading to irritability), and fatigue (lethargy).

References

1. Product Information. *Quazepam*. Atland Pharmaceuticals LLC; 2023.
2. American College of Obstetricians and Gynecologists. Treatment and management of mental health conditions during pregnancy and postpartum. Clinical practice guideline No. 5. *Obstet Gynecol.* 2023;141:1262-1288.
3. Grigoriadis S, Graves L, Peer M, et al. Benzodiazepine use during pregnancy alone or in combination with an antidepressant and congenital malformations: systematic review and meta-analysis. *J Clin Psychiatry.* 2019; 80:18r12412.

4. Tinker SC, Reefhuis J, Bitsko RH, et al. Use of benzodiazepine medications during pregnancy and potential risk for birth defects, National Birth Defects Prevention Study, 1997-2011. *Birth Defects Res.* 2019;111:613-620.
5. Grigoriadis S, Graves L, Peer M, et al. Pregnancy and delivery outcomes following benzodiazepine exposure: a systematic review and meta-analysis. *Can J Psychiatry*. 2020;65:821-834.
6. Szpunar MJ, Freeman MP, Kobylski LA, et al. Risk of major malformations in infants after first trimester exposure to benzodiazepines: results from the Massachusetts General Hospital National Pregnancy Registry for Psychiatric Medications. *Depress Anxiety.* 2022;39:751-759.
7. Chen VCH, Wu SI, Lin CF, et al. Association of prenatal exposure to benzodiazepines with development of autism spectrum and attention-deficit/hyperactivity disorders. *JAMA Netw Open*. 2022;5:e2243282.
8. Hilbert JM, Gural RP, Symchowicz S, Zampaglione N. Excretion of quazepam into human breast milk. *J Clin Pharmacol.* 1984;24:457-462.

QUETIAPINE

Mental Health (Atypical Antipsychotic)

PREGNANCY RECOMMENDATION: Limited Human Data—Animal Data Suggest Risk

BREASTFEEDING RECOMMENDATION: Compatible

PREGNANCY SUMMARY

According to the manufacturer, atypical antipsychotics as a class of drugs do not appear to increase the risk for malformations, small for gestational age, ADHD, or autism spectrum disorders. Several of these reports included patients taking quetiapine. Quetiapine crosses the placenta, so some fetal exposure will occur. Animal studies showed some embryofetal toxicity with malformations in two studies at doses of less than 10 times the RHD. The manufacturer recommends avoiding this medication, if at all possible, during pregnancy. Nevertheless, using this drug during pregnancy should be based on the pros and cons of the mother's clinical need for treatment versus any potential fetal risk that might occur from exposure. ACOG guidelines state that uncontrolled bipolar disorder in pregnancy has increased risks for preterm delivery, fetal growth restriction, adverse neurodevelopmental outcomes, and postpartum psychosis. Women who are pregnant and have taken quetiapine at any time during pregnancy are encouraged to contact the National Pregnancy Registry for Atypical Antipsychotics at 866-961-2388. Quetiapine can prolong the QTc.

BREASTFEEDING SUMMARY

Quetiapine is excreted into human breast milk. The manufacturer reports that no consistent infant adverse effects have been reported when exposed to quetiapine through lactation. Breast milk levels were calculated to range from 0.01 to 0.56 mg/kg/d, producing a relevant infant dose (RID) of less than 1%. However, the long-term effects of this exposure on a nursing infant are unknown. The manufacturer recommends that the developmental and health benefits of breastfeeding should be considered along with the mother's clinical need for quetiapine and any potential adverse effects on the breastfed infant or from the underlying maternal condition. If used while breastfeeding, the infant should be monitored for the most common reported adult side effects of dizziness, abdominal pain, asthenia, and dyspepsia (all leading to irritability), somnolence, constipation, and hypotension.

References

1. Product Information. *Quetiapine Fumarate*. Camber Pharmaceuticals Inc; 2023.
2. American College of Obstetricians and Gynecologists. Treatment and management of mental health conditions during pregnancy and postpartum: ACOG clinical practice guideline No. 5. *Obstet Gynecol*. 2023;141:1262-1288.
3. Rahi M, Heikkinen T, Hartter S, et al. Placental transfer of quetiapine in relation to P-glycoprotein activity. *J Psychopharmacol*. 2007;21:751-756.
4. Newport DJ, Calamaras MR, DeVane CL, et al. Atypical antipsychotic administration during late pregnancy: placental passage and obstetrical outcomes. *Am J Psychiatry*. 2007;164:1214-1220.
5. Viguera A, Freeman MP, Goez-Mogollon L, et al. Reproduction safety of second-generation antipsychotics: updated data from the Massachusetts General Hospital National Pregnancy Registry for atypical antipsychotics. *J Clin Psychiatry*. 2021;82:20m13745.
6. Huybrechts KF, Straub L, Karlsson P, et al. Association of in utero antipsychotic medication exposure with risk of congenital malformations in Nordic countries and the US. *JAMA Psychiatry*. 2023;80:156-166.
7. Cohen LS, Goes-Mogolion L, Sosinsky AZ, et al. Risk of major malformations in infants following first-trimester exposure to quetiapine. *Am J Psychiatry*. 2018;175:1225-1231.
8. Ennis ZN, Damkier P. Pregnancy exposure to olanzapine, quetiapine, risperidone, aripiprazole and risk of congenital malformations. a systematic review. *Basic Clin Pharmacol Toxicol*. 2015;116:315-320.
9. Tenyi T, Trixler M, Keresztes Z. Quetiapine and pregnancy. *Am J Psychiatry*. 2002;159:674.
10. Taylor TM, O'Toole MS, Ohlsen RI, et al. Safety of quetiapine during pregnancy. *Am J Psychiatry*. 2003;160:588-589.
11. Lee A, Giesbrecht E, Dunn E, Ito S. Excretion of quetiapine in breast milk. *Am J Psychiatry*. 2004;161:1715-1716.
12. Misri S, Corral M, Wardrop AA, Kendrick K. Quetiapine augmentation in lactation: a series of case reports. *J Clin Psychopharmacol*. 2006;26:508-511.
13. Gentile S. Quetiapine-fluvoxamine combination during pregnancy and while breastfeeding. *Arch Womens Ment Health*. 2006;9:158-159.
14. Rampono J, Kristensen JH, Ilett KF, et al. Quetiapine and breast feeding. *Ann Pharmacother*. 2007;41:711-714.
15. Grover S, Madam R. Successful use of quetiapine in two successive pregnancies. *J Neuropsychiatry Clin Neurosci*. 2012;24(Winter):E38.
16. Viguera AC, McElheny SA, Caplin PS, et al. Risk of poor neonatal adaptation syndrome among infants exposed to second-generation atypical antipsychotics compared to antidepressants. *J Clin Psychiatry.* 2023;84:22m14492.
17. Wang Z, Chan AYL, Coghill D, et al. Association between prenatal exposure to antipsychotics and attention-deficit/hyperactivity disorder, autism spectrum disorder, preterm birth, and small for gestational age. *JAMA Intern Med*. 2021;181:1332-1340.
18. Westin AA, Brekke M, Molden E, et al. Treatment with antipsychotics in pregnancy: changes in drug disposition. *Clin Pharmacol Ther.* 2018;103:477-484.
19. Leutritz AL, van Braam L, Preis K, et al. Psychotropic medication in pregnancy and lactation and early development of exposed children. *Br J Clin Pharmacol*. 2023;89:737-750.

Q

20. Klier CM, Mossaheb N, Saria A, et al. Pharmacokinetics and elimination of quetiapine, venlafaxine, and trazodone during pregnancy and postpartum. *J Clin Psychopharmacol.* 2007;27:720-722.
21. Park Y, Hernandez-Diaz S, Bateman BT, et al. Continuation of atypical antipsychotic medication during early pregnancy and the risk of gestational diabetes. *Am J Psychiatry.* 2018;175:564-574.
22. Kulkarni J, Gurvich C, Gilbert H, et al. The use of first and second-generation antipsychotic drugs and the potential to develop gestational diabetes mellitus among perinatal patients with psychosis. *Schizophr Res.* 2023;254: 22-26.
23. Heinonen E, Forsberg L, Norby U, et al. Antipsychotic use during pregnancy and risk for gestational diabetes: a national register-based cohort study in Sweden. *CNS Drugs.* 2022;36:529-539.
24. Aydin B, Nayir T, Sahin S, Yildiz A. Olanzapine and quetiapine use during breastfeeding: excretion into breast milk and safe breastfeeding strategy. *J Clin Psychopharmacol.* 2015;35:206-208.
25. Yazdani-Brojeni P, Tamoshima R, Taguchi N, et al. Quetiapine excretion into human breast milk. *J Clin Psychopharmacol.* 2018;38:362-364.

QUINAPRIL

Antihypertensive (ACE—Angiotensin I-Converting Enzyme Inhibitor)

PREGNANCY RECOMMENDATION: Contraindicated (Second and Third Trimesters)

BREASTFEEDING RECOMMENDATION: Probably Compatible

PREGNANCY SUMMARY

No reports describing the specific use of quinapril in human pregnancy have been located. A few large studies have reported the risk for congenital anomalies with first-trimester exposure to angiotensin I-converting enzyme (ACE) inhibitors as a class of drugs. These publications reported overall malformation rates of about 5% to 6%, which is higher than the expected rate of 2% to 4%. However, most of these studies also reported fetal anomaly rates in pregnant patients with hypertension not on treatment to be similar. The impression was that these findings might be related to the disease and not the drug. Likewise, some of these studies also reported an increase in risk for cardiac defects, but again, it was not certain whether this elevated risk was related to the drug or the disease. Furthermore, no pattern to the anomalies has been identified. Regarding the use of ACE inhibitors in the second half of pregnancy, numerous case reports and reviews have reported that these drugs can, in some cases, produce severe fetal renal dysfunction. This can lead to anomalies related to longstanding oligohydramnios and fetal/neonatal death. There are cases, however, where the process reverses itself when the drug is discontinued. These findings are similar to those seen with angiotensin receptor blockers (ARBs). The drug actually carries a boxed warning for these risks. Quinapril probably crosses the placenta, so some fetal exposure will likely occur. Therefore, the absence of the first-trimester human pregnancy experience prevents a complete assessment of the embryofetal risk. Animal studies did not show any embryofetal toxicity in two species at doses of more than 10 times the RHD in one species and less than 10 times the RHD in the second species. Women of reproductive age using quinapril should be informed of these risks, so they can be closely monitored if pregnancy transpires. If a positive pregnancy test occurs, she and her health care providers can modify treatment (if possible) so that the drug is not used in the second or third trimesters. For treating hypertension in pregnancy, ACOG recommends nifedipine and labetalol as first-line agents.

BREASTFEEDING SUMMARY

Quinapril was found to be excreted into human breast milk in a study of six women taking a single 20 mg dose. In one patient, quinapril was never detected in the breast milk. The average maximum breast milk level was about 28 ng/mL. Quinapril was not detected in any breast milk samples after 4 hours. For quinaprilat, the drug was detected in the breast milk of all six patients, but concentrations were below the level for obtaining an exact quantity (<60 ng/mL). The calculated RID for quinapril was 1.6%, and for quinaprilat, it would be below 0.5%. The manufacturer recommends caution in using this drug while breastfeeding. Nevertheless, breastfeeding while using this drug should be based on the mother's clinical need for treatment versus any potential infant risks that might occur. If used, the infant should be monitored for the most common reported adult side effects of headache, nausea, myalgia, and dizziness (all leading to irritability), cough, rash, hypotension, diarrhea, and fatigue (lethargy).

References

1. Prescribing Information. *Accupril*. Parke-Davis Inc; 2019.
2. American College of Obstetricians and Gynecologists' Committee on Practice Bulletins—Obstetrics. ACOG Practice Bulletin No. 203: chronic hypertension in pregnancy. *Obstet Gynecol.* 2019;133:e26-e50.
3. Gestational hypertension and preeclampsia: ACOG Practice Bulletin No. 222. *Obstet Gynecol.* 2020;135:e237-e260.
4. Cooper WO, Hernandez-Diaz C, Arbogast PG, et al. Major congenital malformations after first-trimester exposure to ACE inhibitors. *N Engl J Med.* 2006;354:2443-2451.
5. Li DK, Yang C, Andrade S, et al. Maternal exposure to angiotensin converting enzyme inhibitors in the first trimester and risk of malformations in offspring: a retrospective cohort study. *BMJ.* 2011;343:d5931.
6. Vasilakis-Scaramozza C, Aschengrau A, Cabral HJ, Jick SS. Antihypertensive drugs and the risk of congenital anomalies. *Pharmacotherapy.* 2013;33: 476-482.
7. Bateman BT, Patorno E, Desai RJ, et al. Angiotensin-converting enzyme inhibitors and the risk of congenital malformations. *Obstet Gynecol.* 2017;129: 174-184.
8. Hoeltzenbein M, Tissen-Diabate T, Fiets AK, et al. Increased rate of birth defects after first trimester use of angiotensin converting enzyme inhibitors-treatment or hypertension related? An observational cohort study. *Pregnancy Hypertens.* 2018;13:65-71.
9. Buawangpong N, Teekachunhatean S, Koonrungsesomboon N. Adverse pregnancy outcomes associated with first-trimester exposure to angiotensin-converting enzyme inhibitors or angiotensin II receptor blockers: a systematic review and meta-analysis. *Pharmacol Res Perspect.* 2020;8(5):e00644.
10. Begg EJ, Robson RA, Gardiner SJ, et al. Quinapril and its metabolite quinaprilat in human milk. *Br J Clin Pharm.* 2001;51:478-481.

Q

QUINIDINE

Cardiovascular (Antiarrhythmic)

PREGNANCY RECOMMENDATION: Limited Human Data—No Relevant Animal Data

BREASTFEEDING RECOMMENDATION: Potential Toxicity (Long-Term Use)

PREGNANCY SUMMARY

In the Michigan Medicaid recipient study, 17 newborns had been exposed to quinidine during the first trimester. One (5.9%) major birth defect was observed (one expected). Several case reports have described the use of quinidine in treating maternal and fetal arrhythmias in the second and/or third trimesters. Success has been mixed. Quinidine crosses the placenta, so fetal exposure will occur. Fetal serum levels appear to be similar to maternal levels. No reproductive animal studies have been located. Neonatal thrombocytopenia has been reported after maternal use of quinidine. Additionally, quinidine can induce inhibition of pseudocholinesterase, which is responsible for the metabolism of succinylcholine and ester-type local anesthetics (eg, procaine, tetracaine, cocaine, and chloroprocaine). The quinidine-induced inhibition of this enzyme, which is already significantly decreased by pregnancy itself, could potentially result in toxicity if these drugs were used in a mother being maintained on quinidine. Therefore, this limited human pregnancy experience prevents a complete assessment of embryofetal risk. Using this drug during pregnancy should be based on the pros and cons of the mother's clinical need for treatment versus any potential fetal risk that might occur from exposure. Quinidine can prolong the QTc.

BREASTFEEDING SUMMARY

Quinidine is excreted into human breast milk. A woman taking 1800 mg/d had breast milk concentrations of 6.4 and 8.2 mcg/mL. The calculated RID was about 3% to 4%. The manufacturer notes that nursing infants should be expected to develop quinidine levels at least an order of magnitude lower than maternal levels. However, because infants have lower protein binding of some drugs, they may have an increased risk for toxicity at lower total serum levels. However, quinidine pharmacokinetics and pharmacodynamics in infants have not been adequately studied. Given the boxed warnings, this medication should be limited to short-term use (if at all possible). If the clinical decision is to use this drug while breastfeeding, the infant should be monitored for the most common reported adult side effects of upper gastrointestinal distress, lightheadedness, and headache (all leading to irritability), fatigue (lethargy), and diarrhea.

Q

References

1. Prescribing Information. *Quinidine Sulfate*. Eon Labs Inc; 2019.
2. Killeen AA, Bowers LD. Fetal supraventricular tachycardia treated with high-dose quinidine: toxicity associated with marked elevation of the metabolite, 3(S)-3-hydroxyquinidine. *Obstet Gynecol.* 1987;70:445-449.
3. Hill LM, Malkasian GD Jr. The use of quinidine sulfate throughout pregnancy. *Obstet Gynecol.* 1979;54:366-368.
4. Spinnato JA, Shaver DC, Flinn GS, et al. Fetal supraventricular tachycardia: in utero therapy with digoxin and quinidine. *Obstet Gynecol.* 1984;64:730-735.
5. Guntheroth WG, Cyr DR, Mack LA, et al. Hydrops from reciprocating atrioventricular tachycardia in a 27-week fetus requiring quinidine for conversion. *Obstet Gynecol.* 1985;66(suppl):29S-33S.
6. Sherer DM, Sadovksy E, Menashe M, et al. Fetal ventricular tachycardia associated with nonimmunologic hydrops fetalis: a case report. *J Reprod Med.* 1990;35:292-294.
7. Braverman AC, Bromely BS, Rutherford JD. New onset ventricular tachycardia during pregnancy. *Int J Cardiol.* 1991;33:409-412.
8. Kambam JR, Franks JJ, Smith BE. Inhibitory effect of quinidine on plasma pseudocholinesterase activity in pregnant women. *Am J Obstet Gynecol.* 1987;157:897-899.
9. Wong RD, Murthy ARK, Mathisen GE, et al. Treatment of severe Falciparum malaria during pregnancy with quinidine and exchange transfusion. *Am J Med.* 1992;92:561-562.
10. Domula VM, Weissach G, Lenk H. Über die Auswirkung medikamentöser Behandlung in der Schwangerschaft auf das Gerinnungspotential des Neugeborenen. *Zentralbl Gynaekol.* 1977;99:473.

QUININE

Anti-Infective (Antimalarial)

PREGNANCY RECOMMENDATION: Human Data Suggest Low Risk

BREASTFEEDING RECOMMENDATION: Probably Compatible

PREGNANCY SUMMARY

Some case reports of women taking high doses of quinine during pregnancy described deafness and optic nerve hypoplasia in the exposed children. However, these reports usually concerned the use of quinine in toxic doses as an abortifacient. Two large systematic reviews with meta-analyses did not show an increased risk for major fetal malformations, though most exposures were in the second and third trimesters. Quinine crosses the human placenta and produces fetal levels about

32% of maternal levels. Animal studies showed embryofetal toxicity with malformations in four species at doses less than 10 times the RHD. In a fifth species (monkeys), no embryofetal toxicity or teratogenicity was seen at doses 2 times the RHD. When compared to the general population, *Plasmodium falciparum* malaria during pregnancy is associated with a higher risk of morbidity and mortality. Risks of malaria in pregnancy include fetal loss (both spontaneous abortion and intrauterine fetal demise), preterm delivery, intrauterine growth restriction, low birth weight, and maternal death. Therefore, using this drug during pregnancy should be based on the pros and cons of the mother's clinical need for treatment versus any potential fetal risk that might occur from exposure. QTc prolongation has been observed with quinine. In addition, because quinine stimulates insulin secretion, hypoglycemia can occur.

BREASTFEEDING SUMMARY

Quinine crosses into breast milk at levels of about 31% of maternal plasma. It is estimated that the total daily dose found in breast milk is less than 2 to 3 mg/d (<0.4% of the maternal dose). The drug was detectable in breast milk up to 23 hours after a dose, with concentrations ranging from trace to 2.2 mcg/mL. No adverse effects were reported in the nursing infants. Patients with glucose-6-phosphate dehydrogenase deficiency should not use quinine. Therefore, if an infant is at risk for this disease, testing should be done prior to maternal usage (if breastfeeding the infant is desired). The manufacturer states that although quinine is generally considered compatible with breastfeeding, the risks and benefits should be evaluated, and caution must be exercised if administered during lactation. If an infant is suspected of having malaria, quinine exposure through breastfeeding may not be therapeutic in treating the infant. If the drug is used while breastfeeding, the infant should be monitored for the most common reported adult side effects of headache, nausea, tinnitus, dizziness, and abdominal pain (all leading to irritability), sweating, hearing impairment, vomiting, diarrhea, and disturbances in cardiac rhythm or conduction.

References

1. Product Information. *Quinine sulfate*. Lupin Pharmaceuticals Inc; 2023.
2. Center for Disease Control and Prevention. *Alternatives for pregnant women. Clinical guidance: malaria diagnosis & treatment in the U.S.* Accessed June 14, 2024.https://www.cdc.gov/malaria/hcp/clinical-guidance/pregnant-women.html#
3. Nishimura H, Tanimura T. *Clinical Aspects of the Teratogenicity of Drugs*. American Elsevier; 1976:140-143.
4. Robinson GC, Brummitt JR, Miller JR. Hearing loss in infants and preschool children. II. Etiological considerations. *Pediatrics*. 1963;32:115-124.
5. West RA. Effect of quinine upon auditory nerve. *Am J Obstet Gynecol*. 1938;36:241-248.
6. McKinna AJ. Quinine induced hypoplasia of the optic nerve. *Can J Ophthalmol*. 1966;1:261.
7. Morgon A, Charachon D, Brinquier N. Disorders of the auditory apparatus caused by embryopathy or foetopathy. Prophylaxis and treatment. *Acta Otolaryngol (Stockh)*. 1971;291(suppl):5.
8. Saito M, McGready R, Tinto H, et al. Pregnancy outcomes after first-trimester treatment with artemisinin derivatives versus non-artemisinin antimalarials: a systematic review and individual patient data meta-analysis. *Lancet*. 2023;401:118-130.
9. Saito M, Mansoor R, Kennon K, et al. Pregnancy outcomes and risk of placental malaria after artemisinin-based and quinine-based treatment for uncomplicated falciparum malaria in pregnancy: a WorldWide Antimalarial Resistance Network systematic review and individual patient data meta-analysis. *BMC Med*. 2020;18:138.
10. Saeheng T, Na-Bangchang K. Clinical pharmacokinetics of quinine and its relationship with treatment outcomes in children, pregnant women, and elderly patients, with uncomplicated and complicated malaria: a systematic review. *Malaria J*. 2022;21:41.
11. Mauer MA, DeVaux W, Lahey ME. Neonatal and maternal thrombocytopenic purpura due to quinine. *Pediatrics*. 1957;19:84-87.
12. Glass L, Rajegowda BK, Bowne E, Evans HE. Exposure to quinine and jaundice in a glucose-6-phosphate dehydrogenase-deficient newborn infant. *Pediatrics*. 1973;82:734-735.
13. Terwilliger WG, Hatcher RA. The elimination of morphine and quinine in human milk. *Surg Gynecol Obstet*. 1934;58:823-826.
14. Phillips RE, Looareesuwan S, White NJ, Silamut K, Kietinun S, Warrell DA. Quinine pharmacokinetics and toxicity in pregnant and lactating women with falciparum malaria. *Br J Clin Pharm*. 1986;21:677-683.

QUIZARTINIB

Antineoplastic (Kinase Inhibitor)

PREGNANCY RECOMMENDATION: No Human Data—Animal Data Suggest Potential Risk

BREASTFEEDING RECOMMENDATION: Potential Toxicity

PREGNANCY SUMMARY

No reports describing the use of quizartinib in human pregnancy have been located. The drug and its active metabolite are likely to cross the placenta, so some fetal exposure will probably occur. Therefore, the absence of human pregnancy experience prevents a complete assessment of the embryofetal risk. Animal data showed embryofetal toxicity in one animal species. Based on these animal studies and the drug's mechanism of action, the manufacturer recommends that women with reproductive potential use effective contraception during treatment and for 7 months after the last dose. They also recommend that males with female partners of reproductive potential use effective contraception during treatment and for 4 months after the last dose. Nevertheless, using this drug during pregnancy should be based on the pros and cons of the mother's clinical need for treatment versus any potential fetal risk that might occur from exposure. Quizartinib can prolong the QT interval, and there is a risk for torsades de pointes (an uncommon, distinct form of ventricular tachycardia that can lead to cardiac arrest and sudden death).

BREASTFEEDING SUMMARY

No reports describing the use of quizartinib during human lactation have been located. The drug and its active metabolite will likely be excreted into breast milk, so some infant exposure will probably occur. Due to the concern for potential serious adverse effects that might be seen in a breastfed infant, the manufacturer recommends that women not breastfeed while being treated with this drug and for at least 1 month after the last dose. Nevertheless, breastfeeding while using this drug should be based on the mother's clinical need for treatment. If used, the infant should be monitored for the most common reported adult side effects of nausea, abdominal pain, and headache (all leading to irritability), diarrhea, vomiting, upper respiratory tract infection, and various laboratory abnormalities (see Prescribing Information [PI]).

Reference

1. Prescribing Information. *Vanflyta*. Daiichi Sankyo Company; 2023.

Q

R

RABEPRAZOLE

Gastrointestinal (Proton Pump Inhibitor)

PREGNANCY RECOMMENDATION: Limited Human Data—Animal Data Suggest Potential Risk

BREASTFEEDING RECOMMENDATION: Probably Compatible

PREGNANCY SUMMARY

Several reports describing the use of proton pump inhibitors (PPIs), including rabeprazole, in human pregnancy have been located. PPIs do not appear to increase the risk for malformations. One study evaluated specific agents and did not find an increased risk with rabeprazole. A meta-analysis of PPI in pregnancy compared 1,530 patients exposed to PPI with 133,410 not exposed, and found no increased risk for major congenital malformations, spontaneous abortion, or preterm birth. Rabeprazole is likely to cross the placenta, so some fetal exposure will probably occur. Embryofetal toxicity was observed in one animal species at doses of less than 10 times the recommended human dose (RHD). However, this limited human pregnancy experience for rabeprazole prevents a complete assessment of embryofetal risk. Other publications have reported conflicting data on the risk for childhood asthma and the risk for preeclampsia compared to nonexposed controls. However, it is difficult to fully evaluate these findings because specific rates are not consistently provided for comparison to the expected background risks for these various events. In addition, all of these factors can be influenced by numerous confounding variables. Using this drug during pregnancy should be based on the pros and cons of the mother's clinical need for treatment versus any potential fetal risk that might occur from exposure

BREASTFEEDING SUMMARY

No reports describing the use of rabeprazole during human lactation have been located. The drug will likely be excreted into breast milk, so some infant exposure will likely occur. Breastfeeding while using this drug should be based on the mother's clinical need for treatment versus any potential infant risks that might occur. If used, the infant should be monitored for the most common reported adult side effects of myalgia and arthralgia (both leading to irritability), flatulence, infection, and constipation.

References

1. Prescribing Information. Rabeprazole sodium. Amneal Pharmaceuticals LLC; 2023.
2. Peron A, Ripoche E, Picot C, et al. Use of proton pump inhibitors during pregnancy: a systematic review and meta-analysis of congenital malformations. *Reprod Toxicol*. 2023;119:108419.
3. Li CM, Zhernakova A, Engstrand L, et al. Systematic review with meta-analysis: the risks of proton pump inhibitors during pregnancy. *Ailment Pharmacol Ther*. 2020;51:410-420.
4. Choi A, Noh Y, Jeong HE, et al. Association between proton pump inhibitor use during early pregnancy and risk of congenital malformations. *JAMA Netw Open*. 2023;6:e2250366.
5. Noh Y, Jeong HE, Choi A, et al. Prenatal and infant exposure to acid-suppressive medication and risk of allergic diseases in children. *JAMA Pediatr*. 2023;177:267-277.
6. Lai T, Wu M, Liu J, et al. Acid-suppressive drug use during pregnancy and the risk of childhood asthma: a meta-analysis. *Pediatrics*. 2018;141:e20170889.
7. Choi A, Noh Y, Yon DK, Shin JY. Maternal proton pump inhibitor use during pregnancy and risk of low birth weight in offspring in Korea, 2008-2019. *JAMA Netw Open*. 2023;6:e237962.
8. Choi A, Noh Y, Park SH, et al. Exploration of proton pump inhibitors use during pregnancy and preeclampsia. *JAMA Netw Open*. 2023;4:e2124339.

RADIUM RA 223 DICHLORIDE

Radiopharmaceutical (Prostate Cancer)

PREGNANCY RECOMMENDATION: *Contraindicated

BREASTFEEDING RECOMMENDATION: *Contraindicated

PREGNANCY SUMMARY

No reports describing the use of radium Ra 23 dichloride in human pregnancy have been located. The drug will probably cross the placenta. However, the absence of human pregnancy experience prevents a complete assessment of the

(*continued*)

embryofetal risk. No animal studies have been conducted. The manufacturer recommends that men with female partners of reproductive potential use highly effective contraception during treatment and for at least 6 months after the last dose. *Radium Ra 23 dichloride is not indicated for use in women.

BREASTFEEDING SUMMARY

No reports describing the use of radium Ra 23 dichloride during human lactation have been located. The drug will probably be excreted into breast milk. *However, radium Ra 23 dichloride is not indicated for use in women.

Reference

1. Prescribing Information. Xofigo. Bayer Healthcare Pharmaceuticals; 2013.

RALOXIFENE

Bone Health (Selective Estrogen Receptor Modulator)

PREGNANCY RECOMMENDATION: Contraindicated

BREASTFEEDING RECOMMENDATION: Contraindicated

PREGNANCY SUMMARY

No reports describing the use of raloxifene in human pregnancy have been located. The drug is likely to cross the placenta, so some fetal exposure will probably occur. Embryofetal toxicity with malformations was observed in two species of animals at doses of less than the RHD. The indications for this drug suggest that human pregnancy experience is unlikely. Moreover, raloxifene is an estrogen antagonist in uterine tissue, and estrogen is required to maintain pregnancy. Therefore, the drug is contraindicated for use in pregnancy.

BREASTFEEDING SUMMARY

No reports describing the use of raloxifene during human lactation have been located. The drug will likely be excreted into breast milk, so some infant exposure would probably occur. Raloxifene is an estrogen antagonist in breast tissue. Therefore, it is contraindicated during breastfeeding. If the clinical decision is to use this drug while breastfeeding, the infant should be monitored for the most common reported adult side effects of hot flashes, flu symptoms, arthralgia, and leg cramps (all leading to irritability), peripheral edema, and sweating.

Reference

1. Prescribing Information. Raloxifene hydrochloride. Cadila Pharmaceuticals Limited; 2022.

R

RALTEGRAVIR

Antiretroviral (Integrase Inhibitor)

PREGNANCY RECOMMENDATION: Human Data Suggest Low Risk (Maternal Benefit Outweighs Any Potential Fetal Risk)

BREASTFEEDING RECOMMENDATION: Probably Compatible

PREGNANCY SUMMARY

In 2023, the updated US Department of Health and Human Services AIDS Info guidelines for the use of antiretroviral agents during pregnancy recommend that, in most cases, patients continue their regimen during pregnancy if it is tolerated, safe, and effective in suppressing viral replication. The guideline recommends that discussion and shared decision-making about the known and potential risks, as well as benefits to the mother and fetus, acknowledging limited data, should guide the selection of which antiretrovirals to use during pregnancy. Additionally, treatment initiation should not be delayed due to concerns about teratogenicity with first-trimester exposure. See the guidelines at https://clinicalinfo.hiv.gov/en/guidelines/perinatal/ for the most updated information. If indicated, raltegravir should not be withheld in pregnancy since the expected benefit to the HIV-positive mother outweighs the unknown risk to the fetus.

There are over 1,000 pregnancy exposures to raltegravir. Most of the data have not found an increased risk of malformations with first-trimester raltegravir exposure. Raltegravir crosses the placenta, so fetal exposure will occur. Embryofetal toxicity was observed in one species of animal at doses less than 10 times the RHD. Using this drug during pregnancy should be based on the pros and cons of the mother's clinical need for treatment versus any potential fetal risk that might occur from exposure. Providers caring for pregnant patients with HIV and their infants can call the national Perinatal HIV/AIDS hotline (888-448-8765) for free clinical consultation. Additionally, there is a pregnancy exposure registry that monitors pregnancy outcomes in individuals exposed to antiretroviral medicines during pregnancy. Health care professionals are encouraged to register obstetric patients taking raltegravir in the Antiretroviral Pregnancy Registry (APR) at 800-258-4263.

BREASTFEEDING SUMMARY

In 2023, the updated US Department of Health and Human Services AIDS Info guidelines state that using replacement of breast milk through formula or pasteurized donor human breast milk from a milk bank eliminates the risk of postnatal HIV transmission to the infant. Using antiretroviral therapy to achieve and maintain viral suppression during pregnancy and postpartum decreases the risk for infant transmission to less than 1%, but notes that it is not zero. For patients not on therapy or those without viral load suppression during pregnancy (at a minimum of throughout the third trimester) and at delivery, replacement of breast milk is recommended. Patients on antiretroviral therapy with a sustained undetectable viral load who choose to breastfeed or use replacement of breast milk should be supported with this decision. Raltegravir has been found in human breast milk, so infant exposure will occur. From the available data, a total of 18 women have been evaluated while using this drug during lactation. The estimated infant doses ranged from 0.02 to 0.25 mg/kg/d, and the relative infant doses ranged from about 0.3% to 4.1%. If the clinical decision is to use this drug while breastfeeding, the infant should be monitored for the most common reported adult side effects of headache, dizziness, and nausea (all leading to irritability), insomnia, and fatigue (lethargy).

References

1. Prescribing Information. Isentress. Merck Sharp & Dohme LLC; 2022.
2. Lexi-Comp, Inc. Lexi-Drugs. Lexi-Comp Inc; 2024.
3. Panel on Treatment of HIV During Pregnancy and Prevention of Perinatal Transmission. Recommendations for the use of antiretroviral drugs during pregnancy and interventions to reduce perinatal HIV transmission in the United States. Recommendations for the use of antiretroviral drugs during pregnancy—integrase inhibitors. Accessed July 9, 2024. https://clinicalinfo.hiv.gov/en/guidelines/perinatal/safety-toxicity-arv-agents-integrase-inhibitors-raltegravir-isentress
4. Panel on Treatment of HIV During Pregnancy and Prevention of Perinatal Transmission. Recommendations for the use of antiretroviral drugs during pregnancy and interventions to reduce perinatal HIV transmission in the United States. Recommendations for the use of antiretroviral drugs during pregnancy. Department of Health and Human Services. Accessed July 25, 2023. https://clinicalinfo.hiv.gov/en/guidelines/perinatal
5. McKeown DA, Rosenvinge M, Donaghy S, et al. High neonatal concentrations of raltegravir following transplacental transfer in HIV-1 positive pregnancy women. *AIDS*. 2010;24:2416-2418.
6. Clavel-Osorio C, Cazassus F, Stegman S, et al. One-month transplacental pharmacokinetics of raltegravir in a premature newborn after short-course treatment of the HIV-1-infected mother. *Antimicrob Agents Chemother*. 2013;57:6393-6394.
7. McCormack SA, Best BM. Protecting the fetus against HIV infection: a systemic review of placental transfer of antiretrovirals. *Clin Pharmacokinet*. 2014;53:989-1004.
8. Clarke DF, Acosta EP, Rizk ML, et al. Raltegravir pharmacokinetics in neonates following maternal dosing; International Maternal Pediatric Adolescent AIDS Clinical Trials (IMPAACT) P1097 Study Team. *J Acquir Immune Defic Syndr*. 2014;67:310-315.
9. Watts DH, Stek A, Best BM, et al. Raltegravir pharmacokinetics during pregnancy. *J Acquir Immune Defic Syndr*. 2014;67:375-381.
10. Antiretroviral Pregnancy Registry Steering Committee. Antiretroviral Pregnancy Registry international interim report for 1 January 1989 through 31 January 2024. Registry Coordinating Center. 2023. www.APRegistry.com
11. Rasi V, Cortina-Borja M, Peters H, Sconza R, Thorne C. Surveillance of congenital anomalies after exposure to raltegravir or elvitegravir during pregnancy in the United Kingdom and Ireland, 2008-2018. *J Acquir Immune Defic Syndr*. 2019;80:264-268.
12. Shamsuddin H, Raudenbush CL, Sciba BL, et al. Evaluation of neural tube defects (NTDs) after exposure to raltegravir during pregnancy. *J Acquir Immune Defic Syndr*. 2019;81:247-250.
13. Sibiude J, Le Chenadec J, Mandelbrot L, et al. Risk of birth defects and perinatal outcomes in HIV-infected women exposed to integrase strand inhibitors during pregnancy. *AIDS*. 2021;35:219-226.
14. Smith C, Fought AJ, Sung JF, et al. Congenital malformations and preeclampsia associated with integrase inhibitor use in pregnancy: a single-center analysis. *PLoS One*. 2023;18:e0276473.
15. Pinnetti C, Baroncelli S, Villani P, et al. Rapid HIV-RNA decline following addition of raltegravir and tenofovir to ongoing highly active antiretroviral therapy in a woman presenting with high-level HIV viraemia at week 38 of pregnancy. *J Antimicrob Chemother*. 2010;65:2050-2052.
16. Taylor N, Touzeau V, Geit M, et al. Raltegravir in pregnancy: a case series presentation. *Int J STD AIDS*. 2011;22:358-360.
17. Westling K, Pettersson K, Kaldma A, Naver L. Rapid decline in HIV viral load when introducing raltegravir-containing antiretroviral treatment late in pregnancy. *AIDS Patient Care STDS*. 2012;26:714-717.
18. Hegazi A, Hay P. HIV seroconversion in the third trimester of pregnancy: using raltegravir to prevent mother-to-child transmission. *Int J STD AIDS*. 2013;24:245-246.
19. Cha A, Shaikh R, Williams S, Berkowitz LL. Rapid reduction in HIV vial load in late pregnancy with raltegravir: a case report. *J Int Assoc Provid AIDS Care*. 2013;12:312-314.
20. Nobrega I, Travassos AG, Haguihara T, et al. Short communication: use of raltegravir in late-presenting HIV-infected pregnant women. *AIDS Res Hum Retroviruses*. 2013;29:1451-1454.
21. De Hoffer L, Di Biagio A, Bruzzone B, et al. Use of raltegravir in a late presenter HIV-1 woman in advanced gestational age: case report and literature review. *J Chemother*. 2013;25:181-183.
22. Naver L, Albert J, Bottiger Y, et al. Prophylaxis and treatment of HIV-1 infection in pregnancy: Swedish recommendations 2013. *Scand J Infect Dis*. 2014;46:401-411.
23. Blonk ML, Colbers AP, Hidalgo-Tenorio C, et al. Raltegravir in HIV-1 infected pregnant women: pharmacokinetics, safety, and efficacy. *Clin Infect Dis*. 2015;61:809-816.
24. Boucoiran I, Tulloch K, Pick N, et al. A case series of third-trimester raltegravir initiation: impact on maternal HIV-1 viral load and obstetrical outcomes. *Can J Infect Dis Med Microbiol*. 2015;26:145-150.
25. Rahangdale L, Cates J, Potter J, et al. *Am J Obstet Gynecol*. 2016; 214:385.e1-e7.
26. van Halsema C, Whitfield T, Lin N, et al. Five years' real-life experience with raltegravir in a large HIC centre. *Int J STD AIDS*. 2016;27:387-393.
27. Watts DH, Stek A, Best BM, et al. Raltegravir pharmacokinetics during pregnancy. *J Acquir Immune Defic Syndr*. 2014;67:375-381.
28. Renet S, Closon A, Brochet MS, et al. Increase in transaminase levels following the use of raltegravir in a woman with a high HIV viral load at 35 weeks of pregnancy. *J Obstet Gynaecol Can*. 2013;35:68-72.
29. Feiterna-Sperling C, Bukkems VE, Teulen MJA, et al. Low raltegravir transfer into the breastmilk of a woman living with HIV. *AIDS*. 2020;34:1863-1867.
30. Aebi-Popp K, Kahlert CR, Crisnel PA, et al. Transfer of antiretroviral drugs into breastmilk: a prospective study from the Swiss mother and child HIV cohort study. *J Antimicrob Chemother*. 2022;77:3436-3442.

R

RAMELTEON

Central Nervous System (Melatonin Receptor Agonist)

PREGNANCY RECOMMENDATION: No Human Data—Animal Data Suggest Low Risk

BREASTFEEDING RECOMMENDATION: Probably Compatible

PREGNANCY SUMMARY

No reports describing the use of ramelteon in human pregnancy have been located. The drug will likely cross the placenta, so some fetal exposure will probably occur. However, the absence of human pregnancy experience prevents a complete assessment of embryofetal risk. Animal data did not show embryofetal toxicity in two species at doses of more than 10 times the RHD. Using this drug during pregnancy should be based on the pros and cons of the mother's clinical need for treatment versus any potential fetal risk that might occur from exposure.

BREASTFEEDING SUMMARY

One report describing the use of ramelteon during human lactation has been located. Ramelteon and its metabolite have been found in human breast milk, so some infant exposure will occur. In one lactating woman, the calculated relevant infant dose (RID) was less than 1%, and no infant adverse events were reported. Breastfeeding while using this drug should be based on the mother's clinical need for treatment versus any potential infant risks. If used, the infant should be monitored for the most common reported adult side effects of dizziness and nausea (both leading to irritability), somnolence, and fatigue (lethargy). Patients may consider pumping and discarding milk during treatment with ramelteon and for up to 15 hours after the last dose, which is approximately 5 half-lives, to minimize exposure to the breastfed infant.

References

1. Prescribing Information. Ramelteon. Actavis Pharma Inc; 2022.
2. Saito J, Tachibana Y, Wada YS, et al. Presence of hypnotics in the cord blood and breast milk, with no adverse effects in the infant: a case report. *Breastfeed Med.* 2022;17:349-352.

RAMIPRIL

Antihypertensive (ACE—Angiotensin-1 Converting Enzyme Inhibitor)

PREGNANCY RECOMMENDATION: Contraindicated (Second and Third Trimesters)

BREASTFEEDING RECOMMENDATION: Probably Compatible

PREGNANCY SUMMARY

One case report describing the use of ramipril to treat hypertension in pregnancy with first-trimester exposure was located. The drug was discontinued at 16 weeks of gestation, and the delivered infant at term had no identifiable birth anomalies. No other studies specific to ramipril use in pregnancy were found. Regarding angiotensin-converting enzyme (ACE) inhibitors in general, use during the second and third trimesters of pregnancy has been associated with fetal renal toxicity, as stated by the Boxed Warning for this drug. Numerous cases of severe oligohydramnios leading to findings of limb contractures, craniofacial deformation, and pulmonary hypoplasia with neonatal death have been reported. These fetal renal effects are often permanent, but if the drug is discontinued as soon as possible, they can be reversible in some cases. However, ACE inhibitors should not be used in the second and third trimesters, if at all possible. Regarding first-trimester exposure to ACE inhibitors in general, there was some concern about teratogenicity, especially of the cardiac and central nervous system. However, two large studies of more than 4,450 first-trimester exposures to ACE inhibitors did not find any increased risks for anomalies compared with other pregnant patients with hypertension on treatment with other antihypertensive agents, or on no treatment at all. Therefore, the final summary determined that the use of ACE inhibitors in the first trimester did not increase the risk for fetal malformations compared with other pregnant women with hypertension. Ramipril and its active metabolite, ramiprilat, will likely cross the placenta, so some fetal exposure will probably occur. However, this limited human pregnancy experience with ramipril prevents a complete assessment of the embryofetal risk. Animal reproduction studies did not show any embryofetal toxicity in three species at doses of less than 10 times the RHD in one and more than 10 times the RHD in the other two. Women of reproductive age using ramipril should be informed of these risks, so that they can closely monitor if pregnancy transpires. If a positive pregnancy test occurs, she and her health care providers can modify treatment (if possible) so that the drug is not used in the second or third trimesters. For treating hypertension in pregnancy, the American College of Obstetricians and Gynecologists (ACOG) recommends nifedipine and labetalol as first-line agents.

BREASTFEEDING SUMMARY

No studies have been located that describe the use of ramipril during human lactation. The drug and active metabolite will probably be excreted into breast milk, so some infant exposure will likely occur. Other ACE inhibitors are excreted into human breast milk. Due to a concern for potential serious adverse effects that might be seen in a breastfed infant, the manufacturer recommends that women not breastfeed while being treated with this drug. Nevertheless, breastfeeding while using this drug should be based on the mother's clinical need for treatment. If used, the infant should be monitored for the most common reported adult side effects of headache and dizziness (both leading to irritability), fatigue (lethargy), and cough.

References

1. Prescribing Information. Altace. Pfizer Inc; 2019.
2. Chronic hypertension in pregnancy. ACOG Practice Bulletin No. 203. American College of Obstetricians and Gynecologists. *Obstet Gynecol*. 2019;133:e26-e50.
3. Gestational hypertension and preeclampsia. ACOG Practice Bulletin No. 222. American College of Obstetricians and Gynecologists. *Obstet Gynecol*. 2020;135:e237-e260.
4. Kolagasi O, Sari F, Akar M, Sari R. Normal pregnancy and healthy child after continued exposure to gliclazide and ramipril during pregnancy. *Ann Pharmacother*. 2009;43:147-149.
5. Barr M Jr. Teratogen update: angiotensin-converting enzyme inhibitors. *Teratology*. 1994;50:399-409.
6. Shotan A, Widerhorn J, Hurst A, Elkayam U. Risks of angiotensin-converting enzyme inhibition during pregnancy: experimental and clinical evidence, potential mechanisms, and recommendations for use. *Am J Med*. 1994;96:451-456.
7. Cooper WO, Hernandez-Diaz S, Arbogast PG, et al. Major congenital malformations after first-trimester exposure to ACE inhibitors. *N Engl J Med*. 2006;354:2443-2451.
8. Bateman BT, Patorno E, Desai RJ, et al. Angiotensin-converting enzyme inhibitors and the risk of congenital malformations. *Obstet Gynecol*. 2017;129:174-184.
9. Li DK, Yang C, Andrade S, et al. Maternal exposure to angiotensin converting enzyme inhibitors in the first trimester and risk of malformations in offspring: a retrospective cohort study. *BMJ*. 2011;343:d5931.

RAMUCIRUMAB

Antineoplastic (Vascular Endothelial Growth Factor Receptor 2 Inhibitor)

PREGNANCY RECOMMENDATION: No Human Data and No Relevant Animal Data

BREASTFEEDING RECOMMENDATION: Probably Compatible

PREGNANCY SUMMARY

No reports describing the use of ramucirumab during human pregnancy have been located. Vascular endothelial growth factor (VEGF) is important for the developing fetus, especially in the first trimester. As an immunoglobulin G (IgG) antibody, it likely crosses the placenta, especially during the second half of gestation, so some fetal exposure will probably occur. However, monoclonal antibodies are not expected to cross the placenta until after the first trimester is complete. Therefore, the absence of human pregnancy experience prevents a complete assessment of embryofetal risk. No animal studies with ramucirumab have been conducted. However, in animals with interrupted VEGF signaling or an absent VEGFR2 gene, embryofetal toxicity has been observed. Based on animal studies and the drug's mechanism of action, the manufacturer recommends that women with reproductive potential use effective contraception during treatment and for 3 months after the last dose. Nevertheless, using this drug during pregnancy should be based on the pros and cons of the mother's clinical need for treatment versus any potential fetal risk that might occur from exposure. There is a registry for women who are pregnant and have cancer. For more information, women and health care providers are encouraged to contact the Cancer and Pregnancy Registry at 1-877-635-4499. Hypertension was reported in up to 26% of patients treated with this drug in clinical trials.

R

BREASTFEEDING SUMMARY

No reports describing the use of ramucirumab during human lactation have been located. It is known that IgG antibodies can be found in human breast milk, but are not found in the neonatal or infant circulation. Additionally, if any IgG antibodies were to be ingested through breastfeeding, they would probably be digested in the infant's gastrointestinal tract and not be absorbed. Due to a concern for potential serious adverse effects that might be seen in a breastfed infant, the manufacturer recommends that women not breastfeed while being treated with this drug and for at least 2 months after the last dose. Nevertheless, breastfeeding while using this drug should be based on the mother's clinical need for treatment versus any potential infant risks that might occur. If used, the infant should be monitored for the most common reported adult side effects of abdominal pain and nausea (both leading to irritability), hypertension, diarrhea, fatigue (lethargy), peripheral edema, decreased appetite, ascites, and various laboratory abnormalities (see Prescribing Information [PI]).

Reference

1. Prescribing Information. Cyramza. Eli Lilly and Company; 2022.

RANIBIZUMAB OPHTHALMIC

Ophthalmic (Vascular Endothelial Growth Factor Inhibitor)

PREGNANCY RECOMMENDATION: Limited Human Data—No Relevant Animal Data

BREASTFEEDING RECOMMENDATION: Probably Compatible

PREGNANCY SUMMARY

Five reports describing the use of ranibizumab ophthalmic in 17 patients during human pregnancy have been located. The reported exposures occurred in all trimesters. In the limited data, ranibizumab does not appear to increase maternal or fetal risks. The predicted amount of antibody in the systemic circulation, however, is about 90,000-fold lower than the amounts in the vitreous humor and is below the estimated therapeutic concentration. In addition, for antibodies to cross, the Fc (crystallizable fragment) portion is required. This would suggest that ranibizumab (a Fab only) will not transfer. Based on these issues, exposure to the embryo or fetus is probably close to zero. Thus, if a woman requires ranibizumab, it should not be withheld because of pregnancy. Embryofetal toxicity was observed in one species of animal, but at doses 13 times the RHD and administered every 2 weeks instead of every 4 weeks. Using this drug during pregnancy should be based on the pros and cons of the mother's clinical need for treatment. If used during pregnancy, consider placing pressure over the tear duct in the corner of the eye for at least 1 minute, and then remove any excess solution with absorbent tissue to decrease the amount of drug reaching the systemic circulation even further.

BREASTFEEDING SUMMARY

There are four publications describing six patients using ranibizumab during human lactation. The high molecular weight (MW) suggests that it will not be excreted into human breast milk. However, it is known that IgG antibodies can be found in human breast milk, but are not found in the neonatal or infant circulation. Additionally, if any IgG antibodies were to be ingested through breastfeeding, they would probably be digested in the infant's gastrointestinal tract and not be absorbed. In one case report, ranibizumab levels were not detected in either the breast milk or the infant's blood. The breastfed infant, along with three unexposed infants of the same age, had serum VEGF-A levels checked. In all the infants, plasma VEGF-A levels were below the lower level of quantitation except for the two time points in breastfed infants (~13 pg/mL on day 11 in one infant and ~20 pg/mL on day 9 in the second). Another case report found that breast milk VEGF-A levels significantly decreased within 6 to 12 hours after each injection with a maximum decrease of less than 40%, but then returned to preinjection levels or higher within 24 hours postinjection. Due to a concern for potential serious adverse effects that might be seen in a breastfed infant, the manufacturer recommends that the drug be used with caution during breastfeeding while being treated with this drug. Nevertheless, breastfeeding while using this drug should be based on the mother's clinical need for treatment versus any potential infant risks that might occur. Systemic side effects were not evaluated because of the ophthalmic use. A method to decrease some systemic absorption with ophthalmic use is described above in the Pregnancy Summary.

References

1. Prescribing Information. Byooviz. Biogen Inc; 2023.
2. Sarhianaki A, Katsimpris A, Petropoulos IK, et al. Intravitreal administration of ranibizumab for idiopathic choroidal neovascularization in a pregnant woman. *Klin Monbl Augenheilkd*. 2012;229:451-453.
3. Jouve L, Akesbi J, Nordmann JP. Safety and efficacy of ranibizumab for pregnant women in idiopathic choroidal neovascularization. *Acta Ophthal*. 2015;93:e597-e598.
4. Fossum P, Couret C, Briend B, Weber M, Lagarce L. Safety of intravitreal injection of ranibizumab in early pregnancy: a series of three cases. *Eye*. 2018;32:830-832.
5. Pencak M, Veith M. Intravitreal ranibizumab in pregnant patient with myopic choroidal neovascular membrane. A case report. *Cesk Slov Oftalmol*. 2022;78:79-83.
6. Ong AY, Kiire CA, Frise, et al. Intravitreal anti-vascular endothelial growth factor injections in pregnancy and breastfeeding: a case series and systematic review of the literature. *Eye*. 2024;38:951-963.
7. Ehlken C, Martin G, Stahl A, Agostini HT. Reduction of vascular endothelial growth factor A in human breast milk after intravitreal injection of bevacizumab but not ranibizumab. *Arch Ophthal*. 2012;130:1226-1227.
8. Juncal V, Kohly R, Marafon SB, et al. Levels of systemic VEGF-A and ranibizumab in the infant of a nursing mother receiving intravitreal ranibizumab therapy followed by a 'pump and dump' strategy. *IOVS*. 2021;62:446. https://iovs.arvojournals.org/article.aspx?articleid=2772812
9. Huang Y, Zhou R, Sun Z, et al. Vascular endothelial growth factor-A level in human breast milk after intravitreal injection of ranibizumab: a case report. *Int Breastfeed J*. 2022;17:25.

RANOLAZINE

Cardiovascular (Antianginal Agent)

PREGNANCY RECOMMENDATION: No Human Data—Animal Data Suggest Potential Risk

BREASTFEEDING RECOMMENDATION: Potential Toxicity

PREGNANCY SUMMARY

No reports describing the use of ranolazine in human pregnancy have been located. Ranolazine is likely to cross the placenta, so some fetal exposure will probably occur. However, the absence of human pregnancy experience prevents a complete assessment of embryofetal risk. Animal data showed embryofetal toxicity in two species at doses of less than 10 times the RHD. However, some maternal toxicity also occurred at these dosages. Using this drug during pregnancy should be based on the pros and cons of the mother's clinical need for treatment versus any potential fetal risk that might occur from exposure. Ranolazine can prolong the QTc in a dose-related manner.

BREASTFEEDING SUMMARY

No reports describing the use of ranolazine during human lactation have been located. The drug will likely be excreted into breast milk, so some infant exposure will probably occur. Breastfeeding while using this drug should be based on the mother's clinical need for treatment versus any potential infant risks that might occur. If used, the infant should be monitored for the most common reported adult side effects of dizziness, headache, and nausea (all leading to irritability) and constipation.

Reference

1. Prescribing Information. Ranolazine extended release. Graviti Pharmaceuticals Private Limited; 2021.

RASAGILINE

Central Nervous System (Anti-Parkinson—MAO Type B Inhibitor)

PREGNANCY RECOMMENDATION: Limited Human Data—Animal Data Suggest Potential Risk

BREASTFEEDING RECOMMENDATION: Potential Toxicity

PREGNANCY SUMMARY

One report describing the use of rasagiline in human pregnancy has been located. Seven women were taking rasagiline in combination with other medications at the time of conception. Six women discontinued the drug shortly after pregnancy was diagnosed, while one woman continued throughout pregnancy. Of the seven exposures, there was one spontaneous abortion and one diagnosed with Down syndrome. Of the remaining five infants, no congenital anomalies were identified. Rasagiline is likely to cross the placenta, so some fetal exposure will probably occur. However, this limited human pregnancy experience prevents a complete assessment of embryofetal risk. Embryofetal toxicity was observed in one species of animal, but at doses of about 10 times the RHD. Using this drug during pregnancy should be based on the pros and cons of the mother's clinical need for treatment versus any potential fetal risk that might occur from exposure.

BREASTFEEDING SUMMARY

No reports describing the use of rasagiline during human lactation have been located. The drug will likely be found in breast milk, so some infant exposure will probably occur. Breastfeeding while using this drug should be based on the mother's clinical need for treatment versus any potential infant risks that might occur. If used, the infant should be monitored for the most common reported adult side effects of arthralgia, flu-like symptoms, and dyspepsia (all leading to irritability), peripheral edema, cough, and insomnia.

References

1. Prescribing Information. Rasagiline mesylate. Avet Pharmaceuticals Inc; 2023.
2. Tufekcioglu Z, Hanagasi H, Yalcin Cakmakli G, et al. Use of anti-Parkinson medication during pregnancy: a case series. *J Neurol*. 2018;265:1922-1929.

RASBURICASE

Antineoplastic (Recombinant Urate Oxidase Enzyme)

PREGNANCY RECOMMENDATION: Limited Human Data—Animal Data Suggest Potential Risk

BREASTFEEDING RECOMMENDATION: Probably Compatible

PREGNANCY SUMMARY

One report describing the use of rasburicase during human pregnancy has been located. Exposure occurred in the third trimester near delivery, and the delivered newborn did well with no reported adverse reactions related to the drug. While the MW suggests that the drug will not cross, because it is a protein, it is not known whether some placental transfer might occur in the second half of pregnancy. However, this limited human pregnancy experience prevents a complete assessment of embryofetal risk. Embryofetal toxicity with malformations was observed in one species of animal at doses of about 5 times the RHD. Using this drug during pregnancy should be based on the pros and cons of the mother's clinical need for treatment versus any potential fetal risk that might occur from exposure. There is a registry for women who are pregnant and have cancer. For more information, women and health care providers are encouraged to contact the Cancer and Pregnancy Registry at 1-877-635-4499.

BREASTFEEDING SUMMARY

No reports describing the use of rasburicase during human lactation have been located. The high MW suggests that clinically significant amounts will not be excreted into breast milk. In addition, because it is a protein, if the drug were to be ingested through breastfeeding, it would probably be digested in the infant's gastrointestinal tract and not be absorbed. Due to a concern for potential serious adverse effects that might be seen in a breastfed infant, the manufacturer recommends that women not breastfeed while being treated with this drug and for at least 2 weeks after the last dose. Nevertheless, breastfeeding while using this drug should be based on the mother's clinical need for treatment versus any potential infant risks that might occur. If used, the infant should be monitored for the most common reported adult side effects (when used in combination with other antineoplastic medications) of nausea, headache, abdominal pain, and pharyngeal pain (all leading to irritability), vomiting, fever, peripheral edema, constipation, diarrhea, hypophosphatemia, and increased alanine aminotransferase.

Reference

1. Prescribing Information. Elitek. Sanofi-Aventis U.S. LLC; 2022.

RAVULIZUMAB

Terminal Complement Inhibitor (Monoclonal Antibody)

PREGNANCY RECOMMENDATION: No Human Data—Animal Data Suggest Potential Risk

BREASTFEEDING RECOMMENDATION: Probably Compatible

PREGNANCY SUMMARY

No reports describing the use of ravulizumab in human pregnancy have been located. Because it is an IgG antibody, it probably crosses the placenta, so some fetal exposure is likely to occur. However, the absence of human pregnancy experience prevents a complete assessment of the embryofetal risk. Animal studies did show embryofetal toxicity in male offspring. There is also a theoretical concern that the use of this drug could result in terminal complement inhibition in the fetal circulation. The drug may also increase the risk for life-threatening meningococcal infections. Using this drug during pregnancy should be based on the pros and cons of the mother's clinical need for treatment versus any fetal risk that might occur from exposure.

R

BREASTFEEDING SUMMARY

Ravulizumab probably enters breast milk. However, it is known that IgG antibodies can be found in human breast milk, but are not found in the neonatal or infant circulation. Additionally, if any IgG antibodies were to be ingested through breastfeeding, they would probably be digested in the infant's gastrointestinal tract and not be absorbed. Nevertheless, the manufacturer recommends that women not breastfeed their infants if treated with this drug and for 8 months after the last dose. However, breastfeeding while using ravulizumab should be based on the mother's clinical need for treatment. If used, the infant should be monitored for the most common reported adult side effects of headache (leading to irritability) and upper respiratory tract infections.

Reference

1. Prescribing Information. Ultomiris. Alexion Pharmaceuticals Inc; 2020.

RAXIBACUMAB

Antitoxin (Anthrax—Monoclonal Antibody)

PREGNANCY RECOMMENDATION: No Human Data—Animal Data Suggest Low Risk

BREASTFEEDING RECOMMENDATION: Probably Compatible

PREGNANCY SUMMARY

No reports describing the use of raxibacumab in human pregnancy have been located. As an IgG antibody, raxibacumab likely crosses the placenta, so some fetal exposure will probably occur. However, the absence of human pregnancy experience prevents a complete assessment of embryofetal risk. Animal data did not show any embryofetal toxicity. Using this drug during pregnancy should be based on the pros and cons of the mother's clinical need for treatment versus any potential fetal risk that might occur from exposure.

BREASTFEEDING SUMMARY

No reports describing the use of raxibacumab during human lactation have been located. The drug is likely present in breast milk. However, it is known that IgG antibodies can be found in human breast milk but are not found in the neonatal or infant circulation. Additionally, if any IgG antibodies were to be ingested through breastfeeding, they would probably be digested in the infant's gastrointestinal tract and not be absorbed. Breastfeeding while using this drug should be based on the mother's clinical need for treatment. If used, the infant should be monitored for the most common reported adult side effects of pain and pruritus (both leading to irritability), rash, and somnolence.

Reference

1. Prescribing Information. Raxibacumab. GlaxoSmithKline; 2017.

REGORAFENIB

Antineoplastic (Tyrosine Kinase and VEGF Inhibitor)

PREGNANCY RECOMMENDATION: No Human Data—Animal Data Suggest Risk

BREASTFEEDING RECOMMENDATION: Potential Toxicity

PREGNANCY SUMMARY

No reports describing the use of regorafenib in human pregnancy have been located. Regorafenib is likely to cross the placenta, so some fetal exposure will probably occur. However, the absence of human pregnancy experience prevents a complete assessment of embryofetal risk. Embryofetal toxicity with malformations was observed in two animal species at doses less than the RHD. Based on animal studies and the drug's mechanism of action, the manufacturer recommends that women with reproductive potential use effective contraception during treatment and for 2 months after the last dose. They also recommend that males with female partners of reproductive potential use effective contraception during treatment and for 2 months after the last dose. Nevertheless, using this drug during pregnancy should be based on the pros and cons of the mother's clinical need for treatment versus any potential fetal risk that might occur from exposure. There is a registry for women who are pregnant and have cancer. For more information, women and health care providers are encouraged to contact the Cancer and Pregnancy Registry at 1-877-635-4499. Hypertension was reported in up to 59% of patients treated with this drug in clinical trials.

BREASTFEEDING SUMMARY

No reports describing the use of regorafenib during human lactation have been located. The drug and its metabolites will likely be excreted into breast milk, so some infant exposure will probably occur. Due to a concern for potential serious adverse effects that might be seen in a breastfed infant, the manufacturer recommends that women not breastfeed while being treated with this drug and for at least 2 weeks after the last dose. Nevertheless, breastfeeding while using this drug should be based on the mother's clinical need for treatment versus any potential infant risks that might occur. If used, the infant should be monitored for the most common reported adult side effects of myalgia and nausea (both leading to irritability), fatigue (lethargy), diarrhea, decreased appetite, hypertension, infections, and hyperbilirubinemia.

Reference

1. Prescribing Information. Stivarga. Bayer Healthcare Pharmaceuticals Inc; 2020.

RELATLIMAB (Available With Nivolumab)

Antineoplastic (Anti-LAG-3 Monoclonal Antibody)

PREGNANCY RECOMMENDATION: No Human Data and No Relevant Animal Data

BREASTFEEDING RECOMMENDATION: Probably Compatible

PREGNANCY SUMMARY

Relatlimab is only available in a combination product with nivolumab. No reports describing the use of relatlimab in human pregnancy have been located. Several case reports describing the successful use of nivolumab during pregnancy have been identified (see nivolumab). As IgG antibodies, both drugs are likely to cross the placenta, so some fetal exposure will probably occur. Therefore, the absence of human pregnancy experience prevents a complete assessment of embryofetal risk. No animal studies have been conducted with relatlimab. One of the functions of the programmed death receptor-1 (PD-1) pathway is to preserve pregnancy by maintaining immune tolerance to the fetus. Therefore, there is a theoretical concern for using nivolumab during pregnancy. Animal studies with nivolumab did show embryofetal toxicity, but at doses 9 to 42 times the RHD. Based on animal studies and the drug's mechanism of action, the manufacturer recommends that women with reproductive potential use effective contraception during treatment and for at least 5 months after the last dose. Nevertheless, using this drug during pregnancy should be based on the pros and cons of the mother's clinical need for treatment versus any potential fetal risk that might occur from exposure.

BREASTFEEDING SUMMARY

No reports describing the use of nivolumab or relatlimab during human lactation have been located. It is known that IgG antibodies can be found in human breast milk, but are not found in the neonatal or infant circulation. Additionally, if any IgG antibodies were to be ingested through breastfeeding, they would probably be digested in the infant's gastrointestinal tract and not be absorbed. Regardless, due to the concern for potential serious adverse effects that might be seen in a breastfed infant, the manufacturer recommends that women not breastfeed while being treated with this drug and for at least 5 months after the last dose. Nevertheless, breastfeeding while using this drug should be based on the mother's clinical need for treatment. If used, the infant should be monitored for the most common reported adult side effects of musculoskeletal pain and pruritus (both leading to irritability), lethargy, rash, diarrhea, and various laboratory abnormalities (see PI).

Reference

1. Prescribing Information. Opdualag. Bristol-Myers Squibb; 2022.

RELUGOLIX

Antineoplastic (Gonadotropin-Releasing Hormone Receptor Antagonist)

PREGNANCY RECOMMENDATION: *Contraindicated

BREASTFEEDING RECOMMENDATION: *Contraindicated

PREGNANCY SUMMARY

No reports describing the use of relugolix in human pregnancy have been located. Some amount of the drug will likely cross the placenta. However, the absence of human pregnancy experience prevents a complete assessment of the embryofetal risk. The drug appeared to be fetotoxic in animals at less than the maximum recommended human dose (MRHD). *However, due to drug indication, relugolix should not be used during pregnancy. The manufacturer recommends that males with female partners of reproductive potential use effective contraception while on this drug and for 2 weeks after the last dose. In addition, androgen deprivation may prolong the cardiac QT interval.

R

BREASTFEEDING SUMMARY

Relugolix probably enters breast milk. *However, based on drug indication, it should not be used while breastfeeding.

References

1. Product Information. Orgovyx. Myovant Sciences Inc; 2020.
2. Nakao K, Kuroda K, Horikawa T, et al. Therapeutic effects of an oral gonadotropin-releasing hormone receptor antagonist, relugolix, on preventing premature ovulation in mild ovarian stimulation for IVF. *Reprod Med Biol*. 2022;21:e12422.
3. Hamada M, Michiharu M, Ensaka C, et al. A novel orally active gonadotropin-releasing hormone antagonist, relugolix, is a potential substitute for injectable GnRH antagonists in controlled ovarian stimulation in assisted reproductive technology. *Reprod Med Biol*. 2022;21:e12424.

REMDESIVIR

Antiviral (COVID-19)

PREGNANCY RECOMMENDATION: Limited Human Data—Animal Data Suggest Low Risk

BREASTFEEDING RECOMMENDATION: Probably Compatible

PREGNANCY SUMMARY

One patient with first-trimester exposure to remdesivir at 9 weeks of gestation was located. She delivered at term a healthy newborn. No birth anomalies were identified, and no adverse neonatal events occurred. Some amount of the drug probably crosses the placenta. Animal data did not show any embryofetal toxicity. In a randomized control trial for treating patients with Ebola virus disease, six pregnant patients received the drug, and no fetal toxicity was reported. A large number of studies have reported the use of remdesivir in treating COVID-19 in the second and third trimesters. In 5 large series and 25 case reports and other analyses, more than 200 pregnant women have been treated with remdesivir in the second and third trimesters, and the drug overall was well tolerated with low incidences of serious adverse events. Newborn issues were primarily related to prematurity. Elevated liver transaminases have been reported with the use of remdesivir, and this was mentioned in several studies in this review. However, elevated liver transaminases can occur for pregnancy-related issues and have been reported as a complication of COVID-19 unrelated to drug therapy. Nevertheless, if a pregnant patient is treated with remdesivir, it is recommended that liver transaminases be followed. In addition, one study reported incidental oligohydramnios within 5 days after completing treatment with remdesivir (no other clinical reason for oligohydramnios, such as membrane rupture, hypertension, etc.). Therefore, if a pregnant patient is treated with remdesivir in the latter weeks of the second trimester or third trimester, we recommend that amniotic fluid volume be evaluated posttreatment. The Society for Maternal-Fetal Medicine states that remdesivir can be used in treating both inpatient and outpatient pregnant women with COVID-19. There is a pregnancy exposure registry that monitors pregnancy outcome in patients using this drug during gestation. Health care providers are encouraged to call 1-800-616-3791.

BREASTFEEDING SUMMARY

One case report evaluated the presence of remdesivir in human breast milk. The milk to plasma drug concentrations and relative infant doses for both remdesivir and the predominant active metabolite (GS-441524) were very low (<2%). There is also a report of a newborn treated with remdesivir for Ebola virus disease, and no drug-related issues were reported. Several studies have analyzed human breast milk for the presence of SARS-CoV-2 RNA, and the findings show a rate of less than 5% of breast milk samples. Furthermore, the finding of viral RNA in breast milk does not equate to infectivity. The risk of breastfeeding with bleeding or cracked nipples is unknown. The World Health Organization states that a mother may breastfeed with suspected or confirmed COVID-19. However, they recommend that adherence to infection prevention and control measures should be practiced to prevent contact transmission of the virus to the newborn.

References

1. Prescribing Information. Veklury. Gilead Sciences Inc; 2020
2. Herz-Roiphe R, Kim AY, Kaimal AJ, Goldfarb IT. Utilizing labour and delivery units for remdesivir infusion for high-risk pregnant and postpartum patients with mild-to-moderate disease during a COVID-19 surge. *J Hosp Infect*. 2022;129:38-40.
3. Mulangu S, Didd LE, Davey RT, et al. A randomized controlled trial of Ebola virus disease therapeutics. *N Engl J Med*. 2019;381:2293-2303.
4. Burwick RM, Stephenson KE, Collier AR, et al. Compassionate use of remdesivir in pregnant women with severe coronavirus disease 2019. *Clin Infect Dis*. 2021;73(11):e3996-e4004.
5. Nasrallah S, Nguyen AQ, Hitchings L, et al. Pharmacological treatment in pregnant women with moderate symptoms of coronavirus disease 2019 (COVID-19) pneumonia. *J Matern Fetal Neonatal Med*. 2021;26:1-8.
6. Eid J, Abdelwahab M, Colburn N, et al. Early administration of remdesivir and intensive care unit administration in hospitalized pregnant individuals with coronavirus disease 2019 (COVID-19). *Obstet Gynecol*. 2022;139:619-621.
7. Gutierrez R, Mendez-Figueroa H, Biebighauser JG, et al. Remdesivir use in pregnancy during the SARS-CoV-2 pandemic. *J Matern Fetal Neonatal Med*. 2022;35(25):9445-9451.
8. Marzban-Rad S, Ghafarzadeh M, Bahmani S, Kazemi A. The use of remdesivir among pregnant women and associated clinical outcomes in mother and the child. *Ann Med Surg*. 2022;77:103681.
9. Naqvi M, Zakowski P, Glucksman L, et al. Tocilizumab and remdesivir in a pregnant patient with coronavirus disease 2019 (COVID-19). *Obstet Gynecol*. 2020;136:1025-1029.
10. Igbinosa I, Miller S, Bianco K, et al. Use of remdesivir for pregnant patients with severe novel coronavirus disease 2019. *Am J Obstet Gynecol*. 2020;223:768-770.
11. McCoy JA, Short WR, Srinivas SK, et al. Compassionate use of remdesivir for treatment of severe coronavirus disease 2019 in pregnant women at a United States academic center. *Am J Obstet Gynecol MFM*. 2020;2:100164.
12. Anderson JA, Schauer J, Bryant S, Graves CR. The use of convalescent plasma therapy and remdesivir in the successful management of a critically ill obstetric patient with novel coronavirus 2019 infection: a case report. *Case Rep Womens Health*. 2020;27:e00221.
13. Pierce-Williams RAM, Burd J, Felder L, et al. Clinical course of severe and critical coronavirus disease 2019 in hospitalized pregnancies: a United States cohort study. *Am J Obstet Gynecol MFM*. 2020;2:100134.
14. Maldarelli GA, Savage M, Mazur S, et al. Remdesivir treatment for severe COVID-19 in third trimester pregnancy: case report and management discussion. *Open Forum Infect Dis*. 2020;7:ofaa345.
15. Pelayo J, Pugliese G, Salacup G, et al. Severe COVID-19 in third trimester pregnancy: multidisciplinary approach. *Case Rep Crit Care*. 2020;2020:8889487.
16. Schnettler WT, Al Ahwel Y, Suhag A. Severe acute respiratory distress syndrome in coronavirus disease 2019—infected pregnancy: obstetric and intensive care considerations. *Am J Obstet Gynecol MFM*. 2020;2:100120.
17. Knight M, Bunch K, Vousden N, et al. Characteristics and outcomes of pregnant women admitted to hospital with confirmed SARS-CoV-2 infection in UK: national population- based cohort study, *BMJ*. 2020;369:m2107.
18. Lam H, Lacasse A. Combination of remdesivir, corticosteroid, and convalescent plasma for severe COVID-19 in periviable pregnancy. *Infect Dis Clin Pract*. 2020;28:e21-e23.
19. Lucarelli E, Behn C, Lashley S, et al. Mechanical ventilation in pregnancy due to COVID-19: a cohort of three cases. *Am J Perinatol*. 2020;37:1066-1069.
20. Blitz MJ, Rochelson B, Minkoff H, et al. Maternal mortality among women with coronavirus disease 2019 admitted to the intensive care unit. *Am J Obstet Gynecol*. 2020;223:595-597.
21. Brandt JS, Hill J, Reddy A, et al. Epidemiology of coronavirus disease 2019 in pregnancy: risk factors and associations with adverse maternal and neonatal outcomes. *Am J Obstet Gynecol*. 2021;224:389.e1-389.e9.
22. Rosner-Tenerowicz A, Fuchs T, Zimmer-Stelmach A, et al. Placental pathology in a pregnant woman with severe COVID-19 and successful ECMO treatment: a case report. *BMC Pregnancy Childbirth*. 2021;21(1):760.
23. Singh R, Agrawal A, Asnani M. Remdesivir in pregnant patients with novel coronavirus disease 2019: case series. *J Obstet Gynecol India*. 2022;72(suppl 2):369-371.
24. Yamamoto K, Hagiya H, Maki J, et al. High-dose corticosteroids for a pregnant woman critically ill with coronavirus disease 2019. *Cureus*. 2021;13:e17398.
25. Jacobson J, Antony K, Beninati M, et al. Use of dexamethasone, remdesivir, convalescent plasma and prone positioning in the treatment of severe COVID-19 infection in pregnancy: a case report. *Case Rep Womens Health*. 2021;29:e00273.

R

26. Chinen Y, Kinjyo Y, Mekaru K, et al. Critical respiratory failure in pregnancy complicated with COVID-19: a case report. *Case Rep Womens Health*. 2021;30:e00309.
27. Dande R, Qureshi A, Persaud K, et al. Remdesivir in a pregnant patient with COVID-19 pneumonia. *J Community Hosp Intern Med Perspect*. 2021;11(1):106.
28. Saroyo YB, Rumondang A, Febriana IS, et al. Remdesivir treatment for COVID-19 in pregnant patients with moderate to severe symptoms: serial case report. *Infect Dis Rep*. 2021;13:437-443.
29. Singh V, Choudhary A. Treatment with remdesivir in two pregnant patients with COVID-19 pneumonia. *Cureus*. 2021;13(5):e14986.
30. Pagan ME, Ramseyer AM, Whitcombe DD, et al. Management of critically ill pregnant patients with COVID-19 infection in a rural state. *Am J Perinatol*. 2022;39:165-171.
31. Youssef JG, Bitar MZ, Zahiruddin F, et al. Brief report: rapid clinical recovery from critical coronavirus disease 2019 with respiratory failure in a pregnant patient treated with IV vasoactive intestinal peptide. *Crit Care Explor*. 2022;4:e0607.
32. Alavi SMA, Bahrami S, Najafian M. Severe SARS-CoV-2 infection in a 32-week pregnant woman treated with remdesivir-dexamethasone combination therapy: a case report. *Clin Case Rep*. 2022;10:e06241.
33. Valsecchi C, Winterton D, Fakhr BS, et al. High-dose inhaled nitric oxide for the treatment of spontaneously breathing pregnant patients with severe coronavirus disease 2019 (COVID-19) pneumonia. *Obstet Gynecol*. 2022;140:195-203.
34. Sekkarie A, Woodruff R, Whitaker M, et al. Characteristics of treatment of hospitalized pregnant women with COVID-19. *Am J Obstet Gynecol*. 2022;4:100714.
35. Westhoff WJ, Smith LH, Wyszynski DF, Hernandez-Diaz S. COVID-19 pharmacotherapy utilization patterns during pregnancy: international registry of coronavirus exposure in pregnancy. *Pharmacoepidemiol Drug Saf*. 2022;31:804-809.
36. Society for Maternal-Fetal Medicine. *COVID-19 and Pregnancy: What Maternal-Fetal Medicine Subspecialists Need to Know*. Society for Maternal-Fetal Medicine; 2022.
37. Wada YS, Saito J, Hashii Y, et al. Remdesivir and human milk: a case study. *J Hum Lact*. 2022;38:248-251.
38. Dornemann J, Burzio C, Ronsse A, et al. First newborn baby to receive experimental therapies survives Ebola virus disease. *J Infect Dis*. 2017; 215:171-174.
39. Chen H, Guo J, Wang C, et al. Clinical characteristics and intrauterine vertical transmission potential of COVID-19 infection in nine pregnant women: a retrospective review of medical records. *Lancet*. 2020;395:809-815.
40. Chambers C, Krogstad P, Bertrand K, et al. Evaluation of SARS-CoV-2 in breastmilk from 18 infected women. *JAMA*. 2020;324:1347-1348.
41. World Health Organization. *Breastfeeding and COVID-19*. World Health Organization; 2020.
42. Pace RM, Williams JE, Jarvinen KM, et al. Characterization of SARS-CoV-2 RNA, antibodies, and neutralizing capacity in milk produced by women with COVID-19. *mBio*. 2021;12:e3192.

REMIFENTANIL

Pain (Opioid)

PREGNANCY RECOMMENDATION: Human Data Suggest Potential Risk (Third Trimester)

BREASTFEEDING RECOMMENDATION: Probably Compatible (Hold Breastfeeding)

PREGNANCY SUMMARY

Several reports describing the use of remifentanil in human pregnancy have been located. The drug has mainly been used during labor and delivery. It has been shown to cross the placenta, so some fetal exposure will occur. Therefore, the absence of first-trimester human pregnancy experience prevents a complete assessment of the embryofetal risk. Neonatal respiratory depression and sedation immediately after birth are potential complications of all narcotics when administered to a woman during labor. The short duration of remifentanil and its apparent rapid metabolism by the fetus may lessen these potential effects, but additional studies are needed to demonstrate this benefit. Embryofetal toxicity was observed in one species of animal at doses of less than 10 times the RHD. The manufacturer states that remifentanil use during labor or delivery may result in neonatal respiratory depression, so naloxone should be available if needed. Because of this, it is not recommended for use during or immediately prior to labor when other techniques for analgesia may be more appropriate. Nevertheless, using this drug during pregnancy should be based on the pros and cons of the mother's clinical need for treatment versus any potential fetal risk that might occur from exposure. Being an opioid drug, there is always a risk for addiction and misuse. However, because of the very short elimination half-life, this particular opioid drug is not likely to be one that is chronically used. Remifentanil carries a Boxed Warning for an increased risk of serious life-threatening or fatal respiratory depression; with concomitant use of benzodiazepines or other central nervous system depressants.

BREASTFEEDING SUMMARY

One report describing the use of remifentanil in a lactating woman was located. A 2010 report described the use of propofol, rocuronium, xenon gas, and remifentanil in four breastfeeding women during urgent surgery. No adverse effects were seen in the infants when breastfeeding was resumed at 1.5 to 5 hours postsurgery. The drug will likely be found in breast milk, so some infant exposure is possible. However, if there is any concern, waiting for about an hour and 45 minutes after the last dose administration should result in no relevant infant exposure (5 elimination half-lives if the elimination half-life is 20 minutes). Breastfeeding while using this drug should be based on the mother's clinical need for treatment versus any potential infant risks. If used, the infant should be monitored for the most common reported adult side effects of respiratory depression, bradycardia, hypotension, and skeletal muscle rigidity.

References

1. Prescribing Information. Remifentanil hydrochloride. Hikma Pharmaceuticals USA Inc; 2024.
2. Kan RE, Hughes SC, Rosen MA, et al. Intravenous remifentanil. Placental transfer, maternal and neonatal effects. *Anesthesiology*. 1998;88:1467-1474.
3. Scott H, Bateman C, Price M. The use of remifentanil in general anaesthesia for caesarean section in a patient with mitral valve disease. *Anaesthesia*. 1998;53:691-701.

R

4. Bedard JM, Richardson MG, Wissler RN. General anesthesia with remifentanil for cesarean section in a parturient with an acoustic neuroma. *Can J Anesth*. 1999;46:576-580.
5. Manullang TR, Chun K, Egan TD. The use of remifentanil for cesarean section in a parturient with recurrent aortic coarctation. *Can J Anesth*. 2000;47:454-459.
6. Olufolabi AJ, Booth JV, Wakeling HG, et al. A preliminary investigation of remifentanil as a labor analgesic. *Anesth Analg*. 2000;91:606-608.
7. Thurlow JA, Waterhouse P. Patient-controlled analgesia in labour using remifentanil in two parturients with platelet abnormalities. *Br J Anaesth*. 2000;84:411-413.
8. Evron S, Sadan O, Ezri T, et al. Remifentanil: a new systemic analgesic for labor pain and an alternative to dolestine (abstract). *Am J Obstet Gynecol*. 2001;185:S210.
9. Hammadeh ME, Wilhelm W, Huppert A, et al. Effects of general anaesthesia vs. sedation on fertilization, cleavage and pregnancy rates in an IVF program. *Arch Gynecol Obstet*. 1999;263:56-59.
10. Zhou X, Jin LJ, Hu CY, et al. Efficacy and safety of remifentanil for analgesia in cesarean delivery. *Medicine*. 2017;96:e8341.
11. Wilson MJA, MacArthur C, Hewitt C, et al; RESPITE Trial Collaborative Group. Intravenous remifentanil patient-controlled analgesia versus intramuscular pethidine for pain relief in labour (RESPITE): an open-label, multicenter, randomised controlled trial. *Lancet*. 2018;392:662-672.
12. Stuttmann R, Schafer C, Hilbert P, et al. The breast feeding mother and xenon anaesthesia: four case reports. Breast feeding and xenon anaesthesia. *BMC Anesthesiol*. 2010;10:1-5.

REMIMAZOLAM

Central Nervous System (Benzodiazepine—Hypnotic)

PREGNANCY RECOMMENDATION: No Human Data—Animal Data Suggest Low Risk

BREASTFEEDING RECOMMENDATION: Potential Toxicity

PREGNANCY SUMMARY

No reports describing the use of remimazolam in human pregnancy have been located. The drug probably crosses the placenta. However, the absence of human pregnancy experience prevents a complete assessment of the embryofetal risk. Animal data did not show any embryofetal toxicity in one species at doses less than 10 times the RHD. Observational studies of other benzodiazepine drug exposures during pregnancy have not established a drug-associated risk for fetal malformations. Remimazolam is a controlled substance (Schedule IV). Benzodiazepine use during the second half of pregnancy can lead to changes in the fetal heart monitor tracing with a decrease in variability and loss of accelerations that can be prolonged. If used during labor, neonatal depression can occur immediately post-birth.

BREASTFEEDING SUMMARY

Remimazolam probably enters breast milk. Breastfeeding while using this drug should be based on the mother's clinical need for treatment. If used, the infant should be monitored for the most common reported adult side effects of sedation and hypotension. The manufacturer recommends the option of pumping and discarding breast milk for up to 5 hours (approximately 5 elimination half-lives) after administration, if used while breastfeeding.

Reference

1. Prescribing Information. Byfavo. Acacia Pharma Inc; 2020.

REPAGLINIDE

Antidiabetic (Meglitinide)

PREGNANCY RECOMMENDATION: Limited Human Data—Animal Data Suggest Low Risk

BREASTFEEDING RECOMMENDATION: Probably Compatible

PREGNANCY SUMMARY

There have been eight pregnancy exposures reported with repaglinide use during human pregnancy. In two reports, the mothers were taking the drug prepregnancy and discontinued it by 7 weeks of gestation. The third report did not describe the timing or duration of exposure. No malformations were reported. Repaglinide is likely to cross the placenta, so some fetal exposure will probably occur. However, this limited human pregnancy experience prevents a complete assessment of embryofetal risk. Animal studies did not show any embryofetal toxicity in two species at doses of less than 10 times the RHD in one and more than 10 times the RHD in the second. Using this drug during pregnancy should be based on the pros and cons of the mother's clinical need for treatment versus any potential fetal risk that might occur from exposure. ACOG recommends that insulin be used for types 1 and 2 diabetes occurring during pregnancy and, if diet and exercise alone are not successful, for gestational diabetes. Hypoglycemia has been reported in 31% patients treated with this drug. Therefore, if used during pregnancy, glucose levels should be monitored.

R

BREASTFEEDING SUMMARY

No reports describing the use of repaglinide during human lactation have been located. The drug will likely be excreted into breast milk, so some infant exposure will probably occur. The manufacturer states that repaglinide is not recommended while breastfeeding due to a risk for hypoglycemia in the infant. Nevertheless, breastfeeding while using this drug should be based on the mother's clinical need for treatment versus any potential infant risks that might occur. If used, the infant should be monitored for the most common reported adult side effects of headache, arthralgia, nausea, and back pain (all leading to irritability), hypoglycemia (monitor infant glucose levels), and diarrhea.

References

1. Prescribing Information. Repaglinide. Aurobindo Pharma Limited; 2022.
2. American College of Obstetricians and Gynecologists. ACOG Practice Bulletin No. 201: pregestational diabetes mellitus. *Obstet Gynecol.* 2018;132:e228-e248.
3. American College of Obstetricians and Gynecologists. ACOG Practice Bulletin No. 190: gestational diabetes mellitus. *Obstet Gynecol.* 2018;131:e49-e64.
4. Tertti K, Petsalo A, Niemi M, et al. Transfer of repaglinide in the dually perfused human placenta and the role of the organic anion transporting polypeptides (OATPs). *Eur J Pharm Sci.* 2011;44:181-186.
5. Napoli A, Ciampa F, Colatrella A, Fallucca F. Use of repaglinide during the first weeks of pregnancy in two type 2 diabetic women. *Diabetes Care.* 2006;29:2326-2327.
6. Marshall V, Wilton L, Shakir S. Safety profile of repaglinide as used in general practice in England: results of a prescription-event monitoring study. *Acta Diabetol.* 2006;43:6-13.
7. Mollar-Puchades MA, Martin-Cortes A, Perez-Calvo A, Diaz-Garcia C. Use of repaglinide on a pregnant woman during embryogenesis. *Diabetes Obes Metab.* 2007;9:146-147.

REPOTRECTINIB

Antineoplastic (Tyrosine Kinase Inhibitor)

PREGNANCY RECOMMENDATION: No Human Data—Animal Data Suggest Potential Risk

BREASTFEEDING RECOMMENDATION: Potential Toxicity

PREGNANCY SUMMARY

No reports describing the use of repotrectinib in human pregnancy have been located. The drug will likely cross the placenta, so some fetal exposure will probably occur. Therefore, the absence of human pregnancy experience prevents a complete assessment of the embryofetal risk. Animal studies did show embryofetal toxicity with malformations in one species at doses of less than 10 times the RHD. Based on these animal studies and the drug's mechanism of action, the manufacturer recommends that women with reproductive potential use effective contraception during treatment and for 2 months after the last dose. They also recommend that males with female partners of reproductive potential use effective contraception during treatment and for 4 months after the last dose. Nevertheless, using this drug during pregnancy should be based on the pros and cons of the mother's clinical need for treatment versus any potential fetal risk that might occur from exposure. There is a registry for women who are pregnant and have cancer. For more information, women and health care providers are encouraged to contact the Cancer and Pregnancy Registry at 1-877-635-4499.

R

BREASTFEEDING SUMMARY

No reports describing the use of repotrectinib during human lactation have been located. The drug will likely be found in breast milk, so some infant exposure will probably occur. Due to a concern for potential serious adverse effects that might be seen in a breastfed infant, the manufacturer recommends that women not breastfeed while being treated with this drug and for 10 days after the last dose. Nevertheless, breastfeeding while using this drug should be based on the mother's clinical need for treatment versus any potential infant risk that might occur. If used, the infant should be monitored for the most common reported adult side effects of nausea, peripheral neuropathy, and dizziness (all leading to irritability), fatigue (lethargy), constipation, and various laboratory abnormalities (see PI).

Reference

1. Prescribing Information. Augtyro. Bristol-Meyers Squibb; 2023.

RESLIZUMAB

Respiratory (Monoclonal Antibody—Asthma)

PREGNANCY RECOMMENDATION: No Human Data—Animal Data Suggest Low Risk

BREASTFEEDING RECOMMENDATION: Probably Compatible

PREGNANCY SUMMARY

No reports describing the use of reslizumab in human pregnancy have been located. IgG antibodies are known to cross the placenta, especially during the third trimester, which suggests that some transfer will occur. Therefore, the absence of human pregnancy experience prevents a complete assessment of the embryofetal risk. Animal studies did not show any embryofetal toxicity. It is known that women with poorly controlled asthma are at increased risk of preeclampsia, prematurity, and small for gestational age in the neonate. Asthma control should be closely monitored, and treatment adjusted as necessary in pregnant women. Using this drug during pregnancy should be based on the pros and cons of the mother's clinical need for treatment versus any potential fetal risk that might occur from exposure.

BREASTFEEDING SUMMARY

No reports describing the use of reslizumab during human lactation have been located. It is known that IgG antibodies are excreted into breast milk but are not found in the neonatal or infant circulation. Additionally, if any IgG antibodies were to be ingested through breastfeeding, they would probably be digested in the infant's gastrointestinal tract and not absorbed. Breastfeeding while using this drug should be based on the mother's clinical need for treatment. If used, the infant should be monitored for the most common reported adult side effect of pain (leading to irritability).

Reference

1. Prescribing Information. Cinqair. Teva Respiratory, LLC; 2020.

RESMETIROM

Gastrointestinal (Hepatic)

PREGNANCY RECOMMENDATION: **No Human Data—Animal Data Suggest Low Risk (Maternal Benefit May Outweigh Any Fetal Risk)**

BREASTFEEDING RECOMMENDATION: **Probably Compatible**

PREGNANCY SUMMARY

No reports describing the use of resmetirom in human pregnancy have been located. The drug will likely cross the placenta, so some fetal exposure will probably occur. Therefore, the absence of human pregnancy experience prevents a complete assessment of the embryofetal risk. Animal studies did not show any embryofetal toxicity (in the absence of maternal toxicity) in two species at doses of less than 10 times the RHD in one and more than 10 times the RHD in the second. Using this drug during pregnancy should be based on the pros and cons of the mother's clinical need for treatment versus any potential fetal risk that might occur from exposure. Hepatic fibrosis stages F2 and F3 can produce many adverse effects during pregnancy that can also lead to poor outcomes. Therefore, maternal treatment may outweigh any potential fetal risk.

BREASTFEEDING SUMMARY

No reports describing the use of resmetirom during human lactation have been located. The drug will likely be found in breast milk, so some infant exposure will likely occur. Breastfeeding while using this drug should be based on the mother's clinical need for treatment versus any potential infant risk that might occur. If used, the infant should be monitored for the most common reported adult side effects of nausea, pruritus, dizziness, and abdominal pain (all leading to irritability), vomiting, and diarrhea.

Reference

1. Prescribing Information. Rezdiffra. Madrigal Pharmaceuticals; 2024.

RETAPAMULIN

Antibacterial/Topical (Anti-Impetigo)

PREGNANCY RECOMMENDATION: **No Human Data and No Relevant Animal Data**

BREASTFEEDING RECOMMENDATION: **Probably Compatible**

R

PREGNANCY SUMMARY

No reports describing the use of retapamulin in human pregnancy have been located. Given the very low plasma concentrations after topical administration, retapamulin is not likely to cross the placenta. However, the absence of human pregnancy experience prevents a complete assessment of embryofetal risk. Animal data did show embryofetal toxicity in two species, but the drug was administered orally or intravenously (IV). Using this drug during pregnancy should be based on the pros and cons of the mother's clinical need for treatment versus any potential fetal risk that might occur from exposure.

BREASTFEEDING SUMMARY

No reports describing the use of retapamulin during human lactation have been located. The drug will likely be excreted into breast milk, but the very low plasma concentrations with topical use suggest that clinically significant exposure of a nursing infant is unlikely. Breastfeeding while using this drug should be based on the mother's clinical need for treatment versus any potential infant risks that might occur. Due to the topical use of the drug, systemic side effects were not evaluated.

Reference

1. Prescribing Information. Altabax. Almirall LLC; 2023.

RETEPLASE

Cardiovascular (Thrombolytic Agent)

PREGNANCY RECOMMENDATION: Limited Human Data—Animal Data Suggest Potential Risk (Maternal Benefit May Outweigh Any Embryofetal Risk)

BREASTFEEDING RECOMMENDATION: Probably Compatible

PREGNANCY SUMMARY

One report describing the use of reteplase in human pregnancy was located. The drug was administered at 30 weeks of gestation for an acute pulmonary embolism. Heparin was used in the remainder of the pregnancy. At 36 weeks, she gave birth to a healthy infant. The drug is not likely to cross the placenta; however, because it consists of a protein, it is not known whether some fetal exposure could occur in the second half of gestation. Regardless, this limited human pregnancy experience prevents a complete assessment of the embryofetal risk. Embryofetal toxicity was observed in one animal species at doses less than 10 times the RHD. Using this drug during pregnancy should be based on the pros and cons of the mother's clinical need for treatment versus any potential fetal risk that might occur from exposure. If indicated, the maternal benefit appears to outweigh any potential risk to the embryo or fetus.

BREASTFEEDING SUMMARY

No reports describing the use of reteplase during human lactation have been located. The drug will not likely be found in human breast milk. In addition, because it is a protein, if the drug were to be ingested through breastfeeding, it would probably be digested in the infant's gastrointestinal tract and not be absorbed. Breastfeeding while using this drug should be based on the mother's clinical need for treatment versus any potential infant risks. If used, the infant should be monitored for the most common reported adult side effects of bleeding.

References

1. Prescribing Information. Retavase. Chiesi; 2022.
2. Yap LB, Alp NJ, Forfar JC. Thrombolysis for acute massive pulmonary embolism during pregnancy. *Int J Cardiol*. 2002;82:193-194.

RETIFANLIMAB

Antineoplastic (Monoclonal Antibody—Programmed Death Receptor-1 Inhibitor)

PREGNANCY RECOMMENDATION: No Human Data—Animal Data Suggest Potential Risk

BREASTFEEDING RECOMMENDATION: Probably Compatible

PREGNANCY SUMMARY

No reports describing the use of retifanlimab in human pregnancy have been located. As an IgG antibody, the drug is likely to cross the placenta, so some fetal exposure will probably occur. Therefore, the absence of human pregnancy experience prevents a complete assessment of the embryofetal risk. Animal reproduction studies have not been conducted. However, embryofetal toxicity might occur based on the drug's mechanism of action. The main function of the PD-1 and the PD-1 ligand pathway is to preserve pregnancy by maintaining the maternal immune tolerance to the fetus. Use during pregnancy could theoretically increase the risk for spontaneous abortion and stillbirth. Because of this, the manufacturer recommends that women with reproductive potential who are taking retifanlimab must use effective contraception during treatment and for at least 4 months after the last dose. Nevertheless, using this drug during pregnancy should be based on the pros and cons of the mother's clinical need for treatment versus any potential fetal risk that might occur from exposure. Blockade of the PD-1/PD-1 ligand pathway did not result in an increased risk for fetal malformations.

BREASTFEEDING SUMMARY

No reports describing the use of retifanlimab during human lactation have been located. It is known that IgG antibodies can be found in human breast milk, but are not found in the neonatal or infant circulation. Additionally, if any IgG antibodies were to be ingested through breastfeeding, they would probably be digested in the infant's gastrointestinal tract and not be absorbed. However, due to the potential for adverse effects that might be seen in a breastfed infant, the manufacturer recommends that women should not breastfeed while being treated with retifanlimab and for at least 4 months after the last dose. Nevertheless, breastfeeding while using this drug should be based on the mother's clinical need for treatment. If used, the infant should be monitored for the most common reported adult side effects of musculoskeletal pain, nausea, and pruritus (all leading to irritability), lethargy, diarrhea, rash, and pyrexia.

Reference

1. Prescribing Information. Zynyz. Incyte Corp.; 2023.

REVEFENACIN

Respiratory (COPD—Anticholinergic)

PREGNANCY RECOMMENDATION: No Human Data—Animal Data Suggest Low Risk

BREASTFEEDING RECOMMENDATION: Probably Compatible

PREGNANCY SUMMARY

No reports describing the use of revefenacin in human pregnancy have been located. Some amount of the drug will probably cross the placenta, so fetal exposure will likely occur. However, blood levels are low following systemic absorption after inhalation use. Nevertheless, the absence of human pregnancy experience prevents a complete assessment of the embryofetal risk. Animal data did not show any embryofetal toxicity despite being administered subcutaneously. The use of anticholinergic drugs can worsen narrow-angle glaucoma and urinary retention. Using this drug during pregnancy should be based on the pros and cons of the mother's clinical need for treatment versus any potential fetal risk that might occur from exposure.

BREASTFEEDING SUMMARY

Revefenacin probably enters human breast milk. However, there is likely no effect on a breastfed infant due to the very low bioavailability found with oral use (<3%). If the clinical decision is to use this drug while breastfeeding, the infant should be monitored for the most common reported adult side effects of headache and back pain (both leading to irritability), upper respiratory tract infection, and cough.

Reference

1. Prescribing Information. Yupelri. Theravance Biopharma Ireland Limited for Mylan Specialty L.P; 2018.

REZAFUNGIN

Antifungal

PREGNANCY RECOMMENDATION: No Human Data—Animal Data Suggest Low Risk

BREASTFEEDING RECOMMENDATION: Probably Compatible

PREGNANCY SUMMARY

No reports describing the use of rezafungin in human pregnancy have been located. The drug will likely cross the placenta in limited amounts, so some fetal exposure will probably occur. Therefore, the absence of human pregnancy experience prevents a complete assessment of the embryofetal risk. Animal data did not show any embryofetal toxicity. Using this drug during pregnancy should be based on the pros and cons of the mother's clinical need for treatment versus any potential fetal risk that might occur from exposure.

BREASTFEEDING SUMMARY

No reports describing the use of rezafungin during human lactation have been located. The drug will likely be excreted into breast milk in limited amounts, so some infant exposure will probably occur. Therefore, breastfeeding while using this drug should be based on the mother's clinical need for treatment. If used, the infant should be monitored for the most common reported adult side effects of nausea and abdominal pain (both leading to irritability), diarrhea, vomiting, constipation, pyrexia, and various laboratory abnormalities. (see PI)

Reference

1. Prescribing Information. Rezzayo. Patheon Italia S.p.A.; 2023.

RIBAVIRIN

Antiviral

PREGNANCY RECOMMENDATION: *Contraindicated

BREASTFEEDING RECOMMENDATION: Potential Toxicity

PREGNANCY SUMMARY

There have been several publications describing the use of ribavirin during human pregnancy. *Currently, there is a Boxed Warning for use in pregnancy due to a risk for significant teratogenic and embryocidal effects. Ribavirin is likely to cross the placenta, so some fetal exposure will probably occur. Embryofetal toxicity with malformations was observed in two animal species at doses less than the RHD. Based on animal studies and the drug's mechanism of action, the manufacturer recommends that women with reproductive potential use effective contraception during treatment and for 9 months after the last dose. They also recommend that males with female partners of reproductive potential use effective contraception during treatment and for 6 months after the last dose. It should not be started until a report of a negative pregnancy test, and periodic pregnancy tests are also recommended during treatment.

BREASTFEEDING SUMMARY

No reports describing the use of ribavirin during human lactation have been located. The drug will likely be excreted into breast milk, so some infant exposure will probably occur. Breastfeeding while using this drug should be based on the mother's clinical need for treatment versus any potential infant risks. If used, the infant should be monitored for the most common reported adult side effects of headache, nausea, and myalgia (all leading to irritability), fatigue (lethargy), tremors, and fever.

References

1. Prescribing Information. Ribavirin. Aurobindo Pharma Limited; 2023.
2. Prescribing Information. Virazole. Bausch Health US LLC; 2019.
3. Sinclair SM, Jones JK, Miller RK, et al. Final results from the ribavirin pregnancy registry, 2004-2020. *Birth Defects Res*. 2022;114:1376-1391.
4. Kirshon B, Faro S, Zurawin RK, Samo TC, Carpenter RJ. Favorable outcome after treatment with amantadine and ribavirin in a pregnancy complicated by influenza pneumonia: a case report. *J Reprod Med*. 1988;33:399-401.
5. Centers for Disease Control. Assessing exposures of health-care personnel to aerosols of ribavirin-California. *MMWR Morb Mortal Wkly Rep*. 1988;37:560-563.
6. Atmar RL, Englund JA, Hammill H. Complications of measles during pregnancy. *Clin Infect Dis*. 1992;14:217-226.
7. Rezvani M, Koren G. Pregnancy outcome after exposure to injectable ribavirin during embryogenesis. *Reprod Toxicol*. 2006;21:113-115.
8. Hegenbarth K, Maurer U, Kroisel PM, Fickert P, Trauner M, Stauber RE. No evidence for mutagenic effects of ribavirin: report of two normal pregnancies. *Am J Gastroenterol*. 2001;96:2286-2287.
9. Biana S, Ettore G. Male periconceptional ribavirin—interferon alpha-2B exposure with no adverse fetal effects. *Birth Defects Res A Clin Mol Teratol*. 2003;67:77-78.

RIBOCICLIB

Antineoplastic (Kinase Inhibitor)

PREGNANCY RECOMMENDATION: *Contraindicated

BREASTFEEDING RECOMMENDATION: *Contraindicated

PREGNANCY SUMMARY

No reports describing the use of ribociclib in human pregnancy have been located. Some amount of the drug will probably cross the placenta, so fetal exposure will likely occur. However, the absence of human pregnancy experience prevents a complete assessment of the embryofetal risk. Animal studies showed embryofetal toxicity and teratogenicity. Based on these animal studies and the drug's mechanism of action, the manufacturer recommends that women with reproductive potential use effective contraception during treatment and for 3 weeks after the last dose. *Currently, the drug is contraindicated because its recommended use is in postmenopausal women. The drug was also found to prolong the QT interval.

BREASTFEEDING SUMMARY

No reports describing the use of ribociclib during human lactation have been located. Some of the drug probably enters breast milk, so infant exposure will likely occur. However, due to the concern for potential serious adverse effects in a breastfed infant, the manufacturer recommends that women not breastfeed while being treated with ribociclib and for at least 3 weeks after the last dose. *Currently, the drug is contraindicated because its recommended use is in postmenopausal women.

References

1. Prescribing Information. Kisqali. Novartis Pharmaceuticals Corporation; 2020.
2. James AD, Schiller H, Marvalin C, et al. An integrated assessment of the ADME properties of the CDK4/6 inhibitor ribociclib utilizing preclinical in vitro, in vivo, and human ADME data. *Pharmacol Res Perspect*. 2020;8:e00599.

RIFABUTIN

Anti-Infective (Antitubercular Agent)

PREGNANCY RECOMMENDATION: No Human Data—Animal Data Suggest Potential Risk

BREASTFEEDING RECOMMENDATION: Potential Toxicity

PREGNANCY SUMMARY

No reports describing the use of rifabutin during human pregnancy have been located. Rifabutin and its active metabolite are likely to cross the placenta, so some fetal exposure will probably occur. However, the absence of human pregnancy experience prevents a complete assessment of embryofetal risk. Embryofetal toxicity was observed in one animal species at doses of less than 10 times the RHD. Using this drug during pregnancy should be based on the pros and cons of the mother's clinical need for treatment versus any potential fetal risk that might occur from exposure.

BREASTFEEDING SUMMARY

No reports describing the use of rifabutin during human lactation have been located. The drug will likely be excreted into breast milk, so some infant exposure will probably occur. Because of the potential for serious adverse effects that might be seen in a breastfed infant, including leukopenia and neutropenia, the manufacturer recommends that women not breastfeed while being treated with this drug. Nevertheless, breastfeeding while using this drug should be based on the mother's clinical need for treatment versus any potential infant risks that might occur. If used, the infant should be monitored for the most common reported adult side effects of nausea (leading to irritability), rash, and various laboratory abnormalities (see PI).

Reference

1. Prescribing Information. Rifabutin. Greenstone LLC; 2023.

R

RIFAMPIN

Anti-Infective (Antitubercular Agent)

PREGNANCY RECOMMENDATION: Limited Human Data—Animal Data Suggest Risk

BREASTFEEDING RECOMMENDATION: Probably Compatible

PREGNANCY SUMMARY

Several reports describing the use of rifampin in human pregnancy have been located. The rate of congenital birth defects was about 3.7% in about 230 pregnancies with first-trimester exposure. No pattern to the anomalies was seen.

(*continued*)

The drug has been shown to cross the placenta, so some fetal exposure will occur. At term, the cord blood levels were about 30% of the maternal levels. However, this limited human pregnancy experience prevents a complete assessment of the embryofetal risk. Embryofetal toxicity and malformations were observed in three animal species at doses less than 10 times the RHD. Using this drug during pregnancy should be based on the pros and cons of the mother's clinical need for treatment versus any potential fetal risk that might occur from exposure. Untreated tuberculosis during pregnancy has been associated with an increased risk for poor pregnancy outcomes. The American Thoracic Society (ATS)/Centers for Disease Control and Prevention (CDC)/Infectious Diseases Society of America (IDSA) guidelines recommend that tuberculosis treatment should be initiated when the risk of maternal disease is moderate to high. Rifampin may reduce the efficacy of hormonal contraceptives. Advise patients using hormonal contraceptives to use an alternative nonhormonal contraceptive method during treatment.

BREASTFEEDING SUMMARY

The use of rifampin during human lactation has been reported. The drug was found to be excreted into human breast milk, with milk to maternal plasma levels of about 20%. Calculated RIDs were all less than 4% and in most cases, infant serum levels were undetectable, but the lower limit of quantification (LLOQ) was only 117 µg/mL. No reports describing adverse effects in nursing infants have been located. Because the milk concentrations are too low to produce toxicity in infants, the ATS/CDC/IDSA guidelines state that breastfeeding should not be withheld during tuberculosis treatment using first-line medications, which include rifampin. Additionally, the mothers should use supplemental vitamin B_6 if they are taking a regimen that includes isoniazid. However, the manufacturer recommends that a decision needs to be made whether to discontinue breastfeeding or the drug. Regardless, breastfeeding while using this drug should be based on the mother's clinical need for treatment versus any potential infant risks that might occur. If used, the infant should be monitored for the most common reported adult side effects of heartburn, abdominal cramps, headache, dizziness, extremity pain, and visual disturbances (all leading to irritability), anorexia (monitor feeding patterns and growth), fever, drowsiness, fatigue (lethargy), vomiting, jaundice, diarrhea, and various laboratory abnormalities (see PI).

References

1. Prescribing Information. Rifampin. Chartwell Rx LLC; 2023.
2. Maugans C, Loveday M, Hlangu S, et al. Best practices for the care of pregnant people living with TB. *Int J Tuberc Lung Dis*. 2023;27:357-366.
3. Nahid P, Dorman SE, Alipanah N, et al. ATS/CDC/IDSA guidelines for treatment of drug-susceptible tuberculosis. *Clin Infect Dis*. 2016;63:e147-e195.
4. Centers for Disease Control and Prevention. Tuberculosis (TB). Treatment for TB during pregnancy. Accessed July 30, 2024. https://www.cdc.gov/tb/about/pregnancy.html
5. Rocker I. Rifampicin in early pregnancy. *Lancet*. 1977;2:48.
6. Kenny MT, Strates B. Metabolism and pharmacokinetics of the antibiotic rifampin. *Drug Metab Rev*. 1981;12:159-218.
7. Holdiness MR. Transplacental pharmacokinetics of the antituberculosis drugs. *Clin Pharmacokinet*. 1987;13:125-129.
8. Reimers D. Missbildungen durch Rifampicin. Bericht ueber 2 faelle von normaler fetaler entwicklung nach rifampicin-therapie in der fruehsch wangerschaft. *Munchen Med Wochenschr*. 1971;113:1690.
9. Warkany J. Antituberculous drugs. *Teratology*. 1979;20:133-138.
10. Steen JSM, Stainton-Ellis DM. Rifampicin in pregnancy. *Lancet*. 1977;2:604-605.
11. Eggermont E, Logghe N, Van De Casseye W, et al. Haemorrhagic disease of the newborn in the offspring of rifampicin and isoniazid treated mothers. *Acta Paediatr Belg*. 1976;29:87-90.
12. Singh P, Moulton LH, Barnes GL, et al. Pregnancy in women with HIV in a tuberculosis preventative therapy trial. *J Acquir Immune Defic Syndr*. 2022;91:397-402.
13. Vorherr H. Drug excretion in breast milk. *Postgrad Med J*. 1974;56:97-104.
14. Lenzi E, Santuari S. Preliminary observations on the use of a new semi-synthetic rifamycin derivative in gynecology and obstetrics. *Atti Accad Lancisiana Roma*. 1969;13(suppl 1):87-94. As cited in Snider DE Jr, Powell KE. Should women taking antituberculosis drugs breast-feed? *Arch Intern Med*. 1984;144:589-590.
15. Snider DE Jr, Powell KE. Should women taking antituberculosis drugs breast-feed? *Arch Intern Med*. 1984;144:589-590.

RIFAMYCIN

Antibacterial

PREGNANCY RECOMMENDATION: No Human Data—Animal Data Suggest Low Risk

BREASTFEEDING RECOMMENDATION: Probably Compatible

PREGNANCY SUMMARY

No reports describing the use of rifamycin during human pregnancy have been located. The drug, if present in the maternal vascular system, will probably cross the placenta, but the systemic absorption following oral use of the drug in humans is negligible. However, the absence of human pregnancy experience prevents a complete assessment of embryofetal risk. Animal data did not show any embryofetal toxicity in two species at doses of more than 10 times the RHD. Using this drug during pregnancy should be based on the pros and cons of the mother's clinical need for treatment versus any potential fetal risk that might occur from exposure.

BREASTFEEDING SUMMARY

No reports describing the use of rifamycin during human lactation have been located. The excretion of rifamycin into breast milk is not expected because the systemic absorption following oral use of the drug is negligible. Breastfeeding while using this drug should be based on the mother's clinical need for treatment versus any potential infant risks. If used, the infant should be monitored for the most common reported adult side effects of headache (leading to irritability) and constipation.

Reference

1. Prescribing Information. Aemcolo. RedHill Biopharma Ltd; 2021.

RIFAPENTINE

Anti-Infective (Antitubercular Agent)

PREGNANCY RECOMMENDATION: Limited Human Data—Animal Data Suggest Risk

BREASTFEEDING RECOMMENDATION: Probably Compatible

PREGNANCY SUMMARY

There are over 50 patients reported to have used rifapentine during human pregnancy. In the limited first-trimester exposures, it does not appear that the drug increases the risk for major malformations, but the data are mixed for the risk of early pregnancy loss. Rifapentine and its metabolite are likely to cross the placenta, so some fetal exposure will probably occur. However, this limited human pregnancy experience prevents a complete assessment of embryofetal risk. Embryofetal toxicity and malformations were observed in two animal species at doses of less than 10 times the RHD. Using this drug during pregnancy should be based on the pros and cons of the mother's clinical need for treatment versus any potential fetal risk that might occur from exposure. Untreated tuberculosis during pregnancy has been associated with an increased risk for poor pregnancy outcomes. The ATS/CDC/IDSA guidelines recommend that tuberculosis treatment should be initiated when the risk of maternal disease is moderate to high. Rifapentine may reduce the efficacy of hormonal contraceptives. Advise patients using hormonal contraceptives to use an alternative nonhormonal contraceptive method during treatment.

BREASTFEEDING SUMMARY

No reports describing the use of rifapentine or its metabolite during human lactation have been located. The drug will likely be excreted into breast milk, so some infant exposure is possible. The drug is closely related to rifampin, which has been shown to cross the placenta, but in low amounts. In addition, infant serum levels for rifampin were very low or undetectable. For rifapentine, breastfeeding while using this drug should be based on the mother's clinical need for treatment versus any potential infant risks that might occur. If used, the infant should be monitored for the most common reported adult side effects of heartburn, abdominal cramps, headache, dizziness, extremity pain, and visual disturbances (all leading to irritability), anorexia (monitor feeding patterns and growth), fever, drowsiness, fatigue (lethargy), vomiting, jaundice, diarrhea, and various laboratory abnormalities (see PI). Because rifapentine and rifampin are very similar, and because more is known about rifampin, switching to rifampin is an option if the drug is indicated.

References

1. Prescribing Information. Priftin. Sanofi-aventis U.S. LLC; 2021.
2. Maugans C, Loveday M, Hlangu S, et al. Best practices for the care of pregnant people living with TB. *Int J Tuberc Lung Dis*. 2023;27:357-366.
3. Nahid P, Dorman SE, Alipanah N, et al. ATS/CDC/IDSA guidelines for treatment of drug-susceptible tuberculosis. *Clin Infect Dis*. 2016;63:e147-e195.
4. Centers for Disease Control and Prevention. Tuberculosis (TB). Treatment for TB during pregnancy. Accessed July 30, 2024. https://www.cdc.gov/tb/about/pregnancy.html
5. Moro RN, Scott NA, Vernon A, et al. Exposure to latent tuberculosis treatment during pregnancy. The PREVENT TB and the iAdhere trials. *Ann Am Thorac Soc*. 2018;15:570-580.
6. Mathad JS, Savic R, Britto P, et al. Pharmacokinetics and safety of 3 months of weekly rifapentine and isoniazid for tuberculosis prevention in pregnant women. *Clin Inf Dis*. 2022;74:1604-1613.
7. Singh P, Moulton LH, Barnes GL, et al. Pregnancy in women with HIV in a tuberculosis preventative therapy trial. *J Acquir Immune Defic Syndr*. 2022;91:397-402.

R

RIFAXIMIN

Antibacterial (Rifamycin)

PREGNANCY RECOMMENDATION: No Human Data—Animal Data Suggest Risk

BREASTFEEDING RECOMMENDATION: Probably Compatible

PREGNANCY SUMMARY

No reports describing the use of rifaximin in human pregnancy have been located. Rifaximin is not likely to reach the placenta in significant enough amounts due to low systemic absorption. However, the absence of human pregnancy experience prevents a complete assessment of embryofetal risk. Embryofetal toxicity and malformations were observed in two animal species at doses of less than 10 times the RHD for traveler's diarrhea. Using this drug during pregnancy should be based on the pros and cons of the mother's clinical need for treatment versus any potential fetal risk that might occur from exposure.

BREASTFEEDING SUMMARY

No reports describing the use of rifaximin during human lactation have been located. The drug, if found in the systemic circulation, will likely be excreted into breast milk. However, only small amounts of the drug are absorbed, so overall infant exposure is probably small. Breastfeeding while using this drug should be based on the mother's clinical need for treatment versus any potential infant risks. If used, the infant should be monitored for the most common reported adult side effects of headache, nausea, dizziness, and pruritus (all leading to irritability), peripheral edema, constipation, fatigue (lethargy), insomnia, and anemia.

Reference

1. Prescribing Information. Xifaxan. Salix Pharmaceuticals Inc; 2023.

RILONACEPT

Antineoplastic (Interleukin-1 Inhibitor)

PREGNANCY RECOMMENDATION: No Human Data and No Relevant Animal Data

BREASTFEEDING RECOMMENDATION: Probably Compatible

PREGNANCY SUMMARY

No reports describing the use of rilonacept in pregnancy have been located. As it contains the Fc portion of an IgG antibody, it likely crosses the placenta during the second half of pregnancy, so some fetal exposure will occur. However, the absence of human pregnancy experience prevents a complete assessment of the embryofetal risk. Animal studies showed embryofetal toxicity in two species, but at doses of more than 10 times the RHD. Using this drug during pregnancy should be based on the pros and cons of the mother's clinical need for treatment versus any potential fetal risk that might occur from exposure.

BREASTFEEDING SUMMARY

No reports describing the use of rilonacept during human lactation have been located. The high MW suggests that the drug will not be excreted into breast milk. However, it is known that IgG antibodies can be found in human breast milk, but are not found in the neonatal or infant circulation. Additionally, if any IgG antibodies were to be ingested through breastfeeding, they would probably be digested in the infant's gastrointestinal tract and not be absorbed. Breastfeeding while using this drug should be based on the mother's clinical need for treatment versus any potential infant risks. If used, the infant should be monitored for the most common reported adult side effect of upper respiratory tract infection.

Reference

1. Prescribing Information. Arcalyst. Kiniksa Pharmaceuticals (UK) Ltd; 2021.

RILPIVIRINE

Antiviral (Non-Nucleoside Reverse Transcriptase Inhibitor)

PREGNANCY RECOMMENDATION: Human Data Suggest Low Risk (Maternal Benefit Outweighs Any Embryofetal Risk)

BREASTFEEDING RECOMMENDATION: *Contraindicated

PREGNANCY SUMMARY

Several studies describing the use of rilpivirine during human pregnancy were located. In over 800 first-trimester exposures, the major malformation risk was only 2%. The drug has been shown to cross the placenta, and cord blood levels were about

50% of the maternal serum levels. Animal data did not show any embryofetal toxicity or malformations in two species at doses of more than 10 times the RHD. Using this drug during pregnancy should be based on the pros and cons of the mother's clinical need for treatment versus any potential fetal risk that might occur from exposure. Rilpivirine can prolong the QTc.

In 2024, the updated US Department of Health and Human Services AIDS Info guidelines for the use of antiretroviral agents during pregnancy recommend that, in most cases, patients should continue their regimen during pregnancy if it is tolerated, safe, and effective in suppressing viral replication. Additionally, treatment initiation should not be delayed due to concerns about teratogenicity with first-trimester exposure. See the guidelines at https://clinicalinfo.hiv.gov/en/guidelines/perinatal/ for the most updated information. If indicated, rilpivirine should not be withheld in pregnancy since the expected benefit to the mother with HIV outweighs the unknown risk to the fetus. Providers caring for pregnant patients with HIV and their infants can call the national Perinatal HIV/AIDS hotline (888-448-8765) for free clinical consultation. Additionally, there is a pregnancy exposure registry that monitors pregnancy outcomes in patients exposed to antiretroviral medicines during pregnancy. Health care providers are encouraged to call the APR at 1-800-258-4263.

BREASTFEEDING SUMMARY

Rilpivirine has been shown to be excreted into human breast milk. In two cases, rilpivirine was found in all milk samples that resulted in a calculated RID of about 5.6%. Breastfeeding while using this drug should be based on the mother's clinical need for treatment versus any potential infant risks. If used, the infant should be monitored for the most common reported adult side effects of headache (leading to irritability), insomnia, and rash.

*In 2023, the updated US Department of Health and Human Services AIDS Info guidelines state that using replacement of breast milk through formula or pasteurized donor human breast milk from a milk bank eliminates the risk of postnatal HIV transmission to the infant. Using antiretroviral therapy to achieve and maintain viral suppression during pregnancy and postpartum decreases the risk for infant transmission to less than 1% but notes that it is not zero. For patients not on therapy or those without viral load suppression during pregnancy (at a minimum of throughout the third trimester) and at delivery, replacement of breast milk is recommended. Patients on antiretroviral therapy who have a sustained undetectable viral load and who choose to breastfeed or use replacement of breast milk should be supported with this decision.

References

1. Prescribing Information. Edurant. Janssen Products LP; 2024.
2. Panel on Treatment of HIV During Pregnancy and Prevention of Perinatal Transmission. Recommendations for the use of antiretroviral drugs during pregnancy and interventions to reduce perinatal HIV transmission in the United States. Recommendations for the use of antiretroviral drugs during pregnancy. Department of Health and Human Services. Accessed August 2, 2024. https://clinicalinfo.hiv.gov/sites/default/files/guidelines/documents/perinatal-hiv/guidelines-perinatal.pdf
3. Osiyemi O, Yasin S, Zorrilla C, et al. Pharmacokinetics, antiviral activity, and safety of rilpivirine in pregnant women with HIV-1 infection: results of a phase 3b, multicenter, open-label study. *Infect Dis Ther*. 2018;7:147-159.
4. Tran AH, Best BM, Stek A, et al. Pharmacokinetics of rilpivirine in HIV-infected pregnant women. *J Acquir Immune Defic Syndr*. 2016;72:289-296.
5. Schalkwijk S, Colbers A, Konopnicki D, et al. Lowered rilpivirine exposed during third trimester of pregnancy in human immunodeficiency virus type 1-infected women. *Clin Inf Dis*. 2017;65:1335-1341.
6. Antiretroviral Pregnancy Registry Steering Committee. Antiretroviral Pregnancy Registry International interim report for 1 January 1989 through 31 January 2024. Registry Coordinating Center. 2023. www.APRegistry.com
7. Eke A, Chakhtoura N, Kashuba A, et al. Rilpivirine plasma and cervicovaginal concentrations in women during pregnancy and postpartum. *J Acquir Immune Defic Syndr*. 2018;78:308-313.
8. Frange P, Tubiana R, Sibiude J, et al. Rilpivirine in HIV-1-positive women initiating pregnancy: to switch or not to switch? *J Antimicrob Chemother*. 2020;75:1324-1331.
9. Patel P, Ford SL, Baker M, et al. Pregnancy outcomes and pharmacokinetics in pregnant women living with HIV exposed to long-acting cabotegravir and rilpivirine in clinical trials. *HIV Med*. 2023;24:568-579.
10. Aebi-Popp K, Kahlert CR, Crisinel PA, et al. Transfer of antiretroviral drugs into breastmilk: a prospective study from the Swiss mother and child HIV cohort study. *J Antimicrob Chemother*. 2022;77:3436-3442.

R

RILUZOLE

Central Nervous System (Glutamate Inhibitor—Amyotrophic Lateral Sclerosis)

PREGNANCY RECOMMENDATION: Limited Human Data—Animal Data Suggest Risk

BREASTFEEDING RECOMMENDATION: Potential Toxicity

PREGNANCY SUMMARY

Three case reports describing the use of riluzole in the first trimester of human pregnancy were located. Two of the patients continued therapy throughout gestation, and the other patient discontinued at 9 weeks of gestation. No major anomalies were identified in the newborns. The drug will probably cross the placenta, so some fetal exposure will likely occur. However, this limited human pregnancy experience prevents a complete assessment of embryofetal risk. Embryofetal toxicity was observed in two animal species at doses of less than 10 times the RHD. Using this drug during pregnancy should be based on the pros and cons of the mother's clinical need for treatment versus any potential fetal risk that might occur from exposure.

BREASTFEEDING SUMMARY

One report describing the use of riluzole during human lactation was located. A mother who was diagnosed postpartum with amyotrophic lateral sclerosis (ALS) was started on riluzole. The drug was found in all breast milk samples, and the calculated RID was about 1.6%. Breastfeeding while using this drug should be based on the mother's clinical need for treatment versus any potential infant risks. If used, the infant should be monitored for the most common reported adult side effects of nausea, dizziness, and abdominal pain (all leading to irritability).

References

1. Prescribing Information. Riluzole. Ascend Laboratories LLC; 2021.
2. Sarafov S, Doitchinova M, Karagiozova Z, et al. Two consecutive pregnancies in early and late stage of amyotrophic lateral sclerosis. *Amyotroph Lateral Scler*. 2009;10:483-486.
3. Kawamichi Y, Makino Y, Matsuda Y, et al. Riluzole use during pregnancy in a patient with amyotrophic lateral sclerosis: a case report. *J Int Med Res*. 2010;38:720-726.
4. Scalco RS, Vieira MC, da Cunha Filho EV, et al. Amyotrophic lateral sclerosis and riluzole use during pregnancy: a case report. *Amyotroph Lateral Scler*. 2012;13:471-472.
5. Datta P, Rewers-Felkins K, Aurora N, et al. Estimation of riluzole levels in human milk and infant exposure during its use in a patient with ALS. *J Hum Lact*. 2018;34:355-357.

RIMANTADINE

Antiviral (Anti-Influenza-A)

PREGNANCY RECOMMENDATION: Limited Human Data—Animal Data Suggest Low Risk

BREASTFEEDING RECOMMENDATION: Probably Compatible

PREGNANCY SUMMARY

One report describing the use of rimantadine in human pregnancy has been located. There were 104 patients taking rimantadine, amantadine, or both, and 135 patients taking oseltamivir. The exposure timing for the combined treated groups was 13% in the first trimester, 32% in second trimester, and 55% in the third trimester. When antiviral medications were compared to healthy controls, no difference was observed in major or minor malformations. The drug is likely to cross the placenta, so some fetal exposure will probably occur. However, this limited human pregnancy experience prevents a complete assessment of embryofetal risk. No embryofetal toxicity was observed in one animal species at doses less than the RHD. Using this drug during pregnancy should be based on the pros and cons of the mother's clinical need for treatment versus any potential fetal risk that might occur from exposure.

BREASTFEEDING SUMMARY

No reports describing the use of rimantadine during human lactation have been located. The drug will likely be excreted into breast milk, so some infant exposure will probably occur. Due to a concern for potential serious adverse effects that might be seen in a breastfed infant, the manufacturer recommends that women not breastfeed while being treated with this drug. Nevertheless, breastfeeding while using this drug should be based on the mother's clinical need for treatment versus any potential infant risks that might occur. If used, the infant should be monitored for the most common reported adult side effects of nausea (leading to irritability), vomiting, anorexia (monitor feeding patterns and growth), and insomnia.

References

1. Prescribing Information. Rimantadine hydrochloride. Amneal Pharmaceuticals of New York LLC; 2023.
2. Greer LG, Sheffield JS, Rogers VL, et al. Maternal and neonatal outcomes after antepartum treatment of influenza with antiviral medications. *Obstet Gynecol*. 2010;115:711-716.

R

RIMEGEPANT

Central Nervous System (Antimigraine)

PREGNANCY RECOMMENDATION: No Human Data—Animal Data Suggest Low Risk

BREASTFEEDING RECOMMENDATION: Probably Compatible

PREGNANCY SUMMARY

No reports describing the use of rimegepant in human pregnancy have been located. Some amount of the drug probably crosses the placenta. Animal data did not show any fetotoxic effects. However, the absence of human pregnancy experience prevents a complete assessment of the embryofetal risk. There is a pregnancy exposure registry that monitors pregnancy outcomes in women exposed to this drug during pregnancy. For more information, health care providers or patients are encouraged to call 1-877-366-0324.

BREASTFEEDING SUMMARY

No reports describing the use of rimegepant during human lactation have been located. Some drug is probably excreted into breast milk. Breastfeeding while using this drug should be based on the mother's clinical need for treatment. If used, the infant should be monitored for the most common reported adult side effects of nausea and abdominal pain (both leading to irritability).

Reference

1. Prescribing Information. Nurtec ODT. Biohaven Pharmaceuticals Inc; 2020.

RIOCIGUAT

Cardiovascular (Soluble Guanylate Cyclase Stimulator)

PREGNANCY RECOMMENDATION: No Human Data—Animal Data Suggest Risk (Maternal Benefit May Outweigh Any Embryofetal Risk)

BREASTFEEDING RECOMMENDATION: Potential Toxicity

PREGNANCY SUMMARY

No reports describing the use of riociguat during human pregnancy have been located. Riociguat and its active metabolite are likely to cross the placenta, so some fetal exposure will probably occur. Therefore, the absence of human pregnancy experience prevents a complete assessment of the embryofetal risk. Embryofetal toxicity was observed in two animal species at doses of less than 10 times the RHD. The drug carries a Boxed Warning to avoid administration to pregnant females because of the risk of fetal harm. Riociguat is available to females only through a restricted program called the Adempas Risk Evaluation and Mitigation Strategy (REMS). In this program, females of reproductive potential must use an acceptable method of contraception during use and for 1 month after discontinuation. Patients can choose one highly effective form of contraception (intrauterine device [IUD], implant, or tubal sterilization) or a combination of methods (hormonal method with a barrier method or two barrier methods). If a partner's vasectomy is the chosen method, a hormonal or barrier method must also be utilized. The manufacturer also advises educating patients on pregnancy planning and prevention, including emergency contraception. However, numerous drugs have shown embryofetal toxicity in animals at doses much less than those used with this drug. Furthermore, pregnant women with persistent or recurrent chronic thromboembolic pulmonary hypertension and pulmonary arterial hypertension are high-risk, with an increased risk for poor pregnancy outcomes. Therefore, maternal treatment in many cases may outweigh any embryofetal risk.

BREASTFEEDING SUMMARY

No reports describing the use of riociguat during human lactation have been located. The drug and its active metabolite will likely be excreted into breast milk, so some infant exposure will probably occur. Due to a concern for potential serious adverse effects that might be seen in a breastfed infant, the manufacturer recommends that women not breastfeed while being treated with this drug. Nevertheless, breastfeeding while using this drug should be based on the mother's clinical need for treatment versus any potential infant risks that might occur. If used, the infant should be monitored for the most common reported adult side effects of headache, dizziness, and nausea (all leading to irritability), diarrhea, hypotension, vomiting, anemia, and constipation.

Reference

1. Prescribing Information. Adempas. Bayer Healthcare Pharmaceuticals Inc; 2021.

RIPRETINIB

Antineoplastic (Tyrosine Kinase Inhibitor)

PREGNANCY RECOMMENDATION: No Human Data—Animal Data Suggest Risk

BREASTFEEDING RECOMMENDATION: Potential Toxicity

R

PREGNANCY SUMMARY

No reports describing the use of ripretinib in human pregnancy have been located. The drug will probably cross the placenta, so some fetal exposure will likely occur. However, the absence of human pregnancy experience prevents a complete assessment of the embryofetal risk. Animal studies did show embryofetal toxicity and teratogenicity in two species at doses of less than 10 times the RHD. Based on these animal studies and the drug's mechanism of action, the manufacturer recommends that women with reproductive potential use effective contraception during treatment and for 1 week after the last dose. They also recommend that males with female partners of reproductive potential use effective contraception during treatment and for 1 week after the last dose. Nevertheless, using this drug during pregnancy should be based on the pros and cons of the mother's clinical need for treatment versus any potential fetal risk that might occur from exposure. Hypertension was also reported in up to 14% of patients treated with this drug in clinical trials.

BREASTFEEDING SUMMARY

No reports describing the use of ripretinib during human lactation have been located. The drug will probably enter breast milk, so some infant exposure is likely to occur. However, due to the concern for potential serious adverse effects in a breastfed infant, the manufacturer recommends that women not breastfeed while being treated with this drug and for at least 1 week after the last dose. Nevertheless, breastfeeding while using this drug should be based on the mother's clinical need for treatment. If used, the infant should be monitored for the most common reported adult side effects of nausea, abdominal pain, myalgias, and palmar-plantar erythrodysesthesia (all leading to irritability), alopecia, lethargy, constipation, diarrhea, decreased appetite, and vomiting.

Reference

1. Product Information. Qinlock. Deciphera Pharmaceuticals, LLC; 2021.

RISANKIZUMAB

Immunologic (Interleukin 23 Inhibitor—Monoclonal Antibody)

PREGNANCY RECOMMENDATION: **No Human Data—Animal Data Suggest Potential Risk**

BREASTFEEDING RECOMMENDATION: **Probably Compatible**

PREGNANCY SUMMARY

No reports describing the use of risankizumab during human pregnancy have been located. As an IgG antibody, it likely crosses the placenta, especially during the second half of gestation, so some fetal exposure will probably occur. Therefore, the absence of human pregnancy experience prevents a complete assessment of embryofetal risk. Embryofetal toxicity was observed in one animal species at induction doses of less than 10 times the RHD. Using this drug during pregnancy should be based on the pros and cons of the mother's clinical need for treatment versus any potential fetal risk that might occur from exposure. Women who are pregnant and have taken risankizumab at any time during pregnancy are encouraged to contact the pregnancy registry at 877-302-2161.

BREASTFEEDING SUMMARY

No reports describing the use of risankizumab during human lactation have been located. The very high MW suggests that it will not be excreted into breast milk. However, it is known that IgG antibodies can be found in human breast milk, but are not found in the neonatal or infant circulation. Additionally, if any IgG antibodies were to be ingested through breastfeeding, they would probably be digested in the infant's gastrointestinal tract and not be absorbed. Breastfeeding while using this drug should be based on the mother's clinical need for treatment versus any potential infant risks. If used, the infant should be monitored for the most common reported adult side effects of headache, arthralgia, abdominal pain, back pain, and arthropathy (all leading to irritability), fatigue (lethargy), anemia, pyrexia, rash, and various infections.

Reference

1. Prescribing Information. Skyrizi. AbbVie Inc; 2024.

RISDIPLAM

Central Nervous System (Survival Motor Neuron 2 Splicing Modifier)

PREGNANCY RECOMMENDATION: **No Human Data—Animal Data Suggest Potential Risk**

BREASTFEEDING RECOMMENDATION: **Probably Compatible**

PREGNANCY SUMMARY

No reports describing the use of risdiplam in human pregnancy have been located. The drug will probably cross the placenta, so some fetal exposure will likely occur. However, the absence of human pregnancy experience prevents a complete assessment of the embryofetal risk. Animal studies did show embryofetal toxicity in one species at doses of less than 10 times the RHD. Because of the animal data, the manufacturer recommends effective contraception in women of reproductive age during treatment and for at least 1 month after the last dose. Using this drug during pregnancy should be based on the pros and cons of the mother's clinical need for treatment versus any potential fetal risk that might occur from exposure.

BREASTFEEDING SUMMARY

It is not known if risdiplam is excreted into human breast milk. The drug will probably be found in human breast milk, so some infant exposure will likely occur. Breastfeeding while using this drug should be based on the mother's clinical need for treatment. If used, the infant should be monitored for the most common reported adult side effects of pyrexia, diarrhea, and rash.

Reference

1. Prescribing Information. Evrysdi. Genentech Inc; 2020.

RISEDRONATE

Bone Health (Bisphosphonate)

PREGNANCY RECOMMENDATION: Limited Human Data—Animal Data Suggest Risk

BREASTFEEDING RECOMMENDATION: Potential Toxicity

PREGNANCY SUMMARY

Two patients using risedronate before or during pregnancy were described in a review article. No newborn abnormalities were reported. Risedronate is likely to cross the placenta, so fetal exposure would probably occur. However, the absence of human pregnancy experience prevents a complete assessment of embryofetal risk. Embryofetal toxicity was observed in two animal species at doses of less than 10 times the RHD. Using this drug during pregnancy for glucocorticoid-induced osteoporosis or treatment of Paget disease should be based on the pros and cons of the mother's clinical need for treatment versus any potential fetal risk that might occur from exposure.

BREASTFEEDING SUMMARY

No reports describing the use of risedronate during human lactation have been located. The drug will likely be excreted into breast milk, so some infant exposure will probably occur. However, the mean absolute oral bioavailability is less than 1%. Therefore, the amount of drug that might be found in an infant's circulation is thought to be negligible. Nevertheless, breastfeeding while using this drug should be based on the mother's clinical need for treatment versus any potential infant risks. If used, the infant should be monitored for the most common reported adult side effects of arthralgia, back pain, and abdominal pain (all leading to irritability), diarrhea, and flatulence.

References

1. Prescribing Information. Risedronate sodium. Greenstone LLC; 2023.
2. Djokanovic N, Klieger-Grossmann C, Koren G. Does treatment with bisphosphonates endanger the human pregnancy? *J Obstet Gynaecol Can.* 2008;30:1146-1148.

R

RISPERIDONE

Mental Health (Atypical Antipsychotic)

PREGNANCY RECOMMENDATION: Human Data Suggest Low Risk

BREASTFEEDING RECOMMENDATION: Potential Toxicity

PREGNANCY SUMMARY

Numerous studies that describe the use of risperidone during human pregnancy have been located. In a recent review, there were 2,177 live-born first-trimester exposures with risperidone. The crude pooled rate for malformations was 5.3%.

(*continued*)

However, it is uncertain if all of these were major malformations, and no pattern to the anomalies was seen. Overall, atypical antipsychotics, including risperidone, do not appear to increase the risk for major malformations or small for gestational age newborns. The manufacturer notes that use during the third trimester near delivery increases the risk for extrapyramidal and/or withdrawal symptoms in the neonate after delivery. Risperidone has been shown to cross the placenta, so some fetal exposure will occur. Embryofetal toxicity with malformations was observed in two animal species at doses of less than 10 times the RHD. Using this drug during pregnancy should be based on the pros and cons of the mother's clinical need for treatment versus any potential fetal risk that might occur from exposure. Although elevated glucose levels have been reported with atypical antipsychotic drug use during pregnancy, ACOG recommends checking for gestational diabetes using the standard recommendations. ACOG guidelines from 2023 state that the risks of uncontrolled mental health disorders in pregnancy include preterm delivery, fetal growth restriction, adverse neurodevelopmental outcomes, and postpartum psychosis risk. The manufacturer lists maternal risks for untreated schizophrenia and bipolar disorder as increased risk of relapse, hospitalization, and suicide. There is a pregnancy exposure registry that monitors pregnancy outcomes in women using atypical antipsychotic drugs. Health care providers are encouraged to contact the National Pregnancy Registry for Atypical Antipsychotics at 1-866-961-2388.

BREASTFEEDING SUMMARY

Risperidone and its active metabolite, 9-hydroxyrisperidone, are excreted into breast milk. The manufacturer reports a RID of 2% up to about 5% and that sedation, failure to thrive, jitteriness, and extrapyramidal symptoms have been observed in infants after breastfeeding. Several case reports describe the use of risperidone during lactation, and no abnormal development was noted. Breastfeeding while using this drug should be based on the mother's clinical need for treatment versus any potential infant risks. If used, the infant should be monitored for the most common reported adult side effects of headache, dyspepsia, arthralgia, dizziness, and pruritus (all leading to irritability), diarrhea, fever, and rash.

References

1. Prescribing Information. Risperdal. Janssen Pharmaceuticals Inc; 2022.
2. American College of Obstetricians and Gynecologists. Treatment and management of mental health conditions during pregnancy and postpartum: ACOG clinical practice guideline no. 5. *Obstet Gynecol.* 2023;141:1262-1288.
3. Newport DJ, Calamaras MR, DeVane CL, et al. Atypical antipsychotic administration during late pregnancy: placental passage and obstetrical outcomes. *Am J Psychiatry*. 2007;164:1214-1220.
4. Ratnayake T, Libretto SE. No complications with risperidone treatment before and throughout pregnancy and during the nursing period. *J Clin Psychiatry*. 2002;63:76-77.
5. Yaris F, Yaris E, Kadioglu M, Ulku C, Kesim M, Kalyoncu NI. Use of polypharmacotherapy in pregnancy: a prospective outcome in a case. *Prog Neuro-psychopharmacol Biol Psychiatry*. 2004;28:603-605.
6. Dabbert D, Heinze M. Follow-up of a pregnancy with risperidone microspheres. *Pharmacopsychiatry*. 2006;39:235.
7. Kim SW, Kim KM, Kim JM, et al. Use of long-acting injectable risperidone before and throughout pregnancy in schizophrenia. *Prog Neuropsychopharmacol Biol Psychiatry*. 2007;31:543-545.
8. Ennis ZN, Damkier P. Pregnancy exposure to olanzapine, quetiapine, risperidone, aripiprazole and risk of congenital malformations. A systematic review. *Basic Clin Pharmacol Toxicol*. 2015;116:315-320.
9. Coppola D, Russo LJ, Kwarta RF Jr, Varughese R, Schmider J. Evaluating the postmarketing experience of risperidone use during pregnancy—pregnancy and neonatal outcomes. *Drug Saf*. 2007;30:247-264.
10. Damker P, Videbech P. The safety of second-generation antipsychotics during pregnancy: a clinically focused review. *CNS Drugs*. 2018;32:351-366.
11. Nguyen T, Frayne J, Watson S, et al. Long-acting injectable antipsychotic treatment during pregnancy: outcomes for women at a tertiary maternity hospital. *Psychiatry Res*. 2022;313:114614.
12. Viguera AC, McElheny SA, Caplin PS, et al. Risk of poor neonatal adaption syndrome among infants exposed to second-generation atypical antipsychotics compared to antidepressants. *J Clin Psychiatry*. 2023;84:22m14492.
13. Viguera A, Freeman MP, Goez-Mogollon L, et al. Reproduction safety of second generation antipsychotics: updated data from the Massachusetts General Hospital National Pregnancy Registry for atypical antipsychotics. *J Clin Psychiatry*. 2021;82:20m13745.
14. Huybrechts KF, Straub L, Karlsson P, et al. Association of in utero antipsychotic medication exposure with risk of congenital malformations in Nordic countries and the US. *JAMA Psychiatry*. 2023;80:156-166.
15. Wang Z, Chan AYL, Coghill D, et al. Association between prenatal exposure to antipsychotics and attention-deficit/hyperactivity disorder, autism spectrum disorder, preterm birth, and small for gestational age. *JAMA Intern Med*. 2021;181:1332-1340.
16. Straub L, Hernandez-Diaz S, Bateman BT, et al. Association of antipsychotic drug exposure in pregnancy with risk of neurodevelopmental disorders. A national birth cohort study. *JAMA Intern Med*. 2022;182:522-533.
17. Westin AA, Brekke M, Molden E, et al. Treatment with antipsychotics in pregnancy: changes in drug disposition. *Clin Pharmacol Ther*. 2018;103:477-484.
18. Park Y, Hernandez-Diaz S, Bateman BT, et al. Continuation of atypical antipsychotic medication during early pregnancy and the risk of gestational diabetes. *Am J Psychiatry*. 2018;175:564-574.
19. Kulkarni J, Gurvich C, Gilbert H, et al. The use of first and second generation antipsychotic drugs and the potential to develop gestational diabetes mellitus among perinatal patients with psychosis. *Schizophr Res*. 2023;254:22-26.
20. Heinonen E, Forsberg L, Norby U, et al. Antipsychotic use during pregnancy and risk for gestational diabetes: a national register-based cohort study in Sweden. *CNS Drugs*. 2022;36:529-539.
21. Hill RC, McIvor RJ, Wojnar-Horton RE, Hackett LP, Ilett KF. Risperidone distribution and excretion into human milk: case report and estimated infant exposure during breast-feeding. *J Clin Psychopharmacol*. 2000;20:285-286.
22. Ilett KF, Hackett LP, Kristensen JH, Vaddadi KS, Gardiner SJ, Begg EJ. Transfer of risperidone and 9-hydroxyrisperidone into human milk. *Ann Pharmacother*. 2004;38:273-276.
23. Aichhorn W, Stuppaeck C, Whitworth AB. Risperidone and breast-feeding. *J Psychopharmacol*. 2005;19:211-213.

RITLECITINIB

Antineoplastic (Janus Kinase and Tyrosine Kinase Inhibitor)

PREGNANCY RECOMMENDATION: No Human Data—Animal Data Suggest Low Risk

BREASTFEEDING RECOMMENDATION: Potential Toxicity

PREGNANCY SUMMARY

No reports describing the use of ritlecitinib in human pregnancy have been located. The drug will likely cross the placenta, so some fetal exposure will probably occur. Therefore, the absence of human pregnancy experience prevents a complete assessment of the embryofetal risk. Animal data did not show any embryofetal toxicity in two species at doses of more than 10 times the RHD. Using this drug during pregnancy should be based on the pros and cons of the mother's clinical need for treatment versus any potential fetal risk that might occur from exposure. Pfizer has a pregnancy exposure registry that monitors pregnancy outcomes in women using this drug. Health care providers are encouraged to call 1-877-390-2940 regarding any pregnancy exposure with ritlecitinib.

BREASTFEEDING SUMMARY

No reports describing the use of ritlecitinib during human lactation have been located. The drug will likely be excreted into breast milk, so some infant exposure will probably occur. Due to the concern for potential serious adverse effects that might be seen in a breastfed infant, the manufacturer recommends that women not breastfeed while being treated with this drug and for 14 hours after the last dose. Nevertheless, breastfeeding while using this drug should be based on the mother's clinical need for treatment. If used, the infant should be monitored for the most common reported adult side effects of headache (leading to irritability), diarrhea, rash, pyrexia, urticaria, and various laboratory abnormalities (see PI).

Reference

1. Prescribing Information. Litfulo. Pfizer Labs; 2023.

RITONAVIR

Antiviral (HIV-1 Protease Inhibitor)

PREGNANCY RECOMMENDATION: **Human Data Suggest Low Risk (Maternal Benefit Outweighs Any Potential Embryofetal Risk)**

BREASTFEEDING RECOMMENDATION: **Probably Compatible**

PREGNANCY SUMMARY

In the APR, there were 7,479 pregnancies exposed to ritonavir (3,899 in the first trimester, 2,629 in the second trimester, and 934 in the third trimester) in combination with other antiretroviral agents. First-trimester exposure to ritonavir was associated with a 2.46% (88/3,578) risk for malformations in live births. Ritonavir minimally crosses the placenta (cord blood level 5% of the maternal serum level). Embryofetal toxicity was seen in two animal species at doses of less than 10 times the RHD. If indicated, ritonavir should not be withheld in pregnancy since the expected benefit to the mother with HIV outweighs the unknown risk to the fetus. In 2023, the updated US Department of Health and Human Services AIDS Info guidelines for the use of antiretroviral agents during pregnancy recommend that, in most cases, patients should continue their regimen during pregnancy if it is tolerated, safe, and effective in suppressing viral replication. Treatment initiation should not be delayed due to concerns about teratogenicity with first-trimester exposure. See the guideline at https://clinicalinfo.hiv.gov/en/guidelines/perinatal/ for the most updated information. Providers caring for pregnant patients with HIV and their infants can call the national Perinatal HIV/AIDS hotline (888-448-8765) for free clinical consultation. Additionally, there is a pregnancy exposure registry that monitors pregnancy outcomes in patients using antiretroviral medicines during pregnancy. Health care providers are encouraged to call the APR at 1-800-258-4263. The oral ritonavir and lopinavir/ritonavir solutions are not recommended in pregnancy due to high alcohol content (43% and 42%, respectively). However, the total amount of alcohol is not excessive. Additionally, 15% propylene glycol is also found in the lopinavir/ritonavir solution. Because ritonavir may reduce combined hormonal contraceptive efficacy, women taking these products are advised to use an additional barrier method of contraception or use an effective alternative contraceptive method. Elevated glucose levels, new-onset diabetes, or exacerbation of preexisting diabetes have been reported in patients treated with this drug. Therefore, if used during pregnancy, glucose levels should be monitored.

BREASTFEEDING SUMMARY

Ritonavir is excreted into human breast milk. Two studies found that peak milk levels were 7 to 364 ng/mL. The milk to plasma ratio was about 20%. One study found that about 15% of maternal and milk levels were undetectable at 15 hours post-treatment. The authors calculated a RID of less than 1%. In 2023, the updated US Department of Health and Human Services AIDS Info guidelines state that using replacement of breast milk through formula or pasteurized donor human breast milk from a milk bank eliminates the risk of postnatal HIV transmission to the infant. Using antiretroviral therapy to achieve and maintain viral suppression during pregnancy and postpartum decreases the risk for infant transmission to less than 1% but notes that it is not zero. For patients not on therapy or those without viral load suppression during pregnancy (at a minimum of throughout the third trimester) and at delivery, replacement of breast milk is recommended. Patients on antiretroviral therapy who have a sustained undetectable viral load and who choose to breastfeed or use replacement of breast milk should be supported with this decision.

References

1. Prescribing Information. Ritonavir. Camber Pharmaceuticals Inc; 2023.
2. Panel on Treatment of HIV During Pregnancy and Prevention of Perinatal Transmission. Recommendations for the use of antiretroviral drugs during pregnancy and interventions to reduce perinatal HIV transmission in the United States. Recommendations for the use of antiretroviral drugs during pregnancy. Department of Health and Human Services. Accessed October 24, 2024. https://clinicalinfo.hiv.gov/en/guidelines/perinatal
3. Casey BM, Bawdon RE. Placental transfer of ritonavir with zidovudine in the ex vivo placental perfusion model. *Am J Obstet Gynecol*. 1998;179:758-761.
4. Furco A, Gosrani B, Nicholas S, et al. Successful use of darunavir, etravirine, enfuvirtide and tenofovir/emtricitabine in pregnant woman with multiclass HIV resistance. *AIDS*. 2009;23:434-435.
5. Mirochnick M, Dorenbaum A, Holland D, et al. Concentrations of protease inhibitors in cord blood after in utero exposure. *Pediatr Infect Dis J*. 2002;21:835-838.
6. Antiretroviral Pregnancy Registry Steering Committee. Antiretroviral Pregnancy Registry international interim report for 1 January 1989 through 31 January 2024. Registry Coordinating Center. 2024. www.APRegistry.com
7. Rezk NL, White N, Bridges AS, et al. Studies on antiretroviral drug concentrations in breast milk: validation of a liquid chromatography-tandem mass spectrometric method for the determination of 7 anti-human immunodeficiency virus medications. *Ther Drug Monitor*. 2008;30:611-619.
8. Palombi L, Pirillo MF, Andreotti M, et al. Antiretroviral prophylaxis for breastfeeding transmission in Malawi: drug concentrations, virological efficacy and safety. *Antivir Ther*. 2012;17:1511-1519.
9. Corbett AH, Kayira D, White NR, et al. Antiretroviral pharmacokinetics in mothers and breastfeeding infants from 6 to 24 weeks post-partum: results of the BAN study. *Antivir Ther*. 2014;19:587-595.
10. Ramirez-Ramirez A, Sanchez-Serrano E, Loaiza-Flores G, et al. Simultaneous quantification of four antiretroviral drugs in breast milk samples from HIV-positive women by an ultra-high performance liquid chromatography tandem mass spectrometry (UPLC-MS/MS) method. *PLoS One*. 2018;13:e0191236.
11. Dai J, Furquay T, Huseman S, et al. Low nirmatrelvir and ritonavir exposure through breastmilk: analyzing milk concentrations and infant risk. *Clin Pharmacol Ther*. 2024;16:1217-1221.

RITUXIMAB

Antineoplastic/Immunologic (Anti-CD20—Monoclonal Antibody)

PREGNANCY RECOMMENDATION: Limited Human Data—Animal Data Suggest Potential Risk

BREASTFEEDING RECOMMENDATION: Probably Compatible

PREGNANCY SUMMARY

The use of rituximab in human pregnancy has been described in more than 200 cases. All of the live births were healthy, and none had structural anomalies that were thought to be related to the drug. Use during the second and third trimester may decrease B cell levels, resulting in immunosuppression. As an IgG antibody, it likely crosses the placenta, especially during the second half of gestation, so some fetal exposure will probably occur. However, this limited human pregnancy experience prevents a complete assessment of the embryofetal risk. Animal data did not show any embryofetal toxicity or teratogenicity in one species at doses less than the RHD, but did decrease B cell levels for the first 6 months of life. Using this drug during pregnancy should be based on the pros and cons of the mother's clinical need for treatment versus any potential fetal risk that might occur from exposure. There is a registry for women who are pregnant and have cancer. For more information, women and health care providers are encouraged to contact the Cancer and Pregnancy Registry at 1-877-635-4499. Hypertension was reported in up to 12% of patients in the clinical trials.

BREASTFEEDING SUMMARY

Two reports describing 10 women using rituximab during human lactation were located. Despite the high MW, rituximab was found to be excreted into human breast milk, similar to other IgG antibodies. However, even if it is excreted into breast milk, it will probably be digested in the infant's gastrointestinal tract and not be absorbed. In all cases, milk levels were low at less than 1% maternal levels. Using the maximum milk concentrations, the calculated RIDs were well below 1%. A few minor infant infections were observed, but no other adverse infant effects were noted. Regardless, due to a concern for potential serious adverse effects that might be seen in a breastfed infant, the manufacturer recommends that women not breastfeed while being treated with this drug and for at least 6 months after the last dose. Nevertheless, breastfeeding while using this drug should be based on the mother's clinical need for treatment versus any potential infant risks that might occur. If used, the infant should be monitored for the most common reported adult side effects of nausea and headache (both leading to irritability), fever, diarrhea, lymphopenia, anemia, and various infections.

References

1. Prescribing Information. Riabni. Amgen Inc; 2023.
2. Friedrichs B, Tiemann M, Salwender H, et al. The effects of rituximab treatment during pregnancy on a neonate. *Haematologica*. 2006;91:1426-1427.
3. Herold M, Schnohr S, Bittrich H. Efficacy and safety of combined rituximab chemotherapy during pregnancy. *J Clin Oncol*. 2001;19:3439.
4. Kimby E, Sverrisdottir A, Elinder G. Safety of rituximab therapy during the first trimester of pregnancy; a case history. *Eur J Haematol*. 2004;72:292-293.
5. Decker M, Rothermundt C, Hollander G, Rochlitz C. Rituximab plus CHOP for treatment of diffuse large B-cell lymphoma during second trimester of pregnancy. *Lancet Oncol*. 2006;7:693-694.
6. Scully M, Starke R, Lee R, et al. Successful management of pregnancy in women with a history of thrombotic thrombocytopaenic purpura. *Blood Coagul Fibrinolysis*. 2006;17:459-463.
7. Ojeda-Uribe M, Gilliot C, Jung G, et al. Administration of rituximab during the first trimester of pregnancy without consequences for the newborn. *J Perinatol*. 2006;26:252-255.

8. Klink DT, van Elburg RM, Schreurs MWJ, van Well TJ. Rituximab administration in third trimester of pregnancy suppresses neonatal B-cell development. *Clin Dev Immunol*. 2008;2008:271363.
9. Chakravarty EF, Murray ER, Kelman A, Farmer P. Pregnancy outcomes after maternal exposure to rituximab. *Blood*. 2011;117:1499-1506.
10. Ton E, Tekstra J, Hellmann PM, et al. Safety of rituximab therapy during twins' pregnancy. *Rheumatology*. 2011;50:806-806.
11. Alkaabi J, Alkindi S, Riyami N, et al. Successful treatment of severe thrombocytopenia with romiplostim in a pregnant patient with systemic lupus erythematosus. *Lupus*. 2012;21:1571-1574.
12. Perez CA, Amin J, Aguina L, et al. Primary mediastinal large B-cell lymphoma during pregnancy. *Case Rep Hematol*. 2012;2012:197347.
13. Ojeda-Uribe M, Afif N, Dahan E, et al. Exposure to abatacept or rituximab in the first trimester of pregnancy of three women with autoimmune diseases. *Clin Rheumatol*. 2013;32:695-700.
14. Skorpen CG, Hoeltzenbein M, Tincani A, et al. The EULAR points to consider for the use antirheumatic drugs before pregnancy, and during pregnancy and lactation. *Ann Rheum Dis*. 2016;75:795-810.
15. On S, Chang A. Treatment of lymphoma with rituximab and chemotherapy during pregnancy. *Leuk Lymphoma*. 2022;63:2897-2904.
16. Dernoncourt A, Liabeuf S, Bennis Y, et al. Fetal and neonatal adverse drug reactions associated with biologics taken during pregnancy by women with autoimmune diseases: insights from an analysis of the World Health Organization Pharmacovigilance Database (VigiBase). *BioDrugs*. 2023;37:73-87.
17. Schwanke C, Steinle J, Thiel S, et al. Neonatal B-cell levels and infant health in newborns potentially exposed to anti-CD20 monoclonal antibodies during pregnancy or lactation. *Neurol Neuroimmunol Neuroinflamm*. 2024;11:e200264.
18. Gonzalez Caldito N, Graham EL, Grebenciucova E. Rituximab and pregnancy: late-onset neutropenia in a 2-month infant whose mother received rituximab 2 weeks prior to childbirth. *Mult Scler J*. 2024;30:272-274.
19. Bragnes Y, Boshuizen R, de Vries A, et al. Low level of rituximab in human breast milk in a patient treated during lactation. *Rheumatology*. 2017;56:1047-1048.
20. Krysko KM, LaHue SC, Anderson A, et al. Minimal breast milk transfer of rituximab, a monoclonal antibody used in neurological conditions. *Neurol Neuroimmunol Neuroinflamm*. 2020;7:e637.

RIVAROXABAN

Hematologic (Factor Xa Inhibitor)

PREGNANCY RECOMMENDATION: *Contraindicated

BREASTFEEDING RECOMMENDATION: *Contraindicated

PREGNANCY SUMMARY

Four studies describe the use of rivaroxaban during human pregnancy. In most cases, women were taking the drug prior to pregnancy, and it was discontinued upon pregnancy discovery. One patient continued therapy until 26 weeks of gestation. In the VigiBase analysis, rivaroxaban did not signal an increased risk for spontaneous abortion or malformations after exclusion of cases with confounders. *Nevertheless, the drug crosses the placenta, so fetal exposure will occur. Therefore, there is a theoretical risk for fetal hemorrhage. ACOG recommends low molecular weight heparin and heparin for use during pregnancy. Embryofetal toxicity was observed in two animal species at doses of less than 10 times the RHD. Pregnancy-related hemorrhage and/or emergent delivery are of concern because the drug cannot be reliably monitored with standard laboratory testing. Additionally, dosing during pregnancy has not been studied. Current standard laboratory testing cannot monitor the anticoagulant effect of rivaroxaban, and providers should promptly evaluate any signs or symptoms suggesting blood loss by evaluating hemoglobin and hematocrit.

BREASTFEEDING SUMMARY

Rivaroxaban is excreted into human breast milk. There are four published reports of six women using rivaroxaban during lactation. The calculated RIDs were 0.82% to 5%. In three infants that were exclusively breastfed, infant rivaroxaban levels were undetectable. Rivaroxaban had a half-life in milk of 4.7 hours. Four infants received breast milk, and no health or bleeding problems were reported. *However, the drug is orally administered, and if found in breast milk, it can be absorbed by the infant. This theoretically could produce some anticoagulation in the infant. Therefore, as in pregnancy, if the mother needs anticoagulation, low–molecular-weight heparin or heparin should be used.

References

1. Prescribing Information. Xarelto. Janssen Pharmaceuticals Inc; 2023.
2. American College of Obstetricians and Gynecologists. Thromboembolism in pregnancy. ACOG Practice Bulletin No. 196. *Obstet Gynecol*. 2018;132:e1-e17.
3. American College of Obstetricians and Gynecologists. Inherited thrombophilias in pregnancy. ACOG Practice Bulletin No. 197. *Obstet Gynecol*. 2018;132:e18-e34.
4. Rivaroxaban FDA DDAC document. www.fda.gov. As cited by Huisman MV. Further issues with new oral anticoagulants. *Curr Pharm Des*. 2010;16:3487-3489.
5. Bapat P, Pinto LS, Lubetsky A, et al. Rivaroxaban transfer across the dually perfused isolated human placental cotyledon. *Am J Obstet Gynecol*. 2015;213:710.e1-710.e6.
6. Konigsbrugge O, Langer M, Hayde M, et al. Oral anticoagulation with rivaroxaban during pregnancy: a case report. *Thromb Haemost*. 2014;112:1323-1324.
7. Hoeltzenbein M, Beck E, Meixner K, et al. Pregnancy outcome after exposure to the novel oral anticoagulant rivaroxaban in women at suspected risk for thromboembolic events: a case series from the German Embryotox Pharmacovigilance Centre. *Clin Res Cardiol*. 2016;105:117-126.
8. Sessa M, Mascolo A, Callreus T, et al. Direct-acting oral anticoagulants (DOACs) in pregnancy: new insight from VigiBase. *Nature*. 2019;9:7236.
9. Beyer-Westendorf J, Tittl L, Bistervels I, et al. Safety of direct oral anticoagulant exposure during pregnancy: a retrospective cohort study. *Lancet Haematol*. 2020;7:e884-e891.
10. Wiesen MHJ, Blaich C, Muller C, Streichert T, Pfister R, Michels G. The direct factor Xa inhibitor rivaroxaban passes into human breast milk. *Chest*. 2016;150:e1-e4.
11. Saito J, Kaneko K, Yakuwa N, et al. Rivaroxaban concentration in breast milk during breastfeeding: a case study. *Breastfeed Med*. 2019;14:748-751.
12. Muysson M, Marshall K, Datta P, et al. Rivaroxaban treatment in two breastfeeding mothers: a case series. *Breastfeed Med*. 2020;15:41-43.
13. Yamashita Y, Hira D, Morita M, et al. Potential treatment option of rivaroxaban for breastfeeding women: a case series. *Thromb Res*. 2024;237:141-144.

R

RIVASTIGMINE

Central Nervous System (Central Acetylcholinesterase Inhibitor)

PREGNANCY RECOMMENDATION: No Human Data—Animal Data Suggest Low Risk

BREASTFEEDING RECOMMENDATION: Potential Toxicity

PREGNANCY SUMMARY

No reports describing the use of rivastigmine during human pregnancy have been located. The drug is likely to cross the placenta, so some fetal exposure will probably occur. However, the absence of human pregnancy experience prevents a complete assessment of embryofetal risk. Animal data did not show embryofetal toxicity in two species at doses of less than 10 times the RHD. Using this drug during pregnancy should be based on the pros and cons of the mother's clinical need for treatment versus any potential fetal risk that might occur from exposure.

BREASTFEEDING SUMMARY

No reports describing the use of rivastigmine during human lactation have been located. The drug will likely be excreted into breast milk, so some infant exposure will probably occur. Breastfeeding while using this drug should be based on the mother's clinical need for treatment versus any potential infant risks. If used, the infant should be monitored for the most common reported adult side effects of nausea and dyspepsia (both leading to irritability), vomiting, and anorexia (monitor feeding patterns and growth).

References

1. Prescribing Information. Rivastigmine tartrate. Alembic Pharmaceuticals Inc; 2022.
2. Prescribing Information. Rivastigmine. Amneal Pharmaceuticals LLC; 2024.

RIZATRIPTAN

Central Nervous System (Serotonin 5HT 1B/1D Receptor Agonist)

PREGNANCY RECOMMENDATION: Human Data Suggest Low Risk (First Trimester)

BREASTFEEDING RECOMMENDATION: Probably Compatible

PREGNANCY SUMMARY

There are several reports describing the use of rizatriptan and triptans as a class during human pregnancy. In combined data from a few of the larger studies, 30 major (3.7%) anomalies were seen in about 800 first-trimester exposures. No pattern to the defects was seen. In a few large studies analyzing triptan drugs as a group, the same findings were observed. There was no increase in risk for major anomalies above what was expected, and no pattern to the defects was seen. In addition, triptans were not associated with an increased risk for preterm delivery, preeclampsia, median head circumference, or neurodevelopmental delays. However, it is difficult to fully evaluate these findings because all of these issues can be influenced by numerous confounding variables. Rizatriptan is likely to cross the placenta, so some fetal exposure will probably occur. No embryofetal toxicity was observed in two animal species at doses of less than 10 times the RHD. Using this drug during pregnancy should be based on the pros and cons of the mother's clinical need for treatment versus any potential fetal risk that might occur from exposure. Hypertension was reported in more than 10% of patients treated with this drug in the clinical trials. However, the ACOG clinical practice guideline suggests cautious use of sumatriptan for secondary treatment of persistent headache in pregnancy. It is noted that no studies have evaluated the effects of triptans in pregnancy on uterine or fetal blood flow during the second or third trimester. The publication also advises not to use triptans in pregnant patients with cardiac disease or hypertension due to the rare risk of generalized or cardiac vasoconstriction.

BREASTFEEDING SUMMARY

Rizatriptan is excreted into human breast milk. In one study, the peak milk concentrations ranged from about 15 to 106 ng/mL. The calculated RIDs ranged from less than 1% up to about 6%. A few cases of maternal breast engorgement have been reported when using this drug while breastfeeding, but it is uncertain whether this is related to the drug. Breastfeeding while using this drug should be based on the mother's clinical need for treatment versus any potential infant risks. If used, the infant should be monitored for the most common reported adult side effects of pain or pressure sensation and dizziness (both leading to irritability), fatigue (lethargy), and somnolence. ACOG states in the clinical practice guideline that triptans could be used by lactating patients but recommends a shared decision-making approach regarding the need to avoid breastfeeding for a specific timeframe after use.

References

1. Prescribing Information. Rizatriptan benzoate. Bionpharma Inc; 2021.
2. Phillips K, Clerkin-Oliver C, Nirantharakumar K, et al. How migraine and its associated treatment impact on pregnancy outcomes: umbrella review with updated systematic review and meta-analysis. *Cephalalgia*. 2024;44:3331024241229410.
3. American College of Obstetricians and Gynecologists. Headaches in pregnancy and postpartum. Clinical practice guidelines no. 3. *Obstet Gynecol*. 2021;139:944-972.
4. Evans EW, Lorber KC. Use of 5-HT1 agonists in pregnancy. *Ann Pharmacother*. 2008;42:543-549.
5. Nezvalova-Henriksen K, Spigset O, Nordeng H. Triptan exposure during pregnancy and the risk of major congenital malformations and adverse pregnancy outcomes: results from the Norwegian Mother and Child Cohort Study. *Headache*. 2010;50:563-575.
6. Marchenko A, Etwel F, Olutunfese O, Nickel C, Koren G, Nulman I. Pregnancy outcome following prenatal exposure to triptan medications: a meta-analysis. *Headache*. 2015;55:490-501.
7. Spielmann K, Kayser A, Beck E, et al. Pregnancy outcome after antimigraine triptan use: a prospective observational cohort study. *Cephal*. 2018;38:1081-1092.
8. Berard A, Strom S, Zhao JP, et al. Dihydroergotamine and triptan use to treat migraine during pregnancy and risk of adverse pregnancy outcomes. *Sci Rep*. 2021;11:19302.
9. Dudman DC, Tauqeer F, Kaur M, et al. A systematic review and meta-analysis on the prevalence of pregnancy outcomes in migraine treated patients: a contribution from the IMI2 ConcePTION project. *J Neurol*. 2022;269:742-749.
10. Harris GME, Wood M, Ystrom E, Nordeng H. Prenatal triptan exposure and neurodevelopmental outcomes in 5-year-old children: follow-up from the Norwegian Mother and Child Cohort Study. *Paediatr Perinat Epidemiol*. 2018;32:247-255.
11. Harris GM, Wood M, Ystrom E, Nordeng H. Association of maternal use of triptans during pregnancy with risk of attention-deficit/hyperactivity disorder in offspring. *JAMA Netw Open*. 2022;5:e2215333.
12. Amundsen S, Nordeng H, Ole-Martin F, et al. Transfer of triptans into human breast milk and estimation of infant drug exposure through breastfeeding. *Basic Clin Pharmacol Toxicol*. 2021;128:795-804.
13. Conijn M, Maas V, van Tuyl M, et al. Breastfeeding-related adverse drug reactions of triptans: a descriptive analysis using four pharmacovigilance database. *Breastfeed Med*. 2024;19:645-651.

ROCURONIUM

Central Nervous System (Nondepolarizing Neuromuscular Blocking Agent)

PREGNANCY RECOMMENDATION: Limited Human Data—Animal Data Suggest Potential Risk

BREASTFEEDING RECOMMENDATION: Probably Compatible (Hold Breastfeeding)

PREGNANCY SUMMARY

Human pregnancy experience with rocuronium is mainly in the second and third trimesters. In a study of women undergoing electroconvulsive therapy during pregnancy, there were seven with first-trimester, six with second-trimester, and two with third-trimester exposure. The women received propofol, rocuronium, and sugammadex. Of the seven neonates exposed in the first trimester, two had spontaneous losses. Of the remaining five, no major congenital anomalies were seen at delivery. Small amounts of rocuronium cross the placenta, so some fetal exposure will occur. Embryofetal toxicity was observed in one animal species at doses of less than 10 times the RHD. However, no ventilation was provided, and the fetal toxicity was thought to be due to oxygen deficiency in the dams. However, this limited human pregnancy experience prevents a complete assessment of the embryofetal risk. Using this drug during pregnancy should be based on the pros and cons of the mother's clinical need for treatment versus any potential fetal risk that might occur from exposure. Rocuronium can prolong the QTc interval. The manufacturer states that rocuronium is not recommended for rapid sequence induction for cesarean delivery.

R

BREASTFEEDING SUMMARY

Two reports describing the use of rocuronium in lactating women have been located. In both reports, the drug was used as part of the regimen for general anesthesia. No adverse effects on the infants were reported once breastfeeding was restarted. When used for delivery, there was a delay in initiating breastfeeding. The drug will probably be found in breast milk, so some infant exposure would likely occur. Additionally, rocuronium has poor oral bioavailability, so the amount of rocuronium that might reach the infant's circulation is likely to be small. Breastfeeding while using this drug should be based on the mother's clinical need for treatment versus any potential infant risks. If used, the infant should be monitored for the most common reported adult side effects of blood pressure variations. If there are any concerns, another option would be to hold breastfeeding for about 12 hours after the last dose (5 plus half-lives).

References

1. Prescribing Information. Rocuronium bromide. Almaject Inc; 2022.
2. Abouleish E, Abboud T, Lechevalier T, et al. Rocuronium (Org 9426) for caesarean section. *Br J Anaesth*. 1994;73:336-341.
3. Gaiser RR, Seem EH. Use of rocuronium in a pregnant patient with an open eye injury, receiving magnesium medication, for preterm labour. *Br J Anaesth*. 1996;77:669-671.
4. James MFM. Use of rocuronium in a pregnant patient receiving magnesium medication. *Br J Anaesth*. 1997;78:772.
5. Gaiser K. Use of rocuronium in a pregnant patient receiving magnesium medication (Reply). *Br J Anaesth*. 1997;78:772.
6. Karahan MA, Buyufirat, Binici O, et al. The effects of rocuronium-sugammadex on fetomaternal outcomes in pregnancy undergoing electroconvulsive therapy: a retrospective case series and literature review. *Cureus*. 2019;11:e4820.
7. Kwan WF, Chen BJ, Liao KT. Rocuronium for caesarean section. *Br J Anaesth*. 1995;74:347.
8. Abouleish E, Abboud T. Rocuronium for caesarean section. *Br J Anaesth*. 1995;74:347-348.
9. McSiney M, Edwards C, Wilkins A. Rocuronium for caesarean section. *Br J Anaesth*. 1995;74:348.

10. Swales HA, Gaylord DG. Rocuronium for caesarean section. *Br J Anaesth*. 1995;74:348.
11. Boker A, Ong BY. Anesthesia for cesarean section and posterior fossa craniotomy in a patient with von Hippel-Lindau disease. *Can J Anesth*. 2001;48:387-390.
12. Baraka AS, Sayyid SS, Assaf BA. Thiopental-rocuronium versus ketamine-rocuronium for rapid-sequence intubation in parturients undergoing cesarean section. *Anesth Analg*. 1997;84:1104-1107.
13. Kutlucan L, Seker IS, Demiraran Y, et al. Effects of different anesthesia protocols on lactation in the postpartum period. *J Turk Ger Gynecol Assoc*. 2014;15:233-238.
14. Kosinova M, Stourac P, Adamus M, et al. Rocuronium versus suxamethonium for rapid sequence induction of general anesthesia for caesarean section: influence on neonatal outcome. *Int J Obstet Anesth*. 2017;32:4-10.
15. Blaha J, Noskova, Hlinecka K, et al. Surgical conditions with rocuronium versus suxamethonium in cesarean section: a randomized trial. *Int J Obstet Anesth*. 2020;41:14-21.
16. Stuttmann R, Schafer C, Hilbert P, et al. The breast feeding mother and xenon anaesthesia: four case reports. Breast feeding and xenon anaesthesia. *BMC Anesthesiol*. 2010;10:1-5.
17. Dalal PG, Bosak J, Berlin C. Safety of the breast-feeding infant after maternal anesthesia. *Pediatr Anesth*. 2014;24:359-371.

ROFLUMILAST

Respiratory (Phosphodiesterase-4 Enzyme Inhibitor)

PREGNANCY RECOMMENDATION: No Human Data—Animal Data Suggest Low Risk

BREASTFEEDING RECOMMENDATION: Probably Compatible

PREGNANCY SUMMARY

No reports describing the use of roflumilast in human pregnancy have been located. The drug and its active metabolite are likely to cross the placenta, so some fetal exposure will probably occur. However, the absence of human pregnancy experience prevents a complete assessment of embryofetal risk. Embryofetal toxicity was observed in one animal species, but at doses of about 10 times the RHD. Using this drug during pregnancy should be based on the pros and cons of the mother's clinical need for treatment versus any potential fetal risk that might occur from exposure.

BREASTFEEDING SUMMARY

No reports describing the use of roflumilast during human lactation have been located. The drug and its active metabolite will likely be excreted into breast milk, so some infant exposure will probably occur. Breastfeeding while using this drug should be based on the mother's clinical need for treatment versus any potential infant risks. If used, the infant should be monitored for the most common reported adult side effects of nausea, headache, dizziness, and back pain (all leading to irritability), diarrhea, insomnia, and decreased appetite (monitor feeding patterns and growth).

Reference

1. Prescribing Information. Roflumilast. Camber Pharmaceuticals Inc; 2023.

ROLAPITANT

Gastrointestinal (Antiemetic for Chemotherapy)

PREGNANCY RECOMMENDATION: No Human Data—Animal Data Suggest Potential Risk

BREASTFEEDING RECOMMENDATION: Potential Toxicity

PREGNANCY SUMMARY

No reports describing the use of rolapitant in human pregnancy have been located. The drug and its active metabolite are likely to cross the placenta, so some fetal exposure will probably occur. However, the absence of human pregnancy experience prevents a complete assessment of embryofetal risk. Embryofetal toxicity was observed in one animal species at doses of less than 10 times the RHD. Using this drug during pregnancy should be based on the pros and cons of the mother's clinical need for treatment versus any potential fetal risk that might occur from exposure. Women who are pregnant and have cancer are encouraged to contact the Cancer and Pregnancy Registry at 877-635-4499.

BREASTFEEDING SUMMARY

No reports describing the use of rolapitant during human lactation have been located. The drug and its active metabolite will likely be excreted into human breast milk, so some infant exposure will probably occur. Breastfeeding while using this drug should be based on the mother's clinical need for treatment versus any potential infant risks. If used, the infant should be monitored for the most common reported adult side effects. The side effects, however, are seen when the drug is used in combination with cisplatin-based, highly

R

emetogenic chemotherapy and other chemotherapy agents. Therefore, many of these are probably related to the antineoplastic drugs, but include abdominal pain, dizziness, and dyspepsia (all leading to irritability), hiccups, decreased appetite (monitor feeding patterns and growth), neutropenia, urinary tract infections, stomatitis, and anemia.

Reference

1. Product Information. Varubi. TerSera Therapeutics LLC; 2020.

ROMIDEPSIN

Antineoplastic (Histone Deacetylase Inhibitor)

PREGNANCY RECOMMENDATION: No Human Data—Animal Data Suggest Potential Risk

BREASTFEEDING RECOMMENDATION: Potential Toxicity

PREGNANCY SUMMARY

No reports describing the use of romidepsin in human pregnancy have been located. The drug is likely to cross the placenta, so some fetal exposure will probably occur. However, the absence of human pregnancy experience prevents a complete assessment of embryofetal risk. Embryofetal toxicity was seen in one animal species at doses of less than 10 times the RHD. Based on animal studies and the drug's mechanism of action, the manufacturer recommends that women with reproductive potential use effective contraception during treatment and for 1 month after the last dose. They also recommend that males with female partners of reproductive potential use effective contraception during treatment and for 1 month after the last dose. Nevertheless, using this drug during pregnancy should be based on the pros and cons of the mother's clinical need for treatment versus any potential fetal risk that might occur from exposure. There is a registry for women who are pregnant and have cancer. For more information, women and health care providers are encouraged to contact the Cancer and Pregnancy Registry at 1-877-635-4499. Because romidepsin may reduce the efficacy of estrogen containing contraceptives, alternative methods of non–estrogen-containing products (eg, condoms, intrauterine devices, etc) should be used. Also, elevated glucose levels have been reported in up to about 50% of patients treated with this drug. Therefore, if used during pregnancy, glucose levels should be monitored.

BREASTFEEDING SUMMARY

No reports describing the use of romidepsin during human lactation have been located. The drug will likely be excreted into breast milk, so some infant exposure will probably occur. Due to a concern for potential serious adverse effects that might be seen in a breastfed infant, the manufacturer recommends that women not breastfeed while being treated with this drug. Nevertheless, breastfeeding while using this drug should be based on the mother's clinical need for treatment versus any potential infant risks that might occur. If used, the infant should be monitored for the most common reported adult side effects of nausea and pruritus (both leading to irritability), fatigue (lethargy), infections, vomiting, anorexia (monitor feeding patterns and growth), constipation, and various laboratory abnormalities (see PI).

Reference

1. Prescribing Information. Romidepsin. Teva Parenteral Medicines Inc; 2021.

ROMIPLOSTIM

Hematologic (Thrombopoietic Agent)

PREGNANCY RECOMMENDATION: Limited Human Data—Animal Data Suggest Potential Risk

BREASTFEEDING RECOMMENDATION: *Potential Toxicity

PREGNANCY SUMMARY

Romiplostim use has been described in over 100 human pregnancies. Most exposures are in the third trimester, with only a few first-trimester exposures. One (2.6%) major malformation was seen in about 39 first-trimester users. However, thrombocytopenia and thrombocytosis have been reported in infants where the drug was used close to delivery. The drug has been shown to cross the placenta, so fetal exposure will occur. Therefore, this limited human pregnancy experience, especially early in gestation, prevents a complete assessment of embryofetal risk. Embryofetal toxicity was observed in one animal species at doses of less than 10 times the RHD and in one species at doses of more than 10 times the MRHD. Using this drug during pregnancy should be based on the pros and cons of the mother's clinical need for treatment versus any potential fetal risk that might occur from exposure.

BREASTFEEDING SUMMARY

Romiplostim is excreted into human breast milk; therefore, some infant exposure will occur. However, because it is a protein, if it were to be ingested through breastfeeding, it should at least partially be digested in the infant's gastrointestinal tract and not be absorbed. *Nevertheless, in one case report, an infant had normal platelets at birth. Breastfeeding was stopped at 11 weeks of age due to the infant having thrombocytosis and a peripheral blood smear with rare immature cells, suggestive of blasts. The infant continued to have thrombocytosis until 11 months of age. No infant complications were observed. Maternal romiplostim protein levels were 13.5 times higher than infant levels (as would be expected). Milk levels were higher 1 day postdose when compared with 7 days postdose (where it was barely detectable). It is uncertain whether this is an unusual case or whether the elimination half-life is much longer in infants (the median elimination half-life in adults is 3.5 days). Therefore, the drug should be used with caution in a breastfeeding woman. Further study is needed.

References

1. Prescribing Information. Nplate. Amgen Inc; 2022.
2. Bussel JB, Soff G, Balduzzi A, et al. A review of romiplostim mechanism of action and clinical applicability. *Drug Des Devel Ther*. 2021;15:2243-2268.
3. Labrecque AA, Roy S, Young D, et al. Romiplostim drug presence in pregnancy and lactation. *Blood*. 2023;141:2537-2540.
4. Alkaabi J, Alkindi S, Riyami N, et al. Successful treatment of severe thrombocytopenia with romiplostim in a pregnant patient with systemic lupus erythematosus. *Lupus*. 2012;21:1571-1574.
5. Patil AS, Dotters-Katz SK, Metjian AD, et al. Use of thrombopoietin mimetic for chronic immune thrombocytopenic purpura in pregnancy. *Obstet Gynecol*. 2013;122:483-485.
6. Decroocq J, Marcellin L, Le Ray C, Willems L. Rescue therapy with romiplostim for refractory primary immune thrombocytopenia during pregnancy. *Obstet Gynecol*. 2014;124:481-483.
7. Michel M, Ruggeri M, Gonzalez-Lopez TJ, et al. Use of thrombopoietin receptor agonists for immune thrombocytopenia in pregnancy: results from a multicenter study. *Blood*. 2020;136(26):3056-3061.
8. Rodriguez Nunez RM, Laura RL, Angeles PB, Laura LB. Use of romiplostim during pregnancy as a rescue therapy in primary immune thrombocytopenia: literature review and case description. *Platelets*. 2020;31:403-406.
9. Chon AH, Chan R, Lee RH, et al. Multidrug therapy for refractory immune thrombocytopenia in pregnancy. *Obstet Gynecol*. 2020;135:723-727.
10. Heenan JM. Management of refractory immune thrombocytopaenia in pregnancy. *BMJ Case Rep*. 2021;14:e244656.
11. Bussel JB, Cooper N, Lawrence T, et al. Romiplostim use in pregnant women with immune thrombocytopenia. *Am J Hematol*. 2023;98:31-40.

ROMOSOZUMAB

Bone Health (Sclerostin Inhibitor—Monoclonal Antibody)

PREGNANCY RECOMMENDATION: *Contraindicated

BREASTFEEDING RECOMMENDATION: *Contraindicated

PREGNANCY SUMMARY

No reports describing the use of romosozumab during human pregnancy have been located. As an IgG antibody, it likely crosses the placenta, especially during the second half of gestation, so some fetal exposure would probably occur. However, the absence of human pregnancy experience prevents a complete assessment of embryofetal risk. Embryofetal toxicity was observed in one animal species at doses of less than 10 times the RHD. *Nevertheless, the drug is approved for use in postmenopausal women and, therefore, is contraindicated for use during pregnancy.

R

BREASTFEEDING SUMMARY

No reports describing the use of romosozumab during human lactation have been located. The high MW suggests that the drug will not be excreted into breast milk. However, it is known that IgG antibodies can be found in human breast milk, but are not found in the neonatal or infant circulation. Additionally, if any IgG antibodies were to be ingested through breastfeeding, they would probably be digested in the infant's gastrointestinal tract and not be absorbed. *Nevertheless, the drug is approved for use in postmenopausal women, and, therefore, is contraindicated for use during breastfeeding.

Reference

1. Prescribing Information. Evenity. Amgen Inc; 2024.

ROPEGINTERFERON ALFA-2B

Immunologic (Biologic Response Modulator)

PREGNANCY RECOMMENDATION: No Human Data and No Relevant Animal Data

BREASTFEEDING RECOMMENDATION: Probably Compatible

PREGNANCY SUMMARY

No reports describing the use of ropeginterferon alfa-2b in human pregnancy have been located. The drug is not likely to cross the placenta, so fetal exposure is probably clinically insignificant. Interferon alfa does not appear to cross the placenta (see Interferon). However, the absence of human pregnancy experience prevents a complete assessment of the embryofetal risk. No animal reproduction studies have been conducted with this drug. Regardless, based on the drug's mechanism of action, the manufacturer recommends that women with reproductive potential use effective contraception during treatment and for 8 weeks after the last dose. They also state that ropeginterferon alfa-2b should be assumed to have abortifacient potential if administered to pregnant women in the first trimester. Nevertheless, using this drug during pregnancy should be based on the pros and cons of the mother's clinical need for treatment versus any potential fetal risk that might occur from exposure. Untreated polycythemia vera has been associated with thrombosis, hemorrhage, and spontaneous abortion during pregnancy.

BREASTFEEDING SUMMARY

No reports describing the use of ropeginterferon alfa-2b during human lactation have been located. The drug is not expected to be found in breast milk, but interferon alfa is excreted into breast milk (see Interferon). Regardless, because ropeginterferon alfa-2b is a polypeptide, if it were to be ingested through breastfeeding, it would probably be digested in the infant's gastrointestinal tract and not be absorbed. However, due to the concern for potential serious adverse effects that might be seen in a breastfed infant, the manufacturer recommends that women not breastfeed while being treated with this drug and for 8 weeks after the last dose. Nevertheless, breastfeeding while using this drug should be based on the mother's clinical need for treatment. If used, the infant should be monitored for the most common reported adult side effects of arthralgias, musculoskeletal pain, and pruritus (all leading to irritability), and lethargy.

Reference

1. Prescribing Information. Besremi. PharmaEssentia USA; 2021.

ROPINIROLE

Central Nervous System (Anti-Parkinson Agent—Dopamine Agonist)

PREGNANCY RECOMMENDATION: Limited Human Data—Animal Data Suggest Potential Risk

BREASTFEEDING RECOMMENDATION: Potential Toxicity

PREGNANCY SUMMARY

Three studies describing the use of ropinirole in human pregnancies have been located. Exposures occurred at various times during gestation, but no malformations were observed in the six cases with exposure at the time of conception or with use in the first trimester. The drug will probably cross the placenta, so some fetal exposure will likely occur. Therefore, this limited human pregnancy experience prevents a complete assessment of embryofetal risk. Embryofetal toxicity was observed in one animal species at doses of less than 10 times the RHD. Using this drug during pregnancy should be based on the pros and cons of the mother's clinical need for treatment versus any potential fetal risk that might occur from exposure.

BREASTFEEDING SUMMARY

No reports describing the use of ropinirole during human lactation have been located. The drug will likely be excreted into breast milk, so some infant exposure will probably occur. Breastfeeding while using this drug should be based on the mother's clinical need for treatment versus any potential infant risks that might occur. If used, the infant should be monitored for the most common reported adult side effects of nausea, dizziness, dyspepsia, and headache (all leading to irritability), somnolence, leg edema, vomiting, and sweating. Ropinirole inhibits prolactin secretion and, therefore, may inhibit lactation.

References

1. Prescribing Information. Ropinirole hydrochloride. Alembic Pharmaceuticals Inc; 2024.
2. Dostal M, Weber-Schoendorfer C, Sobesky J, Schaefer C. Pregnancy outcome following use of levodopa, pramipexole, ropinirole, and rotigotine for restless legs syndrome during pregnancy: a case series. *Eur J Neurol*. 2013;20:1241-1246.
3. Lamichhane D, Narayanan NS, Gonzalez-Alegre P. Two cases of pregnancy in Parkinson's disease. *Parkinsonism Relat Disord*. 2014;20:239-240.
4. Tufekcioglu Z, Hanagasi H, Yalcin Cakmakli G, et al. Use of anti-Parkinson medication during pregnancy: a case series. *J Neurol*. 2018;265:1922-1929.

R

ROPIVACAINE

Anesthetic (Local Anesthetic)

PREGNANCY RECOMMENDATION: Human Data Suggest Low Risk (Second and Third Trimesters)

BREASTFEEDING RECOMMENDATION: Probably Compatible

PREGNANCY SUMMARY

The human and animal data suggest that the risk to a human fetus from the use of ropivacaine in pregnancy is very low. However, there are no human pregnancy data for use in the first trimester. The amount of ropivacaine measured in the maternal circulation is very low and does not appear to represent a significant embryofetal risk. The drug has been shown to cross the placenta in low amounts using an ex vivo placental perfusion model. However, the absence of first-trimester human pregnancy experience prevents a complete assessment of embryofetal risk. Animal data did not show any embryofetal toxicity in two species at doses about equal to the RHD. Using this drug during pregnancy should be based on the pros and cons of the mother's clinical need for treatment versus any potential fetal risk that might occur from exposure.

BREASTFEEDING SUMMARY

The manufacturer reports that ropivacaine is excreted into breast milk following administration to women undergoing cesarean delivery. No infant adverse events were reported. Breastfeeding while using this drug should be based on the mother's clinical need for treatment versus any potential infant risks that might occur. If used, the infant should be monitored for the most common reported adult side effects of nausea, headache, pruritus, and back pain (all leading to irritability), hypotension, vomiting, bradycardia, and fever.

References

1. Prescribing Information. Ropivacaine hydrochloride. Amneal Pharmaceuticals LLC; 2024.
2. Johnson RF, Cahana A, Olenick M, et al. A comparison of the placental transfer of ropivacaine versus bupivacaine. *Anesth Analg*. 1999;89:703-708.
3. Datta S, Camann W, Bader A, VanderBurgh L. Clinical effects and maternal and fetal plasma concentrations of epidural ropivacaine versus bupivacaine for cesarean section. *Anesthesiology*. 1995;82:1346-1352.
4. Morton CPJ, Bloomfield S, Magnusson A, et al. Ropivacaine 0.75% for extradural anaesthesia in elective caesarean section: an open clinical and pharmacokinetic study in mother and neonate. *Br J Anaesth*. 1997;79:3-8.
5. Irestedt L, Ekblom A, Olofsson C, et al. Pharmacokinetics and clinical effect during continuous epidural infusion with ropivacaine 2.5 mg/ml or bupivacaine 2.5 mg/ml for labour pain relief. *Acta Anaesthesiol Scand*. 1998;42:890-896.
6. Gaiser RR, Venkateswaren P, Cheek TG, et al. Comparison of 0.25% ropivacaine and bupivacaine for epidural analgesia for labor and vaginal delivery. *J Clin Anesthesia*. 1997;9:564-568.
7. McCrae AF, Jozwiak H, McClure JH. Comparison of ropivacaine and bupivacaine in extradural analgesia for the relief of pain in labour. *Br J Anaesth*. 1995;74:261-265.
8. Eddleston JM, Holland JJ, Griffin RP, et al. A double-blind comparison of 0.25% ropivacaine and 0.25% bupivacaine for extradural analgesia in labour. *Br J Anaesth*. 1996;76:66-71.
9. Irestedt L, Emanuelsson BM, Ekblom A, et al. Ropivacaine 7.5 mg/ml for elective caesarean section. A clinical and pharmacokinetic comparison of 150 mg and 187.5 mg. *Acta Anaesthesiol Scand*. 1997;41:1149-1156.
10. Writer WDR, Stienstra R, Eddleston JM, et al. Neonatal outcome and mode of delivery after epidural analgesia for labour with ropivacaine and bupivacaine: a prospective meta-analysis. *Br J Anaesth*. 1998;81:713-717.
11. Kang T, Tao J, Wang X, et al. Epidural ropivacaine versus bupivacaine for cesarean sections: a system review and meta-analysis. *J Matern Fetal Neonatal Med*. 2024;37:2313356.
12. Takahata K, Horiuchi S, Miyauchi A, et al. A longitudinal study of the association of epidural anesthesia and low-dose synthetic oxytocin regimens with breast milk supply and breastfeeding rates. *Sci Rep*. 2023;13:21146.

ROSUVASTATIN

Antilipemic (Statin, HMG-CoA Reductase Inhibitor)

PREGNANCY RECOMMENDATION: Limited Human Data—Animal Data Suggest Risk

BREASTFEEDING RECOMMENDATION: Potential Toxicity

PREGNANCY SUMMARY

Two studies that analyzed statin drug use in general described more than 1,200 first-trimester exposures. After adjusting for confounders, neither teratogenic effects nor organ-specific malformations were observed with statin use. However, the number of cases that used rosuvastatin was small. The drug is likely to cross the placenta, so some fetal exposure will probably occur. Therefore, this limited human pregnancy experience prevents a complete assessment of embryofetal risk. Embryofetal toxicity was observed in two animal species at doses of less than 10 times the RHD. Cholesterol and other products of cholesterol biosynthesis are essential components for fetal development. Moreover, maternal cholesterol levels increase during pregnancy. Hyperlipidemia treatment is not generally necessary during pregnancy. Atherosclerosis is a chronic process, and stopping lipid-lowering therapy during pregnancy should have little impact on the outcome of long-term therapy of primary hyperlipidemia for most patients. The manufacturer states that it may cause fetal harm when administered during pregnancy due to the mechanism of action, and therefore, recommends discontinuing rosuvastatin when a pregnancy is recognized. Nevertheless, using this drug during pregnancy should be based on the pros and cons of the mother's clinical need for treatment versus any potential fetal risk that might occur from exposure.

BREASTFEEDING SUMMARY

Rosuvastatin is excreted into human breast milk. Two reports describing the use of rosuvastatin during lactation have been located. The calculated RIDs for both cases were 1.5% and 0.8%. Due to a concern for potential serious adverse effects that might be seen in a breastfed infant, the manufacturer recommends that women not breastfeed while being treated with this drug. In addition, hyperlipidemia treatment is not generally necessary during lactation. Atherosclerosis is a chronic process, and stopping lipid-lowering therapy during lactation (at least for a few months) should have little impact on the outcome of long-term therapy of primary hyperlipidemia for most patients. Nevertheless, breastfeeding while using this drug should be based on the mother's clinical need for treatment versus any potential infant risks that might occur. If used, the infant should be monitored for the most common reported adult side effects of headache, nausea, myalgia, and arthralgia (all leading to irritability), and constipation.

References

1. Prescribing Information. Rosuvastatin. Torrent Pharmaceuticals Limited; 2023.
2. Taguchi N, Rubin ET, Hosokawa A, et al. Prenatal exposure to HMG-CoA reductase inhibitors: effects on fetal and neonatal outcomes. *Reprod Toxicol*. 2008;26:175-177.
3. Trakadis Y, Blaser S, Hahn CO, Yoon G. A case report of prenatal exposure to rosuvastatin and telmisartan. *Paediatr Child Health*. 2009;14:450-452.
4. Al-Dughaishi T, Al-Waili K, Banerjee Y, et al. Successful direct adsorption of lipoproteins (DALI) apheresis during pregnancy in an Omani woman with homozygous familial hypercholesterolemia. *Open Cardiovasc Med J*. 2015;9:114-117.
5. Edison RJ, Muenke M. Central nervous system and limb anomalies in case-reports of first trimester statin exposure. *N Engl J Med*. 2004;350:1579-1582.
6. Edison RJ, Muenke M. Mechanistic and epidemiologic considerations in the evaluation of adverse birth outcomes following gestational exposure to statins. *Am J Med Genet*. 2004;131A:287-298.
7. Schutte AE, Symington EA, du Preez JL. Rosuvastatin is transferred into human breast milk: a case report. *Am J Med*. 2013;126:e7-e8.
8. Lwin EMP, Leggett C, Ritchie U, et al. Transfer of rosuvastatin into breast milk: liquid chromatography-mass spectrometry methodology and clinical recommendations. *Drug Des Devel Ther*. 2018;12:3645-3651.

ROZANOLIXIZUMAB

Immunologic (Monoclonal Antibody—Myasthenia Gravis)

PREGNANCY RECOMMENDATION: No Human Data and No Relevant Animal Data

BREASTFEEDING RECOMMENDATION: Probably Compatible

PREGNANCY SUMMARY

No reports describing the use of rozanolixizumab in human pregnancy have been located. As an IgG antibody, it likely crosses the placenta, especially during the second half of pregnancy, but with neonatal Fc receptor blockage, fetal exposure could be minimal. The neonatal Fc receptor is a necessary component for immunoglobulins of the IgG class to cross. However, the absence of human pregnancy experience prevents a complete assessment of the embryofetal risk. Animal reproduction studies showed embryofetal toxicity, but at doses greater than or equal to 10 times the MRHD that also produced maternal toxicity. Using this drug during pregnancy should be based on the pros and cons of the mother's clinical need for treatment versus any potential fetal risk that might occur from exposure. If used up to delivery, the newborn should be evaluated postdelivery for possible low IgG immunoglobulin levels that could increase the risk for infections and decrease the response to vaccines.

BREASTFEEDING SUMMARY

No reports describing the use of rozanolixizumab during human lactation have been located. It is known that IgG antibodies can be found in human breast milk, but are not found in the neonatal or infant circulation. Additionally, if any IgG antibodies were to be ingested through breastfeeding, they would probably be digested in the infant's gastrointestinal tract and not be absorbed. Breastfeeding while using this drug should be based on the mother's clinical need for treatment. If used, the infant should be monitored for the most common reported adult side effects of headache and nausea (both leading to irritability), infections, diarrhea, and pyrexia.

Reference

1. Product Information. Rystiggo. UCB Inc; 2023.

RUCAPARIB

Antineoplastic (Polymerase Inhibitor)

PREGNANCY RECOMMENDATION: No Human Data—Animal Data Suggest Potential Risk

BREASTFEEDING RECOMMENDATION: Potential Toxicity

R

PREGNANCY SUMMARY

No reports describing the use of rucaparib in human pregnancy have been located. The drug will probably cross the placenta, so some fetal exposure will likely occur. Therefore, the absence of human pregnancy experience prevents a complete assessment of the embryofetal risk. Embryofetal toxicity was observed in animal studies. Due to the findings from animal studies and the drug's mechanism of action, the manufacturer recommends that women with reproductive potential use effective contraception during treatment and for at least 6 months after the last dose. They also recommend that males with female partners of reproductive potential use effective contraception during treatment and for at least 3 months after the last dose. Nevertheless, using this drug during pregnancy should be based on the pros and cons of the mother's clinical need for treatment versus any potential fetal risk that might occur from exposure.

BREASTFEEDING SUMMARY

No reports describing the use of rucaparib during human lactation have been located. The drug will probably appear in breast milk, so some infant exposure will likely occur. Due to the concern for potential serious adverse effects that might be seen in a breastfed infant, the manufacturer recommends that women not breastfeed while being treated with rucaparib and for at least 2 weeks after the last dose. Nevertheless, breastfeeding while using this drug should be based on the mother's clinical need for treatment. If used, the infant should be monitored for the most common reported adult side effects of nausea and abdominal pain (both leading to irritability), diarrhea, lethargy, vomiting, constipation, decreased appetite, rash, and various laboratory abnormalities (see PI).

Reference

1. Prescribing Information. Rubraca. Clovis Oncology Inc; 2022.

RUFINAMIDE

Central Nervous System (Antiseizure)

PREGNANCY RECOMMENDATION: No Human Data—Animal Data Suggest Risk

BREASTFEEDING RECOMMENDATION: Potential Toxicity

PREGNANCY SUMMARY

No reports describing the use of rufinamide in human pregnancy have been located. The drug is likely to cross the placenta, so some fetal exposure will probably occur. However, the absence of human pregnancy experience prevents a complete assessment of the embryofetal risk. Embryofetal toxicity was observed in two animal species at doses of less than 10 times the RHD. Using this drug during pregnancy should be based on the pros and cons of the mother's clinical need for treatment versus any potential fetal risk that might occur from exposure. There is a pregnancy exposure registry that monitors pregnancy outcomes in women using antiseizure drugs. Health care providers are encouraged to call the North American Antiepileptic Drug Pregnancy Registry at 1-888-233-2334. Rufinamide may decrease the efficacy of hormonal contraceptives containing ethinyl estradiol or norethindrone. The manufacturer recommends that women of reproductive age use an additional nonhormonal form of contraception if they are taking a contraceptive containing these ingredients.

R

BREASTFEEDING SUMMARY

No reports describing the use of rufinamide during human lactation have been located. The drug will likely be excreted into breast milk, so some infant exposure will probably occur. Breastfeeding while using this drug should be based on the mother's clinical need for treatment versus any potential infant risks that might occur. If used, the infant should be monitored for the most common reported adult side effects of headache, dizziness, and nausea (all leading to irritability), fatigue (lethargy), and somnolence.

Reference

1. Prescribing Information. Rufinamide. Camber Pharmaceuticals Inc; 2021.

RUXOLITINIB

Antineoplastic (Janus Kinase Inhibitor)

PREGNANCY RECOMMENDATION: No Human Data—Animal Data Suggest Risk

BREASTFEEDING RECOMMENDATION: Potential Toxicity

PREGNANCY SUMMARY

No reports describing the use of ruxolitinib during human pregnancy (with reported outcome data) have been located. The drug and its active metabolites are likely to cross the placenta, so some fetal exposure will probably occur. Therefore, the absence of human pregnancy experience prevents a complete assessment of embryofetal risk. Embryofetal toxicity was observed in two animal species at doses of less than 10 times the RHD for oral dosing. Some maternal toxicity also occurred. Using this drug during pregnancy should be based on the pros and cons of the mother's clinical need for treatment versus any potential fetal risk that might occur from exposure. There is a pregnancy exposure registry that monitors pregnancy outcomes in women exposed to ruxolitinib (Opzelura) during pregnancy. For more information, health care providers or patients are encouraged to call 855-463-3463.

BREASTFEEDING SUMMARY

No reports describing the use of ruxolitinib during human lactation have been located. The drug and its metabolites will likely be excreted into breast milk, so some infant exposure will probably occur. Due to a concern for potential serious adverse effects that might be seen in a breastfed infant, the manufacturer recommends that women not breastfeed while being treated with this drug and for at least 2 weeks after the last oral dose or for 4 weeks after the last topical dose. Nevertheless, breastfeeding while using this drug should be based on the mother's clinical need for treatment versus any potential infant risks that might occur. If used, the infant should be monitored for the most common reported adult side effects of dizziness and headache (both leading to irritability), bruising, diarrhea, rash, fever, infections, and various laboratory abnormalities (see PI).

References

1. Prescribing Information. Jakafi. Incyte Corporation; 2023.
2. Product Information. Opzelura. Incyte Corporation; 2023.
3. Wang S, Wu J, Jing X, et al. Etoposide combined with ruxolitinib for refractory hemophagocytic lymphohistiocytosis during pregnancy: a case report and literature review. *Hematology*. 2019;24:751-756.

SACITUZUMAB GOVITECAN

Antineoplastic (Trop-2-Directed Monoclonal Antibody)

PREGNANCY RECOMMENDATION: *Contraindicated

BREASTFEEDING RECOMMENDATION: Contraindicated

PREGNANCY SUMMARY

No reports describing the use of sacituzumab govitecan in human pregnancy have been located. As an immunoglobulin G (IgG) antibody, it probably crosses the placenta. The drug is composed of three components, including the antibody, a topoisomerase inhibitor (SN-38), and a hydrolysable linker that binds the other two together. SN-38 is toxic to rapidly dividing cells by damaging DNA, resulting in cell apoptosis. SN-38 will also probably cross the placenta. Therefore, fetal exposure is likely to occur for both agents. Therefore, the absence of human pregnancy experience prevents a complete assessment of the embryofetal risk. No animal studies have been conducted. Sacituzumab govitecan can cause severe and even life-threatening neutropenia and diarrhea. *Based on the drug's mechanism of action, especially SN-38, the manufacturer recommends that women with reproductive potential use effective contraception during treatment and for 6 months after the last dose. They also recommend that males with female partners of reproductive potential use effective contraception during treatment and for 3 months after the last dose. However, there could be clinical cases where a pregnant woman with advanced breast cancer might consider treatment based on the gestational age and an in-depth discussion of the pros and cons.

BREASTFEEDING SUMMARY

Sacituzumab govitecan is likely present in breast milk. Regarding the antibody, it is known that IgG antibodies can be found in human breast milk, but are not found in neonatal or infant circulation. Additionally, if any IgG antibodies were to be ingested through breastfeeding, they would probably be digested in the infant's gastrointestinal tract and not be absorbed. However, SN-38 is also probably found in breast milk. This drug is toxic to rapidly dividing cells with numerous serious side effects. Therefore, due to the concern for potential serious adverse effects in a breastfed infant, the manufacturer recommends that women not breastfeed while being treated with sacituzumab govitecan and for at least 1 month after the last dose.

Reference

1. Prescribing Information. Trodelvy. Gilead Sciences, Inc; 2021.

SAFINAMIDE

Central Nervous System (Anti-Parkinson Agent)

PREGNANCY RECOMMENDATION: No Human Data—Animal Data Suggest Risk

BREASTFEEDING RECOMMENDATION: Potential Toxicity

PREGNANCY SUMMARY

No reports describing the use of safinamide in human pregnancy have been located. The drug will probably cross the placenta, so some fetal exposure will likely occur. However, the absence of human pregnancy experience prevents a complete assessment of embryofetal risk. Animal studies did show embryofetal toxicity. Using this drug during pregnancy should be based on the pros and cons of the mother's clinical need for treatment versus any potential fetal risk that might occur from exposure.

BREASTFEEDING SUMMARY

No reports describing the use of safinamide during human lactation have been located. The drug will probably enter breast milk, so infant exposure will likely occur. Because of a skin discoloration thought to be due to hyperbilirubinemia seen in rats exposed to the drug through breastfeeding, the manufacturer recommends that women consider not breastfeeding when using this drug. However, breastfeeding should be based on the mother's clinical need for treatment. If used, the infant should be monitored for jaundice and the most common reported adult side effects of involuntary movements, insomnia, and nausea (leading to irritability).

Reference

1. Prescribing Information. Xadago. US WorldMeds, LLC; 2019.

SALMETEROL

Respiratory (Long-Acting β_2-Agonist)

PREGNANCY RECOMMENDATION: Limited Human Data—Animal Data Suggests Low Risk

BREASTFEEDING RECOMMENDATION: Probably Compatible

PREGNANCY SUMMARY

Several studies have been reported on the use of long-acting β_2-agonists (LABAs) in human pregnancy, and overall, there does not appear to be an increased risk for fetal malformations. However, few publications describe the use of salmeterol in the first trimester. In one report, after excluding therapeutic abortions, lost to follow-up, and spontaneous losses, there were no major fetal malformations in 47 first-trimester exposures. However, the very low or undetectable maternal plasma levels that occur with therapeutic inhaled doses suggest that the risk to the fetus from the drug is probably negligible. Conflicting results on the risk for small for gestational age were found. However, it is difficult to fully evaluate these findings because specific rates were not consistently provided for comparison to the expected background risks for these various events. In addition, all of these factors can be influenced by numerous confounding variables, including uncontrolled asthma. Animal data did not show any embryofetal toxicity in one species at doses of more than 10 times the Recommended human inhaled dose (RHID). Embryofetal toxicity was seen, but doses were in excess of 500 times the Maximum recommended human inhaled dose (MRHID). Using this drug during pregnancy should be based on the pros and cons of the mother's clinical need for treatment versus any potential fetal risk that might occur from exposure. Salmeterol can prolong the QT interval in some patients. There is a boxed warning regarding the use of LABAs as monotherapy in patients with asthma, as this can increase the risk for asthma-related death. Uncontrolled asthma during pregnancy can increase the risk for preeclampsia, preterm delivery, and low birth weight newborns. The most recent American College of Obstetricians and Gynecologists (ACOG) publication on asthma in pregnancy (published in 2008—reaffirmed in 2020) and the 2023 Global Initiative for Asthma (GINA) guidelines state that the advantages of actively treating asthma in pregnancy markedly outweigh the potential risks of the medications. Inhaled corticosteroids are usually the first-line treatment for mild to moderate persistent asthma in pregnancy. Listed alternative treatments include cromolyn, theophylline, or leukotriene receptor antagonists. However, ACOG recommends LABAs as the preferred add-on drug when pregnant patients are not controlled with inhaled corticosteroids. The reasoning for this is that LABAs have been shown to be more effective as an add-on treatment in nonpregnant patients.

BREASTFEEDING SUMMARY

No reports describing the use of salmeterol during human lactation have been located. The drug will likely be excreted into breast milk, so some infant exposure will probably occur. Additionally, the maternal plasma levels after an inhaled therapeutic dose are very low or undetectable. Thus, it is unlikely that clinically significant amounts would be found in breast milk. Breastfeeding while using this drug should be based on the mother's clinical need for treatment versus any potential infant risks that might occur. If used, the infant should be monitored for the most common reported adult side effects of headache and musculoskeletal pain (both leading to irritability), nasal congestion, and cough.

References

1. Prescribing Information. Serevent diskus. GlaxoSmithKline LLC; 2022.
2. Wilton LV, Pearce GL, Martin RM, et al. The outcomes of pregnancy in women exposed to newly marketed drugs in general practice in England. *Br J Obstet Gynaecol*. 1998;105:882-889.
3. Buyse ML, ed. *Birth Defects Encyclopedia*. Vol 1. Blackwell Scientific Publications; 1990:1-2.
4. Cossette B, Beauchesne MF, Forget A, et al. Relative perinatal safety of salmeterol vs formoterol and fluticasone vs budesonide use during pregnancy. *Ann Allergy Asthma Immunol*. 2014; 112:459-464.
5. Davies G, Jordan S, Thayer D, et al. Medications prescribed for asthma, discontinuation and perinatal outcomes, including breastfeeding: a population cohort analysis. *PLoS One*. 2020;15:e024289.
6. American College of Obstetricians and Gynecologists. Asthma in pregnancy: ACOG Practice Bulletin No. 90. *Obstet Gynecol*. 2008;111:457-464.
7. Global Initiative for Asthma. Global strategy for asthma management and prevention. Published 2023. Updated July 2023. www.ginasthma.org

S

SAPROPTERIN

Metabolic (Enzyme Cofactor)

PREGNANCY RECOMMENDATION: Limited Human Data—Animal Data Suggest Low Risk (Maternal Benefit May Outweigh Any Embryofetal Risk)

BREASTFEEDING RECOMMENDATION: Probably Compatible

PREGNANCY SUMMARY

Five reports describing 32 patients using sapropterin either before or during pregnancy were identified. No embryofetal adverse effects were attributable to the therapy. The drug is likely to cross the placenta, so some fetal exposure will probably occur. However, this limited human pregnancy experience prevents a complete assessment of embryofetal risk. Animal studies did not show any embryofetal toxicity in two species at doses of less than 10 times the recommended human dose (RHD) in one and at 10 times the RHD in the second. Using this drug during pregnancy should be based on the pros and cons of the mother's clinical need for treatment versus any potential fetal risk that might occur from exposure. The risk of uncontrolled phenylketonuria (PKU) is much greater to the embryo and/or fetus. If diet alone is not adequate to control maternal phenylalanine concentrations, the use of sapropterin appears to be a reasonable option. However, in clinical trials with nonpregnant adults, only about 40% of patients with PKU on average responded to treatment with sapropterin. Elevated phenylalanine levels are associated with developmental delays, microcephaly, congenital heart defects, growth delay, and seizures. The manufacturer recommends that phenylalanine levels should be maintained between 168 and 504 mcg/mL 3 months prior to conception and during pregnancy. ACOG recommends levels less than 600 mcg/mL for at least 3 months prior to conception and 200 to 600 mcg/mL during pregnancy. ACOG states that sapropterin may be an appropriate adjunct to dietary modification during pregnancy and breastfeeding.

BREASTFEEDING SUMMARY

The manufacturer reports that 16 women using sapropterin during lactation were identified from postmarketing registries. These women breastfed their infants for a mean of 3 to 4 months, and no lactation-related safety concerns were reported. In another case, the mother used sapropterin during pregnancy and through 25 months of lactation. The infant had normal development. Breastfeeding while using this drug should be based on the mother's clinical need for treatment versus any potential infant risks that might occur. If used, the infant should be monitored for the most common reported adult side effects of headache and pharyngeal pain (both leading to irritability), rhinorrhea, diarrhea, vomiting, cough, and nasal congestion.

References

1. Prescribing Information. Sapropterin dihydrochloride. Camber Pharmaceuticals Inc; 2022.
2. American College of Obstetricians and Gynecologists. Management of women with phenylalanine hydroxylase deficiency (phenylketonuria). ACOG committee opinion No. 802. *Obstet Gynecol*. 2020;135:167-170.
3. Grange DK, Hillman RE, Burton BK, et al. Sapropterin dihydrochloride use in pregnant women with phenylketonuria: an interim report of the PKU MOMS sub-registry. *Mol Genet Metab*. 2014;112:9-16.
4. Feillet F, Muntau AC, Debray FG, et al. Use of sapropterin dihydrochloride in maternal phenylketonuria. A European experience of eight cases. *J Inherit Metab Dis*. 2014;37:753-762.
5. Aldamiz-Echevarria L, Couce ML, Llarena M, Andrade F. A new case of maternal phenylketonuria treated with sapropterin dihydrochloride (6R-BH4). *Gynecol Endocrinol*. 2014;691-693.
6. Yildiz Y, Dursun A, Tokatli A, et al. Partial hydatidiform mole in a phenylketonuria patient treated with sapropterin dihydrochloride. *Gynecol Endocrinol*. 2017;33:19-20.
7. Nyuzuki H, Yamazaki T, Saito M, Ohtake A. First Japanese case of maternal phenylketonuria treated with sapropterin dihydrochloride and the normal growth and development of the child. *Mol Genet Metab Rep*. 2019;21:100526.

SARECYCLINE

Antibacterial (Tetracycline)

PREGNANCY RECOMMENDATION: Contraindicated—Second and Third Trimesters

BREASTFEEDING RECOMMENDATION: Potential Toxicity

PREGNANCY SUMMARY

No reports describing the use of sarecycline in human pregnancy have been reported. Some amount of the drug will probably cross the placenta, so fetal exposure will likely occur. However, the absence of human pregnancy experience prevents a complete assessment of the embryofetal risk. Animal data did show embryofetal toxicity. Numerous studies on tetracycline drugs have shown a risk for tooth discoloration, tooth enamel hypoplasia, and inhibition of bone growth when used in the second and third trimesters of pregnancy (see Tetracycline). The manufacturer recommends that pregnant women (and women trying to conceive) should not use sarecycline. In addition, based on the drug's approved indication, use during pregnancy is uncertain.

BREASTFEEDING SUMMARY

It is not known if sarecycline is excreted into human breast milk. The drug will probably be found in breast milk, so some infant exposure will likely occur. Tooth discoloration, tooth enamel hypoplasia, and inhibition of bone growth are theoretically possible in an infant if the drug is used during breastfeeding. In addition, based on the drugs approved use in treating acne vulgaris, long-term treatments (≥3 months) are possible. Therefore, the manufacturer recommends that women not breastfeed during treatment with sarecycline.

Reference

1. Prescribing Information. Seysara. Allergan Pharmaceuticals International Limited; 2019

SARGRAMOSTIM

Hematopoietic (Colony-Stimulating Factor)

PREGNANCY RECOMMENDATION: No Human Data—Animal Data Suggest Potential Risk (Maternal Benefit May Outweigh Any Potential Embryofetal Risk—With Some Medical Conditions)

BREASTFEEDING RECOMMENDATION: Probably Compatible

PREGNANCY SUMMARY

No reports describing the use of sargramostim in human pregnancy have been located. The drug appears to cross the placenta at term, but by placental perfusion studies, it was found that only 3% of the maternal blood level crosses. Therefore, the absence of human pregnancy experience prevents a complete assessment of the embryofetal risk. Animal studies did show some embryofetal toxicity in one species at doses of less than 10 times the RHD. Sargramostim differs only slightly from endogenous granulocyte-macrophage colony-stimulating factor (GM-CSF). In addition, maternal serum concentrations of natural GM-CSF increase throughout pregnancy, with the highest levels occurring during term labor. Therefore, it is doubtful if recommended doses of sargramostim will cause direct toxicity to the embryo or fetus. The manufacturer states that the safest course is to avoid sargramostim during gestation. Nevertheless, using this drug during pregnancy should be based on the pros and cons of the mother's clinical need for treatment versus any potential fetal risk that might occur from exposure. Planned or inadvertent pregnancy exposure appears to represent a low risk for the embryo and fetus. It is recommended that if used during pregnancy, the drug be reconstituted only with sterile water without preservatives (avoid benzyl alcohol). Hypertension was reported in up to 34% of patients treated with this drug in the clinical trials. Elevated glucose levels were reported in up to 49% patients treated with this drug. Therefore, if used during pregnancy, glucose levels should be monitored.

BREASTFEEDING SUMMARY

No reports describing the use of sargramostim during human lactation have been located. Endogenous GM-CSF is excreted into breast milk, so sargramostim will also likely be found in breast milk. However, because it is a protein consisting of about 127 amino acids, if the drug were to be ingested through breastfeeding, it would probably be digested in the infant's gastrointestinal tract and not be absorbed. Based on an immunoradiometric assay, breast milk concentrations of GM-CSF (100 pg/mL) are much higher than levels found in cord blood or infant serum. In addition, there was no difference in neutrophil chemotaxis between the groups, suggesting that GM-CSF was either inactivated or not absorbed from the breast milk.

References

1. Prescribing Information. Leukine. Partner Therapeutics Inc; 2023.
2. Vassiliadis S, Ranella A, Papadimitriou L, et al. Serum levels of pro-and anti-inflammatory cytokines in non-pregnant women, during pregnancy, labour and abortion. *Mediators Inflamm*. 1998;7:69-72.
3. Gregor H, Egarter C, Levin D, et al. The passage of granulocyte-macrophage colony-stimulating factor across the human placenta perfused in vitro. *J Soc Gynecol Investig*. 1999;6:307-310.
4. Sjöblom C, Wikland M, Robertson SA. Granulocyte-macrophage colony-stimulating factor (GM-CSF) acts independently of the beta common subunit of the GM-CSF receptor to prevent inner cell mass apoptosis in human embryos. *Biol Reprod*. 2002;67:1817-1823.
5. Salamonsen LA, Dimitriadis E, Robb L. Cytokines in implantation. *Semin Reprod Med*. 2000;18:299-310.
6. Perricone R, De Carolis C, Giacomelli R, et al. GM-CSF and pregnancy: evidence of significantly reduced blood concentrations in unexplained recurrent abortion efficiently reverted by intravenous immunoglobulin treatment. *Am J Reprod Immunol*. 2003;50:232-237.
7. Tranchot-Diallo J, Gras G, Parnet-Mathieu F, et al. Modulations of cytokine expression in pregnant women. *Am J Reprod Immunol*. 1997;37:215-226.
8. Oláh KS, Vince GS, Neilson JP, et al. Interleukin-6, interferon-γ, interleukin-8, and granulocyte-macrophage colony-stimulating factor levels in human amniotic fluid at term. *J Reprod Immunol*. 1996;32:89-98.

9. Bry K, Hallman M, Teramo K, et al. Granulocyte-macrophage colony-stimulating factor in amniotic fluid and in airway specimens of newborn infants. *Pediatr Res*. 1997;41:105-109.
10. Hayashi M, Hamada Y, Ohkura T. Elevation of granulocyte-macrophage colony-stimulating factor in the placenta and blood in preeclampsia. *Am J Obstet Gynecol*. 2004;190:456-461.
11. Gasparoni A, Chirico G, Ciardelli L, et al. Granulocyte-macrophage colony-stimulating factor in human milk. *Eur J Pediatr*. 1996;155:69.
12. Srivastave MD, Srivastava A, Brouhard B, et al. Cytokines in human milk. *Res Commun Mol Pathol Pharmacol*. 1996;93:263-287.

SARILUMAB

Immunologic (Antirheumatic—Monoclonal Antibody)

PREGNANCY RECOMMENDATION: Limited Human Data—Animal Data Suggest Low Risk

BREASTFEEDING RECOMMENDATION: Probably Compatible

PREGNANCY SUMMARY

There is a case report of a woman who conceived while on sarilumab and continued the drug up to delivery. The newborn was delivered at term and was healthy with no abnormalities reported. Blood levels for the drug were not obtained from the neonate after birth; however, as an IgG antibody, it likely crosses the placenta, and some fetal exposure will probably occur. Animal data did not show any embryofetal toxicity. Using this drug during pregnancy should be based on the pros and cons of the mother's clinical need for treatment versus any potential fetal risk that might occur from exposure. There is a pregnancy exposure registry that monitors pregnancy outcomes in women using this drug. Health care providers are encouraged to call the Kevzara Pregnancy Exposure Registry at 1-877-311-8972.

BREASTFEEDING SUMMARY

A single case report of a woman who used sarilumab during human lactation did not report any adverse infant effects. The drug is likely present in breast milk. However, it is known that IgG antibodies can be found in human breast milk, but are not found in the neonatal or infant circulation. Additionally, if any IgG antibodies were to be ingested through breastfeeding, they would probably be digested in the infant's gastrointestinal tract and not be absorbed. The manufacturer recommends that women consider discontinuing the drug while breastfeeding. However, breastfeeding while using this drug should be based on the mother's clinical need for treatment. If used, the infant should be monitored for the most common reported adult side effects of upper respiratory tract infections, urinary tract infections, and various laboratory abnormalities (see PI).

References

1. Product Information. Kevzara. Sanofi-Aventis U.S. LLC; 2018.
2. Mizutani A, Okunishi Y, Tamada T, et al. A woman with rheumatoid arthritis who successfully delivered a healthy child with continuous administration of sarilumab throughout pregnancy. *Intern Med*. 2023;62(4):633-636.

SATRALIZUMAB

Central Nervous System (Interleukin-6 Receptor Antagonist—Monoclonal Antibody)

PREGNANCY RECOMMENDATION: No Human Data—Animal Data Suggest Low Risk

BREASTFEEDING RECOMMENDATION: Probably Compatible

PREGNANCY SUMMARY

No reports describing the use of satralizumab in human pregnancy have been located. Because it is an antibody of the IgG class, it probably crosses the placenta. Animal data did not show fetotoxic effects. However, the absence of human pregnancy experience prevents a complete assessment of the embryofetal risk. There is a pregnancy registry that monitors pregnancy outcomes in women who use this drug during pregnancy. Health care providers are encouraged to register patients by calling 1-833-277-9338. Because the drug is modified from tocilizumab (see Tocilizumab), pregnancy safety issues are probably similar.

BREASTFEEDING SUMMARY

Satralizumab probably enters breast milk. However, it is known that IgG antibodies can be found in human breast milk, but are not found in neonatal or infant circulation. Additionally, if any IgG antibodies were to be ingested through breastfeeding, they would probably be digested in the infant's gastrointestinal tract and not be absorbed. If the clinical decision is to use this drug during breastfeeding, the infant should be monitored for the most common reported adult side effects of arthralgia, headache, pruritus, and nausea (all leading to irritability), rash, lethargy, and neutropenia.

References

1. Prescribing Information. Enspryng. Genentech, Inc; 2020.
2. Costello F, Burton JM. Contemporary management challenges in seropositive NMOSD. *J Neurol*. 2022;269:5674-5681.
3. Holmoy T, Hoglund RA, Illes Z, et al. Recent progress in maintenance of neuromyelitis optica spectrum disorder. *J Neurol*. 2021;268:4522-4536.

SAXAGLIPTIN

Antidiabetic (Dipeptidyl peptidase-4 Inhibitor)

PREGNANCY RECOMMENDATION: Limited Human Data—Animal Data Suggest Low Risk

BREASTFEEDING RECOMMENDATION: Probably Compatible

PREGNANCY SUMMARY

No reports describing the use of saxagliptin in human pregnancy have been located. One study evaluated dipeptidyl peptidase-4 (DPP4) inhibitors as a group during pregnancy. The population-based cohort evaluated the risk for malformations with periconceptional use of antidiabetic medications compared with controls. Patients needed to fill at least one prescription within 90 days prior to pregnancy through the end of the first trimester. Overall, 15,148 were prescribed antidiabetic medication. Exposures included metformin only (*n* = 7,440), insulin (*n* = 5,078), sulfonylureas (*n* = 1,352), DPP4 inhibitors (*n* = 687), glucagon-like peptide 1 (GLP-1) receptor antagonists (*n* = 938), and sodium-glucose cotransporter 2 (SGLT2) inhibitors (*n* = 335). The specific medications used within each class were not provided. When compared to the insulin-exposed group, DPP4 inhibitors had similar rates of any major malformation and cardiac malformations (3.3%). The drug is likely to cross the placenta, so some fetal exposure will probably occur. However, this limited human pregnancy experience prevents a complete assessment of embryofetal risk. Animal studies did not show any embryofetal toxicity in two species at doses of more than 10 times the RHD. Using this drug during pregnancy should be based on the pros and cons of the mother's clinical need for treatment versus any potential fetal risk that might occur from exposure. Uncontrolled diabetes is associated with an increased risk for preeclampsia, spontaneous abortion, preterm delivery, intrauterine fetal demise, delivery complications, and major malformations. Insulin is still the treatment of choice for this disease during pregnancy. Moreover, insulin does not cross the placenta, which eliminates the additional concern that the drug therapy is adversely affecting the fetus. Carefully prescribed insulin therapy will provide better control of the mother's blood glucose, thereby preventing the fetal and neonatal complications that occur with this disease. ACOG recommends that insulin be used for type 1 and 2 diabetes occurring during pregnancy and, if diet therapy alone is not successful, for gestational diabetes. If a woman becomes pregnant while taking saxagliptin, changing the therapy to insulin should be considered.

BREASTFEEDING SUMMARY

No reports describing the use of saxagliptin during human lactation have been located. The drug and its active metabolite will likely be excreted into breast milk, so some infant exposure will probably occur. Breastfeeding while using this drug should be based on the mother's clinical need for treatment versus any potential infant risks that might occur. If used, the infant should be monitored for the most common reported adult side effects of headache (leading to irritability), upper respiratory tract infection, and urinary tract infection.

References

1. Prescribing Information. Saxagliptin. Amneal Pharmaceuticals LLC; 2022.
2. American College of Obstetricians and Gynecologists. ACOG practice bulletin No. 201: pregestational diabetes mellitus. *Obstet Gynecol*. 2018; 132:e228-e248.
3. American College of Obstetricians and Gynecologists. ACOG practice bulletin No. 190: gestational diabetes. *Obstet Gynecol*. 2018;131:e49-e64.
4. Cesta CE, Rotern R, Bateman BT, et al. Safety of GLP-1 receptor agonists and other second-line antidiabetics in early pregnancy. *JAMA Intern Med*. 2024;184:144-152.

SCOPOLAMINE

Gastrointestinal (Anticholinergic—Antimuscarinic)

PREGNANCY RECOMMENDATION: Limited Human Data—No Relevant Animal Data

BREASTFEEDING RECOMMENDATION: Probably Compatible

PREGNANCY SUMMARY

Several reports describing the use of scopolamine during human pregnancy have been located. From the combined data of the Collaborative Perinatal Project and the Michigan Medicaid Surveillance study, there were 336 first-trimester exposures with 3 (0.9%) major birth anomalies identified. Additionally, the manufacturer reports that no increased risk for malformations, spontaneous abortion, or other adverse fetal outcomes was observed in postmarketing reports. The drug appears to cross the placenta, so fetal exposure will occur. Embryofetal toxicity was observed in one animal species, but at doses of about 100 times the RHD. Using this drug during pregnancy should be based on the pros and cons of the mother's clinical need for treatment versus any potential fetal risk that might occur from exposure. Scopolamine, like atropine, can alter the appearance of the fetal heart rate (FHR) tracing by producing an elevation in the baseline and significantly decreasing variability.

BREASTFEEDING SUMMARY

Scopolamine has been shown to be excreted into human breast milk, so infant exposure will occur. Breastfeeding while using this drug should be based on the mother's clinical need for treatment versus any potential infant risks that might occur. If used, the infant should be monitored for the most common reported adult side effects of blurred vision and agitation (both leading to irritability), drowsiness, and somnolence. Because it has anticholinergic effects, use of the drug may decrease breast milk production.

References

1. Prescribing Information. Scopolamine. Mylan Pharmaceuticals Inc; 2024.
2. National Library of Medicine. Scopolamine. Pubchem. Accessed September 13, 2024. https://pubchem.ncbi.nlm.nih.gov/compound/Hyoscine
3. Shenker L. Clinical experiences with fetal heart rate monitoring of one thousand patients in labor. *Am J Obstet Gynecol*. 1973;115:1111-1116.
4. Boehm FH, Growdon JH Jr. The effect of scopolamine on fetal heart rate baseline variability. *Am J Obstet Gynecol*. 1974;120:1099-1104.
5. Ayromlooi J, Tobias M, Berg P. The effects of scopolamine and ancillary analgesics upon the fetal heart rate recording. *J Reprod Med*. 1980;25:323-326.
6. Diaz DM, Diaz SF, Marx GF. Cardiovascular effects of glycopyrrolate and belladonna derivatives in obstetric patients. *Bull NY Acad Med*. 1980; 56:245-248.
7. Heinonen OP, Slone D, Shapiro S. *Birth Defects and Drugs in Pregnancy*. Publishing Sciences Group; 1977.
8. Evens RP, Leopold JC. Scopolamine toxicity in a newborn. *Pediatrics*. 1980; 66:329-330.
9. Larki M, Rasti A, Makvandi S. The effect of hyoscine *N*-butyl bromide rectal on the duration of labour and rate of cervical dilation: a systematic review and meta-analysis. *J Obstet Gynaecol Can*. 2024;46:102292.

SEBELIPASE ALFA

Genetic (Enzyme)

PREGNANCY RECOMMENDATION: No Human Data—Animal Data Suggest Low Risk

BREASTFEEDING RECOMMENDATION: Probably Compatible

PREGNANCY SUMMARY

No reports describing the use of sebelipase alfa in human pregnancy have been located. Based on unlikely placental transfer, fetal exposure is probably negligible. However, the absence of human pregnancy experience prevents a complete assessment of the embryofetal risk. Animal studies did not show any adverse embryofetal toxicity. Patients with a known history of egg allergies should be aware that the drug is produced in egg whites of genetically engineered chickens.

S

BREASTFEEDING SUMMARY

No reports describing the use of sebelipase alfa during human lactation have been located. Excretion into breast milk is probably negligible, so infant exposure is likely to be clinically insignificant. Furthermore, because sebelipase alfa is primarily a protein, if the drug were to be ingested through breastfeeding, it would probably be digested in the infant's gastrointestinal tract and not be absorbed. Breastfeeding while using this drug should be based on the mother's clinical need for treatment. If used while breastfeeding, the infant should be monitored for the most common reported adult side effects of headache and nausea (both leading to irritability), pyrexia, diarrhea, vomiting, constipation, and cough.

Reference

1. Prescribing Information. Kanuma. Alexion Pharmaceuticals, Inc; 2021.

SECNIDAZOLE

Anti-Infective (Nitroimidazole)

PREGNANCY RECOMMENDATION: Limited Human Data—Animal Data Suggest Potential Risk

BREASTFEEDING RECOMMENDATION: Potential Toxicity

PREGNANCY SUMMARY

One study that analyzed pregnancy outcome in women with bacterial vaginosis stated that four women used secnidazole during pregnancy and no adverse newborn effects were reported. However, the gestational age of use and specific pregnancy outcomes for these four cases were not described. The drug will probably cross the placenta, so fetal exposure will likely occur. However, this limited human pregnancy experience prevents a complete assessment of the embryofetal risk. Animal studies did not show any embryofetal toxicity at doses that did not cause maternal toxicity, but maternal toxicity was common. Using this drug during pregnancy should be based on the pros and cons of the mother's clinical need for treatment versus any potential fetal risk that might occur from exposure.

BREASTFEEDING SUMMARY

No reports describing the use of secnidazole during human lactation have been located. The drug will probably enter breast milk, so infant exposure will likely occur. Because of potential adverse reactions that might occur in a breast-fed infant, the manufacturer recommends that women not breastfeed while using this drug and for 96 hours after the last dose. However, breastfeeding should be based on the mother's clinical need for treatment. If used, the infant should be monitored for the most common reported adult side effects of headache, nausea, and abdominal pain (all leading to irritability) and diarrhea.

References

1. Prescribing Information. Solosec. Lupin Pharmaceuticals, Inc; 2021.
2. Soares de Camargo RP, Simoes JA, Cecatti JG, et al. Impact of treatment for bacterial vaginosis on prematurity among Brazilian pregnant women: a retrospective cohort study. *Sao Paula Med J*. 2005;123:108-112.

SECUKINUMAB

Immunologic (Anti-Interleukin 17A—Monoclonal Antibody)

PREGNANCY RECOMMENDATION: Limited Human Data—Animal Data Suggest Low Risk

BREASTFEEDING RECOMMENDATION: Probably Compatible

PREGNANCY SUMMARY

Several studies have been identified that described the use of secukinumab in human pregnancy. A total of 6 (3.0%) major malformations were described in 201 first-trimester exposures. Other uses have been reported during the second and third trimesters without any adverse fetal effects seen. As an IgG antibody, it likely crosses the placenta, especially during the second half of gestation, so some fetal exposure will probably occur. However, this limited human pregnancy experience prevents a complete assessment of embryofetal risk. Animal studies did not show any embryofetal toxicity in two species at doses of more than 10 times the RHD. Using this drug during pregnancy should be based on the pros and cons of the mother's clinical need for treatment versus any potential fetal risk that might occur from exposure.

BREASTFEEDING SUMMARY

No reports describing the use of secukinumab during human lactation have been located. It is known that IgG antibodies can be found in human breast milk, but are not found in the neonatal or infant circulation. Additionally, if any IgG antibodies were to be ingested through breastfeeding, they would probably be digested in the infant's gastrointestinal tract and not be absorbed. Breastfeeding while using this drug should be based on the mother's clinical need for treatment versus any potential infant risks that might occur. If used, the infant should be monitored for the most common reported adult side effects of diarrhea and upper respiratory tract infection.

References

1. Prescribing Information. Cosentyx. Novartis Pharmaceuticals Corporation; 2023.
2. Warren RB, Reich K, Langley RG, et al. Secukinumab in pregnancy: outcomes in psoriasis, psoriatric arthritis and ankylosing spondylitis from the global safety database. *Br J Dermatol*. 2018;179:1205-1207.
3. Chhabra G, Chanana C, Verma P, Saxena A. Impetigo herpetiformis responsive to secukinumab. *Dermatol Ther*. 2019;32:e13040.
4. Liu N, Zhu L, Cheng Y, et al. Successful treatment of recurrent pustular psoriasis of pregnancy with secukinumab: a case report. *Acta Derm Venereol*. 2020;100:adv00251.
5. Ghalandari N, Crijns HJMJ, Bergman EJH, et al. Reported congenital malformations after exposure to non-tumor necrosis factor inhibitor biologics: a retrospective comparative study in EudraVigilance. *Br J Clin Pharmacol*. 2022;88:5378-5388.
6. Zhang J, Xia P, Wan L, et al. Generalized pustular psoriasis of pregnancy successfully treated with secukinumab. *Indian J Dermatol Venereol Leprol*. 2023;89:886-888.
7. Dernoncourt A, Liabeuf S, Bennis Y, et al. Fetal and neonatal adverse drug reactions associated with biologics taken during pregnancy by women with autoimmune diseases: insights from an analysis of the World Health Organization pharmacovigilance database (Vigibase). *BioDrugs*. 2023;37:73-87.
8. Hsieh CY, Tsai YJ, Tsai TF. Use of biologics in Chinese pregnant patients with a deficiency of interleukin-36 receptor antagonist (DITRA): a case series. *Taiwan J Obstet Gynecol*. 2024;63:405-408.

SEGESTERONE ACETATE/ETHINYL ESTRADIOL

Reproductive (Birth Control Vaginal System)

PREGNANCY RECOMMENDATION: *Contraindicated

BREASTFEEDING RECOMMENDATION: Probably Compatible

PREGNANCY SUMMARY

No reports describing the use of the segesterone acetate/ethinyl estradiol vaginal system in human pregnancy have been located. Though placental transfer of both the progestin and estrogen most likely occurs, the overall fetal effect of this combination is unknown. Meta-analyses on combination hormonal contraceptives have not found an increase in birth anomalies overall (see Ethinyl Estradiol and other progestins). Animal reproduction studies have not been performed. *Birth control treatment during pregnancy is contraindicated.

BREASTFEEDING SUMMARY

The manufacturer reports that the segesterone level found in human breast milk was about 5% of the plasma level. In addition, segesterone is poorly absorbed orally. Very small amounts (<1%) of ethinyl estradiol are excreted into human breast milk. Breastfeeding while using this combination of hormonal contraceptive vaginal ring is probably compatible, but there is concern that it might decrease breast milk production in some patients. If used, breast milk production should be monitored, and the infant followed for growth and other reported side effects of headache and nausea (both leading to irritability), vomiting, and diarrhea.

References

1. Prescribing Information. Annovera. Population Council; 2018.
2. Klinger G, Claussen C, Schroder S. Excretion of ethinyloestradiol sulfonate in human milk. *Zentralbl Gynakol*. 1981;103:91-95.

SELADELPAR

Gastrointestinal (Hepatic—Peroxisome Proliferator–Activated Receptor—Delta Agonist)

PREGNANCY RECOMMENDATION: No Human Data—Animal Data Suggest Low Risk

BREASTFEEDING RECOMMENDATION: Probably Compatible

PREGNANCY SUMMARY

No reports describing the use of seladelpar during human pregnancy have been located. The drug will likely cross the placenta, so some fetal exposure will probably occur. Therefore, the absence of human pregnancy experience prevents a complete assessment of the embryofetal risk. Animal studies did not show any embryofetal toxicity in two species at doses of less than 10 times the RHD in one and more than 10 times the RHD in the second. Using this drug during pregnancy should be based on the pros and cons of the mother's clinical need for treatment versus any potential fetal risk that might occur from exposure.

S

BREASTFEEDING SUMMARY

No reports describing the use of seladelpar during human lactation have been located. The drug will likely be found in breast milk, so some infant exposure will likely occur. Breastfeeding while using this drug should be based on the mother's clinical need for treatment versus any potential infant risk that might occur. If used, the infant should be monitored for the most common reported adult side effects of nausea, headache, dizziness, and abdominal pain (all leading to irritability) and abnormal liver function tests.

Reference

1. Prescribing Information. Livdelzi. Gilead Sciences, LLC; 2024.

SELEGILINE

Central Nervous System/Mental Health (MOA Type B Inhibitor)

PREGNANCY RECOMMENDATION: Limited Human Data—Animal Data Suggest Low Risk

BREASTFEEDING RECOMMENDATION: Potential Toxicity

PREGNANCY SUMMARY

Human pregnancy experience with selegiline is limited. Three cases of exposure to selegiline during human pregnancy have been located, and only one of them involved exposure throughout gestation. The exposed child had no birth anomalies and was developing normally at age 10. The drug and its active metabolites are likely to cross the placenta, so some fetal exposure will probably occur. However, this limited human pregnancy experience prevents a complete assessment of embryofetal risk. Animal data did not show any embryofetal toxicity in two species at oral and transdermal doses of less than 10 times the RHD and just above 10 times the RHD. Using this drug during pregnancy should be based on the pros and cons of the mother's clinical need for treatment versus any potential fetal risk that might occur from exposure. Additionally, tyramine-containing foods (some cheeses, meats, dried fruits, fermented foods, and others) should be avoided while taking selegiline and for 2 weeks after the last dose.

BREASTFEEDING SUMMARY

Two reports have described the use of selegiline during human lactation. One exposure was only for 3 days, but no issues were described. In another case, the patient breastfed the infant while continuing her medications. Infant levels were undetectable for selegiline and its metabolite at 12 days postpartum. Normal healthy development was reported at 5 months of age. Because of the potential for serious adverse reactions that might be seen in a breastfed infant, the manufacturer of the patch recommends that women not breastfeed while being treated with selegiline and for 5 days after the last dose. Nevertheless, breastfeeding while using this drug should be based on the mother's clinical need for treatment versus any potential infant risks that might occur. If used, the infant should be monitored for the most common reported adult side effects of nausea, dizziness, abdominal pain, and dyspepsia (all leading to irritability), insomnia, and rash.

References

1. Prescribing Information. Selegiline hydrochloride. Apotex Corp; 2023.
2. Product Information. Emsam. Mylan Specialty LP; 2020.
3. Hagell P, Odin P, Vinge E. Pregnancy in Parkinson's disease: a review of the literature and a case report. *Mov Disord*. 1998;13:34-38.
4. Kupsch A, Oertel WH. Selegiline, pregnancy, and Parkinson's disease. *Mov Disord*. 1998;13:175-194.
5. Bauer RL, Orfei J, Wichman CL. Use of transdermal selegiline in pregnancy and lactation: a case report. *Psychosomatics*. 2017;58:450-452.
6. Huybrechts KF, Palmsten K, Avorn J, et al. Antidepressant use in pregnancy and the risk of cardiac defects. *N Engl J Med*. 2014;370:2397-2407.

SELEXIPAG

Cardiovascular (Vasodilator—Pulmonary Arterial Hypertension)

PREGNANCY RECOMMENDATION: No Human Data—Animal Data Suggest Low Risk

BREASTFEEDING RECOMMENDATION: Potential Toxicity

PREGNANCY SUMMARY

No reports describing the use of selexipag in human pregnancy have been located. The drug probably crosses the placenta, so some fetal exposure will likely occur. Therefore, the absence of human pregnancy experience prevents a complete assessment of the embryofetal risk. Animal data did not show any embryofetal toxicity. Using this drug during pregnancy should be based on the pros and cons of the mother's clinical need for treatment versus any potential fetal risk that might occur from exposure.

BREASTFEEDING SUMMARY

No reports describing the use of selexipag during human lactation have been located. Some amount of the drug will probably appear in breast milk. Due to the concern for potential serious adverse effects that might occur in a breastfed infant, the manufacturer recommends not nursing while using this drug. Nevertheless, breastfeeding while using this drug should be based on the mother's clinical need for treatment. If used, the infant should be monitored for the most common reported adult side effects of nausea, myalgias, headache, jaw pain, and extremity pain (all leading to irritability), diarrhea, and vomiting.

Reference

1. Product Information. Uptravi. Actelion Pharmaceuticals US, Inc; 2021.

SELINEXOR

Antineoplastic (Nuclear Export Inhibitor)

PREGNANCY RECOMMENDATION: Limited Human Data—Animal Data Suggest Potential Risk

BREASTFEEDING RECOMMENDATION: Potential Toxicity

S

PREGNANCY SUMMARY

No reports describing the use of selinexor in human pregnancy have been located. The drug will probably cross the placenta, so some fetal exposure will likely occur. However, the absence of human pregnancy experience prevents a complete assessment of embryofetal risk. Embryofetal toxicity with malformations was observed in one animal study at doses less than the RHD. Based on animal studies and the drug's mechanism of action, the manufacturer recommends that women with reproductive potential use effective contraception during treatment and for 1 week after the last dose. They also recommend that males with female partners of reproductive potential use effective contraception during treatment and for 1 week after the last dose. Nevertheless, using this drug during pregnancy should be based on the pros and cons of the mother's clinical need for treatment versus any potential fetal risk that might occur from exposure. There is a registry for women who are pregnant and have cancer. For more information, women and health care providers are encouraged to contact the Cancer and Pregnancy Registry at 1-877-635-4499. Elevated glucose levels have been reported in 15% patients treated with this drug in the clinical trials. Therefore, if used during pregnancy, glucose levels should be monitored.

BREASTFEEDING SUMMARY

No reports describing the use of selinexor during human lactation have been located. The drug will likely be excreted into human breast milk, so some infant exposure will probably occur. However, due to a concern for potential serious adverse effects that might be seen in a breastfed infant, the manufacturer recommends that women not breastfeed while being treated with this drug and for at least 1 week after the last dose. Nevertheless, breastfeeding while using this drug should be based on the mother's clinical need for treatment versus any potential infant risks that might occur. If used, the infant should be monitored for the most common reported adult side effects of nausea and peripheral neuropathy (both leading to irritability), fatigue (lethargy), decreased appetite (monitor infant growth), diarrhea, vomiting, pyrexia, and various laboratory abnormalities (see PI).

References

1. Prescribing Information. Selinexor. Karyopharm Therapeutics Inc; 2022.

SELPERCATINIB

Antineoplastic (Kinase Inhibitor)

PREGNANCY RECOMMENDATION: No Human Data—Animal Data Suggest Potential Risk

BREASTFEEDING RECOMMENDATION: Potential Toxicity

PREGNANCY SUMMARY

No reports describing the use of selpercatinib in human pregnancy have been located. Some amount of the drug will probably cross the placenta, so fetal exposure will likely occur. However, the absence of human pregnancy experience prevents a complete assessment of the embryofetal risk. Animal studies showed embryofetal toxicity and teratogenicity. Based on these animal studies and the drug's mechanism of action, the manufacturer recommends that women with reproductive potential use effective contraception during treatment and for 1 week after the last dose. They also recommend that males with female partners of reproductive potential use effective contraception during treatment and for 1 week after the last dose. However, using this drug during pregnancy should be based on the pros and cons of the mother's clinical need for treatment versus any potential fetal risk that might occur from exposure. Hypertension was reported in up to 35% of patients treated with selpercatinib in clinical trials. The drug was also found to prolong the QT interval and elevate blood glucose levels.

BREASTFEEDING SUMMARY

No reports describing the use of selpercatinib during human lactation have been located. Some of the drug probably enters breast milk, so infant exposure will likely occur. However, due to the concern for potential serious adverse effects that might be seen in a breastfed infant, the manufacturer recommends that women not breastfeed while being treated with selpercatinib and for at least 1 week after the last dose. Nevertheless, breastfeeding while using this drug should be based on the mother's clinical need for treatment. If used, the infant should be monitored for the most common reported adult side effects of hypertension, diarrhea, lethargy, edema, rash, constipation, elevated glucose, and other laboratory abnormalities (see PI).

Reference

1. Prescribing Information. Retevmo. Eli Lilly and Company; 2021.

SELUMETINIB

Antineoplastic (Kinase Inhibitor)

PREGNANCY RECOMMENDATION: No Human Data—Animal Data Suggest Potential Risk

BREASTFEEDING RECOMMENDATION: Potential Toxicity

PREGNANCY SUMMARY

No reports describing the use of selumetinib in human pregnancy have been located. The drug probably crosses the placenta in small amounts, so some fetal exposure is likely to occur. Therefore, the absence of human pregnancy experience prevents a complete assessment of the embryofetal risk. Animal studies showed embryofetal toxicity. Based on these animal studies and the drug's mechanism of action, the manufacturer recommends that women with reproductive potential use effective contraception during treatment with selumetinib and for 1 week after the last dose. They also recommend that males with female partners of reproductive potential use effective contraception during treatment and for 1 week after the last dose. Using this drug during pregnancy should be based on the pros and cons of the mother's clinical need for treatment versus any potential fetal risk that might occur from exposure. Cardiomyopathy and ocular toxicity may occur in patients treated with this drug. Cardiac ejection fraction and a baseline ophthalmic evaluation should be obtained prior to starting the drug and then assessed periodically while on treatment.

BREASTFEEDING SUMMARY

No reports describing the use of selumetinib during human lactation have been located. The drug is probably excreted into breast milk, so some infant exposure is likely to occur. However, due to the concern for potential adverse effects on a breastfed infant, the manufacturer recommends that women not breastfeed while being treated with selumetinib and for at least 1 week after the last dose. Nevertheless, breastfeeding while using this drug should be based on the mother's clinical need for treatment. If used, the infant should be monitored for the most common reported adult side effects of nausea, headache, abdominal pain, musculoskeletal pain, and pruritus (all leading to irritability), vomiting, diarrhea, rash, lethargy, and pyrexia.

Reference

1. Prescribing Information. Koselugo. AstraZeneca Pharmaceuticals LP; 2021.

SEMAGLUTIDE

Antidiabetic Agent

PREGNANCY RECOMMENDATION: No Human Data and No Relevant Animal Data

BREASTFEEDING RECOMMENDATION: Probably Compatible

PREGNANCY SUMMARY

No reports describing the use of semaglutide in human pregnancy have been located. A negligible amount of the drug may cross the placenta, so fetal exposure will likely not be clinically significant. However, the absence of human pregnancy experience prevents a complete assessment of the embryofetal risk. Animal studies demonstrated embryofetal toxicity, but every dose produced maternal toxicity. Using this drug during pregnancy should be based on the pros and cons of the mother's clinical need for treatment versus any potential fetal risk that might occur from exposure. For fertility purposes, the manufacturer recommends that women and men with reproductive potential discontinue the drug for 2 months before a planned pregnancy.

BREASTFEEDING SUMMARY

No reports describing the use of semaglutide in human lactation have been located. A negligible amount of the drug may be found in breast milk. However, because it is a polypeptide, if the drug were to be ingested through breastfeeding, it probably would be digested in the infant's gastrointestinal tract and not be absorbed. Breastfeeding while using this drug should be based on the mother's clinical need for treatment. If used, the infant should be monitored for the most common reported adult side effects of nausea and abdominal pain (both leading to irritability), vomiting, diarrhea, and constipation.

Reference

1. Prescribing Information. Ozempic. Novo Nordisk A/S; 2022.

SENNA

Gastrointestinal (Stimulant Laxative)

PREGNANCY RECOMMENDATION: Human Data Suggest Low Risk

BREASTFEEDING RECOMMENDATION: Probably Compatible

PREGNANCY SUMMARY

One report describing the use of senna during human pregnancy was located. In 22,843 pregnancies with newborns found to have birth anomalies and 38,151 pregnancies with newborns that did not have birth anomalies, the use of senna in the group with birth anomalies was 506 (2.2%) versus 937 (2.5%) in the group without congenital anomalies. If found in the maternal circulation, some of the drug will probably cross the placenta. However, because senna is activated in the colon, systemic absorption is low. Therefore, overall fetal exposure is likely to be minimal. Using this drug during pregnancy should be based on the pros and cons of the mother's clinical need for treatment versus any potential fetal risk that might occur from exposure.

BREASTFEEDING SUMMARY

Sennosides A and B are not excreted into human breast milk. A 1973 study using colorimetric analysis (sensitivity limit 0.34 mcg/mL) failed to detect the natural agents. The active metabolite, rhein, however, is excreted into breast milk in very small amounts. Lactating women administered 5 g of senna daily for 3 days excreted a mean 0.007% of the dose in their breast milk, and no adverse effects were observed in the nursing infants. This is compatible with the fact that the anthraquinone laxatives are absorbed only slightly after oral administration. Nevertheless, breastfeeding while using this drug should be based on the mother's clinical need for treatment versus any potential infant risks that might occur. If used, the infant should be monitored for the most common reported adult side effects of abdominal discomfort, nausea, and cramps (all leading to irritability), diarrhea, flatulence, and urine discoloration.

References

1. Prescribing Information. Genexa Senna Laxative. Genexa Inc; 2022.
2. Faber P, Strenge-Hesse A. Relevance of rhein excretion into breast milk. *Pharmacology*. 1988;36(suppl 1):212-220.
3. National Library of Medicine. Senna. Pubchem. Accessed August 22, 2024. https://pubchem.ncbi.nlm.nih.gov/compound/Senna
4. Acs N, Banhidy F, Puho EH, Czeizel AE. Senna treatment in pregnant women and congenital abnormalities in their offspring—a population-based case-control study. *Reprod Toxicol*. 2009;28:100-104.
5. Shepard TH. *Catalog of Teratogenic Agents*. 6th ed. The Johns Hopkins University Press; 1989:574-575.
6. Werthmann MW Jr, Krees SV. Quantitative excretion of Senokot in human breast milk. *Med Ann Dist Columbia*. 1973;42:4-5.
7. Baldwin WF. Clinical study of senna administration to nursing mothers: assessment of effects on infant bowel habits. *Can Med Assoc J*. 1963; 89:566-568.
8. Greenhalf JO, Leonard HSD. Laxatives in the treatment of constipation in pregnant and breast-feeding mothers. *Practitioner*. 1973;210:259-263.

SERDEXMETHYLPHENIDATE AND DEXMETHYLPHENIDATE

Central Nervous System (Stimulant)

PREGNANCY RECOMMENDATION: No Human Data—Animal Data Suggest Potential Risk

BREASTFEEDING RECOMMENDATION: Potential Toxicity

S

PREGNANCY SUMMARY

No reports describing the use of serdexmethylphenidate/dexmethylphenidate in human pregnancy have been located. Both drugs will probably cross the placenta, so fetal exposure will likely occur. Therefore, the absence of human pregnancy experience prevents a complete assessment of the embryofetal risk. Animal data did show some embryofetal toxicity with dexmethylphenidate but not with serdexmethylphenidate. Therapeutic doses of methylphenidate during pregnancy have not been associated with fetal/neonatal adverse reactions; whereas premature delivery and low birth weight infants have been associated with amphetamine-dependent mothers (see Methylphenidate). Central nervous system (CNS) stimulants can also cause vasoconstriction. Therefore, a theoretical risk for blood pressure elevation and decreased placental perfusion exists. Using this drug during pregnancy should be based on the pros and cons of the mother's clinical need for treatment versus any potential fetal risk that might occur from exposure. There is a pregnancy exposure registry that monitors pregnancy outcomes in women using psychostimulants. Health care providers and women who are pregnant and have taken serdexmethylphenidate/dexmethylphenidate at any time during pregnancy are encouraged to contact the National Pregnancy Registry for Psychostimulants at 1-866-961-2388.

BREASTFEEDING SUMMARY

No reports describing the use of serdexmethylphenidate/dexmethylphenidate during human lactation have been located. Both drugs are probably excreted into breast milk, so some infant exposure will probably occur. Methylphenidate was present in breast milk, but infant blood levels were low (see Methylphenidate). Breastfeeding while using this drug should be based on the mother's clinical need for treatment. If used, the infant should be monitored for the most common reported adult side effects of nausea and abdominal pain (both leading to irritability), decreased appetite (monitor growth), sleep dysfunction, vomiting, tachycardia, and blood pressure elevation.

Reference

1. Prescribing Information. Azstarys. Corium; 2021.

SERTACONAZOLE

Anti-Infective (Topical—Antifungal)

PREGNANCY RECOMMENDATION: Human Data Suggest Low Risk

BREASTFEEDING RECOMMENDATION: Probably Compatible

PREGNANCY SUMMARY

Two reports describing the use of topical sertaconazole in human pregnancy have been located. There have been over 16,000 pregnancy exposures, including over 5,000 first-trimester exposures. The rate of major birth malformations was 2.68% consistent with the unexposed control group (2.63%) and the expected rate in the United States. The data suggest that sertaconazole does not increase the risk for malformations or other adverse pregnancy outcomes such as preterm delivery and small-for-gestational-age birthweights. The failure to detect the drug in the plasma after multiple topical applications to diseased skin suggests that the human embryofetal risk is negligible. Embryofetal toxicity with malformations was observed in one animal species (and not in a second species) at doses of more than 10 times the RHD. The drug was also administered orally. Using this drug during pregnancy should be based on the pros and cons of the mother's clinical need for treatment versus any potential fetal risk that might occur from exposure.

BREASTFEEDING SUMMARY

No reports describing the use of topical sertaconazole during human lactation have been located. The drug does not produce detectable plasma concentrations after multiple applications to diseased skin. Therefore, the risk to a nursing infant can be considered negligible, and the antifungal agent is probably compatible with breastfeeding. Breastfeeding while using this drug should be based on the mother's clinical need for treatment versus any potential infant risks that might occur. Because it is used topically, systemic side effects were not analyzed.

References

1. Prescribing Information. Ertaczo. Bausch Health US LLC; 2020.
2. Araujo M, Hurault-Delarue C, Sommet A, et al. Topical sertaconazole during pregnancy and risk of adverse pregnancy outcome and major congenital anomalies: comparative study in the EFEMERIS database. *Mycoses*. 2022;65:481-489.
3. Chayachinda C, Thamkhantho M, Rekhawasin, Klerdklinhom C. Sertaconazole 300 mg versus clotrimazole 500 mg vaginal suppository for treating pregnant women with acute vaginal candidiasis: a double-blinded, randomized trial. *BMC Pregnancy Childbirth*. 2024;24:235.

SERTRALINE

Mental Health (Selective Serotonin Reuptake Inhibitor)

PREGNANCY RECOMMENDATION: Human Data Suggest Low Risk (First Trimester) and High Risk (Third Trimester)

BREASTFEEDING RECOMMENDATION: Probably Compatible

PREGNANCY SUMMARY

There are numerous publications describing the use of sertraline during human pregnancy. In two very large analyses involving databases with several million pregnant women, the risk for major birth anomalies with exposure to selective serotonin reuptake inhibitors (SSRIs) in the first trimester is higher than in the control populations, but is not higher than in patients with depression not on SSRI treatment. In addition, the anomaly rate falls within the expected rate of 2% to 4% and no

(*continued*)

pattern to the anomalies has been found. In 2023, ACOG stated that SSRIs do not increase the risk of malformations, cardiovascular malformations, growth restriction, small for gestational age, preterm delivery, gestational diabetes, preeclampsia, or neurodevelopmental delays in speech and language and scholastic or motor disorders. However, its use near delivery is associated with an increased risk for poor neonatal adaptation syndrome. Sertraline crosses the placenta, so some fetal exposure will occur. Embryofetal toxicity was observed in two animal species at doses of less than 10 times the RHD. Using this drug during pregnancy should be based on the pros and cons of the mother's clinical need for treatment versus any potential fetal risk that might occur from exposure. There is a pregnancy exposure registry that monitors pregnancy outcomes in women using antidepressant drugs. Health care providers are encouraged to call the National Pregnancy Registry for Antidepressants at 1-844-405-6185. Sertraline can prolong the QTc interval and should be used with caution in patients with risk factors for QTc prolongation. The manufacturer recommends that the oral solution be avoided during pregnancy because it contains 12% alcohol, and options without alcohol exist (even though the total amount of alcohol is small overall). ACOG states that uncontrolled and undertreated depression is associated with a risk for limited engagement in medical care and self-care, substance use, preterm birth, low birth weight, preeclampsia, postpartum depression, impaired infant attachment (which carries long-term developmental effects), disrupted relationships with partner, and suicide. Additionally, untreated and undertreated mental health disorders should be considered an exposure. Pregnancy and lactation alone should not be a reason to withhold or discontinue mental health medications.

BREASTFEEDING SUMMARY

Several reports describing the use of sertraline during human lactation have been located. Breast milk levels for sertraline and its metabolite are about equal to the maternal plasma levels. However, infant levels for both range from undetectable to 3 ng/mL for sertraline and undetectable to 24 ng/mL for the metabolite, respectively. In the 80 patients in the literature, the calculated RIDs are all below 10% and many are less than 1%. Breastfeeding while using this drug should be based on the mother's clinical need for treatment versus any potential infant risks that might occur. If used, the infant should be monitored for the most common reported adult side effects of nausea and dyspepsia (both leading to irritability), diarrhea, tremors, decreased appetite (monitor infant growth), and sweating.

References

1. Prescribing Information. Sertraline hydrochloride. Greenstone LLC; 2022.
2. American College of Obstetricians and Gynecologists. Treatment and management of mental health conditions during pregnancy and postpartum. Clinical practice guideline No. 5. *Obstet Gynecol*. 2023;141:1262-1288.
3. Hendrick V, Stowe ZN, Altshuler LL, et al. Placental passage of antidepressant medications. *Am J Psychiatry*. 2003;160:993-996.
4. Heinonen E, Blennow M, Blondahl-Wetterholm M, et al. Sertraline concentrations in pregnant women are steady and the drug transfer to their infants is low. *Eur J Clin Pharmacol*. 2021;77:1323-1331.
5. Huybrechts KF, Palmsten K, Avorn J, et al. Antidepressant use in pregnancy and the risk of cardiac defects. *N Engl J Med*. 2014;370:2397-2407.
6. Gao SY, Wu QJ, Sun C, et al. Selective serotonin reuptake inhibitor use during early pregnancy and congenital malformations: a systematic review and meta-analysis of cohort studies of more than 9 million births. *BMC Med*. 2018;16:205.
7. Wang XY, Ying XH, Jiang HY. Antidepressant use during pregnancy and the risk for gestational diabetes: a systematic review and meta-analysis. *J Matern Fetal Neonatal Med*. 2023;36:2162817.
8. Kievet N, Hoppenbrouwers C, Dolman KM, et al. Risk factors for poor neonatal adaptation after exposure to antidepressants in utero. *Acta Paediatr*. 2015;104:384-391.
9. Masarwa R, Bar-Oz B, Gorelik E, et al. Prenatal exposure to selective serotonin reuptake inhibitors and serotonin norepinephrine reuptake inhibitors and risk for persistent pulmonary hypertension of the newborn: a systematic review, meta-analysis, and network meta-analysis. *Am J Obstet Gynecol*. 2019;220:57.e1-57.e13.
10. Altshuler LL, Burt VK, McMullen M, Hendrick V. Breastfeeding and sertraline: a 24-hour analysis. *J Clin Psychiatry*. 1995;56:243-245.
11. Epperson CN, Anerson GM, McDougle CJ. Sertraline and breast-feeding. *N Engl J Med*. 1997;336:1189-1190.
12. Stowe ZN, Owens MJ, Landry JC, et al. Sertraline and desmethylsertraline in human breast milk and nursing infants. *Am J Psychiatry*. 1997;154:1255-1260.
13. Kristensen JH, Ilett KF, Dusci LJ, et al. Distribution and excretion of sertraline and N-desmethylsertraline in human milk. *Br J Clin Pharmacol*. 1998;45:453-457.
14. Wisner KL, Perel JM, Blumer J. Serum sertraline and N-desmethylsertraline levels in breastfeeding mother-infant pairs. *Am J Psychiatry*. 1998;155:690-692.
15. Epperson N, Czarkowski KA, Ward-O'Brien D, et al. Maternal sertraline treatment and serotonin transport in breast-feeding mother-infant pairs. *Am J Psychiatry*. 2001;158:1631-1637.
16. Berle JO, Steen VM, Aamo TO, et al. Breastfeeding during maternal antidepressant treatment with serotonin reuptake inhibitors: infant exposure, clinical symptoms, and cytochrome P450 genotypes. *J Clin Psychiatry*. 2004;65:1228-1234.
17. Marshall AM, Nommsen-Rivers LA, Hernandez LI, et al. Serotonin transport and metabolism in the mammary gland modulates secretory activation and involution. *J Clin Endocrin Metab*. 2010;95:837-846.
18. Schoretsanitis G, Augustin M, Sabmannschausen H, et al. Antidepressants in breast milk; comparative analysis of excretion ratios. *Arch Womens Ment Health*. 2019;22:383-390.

SETMELANOTIDE

Miscellaneous (Melanocortin 4 Receptor Agonist)

PREGNANCY RECOMMENDATION: *Contraindicated

BREASTFEEDING RECOMMENDATION: Probably Compatible

PREGNANCY SUMMARY

No reports describing the use of setmelanotide in human pregnancy have been located. A limited amount of the drug probably crosses the placenta. Animal data did not show fetotoxic effects. *However, based on drug indication, its use during pregnancy is not recommended.

BREASTFEEDING SUMMARY

Setmelanotide probably enters breast milk, but in limited amounts. Multidose vials of setmelanotide contain the preservative benzyl alcohol, which has been associated with serious and possibly fatal reactions in neonates, including "gasping syndrome" when consumed orally. However, benzyl alcohol would be rapidly metabolized to benzoic acid in the maternal liver, and therefore, exposure to a breastfeeding newborn is not likely. The manufacturer does not recommend using setmelanotide while breastfeeding. Nevertheless, breastfeeding while using this drug should be based on the mother's clinical need for treatment. If used, the infant should be monitored for the most common reported adult side effects of headache, abdominal pain, back pain, arthralgias, and extremity pain (all leading to irritability), skin hyperpigmentation, vomiting, diarrhea, and rash.

References

1. Prescribing Information. Imcivree. Rhythm Pharmaceuticals, Inc; 2020.
2. Nair B. Final report on the safety assessment of benzyl alcohol, benzoic acid, and sodium benzoate. *Int J Toxicol*. 2001;20(suppl 3):23-50.

SEVELAMER

Antidote (Phosphate Binder)

PREGNANCY RECOMMENDATION: Human Data Suggest Low Risk

BREASTFEEDING RECOMMENDATION: Probably Compatible

PREGNANCY SUMMARY

No reports describing the use of sevelamer in human pregnancy have been located. Because it is not systemically absorbed, no fetal exposure should occur. However, the absence of human pregnancy experience prevents a complete assessment of embryofetal risk. Embryofetal toxicity was observed in two animal species at doses of less than 10 times the RHD. Because sevelamer can decrease serum levels of fat-soluble vitamins and folic acid in pregnant patients, the manufacturer recommends that providers consider supplementation. Using this drug during pregnancy should be based on the pros and cons of the mother's clinical need for treatment versus any potential fetal risk that might occur from exposure.

BREASTFEEDING SUMMARY

No reports describing the use of sevelamer during human lactation have been located. The drug is not absorbed into the systemic circulation, so it should not be found in breast milk. However, it may decrease serum levels of fat-soluble vitamins and folic acid. Breastfeeding while using this drug should be based on the mother's clinical need for treatment versus any potential infant risks that might occur. Because it does not appear to be absorbed into the maternal circulation, systemic side effects were not evaluated.

Reference

1. Prescribing Information. Sevelamer carbonate. Micro Labs Limited; 2022.

S

SEVOFLURANE

Anesthetic (General Anesthetic)

PREGNANCY RECOMMENDATION: Limited Human Data—Animal Data Suggest Potential Risk

BREASTFEEDING RECOMMENDATION: Probably Compatible

PREGNANCY SUMMARY

Several reports have described the use of sevoflurane immediately prior to delivery. However, the absence of human experience during organogenesis prevents a better assessment of the human embryofetal risk for anomalies. In addition, general anesthesia usually involves the use of multiple pharmacologic agents. Although no teratogenicity has been observed with

(*continued*)

other halogenated general anesthetic agents, only halothane has higher first-trimester human exposure data (see Halothane). The uterine effects of sevoflurane (relaxation and increased blood loss) also appear to be similar to other agents in this class, but the low concentrations used clinically minimize these actions (see Enflurane). All anesthetic agents can cause depression in a newborn, but again, this is lessened by the low doses. In general, inhalational anesthetics are freely transferred to fetal tissues and, in most cases, the maternal and fetal concentrations are equivalent. However, there are no data on whether sevoflurane crosses. Fetal exposure will probably occur. Animal data did show embryofetal toxicity in one animal species with doses of about 1 minimum alveolar concentration (MAC). Nevertheless, this limited human pregnancy experience prevents a complete assessment of embryofetal risk. Using this drug during pregnancy should be based on the pros and cons of the mother's clinical need for treatment versus any potential fetal risk that might occur from exposure. In 2016, the US Food and Drug Administration (FDA) issued a warning regarding the lengthy use of general anesthetic and sedation medications, including sevoflurane, in pregnant women and children less than 3 years old due to the potential impact on the developing brain. It advises that health care professionals should balance the benefits with potential risks, especially in procedures with a duration longer than 3 hours. Single, relatively short use of general anesthetics is unlikely to impact behavior or learning.

BREASTFEEDING SUMMARY

Although sevoflurane has been administered during delivery, the effects of this exposure on the infant who begins nursing immediately after birth have not been described. Sevoflurane is probably excreted into colostrum and breast milk, so some infant exposure might occur. However, the risk to a nursing infant from exposure to sevoflurane via breast milk is probably very low. Because of the short half-life and rapid clearance, the drug should be out of the maternal system by 2 hours after the last dose (five to six half-lives). Breastfeeding while using this drug should be based on the mother's clinical need for treatment versus any potential infant risks that might occur. If used, the infant should be monitored for the most common reported adult side effects of nausea (leading to irritability), vomiting, and increased cough.

References

1. Prescribing Information. Sevoflurane. Baxter Healthcare Corporation; 2023.
2. Behne M, Wilke HJ, Lischke V. Recovery and pharmacokinetic parameters of desflurane, sevoflurane, and isoflurane in patients undergoing urologic procedures. *J Clin Anesth*. 1999;11:460-465.
3. Food and Drug Administration. FDA drug safety communication: FDA review results in new warnings about using general anesthetics and sedation drugs in young children and pregnant women. Accessed August 28, 2024. https://www.fda.gov/drugs/drug-safety-and-availability/fda-drug-safety-communication-fda-review-results-new-warnings-about-using-general-anesthetics-and
4. Friedman JM. Teratogen update: anesthetic agents. *Teratology*. 1988;37:69-77.
5. Kanto J. Risk-benefit assessment of anaesthetic agents in the puerperium. *Drug Saf*. 1991;6:285-301.
6. Kanazawa M, Kinefuchi Y, Suzuki T, et al. The use of sevoflurane anesthesia during early pregnancy. *Tokai J Exp Clin Med*. 1999;24:53-55.
7. Klafta JM. The practice of using sevoflurane inhalation induction for emergency cesarean section and a parturient with no intravenous access. *Anesthesiology*. 1998;88:275.
8. Bhavani-Shankar K, Camann WR. The practice of using sevoflurane inhalation induction for emergency cesarean section and a parturient with no intravenous access. *Anesthesiology*. 1998;88:275-276.
9. Sitzman BT. The practice of using sevoflurane inhalation induction for emergency cesarean section and a parturient with no intravenous access. *Anesthesiology*. 1998;88:276.
10. Gambling DR, Reisner LS. The practice of using sevoflurane inhalation induction for emergency cesarean section and a parturient with no intravenous access. *Anesthesiology*. 1998;88:276-277.
11. Maltby JR. The practice of using sevoflurane inhalation induction for emergency cesarean section and a parturient with no intravenous access. *Anesthesiology*. 1998;88:277-278.
12. Gross JB. The practice of using sevoflurane inhalation induction for emergency cesarean section and a parturient with no intravenous access. *Anesthesiology*. 1998;88:278.
13. Corbett TH. Cancer and congenital anomalies associated with anesthetics. *Ann N Y Acad Sci*. 1976;271:58-66.
14. Shavit CW, Rollins MD, Ferschi MB. Maternal convulsion during high-dose sevoflurane anaesthesia for open foetal surgery. *Br J Anaesth*. 2017;118:634-635.
15. Spigset O. Anaesthetic agents and excretion in breast milk. *Acta Anaesthesiol Scand*. 1994;38:94-103.
16. Mitchell J, Jones W, Winkley E, Kinsella SM. Guideline on anaesthesia and sedation in breastfeeding women 2020. *Anaesth*. 2020;75:1482-1493.

SILDENAFIL

Vasodilator (Phosphodiesterase-5 Inhibitor)

PREGNANCY RECOMMENDATION: Limited Human Data—Animal Data Suggest Low Risk

BREASTFEEDING RECOMMENDATION: Potential Toxicity

PREGNANCY SUMMARY

Several reports describing the use of sildenafil in pregnancy have been located for either the treatment of maternal pulmonary hypertension or for the treatment or prevention of obstetric complications. Most of the exposures have occurred in the second or third trimesters. Sildenafil and its metabolite will likely cross the placenta, so some fetal exposure will probably occur. Animal data did not show any embryofetal toxicity in two species at doses of more than 10 times the RHD. However, this limited human pregnancy experience, especially in the first trimester, prevents a complete assessment of embryofetal risk. Using this drug during pregnancy should be based on the pros and cons of the mother's clinical need for treatment versus any potential fetal risk that might occur from exposure.

BREASTFEEDING SUMMARY

Two reports describing the use of sildenafil during human lactation have been located. Sildenafil and its active metabolite were found to be excreted into human breast milk. The calculated RIDs in both cases were less than 1%. No adverse events were reported in the infants. Breastfeeding while using this drug should be based on the mother's clinical need for treatment versus any potential infant risks that might occur. If used, the infant should be monitored for the most common reported adult side effects of headache, dyspepsia, back pain, myalgia, nausea, dizziness, and limb pain (all leading to irritability), flushing, nasal congestion, diarrhea, and rash.

References

1. Prescribing Information. Sildenafil citrate. Ajanta Pharma USA Inc; 2023.
2. Prescribing Information. Sildenafil citrate. Ascend Laboratories LLC; 2023.
3. Lacassie HJ, Germain AM, Valdes G, Fernandez MS, Allamand F, Lopez H. Management of Eisenmenger syndrome in pregnancy with sildenafil and L-arginine. *Obstet Gynecol*. 2004;103:1118-1120.
4. Molelekwa V, Akhter P, McKenna P, Bowen M, Walsh K. Eisenmenger's syndrome in a 27 week pregnancy—management with bosentan and sildenafil. *Ir Med J*. 2005;98:87-88.
5. Streit M, Speich R, Fischler M, Ulrich S. Successful pregnancy in pulmonary arterial hypertension associated with systemic lupus erythematosus: a case report. *J Med Case Reports*. 2009;3:7255.
6. Turner JM, Russo F, Deprest J, et al. Phosphodiesterase-5 inhibitors in pregnancy: systematic review and meta-analysis of maternal and perinatal safety and clinical outcomes. *BJOG*. 2022;129:1817-1831.
7. Pels A, Kenny LC, Alfirevic Z, et al; International STRIDER Consortium. STRIDER (Sildenafil TheRapy in dismal prognosis early onset fetal growth restriction): an international consortium of randomised placebo-controlled trials. *BMC Pregnancy Childbirth*. 2017;17:440.
8. Groom KM, Ganzevoort W, Alfirevic Z, Lim K, Papgeorghiou AT; STRIDER Consortium. Clinicians should stop prescribing sildenafil for fetal growth restriction (FGR): comment from the STRIDER consortium. *Ultrasound Obstet Gynecol*. 2018;52:295-296.
9. Pels A, Derks J, Evlan-Taspinar A, et al. Maternal sildenafil vs placebo in pregnant women with severe early-onset fetal growth restriction. *JAMA Netw Open*. 2020;3:e205323.
10. Pels A, Onland W, Berger RMF, et al. Neonatal pulmonary hypertension after severe early-onset fetal growth restriction: post hoc reflections on the Dutch STRIDER study. *Eur J Pediatr*. 2022;181:1709-1718.
11. Von Dadelszen P, Audibert F, Bujola E, et al. Halting the Canadian STRIDER randomized controlled trial of sildenafil for severe, early-onset fetal growth restriction: ethical, methodological, and pragmatic considerations. *BMC Res Notes*. 2022;15:244.
12. McKinlay CJD, Anderson C, Cheong JLY, et al. Childhood outcomes after maternal antenatal sildenafil treatment for severe early-onset fetal growth restriction: a randomized trial (STRIDER NZAus). *J Perinat*. 2024;44:396-403.
13. Manouchehri E, Makwandi S, Razi M, et al. Efficient administration of a combination of nifedipine and sildenafil citrate versus only nifedipine on clinical outcomes in women with threatened preterm labor: a systematic review and meta-analysis. *BMC Pediatrics*. 2024;24:106.
14. Maged M, Wageh A, Shams M, Elmetwally A. Use of sildenafil citrate in cases of intrauterine growth restriction (IUGR); a prospective trial. *Taiwan J Obstet Gynecol*. 2018;57:483-486.
15. Marsosi V, Hagighi L, Nasimi PH, et al. Effects of sildenafil on Doppler parameters, maternal and neonatal outcomes in the active labor phase of low-risk pregnancies: a randomized clinical trial. *J Perinat Med*. 2024;52:210-214.
16. Wollein U, Schech B, Schramek N. Determination and quantitation of sildenafil and its major metabolite in the breast milk of a lactating woman. *J Pharm Biomed Anal*. 2016;120:100-105.
17. Nauwelaerts N, Ceulemans M, Defem N, et al. Case report: bosentan and sildenafil exposure in human milk—a contribution from the ConcePTION project. *Front Pharmacol*. 2022;13:881084.

SILTUXIMAB

Antineoplastic (IL-6 Inhibitor—Monoclonal Antibody)

PREGNANCY RECOMMENDATION: No Human Data—Animal Data Suggest Low Risk

BREASTFEEDING RECOMMENDATION: Probably Compatible

PREGNANCY SUMMARY

No reports describing the use of siltuximab during human pregnancy have been located. As an IgG antibody, it likely crosses the placenta, especially during the second half of gestation, so some fetal exposure will occur. However, the absence of human pregnancy experience prevents a complete assessment of the embryofetal risk. Animal data in one species did not show any embryofetal toxicity with doses at less than 10 times the RHD. Based on the drug's mechanism of action, the manufacturer recommends that women with reproductive potential use effective contraception during treatment and for 3 months after the last dose. Nevertheless, using this drug during pregnancy should be based on the pros and cons of the mother's clinical need for treatment versus any potential fetal risk that might occur from exposure. The manufacturer notes that because most antibodies are transferred during the third trimester, infants exposed to siltuximab in utero may be at increased risk for infections. Therefore, providers should consider the risks and benefits of administering live or live-attenuated vaccines to the exposed infants. Hypertension was reported as very common in patients treated with this drug in the clinical trials.

BREASTFEEDING SUMMARY

No reports describing the use of siltuximab during human lactation have been located. It is known that IgG antibodies can be found in human breast milk, but are not found in the neonatal or infant circulation. Additionally, if any IgG antibodies were to be ingested through breastfeeding, they would probably be digested in the infant's gastrointestinal tract and not be absorbed. However, due to a concern for potential serious adverse effects that might be seen in a breastfed infant, the manufacturer recommends that women not breastfeed while being treated with this drug and for at least 3 months

S

after the last dose. Nevertheless, breastfeeding while using this drug should be based on the mother's clinical need for treatment versus any potential infant risks that might occur. If used, the infant should be monitored for the most common reported adult side effects of pruritus (leading to irritability), rash, upper respiratory tract infection, and hypertension.

References

1. Prescribing Information. Sylvant. Recordati Rare Diseases Inc; 2024.
2. National Library of Medicine. Pubchem. Siltuximab. Accessed August 30, 2024. https://pubchem.ncbi.nlm.nih.gov/compound/Siltuximab

SIMETHICONE

Gastrointestinal (Antiflatulent)

PREGNANCY RECOMMENDATION: Human Data Suggest Compatible

BREASTFEEDING RECOMMENDATION: Compatible

PREGNANCY SUMMARY

The Michigan Medicaid Surveillance study identified 248 newborns with exposure to simethicone during the first trimester. A total of 10 (4%) major birth defects were observed. No pattern to the anomalies was seen. Simethicone could not have been a factor in any of these congenital defects because the drug is not absorbed into the systemic circulation with oral use. Thus, the drug can be classified as compatible in pregnancy. No animal reproduction studies have been conducted. Using this drug during pregnancy should be based on the pros and cons of the mother's clinical need for treatment versus any potential fetal risk that might occur from exposure.

BREASTFEEDING SUMMARY

No reports describing the use of simethicone during human lactation have been located. There is no risk to a nursing infant from maternal use of this drug, as it is not systemically absorbed with oral use.

References

1. Prescribers' digital reference. Simethicone—drug summary. Accessed August 30, 2024. https://www.pdr.net/drug-summary/Gas-X-simethicone-2675
2. National Library of Medicine. Simethicone. Pubchem. Accessed August 30, 2024. https://pubchem.ncbi.nlm.nih.gov/compound/Simethicone#section=Depositor-Supplied-Synonyms

SIMVASTATIN

Antilipemic (Statin—HMG-CoA Inhibitor)

PREGNANCY RECOMMENDATION: Reductase Human Data—Animal Data Suggest Potential Risk

BREASTFEEDING RECOMMENDATION: Potential Toxicity

PREGNANCY SUMMARY

There are several publications describing the use of statins, including simvastatin, during human pregnancy. Regarding first-trimester exposure, there were 6 (3.9%) major birth anomalies in 154 exposed pregnancies. No pattern to the anomalies was seen. In a large systematic review, pregnancy outcomes in women exposed to statins during pregnancy (n = 1,655) were compared with unexposed controls (n = 974,159). All exposures were in the first trimester. No significant difference was observed for major malformations. Simvastatin and its active metabolites are likely to cross the placenta, so some fetal exposure will probably occur. However, this limited human pregnancy experience prevents a complete assessment of embryofetal risk for simvastatin specifically. Embryofetal toxicity was observed in one animal species (but not a second species) at doses of less than 10 times the RHD. Cholesterol and other products of cholesterol biosynthesis are essential components for fetal development. Moreover, maternal cholesterol levels increase during pregnancy. The manufacturer states that simvastatin may cause fetal harm when administered during pregnancy due to the mechanism of action. Hyperlipidemia treatment is not generally necessary during pregnancy. Atherosclerosis is a chronic process, and stopping lipid-lowering therapy during pregnancy should have little impact on the long-term outcome of primary hyperlipidemia for most patients. Therefore, the manufacturer recommends discontinuing simvastatin when a pregnancy is recognized. Nevertheless, using this drug during pregnancy should be based on the pros and cons of the mother's clinical need for treatment versus any potential fetal risk that might occur from exposure.

BREASTFEEDING SUMMARY

No reports describing the use of simvastatin during human lactation have been located. The drug will likely be excreted into breast milk, so some infant exposure will probably occur. The manufacturer notes that simvastatin exposure through breast milk may cause harm because it decreases cholesterol synthesis and possibly the synthesis of other cholesterol-derived biologically active substances. Therefore, due to a concern for potential serious adverse effects that might be seen in a breastfed infant, the manufacturer recommends that women not breastfeed while being treated with this drug. Nevertheless, breastfeeding while using this drug should be based on the mother's clinical need for treatment versus any potential infant risks that might occur. If used, the infant should be monitored for the most common reported adult side effects of headache, abdominal pain, and nausea (all leading to irritability), and constipation.

References

1. Prescribing Information. Simvastatin. Camber Pharmaceuticals Inc; 2024.
2. Pollack PS, Shields KE, Burnett DM, et al. Pregnancy outcomes after maternal exposure to simvastatin and lovastatin. *Birth Defects Res A Clin Mol Teratol*. 2005;73:888-896.
3. Edison RJ, Muenke M. Central nervous system and limb anomalies in case reports of first-trimester statin exposure. *N Engl J Med*. 2004;350:1579-1582.
4. Edison RJ, Muenke M. Mechanistic and epidemiologic considerations in the evaluation of adverse birth outcomes following gestational exposure to statins. *Am J Med Genetics*. 2004;131A:287-298.
5. McElhatton P. Preliminary data on exposure to statins during pregnancy (abstract). *Reprod Toxicol*. 2005;20:471-472.
6. Kalyoncu NI, Yaris F, Kadioglu M, et al. Pregnancy outcome following exposure to orlistat, ramipril, glimepiride in a woman with metabolic syndrome. *Saudi Med J*. 2005;26:497-499.
7. Karadas B, Uysal N, Erol H, et al. Pregnancy outcomes following maternal exposure to statins: a systematic review and meta-analysis. *Br J Pharmacol*. 2022;88:3962-3976.

SIPONIMOD

Immunologic (Sphingosine 1-Phosphate Receptor Modulator)

PREGNANCY RECOMMENDATION: No Human Data—Animal Data Suggest Risk

BREASTFEEDING RECOMMENDATION: Potential Toxicity

PREGNANCY SUMMARY

No reports describing the use of siponimod in human pregnancy have been located. Though probably limited, the drug is likely to cross the placenta, so some fetal exposure might occur. However, the absence of human pregnancy experience prevents a complete assessment of embryofetal risk. Embryofetal toxicity with malformations was observed in two animal species at doses of less than 10 times the RHD. Based on animal studies and the drug's mechanism of action, the manufacturer recommends that women with reproductive potential use effective contraception during treatment and for 10 days after the last dose. Nevertheless, using this drug during pregnancy should be based on the pros and cons of the mother's clinical need for treatment versus any potential fetal risk that might occur from exposure. There is a pregnancy exposure registry that monitors pregnancy outcomes in women exposed to siponimod during pregnancy. For more information, health care providers or patients are encouraged to contact MotherToBaby Pregnancy Study in Multiple Sclerosis by calling 877-311-8972. Hypertension was reported in up to 13% of patients treated with this drug in the clinical trials. Siponimod can also prolong the QTc interval.

BREASTFEEDING SUMMARY

No reports describing the use of siponimod during human lactation have been located. A limited amount of the drug may be found in breast milk, so some infant exposure might occur. Breastfeeding while using this drug should be based on the mother's clinical need for treatment versus any potential infant risks that might occur. If used, the infant should be monitored for the most common reported adult side effects of headache (leading to irritability), hypertension, and elevated transaminase levels.

Reference

1. Prescribing Information. Mayzent. Novartis Pharmaceuticals Corporation; 2024.

S

SIROLIMUS

Immunologic (mTOR Inhibitor)

PREGNANCY RECOMMENDATION: Limited Human Data—Animal Data Suggest Risk

BREASTFEEDING RECOMMENDATION: Potential Toxicity

PREGNANCY SUMMARY

There are a few case reports and small series that describe the use of sirolimus in human pregnancy. Overall, 10 first-trimester exposures were reported, with 5 that had spontaneous abortions. Of the remaining five, live births with no congenital anomalies were identified. An additional 10 or more cases describe the use of the drug in the second and third trimesters for treating fetal cardiac tumors and other maternal issues without any adverse effects reported related to the drug. Sirolimus crosses the placenta, so fetal exposure will occur. However, this limited human pregnancy experience prevents a complete assessment of embryofetal risk. Embryofetal toxicity was observed in two animal species at doses of less than 10 times the RHD. Based on animal studies and the drug's mechanism of action, the manufacturer recommends that women with reproductive potential use effective contraception during treatment and for 12 weeks after the last dose. Nevertheless, using this drug during pregnancy should be based on the pros and cons of the mother's clinical need for treatment versus any potential fetal risk that might occur from exposure. Hypertension was reported in over 30% of patients treated with this drug in the clinical trials.

BREASTFEEDING SUMMARY

No reports describing the use of sirolimus during human lactation have been located. The drug will likely be excreted into breast milk, so some infant exposure will probably occur. Breastfeeding while using this drug should be based on the mother's clinical need for treatment versus any potential infant risks that might occur. If used, the infant should be monitored for the most common reported adult side effects of abdominal pain, headache, nausea, arthralgia, dizziness, and myalgia (all leading to irritability), peripheral edema, fever, urinary tract infection, diarrhea, hypertension, and various laboratory abnormalities (see PI).

References

1. Prescribing Information. Sirolimus. Ascend Laboratories LLC; 2022.
2. Barnes BT, Procaccini D, Crino J, et al. Maternal sirolimus therapy for fetal cardiac rhabdomyomas. *N Engl J Med.* 2018;378:1844-1845.
3. Seront E, Biard JM, Van Damme A, et al. A case report of sirolimus use in early fetal management of lymphatic malformation. *Nature Cardio Res.* 2023;2:595-599.
4. Armenti VT, Radomski JS, Moritz MJ, et al. Report from the National Transplantation Pregnancy Registry (NTPR): outcomes of pregnancy after transplantation. *Clin Transpl.* 2003:131-141.
5. Jankowska I, Oldakowska-Jedynak U, Jabiry-Zieniewicz Z, et al. Absence of teratogenicity of sirolimus used during early pregnancy in a liver transplant recipient. *Transplant Proc.* 2004;36:3232-3233.
6. Vachon-Marceau C, Guerra V, Jaeggi E, et al. In-utero treatment of large symptomatic rhabdomyoma with sirolimus. *Ultrasound Obstet Gynecol.* 2019;53:421-422.
7. Shen L, Xu W, Gao J, et al. Pregnancy after the diagnosis of lymphangioleiomyomatosis (LAM). *Orphanet J Rare Dis.* 2021;16:133.
8. Ebrahimi-Fakhari D, Stires G, Hahn E, et al. Prenatal sirolimus treatment for rhabdomyomas in tuberous sclerosis. *Pediatr Neurol.* 2021;125:26-31.
9. Dagge A, Andrade Silva L, Jorge S, et al. Fetal tuberous sclerosis: sirolimus for the treatment of fetal rhabdomyoma. *Fetal Pediatr Path.* 2022;41:800-806.

SITAGLIPTIN

Antidiabetic (Dipeptidyl Peptidase-4 Inhibitor)

PREGNANCY RECOMMENDATION: Limited Human Data—Animal Data Suggest Low Risk

BREASTFEEDING RECOMMENDATION: Probably Compatible

PREGNANCY SUMMARY

No reports describing the use of sitagliptin specifically in human pregnancy have been located. The drug is likely to cross the placenta, so some fetal exposure will probably occur. One observational population-based cohort evaluated the risk for malformations with periconceptional use of antidiabetic medications compared to controls. Patients needed to fill at least one prescription within 90 days prior to pregnancy through the end of the first trimester. There were 3,514,865 pregnancies identified, with 51,826 patients with type 2 diabetes. Of these, 15,148 were prescribed antidiabetic medication. There were 687 DPP4 inhibitors, and when compared to the insulin-exposed group, the rates for any major malformation or cardiac malformations were no different (3.3%). The specific medications used within each class were not provided. In addition, diabetes control was not reported or adjusted for in the analysis. However, the limited human pregnancy experience prevents a complete assessment of embryofetal risk. Animal data did not show any embryofetal toxicity in two species at doses of more than 10 times the RHD. Using this drug during pregnancy should be based on the pros and cons of the mother's clinical need for treatment versus any potential fetal risk that might occur from exposure. Uncontrolled diabetes is associated with an increased risk for preeclampsia, spontaneous abortion, preterm delivery, intrauterine fetal demise, delivery complications, and major malformations. Insulin is still the treatment of choice for this disease during pregnancy. Moreover, insulin does not cross the placenta, which eliminates the additional concern that the drug therapy might adversely affect the fetus. ACOG recommends that insulin be used for type 1 and 2 diabetes occurring during pregnancy and, if diet therapy alone is not successful, for gestational diabetes. If a woman becomes pregnant while taking sitagliptin, changing the therapy to insulin should be considered.

BREASTFEEDING SUMMARY

No reports describing the use of sitagliptin during human lactation have been located. The drug will likely be excreted into breast milk, so some infant exposure will probably occur. Breastfeeding while using this drug should be based on the mother's clinical need for treatment versus any potential infant risks that might occur. If used, the infant should be monitored for the most common reported adult side effects of headache (leading to irritability) and upper respiratory tract infection.

References

1. Prescribing Information. Sitagliptin. Zydus Lifesciences Limited; 2024.
2. American College of Obstetricians and Gynecologists. ACOG practice bulletin No. 201: pregestational diabetes mellitus. *Obstet Gynecol*. 2018;132:e228-e248.
3. American College of Obstetricians and Gynecologists. ACOG practice bulletin No. 190: gestational diabetes. *Obstet Gynecol*. 2018;131:e49-e64.
4. Cesta CE, Rotem R, Bateman BT, et al. Safety of GLP-1 receptor agonist and other second-line antidiabetics in early pregnancy. *JAMA Intern Med*. 2024;184:144-152.

SODIUM BICARBONATE

Gastrointestinal/Antidote (Alkalizing Agent)

PREGNANCY RECOMMENDATION: Limited Human Data—Animal Data Suggest Low Risk

BREASTFEEDING RECOMMENDATION: Probably Compatible

PREGNANCY SUMMARY

There are numerous published reports on the use of sodium bicarbonate during human pregnancy. One case described the use of the drug throughout a pregnancy, delivering at term an infant with no identified anomalies. All the other cases involve the use of the drug in the second and third trimesters. The drug is likely to cross the placenta. However, this limited human pregnancy experience prevents a complete assessment of embryofetal risk. Animal data did not show any embryofetal toxicity in two species. Using this drug during pregnancy should be based on the pros and cons of the mother's clinical need for treatment versus any potential fetal risk that might occur from exposure. Some authors do not recommend the use of sodium bicarbonate (baking soda) for routine gastrointestinal ailments of pregnancy, such as heartburn, due to the potential for metabolic alkalosis and because other alternatives are available.

BREASTFEEDING SUMMARY

No reports describing the use of sodium bicarbonate during human lactation have been located. The drug will likely be excreted into breast milk. Breastfeeding while using this drug should be based on the mother's clinical need for treatment versus any potential infant risks that might occur. If used, the infant should be monitored for the most common reported adult side effects of metabolic alkalosis (associated with muscular twitching, irritability, and tetany) and hypernatremia. Some authors do not recommend the use of sodium bicarbonate (baking soda) for treating gastrointestinal ailments in lactating women, such as heartburn, due to the potential for metabolic alkalosis in the infant and because other alternatives are available.

References

1. Prescribing Information. Sodium bicarbonate. Civica; 2024.
2. Sodium bicarbonate. *Lexi-Drugs*. UpToDate Lexidrug. UpToDate Inc. Accessed September 2, 2024. https://online.lexi.com
3. National Library of Medicine. Sodium bicarbonate. Pubchem. Accessed September 2, 2024. https://pubchem.ncbi.nlm.nih.gov/compound/Sodium-Bicarbonate
4. Thelin CS, Richter JE. Review article: the management of heartburn during pregnancy and lactation. *Ailment Pharmacol Ther*. 2020;51:421-434.
5. Gomes CF, Sousa M, Lourenco, et al. Gastrointestinal diseases during pregnancy: what does the gastroenterologist need to know? *Ann Gastroenterol*. 2018;31:385-394.
6. Grotegut CA, Dandolu V, Katari S, Whiteman VE, Geifman-Holtzman O, Teitelman M. Baking soda pica: a case of hypokalemic metabolic alkalosis and rhabdomyolysis in pregnancy. *Obstet Gynecol*. 2006;107:484-486.
7. Hong YC, O'Boyle CP, Chen IC, et al. Metformin-associated lactic acidosis in a pregnant patient. *Gynecol Obstet Invest*. 2008;66:138-141.
8. Scolari Childress KM, Myles T. Baking soda pica associated with rhabdomyolysis and cardiomyopathy in pregnancy. *Obstet Gynecol*. 2013;122:495-497.
9. Zelner I, Matlow J, Hutson JR, et al. Acute poisoning during pregnancy: observations from the Toxicology Investigators Consortium. *J Med Toxicol*. 2015;11:301-308.
10. Seyedi M, Ghorashi Z, Darijani TS. Randomized controlled trial of oral bicarbonate for labor stagnation. *J Obstet Gynaecol Res*. 2021;47:114-118.
11. Brackett BG, Mastroianni I. Composition of oviductal fluid. In: Johnson AD, Foley CW, eds. *The Oviduct and Its Functions*. Academic Press, Inc; 1974: 135-199.
12. Boatman DE, Robbins RS. Bicarbonate: carbon-dioxide regulation of sperm capacitation, hyperactivated motility, and acrosome reactions. *Biol Reprod*. 1991;44:806-813.
13. Everhardt E, Dony JM, Jansen H, Lemmens WA, Doesburg WH. Improvement of cervical mucus viscoelasticity and sperm penetration with sodium bicarbonate douching. *Hum Reprod*. 1990;5:133-137.
14. Khera KS. Chemically induced alterations in maternal homeostasis and histology of conceptus: their etiologic significance in rat fetal anomalies. *Teratology*. 1991;44:259-297.
15. Mayura K, Hayes AW, Berndt WO. Teratogenicity of secalonic acid D in rats. *Toxicology*. 1982;25:311-322.
16. Nakatsuka T, Fujikake N, Hasebe M, Ikeda H. Effects of sodium bicarbonate and ammonium chloride on the incidence of furosemide-induced fetal skeletal anomaly, wavy rib, in rats. *Teratology*. 1993;48:139-147.
17. Reddy CS, Reddy RV, Hayes AW. Teratogenicity of secalonic acid D in mice. *J Toxicol Environ Health*. 1981;7:445-455.

S

SODIUM IODIDE I 123

(See Sodium Iodide I 131 below)

SODIUM IODIDE I 131

Radiopharmaceutical/Diagnostic (Thyroid)

PREGNANCY RECOMMENDATION: *Contraindicated

BREASTFEEDING RECOMMENDATION: *Contraindicated

PREGNANCY SUMMARY

Sodium iodide I 131 and sodium iodide I 123 are proven human teratogens. Iodine 127 is the natural substance, whereas iodine 131 and iodine 123 are radioactive substances. In the Collaborative Perinatal Project, 19 infants were exposed to sodium iodide I 131, and no major birth anomalies were identified. However, like all iodides, these drugs concentrate in the thyroid gland (up to 50 times higher than blood levels). The fetal thyroid gland does not start accumulating iodine until about 10 to 12 weeks' gestation. At this gestational age and beyond, the fetal thyroid will begin to accumulate and concentrate iodine 131 and iodine 123, which can lead to the loss of thyroid function. *Because of the radioactive effects of even small doses, there is no way to predict infant thyroid function. Therefore, use during pregnancy should be avoided if at all possible. No animal reproduction studies have been conducted. Sodium iodide I 131 emits beta particles and has an elimination half-life of about 8 days. It is most often used in treating thyroid cancer. Sodium iodide I 123 emits gamma rays and has an elimination half-life of about 13 hours. It is most often used for diagnostic procedures, though they can be interchanged.

BREASTFEEDING SUMMARY

Sodium iodide I 131 and sodium iodide I 123 are excreted into human breast milk, so infant exposure will occur. Uptake of iodine 131 by an infant's thyroid gland after breastfeeding has been observed. The time required for the elimination of radioiodine from breast milk may be as long as 14 days. For iodine 123, radioactivity may be present in breast milk for up to 36 hours. *Since exposure to radioactive iodine may result in damage to the nursing infant's thyroid, including an increased risk of thyroid cancer in the future, breastfeeding should be stopped until radioactivity is no longer present in breast milk. It is recommended that patients receiving sodium iodide I 131 should stop breastfeeding a minimum of 4 weeks after a whole body procedure. Patients receiving sodium iodide I 123 should stop breastfeeding for a minimum of 3 to 4 days after the procedure. However, these time limits can vary greatly.

S

References

1. Prescribing Information. Sodium iodide I 131 diagnostic. Jubilant DraxImage Inc, dba Jubilant Radiopharma; 2020.
2. Pauwels EKJ, Thomson WH, Blokland JAK, et al. Aspects of fetal thyroid dose following iodine-131 administration during early stages of pregnancy in patients suffering from benign thyroid disorders. *Eur J Nucl Med*. 1999;26:1453-1457.
3. Chapman EM, Corner GW Jr, Robinson D, Evans RD. The collection of radioactive iodine by the human fetal thyroid. *J Clin Endocrinol Metab*. 1948;8:717-720.
4. Hodges RE, Evans TC, Bradbury JT, Keettel WC. The accumulation of radioactive iodine by human fetal thyroids. *J Clin Endocrinol Metab*. 1955; 15:661-667.
5. Shepard TH. Onset of function in the human fetal thyroid: biochemical and radioautographic studies from organ culture. *J Clin Endocrinol Metab*. 1967;27:945-958.
6. Kearns JE, Hutson W. Tagged isomers and analogues of thyroxine (their transmission across the human placenta and other studies). *J Nucl Med*. 1963;4:453-461.
7. Hollingsworth DR, Austin E. Observations following I131 for Graves' disease during first trimester of pregnancy. *South Med J*. 1969;62:1555-1556.
8. Talbert LM, Thomas CG Jr, Holt WA, Rankin P. Hyperthyroidism during pregnancy. *Obstet Gynecol*. 1970;36:779-785.
9. Valensi G, Nahum A. Action de l'iode radio-actif sur le foetus humain. *Tunisie med*. 1958;36:69. As cited in Nishimura H, Tanimura T. *Clinical Aspects of the Teratogenicity of Drugs*. American Elsevier; 1976:260.
10. Falk W. Beitrag zur Frage der menschlichen Fruchtschadigung durch kunstliche radioaktive Isotope. *Medizinische*. 1959;22:1480. As cited in Nishimura H, Tanimura T. *Clinical Aspects of the Teratogenicity of Drugs*. American Elsevier; 1976:260.
11. Berger M, Briere J. Les dangers de la therapeutique par l'iode radioactif au debut d'une grossesse ignoree. *Bull Med leg Toxicol Med*. 1967;10:37. As cited in Nishimura H, Tanimura T. *Clinical Aspects of the Teratogenicity of Drugs*. American Elsevier; 1976:260.
12. Russell KP, Rose H, Starr P. The effects of radioactive iodine on maternal and fetal thyroid function during pregnancy. *Surg Gynecol Obstet*. 1957; 104:560-564.
13. Ray EW, Sterling K, Gardner LI. Congenital cretinism associated with I131 therapy of the mother. *Am J Dis Child*. 1959;98:506-507.
14. Hamill GC, Jarman JA, Wynne MD. Fetal effects of radioactive iodine therapy in a pregnant woman with thyroid cancer. *Am J Obstet Gynecol*. 1961;81:1018-1023.
15. Fisher WD, Voorhess ML, Gardner LI. Congenital hypothyroidism in infant following maternal I131 therapy. *J Pediatr*. 1963;62:132-146.
16. Pfannenstiel P, Andrews GA, Brown DW. Congenital hypothyroidism from intrauterine 131I damage. In: Cassalino C, Andreoli M, eds. *Current Topics in Thyroid Research*. Academic Press, 1965:749. As cited in Nishimura H, Tanimura T. *Clinical Aspects of the Teratogenicity of Drugs*. American Elsevier; 1976:260.
17. Sirbu P, Macarie E, Isaia V, Zugravesco A. L'influence de l'iode radio-actif sur le foetus. *Bull Fed Soc Gynecol Obstet Franc*. 1968;20:314. As cited in Nishimura H, Tanimura T. *Clinical Aspects of the Teratogenicity of Drugs*. American Elsevier; 1976:260.
18. Hollingsworth DR, Austin E. Thyroxine derivatives in amniotic fluid. *J Pediatr*. 1971;79:923-929.

19. Green HG, Gareis FJ, Shepard TH, Kelley VC. Cretinism associated with maternal sodium iodide I 131 therapy during pregnancy. *Am J Dis Child.* 1971;122:247-249.
20. Jafek BW, Small R, Lillian DL. Congenital radioactive iodine-induced stridor and hypothyroidism. *Arch Otolaryngol.* 1974;99:369-371.
21. Exss R, Graewe B. Congenital athyroidism in the newborn infant from intra-uterine radioiodine action. *Biol Neonate.* 1974;24:289-291.
22. Richards GE, Brewer ED, Conley SB, Saldana LR. Combined hypothyroidism and hypoparathyroidism in an infant after maternal 131I administration. *J Pediatr.* 1981;99:141-143.
23. Berg GEB, Nystrom EH, Jacobsson L, et al. Radioiodine treatment of hyperthyroidism in a pregnant woman. *J Nucl Med.* 1998;39:357-361.
24. Nurnberger CE, Lipscomb A. Transmission of radioiodine (I131) to infants through human maternal milk. *JAMA.* 1952;150:1398-1400.
25. Miller H, Weetch RS. The excretion of radioactive iodine in human milk. *Lancet.* 1955;2:1013.
26. Weaver JC, Kamm ML, Dobson RL. Excretion of radioiodine in human milk. *JAMA.* 1960;173:872-875.
27. Karjalainen P, Penttila IM, Pystynen P. The amount and form of radioactivity in human milk after lung scanning, renography and placental localization by 131I labelled tracers. *Acta Obstet Gynecol Scand.* 1971;50:357-361.
28. Bland EP, Crawford JS, Docker MF, Farr RF. Radioactive iodine uptake by thyroid of breast-fed infants after maternal blood-volume measurements. *Lancet.* 1969;2:1039-1041.
29. Palmer KE. Excretion of 125I in breast milk following administration of labelled fibrinogen. *Br J Radiol.* 1979;52:672-673.
30. Sachs HC, Frattarelli DAC, Galinkin JL, et al; Committee on Drugs, The transfer of drugs and therapeutics into human breast milk: an update on selected topics. *Pediatrics.* 2013;132:e796-e809.
31. Prescribing Information. Sodium iodide 123. Curium US; 2020.

SODIUM OXYBATE

Central Nervous System (CNS Depressant)

PREGNANCY RECOMMENDATION: Limited Human Data—Animal Data Suggest Potential Risk

BREASTFEEDING RECOMMENDATION: Potential Toxicity (Hold Breastfeeding)

PREGNANCY SUMMARY

Four cases of sodium oxybate and/or recreational γ-hydroxybutyrate (GHB) use during pregnancy were located in the literature. Sodium oxybate is the sodium salt of GHB, which is an endogenous compound and metabolite of γ-aminobutyric acid (GABA). Three cases likely had first-trimester exposure, and none of the infants had any identified congenital anomalies described at birth. In the fourth case, the drug was used in the third trimester. The drug crosses the placenta, so some fetal exposure will occur. However, this limited human pregnancy experience prevents a complete assessment of embryofetal risk. Embryofetal toxicity was observed in one animal species (but not a second species) at doses of less than 10 times the RHD. The manufacturer reported that injectable sodium oxybate for obstetric anesthesia resulted in a slight decrease in Apgar scores due to infants being very sleepy. However, cardiac and respiratory parameters were stable. Using this drug during pregnancy should be based on the pros and cons of the mother's clinical need for treatment versus any potential fetal risk that might occur from exposure. Illicit GHB misuse is associated with CNS adverse reactions, including seizures, respiratory depression, decreased consciousness, coma, and even death. Sodium oxybate is only available through a REMS (risk evaluation and mitigation strategies) program called Xywav or Xyrem REMS.

BREASTFEEDING SUMMARY

Three reports describing the use of sodium oxybate (GHB) during human lactation have been located. The drug is found in breast milk, so some infant exposure will occur. In one case, the breast milk drug level was about 20% of the maternal serum level and the calculated RID was about 5%. Breastfeeding while using this drug should be based on the mother's clinical need for treatment versus any potential infant risks that might occur. If used, the infant should be monitored for the most common reported adult side effects of nausea and dizziness (both leading to irritability), vomiting, somnolence, and tremor. Due to the short elimination half-life, waiting for 5 hours after a dose should minimize any infant exposure (5 half-lives).

References

1. Prescribing Information. Sodium oxybate. Amneal Pharmaceuticals NY LLC; 2023.
2. Kuczkowski KM. Liquid ecstasy during pregnancy. *Anaesthesia.* 2004; 59:926.
3. Gashlin LZ, Sullo D, Lawrence RA, Rosen-Carole C. Treatment of narcolepsy with sodium oxybate while breastfeeding: a case report. *Breastfeed Med.* 2016;11:261-263.
4. van Mechelen JC, Dijkstra BAG, Vergouwen ACM. Severe illicit gamma-hydroxybutyric acid withdrawal in a pregnant woman: what to do? *BMC Case Rep.* 2019;12:e230997.
5. Joyce S, Lea S, Woolner M, Leddy A. Treatment of gamma hydroxybutyrate withdrawal in a pregnant female: a case report. *J Addict Med.* 2024;18:342-344.
6. Busardo FP, Berol E, Mannocchi G, et al. Determinations of GHB levels in breast milk and correlation with blood concentrations. *Forensic Sci Int.* 2016;265:172-181.

SODIUM PHENYLBUTYRATE AND TAURURSODIOL

Central Nervous System (Histone Deacetylase Inhibitor)

PREGNANCY RECOMMENDATION: No Human Data—Animal Data Suggest Potential Risk

BREASTFEEDING RECOMMENDATION: Potential Toxicity

PREGNANCY SUMMARY

No reports describing the use of sodium phenylbutyrate and taurursodiol in human pregnancy have been located. Both drugs will likely cross the placenta, so some fetal exposure will probably occur. Therefore, the absence of human pregnancy experience prevents a complete assessment of embryofetal risk. Animal studies did show embryofetal toxicity in one species. Using this drug during pregnancy should be based on the pros and cons of the mother's clinical need for treatment versus any potential fetal risk that might occur from exposure.

BREASTFEEDING SUMMARY

No reports describing the use of sodium phenylbutyrate and taurursodiol during human lactation have been located. Both drugs will likely be found in breast milk, so some infant exposure will probably occur. Breastfeeding while using this drug should be based on the mother's clinical need for treatment. If used, the infant should be monitored for the most common reported adult side effects of nausea and abdominal pain (both leading to irritability), diarrhea, and upper respiratory tract infection.

Reference

1. Prescribing Information. Relyvrio. Amylyx Pharmaceuticals, Inc; 2022.

SODIUM ZIRCONIUM CYCLOSILICATE

Antidote (Potassium Binder)

PREGNANCY RECOMMENDATION: Human Data Suggests Compatible

BREASTFEEDING RECOMMENDATION: Compatible

PREGNANCY SUMMARY

No reports describing the use of sodium zirconium cyclosilicate in human pregnancy have been located. Because the drug is not systemically absorbed, this substance would not be expected to cross the human placenta. In animal studies, the drug was not systemically absorbed.

BREASTFEEDING SUMMARY

Sodium zirconium cyclosilicate is not systemically absorbed and, therefore, would not be expected to enter breast milk.

Reference

1. Prescribing Information. Lokelma. AstraZeneca Pharmaceuticals LP; 2018.

SOFOSBUVIR

Antiviral (Anti-Hepatitis C)

PREGNANCY RECOMMENDATION: Limited Human Data—Animal Data Suggest Low Risk (Contraindicated if Combined With Ribavirin)

BREASTFEEDING RECOMMENDATION: Probably Compatible (Potential Toxicity if Combined With Ribavirin)

PREGNANCY SUMMARY

Four reports describing the use of sofosbuvir in more than 100 human pregnancies have been located. In one study, 96 patients had an unintended pregnancy during hepatitis C treatment that included sofosbuvir, and therapy was discontinued by 4 to 8 weeks' gestation in about 90%, with the remaining 10% continuing to the end of the treatment process. Only one (1%) infant had a major congenital anomaly, an atrial septal defect. It is not known if sofosbuvir crosses the placenta. However, the predominant inactive GS-331007 metabolite has been shown to cross. However, this limited human pregnancy experience prevents a complete assessment of embryofetal risk. Animal data did not show any embryofetal toxicity in two species at doses of more than 10 times the RHD. Using this drug during pregnancy should be based on the pros and cons of the mother's clinical need for treatment versus any potential fetal risk that might occur from exposure. There is a boxed warning for a risk of hepatitis B reactivation in some patients, resulting in fulminant hepatitis, hepatic failure, and even death. If sofosbuvir is combined with ribavirin, this combination is contraindicated in pregnancy (see Ribavirin).

BREASTFEEDING SUMMARY

One report describing the use of sofosbuvir during human pregnancy and lactation has been located. Two mothers received 12 weeks of treatment with either sofosbuvir/ledipasvir or sofosbuvir/velpatasvir starting at 31 weeks and 26 weeks' gestation. The gestational age of delivery was not provided, but both mothers likely completed therapy near the time of delivery or within a few weeks postpartum. Both infants were breastfed, and no adverse newborn effects were described. The drug and its metabolites will likely be excreted into breast milk, so some infant exposure will probably occur. Breastfeeding while using this drug should be based on the mother's clinical need for treatment versus any potential infant risks that might occur. If used, the infant should be monitored for the most common reported adult side effects of headache (leading to irritability) and fatigue (lethargy).

References

1. Prescribing Information. Sovaldi. Gilead Sciences Inc; 2020.
2. Freriksen JJM, Meijerhof M, van Drongelen J, et al. Transfer of daclatasvir and sofosbuvir's main metabolite, GS-331007, across the human placenta ex vivo. *Am J Obstet Gynecol*. 2020;223:941-943.
3. Mandimika C, Ogbuagu O. Successful sofosbuvir lead-in monotherapy for the treatment of hepatitis C virus (HCV) infection in a pregnant woman living with HIV. *BMC Case Rep*. 2019;12:e230529.
4. Chappell CA, Scarsi KK, Kirby BJ, et al. Ledipasvir plus sofosbuvir in pregnant women in hepatitis C virus infection: a phase 1 pharmacokinetic study. *Lancet Microbe*. 2020;1:e200-e208.
5. AbdAllah M, Alboraie M, Abdel-Razek W, et al. Pregnancy outcome of anti-HCV direct-acting antivirals: real-life data from an Egyptian cohort. *Liver Int*. 2021;41:1494-1497.
6. Zeng QL, Yu ZJ, Lv J, et al. Sofosbuvir-based therapy for late pregnant women and infants with severe chronic hepatitis C; a case series. *J Med Virol*. 2022;94:4548-4553.

SOFOSBUVIR/VELPATASVIR

Antiviral (Hepatitis C)

PREGNANCY RECOMMENDATION: Limited Human Data—Animal Data Suggest Low Risk

BREASTFEEDING RECOMMENDATION: Probably Compatible

PREGNANCY SUMMARY

A case series reported the outcomes of two pregnant women on sofosbuvir-based therapy. One woman started sofosbuvir and velpatasvir at 26 weeks' gestation, and the other started sofosbuvir and ledipasvir at 31 weeks' gestation. Both women delivered healthy newborns without any reported abnormalities or adverse consequences. Some amount of each drug will probably cross the placenta, so fetal exposure will likely occur. However, this limited human pregnancy experience prevents a complete assessment of the embryofetal risk. Animal studies did not show any embryofetal toxicity. Current guidance for the treatment of hepatitis C recommends that women who become pregnant while taking direct-acting antivirals (DAAs), like sofosbuvir and velpatasvir, should consult with their physician regarding continuing treatment after a discussion about the potential risks and benefits. DAAs, however, are not recommended for use during pregnancy to reduce mother-to-child transmission. If sofosbuvir/velpatasvir is administered with ribavirin, this combination may be contraindicated (see Ribavirin for further information).

BREASTFEEDING SUMMARY

One case series reported the outcomes of two pregnant women on sofosbuvir-based therapy who breastfed their newborns. One woman received sofosbuvir and velpatasvir, and the other received sofosbuvir and ledipasvir. Both newborns were consistently negative for anti-hepatitis C virus (HCV) antibody and had normal growth during the 1-year follow-up. However, dosage, duration of treatment, and breast milk drug levels were not supplied. Both drugs will probably be found in breast milk, so infant exposure will likely occur. Breastfeeding while using this drug should be based on the mother's clinical need for treatment. If used, the infant should be monitored for the most common reported adult side effects of headache and nausea (both leading to irritability), vomiting, and lethargy.

References

1. Prescribing Information. Epclusa, Gilead Sciences, Inc; 2022.
2. AASLD-IDSA. HCV in pregnancy. Accessed February 19, 2023. http://www.hcvguidelines.org/unique-populations/pregnancy
3. Zeng QL, Yu ZJ, Lv J, et al. Sofosbuvir-based therapy for late pregnant women and infants with severe chronic hepatitis C: a case series study. *J Med Virol*. 2022;94:4548-4553.

S

SOFOSBUVIR/VELPATASVIR/VOXILAPREVIR

Antiviral (Hepatitis C)

PREGNANCY RECOMMENDATION: Limited Human Data—Animal Data Suggest Low Risk

BREASTFEEDING RECOMMENDATION: Probably Compatible

PREGNANCY SUMMARY

No reports describing the use of sofosbuvir/velpatasvir/voxilaprevir combination drug in human pregnancy have been located. Because all three drugs probably cross the placenta (limited amounts for velpatasvir and voxilaprevir), fetal exposure will probably occur. However, the absence of human pregnancy experience prevents a complete assessment of the embryofetal risk. There is one publication of two patients, one who started sofosbuvir/ledipasvir at 31 weeks' gestation, and the other who started sofosbuvir/velpatasvir at 26 weeks' gestation. They both delivered healthy newborns. Animal studies did not show any embryofetal toxicity. There is a risk of developing a reactivation of hepatitis B that can lead to fulminant hepatitis, hepatic failure, and even death when using this drug. Current guidance for the treatment of hepatitis C (HCV) recommends that women who become pregnant while taking DAAs, like sofosbuvir and velpatasvir, should consult with their physician regarding continuing treatment after discussion about the potential risks and benefits. DAAs, however, are not currently recommended during pregnancy to reduce mother-to-child transmission of HCV.

BREASTFEEDING SUMMARY

No reports describing the use of the combination drug of sofosbuvir, velpatasvir, and voxilaprevir in human lactation have been located. Two patients who breastfed with sofosbuvir and one with velpatasvir were not reported to have any adverse effects. However, dosage, duration of treatment, and breast milk drug levels were not supplied. For sofosbuvir, some amount of the drug will probably be found in breast milk. For velpatasvir and voxilaprevir, a minimal amount of both drugs will probably be found in breast milk. Therefore, some infant exposure to all three drugs will likely occur. Breastfeeding while using this drug should be based on the mother's clinical need for treatment. If used, the infant should be monitored for the most common reported adult side effects of headache and nausea (both leading to irritability), diarrhea, and lethargy.

References

1. Prescribing Information. Vosevi. Gilead Sciences, Inc; 2017.
2. AASLD-IDSA. HCV in pregnancy. Accessed February 19, 2023 https://www.hcvguidelines.org/guidance/hcv-in-pregnancy/
3. Zeng QL, Yu ZJ, Lv J, et al. Sofosbuvir-based therapy for late pregnant women and infants with severe chronic hepatitis C: a case series study. *J Med Virol*. 2022;94:4548-4553.

SOFPIRONIUM

Miscellaneous (Topical Skin Product—Axillary Hyperhidrosis)

PREGNANCY RECOMMENDATION: No Human Data—Animal Data Suggest Low Risk

BREASTFEEDING RECOMMENDATION: Probably Compatible

PREGNANCY SUMMARY

No reports describing the use of sofpironium in human pregnancy have been located. Though placental transfer may be possible, fetal exposure is probably small. However, the absence of human pregnancy experience prevents a complete assessment of the embryofetal risk. Animal studies did not find any embryofetal toxicity or malformations in two species at doses more than 10 times the RHD, despite subcutaneous (SC) administration. Using this drug during pregnancy should be based on the pros and cons of the mother's clinical need for treatment versus any potential fetal risk that might occur from exposure. The clinical need for treating axillary hyperhidrosis during pregnancy, especially during the first trimester, is uncertain.

S

BREASTFEEDING SUMMARY

It is not known if sofpironium is excreted into human breast milk. Based on topical use of the drug, the amount of drug found in breast milk is likely to be small. Breastfeeding while using this drug should be based on the mother's clinical need for treatment versus any potential infant risks that might occur. If used, the infant should be monitored for the most common reported adult systemic side effects of blurry vision, pruritus, and dry mouth (all leading to irritability).

Reference

1. Prescribing Information. Sofdra. Botanix SB, Inc; 2024.

SOLIFENACIN

Urinary (Antimuscarinic)

PREGNANCY RECOMMENDATION: No Human Data—Animal Data Suggest Potential Risk

BREASTFEEDING RECOMMENDATION: Potential Toxicity

PREGNANCY SUMMARY

No reports describing the use of solifenacin during human pregnancy have been located. The drug is likely to cross the placenta, so some fetal exposure will probably occur. However, the absence of human pregnancy experience prevents a complete assessment of embryofetal risk. Embryofetal toxicity was observed in one animal species at doses of less than 10 times the RHD. Using this drug during pregnancy should be based on the pros and cons of the mother's clinical need for treatment versus any potential fetal risk that might occur from exposure.

BREASTFEEDING SUMMARY

No reports describing the use of solifenacin during human lactation have been located. The drug will likely be excreted into breast milk, so some infant exposure will probably occur. Breastfeeding while using this drug should be based on the mother's clinical need for treatment versus any potential infant risks that might occur. If used, the infant should be monitored for the most common reported adult side effects of dry mouth and blurred vision (both leading to irritability), constipation, and urinary tract infection. The effects on breast milk production are unknown, but other anticholinergic drugs have been shown to decrease breast milk supply.

Reference

1. Prescribing Information. Solifenacin succinate. Strides Pharma Science Limited; 2020.

SOLRIAMFETOL

Central Nervous System (Dopamine and Norepinephrine Reuptake Inhibitor)

PREGNANCY RECOMMENDATION: No Human Data—Animal Data Suggest Potential Risk

BREASTFEEDING RECOMMENDATION: Potential Toxicity

PREGNANCY SUMMARY

No reports describing the use of solriamfetol in human pregnancy have been located. The drug will likely cross the placenta, so some fetal exposure will probably occur. However, the absence of human pregnancy experience prevents a complete assessment of embryofetal risk. Embryofetal toxicity with malformations was observed in one animal species without maternal toxicity at doses of less than 10 times the RHD. Using this drug during pregnancy should be based on the pros and cons of the mother's clinical need for treatment versus any potential fetal risk that might occur from exposure. There is a pregnancy exposure registry that monitors pregnancy outcomes in women exposed to solriamfetol during pregnancy. For more information, health care providers or patients are encouraged to contact the company by calling 877-283-6220. The manufacturer recommends that the patient's blood pressure be monitored because solriamfetol can elevate blood pressure.

BREASTFEEDING SUMMARY

Solriamfetol has been shown to be excreted into human breast milk. The manufacturer reported on six lactating women who were administered a single 150 mg dose of solriamfetol. The calculated infant dose was about 0.112 mg/kg/d with an RID of about 5.5%. Breastfeeding while using this drug should be based on the mother's clinical need for treatment versus any potential infant risks that might occur. If used, the infant should be monitored for the most common reported adult side effects of headache, nausea, and anxiety (all leading to irritability), decreased appetite (monitor infant growth), and insomnia.

Reference

1. Prescribing Information. Sunosi. Axsome Therapeutics Inc; 2023.

SOMAPACITAN

Endocrine (Human Growth Hormone Analogue)

PREGNANCY RECOMMENDATION: No Human Data—Animal Data Suggest Low Risk

BREASTFEEDING RECOMMENDATION: Probably Compatible

PREGNANCY SUMMARY

No reports describing the specific use of somapacitan in human pregnancy have been located. Placental transfer and embryofetal exposure are likely to be negligible. Animal data did not show fetotoxic effects. However, the absence of human pregnancy experience prevents a complete assessment of the embryofetal risk. Two large reports using other forms of human growth hormone (hGH) replacement therapy at conception and the first trimester found spontaneous abortion rates of 12% and 18% (both within the expected range). In addition, no birth anomalies were identified in 155 newborns. There was one stillbirth (gestational age not supplied) and one delivery in the second trimester for a severe cystic hygroma (genetic testing not reported). Though endocrine societies and organizations state that hGH replacement therapy is not approved for use in pregnancy, there will be women of reproductive age who suffer from growth hormone deficiency and will be on a replacement therapy program where conception will occur. The pregnancy data overall are reassuring. Glucose intolerance has been reported in patients treated with hGH products.

BREASTFEEDING SUMMARY

Somapacitan excretion into breast milk is likely to be negligible. In addition, because it is a protein of 191 amino acids, if the drug were to be ingested through breastfeeding, it probably would be digested in the infant's gastrointestinal tract and not be absorbed. Published data on short-acting recombinant hGH for 7 days during lactation did not demonstrate any adverse effects in infants. Breastfeeding while using this drug should be based on the mother's clinical need for treatment. If used, the infant should be monitored for the most common reported adult side effects of back pain and arthralgias (both leading to irritability).

References

1. Prescribing Information. Sogroya. Novo Nordisk, Inc; 2020.
2. Vila G, Akerblad AC, Mattsson AF, et al. Pregnancy outcomes in women with growth hormone deficiency. *Fertil Steril*. 2015;104(5):1210-1217.
3. Biller BMK, Hoybye C, Carroll P, et al. Pregnancy outcomes in women receiving growth hormone replacement therapy enrolled in the Nordinet International Outcome Study (IOS) and the American Norditropin Studies: Web-Enabled Research (ANSWER) Program. *Pituitary*. 2021;24:611-621.
4. Fleseriu M, Hashim IA, Karavitaki N, et al. Hormonal replacement in hypopituitarism in adults: an endocrine society clinical practice guideline. *J Clin Endocrinol Metab*. 2016;101(11):3888-3921.
5. Vila G, Luger A. Growth hormone deficiency and pregnancy: any role for substitution? *Minerva Endocrinol*. 2018;43(4):451-457.

SOMATROGON

Endocrine (Human Growth Hormone Analogue)

PREGNANCY RECOMMENDATION: No Human Data—Animal Data Suggest Low Risk

BREASTFEEDING RECOMMENDATION: Probably Compatible

PREGNANCY SUMMARY

No reports describing the specific use of somatrogon in human pregnancy have been located. Placental transfer and embryofetal exposure are likely to be negligible. Therefore, the absence of human pregnancy experience prevents a complete assessment of the embryofetal risk. Animal data did not show any embryofetal toxicity. Two large reports using other forms of hGH replacement therapy at conception and the first trimester found spontaneous abortion rates of 12% and 18% (both within the expected range). In addition, no birth anomalies were identified in 155 newborns. There was one stillbirth (gestational age not supplied) and one delivery in the second trimester for a severe cystic hygroma (genetic testing not reported). Though endocrine societies and organizations state that hGH replacement therapy is not approved for use in pregnancy, there will be women of reproductive age who suffer from growth hormone deficiency and will be on a replacement therapy program where conception will occur. The pregnancy data overall are reassuring. Glucose intolerance has been reported in patients treated with hGH products.

BREASTFEEDING SUMMARY

No reports describing the use of somatrogon in human pregnancy have been located. The amount of the drug found in breast milk is likely to be negligible. In addition, because it is primarily a protein, if the drug were to be ingested through breastfeeding, it would probably be digested in the infant's gastrointestinal tract and not be absorbed. Published data on short-acting recombinant hGH for 7 days during lactation did not demonstrate any adverse effects in infants. Breastfeeding while using this drug should be based on the mother's clinical need for treatment. If used, the infant should be monitored for the most common reported adult side effects of headache, abdominal pain, and oropharyngeal pain (all leading to irritability), pyrexia, cough, vomiting, and rash.

References

1. Prescribing Information. Ngenla. Pfizer Labs; 2023.
2. Vila G, Akerblad AC, Mattsson AF, et al. Pregnancy outcomes in women with growth hormone deficiency. *Fertil Steril*. 2015;104(5)1210-1217.
3. Biller BMK, Hoybye C, Carroll P, et al. Pregnancy outcomes in women receiving growth hormone replacement therapy enrolled in the Nordinet International Outcome Study (IOS) and the American Norditropin Studies: Web-Enabled Research (ANSWER) Program. *Pituitary*. 2021;24:611-621.
4. Fleseriu M, Hashim IA, Karavitaki N, et al. Hormonal replacement in hypopituitarism in adults: an endocrine society clinical practice guideline. *J Clin Endocrinol Metab*. 2016;101(11):3888-3921.
5. Vila G, Luger A. Growth hormone deficiency and pregnancy: any role for substitution? *Minerva Endocrinol*. 2018;43(4):451-457.

SONIDEGIB

Antineoplastic (Hedgehog Pathway Inhibitor)

PREGNANCY RECOMMENDATION: No Human Data—Animal Data Suggest Potential Risk

BREASTFEEDING RECOMMENDATION: Potential Toxicity

PREGNANCY SUMMARY

No reports describing the use of sonidegib in human pregnancy have been located. The drug will probably cross the placenta, so some fetal exposure will likely occur. Therefore, the absence of human pregnancy experience prevents a complete assessment of the embryofetal risk. Embryofetal toxicity with significant malformations was observed in animal studies. Based on the animal studies and the drug's mechanism of action, the manufacturer recommends that women with reproductive potential use effective contraception during treatment and for at least 20 months after the last dose. They also recommend that males with female partners of reproductive potential use condoms, even after vasectomy, during treatment, and for at least 8 months after the last dose. If a pregnancy occurs while using this drug, health care providers are encouraged to contact Sun Pharmaceuticals at 1-800-406-7984.

BREASTFEEDING SUMMARY

No reports describing the use of sonidegib during human lactation have been located. The drug will probably be found in breast milk, so some infant exposure will likely occur. However, due to the concern for potential serious adverse effects that might be seen in a breastfed infant, the manufacturer recommends that women not breastfeed while being treated with sonidegib and for at least 20 months after the last dose. Nevertheless, breastfeeding while using this drug should be based on the mother's clinical need for treatment. If used, the infant should be monitored for the most common reported adult side effects of nausea, abdominal pain, musculoskeletal pain, headache, and myalgias (all leading to irritability), vomiting, diarrhea, fatigue, decreased appetite, and pruritus.

Reference

1. Prescribing Information. Odomzo. Sun Pharmaceutical Industries, Inc; 2019.

SORAFENIB

Antineoplastic (Kinase Inhibitor)

PREGNANCY RECOMMENDATION: Limited Human Data—Animal Data Suggest Risk

BREASTFEEDING RECOMMENDATION: Potential Toxicity

S

PREGNANCY SUMMARY

One report describing the use of sorafenib in human pregnancy has been located. A pregnant woman with acute myeloid leukemia was treated with a series of antineoplastic agents, including daunorubicin, cytarabine, fludarabine, and sorafenib in the third trimester. A healthy infant was delivered at 32 weeks' gestation, who overall did well. However, this limited human pregnancy experience prevents a complete assessment of embryofetal risk. Embryofetal toxicity with malformations was observed in two animal species at doses of less than 10 times the RHD. Based on animal studies and the drug's mechanism of action, the manufacturer recommends that women with reproductive potential use effective contraception during treatment and for 6 months after the last dose. They also recommend that males with female partners of reproductive potential use effective contraception during treatment and for 3 months after the last dose. Nevertheless, using this drug during pregnancy should be based on the pros and cons of the mother's clinical need for treatment versus any potential fetal risk that might occur from exposure. There is a registry for women who are pregnant and have cancer. For more information, women and health care providers are encouraged to contact the Cancer and Pregnancy Registry at 1-877-635-4499. Hypertension was reported in up to 17% of patients treated with this drug in the clinical trials. Sorafenib can prolong the QTc interval.

BREASTFEEDING SUMMARY

No reports describing the use of sorafenib during human lactation have been located. The drug will likely be excreted into breast milk, so some infant exposure will probably occur. Due to a concern for potential serious adverse effects that might be seen in a breastfed infant, the manufacturer recommends that women not breastfeed while being treated with this drug and for at least 2 weeks after the last dose. Nevertheless, breastfeeding while using this drug should be based on the mother's clinical need for treatment versus any potential infant risks that might occur. If used, the infant should be monitored for the most common reported adult side effects of nausea and abdominal pain (both leading to irritability), diarrhea, fatigue (lethargy), alopecia, rash, and decreased appetite (monitor infant growth).

References

1. Prescribing Information. Sorafenib. Dr. Reddys Laboratories Inc; 2022.
2. Mahdi AJ, Gosrani D, Chakraborty M, et al. Successful molecular targeted treatment of AML in pregnancy with azacitidine and sorafenib with no adverse fetal outcomes. *Br J Haematol*. 2018;180:578-606.

SOTAGLIFLOZIN

Cardiovascular (SGLT2 Inhibitor)

PREGNANCY RECOMMENDATION: No Human Data—Animal Data Suggest Potential Risk

BREASTFEEDING RECOMMENDATION: Potential Toxicity

PREGNANCY SUMMARY

No reports describing the use of sotagliflozin in human pregnancy have been located. Some amount of the drug and its active metabolite will probably cross the placenta, so fetal exposure will likely occur. Therefore, the absence of human pregnancy experience prevents a complete assessment of the embryofetal risk. Animal studies did not demonstrate any teratogenicity. However, because of the findings in rats administered the drug postnatally (regarding possible renal injury), the manufacturer recommends that the drug not be used in the second and third trimesters of pregnancy. Nevertheless, using this drug during pregnancy should be based on the pros and cons of the mother's clinical need for treatment versus any potential fetal risk that might occur from exposure. In addition, fetal renal status can be monitored by perinatal ultrasound. Lastly, postmarketing surveillance has detected an increase in the incidence of necrotizing fasciitis of the perineum (Fournier gangrene) in both men and women with diabetes using this drug.

BREASTFEEDING SUMMARY

No reports describing the use of sotagliflozin in human lactation have been located. The drug and its active metabolite will probably be found in breast milk, so some infant exposure will likely occur. Because of the findings in rats administered the drug postnatally (regarding possible renal injury), the manufacturer recommends that women not breastfeed while using this drug. However, breastfeeding should be based on the mother's clinical need for treatment. If used, the infant should be monitored for the most common reported adult side effects of diarrhea, volume depletion, and urinary tract infection.

Reference

1. Prescribing Information. Inpefa. Lexicon Pharmaceuticals, Inc; 2023.

SOTALOL

Cardiovascular (Antiarrhythmic)

PREGNANCY RECOMMENDATION: Limited Human Data—Animal data Suggest Low Risk

BREASTFEEDING RECOMMENDATION: Potential Toxicity

PREGNANCY SUMMARY

There are several reports describing the use of sotalol in human pregnancy. Several studies exist where the drug was administered to the mother in treating fetal arrhythmias. A few other reports describe the use in treating maternal arrhythmias and hypertension. Only a few pregnancies had first-trimester exposure, and no fetal anomalies have been described. The drug crosses the placenta, so fetal exposure occurs. However, this limited first-trimester human pregnancy experience prevents a complete assessment of embryofetal risk. Animal data did not show any embryofetal toxicity in two species at doses of less than 10 times the RHD. Using this drug during pregnancy (for maternal disease or off-label use in treating fetal arrhythmias) should be based on the pros and cons of the mother's clinical need for treatment versus any potential fetal risk that might occur from exposure.

BREASTFEEDING SUMMARY

Sotalol has been shown to be excreted into human breast milk. Breast milk levels are often higher than the maternal blood levels, as much as 3 to 8 times. In one case, the infant was consuming about 23% of the maternal dose. No adverse effects were observed in the infant. Due to a concern for potential serious adverse effects that might be seen in a breastfed infant, especially because of these elevated breast milk levels, the manufacturer recommends that women not breastfeed while being treated with this drug. Therefore, breastfeeding while using this drug should be based on the mother's clinical need for treatment versus any potential infant risks that might occur. If used, the infant should be monitored for the most common reported adult side effects of nausea, dizziness, and headache (all leading to irritability), vomiting, bradycardia, fatigue (lethargy), sweating, and hypotension.

References

1. Prescribing Information. Sotalol hydrochloride. Bayshore Pharmaceuticals LLC; 2024.
2. O'Hare MF, Leahey W, Murnaghan GA, McDevitt DG. Pharmacokinetics of sotalol during pregnancy. *Eur J Clin Pharmacol*. 1983;24:521-524.
3. O'Hare MF, Murnaghan GA, Russell CJ, et al. Sotalol as a hypotensive agent in pregnancy. *Br J Obstet Gynaecol*. 1980;87:814-820.
4. Erkkola R, Lammintausta R, Liukko P, Anttila M. Transfer of propranolol and sotalol across the human placenta. Their effect on maternal and fetal plasma renin activity. *Acta Obstet Gynecol Scand*. 1982;61:31-34.
5. Wagner X, Jouglard J, Moulin M, et al. Coadministration of flecainide acetate and sotalol during pregnancy: lack of teratogenic effects, passage across the placenta, and excretion in human breast milk. *Am Heart J*. 1990;119:700-702.
6. Hackett LP, Wojnar-Horton RE, Dusci LJ, et al. Excretion of sotalol in breast milk. *Br J Clin Pharmacol*. 1990;29:277-278.
7. Oudijk MA, Ruskamp JM, Ververs FFT, et al. Treatment of fetal tachycardia with sotalol: transplacental pharmacokinetics and pharmacodynamics. *J Am Coll Cardiol*. 2003;42:765-770.
8. Arnoux P, Seyral P, Llurens M, et al. Amiodarone and digoxin for refractory fetal tachycardia. *Am J Cardiol*. 1987;59:166-167.
9. Sonesson SE, Fouron JC, Wesslen-Eriksson E, Jaeggi E, Winberg P. Foetal supraventricular tachycardia treated with sotalol. *Acta Paediatr*. 1998; 87:584-587.
10. Oudijk MA, Michon MM, Kleinman CS, et al. Sotalol in the treatment of fetal dysrhythmias. *Circulation*. 2000;101:2721-2726.
11. Lisowski LA, Verheijen PM, Benatar AA, et al. Atrial flutter in the perinatal age group: diagnosis, management and outcome. *J Am Coll Cardiol*. 2000;35:771-777.
12. Hill GD, Kovach JR, Saudek DE, et al. Transplacental treatment of fetal tachycardia: a systematic review and meta-analysis. *Perinat Diag*. 2017;37:1076-1083.
13. Alsaied T, Baskar S, Fares M, et al. First-line antiarrhythmic transplacental treatment for fetal tachyarrhythmia: a systematic review and meta-analysis. *J Am Heart Assoc*. 2017;6:e007164.
14. Myoshi T, Maeno Y, Hamasaki T, et al. Antenatal therapy for fetal supraventricular tachyarrhythmias. Multicenter trial. *J Am Coll Cardiol*. 2019;74:874-885.

SOTATERCEPT

Cardiovascular (Activin Signaling Inhibitor—Pulmonary Arterial Hypertension)

PREGNANCY RECOMMENDATION: No Human Data—Animal Data Suggest Risk (Maternal Benefits May Outweigh Any Potential Fetal Risks)

BREASTFEEDING RECOMMENDATION: Probably Compatible

PREGNANCY SUMMARY

No reports describing the use of sotatercept in human pregnancy have been located. As a partial IgG antibody with the Fc portion, it likely crosses the placenta, especially during the second half of gestation, so some fetal exposure will probably occur. Therefore, the absence of human pregnancy experience prevents a complete assessment of the embryofetal risk. Animal studies did show embryofetal toxicity with malformations in two species at doses of less than 10 times the RHD. However, the dosing in humans is usually one injection every 3 weeks. In these animal studies, two injections were administered about 7 days apart. It is not possible to determine if this closer frequency of injections plays any role in the fetal adverse effects. Based on these animal studies and the drug's mechanism of action, the manufacturer recommends that women with reproductive potential use effective contraception during treatment and for 4 months after the last dose. Nevertheless, using this drug during pregnancy should be based on the pros and cons of the mother's clinical need for treatment versus any potential fetal risk that might occur from exposure. There is a pregnancy exposure registry that monitors pregnancy outcomes in women using this drug. Health care providers are encouraged to call Merck Sharp & Dohme at 1-877-888-4231. There are significant maternal and fetal risks associated with pulmonary arterial hypertension in pregnancy, and therefore, maternal treatment may outweigh possible fetal risks in some cases.

S

BREASTFEEDING SUMMARY

No reports describing the use of sotatercept during human lactation have been located. It is known that IgG antibodies can be found in human breast milk, but are not found in the neonatal or infant circulation. Additionally, if any IgG antibodies were to be ingested through breastfeeding, they would probably be digested in the infant's gastrointestinal tract and not be absorbed. Regardless, due to a concern for potential serious adverse effects that might be seen in a breastfed infant, the manufacturer recommends that women not breastfeed while being treated with this drug and for at least 4 months after the last dose. Nevertheless, breastfeeding while using this drug should be based on the mother's clinical need for treatment. If used, the infant should be monitored for the most common reported adult side effects of headache and dizziness (both leading to irritability), diarrhea, rash, and flushing.

Reference

1. Prescribing Information. Winrevair. Merck Sharp & Dohme LLC; 2024.

SOTORASIB

Antineoplastic (KRAS Inhibitor)

PREGNANCY RECOMMENDATION: No Human Data—Animal Data Suggest Potential Risk

BREASTFEEDING RECOMMENDATION: Potential Toxicity

PREGNANCY SUMMARY

No reports describing the use of sotorasib in human pregnancy have been located. Sotorasib will likely cross the placenta, so some fetal exposure will probably occur. Therefore, the absence of human pregnancy experience prevents a complete assessment of embryofetal risk. Animal data did show some embryofetal toxicity, but maternal toxicity also occurred. Using this drug during pregnancy should be based on the pros and cons of the mother's clinical need for treatment versus any potential fetal risk that might occur from exposure. There is a registry for women who are pregnant and have cancer. For more information, women and health care providers are encouraged to contact the Cancer and Pregnancy Registry at 1-877-635-4499.

BREASTFEEDING SUMMARY

No reports describing the use of sotorasib during human lactation have been located. The drug will likely be excreted into breast milk, so some infant exposure will probably occur. Due to the potential for serious adverse effects that might be seen in a breastfed infant, the manufacturer recommends that women not breastfeed while taking sotorasib and for 1 week after the last dose. Nevertheless, breastfeeding while using this drug should be based on the mother's clinical need for treatment. If used, the infant should be monitored for the most common reported adult side effects of nausea and musculoskeletal pain (both leading to irritability), diarrhea, lethargy, cough, and various laboratory abnormalities (see PI).

Reference

1. Prescribing Information. Lumakras. Amgen; 2022.

SPARSENTAN

Renal (Endothelin Type A Receptor and Angiotensin II Receptor Antagonist)

PREGNANCY RECOMMENDATION: No Human Data—Animal Data Suggest Potential Risk

BREASTFEEDING RECOMMENDATION: Potential Toxicity

PREGNANCY SUMMARY

No reports describing the use of sparsentan in human pregnancy have been located. The drug will likely cross the placenta, so some fetal exposure will probably occur. Therefore, the absence of human pregnancy experience prevents a complete assessment of the embryofetal risk. Animal studies did show embryofetal toxicity with malformations. Based on these animal studies and the drug's mechanism of action, the manufacturer recommends that women with reproductive potential use effective contraception during treatment and for 1 month after the last dose. They also recommend a negative pregnancy test prior to drug initiation and every month while on treatment. However, using this drug during pregnancy should be based on the pros and cons of the mother's clinical need for treatment versus any potential fetal risk that might occur from exposure. Sparsentan carries a boxed warning for embryo-fetal toxicity.

BREASTFEEDING SUMMARY

No reports describing the use of sparsentan during human lactation have been located. The drug will likely be excreted into breast milk, so some infant exposure will probably occur. Due to the concern for potential serious adverse effects that might be seen in a breastfed infant, the manufacturer recommends that women not breastfeed while being treated with this drug. Nevertheless, breastfeeding while using this drug should be based on the mother's clinical need for treatment. If used, the infant should be monitored for the most common reported adult side effects of peripheral edema, hypotension, hyperkalemia, and anemia.

Reference

1. Prescribing Information. Filspari. Travere Therapeutics, Inc; 2023.

SPESOLIMAB

Immunologic (Interleukin-36 Receptor Antagonist—Monoclonal Antibody)

PREGNANCY RECOMMENDATION: No Human Data—Animal Data Suggest Low Risk

BREASTFEEDING RECOMMENDATION: Probably Compatible

PREGNANCY SUMMARY

No reports describing the use of spesolimab in human pregnancy have been located. As an IgG antibody, the drug will likely cross the placenta, so some fetal exposure will probably occur. Therefore, the absence of human pregnancy experience prevents a complete assessment of embryofetal risk. Animal data did not show embryofetal toxic effects. Using this drug during pregnancy should be based on the pros and cons of the mother's clinical need for treatment versus any potential fetal risk that might occur from exposure.

BREASTFEEDING SUMMARY

No reports describing the use of spesolimab during human lactation have been located. It is known that IgG antibodies can be found in human breast milk, but are not found in the neonatal or infant circulation. Additionally, if any IgG antibodies were to be ingested through breastfeeding, they would probably be digested in the infant's gastrointestinal tract and not be absorbed. Breastfeeding while using this drug should be based on the mother's clinical need for treatment. If used, the infant should be monitored for the most common reported adult side effects of asthenia, nausea, headache, and pruritus (all leading to irritability), vomiting, and urinary tract infections.

Reference

1. Prescribing Information. Spevigo. Boehringer Ingelheim Pharmaceuticals, Inc; 2022.

SPINOSAD

Dermatologic/Topical (Antiparasitic)

PREGNANCY RECOMMENDATION: Human Data Suggest Low Risk

BREASTFEEDING RECOMMENDATION: Probably Compatible

PREGNANCY SUMMARY

No reports describing the use of spinosad in human pregnancy have been located. Topical use of the drug does not produce quantifiable amounts of spinosad in human plasma, so it is not expected to reach the placental interface. Although the suspension contains an unspecified amount of benzyl alcohol, it is doubtful if sufficient amounts of the additive would be absorbed to cause any embryofetal toxicity. Animal data did show some embryofetal toxicity in two species, but with oral administration. Using this drug during pregnancy should be based on the pros and cons of the mother's clinical need for treatment versus any potential fetal risk that might occur from exposure.

BREASTFEEDING SUMMARY

No reports describing the use of spinosad during human lactation have been located. Excretion of clinically significant amounts of the drug into breast milk is unlikely because plasma concentrations of the drug after topical use are below the level of quantification. Although an unspecified amount of benzyl alcohol is also present in the suspension, it is doubtful if sufficient amounts of the additive would be absorbed to cause toxicity in a nursing infant. Thus, use of the drug during breastfeeding appears to be low risk. The manufacturer recommends educating patients about removing spinosad from the breast tissue area through washing before breastfeeding to avoid any direct infant exposure. Breastfeeding while using this drug should be based on the mother's clinical need for treatment versus any potential infant risks that might occur. Due to the topical use of the drug, systemic side effects were not analyzed.

Reference

1. Prescribing Information. Spinosad. Allegis Pharmaceuticals LLC; 2021.

SPIRONOLACTONE

Cardiovascular (Aldosterone Antagonist—Potassium-Sparing Diuretic)

PREGNANCY RECOMMENDATION: Limited Human Data—Animal Data Suggest Risk

BREASTFEEDING RECOMMENDATION: Probably Compatible

PREGNANCY SUMMARY

There are three reports describing the use of spironolactone in 33 pregnancies. One (3.2%) major anomaly was described in 31 first-trimester exposures. The drug probably crosses the placenta, so some fetal exposure will likely occur. However, this limited human pregnancy experience prevents a complete assessment of embryofetal risk. Embryofetal toxicity was observed in two animal species at doses of less than 10 times the maximum recommended human dose (MRHD), but not in a third species. Due to the potential risks to male fetuses because of the antiandrogenic properties, the manufacturer recommends that spironolactone be avoided in pregnant women or advises pregnant women of the potential risk to a male fetus. Feminization has been observed in male rat fetuses. Congestive heart failure, hypertension, and liver cirrhosis can have numerous pregnancy complications, including intrauterine growth restriction (IUGR), stillbirth, preeclampsia, and preterm delivery. In addition, if these diseases are uncontrolled, there are maternal risks of stroke, myocardial infarction (MI), cardiac failure, and death. Therefore, using this drug during pregnancy should be based on the pros and cons of the mother's clinical need for treatment versus any potential fetal risk that might occur from exposure. In general, however, diuretics are not recommended for the treatment of gestational hypertension because of the potential for maternal hypovolemia characteristic of this disease. Elevated glucose levels have been reported in patients treated with this drug. Therefore, if used during pregnancy, glucose levels should be monitored.

BREASTFEEDING SUMMARY

The manufacturer reports that spironolactone is not found in human breast milk, but canrenone, the principal and active metabolite, is excreted into breast milk. However, the overall amount of canrenone is less than 1% of the maternal plasma levels. The effect on an infant from this ingestion is unknown, but the amount appears to be clinically insignificant. Breastfeeding while using this drug should be based on the mother's clinical need for treatment versus any potential infant risks that might occur. If used, the infant should be monitored for the most common reported adult side effect of gynecomastia.

References

1. Prescribing Information. Spironolactone. Amneal Pharmaceuticals LLC; 2020.
2. Pubchem. Spironolactone. Accessed September 20, 2024. https://pubchem.ncbi.nlm.nih.gov/compound/Spironolactone
3. Kersten M, Hancke K, Janni W, Kraft K. Pregnancy induced Cushing's syndrome and primary aldosteronism: a case report. *BMC Preg Childbirth*. 2020;20:421.
4. Inoue W, Motoki H, Yoshie K, Kuwahara K. Successful management of a pregnant patient with Danon cardiomyopathy. *Intern Med*. 2024;63:681-686.
5. Phelps DL, Karim A. Spironolactone: relationship between concentrations of dethioacetylated metabolite in human serum and milk. *J Pharm Sci*. 1977;66:1203.

STIRIPENTOL

Central Nervous System (Antiseizure)

PREGNANCY RECOMMENDATION: No Human Data—Animal Data Suggest Risk

BREASTFEEDING RECOMMENDATION: Potential Toxicity

PREGNANCY SUMMARY

No reports describing the use of stiripentol in human pregnancy have been located. The drug will probably cross the placenta, so fetal exposure will likely occur. However, the absence of human pregnancy experience prevents a complete assessment of the embryofetal risk. Animal data did show embryofetal toxicity. The drug is used in combination with clobazam (see Clobazam). Using this drug during pregnancy should be based on the pros and cons of the mother's clinical need for treatment versus any potential fetal risk that might occur from exposure. There is a pregnancy exposure registry that monitors pregnancy outcomes in women exposed to antiepileptic drugs. Health care providers are encouraged to call the North American Antiepileptic Drug Pregnancy Registry by calling 1-888-233-2334.

BREASTFEEDING SUMMARY

Stiripentol probably enters breast milk, so infant exposure will likely occur. Breastfeeding while using this drug should be based on the mother's clinical need for treatment. If used, the infant should be monitored for the most common reported adult side effects of nausea and joint pain (both leading to irritability), sedation, decreased appetite, decreased weight, and hypotonia.

Reference

1. Prescribing Information. Diacomit. Biocodex; 2018.

STREPTOMYCIN

Antibacterial (Aminoglycoside)

PREGNANCY RECOMMENDATION: Limited Human Data (First Trimester)—Human Data Suggest Potential Risk (Third Trimester)

BREASTFEEDING RECOMMENDATION: Probably Compatible

PREGNANCY SUMMARY

There are a few reports describing the use of streptomycin in human pregnancy. From the Collaborative Perinatal Project, there were five (3.7%) major anomalies identified with the use of streptomycin in 135 first trimester exposures. There were 7 (2.1%) anomalies seen in 355 cases with anytime use. No pattern to the defects was seen. In another study that analyzed aminoglycoside antibiotics as a group, there were 38 (0.17%) aminoglycoside uses in 22,865 women who had fetuses or newborns with congenital malformations. This was no different than the 42 (0.11%) uses in 38,151 women who had newborns with no structural defects. Very few of these used streptomycin. The drug crosses the placenta, so fetal exposure will occur. However, this limited human pregnancy experience prevents a complete assessment of embryofetal risk. No animal reproduction or fertility studies have been located. From a few case reports, streptomycin may cause fetal ototoxicity resulting in deafness in newborns when used in the third trimester. Due to the harmful effects demonstrated on the fetus, the US Centers of Disease Control and Prevention (CDC) does not recommend using streptomycin during pregnancy for tuberculosis treatment. Nevertheless, using this drug during pregnancy should be based on the pros and cons of the mother's clinical need for treatment versus any potential fetal risk that might occur from exposure.

BREASTFEEDING SUMMARY

Streptomycin has been shown to be excreted into human breast milk, so some infant exposure will occur. Breast milk to plasma ratios are fairly consistent. However, oral absorption of streptomycin is poor, so clinically significant blood levels are not predicted. Thus, ototoxicity in the infant would not be expected. Nevertheless, due to a concern for potential serious adverse effects that might be seen in a breastfed infant, the manufacturer recommends that women not breastfeed while being treated with this drug. Regardless, breastfeeding while using this drug should be based on the mother's clinical need for treatment versus any potential infant risks that might occur. If used, the infant should be monitored for the most common reported adult side effects of nausea and vertigo (both leading to irritability), vomiting, fever, rash, peripheral edema, and eosinophilia.

References

1. Prescribing Information. Streptomycin. XGen Pharmaceuticals DJB Inc; 2023.
2. Centers for Disease Control and Prevention. Treatment for TB during pregnancy. Accessed September 20, 2024. https://www.cdc.gov/tb/topic/treatment/pregnancy.htm
3. Watson E, Stow R. Streptomycin therapy: effects on fetus. *JAMA*. 1948; 137:1599-600.
4. Rubin A, Winston J, Rutledge M. Effects of streptomycin upon the human fetus. *Am J Dis Child*. 1951;82:14-16.
5. Kistner R. The use of streptomycin during pregnancy. *Am J Obstet Gynecol*. 1950;60:422-426.
6. Leroux M. Existe-t-il une surdité congénitale acquise due à la streptomycine? *Ann Otolaryngol*. 1950;67:194-196.
7. Nishimura H, Tanimura T. *Clinical Aspects of the Teratogenicity of Drugs*. Excerpta Medica; 1976:130.
8. Donald PR, Sellars SL. Streptomycin ototoxicity in the unborn child. *S Afr Med J*. 1981;60:316-318.
9. Mann J, Moskowitz R. Plaque and pregnancy. A case report. *JAMA*. 1977;237:1854-1855.
10. Heinonen OP, Slone D, Shapiro S. *Birth Defects and Drugs in Pregnancy*. Publishing Sciences Group; 1977.
11. Marynowski A, Sianozecka E. Comparison of the incidence of congenital malformations in neonates from healthy mothers and from patients treated because of tuberculosis. *Ginekol Pol*. 1972;43:713-715.
12. Lowe C. Congenital defects among children born under supervision or treatment for pulmonary tuberculosis. *Br J Prev Soc Med*. 1964;18:14-16.
13. Czeizel AE, Rockenbauer M, Olsen J, Sorensen HT. A teratological study of aminoglycoside antibiotic treatment during pregnancy. *Scand J Infect Dis*. 2000;32:309-313.
14. Wilson JT. Milk/plasma ratios and contraindicated drugs. In: Wilson JT, ed. *Drugs in Breast Milk*. ADIS Press; 1981:79.

STREPTOZOCIN

Antineoplastic (Alkylating Agent)

PREGNANCY RECOMMENDATION: Limited Human Data—Animal Data Suggest Risk

BREASTFEEDING RECOMMENDATION: Potential Toxicity

PREGNANCY SUMMARY

One report has described the use of streptozocin during the latter half of gestation without apparent fetal harm. The drug will probably cross the placenta, so some fetal exposure will likely occur. However, this limited human pregnancy experience prevents a complete assessment of embryofetal risk. The drug was found to cause embryofetal toxicity in two species at unspecified dosages. Using this drug during pregnancy should be based on the pros and cons of the mother's clinical need for treatment versus any potential fetal risk that might occur from exposure. There is a registry for women who are pregnant and have cancer. For more information, women and health care providers are encouraged to contact the Cancer and Pregnancy Registry at 1-877-635-4499. Elevated blood glucose levels were reported in patients treated with this drug in the clinical trials. Therefore, if used during pregnancy, glucose levels should be monitored.

BREASTFEEDING SUMMARY

No reports describing the use of streptozocin during human lactation have been located. The drug will likely be excreted into breast milk, so some infant exposure will probably occur. However, due to a concern for potential serious adverse effects that might be seen in a breastfed infant, the manufacturer recommends that women not breastfeed while being treated with this drug. Nevertheless, breastfeeding while using this drug should be based on the mother's clinical need for treatment versus any potential infant risks that might occur. If used, the infant should be monitored for the most common reported adult side effects of nausea (leading to irritability), vomiting, diarrhea, and various laboratory abnormalities (see PI).

References

1. Prescribing Information. Zanosar. Teva Parenteral Medicines Inc, 2023.
2. Schapira DV, Chudley AE. Successful pregnancy following continuous treatment with combination chemotherapy before conception and throughout pregnancy. *Cancer*. 1984;54:800-803.

SUCCIMER

Chelating Agent (Heavy Metals)

PREGNANCY RECOMMENDATION: Limited Human Data—Animal Data Suggest Risk (Maternal Benefit May Outweigh Any Embryofetal Risk)

BREASTFEEDING RECOMMENDATION: *Contraindicated

PREGNANCY SUMMARY

Two reports describing the use of succimer in human pregnancy have been located. Both exposures occurred after the first trimester, but no adverse newborn effects were reported. The drug is likely to cross the placenta, so some fetal exposure will probably occur. However, this limited human pregnancy experience prevents a complete assessment of embryofetal risk. Embryofetal toxicity was observed in two animal species, but the extent of the dosing compared with human use was not provided. Using this drug during pregnancy should be based on the pros and cons of the mother's clinical need for treatment versus any potential fetal risk that might occur from exposure.

BREASTFEEDING SUMMARY

No reports describing the use of succimer during human lactation have been located. The drug will likely be excreted into breast milk, so some infant exposure will probably occur. *However, because the use of succimer implies poisoning with lead or other heavy metals, these substances might also be excreted into breast milk and cause infant toxicity as well. Therefore, breastfeeding is probably contraindicated in women receiving succimer until the metal toxicity is reversed. If the clinical decision is to use this drug while breastfeeding, the infant should be monitored for the most common reported adult side effects of nausea, abdominal cramps, headache, and various body pains (all leading to irritability), vomiting, diarrhea, appetite loss (monitor infant growth), and fatigue (lethargy).

References

1. Prescribing Information. Chemet. Recordati Rare Diseases Ince; 2024.
2. Horowitz BZ, Mirkin DB. Lead poisoning and chelation in a mother-neonate pair. J *Toxicol Clin Toxicol*. 2001;39:727-731.
3. Shannon M. Severe lead poisoning in pregnancy. *Ambul Pediatr*. 2003;3:37-39.

SUCCINYLCHOLINE

Pain (Depolarizing Neuromuscular Blocker)

PREGNANCY RECOMMENDATION: Limited Human Data (First Trimester) Human Data Suggest Low Risk (Third Trimester)

BREASTFEEDING RECOMMENDATION: Probably Compatible

PREGNANCY SUMMARY

Succinylcholine has been routinely used in obstetric patients prior to delivery since the 1950s, and no reports of fetal toxicity have been located. However, data on first-trimester use are small. In the Collaborative Perinatal Project, no anomalies were identified in 26 first-trimester exposures. The drug appears to cross the placenta, but measured levels are low at less than 20% maternal levels. In some cases, the drug was not detected in cord blood. This is probably due to the extremely short elimination half-life of about 12 to 70 seconds. However, this limited first-trimester human pregnancy experience prevents a complete assessment of the embryofetal risk. No embryofetal toxicity was seen in two species, but dosing was not supplied. Partial or complete newborn paralysis, with resulting respiratory depression, has been reported when the drug was administered to women with the genetic disorder (autosomal dominant) of atypical cholinesterase deficiency. Prolonged newborn respiratory depression may occur when this trait has been inherited by the infant. The level of cholinesterase activity in the infant will determine the duration of paralysis. Women without the genetic trait rapidly metabolize the drug.

BREASTFEEDING SUMMARY

No reports describing the use of succinylcholine during human lactation have been located. Because the drug is rapidly hydrolyzed by plasma cholinesterase (pseudocholinesterase) to an inactive metabolite, it is doubtful that clinically significant amounts of active drug are transferred into human breast milk. Women with the autosomal dominant genetic trait for atypical cholinesterase deficiency will have high concentrations of succinylcholine, but the effects of the drug on the mother will preclude nursing. Breastfeeding while using this drug should be based on the mother's clinical need for treatment versus any potential infant risks that might occur. If used, the infant should be monitored for the most common reported adult side effects of respiratory depression, hypersensitivity reactions, bradycardia, tachycardia, excessive salivation, and rash.

References

1. Prescribing Information. Succinylcholine chloride. Indoco Remedies Limited; 2020.
2. Donnell GN. Cholinesterase, atypical. In: Buyse ML, ed. *Birth Defects Encyclopedia*. Vol. 1. Blackwell Scientific Publications; 1990:316-317.
3. Moya F, Kvisselgaard N. The placental transmission of succinylcholine. *Anesthesiology*. 1961;22:1-6.
4. Drabkova J, Crul JF, van der Kleijn E. Placental transfer of ^{14}C labelled succinylcholine in near-term Macaca mulatta monkeys. *Br J Anaesthesia*. 1973;45:1087-1096.
5. Owens WD, Zeitlin GL. Hypoventilation in a newborn following administration of succinylcholine to the mother: a case report. *Anesth Analg*. 1975; 54:38-40.
6. Cherala SR, Eddoe DN, Sechzer PH. Placental transfer of succinylcholine causing transient respiratory depression in the newborn. *Anaesthesia Intensive Care*. 1989;17:202-204.
7. Baraka A, Haroun S, Bassili M, Abu-Haider G. Response of the newborn to succinylcholine injection in homozygotic atypical mothers. *Anesthesiology*. 1975;43:115-116.
8. Kvisselgaard N, Moya F. Investigation of placental thresholds to succinylcholine. *Anesthesiology*. 1961;22:7-10.
9. Heinonen OP, Slone D, Shapiro S. *Birth Defects and Drugs in Pregnancy*. Publishing Sciences Group, 1977:358-360.
10. Sener EB, Guldogus F, Karakaya D, et al. Comparison of neonatal effects of epidural and general anesthesia for cesarean section. *Gynecol Obstet Invest*. 2003;55:41-45.
11. Onnis A, Grella P. *The Biochemical Effects of Drugs in Pregnancy*. Vol. 1. Ellis Horwood Limited, 1984:230-231.
12. Spigset O. Anaesthetic agents and excretion in breast milk. *Acta Anaesthesiol Scand*. 1994;38:94-103.

S

SUCRALFATE

Gastrointestinal

PREGNANCY RECOMMENDATION: Human Data Suggest Low Risk—Animal Data Suggest Low Risk

BREASTFEEDING RECOMMENDATION: Probably Compatible

PREGNANCY SUMMARY

In the Michigan Medicaid Surveillance study, 5 (2.7%) major birth anomalies were identified in 183 first-trimester exposures to sucralfate. No pattern to the defects was seen. It is not known if the drug crosses the placenta, but because it has low systemic absorption with oral use (about 2%), sucralfate likely poses little risk for use during pregnancy in patients without kidney dysfunction. In patients with chronic renal failure or those receiving dialysis, sucralfate should be used with caution because aluminum accumulation and toxicity have been reported. However, this limited human pregnancy experience prevents a complete assessment of embryofetal risk. Animal data did not show any embryofetal toxicity in three species at doses of more than 10 times the RHD. Using this drug during pregnancy should be based on the pros and cons of the mother's clinical need for treatment versus any potential fetal risk that might occur from exposure.

BREASTFEEDING SUMMARY

No reports describing the use of sucralfate during human lactation have been located. Minimal, if any, excretion of sucralfate into human breast milk should be expected because only small amounts (2%) of this drug are absorbed systemically with oral use. Breastfeeding while using this drug should be based on the mother's clinical need for treatment versus any potential infant risks that might occur. If used, the infant should be monitored for the most common reported adult side effect of constipation.

References

1. Prescribing Information. Sucralfate. Amneal Pharmaceuticals NY LLC; 2023.
2. Giesing D, Lanman R, Runser D. Absorption of sucralfate in man (abstract). *Gastroenterology*. 1982;82:1066.
3. Dehlink E, Yen E, Leichtner AM, et al. First evidence of a possible association between gastric acid suppression during pregnancy and childhood asthma: a population-based register study. *Clin Exp Allergy*. 2009;39:246-253.

SUFENTANIL

Pain (Opioid)

PREGNANCY RECOMMENDATION: Limited Human Data (First Trimester)—Human Data Suggest Potential Risk (Third Trimester)

BREASTFEEDING RECOMMENDATION: Probably Compatible (Short-Term)

PREGNANCY SUMMARY

Several reports describing the use of sufentanil in human pregnancy have been located. The drug has mainly been used during labor and delivery. Sufentanil has been shown to cross the placenta, so some fetal exposure will occur. However, the absence of the first-trimester human pregnancy experience prevents a complete assessment of the embryofetal risk. Neonatal respiratory depression and sedation immediately after birth are potential complications of all narcotics when administered to a woman during labor. Embryofetal toxicity was observed in two species of animals at doses of less than 10 times the RHD. The manufacturer states that sufentanil use during labor or delivery may result in neonatal respiratory depression, so naloxone should be available if needed. Because of this, it is not recommended for use during or immediately prior to labor when other techniques for analgesia may be more appropriate. Nevertheless, using this drug during pregnancy should be based on the pros and cons of the mother's clinical need for treatment versus any potential fetal risk that might occur from exposure. Being an opioid drug, there is always a risk for addiction and misuse. However, because of the short elimination half-life, this particular opioid drug is not likely to be one that is chronically used. Sufentanil carries a boxed warning for an increased risk of serious life-threatening, or fatal respiratory depression with concomitant use of benzodiazepines or other CNS depressants.

S

BREASTFEEDING SUMMARY

No reports describing the use of sufentanil during human lactation have been located. The drug will likely be excreted into breast milk, so some infant exposure will probably occur. Breastfeeding while using this drug should be based on the mother's clinical need for treatment versus any potential infant risks. If used, the infant should be monitored for the most common reported adult side effects of apnea, rigidity, and bradycardia.

References

1. Prescribing Information. Sufentanil citrate. Akorn; 2022.
2. Johnson RF, Herman N, Arney TL, et al. The placental transfer of sufentanil: effects of fetal pH, protein binding, and sufentanil concentration. *Anesth Analg*. 1997;84:1262-1268.
3. Krishna BR, Zakowski MI, Grant GJ. Sufentanil transfer in the human placenta during in vitro perfusion. *Can J Anaesth*. 1997;44:996-1001.
4. Vertommen JD, Van Aken H, Vandermeulen E, et al. Maternal and neonatal effects of adding epidural sufentanil to 0.5% bupivacaine for cesarean delivery. *J Clin Anesth*. 1991;3:371-376.

5. Loftus JR, Hill H, Cohen SE. Placental transfer and neonatal effects of epidural sufentanil and fentanyl administered with bupivacaine during labor. *Anesthesiology*. 1995;83:300-308.
6. Nielsen PE, Erickson JR, Abouleish EI, et al. Fetal heart rate changes after intrathecal sufentanil or epidural bupivacaine [sic] for labor analgesia: incidence and clinical significance. *Anesth Analg*. 1996;83:742-760.
7. Camann WR, Minzter BH, Denney RA, Datta S. Intrathecal sufentanil for labor analgesia. Effects of added epinephrine. *Anesthesiology*. 1993;78:870-874.
8. Cohen SE, Cherry CM, Holbrook RH Jr, et al. Intrathecal sufentanil for labor analgesia—sensory changes, side effects, and fetal heart rate changes. *Anesth Analg*. 1993;77:1155-1160.
9. Camann WR, Denney RA, Holby ED, Datta S. A comparison of intrathecal, epidural, and intravenous sufentanil for labor analgesia. *Anesthesiology*. 1992;77:884-887.
10. Honet JE, Arkoosh VA, Norris MC, et al. Comparison among intrathecal fentanyl, meperidine, and sufentanil for labor analgesia. *Anesth Analg*. 1992;75:734-739.
11. Russell R, Reynolds F. Epidural infusions for nulliparous women in labour. A randomised double-blind comparison of fentanyl/bupivacaine and sufentanil/bupivacaine. *Anaesthesia*. 1993;48:856-861.
12. Phillips GH. Epidural sufentanil/bupivacaine combinations for analgesia during labor: effect of varying sufentanil doses. *Anesthesiology*. 1987;67:835-838.
13. Van Steenberge A, Debroux HC, Noorduin H. Extradural bupivacaine with sufentanil for vaginal delivery. A double-blind trial. *Br J Anaesth*. 1987;59:1518-1522.
14. Le Polain B, De Kock M, Scholtes JL, Van Lierde M. Clonidine combined with sufentanil and bupivacaine with adrenaline for obstetric analgesia. *Br J Anaesth*. 1993;71:657-660.
15. Grieco WM, Norris MC, Leighton BL, et al. Intrathecal sufentanil labor analgesia: the effects of adding morphine or epinephrine. *Anesth Anal*. 1993;77:1149-1154.
16. D'Angelo R, Anderson MT, Philip J, Eisenach JC. Intrathecal sufentanil compared to epidural bupivacaine for labor analgesia. *Anesthesiology*. 1994;80:1209-1215.
17. Vertommen JD, Lemmens E, Van Aken H. Comparison of the addition of three different doses of sufentanil to 0.125% bupivacaine given epidurally during labour. *Anaesthesia*. 1994;49:678-681.
18. Dahlgren G, Hultstrand C, Jakobsson I, et al. Intrathecal sufentanil, fentanyl, or placebo added to bupivacaine for cesarean section. *Anesth Analg*. 1997;85:1288-1293.
19. Hays RL, Palmer CM. Respiratory depression after intrathecal sufentanil during labor. *Anesthesiology*. 1994;81:511-512.

SUGAMMADEX

Antidote (Neuromuscular Blockade)

PREGNANCY RECOMMENDATION: No Human Data—Animal Data Suggest Low Risk

BREASTFEEDING RECOMMENDATION: Probably Compatible

PREGNANCY SUMMARY

No reports describing the use of sugammadex in human pregnancy have been located. The drug is not likely to cross the placenta, so fetal exposure should be clinically insignificant. However, the absence of human pregnancy experience prevents a complete assessment of the embryofetal risk. Animal data did not show any embryofetal toxicity at doses that did not cause maternal toxicity. Using this drug during pregnancy should be based on the pros and cons of the mother's clinical need for treatment versus any potential fetal risk that might occur from exposure.

BREASTFEEDING SUMMARY

No reports describing the use of sugammadex during human lactation have been located. The drug is not likely to be found in breast milk, so infant exposure should be negligible. Breastfeeding while using this drug should be based on the mother's clinical need for treatment. If used, the infant should be monitored for the most common reported adult side effects of pain, headache, and nausea (all leading to irritability), and vomiting.

Reference

1. Prescribing Information. Bridion. Merck Sharp & Dohme, LLC; 2022

S

SULBACTAM/DURLOBACTAM

Antibacterial

PREGNANCY RECOMMENDATION: Human Data Suggest Low Risk for Sulbactam—No Human Data for Durlobactam—Animal Data Suggest Low Risk

BREASTFEEDING RECOMMENDATION: Probably Compatible

PREGNANCY SUMMARY

Several studies have analyzed the use of sulbactam with ampicillin, and no identified drug-associated embryofetal toxicity or malformations have been identified (see Ampicillin/Sulbactam). Fetal exposure will occur with sulbactam. No human data specific to durlobactam use in pregnancy have been located. In addition, no human studies evaluating the effect of both drugs together during pregnancy have been located. Based on the likely placental transfer of durlobactam, fetal exposure

(*continued*)

will probably occur for this drug, similar to sulbactam. Therefore, the absence of human pregnancy experience prevents a complete assessment of the embryofetal risk for durlobactam, as well as this drug combination. Animal studies on sulbactam and on durlobactam overall did not show any embryofetal toxicity.

BREASTFEEDING SUMMARY

Sulbactam has been shown to enter human breast milk at low concentrations. No reports describing the use of durlobactam during human lactation have been located. However, this drug will also most likely be found in breast milk, so some infant exposure will probably occur. Breastfeeding while using this drug should be based on the mother's clinical need for treatment. If used, the infant should be monitored for the most common reported adult side effects of diarrhea, anemia, hypokalemia, and abnormal liver function tests.

Reference

1. Prescribing Information. Xacduro. Entasis Therapeutics, Ltd; 2023.

SULCONAZOLE

Antifungal (Topical—Imidazole)

PREGNANCY RECOMMENDATION: No Human Data—Animal Data Suggest Low Risk

BREASTFEEDING RECOMMENDATION: Probably Compatible

PREGNANCY SUMMARY

No reports describing the use of sulconazole in human pregnancy have been located. Sulconazole is partially absorbed systemically with topical use (up to 10% of the dose, the highest among imidazole products). The drug is likely to cross the placenta, so some fetal exposure will occur if the drug is at the placental interface. However, the absence of human pregnancy experience prevents a complete assessment of embryofetal risk. No embryofetal toxicity was observed in one animal species with oral doses of more than 10 times the RHD. Embryofetal toxicity was seen in a second species, but again, the oral doses used were more than 10 times the RHD. Using this drug during pregnancy should be based on the pros and cons of the mother's clinical need for treatment versus any potential fetal risk that might occur from exposure. However, because of the higher systemic absorption with topical use, the best course may be to avoid using sulconazole in the first trimester until more data are identified or use a different topical imidazole agent with lower systemic absorption.

BREASTFEEDING SUMMARY

No reports describing the use of sulconazole during human lactation have been located. The drug will likely be excreted into breast milk, so some infant exposure will probably occur. About 10% of the drug is absorbed systemically with topical use. The effect of this exposure on a nursing infant is unknown. Because systemic absorption was the highest known among similar agents, other imidazole antifungals might be more appropriate if a nursing woman requires topical antifungal therapy. Nevertheless, if the clinical decision is to use this drug while breastfeeding, the infant should be monitored for the most common reported adult side effects of itching (leading to irritability).

References

1. Prescribing Information. Sulconazole nitrate. JG Pharma; 2020.
2. Franz TJ, Lehman P. Percutaneous absorption of sulconazole nitrate in humans. *J Pharm Sci*. 1988;77:489-491.
3. Kragie L, Turner SD, Patten CJ, et al. Assessing pregnancy risks of azole antifungals using a high throughput aromatase inhibition assay. *Endocr Res*. 2002;28:129-140.
4. Harada N. Genetic analysis of human placental aromatase deficiency. *J Steroid Biochem Mol Biol*. 1993;44:331-340.

S

SULFACETAMIDE OPHTHALMIC

Ophthalmic/Antibacterial (Sulfonamide)

PREGNANCY RECOMMENDATION: No Human Data—No Relevant Animal Data

BREASTFEEDING RECOMMENDATION: Probably Compatible

PREGNANCY SUMMARY

No reports describing the use of sulfacetamide ophthalmic solution in human pregnancy have been located. If the drug is present at the placental interface, then it will likely cross. However, the amount of systemic absorption following ocular use is minimal; therefore, the overall amount is probably clinically insignificant. Regardless, the absence of human pregnancy experience prevents a complete assessment of embryofetal risk. Animal reproduction and fertility studies have not been conducted. Using this drug during pregnancy should be based on the pros and cons of the mother's clinical need for treatment versus any potential fetal risk that might occur from exposure. If used during pregnancy, consider placing pressure over the tear duct in the corner of the eye for at least 1 minute, and then remove any excess solution with absorbent tissue to decrease the amount of drug reaching the systemic circulation even further.

BREASTFEEDING SUMMARY

No reports describing the use of sulfacetamide during human lactation have been located. Because the amount of systemic absorption with ocular use is low, any risk to a nursing infant should be clinically insignificant. However, because systemically administered sulfonamides may cause kernicterus in infants, the manufacturer recommends not breastfeeding if sulfacetamide is given. Nevertheless, breastfeeding while using this drug should be based on the mother's clinical need for treatment versus any potential infant risks that might occur. Because of the ophthalmic use of the drug, systemic side effects have not been analyzed. A method to decrease some systemic absorption with ophthalmic use is described above in the Pregnancy Summary.

References

1. Prescribing Information. Sulfacetamide sodium. Bausch & Lomb Inc; 2023.
2. National Library of Medicine. Pubchem. Sulfacetamide. https://pubchem.ncbi.nlm.nih.gov/compound/Sulfacetamide

SULFADIAZINE

Antibacterial (Sulfonamide)

PREGNANCY RECOMMENDATION: Limited Human Data—Animal Data Suggest Potential Risk

BREASTFEEDING RECOMMENDATION: Potential Toxicity

PREGNANCY SUMMARY

There are several reports describing the use of sulfadiazine in human pregnancy (primarily in the second and third trimesters). In the Collaborative Perinatal Project, there were 30 (2.1%) major anomalies seen in 1,455 first-trimester exposures to sulfa drugs as a group. Of these, there were 3 (3.2%) congenital defects seen in 95 exposures to sulfadiazine. No pattern to the anomalies was seen. Like other sulfonamides, sulfadiazine crosses the placenta, so fetal exposure will occur. However, this limited first-trimester human pregnancy experience prevents a complete assessment of the embryofetal risk. No animal reproduction studies for sulfadiazine were located, but animal data for other sulfonamides revealed some embryofetal toxicity with malformations in one animal species at doses of about 7 times the RHD. Jaundice has been reported after exposure to sulfa drugs when used near delivery, because sulfa drugs compete with bilirubin binding of albumin. In utero, the fetus clears free bilirubin by the placental circulation; however, after birth, this mechanism is no longer available. Unbound bilirubin is free to cross the blood-brain barrier and may result in kernicterus. Although this toxicity is well known when sulfonamides are administered directly to the neonate, kernicterus in a newborn following in utero exposure to sulfa drugs has not been reported. Taken together, sulfonamides, as single agents, do not appear to pose a significant teratogenic risk. ACOG states that sulfonamides are appropriate for use during the first trimester if no other suitable alternatives are available. Because of the theoretical risk for newborn toxicity and the availability of numerous other antibacterial agents, avoiding sulfa drugs near term is suggested, unless the specific infection highly suggests the use of the sulfa drug. Infant bilirubin levels can be monitored.

BREASTFEEDING SUMMARY

No reports describing the use of sulfadiazine during human lactation have been located. The drug will likely be excreted into breast milk, so some infant exposure will probably occur. Due to a concern for potential serious adverse effects that might be seen in a breastfed infant (including elevated bilirubin levels and risk for kernicterus), the manufacturer recommends that women not breastfeed while being treated with this drug. Nevertheless, breastfeeding while using this drug should be based on the mother's clinical need for treatment versus any potential infant risks that might occur. If used, the infant should be monitored for the most common reported adult side effects of nausea and dyspepsia (both leading to irritability), vomiting, diarrhea, and rash.

References

1. Prescribing Information. Sulfadiazine. Epic Pharma LLC; 2023.
2. American College of Obstetricians and Gynecologists. ACOG committee opinion No. 717: sulfonamides, nitrofurantoin, and risk of birth defects. *Obstet Gynecol*. 2017;130:e150-e152.
3. Center for Disease Control and Prevention. Clinical care of toxoplasmosis. Accessed October 9, 2024. https://www.cdc.gov/toxoplasmosis/hcp/clinical-care/index.html
4. Reiter-Owona I, Hlobil H, Enders M, et al. Sulfadiazine plasma concentrations in women with pregnancy-acquired compared to ocular toxoplasmosis under pyrimethamine and sulfadiazine therapy: a case-control study. *Eur J Med Res*. 2020;25:59.
5. Yu PA, Tran EL, Parker CM, et al. Safety of antimicrobials during pregnancy: a systematic review of antimicrobials considered for treatment and postexposure prophylaxis of plague. *Clin Inf Dis*. 2020;70:537-550.
6. Mandelbrot L, Kieffer F, Sitta R, et al. Prenatal therapy with pyrimethamine + sulfadiazine vs spiramycin to reduce placental transmission of toxoplasmosis: a multicenter, randomized trial. *Am J Obstet Gynecol*. 2018;219:e1-e9.

7. Ardabili S, Kohl J, Gul G, Hodel M. What obstetricians should be aware of: serious side effects of antibiotic toxoplasmosis treatment in pregnancy. *BMJ Case Rep*. 2021;14:e240809.
8. Azad Khan AK, Truelove SC. Placental and mammary transfer of sulphasalazine. *Br Med J*. 1979;2:1553.
9. Heckel GP. Chemotherapy during pregnancy. Danger of fetal injury from sulfanilamide and its derivatives. *JAMA*. 1941;117:1314-1316.
10. Bonze EJ, Fuerstner PG, Falls FH. Use of sulfanilamide derivative in treatment of gonorrhea in pregnant and nonpregnant women. *Am J Obstet Gynecol*. 1939;38:73-79.
11. Carter MP, Wilson F. Antibiotics and congenital malformations. *Lancet*. 1963;1:1267-1268.
12. Little PJ. The incidence of urinary infection in 5000 pregnant women. *Lancet*. 1966;2:925-928.
13. McEwan HP. Anorectal conditions in obstetric patients. *Proc R Soc Med*. 1972;65:279-281.
14. Williams JD, Smith EK. Single-dose therapy with streptomycin and sulfametopyrazine for bacteriuria during pregnancy. *Br Med J*. 1970;4:651-653.
15. Mogadam M, Dobbins WO III, Korelitz BI, Ahmed SW. Pregnancy in inflammatory bowel disease: effect of sulfasalazine and corticosteroids on fetal outcome. *Gastroenterology*. 1981;80:72-76.
16. Richards IDG. A retrospective inquiry into possible teratogenic effects of drugs in pregnancy. *Adv Exp Med Biol*. 1972;27:441-455.
17. Nelson MM, Forfar JO. Association between drugs administered during pregnancy and congenital abnormalities of the fetus. *Br Med J*. 1971;1: 523-527.
18. Saxen I. Associations between oral clefts and drugs taken during pregnancy. *Int J Epidemiol*. 1975;4:37-44.
19. Anonymous. Teratogenic effects of sulphonamides. *Br Med J*. 1965;1:142.
20. Green KG. "Bimez" and teratogenic action. *Br Med J*. 1963;2:56.
21. Ingalls TH, Prindle RA. Esophageal atresia with tracheoesophageal fistula. Epidemiologic and teratologic implications. *N Engl J Med*. 1949;240: 987-995.
22. Harly JD, Farrar JF, Gray JB, Dunlop IC. Aromatic drugs and congenital cataracts. *Lancet*. 1964;1:472-473.
23. Pogorzelska E. A case of multiple congenital anomalies in a child of a mother treated with sulfaguanidine. *Patol Pol*. 1966;17:383-386.
24. Heinonen OP, Slone D, Shapiro S. *Birth Defects and Drugs in Pregnancy*. Publishing Sciences Group; 1977.
25. Crider KS, Cleves MA, Reefhuis J, Berry RJ, Hobbs CA, Hu DJ. Antibacterial medication use during pregnancy and risk of birth defects. *Arch Pediatr Adolesc Med*. 2009;163:978-985.
26. Stewart HL Jr, Pratt JP. Sulfanilamide excretion in human breast milk and effect on breast-fed babies. *JAMA*. 1938;111:1456-1458.
27. Adair FL, Hesseltine HC, Hac LR. Experimental study of the behavior of sulfanilamide. *JAMA*. 1938;111:766-770.
28. Hepburn JS, Paxson NF, Rogers AN. Secretion of ingested sulfanilamide in breast milk and in the urine of the infant. *J Biol Chem*. 1938;123:liv-lv.
29. Pinto SS. Excretion of sulfanilamide and acetylsulfanilamide in human milk. *JAMA*. 1938;111:1914-1916.
30. Hac LR, Adair FL, Hesseltine HC. Excretion of sulfanilamide and acetylsulfanilamide in human breast milk. *Am J Obstet Gynecol*. 1939;38:57-66.
31. Foster FP. Sulfanilamide excretion in breast milk: report of a case. *Proc Staff Meet Mayo Clin*. 1939;14:153-155.
32. Hepburn JS, Paxson NF, Rogers AN. Secretion of ingested sulfanilamide in human milk and in the urine of the nursing infant. *Arch Pediatr*. 1942; 59:413-418.
33. Von Freisen B. A study of small dose sulphamerazine prophylaxis in obstetrics. *Acta Obstet Gynecol Scand*. 1951;31(suppl):75-116.
34. Baskin CG, Law S, Wenger NK. Sulfadiazine rheumatic fever prophylaxis during pregnancy: does it increase the risk of kernicterus in the newborn? *Cardiology*. 1980;65:222-225.
35. Kauffman RE, O'Brien C, Gilford P. Sulfisoxazole secretion into human milk. *J Pediatr*. 1980;97:839-841.
36. Elliott GT, Quinn SI. Sulfisoxazole in human milk. *J Pediatr*. 1981;99:171-172.
37. Kauffman RE. Sulfisoxazole in human milk (reply). *J Pediatr*. 1981;99:172.
38. Ito S, Blajchman A, Stephenson M, Eliopoulos C, Koren G. Prospective follow-up of adverse reactions in breast-fed infants exposed to maternal medication. *Am J Obstet Gynecol*. 1993;168:1393-1399.

SULFAMETHOXAZOLE/TRIMETHOPRIM

Antibacterial (Sulfonamide/Miscellaneous)

PREGNANCY RECOMMENDATION: Human Data Suggest Potential Risk—Animal Data Suggest Potential Risk

BREASTFEEDING RECOMMENDATION: Potential Toxicity

PREGNANCY SUMMARY

There are several reports describing the use of sulfamethoxazole/trimethoprim in human pregnancy. The congenital birth anomaly rate was about 5% in combined data from several large studies that consisted of more than 4,400 first-trimester exposures. Though this rate is a little higher than the expected US rate of 2% to 4%, no pattern to the anomalies was seen. In addition, many of the patients were on other medications for disease states that could affect this rate. Both drugs cross the placenta, so fetal exposure will occur. Embryofetal toxicity with malformations was observed in one animal species at doses of less than 10 times the RHD. Because both components can interfere with folic acid metabolism, the manufacturer recommends only using this combination drug if the potential benefit justifies the potential fetal risk. Sulfonamides also compete with bilirubin for binding to plasma albumin. In utero, the fetus clears free bilirubin by the placental circulation; however, after birth, this mechanism is no longer available. Unbound bilirubin is free to cross the blood-brain barrier and may result in kernicterus. Although this toxicity is well known when sulfonamides are administered directly to the neonate, kernicterus in a newborn following in utero exposure has not been reported.

BREASTFEEDING SUMMARY

The manufacturer reports that sulfamethoxazole and trimethoprim levels in human breast milk are about 2% to 5% of the recommended daily dose for infants over 2 months of age. According to the manufacturer, exposure to sulfamethoxazole/trimethoprim via breast milk should be avoided in premature infants and in infants with hyperbilirubinemia or glucose-6-phosphate dehydrogenase deficiency due to the sulfonamide component. Nevertheless, breastfeeding while using this drug should be based on the mother's clinical need for treatment versus any potential infant risks that might occur. If used, the infant should be monitored for the most common reported adult side effects of nausea (leading to irritability), vomiting, anorexia (monitor infant growth), and rash. Infant bilirubin levels should be monitored.

References

1. Prescribing Information. Bactrim DS, Bactrim. Sun Pharmaceutical Industries Inc; 2024.
2. American College of Obstetricians and Gynecologists. ACOG committee opinion No. 717: sulfonamides, nitrofurantoin, and risk of birth defects. *Obstet Gynecol*. 2017;130:e150-e152.
3. Barker RH. The placental transfer of sulfanilamide. *N Engl J Med*. 1938; 219:41.
4. Speert H. The passage of sulfanilamide through the human placenta. *Bull Johns Hopkins Hosp*. 1938;63:337-339.
5. Stewart HL Jr, Pratt JP. Sulfanilamide excretion in human breast milk and effect on breast-fed babies. *JAMA*. 1938;111:1456-1458.
6. Speert H. The placental transmission of sulfanilamide and its effects upon the fetus and newborn. *Bull Johns Hopkins Hosp*. 1940;66:139-155.
7. Speert H. Placental transmission of sulfathiazole and sulfadiazine and its significance for fetal chemotherapy. *Am J Obstet Gynecol*. 1943;45: 200-207.
8. Von Freisen B. A study of small dose sulphamerazine prophylaxis in obstetrics. *Acta Obstet Gynecol Scand*. 1951;31(suppl):75-116.
9. Sparr RA, Pritchard JA. Maternal and newborn distribution and excretion of sulfamethoxypyridazine (Kynex). *Obstet Gynecol*. 1958;12:131-134.
10. Nishimura H, Tanimura T. *Clinical Aspects of the Teratogenicity of Drugs*. Excerpta Medica; 1976:88.
11. Azad Khan AK, Truelove SC. Placental and mammary transfer of sulphasalazine. *Br Med J*. 1979;2:1553.
12. Heckel GP. Chemotherapy during pregnancy. Danger of fetal injury from sulfanilamide and its derivatives. *JAMA*. 1941;117:1314-1316.
13. Ginzler AM, Cherner C. Toxic manifestations in the newborn infant following placental transmission of sulfanilamide. With a report of 2 cases simulating erythroblastosis fetalis. *Am J Obstet Gynecol*. 1942;44:46-55.
14. Lucey JF, Driscoll TJ Jr. Hazard to newborn infants of administration of long-acting sulfonamides to pregnant women. *Pediatrics*. 1959;24:498-499.
15. Kantor HI, Sutherland DA, Leonard JT, et al. Effect on bilirubin metabolism in the newborn of sulfisoxazole administration to the mother. *Obstet Gynecol*. 1961;17:494-500.
16. Dunn PM. The possible relationship between the maternal administration of sulphamethoxypyridazine and hyperbilirubinaemia in the newborn. *J Obstet Gynaecol Br Commonw*. 1964;71:128-131.
17. Perkins RP. Hydrops fetalis and stillbirth in a male glucose-6-phosphate dehydrogenase-deficient fetus possibly due to maternal ingestion of sulfisoxazole. *Am J Obstet Gynecol*. 1971;111:379-381.
18. Baskin CG, Law S, Wenger NK. Sulfadiazine rheumatic fever prophylaxis during pregnancy: does it increase the risk of kernicterus in the newborn? *Cardiology*. 1980;65:222-225.
19. Ford N, Shubber Z, Jao J, et al. Safety of cotrimoxazole in pregnancy: a systematic review and meta-analysis. *J Acquir Immune Defic Syndr*. 2014; 66:512-521.
20. Williams JD, Condie AP, Brumfitt W, Reeves DS. The treatment of bacteriuria in pregnant women with sulphamethoxazole and trimethoprim. *Postgrad Med J*. 1969;45(suppl):71-76.
21. Ochoa AG. Trimethoprim and sulfamethoxazole in pregnancy. *JAMA*. 1971;217:1244.
22. Brumfitt W, Pursell R. Double-blind trial to compare ampicillin, cephalexin, cotrimoxazole, and trimethoprim in treatment of urinary infection. *Br Med J*. 1972;2:673-676.
23. Brumfitt W, Pursell R. Trimethoprim/sulfamethoxazole in the treatment of bacteriuria in women. *J Infect Dis*. 1973;128(suppl):S657-S663.
24. Brumfitt W, Pursell R. Trimethoprim/sulfamethoxazole in the treatment of urinary infection. *Med J Aust*. 1973;1(suppl):44-48.
25. Bailey RR. Single-dose antibacterial treatment for bacteriuria in pregnancy. *Drugs*. 1984;27:183-186.
26. Soper DE, Merrill-Nach S. Successful therapy of penicillinase-producing Neisseria gonorrhoeae pharyngeal infection during pregnancy. *Obstet Gynecol*. 1986;68:290-291.
27. Cruikshank DP, Warenski JC. First-trimester maternal *Listeria monocytogenes* sepsis and chorioamnionitis with normal neonatal outcome. *Obstet Gynecol*. 1989;73:469-471.
28. Seoud M, Saade G, Awar G, Uwaydah M. Brucellosis in pregnancy. *J Reprod Med*. 1991;36:441-445.
29. Frederiksen B. Maternal septicemia with *Listeria monocytogenes* in second trimester without infection of the fetus. *Acta Obstet Gynecol Scand*. 1992;71:313-315.
30. Ronen GM. Holoprosencephaly and maternal low-calorie weight-reducing diet. *Am J Med Genet*. 1992;42:139.
31. Richardson MP, Osrin D, Donaghy S, et al. Spinal malformations in the fetuses of HIV infected women receiving combination antiretroviral therapy and co-trimoxazole. *Eur J Obstet Gynecol Reprod Biol*. 2000;93:215-217.
32. Hernandez-Diaz S, Werler MM, Walker AM, Mitchell AA. Folic acid antagonists during pregnancy and the risk of birth defects. *N Engl J Med*. 2000;343:1608-1614.
33. Hernandez-Diaz S, Mitchell AA. Folic acid antagonists during pregnancy and risk of birth defects. *N Engl J Med*. 2001;344:934-935.
34. Hernandez-Diaz S, Werler MM, Walker AM, Mitchell AA. Neural tube defects in relation to use of folic acid antagonists during pregnancy. *Am J Epidemiol*. 2001;153:961-968.
35. Czeizel AE, Rockenbauer M, Sorensen HT, Olsen J. The teratogenic risk of trimethoprim-sulfonamides: a population based case-control study. *Reprod Toxicol*. 2001;15:637-646.
36. Crider KS, Cleves MA, Reefhuis J, et al. Antibacterial medication use during pregnancy and risk of birth defects. *Arch Pediatr Adolesc Med*. 2009;163:978-985.
37. Heinonen OP, Slone D, Shapiro S. *Birth Defects and Drugs in Pregnancy*. Publishing Sciences Group; 1977.
38. Bonze EJ, Fuerstner PG, Falls FH. Use of sulfanilamide derivative in treatment of gonorrhea in pregnant and nonpregnant women. *Am J Obstet Gynecol*. 1939;38:73-79.
39. Carter MP, Wilson F. Antibiotics and congenital malformations. *Lancet*. 1963;1:1267-1268.
40. Little PJ. The incidence of urinary infection in 5000 pregnant women. *Lancet*. 1966;2:925-928.
41. McEwan HP. Anorectal conditions in obstetric patients. *Proc R Soc Med*. 1972;65:279-281.
42. Williams JD, Smith EK. Single-dose therapy with streptomycin and sulfametopyrazine for bacteriuria during pregnancy. *Br Med J*. 1970;4: 651-653.
43. Mogadam M, Dobbins WO III, Korelitz BI, Ahmed SW. Pregnancy in inflammatory bowel disease: effect of sulfasalazine and corticosteroids on fetal outcome. *Gastroenterology*. 1981;80:72-76.
44. Richards IDG. A retrospective inquiry into possible teratogenic effects of drugs in pregnancy. *Adv Exp Med Biol*. 1972;27:441-455.
45. Nelson MM, Forfar JO. Association between drugs administered during pregnancy and congenital abnormalities of the fetus. *Br Med J*. 1971;1: 523-527.
46. Saxen I. Associations between oral clefts and drugs taken during pregnancy. *Int J Epidemiol*. 1975;4:37-44.
47. Ito S, Blajchman A, Stephenson M, et al. Prospective follow-up of adverse reactions in breast-fed infants exposed to maternal medication. *Am J Obstet Gynecol*. 1993;168:1393-1399.

SULFASALAZINE

Immunologic (5-ASA Derivative)

PREGNANCY RECOMMENDATION: Limited Human Data—Animal Data Suggest Low Risk

BREASTFEEDING RECOMMENDATION: Potential Toxicity

PREGNANCY SUMMARY

Several reports describing the use of sulfasalazine in human pregnancy have been located. However, limited data exist on first-trimester exposures. In the gastrointestinal tract, sulfasalazine is metabolized to sulfapyridine (SP) and 5-aminosalicylic acid (5-ASA). The drug and its metabolite cross the placenta, so fetal exposure will occur. Therefore, this limited first-trimester human pregnancy experience prevents a complete assessment of the embryofetal risk. Animal data did not show any embryofetal toxicity in two species at doses of less than 10 times the RHD. Sulfasalazine is a folic acid antagonist (dihydrofolate reductase inhibitor). The manufacturer reported that some case reports observed neural tube defects (NTDs) after in utero exposure to the drug; however, the role of sulfasalazine in causing NTDs has not been established. A meta-analysis and systematic review of seven studies that included 1,158 unexposed and 642 exposed to 5-ASA drugs, found no significant increase in birth defects, stillbirths, spontaneous abortion, preterm delivery, or low birth weight. However, specific data on sulfasalazine was not provided. It is difficult to fully evaluate some of these obstetrical complications because the gestational age of exposure was not provided, and many of these factors can be influenced by confounding variables. In another study, concentrations of sulfasalazine and SP in 11 infants were about 5 and 18 mcg/mL at birth, respectively. Neither of these concentrations was sufficient to cause significant displacement of bilirubin from albumin. Kernicterus and severe neonatal jaundice have not been reported following maternal use of sulfasalazine, even when the drug was given up to the time of delivery. Caution is advised, however, because other sulfonamides have caused jaundice in the newborn when given near term. Using this drug during pregnancy should be based on the pros and cons of the mother's clinical need for treatment versus any potential fetal risk that might occur from exposure. In 2017, the European Alliance of Associations for Rheumatology (EULAR) pregnancy guidelines considered sulfasalazine as compatible with use in pregnancy.

BREASTFEEDING SUMMARY

Sulfasalazine has been shown to be excreted into human breast milk, but levels were very low. However, the SP (active metabolite) levels, on average, were about 50% of the maternal levels. Breast milk levels of 5-ASA were undetectable. No adverse effects were observed in the 16 nursing infants exposed in these reports. However, one infant (delivered by a mother who was a slow acetylator) developed bloody diarrhea. The acetylation phenotype of the infant was not determined, but his blood was positive for SP. The manufacturer recommends exercising caution if sulfasalazine is administered to a lactating woman and to monitor the infant for diarrhea and/or bloody stools. Nevertheless, breastfeeding while using this drug should be based on the mother's clinical need for treatment versus any potential infant risks that might occur. If used, the infant should be monitored for the most common reported adult side effects of nausea, headache, and abdominal pain (all leading to irritability), anorexia (monitor infant growth), and vomiting.

S

References

1. Prescribing Information. Sulfasalazine. Actavis Pharma Inc; 2022.
2. Skorpen CG, Hoeltzebein M, Tincani A, et al. The EULAR points to consider for use of antirheumatic drugs before pregnancy, and during pregnancy and lactation. *Ann Rheum Dis*. 2016;75:795-810.
3. Mahadevan U, Robinson C, Bernasko N, et al. Inflammatory bowel disease in pregnancy clinical care pathway: a report from the American Gastroenterological Association IBD Parenthood Project Working Group. *Gastroenterology*. 2019;15:1509-1524.
4. Azad Khan AK, Truelove SC. Placental and mammary transfer of sulphasalazine. *Br Med J*. 1979;2:1553.
5. Jarnerot G, Into-Malmberg MB, Esbjorner E. Placental transfer of sulphasalazine and sulphapyridine and some of its metabolites. *Scand J Gastroenterol*. 1981;16:693-697.
6. Berlin CM Jr, Yaffe SJ. Disposition of salicylazosulfapyridine (Azulfidine) and metabolites in human breast milk. *Dev Pharmacol Ther*. 1980;1:31-39.
7. McEwan HP. Anorectal conditions in obstetric practice. *Proc R Soc Med*. 1972;65:279-281.
8. Willoughby CP, Truelove SC. Ulcerative colitis and pregnancy. *Gut*. 1980;21:469-474.
9. Levy N, Roisman I, Teodor I. Ulcerative colitis in pregnancy in Israel. *Dis Colon Rectum*. 1981;24:351-354.
10. Mogadam M, Dobbins WO III, Korelitz BI, Ahmed SW. Pregnancy in inflammatory bowel disease: effect of sulfasalazine and corticosteroids on fetal outcome. *Gastroenterology*. 1981;80:72-76.
11. Mogadam M. Sulfasalazine, IBD, and pregnancy (reply). *Gastroenterology*. 1981;81:194.
12. Fielding JF. Pregnancy and inflammatory bowel disease. *J Clin Gastroenterol*. 1983;5:107-108.
13. Sorokin JJ, Levine SM. Pregnancy and inflammatory bowel disease: a review of the literature. *Obstet Gynecol*. 1983;62:247-252.
14. Baiocco PJ, Korelitz BI. The influence of inflammatory bowel disease and its treatment on pregnancy and fetal outcome. *J Clin Gastroenterol*. 1984;6:211-216.
15. Fedorkow DM, Persaud D, Nimrod CA. Inflammatory bowel disease: a controlled study of late pregnancy outcome. *Am J Obstet Gynecol*. 1989;160:998-1001.
16. Craxi A, Pagliarello F. Possible embryotoxicity of sulfasalazine. *Arch Intern Med*. 1980;140:1674.
17. Newman NM, Correy JF. Possible teratogenicity of sulphasalazine. *Med J Aust*. 1983;1:528-529.
18. Hoo JJ, Hadro TA, Von Behren P. Possible teratogenicity of sulfasalazine. *N Engl J Med*. 1988;318:1128.
19. Hernandez-Diaz S, Werler MM, Walker AM, Mitchell AA. Folic acid antagonists during pregnancy and the risk of birth defects. *N Engl J Med*. 2000;343:1608-1614.
20. Rahimi R, Nikfar S, Rezaie A, Abdollahi M. Pregnancy outcome in women with inflammatory bowel disease following exposure to 5-aminosalicyclic acid drugs: a meta-analysis. *Reprod Toxicol*. 2008;25:271-275.
21. Howren A, Rebic N, Sayre EC, et al. Perinatal exposure to conventional synthetic disease-modifying anti-rheumatic drugs in women with rheumatic disease and neonatal outcomes: a population-based study. *Clin Exp Rheum*. 2020;38:1080-1087.
22. Perez-Garcia LF, Dolhain RJEM, Vorstenbosch S, et al. The effect of paternal exposure to immunosuppressive drugs on sexual function, reproductive hormone, fertility, pregnancy and offspring outcomes: a systematic review. *Hum Reprod Update*. 2020;26:961-1001.
23. Jarnerot G, Into-Malmberg MB. Sulphasalazine treatment during breast feeding. *Scand J Gastroenterol*. 1979;14:869-871.
24. Branski D, Kerem E, Gross-Kieselstein E, et al. Bloody diarrhea—a possible complication of sulfasalazine transferred through human breast milk. *J Pediatr Gastroenterol Nutr*. 1986;5:316-317.

SULFUR HEXAFLUORIDE

Diagnostic (Ultrasound)

PREGNANCY RECOMMENDATION: No Human Data—Animal Data Suggest Low Risk

BREASTFEEDING RECOMMENDATION: Probably Compatible

PREGNANCY SUMMARY

No reports describing the use of sulfur hexafluoride in human pregnancy have been located. Some of the drug is likely to cross the placenta, so fetal exposure will probably occur. However, the absence of human pregnancy experience prevents a complete assessment of embryofetal risk. Animal data did not show any embryofetal toxicity in two species at doses of more than 10 times the RHD. Using this drug during pregnancy should be based on the pros and cons of the mother's clinical need for treatment versus any potential fetal risk that might occur from exposure. There is a boxed warning for serious cardiopulmonary reactions, including fatalities, during or after the injection of ultrasound contrast agents, including sulfur hexafluoride lipid microspheres. Most of the serious reactions occur within 30 minutes of administration.

BREASTFEEDING SUMMARY

No reports describing the use of sulfur hexafluoride during human lactation have been located. The drug will likely be excreted into breast milk, so some infant exposure will probably occur. Breastfeeding while using this drug should be based on the mother's clinical need for treatment versus any potential infant risks that might occur. If used, the infant should be monitored for the most common reported adult side effects of headache and nausea (both leading to irritability).

Reference

1. Prescribing Information. Lumason. Bracco Diagnostics Inc; 2023.

SULINDAC

Pain (NSAID)

PREGNANCY RECOMMENDATION: Human Data Suggest Risk (Second and Third Trimesters)

BREASTFEEDING RECOMMENDATION: Potential Toxicity

PREGNANCY SUMMARY

There are several reports describing the use of sulindac in human pregnancy, and nearly all were exposures during the second half of pregnancy. A very recent systematic review and meta-analysis included 38 studies with 5,503,3030 patients and evaluated adverse pregnancy outcomes with nonsteroidal anti-inflammatory drug (NSAID) exposure as a group during pregnancy compared to unexposed controls. First-trimester NSAID exposure was associated with an increased risk of overall congenital anomalies and major malformations. However, the overall rate was not higher than the expected rate, and the control groups differed from the case patients in many instances. Both sulindac and the active metabolite, sulindac sulfide, cross the placenta. Embryofetal toxicity was observed in one animal species, but at unspecified dosages. The manufacturer recommends avoiding NSAIDs, including sulindac, at 30 weeks' gestation and beyond due to the risk for premature closure of the fetal ductus arteriosus. Additionally, the manufacturer recommends limiting use to the lowest effective dose and shortest duration possible if NSAIDs are needed between 20 and 30 weeks' gestation due to the risk for fetal renal dysfunction that can lead to oligohydramnios and neonatal renal impairment. There is a boxed warning for an increased risk of serious cardiovascular thrombotic events, including MI and stroke, as well as, an increased risk for gastrointestinal adverse events including bleeding, ulceration, and perforation, both of which can be fatal.

BREASTFEEDING SUMMARY

No reports describing the use of sulindac during human lactation have been located. The drug will likely be excreted into breast milk, so some infant exposure will probably occur. Due to a concern for potential serious adverse effects that might be seen in a breastfed infant, the manufacturer recommends that women not breastfeed while being treated with this drug. Nevertheless, breastfeeding while using this drug should be based on the mother's clinical need for treatment versus any potential infant risks that might occur. If used, the infant should be monitored for the most common reported adult side effects of nausea, dizziness, gastrointestinal pain, and dyspepsia (all leading to irritability), diarrhea, constipation, and rash. Given the longer elimination half-life, using a short-acting NSAID may be preferred.

References

1. Prescribing Information. Sulindac. Actavis Pharma Inc; 2023.
2. National Library of Medicine. Sulindac. Pubchem. Accessed September 27, 2024. https://pubchem.ncbi.nlm.nih.gov/compound/Sulindac
3. Kramer WB, Saade G, Ou CN, et al. Placental transfer of sulindac and its active sulfide metabolite in humans. *Am J Obstet Gynecol.* 1995;172:886-890.
4. Lampela ES, Nuutinen LH, Ala-Kkokko TL, et al. Placental transfer of sulindac, sulindac sulfide, and indomethacin in a human placental perfusion model. *Am J Obstet Gynecol.* 1999;180:174-180.
5. Food and Drug Administration. Nonsteroidal anti-inflammatory drugs (NSAIDs): drug safety communication—avoid use of NSAIDs in pregnancy at 20 weeks or later. Accessed October 8, 2024. https://www.fda.gov/safety/medical-product-safety-information/nonsteroidal-anti-inflammatory-drugs-nsaids-drug-safety-communication-avoid-use-nsaids-pregnancy-20
6. Carlan SJ, O'Brien WF, O'Leary TD, Mastrogiannis D. Randomized comparative trial of indomethacin and sulindac for the treatment of refractory preterm labor. *Obstet Gynecol.* 1992;79:223-228.
7. Kramer WB, Saade GR, Belfort M, et al. A randomized double-blind study comparing the fetal effects of sulindac to terbutaline during the management of preterm labor. *Am J Obstet Gynecol.* 1999;180:396-401.
8. Carlan S, Jones M, Schorr S, et al. Oral sulindac to prevent recurrence of preterm labor (abstract). *Am J Obstet Gynecol.* 1994;170:381.
9. Jones M, Carlan S, Schorr S, et al. Oral sulindac to prevent recurrence of preterm labor (abstract). *Am J Obstet Gynecol.* 1995;172:416.
10. Carlan SJ, O'Brien WF, Jones MH, et al. Outpatient oral sulindac to prevent recurrence of preterm labor. *Obstet Gynecol.* 1995;85:769-774.
11. Peek MJ, McCarthy A, Kyle P, et al. Medical amnioreduction with sulindac to reduce cord complications in monoamniotic twins. *Am J Obstet Gynecol.* 1997;176:334-336.
12. Sciscione A, Leef K, Vakili B, Paul D. Neonatal effects after antenatal treatment with indomethacin vs. sulindac (abstract). *Am J Obstet Gynecol.* 2000;182:S66.
13. Kamath-Rayne, BD, Habli M, Rodriguez Z, et al. Antenatal exposure to sulindac and risk of necrotizing enterocolitis. *Am J Obstet Gynecol.* 2015;212:e1-e7.
14. Chen X, Yang Y, Chen L, et al. Pregnancy outcomes and birth defects in offspring following non-steroidal anti-inflammatory drugs exposure during pregnancy: a systematic review and meta-analysis. *Reprod Tox.* 2024;125:108561.
15. Ying XH, Bao DN, Jiang HY, Shi YD. Maternal non-steroidal anti-inflammatory drug exposure during pregnancy and risk of miscarriage: a systematic review and meta-analysis. *Eur J Clin Pharmacol.* 2022;78:171-180.

SUMATRIPTAN

Central Nervous System (Serotonin 5HT-1B/1D Receptor Agonist—Triptan)

PREGNANCY RECOMMENDATION: Limited Human Data—Animal Data Suggest Risk

BREASTFEEDING RECOMMENDATION: Potential Toxicity

PREGNANCY SUMMARY

There are several reports describing the use of sumatriptan during human pregnancy. The rate of birth anomalies in about 500 first-trimester exposures was about 4%. Triptans were not associated with an increased risk for preterm delivery or preeclampsia. However, it is difficult to fully evaluate these findings because all of these factors can be influenced by numerous confounding variables. The drug is likely to cross the placenta, so some fetal exposure will probably occur. Embryofetal toxicity was observed in two animal species at doses of less than 10 times the RHD. Using this drug during pregnancy should be based on the pros and cons of the mother's clinical need for treatment versus any potential fetal risk that might occur from exposure. Hypertension was reported in patients treated with this drug in the clinical trials. The ACOG clinical practice guideline suggests cautious use of sumatriptan for secondary treatment of persistent headache in pregnancy. It is noted that no studies have evaluated the effects of triptans in pregnancy on uterine or fetal blood flow during the second or third trimester. The publication also advises not to use triptans in pregnant patients with cardiac disease or hypertension due to the rare risk of generalized or cardiac vasoconstriction.

S

BREASTFEEDING SUMMARY

There are two publications describing the use of sumatriptan during human lactation. The drug was found to be excreted into breast milk, so infant exposure will occur. The mean RID based on average concentration throughout the 24-hour sample period was 0.7%, whereas the RID based on the maximum breast milk concentration was 1.8% (1%-3.8%). Many infants are described as having no adverse effects when exposed to sumatriptan through breast milk. However, there are some reports of breast and/or nipple pain, breast milk supply reduction, and breast milk ejection reflex pain. In adults, the mean oral bioavailability of sumatriptan is 15%, suggesting that absorption from the gastrointestinal tract is limited. Thus, oral absorption in infants through breast milk may be small. Breastfeeding while using this drug should be based on the mother's clinical need for treatment versus any potential infant risks that might occur. If used, the infant should be monitored for the most common reported adult side effects of paresthesia, various pains, and vertigo (all leading to irritability) and fatigue (lethargy). If there are any concerns, holding breastfeeding for 12 hours (five elimination half-lives) after administration can help minimize infant exposure. The ACOG clinical practice guideline states that triptans could be used by lactating patients, but recommends a shared decision-making approach regarding the need to avoid breastfeeding for a specific timeframe after use.

References

1. Prescribing Information. Sumatriptan succinate. Dr. Reddy's Laboratories Limited; 2020.
2. Prescribing Information. Sumatriptan. Hikma Pharmaceuticals USA Inc; 2021.
3. Prescribing Information. Sumatriptan. Cipla USA Inc; 2021.
4. Prescribing Information. Onzetra Xsail. Currax Pharmaceuticals LLC; 2024.

5. Phillips K, Clerkin-Oliver C, Nirantharakumar K, et al. How migraine and its associated treatment impact on pregnancy outcomes: umbrella review with updated systematic review and meta-analysis. *Cephalalgia*. 2024;44:3331024241229410.
6. American College of Obstetricians and Gynecologists. Headaches in pregnancy and postpartum. Clinical practice guidelines No. 3. *Obstet Gynecol*. 2021;139:944-972.
7. Ephross SA, Sinclair SM. Final results from the 16-year sumatriptan, naratriptan, and treximet pregnancy registry. *Headache*. 2014;54:1158-1172.
8. Shuhaiber S, Pastuszak A, Schick B, et al. Pregnancy outcome following first trimester exposure to sumatriptan. *Neurology*. 1998;51:581-583.
9. Wilton LV, Pearce GL, Martin RM, Mackay FJ, Mann RD. The outcomes of pregnancy in women exposed to newly marketed drugs in general practice in England. *Br J Obstet Gynaecol*. 1998;105:882-889.
10. Evans EW, Lorber KC. Use of 5-HT1 agonists in pregnancy. *Ann Pharmacother*. 2008;42:543-549.
11. Nezvalova-Henriksen K, Spigset O, Nordeng H. Triptan exposure during pregnancy and the risk of major congenital malformations and adverse pregnancy outcomes: results from the Norwegian Mother and Child Cohort Study. *Headache*. 2010;50:563-575.
12. Marchenko A, Etwel F, Olutunfese O, Nickel C, Koren G, Nulman I. Pregnancy outcome following prenatal exposure to triptan medications: a meta-analysis. *Headache*. 2015;55:490-501.
13. Spielmann K, Kayser A, Beck E, et al. Pregnancy outcome after anti-migraine triptan use: a prospective observational cohort study. *Cephalalgia*. 2018;38:1081-1092.
14. Berard A, Strom S, Zhao JP, et al. Dihydroergotamine and triptan use to treat migraine during pregnancy and risk of adverse pregnancy outcomes. *Sci Rep*. 2021;11:19302.
15. Dudman DC, Tauqeer F, Kaur M, et al. A systematic review and meta-analysis on the prevalence of pregnancy outcomes in migraine treated patients: a contribution from the IMI2 ConcePTION project. *J Neurol*. 2022;269:742-749.
16. Harris GME, Wood M, Ystrom E, Nordeng H. Prenatal triptan exposure and neurodevelopmental outcomes in 5-year-old children: follow-up from the Norwegian Mother and Child Cohort Study. *Paediatr Perinat Epidemiol*. 2018;32:247-255.
17. Harris GM, Wood M, Ystrom E, Nordeng H. Association of maternal use of triptans during pregnancy with risk of attention-deficit/hyperactivity disorder in offspring. *JAMA Netw Open*. 2022;5:e2215333.
18. Wojnar-Horton RE, Hackett LP, Yapp P, Dusci LJ, Paech M, Ilett KF. Distribution and excretion of sumatriptan in human milk. *Br J Clin Pharmacol*. 1996;41:217-221.
19. Fullerton T, Gengo FM. Sumatriptan: a selective 5-hydroxytryptamine receptor agonist for the acute treatment of migraine. *Ann Pharmacother*. 1992;26:800-808.
20. Amundsen S, Nordeng H, Ole-Martin F, et al. Transfer of triptans into human breast milk and estimation of infant drug exposure through breastfeeding. *Basic Clin Pharmacol Toxicol*. 2021;128:795-804.
21. Conijn M, Maas V, van Tuyl M, et al Breastfeeding-related adverse drug reactions of triptans: a descriptive analysis using four pharmacovigilance database. *Breastfeed Med*. 2024;19:645-651.

SUNITINIB

Antineoplastic (Tyrosine Kinase Inhibitor)

PREGNANCY RECOMMENDATION: **No Human Data—Animal Data Suggest Risk**

BREASTFEEDING RECOMMENDATION: **Potential Toxicity**

PREGNANCY SUMMARY

No reports describing the use of sunitinib during human pregnancy have been located. Sunitinib and its active metabolite are likely to cross the placenta, so some fetal exposure will probably occur. However, the absence of human pregnancy experience prevents a complete assessment of embryofetal risk. Embryofetal toxicity with malformations was observed in two animal species at doses of less than 10 times the combined systemic exposure of sunitinib and its metabolite at the RHD. Based on these animal studies and the drug's mechanism of action, the manufacturer recommends that women with reproductive potential use effective contraception during treatment and for 4 weeks after the last dose. They also recommend that males with female partners of reproductive potential use effective contraception during treatment and for 7 weeks after the last dose. Nevertheless, using this drug during pregnancy should be based on the pros and cons of the mother's clinical need for treatment versus any potential fetal risk that might occur from exposure. There is a registry for women who are pregnant and have cancer. For more information, women and health care providers are encouraged to contact the Cancer and Pregnancy Registry at 1-877-635-4499. Hypertension was reported in up to 29% of patients treated with this drug in the clinical trials. Sunitinib can also prolong the QTc interval.

S

BREASTFEEDING SUMMARY

No reports describing the use of sunitinib during human lactation have been located. The drug and its metabolite will likely be excreted into breast milk, so some infant exposure will probably occur. Due to a concern for potential serious adverse effects that might be seen in a breastfed infant, the manufacturer recommends that women not breastfeed while being treated with this drug and for at least 4 weeks after the last dose. Nevertheless, breastfeeding while using this drug should be based on the mother's clinical need for treatment versus any potential infant risks that might occur. If used, the infant should be monitored for the most common reported adult side effects of nausea, dyspepsia, and abdominal pain (all leading to irritability), diarrhea, lethargy, vomiting, decreased appetite (monitor infant growth), hypertension, and thrombocytopenia.

Reference

1. Prescribing Information. Sunitinib Malate. Aurobindo Pharma Limited; 2023.

SUTIMLIMAB

Hematologic (Complement Inhibitor Monoclonal Antibody)

PREGNANCY RECOMMENDATION: No Human Data—Animal Data Suggest Low Risk

BREASTFEEDING RECOMMENDATION: Probably Compatible

PREGNANCY SUMMARY

No reports describing the use of sutimlimab in human pregnancy have been located. As an IgG antibody, the drug will likely cross the placenta in the second half of gestation, so some fetal exposure will probably occur. However, the absence of human pregnancy experience prevents a complete assessment of embryofetal risk. Animal data did not show embryofetal toxic effects. Using this drug during pregnancy should be based on the pros and cons of the mother's clinical need for treatment versus any potential fetal risk that might occur from exposure. Hypertension was reported in up to 23% of patients treated with this drug in the clinical trials.

BREASTFEEDING SUMMARY

No reports describing the use of sutimlimab during human lactation have been located. It is known that IgG antibodies can be found in human breast milk, but are not found in the neonatal or infant circulation. Additionally, if any IgG antibodies were to be ingested through breastfeeding, they would probably be digested in the infant's gastrointestinal tract and not be absorbed. Breastfeeding while using this drug should be based on the mother's clinical need for treatment. If used, the infant should be monitored for the most common reported adult side effects of headache, arthralgia, and nausea (all leading to irritability), rhinitis, hypertension, acrocyanosis, Raynaud phenomenon, urinary tract infection, respiratory tract infection, lethargy, cough, and peripheral edema.

Reference

1. Prescribing Information. Enjaymo. Bioverativ; 2023.

SUVOREXANT

Central Nervous System (Hypnotic—Orexin Antagonist)

PREGNANCY RECOMMENDATION: No Human Data—Animal Data Suggest Low Risk

BREASTFEEDING RECOMMENDATION: Probably Compatible

PREGNANCY SUMMARY

No reports describing the use of suvorexant in human pregnancy have been located. The drug is likely to cross the placenta, so some fetal exposure will probably occur. However, the absence of human pregnancy experience prevents a complete assessment of embryofetal risk. Animal data did not show any embryofetal toxicity in two species at doses of about 10 times or more than the RHD. Using this drug during pregnancy should be based on the pros and cons of the mother's clinical need for treatment versus any potential fetal risk that might occur from exposure.

BREASTFEEDING SUMMARY

No reports describing the use of suvorexant during human lactation have been located. The drug will probably be found in human breast milk, so some infant exposure will likely occur. Breastfeeding while using this drug should be based on the mother's clinical need for treatment. If used, the infant should be monitored for the most common reported adult side effect of somnolence.

Reference

1. Prescribing Information. Belsomra. Merck Sharp & Dohme LLC; 2023.

T

TACROLIMUS

Immunologic (Calcineurin Inhibitor)

PREGNANCY RECOMMENDATION: Human Data Suggest Low Risk—Animal Data Suggest Risk (Maternal Benefit May Outweigh Embryofetal Risk in Some Cases)

BREASTFEEDING RECOMMENDATION: Probably Compatible

PREGNANCY SUMMARY

There are numerous reports describing the use of tacrolimus during human pregnancy. Many are case reports and series with a few larger analyses from the transplant pregnancy registry that may include some of the case reports and series data. When combined, the rate of major birth anomalies was about 5.5% in more than 700 first-trimester exposures. However, most of these involved the use of the drug in renal and liver transplant patients, so more of these had underlying diabetes that may not be well controlled, autoimmune disorders, and other major medical disorders. No pattern to the defects has been identified. Some studies suggest higher rates for cardiac, craniofacial, and skeletal defects, but these were not consistently seen. The drug crosses the placenta, so fetal exposure will occur. Animal data showed embryofetal toxicity in two species at doses of less than 10 times the recommended human dose (RHD). The manufacturer reports that renal dysfunction, transient neonatal hyperkalemia, and low birth weight have been reported at the time of delivery for exposed infants. Also, as expected because of the disease state, several studies have shown an increased rate of intrauterine growth restriction (IUGR), preeclampsia, and preterm delivery. Because of the potential for adverse effects when tacrolimus is used during pregnancy, the manufacturer recommends that female and male patients of reproductive potential speak to their health care providers about family planning options, including appropriate contraception prior to starting treatment with tacrolimus. Also, because of the risk of cytomegalovirus (CMV) infection with organ transplantation, some reviews have advised waiting at least 6 months before conception is attempted (following transplantation), whereas others have recommended waiting a year. Nevertheless, using this drug during pregnancy should be based on the pros and cons of the mother's clinical need for treatment versus any potential fetal risk that might occur from exposure. Tacrolimus can prolong the QT interval and may increase the risk for torsades de pointes. Patients exposed to tacrolimus during pregnancy are encouraged to enroll in the Transplantation Pregnancy Registry International by calling 877-955-6877.

BREASTFEEDING SUMMARY

Tacrolimus has been shown to be excreted into human breast milk in several studies. From a total of about 40 lactating women, the drug and metabolites were found in breast milk in low concentrations with a range from less than 1 to about 3.5 ng/mL. Every calculated relative infant dose (RID) was less than 1%. In addition, the oral bioavailability of tacrolimus in healthy adults is only about 20%, so this should result in even lower systemic infant exposures. Breastfeeding while using this drug should be based on the mother's clinical need for treatment versus any potential infant risks that might occur. If used, the infant should be monitored for the most common reported adult side effects of headache, abdominal pain, nausea, and paresthesia (all leading to irritability), fever, CMV infection, tremor, hyperglycemia, leukopenia, infections, anemia, diarrhea, insomnia, peripheral edema, hyperkalemia, hypomagnesemia, and hyperlipidemia.

References

1. Prescribing Information. *Tacrolimus capsule*. Accord Healthcare, Inc; 2024.
2. Prescribing Information. *Tacrolimus ointment*. Accord Healthcare, Inc; 2024.
3. Laifer SA, Guido RS. Reproductive function and outcome of pregnancy after liver transplantation in women. *Mayo Clin Proc*. 1995;70:388-394.
4. Casele HL, Laifer SA. Pregnancy after liver transplantation. *Semin Perinatol*. 1998;22:149-155.
5. Christopher V, Al-Chalabi T, Richardson PD, et al. Pregnancy outcome after liver transplantation: a single-center experience of 71 pregnancies in 45 recipients. *Liver Transpl*. 2006;12:1138-1143.
6. Peters DH, Fitton A, Plosker GL, Faulds D. Tacrolimus. A review of its pharmacology, and therapeutic potential in hepatic and renal transplantation. *Drugs*. 1993;46:746-794.
7. Farley DE, Shelby J, Alexander D, Scott JR. The effect of two new immunosuppressive agents, FK506 and didemnin B, in murine pregnancy. *Transplantation*. 1991;52:106-110.
8. Jain A, Venkataramanan R, Fung JJ, et al. Pregnancy after liver transplantation under tacrolimus. *Transplantation*. 1997;64:559-565.
9. Winkler ME, Niesert S, Ringe B, Pichlmayr R. Successful pregnancy in a patient after liver transplantation maintained on FK 506. *Transplantation*. 1993;56:751-753.
10. Midtvedt K, Hartmann A, Brekke IB, et al. Successful pregnancies in a combined pancreas and renal allograft recipient and in a renal graft recipient on tacrolimus treatment. *Nephrol Dial Transplant*. 1997;12:2764-2765.
11. Hiramatsu Y, Yoshida S, Kotani T, et al. Changes in the blood level, efficacy, and safety of tacrolimus in pregnancy and the lactation period in patients with systemic lupus erythematosus. *Lupus*. 2018;27:2245-2252.
12. Jain A, Venkataramanan R, Lever J, et al. FK506 and pregnancy in liver transplant patients. *Transplantation*. 1993;56:751.

13. Casele H, Woelkers D, Laifer S. Pregnancy outcome after liver transplantation (abstract). *Am J Obstet Gynecol*. 1997;176:S23.
14. Laifer SA, Yeagley CJ, Armitage JM. Pregnancy after cardiac transplantation. *Am J Perinatol*. 1994;11:217-219.
15. Yoshimura N, Oka T, Fujiwara Y, et al. A case report of pregnancy in a renal transplant recipient treated with FK506 (tacrolimus). *Transplantation*. 1996;61:1552-1553.
16. Resch B, Mache CJ, Windhager T, et al. FK 506 and successful pregnancy in a patient after renal transplantation. *Transplant Proc*. 1998;30: 163-164.
17. Casele HL, Laifer SA. Association of pregnancy complications and choice of immunosuppressant in liver transplant patients. *Transplantation*. 1998;65: 581-583.
18. Armenti VT, McGrory CH, Carter JR, et al. Pregnancy outcomes in female renal transplant recipients. *Transplant Proc*. 1998;30:1732-1734.
19. Armenti VT, Gertner GS, Eisenberg JA, et al. National Transplantation Pregnancy Registry: outcomes of pregnancies in lung recipients. *Transplant Proc*. 1998;30:1528-1530.
20. Armenti VT, Radomski JS, Moritz MJ, et al. Report from the National Transplantation Pregnancy Registry (NTPR): outcomes of pregnancy after transplantation. *Clin Transpl*. 2005:69-83.
21. Pisoni CN, D'Cruz DP. The safety of mycophenolate mofetil in pregnancy. *Expert Opin Drug Saf*. 2008;7:219-222.
22. Vyas S, Kumar A, Piecuch S, et al. Outcome of twin pregnancy in a renal transplant recipient treated with tacrolimus. *Transplantation*. 1999;67: 490-492.
23. Kainz A, Harabacz I, Cowlrick IS, et al. Review of the course and outcome of 100 pregnancies in 84 women treated with tacrolimus. *Transplantation*. 2000;70:1718-1721.
24. Nagy S, Bush MC, Berkowitz R, et al. Pregnancy outcome in liver transplant recipients. *Obstet Gynecol*. 2003;102:121-128.
25. Jain AB, Reyes J, Marcos A, et al. Pregnancy after liver transplantation with tacrolimus immunosuppression: a single center's experience update at 13 years. *Transplantation*. 2003;76:827-832.
26. Bar J, Stahl B, Hod M, et al. Is immunosuppression therapy in renal allograft recipients teratogenic? A single-center experience. *Am J Med Genet*. 2003; 116A:31-36.
27. Jain AB, Shapiro R, Scantlebury VP, et al. Pregnancy after kidney and kidney-pancreas transplantation under tacrolimus: a single center's experience. *Transplantation*. 2004;77:897-902.
28. Garcia-Donaire JA, Acevedo M, Gutierrez MJ, et al. Tacrolimus as basic immunosuppression in pregnancy after renal transplantation. A single-center experience. *Transplant Proc*. 2005;37:3754-3755.
29. Jabiry-Zieniewicz Z, Kaminski P, Pietrzak B, et al. Outcome of four high-risk pregnancies in female liver transplant recipients on tacrolimus immunosuppression. *Transplant Proc*. 2006;38:255-257.
30. Baumgart DC, Sturm A, Wiedenmann B, Dignass AU. Uneventful pregnancy and neonatal outcome with tacrolimus in refractory ulcerative colitis. *Gut*. 2005;54:1822-1823.
31. Ducarme G, Theron-Gerard L, Duvoux C, et al. Pregnancy after liver transplantation with tacrolimus. *Eur J Obstet Gynecol Reprod Biol*. 2007;133:249-250.
32. Olivelra LG, Sass N, Sato JL, et al. Pregnancy after renal transplantation-a five-yr single-center experience. *Clin Transplant*. 2007;21:301-304.
33. Midtvedt K, Bjorang O, Letting AS. Successful pregnancy in renal transplant recipient with previous known polyomavirus nephropathy. *Clin Transplant*. 2007;21:571-573.
34. Gomez-Lobo V, Landy HJ, Matsumoto C, Fishbein TM. Pregnancy in an intestinal transplant recipient. *Obstet Gynecol*. 2012;120:497-500.
35. Drozdowska-Szymczak A, Pietrzak B, Czaplinska N, et al. Immunological status of children born to female liver recipients. *Ann Transplant*. 2018;23: 182-189.
36. French AE, Soldin SJ, Soldin OP, Koren G. Milk transfer and neonatal safety of tacrolimus. *Ann Pharmacother*. 2003;37:815-818.
37. Gardiner SJ, Begg EJ. Breastfeeding during tacrolimus therapy. *Obstet Gynecol*. 2006;107:453-455.
38. Kociszewska-Najman B, Mazanowska N, Pietrzak B, et al. Low transfer of tacrolimus and its metabolites into colostrum of graft recipient mothers. *Nutrients*. 2018;10:E267.

TACROLIMUS TOPICAL

Immunologic (Calcineurin Inhibitor)

PREGNANCY RECOMMENDATION: Limited Human Data—No Relevant Animal Data

BREASTFEEDING RECOMMENDATION: Probably Compatible

PREGNANCY SUMMARY

Only one study was located that described the use of topical tacrolimus during human pregnancy. The drug was used to treat lichen planus after surgery to correct a labial adhesion, and it was administered in the early third trimester. The newborn was delivered at term with no adverse effects identified. Numerous case reports and series with a few larger analyses from the transplant pregnancy registry (that may include some of the case reports and series data) were located with oral and intravenous (IV) tacrolimus use. When data were combined, the rate of major birth anomalies was about 5.5% in more than 700 first-trimester exposures. However, most of these involved the use of the drug in renal and liver transplant patients, so more of these had underlying diabetes that may not be well controlled, autoimmune disorders, and other major medical disorders. No pattern to the defects has been identified. Some studies suggested higher rates for cardiac, craniofacial, and skeletal defects, but these were not consistently seen. Tacrolimus has been shown to cross the placenta with oral and IV use. It will probably cross the placenta with topical use, but the overall amount of drug that is systemically absorbed with topical use would suggest that it would be clinically insignificant. Therefore, this limited human pregnancy experience prevents a complete assessment of the embryofetal risk. Animal reproduction and fertility studies have not been conducted on topical tacrolimus. With systemic use, tacrolimus was found to cause some embryofetal toxicity in animals in two species at doses of less than 10 times the RHD. Using this drug during pregnancy should be based on the pros and cons of the mother's clinical need for treatment versus any potential fetal risk that might occur from exposure.

BREASTFEEDING SUMMARY

Tacrolimus has been shown to be excreted into human breast milk with the oral and IV routes of administration. Therefore, it will probably be excreted into breast milk with topical use. However, because the bioavailability is very low with most plasma levels of 2 ng/mL or less, the amount is probably clinically insignificant. Regardless, due to a concern for potential serious adverse effects that might be seen in a breastfed infant, the manufacturer recommends that women not breastfeed while being treated with this drug. Nevertheless, breastfeeding while using this drug should be based on the mother's clinical need for treatment versus any potential infant risks that might occur. Because of the topical use of the drug, systemic side effects were not fully assessed.

References

1. Prescribing Information. *Tacrolimus ointment*. Accord Healthcare, Inc; 2024.
2. Christopher V, Al-Chalabi T, Richardson PD, et al. Pregnancy outcome after liver transplantation: a single-center experience of 71 pregnancies in 45 recipients. *Liver Transpl*. 2006;12:1138-1143.
3. Peters DH, Fitton A, Plosker GL, Faulds D. Tacrolimus. A review of its pharmacology, and therapeutic potential in hepatic and renal transplantation. *Drugs*. 1993;46:746-794.
4. Taniguchi T, Sasaki M, Segawa K, Otsuki T. Labial adhesion surgery prior to vaginal delivery in a patient with vulvar lichen planus causing labial adhesion: a case report. *Cureus*. 2024;16:e74949.

TAFAMIDIS

Cardiovascular (Transthyretin Stabilizer)

PREGNANCY RECOMMENDATION: No Human Data—Animal Data Suggest Potential Risk

BREASTFEEDING RECOMMENDATION: Potential Toxicity

PREGNANCY SUMMARY

No reports describing the use of tafamidis in human pregnancy have been located. Tafamidis is likely to cross the placenta, so some fetal exposure will probably occur. Embryofetal toxicity was observed in one animal species at doses of less than 10 times the maximum recommended human dose (MRHD). However, the absence of human pregnancy experience prevents a complete assessment of embryofetal risk. Based on animal studies, the manufacturer recommends that women with reproductive potential use effective contraception during treatment. Nevertheless, using this drug during pregnancy should be based on the pros and cons of the mother's clinical need for treatment versus any potential fetal risk that might occur from exposure. Women exposed to tafamidis during pregnancy are encouraged to report exposures to Pfizer by calling 800-438-1985.

BREASTFEEDING SUMMARY

No reports describing the use of tafamidis during human lactation have been located. The drug will likely be excreted into breast milk, so some infant exposure will probably occur. Due to a concern for potential serious adverse effects that might be seen in a breastfed infant, the manufacturer recommends that women not breastfeed while being treated with this drug. Nevertheless, breastfeeding while using this drug should be based on the mother's clinical need for treatment versus any potential infant risks that might occur. The manufacturer reports that adverse events were similar to placebo in the clinical trials.

Reference

1. Prescribing Information. *Vyndaqel, vyndamax*. Pfizer Laboratories Div Pfizer, Inc; 2023.

TAFASITAMAB

Antineoplastic (Monoclonal Antibody)

PREGNANCY RECOMMENDATION: *Contraindicated

BREASTFEEDING RECOMMENDATION: *Contraindicated

PREGNANCY SUMMARY

No reports describing the use of tafasitamab in human pregnancy have been located. Because it is an antibody of the immunoglobulin G (IgG) class, it probably crosses the placenta. Animal studies have not been performed. However, the absence of human pregnancy experience prevents a complete assessment of the embryofetal risk. Tafasitamab is approved for IV infusion in combination with lenalidomide. Clinical studies found that the combination of tafasitamab and lenalidomide resulted in a greater antibody-dependent cellular cytotoxicity when compared to tafasitamab or lenalidomide alone. Lenalidomide is an analogue of thalidomide, which is a well-known potent human teratogen (see Lenalidomide). *Because the drug may cause B cell depletion in pregnant women (and the fetus) and because the drug is used in combination with lenalidomide, the manufacturer recommends that women of reproductive potential use effective contraception when treated with tafasitamab and for at least 3 months after the last dose.

BREASTFEEDING SUMMARY

Tafasitamab probably enters breast milk. However, it is known that IgG antibodies can be found in human breast milk, but are not found in neonatal or infant circulation. Additionally, if any IgG antibodies were to be ingested through breastfeeding, they would probably be digested in the infant's gastrointestinal tract and not be absorbed. *However, because the drug is used in combination with lenalidomide (see Lenalidomide) and the theoretical concern for adverse reactions in a breastfed infant exposed to tafasitamab, the manufacturer recommends that women not breastfeed while using this drug and for at least 3 months after the last dose. The drug by itself may have potential toxicity, but would not be contraindicated.

Reference

1. Prescribing Information. *Monjuvi*. Morphosys US, Inc and Incyte Corporation; 2020.

TAFENOQUINE

Anti-Infective (Antimalarial)

PREGNANCY RECOMMENDATION: No Human Data—Animal Data Suggests Potential Risk

BREASTFEEDING RECOMMENDATION: Potential Toxicity

PREGNANCY SUMMARY

No reports describing the use of tafenoquine in human pregnancy have been located. Tafenoquine is likely to cross the placenta, so some fetal exposure will probably occur. However, the absence of human pregnancy experience prevents a complete assessment of embryofetal risk. Embryofetal toxicity was observed in one animal species at doses of less than 10 times the RHD. Glucose-6-phosphate dehydrogenase (G6PD) deficiency testing is required prior to drug initiation. Infants with a G6PD deficiency who are exposed to tafenoquine can develop hemolytic anemia. Therefore, the manufacturer recommends that women with reproductive potential use effective contraception during treatment and for at least 3 months after the last dose. Nevertheless, adverse pregnancy events such as maternal anemia, prematurity, spontaneous abortion, and intrauterine fetal demise have been associated with malaria during pregnancy. Using this drug during pregnancy should be based on the pros and cons of the mother's clinical need for treatment versus any potential fetal risk that might occur from exposure.

BREASTFEEDING SUMMARY

No reports describing the use of tafenoquine during human lactation have been located. The drug will likely be excreted into breast milk, so some infant exposure will probably occur. Testing for G6PD should occur prior to use. If the infant has G6PD deficiency, the drug should not be used if at all possible. In women and infants with normal G6PD testing, breastfeeding while using this drug should be based on the mother's clinical need for treatment versus any potential infant risks that might occur. If used, the infant should be monitored for the most common reported adult side effects of dizziness, nausea, headache (all leading to irritability), and decreased hemoglobin.

Reference

1. Prescribing Information. *Krintafel*. GlaxoSmithKline LLC; 2023.

TAFLUPROST OPHTHALMIC

Ophthalmic (Prostaglandin Agonist)

PREGNANCY RECOMMENDATION: Limited Human Data—Animal Data Suggest Potential Risk

BREASTFEEDING RECOMMENDATION: Probably Compatible

PREGNANCY SUMMARY

One report describing the use of tafluprost in human pregnancy was located. A pharmacovigilance publication included three pregnancy exposures to tafluprost, and one pregnancy loss was reported (unknown if tafluprost had any role). Very small amounts of the drug are absorbed into the systemic circulation. At a median of 10 minutes postinstillation in each eye of healthy adults, mean plasma concentrations were about 27 pg/mL. At 30 minutes postinstillation, mean plasma concentrations were below the limit of quantification (10 pg/mL). Prostaglandin $F_{2\alpha}$ has been used for pregnancy termination in humans via intrauterine extra-amniotic infusion to treat missed abortion or intrauterine death. However, there is no evidence that the doses given to reduce elevated ophthalmic pressure would lead to any increased risk for significant uterine contractions. Therefore, this limited human pregnancy experience prevents a complete assessment of the embryofetal risk. Embryofetal toxicity was observed in one animal species at doses of less than 10 times the maximum clinical exposure based on body surface area (BSA) comparison. Nevertheless, because the drug will be administered daily for long durations, it may be best to use other antiglaucoma agents that have more human data. Using this drug during pregnancy should be based on the pros and cons of the mother's clinical need for treatment versus any potential fetal risk that might occur from exposure. If used, consider placing pressure over the tear duct in the corner of the eye for at least 1 minute, and then remove any excess solution with absorbent tissue to decrease the amount of drug reaching the systemic circulation even further.

BREASTFEEDING SUMMARY

No reports describing the use of tafluprost ophthalmic during human lactation have been located. With the very small plasma concentrations (27 pg/mL) at 10 minutes after use and below the limit of quantification (10 pg/mL) at 30 minutes postinstillation, it is unlikely that these brief concentrations would have any effect on a nursing infant. A method to decrease some systemic absorption with ophthalmic use is described above in the Pregnancy Summary.

References

1. Prescribing Information. *Tafluprost ophthalmic*. Prasco Laboratories; 2022.
2. Sakai T, Mori C, Koshiba H, et al. Pregnancy loss signal from prostaglandin eye drop use in pregnancy: a disproportionality analysis using Japanese and US Spontaneous reporting databases. *Drugs Real World Outcomes*. 2022;9:43-51.

TAGRAXOFUSP

Antineoplastic (CD123-Directed Cytotoxin)

PREGNANCY RECOMMENDATION: No Human Data and No Relevant Animal Data

BREASTFEEDING RECOMMENDATION: Probably Compatible

PREGNANCY SUMMARY

No reports describing the use of tagraxofusp in human pregnancy have been located. Because the drug consists of proteins, it is not known whether some fetal exposure will occur. Human placental perfusion model studies suggest that there is minimal to no transfer of inflammatory cytokines across the placenta, but the absence of human pregnancy experience prevents a complete assessment of the embryofetal risk. Animal reproduction studies were not performed. The drug has the potential to cause life-threatening capillary leak syndrome. Therefore, because of the mechanism of action, the manufacturer recommends that females of reproductive potential use effective contraception during treatment with tagraxofusp and for 1 week after the last dose. Nevertheless, using this drug during pregnancy should be based on the pros and cons of the mother's clinical need for treatment versus any potential fetal risk that might occur from exposure. Hypertension was reported in up to 14% of patients treated with this drug in clinical trials. There is a registry for women who are pregnant and have cancer. For more information, women and health care providers are encouraged to contact the Cancer and Pregnancy Registry at 1-877-635-4499.

BREASTFEEDING SUMMARY

It is not known if tagraxofusp is excreted into human breast milk. The drug will probably not appear in breast milk, or the levels would be negligible. Furthermore, if ingested through breastfeeding, the drug consists of two large proteins, and most likely these would be digested in the infant's gastrointestinal tract and not be absorbed. However, the manufacturer recommends that women not breastfeed their infants if treated with this drug and for 1 week after the last dose. Nevertheless, breastfeeding while using tagraxofusp should be based on the mother's clinical need for treatment. If used, the infant should be monitored for the most common reported adult side effects of nausea, headache, and back pain (all leading to irritability), vomiting, diarrhea, edema, lethargy, and pyrexia.

References

1. Prescribing Information. *Elzonris*. Stemline Therapeutics, Inc; 2023.
2. Zaretsky MV, Alexander JM, Byrd W, Bawdon RE. Transfer of inflammatory cytokines across the placenta. *Obstet Gynecol*. 2004;103:546-550.
3. Aaltonen R, Heikkinen T, Hakala K, et al. Transfer of proinflammatory cytokines across the term placenta. *Obstet Gynecol*. 2005;106:802-807.

TALAZOPARIB

Antineoplastic (PARP Inhibitor)

PREGNANCY RECOMMENDATION: No Human Data—Animal Data Suggest Potential Risk

BREASTFEEDING RECOMMENDATION: Potential Toxicity

PREGNANCY SUMMARY

No reports describing the use of talazoparib in human pregnancy have been located. The drug will probably cross the placenta, so some fetal exposure will likely occur. Therefore, the absence of human pregnancy experience prevents a complete assessment of the embryofetal risk. Embryofetal toxicity with malformations was observed in one animal species at doses of less than the RHD. Based on animal studies and the drug's mechanism of action, the manufacturer recommends that women with reproductive potential use effective contraception during treatment and for 7 months after the last dose. They also recommend that males with female partners of reproductive potential use effective contraception during treatment and for 4 months after the last dose. Nevertheless, using this drug during pregnancy should be based on the pros and cons of the mother's clinical need for treatment versus any potential fetal risk that might occur from exposure. There is a registry for women who are pregnant and have cancer. For more information, women and health care providers are encouraged to contact the Cancer and Pregnancy Registry at 1-877-635-4499.

BREASTFEEDING SUMMARY

No reports describing the use of talazoparib during human lactation have been located. The drug will likely be excreted into breast milk, so some infant exposure will probably occur. Due to a concern for potential serious adverse effects that might be seen in a breastfed infant, the manufacturer recommends that women not breastfeed while being treated with this drug and for at least 1 month after the last dose. Nevertheless, breastfeeding while using this drug should be based on the mother's clinical need for treatment versus any potential infant risks that might occur. If used, the infant should be monitored for the most common reported adult side effects of nausea and headache (leading to irritability), vomiting, diarrhea, fatigue (lethargy), alopecia, decreased appetite (monitor feeding and growth), and various laboratory abnormalities (see PI).

Reference

1. Prescribing Information. *Talzenna*. Pfizer Laboratories Div Pfizer, Inc; 2024.

TALIGLUCERASE ALFA

Endocrine/Metabolic (Gaucher Disease, Enzyme)

PREGNANCY RECOMMENDATION: Limited Human Data—Animal Data Suggest Low Risk

BREASTFEEDING RECOMMENDATION: Probably Compatible

PREGNANCY SUMMARY

One report describing the use of taliglucerase alfa in human pregnancy has been located. A woman discovered a pregnancy after her seventh taliglucerase alfa infusion, and she continued it throughout pregnancy. She delivered a healthy term infant with no anomalies reported. The drug is not likely to cross the placenta in clinically significant amounts. Animal data did not show any embryofetal toxicity in two species at doses of less than 10 times the MRHD. However, the limited human pregnancy experience prevents a complete assessment of embryofetal risk. If patients with type 1 Gaucher disease are not treated and controlled preconception and during pregnancy, there is a higher risk for spontaneous abortion, as well as other gestational complications. Therefore, treatment may reduce these risks. Therefore, if clinically indicated, taliglucerase alfa should not be withheld because of pregnancy. Using this drug during pregnancy should be based on the pros and cons of the mother's clinical need for treatment versus any potential fetal risk that might occur from exposure.

BREASTFEEDING SUMMARY

One report describing the use of taliglucerase alfa during human lactation was located. Leucocyte activity in breast milk and blood was equivalent to that seen with a similar drug, imiglucerase. Based on the MW and short terminal half-life, clinically significant amounts of the drug are not likely to be excreted into breast milk. Moreover, if excretion does occur, the drug would most likely be digested in the infant's gastrointestinal tract and not absorbed systemically. Breastfeeding while using this drug should be based on the mother's clinical need for treatment versus any potential infant risks that might occur. If used, the infant should be monitored for the most common reported adult side effects of headache, arthralgia, nausea, abdominal pain, pruritus, and extremity pain (all leading to irritability), fatigue (lethargy), flushing, vomiting, and rash.

References

1. Prescribing Information. *Elelyso*. Pfizer Laboratories Div Pfizer, Inc; 2024.
2. Drugbank. *Taliglucerase alfa*. Accessed November 3, 2024. https://www.drugbank.ca/drugs/DB08876
3. Paskulin L, Dornelles AD, Quevedo A, et al. Breastfeeding in patients with Gaucher disease: is taliglucerase alfa safe? *Mol Genet Metab Rep*. 2019;18:30-31.

TAMOXIFEN

Antineoplastic (Antiestrogen)

PREGNANCY RECOMMENDATION: Contraindicated

BREASTFEEDING RECOMMENDATION: Contraindicated

PREGNANCY SUMMARY

There have been over 200 human pregnancies reported that were exposed to tamoxifen. The manufacturer notes that spontaneous abortion, malformations, and fetal deaths have been reported with tamoxifen use in pregnancy. Additionally, patients should be educated about the potential risk of exposure and the potential for a long-term risk of a diethylstilbestrol (DES)-like syndrome. One study reported no anomalies in 85 exposed pregnancies that was followed by a second study that described several birth defects following use. Tamoxifen and its active metabolites will likely cross the placenta, so some fetal exposure will probably occur. However, the limited human pregnancy experience prevents a complete assessment of embryofetal risk. Embryofetal toxicity was found in three animal species at doses of less than the RHD in two and less than 10 times the RHD in the third. The manufacturer recommends that women with reproductive potential who are using tamoxifen should use barrier or nonhormonal contraception during treatment and for 2 months after the last dose. Because of its antiestrogenic effect, using an alternative drug is recommended, if possible. Hypertension was reported in up to 13% of patients treated with this drug in clinical trials. Tamoxifen can also prolong the QT interval. There is a registry for women who are pregnant and have cancer. For more information, women and health care providers are encouraged to contact the Cancer and Pregnancy Registry at 1-877-635-4499.

BREASTFEEDING SUMMARY

Tamoxifen and its active metabolites are excreted into breast milk. Tamoxifen was detected on day 2, *N*-desmethyl tamoxifen on day 6, and 4-hydroxy tamoxifen and endoxifen were detected on day 18. It has also been shown to inhibit lactation. Because tamoxifen inhibits lactation and because of the adverse effects noted in newborn animals and human adults when administered directly, the drug is contraindicated during nursing. However, if the clinical decision is to use this drug while breastfeeding, the infant should be monitored for the most common reported adult side effects of nausea, back pain, and headache (all leading to irritability), flushing, fluid retention, weight loss, and rash.

References

1. Prescribing Information. *Tamoxifen citrate*. Actavis Pharma, Inc; 2022.
2. Clark S. Prophylactic tamoxifen. *Lancet*. 1993;342:168.
3. Cullins SL, Pridjian G, Sutherland CM. Goldenhar's syndrome associated with tamoxifen given to the mother during gestation. *JAMA*. 1994;271:1905-1906.
4. Rollnick BR, Kaye CI. Oculo-auriculo-vertebral anomaly. In: Buyse ML, ed. *Birth Defects Encyclopedia*. Vol II. Blackwell Scientific Publications; 1990:1272-1274.
5. Tewari K, Bonebrake RG, Asrat T, Shanberg AM. Ambiguous genitalia in infant exposed to tamoxifen in utero. *Lancet*. 1997;350:183.
6. Koizumi K, Aono T. Pregnancy after combined treatment with bromocriptine and tamoxifen in two patients with pituitary prolactinomas. *Fert Steril*. 1986;46:312-314.
7. Lai C-H, Hsueh S, Chao A-S, Soong Y-K. Successful pregnancy after tamoxifen and megestrol acetate therapy for endometrial carcinoma. *Br J Obstet Gynaecol*. 1994;101:547-549.
8. Schuurman TN, Witteveen PO, van der Wall E, et al. Tamoxifen and pregnancy: an absolute contraindication? *Breast Cancer Res Treat*. 2019;175:17-25.
9. Ruiz-Velasco V, Rosas-Arceo J, Matute MM. Chemical inducers of ovulation: comparative results. *Int J Fertil*. 1979;24:61-64.
10. Messinis IE, Nillius SJ. Comparison between tamoxifen and clomiphene for induction of ovulation. *Acta Obstet Gynecol Scand*. 1982;61:377-379.
11. Fukushima T, Tajima C, Fukuma K, Maeyama M. Tamoxifen in the treatment of infertility associated with luteal phase deficiency. *Fertil Steril*. 1982;37:755-761.
12. Tajima C, Fukushima T. Endocrine profiles in tamoxifen-induced ovulatory cycles. *Fertil Steril*. 1983;40:23-30.
13. Tsuiki A, Uehara S, Kyono K, et al. Induction of ovulation with an estrogen antagonist, tamoxifen. *Tohoku J Exp Med*. 1984;144:21-31.
14. Weseley AC, Melnick H. Tamoxifen in clomiphene-resistant hypothalamic anovulation. *Int J Fertil*. 1987;32:226-228.
15. Suginami H, Yano K, Kitagawa H, et al. A clomiphene citrate and tamoxifen citrate combination therapy: a novel therapy for ovulation induction. *Fertil Steril*. 1993;59:976-979.
16. Lunglmayr G. Potentialities and limitations of endocrine treatment in idiopathic oligozoospermia. *Acta Eur Fertil*. 1983;14:401-404.
17. Schill WB, Schillinger R. Selection of oligozoospermic men for tamoxifen treatment by an antiestrogen test. *Andrologia*. 1987;19:266-272.
18. Brake A, Krause W. Treatment of idiopathic oligozoospermia with tamoxifen—a follow-up report. *Int J Androl*. 1992;15:507-508.

19. Breznik R, Borko E. Effectiveness of antiestrogens in infertile men. *Arch Androl.* 1993;31:43-48.
20. Kotoulas I-G, Mitropoulos D, Cardamakis E, et al. Tamoxifen treatment in male infertility. I. Effect on spermatozoa. *Fertil Steril.* 1994;61:911-914.
21. Sigman M, Vance ML. Medical treatment of idiopathic infertility. *Urol Clin North Am.* 1987;14:459-469.
22. Peccatori FA, Codacci-Pisanelli G, Mellgren G, et al. First-in-human pharmacokinetics of tamoxifen and its metabolites in the milk of a lactation mother: a case study. *ESMO Open.* 2020;5:e000859.
23. Shaaban MM. Suppression of lactation by an antiestrogen, tamoxifen. *Eur J Obstet Gynecol Reprod Biol.* 1975;4:167-169.
24. Masala A, Delitala G, Lo Dico G, et al. Inhibition of lactation and inhibition of prolactin release after mechanical breast stimulation in puerperal women given tamoxifen or placebo. *Br J Obstet Gynecol.* 1978;85:134-137.

TAMSULOSIN

Urinary (Selective α_{1A} Antagonist)

PREGNANCY RECOMMENDATION: Limited Human Data—Animal Data Suggest Low Risk

BREASTFEEDING RECOMMENDATION: Probably Compatible

PREGNANCY SUMMARY

There are two reports describing the use of tamsulosin in 96 human pregnancies. Most of the exposures occurred during the second or third trimesters. Tamsulosin did not appear to increase the risk for adverse outcomes. The drug will likely cross the placenta, so some fetal exposure will probably occur. However, the limited human pregnancy experience prevents a complete assessment of embryofetal risk. Animal data did not show any embryofetal toxicity in one species at doses of more than 10 times the RHD. Using this drug during pregnancy should be based on the pros and cons of the mother's clinical need for treatment versus any potential fetal risk that might occur from exposure.

BREASTFEEDING SUMMARY

No reports describing the use of tamsulosin during human lactation have been located. The drug will likely be excreted into breast milk, so some infant exposure will probably occur. Breastfeeding while using this drug should be based on the mother's clinical need for treatment versus any potential infant risks that might occur. If used, the infant should be monitored for the most common reported adult side effects of headache, dizziness, asthenia, back pain, and nausea (all leading to irritability), infections, diarrhea, cough, somnolence, and insomnia.

References

1. Prescribing Information. *Tamsulosin hydrochloride*. Aurobindo Pharma Limited; 2021.
2. Bailey G, Vaughan L, Rose C, Krambeck A. Perinatal outcomes with tamsulosin therapy for symptomatic urolithiasis. *J Urol.* 2016;195:99-103.
3. Theriault B, Morin F, Cloutier J. Safety and efficacy of tamsulosin as medical expulsive therapy in pregnancy. *World J Urol.* 2020;38:2301-2306.

TAPENTADOL

Pain (Opioid)

PREGNANCY RECOMMENDATION: Limited Human Data—Animal Data Suggest Risk

BREASTFEEDING RECOMMENDATION: Potential Toxicity

PREGNANCY SUMMARY

One report was located that described the use of tapentadol in human pregnancy. Excluding lost to follow-up, ongoing pregnancies, and elective terminations, of 15 pregnancies, there was 1 early spontaneous abortion and 14 infants with no identified birth anomalies. However, the number of those exposed in the first trimester was not fully supplied. There were two cases of neonatal opioid withdrawal syndrome. The drug will probably cross the placenta, so some fetal exposure will likely occur. Therefore, this limited human pregnancy experience prevents a complete assessment of the embryofetal risk. Embryofetal toxicity with malformations and maternal toxicity were observed in two animal species at doses of about equal to and less than the MRHD. Use of opioid drugs for prolonged periods or with high doses at term has the potential to cause neonatal abstinence syndrome and respiratory depression in the newborn. The drug has a risk of producing dependence, leading to misuse. It is a Schedule II controlled substance. Using this drug during pregnancy should be based on the pros and cons of the mother's clinical need for treatment versus any potential fetal risk that might occur from exposure. Orthostatic hypotension and syncope were reported in patients treated with this drug during the clinical trials. There are several boxed warnings with tapentadol, which include increased risks of addiction and misuse that can lead to overdose and death;

T

serious, life-threatening, or fatal respiratory depression, especially with concomitant use of other opioid drugs, benzodiazepines, or other central nervous system (CNS) depressants; coma; and neonatal abstinence syndrome.

BREASTFEEDING SUMMARY

One report describing the use of tapentadol during human lactation was located. There were four exposures through breast milk, and no adverse events in infants were reported. No other information was provided. The drug will likely be excreted into breast milk, so some infant exposure will probably occur. The manufacturer recommends monitoring for excessive sedation and respiratory depression if the infant is exposed through breast milk. Additionally, the infant should be monitored for withdrawal symptoms after maternal administration of the opioid or breastfeeding is discontinued. If the clinical decision is to use this drug while breastfeeding, the infant should be monitored for the most common reported adult side effects of nausea and dizziness (both leading to irritability), vomiting, and somnolence.

References

1. Prescribing Information. *Nucynta*. Collegium Pharmaceutical, Inc; 2023.
2. Stollenwerk A, Sohns M, Heisig F, et al. Review of post-marketing safety data on tapentadol, a centrally acting analgesic. *Adv Ther*. 2018;35:12-30.

TAPINAROF

Dermatologic (Aryl Hydrocarbon Receptor Agonist)

PREGNANCY RECOMMENDATION: No Human Data—Animal Data Suggest Low Risk

BREASTFEEDING RECOMMENDATION: Probably Compatible

PREGNANCY SUMMARY

No reports describing the use of tapinarof in human pregnancy have been located. Based on likely limited placental transfer, fetal exposure is probably negligible. However, the absence of human pregnancy experience prevents a complete assessment of the embryofetal risk. Animal data did not show any embryofetal toxicity despite subcutaneous (SC) administration. Using this drug during pregnancy should be based on the pros and cons of the mother's clinical need for treatment versus any potential fetal risk that might occur from exposure.

BREASTFEEDING SUMMARY

No reports describing the use of tapinarof during human lactation have been located. A very limited amount of the drug may be found in breast milk, but the level would probably be clinically insignificant. Breastfeeding while using this drug should be based on the mother's clinical need for treatment. If used, the infant should be monitored for the most common reported adult side effects of headache and pruritus (both leading to irritability), folliculitis, nasopharyngitis, contact dermatitis, and influenza.

Reference

1. Prescribing Information. *Vtama*. Dermavant Sciences, Inc; 2022.

TALQUETAMAB

Antineoplastic (Bispecific Antibody—CD3 T-Cell Engager)

PREGNANCY RECOMMENDATION: No Human Data and No Relevant Animal Data

BREASTFEEDING RECOMMENDATION: Probably Compatible

PREGNANCY SUMMARY

No reports describing the use of talquetamab in human pregnancy have been located. As an IgG antibody, it likely crosses the placenta, especially during the second half of gestation, so some fetal exposure will probably occur. Therefore, the absence of human pregnancy experience prevents a complete assessment of the embryofetal risk. Animal reproduction and fertility studies have not been conducted with talquetamab. Based on the drug's mechanism of action, the manufacturer recommends that women with reproductive potential use effective contraception during treatment and for 3 months after the last dose. Nevertheless, using this drug during pregnancy should be based on the pros and cons of the mother's clinical need for treatment versus any potential fetal risk that might occur from exposure. There is a registry for women who are pregnant and have cancer. For more information, women and health care providers are encouraged to contact the Cancer and Pregnancy Registry at 1-877-635-4499.

BREASTFEEDING SUMMARY

No reports describing the use of talquetamab during human lactation have been located. It is known that IgG antibodies can be found in human breast milk, but are not found in the neonatal or infant circulation. Additionally, if any IgG antibodies were to be ingested through breastfeeding, they would probably be digested in the infant's gastrointestinal tract and not be absorbed. However, due to a concern for potential serious adverse effects that might be seen in a breastfed infant, the manufacturer recommends that women not breastfeed while being treated with this drug and for at least 4 months after the last dose. Nevertheless, breastfeeding while using this drug should be based on the mother's clinical need for treatment versus any potential infant risks that might occur. If used, the infant should be monitored for the most common reported adult side effects of musculoskeletal pain, headache, and abdominal pain (all leading to irritability), fatigue (lethargy), fever, rash, diarrhea, and various laboratory abnormalities (see PI).

Reference

1. Prescribing Information. *Talvey*. Janssen Biotech, Inc; 2023.

TARLATAMAB

Antineoplastic (Bispecific T-Cell Engager Antibody)

PREGNANCY RECOMMENDATION: No Human Data and No Relevant Animal Data

BREASTFEEDING RECOMMENDATION: Probably Compatible

PREGNANCY SUMMARY

No reports describing the use of tarlatamab in human pregnancy have been located. This antibody is a bispecific T-cell engager antibody, and it is not known if it is transported across the placenta similar to IgG antibodies (though it does contain an Fc fragment). Because it might cross the placenta (especially later in gestation), some fetal exposure may occur. Therefore, the absence of human pregnancy experience prevents a complete assessment of the embryofetal risk. Animal reproduction and fertility studies have not been conducted. Based on the drug's mechanism of action, the manufacturer recommends that women with reproductive potential use effective contraception during treatment and for 2 months after the last dose. Nevertheless, using this drug during pregnancy should be based on the pros and cons of the mother's clinical need for treatment versus any potential fetal risk that might occur from exposure. There is a registry for women who are pregnant and have cancer. For more information, women and health care providers are encouraged to contact the Cancer and Pregnancy Registry at 1-877-635-4499.

BREASTFEEDING SUMMARY

No reports describing the use of tarlatamab during human lactation have been located. It is known that IgG antibodies can be found in human breast milk, but are not found in the neonatal or infant circulation. However, this antibody is a bispecific T-cell engager antibody, and it is not known if it is excreted into breast milk, similar to IgG antibodies. Regardless, because it is an antibody with 982 amino acids, if it were to be ingested through breastfeeding, it would probably be digested in the infant's gastrointestinal tract and not be absorbed. However, due to a concern for potential serious adverse effects that might be seen in a breastfed infant, the manufacturer recommends that women not breastfeed while being treated with this drug and for at least 2 months after the last dose. Nevertheless, breastfeeding while using this drug should be based on the mother's clinical need for treatment versus any potential infant risks that might occur. If used, the infant should be monitored for the most common reported adult side effects of nausea and musculoskeletal pain (both leading to irritability), fatigue (lethargy), fever, decreased appetite (monitor infant growth), constipation, and various laboratory abnormalities (see PI).

Reference

1. Prescribing Information. *Imdelltra*. Amgen, Inc; 2024.

TASIMELTEON

Central Nervous System (Hypnotic—Melatonin Receptor Agonist)

PREGNANCY RECOMMENDATION: No Human Data—Animal Data Suggest Low Risk

BREASTFEEDING RECOMMENDATION: Probably Compatible

PREGNANCY SUMMARY

No reports describing the use of tasimelteon in human pregnancy have been located. The drug is likely to cross the placenta, so some fetal exposure will probably occur. Therefore, the absence of human pregnancy experience prevents a complete assessment of embryofetal risk. Animal data did not show any embryofetal toxicity in one species at doses of more than 10 times the MRHD. Using this drug during pregnancy should be based on the pros and cons of the mother's clinical need for treatment versus any potential fetal risk that might occur from exposure.

BREASTFEEDING SUMMARY

No reports describing the use of tasimelteon during human lactation have been located. The drug will likely be excreted into breast milk, so some infant exposure will probably occur. Breastfeeding while using this drug should be based on the mother's clinical need for treatment versus any potential infant risks that might occur. If used, the infant should be monitored for the most common reported adult side effects of headache and nightmares or unusual dreams (both leading to irritability), increased alanine aminotransferase levels, and upper respiratory or urinary tract infections.

Reference

1. Prescribing Information. *Tasimelteon*. Amneal Pharmaceuticals NY LLC; 2023.

TAUROLIDINE AND HEPARIN

Miscellaneous (Catheter Lock Solution)

PREGNANCY RECOMMENDATION: No Human Data and No Relevant Animal Data

BREASTFEEDING RECOMMENDATION: Probably Compatible

PREGNANCY SUMMARY

No reports describing the use of taurolidine in human pregnancy have been located. The drug will probably not cross the placenta in amounts that would have any clinical significance. However, the absence of human pregnancy experience prevents a complete assessment of the embryofetal risk. No animal reproduction or fertility studies have been conducted. Using this product during pregnancy should be based on the pros and cons of the mother's clinical need for use versus any potential fetal risk that might occur.

BREASTFEEDING SUMMARY

No reports describing the use of taurolidine during human lactation have been located. The drug would probably be excreted into breast milk if found in the systemic circulation. However, if used properly, the product is for catheter lock use only and should not be injected. Therefore, any amount that might be in the systemic circulation for possible excretion into breast milk should be clinically insignificant. Heparin is not found in breast milk in clinically significant amounts (see Heparin). Breastfeeding while using this product should be based on the mother's clinical need for treatment.

Reference

1. Prescribing Information. *Defencath*. CorMedix, Inc; 2023.

T

TAVABOROLE

Anti-Infective (Topical Antifungal)

PREGNANCY RECOMMENDATION: No Human Data—Animal Data Suggest Low Risk

BREASTFEEDING RECOMMENDATION: Probably Compatible

PREGNANCY SUMMARY

No reports describing the use of tavaborole in human pregnancy have been located. The drug is absorbed systemically, but blood levels are very low. Therefore, some tavaborole may cross the placenta, but this exposure is probably not clinically significant. However, the absence of human pregnancy experience prevents a complete assessment of embryofetal risk. Animal

(continued)

data did not show any embryofetal toxicity in two species at doses of more than 10 times the MRHD. Using this drug during pregnancy should be based on the pros and cons of the mother's clinical need for treatment versus any potential fetal risk that might occur from exposure.

BREASTFEEDING SUMMARY

No reports describing the use of tavaborole during human lactation have been located. The drug may be found in breast milk, but the very low systemic absorption following topical use would suggest that the amount would be clinically insignificant.

Breastfeeding while using this drug should be based on the mother's clinical need for treatment versus any potential infant risks that might occur. Because of the topical use of the drug, systemic side effects were not evaluated.

Reference

1. Prescribing Information. *Tavaborole*. Alembic Pharmaceuticals, Inc; 2023.

TAZAROTENE

Dermatologic (Retinoid—Topical)

PREGNANCY RECOMMENDATION: *Contraindicated

BREASTFEEDING RECOMMENDATION: Potential Toxicity

PREGNANCY SUMMARY

No reports describing the use of tazarotene in human pregnancy have been located. The drug is likely to cross the placenta. But the amounts absorbed systemically with topical use are low, at less than 2 ng/mL. However, some fetal exposure may occur. It is not known if these low plasma levels can produce any fetal anomalies or toxicity. Therefore, the absence of human pregnancy experience prevents a complete assessment of embryofetal risk. Embryofetal toxicity with malformations was observed in one animal species with topical administration and in two species with oral administration at doses of less than 10 times the MRHD exposure. *Systemic retinoids are known teratogens producing numerous fetal anomalies of the CNS, eye, face, skeletal system, and others. Based on the animal studies and the drug's mechanism of action, the manufacturer recommends that women with reproductive potential use effective contraception during treatment. Tazarotene should be started during menses whenever possible. If an acceptable substitution can be used during pregnancy, this should be considered.

BREASTFEEDING SUMMARY

No reports describing the use of tazarotene during human lactation have been located. The drug may be excreted into breast milk, but the amounts absorbed systemically following topical use are low, at less than 2 ng/mL. However, some fetal exposure may occur. Breastfeeding while using this drug should be based on the mother's clinical need for treatment versus any potential infant risks that might occur. The most common adverse events in nonpregnant adults were related to topical application. Systemic side effects were not evaluated.

Reference

1. Prescribing Information. *Tazarotene*. Cosette Pharmaceuticals, Inc; 2022.

TAZEMETOSTAT

Antineoplastic (Methyltransferase Inhibitor)

PREGNANCY RECOMMENDATION: No Human Data—Animal Data Suggest Risk

BREASTFEEDING RECOMMENDATION: Potential Toxicity

PREGNANCY SUMMARY

No reports describing the use of tazemetostat in human pregnancy have been located. Some of the drug probably crosses the placenta. Therefore, the absence of human pregnancy experience prevents a complete assessment of the embryofetal risk. Teratogenicity was observed in animal studies. Due to the findings from animal studies and its mechanism of action, the manufacturer recommends that women with reproductive potential who are taking tazemetostat use effective nonhormonal contraception during treatment and for at least 6 months after the last dose. They also recommend that males with female partners of reproductive potential use effective contraception during treatment and for 3 months after the last dose. Using this drug during pregnancy should be based on the pros and cons of the mother's clinical need for treatment versus any potential fetal risk that might occur from exposure.

BREASTFEEDING SUMMARY

No reports describing the use of tazemetostat during human lactation have been located. Some drug probably enters breast milk, so infant exposure will likely occur. However, due to the concern of potential adverse effects for a breastfed infant, the manufacturer recommends that women not breastfeed while being treated with tazemetostat and for at least 1 week after the last dose. Nevertheless, breastfeeding while using this drug should be based on the mother's clinical need for treatment. If used, the infant should be monitored for the most common reported adult side effects of musculoskeletal pain, abdominal pain, and nausea (all leading to irritability), lethargy, vomiting, decreased appetite, and constipation.

Reference

1. Prescribing Information. *Tazverik*. Epizyme, Inc; 2020.

TEBENTAFUSP

Antineoplastic (CD3 T-Cell Engager)

PREGNANCY RECOMMENDATION: No Human Data and No Relevant Animal Data

BREASTFEEDING RECOMMENDATION: Probably Compatible

PREGNANCY SUMMARY

No reports describing the use of tebentafusp in human pregnancy have been located. Because the drug consists of proteins, it is not known whether some fetal exposure could occur. However, the absence of human pregnancy experience prevents a complete assessment of the embryofetal risk. Animal reproduction studies have not been performed. Because of the mechanism of action, the manufacturer recommends that females of reproductive potential use effective contraception during treatment with tebentafusp and for 1 week after the last dose. Nevertheless, using this drug during pregnancy should be based on the pros and cons of the mother's clinical need for treatment versus any potential fetal risk that might occur from exposure.

BREASTFEEDING SUMMARY

It is not known if tebentafusp is excreted into human breast milk. The drug will probably not appear in breast milk, or the levels would be negligible. Furthermore, if ingested through breastfeeding, the drug is a peptide and most likely would be digested in the infant's gastrointestinal tract and not be absorbed. However, the manufacturer recommends that women not breastfeed their infants if treated with this drug and for 1 week after the last dose. Nevertheless, breastfeeding while using tebentafusp should be based on the mother's clinical need for treatment. If used, the infant should be monitored for the most common reported adult side effects of nausea, headache, abdominal pain, and pruritus (all leading to irritability), vomiting, rash, edema, lethargy, pyrexia, and several laboratory abnormalities (see PI).

Reference

1. Prescribing Information. *Kimmtrak*. Immunocore Commercial LLC; 2022.

TECHNETIUM TC 99M

Diagnostic (Radiography)

PREGNANCY RECOMMENDATION: Limited Human Data—No Relevant Animal Data

BREASTFEEDING RECOMMENDATION: Probably Compatible (Hold Breastfeeding)

PREGNANCY SUMMARY

There are 220 human pregnancy exposures to technetium Tc 99m across all trimesters of pregnancy. High-dose radiation exposure to the embryo or fetus is known to be associated with risks for IUGR, embryofetal loss, mental deficiency, and cancer. However, it is generally accepted that doses less than 5 Gy to the embryo or fetus are not teratogenic. To evaluate potential risks for diagnostic procedures that utilize technetium Tc 99m, estimates of the radiation dose to the human embryo or fetus have been calculated under various scenarios, and these estimates are under the 5 Gy limit. This suggests a low level of concern in situations where the diagnostic procedure is necessary in pregnancy or has been inadvertently performed in an unrecognized pregnancy. It does not appear to increase the risk for adverse pregnancy outcomes. Technetium Tc 99m is likely to cross the placenta, so some fetal exposure will probably occur. However, this limited human pregnancy experience still prevents a complete assessment of embryofetal risk. No animal reproduction studies have been conducted. Using this diagnostic agent during pregnancy should be based on the pros and cons of the mother's clinical need for treatment versus any potential fetal risk that might occur from exposure.

BREASTFEEDING SUMMARY

Technetium Tc 99m has been shown to be excreted into breast milk. The Academy of Breastfeeding Medicine states that breastfeeding does not need to be interrupted when using technetium Tc 99m in some radiography procedures. However, breastfeeding should be held with technetium Tc 99m ventilation-perfusion ($\dot{V}/\dot{Q}$) scans. When breastfeeding is held, the breast milk can be collected, refrigerated, and then fed to the infant after 10 physical half-lives (about 60 hours).

References

1. Prescribing Information. *Ultra-technekow V4*. Curium US LLC; 2024.
2. Prescribing Information. *Myoview*. Medi-Physics, Inc dba GE Healthcare; 2022.
3. National Library of Medicine. *StatPearls*. Technetium-99m. Accessed November 11, 2024. https://www.ncbi.nlm.nih.gov/books/NBK559013/
4. National Library of Medicine. *Pubchem*. Technetium (99Mtc) Medronic Acid. Accessed November 11, 2024. https://pubchem.ncbi.nlm.nih.gov/compound/Tc-99m-Mdp
5. Adelstein SJ. Administered radionuclides in pregnancy. *Teratology*. 1999;59:236-239.
6. International Commission on Radiological Protection Pregnancy and medical radiation. *Ann ICRP*. 2000;30:1-43.
7. Taskar-Pandit N, Dauer LT, Montgomery L, et al. Organ and fetal absorbed dose estimates from 99mTc-sulfur colloid lymphoscintigraphy and sentinel node localization in breast cancer patients. *J Nucl Med*. 2006;47:1202-1208.
8. Schaefer C, Meister R, Wentzeck R, Weber-Schoendorfer C. Fetal outcome after technetium scintigraphy in early pregnancy. *Reprod Toxicol*. 2009;28:161-166.
9. Balan KK, Critchley M, Vedavathy KK, et al. The value of ventilation-perfusion imaging in pregnancy. *Br J Radiol*. 1997;70:338-340.
10. Gropper AB, Zabicki Calvillo K, Dominici L, et al. Sentinel lymph node biopsy in pregnant women with breast cancer. *Ann Surg Oncol*. 2014;21:2506-2511.
11. Mitchell KB, Fleming MM, Anderson PO, et al. ABM clinical protocol #31: radiology and nuclear medicine studies in lactating women. *Breastfeed Med*. 2019;14:290-294.
12. Rubow S, Klopper J, Wasserman H, et al. The excretion of radiopharmaceuticals in human breast milk: additional data and dosimetry. *Eur J Nucl Med*. 1994;21:144-153.
13. Khan MT, Sultan FAT. Diffuse breast uptake of technetium-99m tetrofosmin during myocardial perfusion imaging in a lactating mother. *BMJ Case Rep*. 2021;14:e236770.
14. Malhotra G, Phadke MS, Rakshit S, et al. Unilateral breast uptake of 99mTc-MIBI in a lactating woman during myocardial perfusion imaging. *Clin Nucl Med*. 2022;47:e6-e8.

TECLISTAMAB

Antineoplastic (Anti-CD3 Monoclonal Antibody)

PREGNANCY RECOMMENDATION: No Human Data and No Relevant Animal Data

BREASTFEEDING RECOMMENDATION: Probably Compatible

T

PREGNANCY SUMMARY

No reports describing the use of teclistamab in human pregnancy have been located. As an IgG antibody, it likely crosses the placenta, so some fetal exposure will probably occur. Therefore, the absence of human pregnancy experience prevents a complete assessment of the embryofetal risk. No animal reproduction studies have been conducted. Because the drug causes T-cell activation and cytokine release, immune activation could theoretically compromise pregnancy maintenance. Based on the drug's mechanism of action, the manufacturer recommends that women with reproductive potential use effective contraception during treatment and for 5 months after the last dose. Nevertheless, using this drug during pregnancy should be based on the pros and cons of the mother's clinical need for treatment versus any potential fetal risk that might occur from exposure. Women who are pregnant and have cancer are encouraged to contact the Cancer and Pregnancy Registry at 877-635-4499.

BREASTFEEDING SUMMARY

No reports describing the use of teclistamab during human lactation have been located. It is known that IgG antibodies can be found in human breast milk, but are not found in the neonatal or infant circulation. Additionally, if any IgG antibodies were to be ingested through breastfeeding, they would probably be digested in the infant's gastrointestinal tract and not be absorbed. Regardless, due to the potential for adverse effects that might be seen in a breastfed infant, the manufacturer recommends that women should not breastfeed while being treated with teclistamab and for at least 5 months after the last dose. Nevertheless, breastfeeding while using this drug should be based on the mother's clinical need for treatment. If used, the infant should be monitored for the most common reported adult side effects of musculoskeletal pain, nausea, and headache (all leading to irritability), pyrexia, cytokine release syndrome, lethargy, upper respiratory tract infection, pneumonia, and diarrhea.

Reference

1. Prescribing Information. *Tecvayli*. Janssen Biotech, Inc; 2022.

TECOVIRIMAT

Antiviral (Orthopoxvirus)

PREGNANCY RECOMMENDATION: Limited Human Data—Animal Data Suggest Low Risk (Maternal Benefit May Outweigh Embryo–Fetal Risk)

BREASTFEEDING RECOMMENDATION: Probably Compatible

PREGNANCY SUMMARY

Two studies were located that describe the use of tecovirimat during human pregnancy. A total of 12 pregnant women with monkeypox infections were treated in all three trimesters. No medication-related adverse events were reported. Some amount of the drug will likely cross the placenta, so fetal exposure will probably occur. However, this limited human pregnancy experience prevents a complete assessment of embryofetal risk. Animal data did not show any embryofetal toxicity in two species: one at doses more than 10 times the RHD and one at less than the RHD. Using this drug during pregnancy should be based on the pros and cons of the mother's clinical need for treatment versus any potential fetal risk that might occur from exposure. There are limited data regarding monkeypox infections during pregnancy; however, maternal infections have been associated with an increased risk for spontaneous pregnancy loss, preterm delivery, fetal transmission, and neonatal infections. Because there is a potential for serious disease and vertical transmission, the Centers for Disease Control and Prevention (CDC) recommends that treatment be offered to pregnant patients and that providers discuss the risks and benefits of using the drug. See the CDC website for additional recommendations. Tecovirimat can cause prolongation of the QT interval. One publication recommended a baseline electrocardiogram and being aware of torsade de pointes, especially if this medication is used with other QT-prolonging medications, such as erythromycin.

BREASTFEEDING SUMMARY

No reports describing the use of tecovirimat during human lactation have been located. The drug will likely be excreted into breast milk, so some infant exposure will probably occur. The manufacturer recommends avoiding breastfeeding in mothers with monkeypox because of the transmission through direct contact. Monkeypox can also be present in breast milk, and it is recommended that breastfeeding be delayed until scabs appear on the rash. Additionally, the CDC recommends that newborns not have direct contact with people who have an active monkeypox infection. See the CDC website for more information on management and precautions. If the clinical decision is to use this drug while breastfeeding, the infant should be monitored for the most common reported adult side effects of headache, nausea, and abdominal pain (all leading to irritability), and vomiting.

References

1. Prescribing Information. *Tpoxx*. SIGA Technologies, Inc; 2024.
2. Centers for Disease Control and Prevention. *Mpox considerations for people who are pregnant or breastfeeding*. Accessed November 7, 2025. https://www.cdc.gov/monkeypox/hcp/clinical-care/pregnancy.html
3. Dashraath P, Nielsen-Saines K, Rimoin A. Monkeypox in pregnancy: virology, clinical presentation, and obstetric management. *Am J Obstet Gynecol*. 2022;227:849-861e7.
4. Oakley LP, Hufstetler K, O'Shea J, et al. Mpox cases among cisgender women and pregnant persons—United States, May 11-November 7, 2022. *MMWR Morb Mortal Wkly Rep*. 2023;72:9-14.
5. Sampson MM, Magee G, Schrader EA, et al. Mpox (monkeypox) infection during pregnancy. *Obstet Gynecol*. 2023;141:1007-1010.

T

TEDIZOLID

Antibacterial (Oxazolidinone)

PREGNANCY RECOMMENDATION: No Human Data—Animal Data Suggest Potential Risk

BREASTFEEDING RECOMMENDATION: Probably Compatible

PREGNANCY SUMMARY

No reports describing the use of tedizolid in human pregnancy have been located. The drug will likely cross the placenta, so some fetal exposure will probably occur. However, the absence of human pregnancy experience prevents a complete assessment of embryofetal risk. No embryofetal toxicity was seen in mice and rats at doses approximately equal to the RHD. However, embryofetal toxicity was seen in one species without maternal toxicity at higher doses that were less than 10 times the RHD. Using this drug during pregnancy should be based on the pros and cons of the mother's clinical need for treatment versus any potential fetal risk that might occur from exposure.

BREASTFEEDING SUMMARY

No reports describing the use of tedizolid during human lactation have been located. The drug will likely be excreted into breast milk, so some infant exposure will probably occur. Breastfeeding while using this drug should be based on the mother's clinical need for treatment versus any potential infant risks that might occur. If used, the infant should be monitored for the most common reported adult side effects of nausea, headache, and dizziness (all leading to irritability), diarrhea, and vomiting.

Reference

1. Prescribing Information. *Sivextro*. Merck Sharp & Dohme LLC; 2023.

TEDUGLUTIDE

Gastrointestinal (Glucagon-Like Peptide-2 Analogue)

PREGNANCY RECOMMENDATION: **No Human Data—Animal Data Suggest Low Risk (Maternal Benefit May Outweigh Any Embryofetal Risk)**

BREASTFEEDING RECOMMENDATION: **Probably Compatible**

PREGNANCY SUMMARY

No reports describing the use of teduglutide in human pregnancy have been located. Clinically significant amounts of teduglutide are not likely to cross the placenta at least during early gestation. However, the absence of human pregnancy experience prevents a complete assessment of embryofetal risk. Animal data did not show any embryofetal toxicity in two species at doses of more than 10 times the MRHD. Using this drug during pregnancy should be based on the pros and cons of the mother's clinical need for treatment versus any potential fetal risk that might occur from exposure. Moreover, the drug is an analogue of a naturally occurring peptide secreted by L-cells of the distal intestine. Consequently, if indicated, the drug should not be withheld because of pregnancy.

BREASTFEEDING SUMMARY

One abstract from 2022 was found that described the use of teduglutide during human lactation. A patient started teduglutide at one month postpartum and continued to breastfeed for 4 months. No infant adverse events were reported. The drug is not likely to be excreted into breast milk in any clinically significant amounts. In addition, even if some excretion did occur, the peptide would probably be digested in the infant's gastrointestinal tract and not be absorbed. However, the manufacturer states that women receiving teduglutide should not breastfeed because of the tumorigenicity seen in rats. Nevertheless, breastfeeding while using this drug should be based on the mother's clinical need for treatment versus any potential infant risks that might occur. If used, the infant should be monitored for the most common reported adult side effects of abdominal pain and nausea (both leading to irritability), upper respiratory tract infection, vomiting, fluid overload, and hypersensitivity.

References

1. Prescribing Information. *Gattex*. Takeda Pharmaceuticals American, Inc; 2024.
2. Lillienau J, Nilsson E, Vulcan A, Nilsson A. Use of teduglutide during breastfeeding after pregnancy in a patient with severe intestinal failure. *Transplantation*. 2023;107:53.

TELAVANCIN

Antibacterial (Glycopeptide)

PREGNANCY RECOMMENDATION: **No Human Data—Animal Data Suggest Risk**

BREASTFEEDING RECOMMENDATION: **Potential Toxicity**

T

PREGNANCY SUMMARY

No reports describing the use of telavancin, a synthetic derivative of vancomycin, in human pregnancy have been located. The drug was shown to cross the placenta in small amounts at term in an ex vivo placental perfusion study. Transplacental passage in the first trimester should be limited. However, the absence of human pregnancy experience prevents a complete assessment of embryofetal risk. Embryofetal toxicity with malformations was seen in three animal species at doses of less than 10 times the MRHD. Based on animal studies, the manufacturer recommends that women with reproductive potential use effective contraception during treatment and for 2 weeks after the last dose. Nevertheless, using this drug during pregnancy should be based on the pros and cons of the mother's clinical need for treatment versus any potential fetal risk that might occur from exposure. Because other antibacterial options are available, not using this drug, at least until further human pregnancy data are available, might be considered. The drug carries a boxed warning for embryofetal toxicity (seen in the animal studies) along with other potential risks. Telavancin was also found to prolong the QTc interval in the clinical trials.

BREASTFEEDING SUMMARY

No reports describing the use of telavancin during human lactation have been located. The drug may be found in breast milk, but the amount should be limited. However, the high fat solubility could increase concentrations. Breastfeeding while using this drug should be based on the mother's clinical need for treatment versus any potential infant risks that might occur. If used, the infant should be monitored for the most common reported adult side effects of nausea and taste disturbance (both leading to irritability), diarrhea, vomiting, and foamy urine.

References

1. Prescribing Information. *Vibativ*. Cumberland Pharmaceuticals, Inc; 2023.

TELMISARTAN

Antihypertensive (Angiotensin II Receptor Blocker—ARB)

PREGNANCY RECOMMENDATION: Human Data Suggest Risk (Second and Third Trimesters)

BREASTFEEDING RECOMMENDATION: Probably Compatible

PREGNANCY SUMMARY

Two reports describing the use of telmisartan during the third trimester in human pregnancy were located. Both resulted in oligohydramnios and anuria that resolved postdelivery. Telmisartan crosses the placenta, so fetal exposure will occur. However, this limited first-trimester human pregnancy experience prevents a complete assessment of embryofetal risk. Decreased fetal renal function leading to anuria and oligohydramnios is commonly known as a major risk in the use of angiotensin II receptor blockers (ARBs) and angiotensin-converting enzyme (ACE) inhibitors, and this can lead to fetal lung hypoplasia, skeletal malformations, and death in some cases. However, it is not universally fatal, as seen in the two cases described earlier. Therefore, use in the second and third trimesters should be avoided if at all possible. The drug carries a boxed warning regarding these fetal risks and to discontinue telmisartan as soon as possible when pregnancy is detected. If a mother has no appropriate alternative therapy, the manufacturer recommends educating the patient about the potential fetal risks. If used, serial ultrasounds to monitor amniotic fluid volume should be performed. No embryofetal toxicity or malformations were seen in two species at doses of less than 10 times the MRHD. Some embryofetal toxicity was seen in one of these species at doses that were still below 10 times the MRHD, but maternal toxicity also occurred. Uncontrolled maternal hypertension is associated with an increased risk for preeclampsia, gestational diabetes, placental abruption, preterm delivery, IUGR, and intrauterine death.

BREASTFEEDING SUMMARY

No reports describing the use of telmisartan during human lactation have been located. The drug will likely be excreted into breast milk, so some infant exposure will probably occur. Breastfeeding while using this drug should be based on the mother's clinical need for treatment versus any potential infant risks that might occur. If used, the infant should be monitored for the most common reported adult side effects of back pain (leading to irritability) and diarrhea.

References

1. Prescribing Information. *Telmisartan*. Alembic Pharmaceuticals, Inc; 2022.
2. Pietrement C, Malot L, Santerne B, et al. Neonatal acute renal failure secondary to maternal exposure to telmisartan, angiotensin II receptor antagonist. *J Perinatol*. 2003;23:254-255.
3. Polifka JE. Is there an embryopathy associated with first-trimester exposure to angiotensin-converting enzyme inhibitors and angiotensin receptor antagonists? A critical review of the evidence. *Birth Defects Res (Part A)*. 2012;94:576-598.
4. Marchetto L, Sordino D, De Bernardo G, Trevisanuto D. Postnatal acute renal failure after fetal exposure to angiotensin receptor blockers. *BMJ Case Rep*. 2015;2:bcr2014207450.

T

TELOTRISTAT ETHYL

Miscellaneous (Tryptophan Hydroxylase Inhibitor—Carcinoid Syndrome)

PREGNANCY RECOMMENDATION: No Human Data—Animal Data Suggest Low Risk

BREASTFEEDING RECOMMENDATION: Probably Compatible

PREGNANCY SUMMARY

No reports describing the use of telotristat ethyl in human pregnancy have been located. The drug will probably cross the placenta, so fetal exposure will likely occur. However, the absence of human pregnancy experience prevents a complete assessment of the embryofetal risk. Animal studies did not show any embryofetal toxicity. Using this drug during pregnancy should be based on the pros and cons of the mother's clinical need for treatment versus any potential fetal risk that might occur from exposure.

BREASTFEEDING SUMMARY

No reports describing the use of telotristat ethyl during human lactation have been located. The drug will probably enter breast milk, so some infant exposure will likely occur. Breastfeeding should be based on the mother's clinical need for treatment. If used, the infant should be monitored for the most common reported adult side effects of headache and nausea (both leading to irritability), constipation, decreased appetite, peripheral edema, and pyrexia.

Reference

1. Prescribing Information. *Xermelo*. Lexicon Pharmaceuticals, Inc; 2017.

TEMAZEPAM

Central Nervous System (Benzodiazepine—Insomnia)

PREGNANCY RECOMMENDATION: Human Data Suggest Low Risk (First Trimester)/Human Data Suggest Risk (Third Trimester)

BREASTFEEDING RECOMMENDATION: Potential Toxicity

PREGNANCY SUMMARY

Two large studies totaling 525 pregnant women exposed to temazepam in the first trimester found no increase in the number of major birth defects (17 in 525 pregnancies or 3.2%). No pattern to the defects was seen. A few larger studies have analyzed the use of benzodiazepine drugs as a group, and again, no increased risk for birth defects was identified. However, the use of temazepam in these evaluations was minimal. The drug has been shown to cross the placenta, so fetal exposure will occur. Embryofetal toxicity was observed in two species of animal studies, but the equivalent human dose was not provided. Using this drug during pregnancy should be based on the pros and cons of the mother's clinical need for treatment versus any potential fetal risk that might occur from exposure. Health care providers are encouraged to register women who are pregnant and have taken temazepam at any time during pregnancy by contacting the National Pregnancy Registry for Psychiatry Medications at 866-961-2388. The drug carries a boxed warning for an increased risk of with concomitant use with opioid drugs. Due to the adverse event profile and addictive potential, the American College of Obstetricians and Gynecologists (ACOG) recommends avoiding benzodiazepines or using them sparingly as an anxiety treatment. If prescribed, ACOG recommends using the lowest effective dose and states that doses can be tapered down by 25% to 50% per week. Withdrawal symptoms can occur with abrupt cessation, including seizures. Neonatal sedation, decreased muscle tone, respiratory compromise, and neonatal intensive care unit (NICU) admission have been associated with benzodiazepine use near delivery. Because temazepam is not indicated for use in treating anxiety, consider using other agents for insomnia during pregnancy.

BREASTFEEDING SUMMARY

Temazepam has been shown to be excreted into human breast milk. Sedation, poor feeding, and poor weight gain have been observed in infants exposed through breast milk. Ten lactating women were evaluated while using temazepam. The drug was detected in the breast milk of only one woman with before- and after-feed levels of 28 and 26 ng/mL, respectively. The breast milk to maternal plasma ratio in this patient was about 12%. The calculated RID was about 1.5%. Breastfeeding while using this drug should be based on the mother's clinical need for treatment versus any potential infant risks that might occur. If used, the infant should be monitored for the most common reported adult side effects of headache and dizziness (both leading to irritability), drowsiness, fatigue (lethargy), sedation, and poor feeding (monitor infant growth).

References

1. Prescribing Information. *Temazepam*. Alembic Pharmaceuticals, Inc; 2023.
2. Pubchem. *Temazepam*. Accessed November 17, 2024. https://pubchem.ncbi.nlm.nih.gov/compound/Temazepam
3. American College of Obstetricians and Gynecologists. Treatment and management of mental health conditions during pregnancy and postpartum: ACOG Clinical Practice Guideline No. 5. *Obstet Gynecol*. 2023;141:1262-1288.
4. Cooper J, Jauniaux E, Gulbis B, Bromley L. Placental transfer of temazepam and fentanyl in early human pregnancy. *Reprod Biomed Online*. 2001; 2:165-171.
5. Ban L, West J, Gibson JE, et al. First trimester exposure to anxiolytic and hypnotic drugs and the risks of major congenital anomalies: a United Kingdom population-based cohort study. *PLoS One*. 2014;9:e100996.
6. Kargas GA, Kargas SA, Bruyere HJ Jr, et al. Perinatal mortality due to interaction of diphenhydramine and temazepam. *N Engl J Med*. 1985;313:1417.
7. Damen L, Visser DH, Sie SD, van Weissenbruch MM. Apparent life-threatening event following maternal use of temazepam during labour. *Case Rep Pediatr*. 2014;2014:650605.
8. Grigoriadis S, Graves L, Peer M, et al. Benzodiazepine use during pregnancy alone or in combination with an antidepressant and congenital malformations: systematic review and meta-analysis. *J Clin Psychiatry*. 2019;80: 18r12412.
9. Tinker SC, Reefhuis J, Bitsko RH, et al. Use of benzodiazepine medications during pregnancy and potential risk for birth defects, National Birth Defects Prevention Study, 1997-2011. *Birth Defects Res*. 2019;111:613-620.
10. Grigoriadis S, Graves L, Peer M, et al. Pregnancy and delivery outcomes following benzodiazepine exposure: a systematic review and meta-analysis. *Can J Psych*. 2020;65:821-834.
11. Szpunar MJ, Freeman MP, Kobylski LA, et al. Risk of major malformations in infants after first trimester exposure to benzodiazepines: results from the Massachusetts General Hospital National Pregnancy Registry for Psychiatric Medications. *Depress Anxiety*. 2022;39:751-759.
12. Chen VCH, Wu SI, Lin CF, et al. Association of prenatal exposure to benzodiazepines with development of autism spectrum and attention-deficit/hyperactivity disorders. *JAMA Netw Open*. 2022;5:e2243282.

TEMOZOLOMIDE

Antineoplastic (Alkylating Agent)

PREGNANCY RECOMMENDATION: Limited Human Data—Animal Data Suggest Risk

BREASTFEEDING RECOMMENDATION: Potential Toxicity

PREGNANCY SUMMARY

Two reports described temozolomide exposure in human pregnancy. In one case, exposure occurred at the time of conception and early first trimester, and in the second case, exposure occurred in the second trimester. Both infants were healthy at delivery with no identified anomalies. Temozolomide and its active metabolite, MTIC, will likely cross the placenta, so some fetal exposure will probably occur. However, this limited human pregnancy experience prevents a complete assessment of embryofetal risk. Embryofetal toxicity with malformations were observed in two animal species at doses less than the RHD. Based on animal studies and the drug's mechanism of action, the manufacturer recommends that women with reproductive potential use effective contraception during treatment and for 6 months after the last dose. They also recommend that males with female partners of reproductive potential use effective contraception during treatment and for 3 months after the last dose. Nevertheless, using this drug during pregnancy should be based on the pros and cons of the mother's clinical need for treatment versus any potential fetal risk that might occur from exposure. There is a registry for women who are pregnant and have cancer. For more information, women and health care providers are encouraged to contact the Cancer and Pregnancy Registry at 1-877-635-4499.

BREASTFEEDING SUMMARY

No reports describing the use of temozolomide during human lactation have been located. The drug and its active metabolite will likely be excreted into breast milk, so some infant exposure will probably occur. However, due to a concern for potential serious adverse effects that might be seen in a breastfed infant, the manufacturer recommends that women not breastfeed while being treated with this drug and for at least 1 week after the last dose. Nevertheless, breastfeeding while using this drug should be based on the mother's clinical need for treatment versus any potential infant risks that might occur. If used, the infant should be monitored for the most common reported adult side effects of nausea and headache (both leading to irritability), alopecia, fatigue (lethargy), vomiting, constipation, anorexia (monitor infant feeding patterns and growth), and various laboratory abnormalities (see PI).

References

1. Prescribing Information. *Temodar*. Merck Sharp & Dohme LLC; 2023.
2. McGrane J, Bedford T, Kelly S. Successful pregnancy and delivery after concomitant temozolomide and radiotherapy treatment of glioblastoma multiforme. *Clin Oncol (R Coll Radiol)*. 2012;24:311.
3. Evans AC, Nelson MB, Dhall G. Pregnancy in a patient with a malignant brain tumor taking temozolomide: case report and review of the literature. *J Pediatr Oncol Nurs*. 2015;32:326-328.

T

TEMSIROLIMUS

Antineoplastic (mTOR Inhibitor)

PREGNANCY RECOMMENDATION: No Human Data—Animal Data Suggest Risk

BREASTFEEDING RECOMMENDATION: Potential Toxicity

PREGNANCY SUMMARY

No reports describing the use of temsirolimus in human pregnancy have been located. The active metabolite, sirolimus, crosses the placenta (see Sirolimus), so fetal exposure will occur. However, the absence of human pregnancy experience prevents a complete assessment of embryofetal risk. Embryofetal toxicity was observed in two animal species at doses less than the RHD. Based on animal studies and the drug's mechanism of action, the manufacturer recommends that women with reproductive potential use effective contraception during treatment and for 3 months after the last dose. They also recommend that males with female partners of reproductive potential use effective contraception during treatment and for 3 months after the last dose. Nevertheless, using this drug during pregnancy should be based on the pros and cons of the mother's clinical need for treatment versus any potential fetal risk that might occur from exposure. There is a registry for women who are pregnant and have cancer. For more information, women and health care providers are encouraged to contact the Cancer and Pregnancy Registry at 1-877-635-4499. Elevated glucose levels have been reported in up to 89% patients treated with this drug. Therefore, if used during pregnancy, glucose levels need to be monitored.

BREASTFEEDING SUMMARY

No reports describing the use of temsirolimus or the active metabolite, sirolimus, during human lactation have been located. The drug and its active metabolite will likely be excreted into breast milk, so some infant exposure will probably occur. However, due to a concern for potential serious adverse effects that might be seen in a breastfed infant, the manufacturer recommends that women not breastfeed while being treated with this drug and for at least 3 weeks after the last dose. Nevertheless, breastfeeding while using this drug should be based on the mother's clinical need for treatment versus any potential infant risks that might occur. If used, the infant should be monitored for the most common reported adult side effects of nausea (leading to irritability), rash, peripheral edema, anorexia (monitor infant feeding patterns and growth), and various laboratory abnormalities (see PI).

Reference

1. Prescribing Information. *Temsirolimus*. Accord Healthcare, Inc; 2023.

TENAPANOR

Gastrointestinal (Laxative—Sodium/Hydrogen Exchanger 3 Inhibitor)

PREGNANCY RECOMMENDATION: Limited Human Data—Animal Data Suggest Low Risk

BREASTFEEDING RECOMMENDATION: Probably Compatible

PREGNANCY SUMMARY

The manufacturer reports that a small number of pregnant women have been exposed to tenapanor during pregnancy. Exposure was not associated with increased risk for malformations, spontaneous abortions, or adverse maternal or fetal outcomes. No other information was provided. Systemic absorption is negligible with oral use, resulting in plasma concentrations below the detectable level of 0.5 ng/mL. Its inactive metabolite, M1, has a maximum plasma concentration at steady state of about 15 ng/mL. Tenapanor may cross the placenta in the latter part of gestation; however, the amount found in the systemic circulation with oral use is negligible. Therefore, any fetal exposure is likely to be clinically insignificant. However, the limited human pregnancy experience prevents a complete assessment of embryofetal risk. No embryofetal toxicity was seen in three animal species at doses of less than 10 times the RHD. Using this drug during pregnancy should be based on the pros and cons of the mother's clinical need for treatment versus any potential fetal risk that might occur from exposure.

BREASTFEEDING SUMMARY

No reports describing the use of tenapanor during human lactation have been located. The drug may be found in breast milk, but the amount found in the systemic circulation with oral use is negligible. Therefore, any infant exposure is likely to be clinically insignificant. Breastfeeding while using this drug should be based on the mother's clinical need for treatment versus any potential infant risks that might occur. If used, the infant should be monitored for the most common reported adult side effects of dizziness and abdominal cramps (both leading to irritability), diarrhea, and flatulence.

Reference

1. Prescribing Information. *Ibsrela*. Ardelyx, Inc; 2022.

TENECTEPLASE

Cardiovascular (Thrombolytic)

PREGNANCY RECOMMENDATION: Limited Human Data—Animal Data Suggest Low Risk (Maternal Benefit May Outweigh Any Embryofetal Risk)

BREASTFEEDING RECOMMENDATION: Probably Compatible

PREGNANCY SUMMARY

Three case reports describing the use of tenecteplase in human pregnancy were located. Exposures were at 6 weeks, 29 weeks, and unspecified gestational ages. All the infants were healthy with no identified fetal anomalies. The drug should not cross the placenta in clinically significant amounts, but because it is a protein, it is not known whether some placental transfer might occur in the second half of gestation. However, the limited human pregnancy experience prevents a complete assessment of embryofetal risk. Animal data did not show any embryofetal toxicity in one species at doses of less than 10 times the RHD. Using this drug during pregnancy should be based on the pros and cons of the mother's clinical need for treatment versus any potential fetal risk that might occur from exposure. Because myocardial infarction during pregnancy is a medical emergency that can be fatal if untreated, life-sustaining therapy should not be withheld because of potential fetal concerns.

BREASTFEEDING SUMMARY

No reports describing the use of tenecteplase during human lactation have been located. It is not known whether this drug will be excreted into human breast milk. However, because it is a 527-amino acid protein, if the drug were to be ingested through breastfeeding, it would probably be digested in the infant's gastrointestinal tract and not be absorbed. Breastfeeding while using this drug should be based on the mother's clinical need for treatment versus any potential infant risks that might occur. If used, the infant should be monitored for the most common reported adult side effects of bleeding and hypersensitivity. Because of the indication for use of this drug, using tenecteplase should not be withheld due to breastfeeding.

References

1. Prescribing Information. *TNKASE*. Genentech, Inc; 2023.
2. Bessereau J, Desvignes O, Huon B, et al. Case report of a successful pregnancy following thrombolysis for acute myocardial infarction. *Arch Mal Coeur Vaiss*. 2007;100:955-958.
3. Maegdefessel L, Issa H, Scheler C, et al. 27-year-old pregnant woman with syncope and dyspnea after aortic alloplastic heart valve replacement 15 years ago. *Internist (Berl)*. 2008;49:868-872.
4. dos Santos LF, Andrade C, Rodrigues B, et al. Pregnancy and acute pulmonary embolism: a case report. *Rev Port Cardiol*. 2012;31:389-394.

TENOFOVIR ALAFENAMIDE

Antiviral (Reverse Transcriptase Inhibitor HIV-1/Hepatitis B)

PREGNANCY RECOMMENDATION: Human and Animal Data Suggest Low Risk

BREASTFEEDING RECOMMENDATION: *Contraindicated (HIV)/Probably Compatible (Hepatitis B)

PREGNANCY SUMMARY

Tenofovir is available as two different prodrugs, tenofovir disoproxil fumarate (DF) (see Tenofovir DF) and tenofovir alafenamide (AF). Several reports describing the use of tenofovir AF in human pregnancy have been located. In the Antiretroviral Pregnancy Registry (APR) interim report up to January 2024, there were 1,633 pregnancies exposed to tenofovir AF. A total of 49 (3.9%) were identified to have a major birth anomaly in 1,242 first-trimester pregnancy exposures. No pattern to the defects was seen. The drug crosses the placenta, so fetal exposure will occur. Animal data did not show any embryofetal toxicity in two species at doses of more than 10 times the MRHD. Using this drug during pregnancy should be based on the pros and cons of the mother's clinical need for treatment versus any potential fetal risk that might occur from exposure. In 2024, the updated US Department of Health and Human Services AIDS Info guidelines for the use of antiretroviral agents during pregnancy recommend that, in most cases, patients continue their regimen during pregnancy if it is tolerated, safe, and effective in suppressing viral replication. Additionally, treatment initiation should not be delayed due to concerns about teratogenicity with first-trimester exposure. See the guidelines for the most updated information. If indicated, tenofovir AF

(continued)

T

should not be withheld in pregnancy since the expected benefit to the mother with HIV or infected with hepatitis B outweighs any unknown risk to the fetus. Providers caring for pregnant patients with HIV and their infants can call the national Perinatal HIV/AIDS hotline (888-448-8765) for free clinical consultation. Additionally, there is a pregnancy exposure registry that monitors pregnancy outcomes in patients using antiretroviral medicines during pregnancy. Health care providers are encouraged to call the APR at 1-800-258-4263.

BREASTFEEDING SUMMARY

Tenofovir AF has been shown to be excreted into human breast milk. No adverse effects have been reported in the infant. Breast milk levels have ranged from undetectable to a peak level of about 100 ng/mL at 4 hours postdose. Another study found a median peak tenofovir AF level of 1.7 ng/mL. Calculated RIDs were all less than 1%. *In 2023, the updated US Department of Health and Human Services AIDS Info guidelines state that using replacement of breast milk through formula or pasteurized donor human breast milk from a milk bank eliminates the risk of postnatal HIV transmission to the infant. Using antiretroviral therapy to achieve and maintain viral suppression during pregnancy and postpartum decreases the risk for infant transmission to less than 1%, but notes that it is not zero. For patients not on therapy or those without viral load suppression during pregnancy (at a minimum of throughout the third trimester) and at delivery, replacement of breast milk is recommended. Patients on antiretroviral therapy who have a sustained undetectable viral load and who choose to breastfeed or use replacement of breast milk should be supported with this decision. Breastfeeding in patients with hepatitis B can be performed as long as the infant has received appropriate treatment with hepatitis B immunoglobulin and hepatitis B vaccine postdelivery.

References

1. Prescribing Information. *Vemlidy*. Gilead Sciences, Inc; 2024.
2. Panel on Treatment of HIV During Pregnancy and Prevention of Perinatal Transmission. Recommendations for the use of antiretroviral drugs during pregnancy and interventions to reduce perinatal HIV transmission in the United States. Department of Health and Human Services. Accessed July 25, 2023. https://clinicalinfo.hiv.gov/en/guidelines/perinatal
3. Antiretroviral Pregnancy Registry Steering Committee. *Antiretroviral Pregnancy Registry International Interim Report for 1 January 1989 through 31 January 2023*. Registry Coordinating Center; 2023. www.APRegistry.com
4. Eke AC, Ramaiyer M, Eleje GU, et al. A systematic review and meta-analysis of maternal weight changes and pregnancy outcomes associated with integrase inhibitors and tenofovir alafenamide in pregnant women with HIV. *Am J Obstet Gynecol MFM*. 2024;6:101406.
5. Kayes T, Crane H, Symonds A, et al. Plasma and breast milk pharmacokinetics of tenofovir alafenamide in mothers with chronic hepatitis B. *Aliment Pharmacol Ther*. 2022;56:510-518.
6. Yang N, Zhou G, Cheng X, et al. Distribution evaluation of tenofovir in the breast milk of mothers with HBeAg-positive chronic HBV infection after treatment with tenofovir alafenamide and tenofovir disoproxil fumarate by a sensitive UPLC-MS/MS method. *Front Pharmacol*. 2021;12:734760.
7. Bojun L, Ye G, Yan W, et al. Tenofovir (TFV) or tenofovir alafenamide (TAF) concentration in breast milk and infants' cord blood, with tenofovir disoproxil fumarate (TDF) or TAF treatment in pregnancy. *Hepatol Int*. 2020; 14(suppl 1):S78.
8. Aebi-Popp K, Kahlert CR, Crisinel PA, et al. Transfer of antiretroviral drugs into breastmilk: a prospective study from the Swiss Mother and Child HIV Cohort Study. *J Antimicrob Chemother*. 2022;77:3436-3442.

TENOFOVIR DISOPROXIL FUMARATE

Antiviral (Reverse Transcriptase Inhibitor HIV-1/Hepatitis B)

PREGNANCY RECOMMENDATION: Human and Animal Data Suggest Low Risk

BREASTFEEDING RECOMMENDATION: *Contraindicated (HIV)/Probably Compatible (Hepatitis B)

PREGNANCY SUMMARY

Tenofovir is available as two different prodrugs, tenofovir disoproxil fumarate (DF) and tenofovir alafenamide (AF) (see Tenofovir AF). Several reports describing the use of tenofovir DF in human pregnancy have been located. In the APR interim report up through January 2024, there were 7,806 pregnancies exposed to tenofovir DF. A total of 129 (2.6%) were identified to have a major birth anomaly in 5,014 first-trimester pregnancy exposures. No pattern to the defects was seen. The drug crosses the placenta, so fetal exposure will occur. Animal data did not show any embryofetal toxicity in two species at doses of more than 10 times the MRHD. Using this drug during pregnancy should be based on the pros and cons of the mother's clinical need for treatment versus any potential fetal risk that might occur from exposure. In 2024, the updated US Department of Health and Human Services AIDS Info guidelines for the use of antiretroviral agents during pregnancy recommend that, in most cases, patients continue their regimen during pregnancy if it is tolerated, safe, and effective in suppressing viral replication. Additionally, treatment initiation should not be delayed due to concerns about teratogenicity with first -trimester exposure. See the guidelines for the most updated information. If indicated, tenofovir DF should not be withheld in pregnancy since the expected benefit to the mother with HIV or infected with hepatitis B outweighs any unknown risk to the fetus. Providers caring for pregnant patients with HIV and their infants can call the national Perinatal HIV/AIDS hotline (888-448-8765) for free clinical consultation. Additionally, there is a pregnancy exposure registry that monitors pregnancy outcomes in patients using antiretroviral medicines during pregnancy. Health care providers are encouraged to call the APR at 1-800-258-4263.

T

BREASTFEEDING SUMMARY

Tenofovir DF has been shown to be excreted into human breast milk. No adverse effects have been reported in the infants. Breast milk levels are low, ranging from undetectable to 10 ng/mL in most cases. The calculated RIDs were all less than 1%. *In 2023, the updated US Department of Health and Human Services AIDS Info guidelines state that using replacement of breast milk through formula or pasteurized donor human breast milk from a milk bank eliminates the risk of postnatal HIV transmission to the infant. Using antiretroviral therapy to achieve and maintain viral suppression during pregnancy and postpartum decreases the risk for infant transmission to less than 1%, but notes that it is not zero. For patients not on therapy or those without viral load suppression during pregnancy (at a minimum of throughout the third trimester) and at delivery, replacement milk is recommended. Patients on antiretroviral therapy who have a sustained undetectable viral load and who choose to breastfeed or use replacement of breast milk should be supported with this decision. Breastfeeding in patients with hepatitis B can be performed as long as the infant has received appropriate treatment with hepatitis B immunoglobulin and hepatitis B vaccine postdelivery.

References

1. Prescribing Information. *Viread*. Gilead Sciences, Inc; 2019.
2. Panel on Treatment of HIV During Pregnancy and Prevention of Perinatal Transmission. Recommendations for the use of antiretroviral drugs during pregnancy and interventions to reduce perinatal HIV transmission in the United States. Department of Health and Human Services. Accessed December 29, 2024. https://clinicalinfo.hiv.gov/en/guidelines/perinatal
3. Antiretroviral Pregnancy Registry Steering Committee. *Antiretroviral Pregnancy Registry International Interim Report for 1 January 1989 through 31 January 2023*. Registry Coordinating Center; 2023. www.APRegistry.com
4. Siberry GK, Williams PL, Mendez H, et al; for the Pediatric HIV/AIDS Cohort Study (PHACS). Safety of tenofovir use during pregnancy: early growth outcomes in HIV-exposed uninfected infants. *AIDS*. 2012;26:1151-1159.
5. Kourtis AP, Wiener J, Wang L, et al. Tenofovir disoproxil fumarate use during pregnancy and infant bone health: the tenofovir in pregnancy pilot study. *Pediatr Infect Dis J*. 2018;37:e264-e268.
6. Pan CQ, Dai E, Duan Z, et al. Long-term safety of infants from mothers with chronic hepatitis B treated with tenofovir disoproxil in China. *Gut*. 2022; 71:798-806.
7. Li S, Jin J, Jian Y, et al. Low levels of tenofovir in breast milk support breastfeeding in HBV-infected mothers treated with tenofovir disoproxil fumarate. *Int J Antimicrob Agents*. 2023;61:106726.
8. Yang N, Zhou G, Cheng X, et al. Distribution evaluation of tenofovir in the breast milk of mothers with HBeAg-positive chronic HBV infection after treatment with tenofovir alafenamide and tenofovir disoproxil fumarate by a sensitive UPLC-MS/MS method. *Front Pharmacol*. 2021;12:734760.
9. Bojun L, Ye G, Yan W, et al. Tenofovir (TFV) or tenofovir alafenamide (TAF) concentration in breast milk and infants' cord blood, with tenofovir disoproxil fumarate (TDF) or TAF treatment in pregnancy. *Hepatol Int*. 2020; 14(suppl 1):S78.
10. Kapito-Tembo AP, Bauleni A, Wesevich A, et al. Growth and neurodevelopment outcomes in HIV-, tenofovir-, and efavirenz-exposed breastfed infants in the PMTCT option B+ program in Malawi. *J Acquir Immune Defic Syndr*. 2021;86:81-90.
11. Nabwire F, Hamil MM, Fowler MG, et al. Milk calcium and phosphorus in Ugandan women with HIV on tenofovir-based antiretroviral therapy. *J Human Lact*. 2023;39:288-299.
12. Erturk US, Mete B, Ozaras R, et al. Plasma and breast milk pharmacokinetics of tenofovir disoproxil fumarate in nursing mother with chronic hepatitis B-infant pairs. *Antimicrob Agents Chemother*. 2021;65:e01110-e01121.

TEPLIZUMAB

Antineoplastic (Anti-CD3 Monoclonal Antibody)

PREGNANCY RECOMMENDATION: No Human Data—Animal Data Suggest Potential Risk

BREASTFEEDING RECOMMENDATION: Probably Compatible

PREGNANCY SUMMARY

No reports describing the use of teplizumab in human pregnancy have been located. As an IgG, the drug will likely cross the placenta, so some fetal exposure will probably occur. Therefore, the absence of human pregnancy experience prevents a complete assessment of embryofetal risk. No animal reproduction studies have been conducted with teplizumab. However, reduced T cells, increased B cells, and a reduction in the adaptive immune response were observed in mouse pups at high doses. Using this drug during pregnancy should be based on the pros and cons of the mother's clinical need for treatment versus any potential fetal risk that might occur from exposure. Women who are pregnant and have taken teplizumab at any time during pregnancy are encouraged to contact Provention Bio, Inc.'s adverse event reporting line at 844-778-2246.

BREASTFEEDING SUMMARY

No reports describing the use of teplizumab during human lactation have been located. It is known that IgG antibodies can be found in human breast milk, but are not found in the neonatal or infant circulation. Additionally, if any IgG antibodies were to be ingested through breastfeeding, they would probably be digested in the infant's gastrointestinal tract and not be absorbed. To minimize newborn exposure, the manufacturer recommends that breastfeeding be interrupted and the lactating woman pump and discard the breast milk during treatment and for 20 days after the last dose. Nevertheless, breastfeeding while using this drug should be based on the mother's clinical need for treatment. If used, the infant should be monitored for the most common reported adult side effects of lymphopenia, rash, leukopenia, and headache (leading to irritability).

Reference

1. Prescribing Information. *Tzield*. Provention Bio, Inc; 2022.

TEPOTINIB

Antineoplastic (Kinase Inhibitor)

PREGNANCY RECOMMENDATION: No Human Data—Animal Data Suggest Potential Risk

BREASTFEEDING RECOMMENDATION: Potential Toxicity

PREGNANCY SUMMARY

No reports describing the use of tepotinib in human pregnancy have been located. The drug will likely cross the placenta, so some fetal exposure will probably occur. However, the absence of human pregnancy experience prevents a complete assessment of the embryofetal risk. Embryofetal toxicity with malformations was observed in animal studies. Based on animal studies, the manufacturer recommends that women with reproductive potential use effective contraception during treatment and for 1 week after the last dose. They also recommend that males with female partners of reproductive potential use effective contraception during treatment and for 1 week after the last dose. Nevertheless, using this drug during pregnancy should be based on the pros and cons of the mother's clinical need for treatment versus any potential fetal risk that might occur from exposure.

BREASTFEEDING SUMMARY

No reports describing the use of tepotinib during human lactation have been located. Some amount of the drug will likely be excreted into breast milk, so infant exposure will probably occur. Due to the concern for potential serious adverse effects that might be seen in a breastfed infant, the manufacturer recommends that women not breastfeed while being treated with this drug and for at least 1 week after the last dose. Nevertheless, if the clinical decision is to use this drug while breastfeeding, the infant should be monitored for the most common reported adult side effects of nausea and musculoskeletal pain (both leading to irritability), edema, lethargy, diarrhea, dyspnea, and various laboratory abnormalities (see PI).

Reference

1. Prescribing Information. *Tepmetko*. EMD Serono; 2021.

TEPROTUMUMAB

Miscellaneous Insulin-Like Growth Factor-1 Receptor Antagonist (Monoclonal Antibody)

PREGNANCY RECOMMENDATION: No Human Data—Animal Suggest Potential Risk

BREASTFEEDING RECOMMENDATION: Probably Compatible

PREGNANCY SUMMARY

No reports describing the use of teprotumumab in human pregnancy have been located. As an IgG antibody, it likely crosses the placenta, so some fetal exposure will probably occur. Therefore, the absence of human pregnancy experience prevents a complete assessment of the embryofetal risk. Embryofetal toxicity was observed in animal studies. Due to the findings from animal studies and the drug's mechanism of action, the manufacturer recommends that women with reproductive potential use effective contraception prior to initiation, during treatment, and for 6 months after the last dose. Nevertheless, using this drug during pregnancy should be based on the pros and cons of the mother's clinical need for treatment versus any potential fetal risk that might occur from exposure. Hyperglycemia may occur in patients treated with teprotumumab. Glucose levels should be monitored while on treatment.

T

BREASTFEEDING SUMMARY

Teprotumumab is likely present in breast milk in small amounts. However, it is known that IgG antibodies can be found in human breast milk, but are not found in the neonatal or infant circulation. Additionally, if any IgG antibodies were to be ingested through breastfeeding, they would probably be digested in the infant's gastrointestinal tract and not be absorbed. Breastfeeding while using this drug should be based on the mother's clinical need for treatment. If used, the infant should be monitored for the most common reported adult side effects of muscle spasm, nausea, and headache (all leading to irritability), alopecia, diarrhea, fatigue, and dry skin.

Reference

1. Prescribing Information. *Tepezza*. Horizon Therapeutics USA, Inc; 2020.

TERAZOSIN

Antihypertensive (α_1-Adrenergic Blocker)

PREGNANCY RECOMMENDATION: No Human Data and No Relevant Animal Data

BREASTFEEDING RECOMMENDATION: Probably Compatible

PREGNANCY SUMMARY

No reports describing the use of terazosin in human pregnancy have been located. The drug will likely cross the placenta, so some fetal exposure will probably occur. However, the absence of human pregnancy experience prevents a complete assessment of embryofetal risk. Animal data did show some embryofetal toxicity in two species, but at doses well above 10 times the MRHD. Using this drug during pregnancy should be based on the pros and cons of the mother's clinical need for treatment versus any potential fetal risk that might occur from exposure.

BREASTFEEDING SUMMARY

No reports describing the use of terazosin during human lactation have been located. The drug will likely be excreted into breast milk, so some infant exposure will probably occur. Breastfeeding while using this drug should be based on the mother's clinical need for treatment. If used, the infant should be monitored for the most common reported adult side effects of headache, paresthesia, and dizziness (leading to irritability), somnolence, peripheral edema, and nasal congestion.

Reference

1. Prescribing Information. *Terazosin*. Bionpharma, Inc; 2024.

TERBINAFINE

Anti-Infective (Antifungal)

PREGNANCY RECOMMENDATION: Human Data and Animal Data Suggest Low Risk

BREASTFEEDING RECOMMENDATION: Potential Toxicity (Oral)/Probably Compatible (Topical)

PREGNANCY SUMMARY

There are two publications describing the use of terbinafine during pregnancy. The rate of major congenital birth anomalies was 3.8% in 522 first-trimester exposures to oral terbinafine and 3.8% in the control group of 5,220 first-trimester unexposed pregnancies. In addition, the rate of major congenital anomalies with first-trimester topical exposure was 3.6% in 1,476 cases. Again, this was no different from the 3.3% rate in the 14,760 first-trimester unexposed controls. No pattern to the defects was seen. The drug is likely to cross the placenta, so some fetal exposure will probably occur. Animal data did not show any embryofetal toxicity in two species at doses of more than 10 times the MRHD. Using this drug during pregnancy should be based on the pros and cons of the mother's clinical need for treatment versus any potential fetal risk that might occur from exposure.

BREASTFEEDING SUMMARY

Terbinafine is excreted into breast milk. The effect of this exposure on a nursing infant is unknown. Because the duration of oral therapy is usually prolonged (6-12 weeks for patients with fingernail or toenail onychomycosis, respectively), and the drug may accumulate in breast milk, the potential for toxicity in a nursing infant may be increased. Based on the accumulation and possible prolonged exposure, women taking oral terbinafine should consider not breastfeeding. However, less than 5% of topical terbinafine is systemically absorbed. Therefore, it is not likely to have clinically significant amounts excreted into breast milk. This topical form should not be applied to the breasts. If the clinical decision is to use this drug while breastfeeding, the infant should be monitored for the most common reported adult side effects of headache, pruritus, nausea, abdominal pain, and dyspepsia (all leading to irritability), diarrhea, rash, liver enzyme abnormalities, and flatulence.

References

1. Prescribing Information. *Terbinafine hydrochloride*. Bionpharma, Inc; 2023.
2. Terbinafine. *Lexi-Drugs*. UpToDate Lexidrug. UpToDate, Inc. Accessed November 22, 2024. https://online.lexi.com
3. Andersson NW, Thomsen SF, Andersen JT. Evaluation of association between oral and topical terbinafine use in pregnancy and risk of major malformations and spontaneous abortion. *JAMA Dermatol*. 2020;156:375-383.
4. Andersson NW, Thomsen SF, Andersen JT. Exposure to terbinafine in pregnancy and risk of preterm birth, small for gestational age, low birth weight, and stillbirth: a nationwide cohort study. *J Am Acad Dermatol*. 2021; 84:763-767.

TERBUTALINE

Respiratory; Reproductive (β_2-Agonist)

PREGNANCY RECOMMENDATION: Limited Human Data (First Trimester)—Animal Data Suggest Low Risk/*Human Data Low Risk (Second/Third Trimester)

BREASTFEEDING RECOMMENDATION: Probably Compatible

PREGNANCY SUMMARY

Numerous studies have been located that describe the use of terbutaline in human pregnancy. Most publications involve the use of the drug in the late second and early third trimesters as a tocolytic agent. In addition, most evaluations regarding patients with asthma who are on chronic medications, who become pregnant, use inhalers or other oral medicines, not terbutaline. From the Michigan Medicaid Surveillance study, there were 7 (4.7%) anomalies (6 expected) in 149 pregnancies with first-trimester exposure. No pattern to the defects was seen. The drug crosses the placenta, so some fetal exposure will occur. However, the limited first-trimester human pregnancy experience prevents a complete assessment of the embryofetal risk. Animal studies did not show any embryofetal toxicity or malformations in one species at doses well above 10 times the MRHD. In a second species, embryofetal toxicity with malformations was seen, but the doses were above 10 times the MRHD. Longer use of the drug can lead to hyperglycemia, and this can lead to neonatal hypoglycemia when used near delivery. *If administered as a tocolytic agent, its use is recommended to be limited to short-term treatment. Using this drug during pregnancy should be based on the pros and cons of the mother's clinical need for treatment versus any potential fetal risk that might occur from exposure. Terbutaline can prolong the QTc interval. The drug carries a boxed warning to avoid using terbutaline for prolonged tocolysis (beyond 48-72 hours). It also states that the drug should not be used as an outpatient or at home as a maintenance tocolytic. Prolonged use has been associated with tachycardia, hyperglycemia, hypokalemia, cardiac arrhythmias, pulmonary edema, myocardial ischemia, fetal tachycardia, and neonatal hypoglycemia.

BREASTFEEDING SUMMARY

Terbutaline has been shown to be excreted into human breast milk. In four cases, maternal levels ranged from about 1 to about 5 ng/mL, depending on the daily doses. Breast milk concentrations range from about 2.5 to 4 ng/mL. All of the calculated RIDs were less than 1%. Infant serum levels have also been assessed in a few cases, and the drug was not detected (LLQ of 1 ng/mL). No symptoms of adrenergic stimulation were observed in the four infants, and all exhibited normal development. Breastfeeding while using this drug should be based on the mother's clinical need for treatment versus any potential infant risks that might occur. If used, the infant should be monitored for the most common reported adult side effects of nervousness and dizziness (leading to irritability), tachycardia, and hyperglycemia.

References

1. Prescribing Information. *Terbutaline sulfate*. Areva Pharmaceuticals; 2024.
2. Food and Drug Administration. *FDA drug safety communication: new warnings against use of terbutaline to treat preterm labor*. Accessed February 23, 2020. https://www.fda.gov/drugs/drug-safety-and-availability/fda-drug-safety-communication-new-warnings-against-use-terbutaline-treat-preterm-labor
3. American College of Obstetricians and Gynecologists. Asthma in pregnancy: ACOG Practice Bulletin No. 90. *Obstet Gynecol*. 2008;111:457-464.
4. Global Initiative for Asthma. *2024 Global strategy for asthma management and prevention*. Accessed November 22, 2024. chrome-extension://efaidnbmnnnibpcajpcglclefindmkaj/https://ginasthma.org/wp-content/uploads/2024/05/GINA-2024-Strategy-Report-24_05_22_WMS.pdf
5. Ingemarsson I, Westgren M, Lindberg C, et al. Single injection of terbutaline in term labor: placental transfer and effects on maternal and fetal carbohydrate metabolism. *Am J Obstet Gynecol*. 1981;139:697-701.
6. Haller DL. The use of terbutaline for premature labor. *Drug Intell Clin Pharm*. 1980;14:757-764.
7. Ingemarsson I. Cardiovascular complications of terbutaline for preterm labor. *Am J Obstet Gynecol*. 1982;142:117.
8. Andersson KE, Bengtsson LP, Gustafson I, et al. The relaxing effect of terbutaline on the human uterus during term labor. *Am J Obstet Gynecol*. 1975; 121:602-609.
9. Ingermarrson I. Effect of terbutaline on premature labor. A double-blind placebo-controlled study. *Am J Obstet Gynecol*. 1976;125:520-524.
10. Ravindran R, Viegas OJ, Padilla LM, et al. Anesthetic considerations in pregnant patients receiving terbutaline therapy. *Anesth Analg (Cleve)*. 1980;59:391-392.
11. Katz M, Robertson PA, Creasy RK. Cardiovascular complications associated with terbutaline treatment for preterm labor. *Am J Obstet Gynecol*. 1981; 139:605-608.
12. Ingemarsson I, Bengtsson B. A five-year experience with terbutaline for preterm labor: low rate of severe side effects. *Obstet Gynecol*. 1985;66:176-180.
13. Benedetti TJ. Maternal complications of parenteral β-sympathomimetic therapy for premature labor. *Am J Obstet Gynecol*. 1983;145:1-6.
14. Vargas GC, Macedo GJ, Amved AR, Lowenberg FE. Terbutaline, a new uterine inhibitor. *Ginecol Obstet Mex*. 1974;36:75-88.
15. Epstein MF, Nicholls RN, Stubblefield PG. Neonatal hypoglycemia after beta-sympathomimetic tocolytic therapy. *J Pediatr*. 1979;94:449-453.
16. Westgren M, Carlsson C, Lindholm T, et al. Continuous maternal glucose measurements and fetal glucose and insulin levels after administration of terbutaline in term labor. *Acta Obstet Gynecol Scand*. 1982;108:63-65.
17. Main EK, Main DM, Gabbe SG. Chronic oral terbutaline tocolytic therapy is associated with maternal glucose intolerance. *Am J Obstet Gynecol*. 1987;157: 644-647.
18. Lenke RR, Trupin S. Sudden, unforeseen fetal death in a woman being treated for premature labor: a case report. *J Reprod Med*. 1984;29:872-874.
19. Fletcher SE, Fyfe DA, Case CL, et al. Myocardial necrosis in a newborn after long-term maternal subcutaneous terbutaline infusion for suppression of preterm labor. *Am J Obstet Gynecol*. 1991;165:1401-1404.
20. Queisser-Luft A, Eggers I, Stolz G, et al. Serial examination of 20,248 newborn fetuses and infants: correlations between drug exposure and major malformations. *Am J Med Genet*. 1996;63:268-276.
21. Suzuki M, Inagaki K, Kihira M, et al. Maternal liver impairment associated with prolonged high-dose administration of terbutaline for premature labor. *Obstet Gynecol*. 1985;66:14S-15S.
22. Bhat N, Seifer D, Hensleigh P. Paradoxical response to intravenous terbutaline. *Am J Obstet Gynecol*. 1985;153:310-311.

T

23. Tejani NA, Verma UL, Chatterjee S, Mittelmann S. Terbutaline in the management of acute intrapartum fetal acidosis. *J Reprod Med.* 1983;28:857-861.
24. Barrett JM. Fetal resuscitation with terbutaline during eclampsia-induced uterine hypertonus. *Am J Obstet Gynecol.* 1984;150:895.
25. Ingemarsson I, Arulkumaran S, Ratnam SS. Single injection of terbutaline in term labor. I. Effect on fetal pH in cases with prolonged bradycardia. *Am J Obstet Gynecol.* 1985;153:859-865.
26. Ingemarsson I, Arulkumaran S, Ratnam SS. Single injection of terbutaline in term labor. II. Effect on uterine activity. *Am J Obstet Gynecol.* 1985;153:865-869.
27. Mendez-Bauer C, Shekarloo A, Cook V, Freese U. Treatment of acute intrapartum fetal distress by β2-sympathomimetics. *Am J Obstet Gynecol.* 1987;156:638-642.
28. Stubblefield PG, Heyl PS. Treatment of premature labor with subcutaneous terbutaline. *Obstet Gynecol.* 1982;59:457-462.
29. Caritis SN, Carson D, Greebon D, et al. A comparison of terbutaline and ethanol in the treatment of preterm labor. *Am J Obstet Gynecol.* 1982; 142:183-190.
30. Kaul AF, Osathanondy R, Safon LE, et al. The management of preterm labor with the calcium channel–blocking agent nifedipine combined with the β-mimetic terbutaline. *Drug Intell Clin Pharm.* 1985;19:369-371.
31. O'Leary JA. Prophylactic tocolysis of twins. *Am J Obstet Gynecol.*1986;154: 904-905.
32. Arias F, Knight AB, Tomich PB. A retrospective study on the effects of steroid administration and prolongation of the latent phase in patients with preterm premature rupture of the membranes. *Am J Obstet Gynecol.* 1986; 154:1059-1063.
33. Bergman B, Hedner T. Antepartum administration of terbutaline and the incidence of hyaline membrane disease in preterm infants. *Acta Obstet Gynecol Scand.* 1978;57:217-221.
34. Wallace R, Caldwell D, Ansbacher R, Otterson W. Inhibition of premature labor by terbutaline. *Obstet Gynecol.* 1978;51:387-393.
35. Svenningsen NW. Follow-up studies on preterm infants after maternal β-receptor agonist treatment. *Acta Obstet Gynecol Scand Suppl.* 1982; 108:67-70.
36. Karlsson K, Krantz M, Hamberger L. Comparison of various β-mimetics on preterm labor, survival and development of the child. *J Perinat Med.* 1980;8:19-26.
37. Thorkelsson T, Loughead JL. Long-term subcutaneous terbutaline tocolysis: report of possible neonatal toxicity. *J Perinatol.* 1991;11:235-238.
38. Connors SL, Crowell DE, Eberhart CG, et al. Beta2-adrenergic receptor activation and genetic polymorphisms in autism: data from dizygotic twins. *J Clin Neurol.* 2005;20:876-884.
39. Witter FR, Zimmerman AW, Reichmann JP, Connors SL. In utero beta 2 adrenergic agonist exposure and adverse neurophysiologic and behavioral outcomes. *Am J Obstet Gynecol.* 2009;210:553-559.
40. Lonnerholm G, Lindstrom B. Terbutaline excretion into breast milk. *Br J Clin Pharmacol.* 1982;13:729-730.
41. Boreus LO, de Chateau P, Lindberg C, Nyberg L. Terbutaline in breast milk. *Br J Clin Pharmacol.* 1982;13:731-732.

TERCONAZOLE

Anti-Infective (Antifungal)

PREGNANCY RECOMMENDATION: Human Data and Animal Data Suggest Low Risk

BREASTFEEDING RECOMMENDATION: Probably Compatible

PREGNANCY SUMMARY

One report describing the use of terconazole in human pregnancy was located. From the Michigan Medicaid Surveillance study, 1,167 newborns had been exposed to terconazole during the first trimester. A total of 34 (2.9%) major birth defects were observed (47 expected). No pattern to the defects was seen. The drug will probably cross the placenta, so some fetal exposure will likely occur. Animal studies did not show any embryofetal toxicity in one species at doses of more than 10 times the intravaginal human dose. About 70% of the antifungal agent remained in the vaginal area after administration of a single suppository, and about 10% was systemically absorbed over 7 days. Using this drug during pregnancy should be based on the pros and cons of the mother's clinical need for treatment versus any potential fetal risk that might occur from exposure.

BREASTFEEDING SUMMARY

No reports describing the use of terconazole during human lactation have been located. The drug will likely be excreted into breast milk, so some infant exposure may occur. However, about 70% of the antifungal agent remained in the vaginal area after administration of a single suppository, and only about 10% was systemically absorbed over 7 days. Therefore, overall infant exposure is likely to be small. If the clinical decision is to use this drug while breastfeeding, the infant should be monitored for the most common reported adult side effect of headache (leading to irritability).

References

1. Prescribing Information. *Terconazole*. E. Fougera & Co. a division of Fougera Pharmaceuticals, Inc; 2021.
2. Centers for Disease Control and Prevention. *Sexually transmitted infections treatment guidelines, 2021. Vulvovaginal candidiasis (VVC)*. Accessed November 23, 2024. https://www.cdc.gov/std/treatment-guidelines/candidiasis.htm

TERIFLUNOMIDE

Immunologic (Pyrimidine Synthesis Inhibitor—Multiple Sclerosis)

PREGNANCY RECOMMENDATION: Limited Human Data—Animal Data Suggest Risk

BREASTFEEDING RECOMMENDATION: Potential Toxicity

T

PREGNANCY SUMMARY

Five reports describing the use of teriflunomide in human pregnancy were located. The manufacturer reports that there are over 150 prospectively collected teriflunomide pregnancy exposures. The rates of major malformations or spontaneous abortions were not increased with first-trimester exposure followed by an accelerated elimination procedure. No specific pattern of malformations has been identified in humans. However, limitations of this data include small numbers of reported pregnancies, short duration of exposure, and inability to control for confounders. The drug will probably cross the placenta, so some fetal exposure will likely occur. Therefore, this limited human pregnancy experience prevents a complete assessment of the embryofetal risk. Embryofetal toxicity with malformations was observed in two animal species at doses of less than 10 times the MRHD. Based on animal studies and the drug's mechanism of action, the manufacturer recommends that women with reproductive potential use effective contraception during treatment. Using this drug during pregnancy should be based on the pros and cons of the mother's clinical need for treatment versus any potential fetal risk that might occur from exposure. The manufacturer states that fetal risks are negligible with maternal plasma levels of less than 20 ng/mL. The drug carries a boxed warning for teratogenicity and embryolethality, as well as life-threatening liver injury, including acute liver failure requiring transplant.

BREASTFEEDING SUMMARY

No reports describing the use of teriflunomide during human lactation have been located. The drug will likely be excreted into breast milk, so some infant exposure will probably occur. Because of the severe toxicity that has occurred in adults taking the drug (severe hepatotoxicity, bone marrow depression, immunosuppression, etc), the manufacturer states that the drug should not be used by women who are nursing. Nevertheless, if the clinical decision is to use this drug while breastfeeding, the infant should be monitored for the most common reported adult side effects of headache and nausea (both leading to irritability), diarrhea, alopecia, and elevated liver enzyme levels.

References

1. Prescribing Information. *Teriflunomide*. Aurobindo Pharma Limited; 2024.
2. Kieseier B, Benamor M, Benzerdjeb H, Stuve O. Pregnancy outcomes from the teriflunomide clinical development programme: retrospective analysis of the teriflunomide clinical trial database. *Multi Scler*. 2012;18(suppl 4):P737. As cited by Lu E, Wang BW, Guimond C, et al. Safety of disease-modifying drugs for multiple sclerosis in pregnancy: current challenges and future considerations for effective pharmacovigilance. *Expert Rev Neurother*. 2013;13: 251-261.
3. Andersen JB, Moberg JY, Spelman T, Magyari M. Pregnancy outcomes in men and women treated with teriflunomide. A population-based nationwide Danish register study. *Front Immunol*. 2018;9:2706.
4. D'Aleo G, Rifici C, Donato A, et al. Twin pregnancy outcome following teriflunomide treatment in a relapsing-remitting multiple sclerosis patient: a case report. *Medicine*. 2020;99:e21212.
5. Vukusic S, Coyle PK, Jurgensen S, et al. Pregnancy outcomes in patients with multiple sclerosis treated with teriflunomide: clinical study data and 5 years of post-marketing experience. *Mult Scler*. 2020;26:829-836.
6. Platzbecker K, Wentzell N, Kollhorst B, Haug U. Fingolimod, teriflunomide and cladribine for the treatment of multiple sclerosis in women of childbearing age: description of drug utilization and exposed pregnancies in Germany. *Mult Scler Relat Disord*. 2022;67:104184.

TERLIPRESSIN

Endocrine (Pituitary Hormone)

PREGNANCY RECOMMENDATION: Limited Human Data—Animal Data Suggest Risk

BREASTFEEDING RECOMMENDATION: Probably Compatible

PREGNANCY SUMMARY

No reports describing the use of terlipressin in human pregnancy regarding teratogenesis have been located. Based on likely limited placental transfer, fetal exposure will probably be small. However, the absence of human pregnancy experience prevents a complete assessment of the embryofetal risk. The manufacturer described a small study that included patients receiving a single dose of terlipressin during the first trimester that resulted in uterine contractions and endometrial ischemia. Embryofetal toxicity was observed in animal studies. Using this drug during pregnancy should be based on the pros and cons of the mother's clinical need for treatment versus any potential fetal risk that might occur from exposure.

BREASTFEEDING SUMMARY

No reports describing the use of terlipressin during human lactation have been located. A limited amount of both drugs will probably be found in breast milk, so some infant exposure may occur. However, because it is a peptide, if the drug were to be ingested through breastfeeding, it would probably be digested in the infant's gastrointestinal tract and not be absorbed. Breastfeeding while using this drug should be based on the mother's clinical need for treatment. If used, the infant should be monitored for the most common reported adult side effects of abdominal pain and nausea (both leading to irritability), respiratory failure, diarrhea, and dyspnea.

Reference

1. Prescribing Information. *Terlivaz*. Mallinckrodt Company; 2023.

T

TESAMORELIN

Endocrine/Metabolic (Growth Hormone–Releasing Factor Analogue)

PREGNANCY RECOMMENDATION: *Contraindicated

BREASTFEEDING RECOMMENDATION: *Contraindicated

PREGNANCY SUMMARY

No reports describing the use of tesamorelin in human pregnancy have been located. Tesamorelin is not likely to cross the placenta in clinically significant amounts. However, because it consists of a protein, it is not known whether some fetal exposure could occur in the second half of gestation. Nevertheless, the absence of human pregnancy experience prevents a complete assessment of the embryofetal risk. Animal data showed embryofetal toxicity in one species at doses less than the RHD, but no embryofetal toxicity was seen in the second species at doses well above 10 times the RHD. *However, because of the approved use for the drug, tesamorelin is contraindicated for use in pregnancy. During human pregnancy, visceral adipose tissue increases due to normal hormonal and metabolic changes. Altering these changes with tesamorelin offers no known benefit and could result in fetal harm.

BREASTFEEDING SUMMARY

No reports describing the use of tesamorelin during human lactation have been located. The drug is not likely to be found in human breast milk in significant amounts. Moreover, any drug that might be in breast milk would most likely be digested in the infant's gastrointestinal tract and not be absorbed. *However, because the approved use for this drug is in patients with HIV, the manufacturer recommends not using it during breastfeeding due to the potential for HIV transmission, developing HIV resistance in patients with HIV, and possible adverse effects. In 2023, the updated US Department of Health and Human Services AIDS Info guidelines state that using replacement of breast milk through formula or pasteurized donor human breast milk from a milk bank eliminates the risk of postnatal HIV transmission to the infant. Using antiretroviral therapy to achieve and maintain viral suppression during pregnancy and postpartum decreases the risk for infant transmission to less than 1%, but notes that the risk is not zero. For patients not on therapy or those without viral load suppression during pregnancy (at a minimum of throughout the third trimester) and at delivery, replacement of breast milk is recommended. Patients on antiretroviral therapy who have a sustained undetectable viral load and who choose to breastfeed or use replacement of breast milk should be supported with this decision.

References

1. Prescribing Information. *Egrifta SV*. Theratechnologies, Inc; 2024.
2. Panel on Treatment of HIV During Pregnancy and Prevention of Perinatal Transmission. Recommendations for the use of antiretroviral drugs during pregnancy and interventions to reduce perinatal HIV transmission in the United States. Department of Health and Human Services. Accessed July 25, 2023. https://clinicalinfo.hiv.gov/en/guidelines/perinatal

TESTOSTERONE

Reproductive (Androgen)

PREGNANCY RECOMMENDATION: Contraindicated

BREASTFEEDING RECOMMENDATION: Contraindicated

PREGNANCY SUMMARY

Numerous case reports and series have been located that describe the use of testosterone during human pregnancy. From the Collaborative Perinatal Project, 10 testosterone/testosterone derivatives were used in the first trimester, and no major anomalies were identified. However, many other publications regarding pregnancy exposure describe clitoral hypertrophy, fused or partially fused labia, and, possibly, an absent vagina. These varying degrees of masculinization are referred to as nonadrenal female pseudohermaphroditism. Exposure to testosterone hormones at any gestational age is associated with clitoral hypertrophy. However, to cause labial-scrotal fusion, exposure must occur before the 10th or 11th fetal week when female differentiation of external genitalia is complete. Other than these genital abnormalities, testosterone and its derivatives do not appear to cause structural defects, though the numbers are very limited. The drug crosses the placenta, so fetal exposure will occur. Embryofetal toxicity was observed in five animal species at doses approximately equal to the RHD used for testosterone replacement therapy. Testosterone and its derivatives are contraindicated at any time during pregnancy.

BREASTFEEDING SUMMARY

Testosterone has been shown to be excreted into human breast milk. Therefore, fetal exposure will occur. The manufacturer recommends that women should not breastfeed while being treated with this drug. If the clinical decision is to use this drug while breastfeeding, the infant should be monitored for the most common reported adult side effects of headache (leading to irritability), hypertension, acne, and various abnormal laboratory tests (see PI).

References

1. Product Information. *Testosterone Gel, 1%*. Encube Ethicals Private Limited; 2024.
2. Product Information. *Depo-Testosterone*. Pharmacia and Upjohn Company LLC; 2020.
3. Product Information. *Jatenzo*. Tolmar, Inc; 2023.
4. Product Information. *Testosterone*. Deseret Biologicals, Inc; 2024.
5. Product Information. *Testosterone*. Zoe Processing; 2019.
6. Product Information. *Natesto Nasal Gel*. Acerus Pharmaceuticals Corporation; 2021.
7. Product Information. *Testopel*. Endo USA, Inc; 2024.
8. Product Information. *Xyosted*. Antares Pharma, Inc; 2023.
9. Grumbach MM, Ducharme JR. The effects of androgens on fetal sexual development. *Fertil Steril*. 1960;11:157-180.
10. Hayles AB, Nolan RB. Female pseudohermaphroditism: report of case in an infant born of a mother receiving methyltestosterone during pregnancy. *Proc Staff Meet Mayo Clin*. 1957;32:41-44.
11. Zander J, Muller HA. Uber die methylandrosteniolbehandlung wahrend emer schwangerschaft. *Geburtschilfe Frauenheilkd*. 1953;13:216-224. As cited by Schardein JL. Chemically Induced Birth Defects. 3rd ed. Marcel Dekker; 2000:286.
12. Hoffman F, Overzier C, Uhde G. Zur frage der hormonanlen frzeugung fataler zwittenbildungen beim menschen. *Geburtschilfe Frauenheilkd*. 1955;15:1061-1070. As cited by Schardein JL. Chemically Induced Birth Defects. 3rd ed. Marcel Dekker; 2000:286.
13. Grunwaldt E, Bates T. Nonadrenal female pseudohermaphrodism after administration of testosterone to mother during pregnancy. *Pediatrics*. 1957; 20:503-505.
14. Nellhaus G. Artificially induced female pseudohermaphroditism. *N Engl J Med*. 1958;258:935-938.
15. Gold AP, Michael AF Jr. Testosterone-induced female pseudrohermaphrodism. *J Pediatr*. 1958;52:279-283.
16. Moncrieff A. Non-adrenal female pseudohermaphroditism associated with hormone administration in pregnancy. *Lancet*. 1958;2:267-268.
17. Black JA, Bentley JFR. Effect on the foetus of androgens given during pregnancy. *Lancet*. 1959;1:21-24.
18. Dewhurst CJ, Gordon RR. Change of sex. *Lancet*. 1963;2:1213-1216.
19. Reschini E, Giustina G, D'Alberton A, Candiani GB. Female pseudohermaphroditism due to maternal androgen administration: 25-year follow-up. *Lancet*. 1985;1:1226.
20. Dewhurst J, Gordon RR. Fertility following change of sex: a follow-up. *Lancet*. 1984;2:1461-1462.
21. Bisset WH, Bain AD, Gauld IK. Female pseudo-hermaphrodite presenting with bilateral cryptorchidism. *Br Med J*. 1966;1:279-280.
22. Martinie-Dubousquet J. Embryopathy entailed by administration of sex hormones to the mother. *Rev Pathol Gen Comp*. 1953;53:1065-1076. As cited by Schardein JL. Chemically Induced Birth Defects. 3rd ed. Marcel Dekker; 2000:289.
23. Heinonen OP, Slone D, Shapiro S. *Birth Defects and Drugs in Pregnancy*. Publishing Sciences Group, 1977:389-390.
24. Oberhelman-Eaton S, Chang A, Gonzalez C, et al. Initiation of gender-affirming testosterone therapy in a lactating transgender man. *J Hum Lact*. 2022;38:339-343.
25. MacDonald T, Noel-Weiss J, West D, et al. Transmasculine individuals' experiences with lactation, chestfeeding, and gender identity: a qualitative study. *BMC Pregnancy Childbirth*. 2016;16:106.

TETRABENAZINE

Central Nervous System (Vesicular Monoamine Transporter 2 Inhibitor)

PREGNANCY RECOMMENDATION: Limited Human Data—Animal Data Suggest Potential Risk

BREASTFEEDING RECOMMENDATION: Potential Toxicity

PREGNANCY SUMMARY

One report describing the use of tetrabenazine in human pregnancy was located. The drug was started in the late second trimester. No drug-induced fetal or newborn effects were observed. Tetrabenazine and its three active metabolites are likely to cross the placenta, so some fetal exposure will probably occur. However, the limited human pregnancy experience prevents a complete assessment of embryofetal risk. Embryofetal toxicity was observed in one animal species at doses less than the MRHD, but no embryofetal toxicity was seen in a second species at doses of more than 10 times the MRHD. Using this drug during pregnancy should be based on the pros and cons of the mother's clinical need for treatment versus any potential fetal risk that might occur from exposure. Tetrabenazine can prolong the QTc interval.

T

BREASTFEEDING SUMMARY

No reports describing the use of tetrabenazine during human lactation have been located. The drug and its three active metabolites will likely be excreted into breast milk, so some infant exposure will probably occur. Breastfeeding while using this drug should be based on the mother's clinical need for treatment versus any potential infant risks that might occur. If used, the infant should be monitored for the most common reported adult side effects of anxiety and nausea (both leading to irritability), sedation/somnolence, fatigue (lethargy), and sleeping disorders.

References

1. Prescribing Information. *Tetrabenazine*. Ajanta Pharma USA, Inc; 2021.
2. Lubbe WF, Walker EB. Chorea gravidarum associated with circulating lupus anticoagulant: successful outcome of pregnancy with prednisone and aspirin therapy. Case report. *Br J Obstet Gynaecol*. 1983;90:487-490.

TETRACAINE

Anesthetic (Local Anesthetic)

PREGNANCY RECOMMENDATION: Limited Human Data and No Relevant Animal Data

BREASTFEEDING RECOMMENDATION: Probably Compatible

PREGNANCY SUMMARY

There are three publications describing the use of tetracaine during human pregnancy. One publication described one major anomaly in 23 first-trimester exposures. The other two publications described the use of the drug near delivery for anesthesia purposes. No adverse fetal effects were seen with use of the drug. The drug will likely cross the placenta, so some fetal exposure will occur. However, the elimination half-life is extremely short, so most exposures will probably be clinically insignificant. However, the limited human pregnancy experience prevents a complete assessment of embryofetal risk. No animal reproductive studies have been conducted. Using this drug during pregnancy should be based on the pros and cons of the mother's clinical need for treatment versus any potential fetal risk that might occur from exposure.

BREASTFEEDING SUMMARY

No reports describing the use of tetracaine during human lactation have been located. The drug might be excreted into breast milk, but the extremely rapid metabolism would suggest that any exposure is probably clinically insignificant. Breastfeeding while using this drug should be based on the mother's clinical need for treatment versus any potential infant risks that might occur. Due to the short systemic effect, clinical side effects were not evaluated.

References

1. Prescribing Information. *Tetracaine HCl*. BPI Labs LLC; 2024.
2. Prescribing Information. *Tetracaine*. Bellus Medical LLC; 2024.
3. National Library of Medicine. *Pubchem*. Tetracaine. Accessed November 29, 2024. https://pubchem.ncbi.nlm.nih.gov/compound/Tetracaine
4. Heinonen OP, Slone D, Shapiro S. *Birth Defects and Drugs in Pregnancy*. Publishing Sciences Group; 1977.
5. Datta S, Ostheimer GW, Weiss JB, et al. Neonatal effect of prolonged anesthetic induction for cesarean section. *Obstet Gynecol*. 1981;58:331-335.
6. Kavanagh T, Dube A, Albert A, Gunka V. A randomized controlled trial comparing Ametop™ with placebo for reducing pain associated with local anesthetic skink infiltration before neuraxial anesthesia in parturient. *Int J Obstet Anesth*. 2016;27:41-45.

TETRACAINE OPHTHALMIC

Ophthalmic/Anesthetic (Topical)

PREGNANCY RECOMMENDATION: No Human Data and No Relevant Animal Data

BREASTFEEDING RECOMMENDATION: Probably Compatible

PREGNANCY SUMMARY

No reports describing the use of tetracaine ophthalmic in human pregnancy have been located. The drug is not likely to cross the placenta in clinically significant amounts. However, the absence of human pregnancy experience prevents a complete assessment of embryofetal risk. No animal reproduction or fertility studies have been conducted. Using this drug during pregnancy should be based on the pros and cons of the mother's clinical need for treatment versus any potential fetal risk that might occur from exposure. If used during pregnancy, consider placing pressure over the tear duct in the corner of the eye for at least 1 minute, and then remove any excess solution with absorbent tissue to decrease the amount of drug reaching the systemic circulation even further.

BREASTFEEDING SUMMARY

No reports describing the use of tetracaine ophthalmic during human lactation have been located. The drug may be excreted into breast milk, if found in the systemic circulation. However, any amount is likely to be clinically insignificant due to the topical ocular use of the drug. A method to decrease some systemic absorption with ophthalmic use is described above in the Pregnancy Summary.

Reference

1. Prescribing Information. *Tetracaine hydrochloride*. Bausch Health US LLC; 2020.

TETRACYCLINE

Antibacterial (Tetracycline)

PREGNANCY RECOMMENDATION: *Contraindicated

BREASTFEEDING RECOMMENDATION: Potential Toxicity

PREGNANCY SUMMARY

Numerous publications have been located describing the use of tetracycline in human pregnancy. From three large studies, there were 60 (3.9%) major malformations identified in 1,538 first-trimester exposures. No pattern to the defects was seen. However, tetracyclines are a class of antibiotics that should be used with extreme caution, if at all, in pregnancy. These agents can cause permanent tooth discoloration and bone stippling that can lead to bone weakening and possibly bone growth. This occurs primarily in the second half of gestation, but fetal tooth and bone development in the fetus starts around 8 to 10 weeks of gestation. The drug crosses the placenta, so some fetal exposure will occur. Animal reproduction studies have not been conducted. The drug also poses a risk for tetracycline-induced hepatotoxicity that can be fatal in some cases. It is similar to but different from fatty liver of pregnancy. The manufacturer reports that the tetracycline class drugs may cause permanent tooth discoloration (yellow-gray-brown) and enamel hypoplasia when used during pregnancy up to 8 years of age. This is more common with long-term use but has been observed with repeated short-term courses. *Unless used for anthrax or infections where other antibiotics are not likely to be effective or are contraindicated, tetracycline medications should not be used during pregnancy or early childhood, if at all possible.

BREASTFEEDING SUMMARY

Tetracycline has been shown to be excreted into human breast milk in low concentrations. Theoretically, dental staining and inhibition of bone growth could occur in breastfed infants whose mothers were consuming tetracycline. However, this theoretical possibility seems small because tetracycline serum levels in infants exposed in such a manner were undetectable (LLQ of 50 ng/mL). However, due to a concern for potential serious adverse effects that might be seen in a breastfed infant, the manufacturer recommends that women not breastfeed while being treated with this drug. Nevertheless, if the clinical decision is to use this drug during lactation, the infant should be monitored for the most common adult side effects of nausea, and epigastric pain (both leading to irritability), anorexia (monitor infant growth), vomiting, diarrhea, black hairy tongue, Candida overgrowth, rash, and various laboratory abnormalities (see PI).

References

1. Prescribing Information. *Tetracycline hydrochloride*. Amneal Pharmaceuticals NY LLC; 2023.
2. Tetracycline. *Lexi-Drugs*. UpToDate Lexidrug. UpToDate, Inc. Accessed November 29, 2024. https://online.lexi.com
3. Guilbeau JA, Schoenbach EG, Schaub IG, Latham DV. Aureomycin in obstetrics: therapy and prophylaxis. *JAMA*. 1950;143:520-526.
4. Charles D. Placental transmission of antibiotics. *J Obstet Gynaecol Br Emp*. 1954;61:750-757.
5. Gibbons RJ, Reichelderfer TE. Transplacental transmission of demethylchlortetracycline and toxicity studies in premature and full term, newly born infants. *Antibiot Med Clin Ther*. 1960;7:618-622.
6. Posner AC, Prigot A, Konicoff NG. Further observations on the use of tetracycline hydrochloride in prophylaxis and treatment of obstetric infections. In: *Antibiotics Annual, 1954-55*. Medical Encyclopedia; 1955:594-598.
7. Posner AC, Konicoff NG, Prigot A. Tetracycline in obstetric infections. In: *Antibiotics Annual, 1955-56*. Medical Encyclopedia; 1956:345-348.
8. Cohlan SQ, Bevelander G, Bross S. Effect of tetracycline on bone growth in the premature infant. *Antimicrob Agents Chemother*. 1961:340-347.
9. Harcourt JK, Johnson NW, Storey E. In vivo incorporation of tetracycline in the teeth of man. *Arch Oral Biol*. 1962;7:431-437.
10. Rendle-Short TJ. Tetracycline in teeth and bone. *Lancet*. 1962;1:1188.
11. Douglas AC. The deposition of tetracycline in human nails and teeth: a complication of long term treatment. *Br J Dis Chest*. 1963;57:44-47.
12. Kutscher AH, Zegarelli EV, Tovell HM, Hochberg B. Discoloration of teeth induced by tetracycline. *JAMA*. 1963;184:586-587.
13. Kline AH, Blattner RJ, Lunin M. Transplacental effect of tetracyclines on teeth. *JAMA*. 1964;188:178-180.
14. Macaulay JC, Leistyna JA. Preliminary observations on the prenatal administration of demethylchlortetracycline HCl. *Pediatrics*. 1964;34:423-424.
15. Stewart DJ. The effects of tetracyclines upon the dentition. *Br J Dermatol*. 1964;76:374-378.
16. Swallow JN. Discoloration of primary dentition after maternal tetracycline ingestion in pregnancy. *Lancet*. 1964;2:611-612.
17. Porter PJ, Sweeney EA, Golan H, Kass EH. Controlled study of the effect of prenatal tetracycline on primary dentition. *Antimicrob Agents Chemother*. 1965;5:668-671.
18. Toaff R, Ravid R. Tetracyclines and the teeth. *Lancet*. 1966;2:281-282.
19. Kutscher AH, Zegarelli EV, Tovell HM, et al. Discoloration of deciduous teeth induced by administrations of tetracycline antepartum. *Am J Obstet Gynecol*. 1966;96:291-292.
20. Brearley LJ, Stragis AA, Storey E. Tetracycline-induced tooth changes. Part 1. Prevalence in preschool children. *Med J Aust*. 1968;2:653-658.
21. Brearley LJ, Storey E. Tetracycline-induced tooth changes. Part 2. Prevalence, localization and nature of staining in extracted deciduous teeth. *Med J Aust*. 1968;2:714-719.
22. Baker KL, Storey E. Tetracycline-induced tooth changes. Part 3. Incidence in extracted first permanent molar teeth. *Med J Aust*. 1970;1:109-113.
23. Anthony JR. Effect on deciduous and permanent teeth of tetracycline deposition in utero. *Postgrad Med*. 1970;48:165-168.
24. Genot MT, Golan HP, Porter PJ, Kass EH. Effect of administration of tetracycline in pregnancy on the primary dentition of the offspring. *J Oral Med*. 1970;25:75-79.
25. Schultz JC, Adamson JS Jr, Workman WW, Normal TD. Fatal liver disease after intravenous administration of tetracycline in high dosage. *N Engl J Med*. 1963;269:999-1004.
26. Bruno M, Ober WB. Clinicopathologic conference: jaundice at the end of pregnancy. *NY State J Med*. 1962;62:3792-3800.
27. Lewis PL, Takeda M, Warren MJ. Obstetric acute yellow atrophy. Report of a case. *Obstet Gynecol*. 1963;22:121-127.
28. Briggs RC. Tetracycline and liver disease. *N Engl J Med*. 1963;269:1386.
29. Leonard GL. Tetracycline and liver disease. *N Engl J Med*. 1963;269:1386.
30. Gough GS, Searcy RL. Additional case of fatal liver disease with tetracycline therapy. *N Engl J Med*. 1964;270:157-158.
31. Whalley PJ, Adams RH, Combes B. Tetracycline toxicity in pregnancy. *JAMA*. 1964;189:357-362.

T

32. Kunelis CT, Peters JL, Edmondson HA. Fatty liver of pregnancy and its relationship to tetracycline therapy. *Am J Med*. 1965;38:359-377.
33. Lew HT, French SW. Tetracycline nephrotoxicity and nonoliguric acute renal failure. *Arch Intern Med*. 1966;118:123-128.
34. Meihoff WE, Pasquale DN, Jacoby WJ Jr. Tetracycline-induced hepatic coma, with recovery. A report of a case. *Obstet Gynecol*. 1967;29:260-265.
35. Aach R, Kissane J. Clinicopathologic conference: a seventeen year old girl with fatty liver of pregnancy following tetracycline therapy. *Am J Med*. 1967;43:274-283.
36. Whalley PJ, Martin FG, Adams RH, Combes B. Disposition of tetracycline by pregnant women with acute pyelonephritis. *Obstet Gynecol*. 1970;36:821-826.
37. Pride GL, Cleary RE, Hamburger RJ. Disseminated intravascular coagulation associated with tetracycline-induced hepatorenal failure during pregnancy. *Am J Obstet Gynecol*. 1973;115:585-586.
38. Wenk RE, Gebhardt FC, Behagavan BS, et al. Tetracycline-associated fatty liver of pregnancy, including possible pregnancy risk after chronic dermatologic use of tetracycline. *J Reprod Med*. 1981;26:135-141.
39. King TM, Bowe ET, D'Esopo DA. Toxic effects of the tetracyclines. *Bull Sloane Hosp Women*. 1964;10:35-41.
40. Kaplan MM. Acute fatty liver of pregnancy. *N Engl J Med*. 1985;313:367-370.
41. Allen ES, Brown WE. Hepatic toxicity of tetracycline in pregnancy. *Am J Obstet Gynecol*. 1966;95:12-18.
42. Heinonen O, Slone D, Shapiro S. *Birth Defects and Drugs in Pregnancy*. Publishing Sciences Group; 1977.
43. Wilson F. Congenital defects in the newborn. *Br Med J*. 1962;2:255.
44. Carter MP, Wilson F. Tetracycline and congenital limb abnormalities. *Br Med J*. 1962;2:407-408.
45. Mennie AT. Tetracycline and congenital limb abnormalities. *Br Med J*. 1962;2:480.
46. Harley JD, Farrar JF, Gray JB, Dunlop IC. Aromatic drugs and congenital cataracts. *Lancet*. 1964;1:472.
47. Corcoran R, Castles JM. Tetracycline for acne vulgaris and possible teratogenesis. *Br Med J*. 1977;2:807-808.
48. Horne HW Jr, Kundsin RB. The role of mycoplasma among 81 consecutive pregnancies: a prospective study. *Int J Fertil*. 1980;25:315-317.
49. Coppes JB. Bubonic plague in pregnancy. *J Reprod Med*. 1980;25:91-95.
50. Czeizel AE, Rockenbauer M. Teratogenic study of doxycycline. *Obstet Gynecol*. 1997;89:524-528.
51. Cooper WO, Hernandez-Diaz S, Arbogast PG, et al. Antibiotics potentially used in response to bioterrorism and the risk of major congenital malformations. *Paediatr Perinat Epidemiol*. 2009;23:18-28.
52. Czeizel AE, Rockenbauer M. A population-based case-control teratologic study of oral oxytetracycline treatment during pregnancy. *Eur J Obstet Gynecol Reprod Biol*. 2000;88:27-33.
53. Nakitanda AO, Odsbu I, Cesta CE, et al. First trimester tetracycline exposed and risk of major congenital malformations. *JAMA Netw Open*. 2024;7:e2445055.
54. Briggs M. Tetracycline and steroid hormone binding to human spermatozoa. *Acta Endocrinol*. 1974;75:785-792.
55. Knowles JA. Drugs in milk. *Pediatr Curr*. 1972;21:28-32.
56. Graf VH, Reimann S. Untersuchungen uber die Konzentration von Pyrrolidino-methyl-tetracycline in der Muttermilch. *Dtsch Med Wochenschr*. 1959;84:1694.
57. Hunt MJ, Salisbury ELC, Grace J, Armati R. Black breast milk due to minocycline therapy. *Br J Dermatol*. 1996;134:943-944.

TETRAHYDROZOLINE OPHTHALMIC

Ophthalmic (α-Agonist—Topical)

PREGNANCY RECOMMENDATION: No Human Data and No Relevant Animal Data

BREASTFEEDING RECOMMENDATION: Probably Compatible

PREGNANCY SUMMARY

No reports describing the use of tetrahydrozoline ophthalmic in human pregnancy have been located. The drug is likely to cross the placenta, but the low systemic absorption after ocular administration suggests that the amount is likely to be minimal. However, the absence of human pregnancy experience prevents a complete assessment of embryofetal risk. No animal reproduction or fertility studies have been conducted. Using this drug during pregnancy should be based on the pros and cons of the mother's clinical need for treatment versus any potential fetal risk that might occur from exposure. If used during pregnancy, consider placing pressure over the tear duct in the corner of the eye for at least 1 minute, and then remove any excess solution with absorbent tissue to decrease the amount of drug reaching the systemic circulation even further.

BREASTFEEDING SUMMARY

No reports describing the use of tetrahydrozoline ophthalmic during human lactation have been located. The drug will likely be excreted into breast milk if present in the systemic circulation. However, the amount should be minimal due to the low absorption following topical ocular use. A method to decrease some systemic absorption with ophthalmic use is described above in the Pregnancy Summary.

References

1. Tetrahydrozoline (ophthalmic). *Lexi-Drugs*. UpToDate Lexidrug. UpToDate, Inc. Accessed November 30, 2024. https://online.lexi.com
2. National Library of Medicine—Pubchem. *Tetrahydrozoline*. Accessed November 30, 2024. https://pubchem.ncbi.nlm.nih.gov/compound/Tetrahydrozoline
3. Prescribing Information. *Careall eyedrop original*. New World Imports, Inc; 2024.

TEZACAFTOR/IVACAFTOR

Genetic (Cystic Fibrosis)

PREGNANCY RECOMMENDATION: No Human Data—Animal Data Suggest Low Risk

BREASTFEEDING RECOMMENDATION: Probably Compatible

PREGNANCY SUMMARY

No reports describing the use of tezacaftor and ivacaftor in human pregnancy have been located. Both drugs will probably cross the placenta, so some fetal exposure will likely occur for both agents. However, the absence of human pregnancy experience prevents a complete assessment of the embryofetal risk. Animal studies did not show any embryofetal toxicity for either drug. Because cystic fibrosis is a chronic, debilitating genetic disorder, this drug should not be withheld because of pregnancy.

BREASTFEEDING SUMMARY

Tezacaftor and ivacaftor are probably excreted into human breast milk. Breastfeeding while using this drug should be based on the mother's clinical need for treatment. If used, the infant should be monitored for the most common reported adult side effects of headache and nausea (both leading to irritability) and nasal congestion.

Reference

1. Prescribing Information. *Symdeko*. Vertex Pharmaceuticals, Inc; 2018.

TEZEPELUMAB

Respiratory (Monoclonal Antibody)

PREGNANCY RECOMMENDATION: No Human Data—Animal Data Suggest Low Risk

BREASTFEEDING RECOMMENDATION: Probably Compatible

PREGNANCY SUMMARY

No reports describing the use of tezepelumab in human pregnancy have been located. As an IgG antibody, the drug will likely cross the placenta at least during the second half of pregnancy, so some fetal exposure will probably occur. Therefore, the absence of human pregnancy experience prevents a complete assessment of the embryofetal risk. The animal data did not show any embryofetal toxicity. Using this drug during pregnancy should be based on the pros and cons of the mother's clinical need for treatment versus any potential fetal risk that might occur from exposure.

BREASTFEEDING SUMMARY

No reports describing the use of tezepelumab during human lactation have been located. It is known that IgG antibodies can be found in human breast milk, but are not found in the neonatal or infant circulation. Additionally, if any IgG antibodies were to be ingested through breastfeeding, they would probably be digested in the infant's gastrointestinal tract and not be absorbed. Breastfeeding while using this drug should be based on the mother's clinical need for treatment. If used, the infant should be monitored for the most common reported adult side effects of arthralgia and back pain (both leading to irritability) and pharyngitis.

Reference

1. Prescribing Information. *Tezspire*. Amgen, Inc and AstraZeneca AB; 2021.

THALIDOMIDE

Immunologic (Multiple Myeloma/Erythema Nodosum Leprosum)

PREGNANCY RECOMMENDATION: Contraindicated (Mainly First Trimester)

BREASTFEEDING RECOMMENDATION: Potential Toxicity

PREGNANCY SUMMARY

Thalidomide is a well-known potent human teratogen. It was introduced into clinical medicine in West Germany in 1956. Although a wide range of indications was promoted for the drug, it was primarily used as a sedative and an antinausea agent. However, it became apparent over time that it could produce serious defects of the limbs, digits, head, face, eyes, ears, tongue, teeth, and in some cases the CNS, cardiac, gastrointestinal tract, and genitourinary tract. Because of these findings, thalidomide was withdrawn from the market in most countries in late 1961. However, it is now available as an immunomodulatory agent approved for oral use in combination with dexamethasone for the treatment of newly diagnosed multiple myeloma. It can also be used in the acute treatment of the cutaneous manifestations of moderate to severe erythema nodosum leprosum (a cutaneous manifestation of leprosy). The critical period of exposure is about 5 to 7 weeks' gestation (after the first day of the last menstrual period) or about 20 to 36 days postconception. The drug is contraindicated in pregnancy. It carries a boxed warning for this embryofetal toxicity, as well as venous thromboembolism. This medication is only available through a Risk Evaluation and Mitigation Strategies (REMS) program. There is a very strict protocol that should be followed if using thalidomide in women that have reproductive potential. Women should use two methods of reliable birth control simultaneously: tubal ligation, intrauterine device (IUD), hormonal birth control pills, vaginal rings, or implants; or a partner's vasectomy with one additional effective contraceptive method (male latex or synthetic condom, female diaphragm, or cervical cap). Contraception must begin 4 weeks prior to initiating therapy. The woman must have two negative pregnancy tests before initiating thalidomide. The first test should be performed within 10 to 14 days, and the second test within 24 hours prior to prescribing thalidomide. Once treatment has started and during dose interruptions, pregnancy testing for females of reproductive potential should occur weekly during the first 4 weeks of use, then pregnancy testing can be repeated every 4 weeks in females with regular menstrual cycles. If menstrual cycles are irregular, the pregnancy testing should occur every 2 weeks. Contraception should continue for at least 4 weeks after completing therapy. Pregnancy testing and counseling should be performed if a patient misses her period or if there is any abnormality in her menstrual bleeding. Thalidomide treatment must be discontinued during this evaluation. Thalidomide is present in the semen of males who take thalidomide. Therefore, males must always use a latex or synthetic condom during any sexual contact with females of reproductive potential, even if they have undergone a successful vasectomy. Male patients taking thalidomide must not donate sperm. There is a pregnancy exposure registry that monitors pregnancy outcomes in women exposed to thalidomide during pregnancy, as well as female partners of male patients who are exposed to thalidomide. This registry is also used to understand the root cause of the pregnancy. Report any suspected fetal exposure to thalidomide to the US Food and Drug Administration (FDA) via the MedWatch program at 800-FDA-1088 and to the REMS Call Center at 888-423-5436.

BREASTFEEDING SUMMARY

No reports describing the use of thalidomide during human lactation have been located. The drug will likely be excreted into breast milk, so some infant exposure will probably occur. However, due to a concern for potential serious adverse effects that might be seen in a breastfed infant, the manufacturer recommends that women not breastfeed while being treated with this drug and for at least 1 week after the last dose. Nevertheless, if the clinical decision is to use this drug while breastfeeding, the infant should be monitored for the most common reported adult side effects of nausea, agitation, dizziness, and neuropathy (all leading to irritability), fatigue (lethargy), peripheral edema, constipation, rash/desquamation, anorexia (monitor infant growth), tremor, fever, and various laboratory abnormalities (see PI).

References

1. Prescribing Information. *Thalomid*. Celegene Corporation; 2023.
2. Mellin GW, Katzenstein M. The saga of thalidomide. Neuropathy to embryopathy, with case reports of congenital anomalies. *N Engl J Med*. 1962; 267:1184-1193.
3. Mellin GW, Katzenstein M. The saga of thalidomide (concluded). Neuropathy to embryopathy, with case reports of congenital anomalies. *N Engl J Med*. 1962;267:1238-1244.
4. Taussig HB. A study of the German outbreak of phocomelia. *JAMA*. 1962;180:1106-1114.
5. Nowack E. The sensitive period of thalidomide embryopathy (in German). *Humangenetik*. 1965;1:516-536.
6. Smithells RW. The thalidomide legacy. *Proc R Soc Med*. 1965;58:491-492.
7. Newman CGH. Clinical observations on the thalidomide syndrome. *Proc R Soc Med*. 1977;70:225-227.
8. Newman CGH. Teratogen update: clinical aspects of thalidomide embryopathy—a continuing preoccupation. *Teratology*. 1985;32:133-144.
9. Newman CGH. The thalidomide syndrome: risks of exposure and spectrum of malformations. *Clin Perinatol*. 1986;13:555-573.
10. Miller MT, Stromland K. Teratogen update: thalidomide: a review, with focus on ocular findings and new potential uses. *Teratology*. 1999;60:306-321.
11. Brent RL, Holmes LB. Clinical and basic science lessons from the thalidomide tragedy: what have we learned about the causes of limb defects? *Teratology*. 1988;38:241-251.
12. Lenz W. A short history of thalidomide embryopathy. *Teratology*. 1988; 38:203-215.
13. Hayman DJ. Distaval. *Lancet*. 1961;2:1262.
14. Lenz W. Thalidomide and congenital abnormalities. *Lancet*. 1962;1:45.
15. McBride WG. Thalidomide and congenital abnormalities. *Lancet*. 1961;2: 1358.
16. Pfeiffer RA, Kosenow W. Thalidomide and congenital abnormalities. *Lancet*. 1962;1:45-46.
17. Jones EE, Williamson DAJ. Thalidomide and congenital abnormalities. *Lancet*. 1962;1:222.
18. Burley DM. Thalidomide and congenital abnormalities. *Lancet*. 1962;1:271.
19. Lenz W. Thalidomide and congenital abnormalities. *Lancet*. 1962;1:271-272.
20. Speirs AL. Thalidomide and congenital abnormalities. *Lancet*. 1962;1:303-305.
21. Anonymous. Thalidomide and congenital malformations. *Lancet*. 1962;1: 307-308.
22. Kohler HG, Fisher AM, Dunn PM. Thalidomide and congenital abnormalities. *Lancet*. 1962;1:326.
23. Willman A, Dumoulin JG. Thalidomide ("Distaval") and foetal abnormalities. *Br Med J*. 1962;1:477.
24. Pliess G. Thalidomide and congenital abnormalities. *Lancet*. 1962;1: 1128-1129.
25. Rodin AE, Koller LA, Taylor JD. Association of thalidomide (Kevadon) with congenital anomalies. *Can Med Assoc J*. 1962;86:744-746.
26. Smithells RW. Thalidomide and malformations in Liverpool. *Lancet*. 1962;1:1270-1273.
27. Kajii T. Thalidomide and congenital deformities. *Lancet*. 1962;2:151.
28. Leck IM, Millar ELM. Incidence of malformations since the introduction of thalidomide. *Br Med J*. 1962;2:16-20.
29. Jacobs J. Drugs and foetal abnormalities. *Br Med J*. 1962;2:407.
30. Pfeiffer RA, Nessel E. Multiple congenital abnormalities. *Lancet*. 1962;2:349-350.
31. Ward SP. Thalidomide and congenital abnormalities. *Br Med J*. 1962;2: 646-647.
32. Knapp K, Lenz W, Nowack E. Multiple congenital abnormalities. *Lancet*. 1962;2:725.
33. Owen R, Smith A. Cor triloculare and thalidomide. *Lancet*. 1962;2:836.
34. Rosendal T. Thalidomide and aplasia-hypoplasia of the otic labyrinth. *Lancet*. 1963;1:724-725.
35. Kajii T, Goto M. Cleft lip and palate after thalidomide. *Lancet*. 1963;2: 151-152.
36. McBride WG. The teratogenic action of drugs. *Med J Aust*. 1963;2:689-693.
37. Cullen JF. Ocular defects in thalidomide babies. *Br J Ophthalmol*. 1964;48: 151-153.
38. Cant JS. Minor ocular abnormalities associated with thalidomide. *Lancet*. 1966;1:1134.

T

39. Fogh-Andersen P. Thalidomide and congenital cleft deformities. *Acta Chir Scand*. 1966;131:197-200.
40. Kajii T, Kida M, Takahashi K. The effect of thalidomide intake during 113 human pregnancies. *Teratology*. 1973;8:163-166.
41. Murphy R, Mohr P. Two congenital neurological abnormalities caused by thalidomide. *Br Med J*. 1977;2:1191.
42. Stainsby GD, Quibell EP. Perthes-like changes in the hips of children with thalidomide deformities. *Lancet*. 1967;2:242-243.
43. Smithells RW. Thalidomide, absent appendix, and sweating. *Lancet*. 1978;1:1042.
44. Bremner DN, Mooney G. Agenesis of appendix: a further thalidomide anomaly. *Lancet*. 1978;1:826.
45. McBride WG. Excessive sweating and reduction deformities. *Lancet*. 1978; 1:826.
46. McBride WG. Another, late thalidomide abnormality. *Lancet*. 1981;2:368.
47. Gollop TR, Eigier A, Guidugli-Neto J. Prenatal diagnosis of thalidomide syndrome. *Prenat Diag*. 1987;7:295-298.
48. Hagen EO. Congenital malformations in a thalidomide baby: a postmortem anatomical study. *Can Med Assoc J*. 1965;92:283-286.
49. Hammarstrom L, Henrikson CO, Larsson KS. Anomalies of the teeth in a child with upper phocomelia. Report of a case. *Oral Surg*. 1970;29:191-196.
50. Shand JEG, Bremner DN. Agenesis of the vermiform appendix in a thalidomide child. *Br J Surg*. 1977;64:203-204.
51. Axrup K, d'Avignon M, Hellgren K, et al. Children with thalidomide embryopathy: odontologic observations and aspects. *Dental Digest*. 1966;72:403-405, 425.
52. Ruffing L. Evaluation of thalidomide children. *Birth Defects Orig Article Series*. 1977;13:287-300.
53. Lenz W, Knapp K. Thalidomide embryopathy. *Arch Environ Health*. 1962;5: 100-105.
54. Lenz W. Malformations caused by drugs in pregnancy. *Am J Dis Child*. 1966;112:99-106.
55. Lenz W. How can the teratogenic action of a factor be established in man? *South Med J*. 1971;64(suppl 1):41-47.
56. Tabuchi A, Yamada A, Umisa H, et al. Phocomelia-like deformity and thalidomide preparations. *Hiroshima J Med Sci*. 1963;12:11-35.
57. Kajii T. Thalidomide experience in Japan. *Ann Paediatr*. 1965;205:341-354.
58. Livingstone G. Congenital ear abnormalities due to thalidomide. *Proc R Soc Med*. 1965;58:493-497.
59. Takemori S, Tanaka Y, Suzuki J-I. Thalidomide anomalies of the ear. *Arch Otolaryngol*. 1976;102:425-427.
60. Stahl A. Clinical, orthodontic, and radiological findings in the jaws and face of children with dysmelia associated with thalidomide-embryopathy. *Int Dental J*. 1968;18:631-638.
61. Smithells RW. Defects and disabilities of thalidomide children. *Br Med J*. 1973;1:269-272.
62. Gilkes MJ, Strode M. Ocular anomalies in association with developmental limb abnormalities of drug origin. *Lancet*. 1963;1:1026-1027.
63. Zetterstrom B. Ocular malformations caused by thalidomide. *Acta Ophthalmol*. 1966;44:391-395.
64. Rafuse EV, Arstikaitis M, Brent HP. Ocular findings in thalidomide children. *Can J Ophthalmol*. 1967;2:222-225.
65. Miller MT, Stromland K. Ocular motility in thalidomide embryopathy. *J Pediatr Ophthalmol Strab*. 1991;28:47-54.
66. Stromland K, Miller MT. Thalidomide embryopathy: revisited 27 years later. *Acta Ophthalmol*. 1993;71:238-245.
67. Stephenson JBP. Epilepsy: a neurological complication of thalidomide embryopathy. *Devel Med Child Neurol*. 1976;18:189-197.
68. Stromland K, Nordin V, Miller M, et al. Autism in thalidomide embryopathy: a population study. *Dev Med Child Neurol*. 1994;36:351-356.
69. Edwards DH, Nichols PJR. The spinal abnormalities in thalidomide embryopathy. *Acta Orthop Scand*. 1977;48:273-276.
70. Nichols PJR, Boldero JL, Goodfellow JW, Hamilton A. Abnormalities of the vertebral column associated with thalidomide-induced limb deformities. *Orthop (Oxford)*. 1968;1:71-90. As cited by Edwards DH, Nichols PJR. The spinal abnormalities in thalidomide embryopathy. Acta Orthop Scand. 1977;48:273-276.
71. Maouris PG, Hirsch PJ. Pregnancy in women with thalidomide-induced disabilities. Case report and a questionnaire study. *Br J Obstet Gynecol*. 1988;95:717-719.
72. Brown MA, Farrell C, Newton P, Child RP. Thalidomide, pregnancy and renal failure. *Med J Aust*. 1990;152:148-149.

THEOPHYLLINE

Respiratory (Bronchodilator)

PREGNANCY RECOMMENDATION: Human Data Suggest Low Risk

BREASTFEEDING RECOMMENDATION: Potential Toxicity

PREGNANCY SUMMARY

Numerous publications regarding the use of theophylline during human pregnancy were located. From the Collaborative Perinatal Project and the Michigan Medicaid Surveillance study, there were 46 (3.1%) major congenital anomalies in 1,469 first-trimester exposures to theophylline and aminophylline. No pattern to the defects was seen. The drug crosses the placenta, so fetal exposure will occur. Embryofetal toxicity was observed in three animal species at IV doses of less than, intraperitoneal doses of about equal to, and SC doses at about 2 times the MRHD. Using this drug during pregnancy should be based on the pros and cons of the mother's clinical need for treatment versus any potential fetal risk that might occur from exposure. According to the 2008 ACOG asthma guidelines, theophylline is not a preferred candidate for asthma therapy but is considered an alternative agent. However, the 2024 Global Initiative for Asthma states that oral theophylline should not be used for the treatment of asthma in any age group. However, risks of uncontrolled asthma during pregnancy include preterm delivery, low birth weight, and preeclampsia.

T

BREASTFEEDING SUMMARY

Theophylline has been shown to be excreted into human breast milk. The manufacturer reports that breast milk and maternal serum concentrations are about equivalent. Whereas a separate study reported levels of about 70% in breast milk when compared to maternal serum concentrations. The target adult blood level for theophylline is 10 to 20 mcg/mL, and an exclusively breastfed infant could achieve these concentrations in some cases. As long as the mother does not have elevated blood toxic levels, serious adverse events in infants are unlikely. If the clinical decision is to use this drug while breastfeeding, the infant should be monitored for the most common reported adult side effects of nausea and headache (both leading to irritability), vomiting, and insomnia.

References

1. Prescribing Information. *Theophylline*. Alembic Pharmaceuticals, Inc; 2021.
2. American College of Obstetricians and Gynecologists. Asthma in pregnancy: ACOG Practice Bulletin No. 90. *Obstet Gynecol*. 2008;111:457-464.
3. Global Initiative for Asthma. *2024 Global strategy for asthma management and prevention*. Accessed November 30, 2024. https://ginasthma.org/wp-content/uploads/2024/05/GINA-2024-Strategy-Report-24_05_22_WMS.pdf
4. Arwood LL, Dasta JF, Friedman C. Placental transfer of theophylline: two case reports. *Pediatrics*. 1979;63:844-846.
5. Yeh TF, Pildes RS. Transplacental aminophylline toxicity in a neonate. *Lancet*. 1977;1:910.
6. Labovitz E, Spector S. Placental theophylline transfer in pregnant asthmatics. *JAMA*. 1982;247:786-788.
7. Horowitz DA, Jablonski W, Mehta KA. Apnea associated with theophylline withdrawal in a term neonate. *Am J Dis Child*. 1982;136:73-74.
8. Ron M, Hochner-Celnikier D, Menczel J, et al. Maternal-fetal transfer of aminophylline. *Acta Obstet Gynecol Scand*. 1984;63:217-218.
9. Heinonen OP, Slone D, Shapiro S. *Birth Defects and Drugs in Pregnancy*. Publishing Sciences Group; 1977:367, 370.
10. Hadjigeorgiou E, Kitsiou S, Psaroudakis A, et al. Antepartum aminophylline treatment for prevention of the respiratory distress syndrome in premature infants. *Am J Obstet Gynecol*. 1979;135:257-260.
11. Granati B, Grella PV, Pettenazzo A, et al. The prevention of respiratory distress syndrome in premature infants: efficacy of antenatal aminophylline treatment versus prenatal glucocorticoid administration. *Pediatr Pharmacol (New York)*. 1984;4:21-24.
12. Lipshitz J. Uterine and cardiovascular effects of aminophylline. *Am J Obstet Gynecol*. 1978;131:716-718.
13. Bird LM, Anderson NC Jr, Chandler ML, et al. The effects of aminophylline and nifedipine on contractility of isolated pregnant human myometrium. *Am J Obstet Gynecol*. 1987;157:171-177.
14. Dombrowski MP, Bottoms SF, Boike GM, Wald J. Incidence of preeclampsia among asthmatic patients lower with theophylline. *Am J Obstet Gynecol*. 1986;155:265-267.
15. Volpe JJ. Effects of methylxanthines on lipid synthesis in developing neural systems. *Semin Perinatol*. 1981;5:395-405.
16. Aranda JV, Dupont C. Metabolic effects of methylxanthines in premature infants. *J Pediatr*. 1976;89:833-834.
17. Nelson RM, Resnick MB, Holstrum WJ, Eitzman DV. Development outcome of premature infants treated with theophylline. *Dev Pharmacol Ther*. 1980;1:274-280.
18. Halbrecht I, Komlos L, Shabtay F, et al. Triploidy 69, XXX in a stillborn girl. *Clin Genet*. 1973;4:210-212.
19. Weinstein D, Mauer I, Katz ML, Kazmer S. The effect of methylxanthines on chromosomes of human lymphocytes in culture. *Mutat Res*. 1975;31:57-61.
20. Sutton PL, Koup JR, Rose JQ, Middleton E. The pharmacokinetics of theophylline in pregnancy. *J Allergy Clin Immunol*. 1978;61:174.
21. Carter BL, Driscoll CE, Smith GD. Theophylline clearance during pregnancy. *Obstet Gynecol*. 1986;68:555-559.
22. Yurchak AM, Jusko WJ. Theophylline secretion into breast milk. *Pediatrics*. 1976;57:518-525.
23. Stec GP, Greenberger P, Ruo TI, et al. Kinetics of theophylline transfer to breast milk. *Clin Pharmacol Ther*. 1980;28:404-408.
24. Berlin CM. Excretion of methylxanthines in human milk. *Semin Perinatol*. 1981;5:389-394.

THIOGUANINE

Antineoplastic (Purine Analogue)

PREGNANCY RECOMMENDATION: Limited Human Data—Animal Data Suggest Potential Risk

BREASTFEEDING RECOMMENDATION: Potential Toxicity

PREGNANCY SUMMARY

Several reports describing the use of thioguanine in human pregnancy have been located. From about 130 pregnancies with first-trimester exposure, the major birth anomaly rate was about 2.5%, and no pattern to the defects was seen. The drug appears to cross the placenta, so some fetal exposure will occur. However, the absence of human pregnancy experience prevents a complete assessment of the embryofetal risk. Embryofetal toxicity was seen in one species at doses of less than 10 times the RHD. Based on animal studies and the drug's mechanism of action, the manufacturer recommends that women with reproductive potential use effective contraception during treatment. Nevertheless, using this drug during pregnancy should be based on the pros and cons of the mother's clinical need for treatment versus any potential fetal risk that might occur from exposure. In 2024, the FDA issued an alert that thiopurine (azathioprine, 6-mercaptopurine, and 6-thioguanine) use in pregnancy is associated with a rare risk of intrahepatic cholestasis of pregnancy. Thiopurine should be discontinued if this develops. There is a registry for women who are pregnant and have cancer. For more information, women and health care providers are encouraged to contact the Cancer and Pregnancy Registry at 1-877-635-4499.

BREASTFEEDING SUMMARY

One report describing the use of thioguanine during human lactation was located. In a study of patients with inflammatory bowel disease, 98 women continued thioguanine postpartum, and 38% breastfed their infant. No adverse events were reported in the nursing infants. The drug and its active metabolites will likely be excreted into human breast milk, so some infant exposure will probably occur. Due to a concern for potential serious adverse effects that might be seen in a breastfed infant, the manufacturer recommends that women not breastfeed while being treated with this drug. Nevertheless, if the clinical decision is to use this drug while breastfeeding, the infant should be monitored for the most common reported adult side effects of various laboratory abnormalities (see PI).

References

1. Prescribing Information. *Tabloid*. Aspen Global, Inc; 2022.
2. Thioguanine. *Lexi-Drugs*. UpToDate Lexidrug. UpToDate, Inc. Accessed December 6, 2024. https://online.lexi.com
3. National Library of Medicine—Pubchem. *Thioguanine*. Accessed December 6, 2024. https://pubchem.ncbi.nlm.nih.gov/compound/Thioguanine
4. Food and Drug Administration. *FDA alerts health care professionals of pregnancy problems associated with thiopurines*. Accessed December 6, 2024. https://www.fda.gov/drugs/drugsafety-and-availability/fda-alerts-health-care-professionals-pregnancy-problems-associatedthiopurines#:~:text=Thiopurines%20are%20immunosuppressants%20with%20a,thiopurines%20
5. if%20they%20develop%20ICP

6. Pavlidis P, Ansari A, Duley J, et al. Splitting a therapeutic dose of thioguanine may avoid liver toxicity and be an efficacious treatment for severe inflammatory bowel disease: a 2-center observational cohort study. *Inflamm Bowel Dis*. 2014;20:2239-2246.
7. Crouwel F, Simsek M, de Boer MA, et al. Exposure to thioguanine during 117 pregnancies in women with inflammatory bowel disease. *J Crohns Colitis*. 2023;17:738-745.
8. Maurer LH, Forcier RJ, McIntyre OR, Benirschke K. Fetal group C trisomy after cytosine arabinoside and thioguanine. *Ann Intern Med*. 1971;75:809-810.
9. Schafer AI. Teratogenic effects of antileukemic chemotherapy. *Arch Intern Med*. 1981;141:514-515.
10. Au-Yong R, Collins P, Young JA. Acute myeloblastic leukaemia during pregnancy. *Br Med J*. 1972;4:493-494.
11. Raich PC, Curet LB. Treatment of acute leukemia during pregnancy. *Cancer*. 1975;36:861-862.
12. Gokal R, Durrant J, Baum JD, Bennett MJ. Successful pregnancy in acute monocytic leukaemia. *Br J Cancer*. 1976;34:299-302.
13. Lilleyman JS, Hill AS, Anderton KJ. Consequences of acute myelogenous leukemia in early pregnancy. *Cancer*. 1977;40:1300-1303.
14. Moreno H, Castleberry RP, McCann WP. Cytosine arabinoside and 6-thioguanine in the treatment of childhood acute myeloblastic leukemia. *Cancer*. 1977;40:998-1004.
15. Manoharan A, Leyden MJ. Acute nonlymphocytic leukaemia in the third trimester of pregnancy. *Aust NZ J Med*. 1979;9:71-74.
16. Taylor G, Blom J. Acute leukemia during pregnancy. *South Med J*. 1980;73:1314-1315.
17. Tobias JS, Bloom HJG. Doxorubicin in pregnancy. *Lancet*. 1980;1:776.
18. Pawliger DF, McLean FW, Noyes WD. Normal fetus after cytosine arabinoside therapy. *Ann Intern Med*. 1971;74:1012.
19. Plows CW. Acute myelomonocytic leukemia in pregnancy: report of a case. *Am J Obstet Gynecol*. 1982;143:41-43.
20. Lowenthal RM, Marsden KA, Newman NM, et al. Normal infant after treatment of acute myeloid leukaemia in pregnancy with daunorubicin. *Aust NZ J Med*. 1978;8:431-432.
21. O'Donnell R, Costigan C, O'Connell LG. Two cases of acute leukaemia in pregnancy. *Acta Haematol*. 1979;61:298-300.
22. Hamer JW, Beard MEJ, Duff GB. Pregnancy complicated by acute myeloid leukaemia. *NZ Med J*. 1979;89:212-213.
23. Doney KC, Kraemer KG, Shepard TH. Combination chemotherapy for acute myelocytic leukemia during pregnancy: three case reports. *Cancer Treat Rep*. 1979;63:369-371.
24. Volkenandt M, Buchner T, Hiddemann W, Van De Loo J. Acute leukaemia during pregnancy. *Lancet*. 1987;2:1521-1522.
25. Feliu J, Juarez S, Ordonez A, Garcia-Paredes ML, Gonzalez-Baron M, Montero JM. Acute leukemia and pregnancy. *Cancer*. 1988;61:580-584.
26. Nicholson HO. Cytotoxic drugs in pregnancy: review of reported cases. *J Obstet Gynaecol Br Commonw*. 1968;75:307-312.
27. Dobbing J. Pregnancy and leukaemia. *Lancet*. 1977;1:1155.
28. Russell JA, Powles RL, Oliver RTD. Conception and congenital abnormalities after chemotherapy of acute myelogenous leukaemia in two men. *Br Med J*. 1976;1:1508.
29. Evenson DP, Arlin Z, Welt S, et al. Male reproductive capacity may recover following drug treatment with the L-10 protocol for acute lymphocytic leukemia. *Cancer*. 1984;53:30-36.
30. Matthews JH, Wood JK. Male fertility during chemotherapy for acute leukemia. *N Engl J Med*. 1980;303:1235.

THIORIDAZINE

Mental Health (Phenothiazine—First Generation Antipsychotic)

PREGNANCY RECOMMENDATION: Limited Human Data—No Relevant Animal Data

BREASTFEEDING RECOMMENDATION: Potential Toxicity

PREGNANCY SUMMARY

A total of 96 first-trimester pregnancy exposures to thioridazine were reported in three studies. Of these, there were three (3.1%) major congenital anomalies identified. No pattern to the defects was seen. The drug will likely cross the placenta, so some fetal exposure will probably occur. However, this limited human pregnancy experience prevents a complete assessment of embryofetal risk. No animal studies were located. Using this drug during pregnancy should be based on the pros and cons of the mother's clinical need for treatment versus any potential fetal risk that might occur from exposure. Extrapyramidal and/or withdrawal symptoms have been reported in a few infants exposed to the drug up to delivery. Symptoms included agitation, hypertonia, hypotonia, tremor, somnolence, apnea, and feeding disorders. The drug carries a boxed warning for prolongation of the QT interval and an increased risk of mortality in older patients with dementia-related psychosis.

T

BREASTFEEDING SUMMARY

No reports describing the use of thioridazine during human lactation have been located. The drug will likely be excreted into breast milk, so some infant exposure will probably occur. Other phenothiazines have been shown to be excreted into breast milk and have caused symptoms in some infants. The drug can increase prolactin levels, but this should not adversely affect breastfeeding. Breastfeeding while using this drug should be based on the mother's clinical need for treatment versus any potential infant risks that might occur. If used, the infant should be monitored for the most common reported adult side effects of nausea and mouth dryness (both leading to irritability), drowsiness, constipation, diarrhea, nasal stuffiness, and peripheral edema.

References

1. Prescribing Information. *Thioridazine*. Mylan Pharmaceuticals, Inc; 2024.
2. Moya F, Thorndike V. Passage of drugs across the placenta. *Am J Obstet Gynecol*. 1962;84:1778-1798.
3. Hill RM, Desmond MM, Kay JL. Extrapyramidal dysfunction in an infant of a schizophrenic mother. *J Pediatr*. 1966;69:589-595.
4. Vince DJ. Congenital malformations following phenothiazine administration during pregnancy. *Can Med Assoc J*. 1969;100:223.
5. Scanlan FJ. The use of thioridazine (Mellaril) during the first trimester. *Med J Aust*. 1972;1:1271-1272.
6. Seifritz E, Holsboer-Trachsler E, Haberthur F, Hemmeter U, Poldinger W. Unrecognized pregnancy during citalopram treatment. *Am J Psychiatry*. 1993;150:1428-1429.
7. Heinonen OP, Slone D, Shapiro S. *Birth Defects and Drugs in Pregnancy*. Publishing Sciences Group; 1983:323.

THIOTEPA

Antineoplastic (Alkylating Agent)

PREGNANCY RECOMMENDATION: Limited Human Data—Animal Data Suggest Risk

BREASTFEEDING RECOMMENDATION: Potential Toxicity

PREGNANCY SUMMARY

One report describing the use of thiotepa in human pregnancy was located. Exposure occurred in the second and third trimesters, and no apparent fetal harm was observed. The drug will likely cross the placenta, so some fetal exposure will probably occur. However, the limited human pregnancy experience prevents a complete assessment of embryofetal risk. Embryofetal toxicity with malformations was observed in three animal species at doses of less than or equal to the RHD, but the drug was administered intraperitoneally. It is not known how this compares with use in humans. Based on animal studies and the drug's mechanism of action, the manufacturer recommends that women with reproductive potential use effective contraception during treatment and for 6 months after the last dose. They also recommend that males with female partners of reproductive potential use effective contraception during treatment and for 1 year after the last dose. Nevertheless, using this drug during pregnancy should be based on the pros and cons of the mother's clinical need for treatment versus any potential fetal risk that might occur from exposure. There is a registry for women who are pregnant and have cancer. For more information, women and health care providers are encouraged to contact the Cancer and Pregnancy Registry at 1-877-635-4499.

BREASTFEEDING SUMMARY

No reports describing the use of thiotepa during human lactation have been located. The drug and active metabolite will likely be excreted into breast milk, so some infant exposure will probably occur. However, due to a concern for potential serious adverse effects that might be seen in a breastfed infant, the manufacturer recommends that women not breastfeed while being treated with this drug. Nevertheless, breastfeeding while using this drug should be based on the mother's clinical need for treatment versus any potential infant risks that might occur. If used, the infant should be monitored for the most common reported adult side effects of diarrhea, hemorrhage, hematuria, rash, CMV infection, and various laboratory abnormalities (see PI).

References

1. Prescribing Information. *Thiotepa*. Meitheal Pharmaceuticals, Inc; 2023.
2. Gililland J, Weinstein L. The effects of cancer chemotherapeutic agents on the developing fetus. *Obstet Gynecol Surv*. 1983;38:6-13.
3. Dobbing J. Pregnancy and leukaemia. *Lancet*. 1977;1:1155.

THIOTHIXENE

Antipsychotic (Phenothiazine Derivative—First Generation Antipsychotic)

PREGNANCY RECOMMENDATION: Limited Human Data—Animal Data Suggest Potential Risk

BREASTFEEDING RECOMMENDATION: Potential Toxicity

PREGNANCY SUMMARY

The Michigan Medicaid Surveillance study reported first-trimester use of thiothixene in 38 human pregnancies. One (2.6%) major malformation was observed. The manufacturer reports that neonatal extrapyramidal and/or withdrawal symptoms have been observed after exposure during the third trimester near delivery. Symptoms observed include agitation, hypertonia, hypotonia, tremor, somnolence, apnea, and feeding disorders. The drug will likely cross the placenta, so fetal exposure will probably occur. However, the limited human pregnancy experience prevents a complete assessment of embryofetal risk. Embryofetal toxicity was observed in two animal species at unknown human equivalent doses. Using this drug during pregnancy should be based on the pros and cons of the mother's clinical need for treatment versus any potential fetal risk that might occur from exposure.

BREASTFEEDING SUMMARY

No reports describing the use of thiothixene during human lactation have been located. The drug will likely be excreted into breast milk, so some infant exposure will probably occur. Thiothixene can increase serum prolactin levels, but this should not adversely affect breastfeeding. Breastfeeding while using this drug should be based on the mother's clinical need for treatment versus any potential infant risks that might occur. If used, the infant should be monitored for the most common reported adult side effects of dizziness (leading to irritability), increased heart rate, decreased blood pressure, and drowsiness.

References

1. Prescribing Information. *Thiothixene*. Amneal Pharmaceuticals NY LLC; 2023.

THYROTROPIN ALFA

Diagnostic/Radiopharmaceutical

PREGNANCY RECOMMENDATION: Human Data Suggest Compatible/(Contraindicated if Used With Radioactive Iodine)

BREASTFEEDING RECOMMENDATION: Probably Compatible/Contraindicated if Used With Radioactive Iodine

PREGNANCY SUMMARY

No reports describing the use of thyrotropin alfa, a recombinant thyroid-stimulating hormone (TSH), in human pregnancy have been located. Endogenous TSH does not cross the placenta, so thyrotropin alfa is not likely to cross the placenta. However, the absence of human pregnancy experience prevents a complete assessment of embryofetal risk. Animal reproduction studies have not been conducted. Using this drug during pregnancy should be based on the pros and cons of the mother's clinical need for treatment versus any potential fetal risk that might occur from exposure. However, because it does not appear to cross the placenta, it is likely compatible for use in pregnancy. If used in combination with radioactive iodine (RAI), the combination is contraindicated during pregnancy because of the potential risk of radiation and irreversible neonatal hypothyroidism. There is a registry for women who are pregnant and have cancer. For more information, women and health care providers are encouraged to contact the Cancer and Pregnancy Registry at 1-877-635-4499.

BREASTFEEDING SUMMARY

No reports describing the use of thyrotropin during human lactation have been located. Breast milk does not provide sufficient levothyroxine (T_4) or liothyronine (T_3) to prevent the effects of congenital hypothyroidism. As a consequence, serum levels of TSH in breastfed hypothyroid infants are markedly elevated. In euthyroid babies, serum levels of this hormone have been measured and compared in breastfed and bottle-fed infants. No differences in TSH levels have been discovered between breastfed and bottle-fed infants. If used alone, breastfeeding while using this drug should be based on the mother's clinical need for treatment versus any potential infant risks that might occur. If used, the infant should be monitored for the most common reported adult side effects of nausea and headache (both leading to irritability). If used in combination with RAI, it is contraindicated.

References

1. Prescribing Information. *Thyrogen*. Genzyme Corporation; 2023.
2. Cohlan SQ. Fetal and neonatal hazards from drugs administered during pregnancy. *NY State J Med*. 1964;64:493-499.
3. Feely J. The physiology of thyroid function in pregnancy. *Postgrad Med J*. 1979;55:336-339.
4. Abbassi V, Steinour TA. Successful diagnosis of congenital hypothyroidism in four breast-fed neonates. *J Pediatr*. 1980;97:259-261.
5. Letarte J, Guyda H, Dussault JH, Glorieux J. Lack of protective effect of breast-feeding in congenital hypothyroidism: report of 12 cases. *Pediatrics*. 1980;65:703-705.
6. Mizuta H, Amino N, Ichihara K, et al. Thyroid hormones in human milk and their influence on thyroid function of breast-fed babies. *Pediatr Res*. 1983;17:468-471.
7. Hahn HB Jr, Spiekerman M, Otto WR, Hossalla DE. Thyroid function tests in neonates fed human milk. *Am J Dis Child*. 1983;137:220-222.
8. Franklin R, O'Grady C, Carpenter L. Neonatal thyroid function: comparison between breast-fed and bottle-fed infants. *J Pediatr*. 1985;106:124-126.

TIAGABINE

Central Nervous System (Antiseizure)

PREGNANCY RECOMMENDATION: Limited Human Data—Animal Data Suggest Potential Risk

BREASTFEEDING RECOMMENDATION: Potential Toxicity

PREGNANCY SUMMARY

Three studies were located that describe the use of tiagabine in human pregnancy. Of 14 first-trimester exposures, there was 1 spontaneous abortion and 1 minor anomaly in the 13 remaining pregnancies. The drug will probably cross the placenta, so some fetal exposure will likely occur. Therefore, this limited human pregnancy experience prevents a complete assessment of the embryofetal risk. Embryofetal toxicity was not seen in two species at doses of less than 10 times the MRHD. However, in these two species, there was some embryofetal toxicity at higher doses (one at doses still less than 10 times the MRHD and the other at doses of more than 10 times the MRHD). Using this drug during pregnancy should be based on the pros and cons of the mother's clinical need for treatment versus any potential fetal risk that might occur from exposure. There is a pregnancy exposure registry that monitors pregnancy outcomes in women using antiseizure drugs. Health care providers are encouraged to call the North American Antiepileptic Drug Pregnancy Registry at 1-888-233-2334.

BREASTFEEDING SUMMARY

No reports describing the use of tiagabine during human lactation have been located. The drug will likely be excreted into breast milk, so some infant exposure will probably occur. The manufacturer recommends that tiagabine only be used during lactation if the benefits clearly outweigh the risks. If the clinical decision is to use this drug while breastfeeding, the infant should be monitored for the most common reported adult side effects of dizziness/lightheadedness, nausea, nervousness/irritability, and abdominal pain (all leading to irritability), fatigue (lethargy), somnolence, and tremor.

References

1. Prescribing Information. *Tiagabine hydrochloride*. Amneal Pharmaceuticals NY LLC; 2023.
2. Morrell MJ. The new antiepileptic drugs and women: efficacy, reproductive health, pregnancy, and fetal outcome. *Epilepsia*. 1996;37(suppl 6):S34-S44.
3. Leppik IE, Gram L, Deaton R, Sommerville KW. Safety of tiagabine: summary of 53 trials. *Epilepsy Res*. 1999;33:235-246.
4. The Lamotrigine Pregnancy Registry. *Final Report: September 1, 1992 through March 31, 2010*. GlaxoSmithKline; July 2010.
5. Yerby MS. Clinical care of pregnant women with epilepsy: neural tube defects and folic acid supplementation. *Epilepsia*. 2003;44(suppl 3):33-40.

TICAGRELOR

Cardiovascular (Antiplatelet)

PREGNANCY RECOMMENDATION: Limited Human Data—Animal Data Suggest Risk

BREASTFEEDING RECOMMENDATION: Potential Toxicity

PREGNANCY SUMMARY

Two case reports describing the use of ticagrelor in human pregnancy were located. One involved first-trimester exposure (along with numerous other drugs) and she delivered at term a healthy newborn with no identified birth defects. The second case involved treatment in the early third trimester, and no adverse newborn effects were reported related to the medication. The drug will probably cross the placenta, so some fetal exposure will likely occur. Therefore, this limited human pregnancy experience prevents a complete assessment of the embryofetal risk. Embryofetal toxicity was observed in two animal species at doses of less than 10 times the MRHD. Using this drug during pregnancy should be based on the pros and cons of the mother's clinical need for treatment versus any potential fetal risk that might occur from exposure. There is a boxed warning for an increased risk of bleeding and reduced effectiveness of ticagrelor when combined with more than 100 mg of aspirin per day.

BREASTFEEDING SUMMARY

No reports describing the use of ticagrelor during human lactation have been located. The drug and its active metabolite will likely be excreted into breast milk, so some infant exposure will probably occur. Due to a concern for potential serious adverse effects that might be seen in a breastfed infant, the manufacturer recommends that women not breastfeed while being treated with this drug. Nevertheless, breastfeeding while using this drug should be based on the mother's clinical need for treatment versus any potential infant risks that might occur. If used, the infant should be monitored for the most common reported adult side effects of bleeding and dyspnea.

References

1. Prescribing Information. *Ticagrelor*. Amneal Pharmaceuticals NY LLC; 2020.
2. Verbruggen M, Mannaerts D, Muys J, Jacquemyn Y. Use of ticagrelor in human pregnancy, the first experience. *BMJ Case Rep*. 2015;2015:bcr2015212217.
3. Argentiero D, Savonitto S, D'Andrea P, Iacovelli F. Ticagrelor and tirofiban in pregnancy and delivery: beyond labels. *J Thromb Thrombolysis*. 2020;49:145-148.

TIGECYCLINE

Antibacterial (Tetracycline)

PREGNANCY RECOMMENDATION: *Contraindicated

BREASTFEEDING RECOMMENDATION: Potential Toxicity

T

PREGNANCY SUMMARY

No reports describing the use of tigecycline in human pregnancy have been located. The drug will probably cross the placenta, so some fetal exposure will likely occur. Therefore, the absence of human pregnancy experience prevents a complete assessment of the embryofetal risk. Embryofetal and maternal toxicity were observed in two animal species at doses of less than 10 times the MRHD. *Because tigecycline is a tetracycline, this drug may result in permanent tooth discoloration of deciduous teeth and bone stippling when used in the second and third trimesters of pregnancy. Although this risk is more common with long-term use of tetracyclines, it has also been observed with repeated short courses. *However, in a meta-analysis of the phase three and four clinical trials, there was an increase in all-cause mortality. The drug carries a boxed warning for this risk. The etiology for this is not known. Therefore, using this drug during pregnancy should be based on the pros and cons of the mother's clinical need for treatment versus any potential fetal risk that might occur from exposure. If possible, an alternative drug should be considered for use during pregnancy.

BREASTFEEDING SUMMARY

No reports describing the use of tigecycline during human lactation have been located. The drug will probably be excreted into breast milk, so some infant exposure will likely occur. However, the oral bioavailability of tigecycline is such that there might be little or no systemic exposure. Even if the oral bioavailability in infants is negligible, the presence of the antibiotic in breast milk could cause a modification of bowel flora. However, due to a concern for potential adverse effects on a breastfeeding infant, including tooth discoloration and inhibition of bone growth, the manufacturer recommends that women taking tigecycline avoid nursing if it is used for longer than 3 weeks. If the clinical decision is to use this drug during lactation, to reduce infant exposure, consider pumping and dumping breast milk while taking tigecycline and for 9 days (five half-lives) after the last dose. If used, the infant should be monitored for the most common reported adult side effects of abdominal pain and headache (both leading to irritability), vomiting, and diarrhea.

Reference

1. Prescribing Information. *Tigecycline*. Amneal Pharmaceuticals LLC; 2020.

TILDRAKIZUMAB

Dermatologic/Immunologic (Monoclonal Antibody—IL-23 Antagonist)

PREGNANCY RECOMMENDATION: Limited Human Data—Animal Data Suggest Low Risk

BREASTFEEDING RECOMMENDATION: Probably Compatible

PREGNANCY SUMMARY

One report describing the use of tildrakizumab in human pregnancy has been located. From the clinical trials, excluding elective terminations, there were 10 pregnancies with first-trimester exposure that resulted in 2 spontaneous abortions and 8 live births with no fetal anomalies described. As an IgG antibody, it likely crosses the placenta, especially during the second half of gestation, so some fetal exposure will probably occur. However, this limited human pregnancy experience prevents a complete assessment of embryofetal risk. Animal data did not show any embryofetal toxicity in one species at doses of more than 10 times the MRHD. Using this drug during pregnancy should be based on the pros and cons of the mother's clinical need for treatment versus any potential fetal risk that might occur from exposure.

BREASTFEEDING SUMMARY

No reports describing the use of tildrakizumab during human lactation have been located. It is known that IgG antibodies can be found in human breast milk, but are not found in the neonatal or infant circulation. Additionally, if any IgG antibodies were to be ingested through breastfeeding, they would probably be digested in the infant's gastrointestinal tract and not be absorbed. Breastfeeding while using this drug should be based on the mother's clinical need for treatment versus any potential infant risks that might occur. If used, the infant should be monitored for the most common reported adult side effects of upper respiratory tract infections and diarrhea.

References

1. Prescribing Information. *Ilumya*. Sun Pharmaceutical Industries, Inc; 2024.
2. Haycraft K, DiRuggiero D, Rozzo SJ, et al. Outcomes of pregnancies from the tildrakizumab phase I-III clinical development programme. *Br J Dermatol*. 2020;183:184-186.

TIMOLOL

Cardiovascular (Nonselective β-Blocker)

PREGNANCY RECOMMENDATION: Limited Human Data—Animal Data Suggest Low Risk

BREASTFEEDING RECOMMENDATION: Probably Compatible

PREGNANCY SUMMARY

One case report describing the use of timolol in the third trimester of human pregnancy was located. No adverse effects on the fetus or newborn were seen related to the drug. The drug appears to cross the placenta, so some fetal exposure will occur. Therefore, this limited human pregnancy experience prevents a complete assessment of the embryofetal risk. Animal studies did not show any embryofetal toxicity in three species at doses of more than 10 times the MRHD. Using this drug during pregnancy should be based on the pros and cons of the mother's clinical need for treatment versus any potential fetal risk that might occur from exposure. Systemic use of some β-blockers has been associated with an increased risk for IUGR and reduced placental weight (see Atenolol). Although IUGR is a serious concern, the benefits of maternal therapy with β-blockers, in some cases, might outweigh the risks to the fetus and must be judged on a case-by-case basis.

BREASTFEEDING SUMMARY

Timolol has been shown to be excreted into human breast milk. In nine lactating women given 5 mg orally 3 times daily, the mean breast milk concentration of timolol about 2 hours after a dose was about 16 ng/mL. When a dose of 10 mg 3 times daily was given to four patients, mean breast milk levels were about 41 ng/mL. The breast milk to maternal plasma ratios for the two regimens were both about 80%. No adverse reactions were noted in the nursing infants. However, due to a concern for potential serious adverse effects that might be seen in a breastfed infant, the manufacturer recommends that women not breastfeed while being treated with this drug. Nevertheless, breastfeeding while using this drug should be based on the mother's clinical need for treatment versus any potential infant risks that might occur. If used, the infant should be monitored for the most common reported adult side effects of fatigue/tiredness (lethargy) and bradycardia.

References

1. Prescribing Information. *Timolol maleate*. Athem LLC; 2022.
2. Schneider H, Proegler M. Placental transfer of β-adrenergic antagonists studied in an in vitro perfusion system of human placental tissue. *Am J Obstet Gynecol*. 1988;159:42-47.
3. Devoe LD, O'Dell BE, Castillo RA, et al. Metastatic pheochromocytoma in pregnancy and fetal biophysical assessment after maternal administration of alpha-adrenergic, beta-adrenergic, and dopamine antagonists. *Obstet Gynecol*. 1986;68:15S-18S.
4. Fidler J, Smith V, DeSwiet M. Excretion of oxprenolol and timolol in breast milk. *Br J Obstet Gynaecol*. 1983;90:961-965.

TIMOLOL OPHTHALMIC

Ophthalmic (Nonselective β-Blocker)

PREGNANCY RECOMMENDATION: Limited Human Data—Animal Data Suggest Low Risk

BREASTFEEDING RECOMMENDATION: Probably Compatible

PREGNANCY SUMMARY

Five reports describing the use of timolol ophthalmic in more than 80 pregnancies were located. Most of these were first-trimester exposures, and no increased risk for major birth anomalies was described. The amounts that are absorbed into the systemic circulation are low (mean peak plasma level <5 ng/mL). However, fetal bradycardia, which resolved when the timolol dose was decreased, has been described. The drug appears to cross the placenta, so some fetal exposure will occur. Therefore, this limited human pregnancy experience prevents a complete assessment of the embryofetal risk. Animal studies did not show any embryofetal toxicity in three species at doses of more than 10 times the maximum recommended human oral dose. Using this drug during pregnancy should be based on the pros and cons of the mother's clinical need for treatment versus any potential fetal risk that might occur from exposure. If used during pregnancy, consider placing pressure over the tear duct in the corner of the eye for at least 1 minute, and then remove any excess solution with absorbent tissue to decrease the amount of drug reaching the systemic circulation even further.

BREASTFEEDING SUMMARY

Timolol ophthalmic has been shown to be excreted into human breast milk. Two patients used timolol ophthalmic while breastfeeding. The mean timolol breast milk levels were 0.93 and 0.12 ng/mL. The calculated RIDs were less than 1%. In addition, these concentrations were below those expected to produce cardiac effects in the infant. No adverse reactions were noted in the nursing infants described in the above reports. Breastfeeding while using this drug should be based on the mother's clinical need for treatment versus any potential infant risks that might occur. If used, the infant should be closely observed for a decrease in heart rate and other symptoms related to β-blockade.

References

1. Prescribing Information. *Timolol hemihydrate*. Somerset Therapeutics LLC; 2024.
2. Prescribing Information. *Timolol GFS*. Sandoz, Inc; 2024.
3. Schneider H, Proegler M. Placental transfer of β-adrenergic antagonists studied in an in vitro perfusion system of human placental tissue. *Am J Obstet Gynecol*. 1988;159:42-47.
4. Merlob P, Litwin A, Mor N. Possible association between acetazolamide administration during pregnancy and metabolic disorders in the newborn. *Eur J Obstet Gynecol Reprod Biol*. 1990;35:85-88.
5. Wagenvoort AM, Van Vugt JMG, Sobotka M, Van Geijn HP. Topical timolol therapy in pregnancy: is it safe for the fetus? *Teratology*. 1998;58:258-262.
6. Johnson SM, Martinez M, Freedman S. Management of glaucoma in pregnancy and lactation. *Surv Ophthalmol*. 2001;45:449-454.
7. Mendez-Hernandez C, Garcia-Feijoo J, Saenz-Frances F, et al. Topical intraocular pressure therapy effects on pregnancy. *Clin Ophthalmol*. 2012;6:1629-1632.
8. Pellegrino M, D'Oria L, De Luca C, et al. Glaucoma drug therapy in pregnancy: literature review and teratology information service (TIS) case series. *Curr Drug Saf*. 2018;13:3-11.
9. Lustgarten JS, Podos SM. Topical timolol and the nursing mother. *Arch Ophthalmol*. 1983;101:1381-1382.
10. Madadi P, Koren G, Freeman DJ, et al. Timolol concentrations in breast milk of a woman treated for glaucoma: calculation of neonatal exposure. *J Glaucoma*. 2008;17:329-331.
11. Novack GD. Timolol concentrations in breast milk of a woman treated for glaucoma: calculation of neonatal exposure. *J Glaucoma*. 2008;17:510.
12. Madadi P, Koren G, Campbell RJ, Trope GE. Timolol concentrations in breast milk of a woman treated for glaucoma: calculation of neonatal exposure. *J Glaucoma*. 2008;17:511.
13. Razeghinejad MR, Tania Tai TY, Fudemberg SJ, Katz LJ. Pregnancy and glaucoma. *Surv Ophthalmol*. 2011;56:324-335.

TINIDAZOLE

Anti-Infective (Nitroimidazole—Antiprotozoal, Antibiotic, and Amebicide)

PREGNANCY RECOMMENDATION: Limited Human Data—Animal Data Suggest Potential Risk

BREASTFEEDING RECOMMENDATION: Hold Breastfeeding (Single Dose), Potential Toxicity (Divided Dose)

PREGNANCY SUMMARY

Two reports describing the use of tinidazole in human pregnancy were located. In the first study, of 22,843 cases with congenital anomalies, 10 (0.04%) used tinidazole, which was no different in the 38,151 controls (no birth defects), where 16 (0.04%) had used the drug. There were six uses in the first trimester for both groups. The second study involved use at about 20 weeks' gestation to treat resistant trichomoniasis. No adverse effects due to the drug were seen. It appears that tinidazole crosses the placenta, so some fetal exposure may occur. However, this limited human pregnancy experience prevents a complete assessment of embryofetal risk. Embryofetal toxicity was observed in one animal species at doses less than 10 times the MRHD, but no adverse effects were seen in a second species at doses less than 10 times the MRHD. Using this drug during pregnancy should be based on the pros and cons of the mother's clinical need for treatment versus any potential fetal risk that might occur from exposure. According to the CDC's 2021 Sexually Transmitted Diseases Treatment Guidelines, trichomoniasis during pregnancy should be treated with metronidazole.

T

BREASTFEEDING SUMMARY

Tinidazole was found to be excreted into human breast milk. In more than 30 lactating women, the breast milk to maternal serum levels ranged from about 60% to 160%. In one group of 24 women, the mean peak breast milk level was 5.8 mcg/mL. Nearly all of the calculated RIDs were above 10%. The manufacturer stated that there are no reports of adverse effects on breastfed infants, but recommended withholding breastfeeding during treatment and for 72 hours after the last dose. The CDC recommends withholding breastfeeding for 72 hours after a 2-g single dose of tinidazole. Breastfeeding while using this drug should be based on the mother's clinical need for treatment versus any potential infant risks that might occur. If used, the infant should be monitored for the most common reported adult side effects of metallic or bitter taste, nausea, dyspepsia, abdominal cramps, headache, and dizziness (all leading to irritability), weakness or fatigue (lethargy), vomiting, anorexia (monitor infant growth), and constipation.

References

1. Prescribing Information. *Tinidazole*. Edenbridge Pharmaceuticals LLC; 2022.
2. National Library of Medicine—Pubchem. Tinidazole. Accessed December 13, 2024. https://pubchem.ncbi.nlm.nih.gov/compound/Tinidazole
3. Karhunen M. Placental transfer of metronidazole and tinidazole in early human pregnancy after a single infusion. *Br J Clin Pharmacol*. 1984;18:254-257.
4. Czeizel AE, Kazy Z, Vargha P. Oral tinidazole treatment during pregnancy and teratogenesis. *Int J Gynecol Obstet*. 2003;83:305-306.
5. Forbes GL, Drayton R, Forbes GD. A case of metronidazole-resistant Trichomonas vaginalis in pregnancy. *Int J STD AIDS*. 2016;27:906-908.

6. Centers for Disease Control and Prevention. *Sexually transmitted infections treatment guidelines, 2021*. Trichomoniasis. Accessed December 13, 2024. https://www.cdc.gov/std/treatment-guidelines/STI-Guidelines-2021.pdf
7. Welling PG, Monro AM. The pharmacokinetics of metronidazole and tinidazole in man. *Arzneimittelforsch*. 1972;22:2128-2132. As cited in Mannisto PT, Karhunen M, Koskela O, et al. Concentrations of tinidazole in breast milk. Acta Pharmacol Toxicol (Copenh). 1983;53:254-256.
8. Mannisto PT, Karhunen M, Koskela O, Suikkari AM, Mattila J, Haataja H. Concentrations of tinidazole in breast milk. *Acta Pharmacol Toxicol (Copenh)*. 1983;53:254-256.
9. Evaldson GR, Lindgren S, Nord CE, Rane AT. Tinidazole milk excretion and pharmacokinetics in lactating women. *Br J Clin Pharmacol*. 1985;19:503-507.

TIOCONAZOLE

Anti-Infective (Topical Antifungal)

PREGNANCY RECOMMENDATION: Limited Human Data—No Relevant Animal Data

BREASTFEEDING RECOMMENDATION: Probably Compatible

PREGNANCY SUMMARY

One report describing the use of tioconazole in human pregnancy was located. The gestational ages of exposure were not provided, but 45 women with intractable vaginal candidiasis were treated during pregnancy. All 45 women delivered normal, healthy infants with no reported anomalies. The drug will probably cross the placenta, so some fetal exposure may occur. However, systemic absorption of the drug following vaginal use is low, suggesting that any exposure might be clinically insignificant. Regardless, human pregnancy experience prevents a complete assessment of the embryofetal risk. Animal reproduction studies have not been conducted. Using this drug during pregnancy should be based on the pros and cons of the mother's clinical need for treatment versus any potential fetal risk that might occur from exposure. The CDC recommends treating vulvovaginal candidiasis during pregnancy with 7 days of a topical azole medication.

BREASTFEEDING SUMMARY

No reports describing the use of tioconazole during human lactation have been located. The drug may be excreted into breast milk. However, systemic absorption of the drug following vaginal use is low, suggesting that any amount that might be present would be clinically insignificant. Moreover, a 1% tioconazole cream has been used safely in neonates and infants to treat candidiasis diaper rash. Thus, the effect of maternal use of intravaginal tioconazole on a nursing infant appears to be negligible.

References

1. Prescribing Information. *Basic care tioconazole*. Amazon.com Services LLC; 2021.
2. National Library of Medicine—Pubchem. *Tioconazole*. Accessed December 13, 2024. https://pubchem.ncbi.nlm.nih.gov/compound/Tioconazole#section=Carcinogen-Classification
3. Gjonnaess H, Jerve F, Bergen T. Tioconazole 2% cream in vaginal candidosis: systemic absorption and results of three days treatment compared to clotrimazole vaginal tablets. *Curr Ther Res*. 1981;30:995-1004.
4. Houang ET, Lawrence AG. Systemic absorption and persistence of tioconazole in vaginal fluid after insertion of a single 300-mg tioconazole ovule. *Antimicrob Agents Chemother*. 1985;27:964-965.
5. Centers for Disease Control and Prevention. *Sexually transmitted infections treatment guidelines, 2021*. Trichomoniasis. Accessed December 13, 2024. https://www.cdc.gov/std/treatment-guidelines/STI-Guidelines-2021.pdf
6. Adetoro OO. Tioconazole in the management of recurrent vaginal candidosis during pregnancy in Ilorin, Nigeria. *Curr Ther Res*. 1987;41:647-650.
7. Gibbs DL, Kashin P, Jevons S. Comparative and non-comparative studies on the efficacy and tolerance of tioconazole cream 1% versus another imidazole and/or placebo in neonates and infants with candidal diaper rash and/or impetigo. *J Intern Med Res*. 1987;15:23-31.

TIOTROPIUM

Respiratory (Long-Acting Antimuscarinic)

PREGNANCY RECOMMENDATION: No Human Data—Animal Data Suggest Low Risk

BREASTFEEDING RECOMMENDATION: Probably Compatible

PREGNANCY SUMMARY

No reports describing the use of tiotropium in human pregnancy have been located. About 33% of tiotropium is systemically absorbed with the Respimat device, and about 19% with the HandiHaler device. Therefore, the drug will probably cross the placenta, so some fetal exposure will likely occur. However, the absence of human pregnancy experience prevents a complete assessment of embryofetal risk. Animal data did not show any embryofetal toxicity in two species at doses of more than 10 times the maximum recommended human daily inhalation dose (MRHDID). Using this drug during

(*continued*)

pregnancy should be based on the pros and cons of the mother's clinical need for treatment versus any potential fetal risk that might occur from exposure. Uncontrolled asthma can increase the risk for preeclampsia, preterm delivery, and low birth weight.

BREASTFEEDING SUMMARY

No reports describing the use of tiotropium during human lactation have been located. Some amount of the drug will likely be excreted into breast milk, so infant exposure may occur. However, if it is found in breast milk, oral absorption is low at less than 3%. Therefore, any exposure is likely to be clinically insignificant. Breastfeeding while using this drug should be based on the mother's clinical need for treatment versus any potential infant risks that might occur. If used, the infant should be monitored for the most common reported systemic side effects of headache (leading to irritability) and bronchitis.

References

1. Prescribing Information. *Spiriva respimat*. Boehringer Ingelheim Pharmaceuticals, Inc; 2021.
2. Prescribing Information. *Spiriva handihaler*. Boehringer Ingelheim Pharmaceuticals, Inc; 2021.

TIPRANAVIR

Antiretroviral (Protease Inhibitor)

PREGNANCY RECOMMENDATION: Limited Human Data—Animal Data Suggest Potential Risk

EASTFEEDING RECOMMENDATION: *Contraindicated

PREGNANCY SUMMARY

The APR and expanded access program reported about 17 live births with exposure to tipranavir-containing regimens with 13 exposed in the first trimester and 4 exposed in the second/third trimester. No congenital malformations were observed. Tipranavir has been shown to cross the placenta, so some fetal exposure will occur. However, this limited human pregnancy experience prevents a complete assessment of embryofetal risk. Embryofetal toxicity was seen in two animal species at doses well below the RHD, but maternal toxicity also occurred. Using this drug during pregnancy should be based on the pros and cons of the mother's clinical need for treatment versus any potential fetal risk that might occur from exposure. In 2023, the updated US Department of Health and Human Services AIDS Info guidelines for the use of antiretroviral agents during pregnancy recommend that, in most cases, patients continue their regimen during pregnancy if it is tolerated, safe, and effective in suppressing viral replication. Additionally, treatment initiation should not be delayed due to concerns about teratogenicity with first-trimester exposure. See the guideline for the most updated information. Currently, the HIV guidelines do not recommend using tipranavir during pregnancy, primarily due to a very limited number of exposures. Providers caring for pregnant patients with HIV and their infants can call the national Perinatal HIV/AIDS hotline (888-448-8765) for a free clinical consultation. There is a pregnancy exposure registry that monitors pregnancy outcomes in patients using antiretroviral medicines during pregnancy. Health care providers are encouraged to call APR at 1-800-258-4263.

BREASTFEEDING SUMMARY

No reports describing the use of tipranavir during human lactation have been located. The drug will likely be excreted into breast milk, so some infant exposure will probably occur. *In 2023, the updated US Department of Health and Human Services AIDS Info guidelines state that using replacement of breast milk through formula or pasteurized donor human breast milk from a milk bank eliminates the risk of postnatal HIV transmission to the infant. Using antiretroviral therapy to achieve and maintain viral suppression during pregnancy and postpartum decreases the risk for infant transmission to less than 1% but notes that it is not zero. For patients not on therapy or those without viral load suppression during pregnancy (at a minimum of throughout the third trimester) and at delivery, replacement of breast milk is recommended. Patients on antiretroviral therapy who have a sustained undetectable viral load and who choose to breastfeed or use replacement of breast milk should be supported in this decision. If the clinical decision is to use this drug while breastfeeding, the infant should be monitored for the most common reported adult side effects of nausea, headache, and abdominal pain (all leading to irritability), diarrhea, pyrexia, vomiting, and fatigue (lethargy).

References

1. Prescribing Information. *Aptivus*. Boehringer Ingelheim Pharmaceuticals, Inc; 2024.
2. Panel on Treatment of HIV During Pregnancy and Prevention of Perinatal Transmission. Recommendations for the use of antiretroviral drugs during pregnancy and interventions to reduce perinatal HIV transmission in the United States. Department of Health and Human Services. Accessed July 25, 2023. https://clinicalinfo.hiv.gov/en/guidelines/perinatal
3. Wensing AMJ, Boucher CAB, van Kasteren M, et al. Prevention of mother-to-child transmission of multi-drug resistant HIV-1 using maternal therapy with both enfuvirtide and tipranavir. *AIDS*. 2006;20:1465-1467.
4. Weizsaecker K, Kurowski M, Hoffmeister B, et al. Pharmacokinetic profile in late pregnancy and cord blood concentration of tipranavir and enfuvirtide. *Int J STD AIDS*. 2011;22:294-295.

T

TIRBANIBULIN

Dermatologic (Topical Skin Product)

PREGNANCY RECOMMENDATION: No Human Data—Animal Data Suggest Low Risk

BREASTFEEDING RECOMMENDATION: Probably Compatible

PREGNANCY SUMMARY

No reports describing the use of tirbanibulin in human pregnancy have been located. The drug will probably cross the placenta in minimal amounts. However, the absence of human pregnancy experience prevents a complete assessment of the embryofetal risk. Animal data did not show any embryofetal toxicity, even when administered orally. Based on drug indication, use during pregnancy is uncertain.

BREASTFEEDING SUMMARY

Tirbanibulin probably enters breast milk. However, because the drug is used topically with low plasma levels found following systemic absorption, the total drug amount in breast milk is likely to be negligible. Breastfeeding while using tirbanibulin should be based on the mother's clinical need for treatment.

Reference

1. Prescribing Information. *Klisyri*. Almirall, Inc; 2020.

TIROFIBAN

Cardiovascular (IIb/IIIa Receptor Antagonist—Antiplatelet)

PREGNANCY RECOMMENDATION: Limited Human Data—Animal Data Suggest Low Risk (Maternal Benefit May Outweigh Embryo–Fetal Risk)

BREASTFEEDING RECOMMENDATION: Potential Toxicity (Hold Breastfeeding)

PREGNANCY SUMMARY

Three case reports describing the successful use of tirofiban in the second and third trimesters of human pregnancy were located. No adverse fetal effects related to the drug were identified. The drug will probably cross the placenta, so some fetal exposure will likely occur. Therefore, this limited human pregnancy experience prevents a complete assessment of the embryofetal risk. Animal data did not show any embryofetal toxicity in one species at doses of less than 10 times the RHD and in a second species at more than 10 times the RHD. The primary concern with use during pregnancy, however, appears to be the potential for maternal hemorrhage. If this is adequately controlled, the benefits of the drug to the mother appear to outweigh any unknown risks to the fetus. Using this drug during pregnancy should be based on the pros and cons of the mother's clinical need for treatment versus any potential fetal risk that might occur from exposure.

BREASTFEEDING SUMMARY

No reports describing the use of tirofiban during human lactation have been located. The drug will likely be excreted into breast milk, so some infant exposure will probably occur. The drug is commonly combined with heparin and sometimes with aspirin. The effect of this exposure on a nursing infant is not fully known. Breastfeeding while using this drug should be based on the mother's clinical need for treatment versus any potential infant risks that might occur. If used, the infant should be monitored for the most common reported adult side effect of bruising or bleeding. Another possibility is to hold breastfeeding for 10 to 12 hours (about five to six half-lives).

References

1. Prescribing Information. *Tirofiban hydrochloride*. Nexus Pharmaceuticals LLC; 2023.
2. Boztosun B, Olcay A, Avci A, Kirma C. Treatment of acute myocardial infarction in pregnancy with coronary artery balloon angioplasty and stenting: use of tirofiban and clopidogrel. *Int J Cardiol*. 2008;127:413-416.
3. Hajj-Chahine J, Jayle C, Tomasi J, Corbi P. Successful surgical management of massive pulmonary embolism during the second trimester in a parturient with heparin-induced thrombocytopenia. *Interact Cardio Vasc Thorac Surg*. 2010;11:679-681.
4. Argentiero D, Savonitto S, D'Andrea P, Iacovelli F. Ticagrelor and tirofiban in pregnancy and delivery: beyond labels. *J Thromb Thrombolysis*. 2020;49:145-148.

T

TIRZEPATIDE

Antidiabetic (Glucagon-Like Peptide-1 Receptor Agonist)

PREGNANCY RECOMMENDATION: No Human Data—Animal Data Suggest Potential Risk

BREASTFEEDING RECOMMENDATION: Probably Compatible

PREGNANCY SUMMARY

No reports describing the use of tirzepatide in human pregnancy have been located. Tirzepatide is not likely to cross the placenta, so fetal exposure will probably not occur, or at most be negligible. However, the absence of human pregnancy experience prevents a complete assessment of embryofetal risk. Embryofetal toxicity with malformations was observed in animal studies, but in conjunction with maternal toxicity. Using this drug during pregnancy should be based on the pros and cons of the mother's clinical need for treatment versus any potential fetal risk that might occur from exposure. Insulin is still the treatment of choice for this disease during pregnancy. Moreover, insulin does not cross the placenta, which eliminates the additional concern that the drug therapy is adversely affecting the fetus. Carefully prescribed insulin therapy will provide better control of the mother's blood glucose, thereby preventing the fetal and neonatal complications that occur with this disease. High maternal glucose levels, as might occur in diabetes, are associated with a number of maternal and fetal adverse effects, including fetal structural anomalies if the hyperglycemia occurs early in gestation. To prevent this toxicity, ACOG recommends that insulin be used for type 1 and type 2 diabetes occurring during pregnancy and, if diet therapy alone is not successful, for gestational diabetes. If a woman becomes pregnant while taking tirzepatide, changing the therapy to insulin should be considered. Due to the delayed gastric emptying, tirzepatide can decrease the efficacy of oral hormonal contraceptives. This effect does diminish over time. The manufacturer recommends that patients using oral hormonal contraceptives switch to a non-oral contraceptive or add a barrier method of contraception for at least 4 weeks after initiation and for 4 weeks after each dose escalation.

BREASTFEEDING SUMMARY

No reports describing the use of tirzepatide during human lactation have been located. The drug will likely not be found in breast milk. Additionally, because tirzepatide is a polypeptide, if any drug were to be ingested through breastfeeding, it would probably be digested in the infant's gastrointestinal tract and not be absorbed. Breastfeeding while using this drug should be based on the mother's clinical need for treatment. If used, the infant should be monitored for the most common reported adult side effects of nausea, dyspepsia, and abdominal pain (all leading to irritability), diarrhea, decreased appetite, vomiting, and constipation.

References

1. Prescribing Information. *Mounjaro*. Eli Lilly and Company; 2023.
2. American College of Obstetricians and Gynecologists. ACOG Practice Bulletin No. 201: pregestational diabetes mellitus. *Obstet Gynecol*. 2018;132:e228-e248.
3. American College of Obstetricians and Gynecologists. ACOG Practice Bulletin No. 190: gestational diabetes. *Obstet Gynecol*. 2018;131:e49-e64.

TISLELIZUMAB

Antineoplastic (Monoclonal Antibody—Programmed Death Receptor 1 Inhibitor)

PREGNANCY RECOMMENDATION: No Human Data and No Relevant Animal Data

BREASTFEEDING RECOMMENDATION: Probably Compatible

PREGNANCY SUMMARY

No reports describing the use of tislelizumab in human pregnancy have been located. As an IgG antibody, it likely crosses the placenta, especially during the second half of gestation, so some fetal exposure will probably occur. Therefore, the absence of human pregnancy experience prevents a complete assessment of the embryofetal risk. A primary function of the programmed death receptor 1 (PD-1)/PD-1 ligand pathway is to preserve pregnancy by maintaining maternal tolerance to a fetus. Therefore, there are theoretical risks to using this drug, especially in the first trimester. Animal reproduction and fertility studies have not been conducted with tislelizumab. Based on the drug's mechanism of action, the manufacturer recommends that women with reproductive potential use effective contraception during treatment and for 4 months after the last dose. Nevertheless, using this drug during pregnancy should be based on the pros and cons of the mother's clinical need for treatment versus any potential fetal risk that might occur from exposure. There is a registry for women who are pregnant and have cancer. For more information, women and health care providers are encouraged to contact the Cancer and Pregnancy Registry at 1-877-635-4499.

BREASTFEEDING SUMMARY

No reports describing the use of tislelizumab during human lactation have been located. It is known that IgG antibodies can be found in human breast milk, but are not found in the neonatal or infant circulation. Additionally, if any IgG antibodies were to be ingested through breastfeeding, they would probably be digested in the infant's gastrointestinal tract and not be absorbed. However, due to a concern for potential serious adverse effects that might be seen in a breastfed infant, the manufacturer recommends that women not breastfeed while being treated with this drug and for at least 4 months after the last dose. Nevertheless, breastfeeding while using this drug should be based on the mother's clinical need for treatment versus any potential infant risks that might occur. If used, the infant should be monitored for the most common reported adult side effects of musculoskeletal pain (leading to irritability), fatigue (lethargy), cough, and various laboratory abnormalities (see PI).

Reference

1. Prescribing Information. *Tevimbra*. Beigene; 2024.

TISOTUMAB VEDOTIN

Antineoplastic (Monoclonal Antibody Drug Conjugate)

PREGNANCY RECOMMENDATION: No Human Data—Animal Data Suggest Potential Risk

BREASTFEEDING RECOMMENDATION: Potential Toxicity

PREGNANCY SUMMARY

No reports describing the use of tisotumab vedotin in human pregnancy have been located. Tisotumab vedotin likely crosses the placenta, so some fetal exposure will probably occur. Unconjugated monomethyl auristatin E (MMAE) is also likely to cross the placenta, but maternal blood levels are low. The clinical significance of the amount of this drug in the fetal circulation is unknown. Therefore, the absence of human pregnancy experience prevents a complete assessment of embryofetal risk. Animal data did show embryofetal toxicity for MMAE. Based on these animal studies and the drug's mechanism of action, the manufacturer recommends that women with reproductive potential use effective contraception during treatment and for 2 months after the last dose. They also recommend that males with female partners of reproductive potential use effective contraception during treatment and for 4 months after the last dose. Nevertheless, using this drug during pregnancy should be based on the pros and cons of the mother's clinical need for treatment versus any potential fetal risk that might occur from exposure.

BREASTFEEDING SUMMARY

No reports describing the use of tisotumab vedotin during human lactation have been located. It is known that IgG antibodies can be found in human breast milk, but are not found in the neonatal or infant circulation. Additionally, if any IgG antibodies were to be ingested through breastfeeding, they would probably be digested in the infant's gastrointestinal tract and not be absorbed. Very small amounts of unconjugated MMAE may also be found in milk. The clinical significance of this is unknown. Due to the potential for serious adverse effects that might be seen in a breastfed infant, the manufacturer recommends that women not breastfeed while using tisotumab vedotin and for 3 weeks after the last dose. Nevertheless, breastfeeding while using this drug should be based on the mother's clinical need for treatment. If used, the infant should be monitored for the most common reported adult side effects of nausea and neuropathy (both leading to irritability), diarrhea, lethargy, rash, conjunctival reactions, and various laboratory abnormalities (see PI).

References

1. Prescribing Information. *Tivdak*. Seagen, Inc; 2022.
2. National Library of Medicine—PubChem. *MMAE*. https://pubchem.ncbi.nlm.nih.gov/compound/MMAE

TIVOZANIB

Antineoplastic (Tyrosine Kinase Inhibitor)

PREGNANCY RECOMMENDATION: No Human Data—Animal Data Suggest Potential Risk

BREASTFEEDING RECOMMENDATION: Potential Toxicity

T

PREGNANCY SUMMARY

No reports describing the use of tivozanib in human pregnancy have been located. Tivozanib is likely to cross the placenta, so some fetal exposure will probably occur. Therefore, the absence of human pregnancy experience prevents a complete assessment of the embryofetal risk. Embryofetal toxicity was observed in animal studies. Based on the animal studies and the drug's mechanism of action, the manufacturer recommends that women with reproductive potential use effective contraception during treatment and for 1 month after the last dose. They also recommend that males with female partners of reproductive potential use effective contraception during treatment and for 1 month after the last dose. Nevertheless, using this drug during pregnancy should be based on the pros and cons of the mother's clinical need for treatment versus any potential fetal risk that might occur from exposure. Elevated glucose levels have been reported in patients treated with this drug. Hypertension was also reported in up to 45% of patients treated with tivozanib in the clinical trials.

BREASTFEEDING SUMMARY

No reports describing the use of tivozanib during human lactation have been located. It is likely that some amount of the drug will be excreted into breast milk, so infant exposure will probably occur. Due to the potential for serious adverse effects that might be seen in a breastfed infant, the manufacturer recommends that women not breastfeed while taking tivozanib and for 1 month after the last dose. Nevertheless, breastfeeding while using this drug should be based on the mother's clinical need for treatment. If used, the infant should be monitored for the most common reported adult side effects of nausea (leading to irritability), lethargy, elevated blood pressure, diarrhea, decreased appetite (monitor growth), cough, and various laboratory abnormalities (see PI).

Reference

1. Prescribing Information. *Fotivda*. AVEO Pharmaceuticals; 2021.

TIZANIDINE

Central Nervous System (Skeletal Muscle Relaxant)

PREGNANCY RECOMMENDATION: No Human Data—Animal Data Suggest Risk

BREASTFEEDING RECOMMENDATION: Potential Toxicity

PREGNANCY SUMMARY

No reports describing the use of tizanidine in human pregnancy have been located. The drug will probably cross the placenta, so some fetal exposure will likely occur. Therefore, the absence of human pregnancy experience prevents a complete assessment of the embryofetal risk. Embryofetal toxicity was observed in two animal species at doses of less than 10 times the MRHD. Using this drug during pregnancy should be based on the pros and cons of the mother's clinical need for treatment versus any potential fetal risk that might occur from exposure. Dose-related hypotension has been observed in humans with this drug, and this could potentially have a serious adverse effect in pregnant women. Single doses of the recommended dose (8 mg) have caused a 20% reduction in either the systolic or diastolic blood pressure in up to two-thirds of patients. This effect may be minimized by titration of the dose, but close monitoring of the maternal blood pressure is needed. The manufacturer states that with discontinuation of the drug, rebound hypertension, tachycardia, and hypertonia can occur, especially in patients on high doses (≥20 mg/d) for long periods (≥9 weeks) or on concomitant narcotics. To minimize this risk, the dose should be slowly tapered (2-4 mg daily).

BREASTFEEDING SUMMARY

No reports describing the use of tizanidine during human lactation have been located. The drug will likely be excreted into breast milk, so some infant exposure will probably occur. However, due to a concern for potential serious adverse effects that might be seen in a breastfed infant, the manufacturer recommends caution if used by a nursing woman. Breastfeeding while using this drug should be based on the mother's clinical need for treatment versus any potential infant risks that might occur. If used, the infant should be monitored for the most common reported adult side effects of dry mouth and dizziness (both leading to irritability), somnolence, and urinary tract infection.

Reference

1. Prescribing Information. *Tizanidine*. Direct Rx; 2022.

TOBRAMYCIN

Antibacterial (Aminoglycoside)

PREGNANCY RECOMMENDATION: Limited Human Data—Animal Data Suggest Low Risk

BREASTFEEDING RECOMMENDATION: Probably Compatible

PREGNANCY SUMMARY

A few studies were located that describe the use of tobramycin during human pregnancy. From the Michigan Medicaid Surveillance study, 3 (3.7%) major anomalies (all different) were seen in 81 first-trimester exposures. In a second study of 22,843 cases with congenital anomalies, 38 (0.17%) used aminoglycoside drugs, which was no different in the 38,151 controls (no birth defects) where 42 (0.11%) had used the drug. In 6 of the 80 cases, tobramycin was used. The drug crosses the placenta, so fetal exposure will occur. However, this limited human pregnancy experience prevents a complete assessment of embryofetal risk. Animal data did not show any embryofetal toxicity in two species at doses of less than 10 times the MRHD in one species and more than 10 times the MRHD in the second species. In the first species, maternal toxicity was seen. Using this drug during pregnancy should be based on the pros and cons of the mother's clinical need for treatment versus any potential fetal risk that might occur from exposure. However, for systemic tobramycin use, the manufacturer states that aminoglycosides can cause fetal injury with use during pregnancy. There have been several reports of total irreversible bilateral congenital deafness and severe nephrotoxicity in children whose mothers received streptomycin during pregnancy. Serious side effects to the mother, fetus, or newborn have not been consistently reported with other aminoglycosides. If tobramycin is used during pregnancy or the patient becomes pregnant while taking it, using the drug for a short treatment period is recommended.

BREASTFEEDING SUMMARY

Tobramycin has been shown to be excreted into human breast milk. Following an 80-mg intramuscular (IM) dose given to five lactating women, breast milk levels varied from a trace to about 0.5 mcg/mL over 8 hours. Peak levels occurred at 4 hours after injection. Because oral absorption of this antibiotic is poor, ototoxicity in the infant would not be expected. However, modification of bowel flora can occur in a nursing infant. Breastfeeding while using this drug should be based on the mother's clinical need for treatment versus any potential infant risks that might occur. If used, the infant should be monitored for the most common reported adult side effects of nausea, headache, and blurred vision (all leading to irritability), diarrhea, rash, and cough.

References

1. Prescribing Information. *Tobramycin*. Baxter Healthcare Corporation; 2023.
2. Prescribing Information. *Tobramycin inhalation solution*. Dr. Reddy's Laboratories, Inc; 2023.
3. Bernard B, Garcia-Cazares S, Ballard C, et al. Tobramycin: maternal-fetal pharmacology. *Antimicrob Agents Chemother*. 1977;11:688-694.
4. Fernandez H, Bourget P, Delouis C. Fetal levels of tobramycin following maternal administration. *Obstet Gynecol*. 1990;76:992-994.
5. Olsen J, Sorensen HT. A teratological study of aminoglycoside antibiotic treatment during pregnancy. *Scand J Infect Dis*. 2000;32:309-313.
6. Yu PA, Tran EL, Parker CM, et al. Safety of antimicrobials during pregnancy: a systematic review of antimicrobials considered for treatment and postexposure prophylaxis of plague. *Clin Infect Dis*. 2020;70:S37-S50.
7. Takase Z. Laboratory and clinical studies on tobramycin in the field of obstetrics and gynecology. *Chemotherapy (Tokyo)*. 1975;23:1402.

TOBRAMYCIN OPHTHALMIC

Ophthalmic/Antibacterial (Aminoglycoside—Topical)

PREGNANCY RECOMMENDATION: No Human Data—Animal Data Suggest Low Risk

BREASTFEEDING RECOMMENDATION: Probably Compatible

PREGNANCY SUMMARY

No reports describing the use of tobramycin ophthalmic in human pregnancy have been located. Systemic levels were undetectable (LLQ of 200 ng/mL) after topical ocular administration. The drug has been shown to cross the placenta with systemic use, so some fetal exposure can occur if the drug is present in the circulation. However, the absence of human pregnancy experience prevents a complete assessment of embryofetal risk. No embryofetal toxicity was seen in three animal species at doses of more than 10 times the MRHD. Using this drug during pregnancy should be based on the pros and cons of the mother's clinical need for treatment versus any potential fetal risk that might occur from exposure. If used during pregnancy, consider placing pressure over the tear duct in the corner of the eye for at least 1 minute, and then remove any excess solution with absorbent tissue to decrease the amount of drug reaching the systemic circulation even further.

T

BREASTFEEDING SUMMARY

No reports describing the use of tobramycin ophthalmic during human lactation have been located. Systemic exposure is negligible with ocular use. In addition, oral absorption of this antibiotic is poor. Therefore, any infant exposure is likely to be clinically insignificant. Breastfeeding while using this drug should be based on the mother's clinical need for treatment versus any potential infant risks that might occur.

References

1. Prescribing Information. *Tobramycin ophthalmic solution*. Alembic Pharmaceuticals, Inc; 2024.

TOCILIZUMAB

Immunologic (Monoclonal Antibody—IL-6 Receptor Antagonist)

PREGNANCY RECOMMENDATION: Limited Human Data—Animal Data Suggest Potential Risk

BREASTFEEDING RECOMMENDATION: Probably Compatible

PREGNANCY SUMMARY

Numerous case reports and small series were located that describe the use of tocilizumab in human pregnancy. From about 10 first-trimester exposures, no major malformations were reported. In addition, no adverse fetal effects were described with the use of the drug in the second and third trimesters. The drug has been shown to cross the placenta, so fetal exposure will occur. However, the limited human pregnancy experience prevents a complete assessment of embryofetal risk. Embryofetal toxicity with malformations was observed in one animal species at doses of less than 10 times the MRHD. Using this drug during pregnancy should be based on the pros and cons of the mother's clinical need for treatment versus any potential fetal risk that might occur from exposure.

BREASTFEEDING SUMMARY

Two studies have shown that tocilizumab is excreted into breast milk in low amounts (<1% maternal serum levels). This is consistent with other studies analyzing breast milk levels for IgG antibodies. However, IgG antibodies are known to be found in human breast milk, but are not found in the neonatal or infant circulation. Additionally, if any IgG antibodies were to be ingested through breastfeeding, they would probably be digested in the infant's gastrointestinal tract and not be absorbed. Breastfeeding while using this drug should be based on the mother's clinical need for treatment versus any potential infant risks that might occur. If used, the infant should be monitored for the most common reported adult side effects of headache (leading to irritability), upper respiratory tract infections, and increased liver enzyme levels.

References

1. Prescribing Information. *Actemra*. Genentech, Inc; 2024.
2. Saito J, Yakuwa N, Kaneko K, et al. Tocilizumab during pregnancy and lactation: drug levels in maternal serum, cord blood, breast milk and infant serum. *Rheumatol*. 2019;58:1505-1507.
3. Tada Y, Sakai M, Nakao Y, et al. Placental transfer of tocilizumab in a patient with rheumatoid arthritis. *Rheumatol*. 2019;58:1694-1695.

TOFACITINIB

Immunologic (JAK Inhibitor)

PREGNANCY RECOMMENDATION: Limited Human Data—Animal Data Suggest Potential Risk

BREASTFEEDING RECOMMENDATION: Potential Toxicity

PREGNANCY SUMMARY

Several case reports and small series have described the use of tofacitinib during human pregnancy. Of 40 first-trimester exposures, 2 (5%) major birth anomalies were described. Both defects were different. Based on ex vivo placental perfusion studies, the drug appears to cross the placenta, so some fetal exposure will occur. However, the limited human pregnancy experience prevents a complete assessment of embryofetal risk. Embryofetal toxicity was not seen in two animal species at doses of less than 10 times the MRHD. However, in one of these, embryofetal toxicity with malformations was seen with higher doses that were still less than 10 times the MRHD. Based on animal studies and the drug's mechanism of action, the manufacturer recommends that women with reproductive potential use effective contraception during treatment.

Nevertheless, using this drug during pregnancy should be based on the pros and cons of the mother's clinical need for treatment versus any potential fetal risk that might occur from exposure. Uncontrolled rheumatoid arthritis or ulcerative colitis is associated with adverse pregnancy outcomes such as preterm delivery, IUGR, and preeclampsia. There is a pregnancy exposure registry that monitors pregnancy outcomes in women using this drug. Health care providers are encouraged to call the Tofacitinib Pregnancy Exposure Registry at 1-877-311-8972.

BREASTFEEDING SUMMARY

One report describing the use of tofacitinib during human lactation was located. A woman continued tofacitinib therapy after delivery and while breastfeeding. No adverse infant events were reported. The drug will likely be excreted into human breast milk, so some infant exposure will probably occur. Because of the risk for serious infections, the manufacturer recommends that women not breastfeed while being treated with this drug and for at least 18 hours after the last dose of the tablet and oral solution or after 36 hours after the last extended-release tablet. Nevertheless, if the clinical decision is to use this drug while breastfeeding, the infant should be monitored for the most common reported adult side effects of headache (leading to irritability), upper respiratory tract infections, diarrhea, and various laboratory abnormalities (see PI).

References

1. Prescribing Information. *Xeljanz*. U.S. Pharmaceuticals; 2024.
2. Mitrova K, Julsgaard M, Augustijns P, et al. Tofacitinib in pregnancy: assessing pregnancy and infant outcomes, cord blood, and breast milk concentrations. *Clin Gastroenterol Hepatol*. 2025;23:163-165.
3. Elieson GAM, Fransen M, van Hove H, et al. Placental transfer of tofacitinib in the ex vivo dual-side human perfusion model. *Curr Res Toxicol*. 2024; 6:100149.
4. Mahadevan U, Dubinsky MC, Su C, et al. Outcomes of pregnancies with maternal/paternal exposure in the tofacitinib safety databases for ulcerative colitis. *Inflamm Bowel Dis*. 2018;24:2494-2500.
5. Fernandez-Sanches M, Ribes-Artero H, Roma-Sanche E, et al. Fetal exposure to tofacitinib during the first trimester: a healthy newborn case report. *Birth Defects Res*. 2021;113:1275-1279.
6. Arzivian A, Zhang E, Laube R, Leong R. First-trimester exposure to tofacitinib in ulcerative colitis: a case report of a healthy newborn and literature review. *Clin Case Rep*. 2024;12:e8764.
7. Rowan C, Yeaman F, Ernest-Suarez K, et al. Tofacitinib as a rescue therapy for ulcerative colitis in pregnancy. *Inflamm Bowel Dis*. 2024;30:868-870.
8. Ernest-Suarez K, Murguia-Favela LE, Novak KL, et al. Continuous tofacitinib exposure in utero and during breastfeeding. *Crohns Colitis 360*. 2024;6: otae006.

TOFERSEN

Central Nervous System (Antisense Oligonucleotide)

PREGNANCY RECOMMENDATION: No Human Data—Animal Data Suggest Low Risk

BREASTFEEDING RECOMMENDATION: Probably Compatible

PREGNANCY SUMMARY

No reports describing the use of tofersen in human pregnancy have been located. Though placental transfer is possible, fetal exposure is probably negligible. However, the absence of human pregnancy experience prevents a complete assessment of the embryofetal risk. Animal data did not show any embryofetal toxicity despite being administered subcutaneously. Using this drug during pregnancy should be based on the pros and cons of the mother's clinical need for treatment versus any potential fetal risk that might occur from exposure.

BREASTFEEDING SUMMARY

No reports describing the use of tofersen in human lactation have been located. Though a negligible amount of the drug may be found in breast milk, a clinical effect is unlikely. However, breastfeeding while using this drug should be based on the mother's clinical need for treatment. If used, the infant should be monitored for the most common reported adult side effects of arthralgias and myalgias (both leading to irritability) and lethargy.

Reference

1. Prescribing Information. *Qalsody*. Biogen MA, Inc; 2023.

TOLCAPONE

Central Nervous System (Anti-Parkinson—COMT Inhibitor)

PREGNANCY RECOMMENDATION: No Human Data—Animal Data Suggest Risk

BREASTFEEDING RECOMMENDATION: Potential Toxicity

PREGNANCY SUMMARY

No reports describing the use of tolcapone in human pregnancy have been located. The drug will probably cross the placenta, so some fetal exposure will likely occur. Therefore, the absence of human pregnancy experience prevents a complete assessment of the embryofetal risk. Embryofetal toxicity was observed in two animal species at doses of less than 10 times the RHD for tolcapone by itself. However, the drug is always used in combination with levodopa/carbidopa. Increased embryofetal toxicity was observed with the combination compared to levodopa/carbidopa alone in two animal species at doses of less than the RHD. Using this drug during pregnancy should be based on the pros and cons of the mother's clinical need for treatment versus any potential fetal risk that might occur from exposure. The drug carries a boxed warning for potentially fatal, acute fulminant liver failure. Because of this risk, the manufacturer recommends that it should only be used in patients who are not appropriate candidates for other adjunctive therapies. Additionally, the manufacturer reports that if the patient fails to show substantial clinical benefit within 3 weeks of treatment initiation, therapy with tolcapone should be withdrawn.

BREASTFEEDING SUMMARY

No reports describing the use of tolcapone during human lactation have been located. The drug will likely be excreted into breast milk, so some infant exposure will probably occur. However, due to a concern for potential serious adverse effects (including potentially fatal, acute fulminant liver failure) that might be seen in a breastfed infant, the manufacturer recommends that women not breastfeed while being treated with this drug. Nevertheless, breastfeeding while using this drug should be based on the mother's clinical need for treatment versus any potential infant risks that might occur. If used, the infant should be monitored for the most common reported adult side effects of nausea (leading to irritability), diarrhea, anorexia (monitor infant growth), vomiting, urine discoloration, somnolence, and sweating.

Reference

1. Prescribing Information. *Tolcapone*. Oceanside Pharmaceuticals; 2020.

TOLMETIN

Pain (Nonsteroidal Anti-Inflammatory Drug)

PREGNANCY RECOMMENDATION: Human Data Suggest Risk (Second and Third Trimesters)

BREASTFEEDING RECOMMENDATION: Probably Compatible

PREGNANCY SUMMARY

One report describing the use of tolmetin in human pregnancy was located. Of the 99 newborns with first-trimester exposure, 1 (1%) had a major birth defect (4 expected). The drug will probably cross the placenta, so some fetal exposure will likely occur. Therefore, this limited human pregnancy experience with tolmetin prevents a complete assessment of the embryofetal risk. Animal data did not show any embryofetal toxicity in two species at doses of less than 10 times the MRHD. Regarding nonsteroidal anti-inflammatory drug (NSAID) use as a group, some studies have suggested an increased risk for cardiac anomalies and cleft lip and palate, but again, these findings have not been consistently found. Data from other evaluations analyzing NSAIDs as a group have not found any pattern to the defects. NSAIDs can cause premature stricture or closure of the fetal ductus arteriosus when used in the latter portion of gestation. In some instances, this can produce persistent pulmonary hypertension in the neonate. These drugs have also been reported to produce fetal renal dysfunction leading to oligohydramnios when used after 20 weeks' gestation. The FDA recommends that NSAIDs be avoided in women at 20 weeks or later in pregnancy. If deemed necessary by a health care provider, the use of NSAIDs between 20 and 30 weeks should be limited to the lowest effective dose and shortest duration. If treatment extends beyond 48 hours, providers should consider an ultrasound to monitor amniotic fluid levels. Using this drug during pregnancy should be based on the pros and cons of the mother's clinical need for treatment versus any potential fetal risk that might occur from exposure.

BREASTFEEDING SUMMARY

Tolmetin has been shown to be excreted into human breast milk. Breast milk levels ranged from about 60 to 180 ng/mL. The calculated RID was less than 1%. The clinical significance of these levels to the nursing infant is unknown. However, due to a concern for potential serious adverse effects that might be seen in a breastfed infant, the manufacturer recommends that women not breastfeed while being treated with this drug. Nevertheless, if the clinical decision is to use this drug while breastfeeding, the infant should be monitored for the most common reported adult side effects of nausea, dyspepsia, gastrointestinal distress, abdominal pain, headache, and dizziness (all leading to irritability), diarrhea, flatulence, vomiting, and peripheral edema.

References

1. Prescribing Information. *Tolmetin sodium*. Atland Pharmaceuticals LLC; 2024.
2. Medscape. *Tolmetin*. Accessed December 21, 2024. https://reference.medscape.com/drug/tolmetin-343306#0
3. Food and Drug Administration. *Nonsteroidal anti-inflammatory drugs (NSAIDs): drug safety communication—avoid use of NSAIDs in pregnancy at 20 weeks or later*. Accessed October 8, 2024. https://www.fda.gov/safety/medical-product-safety-information/nonsteroidal-antiinflammatory-drugs-nsaids-drug-safety-communication-avoid-use-nsaids-pregnancy-20
4. Chen X, Yang Y, Chen L, et al. Pregnancy outcomes and birth defects in offspring following non-steroidal anti-inflammatory drugs exposure during pregnancy: a systematic review and meta-analysis. *Reprod Tox*. 2024;125:108561.
5. Ying XH, Bao DN, Jiang HY, Shi YD. Maternal non-steroidal anti-inflammatory drug exposure during pregnancy and risk of miscarriage: a systematic review and meta-analysis. *Eur J Clin Pharmacol*. 2022;78:171-180.
6. Sagraves R, Waller ES, Goehrs HR. Tolmetin in breast milk. *Drug Intell Clin Pharm*. 1985;19:55-56.

TOLNAFTATE

Anti-Infective (Topical Antifungal)

PREGNANCY RECOMMENDATION: Limited Human Data—No Relevant Animal Data

BREASTFEEDING RECOMMENDATION: Probably Compatible

PREGNANCY SUMMARY

One report described nine pregnancies exposed to tolnaftate spray in the first trimester. There were 5 (0.02%) uses in 22,843 with birth anomalies and 4 (0.01%) in 38,151 controls without birth defects. The drug will probably cross the placenta if found in the systemic circulation. However, less than 1% of the drug is absorbed following topical use. Therefore, the overall exposure with topical use is likely to be clinically insignificant. However, the limited human pregnancy experience prevents a complete assessment of embryofetal risk. Embryofetal toxicity was seen in two species, but with oral or SC doses of more than 10 times the MRHD. Using this drug during pregnancy should be based on the pros and cons of the mother's clinical need for treatment versus any potential fetal risk that might occur from exposure. Tolnaftate is available over the counter.

BREASTFEEDING SUMMARY

No reports describing the use of tolnaftate during human lactation have been located. The drug will likely be excreted into breast milk if found in the systemic circulation. However, less than 1% of the drug is systemically absorbed following topical administration. Therefore, the overall exposure is likely to be clinically insignificant. Breastfeeding while using this drug should be based on the mother's clinical need for treatment versus any potential infant risks that might occur. Because of the topical use of the drug, systemic side effects were not fully analyzed.

References

1. Czeizel AE, Kazy Z, Puho E. Tolnaftate spray treatment during pregnancy. *Reprod Toxicol*. 2004;18:443-444.
2. National Library of Medicine—Pubchem. *Tolnaftate*. Accessed December 21, 2024. https://pubchem.ncbi.nlm.nih.gov/compound/5510
3. Czeizel AE, Kazy Z, Puho E. Tolnaftate spray treatment during pregnancy. *Reprod Toxicol*. 2004;18:443-444.
4. Noguchi T, Hashimoto Y, Makita T, Tanimura T. Teratogenesis study of tolnaftate, an antitrichophyton agent. *Toxicol Appl Pharmacol*. 1966;8:386-397.

TOLTERODINE

Urinary (Selective Antimuscarinic)

PREGNANCY RECOMMENDATION: No Human Data—Animal Data Suggest Low Risk

BREASTFEEDING RECOMMENDATION: Potential Toxicity

PREGNANCY SUMMARY

No reports describing the use of tolterodine in human pregnancy have been located. The drug and active metabolite will probably cross the placenta, so some fetal exposure will likely occur. Therefore, the absence of human pregnancy experience prevents a complete assessment of the embryofetal risk. Animal data did not show any embryofetal toxicity in two species at doses of less than (in one) and more than (in the second) 10 times the RHD. Using this drug during pregnancy should be based on the pros and cons of the mother's clinical need for treatment versus any potential fetal risk that might occur from exposure. Tolterodine was found to prolong the QT interval in the clinical trials.

T

BREASTFEEDING SUMMARY

No reports describing the use of tolterodine during human lactation have been located. The drug and active metabolite will likely be excreted into breast milk, so some infant exposure will probably occur. Due to the anticholinergic effects, tolterodine may decrease breast milk supply. Due to a concern for potential serious adverse effects that might be seen in a breastfed infant, the manufacturer recommends that women not breastfeed while being treated with this drug. However, if the clinical decision is to use this drug while breastfeeding, the infant should be monitored for the most common reported adult side effects of headache, dry mouth, dizziness, and abdominal pain (all leading to irritability), and constipation.

Reference

1. Prescribing Information. *Tolterodine tartrate*. Macleods Pharmaceuticals Limited; 2022.

TOLVAPTAN

Urinary (Vasopressin Receptor Antagonist)

PREGNANCY RECOMMENDATION: No Human Data—Animal Data Suggest Low Risk

BREASTFEEDING RECOMMENDATION: Potential Toxicity

PREGNANCY SUMMARY

No reports describing the use of tolvaptan in human pregnancy have been located. The drug will probably cross the placenta, so some fetal exposure will likely occur. Therefore, the absence of human pregnancy experience prevents a complete assessment of the embryofetal risk. Animal data did not show any embryofetal toxicity in two species at doses of less than 10 times the MRHD. Some embryofetal toxicity with maternal toxicity was seen in one of these species at higher doses, but still less than 10 times the MRHD. Using this drug during pregnancy should be based on the pros and cons of the mother's clinical need for treatment versus any potential fetal risk that might occur from exposure.

BREASTFEEDING SUMMARY

No reports describing the use of tolvaptan during human lactation have been located. The drug will likely be excreted into breast milk, so some infant exposure will probably occur. However, due to a concern for potential serious adverse effects (including electrolyte abnormalities) that might be seen in a breastfed infant, the manufacturer recommends that women not breastfeed while being treated with this drug. Nevertheless, if the clinical decision is to use this drug while breastfeeding, the infant should be monitored for the most common reported adult side effects of dry mouth and thirst (leading to irritability), fatigue (lethargy), constipation, polyuria, and hyperglycemia.

Reference

1. Prescribing Information. *Tolvaptan*. Apotex Corp; 2022.

TOPIRAMATE

Central Nervous System (Antiseizure)

PREGNANCY RECOMMENDATION: Human Data Suggest Potential Risk (First Trimester)—Animal Data Suggest Risk

BREASTFEEDING RECOMMENDATION: Potential Toxicity

T

PREGNANCY SUMMARY

There are several reports describing the use of topiramate in human pregnancy. In combined data from several studies, the rate of major birth anomalies in more than 250 first-trimester exposures was about 6.5%. Of these, there was a higher-than-expected rate for cleft lip and/or cleft palate (1.5%). In addition, there are some studies that suggest an adverse effect on childhood neurodevelopment, though this disorder has numerous factors that are difficult to control for and isolate as to absolute risk. The drug crosses the placenta with levels about equivalent to maternal serum concentrations, so some fetal exposure will occur. Embryofetal toxicity with malformations was observed in three animal species at doses of less than the MRHD for two species and less than 10 times the MRHD for the third. However, the limited human pregnancy experience still prevents a complete assessment of embryofetal risk. Based on the animal studies and human data, the manufacturer recommends that women with reproductive potential use effective contraception during treatment. Nevertheless, using this drug during pregnancy should be based on the pros and cons of the mother's clinical need for treatment versus any potential fetal risk that might occur from exposure. There is a pregnancy exposure registry that monitors pregnancy outcomes in women using antiseizure drugs. Health care providers are encouraged to call the North American Antiepileptic Drug Pregnancy Registry at 1-888-233-2334.

BREASTFEEDING SUMMARY

Topiramate has been shown to be excreted into human breast milk with levels similar to maternal plasma levels. Infant serum levels appear to be lower. Mean maternal and breast milk levels were similar at 3.8 and 3.5 mcg/mL, respectively. The breast milk to maternal ratio was about one. However, infant levels had a mean of about 1.1 mcg/mL. None of the infants had therapeutic blood levels. Breastfeeding while using this drug should be based on the mother's clinical need for treatment versus any potential infant risks that might occur. If the clinical decision is to use this drug while breastfeeding, the infant should be monitored for the most common reported adult side effects of paresthesia, nausea, abdominal pain, dizziness, and nervousness (all leading to irritability), fatigue (lethargy), somnolence, anorexia (monitor infant growth), and diarrhea.

References

1. Prescribing Information. *Topiramate*. Ascend Laboratories LLC; 2023.
2. Pack AM, Oskoui M, Williams Roberson S, et al. Teratogenesis, perinatal, and neurodevelopmental outcomes after in utero exposure to antiseizure medication: practice guidelines from the AAN, AES, and SMFM. *Neurology*. 2024;102:e209279.
3. Yerby MS. Clinical care of pregnant women with epilepsy: neural tube defects and folic acid supplements. *Epilepsia*. 2003;44(suppl 3):33-40.
4. Ohman I, Vitols S, Luef G, et al. Topiramate kinetics during delivery, lactation, and in the neonate: preliminary observations. *Epilepsia*. 2002; 43:1157-1160.
5. Kacirova I, Grundmann M, Brozmanova H, Koristkova B. Monitoring topiramate concentrations at delivery and during lactation. *Biomed Pharmacol*. 2021;138:111446.
6. Hunt S, Russell A, Smithson WH, et al. Topiramate in pregnancy: preliminary experience from the UK Epilepsy and Pregnancy Register. *Neurology*. 2008;71:272-276.
7. Ornoy A, Zvi N, Arnon J, et al. The outcome of pregnancy following topiramate treatment: a study on 52 pregnancies. *Reprod Toxicol*. 2008;25:388-389.
8. The Lamotrigine Pregnancy Registry. *Final Report: 1 September 1992 through 31 March 2010*. GlaxcoSmithKline; July 2010.
9. Hernandez-Diaz S, Huybrechts KF, Desai RJ, et al. Topiramate use early in pregnancy and the risk of oral clefts. *Neurology*. 2018;90:e342-e351.
10. Vajda F, O'Brien T, Graham J, et al. Specific fetal malformations following intrauterine exposure to antiseizure medication. *Epilepsy Behav*. 2023;142: 109219.
11. Rihtman T, Parush S, Ornoy A. Preliminary findings of the developmental effects of in utero exposure to topiramate. *Reprod Toxicol*. 2012;34:308-311.
12. Dreier JW, Bjork MH, Alvestad S, et al. Prenatal exposure to antiseizure medication and incidence of childhood- and adolescence-onset of psychiatric disorders. *JAMA Neurol*. 2023;80:568-577.
13. Honybun E, Cockle E, Malpas CB, et al. Neurodevelopmental and functional outcomes following in utero exposure to antiseizure medication: a systematic review. *Neurology*. 2024;102:e209175.
14. Pennell PB, Karanam A, Meador KJ, et al. Antiseizure medication concentrations during pregnancy: results from the maternal outcomes and neurodevelopmental effects of antiepileptic drugs (MONEAD) study. *JAMA Neurol*. 2022;79:370-379.
15. Panchaud A, Cohen JM, Patorno E, et al. Anticonvulsants and the risk of perinatal bleeding complications. *Neurology*. 2018;91:e533-e542.
16. Morrell MJ. The new antiepileptic drugs and women: efficacy, reproductive health, pregnancy, and fetal outcome. *Epilepsia*. 1996;37(suppl 6):S34-S44.
17. Birnbaum AK, Meador KJ, Karanam A, et al. Antiepileptic drug exposure in infants of breastfeeding mothers with epilepsy. *JAMA Neurol*. 2020; 77:441-450.

TOPOTECAN

Antineoplastic (Topoisomerase Inhibitor)

PREGNANCY RECOMMENDATION: No Human Data—Animal Data Suggest Risk

BREASTFEEDING RECOMMENDATION: Potential Toxicity

PREGNANCY SUMMARY

No reports describing the use of topotecan in human pregnancy have been located. The drug will probably cross the placenta, so some fetal exposure will likely occur. Therefore, the absence of human pregnancy experience prevents a complete assessment of the embryofetal risk. Embryofetal toxicity with malformations was observed in two animal species at doses approximately equal to the RHD. Maternal toxicity also occurred in one of these species. Based on animal studies and the drug's mechanism of action, the manufacturer recommends that women with reproductive potential use effective contraception during treatment and for 6 months after the last dose. They also recommend that males with female partners of reproductive potential use effective contraception during treatment and for 3 months after the last dose. Nevertheless, using this drug during pregnancy should be based on the pros and cons of the mother's clinical need for treatment versus any potential fetal risk that might occur from exposure. There is a registry for women who are pregnant and have cancer. For more information, women and health care providers are encouraged to contact the Cancer and Pregnancy Registry at 1-877-635-4499.

BREASTFEEDING SUMMARY

No reports describing the use of topotecan during human lactation have been located. The drug will likely be excreted into breast milk, so some infant exposure will probably occur. However, due to a concern for potential serious adverse effects that might be seen in a breastfed infant, the manufacturer recommends that women not breastfeed while being treated with this drug and for at least 1 week after the last dose. Nevertheless, if the clinical decision is to use this drug while breastfeeding, the infant should be monitored for the most common reported adult side effects of nausea and abdominal pain (both leading to irritability), vomiting, fatigue (lethargy), diarrhea, dyspnea, and various laboratory abnormalities (see PI).

References

1. Prescribing Information. *Topotecan hydrochloride*. Accord Healthcare, Inc; 2023.
2. Prescribing Information. *Hycamtin*. Novartis Pharmaceuticals Corporation; 2018.

TORIPALIMAB

Antineoplastic (Monoclonal Antibody—Programmed Death Receptor 1 Inhibitor)

PREGNANCY RECOMMENDATION: No Human Data and No Relevant Animal Data

BREASTFEEDING RECOMMENDATION: Probably Compatible

PREGNANCY SUMMARY

No reports describing the use of toripalimab in human pregnancy have been located. As an IgG antibody, it likely crosses the placenta, especially during the second half of gestation, so some fetal exposure will probably occur. Therefore, the absence of human pregnancy experience prevents a complete assessment of the embryofetal risk. A primary function of the PD-1/PD-1 ligand pathway is to preserve pregnancy by maintaining maternal tolerance to a fetus. Therefore, there are theoretical risks to using this drug, especially in the first trimester. Animal reproduction and fertility studies have not been conducted with toripalimab. Based on the drug's mechanism of action, the manufacturer recommends that women with reproductive potential use effective contraception during treatment and for 4 months after the last dose. Nevertheless, using this drug during pregnancy should be based on the pros and cons of the mother's clinical need for treatment versus any potential fetal risk that might occur from exposure. There is a registry for women who are pregnant and have cancer. For more information, women and health care providers are encouraged to contact the Cancer and Pregnancy Registry at 1-877-635-4499.

BREASTFEEDING SUMMARY

No reports describing the use of toripalimab during human lactation have been located. It is known that IgG antibodies can be found in human breast milk, but are not found in the neonatal or infant circulation. Additionally, if any IgG antibodies were to be ingested through breastfeeding, they would probably be digested in the infant's gastrointestinal tract and not be absorbed. However, due to a concern for potential serious adverse effects that might be seen in a breastfed infant, the manufacturer recommends that women not breastfeed while being treated with this drug and for at least 4 months after the last dose. Nevertheless, breastfeeding while using this drug should be based on the mother's clinical need for treatment versus any potential infant risks that might occur. If used, the infant should be monitored for the most common reported adult side effects of musculoskeletal pain, nausea, and dizziness (all leading to irritability), lethargy, vomiting, fever, decreased appetite (monitor infant growth), cough, insomnia, rash, and diarrhea.

Reference

1. Prescribing Information. *Loqtorzi*. Coherus BioSciences, Inc; 2023.

TORSEMIDE

Cardiovascular (Loop Diuretic)

PREGNANCY RECOMMENDATION: No Human Data—Animal Data Suggest Potential Risk

BREASTFEEDING RECOMMENDATION: Potential Toxicity

PREGNANCY SUMMARY

No reports describing the use of torsemide in human pregnancy have been located. The drug will probably cross the placenta, so some fetal exposure will likely occur. Therefore, the absence of human pregnancy experience prevents a complete assessment of the embryofetal risk. Maternal and embryofetal toxicity with malformations were observed in two animal species at doses of less than 10 times the RHD. Using this drug during pregnancy should be based on the pros and cons of the mother's clinical need for treatment versus any potential fetal risk that might occur from exposure. Elevated glucose levels have been reported in patients (specific rate not provided) treated with this drug. Therefore, if used during pregnancy, glucose levels should be monitored.

BREASTFEEDING SUMMARY

One publication reported the use of torsemide during human lactation. The study evaluated the use of the drug (n = 59) compared with placebo (n = 59) in treating persistent postpartum hypertension. Overall, 80% and 75% of the torsemide and placebo groups breastfed their infants. No reports of adverse infant effects from the drug were described. One patient described a decrease in breast milk supply in the torsemide group. The drug will likely be excreted into breast milk, so some infant exposure will probably occur. Breastfeeding while using this drug should be based on the mother's clinical need for treatment versus any potential infant risks that might occur. If used, the infant should be monitored for the most common reported adult side effect of increased urination.

References

1. Prescribing Information. *Torsemide*. Aurobindo Pharma Limited; 2022.
2. Viteri OA, Alrais MA, Pedroza C, et al. Torsemide for prevention of persistent postpartum hypertension in women with preeclampsia: a randomized controlled trial. *Obstet Gynecol*. 2018;132:1185-1191.

TOVORAFENIB

Antineoplastic (Type II RAF Kinase Inhibitor)

PREGNANCY RECOMMENDATION: No Human Data—Animal Data Suggest Potential Risk

BREASTFEEDING RECOMMENDATION: Potential Toxicity

PREGNANCY SUMMARY

No reports describing the use of tovorafenib in human pregnancy have been located. The drug will likely cross the placenta, so some fetal exposure will probably occur. Therefore, the absence of human pregnancy experience prevents a complete assessment of the embryofetal risk. Animal studies did show embryofetal toxicity with malformations in one species at doses of less than the RHD. However, treatment was daily for about 11 days. It is not possible to determine if there was any additional effect of this greater dosing frequency. Based on these animal studies and the drug's mechanism of action, the manufacturer recommends that women with reproductive potential use effective contraception during treatment and for 4 weeks after the last dose. They also recommend that males with female partners of reproductive potential use effective contraception during treatment and for 2 weeks after the last dose. Nevertheless, using this drug during pregnancy should be based on the pros and cons of the mother's clinical need for treatment versus any potential fetal risk that might occur from exposure. There is a registry for women who are pregnant and have cancer. For more information, women and health care providers are encouraged to contact the Cancer and Pregnancy Registry at 1-877-635-4499.

BREASTFEEDING SUMMARY

No reports describing the use of tovorafenib during human lactation have been located. The drug will likely be found in breast milk, so some infant exposure will probably occur. Due to a concern for potential serious adverse effects that might be seen in a breastfed infant, the manufacturer recommends that women not breastfeed while being treated with this drug and for 2 weeks after the last dose. Nevertheless, breastfeeding while using this drug should be based on the mother's clinical need for treatment versus any potential infant risk that might occur. If used, the infant should be monitored for the most common reported adult side effects of nausea and headache (both leading to irritability), fatigue (lethargy), rash, vomiting, fever, constipation, and various laboratory abnormalities (see PI).

Reference

1. Prescribing Information. *Ojemda*. Day One Pharmaceuticals; 2024.

TRABECTEDIN

Antineoplastic (Alkylating Agent)

PREGNANCY RECOMMENDATION: No Human Data and No Relevant Animal Data

BREASTFEEDING RECOMMENDATION: Potential Toxicity

PREGNANCY SUMMARY

No reports describing the use of trabectedin in human pregnancy have been located. Some amount of the drug will probably cross the placenta, so fetal exposure will likely occur. Therefore, the absence of human pregnancy experience prevents a complete assessment of the embryofetal risk. No relevant animal studies have been conducted. Based on trabectedin's mechanism of action, the manufacturer recommends that women with reproductive potential use effective contraception during treatment and for at least 2 months after the last dose. They also recommend that males with female partners of reproductive potential use effective contraception during treatment and for at least 5 months after the last dose. Using this drug during pregnancy should be based on the pros and cons of the mother's clinical need for treatment versus any potential fetal risk that might occur from exposure. In the clinical trials, 6% of patients developed cardiomyopathy, with the ejection fraction dropping below 50%. It is recommended that patients obtain a baseline echocardiogram prior to drug initiation.

BREASTFEEDING SUMMARY

No reports describing the use of trabectedin during human lactation have been located. Some amount of the drug will probably be excreted into breast milk, so infant exposure will likely occur. Due to the concern for potential serious adverse effects that might be seen in a breastfed infant, the manufacturer recommends that women not breastfeed during treatment with this drug. Nevertheless, breastfeeding while using this drug should be based on the mother's clinical need for treatment. If used, the infant should be monitored for the most common reported adult side effects of nausea and headache (both leading to irritability), decreased appetite, vomiting, diarrhea, fatigue, peripheral edema, and numerous laboratory abnormalities (see PI).

Reference

1. Prescribing Information. *Yondelis*. Janssen Pharmaceutical Companies; 2020.

TRALOKINUMAB

Dermatologic (Monoclonal Antibody)

PREGNANCY RECOMMENDATION: No Human Data—Animal Data Suggest Low Risk

BREASTFEEDING RECOMMENDATION: Probably Compatible

PREGNANCY SUMMARY

No reports describing the use of tralokinumab in human pregnancy have been located. As an IgG antibody, the drug will likely cross the placenta at least during the second half of pregnancy, so some fetal exposure will probably occur. Therefore, the absence of human pregnancy experience prevents a complete assessment of the embryofetal risk. Animal data did not show any embryofetal toxicity. Using this drug during pregnancy should be based on the pros and cons of the mother's clinical need for treatment versus any potential fetal risk that might occur from exposure.

BREASTFEEDING SUMMARY

No reports describing the use of tralokinumab during human lactation have been located. It is known that IgG antibodies can be found in human breast milk, but are not found in the neonatal or infant circulation. Additionally, if any IgG antibodies were to be ingested through breastfeeding, they would probably be digested in the infant's gastrointestinal tract and not be absorbed. Breastfeeding while using this drug should be based on the mother's clinical need for treatment. If used, the infant should be monitored for the most common reported adult side effects of conjunctivitis, upper respiratory tract infection, and eosinophilia.

Reference

1. Prescribing Information. *Adbry*. Leo Pharma A/S; 2022.

T

TRAMADOL

Pain (Opioid)

PREGNANCY RECOMMENDATION: Human and Animal Data Suggest Potential Risk

BREASTFEEDING RECOMMENDATION: Potential Toxicity

PREGNANCY SUMMARY

Several reports describing the use of tramadol in human pregnancy have been located. Of the three large cohort studies involving over 6,000 first-trimester exposures to tramadol, two found an increased risk for major malformations in general when compared with controls. However, the rates of congenital defects in the three studies were 4% in 1,751 pregnancies, 4% in 3,796 pregnancies, and about 3% in 781 pregnancies. Therefore, the rates fell within the expected range of 2% to 4% for the general population. In addition, no specific pattern in the defects was identified. Therefore, this slight increase in risk when compared with controls could be related to the patient's disease state. The drug crosses the placenta, so fetal exposure will occur. Maternal and embryofetal toxicity were observed in three animal species at doses of less than 10 times the MRHD. Prolonged use of opioid analgesics, including tramadol, during pregnancy for medical or nonmedical purposes can result in respiratory depression and physical dependence in the neonate and produce neonatal opioid withdrawal syndrome (NOWS) shortly after birth. Symptoms can include irritability, hyperactivity, abnormal sleep patterns, high-pitched cry, tremor, vomiting, diarrhea, and failure to gain weight. The onset, duration, and severity of NOWS vary based on the specific opioid used, duration of use, timing and amount of last maternal use, and rate of elimination of the drug by the newborn. Tramadol is not recommended for use in pregnant women during or immediately prior to labor, when other analgesic techniques are more appropriate. The drug can prolong the QT interval. There is also a boxed warning for the risk of addiction and misuse. The drug is classified as a Schedule IV controlled substance.

BREASTFEEDIN SUMMARY

Tramadol and the active metabolite, M1, have been shown to be excreted into human breast milk. The drug has been found in nearly every breast milk sample tested. However, the calculated RIDs for the drug and the active metabolite are all less than 10% and most are less than 1%. The manufacturer states that tramadol is not recommended for obstetrical preoperative medication or for postdelivery analgesia in nursing mothers because its safety has not been studied. Additionally, if the woman is an ultrarapid metabolizer, M1 levels may be higher than expected in the serum and breast milk, which could be dangerous to the breastfed infant. Due to a concern for potential serious adverse effects that might be seen in a breastfed infant, the manufacturer recommends that women not breastfeed while being treated with this drug. If the clinical decision is to use this drug while breastfeeding, the infant should be monitored for excess sedation and respiratory depression, as well as the most common reported adult side effects of dizziness, nausea, headache, pruritus, and dyspepsia (all leading to irritability), somnolence, vomiting, CNS stimulation (agitation, tremor, and spasticity), and diarrhea.

References

1. Prescribing Information. *Tramadol*. ACI Healthcare USA, Inc; 2023.
2. Prescribing Information. *Tramadol HCl ER, tramadol hydrochloride*. Direct Rx; 2024.
3. Kallen B, Reis M. Use of tramadol in early pregnancy and congenital malformation risk. *Reprod Toxicol*. 2015;58:246-251.
4. Sorensen AMS, Noergaard MM, Gotfredsen DR, et al. Exposure to tramadol during early pregnancy and the risk of spontaneous abortion or major congenital malformations. *Obstet Gynecol*. 2022;39:545-553.
5. Bowie AC, Werler MM, Velez MP, et al. Prescribed opioid analgesics in early pregnancy and the risk of congenital anomalies: a population-based cohort study. *CMAJ*. 2022;194:e152-e162.
6. Husslein P, Kubista E, Egarter C. Obstetrical analgesia with tramadol—results of a prospective randomized comparative study with pethidine. *Z Geburtshilfe Perinatol*. 1987;191:234-237.
7. Bitsch M, Emmrich J, Hary J, Lippach G, Rindt W. Obstetrical analgesia with tramadol. *Fortschr Med*. 1980;98:632-634.
8. Bredow V. Use of tramadol versus pethidine versus denaverine suppositories in labor—a contribution to noninvasive therapy of labor pain. *Zentralbl Gynakol*. 1992;114:551-554.
9. Suvonnakote T, Thitadilok W, Atisook R. Pain relief during labour. *J Med Assoc Thailand*. 1986;69:575-580.
10. Viegas OAC, Khaw B, Ratnam SS. Tramadol in labour pain in primiparous patients: a prospective comparative clinical trial. *Eur J Obstet Gynecol Reprod Biol*. 1993;49:131-135.
11. Prasertsawat PO, Herabutya Y, Chaturachinda K. Obstetric analgesia: comparison between tramadol, morphine, and pethidine. *Curr Ther Res Clin Exp*. 1986;40:1022-1028.
12. Kainz C, Joura E, Obwegeser R, Plockinger B, Gruber W. Effectiveness and tolerance of tramadol with or without an antiemetic and pethidine in obstetric analgesia. *Z Geburtshilfe Perinatol*. 1992;196:78-82.
13. Keskin HL, Keskin EA, Avsar AF, Tabuk M, Caglar GS. Pethidine versus tramadol for pain relief during labor. *Int J Gynaecol Obstet*. 2003;82:11-16.
14. Khooshideh M, Shahriari A. A comparison of tramadol and pethidine analgesia on the duration of labour: a randomised clinical trial. *Aust N Z J Obstet Gynaecol*. 2009;49:59-63.
15. Rao ZA, Choudhri A, Naqvi S, Ehsan-ul-Haq. Walking epidural with low dose bupivacaine plus tramadol on normal labour in primipara. *J Coll Physicians Surg Pak*. 2010;20:295-298.
16. Meyer FP, Rimasch H, Blaha B, Banditt P. Tramadol withdrawal in a neonate. *Eur J Clin Pharmacol*. 1997;53:159-160.
17. Willaschek C, Wolter E, Buchhorn R. Tramadol withdrawal in a neonate after long-term analgesic treatment of the mother. *Eur J Clin Pharmacol*. 2009;65:429-430.
18. Hartenstein S, Proquitte H, Bauer S, et al. Neonatal abstinence syndrome (NAS) after intrauterine exposure to tramadol. *J Perinat Med*. 2010;38:695-696.
19. O'Mara K, Gal P, DaVanzo C. Treatment of neonatal withdrawal with clonidine after long-term, high-dose maternal use of tramadol. *Ann Pharmacother*. 2010;44:1342-1344.
20. Anonymous. Tramadol withdrawal symptoms in infants exposed in utero. *Prescribe Int*. 2012;21:71-72.
21. Esposito DB, Huybrechts KF, Werler MM, et al. Characteristics of prescription opioid analgesics in pregnancy and risk of neonatal withdrawal syndrome in newborns. *JAMA Netw Open*. 2022;5:e2228588.
22. Ilett KF, Paech MJ, Page-Sharp M, et al. Use of a sparse sampling study design to assess transfer of tramadol and its O-desmethyl metabolite into transitional breast milk. *Br J Clin Pharmacol*. 2008;65:661-666.
23. Gesseck AM, Peace MR, Nanco CR, et al. Neonatal exposure to tramadol through mother's breast milk. *J Anal Toxicol*. 2021;45:840-846.

TRAMETINIB

Antineoplastic (MEK Inhibitor)

PREGNANCY RECOMMENDATION: No Human Data—Animal Data Suggest Risk

BREASTFEEDING RECOMMENDATION: Potential Toxicity

PREGNANCY SUMMARY

No reports describing the use of trametinib in human pregnancy have been located. The drug will probably cross the placenta, so some fetal exposure will likely occur. Therefore, the absence of human pregnancy experience prevents a complete assessment of the embryofetal risk. Embryofetal toxicity was seen in two animal species at doses of less than the RHD. Based on these animal studies and the drug's mechanism of action, the manufacturer recommends that women with reproductive potential use effective contraception during treatment and for 4 months after the last dose. They also recommend that males with female partners of reproductive potential use effective contraception during treatment and for 4 months after the last dose (even males who have had a vasectomy). Nevertheless, using this drug during pregnancy should be based on the pros and cons of the mother's clinical need for treatment versus any potential fetal risk that might occur from exposure. There is a registry for women who are pregnant and have cancer. For more information, women and health care providers are encouraged to contact the Cancer and Pregnancy Registry at 1-877-635-4499. Hypertension was reported in up to 15% of patients treated with this drug in the clinical trials. Elevated glucose levels have also been reported in up to 71% of patients treated with this drug in combination with dabrafenib. Therefore, if used during pregnancy, glucose levels should be monitored.

BREASTFEEDING SUMMARY

No reports describing the use of trametinib during human lactation have been located. The drug will likely be excreted into breast milk, so some infant exposure will probably occur. However, due to a concern for potential serious adverse effects that might be seen in a breastfed infant, the manufacturer recommends that women not breastfeed while being treated with this drug and for at least 4 months after the last dose. Nevertheless, if the clinical decision is to use this drug while breastfeeding, the infant should be monitored for the most common reported adult side effects of rash, diarrhea, and lymphedema.

References

1. Prescribing Information. *Mekinist*. Novartis Pharmaceuticals Corporation; 2024.
2. Cocorocchio E, Pala L, Battaglia A, et al. Fatherhood during dabrafenib and trametinib therapy for metastatic melanoma. *Acta Oncol*. 2018;8: 1131-1133.

TRANDOLAPRIL

Antihypertensive (ACE—Angiotensin-I-Converting Enzyme Inhibitor)

PREGNANCY RECOMMENDATION: Contraindicated (Second and Third Trimesters)

BREASTFEEDING RECOMMENDATION: Probably Compatible

PREGNANCY SUMMARY

T

No reports describing the specific use of trandolapril in human pregnancy have been located. A few large studies have reported the risk for congenital anomalies with first-trimester exposure to ACE inhibitors as a class of drugs. These publications reported overall malformation rates of about 5% to 6%, which is higher than the expected rate of 2% to 4%. However, most of these studies also reported fetal anomaly rates in pregnant patients with hypertension not on treatment to be similar. The impression was that these findings might be related to the disease and not the drug. Likewise, some of these studies also reported an increase in risk for cardiac defects, but again, it was not certain as to whether this elevated risk was related to the drug or the disease. Furthermore, no pattern to the anomalies has been identified. Regarding the use of ACE inhibitors in the second half of gestation, numerous case reports and reviews have reported that these drugs can, in some cases, produce severe fetal renal dysfunction. This can lead to anomalies related to longstanding oligohydramnios and fetal/neonatal death. There are cases, however, where the process reverses itself when the drug is discontinued. These findings are similar to those seen with ARBs. The drug actually carries a boxed warning for these risks. Trandolapril probably crosses the placenta, so some fetal exposure will likely occur. Therefore, the absence of first-trimester human pregnancy experience prevents a complete assessment of the embryofetal risk. Animal studies did not show any embryofetal toxicity in three species at doses of more than 10 times the RHD in two species and less than 10 times the RHD in the third species. Women of reproductive age using trandolapril should be informed of these risks, so they can closely monitor if pregnancy transpires. If a positive pregnancy test occurs, she and her health care providers can modify treatment (if possible) so that the drug is not used in the second or third trimesters. For treating hypertension in pregnancy, ACOG recommends nifedipine and labetalol as first-line agents.

BREASTFEEDING SUMMARY

No reports describing the use of trandolapril during human lactation have been located. The drug and active metabolite (trandolaprilat) will likely be excreted into breast milk, so some infant exposure will probably occur. However, due to a concern for potential serious adverse effects that might be seen in a breastfed infant, the manufacturer recommends that women not breastfeed while being treated with this drug. Nevertheless, breastfeeding while using this drug should be based on the mother's clinical need for treatment versus any potential infant risks that might occur. If used, the infant should be monitored for the most common reported adult side effects of headache, nausea, myalgia, and dizziness (all leading to irritability), cough, rash, hypotension, diarrhea, and fatigue (lethargy).

References

1. Prescribing Information. *Trandolapril*. Aurobindo Pharma Limited; 2024.
2. American College of Obstetricians and Gynecologists. ACOG Practice Bulletin No. 203: chronic hypertension in pregnancy. *Obstet Gynecol*. 2019;133: e26-e50.
3. American College of Obstetricians and Gynecologists. Gestational hypertension and preeclampsia. ACOG Practice Bulletin No. 222. *Obstet Gynecol*. 2020;135:e237-e260.
4. Cooper WO, Hernandez-Diaz C, Arbogast PG, et al. Major congenital malformations after first-trimester exposure to ACE inhibitors. *N Engl J Med*. 2006;354:2443-2451.
5. Li DK, Yang C, Andrade S, et al. Maternal exposure to angiotensin converting enzyme inhibitors in the first trimester and risk of malformations in offspring: a retrospective cohort study. *BMJ*. 2011;343:d5931.
6. Vasilakis-Scaramozza C, Aschengrau A, Cabral HJ, Jick SS. Antihypertensive drugs and the risk of congenital anomalies. *Pharmacotherapy*. 2013; 33:476-482.
7. Bateman BT, Patorno E, Desai RJ, et al. Angiotensin-converting enzyme inhibitors and the risk of congenital malformations. *Obstet Gynecol*. 2017; 129:174-184.
8. Hoeltzenbein M, Tissen-Diabate T, Fiets AK, et al. Increased rate of birth defects after first trimester use of angiotensin converting enzyme inhibitors-treatment or hypertension related? An observational cohort study. *Pregnancy Hypertens*. 2018;13:65-71.
9. Buawangpong N, Teekachunhatean S, Koonrungsesomboon N. *Adverse pregnancy outcomes associated with first-trimester exposure to angiotensin-converting enzyme inhibitors or angiotensin II receptor blockers: a systematic review and meta-analysis*. Pharmacol Res Perspect. 2020 Oct;8(5):e00644.

TRANEXAMIC ACID

Hematologic (Hemostatic—Antifibrinolytic)

PREGNANCY RECOMMENDATION: Limited Human Data—Animal Data Suggest Low Risk (Maternal Benefit May Outweigh Embryo–Fetal Risk)

BREASTFEEDING RECOMMENDATION: Probably Compatible

PREGNANCY SUMMARY

Several reports describing the use of tranexamic acid in human pregnancy have been located. Nearly all of the exposures have occurred in the second and third trimesters. One case report described use in the late first trimester, and at delivery, no major birth anomalies were identified. The manufacturer reported on two other cases, with exposure at conception and the first trimester, where some structural defects were present, but no further information was supplied. In about 90 uses in the second and third trimesters, no significant fetal/neonatal adverse effects related to the drug were reported. The drug has been shown to cross the placenta, so some fetal exposure will occur. However, this limited human pregnancy experience, especially first-trimester use, prevents a complete assessment of the embryofetal risk. Animal data did not show any embryofetal toxicity in three species at doses of less than 10 times the MRHD. Using this drug during pregnancy should be based on the pros and cons of the mother's clinical need for treatment versus any potential fetal risk that might occur from exposure. In addition, several studies have described the use of the drug postdelivery (after cord clamping) in treating postpartum hemorrhage, many with good success.

BREASTFEEDING SUMMARY

Tranexamic acid is excreted into human breast milk. More than 30 lactating women have been studied, and breast milk concentrations of the drug were 1% of the peak maternal serum concentrations. Breast milk levels ranged from about 60 to about 470 ng/mL. In another study of 21 breastfeeding women using tranexamic acid, no difference was observed between exposed and unexposed for any infant growth parameter, adverse effects, or abnormal medical conditions at the time of follow-up. In adults, approximately 30% to 50% of an oral dose is absorbed. The amount of drug a nursing infant would systemically absorb from breast milk is unknown, but it is most likely small. If the clinical decision is to use this drug while breastfeeding, the infant should be monitored for the most common reported adult side effects of nausea (leading to irritability), vomiting, diarrhea, rash, hypotension, and thromboembolic events.

T

References

1. Prescribing Information. *Tranexamic acid*. Armas Pharmaceuticals, Inc; 2021.
2. Prescribing Information. *Tranexamic acid*. Advagen Pharma Limited; 2024.
3. Svanberg L, Åstedt B, Nilsson IM. Abruptio placentae—treatment with the fibrinolytic inhibitor tranexamic acid. *Acta Obstet Gynecol Scand*. 1980; 59:127-130.
4. Lindoff C, Rybo G, Åstedt B. Treatment with tranexamic acid during pregnancy and the risk of thrombo-embolic complications. *Thromb Haemost*. 1993;70:238-240.
5. Kullander S, Nilsson IM. Human placental transfer of an antifibrinolytic agent (AMCA). *Acta Obstet Gynecol Scand*. 1970;49:241-242.
6. Walzman M, Bonnar J. Effects of tranexamic acid on the coagulation and fibrinolytic systems in pregnancy complicated by placental bleeding. *Arch Toxicol*. 1982;5:214-220.
7. Storm O, Weber J. Prolonged treatment with tranexamic acid (Cyklokapron) during pregnancy. *Ugeskr Laeg*. 1976;138:1781-1782.
8. Åstedt B, Nilsson IM. Recurrent abruptio placentae treated with the fibrinolytic inhibitor tranexamic acid. *Br Med J*. 1978;1:756-757.
9. Sundqvist S-B, Nilsson IM, Svanberg L, Cronberg S. Glanzmann's thrombasthenia: pregnancy and parturition (abstract). *Thromb Haemost*. 1981; 46:225.
10. Svanberg L, Åstedt B, Nilsson IM. Abruptio placentae—treatment with the fibrinolytic inhibitor tranexamic acid. *Acta Obstet Gynecol Scand*. 1980;59:127-130.
11. Loli-Ausejo D, Hernandez-Martin I, Cabanas R, et al. Tranexamic acid plus bemiparin sodium as long-term prophylaxis in a patient with FXII-HAE during pregnancy: a case report. *J Investig Allergol Clin Immunol*. 2020;30: 464-465.
12. Fagher B, Ahlgren M, Åstedt B. Acute massive pulmonary embolism treated with streptokinase during labor and the early puerperium. *Acta Obstet Gynecol Scand*. 1990;69:659-662.
13. Castle D, Desborough MJR, Kemp M, et al. Outcomes and management of pregnancy in women with bleeding disorder of unknown cause. *J Thromb Haemost*. 2022;20:2519-2525.
14. Eriksson O, Kjellman H, Nilsson L. *Tranexamic acid in human milk after oral administration of Cyklokapron to lactating women. Data on file, KabiVitrum AB, Stockholm, Sweden (Data supplied by R.G. Leonardi, Ph.D., KabiVitrum)*, 1987.
15. Gilad O, Merlob P, Stahl B, Klinger G. Outcome following tranexamic acid exposure during breastfeeding. *Breastfeed Med*. 2014;9:407-410.
16. Ahmadzia HK, Luban NC, Li S, et al. Optimal use of intravenous tranexamic acid for hemorrhage prevention in pregnant women. *Am J Obstet Gynecol*. 2021;225:85.e1-11.

TRANYLCYPROMINE

Mental Health (Antidepressant—MAO Inhibitor)

PREGNANCY RECOMMENDATION: Limited Human Data—No Relevant Animal Data

BREASTFEEDING RECOMMENDATION: Potential Toxicity

PREGNANCY SUMMARY

In the Collaborative Perinatal Project, 21 first-trimester exposures to monoamine oxidase inhibitors were reported, 13 of which were tranylcypromine. Overall, there were 3 (14%) major malformations, but specific details on the 13 tranylcypromine cases were not provided. A second case report described two individual pregnancies in the same patient who was being treated with tranylcypromine. The first was complicated by an intrauterine fetal death (IUFD) that was thought to have some facial anomalies. The second was delivered at term and had numerous birth anomalies (including the face). Chromosomal microarray was normal, but at the last assessment (age 7), the child was physically and developmentally delayed. It is uncertain if these two pregnancies were affected by the drug. The drug will probably cross the placenta, so some fetal exposure will likely occur. Therefore, this limited human pregnancy experience prevents a complete assessment of the embryofetal risk. Animal reproduction studies have not been conducted. Using this drug during pregnancy should be based on the pros and cons of the mother's clinical need for treatment versus any potential fetal risk that might occur from exposure. There is a pregnancy exposure registry that monitors pregnancy outcomes in women using antidepressant drugs. Health care providers are encouraged to call the National Pregnancy Registry for Antidepressants at 1-844-405-6185.

BREASTFEEDING SUMMARY

One report describing the use of tranylcypromine during human lactation has been located. The mother breastfed her infant while taking tranylcypromine, pimozide, diazepam, and alprazolam. The infant experienced abdominal distention and feeding intolerance that resolved after the infant was switched to formula feeding. Due to a concern for potential serious adverse effects that might be seen in a breastfed infant, the manufacturer recommends that women not breastfeed while being treated with this drug. Nevertheless, if the clinical decision is to use this drug while breastfeeding, the infant should be monitored for the most common reported adult side effects of dizziness, headache, and dry mouth (all leading to irritability), insomnia, sedation, constipation, and tremor.

References

1. Prescribing Information. *Tranylcypromine sulfate*. Actavis Pharma, Inc; 2021.
2. American College of Obstetricians and Gynecologists. Treatment and management of mental health conditions during pregnancy and postpartum: ACOG Clinical Practice Guideline No. 5. *Obstet Gynecol*. 2023;141: 1262-1288.
3. Heinonen OP, Slone D, Shapiro S. *Birth Defects and Drugs in Pregnancy*. Publishing Sciences Group; 1977:336-337.
4. Kennedy D, Webster WS, Hill M, Ritchie HE. Abnormal pregnancy outcome associated with high-dose maternal tranylcypromine therapy: case report and literature review. *Reprod Toxicol*. 2007;69:146-149.

T

TRASTUZUMAB

Antineoplastic (HER2 Receptor Antagonist)

PREGNANCY RECOMMENDATION: Contraindicated (Second and Third Trimesters)

BREASTFEEDING RECOMMENDATION: Probably Compatible

PREGNANCY SUMMARY

There are over 30 pregnancies with exposure to trastuzumab during human pregnancy. This human data describes a high rate of fetal renal toxicity that is primarily seen in the second half of gestation. Oligohydramnios is often seen (in nearly 70% of reported cases) after 20 weeks' gestation, which can lead to obstetrical complications related to decreased amniotic fluid volume. Postdelivery, there does not appear to be any common renal pathology identified. However, trastuzumab does not appear to cause structural anomalies when exposure occurs during organogenesis. In some cases, the renal toxicity was reversible when the drug was stopped. As an IgG antibody, it likely crosses the placenta, especially during the second half of gestation, so some fetal exposure will probably occur. However, this limited human pregnancy experience prevents a complete assessment of the embryofetal risk. Embryofetal toxicity was observed in one species, but at doses of more than 10 times the RHD. Based on animal studies and the drug's mechanism of action, the manufacturer recommends that women with reproductive potential use effective contraception during treatment and for 7 months after the last dose. Because this drug is prescribed for serious malignancies, using this drug during pregnancy should be based on the pros and cons of the mother's clinical need for treatment versus any potential fetal risk that might occur from exposure. There is a pregnancy exposure registry that monitors pregnancy outcomes in women using this drug. Health care providers are encouraged to call Genentech at 888-835-2555. The drug also carries a boxed warning for an increased risk of cardiomyopathy, pulmonary toxicity, infusion reactions, and embryofetal toxicity.

BREASTFEEDING SUMMARY

No reports describing the use of trastuzumab during human lactation have been located. It is known that IgG antibodies can be found in human breast milk, but are not found in the neonatal or infant circulation. Additionally, if any IgG antibodies were to be ingested through breastfeeding, they would probably be digested in the infant's gastrointestinal tract and not be absorbed. Breastfeeding while using this drug should be based on the mother's clinical need for treatment versus any potential infant risks that might occur. If used, the infant should be monitored for the most common reported adult side effects of headache and nausea (both leading to irritability), diarrhea, fever, infections, insomnia, cough, rash, and fatigue (lethargy).

References

1. Prescribing Information. *Herceptin*. Genentech, Inc; 2024.
2. National Library of Medicine—Pubchem. *Trastuzumab*. Accessed December 24, 2024. https://pubchem.ncbi.nlm.nih.gov/compound/Trastuzumab
3. Bader AA, Schiembach D, Tamussino KF, et al. Anhydramnios associated with administration of trastuzumab and paclitaxel for metastatic breast cancer during pregnancy. *Lancet Oncol*. 2007;8:79-81.
4. Xia LY, Hu QL, Zhou Q. Use of trastuzumab in treating breast cancer during pregnancy: a systematic review and meta-analysis. *BMC Womens Health*. 2021;21:169.
5. Lambertini M, Martel S, Campbell C, et al. Pregnancies during and after trastuzumab and/or lapatinib in patients with human epidermal growth factor receptor 2-positive early breast cancer: analysis from the NeoALLTO (BIG 1-06) and ALTTO (BIG 2-06) trials. *Cancer*. 2019;125:307-316.
6. Berveiller P, Mir O, Sauvanet E, Antoine EC, Goldwasser F. Ectopic pregnancy in a breast cancer patient receiving trastuzumab. *Reprod Toxicol*. 2008;25:286-288.
7. Pant S, Landon MB, Blumenfeld M, Farrar W, Shapiro CL. Treatment of breast cancer with trastuzumab during pregnancy. *J Clin Oncol*. 2008;26:1567-1569.
8. Yildirim N, Bahceci A. Use of pertuzumab and trastuzumab during pregnancy. *Anticancer Drugs*. 2018;29:810-813.

TRAVOPROST OPHTHALMIC

Ophthalmic (Prostaglandin Analogue)

PREGNANCY RECOMMENDATION: No Human Data and No Relevant Animal Data

BREASTFEEDING RECOMMENDATION: Probably Compatible

PREGNANCY SUMMARY

No reports describing the use of travoprost ophthalmic in human pregnancy have been located. The drug will probably cross the placenta, so some fetal exposure might occur. However, systemic absorption is negligible with ocular use, so any amount is likely to be clinically insignificant. However, the absence of human pregnancy experience prevents a complete assessment of the embryofetal risk. Animal data were found to cause some embryofetal toxicity in two species at doses of less than

(*continued*)

10 times the MRHOD, but the drug was administered SC. When administered topically for ocular use in humans, little to no drug is absorbed systemically. Using this drug during pregnancy should be based on the pros and cons of the mother's clinical need for treatment versus any potential fetal risk that might occur from exposure. Nevertheless, because the drug will be administered daily for long time periods, using a different antiglaucoma medication might be considered. If used during pregnancy, consider placing pressure over the tear duct in the corner of the eye for at least 1 minute, and then remove any excess solution with absorbent tissue to decrease the amount of drug reaching the systemic circulation even further.

BREASTFEEDING SUMMARY

No reports describing the use of travoprost ophthalmic during human lactation have been located. The drug might be excreted into breast milk, but systemic absorption with ocular use is negligible, so any amount found in breast milk is likely to be clinically insignificant. Breastfeeding while using this drug should be based on the mother's clinical need for treatment versus any potential infant risks that might occur. A method to decrease some systemic absorption with ophthalmic use is described above in the Pregnancy Summary.

Reference

1. Prescribing Information. *Travoprost ophthalmic solution, 0.004%*. Mylan Pharmaceuticals, Inc; 2023.

TRAZODONE

Mental Health (Serotonin Modulator—Antidepressant)

PREGNANCY RECOMMENDATION: Limited Human Data—Animal Data Suggest Risk

BREASTFEEDING RECOMMENDATION: Potential Toxicity

PREGNANCY SUMMARY

There are several reports describing the use of trazodone in human pregnancy. First-trimester exposure has been reported in over 290 pregnancies with a major malformation rate of only 0.5%. In addition, the manufacturer reports that published prospective cohort studies, case series, and case reports over several decades have not identified any drug-associated risks of major malformation, miscarriage, or adverse maternal or fetal outcomes. Both trazodone and its active metabolite, 1-m-chlorophenylpiperazine (mCPP), cross the placenta and have levels nearly equal to maternal levels. Embryofetal toxicity was observed in two animal species at doses of less than 10 times the MRHD. However, this limited human pregnancy experience still prevents a complete assessment of embryofetal risk. Using this drug during pregnancy should be based on the pros and cons of the mother's clinical need for treatment versus any potential fetal risk that might occur from exposure. There is a pregnancy exposure registry that monitors pregnancy outcomes in women using antidepressant drugs. Health care providers are encouraged to call the National Pregnancy Registry for Antidepressants at 1-844-405-6185. Hypertension was reported in up to 20% of patients treated with this drug in the clinical trials. Trazodone can also prolong the QT interval.

BREASTFEEDING SUMMARY

Trazodone and its active metabolite, mCPP, have been found in human breast milk. The breast milk of 13 lactating women was tested, and the drug and active metabolite were found in most samples. Trazodone levels ranged from undetectable to a peak of about 50 ng/mL. The breast milk levels for trazodone were about 10% of the maternal serum values. Calculated RIDs were less than 1%. Breastfeeding while using this drug should be based on the mother's clinical need for treatment versus any potential infant risks that might occur. If used, the infant should be monitored for the most common reported adult side effects of peripheral edema, drowsiness, fatigue (lethargy), diarrhea, nasal congestion, and weight loss (monitor infant growth).

References

1. Prescribing Information. *Trazodone hydrochloride*. Accord Healthcare, Inc; 2024.
2. National Library of Medicine—PubChem. *Trazodone*. Accessed December 25, 2024. https://pubchem.ncbi.nlm.nih.gov/compound/Trazodone
3. Saito J, Ishii M, Mito A, et al. Trazodone levels in maternal serum, cord blood, breast milk, and neonatal serum. *Breastfeed Med*. 2021;16:922-925.
4. Jacobson SJ, Jones K, Johnson K, et al. Prospective multicentre study of pregnancy outcome after lithium exposure during first trimester. *Lancet*. 1992;339:530-533.
5. McElhatton PR, Garbis HM, Elefant E, et al. The outcome of pregnancy in 689 women exposed to therapeutic doses of antidepressants. A collaborative study of the European Network of Teratology Information Services (ENTIS). *Reprod Toxicol*. 1996;10:285-294.
6. Einarson A, Bonari L, Voyer-Lavigne S, et al. A multicentre prospective controlled study to determine the safety of trazodone and nefazodone use during pregnancy. *Can J Psychiatry*. 2003;48:106-109.
7. Einarson TR, Einarson A. Newer antidepressants in pregnancy and rates of major malformations: a meta-analysis of prospective comparative studies. *Pharmacoepidemiol Drug Saf*. 2005;14:823-827.
8. Einarson A, Choi J, Einarson TR, Koren G. Incidence of major malformations in infants following antidepressant exposure in pregnancy: results of a large prospective cohort study. *Can J Psychiatry*. 2009;54:242-246.
9. Dao K, Shechtman S, Diav-Citrin O, et al. Reproductive safety of trazodone after maternal exposure in early pregnancy. *J Clin Psychopharmacol*. 2023;43:12-19.
10. Verbeeck RK, Ross SG, McKenna EA. Excretion of trazodone in breast milk. *Br J Clin Pharmacol*. 1986;22:367-370.
11. Misri S, Corral M, Wardrop AA, Kendrick K. Quetiapine augmentation in lactation: a series of case reports. *J Clin Psychopharm*. 2006;26:508-511.

TREMELIMUMAB

Antineoplastic (Anti-CTLA4 Monoclonal Antibody)

PREGNANCY RECOMMENDATION: No Human Data—Animal Data Suggest Potential Risk

BREASTFEEDING RECOMMENDATION: Probably Compatible

PREGNANCY SUMMARY

No reports describing the use of tremelimumab in human pregnancy have been located. As an IgG antibody, the drug will likely cross the placenta, so some fetal exposure will probably occur. Therefore, the absence of human pregnancy experience prevents a complete assessment of the embryofetal risk. Animal studies did not show embryofetal toxic effects. However, cytotoxic T-lymphocyte-associated antigen 4 (CTLA-4) is involved in maintaining maternal immune tolerance to the fetus to preserve the pregnancy, as well as immune regulation in the newborn. In a murine pregnancy model, CTLA-4 blockade resulted in increased resorptions and reduced live fetuses. Based on these animal studies and the drug's mechanism of action, the manufacturer recommends that women with reproductive potential use effective contraception during treatment and for 3 months after the last dose. Nevertheless, using this drug during pregnancy should be based on the pros and cons of the mother's clinical need for treatment versus any potential fetal risk that might occur from exposure. Women who are pregnant and have cancer are encouraged to contact the Cancer and Pregnancy Registry at 877-635-4499 if using this drug is contemplated.

BREASTFEEDING SUMMARY

No reports describing the use of tremelimumab during human lactation have been located. It is known that IgG antibodies can be found in human breast milk, but are not found in the neonatal or infant circulation. Additionally, if any IgG antibodies were to be ingested through breastfeeding, they would probably be digested in the infant's gastrointestinal tract and not absorbed. However, due to the concern for potential serious adverse effects that might be seen in a breastfed infant, the manufacturer recommends that women not breastfeed while being treated with this drug and for at least 3 months after the last dose. Nevertheless, breastfeeding while using this drug should be based on the mother's clinical need for treatment. If used, the infant should be monitored for the most common reported adult side effects of musculoskeletal pain, abdominal pain, and pruritus (all leading to irritability), rash, diarrhea, lethargy, and various laboratory abnormalities (see PI).

Reference

1. Prescribing Information. *Imjudo*. AstraZeneca; 2023.

TREPROSTINIL

Cardiovascular (Prostacyclin Analogue—Vasodilator)

PREGNANCY RECOMMENDATION: Limited Human Data—Animal Data Suggest Low Risk (Maternal Benefit May Outweigh Any Embryofetal Risk)

BREASTFEEDING RECOMMENDATION: Potential Toxicity

PREGNANCY SUMMARY

Several studies were located that describe the use of treprostinil in more than 40 human pregnancies. All of the exposures were in the second and third trimesters or during delivery in the treatment of pulmonary arterial hypertension (PAH). PAH is a serious medical condition with a maternal mortality rate in pregnancy that approaches 20%. The drug will probably cross the placenta, so some fetal exposure will likely occur. Therefore, the absence of the first-trimester human pregnancy experience prevents a complete assessment of the embryofetal risk. Animal data did not show any embryofetal toxicity in one species at doses of more than 10 times the MRHD. There was some embryofetal toxicity in a second species at 5 times the MRHD, but maternal toxicity also occurred. Treprostinil can prolong the QT interval. Using this drug during pregnancy should be based on the pros and cons of the mother's clinical need for treatment versus any potential fetal risk that might occur from exposure. However, due to the severity of PAH in pregnancy, the drug should not be withheld for potential unknown fetal risks.

T

BREASTFEEDING SUMMARY

No reports describing the use of treprostinil during human lactation have been located. The drug will likely be excreted into breast milk, so some infant exposure will probably occur. Breastfeeding while using this drug should be based on the mother's clinical need for treatment. If used, the infant should be monitored for the most common reported adult side effects of headache and nausea (both leading to irritability), diarrhea, peripheral edema, and hypotension. However, due to the severity of PAH in pregnancy and the postpartum period, the drug should probably not be withheld.

References

1. Prescribing Information. *Treprostinil*. Alembic Pharmaceuticals, Inc; 2023.
2. Prescribing Information. *Orenitram*. United Therapeutics Corporation; 2023.
3. Prescribing Information. *Tyvaso DPI*. United Therapeutics Corporation; 2024.
4. Rosengarten D, Kramer MR. Pregnancy in a woman with pulmonary hypertension: favorable outcome with intravenous treprostinil. *Clin Exp Obstet Gynecol*. 2015;42:390-391.
5. Xiang Y, Li J, Sun Y. A case report of pulmonary arterial hypertension in pregnancy and complications of anticoagulation therapy. *Medicine*. 2018;97:e11810.
6. Zhang J, Lu J, Zhou X, et al. Perioperative management of pregnant women with idiopathic pulmonary arterial hypertension: an observational case series study from China. *J Cardiothorac Vasc Anesth*. 2018;32:2547-2559.
7. Ye J, Chen JY, Xu N, et al. Bilateral lung transplantation after caesarean section in pregnancy with severe pulmonary arterial hypertension. *Medicine*. 2019;98:47(e18109).
8. Luo J, Shi H, Xu L, et al. Pregnancy outcomes in patients with pulmonary arterial hypertension. *Medicine*. 2020;99:23(e20285).

TRETINOIN (SYSTEMIC)

Antineoplastic (Retinoid)

PREGNANCY RECOMMENDATION: Contraindicated (Mainly First Trimester)

BREASTFEEDING RECOMMENDATION: Potential Toxicity

PREGNANCY SUMMARY

Oral tretinoin, as with other systemic retinoids, taken during early pregnancy can produce a pattern of birth defects termed retinoic acid embryopathy. These defects consist of CNS, craniofacial, cardiovascular, skeletal, ear, eye, and other anomalies. There are about 20 cases where women were treated with the drug for acute promyelocytic leukemia in the second and third trimesters, and no significant adverse fetal effects were described. Based on its proven teratogenic effect, the drug crosses the placenta. Therefore, fetal exposure will occur. Embryofetal toxicity was observed in four animal species at doses of less than the RHD in three and less than 10 times the RHD in the fourth. Women with reproductive potential who are taking tretinoin are advised to continuously abstain from sexual intercourse or to use two effective methods of contraception during treatment and for 1 month after the last dose. The manufacturer also recommends that males with female partners of reproductive potential use effective contraception during and for 1 week after the last dose. The drug carries a boxed warning for the increased risk of retinoic acid embryopathy. Using this drug to treat malignancy in the second half of gestation should be based on the pros and cons of the mother's clinical need for treatment versus any potential fetal risk that might occur from exposure

BREASTFEEDING SUMMARY

No reports describing the use of systemic tretinoin during human lactation have been located. The drug will likely be excreted into breast milk, so some infant exposure will probably occur. However, due to a concern for potential serious adverse effects that might be seen in a breastfed infant, the manufacturer recommends that women not breastfeed while being treated with this drug and for at least 1 week after the last dose. Nevertheless, if the clinical decision is to use this drug while breastfeeding, the infant should be monitored for the most common reported adult side effects of headache, nausea, bone pain, chest discomfort, and abdominal pain (all leading to irritability), vomiting, malaise (lethargy), upper respiratory tract infections, dyspnea, infections, rash, peripheral edema, and leukocytosis.

References

1. Prescribing Information. *Tretinoin*. Endo USA; 2023.
2. Morriss-Kay G. Retinoic acid and development. *Pathobiology*. 1992;60:264-270.
3. Simone MD, Stasi R, Venditti A, et al. All-trans retinoic acid (ATRA) administration during pregnancy in relapsed acute promyelocytic leukemia. *Leukemia*. 1995;9:1412-1413.
4. Stentoft J, Lanng Nielsen J, et al. All-trans retinoic acid in acute promyelocytic leukemia in late pregnancy. *Leukemia*. 1994;8(suppl 2):S77-S80.
5. Harrison P, Chipping P, Fothergill GA. Successful use of all-trans retinoic acid in acute promyelocytic leukaemia presenting during the second trimester of pregnancy. *Br J Haematol*. 1994;86:681-682.
6. Lin C-P, Huang M-J, Liu H-J, et al. Successful treatment of acute promyelocytic leukemia in a pregnant Jehovah's Witness with all-trans retinoic acid, rhG-CSF, and erythropoietin. *Am J Hematol*. 1996;51:251-252.
7. Incerpi MH, Miller DA, Posen R, Byrne JD. All-trans retinoic acid for the treatment of acute promyelocytic leukemia in pregnancy. *Obstet Gynecol*. 1997;89:826-828.
8. Morton J, Taylor K, Wright S, et al. Successful maternal and fetal outcome following the use of ATRA for the induction APML late in the first trimester (abstract). *Blood*. 1995;86(suppl 1):772a.
9. Giagounidis AAN, Beckman MW, Giagoundis AS, et al. Acute promyelocytic leukemia and pregnancy. *Eur J Haematol*. 2000;64:267-271.
10. Watanabe R, Okamoto S, Moriki T, et al. Treatment of acute promyelocytic leukemia with all-trans retinoic acid during the third trimester of pregnancy. *Am J Hematol*. 1995;48:210-211.
11. Nakamura K, Dan K, Iwakiri R, et al. Successful treatment of acute promyelocytic leukemia in pregnancy with all-trans retinoic acid. *Ann Hematol*. 1995;71:263-264.

12. Lipovsky MM, Biesma DH, Christiaens GCML, Petersen EJ. Successful treatment of acute promyelocytic leukaemia with all-trans-retinoic-acid during late pregnancy. *Br J Haematol*. 1996;94:699-701.
13. Consoli U, Figuera A, Milone G, et al. Acute promyelocytic leukemia during pregnancy: report of 3 cases. *Int J Hematol*. 2004;79:31-36.
14. Dang CC, Guan YK, Lau NS, Chan SY. Two successful deliveries of healthy children by a young woman diagnosed and treated during induction and relapsed therapy for acute promyelocytic leukemia. *J Oncol Pharm Practice*. 2020;26:2034-2037.
15. Li H, Han C, Li K, et al. New onset acute promyelocytic leukemia during pregnancy: report of 2 cases. *Cancer Biol Ther*. 2019;20:397-401.
16. Li YW, Xu YF, Hu W, et al. Acute myeloid leukemia during pregnancy: a single institutional experience with 17 patients and literature review. *Int J Hematol*. 2020;112:487-495.

TRETINOIN (TOPICAL)

Dermatologic (Retinoid)

PREGNANCY RECOMMENDATION: Limited Human Data—No Relevant Animal Data

BREASTFEEDING RECOMMENDATION: Probably Compatible

PREGNANCY SUMMARY

From two studies, there were 6 (1.9%) major malformations reported in 311 first-trimester exposures. No pattern to the defects was seen. However, from the manufacturer and other isolated case reports, several retinoid-like malformations have been described with this topical agent. Elevated serum concentrations of all-*trans* retinoic acid in early gestation are considered teratogenic in humans. However, because of tretinoin topical's relatively poor systemic absorption (if occlusive dressings are not used), it is not thought to present a significant fetal risk. Because some absorption does occur, it is not possible to fully exclude any teratogenic risk. These case reports may reflect a greater-than-normal fetal exposure from higher-than-usual maternal use or enhanced systemic absorption. It may also involve selective reporting of adverse outcomes that are not caused by topical tretinoin. Until more data are available, however, the safest course is to avoid the use of this topical agent, especially in the first trimester. Regardless, if inadvertent exposure does occur during early pregnancy, the fetal risk, if any, appears to be low. Topical tretinoin has the potential to cross the placenta, so some fetal exposure may occur. Embryofetal toxicity with malformations was observed in two animal species with topical exposure, but at doses of well above 10 times the RHD. Nevertheless, this human pregnancy data are too limited to provide a complete assessment of embryofetal risk. Using this drug during pregnancy should be based on the pros and cons of the mother's clinical need for treatment versus any potential fetal risk that might occur from exposure.

BREASTFEEDING SUMMARY

No reports describing the use of topical tretinoin during human lactation have been located. Although other retinoids are excreted into human breast milk, the minimal absorption that occurs following topical application of tretinoin probably produces clinically insignificant amounts in human breast milk. Thus, use of tretinoin while breastfeeding does not appear to represent a significant risk to a nursing infant. However, the drug should not be applied directly to the breast.

References

1. Prescribing Information. *Tretinoin*. Actavis Pharma, Inc; 2024.
2. Prescribing Information. *Tretinoin*. Encube Ethicals Private Limited; 2023.
3. Camera G, Pregliasco P. Ear malformation in baby born to mother using tretinoin cream. *Lancet*. 1992;339:687.
4. Lipson AH, Collins F, Webster WS. Multiple congenital defects associated with maternal use of topical tretinoin. *Lancet*. 1993;341:1352-1353.
5. Navarre-Belhassen C, Blanchet P, Hillaire-Buys D, et al. Multiple congenital malformations associated with topical tretinoin. *Ann Pharmacother*. 1998;32:505-506.
6. Colley SMJ, Walpole I, Fabian VA, Kakulas BA. Topical tretinoin and fetal malformations. *Med J Aust*. 1998;168:467.
7. Selcen D, Seidman S, Nigro MA. Otocerebral anomalies associated with topical tretinoin use. *Brain Dev*. 2000;22:218-220.
8. Johnson KA, Chambers CD, Felix R, et al. Pregnancy outcome in women prospectively ascertained with Retin-A exposures: an ongoing study (abstract). *Teratology*. 1994;49:375.
9. Rosa F, Piazza-Hepp T, Goetsch R. Holoprosencephaly with 1st trimester topical tretinoin (abstract). *Teratology*. 1994;49:418-419.
10. Jick SS, Terris BZ, Jick H. First trimester topical tretinoin and congenital disorders. *Lancet*. 1993;341:1181-1182.
11. Jick H. Retinoids and teratogenicity. *J Am Acad Dermatol*. 1998;39:S118-S122.
12. Shapiro L, Pastuszak A, Curto G, Koren G. Safety of first-trimester exposure to topical tretinoin: prospective cohort study. *Lancet*. 1997;350:1143-1144.
13. Martinez-Frias ML, Rodriguez-Pinilla E. First-trimester exposure to topical tretinoin: its safety is not warranted. *Teratology*. 1999;60:5.

TRIAMCINOLONE

Corticosteroid

PREGNANCY RECOMMENDATION: Limited Human Data—Animal Data Suggest Risk

BREASTFEEDING RECOMMENDATION: Probably Compatible

PREGNANCY SUMMARY

There are several reports describing the use of triamcinolone in human pregnancy. It has numerous approved methods of administration, including intranasal, IM, intra-articular, intralesional, and topical use for a wide range of indications. Regarding systemic administration, a total of nine first-trimester exposures were identified, and no major malformations were seen. A few case reports exist for use with other forms of administration, and no distinct birth defect patterns have been identified. The drug will probably cross the placenta, so some fetal exposure will likely occur. Therefore, this limited human pregnancy experience prevents a complete assessment of the embryofetal risk. As seen with other corticosteroids, embryofetal toxicity was observed in three animal species at doses approximately equal to the RHD. Using this drug during pregnancy should be based on the pros and cons of the mother's clinical need for treatment versus any potential fetal risk that might occur from exposure. Hypertension has been reported in patients treated with this drug, as well as elevated glucose levels, primarily with injectable use. Therefore, if used during pregnancy, glucose levels should be monitored. Systemic exposure to the drug is less with topical, intranasal, intra-articular, and intralesional use when compared with IM use.

BREASTFEEDING SUMMARY

Three reports describing the use of triamcinolone injection during human lactation have been located. Small amounts of the drug have been detected in human breast milk, but some samples have no detectable concentrations. Calculated RIDs were all less than 1%. Small amounts of other corticosteroids (see Hydrocortisone and Prednisone) are excreted into breast milk. Breastfeeding while using this drug should be based on the mother's clinical need for treatment versus any potential infant risks that might occur. If used, the infant should be monitored for the most common reported adult side effects of headache (leading to irritability), peripheral edema, cough, and weakness (lethargy).

References

1. Prescribing Information. *Triamcinolone acetonide*. Direct Rx; 2022.
2. Prescribing Information. *Kenalog-10*. E.R. Squibb & Sons LLC; 2024.
3. Prescribing Information. *Nasacort allergy 24HR*. Chattem, Inc; 2024.
4. Prescribing Information. *Kenalog-40, kenalog-80*. E.R. Squibb & Sons LLC; 2024.
5. Berard A, Sheehy O, Kurzinger ML, Juhaeri J. Intranasal triamcinolone use during pregnancy and the risk of adverse pregnancy outcomes. *J Allergy Clin Immunol*. 2016;138:97-104.
6. Katz VL, Thorp JM Jr, Bowes WA Jr. Severe symmetric intrauterine growth retardation associated with the topical use of triamcinolone. *Am J Obstet Gynecol*. 1990;162:396-397.
7. Heinonen OP, Slone D, Shapiro S. *Birth Defects and Drugs in Pregnancy*. Publishing Sciences Group; 1977:388-400.
8. Rolf BB. Corticosteroids and pregnancy. *Am J Obstet Gynecol*. 1966;95: 339-344.
9. Carmichael SL, Shaw GM. Maternal corticosteroid use and risk of selected congenital anomalies. *Am J Med Genet*. 1999;86:242-244.
10. Vincent R, Blackburn J, Wienecke G, Bautista A. Sacroiliac joint pain in pregnancy: a case report. *A Pract*. 2019;13:51-53.
11. Rosen-Carole C, Datta P, Palmiter K, et al. Transfer of injected triamcinolone into human milk of a lactating patient suffering from idiopathic granulomatous mastitis. *Breastfeed Med*. 2023;18:74-77.
12. Mitchell K, Krutsch K, Datta P, Hale TW. Evaluating the transfer of injected triamcinolone acetonide into human milk: confirmatory results. *Breastfeed Med*. 2024;19:309-310.
13. McGuire E. Sudden loss of milk supply following high-dose triamcinolone (Kenacort) injection. *Breastfeed Rev*. 2012;20:32-34.

TRIAMCINOLONE OPTHALMIC

Ophthalmic (Corticosteroid)

PREGNANCY RECOMMENDATION: Limited Human Data—No Relevant Animal Data

BREASTFEEDING RECOMMENDATION: Probably Compatible

PREGNANCY SUMMARY

Three reports describing the use of triamcinolone ophthalmic in human pregnancy were located. The uses were administered during the second and third trimesters, and no pregnancy or infant complications were reported. The drug might cross the placenta, so some fetal exposure may occur. However, the amount of drug absorbed systemically with ocular use is negligible, so any exposure is probably clinically insignificant. Therefore, this limited human pregnancy experience prevents a complete assessment of the embryofetal risk. No animal reproduction studies have been conducted with ophthalmic triamcinolone. Using this drug during pregnancy should be based on the pros and cons of the mother's clinical need for treatment versus any potential fetal risk that might occur from exposure.

BREASTFEEDING SUMMARY

No reports describing the use of triamcinolone ophthalmic during human lactation have been located. The drug might be excreted into breast milk, but systemic absorption with ocular use is negligible, so any amount found in breast milk is likely to be clinically insignificant. Breastfeeding while using this drug should be based on the mother's clinical need for treatment versus any potential infant risks that might occur.

References

1. Prescribing Information. *Xipere*. Bausch & Lomb, Inc; 2022.
2. Prescribing Information. *Triesence*. Novartis Pharmaceuticals Corporation; 2022.
3. Fazelat A, Lashkan K. Off-label use of intravitreal triamcinolone acetonide for diabetic macular edema in a pregnant patient. *Clin Ophthalmol*. 2011;5:439-441.
4. Nakamura T, Keino H, Okada A. Sub-Tenon triamcinolone acetonide injection in a pregnant patient with Vogt-Koyanagi-Harada disease. *Retin Cases Brief Rep*. 2018;12:375-378.
5. Maggio E, Mete M, Polito A, et al. Retrobulbar triamcinolone for inflammatory choroidal neovascularization in pregnancy. *BMC Ophthal*. 2020;20:483.

TRIAMTERENE

Diuretic (Potassium-Sparing Diuretic)

PREGNANCY RECOMMENDATION: Limited Human Data—Animal Data Suggest Low Risk

BREASTFEEDING RECOMMENDATION: Potential Toxicity

PREGNANCY SUMMARY

From two studies (the Collaborative Perinatal Project and Michigan Medicaid Surveillance study), there were 325 first-trimester pregnancy exposures to triamterene. A total of 15 (4.6%) major birth defects were identified, but no pattern to the defects was seen. The drug is a weak folic acid inhibitor, but neural tube defects have not been associated with the use of this drug. Per the manufacturer, the drug appears to cross the placenta, so some fetal exposure will occur. However, the limited human pregnancy experience prevents a complete assessment of embryofetal risk. Animal data did not show embryofetal toxicity in one species at doses of less than 10 times the MRHD. Using this drug during pregnancy should be based on the pros and cons of the mother's clinical need for treatment versus any potential fetal risk that might occur from exposure. There is a boxed warning for hyperkalemia with prolonged use of this drug. Diuretics are indicated in pregnancy when edema is due to pathologic causes, just as they are in the absence of pregnancy.

BREASTFEEDING SUMMARY

No reports describing the use of triamterene during human lactation have been located. The drug will likely be excreted into breast milk, so some infant exposure will probably occur. Because it is a diuretic, it theoretically could decrease breast milk supply. Therefore, due to a concern for potential serious adverse effects that might be seen in a breastfed infant, the manufacturer recommends that women not breastfeed while being treated with this drug. Nevertheless, if the clinical decision is to use this drug while breastfeeding, the infant should be monitored for the most common reported adult side effects of rash and various laboratory abnormalities (see PI).

References

1. Prescribing Information. *Triamterene*. Prasco Laboratories; 2023.
2. Heinonen OP, Slone D, Shapiro S. *Birth Defects and Drugs in Pregnancy*. Publishing Sciences Group; 1977.
3. Hernandez-Diaz S, Werler MM, Walker AM, Mitchell AA. Folic acid antagonists during pregnancy and the risk of birth defects. *N Engl J Med*. 2000;343:1608-1614.

TRIAZOLAM

Central Nervous System (Benzodiazepine—Insomnia)

PREGNANCY RECOMMENDATION: Limited Human Data (First Trimester)/Human Data Suggest Risk (Third Trimester)

BREASTFEEDING RECOMMENDATION: Potential Toxicity

PREGNANCY SUMMARY

Limited studies specific to triazolam use in human pregnancy were located. In the Michigan Medicaid Surveillance study, there were 7 total anomalies, of which 5 (3.6%) were major defects in 138 first-trimester exposures. No pattern to the defects was seen. A few larger studies have analyzed the use of benzodiazepine drugs as a group, and again, no increased risk for birth defects was identified. However, the use of triazolam in these studies was minimal. The drug will probably cross the placenta, so some fetal exposure will likely occur. Therefore, this limited human pregnancy experience, with triazolam specifically, prevents a complete assessment of the embryofetal risk. Embryofetal toxicity with malformations was observed

(*continued*)

T

in two animal species, but at doses of more than 10 times the MRHD. Using this drug during pregnancy should be based on the pros and cons of the mother's clinical need for treatment versus any potential fetal risk that might occur from exposure. Health care providers are encouraged to register women who are pregnant and have taken triazolam at any time during pregnancy by contacting the National Pregnancy Registry for Psychiatry Medications at 866-961-2388. The drug carries a boxed warning for an increased risk of misuse and addiction, and dependence and withdrawal with concomitant use with opioid drugs. Due to the adverse event profile and addictive potential, ACOG recommends avoiding benzodiazepines, or use sparingly, as an anxiety treatment. If prescribed, ACOG recommends using the lowest effective dose, and states that doses can be tapered down by 25% to 50% per week. Withdrawal symptoms can occur with abrupt cessation, including seizures. Neonatal sedation, decreased muscle tone, respiratory compromise, and NICU admission have been associated with benzodiazepine use near delivery. Because triazolam is not indicated for use in treating anxiety, consider using other agents for insomnia during pregnancy.

BREASTFEEDING SUMMARY

No reports describing the use of triazolam during human lactation have been located. The drug will likely be excreted into breast milk, so some infant exposure will probably occur. Breastfeeding while using this drug should be based on the mother's clinical need for treatment versus any potential infant risks that might occur. If used, the infant should be monitored for the most common reported adult side effects of sedation, poor feeding, and poor weight gain, as well as dizziness and lightheadedness (both leading to irritability).

References

1. Prescribing Information. *Triazolam*. Greenstone LLC; 2023.
2. American College of Obstetricians and Gynecologists. Treatment and management of mental health conditions during pregnancy and postpartum: ACOG Clinical Practice Guideline No. 5. *Obstet Gynecol*. 2023;141:1262-1288.
3. Grigoriadis S, Graves L, Peer M, et al. Benzodiazepine use during pregnancy alone or in combination with an antidepressant and congenital malformations: systematic review and meta-analysis. *J Clin Psychiatry*. 2019;80:18r12412.
4. Tinker SC, Reefhuis J, Bitsko RH, et al. Use of benzodiazepine medications during pregnancy and potential risk for birth defects, National Birth Defects Prevention Study, 1997-2011. *Birth Defects Res*. 2019;111:613-620.
5. Grigoriadis S, Graves L, Peer M, et al. Pregnancy and delivery outcomes following benzodiazepine exposure: a systematic review and meta-analysis. *Can J Psych*. 2020;65:821-834.
6. Szpunar MJ, Freeman MP, Kobylski LA, et al. Risk of major malformations in infants after first trimester exposure to benzodiazepines: results from the Massachusetts General Hospital National Pregnancy Registry for Psychiatric Medications. *Depress Anxiety*. 2022;39:751-759.
7. Chen VCH, Wu SI, Lin CF, et al. Association of prenatal exposure to benzodiazepines with development of autism spectrum and attention-deficit/hyperactivity disorders. *JAMA Netw Open*. 2022;5:e2243282.

TRICLABENDAZOLE

Anti-Infective (Antihelminthic)

PREGNANCY RECOMMENDATION: No Human Data—Animal Data Suggest Low Risk

BREASTFEEDING RECOMMENDATION: Probably Compatible

PREGNANCY SUMMARY

No reports describing the use of triclabendazole in human pregnancy have been located. The drug and active metabolites will probably cross the placenta, so some fetal exposure will likely occur. Therefore, the absence of human pregnancy experience prevents a complete assessment of the embryofetal risk. Animal data did not show any embryofetal toxicity (despite maternal toxicity) in two species at doses of less than 10 times the MRHD. Using this drug during pregnancy should be based on the pros and cons of the mother's clinical need for treatment versus any potential fetal risk that might occur from exposure. Triclabendazole can prolong the QT interval.

T

BREASTFEEDING SUMMARY

No reports describing the use of triclabendazole during human lactation have been located. The drug and its active metabolites will likely be excreted into breast milk, so some infant exposure will probably occur. Breastfeeding while using this drug should be based on the mother's clinical need for treatment versus any potential infant risks that might occur. If used, the infant should be monitored for the most common reported adult side effects of abdominal pain, nausea, headache, musculoskeletal pain, and pruritus (all leading to irritability), hyperhidrosis, decreased appetite (monitor infant growth), rash, and vomiting.

Reference

1. Prescribing Information. *Egaten*. Novartis Pharmaceuticals Corporation; 2022.

TRIENTINE

Chelating Agent (Copper Chelating)

PREGNANCY RECOMMENDATION: Limited Human Data—Animal Data Suggest Potential Risk

BREASTFEEDING RECOMMENDATION: Potential Toxicity

PREGNANCY SUMMARY

Several studies describing the use of trientine in human pregnancy were located. In every study, the drug was used in patients with Wilson disease. Excluding elective pregnancy terminations and first-trimester spontaneous abortions, no major birth anomalies were reported in 39 first-trimester exposures. The drug will probably cross the placenta, so some fetal exposure will likely occur. However, this limited human pregnancy experience prevents a complete assessment of the embryofetal risk. Animal data did show some embryofetal toxicity in one species at doses approximately equal to the MRHD. Using this drug during pregnancy should be based on the pros and cons of the mother's clinical need for treatment versus any potential fetal risk that might occur from exposure.

BREASTFEEDING SUMMARY

The drug will be found in human breast milk in low amounts. Breast milk was analyzed for the drug (in four cases) and for the drug-copper complex (in six cases), and neither was detected. Numerous infants have been breastfed during maternal trientine treatment of Wilson disease. Overall, the serum zinc and copper levels were normal, and no adverse infant effects were described. If the clinical decision is to use this drug while breastfeeding, the infant should be monitored for the most common reported adult side effects of heartburn, epigastric pain, aphthous ulcers, abdominal cramps, and myalgia (all leading to irritability), rash, anorexia (monitor infant growth), and weakness (lethargy).

References

1. Prescribing Information. *Trientine hydrochloride*. Accord Healthcare, Inc; 2021.
2. Nunns D, Hawthorne B, Goulding P, Maresh M. Wilson's disease in pregnancy. *Eur J Obstet Gynecol Reprod Biol*. 1995;62:141-143.
3. Walshe JM. The management of pregnancy in Wilson's disease treated with trientine. *Q J Med*. 1986;58;81-87.
4. Desbriere R, Roquelaure B, Sarles J, Boubli L. Pregnancy in a patient treated with trientine dihydrochloride for Wilson's disease. *Presse Med*. 1998;27:806.
5. Dathe K, Beck E, Schaefer C. Pregnancy outcome after chelation therapy in Wilson disease. Evaluation of the German Embryotox Database. *Reprod Toxicol*. 2016;65:39-45.
6. Pfeiffenberger J, Beinhardt S, Gotthardt DN, et al. Pregnancy in Wilson's disease: management and outcome. *Hepatology*. 2018;67:1261-1269.
7. Izumi Y. [Can mothers with Wilson's disease give her breast milk to their infant?]. *Teikyo Med J*. 2012;35:17-24.
8. Shiga K, Kaga H, Kodama H, et al. Copper and zinc concentrations in the breast milk of mothers with Wilson disease and effects on infants. *J Inherit Metab Dis*. 2006;29(suppl 1):139. Abstract. doi: 10.1007/s10545-006-9995-6.
9. Demir K, Soyer OM, Karaca C, et al. The course of pregnancy in Wilson's disease-one center, 20 years' experience. *Gastroenterology*. 2014;146: S-1009. Abstract TU1834.

TRIFAROTENE

Dermatologic (Retinoid—Topical)

PREGNANCY RECOMMENDATION: No Human Data and No Relevant Animal Data

BREASTFEEDING RECOMMENDATION: Probably Compatible

PREGNANCY SUMMARY

No reports describing the use of trifarotene in human pregnancy have been located. Systemic absorption is negligible with topical use (undetectable to 10 pg/mL). Therefore, any transplacental transfer is likely to be clinically insignificant. The manufacturer reports that data from clinical trials regarding the use of trifarotene cream during pregnancy has not demonstrated an increased risk for malformations, spontaneous abortion, or adverse maternal or fetal outcomes. However, there are case reports of major birth defects, similar to those seen in fetuses exposed to oral retinoids, when pregnant women have been exposed to other topical retinoids. However, the absence of human pregnancy experience prevents a complete assessment of the embryofetal risk. Animal data showed embryofetal toxicity in two species, but with oral doses of more than 500 times the MRHD of topical therapy. Using this drug during pregnancy should be based on the pros and cons of the mother's clinical need for treatment versus any potential fetal risk that might occur from exposure. Regardless, because isotretinoin (a systemic retinoid) is such a terrible teratogen, if an alternative nonretinoid drug can be used (especially in the first trimester), this might be considered.

BREASTFEEDING SUMMARY

No reports describing the use of trifarotene during human lactation have been located. Systemic absorption is negligible with topical use (undetectable to 10 pg/mL). Therefore, any excretion into human breast milk is likely to be clinically insignificant. Breastfeeding while using this drug should be based on the mother's clinical need for treatment versus any potential infant risks that might occur. Because of the negligible absorption, systemic side effects were not evaluated. However, it is recommended that application to the smallest area of skin for the shortest duration possible should occur while breastfeeding. Advise breastfeeding women not to apply directly to the nipple or areola to avoid direct infant contact.

Reference

1. Prescribing Information. *Aklief*. Galderma Laboratories LP; 2023.

TRIFLUOPERAZINE

Mental Health (First Generation Typical Antipsychotic)

PREGNANCY RECOMMENDATION: Limited Human Data—Animal Data Suggest Low Risk

BREASTFEEDING RECOMMENDATION: Potential Toxicity

PREGNANCY SUMMARY

There are several reports describing the use of trifluoperazine in human pregnancy. The data about the risk are mixed. From three studies, the rate of major birth anomalies was about 3.2% in more than 100 first-trimester exposures. In addition, no pattern to the defects was seen. However, a few case reports and small series have described a risk for limb defects, including phocomelia, though this was not seen in the larger studies. When used near term, the use of this drug has been associated with neonates experiencing prolonged jaundice, extrapyramidal signs and/or withdrawal symptoms, hyperreflexia, and hyporeflexia. Trifluoperazine has been shown to cross the placenta, so fetal exposure will occur. However, the limited human pregnancy experience prevents a complete assessment of the embryofetal risk. Animal data did not show any embryofetal toxicity in two species at doses or more than 10 times the MRHD. Using this drug during pregnancy should be based on the pros and cons of the mother's clinical need for treatment versus any potential fetal risk that might occur from exposure. Elevated glucose levels have been reported in patients treated with this drug. Therefore, if used during pregnancy, glucose levels should be monitored.

BREASTFEEDING SUMMARY

Two reports have been located that describe trifluoperazine use during lactation. Three women were taking 5 to 10 mg daily, and no infant adverse events were reported. Breast milk levels were low with calculated RIDs of 3% or less. In one case, the infant's serum concentration was only 1 ng/mL. As an antipsychotic, trifluoperazine can increase prolactin levels, but this should not adversely affect breastfeeding. However, due to a concern for potential serious adverse effects that might be seen in a breastfed infant, the manufacturer recommends that women not breastfeed while being treated with this drug. Nevertheless, breastfeeding while using this drug should be based on the mother's clinical need for treatment versus any potential infant risks that might occur. If used, the infant should be monitored for the most common reported adult side effects of dizziness, dry mouth, and blurred vision (all leading to irritability), drowsiness, insomnia, rash, fatigue (lethargy), anorexia (monitor infant growth), and extrapyramidal reactions.

References

1. Prescribing Information. *Trifluoperazine*. Mylan Pharmaceuticals, Inc; 2024.
2. Moya F, Thorndike V. Passage of drugs across the placenta. *Am J Obstet Gynecol*. 1962;84:1778-1798.
3. Canadian Department of National Health and Welfare, Food and Drug Directorate. *Letter of notification to Canadian physicians*. Ottawa, December 7, 1962.
4. Moriarity AJ. Trifluoperazine and congenital malformations. *Can Med Assoc J*.1963;88:97.
5. Moriarty AJ, Nance MR. Trifluoperazine and pregnancy. *Can Med Assoc J*. 1963;88:375-376.
6. Schrire I. Trifluoperazine and foetal abnormalities. *Lancet*. 1963;1:174.
7. Corner BD. Congenital malformations. Clinical considerations. *Med J Southwest*. 1962;77:46-52.
8. Hall G. A case of phocomelia of the upper limbs. *Med J Aust*. 1963;1:449-450.
9. Vince DJ. Congenital malformations following phenothiazine administration during pregnancy. *Can Med Assoc J*. 1969;100:223.
10. Hill RM, Desmond MM, Kay JL. Extrapyramidal dysfunction in an infant of a schizophrenic mother. *J Pediatr*. 1966;69:589-595.
11. Slone D, Siskind V, Heinonen OP, et al. Antenatal exposure to the phenothiazines in relation to congenital malformations, perinatal mortality rate, birth weight, and intelligence quotient score. *Am J Obstet Gynecol*. 1977;128:486-488.
12. Bond GR, Zee AV. Overdosage of misoprostol in pregnancy. *Am J Obstet Gynecol*. 1994;171:561-562.
13. Yoshida K, Smith B, Craggs M, Kumar R. Neuroleptic drugs in breast-milk: a study of pharmacokinetics and of possible adverse effects in breast-fed infants. *Psychol Med*. 1998;28:81-91.
14. Birnbaum CS, Cohen LS, Bailey JW, et al. Serum concentrations of antidepressants and benzodiazepines in nursing infants: a case series. *Pediatrics*. 1999;104:1-6.

TRIFLURIDINE AND TIPIRACIL

Antineoplastic (Nucleoside Metabolic Inhibitor/Thymidine Phosphorylase Inhibitor)

PREGNANCY RECOMMENDATION: No Human Data—Animal Data Suggest Potential Risk

BREASTFEEDING RECOMMENDATION: Potential Toxicity

PREGNANCY SUMMARY

No reports describing the use of trifluridine and tipiracil in human pregnancy have been located. Both drugs will probably cross the placenta, so some fetal exposure will likely occur. Therefore, the absence of human pregnancy experience prevents a complete assessment of the embryofetal risk. Animal studies did show embryofetal toxicity. Due to the findings from the animal studies and the drug's mechanism of action, the manufacturer recommends that women with reproductive potential use effective contraception during treatment and for at least 6 months after the last dose. They also recommend that males with female partners of reproductive potential use condoms during treatment and for at least 3 months after the last dose. Nevertheless, using this drug during pregnancy should be based on the pros and cons of the mother's clinical need for treatment versus any potential fetal risk that might occur from exposure.

BREASTFEEDING SUMMARY

No reports describing the use of trifluridine and tipiracil during human lactation have been located. Both drugs will probably appear in breast milk, so infant exposure will likely occur. However, due to the concern for potential serious adverse effects that might be seen in a breastfed infant, the manufacturer recommends that women not breastfeed while being treated with this drug combination and for at least 1 day after the last dose. Nevertheless, breastfeeding while using this drug should be based on the mother's clinical need for treatment. If used, the infant should be monitored for the most common reported adult side effects of nausea (leading to irritability), diarrhea, vomiting, pyrexia, lethargy, decreased appetite, and various laboratory abnormalities (see PI).

Reference

1. Prescribing Information. *Lonsurf*. Taiho Pharmaceutical Co., Ltd; 2019.

TRIFLURIDINE OPHTHALMIC

Ophthalmic (Antiviral—Topical)

PREGNANCY RECOMMENDATION: No Human Data—Animal Data Suggest Low Risk

BREASTFEEDING RECOMMENDATION: Probably Compatible

PREGNANCY SUMMARY

No reports describing the use of trifluridine in human pregnancy have been located. If found in the maternal circulation, the drug will probably cross the placenta, so some fetal exposure could occur. However, systemic absorption of the drug has not been detected following ocular use. Therefore, any exposure is likely to be clinically insignificant. Regardless, the absence of human pregnancy experience prevents a complete assessment of the embryofetal risk. Animal data did not show any embryofetal toxicity in one species with ocular administration at doses of less than 10 times the MRHD. Some embryofetal toxicity was seen in two animal species, but with SC doses of more than 10 times the MRHD. Using this drug during pregnancy should be based on the pros and cons of the mother's clinical need for treatment versus any potential fetal risk that might occur from exposure. If used during pregnancy, consider placing pressure over the tear duct in the corner of the eye for at least 1 minute, and then remove any excess solution with absorbent tissue to decrease the amount of drug reaching the systemic circulation even further.

BREASTFEEDING SUMMARY

No reports describing the use of trifluridine during human lactation have been located. If found in the maternal circulation, the drug will probably be found in breast milk. However, systemic absorption of the drug has not been detected following ocular use. Therefore, any exposure is likely to be clinically insignificant. Breastfeeding while using this drug should be based on the mother's clinical need for treatment versus any potential infant risks that might occur. Because of the lack of absorption into the circulation, systemic side effects have not been evaluated.

Reference

1. Prescribing Information. *Trifluridine*. Sandoz, Inc; 2024.

TRIHEPTANOIN

Nutritional Supplement

PREGNANCY RECOMMENDATION: No Human Data—Animal Data Suggest Low Risk

BREASTFEEDING RECOMMENDATION: Probably Compatible

PREGNANCY SUMMARY

No reports describing the use of triheptanoin in human pregnancy have been located. The drug will probably cross the placenta, so some fetal exposure will likely occur. However, the absence of human pregnancy experience prevents a complete assessment of embryofetal risk. Animal data did not show embryofetal toxicity. There is a pregnancy safety study that monitors pregnancy outcomes in women exposed to triheptanoin during pregnancy. Health care providers or patients are encouraged to contact the manufacturer at 1-888-0756-8657.

BREASTFEEDING SUMMARY

No reports describing the use of triheptanoin during human lactation have been located. The drug will probably enter breast milk, so some infant exposure will likely occur. Medium-chain triglycerides and other fatty acids are normal components of breast milk. If the clinical decision is to use this drug while breastfeeding, the infant should be monitored for the most common reported adult side effects of abdominal pain and nausea (both leading to irritability), diarrhea, and vomiting.

Reference

1. Prescribing Information. *Dojolvi*. Ultragenyx Pharmaceutical, Inc; 2020.

TRIHEXYPHENIDYL

Central Nervous System (Parasympatholytic—Anti-Parkinson)

PREGNANCY RECOMMENDATION: Limited Human Data—No Relevant Animal Data

BREASTFEEDING RECOMMENDATION: Probably Compatible

PREGNANCY SUMMARY

Three reports describing the use of trihexyphenidyl in human pregnancy were located. A total of 17 first-trimester exposures were described, and no major malformations were identified. The drug will probably cross the placenta, so some fetal exposure will likely occur. However, the limited human pregnancy experience prevents a complete assessment of the embryofetal risk. Animal reproduction studies have not been conducted. Using this drug during pregnancy should be based on the pros and cons of the mother's clinical need for treatment versus any potential fetal risk that might occur from exposure.

BREASTFEEDING SUMMARY

T

Two reports describing the use of trihexyphenidyl during human lactation have been located. Breast milk was not evaluated for trihexyphenidyl drug levels. However, none of the children exhibited any apparent adverse effects. The drug will likely be excreted into breast milk, so some infant exposure will probably occur. Breastfeeding while using this drug should be based on the mother's clinical need for treatment versus any potential infant risks that might occur. If used, the infant should be monitored for the most common reported adult side effects of dizziness, dry mouth, nausea, nervousness, and blurred vision (all leading to irritability). Because it has some anticholinergic properties, it may decrease breast milk supply.

References

1. Prescribing Information. *Trihexyphenidyl hydrochloride*. Actavis Pharma, Inc; 2024.
2. Heinonen OP, Slone D, Shapiro S. *Birth Defects and Drugs in Pregnancy*. Publishing Sciences Group; 1977:346-353.
3. Mendhekar DN, Andrade C. Uneventful use of haloperidol and trihexyphenidyl during three consecutive pregnancies. *Arch Womens Ment Health*. 2011; 14:83-84.
4. Mendhekar D, Andrade C. A 26-year follow-up of a woman with 5 consecutive children exposed to risperidone during pregnancy and breastfeeding. *Prim Care Companion CNS Disord*. 2024;26:23cr03660.

TRILACICLIB

Antineoplastic (Cyclin-Dependent Kinase Inhibitor)

PREGNANCY RECOMMENDATION: **No Human Data and No Relevant Animal Data**

BREASTFEEDING RECOMMENDATION: **Potential Toxicity**

PREGNANCY SUMMARY

No reports describing the use of trilaciclib in human pregnancy have been located. Trilaciclib will probably cross the placenta, so some fetal exposure will likely occur. Therefore, the absence of human pregnancy experience prevents a complete assessment of the embryofetal risk. Animal reproduction studies have not been performed. Based on the drug's mechanism of action, the manufacturer recommends that women with reproductive potential use effective contraception during treatment and for at least 3 weeks after the last dose. Nevertheless, using this drug during pregnancy should be based on the pros and cons of the mother's clinical need for treatment versus any potential fetal risk that might occur from exposure. Elevated glucose levels have been reported in patients treated with this drug. Additionally, trilaciclib was associated with the prolongation of the QT interval.

BREASTFEEDING SUMMARY

No reports describing the use of trilaciclib during human lactation have been located. The drug will likely be excreted into breast milk. Based on the drug's mechanism of action, the manufacturer recommends that women not breastfeed while taking trilaciclib and for at least 3 weeks after the last dose. Nevertheless, breastfeeding while using this drug should be based on the mother's clinical need for treatment. If used, the infant should be monitored for the most common reported adult side effects of headache (leading to irritability), lethargy, pneumonia, and various laboratory abnormalities (see PI).

Reference

1. Prescribing Information. *Cosela*. G1 Therapeutics; 2021.

TRIMETHOBENZAMIDE

Gastrointestinal (Antinausea)

PREGNANCY RECOMMENDATION: **Human Data Suggest Low Risk**

BREASTFEEDING RECOMMENDATION: **Probably Compatible**

PREGNANCY SUMMARY

Six reports were located that described the use of trimethobenzamide in human pregnancy. In more than 750 first-trimester exposures, the rate of major birth defects was only about 2.3%. No pattern to the defects was seen. Trimethobenzamide has been used in pregnancy to treat nausea and vomiting for more than four decades. The drug will probably cross the placenta, so some fetal exposure will likely occur. Embryofetal toxicity was observed in two animal species at doses of less than 10 times the RHD. Using this drug during pregnancy should be based on the pros and cons of the mother's clinical need for treatment versus any potential fetal risk that might occur from exposure.

BREASTFEEDING SUMMARY

No reports describing the use of trimethobenzamide during human lactation have been located. The drug will likely be excreted into breast milk, so some infant exposure will probably occur. Breastfeeding while using this drug should be based on the mother's clinical need for treatment versus any potential infant risks that might occur. If used, the infant should be monitored for the most common reported adult side effects of dizziness, headache, and muscle cramps (all leading to irritability), diarrhea, and sedation.

References

1. Prescribing Information. *Trimethobenzamide*. Chartwell Rx LLC; 2023.
2. Prescribing Information. *Tigan®*. HF Acquisition Co LLC, DBA HealthFirst; 2024.
3. Breslow S, Belafsky HA, Shangold JE, et al. Antiemetic effect of trimethobenzamide in pregnant patients. *Clin Med*. 1961;8:2153-2155.
4. Winters HS. Antiemetics in nausea and vomiting of pregnancy. *Obstet Gynecol*. 1961;18:753-756.
5. Milkovich L, van den Berg BJ. An evaluation of the teratogenicity of certain antinauseant drugs. *Am J Obstet Gynecol*. 1976;125:244-248.
6. Jick H, Holmes LB, Hunter JR, et al. First-trimester drug use and congenital disorders. *JAMA*. 1981;246:343-346.
7. Aselton P, Jick H, Milunsky A, et al. First-trimester drug use and congenital disorders. *Obstet Gynecol*. 1985;65:451-455.
8. Heinonen OP, Slone D, Shapiro S. *Birth Defects and Drugs in Pregnancy*. Wright PSB; 1983:330.

TRIMETHOPRIM

Anti-Infective

PREGNANCY RECOMMENDATION: Human Data Suggest Potential Risk (First Trimester)

BREASTFEEDING RECOMMENDATION: Potential Toxicity

PREGNANCY SUMMARY

Several reports describing the use of trimethoprim in human pregnancy have been located. In one large study analyzing the use of trimethoprim (in prescriptions filled 1-3 months prior to conception), the overall congenital malformation rate was higher than that of the control group. However, no distinct pattern to the defects was seen. Because trimethoprim is a weak folic acid inhibitor, a few studies have analyzed these drugs as a group. The risk for neural tube defect (NTD), cardiovascular, and other anomalies was higher, though numbers for just trimethoprim use only were small. The drug appears to cross the placenta, so some fetal exposure will occur. However, the limited data specific to trimethoprim use in human pregnancy prevent a complete assessment of the embryofetal risk. Embryofetal toxicity was observed in one animal species at doses of less than 10 times the MRHD. Using this drug during pregnancy should be based on the pros and cons of the mother's clinical need for treatment versus any potential fetal risk that might occur from exposure. The manufacturer states that trimethoprim should be used during pregnancy only if the potential benefit justifies the potential risk to the fetus because trimethoprim may interfere with folic acid metabolism. As with all pregnancies, folic acid supplementation, at least 0.4 mg/d, started before conception may reduce some of the risk for these congenital defects.

BREASTFEEDING SUMMARY

Trimethoprim has been shown to be excreted in human breast milk. Following a daily dose of 320 mg for 5 days, breast milk concentrations ranged between 1.2 and 2.4 mcg/mL (average 1.8 mcg/mL), with peak levels occurring at 2 to 3 hours. No adverse effects were reported in the infants. The calculated RID was about 6%. Nearly identical results were found in a second study with 50 patients. Mean breast milk levels were 2.0 mcg/mL, representing a breast milk to maternal plasma ratio of 1.25. The manufacturer states that caution should be exercised when trimethoprim is administered to a nursing woman because it may interfere with folic acid metabolism. Breastfeeding while using this drug should be based on the mother's clinical need for treatment. If used, the infant should be monitored for the most common reported adult side effects of pruritus, epigastric pain, nausea, and glossitis (all leading to irritability), rash, vomiting, pyrexia, and various laboratory abnormalities (see PI).

References

1. Prescribing Information. *Trimethoprim*. Dr. Reddy's Laboratories, Inc; 2024.
2. Ylikorkala O, Sjostedt E, Jarvinen PA, et al. Trimethoprim-sulfonamide combination administered orally and intravaginally in the 1st trimester of pregnancy: its absorption into serum and transfer to amniotic fluid. *Acta Obstet Gynecol Scand*. 1973;52:229-234.
3. Reid DWJ, Caille G, Kaufmann NR. Maternal and transplacental kinetics of trimethoprim and sulfamethoxazole, separately and in combination. *Can Med Assoc J*. 1975;112:67s-72s.
4. Reeves DS, Wilkinson PJ. The pharmacokinetics of trimethoprim and trimethoprim/sulfonamide combinations, including penetration into body tissues. *Infection*. 1979;7(suppl 4):S330–S341.
5. Bawdon RE, Maberry MC, Fortunato SJ, et al. Trimethoprim and sulfamethoxazole transfer in the in vitro perfused human cotyledon. *Gynecol Obstet Invest*. 1991;31:240-242.
6. Hernandez-Diaz S, Werler MM, Walker AM, Mitchell AA. Folic acid antagonists during pregnancy and the risk of birth defects. *N Engl J Med*. 2000; 343:1608-1614.
7. Hernandez-Diaz S, Mitchell AA. Folic acid antagonists during pregnancy and risk of birth defects. *N Engl J Med*. 2001;344:934-935.
8. Hernandez-Diaz S, Werler MM, Walker AM, Mitchell AA. Neural tube defects in relation to use of folic acid antagonists during pregnancy. *Am J Epidemiol*. 2001;153:961-968.
9. Sun Y, Wu CS, Olsen J. Trimethoprim use before pregnancy and risk of congenital malformation: reanalyzed using a case-crossover design and a case-time-control design. *Pharmacoepid Drug Saf*. 2014;23:1076-1083.
10. Arnauld R, Soutoul JH, Gallier J, et al. A study of the passage of trimethoprim into the maternal milk. *Quest Med*. 1972;25:959-964.
11. Miller RD, Salter AJ. The passage of trimethoprim/sulphamethoxazole into breast milk and its significance. In: Daikos GK, ed. Progress in Chemotherapy, Proceedings of the Eighth International Congress of Chemotherapy, Athens, 1973. Hellenic Society for Chemotherapy, 1974:687-691.
12. Ito S, Blajchman A, Stephenson M, et al. Prospective follow-up of adverse reactions in breast-fed infants exposed to maternal medication. *Am J Obstet Gynecol*. 1993;168:1393-1399.

TRIMIPRAMINE

Mental Health (Tricyclic Antidepressant)

PREGNANCY RECOMMENDATION: Limited Human Data-No Relevant Animal Data

BREASTFEEDING RECOMMENDATION: Probably Compatible

PREGNANCY SUMMARY

One report of nine women taking trimipramine in human pregnancy was located. No major malformations were described. The drug will probably cross the placenta, so some fetal exposure will likely occur. Therefore, the absence of human pregnancy experience prevents a complete assessment of the embryofetal risk. Embryofetal toxicity with malformations was observed in two animal species, but at doses of more than 10 times the RHD. In general, though, most tricyclic antidepressants do not have a known teratogenic effect in humans; however, there have been reports of neonatal withdrawal when used near delivery. Using this drug during pregnancy should be based on the pros and cons of the mother's clinical need for treatment versus any potential fetal risk that might occur from exposure. There is a pregnancy exposure registry that monitors pregnancy outcomes in women using antidepressant drugs. Health care providers are encouraged to call the National Pregnancy Registry for Antidepressants at 1-844-405-6185. ACOG states that uncontrolled and undertreated depression is associated with a risk for limited engagement in medical care, self-care, substance use, preterm birth, low birth weight, postpartum depression, impaired infant attachment (which carries long-term developmental effects), disrupted relationships with partner, and suicide. Additionally, untreated and undertreated mental health disorders should be considered an exposure. Therefore, pregnancy alone should not be a reason to withhold or discontinue mental health medications.

BREASTFEEDING SUMMARY

No reports describing the use of trimipramine during human lactation have been located. The drug will likely be excreted into breast milk, so some infant exposure will probably occur. Breastfeeding while using this drug should be based on the mother's clinical need for treatment. If used, the infant should be monitored for the most common reported adult side effects of anxiety, paresthesia, and dry mouth (all leading to irritability), and insomnia. Due to some anticholinergic effects, the drug can decrease breast milk supply. Lactation alone should not be a reason to withhold or discontinue mental health medications.

References

1. Prescribing Information. *Trimipramine maleate*. Breckenridge Pharmaceutical, Inc; 2024.
2. American College of Obstetricians and Gynecologists. Treatment and management of mental health conditions during pregnancy and postpartum: ACOG Clinical Practice Guideline No. 5. *Obstet Gynecol*. 2023;141:1262-1288.
3. McElhatton PR, Garbis HM, Elefant E, et al. The outcome of pregnancy in 689 women exposed to therapeutic doses of antidepressants. A collaborative study of the European Network of Teratology Information Services (ENTIS). *Reprod Toxicol*. 1996;10:285-294.

TRIPROLIDINE

Antihistamine (First Generation—H_1 Inhibitor)

PREGNANCY RECOMMENDATION: Human Data Suggest Low Risk

BREASTFEEDING RECOMMENDATION: Probably Compatible

PREGNANCY SUMMARY

From three studies, four publications (Collaborative Perinatal Project, Michigan Medicaid Surveillance study, and Group Health Cooperative of Puget Sound), a total of 1,554 pregnancies with first-trimester exposure to triprolidine were located. Of these, there were 45 (2.9%) major birth anomalies. No pattern to the defects was seen. In general, antihistamines are considered low risk in pregnancy. The drug will probably cross the placenta, so some fetal exposure will likely occur. Animal reproduction studies have not been conducted. Using this drug during pregnancy should be based on the pros and cons of the mother's clinical need for treatment versus any potential fetal risk that might occur from exposure.

BREASTFEEDING SUMMARY

Triprolidine was found to be excreted into human breast milk in three lactating women. The drug was found in all samples, with milk levels of about 50% to 70% maternal serum concentrations. The calculated RIDs were less than 1%. Given the anticholinergic properties of triprolidine, it may decrease breast milk supply. Breastfeeding while using this drug should be based on the mother's clinical need for treatment versus any potential infant risks that might occur. If used, the infant should be monitored for the most common reported adult side effects of nausea, headache, dizziness, and dry mouth (all leading to irritability), sedation, constipation, vomiting, and decreased appetite (monitor infant growth).

References

1. National Library of Medicine—Pubchem. *Triprolidine*. Accessed December 29, 2024. https://pubchem.ncbi.nlm.nih.gov/compound/Triprolidine
2. Heinonen OP, Slone D, Shapiro S. *Birth Defects and Drugs in Pregnancy*. Publishing Sciences Group; 1977:323.
3. Nelson MM, Forfar JO. Associations between drugs administered during pregnancy and congenital abnormalities of the fetus. *Br Med J*. 1971;1:523-527.

T

4. Jick H, Holmes LB, Hunter JR, et al. First-trimester drug use and congenital disorders. *JAMA*. 1981;246:343-346.
5. Aselton P, Jick H, Milunsky A, et al. First-trimester drug use and congenital disorders. *Obstet Gynecol*. 1985;65:451-455.
6. Findlay JWA, Butz RF, Sailstad JM, et al. Pseudoephedrine and triprolidine in plasma and breast milk of nursing mothers. *Br J Clin Pharmacol*. 1984;18:901-906.

TROFINETIDE

Genetic (Glypromate Analogue)

PREGNANCY RECOMMENDATION: No Human Data—Animal Data Suggest Low Risk

BREASTFEEDING RECOMMENDATION: Probably Compatible

PREGNANCY SUMMARY

No reports describing the use of trofinetide in human pregnancy have been located. The drug will likely cross the placenta, so some fetal exposure will probably occur. Therefore, the absence of human pregnancy experience prevents a complete assessment of the embryofetal risk. Animal data did not show any embryofetal toxicity, but the doses used were less than the MRHD. Using trofinetide during pregnancy should be based on the pros and cons of the mother's clinical need for treatment versus any potential fetal risk that might occur from exposure.

BREASTFEEDING SUMMARY

No reports describing the use of trofinetide during human lactation have been located. The drug will likely be excreted into breast milk, so some infant exposure will probably occur. Because trofinetide is a tripeptide, if the drug were to be ingested through breastfeeding, it might be digested in the infant's gastrointestinal tract and not be absorbed. Breastfeeding while using this drug should be based on the mother's clinical need for treatment. If used, the infant should be monitored for the most common reported adult side effects of diarrhea and vomiting.

Reference

1. Prescribing Information. *Daybue*. Acadia Pharmaceuticals, Inc; 2023.

TROPICAMIDE OPHTHALMIC

Ophthalmic (Anticholinergic)

PREGNANCY RECOMMENDATION: No Human Data and No Relevant Animal Data

BREASTFEEDING RECOMMENDATION: Probably Compatible

PREGNANCY SUMMARY

No reports describing the use of tropicamide ophthalmic in human pregnancy have been located. Because of the topical ophthalmic use, the amount of systemic absorption is likely to be minimal, but no data exist regarding this issue. If the drug is absorbed systemically, tropicamide is likely to cross the placenta, so fetal exposure could occur. However, the absence of human pregnancy experience prevents a complete assessment of embryofetal risk. Animal reproduction studies have not been conducted. Using this drug during pregnancy should be based on the pros and cons of the mother's clinical need for treatment versus any potential fetal risk that might occur from exposure. In general, anticholinergic medications are not thought to present a clinically significant risk of developmental toxicity. If used during pregnancy, consider placing pressure over the tear duct in the corner of the eye for at least 1 minute, and then remove any excess solution with absorbent tissue to decrease the amount of drug reaching the systemic circulation even further.

BREASTFEEDING SUMMARY

No reports describing the use of tropicamide ophthalmic during human lactation have been located. Because of the topical ocular use, the amount of systemic absorption is likely to be minimal, but no data exist regarding this issue. Therefore, the drug might be excreted into breast milk if found in the circulation. Breastfeeding while using this drug should be based on the mother's clinical need for treatment versus any potential infant risks that might occur. Due to the topical use, systemic side effects were not analyzed.

Reference

1. Prescribing Information. *Tropicamide*. Bausch & Lomb, Inc; 2023.

TROSPIUM

Urinary (Antispasmodic—Antimuscarinic)

PREGNANCY RECOMMENDATION: No Human Data—Animal Data Suggest Low Risk

BREASTFEEDING RECOMMENDATION: Probably Compatible

PREGNANCY SUMMARY

No reports describing the use of trospium in human pregnancy have been located. The drug will probably cross the placenta, so some fetal exposure will likely occur. Therefore, the absence of human pregnancy experience prevents a complete assessment of the embryofetal risk. Animal studies did not show any embryofetal toxicity in two species at doses of more than 10 times the MRHD. Using this drug during pregnancy should be based on the pros and cons of the mother's clinical need for treatment versus any potential fetal risk that might occur from exposure.

BREASTFEEDING SUMMARY

No reports describing the use of trospium during human lactation have been located. The drug will likely be excreted into breast milk, so some infant exposure will probably occur. Breastfeeding while using this drug should be based on the mother's clinical need for treatment. If used, the infant should be monitored for the most common reported adult side effects of dry mouth and headache (leading to irritability), and constipation. Given the anticholinergic effects, this medication may decrease breast milk supply.

Reference

1. Prescribing Information. *Trospium chloride*. Actavis Pharma, Inc; 2024.

TUCATINIB

Antineoplastic (Tyrosine Kinase Inhibitor)

PREGNANCY RECOMMENDATION: No Human Data—Animal Data Suggest Potential Risk

BREASTFEEDING RECOMMENDATION: Potential Toxicity

PREGNANCY SUMMARY

No reports describing the use of tucatinib in human pregnancy have been located. The drug will probably cross the placenta, so some fetal exposure will likely occur. Therefore, the absence of human pregnancy experience prevents a complete assessment of the embryofetal risk. Animal studies did show embryofetal toxicity. Based on these animal studies and the drug's mechanism of action, the manufacturer recommends that women with reproductive potential use effective contraception during treatment and for 1 week after the last dose. They also recommend that males with female partners of reproductive potential use effective contraception during treatment and for 1 week after the last dose. Using this drug during pregnancy should be based on the pros and cons of the mother's clinical need for treatment versus any potential fetal risk that might occur from exposure. The drug is used in combination with trastuzumab and capecitabine (see Trastuzumab and Capecitabine).

BREASTFEEDING SUMMARY

No reports describing the use of tucatinib during human lactation have been located. The drug will probably be excreted into breast milk, so some infant exposure will likely occur. However, due to the concern for potential adverse effects in a breastfed infant, the manufacturer recommends that women not breastfeed while being treated with tucatinib and for at least 1 week after the last dose. Nevertheless, if the clinical decision is to use this drug while breastfeeding, the infant should be monitored for the most common reported adult side effects of abdominal pain, headache, and nausea (all leading to irritability), vomiting, diarrhea, lethargy, decreased appetite, and rash. The drug is used in combination with trastuzumab and capecitabine (see Trastuzumab and Capecitabine).

Reference

1. Prescribing Information. *Tukysa*. Seagen, Inc; 2020.

U

UBLITUXIMAB

Central Nervous System (Anti-CD20—Monoclonal Antibody)

PREGNANCY RECOMMENDATION: **No Human Data and No Relevant Animal Data**

BREASTFEEDING RECOMMENDATION: **Probably Compatible**

PREGNANCY SUMMARY

No reports describing the use of ublituximab in human pregnancy have been located. As an immunoglobulin G (IgG) antibody, the drug will likely cross the placenta, especially in the third trimester, so fetal exposure will probably occur. Therefore, the absence of human pregnancy experience prevents a complete assessment of the embryofetal risk. Administration of other anti-CD20 antibodies during pregnancy has resulted in transient peripheral B-cell depletion and lymphocytopenia in exposed infants. The manufacturer recommends that live vaccines should not be administered to infants exposed to ublituximab in utero until B-cell recovery occurs. Animal studies showed embryofetal toxicity with significant maternal toxicity, but at doses above 10 times the recommended human dose (RHD). Based on these animal studies, the manufacturer recommends that women with reproductive potential use effective contraception during treatment and for 6 months after the last dose. Nevertheless, using this drug during pregnancy should be based on the pros and cons of the mother's clinical need for treatment versus any potential fetal risk that might occur from exposure.

BREASTFEEDING SUMMARY

No reports describing the use of ublituximab during human lactation have been located. It is known that IgG antibodies can be found in human breast milk, but are not found in the neonatal or infant circulation. Additionally, if any IgG antibodies were to be ingested through breastfeeding, they would probably be digested in the infant's gastrointestinal tract and not be absorbed. Breastfeeding while using this drug should be based on the mother's clinical need for treatment versus any potential infant risks that might occur. If used, the infant should be monitored for the most common reported adult side effects of upper respiratory tract infections.

Reference

1. Prescribing Information. Briumvi. TG Therapeutics, Inc; 2022.

UBROGEPANT

Central Nervous System (Antimigraine)

PREGNANCY RECOMMENDATION: **No Human Data—Animal Data Suggest Low Risk**

BREASTFEEDING RECOMMENDATION: **Probably Compatible**

PREGNANCY SUMMARY

No reports describing the use of ubrogepant in human pregnancy have been located. The drug will likely cross the placenta, so some fetal exposure will probably occur. Animal data did not show any embryofetal toxicity in two species at doses 8 and 15 times the RHD. However, the absence of human pregnancy experience prevents a complete assessment of embryofetal risk. Using this drug during pregnancy should be based on the pros and cons of the mother's clinical need for treatment versus any potential fetal risk that might occur from exposure. Women who are pregnant and have taken ubrogepant at any time during pregnancy are encouraged to contact the Ubrelvy pregnancy registry at 833-277-0206. During pregnancy, women with migraines may be at increased risk for preeclampsia and gestational hypertension.

BREASTFEEDING SUMMARY

No reports describing the use of ubrogepant during human lactation have been located. The drug will probably be found in breast milk, so some infant exposure will likely occur. The manufacturer recommends that the developmental and health benefits of breastfeeding should be considered along with the mother's clinical need for ubrogepant and any potential adverse effects on the breastfed infant or from the underlying maternal condition. If used while breastfeeding, the infant should be monitored for the most common reported adult side effects of nausea (leading to irritability) and somnolence.

References

1. Prescribing Information. Ubrelvy. Allergan, Inc; 2023.
2. Vig SJ, Garza J, Tao Y. The use of erenumab for migraine prophylaxis during pregnancy: a case report and narrative review. *Headache*. 2022;62: 1256-1263.

ULIPRISTAL

Reproductive (Emergency Contraceptive, Progestin Receptor Modulator)

PREGNANCY RECOMMENDATION: *Contraindicated

BREASTFEEDING RECOMMENDATION: Probably Compatible

PREGNANCY SUMMARY

Data from the manufacturer reported 462 pregnancy exposures, of which 302 had elective terminations, 63 spontaneously aborted, and 13 were ectopic pregnancies. Of the remaining 84 pregnancies, 1 minor and 4 major (2 with genetic syndromes) malformations were observed. From two other reports, a total of 65 pregnancies were reported with first-trimester exposure to the drug, and of these, 12 had elective terminations. Of the remaining 53, there were 9 (17%) spontaneous abortions and 42 deliveries of infants without any major anomalies. It is likely that ulipristal and its active metabolite will cross the placenta, so fetal exposure will probably occur. In animal studies, embryofetal toxicity was observed in several species at doses of 3 times (or less) the RHD (in two species, exposure was less than the RHD). *The drug is approved for use in preventing pregnancy and, therefore, is contraindicated. If pregnancy occurs, the data, though limited, do not show an increased risk for major birth anomalies.

BREASTFEEDING SUMMARY

Ulipristal and its active metabolite were found in human breast milk. Breast milk levels were sampled in 12 lactating women after administration of ulipristal. Mean breast milk ulipristal and active metabolite levels were highest in the first 24 hours (22.7 and 4.49 ng/mL, respectively) and decreased each sampled day. On day 5, levels were 0.69 and 0.10 ng/mL for ulipristal and the active metabolite, respectively. It is estimated that 4.1 mcg/kg of ulipristal and active metabolite would be present in breast milk on day 1, and total administration over 5 days would be 5.2 mcg/kg in a fully breastfed child. The manufacturer estimates that the relative infant dose is about 0.8% for both ulipristal and the active metabolite on day 1 of drug administration and is about 1% over 5 days after administration. No information is available about effects on breast milk production or the breastfed child. The manufacturer recommends that the developmental and health benefits of breastfeeding should be considered along with the mother's clinical need for ulipristal versus any potential adverse effects that might be seen in a breastfed infant. If used while breastfeeding, the infant should be monitored for the most common reported adult side effects of headache, abdominal pain, dizziness, and nausea (all leading to irritability) and fatigue (lethargy).

References

1. Prescribing Information. Ella. HRA Pharma America, Inc; 2023.
2. Hrgovic Z, Habek D, Cerkez Habek J. Spontaneous pregnancy during ulipristal treatment of giant uterine leiomyoma. *J Clin Pharm Ther*. 2018;43: 121-123.
3. De Gasperis-Brigante C, Singh SS, Vilos G, et al. Pregnancy outcomes following ulipristal acetate for uterine fibroids: a systematic review. *J Obstet Gynaecol Can*. 2018;40:1066-1076.
4. Wagner JK, Dathe K, Schaefer C, Hoeltzenbein M. Ulipristal acetate and pregnancy outcome-an observational study. *Hum Reprod*. 2020;35:751-758.

UMBRALISIB

Antineoplastic (Phosphatidylinositol 3-Kinase Inhibitor)

PREGNANCY RECOMMENDATION: No Human Data—Animal Data Suggest Risk

BREASTFEEDING RECOMMENDATION: Potential Toxicity

PREGNANCY SUMMARY

No reports describing the use of umbralisib in human pregnancy have been located. It is likely that some amount of the drug will cross the placenta, so fetal exposure will probably occur. Therefore, the absence of human pregnancy experience prevents a complete assessment of the embryofetal risk. In animal studies, embryofetal toxicity with malformations was observed in one species at doses about equal to the RHD. In a second species, there was embryofetal toxicity and maternal toxicity, but the doses were well below the RHD. Based on the animal studies and the drug's mechanism of action, the manufacturer recommends that women with reproductive potential use effective contraception during treatment and for 1 month after the last dose. They also recommend that males with female partners of reproductive potential use effective contraception during treatment and for 1 month after the last dose. Nevertheless, using this drug during pregnancy should be based on the pros and cons of the mother's clinical need for treatment versus any potential fetal risk that might occur from exposure. There is a registry for women who are pregnant and have cancer. For more information, women and health care providers are encouraged to contact the Cancer and Pregnancy Registry at 1-877-635-4499.

BREASTFEEDING SUMMARY

No reports describing the use of umbralisib during human lactation have been located. It is likely that some amount of the drug will be excreted into breast milk, so infant exposure will probably occur. Based on the potential for serious adverse effects that might be seen in a breastfed infant, the manufacturer recommends that women not breastfeed while taking umbralisib and for one month after the last dose. Nevertheless, if the clinical decision is to use this drug while breastfeeding, the infant should be monitored for the most common reported adult side effects of nausea, musculoskeletal pain and abdominal pain (all leading to irritability), decreased appetite (monitor growth), rash, diarrhea, lethargy, upper respiratory tract infection, vomiting, and various laboratory abnormalities (see Prescribing Information [PI]).

Reference

1. Prescribing Information. Ukoniq. TG Therapeutics; 2021.

UMECLIDINIUM AND VILANTEROL INHALATION POWDER

Autonomic (Anticholinergic/β-2 Agonist)

PREGNANCY RECOMMENDATION: No Human Data—Animal Data Suggest Low Risk

BREASTFEEDING RECOMMENDATION: Probably Compatible

PREGNANCY SUMMARY

No reports describing the use of umeclidinium and vilanterol in human pregnancy have been located. Some amount of both drugs will probably cross the placenta, so fetal exposure will likely occur. However, the absence of human pregnancy experience prevents a complete assessment of the embryofetal risk. Animal studies did not show any embryofetal toxicity. Therefore, using this drug during pregnancy should be based on the pros and cons of the mother's clinical need for treatment versus any potential fetal risk that might occur from exposure. β-2-Adrenergic stimulation can decrease uterine contractions.

BREASTFEEDING SUMMARY

No reports describing the use of umeclidinium and vilanterol during human lactation have been located. Some amount of both drugs will probably be found in breast milk. Breastfeeding while using this drug should be based on the mother's clinical need for treatment. If used, the infant should be monitored for the most common reported adult side effects of neck pain, muscle pain, and extremity pain (all leading to irritability), upper and lower respiratory tract infections, constipation, and diarrhea.

Reference

1. Prescribing Information. Anoro Ellipta. GlaxoSmithKline; 2018.

U

UNDECYLENIC ACID

Anti-Infective (Antifungal—Topical)

PREGNANCY RECOMMENDATION: No Human Data and No Relevant Animal Data

BREASTFEEDING RECOMMENDATION: Probably Compatible

PREGNANCY SUMMARY

No reports describing the use of undecylenic acid in human pregnancy have been located. If systemic absorption occurs after topical administration, the drug is likely to cross the placenta. No studies have been located to determine the level of systemic absorption. Animal reproduction studies have not been conducted. Therefore, the absence of human pregnancy experience prevents a complete assessment of embryofetal risk. Using this drug during pregnancy should be based on the pros and cons of the mother's clinical need for treatment versus any potential fetal risk that might occur from exposure.

BREASTFEEDING SUMMARY

No reports describing the use of undecylenic acid during human lactation have been located. If systemic absorption occurs after topical administration, the drug may be found in breast milk, so infant exposure would be possible. Because studies evaluating whether the drug is absorbed into the bloodstream following topical use were not located, systemic adverse reactions have not been evaluated. Breastfeeding while using this drug should be based on the mother's clinical need for treatment versus any potential infant risks that might occur. However, no adverse events were noted when compared to placebo in adults.

References

1. Prescribing Information. Undecylenic Acid. Oakhurst Pharmaceuticals; 2023.
2. Chretien JH, Esswein JG, Sharpe LM, et al. Efficacy of undecylenic acid-zinc undecylenate powder in culture positive tinea pedis. *Int J Dermatol*. 1980; 19:51-54.

UPADACITINIB

Immunologic (Janus Kinase Inhibitor)

PREGNANCY RECOMMENDATION: No Human Data—Animal Data Suggest Risk

BREASTFEEDING RECOMMENDATION: Potential Toxicity

PREGNANCY SUMMARY

No reports describing the use of upadacitinib in human pregnancy have been located. The drug will likely cross the placenta, so some fetal exposure will probably occur. Therefore, the absence of human pregnancy experience prevents a complete assessment of embryofetal risk. In animal studies, embryofetal toxicity with malformations was observed in two species at doses of less than 10 times the RHD. Based on animal studies and the drug's mechanism of action, the manufacturer recommends that women with reproductive potential use effective contraception during treatment and for 4 weeks after the last dose. Nevertheless, using this drug during pregnancy should be based on the pros and cons of the mother's clinical need for treatment versus any potential fetal risk that might occur from exposure. Pregnancies in women with rheumatoid arthritis, especially if uncontrolled, are associated with increased risks for adverse pregnancy outcomes. There is a pregnancy exposure registry that monitors pregnancy outcomes in patients using this drug during gestation. Health care providers are encouraged to call AbbVie at 800-633-9110.

BREASTFEEDING SUMMARY

No reports describing the use of upadacitinib during human lactation have been located. The drug will probably be found in breast milk, so some infant exposure will likely occur. Due to the potential for serious adverse effects that might be seen in a nursing infant, the manufacturer recommends that patients not breastfeed while taking upadacitinib and for 6 days (approximately 10 half-lives) after the last dose. Nevertheless, breastfeeding while using this drug should be based on the mother's clinical need for treatment versus any potential infant risks that might occur. If used, the infant should be monitored for the most common reported adult side effects of nausea, headache, abdominal pain, and myalgia (all leading to irritability), upper respiratory tract infections, rash, cough, pyrexia, fatigue (lethargy), and various laboratory abnormalities (see PI).

Reference

1. Prescribing Information. Rinvoq. AbbVie, Inc; 2023.

U

UREA

Urinary/Dermatologic/Diagnostic

PREGNANCY RECOMMENDATION: No Human Data and No Relevant Animal Data

BREASTFEEDING RECOMMENDATION: Probably Compatible

PREGNANCY SUMMARY

No reports describing the use of urea in human pregnancy have been located. Urea will probably cross the placenta, so some fetal exposure will likely occur. Animal data for topical use did not show any embryofetal toxicity, but specifics were not provided. No animal reproduction studies were located for the oral uses. Therefore, the absence of human pregnancy experience prevents a complete assessment of embryofetal risk. Using this drug during pregnancy should be based on the pros and cons of the mother's clinical need for treatment versus any potential fetal risk that might occur from exposure.

BREASTFEEDING SUMMARY

No reports describing the use of urea during human lactation have been located. The drug will likely be excreted into breast milk, so some infant exposure will probably occur. Breastfeeding while using this drug should be based on the mother's clinical need for treatment versus any potential infant risks that might occur. If used, the infant should be monitored for the most common reported adult side effects of nausea (leading to irritability) and hypernatremia.

References

1. Prescribing Information. CEM-UREA. PruGen, Inc; 2017.
2. Prescribing Information. Pytest. Avent, Inc; 2022.

URIDINE TRIACETATE

Genetic

PREGNANCY RECOMMENDATION: No Human Data—Animal Data Suggest Low Risk

BREASTFEEDING RECOMMENDATION: Probably Compatible

PREGNANCY SUMMARY

No reports describing the use of uridine triacetate in human pregnancy have been located. The drug will probably cross the placenta, so some fetal exposure will likely occur. Therefore, the absence of human pregnancy experience prevents a complete assessment of the embryofetal risk. Animal data did not show any embryofetal toxicity in one species at doses of less than 10 times the RHD. Using this drug during pregnancy should be based on the pros and cons of the mother's clinical need for treatment versus any potential fetal risk that might occur from exposure.

BREASTFEEDING SUMMARY

No reports describing the use of uridine triacetate during human lactation have been located. Some amount of the drug will probably be found in breast milk, so some infant exposure will likely occur. Breastfeeding while using this drug should be based on the mother's clinical need for treatment. If used, the infant should be monitored for the most common reported adult side effects of nausea (leading to irritability), vomiting, and diarrhea.

Reference

1. Prescribing Information. Xuriden. Wellstat Therapeutics Corporation; 2018.

URSODIOL

Gastrointestinal (Gallstone Dissolution Agent)

PREGNANCY RECOMMENDATION: Compatible (Second and Third Trimesters)

BREASTFEEDING RECOMMENDATION: Probably Compatible

U

PREGNANCY SUMMARY

Two systematic reviews and meta-analyses evaluated ursodiol during the second half of pregnancy in over 5,000 women. No adverse events were observed with ursodiol treatment. In the analysis of the randomized controlled trials of one article, ursodiol reduced the risk for the composite outcome of preterm birth and stillbirth. During the clinical trials, inadvertent exposure during the first trimester to therapeutic doses of ursodiol occurred in four women. No effect on their fetuses or newborns was found. Ursodiol may cross the placenta, but the amount is thought to be negligible. Animal studies did not show any embryofetal toxicity in two species at doses of 5 and 100 times the RHD. Therefore, the absence of first-trimester human pregnancy experience prevents a complete assessment of this embryofetal risk. Using this drug during pregnancy should be based on the pros and cons of the mother's clinical need for treatment versus any potential fetal risk that might occur from exposure. The Society of Maternal Fetal Medicine consult series states that intrahepatic cholestasis of pregnancy increases the risk for preterm delivery, meconium-stained amniotic fluid, and intrauterine fetal demise and recommends first-line treatment with ursodeoxycholic acid for the treatment of maternal symptoms.

BREASTFEEDING SUMMARY

Three publications described the use of ursodiol during human lactation in 28 women. Based on an average breast milk consumption of 1000 mL/d, the authors estimated that the daily intake of ursodiol for a breastfeeding infant is about 27 mcg. In full-term infants, the total bile acid pool is approximately 60 mg, and the estimated daily intake of ursodiol from breast milk is about 0.0005% of the total newborn bile acid pool. Neither adverse events in the early infant period nor abnormal development was observed up to age 1. However, the manufacturer recommends exercising caution when ursodiol is administered to a breastfeeding mother. If used while breastfeeding, the infant should be monitored for the most common reported adult side effects of headache, nausea, and abdominal pain (all leading to irritability), diarrhea, and constipation.

References

1. Prescribing Information. Ursodiol. Amneal Pharmaceuticals NY LLC; 2023.
2. Society for Maternal-Fetal Medicine Consult Series #53: Intrahepatic cholestasis of pregnancy. Am J Obstet Gynecol. 2021 Feb;224(2):B2-B9.
3. Bachrach WH, Hofmann AF. Ursodeoxycholic acid in the treatment of cholesterol cholelithiasis. Part I. *Dig Dis Sci*. 1982;27:737-761.
4. Walker KF, Chappell LC, Hague WM, et al. Pharmacological interventions for treating intrahepatic cholestasis of pregnancy. *Cochrane Database Syst Rev*. 2020;7:CD000493.
5. Ovadia C, Sajous J, Seed JT, et al. Ursodeoxycholic acid in intrahepatic cholestasis of pregnancy: a systematic review and individual participant data meta-analysis. *Lancet Gastroenterol Hepatol*. 2021;6:547-558.
6. Melo D, Areia AL, Moura P. Primary biliary cholangitis first demonstrated in pregnancy: a case report. *J Med Case Rep*. 2022;16:38.
7. Brites D, Rodrigues CMP. Elevated levels of bile acids in colostrum of patients with cholestasis of pregnancy are decreased following ursodeoxycholic acid therapy. *J Hepatol*. 1998;29:743-751.
8. Vitek L, Zelenkova M, Bruha R. Safe use of ursodeoxycholic acid in a breast-feeding patient with primary biliary cirrhosis. *Dig Liver Dis*. 2010;42:911-912.
9. Simjak P, Petr T, Kaslova B, et al. Ursodeoxycholic acid use in lactation female patients is associated with clinically negligible concentrations of this bile acid in breast milk. *Nature*. 2022;12:19543.

USTEKINUMAB

Immunologic (IL-12/IL-23 Antagonist—Monoclonal Antibody)

PREGNANCY RECOMMENDATION: Human Data Suggest Low Risk

BREASTFEEDING RECOMMENDATION: Probably Compatible

PREGNANCY SUMMARY

Several studies were located that combined a total of more than 800 women exposed to ustekinumab during human pregnancy, most often for inflammatory bowel disease. Exposures included preconception, early pregnancy, entire pregnancy, and third trimester. It did not appear to increase the risk for fetal malformations. Ustekinumab crosses the placenta at term and has higher levels in the cord blood compared to maternal serum. Animal studies did not show any embryofetal toxicity in one species at doses of 100 times the RHD. Using this drug during pregnancy should be based on the pros and cons of the mother's clinical need for treatment versus any potential fetal risk that might occur from exposure. There is a pregnancy exposure registry that monitors pregnancy outcomes in women exposed to ustekinumab during pregnancy. Health care providers and patients are encouraged to contact MotherToBaby at 877-311-8972.

BREASTFEEDING SUMMARY

There are four reports describing 13 women using ustekinumab during breastfeeding. As expected, ustekinumab (being an IgG1 antibody) was found in breast milk. However, IgG antibodies found in human breast milk are not found in the neonatal or infant circulation. Additionally, if any IgG antibodies were to be ingested through breastfeeding, they would probably be digested in the infant's gastrointestinal tract and not be absorbed. The manufacturer recommends that the developmental and health benefits of breastfeeding be considered along with the mother's clinical need for ustekinumab versus any potential adverse effects that might be seen in a breastfed infant. If used while breastfeeding, the infant should be monitored for the most common reported adult side effects of headache, pruritus, abdominal pain, and nausea (all leading to irritability), fatigue (lethargy), upper respiratory tract infection and other infections, vomiting, fever, and diarrhea.

References

1. Prescribing Information. Stelara. Janssen Biotech, Inc; 2022.
2. Klenske E, Osaba L, Nagore D, et al. Drug levels in the maternal serum, cord blood and breast milk of ustekinumab-treated patient with Crohn's disease. *J Crohns Col*. 2019;13:267-269.
3. Mitrova K, Pipek B, Bortlik M, et al. Safety of ustekinumab and vedolizumab during p regnancy—pregnancy, neonatal, and infant outcome: a prospective multicentre study. *J Crohns Colitis*. 2022;16:1808-1815.
4. Galluzo M, D'Adamio S, Bianchi L, Talamonti M. Psoriasis in pregnancy: case series and literature review of data concerning exposure during pregnancy to ustekinumab. *J Dermatol Treat*. 2019;30:40-44.
5. Wils P, Seksik P, Stefanescu C, et al. Safety of ustekinumab or vedolizumab in pregnant inflammatory bowel disease patients: a multicentre cohort study. *Aliment Pharmacol Ther*. 2020;53:460-470.
6. Ghalandari N, Crijns HJMJ, Bergman EJH, et al. Reported congenital malformations after exposure to non-tumor necrosis factor inhibitor biologics: a retrospective comparative study n EudraVigilance. *Br J Clin Pharmacol*. 2022;88:5378-5388.
7. Honap S, Meade S, Ibraheim H, et al. Effectiveness and safety of ustekinumab in inflammatory bowel disease: a systematic review and meta-analysis. *Dig Dis Sci*. 2022;67:1018-1035.
8. Avni-Biron I, Mishael T, Zittan E, et al. Ustekinumab during pregnancy in patients with inflammatory bowel disease: a prospective multicentre cohort study. *Aliment Pharmacol Ther*. 2022;56:1361-1369.
9. Dernoncourt A, Liabeuf S, Bennis Y, et al. Fetal and neonatal adverse drug reactions associated with biologics taken during pregnancy by women with autoimmune diseases: insights from an analysis of the World Health Organization pharmacovigilance database (Vigibase). *BioDrugs*. 2023;37:73-87.
10. Sanchez-Garcia V, Hernandez-Quiles R, de-Miguel-Balsa E, et al. Exposure to biologic therapy before and during pregnancy in patients with psoriasis: systematic review and meta-analysis. *J Eur Acad Dermatol Venererol*. 2023;37:1971-1990.
11. Skejo C, Thim S, Sellmer An, Julsgaard M. Early onset sepsis and lobar pneumonia in a newborn exposed in utero to ustekinumab and azathioprine. *Inflamm Bowel Dis*. 2024;30:314-315.
12. Lund T, Thomsen SF. Use of TNF-inhibitors and ustekinumab for psoriasis during pregnancy: a patient series. *Dermatol Ther*. 2017;30.
13. Matro R, Martin CF, Wolf D, et al. Exposure concentrations of infants breastfed by women receiving biologic therapies for inflammatory bowel diseases and effects of breastfeeding on infections and development. *Gastroenterol*. 2018;155:696-704.
14. Mugheddu C, Atzori L, Lappi A, et al. Biologics exposure during pregnancy and breastfeeding in a psoriasis patient. *Dermatol Ther*. 2019;32:e12895.

V

VACCINE, ADENOVIRUS TYPE 4 AND TYPE 7, LIVE

Vaccine (Live Vaccine)

PREGNANCY RECOMMENDATION: *Contraindicated

BREASTFEEDING RECOMMENDATION: Potential Toxicity

PREGNANCY SUMMARY

No apparent embryo or fetal harm was observed in four pregnancies inadvertently exposed to the vaccine at an estimated 21 weeks preconception or 2 to 13 days after conception. *However, because naturally occurring infections with adenoviruses have been associated with fetal harm, this live vaccine is contraindicated in pregnancy. Animal reproduction studies have not been conducted. However, this limited human pregnancy experience prevents a complete assessment of embryofetal risk. Using this drug during pregnancy should be based on the pros and cons of the mother's clinical need for treatment versus any potential fetal risk that might occur from exposure. Women with reproductive potential who are taking this vaccine are advised to use effective contraception for 6 weeks after the last dose. Because viral shedding lasts 28 days, persons receiving the vaccine should exercise caution when in close contact with pregnant women during this time period.

BREASTFEEDING SUMMARY

No reports describing exposure to this vaccine during lactation have been located. This live, nonattenuated virus can be shed in the stool over 28 days postinoculation. Close contacts of those vaccinated may be exposed to the virus and theoretically could develop an infection. The potential for a febrile respiratory disease in a nursing infant from exposure is unknown. Therefore, the safest course is to avoid the vaccine during breastfeeding and for at least 28 days after vaccination. If the clinical decision is to use this drug while breastfeeding, the infant should be monitored for the most common reported adult side effects of headache, throat pain, arthralgia, nausea, and abdominal pain (all leading to irritability), upper respiratory tract infections, nasal congestion, cough, diarrhea, and vomiting.

References

1. Product information. Adenovirus type 4 and type 7 vaccine, live. Teva Pharmaceuticals; 2022.
2. Towbin JA, Griffin LD, Martin AB, et al. Intrauterine adenoviral myocarditis presenting as nonimmune hydrops fetalis: diagnosis by polymerase chain reaction. *Pediatr Infect Dis J*. 1994;13:144-150.
3. Forsnes EV, Eggleston MK, Wax JR. Differential transmission of adenovirus in a twin pregnancy. *Obstet Gynecol*. 1998;91:817-818.

VACCINE, ANTHRAX

Vaccine (Inactivated Vaccine)

PREGNANCY RECOMMENDATION: No Human Data and No Relevant Animal Data

BREASTFEEDING RECOMMENDATION: Probably Compatible

PREGNANCY SUMMARY

There are two formulations of the anthrax vaccine available in the United States: anthrax vaccine adsorbed (AVA) and anthrax vaccine adsorbed, adjuvanted (AVA-adjuvanted). Although animal reproduction studies with the anthrax vaccine have not been conducted, there appears to be no plausible biological mechanism for adverse pregnancy effects. The human reproduction data, limited to vaccination before conception, do not appear to suggest a risk from vaccination to either a woman's subsequent fertility or a subsequent pregnancy outcome. According to the US Centers for Disease Control and Prevention (CDC) guidelines for vaccinating pregnant women, preexposure administration of the vaccine, when the risk for exposure to aerosolized *Bacillus anthracis* spores is presumably low, is not recommended and should be delayed until after pregnancy. For postexposure and when the risk for exposure to aerosolized *B. anthracis* is high, pregnancy is not a contraindication.

(continued)

The vaccine and 60 days of antimicrobial therapy should be used if a woman is at risk of exposure. Because of the limited human pregnancy experience, routine use of this vaccine during gestation is not recommended. Using this vaccine during pregnancy should be based on the pros and cons of the mother's clinical need for treatment versus any potential fetal risk that might occur from exposure. If exposure to AVA or AVA-adjuvanted occurs during pregnancy, health care professionals are encouraged to contact the BioThrax Vaccine in Pregnancy Registry at 619-553-9255.

BREASTFEEDING SUMMARY

No reports describing the use of anthrax vaccine in lactating women have been located. It is not known if the vaccine antigen or the antibodies induced by the vaccine are excreted into human breast milk. Because of the nature of the anthrax vaccine, the potential for adverse effects in a nursing infant appears to be negligible. The CDC states that the anthrax vaccine is safe for use during lactation. If the clinical decision is to use this vaccine while breastfeeding, the infant should be monitored for the most common reported adult side effects not related to injection site reactions, including muscle aches and headache (both leading to irritability) and fatigue (lethargy).

References

1. Product information. Biothrax-bacillus anthracis injection, suspension. Emergent BioDefense Operations Lansing, LLC; 2015.
2. Product information. Cyfendus. Emergent Product Development Gaithersburg, Inc; 2023.
3. Centers for Disease Control and Prevention. Use of anthrax vaccine in the United States: recommendations of the Advisory Committee on Immunization Practices, 2019. *MMWR Recomm Rep*. 2019;68(No. RR-4):1-14.
4. Centers for Disease Control and Prevention. Guidelines for vaccinating pregnant women. Accessed July 31, 2023. https://www.cdc.gov/vaccines/pregnancy/hcp-toolkit/guidelines.html
5. Wiesen AR, Little CT. Relationship between prepregnancy anthrax vaccination and pregnancy and birth outcomes among US Army women. *JAMA*. 2002;287:1556-1560.
6. Conlin AMS, Bukowinski AT, Gumbs GR; for the Department of Defense Birth and Infant Health Registry Team. Analysis of pregnancy and infant health outcomes among women in the national smallpox vaccine in pregnancy registry who received anthrax vaccine adsorbed. *Vaccine*. 2015;33:4387-4390.
7. Conlin AMS, Sevick CJ, Gumbs GR, et al. Safety of inadvertent anthrax vaccination during pregnancy: an analysis of birth defects in the U.S. military population, 2003-2010. *Vaccine*. 2017;35:4414-4420.
8. Centers for Disease Control and Prevention. Notice to readers: status of U.S. Department of defense preliminary evaluation of the association of anthrax vaccination and congenital anomalies. *MMWR Morb Mortal Wkly Rep*. 2002;51:127.
9. Centers for Disease Control and Prevention. Vaccinations: vaccination safety for breastfeeding mothers. Accessed April 7, 2024. https://www.cdc.gov/breastfeeding/breastfeeding-special-circumstances/vaccinations-medications-drugs/vaccinations.html

VACCINE, BCG

Vaccine (Live Vaccine)

PREGNANCY RECOMMENDATION: *Contraindicated

BREASTFEEDING RECOMMENDATION: Potential Toxicity

PREGNANCY SUMMARY

The BCG vaccine is a live, attenuated bacterial vaccine used to provide immunity to tuberculosis in persons not previously infected with *Mycobacterium tuberculosis* who are at high risk for exposure. It is not known if the vaccine antigen crosses the placenta. No animal reproduction studies have been located. The risk to the fetus from maternal vaccination is unknown. Therefore, the absence of human pregnancy experience prevents a complete assessment of embryofetal risk. *Because it is a live preparation, the CDC and manufacturer recommend that it not be used in pregnancy.

BREASTFEEDING SUMMARY

One case report describing the use of the BCG vaccine in human lactation was located. A woman was diagnosed with pT1 urothelial carcinoma at 2 months postpartum. She decided to treat this with intravesical BCG therapy while breastfeeding. She was determined to breastfeed while receiving this treatment. The infant received the BCG vaccine 2 weeks prior to the mother's treatment. The pediatrician advised holding breastfeeding during the first 24 hours after administration; however, the patient resumed breastfeeding that evening due to extreme breast tenderness. She continued to breastfeed successfully through the six courses of induction therapy and the first 3 weeks of weekly maintenance therapy. No adverse events were reported with the mother or infant. Breastfeeding while using this drug should be based on the mother's clinical need for treatment. If used, the infant should be monitored for adverse events; however, the most common reported adult side effect is injection site reaction.

V

References

1. Product information. BCG vaccine. Merck Sharp & Dohme, LLC; 2023.
2. Centers for Disease Control and Prevention. Guidelines for vaccinating pregnant women. Accessed July 31, 2023. https://www.cdc.gov/vaccines/pregnancy/hcp-toolkit/guidelines.html
3. Barbur E, Doganca T, Obek C. Safe use of intravesical bacillus Calmette-Guerin immunotherapy for bladder cancer during breastfeeding: a case report. *Immunotherapy*. 2022;14:759-764.

VACCINE, CHOLERA

Vaccine (Live Vaccine)

PREGNANCY RECOMMENDATION: Human Data Suggest Low Risk

BREASTFEEDING RECOMMENDATION: Probably Compatible

PREGNANCY SUMMARY

Cholera infection during pregnancy may result in significant morbidity and mortality to the mother and the fetus, particularly during the third trimester. Only one cholera vaccine is available in the United States, but other products are available globally. It is given orally but is not absorbed systemically. After vaccination, the vaccine strain may be shed in the stool for at least 7 days and has potential for transmission of the vaccine strain to the infant during vaginal delivery. In 2022, the CDC stated that no data are available for the cholera vaccine currently licensed in the United States, and travelers should consider the risks of traveling to locations with active cholera infections. In 2017, the World Health Organization (WHO) stated that the available data for the cholera vaccine suggest that it is safe for use in pregnancy. No difference in birth defects, spontaneous abortion, intrauterine fetal demise, and low birth weight was observed between those who received the vaccine and those who did not in the six published trials.

BREASTFEEDING SUMMARY

Maternal vaccination with cholera vaccine has increased specific immunoglobulin A (IgA) antibody titers in human breast milk. In a second study, cholera vaccine (whole cell plus toxoid) was administered to six lactating mothers, resulting in a significant rise in breast milk anticholera toxin IgA titers in five of the patients. Breast milk from three of these five mothers also had a significant increase in anticholera toxin immunoglobulin G (IgG) titers. Since the vaccine is not systemically absorbed, exposure to the vaccine through breast milk is not expected.

References

1. Product information. Vaxchora. Emergent Travel Health, Inc; 2023.
2. Collins JP, Ryan ET, Wong KK, et al. Cholera vaccine: recommendations of the advisory committee on immunization practices, 2022. *MMWR Recomm Rep*. 2022;71:1-8. https://www.cdc.gov/mmwr/volumes/71/rr/rr7102a1.htm
3. World Health Organization. Cholera vaccines: WHO position paper—August 2017. Accessed April 7, 2024. https://apps.who.int/iris/bitstream/handle/10665/258764/WER9234-477-498.pdf?sequence=1
4. Hashim R, Khatib AM, Enwere G, et al. Safety of the recombinant cholera toxin B subunit, killed whole-cell (rBS-WC) oral cholera vaccine in pregnancy. *PLoS Negl Trop Dis*. 2012;6:e1743.
5. Khan AI, Chowdhury F, Leung DT, L, et al. Cholera in pregnancy: clinical and immunological aspects. *Int J Infect Dis*. 2015;39:20-24.
6. Merson MH, Black RE, Sack DA, et al. Maternal cholera immunisation and secretory IgA in breast milk. *Lancet*. 1980;1:931-932.
7. Ali M, Nelson A, Luquero FJ, et al. Safety of a killed oral cholera vaccine (Shanchol) in pregnant women in Malawi: an observational cohort study. *Lancet Infect Dis*. 2017;17:538-544.
8. Khan AI, Ali M, Chowdhury F, et al. Safety of the oral cholera vaccine in pregnancy: retrospective findings from a subgroup following mass vaccination campaign in Dhaka, Bangladesh. *Vaccine*. 2017;35:1538-1543.
9. Zhang Y, Zhang H, Wang B, et al. Pregnancy outcomes after a mass vaccination campaign with an oral cholera vaccine: a systematic review and meta-analysis. *BJOG*. 2020;127:1066-1073.
10. Grout L, Martinez-Pino I, Ciglenecki I, et al. Pregnancy outcomes after a mass vaccination campaign with an oral cholera vaccine in Guinea: a retrospective cohort study. *PLoS Negl Trop Dis*. 2015;9:e0004274.
11. Svennerholm AM, Holmgren J, Hanson LA, et al. Boosting of secretory IgA antibody responses in man by parenteral cholera vaccination. *Scand J Immunol*. 1977;6:134549.

VACCINE, HAEMOPHILUS B CONJUGATE

Vaccine (Inactive Vaccine)

PREGNANCY RECOMMENDATION: Limited Human Data and No Relevant Animal Data

BREASTFEEDING RECOMMENDATION: Probably Compatible

PREGNANCY SUMMARY

Commercially available *Haemophilus* B conjugate vaccine is a combination of the capsular polysaccharides purified from *Haemophilus influenzae* type B bound with various proteins, including tetanus toxoid and meningococcal protein. It is a non-live vaccine. The human pregnancy experience is limited to third-trimester exposures in 151 women and did not reveal adverse effects. The vaccine is probably compatible for use in pregnancy. No animal reproduction studies have been located. However, this limited first-trimester human pregnancy experience prevents a complete assessment of the embryofetal risk. Using this drug during pregnancy should be based on the pros and cons of the mother's clinical need for treatment versus any potential fetal risk that might occur from exposure.

BREASTFEEDING SUMMARY

Women who were vaccinated with *Haemophilus* B conjugate vaccine at 34 to 36 weeks' gestation had significantly higher antibody titers (>20 times) in their colostrum than either nonimmunized women or those who were vaccinated before pregnancy. Breast milk antibody titers were also significantly higher (>20 times) than the comparison groups at 3 and 6 months after delivery. It is not known if the vaccine antigen or the antibodies induced by the vaccine are excreted into human breast milk. According to the Advisory Committee on Immunization Practices (ACIP) general best practice guidelines for immunizations in special situations, administering live or non-live vaccines (except smallpox and yellow fever vaccines) does not affect the safety of breastfeeding for women or their infants. Additionally, the CDC states that this vaccine is safe for use during lactation.

References

1. Briere EC, Rubin L, Moro PL, et al. Prevention and control of *Haemophilus influenza* type b disease: recommendations of the Advisory Committee on Immunization Practices (ACIP). *MMWR Recomm Rep*. 2014;63:1-14.
2. Product information. ActHib. Sanofi Pasteur, Inc; 2023.
3. Product information. Hiberex. GlaxoSmithKline Biologics SA; 2023.
4. Product information. PedvaxHib. Merck Sharp & Dohme, LLC; 2023.
5. Glezen WP, Englund JA, Siber GR, et al. Maternal immunization with the capsular polysaccharide vaccine for *Haemophilus influenzae* type b. *J Infect Dis*. 1992;165(suppl 1):S134-S136.
6. Amstey MS, Insel R, Munoz J, et al. Fetal-neonatal passive immunization against *Hemophilus influenzae*, type b. *Am J Obstet Gynecol*. 1985;153:607-611.
7. Linder N, Ohel G. In utero vaccination. *Clin Perinatol*. 1994;21:663-674.
8. Insel RA, Amstey M, Pichichero ME. Postimmunization antibody to the *Haemophilus influenzae* type B capsule in breast milk. *J Infect Dis*. 1985;152:407-408.
9. Centers for Disease Control and Prevention. Vaccinations. Vaccination safety for breastfeeding mothers. Accessed April 7, 2024. https://www.cdc.gov/breastfeeding/breastfeeding-special-circumstances/vaccinations-medications-drugs/vaccinations.html

VACCINE, HEPATITIS A

Vaccine (Inactive Vaccine)

PREGNANCY RECOMMENDATION: Human Data Suggest Low Risk

BREASTFEEDING RECOMMENDATION: Probably Compatible

PREGNANCY SUMMARY

Hepatitis A virus vaccine is an inactive, noninfectious vaccine. Several reports describing the use of the vaccine in over 1,400 pregnant humans have been located. Similar to other non-live vaccines, the risk to the fetus from maternal vaccination appears to be minimal. One report found an increased risk for small for gestational age birthweight with vaccine exposure in pregnancy. No animal reproduction studies have been conducted. The CDC considers the theoretical risk to the developing fetus to be low and recommends that hepatitis A vaccine should be administered to pregnant women who might be at risk for infection. Using this drug during pregnancy should be based on the pros and cons of the mother's clinical need for treatment versus any potential fetal risk that might occur from exposure.

BREASTFEEDING SUMMARY

No reports describing the use of hepatitis A vaccine during human lactation have been located. It is not known if the vaccine antigen or the antibodies induced by the vaccine are excreted into human breast milk. According to the ACIP general best practice guidelines for immunizations in special situations, administering live or non-live vaccines (except for smallpox and yellow fever vaccines) does not affect the safety of breastfeeding for women or their infants. Additionally, the CDC states that this vaccine is safe for use in lactation.

References

1. Product information. Havrix. GlaxoSmithKline Biologicals SA; 2023.
2. Product information. Vaqta. Merck Sharp & Dohme; 2023.
3. Centers for Disease Control and Prevention. Guidelines for vaccinating pregnant women. Accessed April 7, 2024. https://www.cdc.gov/vaccines/pregnancy/hcp-toolkit/guidelines.html
4. Moro PL, Museru OI, Niu M, et al. Reports to the vaccine adverse event reporting system after hepatitis A and hepatitis AB vaccines in pregnant women. *Am J Obstet Gynecol*. 2014;210:e1-e6.
5. Groom HC, Smith N, Irving SA, et al. Uptake and safety of hepatitis A vaccination during pregnancy: a vaccine safety datalink study. *Vaccine*. 2019;37:6648-6655.
6. Centers for Disease Control and Prevention. Vaccinations: vaccination safety for breastfeeding mothers. Accessed April 7, 2024. https://www.cdc.gov/breastfeeding/breastfeeding-special-circumstances/vaccinations-medications-drugs/vaccinations.html

VACCINE, HEPATITIS B RECOMBINANT

Vaccine (Inactive Vaccine)

PREGNANCY RECOMMENDATION: Human Data—Compatible Human Data Suggest Compatible

BREASTFEEDING RECOMMENDATION: Probably Compatible

PREGNANCY SUMMARY

There are two types of the inactive hepatitis B vaccine approved in the United States, a recombinant and recombinant adjuvanted (see Vaccine, Hepatitis B Recombinant Adjuvanted). From the published data on the hepatitis B recombinant vaccine during pregnancy, vaccination does not appear to increase any risk to the fetus. Additionally, the CDC states that if the woman has not been previously vaccinated with hepatitis B, the pregnant woman should be vaccinated during pregnancy since all adults 19 to 59 years old are recommended to receive this vaccine. No animal reproduction studies have been conducted. Using this vaccine during pregnancy should be based on the pros and cons of the mother's clinical need for treatment versus any potential fetal risk that might occur from exposure.

BREASTFEEDING SUMMARY

No reports describing the use of hepatitis B recombinant vaccine during human lactation have been located. It is not known if the vaccine antigen or the antibodies induced by the vaccine are excreted into human breast milk. According to the ACIP general best practice guidelines for immunizations in special situations, administering live or non-live vaccines (except smallpox and yellow fever vaccines) does not affect the safety of breastfeeding for women or their infants. Additionally, the CDC states that this vaccine is safe for use in lactation.

References

1. Product information. Engerix-B. GlaxoSmithKline Biologicals SA; 2023.
2. Product information. Recombivax HB. Merck Sharp & Dohme, LLC; 2023.
3. Product information. PreHevbrio. VBI Vaccines (Delaware), Inc; 2021.
4. Centers for Disease Control and Prevention. Guidelines for vaccinating pregnant women. Accessed April 7, 2024. https://www.cdc.gov/vaccines/pregnancy/hcp-toolkit/guidelines.html
5. Moro PL, Museru OI, Niu M, et al. Reports to the vaccine adverse event reporting system after hepatitis A and hepatitis AB vaccines in pregnant women. *Am J Obstet Gynecol*. 2014;210:e1-e6.
6. Moro PL, Zheteyeva Y, Barash F, et al. Assessing the safety of hepatitis B vaccination during pregnancy in the vaccine adverse event reporting system (VAERS), 1990-2016. *Vaccine*. 2018;36:50-54.
7. Groom HC, Irving SA, Koppolu P, et al. Uptake and safety of hepatitis B vaccination during pregnancy: a vaccine safety datalink study. *Vaccine*. 2018;36:6111-6116.
8. Centers for Disease Control and Prevention. Vaccinations: vaccination safety for breastfeeding mothers. Accessed April 7, 2024. https://www.cdc.gov/breastfeeding/breastfeeding-special-circumstances/vaccinations-medications-drugs/vaccinations.html

VACCINE, HEPATITIS B RECOMBINANT ADJUVANTED

Vaccine (Inactive Vaccine)

PREGNANCY RECOMMENDATION: No Human Data—Animal Data Suggest Low Risk

BREASTFEEDING RECOMMENDATION: Probably Compatible

PREGNANCY SUMMARY

There are two types of the inactive hepatitis B vaccine approved in the United States, a recombinant (see Vaccine, Hepatitis B Recombinant) and recombinant adjuvanted. No human data is available for the adjuvanted formulation. Animal studies did not show any embryofetal toxicity. The CDC states that if the woman has not been previously vaccinated with hepatitis B, the pregnant woman should be vaccinated during pregnancy, since all adults 19 to 59 years old are recommended to receive this vaccine. Therefore, this limited human pregnancy experience prevents a complete assessment of embryofetal risk. Women who have received Heplisav-B during pregnancy are encouraged to contact the Heplisav-B pregnancy registry at 844-443-7734.

BREASTFEEDING SUMMARY

No reports describing the use of hepatitis B recombinant adjuvanted vaccine during human lactation have been located. It is not known if the vaccine antigen or the antibodies induced by the vaccine are excreted into human breast milk. According to the ACIP general best practice guidelines for immunizations in special situations, administering live or non-live vaccine (except smallpox and yellow fever vaccines) does not affect the safety of breastfeeding for women or their infants. Additionally, the CDC states that this vaccine is safe for use in lactation.

References

1. Product information. Heplisav-B. Dynavax Technologies Corporation; 2024.
2. Centers for Disease Control and Prevention. Guidelines for vaccinating pregnant women. Accessed April 7, 2024. https://www.cdc.gov/vaccines/pregnancy/hcp-toolkit/guidelines.html
3. Centers for Disease Control and Prevention. Vaccinations: vaccination safety for breastfeeding mothers. Accessed April 7, 2024. https://www.cdc.gov/breastfeeding/breastfeeding-special-circumstances/vaccinations-medications-drugs/vaccinations.html

VACCINE, HUMAN PAPILLOMAVIRUS 9-VALENT, RECOMBINANT

Vaccine (Inactive Vaccine)

PREGNANCY RECOMMENDATION: *Limited Human Data—Animal Data Suggest Low Risk

BREASTFEEDING RECOMMENDATION: Probably Compatible

PREGNANCY SUMMARY

One report from the manufacturer for human papillomavirus 9-valent (HPV-9) vaccination during pregnancy found a spontaneous abortion rate of 27.4% in women that became pregnant within 30 days before or after receiving the HPV-9 vaccination. Animal data in one species receiving a single human dose did not show any embryofetal toxicity. However, the limited human pregnancy experience prevents a complete assessment of embryofetal risk. The manufacturer states that studies conducted with the previous version of the vaccine (HPV-4) are relevant to the 9-valent vaccine because it was manufactured by the same process and has overlapping compositions. The data describing human pregnancy experience with the HPV-4 vaccination supports the lack of toxicity for the embryo and/or fetus. Moreover, the vaccine is noninfectious and preservative- and antibiotic-free. However, *the CDC and the American College of Obstetricians and Gynecologists (ACOG) state that the vaccine is not recommended during pregnancy. If a woman becomes pregnant before completion of the two- or three-dose schedule, completion of the series should be delayed until the pregnancy is completed. If the vaccine is given during an ongoing pregnancy, patients are encouraged to enroll in the Gardasil 9 pregnancy registry at 800-986-8999.

BREASTFEEDING SUMMARY

It is not known if HPV antigens or antibodies induced by the vaccine are excreted into human breast milk. Five hundred nursing mothers were given the vaccine during clinical trials and compared with 495 women who received a placebo vaccine. The number of nursing infants experiencing a serious adverse experience was higher in mothers receiving the vaccine than in those receiving a placebo, 4.2% ($n = 21$) versus 2.0% ($n = 10$), respectively. However, none of the adverse experiences were judged to be related to the vaccine. In clinical studies, more nursing infants with acute respiratory illnesses were found in the group of mothers who had received the vaccine within 30 days ($n = 6$) than in the control group ($n = 2$). According to the ACIP general best practice guidelines for immunizations in special situations, administering live or non-live vaccines (except smallpox and yellow fever vaccines) does not affect the safety of breastfeeding for women or their infants. Additionally, the CDC states that this vaccine is safe for use in lactation.

References

1. Product information. Gardasil 9. Merck Sharp & Dohme, LLC; 2024.
2. American College of Obstetricians and Gynecologists. Human papillomavirus vaccination. Committee opinion no. 809. *Obstet Gynecol*. 2020;136:e15-e21.
3. Centers for Disease Control and Prevention. Guidelines for vaccinating pregnant women. Accessed April 7, 2024. https://www.cdc.gov/vaccines/pregnancy/hcp-toolkit/guidelines.html
4. Garland SM, Ault KA, Gall SA, et al. Pregnancy and infant outcomes in the clinical trials of a human papillomavirus type 6/11/16/18 vaccine—a combined analysis of five randomized controlled trials. *Obstet Gynecol*. 2009;114:1179-1188.
5. Smith-McCune K, Sawaya GF. Update on quadrivalent human papillomavirus vaccination and pregnancy outcomes. *Obstet Gynecol*. 2009;114:1168-1169.
6. Smith-McCune K. Quadrivalent HPV vaccine administered to women who became pregnant during trials did not appear to adversely affect pregnancy outcome; however, use during pregnancy is not recommended. *Evid Based Med*. 2010;15:80-81.
7. Scheller NM, Pasternak B, Molgaard-Nielsen D, et al. Quadrivalent HPV vaccination and the risk of adverse pregnancy outcomes. *N Engl J Med*. 2017;376:1223-1233.
8. Lipkind HS, Vazquez-Benitez G, Nordin JD, et al. Maternal and infant outcomes after human papillomavirus vaccination in the periconceptional period or during pregnancy. *Obstet Gynecol*. 2017;130:599-608.
9. Centers for Disease Control and Prevention. Vaccinations: vaccination safety for breastfeeding mothers. Accessed April 7, 2024. https://www.cdc.gov/breastfeeding/breastfeeding-special-circumstances/vaccinations-medications-drugs/vaccinations.html

VACCINE, INFLUENZA QUADRIVALENT NASAL SPRAY

Vaccine (Live Vaccine)

PREGNANCY RECOMMENDATION: Contraindicated

BREASTFEEDING RECOMMENDATION: Probably Compatible

The nasal spray influenza vaccine is available as a live, attenuated vaccine used to provide immunity to influenza. The vaccine is not systemically absorbed after nasal administration so placental transfer is not expected. *Because it is a live preparation, the CDC and manufacturer recommend that it not be used in pregnancy.

VACCINE, INFLUENZA INACTIVATED/RECOMBINANT

Vaccine (Inactive Vaccine)

PREGNANCY RECOMMENDATION: Human Data Suggest Compatible

BREASTFEEDING RECOMMENDATION: Compatible

PREGNANCY SUMMARY

Influenza quadrivalent vaccine is a non-live vaccine available as an inactivated or recombinant vaccine. The vaccine is considered compatible during all stages of pregnancy. Neonatal passive immunization of short duration has been documented in some studies. Animal data did not show embryofetal toxicity in one species receiving a human dose. Because of the cardiovascular and respiratory tract changes that occur during pregnancy, along with a decreased immune system, women are at a higher risk for severe illness and complications from influenza during pregnancy and the postpartum period compared to nonpregnant women. ACOG and the CDC recommend that the inactive or recombinant influenza vaccine be administered to women who are or will be pregnant during the flu season. However, the intranasal vaccine spray contains a live, attenuated virus and should not be used during pregnancy. There are pregnancy exposure registries that monitor pregnancy outcomes in women exposed to certain brands of the influenza vaccine during pregnancy:

BREASTFEEDING SUMMARY

One report describing the use of the influenza vaccine during human lactation has been located. A 2018 publication compared the safety and antibody response between the live, attenuated and inactivated influenza vaccines in breastfeeding women. Overall, 248 women and 249 infants were enrolled. The median age of the infants was 76 days. Irritability/fussiness occurred significantly more often in infants whose mothers received the live, attenuated vaccine compared to those mothers who received the inactivated vaccine (59.7% and 44.8%, respectively). Neither the vaccine nor wild-type influenza virus was found in breast milk. One infant was positive by polymerase chain reaction (PCR) nasal swab and cell culture for the influenza A vaccine strain on day 2 after the mother received the live, attenuated vaccine. The mother was negative for influenza by nasal PCR on day 2. Breast milk IgA response to H1N1 and IgG titers to all five strains was significantly higher in mothers who received the inactive vaccine compared to the live, attenuated vaccine. Similarly, maternal serum IgG antibody in all comparisons was significantly higher in the inactive vaccine group compared with the live, attenuated vaccine group. According to the ACIP general best practice guidelines for immunizations in special situations, administering live or non-live vaccines (except smallpox and yellow fever vaccines) does not affect the safety of breastfeeding for women or their infants. Additionally, the CDC states that the inactive and live, attenuated influenza vaccines are safe for use during lactation.

References

1. Product information. Afluria quadrivalent. Seqirus Pty. Ltd; 2023.
2. Product information. Flucelvax quadrivalent. Seqirus, Inc; 2023.
3. Product information. Fluarix quadrivalent. GlaxoSmithKline Biologicals SA; 2023.
4. Product information. Flublok quadrivalent Northern hemisphere. Sanofi Pasteur, Inc; 2023.
5. Centers for Disease Control and Prevention. Guidelines for vaccinating pregnant women. Accessed August 14, 2023. https://www.cdc.gov/vaccines/pregnancy/hcp-toolkit/guidelines.html
6. American College of Obstetricians and Gynecologists. Influenza vaccination during pregnancy. ACOG Committee Opinion No. 732. *Obstet Gynecol*. 2018;131:e109-e114.
7. Linder N, Ohel G. In utero vaccination. *Clin Perinatol*. 1994;21:663-674.
8. Centers for Disease Control and Prevention. Flu vaccine safety and pregnancy: questions and answers. Accessed April 7, 2024. https://www.cdc.gov/flu/highrisk/qa_vacpregnant.htm#:~:text=A%20Flu%20Vaccine%20is%20the,and%20the%20baby%20from%20flu
9. Omer SB, Clark DR, Madhi SA, et al. Efficacy, duration of protection, birth outcomes, and infant growth associated with influenza vaccination in pregnancy: a pooled analysis of three randomised controlled trials. *Lancet Respir Med*. 2020;8:597-608.
10. Munoz FM, Greisinger AJ, Wehmanen OA, et al. Safety of influenza vaccination during pregnancy. *Am J Obstet Gynecol*. 2005;192:1098-1106.
11. Ledlie S, Gandhi-Banga S, Shrestha A, et al. Exposure to quadrivalent influenza vaccine during pregnancy: results from a global pregnancy registry. *Influenza Other Respir Viruses*. 2022;16:90-100.
12. Nwoji U. Seasonal influenza vaccine exposure in pregnancy: 5-year results from a pregnancy registry. *Hum Vaccin Immunother*. 2022;18:e1932213.
13. Brady RC, Jackson LA, Frey SE, et al. Randomized trial comparing the safety and antibody responses to live attenuated versus inactivated influenza vaccine when administered to breastfeeding women. *Vaccine*. 2018;36:4663-4671.
14. Centers for Disease Control and Prevention. Vaccinations: vaccination safety for breastfeeding mothers. Accessed April 7, 2024. https://www.cdc.gov/breastfeeding/breastfeeding-special-circumstances/vaccinations-medications-drugs/vaccinations.html

VACCINE, MEASLES, MUMPS, AND RUBELLA

Vaccine (Live Vaccine)

PREGNANCY RECOMMENDATION: *Contraindicated

BREASTFEEDING RECOMMENDATION: Probably Compatible

PREGNANCY SUMMARY

*The measles, mumps, and rubella (MMR) vaccine is a live, attenuated virus vaccine that should not be administered during pregnancy. The rubella vaccine virus can cross the placenta and may result in an asymptomatic fetal infection. The mumps vaccine virus can also cross the placenta, but no malformations or fetal/infant disease has been observed. Lastly, the measles virus can infect the placenta and potentially lead to fetal harm. It is not known if the measles vaccine virus can infect the placenta. Human IgG antibodies are known to cross the placenta, especially during the third trimester, which suggests that some transfer of the MMR antibodies induced by the vaccine will likely occur. There have been 425 prospectively identified pregnancies with inadvertent MMR vaccine administration within 30 days prior to conception or during pregnancy. Of these, there were 16 malformations (3.8%), 4 fetal deaths (0.9%), and 50 spontaneous abortions (11.8%). No cases of congenital rubella syndrome have been identified. No animal reproduction studies have been conducted. Women with reproductive potential should avoid pregnancy for 28 days after vaccination per the manufacturer and CDC. Using this drug during pregnancy should be based on the pros and cons of the mother's clinical need for treatment versus any potential fetal risk that might occur from exposure.

BREASTFEEDING SUMMARY

No reports describing the use of the MMR vaccine during human lactation have been located. According to the ACIP general best practice guidelines for immunizations in special situations, administering live or non-live vaccines (except smallpox and yellow fever vaccines) does not affect the safety of breastfeeding for women or their infants. Additionally, the CDC states that the MMR vaccine is safe for use during lactation. The manufacturer reports that a previously available live vaccine that only contained rubella has been administered during lactation. The vaccine rubella virus may be found in breast milk and can be transmitted to infants. Some infants had serologic evidence of rubella virus vaccine strain antibodies. However, none exhibited severe disease. In only one case, a mild clinical illness typical of acquired rubella was observed.

References

1. Product information. M-M-R II. Merck Sharp & Dohme; 2023.
2. Centers for Disease Control and Prevention. Guidelines for vaccinating pregnant women. Accessed April 7, 2024. https://www.cdc.gov/vaccines/pregnancy/hcp-toolkit/guidelines.html
3. Centers for Disease Control and Prevention. Rubella vaccination during pregnancy—United States, 1971-1982. *MMWR Morb Mortal Wkly Rep*. 1983;32:429-432.
4. Burgess MA. Rubella reinfection—what risk to the fetus? *Med J Aust*. 1992;156:824-825.
5. Condon R, Bower, C. Congenital rubella after previous maternal vaccination. *Med J Aust*. 1992;156:882.
6. Centers for Disease Control and Prevention. Rubella vaccination during pregnancy—United States, 1971-1988. *MMWR Morb Mortal Wkly Rep*. 1989;38:289-293.
7. Preblud SR, Williams NM. Fetal risk associated with rubella vaccine: implications for vaccination of susceptible women. *Obstet Gynecol*. 1985;66:121-123.
8. Hofmann J, Kortung M, Pustowoit B, et al. Persistent fetal rubella vaccine virus infection following inadvertent vaccination during early pregnancy. *J Med Virol*. 2000;61:155-158.
9. Centers for Disease Control and Prevention. Vaccinations: vaccination safety for breastfeeding mothers. Accessed April 7, 2024. https://www.cdc.gov/breastfeeding/breastfeeding-special-circumstances/vaccinations-medications-drugs/vaccinations.html
10. Centers for Disease Control and Prevention. Prevention of measles, rubella, congenital rubella syndrome, and mumps: 2013: summary recommendations of the Advisory Committee on Immunization Practices (ACIP). *MMWR Recomm Rep*. 2013;62(RR04):1-34.
11. Isacson P, Kehrer AF, Wilson H, et al. Comparative study of live, attenuated rubella virus vaccines during the immediate puerperium. *Obstet Gynecol*. 1971;37:332-337.
12. Grillner L, Hedstrom CE, Bergstrom H, et al. Vaccination against rubella of newly delivered women. *Scand J Infect Dis*. 1973;5:237-241.
13. Buimovici-Klein E, Hite RL, Byrne T, et al. Isolation of rubella virus in milk after postpartum immunization. *J Pediatr*. 1977;91:939-941.
14. Losonsky GA, Fishaut JM, Strussenberg J, et al. Effect of immunization against rubella on lactation products. I. Development and characterization of specific immunologic reactivity in breast milk. *J Infect Dis*. 1982;145:654-660.
15. Losonsky GA, Fishaut JM, Strussenberg J, et al. Effect of immunization against rubella on lactation products. II. Maternal-neonatal interactions. *J Infect Dis*. 1982;145:661-666.
16. Landes RD, Bass JW, Millunchick EW, et al. Neonatal rubella following postpartum maternal immunization. *J Pediatr*. 1980;97:465-467.
17. Lerman SJ. Neonatal rubella following maternal immunization. *J Pediatr*. 1981;98:668.
18. Bass JW, Landes RD. Neonatal rubella following maternal immunization (reply). *J Pediatr*. 1981;98:668-669.

VACCINE, MENINGOCOCCAL GROUP B

Vaccine (Inactive Vaccine)

PREGNANCY RECOMMENDATION: No Human Data—Animal Data Suggest Low Risk

BREASTFEEDING RECOMMENDATION: Probably Compatible

V

PREGNANCY SUMMARY

Meningococcal vaccine is available in two types: a polysaccharide ACYW (MenACYW—see Vaccine, Meningococcal Groups A, C, Y, and W-135) and group B specific (MenB). No reports describing the use of MenB vaccine in human pregnancy have been located. Animal data did not show any embryofetal toxicity in one species receiving a single human dose. However, the absence of human pregnancy experience prevents a complete assessment of embryofetal risk. Using this vaccine drug during pregnancy should be based on the pros and cons of the mother's clinical need for treatment versus any potential fetal risk that might occur from exposure. The CDC recommends deferring the MenB vaccine in pregnant women unless, after a discussion with her health care providers, the patient is at increased risk, and the vaccine benefits outweigh the potential risks.

BREASTFEEDING SUMMARY

No reports describing the use of MenB during human lactation have been located. According to the ACIP general best practice guidelines for immunizations in special situations, administering live or non-live vaccines (except smallpox and yellow fever vaccines) does not affect the safety of breastfeeding for women or their infants. Additionally, the CDC states that the MenB vaccine is safe for use in lactation.

References

1. Product information. Trumenba. Wyeth Pharmaceutical Division of Wyeth Holdings, LLC; 2021.
2. Product information. Bexsero. GlaxoSmithKline Biologicals SA; 2023.
3. Centers for Disease Control and Prevention. Vaccinations: vaccination safety for breastfeeding mothers. Accessed August 13, 2023. https://www.cdc.gov/breastfeeding/breastfeeding-special-circumstances/vaccinations-medications-drugs/vaccinations.html

VACCINE, MENINGOCOCCAL GROUPS A, C, Y, AND W-135

Vaccine (Inactive Vaccine)

PREGNANCY RECOMMENDATION: Limited Human Data - Animal Data Suggest Low Risk

BREASTFEEDING RECOMMENDATION: Probably Compatible

PREGNANCY SUMMARY

Meningococcal vaccine is available in two types: MenACYW and MenB (see Vaccine, Meningococcal Group B). The CDC recommends that the MenACYW can be administered during pregnancy if otherwise indicated, but that MenB should be delayed until postpartum. The vaccine does not appear to increase the risk for adverse pregnancy or fetal outcomes. In one study, MenACYW vaccination resulted in the transfer of maternal antibodies to the fetus, but the transfer was irregular and was not dependent on maternal titer or the period in pregnancy when vaccination occurred. Animal studies have not shown any embryofetal toxicity. However, this limited human pregnancy experience prevents a complete assessment of embryofetal risk. Using this vaccine during pregnancy should be based on the pros and cons of the mother's clinical need for treatment versus any potential fetal risk that might occur from exposure. Health care providers and women who are pregnant and have taken Menactra or MenQuadfi at any time during pregnancy are encouraged to contact Sanofi Pasteur at 800-822-2463.

BREASTFEEDING SUMMARY

No reports describing the use of MenACWY during human lactation have been located. According to the ACIP general best practice guidelines for immunizations in special situations, administering live or non-live vaccines (except smallpox and yellow fever vaccines) does not affect the safety of breastfeeding for women or their infants. Additionally, the CDC states that the MenACWY vaccine is safe for use in lactation.

References

1. Product information. Menveo. GlaxoSmithKline Biologics SA; 2023.
2. Product information. Menactra. Sanofi Pasteur, Inc; 2019.
3. Product information. Menquadfi. Sanofi Pasteur, Inc; 2023.
4. Centers for Disease Control and Prevention. Guidelines for vaccinating pregnant women. Accessed April 7, 2024. https://www.cdc.gov/vaccines-pregnancy/hcp/vaccination-guidelines/
5. Letson GW, Little JR, Ottman J, Miller GL. Meningococcal vaccine in pregnancy: an assessment of infant risk. *Pediatr Infect Dis*. 1998;17:261-263.
6. Becerra-Culqui TA, Sy LS, Ackerson BK, et al. Safety of MenACWY-CRM vaccine exposure during pregnancy. *Vaccine*. 2020;38:2683-2690.
7. Nasser R, Rakedzon S, Dickstein Y, et al. Are all vaccines safe for the pregnant traveller? A systematic review and meta-analysis. *J Trav Med*. 2019;27:1-16.
8. Clark DR, Omer SB, Tapia MD, et al. Influenza or meningococcal immunization during pregnancy and mortality in women and infants. *Pediatr Infect Dis J*. 2020;39:641-644.
9. Carvalho ADA, Giampaglia CMS, Kimura H, et al. Maternal and infant antibody response to meningococcal vaccination in pregnancy. *Lancet*. 1977; 2:809-811.
10. Centers for Disease Control and Prevention. Vaccinations: vaccination safety for breastfeeding mothers. Accessed April 7, 2024. https://www.cdc.gov/breastfeeding/breastfeeding-special-circumstances/vaccinations-medications-drugs/vaccinations.html

VACCINE, PNEUMOCOCCAL 13-, 15-, AND 20-VALENT CONJUGATE

Vaccine (Inactive Vaccine)

PREGNANCY RECOMMENDATION: No Human Data—Animal Data Suggest Low Risk

BREASTFEEDING RECOMMENDATION: Probably Compatible

PREGNANCY SUMMARY

Pneumococcal conjugate vaccine is available as a 13-, 15-, and 20-valent inactive vaccine. No reports describing the use of pneumococcal conjugate vaccines in human pregnancy have been located. Animal data did not show any embryofetal toxicity in two species receiving doses of more than 10 times the recommended human dose (RHD). Therefore, the absence of human pregnancy experience prevents a complete assessment of the embryofetal risk. Using this vaccine during pregnancy should be based on the pros and cons of the mother's clinical need for treatment versus any potential fetal risk that might occur from exposure. The CDC has not published recommendations for the pneumococcal conjugate vaccines in pregnancy.

BREASTFEEDING SUMMARY

No reports describing the use of pneumococcal conjugate vaccines during human lactation have been located. According to the ACIP general best practice guidelines for immunizations in special situations, administering live or non-live vaccines (except smallpox and yellow fever vaccines) does not affect the safety of breastfeeding for women or their infants. However, only the pneumococcal 13-valent vaccine is listed in the "safe for use in lactation" list. The 15- and 20-valent vaccines were not listed.

References

1. Product information. Prevnar 13. Wyeth Pharmaceutical Division of Wyeth Holdings, LLC; 2019.
2. Product information. Vaxneuvance. Merck Sharp & Dohme, LLC; 2023.
3. Product information. Prevnar 20. Wyeth Pharmaceutical Division of Wyeth Holdings, LLC; 2023.
4. Centers for Disease Control and Prevention. Guidelines for vaccinating pregnant women. Accessed April 16, 2024. https://www.cdc.gov/vaccines-pregnancy/hcp/vaccination-guidelines/
5. Centers for Disease Control and Prevention. Vaccinations: vaccination safety for breastfeeding mothers. Accessed April 16, 2024. https://www.cdc.gov/breastfeeding/breastfeeding-special-circumstances/vaccinations-medications-drugs/vaccinations.html

VACCINE, PNEUMOCOCCAL 23-VALENT POLYSACCHARIDE

Vaccine (Inactive Vaccine)

PREGNANCY RECOMMENDATION: Limited Human Data - No Relevant Animal Data

BREASTFEEDING RECOMMENDATION: Probably Compatible

PREGNANCY SUMMARY

Pneumococcal 23-valent polysaccharide vaccine (PPSV23) does not appear to increase harm when administered during the second half of pregnancy. No data is available for early pregnancy exposure. It is unknown if the antigens in PPSV23 cross the placenta. Transplacental passage of maternal antibodies does occur. No animal reproduction data have been located. However, this limited human pregnancy experience prevents a complete assessment of embryofetal risk. Using this vaccine during pregnancy should be based on the pros and cons of the mother's clinical need for treatment versus any potential fetal risk that might occur from exposure. The CDC notes that the risk to the fetus from pneumococcal polysaccharide vaccine use during the first trimester of pregnancy is unknown, but no reports of adverse consequences in newborns whose mothers were inadvertently vaccinated with PPSV23 during pregnancy have been described.

BREASTFEEDING SUMMARY

In a study conducted in Bangladesh, marked increases of specific IgA antibody titers were measured in the colostrum of mothers who had received pneumococcal polyvalent vaccine at 30 to 34 weeks' gestation. Antibody titers remained higher than controls up to 5 months after delivery. According to the ACIP general best practice guidelines for immunizations in special situations, administering live or non-live vaccines (except smallpox and yellow fever vaccines) does not affect the safety of breastfeeding for women or their infants. Additionally, the CDC states that the PPSV23 vaccine is safe for use in lactation.

References

1. Product information. Pneumovax 23. Merck Sharp & Dohme, LLC; 2023.
2. Centers for Disease Control and Prevention. Guidelines for vaccinating pregnant women. Accessed April 16, 2024. https://www.cdc.gov/vaccines-pregnancy/hcp/vaccination-guidelines/
3. Faix RG. Maternal immunization to prevent fetal and neonatal infection. *Clin Obstet Gynecol*. 1991;34:277-287.
4. Weinberg A, Muresan P, Laimon L, et al. Safety, immunogenicity and transplacental antibody transport of conjugated and polysaccharide pneumococcal vaccines administered to pregnant women with HIV: a multicenter randomized controlled trial. *Lancet HIV*. 2021;8:e408-e419.
5. Shahid NS, Steinhoff MC, Hoque SS, et al. Serum, breast milk, and infant antibody after maternal immunisation with pneumococcal vaccine. *Lancet*. 1995;346:1252-1257.
6. O'Dempsey TJD, McArdle T, Ceesay SJ, et al. Immunization with a pneumococcal capsular polysaccharide vaccine during pregnancy. *Vaccine*. 1996;14:963-970.
7. Mulholland K. Maternal immunization for the prevention of bacterial infection in young infants. *Vaccine*. 1998;16:1464-1466.
8. Glezen WP. Pneumococcal polysaccharide vaccine in pregnancy. *Pediatrics*. 1999;104:1417-1418.
9. Chaithongwongwatthana S, Yamasmit W, Limpongsanurak S, et al. Pneumococcal vaccination during pregnancy for preventing infant infection. *Cochrane Database Syst Rev*. 2015;1:CD004903.
10. Berezin EN, Lopes CC, Cardoso MRA. Maternal immunization with pneumococcal polysaccharide vaccine: persistence of maternal antibodies in infants. *J Trop Pediatr*. 2017;63:118-123.
11. Binks MJ, Moberley SA, Balloch A, et al. PneuMum: impact from a randomised controlled trial of maternal 23-valent pneumococcal polysaccharide vaccination on middle ear disease amongst Indigenous infants, Northern Territory, Australia. *Vaccine*. 2015;33:6579-6587.
12. McHugh L, Binks M, Ware RS, et al. Birth outcomes in Aboriginal mother-infant pairs from the Northern Territory, Australia, who received 23-valent polysaccharide pneumococcal vaccination during pregnancy, 2006-2011: the PneuMum randomised controlled trial. *Aust N Z J Obstet Gynaecol*. 2020;60:82-87.
13. Mossi-Pinhata MM, Ward S, Laimon L, et al. Effect of maternal immunization with 10-valent pneumococcus conjugate vaccine (PCV-10), 23-valent pneumococcus polysaccharide vaccine, or placebo on the immunogenicity of PCV-10 in human immunodeficiency virus-exposed uninfected infants: a randomized clinical trial. *Clin Infect Dis*. 2022;75:996-1005.
14. Centers for Disease Control and Prevention. Vaccinations: vaccination safety for breastfeeding mothers. Accessed April 16, 2024. https://www.cdc.gov/breastfeeding/breastfeeding-special-circumstances/vaccinations-medications-drugs/vaccinations.html

VACCINE, POLIOVIRUS INACTIVATED

Vaccine (Inactive Vaccine)

PREGNANCY RECOMMENDATION: *Limited Human Data and No Relevant Animal Data (Maternal Benefit May Outweight Embryo-Fetal Risk)

BREASTFEEDING RECOMMENDATION: Probably Compatible

PREGNANCY SUMMARY

Fetal damage may occur if a mother contracts the disease during pregnancy. However, the risk to the embryo-fetus from the inactivated polio vaccine (IPV) appears to be low, if at all. No animal reproduction studies have been performed. *The CDC recommends the use of the vaccine during pregnancy only if the mother is at an increased risk of exposure and requires immediate protection. Otherwise, vaccination during pregnancy is not recommended. However, the limited human pregnancy experience prevents a complete assessment of embryofetal risk. Using this vaccine during pregnancy should be based on the pros and cons of the mother's clinical need for treatment versus any potential fetal risk that might occur from exposure.

BREASTFEEDING SUMMARY

No reports describing the use of IPV during human lactation have been located. According to the ACIP general best practice guidelines for immunizations in special situations, administering live or non-live vaccines (except smallpox and yellow fever vaccines) does not affect the safety of breastfeeding for women or their infants. Additionally, the CDC states that the IPV vaccine is safe for use in lactation.

References

1. Product information. IPOL. Sanofi Pasteur, Inc; 2022.
2. Centers for Disease Control and Prevention. Guidelines for vaccinating pregnant women. Accessed August 20, 2023. https://www.cdc.gov/vaccines-pregnancy/hcp/vaccination-guidelines/
3. Linder N, Ohel G. In utero vaccination. *Clin Perinatol*. 1994;21:663-674.
4. Heinonen OP, Slone D, Shapiro S. *Birth Defects and Drugs in Pregnancy*. Publishing Sciences Group; 1977.
5. Centers for Disease Control and Prevention. Guidelines for vaccinating pregnant women. Accessed August 19, 2023. https://www.cdc.gov/vaccines/pregnancy/hcp-toolkit/guidelines.html

VACCINE, RABIES

Vaccine (Inactive Vaccine)

PREGNANCY RECOMMENDATION: Limited Human Data - No Relevant Animal Data (Maternal Benefit Probably Outweighs Any Embryofetal Risk)

BREASTFEEDING RECOMMENDATION: Probably Compatible

PREGNANCY SUMMARY

There have been 244 published cases of using several types of rabies vaccines during pregnancy. No adverse events have been attributed to vaccine administration during pregnancy. Currently, chicken egg fibroblast and human diploid-based vaccines are available in the United States. No animal reproduction studies have been conducted. However, this limited human pregnancy experience prevents a complete assessment of embryofetal risk. Using this vaccine during pregnancy should be based on the pros and cons of the mother's clinical need for treatment versus any potential fetal risk that might occur from exposure. Because rabies is nearly 100% fatal if contracted, the vaccine should be given for postexposure prophylaxis regardless of pregnancy. Additionally, preexposure prophylaxis might also be indicated during pregnancy if the risk of rabies exposure is substantial.

BREASTFEEDING SUMMARY

No reports describing the use of the rabies vaccine during human lactation have been located. According to the ACIP general best practice guidelines for immunizations in special situations, administering live or non-live vaccines (except smallpox and yellow fever vaccines) does not affect the safety of breastfeeding for women or their infants. Additionally, the CDC states that the rabies vaccine is safe for use during lactation.

References

1. Product information. RabAvert. Bavarian Nordic A/S; 2023.
2. Product information. Imovax Rabies. Sanofi Pasteur, Inc; 2023.
3. Centers for Disease Control and Prevention. Guidelines for vaccinating pregnant women. Accessed August 20, 2023. https://www.cdc.gov/vaccines-pregnancy/hcp/vaccination-guidelines/
4. Amstey MS. Vaccination in pregnancy. *Clin Obstet Gynaecol*. 1983;10:13-22.
5. Varner MW, McGuinness GA, Galask RP. Rabies vaccination in pregnancy. *Am J Obstet Gynecol*. 1982;143:717-718.
6. Fescharek R, Quast U, Dechert G. Postexposure rabies vaccination during pregnancy: experience from post-marketing surveillance with 16 patients. *Vaccine*. 1990;8:409-410.
7. Spence MR, Davidson DE, Dill GS Jr, Boonthai P, Sagartz JW. Rabies exposure during pregnancy. *Am J Obstet Gynecol*. 1975;123:655-656.
8. Klietmann W, Domres B, Cox JH. Rabies post-exposure treatment and side-effects in man using HDC (MRC 5) vaccine. *Dev Biol Stand*. 1978;40:109-113.
9. Cates W Jr. Treatment of rabies exposure during pregnancy. *Obstet Gynecol*. 1974;44:893-896.
10. Chutivongse S, Wilde H. Postexposure rabies vaccination during pregnancy: experience with 21 patients. *Vaccine*. 1989;7:546-548.
11. Chutivongse S, Wilde H, Benjavongkulchai M, et al. Postexposure rabies vaccination during pregnancy: effect on 202 women and their infants. *Clin Infect Dis*. 1995;20:818-820.
12. Windrim C, McGreer AJ, Murphy KE. Exposure to rabies during pregnancy. *CMAJ*. 2018;190:e1281-e1283.

VACCINE, SMALLPOX

Vaccine (Live Vaccine)

PREGNANCY RECOMMENDATION: *Contraindicated

BREASTFEEDING RECOMMENDATION: *Contraindicated

PREGNANCY SUMMARY

A 2015 systematic review and meta-analysis involving 12,201 smallpox vaccine pregnancy exposures found that spontaneous abortion, intrauterine fetal demise, and preterm delivery rates were not increased. However, first-trimester vaccine exposure was associated with an increased risk for malformations compared to controls (2.4% and 1.5%, respectively). Regardless, the 2.4% rate falls within the expected rate for major anomalies in pregnancy in the United States. In addition, no pattern to the defects has been described. Fetal virus transmission has been reported after maternal vaccination during pregnancy. The manufacturer also notes that fetal vaccinia and death may occur after exposure to the vaccine. No animal reproduction studies have been conducted. Using this vaccine during pregnancy should be based on the pros and cons of the mother's clinical need for treatment versus any potential fetal risk that might occur from exposure. Although smallpox infections had a high mortality rate, smallpox was declared eradicated by the World Health Assembly in 1980. Since this time, no naturally occurring smallpox has been observed. *The CDC classifies smallpox vaccine as contraindicated during pregnancy, within 28 days of conception, and in persons who might have close contact with pregnant women within 28 days of their vaccination due to the limited risk but severe consequences of fetal infection. However, because the risk for fetal vaccinia is low, inadvertent exposure to the vaccine during or before pregnancy should not be a reason for pregnancy termination. If the pregnant woman has definite smallpox virus exposure, she should be vaccinated due to the high risk of contracting the disease. The risks of clinical smallpox to the mother and fetus substantially outweigh any potential risk of vaccination. The manufacturer reports that pregnant women should avoid contact with persons with an active vaccine lesion because there is a potential of having inadvertent transmission after changing bandages or contact with vaccine sites. The CDC has a prospective pregnant registry for women with inadvertent vaccine administration during pregnancy. Health care providers are encouraged to call the CDC at 404-639-8253. Again, because this virus is not found naturally in the environment, infections can only come from laboratories that still maintain active virus cultures or through bioterrorism. If infections occur through these avenues, health care professionals should call the Department of Defense at 619-553-9255.

BREASTFEEDING SUMMARY

No reports describing the use of the smallpox vaccine during human lactation have been located. In an unusual report, however, tertiary contact vaccinia transmission from a mother to her nursing infant through direct skin-to-skin and skin-to-mucous membrane contact was documented. The father, a soldier in the United States Army, had received smallpox vaccination but had reportedly taken standard precautions to avoid spread to his family. Approximately 1 to 2 weeks later, his wife developed vesicles on both areolas. About 2 weeks later, a papule developed on the philtrum of the breastfeeding infant. PCR and culture for vaccinia of the mother and infant confirmed contact vaccinia. *Because of the theoretical risk of contact transmission in a nursing infant, the CDC states that breastfeeding is contraindicated. However, based on the recommendations during pregnancy, if a nursing woman is exposed to smallpox or monkeypox, she should receive the vaccine, but should probably stop breastfeeding.

References

1. Product information. ACAM2000. Emergent Product Development Gaithersburg, Inc; 2018.
2. Petersen BW, Harms TJ, Reynolds MG, et al. Use of vaccinia virus smallpox vaccine in laboratory and health care personnel at risk for occupational exposure to orthopoxviruses—recommendations of Advisory Committee on Immunization Practices (ACIP), 2015. *MMWR Morb Mortal Wkly Rep*. 2016;65:257-262.
3. Centers for Disease Control and Prevention. Smallpox. Accessed September 2, 2023. https://www.cdc.gov/smallpox/index.html
4. Badell ML, Meaney-Delman D, Tuuli MG, et al. Risks associate with smallpox vaccination in pregnancy: a systematic review and meta-analysis. *Obstet Gynecol*. 2015;125:1439-1451.
5. Centers for Disease Control and Prevention. Guidelines for vaccinating pregnant women. Accessed August 20, 2023. https://www.cdc.gov/vaccines-pregnancy/hcp/vaccination-guidelines/
6. Levine MM. Live-virus vaccines in pregnancy. Risks and recommendations. *Lancet*. 1974;2:34-38.
7. Napolitano PG, Ryan MAK, Grabenstein JD. Pregnancy discovered after smallpox vaccination: is vaccinia immune globulin appropriate? *Am J Obstet Gynecol*. 2004;191:1863-1867.
8. Centers for Disease Control and Prevention. Women with smallpox vaccine exposure during pregnancy reported to the national smallpox vaccine in pregnancy registry—United States, 2003. *MMWR Morb Mortal Wkly Rep*. 2003;52:386-388.
9. Conlin AMS, Bukowinski AT, Gumbs GR; for the Department of Defense Birth and Infant Health Registry Team. Analysis of pregnancy and infant health outcomes among women in the national smallpox vaccine in pregnancy registry who received anthrax vaccine adsorbed. *Vaccine*. 2015;33:4387-4390.
10. Garde V, Harper D, Fairchok MP. Tertiary contact vaccinia in a breastfeeding infant. *JAMA*. 2004;291:725-727.

VACCINE, TETANUS TOXOID, REDUCED DIPHTHERIA TOXOID, ACELLULAR PERTUSSIS

Vaccine (Inactive Vaccine)

PREGNANCY RECOMMENDATION: Human Data Suggest Compatible

BREASTFEEDING RECOMMENDATION: Probably Compatible

PREGNANCY SUMMARY

The tetanus toxoid/reduced diphtheria toxoid/acellular pertussis adsorbed vaccine (Tdap) has not been associated with increased risks during pregnancy. Both the CDC and ACOG recommend a Tdap vaccine for all pregnant women between 27 and 36 weeks' gestation, regardless of previous vaccination. Tdap IgG antibodies cross the placenta. Animal data did not show any embryofetal toxicity in one species receiving a single human dose.

BREASTFEEDING SUMMARY

No reports describing the administration of Tdap during human lactation have been located. Tdap should present no risk to a nursing infant because antibodies to pertussis, tetanus, and diphtheria should be present in both the mother and the infant. Moreover, diphtheria toxoid/tetanus toxoid/acellular pertussis vaccine adsorbed (DTaP) is indicated for infants and children 2 months through 6 years of age (before the seventh birthday). The CDC recommends administering Tdap immediately postpartum if the woman was not vaccinated during pregnancy, and it is considered safe with lactation.

References

1. Product information. Adacel Tdap. Sanofi Pasteur, Inc; 2023.
2. Product information. Boostrix. GlaxoSmithKline Biologics SA; 2023.
3. Amstey MS. Vaccination in pregnancy. *Clin Obstet Gynaecol*. 1983;10:13-22.
4. Centers for Disease Control and Prevention. Tdap (Pertussis) vaccine and pregnancy. Accessed September 4, 2023. https://www.cdc.gov/vaccines/pregnancy/hcp-toolkit/tdap-vaccine-pregnancy.html
5. American College of Obstetricians and Gynecologists. Update on immunization and pregnancy: tetanus, diphtheria, and pertussis vaccination. Committee Opinion, Number 718. *Obstet Gynecol*. 2017;130:e153-e157.
6. Centers for Disease Control and Prevention. Guidelines for vaccinating pregnant women. Accessed August 20, 2023. https://www.cdc.gov/vaccines-pregnancy/hcp/vaccination-guidelines/

7. Post AL, Li SH, Berry M, et al. Efficiency of placental transfer of vaccine-elicited antibodies relative to prenatal Tdap vaccination status. *Vaccine*. 2020;38: 4869-4876.
8. Van Savage J, Decker MD, Edwards KM, et al. Natural history of pertussis antibody in the infant and effect on vaccine response. *J Infect Dis*. 1990;161: 487-492.
9. Edwards KM. Pertussis: an important target for maternal immunization. *Vaccine*. 2003;21:3483-3486.
10. Munoz FM, Bond NH, Maccato M, et al. Safety and immunogenicity of tetanus diphtheria and acellular pertussis (Tdap) immunization during pregnancy in mothers and infants: a randomized clinical trial. *JAMA*. 2014;311: 1760-1769.
11. Halperin SA, Langley JM, Ye L, et al. A randomized controlled trial of the safety and immunogenicity of tetanus, diphtheria, and acellular pertussis vaccine immunization during pregnancy and subsequent infant immune response. *Clin Inf Dis*. 2018;67:1063-1071.
12. Griffin JB, Yu L, Watson D, et al. Pertussis immunisation in pregnancy safety (PIPS) study: a retrospective cohort study of safety outcomes in pregnant women vaccinated with Tdap vaccine. *Vaccine*. 2018;36:5173-5179.
13. Vygen-Bonnet S, Hellenbrand W, Garbe E, et al. Safety and effectiveness of acellular pertussis vaccination during pregnancy: a systematic review. *BMC Infect Dis*. 2020;20:136.
14. Czeizel AE, Rockenbauer M. Tetanus toxoid and congenital abnormalities. *Int J Gynecol Obstet*. 1999;64:253-258.
15. Centers for Disease Control and Prevention. Diphtheria vaccine recommendations. Accessed September 3, 2023. https://www.cdc.gov/vaccines/vpd/dtap-tdap-td/hcp/recommendations.html

VACCINE, TYPHOID

Vaccine (Inactive Vaccine)

PREGNANCY RECOMMENDATION: No Human Data and No Relevant Animal Data (Maternal Benefit Probably Outweighs Any Potential Fetal Risk)

BREASTFEEDING RECOMMENDATION: Probably Compatible

PREGNANCY SUMMARY

Two typhoid vaccines are available in the United States. Typhim Vi is a polysaccharide inactive vaccine administered intramuscularly (IM). Vivotif is a live, attenuated virus vaccine administered orally (see Vaccine, Typhoid Live Vaccine). No reports describing the use of typhoid vaccine in human pregnancy have been located. No animal reproduction studies have been conducted. Therefore, the absence of human pregnancy experience prevents a complete assessment of embryofetal risk. Typhoid is a serious infectious disease with high morbidity and mortality. The risk to the fetus from the vaccine is unknown. Regardless, the CDC and manufacturer recommend that the typhoid Vi polysaccharide vaccine be administered to pregnant women only if clearly needed. Additionally, the manufacturer recommends delaying administration to the second or third trimester when possible as a reasonable precaution to reduce the possibility of fetal harm.

BREASTFEEDING SUMMARY

No reports describing the use of typhoid Vi vaccine during human lactation have been located. According to the ACIP general best practice guidelines for immunizations in special situations, administering live or non-live vaccines (except smallpox and yellow fever vaccines) does not affect the safety of breastfeeding for women or their infants. Additionally, the CDC states that typhoid Vi vaccine is safe for use during lactation.

References

1. Product information. Typhim Vi. Sanofi Pasteur, Inc; 2023.
2. Centers for Disease Control and Prevention. Guidelines for vaccinating pregnant women. Accessed August 20, 2023. https://www.cdc.gov/vaccines/pregnancy/hcp-toolkit/guidelines.html
3. Centers for Disease Control and Prevention. Guidelines for vaccinating pregnant women. Accessed August 19, 2023. https://www.cdc.gov/vaccines-pregnancy/hcp/vaccination-guidelines/

VACCINE, TYPHOID

Vaccine (Live Vaccine)

PREGNANCY RECOMMENDATION: *Contraindicated

BREASTFEEDING RECOMMENDATION: *Contraindicated

PREGNANCY SUMMARY

Two typhoid vaccines are available in the United States. Typhim Vi (typhoid Vi) is a polysaccharide inactive vaccine administered IM. Vivotif (typhoid Ty21a) is a live, attenuated virus vaccine administered orally. No reports describing the use of typhoid vaccine in human pregnancy have been located. No animal reproduction studies have been conducted. Therefore, the absence of human pregnancy experience prevents a complete assessment of embryofetal risk. Typhoid is a serious infectious disease with high morbidity and mortality. The risk to the fetus from the vaccine is unknown. *The CDC states that live virus vaccines such as the typhoid Ty21a are contraindicated for use in pregnancy. The manufacturer states that typhoid Ty21a should be administered to a pregnant woman only if clearly needed, but the inactive virus vaccine can be used as an alternative.

BREASTFEEDING SUMMARY

No reports describing the use of typhoid Ty21a vaccine during human lactation have been located. According to the ACIP general best practice guidelines for immunizations in special situations, administering live or non-live vaccines (except smallpox and yellow fever vaccines) does not affect the safety of breastfeeding for women or their infants. *However, because there is an inactive virus vaccine available, the typhoid Ty21a live virus vaccine is not indicated.

References

1. Product information. Vivotif. Emergent Travel Health, Inc; 2021.
2. Centers for Disease Control and Prevention. Guidelines for vaccinating pregnant women. Accessed August 20, 2023. https://www.cdc.gov/vaccines/pregnancy/hcp-toolkit/guidelines.html
3. Centers for Disease Control and Prevention. Guidelines for vaccinating pregnant women. Accessed August 19, 2023. https://www.cdc.gov/vaccines-pregnancy/hcp/vaccination-guidelines/

VACCINE, VARICELLA

Vaccine (Live Vaccine)

PREGNANCY RECOMMENDATION: *Contraindicated

BREASTFEEDING RECOMMENDATION: Compatible

PREGNANCY SUMMARY

The Varivax pregnancy registry described over 900 exposures within 3 months before conception or during pregnancy. The varicella vaccine did not appear to increase the risk for malformations or congenital varicella syndrome. However, the registry states that it does not have sufficient power to rule out a low risk for congenital varicella syndrome. No animal reproduction studies have been conducted. The risk of congenital varicella syndrome (with an active varicella infection) is approximately 1% during the first 20 weeks of gestation. Moreover, there is a significant risk for infectious morbidity and possible mortality in the neonate and young child when maternal varicella infection occurs after the first trimester. *The CDC recommends that the varicella vaccine (because it is a live virus vaccine) should not be administered during pregnancy. However, the risk from the vaccine is thought to be much less because the virulence of the attenuated virus used in the vaccine is less than that of the natural virus. Although varicella virus vaccine is contraindicated immediately before and during pregnancy because of unknown fetal effects, the potential for harmful fetal effects appears to be low. No cases of varicella vaccine–induced fetal harm have been identified to date. Routine pregnancy testing prior to vaccine administration is not recommended. If the patient becomes pregnant within 4 weeks of vaccine administration or if administered inadvertently in a pregnant woman, it is recommended to counsel the patient about the theoretical basis for fetal concern, but this should not be a reason for termination. The ACIP and American Academy of Pediatrics (AAP) recommend women avoid pregnancy for 1 month after each dose of the vaccine, whereas the manufacturer recommends 3 months. Vaccination of a child is not contraindicated if the child's nonimmune mother or other nonimmune household member is pregnant.

BREASTFEEDING SUMMARY

In women with varicella-zoster infections, it does not appear that the virus is found in breast milk. A 2003 study reported that varicella DNA was not detected in 217 postvaccination samples of breast milk from 12 women who had received two doses of the vaccine. Because there was no evidence of varicella vaccine virus excretion into breast milk, the investigators concluded that there was no need to delay vaccination in breastfeeding women. According to the ACIP general best practice guidelines for immunizations in special situations, administering live or non-live vaccines (except smallpox and yellow fever vaccines) does not affect the safety of breastfeeding for women or their infants. Additionally, the CDC states that the varicella vaccine is safe for use during lactation.

References

1. Product information. Varivax. Merck Sharp & Dohme, LLC; 2023.
2. Centers for Disease Control and Prevention. Prevention of varicella. Recommendations of Advisory Committee on Immunization Practices (ACIP). *MMWR*. 2007;56(RR04):1-40.
3. Centers for Disease Control and Prevention. Guidelines for vaccinating pregnant women. Accessed August 20, 2023. https://www.cdc.gov/vaccines-pregnancy/hcp/vaccination-guidelines/
4. American Academy of Pediatrics. Immunization in pregnancy. In: Kimberlin DW, Brady MT, Jackson MA, Long SS, eds. *Red Book: 2018 Report of the Committee on Infectious Diseases*. 31st ed. American Academy of Pediatrics; 2018:67-112.
5. Pastuszak AL, Levy M, Schick B, et al. Outcome after maternal varicella infection in the first 20 weeks of pregnancy. *N Engl J Med*. 1994;330:901-905.
6. Dickinson J, Gonik B. Teratogenic viral infections. *Clin Obstet Gynecol*. 1990;33:242-252.
7. Birthistle K, Carrington D. Fetal varicella syndrome—a reappraisal of the literature. *J Infect*. 1998;36(suppl 1):25-29.

V

8. Siegel M. Congenital malformations following chickenpox, measles, mumps, and hepatitis. Results of a cohort study. *JAMA*. 1973;226:1521-1524.
9. Paryani SG, Arvin AM. Intrauterine infection with varicella-zoster virus after maternal varicella. *N Engl J Med*. 1986;314:1542-1546.
10. Balducci J, Rodis JF, Rosengren S, et al. Pregnancy outcome following first-trimester varicella infection. *Obstet Gynecol*. 1992;79:5-6.
11. Enders G, Miller E, Cradock-Watson J, et al. Consequences of varicella and herpes zoster in pregnancy: prospective study of 1739 cases. *Lancet*. 1994; 343:1547-1550.
12. Laforet EG, Lynch CL Jr. Multiple congenital defects following maternal varicella. Report of a case. *N Engl J Med*. 1947;236:534-537.
13. Harris RE, Rhoades ER. Varicella pneumonia complicating pregnancy. Report of a case and review of literature. *Obstet Gynecol*. 1965;25:734-740.
14. Sever J, White LR. Intrauterine viral infections. *Annu Rev Med*. 1968;19: 471-486.
15. McKendry JBJ, Bailey JD. Congenital varicella associated with multiple defects. *Can Med Assoc J*. 1973;108:66-68.
16. Savage MO, Moosa A, Gordon RR. Maternal varicella infection as a cause of fetal malformations. *Lancet*. 1973;1:352-354.
17. Srabstein JC, Morris N, Larke RPB, et al. Is there a congenital varicella syndrome? *J Pediatr*. 1974;84:239-243.
18. Frey HM, Bialkin G, Gershon AA. Congenital varicella: case report of a serologically proved long-term survivor. *Pediatrics*. 1977;59:110-112.
19. Bai PVA, John TJ. Congenital skin ulcers following varicella in late pregnancy. *J Pediatr*. 1979;94:65-67.
20. Enders G. Varicella-zoster virus infection in pregnancy. *Prog Med Virol*. 1984;29:166-196.
21. Landsberger EJ, Hager WD, Grossman JH III. Successful management of varicella pneumonia complicating pregnancy. A report of three cases. *J Reprod Med*. 1986;31:311-314.
22. Hockberger RS, Rothstein RJ. Varicella pneumonia in adults: a spectrum of disease. *Ann Emerg Med*. 1986;15:931-934.
23. Glaser JB, Loftus J, Ferragamo V, et al. Varicella-zoster infection in pregnancy. *N Engl J Med*. 1986;315:1416.
24. Preblud SR, Cochi SL, Orenstein WA. Varicella-zoster infection in pregnancy. *N Engl J Med*. 1986;315:1416-1417.
25. Trlifajova J, Benda R, Benes C. Effect of maternal varicella-zoster virus infection on the outcome of pregnancy and the analysis of transplacental virus transmission. *Acta Virol*. 1986;30:249-255.
26. Alkalay AL, Pomerance JJ, Rimoin DL. Fetal varicella syndrome. *J Pediatr*. 1987;111:320-323.
27. Higa K, Dan K, Manabe H. Varicella-zoster virus infections during pregnancy: hypothesis concerning the mechanisms of congenital malformations. *Obstet Gynecol*. 1987;69:214-222.
28. Hankins GDV, Gilstrap LC III, Patterson AR. Acyclovir treatment of varicella pneumonia in pregnancy. *Crit Care Med*. 1987;15:336-337.
29. Eder SE, Apuzzio JJ, Weiss G. Varicella pneumonia during pregnancy. Treatment of two cases with acyclovir. *Am J Perinatol*. 1988;5:16-18.
30. Boyd K, Walder E. Use of acyclovir to treat chickenpox in pregnancy. *Br Med J*. 1988;296:393-394.
31. Smego RA Jr, Asperilla MO. Use of acyclovir for varicella pneumonia during pregnancy. *Obstet Gynecol*. 1991;78:1112-1116.
32. Broussard RC, Payne K, George RB. Treatment with acyclovir of varicella pneumonia in pregnancy. *Chest*. 1991;99:1045-1047.
33. Michie CA, Acolet D, Charlton R, et al. Varicella-zoster contracted in the second trimester of pregnancy. *Pediatr Infect Dis J*. 1992;11:1050-1053.
34. Pretorius DH, Hayward I, Jones KL, et al. Sonographic evaluation of pregnancies with maternal varicella infection. *J Ultrasound Med*. 1992;11:459-463.
35. Whitty JE, Renfroe YR, Bottoms SF, et al. Varicella pneumonia in pregnancy: clinical experience (abstract). *Am J Obstet Gynecol*. 1993;168:427.
36. Martin KA, Junker AK, Thomas EE, et al. Occurrence of chickenpox during pregnancy in women seropositive for varicella-zoster virus. *J Infect Dis*. 1994;170:991-995.
37. Jones KL, Johnson KA, Chambers CD. Offspring of women infected with varicella during pregnancy: a prospective study. *Teratology*. 1994;49:29-32.
38. Andreou A, Basiakos H, Hatzikoumi I, et al. Fetal varicella syndrome with manifestations limited to the eye. *Am J Perinatol*. 1995;12:347-348.
39. Figueroa-Damian R, Arredondo-Garcia JL. Perinatal outcome of pregnancies complicated with varicella infection during the first 20 weeks of gestation. *Am J Perinatol*. 1997;14:411-414.
40. Nathwani D, Maclean A, Conway S, et al. Varicella infections in pregnancy and the newborn. A review prepared for the UK Advisory Group on Chickenpox on behalf of the British Society for the Study of Infection. *J Infect*. 1998;36(suppl 1):59-71.
41. Centers for Disease Control and Prevention. Unintentional administration of varicella virus vaccine—United States, 1996. *MMWR*. 1996;45:1017-1018.
42. Merck/CDC Pregnancy Registry for varicella-containing vaccines (Varivax, Proquad, & Zostavax). The 14th annual report: 2009. *Covering the Period from Approval of Varivax (March 17, 1995) through March 16, 2009*.
43. Salzman MB, Sharrar RG, Steinberg S, et al. Transmission of varicella-vaccine virus from a healthy 12-month-old child to his pregnant mother. *J Pediatr*. 1997;131:151-154.
44. Long SS. Toddler-to-mother transmission of varicella-vaccine virus: how bad is that? *J Pediatr*. 1997;131:10-12.
45. Wald ER. Transmission of varicella-vaccine virus: what is the risk? *J Pediatr*. 1998;133:310.
46. Frederick IB, White RJ, Braddock SW. Excretion of varicella-herpes zoster virus in breast milk. *Am J Obstet Gynecol*. 1986;154:1116-1117.
47. Bohlke K, Galil K, Jackson LA, et al. Postpartum varicella vaccination: is the vaccine virus excreted in breast milk? *Obstet Gynecol*. 2003;102:970-977.

VACCINE, YELLOW FEVER

Vaccine (Live Vaccine)

PREGNANCY RECOMMENDATION: *Human Data Suggest Low Risk (Maternal Benefit May Outweigh Any Embryofetal Risk)

BREASTFEEDING RECOMMENDATION: Contraindicated

PREGNANCY SUMMARY

There are over 1,500 women in the literature with yellow fever vaccination within 28 days of conception or during pregnancy. The study authors concluded that although their sample was too small to rule out a moderately increased risk of adverse outcome, their data do not support such an association and could be used to reassure pregnant women who have inadvertently received the vaccine. In a publication of 1,347 US active military women vaccinated before or during pregnancy, no increased risk for malformations, spontaneous abortion, preeclampsia, spontaneous preterm labor/delivery, or low birth weight was found. It appears that the vaccine antigen can cross the placenta. It is not known if the antibodies induced by the vaccine cross the placenta. However, human IgG antibodies are known to cross the placenta, especially during the third trimester, which suggests that some transfer will occur. No animal reproduction studies have been conducted. Using

V

this vaccine during pregnancy should be based on the pros and cons of the mother's clinical need for treatment versus any potential fetal risk that might occur from exposure. Yellow fever is a serious infectious disease with high morbidity and mortality. *The CDC states that the vaccine should not be used in pregnancy except if exposure to yellow fever is unavoidable. Serologic testing to confirm an immune response should also be considered since pregnancy may affect immunologic function. Additionally, the CDC advises women to wait 4 weeks before attempting to conceive after receiving the yellow fever vaccine.

BREASTFEEDING SUMMARY

Three reports describing the administration of yellow fever vaccine during human lactation in women have been located. Of the 13 women who received the vaccine, IgM for yellow fever was detected in the breast milk samples of 3 women. Additionally, two infants developed meningoencephalitis, which the authors attributed to maternal vaccination. The CDC states that the yellow fever vaccine is contraindicated in breastfeeding women.

References

1. Product information. YF-VAX. Sanofi Pasteur, Inc; 2023.
2. Amstey MS. Vaccination in pregnancy. *Clin Obstet Gynaecol*. 1983;10:13-22.
3. Centers for Disease Control and Prevention. Guidelines for vaccinating pregnant women. Accessed September 15, 2023. https://www.cdc.gov/vaccines-pregnancy/hcp/vaccination-guidelines/
4. Heinonen OP, Slone D, Shapiro S. *Birth Defects and Drugs in Pregnancy*. Publishing Sciences Group; 1977:315.
5. Nasidi A, Monath TP, Vandenberg J, et al. Yellow fever vaccination and pregnancy: a four-year prospective study. *Trans R Soc Trop Med Hyg*. 1993; 87:337-339.
6. Tsai TF, Paul R, Lynberg MC, et al. Congenital yellow fever virus infection after immunization in pregnancy. *J Infect Dis*. 1993;168:1520-1523.
7. Robert E, Vial T, Schaefer C, et al. Exposure to yellow fever vaccine in early pregnancy. *Vaccine*. 1999;17:283-285.
8. Linder N, Ohel G. In utero vaccination. *Clin Perinatol*. 1994;21:663-674.
9. Hall C, Khodr ZG, Chang RN, et al. Safety of yellow fever vaccination in pregnancy: findings from a cohort of active duty US military women. *J Travel Med*. 2020;27:1-8.
10. Kuhn S, Twele-Montecinos L, MacDonald J, et al. Case report: probable transmission of vaccine strain of yellow fever virus to an infant via breast milk. *CMAJ*. 2011;183:e243-e245.
11. Traiber C, Coelho-Amaral P, Ritter VRF, Winge A. Infant meningoencephalitis caused by yellow fever vaccine virus transmitted via breastmilk. *J Pediatr (Rio J)*. 2011;87:269-272.
12. Fernandes EG, Nogueira JS, Gomes VB, et al. The search for yellow fever virus vaccine in breast milk of inadvertently vaccinated women in Brazil. *Rev Inst Med Trop Sao Paulo*. 2020;62:e33.

VADADUSTAT

Hematologic (HIF-Prolyl Hydroxylase Inhibitor)

PREGNANCY RECOMMENDATION: No Human Data—Animal Data Suggest Potential Risk (Maternal Benefit May Outweigh Any Embryofetal Risk)

BREASTFEEDING RECOMMENDATION: Potential Toxicity

PREGNANCY SUMMARY

No reports describing the use of vadadustat in human pregnancy have been located. The drug will probably cross the placenta, so some fetal exposure will likely occur. Therefore, the absence of human pregnancy experience prevents a complete assessment of the embryofetal risk. Animal reproduction studies did show some embryofetal toxicity in one species at doses of less than 10 times the RHD, but not in a second species. Using this drug during pregnancy should be based on the pros and cons of the mother's clinical need for treatment versus any potential fetal risk that might occur from exposure. In the clinical trials, about 14% of patients developed hypertension.

BREASTFEEDING SUMMARY

No reports describing the use of vadadustat during human lactation have been located. The drug will likely be found in human breast milk, so some infant exposure will probably occur. Due to a concern for potential serious adverse effects that might be seen in a breastfed infant, the manufacturer recommends that women not breastfeed while being treated with this drug and for at least 2 days after the last dose. Nevertheless, breastfeeding while using this drug should be based on the mother's clinical need for treatment versus any potential infant risks that might occur. If used, the infant should be monitored for the most common reported adult side effects of hypertension and diarrhea.

Reference

1. Prescribing Information. Vafseo. Akebia Therapeutics, Inc; 2024.

VALACYCLOVIR

Antiviral (Antiherpetic Virus)

PREGNANCY RECOMMENDATION: Human Data Suggest Compatible

BREASTFEEDING RECOMMENDATION: Probably Compatible

PREGNANCY SUMMARY

Over 2,000 pregnancies with valacyclovir exposure have been located. Although the experience with valacyclovir in early pregnancy is limited, many studies have reported the use of acyclovir during all stages of pregnancy (see also Acyclovir). Based on the combined data, there is no evidence of a major risk to the human fetus from valacyclovir or acyclovir. Valacyclovir and its active metabolite, acyclovir, cross the placenta. Animal data did not show any embryofetal toxicity in two species receiving doses less than 10 times the RHD. Using this drug during pregnancy should be based on the pros and cons of the mother's clinical need for treatment versus any potential fetal risk that might occur from exposure. First-trimester primary herpes infection is associated with neonatal chorioretinitis, microcephaly, and skin lesions. For the management of herpes in pregnancy, ACOG recommends either valacyclovir or acyclovir for primary or first-episode infections, symptomatic recurrent episodes, and daily suppression (from 36 weeks until delivery). However, only acyclovir is recommended for severe or disseminated disease. Because of increased renal elimination during pregnancy, the doses for suppressive therapy are usually higher than nonpregnant women.

BREASTFEEDING SUMMARY

Valacyclovir is rapidly and nearly completely converted to acyclovir and the amino acid L-valine. Acyclovir is concentrated in human breast milk with breast milk to plasma ratios in the range of 3 to 4 (see Acyclovir). In a 2002 study, five healthy postpartum women who were breastfeeding were given valacyclovir (500 mg) twice daily for 7 days. The peak breast milk concentration occurred 4 hours after the first dose (breast milk to serum ratio of 3.4), whereas the peak serum level occurred at 2 hours. At steady state, the breast milk to serum ratio was about 1.9. The median infant urine acyclovir concentration was 0.74 mcg/mL. Twenty-four hours after the last dose, the breast milk to serum ratio was 0.25. The calculated relative infant dose (RID) was less than 1%. Acyclovir has been used to treat herpesvirus infections in the neonate, and no adverse effects have been reported when acyclovir was used during breastfeeding (see Acyclovir). Valacyclovir also appears to be compatible with breastfeeding. If used while breastfeeding, the infant should be monitored for the most common reported adult side effects of headache, nausea, and abdominal pain (all leading to irritability).

References

1. Product information. Valtrex. GlaxoSmithKline, LLC; 2022.
2. American College of Obstetricians and Gynecologists. ACOG Practice Bulletin No. 220: management of genital herpes in pregnancy. *Obstet Gynecol.* 2020;135:e193-e202.
3. Kimberlin DF, Weller S, Andrews WW, et al. Valaciclovir pharmacokinetics in late pregnancy (abstract). *Am J Obstet Gynecol.* 1998;178:S12.
4. Kimberlin DF, Weller S, Whitley RJ, et al. Pharmacokinetics of oral valacyclovir and acyclovir in late pregnancy. *Am J Obstet Gynecol.* 1998;179:846-851.
5. Acyclovir Pregnancy Registry and Valacyclovir Pregnancy Registry. *Final Study Report. 1 June 1984 through 30 April 1999.* Glaxo Wellcome; 1999.
6. Anderson R, Lundqvist A, Bergstrom T. Successful treatment of generalized primary herpes simplex type 2 infection during pregnancy. *Scand J Infect Dis.* 1999;31:201-202.
7. Sheffield JS, Hill JB, Hollier LM, et al. Valacyclovir prophylaxis to prevent recurrent herpes at delivery. *Obstet Gynecol.* 2006;108:141-147.
8. Nath AK, Thappa DM. Newer trends in the management of genital herpes. *Indian J Dermatol Venereol Leprol.* 2009;75:566-574.
9. Pasternak B, Hviid A. Use of acyclovir, valacyclovir, and famciclovir in the first trimester of pregnancy and the risk of birth defects. *JAMA.* 2010;304:859-866.
10. Mills JL, Carter TC. Acyclovir exposure and birth defects-an important advance, but more are needed. *JAMA.* 2010;304:905-906.
11. Shahar-Nissan K, Pardo J, Peled O, et al. Valaciclovir to prevent vertical transmission of cytomegalovirus after maternal primary infection during pregnancy: a randomised, double-blind, placebo-controlled trial. *Lancet.* 2020;396:779-785.
12. Zammarchi L, Lazzarotto T, Andreoni M, et al. Management of cytomegalovirus infection in pregnancy: is it time for valacyclovir? *Clin Microbiol Inf.* 2020;26:1151-1154.
13. Sheffield JS, Fish DN, Hollier LM, et al. Acyclovir concentrations in human breast milk after valaciclovir administration. *Am J Obstet Gynecol.* 2002;186:100-102.

V

VALBENAZINE

Central Nervous System (Vesicular Monoamine Transporter-2 Inhibitor)

PREGNANCY RECOMMENDATION: No Human Data—Animal Data Suggest Potential Risk

BREASTFEEDING RECOMMENDATION: Potential Toxicity

PREGNANCY SUMMARY

No reports describing the use of valbenazine in human pregnancy have been located. The drug and its active metabolite will probably cross the placenta, so fetal exposure will likely occur. However, the absence of human pregnancy experience prevents a complete assessment of embryofetal risk. Animal studies did show embryofetal toxicity. Using this drug during pregnancy should be based on the pros and cons of the mother's clinical need for treatment versus any potential fetal risk that might occur from exposure.

BREASTFEEDING SUMMARY

No reports describing the use of valbenazine during human lactation have been located. The drug and its active metabolite will probably enter breast milk, so infant exposure will likely occur. Because of the animal data, the manufacturer recommends that a woman not breastfeed while using this drug and for 5 days after the last dose. However, breastfeeding should be based on the mother's clinical need for treatment. If used, the infant should be monitored for the most common reported adult side effect of somnolence.

Reference

1. Prescribing Information. Ingrezza. Neurocrine Biosciences, Inc; 2021.

VALGANCICLOVIR

Antiviral (Anticytomegalovirus)

PREGNANCY RECOMMENDATION: Limited Human Data—Animal Data Suggest Potential Risk

BREASTFEEDING RECOMMENDATION: Potential Toxicity

PREGNANCY SUMMARY

Valganciclovir is a prodrug that is rapidly converted to ganciclovir after oral administration (See Ganciclovir). Two publications described the use of valganciclovir in pregnancy. In a case series of two patients, both infants were negative for cytomegalovirus (CMV) at birth but developed infections within the first few weeks of life. One infant was found to have slight ventricle asymmetry within the normal range and a small subependymal cyst. In the WHO VigiBase, 34 adverse pregnancy reports were located for valganciclovir. The only disproportionality signal found was an increased risk for small weight for gestational age. The malformation rate was 35% with valganciclovir, but gestational age of exposure was not provided, and most patients took concomitant medications. For ganciclovir, human pregnancy experience has not shown toxicity, but the number of cases is very limited. The animal data for ganciclovir are suggestive of embryofetal risk. Therefore, this limited human pregnancy experience prevents a complete assessment of embryofetal risk. Based on the animal studies, the manufacturer recommends that women with reproductive potential use effective contraception during treatment and for 1 month after the last dose. They also recommend that males with female partners of reproductive potential use effective contraception during treatment and for 3 months after the last dose. Nevertheless, using this drug during pregnancy should be based on the pros and cons of the mother's clinical need for treatment versus any potential fetal risk that might occur from exposure. Primary CMV infections occurring in pregnancy have a high risk of transplacental passage of the virus to the fetus. Unfortunately, some of these newborns can present with central nervous system (CNS) damage resulting in developmental delay. However, the prevention of these in utero infections by ganciclovir (valganciclovir) has not been proven.

BREASTFEEDING SUMMARY

No reports describing the use of valganciclovir during human lactation have been located. The drug will likely be excreted into breast milk, so some infant exposure will probably occur. Due to a concern for potential serious adverse effects that might be seen in a breastfed infant, the manufacturer recommends that women not breastfeed while being treated with this drug. Nevertheless, breastfeeding while using this drug should be based on the mother's clinical need for treatment versus any potential infant risks that might occur. If used, the infant should be monitored for the most common reported adult side effects of nausea and headache (both leading to irritability), diarrhea, vomiting, pyrexia, fatigue (lethargy), and tremor.

References

1. Product information. Valganciclovir hydrochloride. Aurobindo Pharma Limited; 2022.
2. Seidel V, Feiterna-Sperling C, Siedentopf JP, et al. Intrauterine therapy of cytomegalovirus infection with valganciclovir: review of the literature. *Med Microbiol Immunol*. 2017;206:347-354.
3. Contejean A, Leruez-Ville M, Treluyer JM, et al. Assessing the risk of adverse pregnancy outcomes and birth defects reporting in women exposed to ganciclovir or valganciclovir during pregnancy: a pharmacovigilance study. *J Antimicrob Chemother*. 2023;78:1265-1269.

VALPROIC ACID

Central Nervous System (Antiseizure/Antimania)

PREGNANCY RECOMMENDATION: Human Data Suggest Risk

BREASTFEEDING RECOMMENDATION: Potential Toxicity

PREGNANCY SUMMARY

Valproic acid and the salt form, sodium valproate, are human teratogens. The absolute risk of producing a child with neural tube defects (NTDs) when these agents are used between the 17th and 30th days after fertilization is 1% to 2%. A characteristic pattern of minor facial defects is apparently also associated with valproic acid. Studies have suggested that a distinct constellation of defects and fetal growth restriction may exist for infants exposed in utero to the anticonvulsant. These defects involve the head and face, digits, urogenital tract, and neurodevelopmental and physical growth. A correlation between maternal dose and major and minor anomalies has been reported. Valproic acid crosses the placenta. Women with reproductive potential who are taking valproic acid are advised to use effective contraception during treatment, especially when valproate use is considered for a condition not usually associated with permanent injury or death, such as prophylaxis of migraine headaches. Due to the risk for malformations, child cognition, and neurodevelopment disorders, the International League Against Epilepsy 2019 guidelines note that valproic acid should be avoided in the treatment of women who can become pregnant whenever possible. In 2023, ACOG recommended against the use of valproic acid as a first-line bipolar treatment, and it should be avoided in pregnancy because reasonable alternatives exist. Similarly, it is not recommended for headache prevention by the US Food and Drug Administration (FDA) and ACOG. Women who are pregnant and have taken antiseizure medications such as valproic acid at any time during pregnancy are encouraged to contact the North American Antiepileptic Drug (NAAED) Pregnancy Registry at 888-233-2334.

BREASTFEEDING SUMMARY

Valproic acid and its salt, sodium valproate, are excreted into human breast milk in low concentrations. Breast milk concentrations up to 15% of the corresponding level in the mother's serum have been measured. The manufacturer reports breast milk concentrations of 0.4 to 3.9 mcg/mL. Breastfed infants who were 3 days to 12 weeks old had blood levels of 0.7 to 4 mcg/mL, which were 1% to 6% of maternal levels. In a study of 199 children who had been breastfed while their mothers were taking a single antiepileptic drug (carbamazepine, phenytoin, lamotrigine, or valproic acid) were evaluated at 3 years of age regarding cognitive outcome. Mean adjusted intelligence quotient (IQ) scores were similar for exposed versus unexposed children. If the clinical decision is to use this drug while breastfeeding, the infant should be monitored for the most common reported adult side effects of abdominal pain, dizziness, headache, and nausea (all leading to irritability), anorexia, diarrhea, vomiting, ecchymosis, fever, peripheral edema, somnolence (fatigue), and tremor.

References

1. Product information. Valproic acid. Eywa Pharma, Inc; 2022.
2. Tomson T, Battino D, Bromley R, et al. Management of epilepsy in pregnancy: a report from the international league against epilepsy task force on women and pregnancy. *Epilepsia*. 2019;00:1-3.
3. American College of Obstetricians and Gynecologists. Treatment and management of mental health conditions during pregnancy and postpartum. Clinical Practice Guideline No. 5. *Obstet Gynecol*. 2023;141:1262-1288.
4. American College of Obstetricians and Gynecologists. Headaches in pregnancy and postpartum. Clinical Practice Guideline No. 3. *Obstet Gynecol*. 2021;139:944-972.
5. Food and Drug Administration. FDA drug safety communication: valproate anti-seizure products contraindicated for migraine prevention in pregnant women due to decreased IQ scores in exposed children. Accessed September 18, 2023. https://www.fda.gov/drugs/drug-safety-and-availability/fda-drug-safety-communication-valproate-anti-seizure-products-contraindicated-migraine-prevention
6. Alexander FW. Sodium valproate and pregnancy. *Arch Dis Child*. 1979; 54:240.
7. Dickinson RG, Harland RC, Lynn RK, et al. Transmission of valproic acid (Depakene) across the placenta: half-life of the drug in mother and baby. *J Pediatr*. 1979;94:832-835.
8. Simila S, von Wendt L, Hartikainen-Sorri A-L, et al. Sodium valproate, pregnancy, and neonatal hyperglycinaemia. *Arch Dis Child*. 1979;54:985-986.
9. Nau H, Rating D, Koch S, et al. Valproic acid and its metabolites: placental transfer, neonatal pharmacokinetics, transfer via mother's milk and clinical status in neonates of epileptic mothers. *J Pharmacol Exp Ther*. 1981;219: 768-777.
10. Froescher W, Eichelbaum M, Niesen M, et al. Antiepileptic therapy with carbamazepine and valproic acid during pregnancy and lactation period. In: Dam M, Gram L, Penry JK, eds. *Advances in Epileptology: The XIIth Epilepsy International Symposium*. Raven Press; 1981:581-588.
11. Froescher W, Niesen M, Altmann D, et al. Antiepileptika-Therapie wahrend Schwangerschaft und Geburt. In: Remschmidt H, Rentz R, Jungmann J, eds. *Epilepsie 1980*. Georg Thieme Publishers; 1981:152-163.
12. Iskizaki T, Yokochi K, Chiba K, et al. Placental transfer of anticonvulsants (phenobarbital, phenytoin, valproic acid) and the elimination from neonates. *Pediatr Pharmacol*. 1981;1:291-303.
13. Nau H, Kuhnz W, Egger H-J, et al. Anticonvulsants during pregnancy and lactation: transplacental, maternal and neonatal pharmacokinetics. *Clin Pharmacokinet*. 1982;7:508-543.
14. Kaneko S, Otani K, Fukushima Y, et al. Transplacental passage and half-life of sodium valproate in infants born to epileptic mothers. *Br J Clin Pharmacol*. 1983;15:503-506.
15. Nau H, Helge H, Luck W. Valproic acid in the perinatal period: decreased maternal serum protein binding results in fetal accumulation and neonatal displacement of the drug and some metabolites. *J Pediatr*. 1984;104:627-634.
16. Froescher W, Gugler R, Niesen M, et al. Protein binding of valproic acid in maternal and umbilical cord serum. *Epilepsia*. 1984;25:244-249.
17. Philbert A, Pedersen B, Dam M. Concentration of valproate during pregnancy, in the newborn and in breast milk. *Acta Neurol Scand*. 1985;72:460-463.
18. Nau H, Schafer H, Rating D, et al. Placental transfer and neonatal pharmacokinetics of valproic acid and some of its metabolites. In: Janz D, Bossi L, Dam M, et al, eds. *Epilepsy, Pregnancy, and the Child*. Raven Press, 1982:367-372.
19. Perucca E, Ruprah M, Richens A. Altered drug binding to serum proteins in pregnant women: therapeutic relevance. *J R Soc Med*. 1981;74:422-426.

V

20. Rating D, Jager-Roman E, Koch S, et al. Enzyme induction in neonates due to antiepileptic therapy during pregnancy. In: Janz D, Bossi L, Dam M, Helge H, Richens A, Schmidt D, eds. *Epilepsy, Pregnancy, and the Child*. Raven Press; 1982:349-355.
21. Dalens B, Raynaud EJ, Gaulme J. Teratogenicity of valproic acid. *J Pediatr*. 1980;97:332-333.
22. Gomez MR. Possible teratogenicity of valproic acid. *J Pediatr*. 1981;98: 508-509.
23. Thomas D, Buchanan N. Teratogenic effects of anticonvulsants. *J Pediatr*. 1981;99:163.
24. Weinbaum PJ, Cassidy SB, Vintzileos AM, et al. Prenatal detection of a neural tube defect after fetal exposure to valproic acid. *Obstet Gynecol*. 1986;67:31S-33S.
25. Clay SA, McVie R, Chen H. Possible teratogenic effect of valproic acid. *J Pediatr*. 1981;99:828.
26. Robert E, Guibaud P. Maternal valproic acid and congenital neural tube defects. *Lancet*. 1982;2:937.
27. Blaw ME, Woody RC. Valproic acid embryopathy? *Neurology*. 1983;33:255.
28. Bailey CJ, Pool RW, Poskitt EME, et al. Valproic acid and fetal abnormality. *Br Med J*. 1983;286:190.
29. Koch S, Jager-Roman E, Rating D, et al. Possible teratogenic effect of valproate during pregnancy. *J Pediatr*. 1983;103:1007-1008.
30. Bantz EW. Valproic acid and congenital malformations: a case report. *Clin Pediatr*. 1984;23:353-354.
31. Jager-Roman E, Deichi A, Jakob S, et al. Fetal growth, major malformations, and minor anomalies in infants born to women receiving valproic acid. *J Pediatr*. 1986;108:997-1004.
32. Shakir RA, Johnson RH, Lambie DG, et al. Comparison of sodium valproate and phenytoin as single drug treatment in epilepsy. *Epilepsia*. 1981; 22:27-33.
33. Hatjis CG, Rose JC, Pippitt C, et al. Effect of treatment with sodium valproate on plasma adrenocorticotropic hormone and cortisol concentrations in pregnancy. *Am J Obstet Gynecol*. 1985;152:315-316.
34. Product information. Depakene. Abbott Laboratories; 2000.
35. Anonymous. Teratogenic risks of antiepileptic drugs. *Br Med J*. 1981; 283;515-516.
36. Paulson GW, Paulson RR. Teratogenic effects of anticonvulsants. *Arch Neurol*. 1981;38:140-143.
37. 37 Brown NA, Kao J, Fabro S. Teratogenic potential of valproic acid. *Lancet*. 1980;1:660-661.
38. Whittle BA. Pre-clinical teratological studies on sodium valproate (Epilim) and other anticonvulsants. In: Legg NJ, ed. *Clinical and Pharmacological Aspects of Sodium Valproate (Epilim) in the Treatment of Epilepsy*. MCS Consultants; 1976:105-111.
39. Hiilesmaa VK, Bardy AH, Granstrom ML, et al. Valproic acid during pregnancy. *Lancet*. 1980;1:883.
40. Nakane Y, Okuma T, Takahashi R, et al. Multi-institutional study on the teratogenicity and fetal toxicity of antiepileptic drugs: a report of a collaborative study group in Japan. *Epilepsia*. 1980;21:663-680.
41. Jeavons PM. Non-dose-related side effects of valproate. *Epilepsia*. 1984; 25(suppl 1):S50-S55.
42. Centers for Disease Control and Prevention. Valproate: a new cause of birth defects-report from Italy and follow-up from France. *MMWR Morb Mortal Wkly Rep*. 1983;32:438-439.
43. Bossi L, Battino D, Boldi B, et al. Anthropometric data and minor malformations in newborns of epileptic mothers. In: Janz D, Bossi L, Dam M, Helge H, Richens A, Schmidt D, eds. *Epilepsy, Pregnancy, and the Child*. Raven Press; 1982:299-301.
44. American Academy of Pediatrics Committee on Drugs. Valproic acid: benefits and risks. *Pediatrics*. 1982;70:316-319.
45. Bjerkedal T, Czeizel A, Goujard J, et al. Valproic acid and spina bifida. *Lancet*. 1982;2:1096-1172.
46. Stanely OH, Chambers TL. Sodium valproate and neural tube defects. *Lancet* 1982;2:1282.
47. Jeavons PM. Sodium valproate and neural tube defects. *Lancet*. 1982; 2:1282-1283.
48. Castilla E. Valproic acid and spina bifida. *Lancet*. 1983;2:683.
49. Robert E, Rosa F. Valproate and birth defects. *Lancet*. 1983;2:1142.
50. 5-. Mastroiacovo P, Bertollini R, Morandini S, et al. Maternal epilepsy, valproate exposure, and birth defects. *Lancet*. 1983;2:1499.
51. Lindhout D, Meinardi H. Spina bifida and in-utero exposure to valproate. *Lancet*. 1984;2:396.
52. Felding I, Rane A. Congenital liver damage after treatment of mother with valproic acid and phenytoin? *Acta Paediatr Scand*. 1984;73:565-568.
53. Legius E, Jaeken J, Eggermont E. Sodium valproate, pregnancy, and infantile fatal liver failure. *Lancet*. 1987;2:1518-1519.
54. Rating D, Jager-Roman E, Koch S, et al. Minor anomalies in the offspring of epileptic parents. In: Janz D, Bossi L, Dam M, Helge H, Richens A, Schmidt D, eds. *Epilepsy, Pregnancy, and the Child*. Raven Press; 1982:283-288.
55. DiLiberti JH, Farndon PA, Dennis NR, et al. The fetal valproate syndrome. *Am J Med Genet*. 1984;19:473-481.
56. Lindhout D, Meinardi H, Barth PG. Hazards of fetal exposure to drug combinations. In: Janz D, Bossi L, Dam M, Helge H, Richens A, Schmidt D, eds. *Epilepsy, Pregnancy, and the Child*. Raven Press; 1982:275-281.
57. Koch S, Hartmann A, Jager-Roman E, et al. Major malformations in children of epileptic parents-due to epilepsy or its therapy? In: Janz D, Bossi L, Dam M, Helge H, Richens A, Schmidt D, eds. *Epilepsy, Pregnancy, and the Child*. Raven Press; 1982:313-315.
58. Ardinger HH, Atkin JF, Blackston RD, et al. Verification of the fetal valproate syndrome phenotype. *Am J Med Genet*. 1988;29:171-185.
59. Staunton H. Valproate, spina bifida, and birth defect registries. *Lancet*. 1989; 1:381.
60. Oakeshott P, Hunt GM. Valproate and spina bifida. *Br Med J*. 1989; 298:1300-1301.
61. Oakeshott P, Hunt G. Valproate and spina bifida. *Lancet*. 1989;1:611.
62. Martinez-Frias ML, Rodriguez-Pinilla E, Salvador J. Valproate and spina bifida. *Lancet*. 1989;1:611-612.
63. Carter BS, Stewart JM. Valproic acid prenatal exposure: association with lipomyelomeningocele. *Clin Pediatr*. 1989;28:81-85.
64. Boussemart T, Bonneau D, Levard G, et al. Omphalocele in a newborn baby exposed to sodium valproate in utero. *Eur J Pediatr*. 1995;154:220-221.
65. Hubert A, Bonneau D, Couet D, et al. Aplasia cutis congenita of the scalp in an infant exposed to valproic acid in utero. *Acta Paediatr*. 1994;83:789-790.
66. Centers for Disease Control and Prevention. Valproic acid and spina bifida: a preliminary report—France. *MMWR Morb Mortal Wkly Rep*. 1982;31: 565-566.
67. Lammer EJ, Sever LE, Oakley GP Jr. Teratogen update: valproic acid. *Teratology*. 1987;35:465-473.
68. Anonymous. Valproate and malformations. *Lancet*. 1982;2:1313-1314.
69. Lemire RJ. Neural tube defects. *JAMA*. 1988;259:558-562.
70. Jager-Roman E, Rating D, Koch S, et al. Somatic parameters, diseases, and psychomotor development in the offspring of epileptic parents. In: Janz D, Bossi L, Dam M, Helge H, Richens A, Schmidt D, eds. *Epilepsy, Pregnancy, and the Child*. Raven Press; 1982:425-432.
71. Jentink J, Loane MA, Dolk H, et al; EUROCAT Antiepileptic Study Working Group. Valproic acid monotherapy in pregnancy and major congenital malformations. *N Engl J Med*. 2010;362:2185-2193.
72. Granstrom M-L. Development of the children of epileptic mothers: preliminary results from the prospective Helsinki study. In: Janz D, Bossi L, Dam M, Helge H, Richens A, Schmidt D, eds. *Epilepsy, Pregnancy, and the Child*. Raven Press; 1982:403-408.
73. Clayton-Smith J, Donnai D. Fetal valproate syndrome. *J Med Genet*. 1995; 32:724-727.
74. Arpino C, Brescianini S, Robert E, et al. Teratogenic effects of antiepileptic drugs: use of an international database on malformations and drug exposure (MADRE). *Epilepsia*. 2000;41:1436-1443.
75. Rodriguez-Pinilla E, Arroyo I, Fondevilla J, et al. Prenatal exposure to valproic acid during pregnancy and limb deficiencies: a case-control study. *Am J Med Genet*. 2000;90:376-381.
76. Canger R, Battino D, Canevini MP, et al. Malformations in offspring of women with epilepsy: a prospective study. *Epilepsia*. 1999;40:1231-1236.
77. The Lamotrigine Pregnancy Registry. Final report. September 1, 1992 through March 31, 2010. GlaxoSmithKline; 2010.
78. Williams PG, Hersh JH. A male with fetal valproate syndrome and autism. *Dev Med Child Neurol*. 1997;39:632-634.
79. Christensen J, Gronborg TK, Sorensen MJ, et al. Prenatal valproate exposure and risk of autism spectrum disorders and childhood autism. *JAMA*. 2013;309:1696-703.
80. Moore SJ, Turnpenny P, Quinn A, et al. A clinical study of 57 children with fetal anticonvulsant syndromes. *J Med Genet*. 2000;37:489-497.
81. Williams G, King J, Cunningham M, et al. Fetal valproate syndrome and autism: additional evidence of an association. *Dev Med Child Neurol*. 2001;43: 202-206.
82. Ornoy A. Valproic acid in pregnancy: how much are we endangering the embryo and fetus? *Reprod Toxicol*. 2009;28:1-10.
83. Koch S, Jager-Roman E, Losche G, et al. Antiepileptic drug treatment in pregnancy: drug side effects in the neonate and neurological outcome. *Acta Paediatr*. 1996;84:739-746.

84. Meador KJ, Baker GA, Browning N, et al; NEAD Study Group. Fetal antiepileptic drug exposure and cognitive outcomes at age 6 years (NEAD study): a prospective observational study. *Lancet Neurol*. 2013;12:244-252.
85. Vajda FJ, O'Brien TJ, Hitchcock A, et al. Critical relationship between sodium valproate dose and human teratogenicity: results of the Australian register of anti-epileptic drugs in pregnancy. *J Clin Neurosci*. 2004;11:854-858.
86. Vajda FJE, Eadie MJ. Maternal valproate dosage and foetal malformations. *Acta Neurol Scand*. 2005;112:137-143.
87. Vajda FJE, Hitchcock A, Graham J, et al. Foetal malformations and seizure control: 52 months data of the Australian Pregnancy Registry. *Eur J Neurol*. 2006;13:645-654.
88. Granstrom ML, Hiilesmaa VK. Physical growth of the children of epileptic mothers: preliminary results from the prospective Helsinki study. In: Janz D, Bossi L, Dam M, Helge H, Richens A, Schmidt D, eds. *Epilepsy, Pregnancy, and the Child*. Raven Press; 1982:397-401.
89. Hurd RW, Wilder BJ, Van Rinsvelt HA. Valproate, birth defects, and zinc. *Lancet*. 1983;1:181.
90. Almgren M, Kallen B, Lavebratt C. Population-based study of antiepileptic drug exposure *in utero*-influence on head circumference in newborns. *Seizure*. 2009;18:672-675.
91. Kerr BM, Levy RH. Inhibition of epoxide hydrolase by anticonvulsants and risk of teratogenicity. *Lancet*. 1989;1:610-611.
92. Majer RV, Green PJ. Neonatal afibrinogenaemia due to sodium valproate. *Lancet*. 1987;2:740-741.
93. Swanson BN, Harland RC, Dickinson RG, et al. Excretion of valproic acid into semen of rabbits and man. *Epilepsia*. 1978;19:541-546.
94. Frew J. Valproate link to spina bifida. *Med J Aust*. 1983;1:150.
95. American Academy of Pediatrics Committee on Drugs. Valproate teratogenicity. *Pediatrics*. 1983;71:980.
96. Bardy AH, Granstrom ML, Hiilesmaa VK. Valproic acid and breast-feeding. In: Janz D, Bossi L, Dam M, Helge H, Richens A, Schmidt D, eds. *Epilepsy, Pregnancy, and the Child*. Raven Press; 1982:359-360.
97. Wisner KL, Perel JM. Serum levels of valproate and carbamazepine in breast-feeding mother-infant pairs. *J Clin Psychopharmacol*. 1998;18:167-169.
98. Stahl MMS, Neiderud J, Vinge E. Thrombocytopenic purpura and anemia in a breast-fed infant whose mother was treated with valproic acid. *J Pediatr*. 1997;130:1001-1003.
99. Meador KJ, Baker GA, Browning N, et al; NEAD Study Group. Effects of breastfeeding in children of women taking antiepileptic drugs. *Neurology*. 2010;75:1954-1960.

VALRUBICIN

Antineoplastic (Anthracycline)

PREGNANCY RECOMMENDATION: No Human Data and No Relevant Animal Data

BREASTFEEDING RECOMMENDATION: Probably Compatible (With Bladder Intact)

PREGNANCY SUMMARY

No reports describing the use of valrubicin in human pregnancy have been located. Only nanogram quantities of valrubicin are absorbed into the systemic circulation from the bladder, and valrubicin metabolites have been measured in blood. If valrubicin reaches the systemic circulation, it will likely cross the placenta. The animal data resulted in embryofetal toxicity, including malformations in one species at doses of about 0.2 times the RHD, but the drug was given intravenously (IV) on a daily basis, and systemic concentrations were not provided. However, the systemic levels in these animals had to be much higher than those seen in humans, that only have absorption from the bladder wall. Thus, these results are not relevant to human exposure. However, the absence of human pregnancy experience prevents a complete assessment of embryofetal risk. Based on animal studies and the drug's mechanism of action, the manufacturer recommends that women with reproductive potential use effective contraception during treatment and for 6 months after the last dose. They also recommend that males with female partners of reproductive potential use effective contraception during treatment and for 3 months after the last dose. Nevertheless, using this drug during pregnancy should be based on the pros and cons of the mother's clinical need for treatment versus any potential fetal risk that might occur from exposure. If indicated and the bladder wall is intact, the drug should probably not be withheld just because of pregnancy. There is a registry for women who are pregnant and have cancer. For more information, women and health care providers are encouraged to contact the Cancer and Pregnancy Registry at 1-877-635-4499.

BREASTFEEDING SUMMARY

No reports describing the use of valrubicin during human lactation have been located. The drug, if it reaches the systemic circulation, will probably be excreted into breast milk, so some infant exposure may occur. However, due to low systemic absorption levels, the amount is likely to be minimal. Breastfeeding while using this drug should be based on the mother's clinical need for treatment versus any potential infant risks that might occur. If used, the infant should be monitored for the most common reported adult side effects of abdominal pain and nausea (both leading to irritability).

Reference

1. Product information. Valrubicin intravesical solution. Hikma Pharmaceuticals USA, Inc; 2022.

V

VALSARTAN

Antihypertensive (Angiotensin II Receptor Blocker)

PREGNANCY RECOMMENDATION: Human Data Suggest Risk (Second & Third Trimesters)

BREASTFEEDING RECOMMENDATION: Probably Compatible

PREGNANCY SUMMARY

Valsartan use during the second half of pregnancy is associated with fetal toxic effects of fetal renal dysfunction leading to anuria and oligohydramnios. The decrease in amniotic fluid can lead to fetal limb contractures, craniofacial deformation, and pulmonary hypoplasia. However, this finding is not absolute, and, in some cases, fetal renal function and amniotic fluid volume can return to normal with discontinuation of the drug. A few studies have also suggested a possible increased risk for birth defects with first-trimester use, but most large studies have not confirmed this finding. Valsartan carries a boxed warning for use in pregnancy, and the manufacturer recommends discontinuing the medication as soon as a pregnancy is detected. Valsartan is likely to cross the placenta, so some fetal exposure will probably occur. Animal studies did not show any embryofetal toxicity in two species at doses of 9 times or more than the RHD. Hypertension in pregnancy is associated with numerous obstetrical complications, and therefore, good blood pressure control is recommended. However, a suitable antihypertensive medication alternative can probably be identified.

BREASTFEEDING SUMMARY

No reports describing the use of valsartan during human lactation have been located. The drug will likely be excreted into breast milk, so some infant exposure will probably occur. Breastfeeding while using this drug should be based on the mother's clinical need for treatment versus any potential infant risks that might occur. If used, the infant should be monitored for the most common reported adult side effects of headache, dizziness, abdominal pain, arthralgia, and back pain (all leading to irritability), fatigue (lethargy), hypotension, and hyperkalemia.

References

1. Product information. Valsartan. Alembic Pharmaceuticals, Inc; 2021.
2. Briggs GG, Nageotte MP. Fatal fetal outcome with the combined use of valsartan and atenolol. *Ann Pharmacother*. 2001;35:859-861.
3. Chung NA, Lip GYH, Beevers M, et al. Angiotensin-II-receptor inhibitors in pregnancy. *Lancet*. 2001;357:1620-1621.
4. Martinovic J, Benachi A, Laurent N, et al. Fetal toxic effects and angiotensin-II-receptor antagonists. *Lancet*. 2001;358:241-242.
5. Berkane N, Carlier P, Verstraete L, et al. Fetal toxicity of valsartan and possible reversible adverse side effects. *Birth Defects Res A Clin Mol Teratol*. 2004;70:547-549.
6. Schaefer C. Angiotensin II-receptor-antagonists: further evidence of fetotoxicity but not teratogenicity. *Birth Defects Res A Clin Mol Teratol*. 2003;67:591-594.
7. Bos-Thompson MA, Hillaire-Buys D, Muller F, et al. Fetal toxic effects of angiotensin II receptor antagonists: case report and follow-up after birth. *Ann Pharmacother*. 2005;39:157-161.
8. Vendemmia M, Garcia-Meric P, Rizzotti A, et al. Fetal and neonatal consequences of antenatal exposure to type 1 angiotensin II receptor-antagonists. *J Matern Fetal Neonatal Med*. 2005;19:137-140.
9. Velazquez-Armenta EY, Han JY, Choi JS, et al. Angiotensin II receptor blockers in pregnancy: a case report and systematic review of the literature. *Hypertens Pregnancy*. 2007;26:51-66.
10. Polifka JE. Is there an embryopathy associated with first-trimester exposure to angiotensin-converting enzyme inhibitors and angiotensin receptor antagonists? A critical review of the evidence. *Birth Defects Res A Clin Mol Teratol*. 2012;94:576-598.
11. Hoeltzenbein M, Tissen-Diabate T, Fietz AK, et al. Pregnancy outcome after first trimester use of angiotensin AT1 receptor blockers: an observational cohort study. *Clin Res Cardiol*. 2018;107:679-687.

VAMOROLONE

Corticosteroid

PREGNANCY RECOMMENDATION: No Human Data and No Relevant Animal Data (Maternal Benefit May Outweigh Any Embryofetal Risk)

BREASTFEEDING RECOMMENDATION: Potential Toxicity

PREGNANCY SUMMARY

No reports describing the use of vamorolone in human pregnancy have been located. The drug will probably cross the placenta, so some fetal exposure will likely occur. Therefore, the absence of human pregnancy experience prevents a complete assessment of the embryofetal risk. Some studies have suggested that corticosteroid use in the first trimester can increase the risk for cleft lip and palate (CLP). However, this risk has not been found in other analyses. Animal reproduction and fertility studies have not been conducted. Duchenne muscular dystrophy (DMD) is primarily seen in males (X-linked recessive genetic disorder). Females with severe DMD who are of reproductive age potential are exceedingly rare. Using this drug during pregnancy should be based on the pros and cons of the mother's clinical need for treatment versus any potential fetal risk that might occur from exposure. In the clinical trials, vamorolone (consistent with other corticosteroids) was associated with producing hyperglycemia.

BREASTFEEDING SUMMARY

No reports describing the use of vamorolone during human lactation have been located. The drug will likely be found in human breast milk, so some infant exposure will probably occur. Breastfeeding while using this drug should be based on the mother's clinical need for treatment versus any potential infant risks that might occur. If used, the infant should be monitored for the most common reported adult side effects of irritability and vomiting.

Reference

1. Prescribing Information. Agamree. Santhera Pharmaceuticals, Ltd; 2023.

VANCOMYCIN

Antibiotic (Glycopeptide)

PREGNANCY RECOMMENDATION: Limited Human Data—Animal Data Suggest Low Risk

BREASTFEEDING RECOMMENDATION: Probably Compatible

PREGNANCY SUMMARY

Vancomycin has been used in over 50 pregnant patients in the published literature, and no adverse fetal/neonatal findings were reported. Vancomycin has been shown to cross the placenta at term, so some fetal exposure will occur. However, this limited human pregnancy experience prevents a complete assessment of the embryofetal risk. Animal data did not show any embryofetal toxicity in two species receiving doses at about equal to the RHD. Using this drug during pregnancy should be based on the pros and cons of the mother's clinical need for treatment versus any potential fetal risk that might occur from exposure.

BREASTFEEDING SUMMARY

Vancomycin is excreted into human breast milk. In one woman treated with IV vancomycin (dosage 2 g/d), the breast milk level 4 hours after a dose was 12.7 mcg/mL. This value was nearly identical to the maternal serum trough concentration. Regardless, vancomycin is poorly absorbed from the gastrointestinal tract, and thus, systemic absorption by the infant is likely to be negligible. However, one potential problem that could exist for a nursing infant would be modification of bowel flora.

References

1. Product information. Vancomycin hydrochloride. BluePoint Laboratories; 2022.
2. Product information. Firvanq. Azurity Pharmaceuticals; 2023.
3. Lexi-Comp, Inc. (Lexi-drugs). Lexi-Comp, Inc; 2023.
4. Bourget P, Fernandez H, Delouis C, et al. Transplacental passage of vancomycin during the second trimester of pregnancy. *Obstet Gynecol*. 1991;78:908-911.
5. Towers CV, Weitz B. Transplacental passage of vancomycin. *J Matern Fetal Neonatal Med*. 2018;31:1021-1024.
6. Laiprasert J, Klein K, Mueller BA, et al. Transplacental passage of vancomycin in noninfected term pregnant women. *Obstet Gynecol*. 2007;109:1105-1110.
7. Hill LM. Fetal distress secondary to vancomycin-induced maternal hypotension. *Am J Obstet Gynecol*. 1985;153:74-75.
8. Reyes MP, Ostrea EM Jr, Cabinian AE, et al. Vancomycin during pregnancy: does it cause hearing loss or nephrotoxicity in the infant? *Am J Obstet Gynecol*. 1989;161:977-981.
9. Gouyon JB, Petion AM. Toxicity of vancomycin during pregnancy. *Am J Obstet Gynecol*. 1990;163:1375-1376.
10. Reyes MP, Ostrea EM Jr. Toxicity of vancomycin during pregnancy. Reply. *Am J Obstet Gynecol*. 1990;163:1376.

VANDETANIB

Antineoplastic (Tyrosine Kinase Inhibitor)

PREGNANCY RECOMMENDATION: Limited Human Data—Animal Data Suggest Potential Risk

BREASTFEEDING RECOMMENDATION: Potential Toxicity

PREGNANCY SUMMARY

One report describing the use of vandetanib in human pregnancy was located. A patient with multiple endocrine neoplasia type 2B and metastatic medullary thyroid cancer took vandetanib until about 6 weeks' gestation. A healthy newborn was delivered at 34 weeks' gestation with no identified anomalies. Vandetanib is likely to cross the placenta, so some fetal exposure will probably occur. In animal studies, embryofetal toxicity with malformations was observed in one species receiving doses less than the RHD. However, the absence of human pregnancy experience prevents a complete assessment of embryofetal risk. Based on animal studies and the drug's mechanism of action, the manufacturer recommends that women with reproductive potential use effective contraception during treatment and for 4 months after the last dose. Nevertheless, using this drug during pregnancy should be based on the pros and cons of the mother's clinical need for treatment versus any potential fetal risk that might occur from exposure. Vandetanib can prolong the QT interval. Hypertension was also reported in greater than 10% of patients treated with this drug in the clinical trials. There is a registry for women who are pregnant and have cancer. For more information, women and health care providers are encouraged to contact the Cancer and Pregnancy Registry at 1-877-635-4499.

BREASTFEEDING SUMMARY

No reports describing the use of vandetanib during human lactation have been located. The drug will likely be excreted into breast milk, so some infant exposure will probably occur. The manufacturer recommends that women not breastfeed while taking vandetanib and for 4 months after the last dose. Nevertheless, breastfeeding while using this drug should be based on the mother's clinical need for treatment versus any potential infant risks that might occur. If used, the infant should be monitored for the most common reported adult side effects of nausea, headache, and abdominal pain (both leading to irritability), diarrhea, rash, hypertension, upper respiratory tract infections, and decreased appetite (monitor infant growth).

References

1. Product information. Caprelsa. Genzyme Corporation; 2024.
2. Thomas N, Glod J, Derse-Anthony C, et al. Pregnancy on vandetanib in metastatic medullary thyroid carcinoma associated with multiple endocrine neoplasia type 2B. *Clin Endocrinol*. 2018;88:754-756.

VARENICLINE

Smoking Cessation Aid (Partial Nicotine Agonist)

PREGNANCY RECOMMENDATION: Human Data Suggest Low Risk

BREASTFEEDING RECOMMENDATION: Probably Compatible

PREGNANCY SUMMARY

Over 1,500 pregnancies have reported varenicline exposure during pregnancy. Although many were preconception and/or first-trimester exposures, the duration of exposure was not reported in some publications. No increased risk for malformations was observed with first-trimester exposure. One study found an increased risk for small for gestational age birthweight compared to nonsmoking controls. Another study found a reduced risk for preterm delivery, small for gestational age, severe neonatal morbidity complications, and an Apgar score less than 7 at 5 minutes compared to smoking controls. A third study found that cessation rates during pregnancy were significantly higher for varenicline compared to nicotine replacement therapy patches. Varenicline is likely to cross the placenta, so some fetal exposure will probably occur. Animal studies did not show any embryofetal toxicity in two species receiving doses of more than 10 times the RHD. Using this drug during pregnancy should be based on the pros and cons of the mother's clinical need for treatment versus any potential fetal risk that might occur from exposure. Smoking is known to cause significant developmental toxicity (as well as toxicity in the smoker). Thus, the benefit to the woman and her pregnancy appears to outweigh the limited known risk to the embryo and/or fetus with the use of this drug. If nonpharmacologic methods for smoking cessation have failed, and the use of varenicline is indicated, it should not be withheld because of pregnancy.

BREASTFEEDING SUMMARY

No reports describing the use of varenicline during human lactation have been located. The drug will likely be excreted into breast milk, so some infant exposure will probably occur. However, smoking during breastfeeding is known to represent a significant risk to the nursing infant, as well as to the mother. Thus, the benefit to the woman and her infant appears to outweigh the unknown risk to the infant. If the clinical decision is to use this drug while breastfeeding, the infant should be monitored for the most common reported adult side effects of nausea (leading to irritability), vomiting, constipation, and flatulence.

References

1. Product information. Varenicline. Apotex Corp; 2024.
2. Harrison-Woolrych M, Paterson H, Tan M. Exposure to the smoking cessation medicine varenicline during pregnancy: a prospective nationwide cohort study. *Pharmacoepidemiol Drug Saf*. 2013;22:1086-1092.
3. Kaplan YC, Olgac Dundar N, Kasap B, Karadas B. Pregnancy outcome after varenicline exposure in the first trimester. *Case Rep Obstet Gynecol*. 2014;2014:263981.
4. Richardson JL, Stephens S, Yates LM, et al. Pregnancy outcomes after maternal varenicline use; analysis of surveillance data collected by the European Network of Teratology Information Services. *Reprod Toxicol*. 2017;67:26-34.
5. Tran DT, Preen DB, Einarsdottir K et al. Use of smoking cessation pharmacotherapies during pregnancy is not associated with increased risk of adverse pregnancy outcomes: a population-based cohort study. *BMC Med*. 2020;18:15.
6. Pedersen L, Petronis KR, Norgaard M, et al. Risk of adverse birth outcomes after maternal varenicline use: a population-based observational study in Denmark and Sweden. *Pharmacoepidemiol Drug Saf*. 2020;29:94-102.
7. Choi SK, Tran DT, Kemp-Casey A, et al. The comparative effectiveness of varenicline and nicotine patches for smoking abstinence during pregnancy: evidence from a population-based cohort study. *Nicotine Tob Res*. 2021;23:1664-1672.

VARENICLINE NASAL SPRAY

Autonomic (Cholinergic Agonist)

PREGNANCY RECOMMENDATION: No Human Data—Animal Data Suggest Low Risk

BREASTFEEDING RECOMMENDATION: Probably Compatible

PREGNANCY SUMMARY

No reports describing the use of varenicline nasal spray in human pregnancy have been located. The drug will likely cross the placenta, but the low systemic absorption with nasal spray use should limit transfer. Therefore, the overall exposure is probably negligible. However, the absence of human pregnancy experience prevents a complete assessment of embryofetal risk. Animal data did not show any embryofetal toxicity in two species at doses of more than 10 times the maximum recommended human dose (MRHD). Using this drug during pregnancy should be based on the pros and cons of the mother's clinical need for treatment versus any potential fetal risk that might occur from exposure.

BREASTFEEDING SUMMARY

No reports describing the use of varenicline nasal spray during human lactation have been located. The drug may be found in human breast milk, but the low systemic absorption after nasal administration should limit excretion. Overall exposure to an infant through breast milk is likely to be negligible. Breastfeeding while using this drug should be based on the mother's clinical need for treatment versus any potential infant risks that might occur. If used, the infant should be monitored for adverse effects. However, because the product is a nasal spray, systemic side effects were not analyzed.

Reference

1. Product information. Tyrvaya. Oyster Point Pharma; 2024.

VASOPRESSIN

Cardiovascular (Antidiuretic Hormone Analogue)

PREGNANCY RECOMMENDATION: Limited Human Data—No Relevant Animal Data (Maternal Benefit Probably Outweighs Any Potential Fetal Risk)

BREASTFEEDING RECOMMENDATION: Probably Compatible

PREGNANCY SUMMARY

No reports linking the use of vasopressin with congenital defects have been located. The manufacturer notes that it may cause uterine contractions. Vasopressin and the structurally related synthetic polypeptide desmopressin have been used during pregnancy to treat diabetes insipidus (see Desmopressin). Vasopressin likely has limited passage across the placenta due to its very short elimination half-life (≤10 minutes). No animal reproduction studies have been conducted. However, this limited human pregnancy experience prevents a complete assessment of embryofetal risk. Using this drug during pregnancy should be based on the pros and cons of the mother's clinical need for treatment versus any potential fetal risk that might occur from exposure.

BREASTFEEDING SUMMARY

No reports describing the use of vasopressin during human lactation have been located. Experimental work in lactating women suggests that suckling almost doubles the maternal blood concentration of vasopressin. Vasopressin may be found in breast milk, so some infant exposure is possible. However, due to the very short elimination half-life (≤10 minutes) and the fact that it is a peptide of nine amino acids, the amount of drug absorbed from the infant's gastrointestinal tract is likely to be clinically insignificant. In addition, the approved use for the drug suggests that it should not be withheld in a postpartum woman due to breastfeeding. If the clinical decision is to use this drug while breastfeeding, the infant should be monitored for the most common reported adult side effects of decreased cardiac output, bradycardia, tachyarrhythmias, hyponatremia, and ischemia.

References

1. Product information. Vasopressin. Amneal Pharmaceuticals, LLC; 2023.
2. Hime MC, Richardson JA. Diabetes insipidus and pregnancy. *Obstet Gynecol Surv*. 1978;33:375-379.
3. Hadi HA, Mashini IS, Devoe LD. Diabetes insipidus during pregnancy complicated by preeclampsia. A case report. *J Reprod Med*. 1985;30:206-208.
4. Phelan JP, Guay AT, Newman C. Diabetes insipidus in pregnancy: a case review. *Am J Obstet Gynecol*. 1978;130:365-366.
5. van der Wildt B, Drayer JIM, Eske TKAB. Diabetes insipidus in pregnancy as a first sign of a craniopharyngioma. *Eur J Obstet Gynecol Reprod Biol*. 1980;10:269-274.

6. Ford SM Jr. Transient vasopressin-resistant diabetes insipidus of pregnancy. *Obstet Gynecol*. 1986;68:288-289.
7. Ford SM Jr, Lumpkin HL III. Transient vasopressin-resistant diabetes insipidus of pregnancy. *Obstet Gynecol*. 1986;68:726-728.
8. Rubens R, Thiery M. Case report: diabetes insipidus and pregnancy. *Eur J Obstet Gynecol Reprod Biol*. 1987;26:265-270.
9. Hughes JM, Barron WM, Vance ML. Recurrent diabetes insipidus associated with pregnancy: pathophysiology and therapy. *Obstet Gynecol*. 1989;73:462-464.
10. Goolsby L, Harlass F. Central diabetes insipidus: a complication of ventriculoperitoneal shunt malfunction during pregnancy. *Am J Obstet Gynecol*. 1996;174:1655-1657.
11. Stubbe E. Pregnancies in diabetes insipidus. *Geburtsh und Frauenheilk*. 1994;54:111-113.
12. Swanbeck J, Baxi L, Hurlet AM. DDAVP in the management of Von Willebrand's disease in pregnancy (abstract). *Am J Obstet Gynecol*. 1992;166:427.
13. Robinson KW, Hawker RW, Robertson PA. Antidiuretic hormone (ADH) in the human female. *J Clin Endocrinol Metab*. 1957;17:320-322.
14. Oravec D, Lichardus B. Management of diabetes insipidus in pregnancy. *Br Med J*. 1972;4:114-115.
15. Gaffney PR, Jenkins DM. Vasopressin: mediator of the clinical signs of fetal distress. *Br J Obstet Gynaecol*. 1983;90:987.

VECURONIUM

Miscellaneous (Neuromuscular Blocker Agent, Nondepolarizing)

PREGNANCY RECOMMENDATION: Limited Human Data—No Relevant Animal Data

BREASTFEEDING RECOMMENDATION: Probably Compatible

PREGNANCY SUMMARY

Over 40 obstetric patients have used vecuronium in the third trimester or as adjunct therapy during gamete intrafallopian transfer (GIFT) procedures. Additionally, it has been used in the second and third trimesters by direct IV and IM fetal dosing to produce paralysis during various procedures. No adverse effects attributable to vecuronium on pregnancy rates, the fetus, or the newborn have been reported in these studies. Small amounts of vecuronium cross the placenta. Based on a lack of information regarding embryo risk from exposure to vecuronium during organogenesis, the teratogenicity potential cannot be determined. Use in the latter half of gestation, however, appears to carry little, if any, risk to the fetus or newborn. However, this limited human pregnancy experience prevents a complete assessment of embryofetal risk. No animal reproduction studies have been conducted. Using this drug during pregnancy should be based on the pros and cons of the mother's clinical need for treatment versus any potential fetal risk that might occur from exposure. The manufacturer also notes that magnesium sulfate, which is often used for preeclampsia management, may enhance the neuromuscular blockade of vecuronium.

BREASTFEEDING SUMMARY

No reports describing the use of vecuronium during human lactation have been located. However, even if such use was reported, it is doubtful if clinically significant amounts of vecuronium would be excreted into breast milk. In theory, if the drug were to be found in the maternal vascular system, some vecuronium could be found in breast milk. However, for a lactating woman, its use would primarily be as an adjunct to endotracheal intubation for general anesthesia. Therefore, once the procedure is complete, vecuronium would be gone from the mother's system due to the very short elimination half-life (~ 4 minutes). This suggests that vecuronium represents no risk to a breastfeeding infant. If the clinical decision is to use this drug while breastfeeding, the infant should be monitored for the most common reported adult side effects of prolonged pharmacological action, producing skeletal muscle weakness or apnea.

References

1. Product information. Vecuronium. Hikma Pharmaceuticals USA, Inc; 2019.
2. Guay J, Grenier Y, Varin F. Clinical pharmacokinetics of neuromuscular relaxants in pregnancy. *Clin Pharmacokinet*. 1998;483-496.
3. Demetriou M, Depoix JP, Diakite B, et al. Placental transfer of ORG NC45 in women undergoing caesarean section. *Br J Anaesth*. 1982;54:643-645.
4. Dailey PA, Fisher DM, Shnider SM, et al. Pharmacokinetics, placental transfer, and neonatal effects of vecuronium (ORG NC45) administered prior to delivery (abstract). *Anesthesiology*. 1982;57:A391.
5. Dailey PA, Fisher DM, Shnider SM, et al. Pharmacokinetics, placental transfer, and neonatal effects of vecuronium and pancuronium administered during cesarean section. *Anesthesiology*. 1984;60:569-574.
6. Hawkins JL, Johnson TD, Kubicek MA, et al. Vecuronium for rapid-sequence intubation for cesarean section. *Anesth Analg*. 1990;71:185-190.
7. Iwama H, Kaneko T, Tobishima S, et al. Time dependency of the ratio of umbilical vein/maternal artery concentrations of vecuronium in caesarean section. *Acta Anaesthesiol Scand*. 1999;43:9-12.
8. Baraka A, Jabbour S, Tabboush Z, et al. Onset of vecuronium neuromuscular block is more rapid in patients undergoing caesarean section. *Can J Anaesth*. 1992;39:135-138.
9. Teviotdale BM. Vecuronium-thiopentone induction for emergency caesarean section under general anaesthesia. *Anaesth Intensive Care*. 1993;21:288-291.
10. Brimacombe J, Berry A. Vecuronium for emergency caesarean section. *Anaesth Intensive Care*. 1994;22:119.
11. Das S, Bhattacharjee M, Maitra S. Study of neonatal status after use of vecuronium as a muscle relaxant in caesarean section. *J Indian Med Assoc*. 1993;91:54-56.
12. Pierce ET, Smalky M, Alper MM, et al. Comparison of pregnancy rates following gamete intrafallopian transfer (GIFT) under general anesthesia with thiopental sodium or propofol. *J Clin Anesth*. 1992;4:394-398.
13. Baraka A, Noueihed R, Sinno H, et al. Succinylcholine-vecuronium (ORG NC 45) sequence for cesarean section. *Anesth Analg*. 1983;62:909-913.
14. Daffos F, Forestier F, MacAleese J, et al. Fetal curarization for prenatal magnetic resonance imaging. *Prenat Diagn*. 1988;8:312-314.
15. Rowbottom SJ, Gin T, Cheung LP. General anaesthesia for caesarean section in a patient with uncorrected complex cyanotic heart disease. *Anaesth Intensive Care*. 1994;22:74-78.

16. Liu SS, Forrester RM, Murphy GS, et al. Anaesthetic management of a parturient with myocardial infarction related to cocaine use. *Can J Anaesth*. 1992;39:858-861.
17. Lindemann R. Respiratory muscle rigidity in a preterm infant after use of fentanyl during caesarean section. *Eur J Pediatr*. 1998;157:1012-1013.
18. Leveque C, Murat I, Toubas F, et al. Fetal neuromuscular blockade with vecuronium bromide: studies during intravascular intrauterine transfusion in isoimmunized pregnancies. *Anesthesiology*. 1992;76:642-644.
19. Watson WJ, Atchison SR, Harlass FE. Comparison of pancuronium and vecuronium for fetal neuromuscular blockade during invasive procedures. *J Matern Fetal Med*. 1996;5:151-154.
20. Cherala S, Eddie D, Halpern M, et al. Priming with vecuronium in obstetrics. *Anaesthesia*. 1987;42:1021.

VEDOLIZUMAB

Immunologic (Monoclonal Antibody)

PREGNANCY RECOMMENDATION: Limited Human Data—Animal Data Suggest Low Risk

BREASTFEEDING RECOMMENDATION: Probably Compatible

PREGNANCY SUMMARY

Over 350 pregnancies have been exposed to vedolizumab. In observational cohort studies, no differences were observed between vedolizumab and patients with inflammatory bowel disease without biologic therapy control. However, a systematic review and meta-analysis found an increased risk for overall complications of preterm delivery and spontaneous abortion rates among pregnancies exposed to vedolizumab compared to unexposed. However, the control and severity of the inflammatory bowel disease were not provided. Vedolizumab crosses the placenta (consistent with being an IgG antibody), so some infant exposure will occur in the second half of gestation. However, this limited human pregnancy experience still prevents a complete assessment of embryofetal risk. Animal reproduction studies did not show any embryofetal toxicity in one species at doses of about 10 times the RHD. Using this drug during pregnancy should be based on the pros and cons of the mother's clinical need for treatment versus any potential fetal risk that might occur from exposure. Women who are pregnant and have taken vedolizumab at any time during pregnancy are encouraged to contact Takeda at 877-TAKEDA7 (877-825-3327). Uncontrolled inflammatory bowel disease is associated with increased disease activity, preterm delivery, and low birth weight in pregnancy. Therefore, maternal treatment for control will likely improve the odds for a better pregnancy outcome.

BREASTFEEDING SUMMARY

Three reports describing the use of vedolizumab during human lactation have been located. Vedolizumab is excreted into human breast milk, consistent with being an IgG antibody. Peak breast milk levels were about 0.2 to 0.5 mcg/mL, found 3 to 7 days after infusion. In one study, maternal levels were 18 mcg/mL. The calculated infant doses were about 0.02 to 0.05 mg/kg/d. However, it is known that IgG antibodies can be found in human breast milk, but are not found in the neonatal or infant circulation. Additionally, these IgG antibodies, when ingested through breastfeeding, would probably be digested in the infant's gastrointestinal tract and not be absorbed. Breastfeeding while using this drug should be based on the mother's clinical need for treatment versus any potential infant risks that might occur. If used, the infant should be monitored for the most common reported adult side effects of headache, arthralgia, nausea, pruritus, back pain, oropharyngeal pain, and pain in the extremities (all leading to irritability), pyrexia, upper respiratory tract infections, fatigue (lethargy), rash, and sinusitis.

V

References

1. Product information. Entyvio. Takeda Pharmaceuticals America; 2022.
2. Flannagan E, Gibson PR, Wright EK, et al. Infliximab, adalimumab, and vedolizumab concentrations across pregnancy and vedolizumab concentrations in infants following intrauterine exposure. *Aliment Pharmacol Ther*. 2020;52:1551-1562.
3. Mitrova K, Pipek B, Bortlik M, et al. Safety of ustekinumab and vedolizumab during pregnancy-pregnancy, neonatal, and infant outcome: a prospective multicentre study. *J Crohns Colitis*. 2022;16:1808-1815.
4. Mahadevan U, Vermeire S, Lasch K, et al. Vedolizumab exposure in pregnancy: outcomes from clinical studies in inflammatory bowel disease. *Aliment Pharmacol Ther*. 2017;45:941-950.
5. Julsgaard M, Kjedlsen J, Baumgart DC. Vedolizumab safety in pregnancy and newborn outcomes. *Gut*. 2017;66:1866-1867.
6. Beaulieu DB, Ananthakrishnan AN, Martin C, et al. Use of biologic therapy by pregnant women with inflammatory bowel disease does not affect infant response to vaccines. *Clin Gastroenterol Hepatol*. 2018;16:99-105.
7. Moens A, van der Woude CJ, Julsgaard M, et al. Pregnancy outcomes in inflammatory bowel disease patients treated with vedolizumab, anti-TNF or conventional therapy: results of the European CONCEIVE study. *Ailment Pharmacol Ther*. 2020;51:129-138.
8. Bell C, Tandon P, Lentz E, et al. Systematic review and meta-analysis: safety of vedolizumab during pregnancy in patients with inflammatory bowel disease. *J Gastroenterol Hepatol*. 2021;36:2640-2648.
9. Lahat A, Shitrit AB, Naftali T, et al. Vedolizumab levels in breast milk or nursing mothers with inflammatory bowel disease. *J Crohns Colitis*. 2018;12:120-123.
10. Julsgaard M, Kjedlsen J, Bibby BM, et al. Vedolizumab concentrations in the breast milk of nursing mothers with inflammatory bowel disease. *Gastroenterology*. 2018;154:752-754.

VELAGLUCERASE ALFA

Genetic (Enzyme)

PREGNANCY RECOMMENDATION: Limited Human Data—Animal Data Suggest Low Risk (Maternal Benefit May Outweigh Any Embryofetal Risk)

BREASTFEEDING RECOMMENDATION: Probably Compatible

PREGNANCY SUMMARY

The limited human pregnancy reports describing exposure to velaglucerase alfa for Gaucher disease do not suggest any embryofetal risk. Moreover, the limited information available with a similar enzyme-replacement therapy, imiglucerase, also does not suggest risk. Velaglucerase alfa is likely to have limited placental passage. However, this limited human pregnancy experience prevents a complete assessment of embryofetal risk. Animal reproduction studies did not show any embryofetal toxicity in two species at doses of less than 10 times the RHD. Using this drug during pregnancy should be based on the pros and cons of the mother's clinical need for treatment versus any potential fetal risk that might occur from exposure. Gaucher disease increases the risk for spontaneous abortion, thrombocytopenia, and hepatosplenomegaly. Therefore, treatment may improve the overall pregnancy outcome.

BREASTFEEDING SUMMARY

No reports describing the use of velaglucerase alfa during human lactation have been located. A limited amount of the drug may be found in human breast milk. The manufacturer notes that endogenous β-glucocerebrosidase is found in human breast milk. Regardless, the glycoprotein will probably be destroyed in the infant's gastrointestinal tract and not be absorbed. Breastfeeding while using this drug should be based on the mother's clinical need for treatment versus any potential infant risks that might occur. If used, the infant should be monitored for the most common reported adult side effects of headache, dizziness, abdominal pain, nausea, back pain, and joint pain (all leading to irritability), prolonged activated partial thromboplastin time (PTT), fatigue (lethargy), and pyrexia.

References

1. Product information. VPRIV, Takeda Pharmaceuticals American; 2021.
2. Elstein D, Hughes D, Goker-Alpan O, et al. Outcome of pregnancies in women receiving velaglucerase alfa for Gaucher disease. *J Obstet Gynaecol Res*. 2014;40:968-975.
3. Lau H, Belmatoug N, Deegan P, et al. Reported outcomes of 453 pregnancies in patients with Gaucher disease: an analysis from the Gaucher outcome survey. *Blood Cells Mol Dis*. 2018;68:226-231.
4. Zimran A, Morris E, Mengel E, et al. The female Gaucher patient: the impact of enzyme replacement therapy around key reproductive events (menstruation, pregnancy and menopause). *Blood Cells Mol Dis*. 2009;43:264-288.
5. Granovsky-Grisaru S, Belmatoug N, vom Dahl S, et al. The management of pregnancy in Gaucher disease. *Eur J Obstet Gynecol Reprod Biol*. 2011; 156:3-8.

VELMANASE ALFA

Genetic (Enzyme)

PREGNANCY RECOMMENDATION: No Human Data—Animal Data Suggest Risk

BREASTFEEDING RECOMMENDATION: Probably Compatible

PREGNANCY SUMMARY

No reports describing the use of velmanase alfa in human pregnancy have been located. The drug is not likely to cross the placenta; however, because it consists of a protein, it is not known whether some fetal exposure could occur. Therefore, the absence of human pregnancy experience prevents a complete assessment of the embryofetal risk. Animal studies did show embryofetal toxicity with malformations. Based on these animal studies, the manufacturer recommends that women with reproductive potential use effective contraception during treatment and for 14 days after the last dose.

BREASTFEEDING SUMMARY

No reports describing the use of velmanase alfa during human lactation have been located. The drug most likely will not appear in breast milk. Furthermore, because it is an enzyme, if any drug were to be present in breast milk, it would most likely be digested in the infant's gastrointestinal tract and not be absorbed. Breastfeeding while using this drug should be based on the mother's clinical need for treatment. If used, the infant should be monitored for the most common reported adult side effects of headache and arthralgias (both leading to irritability), and pyrexia.

Reference

1. Prescribing Information. Lamzede. Chiesi Farmaceutici S.p.A; 2023.

VEMURAFENIB

Antineoplastic (BRAF Kinase Inhibitor)

PREGNANCY RECOMMENDATION: Limited Human Data—Animal Data Suggest Low Risk (but at Low Doses)

BREASTFEEDING RECOMMENDATION: Potential Toxicity

PREGNANCY SUMMARY

Three case reports have described the use of vemurafenib during the second half of pregnancy. No adverse effects related to the drug were described. The drug has been shown to cross the placenta, so infant exposure will occur. However, this limited human pregnancy experience prevents a complete assessment of embryofetal risk. Animal data did not show any embryofetal toxicity in two species, but at doses of less than or equal to adult dosing. Based on the drug's mechanism of action, the manufacturer recommends that women with reproductive potential use effective contraception during treatment and for 2 weeks after the last dose. Nevertheless, using this drug during pregnancy should be based on the pros and cons of the mother's clinical need for treatment versus any potential fetal risk that might occur from exposure. Women who are pregnant and have cancer are encouraged to contact the Cancer and Pregnancy Registry at 877-635-4499. Hypertension was reported in up to 36% of patients treated with this drug in the clinical trials. Vemurafenib has also been shown to prolong the QTc interval.

BREASTFEEDING SUMMARY

No reports describing the use of vemurafenib during human lactation have been located. The drug will likely be excreted into breast milk, so some infant exposure will probably occur. Due to a concern for potential serious adverse effects that might be seen in a breastfed infant, the manufacturer recommends that women not breastfeed while being treated with this drug. Nevertheless, breastfeeding while using this drug should be based on the mother's clinical need for treatment versus any potential infant risks that might occur. If used, the infant should be monitored for the most common reported adult side effects of arthralgia, nausea, and pruritus (all leading to irritability), rash, alopecia, fatigue (lethargy), and photosensitivity.

References

1. Product information. Zelboraf. Genentech; 2020.
2. Maleka A, Enblad G, Sjörs G, Lindqvist A, Ullenhag GJ. Treatment of metastatic malignant melanoma with vemurafenib during pregnancy. *J Clin Oncol*. 2013;31:e192-e193.
3. de Haan J, van Thienen JV, Casaer M, et al. Severe adverse reaction to vemurafenib in a pregnant woman with metastatic melanoma. *Case Rep Oncol*. 2018;11:119-124.
4. Marce D, Cornillier H, Denis C, et al. Partial response of metastatic melanoma to BRAF-inhibitor-monotherapy in a pregnant patient with no fetal toxicity. *Melanoma Res*. 2019;29:446-447.

VENETOCLAX

Antineoplastic (BCL-2 Inhibitor)

PREGNANCY RECOMMENDATION: No Human Data—Animal Data Suggest Potential Risk

BREASTFEEDING RECOMMENDATION: Potential Toxicity

PREGNANCY SUMMARY

No reports describing the use of venetoclax in human pregnancy have been located. Some amount of the drug will probably cross the placenta, so some fetal exposure will likely occur. Therefore, the absence of human pregnancy experience prevents a complete assessment of the embryofetal risk. Embryofetal toxicity was observed in animal studies. Due to the findings from animal studies and the drug's mechanism of action, the manufacturer recommends that women with reproductive potential use effective contraception during treatment and for at least 30 days after the last dose. Nevertheless, using this drug during pregnancy should be based on the pros and cons of the mother's clinical need for treatment versus any potential fetal risk that might occur from exposure.

BREASTFEEDING SUMMARY

No reports describing the use of venetoclax during human lactation have been located. The drug will probably appear in breast milk, so some infant exposure will likely occur. However, due to the concern for potential serious adverse effects that might be seen in a breastfed infant, the manufacturer recommends that women not breastfeed while being treated with venetoclax and for at least 1 week after the last dose. Nevertheless, breastfeeding while using this drug should be based on the mother's clinical need for treatment. If used, the infant should be monitored for the most common reported adult side effects of nausea and musculoskeletal pain (both leading to irritability), diarrhea, lethargy, vomiting, constipation, cough, rash, and various laboratory abnormalities (see Prescribing Information [PI]).

Reference

1. Prescribing Information. Venclexta. AbbVie, Inc; 2022.

VENLAFAXINE

Mental Health (SNRI)

PREGNANCY RECOMMENDATION: Human Data Suggest Compatible (First Trimester) / Human Data Suggest Potential Risk (Third Trimester)

BREASTFEEDING RECOMMENDATION: Potential Toxicity

PREGNANCY SUMMARY

There are several publications describing the use of venlafaxine in human pregnancy. A recent systematic review found that first-trimester use of venlafaxine (n = 3,186) did not increase the risk for major congenital malformations. However, ACOG states that use of antidepressants, including venlafaxine, during pregnancy increases the risk for persistent pulmonary hypertension and transient neonatal adaption syndrome when used near delivery. Venlafaxine and its active metabolite (*O*-desmethylvenlafaxine) cross the placenta, so fetal exposure will occur. Animal data found embryofetal toxicity in one of two tested species with doses less than 5 times the RHD. Using this drug during pregnancy should be based on the pros and cons of the mother's clinical need for treatment versus any potential fetal risk that might occur from exposure. There is a pregnancy exposure registry that monitors pregnancy outcomes in women exposed to antidepressants during pregnancy. For more information, health care providers or patients are encouraged to contact the National Pregnancy Registry for Antidepressants at 844-405-6185. The manufacturer recommends closely monitoring all antidepressant-treated patients for clinical worsening and the emergence of suicidal thoughts and behaviors. ACOG, however, states that uncontrolled and undertreated depression during pregnancy is associated with a risk for limited engagement in medical care and self-care, substance use, preterm birth, low birth weight, postpartum depression, impaired infant attachment (which carries long-term developmental effects), disrupted relationships with partner, and suicide. Additionally, untreated and undertreated mental health disorders should be considered an exposure. Pregnancy and lactation alone should not be a reason to withhold or discontinue mental health medications.

BREASTFEEDING SUMMARY

There have been 27 infants reported in the literature with exposure to venlafaxine through breast milk. Venlafaxine breast milk levels are about 3% to 8% of the maternal weight-adjusted dose. Additionally, the active metabolite, desvenlafaxine, has a RID of about 3% to 6%. However, no adverse events were reported with exposure. Breastfeeding while using this drug should be based on the mother's clinical need for treatment versus any potential infant risks that might occur. If used, the infant should be monitored for the most common reported adult side effects of nausea (leading to irritability), somnolence, sweating, decreased appetite (monitor infant growth), and constipation.

References

1. Product information. Venlafaxine. Advagen Pharma Ltd; 2023.
2. American College of Obstetricians and Gynecologists. Treatment and management of mental health conditions during pregnancy and postpartum. Clinical practice guideline No. 5. *Obstet Gynecol*. 2023;141:1262-1288.
3. Rampono J, Simmer K, Ilett KF, et al. Placental transfer of SSRI and SNRI antidepressants and effects on the neonate. *Pharmacopsychiatry*. 2009;42:95-100.
4. Ellingrod VL, Perry PJ. Venlafaxine: a heterocyclic antidepressant. *Am J Hosp Pharm*. 1994;51:3033-3046.
5. Einarson A, Fatoye B, Sarkar M, et al. Pregnancy outcome following gestational exposure to venlafaxine: a multicenter prospective controlled study. *Am J Psychiatry*. 2001;158:1728-1730.
6. Broy P, Berard A. Gestational exposure to antidepressants and the risk of spontaneous abortion: a review. *Curr Drug Deliv*. 2010;7:76-92.
7. Yaris F, Kadioglu M, Kesim M, et al. Newer antidepressants in pregnancy: prospective outcome of a case series. *Reprod Toxicol*. 2004;19:235-238.
8. Bellantuono C, Migliarese G, Gentile S. Serotonin reuptake inhibitors in pregnancy and the risk of major malformations: a systematic review. *Hum Psychopharmacol Clin Exp*. 2007;22:121-128.
9. Chambers CD, Hernandez-Diaz S, Van Marter LJ, et al. Selective serotonin-reuptake inhibitors and risk of persistent pulmonary hypertension of the newborn. *N Engl J Med*. 2006;354:579-587.
10. Lennestal R, Kallen B. Delivery outcome in relation to maternal use of some recently introduced antidepressants. *J Clin Psychopharmacol*. 2007;27:607-613.
11. Einarson A, Choi J, Einarson TR, et al. Incidence of major malformations in infants following antidepressant exposure in pregnancy: results of a large prospective cohort study. *Can J Psychiatry*. 2009;54:242-246.
12. Berard A, Zhao JP, Sheehy O. Antidepressant use during pregnancy and the risk of major congenital malformations in a cohort of depressed pregnant women: an updated analysis of the Quebec Pregnancy Cohort. *BMJ Open*. 2017;7:e013372.
13. Berard A, Sheehy O, Zhao JP, et al. SSRI and SNRI use during pregnancy and the risk of persistent pulmonary hypertension of the newborn. *Br J Clin Pharmacol*. 2017;83:1126-1133.
14. Lassen D, Ennis ZN, Damkier P. First-trimester pregnancy exposure to venlafaxine or duloxetine and risk of major congenital malformations: a systematic review. *Basic Clin Pharmacol Toxicol*. 2016;118:32-36.
15. Moses-Kolko EL, Bogen D, Perel J, et al. Neonatal signs after late in utero exposure to serotonin reuptake inhibitors. Literature review and implications for clinical applications. *JAMA*. 2005;293:2372-2383.
16. Levinson-Castiel R, Merlob P, Linder N, et al. Neonatal abstinence syndrome after in utero exposure to selective serotonin reuptake inhibitors in term infants. *Arch Pediatr Adoles Med*. 2006;160:173-176.

17. Koren G, Moretti M, Kapur B. Can venlafaxine in breast milk attenuate the norepinephrine and serotonin reuptake neonatal withdrawal syndrome? *J Obstet Gynaecol Can*. 2006;28:299-302.
18. Pakalapati RK, Bolisetty S, Austin MP, et al. Neonatal seizures from in utero venlafaxine exposure. *J Paediatr Child Health*. 2006;42:737-738.
19. Ferreira E, Carceller AM, Agogue C, et al. Effects of selective serotonin reuptake inhibitors and venlafaxine during pregnancy in term and preterm neonates. *Pediatrics*. 2007;119:52-59.
20. Ilett KF, Hackett LP, Dusci LJ, et al. Distribution and excretion of venlafaxine and O-desmethylvenlafaxine in human milk. *Br J Clin Pharmacol*. 1998;45:459-462.
21. Hendrick V, Altshuler L, Wertheimer A, Dunn WA. Venlafaxine and breast-feeding. *Am J Psychiatry*. 2001;158:2089-2090.
22. Berle JO, Steen VM, Aamo TO, et al. Breastfeeding during maternal antidepressant treatment with serotonin reuptake inhibitors: infant exposure, clinical symptoms, and cytochrome P450 genotypes. *J Clin Psychiatry*. 2004;65:1228-1234.
23. Ilett KF, Kristensen JH, Hackett LP, et al. Distribution of venlafaxine and its O-desmethyl metabolite in human milk and their effects in breastfed infants. *Br J Clin Pharmacol*. 2002;53:17-22.
24. Newport DJ, Ritchie JC, Knight BT, et al. Venlafaxine in human breast milk and nursing infant plasma: determination of exposure. *J Clin Psychiatry*. 2009;70:1304-1310.
25. Preskorn S, Patroneva A, Silman H, et al. Comparison of the pharmacokinetics of venlafaxine extended release and desvenlafaxine in extensive and poor cytochrome P450 2D6 metabolizers. *J Clin Psychopharmacol*. 2009;29:39-43.

VERAPAMIL

Antihypertensive (Nondihydropyridine Calcium Channel Blocker)

PREGNANCY RECOMMENDATION: Limited Human Data—Animal Data Suggest Potential Risk

BREASTFEEDING RECOMMENDATION: Probably Compatible

PREGNANCY SUMMARY

Several case reports and two cohort studies have evaluated verapamil use during pregnancy. There are over 160 first-trimester exposures. It does not appear to increase the risk for malformations. One study found an increased risk for miscarriage, preterm delivery, and decreased birth weight compared to healthy controls; however, it is unclear if the authors adjusted for maternal hypertension. Verapamil has been shown to cross the placenta. However, the human pregnancy experience still prevents a complete assessment of the full embryofetal risk. In animal studies, embryofetal toxicity was observed in one species (but not in a second species) at doses of less than 10 times the RHD. Using this drug during pregnancy should be based on the pros and cons of the mother's clinical need for treatment versus any potential fetal risk that might occur from exposure. ACOG states that uncontrolled chronic hypertension has maternal risks of cerebrovascular accidents, pulmonary edema, renal insufficiency, myocardial infarction, preeclampsia, placental abruption, postpartum hemorrhage, gestational diabetes, and mortality. It has fetal risks of stillbirth or perinatal death, growth restriction, preterm birth, and congenital anomalies. For treating hypertension in pregnancy, ACOG recommends nifedipine and labetalol as first-line agents.

BREASTFEEDING SUMMARY

Three case reports describe the use of verapamil in human lactation. Verapamil and its metabolite, norverapamil, are excreted into human breast milk, and levels were up to 60% and 16% of maternal levels, respectively, with maternal doses up to 320 mg daily. Infant verapamil levels were not detectable or were at low levels. In one publication, the investigators estimated that the breastfed child received less than 0.01% of the mother's dose. Neither verapamil nor its metabolite could be detected in the plasma of the child. No adverse events were reported. The manufacturer recommends discontinuing verapamil while breastfeeding due to the potential for adverse events. Nevertheless, breastfeeding while using this drug should be based on the mother's clinical need for treatment versus any potential infant risks that might occur. If used, the infant should be monitored for the most common reported adult side effects of headache, dizziness, and myalgia (all leading to irritability), constipation, lethargy, rash, ankle edema, and sleep disturbances.

V

References

1. Product information. Verapamil hydrochloride. Teva Pharmaceuticals, Inc; 2022.
2. American College of Obstetricians and Gynecologists. Chronic hypertension in pregnancy. Practice bulletin No. 203. *Obstet Gynecol*. 2019;133:e26-e50.
3. Wolff F, Breuker KH, Schlensker KH, et al. Prenatal diagnosis and therapy of fetal heart rate anomalies: with a contribution on the placental transfer of verapamil. *J Perinat Med*. 1980;8:203-208.
4. Strigl R, Gastroph G, Hege HG, et al. Nachweis von verapamil in mutterlichen und fetalen blut des menschen. *Geburtshilfe Frauenheilkd*. 1980;40:496-499.
5. Lilja H, Karlsson K, Lindecrantz K, et al. Treatment of intrauterine supraventricular tachycardia with digoxin and verapamil. *J Perinat Med*. 1984;12:151-154.
6. Rey E, Duperron L, Gauthier R, et al. Transplacental treatment of tachycardia-induced fetal heart failure with verapamil and amiodarone: a case report. *Am J Obstet Gynecol*. 1985;153:311-312.
7. Maxwell DJ, Crawford DC, Curry PVM, et al. Obstetric importance, diagnosis, and management of fetal tachycardias. *Br Med J*. 1988;297:107-110.
8. Weiner CP, Thompson MIB. Direct treatment of fetal supraventricular tachycardia after failed transplacental therapy. *Am J Obstet Gynecol*. 1988;158:570-573.
9. Owen J, Colvin EV, Davis RO. Fetal death after successful conversion of fetal supraventricular tachycardia with digoxin and verapamil. *Am J Obstet Gynecol*. 1988;158:1169-1170.
10. Klein V, Repke JT. Supraventricular tachycardia in pregnancy: cardioversion with verapamil. *Obstet Gynecol*. 1984;63:16S-18S.
11. Brittinger WD, Schwarzbeck A, Wittenmeier KW, et al. Klinisch-Experimentelle Untersuchungen uber die Blutdruckendende Wirkung von Verapamil. *Dtsch Med Wochenschr*. 1970;95:1871-1877.
12. Mosler KH, Rosenboom HG. Neuere Moglichkeiten einer tokolytischen Behandlung in de Geburtshilfe. *Z Geburtshilfe Perinatol*. 1972;176:85-96.

13. Gummerus M. Prevention of premature birth with nylidrin and verapamil. *Z Geburtshilfe Perinatol*. 1975;179:261-266.
14. Gummerus M. Treatment of premature labor and antagonization of the side effects of tocolytic therapy with verapamil. *Z Geburtshilfe Perinatol*. 1977;181:334-340.
15. Shen O, Entebi E, Yagel S. Congenital hypertrophic cardiomyopathy associated with in utero verapamil exposure. *Prenat Diagn*. 1995;15:1088-1089.
16. Goodnick PJ. Verapamil prophylaxis in pregnant women with bipolar disorder. *Am J Psychiatry*. 1993;150:1560.
17. Magee LA, Schick B, Donnenfeld AE, et al. The safety of calcium channel blockers in human pregnancy: a prospective, multicenter cohort study. *Am J Obstet Gynecol*. 1996;174:823-828.
18. Rotmensch HH, Rotmensch S, Elkayam U. Management of cardiac arrhythmias during pregnancy: current concepts. *Drugs*. 1987;33:623-633.
19. Weber-Schoendorfer C, Hannemann D, Meister R, et al. The safety of calcium channel blockers during pregnancy: a prospective, multicenter, observational study. *Reprod Toxicol*. 2008;26:24-30.
20. Andersen HJ. Excretion of verapamil in human milk. *Eur J Clin Pharmacol*. 1983;25:279-280.
21. Inoue H, Unno N, Ou MC, et al. Level of verapamil in human milk. *Eur J Clin Pharmacol*. 1984;26:657-658.
22. Anderson P, Bondesson U, Mattiasson I, et al. Verapamil and norverapamil in plasma and breast milk during breast feeding. *Eur J Clin Pharmacol*. 1987; 31:625-627.

VERICIGUAT

Cardiovascular (Guanylate Cyclase Stimulator)

PREGNANCY RECOMMENDATION: No Human Data—Animal Data Suggest Potential Risk

BREASTFEEDING RECOMMENDATION: Potential Toxicity

PREGNANCY SUMMARY

No reports describing the use of vericiguat in human pregnancy have been located. It is likely that some amount of the drug will cross the placenta, so fetal exposure will probably occur. Therefore, the absence of human pregnancy experience prevents a complete assessment of the embryofetal risk. Embryofetal toxicity with malformations was observed in one animal species, but this was also seen with maternal toxicity. However, due to findings in the animal studies, the manufacturer recommends that women with reproductive potential use effective contraception during treatment and for 1 month after the last dose. Nevertheless, using this drug during pregnancy should be based on the pros and cons of the mother's clinical need for treatment versus any potential fetal risk that might occur from exposure. Women who are pregnant and have taken vericiguat at any time during pregnancy are encouraged to contact 877-888-4231.

BREASTFEEDING SUMMARY

No reports describing the use of vericiguat during human lactation have been located. Some amount of the drug will probably appear in breast milk, so infant exposure will likely occur. Due to the potential for serious adverse reactions that might be seen in a breastfed infant, the manufacturer recommends that women refrain from breastfeeding while taking vericiguat. Nevertheless, breastfeeding while using this drug should be based on the mother's clinical need for treatment. If used, the infant should be monitored for the most common reported adult side effects of hypotension and anemia.

Reference

1. Prescribing Information. Verquvo. Merck Sharp & Dohme; 2021.

VERTEPORFIN OPHTHALMIC

Ophthalmic (Photoenhancer)

PREGNANCY RECOMMENDATION: Limited Human Data—Animal Data Suggest Low Risk

BREASTFEEDING RECOMMENDATION: Potential Toxicity (Hold Breastfeeding)

PREGNANCY SUMMARY

Three case reports with first-trimester exposure of verteporfin ophthalmic in human pregnancy have been located. No fetal anomalies or adverse reactions to the drug were described. The drug is likely to cross the placenta, so some fetal exposure will probably occur. However, this limited human pregnancy experience prevents a complete assessment of embryofetal risk. Animal data did not show any embryofetal toxicity in two species at doses of more than 6 times the RHD. Using this drug during pregnancy should be based on the pros and cons of the mother's clinical need for treatment versus any potential fetal risk that might occur from exposure.

BREASTFEEDING SUMMARY

Verteporfin ophthalmic and its diacid metabolite are excreted into human breast milk. After a 6 mg/m^2 infusion, breast milk concentrations of the drug were 66% of the corresponding maternal plasma concentration. Verteporfin was undetectable in breast milk after 24 hours, but the metabolite was measured in breast milk up to at least 48 hours. The effect of this exposure on a nursing infant is unknown, but adverse effects affecting many organ systems are common in adults treated with IV infusions of the drug. Withholding breastfeeding for about 48 hours should lessen the exposure and potential risk of toxicity to the infant. Due to a concern for potential serious adverse effects that might be seen in a breastfed infant, the manufacturer recommends that women not breastfeed while being treated with this drug. Nevertheless, breastfeeding while using this drug should be based on the mother's clinical need for treatment versus any potential infant risks that might occur. If used, the infant should be monitored for the most common reported adult side effects of irritability.

References

1. Product information. Visudyne. Bausch Health US, LLC; 2021.
2. De Santis M, Carducci B, De Santis L, Lucchese A, Straface G. First case of post-conception verteporfin exposure: pregnancy and neonatal outcome. *Acta Ophthalmol Scand*. 2004;82:623-624.
3. Rosen E, Rubowitz A, Ferencz JR. Exposure to verteporfin and bevacizumab therapy for choroidal neovascularization secondary to punctate inner choroidopathy during pregnancy. *Eye (Lond)*. 2009;23:1479.
4. Rodrigues M, Meira D, Batista S, Carrilho MM. Accidental pregnancy exposure to verteporfin: obstetrical and neonatal outcomes: a case report. *Aust NZ J Obstet Gynaecol*. 2009;49:236-237.

VESTRONIDASE ALFA

Genetic (Lysosomal β-Glucuronidase Enzyme)

PREGNANCY RECOMMENDATION: No Human Data—Animal Data Suggest Low Risk

BREASTFEEDING RECOMMENDATION: Probably Compatible

PREGNANCY SUMMARY

No reports describing the use of vestronidase alfa in human pregnancy have been located. The drug most likely does not cross the placenta; therefore, fetal exposure is probably nonexistent or extremely limited. However, the absence of human pregnancy experience prevents a complete assessment of the embryofetal risk. Animal studies did not show embryofetal toxicity.

BREASTFEEDING SUMMARY

No reports describing the use of vestronidase alfa during human lactation have been located. The drug most likely will not appear in breast milk. Furthermore, because it is an enzyme, if any drug were to be present in breast milk, it would most likely be digested in the infant's gastrointestinal tract and not be absorbed. Breastfeeding while using this drug should be based on the mother's clinical need for treatment. If used, the infant should be monitored for the most common reported adult side effects of diarrhea, rash, peripheral swelling, and pruritus (leading to irritability).

Reference

1. Prescribing Information. Mepsevii. Ultragenyx Pharmaceutical, Inc; 2020.

VIBEGRON

Urinary (β_3-Adrenergic Agonist)

PREGNANCY RECOMMENDATION: No Human Data—Animal Data Suggest Low Risk

BREASTFEEDING RECOMMENDATION: Probably Compatible

V

PREGNANCY SUMMARY

No reports describing the use of vibegron in human pregnancy have been located. The drug probably crosses the placenta. Animal data did not show fetotoxic effects. However, the absence of human pregnancy experience prevents a complete assessment of the embryofetal risk. β_3-Adrenergic receptors are primarily found in the bladder, gallbladder, and intestines; however, cross-reactivity with other β-receptors might be postulated. In one large randomized placebo-controlled trial, no effect on ambulatory blood pressure was found. Based on drug indication, use during pregnancy is uncertain.

BREASTFEEDING SUMMARY

Vibegron probably enters breast milk. Breastfeeding while using this drug should be based on the mother's clinical need for treatment. If used, the infant should be monitored for the most common reported adult side effects of headache (leading to irritability), vomiting, and diarrhea.

Reference

1. Product Information. Gemtesa. Urovant Sciences, Inc; 2020.

VIGABATRIN

Central Nervous System (Antiseizure)

PREGNANCY RECOMMENDATION: Limited Human Data—Animal Data Suggest Risk

BREASTFEEDING RECOMMENDATION: Potential Toxicity

PREGNANCY SUMMARY

There were over 100 pregnancy exposures from a cohort trial, postmarketing experience, lamotrigine registry, and case reports. Although adverse outcomes have been described, the drug was always combined with older antiepileptic drugs known to cause structural anomalies and other forms of developmental toxicity. The contribution of vigabatrin to this toxicity has not been determined. Because the drug can cause vision loss that may be permanent in a high percentage of patients, it should be reserved for resistant cases and is only available through the REMS program. Vision abnormalities were not found in six children exposed in utero who were examined for this toxicity. Vigabatrin crosses the placenta, so fetal exposure will occur. However, this limited human pregnancy experience prevents a complete assessment of embryofetal risk. In animal studies, embryofetal toxicity with malformations was observed in two species at doses of less than 10 times the RHD. Using this drug during pregnancy should be based on the pros and cons of the mother's clinical need for treatment versus any potential fetal risk that might occur from exposure. Women who are pregnant and have taken vigabatrin at any time during pregnancy are encouraged to contact the NAAED Pregnancy Registry at 888-233-2334. The drug carries a boxed warning for permanent bilateral concentric visual field constriction, including tunnel vision, that can result in disability and may decrease visual acuity. It is only available through the vigabatrin REMS program.

BREASTFEEDING SUMMARY

Vigabatrin has been shown to be excreted into human breast milk. In two women, 7 days postpartum, and both taking vigabatrin (1,000 mg twice daily), the predose breast milk to plasma ratio was less than 1. The ratio was also less than 1 in the one woman tested at 3- and 6-hours postdose. The estimated daily maximum doses that a nursing infant would receive as a percentage of the mother's daily weight-adjusted dose were 1% for the active enantiomer. Due to a concern for potential serious adverse effects that might be seen in a breastfed infant, the manufacturer recommends that women not breastfeed while being treated with this drug. Nevertheless, breastfeeding while using this drug should be based on the mother's clinical need for treatment versus any potential infant risks that might occur. If used, the infant should be monitored for the most common reported adult side effects of dizziness and blurred vision (both leading to irritability), somnolence, tremor, and fatigue (lethargy). An important side note is that vigabatrin is approved for use in infants as young as 1 month of age. In pediatric patients, the most common adverse event was weight gain.

References

1. Product information. Vigabatrin. Amneal Pharmaceuticals NY, LLC; 2022.
2. Challier JC, Rey E, Bintein T, et al. Passage of S(+) and R(−) γ-vinyl-GABA across the human isolated perfused placenta. *Br J Clin Pharmacol*. 1992;34:139-143.
3. Tran A, O'Mahoney T, Rey E, et al. Vigabatrin: placental transfer in vivo and excretion into breast milk of the enantiomers. *Br J Clin Pharmacol*. 1998;45:409-411.
4. Lindhout D, Omtzigt JGC. Teratogenic effects of antiepileptic drugs: implications for the management of epilepsy in women of childbearing age. *Epilepsia*. 1994;35(suppl 4):S19-S28.
5. Morrell MJ. The new antiepileptic drugs and women: efficacy, reproductive health, pregnancy, and fetal outcome. *Epilepsia*. 1996;37(suppl 6):S34-S44.
6. Wilton LV, Pearce GL, Martin RM, et al. The outcomes of pregnancy in women exposed to newly marketed drugs in general practice in England. *Br J Obstet Gynaecol*. 1998;105:882-889.
7. Calzolari E, Calabrese O, Cocchi G, et al. Anophthalmia and situs viscerum inversus in an infant exposed to vigabatrin. *Teratology*. 1997;56:397.
8. Gosakan R, von Knorring N, Stewart P. Successful pregnancy in a patient with hyperoxaluria and combined liver and renal transplant. *J Obstet Gynaecol*. 2003;23:434-435.
9. Sorri I, Herrgard E, Viinikainen K, et al. Ophthalmologic and neurologic findings in two children exposed to vigabatrin in utero. *Epilepsy Res*. 2005;65:117-120.
10. Lawthom C, Smith PEM, Wild JM. In utero exposure to vigabatrin: no indication of visual field loss. *Epilepsia*. 2009;50:318-321.
11. The Lamotrigine Pregnancy Registry. Final report. 1 September 1992 through 31 March 2010. GlaxoSmithKline; 2010.
12. Bar-Oz B, Nulman I, Koren G, et al. Anticonvulsants and breast feeding—a critical review. *Paediatr Drugs*. 2000;2:113-126.

VILAZODONE

Mental Health (SSRI/5-HT_{1A} Receptor Partial Agonist)

PREGNANCY RECOMMENDATION: Limited Human Data (First Trimester) / Human Data Suggest Risk (Third Trimester)

BREASTFEEDING RECOMMENDATION: Potential Toxicity

PREGNANCY SUMMARY

One report describing the use of vilazodone in human pregnancy was located. The woman used vilazodone 40 mg daily throughout the pregnancy and 6 months postpartum. No adverse events or malformations were reported in the infant. Vilazodone is likely to cross the placenta, so some fetal exposure will probably occur. However, the limited human pregnancy experience prevents a complete assessment of embryofetal risk. Animal data did not show any embryofetal toxicity in two species at doses of more than 10 times the RHD. Using this drug during pregnancy should be based on the pros and cons of the mother's clinical need for treatment versus any potential fetal risk that might occur from exposure. ACOG states that antidepressants, including selective serotonin reuptake inhibitors (SSRIs), during pregnancy increase the risk for persistent pulmonary hypertension and transient neonatal adaption syndrome when used in the third trimester prior to birth. There is a pregnancy exposure registry that monitors pregnancy outcomes in women exposed to antidepressants during pregnancy. For more information, health care providers or patients are encouraged to contact the National Pregnancy Registry for Antidepressants at 844-405-6185. The drug carries a boxed warning for an increased risk of suicidal thoughts and behaviors in pediatric patients and young adults taking antidepressants. The manufacturer recommends closely monitoring all antidepressant-treated patients for clinical worsening and the emergence of suicidal thoughts and behaviors. ACOG states that uncontrolled and undertreated depression is associated with a risk for limited engagement in medical care and self-care, substance use, preterm birth, low birth weight, preeclampsia, postpartum depression, impaired infant attachment (which carries long-term developmental effects), disrupted relationships with partner, and suicide. Additionally, untreated and undertreated mental health disorders should be considered an exposure. Pregnancy should not be a reason to withhold or discontinue mental health medications.

BREASTFEEDING SUMMARY

One report describing the use of vilazodone during human lactation has been located. The woman breastfed her infant until 6 months of age. No adverse events were described, and the infant was meeting all developmental milestones. The drug will likely be excreted into breast milk, so some infant exposure will probably occur. Breastfeeding while using this drug should be based on the mother's clinical need for treatment versus any potential infant risks that might occur. If used, the infant should be monitored for the most common reported adult side effects of nausea (leading to irritability), diarrhea, vomiting, and insomnia.

References

1. Product information. Vilazodone. Accord Healthcare, Inc; 2022.
2. American College of Obstetricians and Gynecologists. Treatment and management of mental health conditions during pregnancy and postpartum. Clinical practice guideline No. 5. *Obstet Gynecol*. 2023;141:1262-1288.
3. Morrison CM. A case report of the use of vilazodone in pregnancy. *Prim Care Companion CNS Disord*. 2014;16:PCC.13l01612.
4. Marshall AM, Nommsen-Rivers LA, Hernandez LI, et al. Serotonin transport and metabolism in the mammary gland modulates secretory activation and involution. *J Clin Endocrin Metab*. 2010;95:837-846

VILOXAZINE

Mental Health (Selective Norepinephrine Reuptake Inhibitor)

PREGNANCY RECOMMENDATION: No Human Data—Animal Data Suggest Potential Risk

BREASTFEEDING RECOMMENDATION: Potential Toxicity

V

PREGNANCY SUMMARY

No reports describing the use of viloxazine in human pregnancy have been located. Viloxazine is likely to cross the placenta, so fetal exposure will probably occur. However, the absence of human pregnancy experience prevents a complete assessment of the embryofetal risk. Embryofetal toxicity with malformations was observed in animal studies. The manufacturer recommends discontinuing the drug when a pregnancy is discovered unless the benefits of continuing the medication outweigh the potential risk. Therefore, using this drug during pregnancy should be based on the pros and cons of the mother's clinical need for treatment versus any potential fetal risk that might occur from exposure. There is a pregnancy exposure registry that monitors pregnancy outcomes in women using this drug. Health care providers and women who are pregnant and have taken viloxazine at any time during pregnancy are encouraged to contact the National Pregnancy Registry for Psychiatric Medications at 1-866-961-2388. Hypertension was reported in up to 13% of adult patients treated with this drug in the clinical trials.

BREASTFEEDING SUMMARY

No reports describing the use of viloxazine during human lactation have been located. The drug will likely be excreted into breast milk, so some infant exposure will probably occur. Breastfeeding while using this drug should be based on the mother's clinical need for treatment. If used, the infant should be monitored for the most common reported side effects of headache and nausea (both leading to irritability), sleep dysfunction, decreased appetite (monitor growth), lethargy, and vomiting.

Reference

1. Prescribing Information. Qelbree. Supernus Pharmaceuticals, Inc; 2021.

VILTOLARSEN

Genetic (Antisense Oligonucleotide)

PREGNANCY RECOMMENDATION: No Human Data and No Relevant Animal Data

BREASTFEEDING RECOMMENDATION: Probably Compatible

PREGNANCY SUMMARY

No reports describing the use of viltolarsen in human pregnancy have been located. Placental transfer and embryofetal exposure are likely to be negligible. However, the absence of human pregnancy experience prevents a complete assessment of the embryofetal risk. Animal studies have not been performed. Duchenne muscular dystrophy (DMD) is primarily seen in males (X-linked recessive genetic disorder). Females with severe DMD who are of reproductive age potential are exceedingly rare. Using this drug during pregnancy should be based on the pros and cons of the mother's clinical need for treatment versus any potential fetal risk that might occur from exposure.

BREASTFEEDING SUMMARY

Viltolarsen excretion into breast milk is likely to be negligible. Breastfeeding while using this drug should be based on the mother's clinical need for treatment. If used, the infant should be monitored for the most common reported adult side effects of upper respiratory tract infection, cough, and pyrexia.

Reference

1. Prescribing Information. Viltepso. NS Pharma, Inc; 2020.

VINBLASTINE

Antineoplastic (Vinca Alkaloid)

PREGNANCY RECOMMENDATION: Limited Human Data—Animal Data Suggest Risk

BREASTFEEDING RECOMMENDATION: Potential Toxicity

PREGNANCY SUMMARY

Several cases have described the use of vinblastine during human pregnancy, and these limited human data do not support a significant association with developmental toxicity. The drug is likely to cross the placenta, so some fetal exposure will probably occur. However, this limited human pregnancy experience prevents a complete assessment of embryofetal risk. Animal studies did show some embryofetal toxicity with malformations in two studies, but at unspecified doses. Using this drug during pregnancy should be based on the pros and cons of the mother's clinical need for treatment versus any potential fetal risk that might occur from exposure. Women who are pregnant and have cancer are encouraged to contact the Cancer and Pregnancy Registry at 877-635-4499. Hypertension was reported in several patients treated with this drug in the clinical trials. The drug also carries a boxed warning for the risk of extravasation injury.

BREASTFEEDING SUMMARY

No reports describing the use of vinblastine during human lactation have been located. The drug will likely be excreted into breast milk, so some infant exposure will probably occur. Breastfeeding while using this drug should be based on the mother's clinical need for treatment versus any potential infant risks that might occur. If used, the infant should be monitored for the most common reported adult side effects of bone pain and jaw pain (both leading to irritability), leukopenia, alopecia, constipation, hypertension, and lethargy.

References

1. Product information. Vinblastine sulfate. Fresenius Kabi USA; 2019.
2. Armstrong JG, Dyke RW, Fouts PJ, et al. Delivery of a normal infant during the course of oral vinblastine sulfate therapy for Hodgkin's disease. *Ann Intern Med*. 1964;61:106-107.
3. Rosenzweig AI, Crews QE Jr, Hopwood HG. Vinblastine sulfate in Hodgkin's disease in pregnancy. *Ann Intern Med*. 1964;61:108-112.
4. Lacher MJ. Use of vinblastine sulfate to treat Hodgkin's disease during pregnancy. *Ann Intern Med*. 1964;61:113-115.
5. Lacher MJ, Geller W. Cyclophosphamide and vinblastine sulfate in Hodgkin's disease during pregnancy. *JAMA*. 1966;195:192-194.
6. Nordlund JJ, DeVita VT Jr, Carbone PP. Severe vinblastine-induced leukopenia during late pregnancy with delivery of a normal infant. *Ann Intern Med*. 1968;69:581-582.
7. Goguei A. Hodgkin's disease and pregnancy. *Nouv Presse Med*. 1970;78:1507-1510.
8. Johnson IR, Filshie GM. Hodgkin's disease diagnosed in pregnancy: case report. *Br J Obstet Gynaecol*. 1977;84:791-792.
9. Nisce LZ, Tome MA, He S, Lee BJ III, Kutcher GJ. Management of coexisting Hodgkin's disease and pregnancy. *Am J Clin Oncol*. 1986;9:146-151.
10. Malone JM, Gershenson DM, Creasy RK, et al. Endodermal sinus tumor of the ovary associated with pregnancy. *Obstet Gynecol*. 1986;68(suppl):86S-89S.
11. Garrett MJ. Teratogenic effects of combination chemotherapy. *Ann Intern Med*. 1974;80:667.
12. Thomas RPM, Peckham MJ. The investigation and management of Hodgkin's disease in the pregnant patient. *Cancer*. 1976;38:1443-1451.
13. Rustin GJS, Booth M, Dent J, et al. Pregnancy after cytotoxic chemotherapy for gestational trophoblastic tumours. *Br Med J*. 1984;288:103-106.
14. Nicholson HO. Cytotoxic drugs in pregnancy: review of reported cases. *J Obstet Gynaecol Br Commonw*. 1968;75:307-312.
15. Dobbing J. Pregnancy and leukaemia. *Lancet*. 1977;1:1155.
16. Maggen C, Dierickx D, Lugtenburg P, et al; for the International Network on Cancer, Infertility, and Pregnancy. Obstetric and maternal outcomes in patients diagnosed with Hodgkin lymphoma during pregnancy: a multicentre, retrospective, cohort study. *Lancet Haematol*. 2019;6:e551-e561.
17. Morgenfeld MC, Goldberg V, Parisier H, et al. Ovarian lesions due to cytostatic agents during the treatment of Hodgkin's disease. *Surg Gynecol Obstet*. 1972;134:826-828.
18. Ross GT. Congenital anomalies among children born of mothers receiving chemotherapy for gestational trophoblastic neoplasms. *Cancer*. 1976;37:1043-1047.
19. Schilsky RL, Lewis BJ, Sherins RJ, et al. Gonadal dysfunction in patients receiving chemotherapy for cancer. *Ann Intern Med*. 1980;93:109-114.
20. Rubery ED. Return of fertility after curative chemotherapy for disseminated teratoma of testis. *Lancet*. 1983;1:186.
21. Shalet SM, Vaughan Williams CA, Whitehead E. Pregnancy after chemotherapy induced ovarian failure. *Br Med J*. 1985;290:898.
22. Gershenson DM. Menstrual and reproductive function after treatment with combination chemotherapy for malignant ovarian germ cell tumors. *J Clin Oncol*. 1988;6:270-275.
23. Gaudio F, Nardelli C, Masciandaro P, et al. Pregnancy rate and outcome of pregnancies in long-term survivors of Hodgkin's lymphoma. *Ann Hematol*. 2019;98:1947-1952.

VINCRISTINE

Antineoplastic (Vinca Alkaloid)

PREGNANCY RECOMMENDATION: Limited Human Data—Animal Data Suggest Risk

BREASTFEEDING RECOMMENDATION: Potential Toxicity

PREGNANCY SUMMARY

The use of vincristine, always in combination with other antineoplastics, has been described in at least 36 pregnancies (1 with twins), 9 during the first trimester. Developmental toxicity was observed in some of these pregnancies, but the relationship to vincristine is unknown. (See Rituximab for additional data.) It is likely that some amount of vincristine crosses the placenta, so some fetal exposure will probably occur. However, this limited human pregnancy experience prevents a complete assessment of embryofetal risk. Embryofetal toxicity with malformations was observed in three animal species, but the doses were not specified. Using this drug during pregnancy should be based on the pros and cons of the mother's clinical need for treatment versus any potential fetal risk that might occur from exposure. Women who are pregnant and have cancer are encouraged to contact the Cancer and Pregnancy Registry at 877-635-4499. Hypertension was reported in patients treated with this drug during the clinical trials.

BREASTFEEDING SUMMARY

No reports describing the use of vincristine during human lactation have been located. The drug will likely be excreted into breast milk, so some infant exposure may occur. Breastfeeding while using this drug should be based on the mother's clinical need for treatment versus any potential infant risks that might occur. If used, the infant should be monitored for the most common reported adult side effects of neuropathy and paresthesia (both leading to irritability), alopecia, leukopenia, constipation, and loss of deep tendon reflexes.

References

1. Product information. Vincristine sulfate. Hospira, Inc; 2023.
2. Pizzuto J, Aviles A, Noriega L, et al. Treatment of acute leukemia during pregnancy: presentation of nine cases. *Cancer Treat Rep*. 1980;64:679-683.

3. Colbert N, Najman A, Gorin NC, et al. Acute leukaemia during pregnancy: favourable course of pregnancy in two patients treated with cytosine arabinoside and anthracyclines. *Nouv Presse Med*. 1980;9:175-178.
4. Daly H, McCann SR, Hanratty TD, et al. Successful pregnancy during combination chemotherapy for Hodgkin's disease. *Acta Haematol (Basel)*. 1980;64: 154-156.
5. Tobias JS, Bloom HJG. Doxorubicin in pregnancy. *Lancet*. 1980;1:776.
6. Garcia V, San Miguel J, Borrasea AL. Doxorubicin in the first trimester of pregnancy. *Ann Intern Med*. 1981;94:547.
7. Dara P, Slater LM, Armentrout SA. Successful pregnancy during chemotherapy for acute leukemia. *Cancer*. 1981;47:845-846.
8. Burnier AM. Discussion. In Plows CW. Acute myelomonocytic leukemia in pregnancy: report of a case. *Am J Obstet Gynecol*. 1982;143:41-43.
9. Lilleyman JS, Hill AS, Anderton KJ. Consequences of acute myelogenous leukemia in early pregnancy. *Cancer*. 1977;40:1300-1303.
10. Thomas PRM, Peckham MJ. The investigation and management of Hodgkin's disease in the pregnant patient. *Cancer*. 1976;38:1443-1451.
11. Pawliger DF, McLean FW, Noyes WD. Normal fetus after cytosine arabinoside therapy. *Ann Intern Med*. 1971;74:1012.
12. Lowenthal RM, Funnell CF, Hope DM, et al. Normal infant after combination chemotherapy including teniposide for Burkitt's lymphoma in pregnancy. *Med Pediatr Oncol*. 1982;10:165-169.
13. Sears HF, Reid J. Granulocytic sarcoma: local presentation of a systemic disease. *Cancer*. 1976;37:1808-1813.
14. Durie BGM, Giles HR. Successful treatment of acute leukemia during pregnancy: combination therapy in the third trimester. *Arch Intern Med*. 1977; 137:90-91.
15. Newcomb M, Balducci L, Thigpen JT, et al. Acute leukemia in pregnancy: successful delivery after cytarabine and doxorubicin. *JAMA*. 1978;239:2691-2692.
16. Mennuti MT, Shepard TH, Mellman WJ. Fetal renal malformation following treatment of Hodgkin's disease during pregnancy. *Obstet Gynecol*. 1975;46:194-196.
17. Coopland AT, Friesen WJ, Galbraith PA. Acute leukemia in pregnancy. *Am J Obstet Gynecol*. 1969;105:1288-1289.
18. Doney KC, Kraemer KG, Shepard TH. Combination chemotherapy for acute myelocytic leukemia during pregnancy: three case reports. *Cancer Treat Rep*. 1979;63:369-371.
19. Okun DB, Groncy PK, Sieger L, et al. Acute leukemia in pregnancy: transient neonatal myelosuppression after combination chemotherapy in the mother. *Med Pediatr Oncol*. 1979;7:315-319.
20. Weed JC Jr, Roh RA, Mendenhall HW. Recurrent endodermal sinus tumor during pregnancy. *Obstet Gynecol*. 1979;54:653-656.
21. Kim DS, Park MI. Maternal and fetal survival following surgery and chemotherapy of endodermal sinus tumor of the ovary during pregnancy: a case report. *Obstet Gynecol*. 1989;73:503-507.
22. Karp GI, von Oeyen P, Valone F, et al. Doxorubicin in pregnancy: possible transplacental passage. *Cancer Treat Rep*. 1983;67:773-777.
23. Haerr RW, Pratt AT. Multiagent chemotherapy for sarcoma diagnosed during pregnancy. *Cancer*. 1985;56:1028-1033.
24. Volkenandt M, Buchner T, Hiddemann W, et al. Acute leukaemia during pregnancy. *Lancet*. 1987;2:1521-1522.
25. Schleuning M, Clemm C. Chromosomal aberrations in a newborn whose mother received cytotoxic treatment during pregnancy. *N Engl J Med*. 1987; 317:1666-1667.
26. Feliu J, Juarez S, Ordonez A, et al. Acute leukemia and pregnancy. *Cancer*. 1988;61:580-584.
27. Turchi JJ, Villasis C. Anthracyclines in the treatment of malignancy in pregnancy. *Cancer*. 1988;61:435-440.
28. Weinrach RS. Leukemia in pregnancy. *Ariz Med*. 1972;29:326-329.
29. Ortega J. Multiple agent chemotherapy including bleomycin of non-Hodgkin's lymphoma during pregnancy. *Cancer*. 1977;40:2829-2835.
30. Jones RT, Weinerman ER. MOPP (nitrogen mustard, vincristine, procarbazine, and prednisone) given during pregnancy. *Obstet Gynecol*. 1979;54: 477 478.
31. Giacalone PL, Laffargue F, Benos P. Chemotherapy for breast carcinoma during pregnancy. *Cancer*. 1999;86:2266-2272.
32. Nicholson HO. Cytotoxic drugs in pregnancy: review of reported cases. *J Obstet Gynaecol Br Commonw*. 1968;75:307-312.
33. Dobbing J. Pregnancy and leukaemia. *Lancet*. 1977;1:1155.
34. Schilsky RL, Sherins RJ, Hubbard SM, et al. Long-term follow-up of ovarian function in women treated with MOPP chemotherapy for Hodgkin's disease. *Am J Med*. 1981;71:552-556.
35. Schwartz PE, Vidone RA. Pregnancy following combination chemotherapy for a mixed germ cell tumor of the ovary. *Gynecol Oncol*. 1981;12:373-378.
36. Estiu M. Successful pregnancy in leukaemia. *Lancet*. 1977;1:433.
37. Johnson SA, Goldman JM, Hawkins DF. Pregnancy after chemotherapy for Hodgkin's disease. *Lancet*. 1979;2:93.
38. Schilsky RL, Lewis BJ, Sherins RJ, et al. Gonadal dysfunction in patients receiving chemotherapy for cancer. *Ann Intern Med*. 1980;93:109-114.
39. Sherins RJ, DeVita VT Jr. Effect of drug treatment for lymphoma on male reproductive capacity. *Ann Intern Med*. 1973;79:216-220.
40. Sherins RJ, Olweny CLM, Ziegler JL. Gynecomastia and gonadal dysfunction in adolescent boys treated with combination chemotherapy for Hodgkin's disease. *N Engl J Med*. 1978;299:12-16.
41. Lendon PRM, Peckham MJ. The investigation and management of Hodgkin's disease in the pregnant patient. *Cancer*. 1976;38:1944-1951.
42. Lee RB, Kelly J, Elg SA, et al. Pregnancy following conservative surgery and adjunctive chemotherapy for stage III immature teratoma of the ovary. *Obstet Gynecol*. 1989;73:853-855.
43. Gershenson DM. Menstrual and reproductive function after treatment with combination chemotherapy for malignant ovarian germ cell tumors. *J Clin Oncol*. 1988;6:270-275.
44. Rustin GJS, Booth M, Dent J, et al. Pregnancy after cytotoxic chemotherapy for gestational trophoblastic tumours. *Br Med J*. 1984;288:103-106.

VINORELBINE

Antineoplastic (Vinca Alkaloid)

PREGNANCY RECOMMENDATION: Limited Human Data—Animal Data Suggest Risk

BREASTFEEDING RECOMMENDATION: Potential Toxicity

PREGNANCY SUMMARY

The human pregnancy experience with vinorelbine is limited to 10 cases, all in the second and third trimesters, and other antineoplastic agents were used in each case. Transient anemia was observed in one infant, and another had mild leukopenia. Some vinorelbine is likely to cross the placenta, so fetal exposure will probably occur. However, this limited human pregnancy experience prevents a complete assessment of embryofetal risk. Embryofetal toxicity was observed in two animal species at doses less than the RHD. Based on the animal studies and the drug's mechanism of action, the manufacturer recommends that women with reproductive potential use effective contraception during treatment and for 6 months after the last dose. They also recommend that males with female partners of reproductive potential use effective contraception during treatment and for 3 months after the last dose. Nevertheless, using this drug during pregnancy should be based on the pros and cons of the mother's clinical need for treatment versus any potential fetal risk that might occur from exposure. Women who are pregnant and have cancer are encouraged to contact the Cancer and Pregnancy Registry at 877-635-4499.

V

BREASTFEEDING SUMMARY

No reports describing the use of vinorelbine during human lactation have been located. The drug will probably be excreted into breast milk (though likely limited), so some infant exposure may occur. Due to a concern for potential serious adverse effects that might be seen in a breastfed infant, the manufacturer recommends that women not breastfeed while being treated with this drug and for at least 9 days after the last dose. Nevertheless, breastfeeding while using this drug should be based on the mother's clinical need for treatment versus any potential infant risks that might occur. If used, the infant should be monitored for the most common reported adult side effects of nausea, asthenia, and peripheral neuropathy (all leading to irritability), vomiting, constipation, and various laboratory abnormalities (see PI).

References

1. Product information. Vinorelbine. Actavis Pharma, Inc; 2022.
2. Cuvier C, Espie M, Extra JM, et al. Vinorelbine in pregnancy. *Eur J Cancer*. 1997;33:168-169.
3. Giacalone PL, Laffargue F, Benos P. Chemotherapy for breast carcinoma during pregnancy. *Cancer*. 1999;86:2266-2272.
4. De Santos M, Lucchese A, De Carolis S, et al. Metastatic breast cancer in pregnancy: first case of chemotherapy with docetaxel. *Eur J Cancer Care (Engl)*. 2000;9:235-237.
5. Jänne PA, Rodriguez-Thompson D, Metcalf DR, et al. Chemotherapy for a patient with advanced non-small-cell lung cancer during pregnancy: a case report and a review of chemotherapy treatment during pregnancy. *Oncology*. 2001;61:175-183.
6. Fanale MA, Uyei AR, Therialult RL, et al. Treatment of metastatic breast cancer with trastuzumab and vinorelbine during pregnancy. *Clin Breast Cancer*. 2005;6:354-356.

VISMODEGIB

Antineoplastic (Hedgehog Pathway Inhibitor)

PREGNANCY RECOMMENDATION: No Human Data—Animal Data Suggest Potential Risk

BREASTFEEDING RECOMMENDATION: Potential Toxicity

PREGNANCY SUMMARY

No reports describing the use of vismodegib during human pregnancy have been located. Vismodegib is likely to cross the placenta, so some fetal exposure will probably occur. Therefore, the absence of human pregnancy experience prevents a complete assessment of embryofetal risk. Embryofetal toxicity with malformations was observed in one animal species at doses of less than the RHD. The drug actually carries a boxed warning for this risk. Based on animal studies and the drug's mechanism of action, the manufacturer recommends that women with reproductive potential use effective contraception during treatment and for 1 week after the last dose. They also recommend that males with female partners of reproductive potential use effective contraception during treatment and for 24 months after the last dose. Additionally, because vismodegib is found in semen, the manufacturer also recommends that males with female partners of reproductive potential use condoms, even after a vasectomy, during treatment, and should not donate semen during treatment or for 3 months after the last dose. Nevertheless, using this drug during pregnancy should be based on the pros and cons of the mother's clinical need for treatment versus any potential fetal risk that might occur from exposure. There is a pregnancy exposure registry for vismodegib, and the manufacturer recommends calling Genentech at 888-835-2555 to report pregnancies. Additionally, women who are pregnant and have cancer are encouraged to contact the Cancer and Pregnancy Registry at 877-635-4499.

BREASTFEEDING SUMMARY

No reports describing the use of vismodegib during human lactation have been located. The drug will likely be excreted into breast milk, so some infant exposure will probably occur. Due to a concern for potential serious adverse effects that might be seen in a breastfed infant, the manufacturer recommends that women not breastfeed while being treated with this drug and for at least 24 months after the last dose. Nevertheless, breastfeeding while using this drug should be based on the mother's clinical need for treatment versus any potential infant risks that might occur. If used, the infant should be monitored for the most common reported adult side effects of nausea, arthralgias, and muscle spasms (all leading to irritability), decreased appetite (monitor weight gain), alopecia, fatigue (lethargy), constipation, and vomiting.

V

Reference

1. Product information. Erivedge. Genentech, Inc; 2023.

VITAMIN A (RETINOL)

Vitamin (Fat-Soluble Vitamin)

PREGNANCY RECOMMENDATION: Human Data Suggest Compatible/Contraindicated (With Doses Above the US RDA)

BREASTFEEDING RECOMMENDATION: Compatible

PREGNANCY SUMMARY

Several reports are available evaluating the safety of vitamin A during pregnancy. The recommended daily allowance (RDA), as well as the ACOG and AAP recommendations for daily intake of vitamin A for obstetric patients who are 18 years of age or less, is 750 mcg retinol activity equivalents (RAE) (which is about 2,500 IU). For pregnant women 19 years or older, it is 770 mcg of RAE (about 2,567 IU). Doses exceeding the RDA should be avoided by women who are pregnant or who may become pregnant. ACOG states that daily vitamin A intake of more than 10,000 IU may be associated with malformations such as anomalies of the bones, urinary tract, and CNS. β-Carotene, a precursor to vitamin A, has not been associated with vitamin A toxicity in humans or animals (see β-Carotene). Vitamin A crosses the placenta. Two synthetic isomers of vitamin A, isotretinoin and etretinate, have been shown to be potent human teratogens (see Isotretinoin and Etretinate). Lastly, vitamin A is fat soluble and some is stored in the body's fatty tissues and liver. Because of the combined animal and human data showing that excess amounts of vitamin A are stored in the body's fatty tissues and liver, and because of the human experience with isotretinoin and etretinate, large doses of vitamin A must be viewed as harmful to the human fetus.

BREASTFEEDING SUMMARY

Vitamin A is a natural constituent of breast milk. Deficiency of this vitamin in breastfed infants is rare. The RDA of vitamin A during lactation is 1,200 and 1,300 mcg RAE for patients 18 years of age or less and for patients 19 years of age or older, respectively. The IU equivalent is about 4,000 and 4,333, respectively. It is not known whether high maternal doses of vitamin A represent a danger to a nursing infant.

References

1. AAP Committee on Fetus and Newborn and ACOG Committee on Obstetric Practice. Antepartum care. In: Kilpatrick SJ, Papile LA, Macones GA, eds. *Guidelines for Perinatal Care*. 8th ed. American Academy of Pediatrics; 2017.
2. National Institutes of Health. Office of dietary supplements. Vitamin A. Accessed October 1, 2023. https://ods.od.nih.gov/factsheets/VitaminA-HealthProfessional/
3. National Library of Medicine. Pubchem. Retinol. Accessed September 30, 2023. https://pubchem.ncbi.nlm.nih.gov/compound/Retinol
4. Spiegler E, Kim YK, Wassef L, et al. Maternal-fetal transfer and metabolism of vitamin A and its precursor β-carotene in the developing tissues. *Biochim Biophys Acta*. 2012;1821:88-98.
5. Smithells RW. Spina bifida and vitamins. *Br Med J*. 1983;286:388-389.
6. Houet R, Ramioul-Lecomte S. Repercussions sur l'enfant des avitaminoses de la mere pendant la grossesse. *Ann Paediatr*. 1950;175:378. As cited in Warkany J. *Congenital Malformations. Notes and Comments*. Year Book Medical Publishers; 1971:127-128.
7. Sarma V. Maternal vitamin A deficiency and fetal microcephaly and anophthalmia. *Obstet Gynecol*. 1959;13:299-301.
8. Lamba PA, Sood NN. Congenital microphthalmos and colobomata in maternal vitamin A deficiency. *J Pediatr Ophthalmol*. 1968;115-117. As cited in Warkany J. *Congenital Malformation. Notes and Comments*. Year Book Medical Publishers; 1971:127-128.
9. Rosa FW, Wilk AL, Kelsey FO. Teratogen update: vitamin A congeners. *Teratology*. 1986;33:355-364.
10. Rosa FW. Teratogenicity of isotretinoin. *Lancet*. 1983;2:513.
11. Rosa FW. Retinoic acid embryopathy. *N Engl J Med*. 1986;315:262.
12. Pilotti G, Scorta A. Ipervitaminosi A gravidica e malformazioni neonatali dell'apparato urinaria. *Minerva Ginecol*. 1965;17:1103-1108. As cited in Nishimura H, Tanimura T. *Clinical Aspects of the Teratogenicity of Drugs*. American Elsevier; 1976:251-252.
13. Bernhardt IB, Dorsey DJ. Hypervitaminosis A and congenital renal anomalies in a human infant. *Obstet Gynecol*. 1974;43:750-755.
14. Stange L, Carlstrom K, Eriksson M. Hypervitaminosis A in early human pregnancy and malformations of the central nervous system. *Acta Obstet Gynecol Scand*. 1978;57:289-291.
15. Morriss GM, Thomson AD. Vitamin A and rat embryos. *Lancet*. 1974;2:899-900.
16. Mounoud RL, Klein D, Weber F. A propos d'un cas de syndrome de Goldenhar: intoxication aigue a la vitamine A chez la mere pendant la grossesse. *J Genet Hum*. 1975;23:135-154.
17. Von Lennep E, El Khazen N, De Pierreux G, et al. A case of partial sirenomelia and possible vitamin A teratogenesis. *Prenat Diagn*. 1985;5:35-40.
18. Centers for Disease Control and Prevention. Use of supplements containing high-dose vitamin A—New York State, 1983-1984. *MMWR*. 1987;36:80-82.
19. Martinez-Frias ML, Salvador J. Megadose vitamin A and teratogenicity. *Lancet*. 1988;1:236.
20. Martinez-Frias ML, Salvador J. Epidemiological aspects of prenatal exposure to high doses of vitamin A in Spain. *Eur J Epidemiol*. 1990;6:118-123.
21. Werler MM, Lammer EJ, Rosenberg L, et al. Maternal vitamin A supplementation in relation to selected birth defects. *Teratology*. 1990;42:497-503.
22. Evans K, Hickey-Dwyer MU. Cleft anterior segment with maternal hypervitaminosis A. *Br J Ophthalmol*. 1991;75:691-692.
23. Dudas I, Czeizel AE. Use of 6,000 IU vitamin A during early pregnancy without teratogenic effect. *Teratology*. 1992;45:335-336.
24. Rothman KJ, Moore LL, Singer MR, et al. Teratogenicity of high vitamin A intake. *N Engl J Med*. 1995;333:1369-1373.
25. Oakley GP Jr, Erickson JD. Vitamin A and birth defects. Continuing caution is needed. *N Engl J Med*. 1995;333:1414-1415.
26. Werler M, Lammer EJ, Mitchell AA. Teratogenicity of high vitamin A intake. *N Engl J Med*. 1996;334:1195.
27. Brent RL, Hendrickx AG, Holmes LB, et al. Teratogenicity of high vitamin A intake. *N Engl J Med*. 1996;334:1196.
28. Watkins M, Moore C, Mulinare J. Teratogenicity of high vitamin A intake. *N Engl J Med*. 1996;334:1196.
29. Challem JJ. Teratogenicity of high vitamin A intake. *N Engl J Med*. 1996;334:1196-1197.
30. Hunt JR. Teratogenicity of high vitamin A intake. *N Engl J Med*. 1996;334:1197.
31. Rothman KJ, Moore LL, Singer MR, et al. Teratogenicity of high vitamin A intake. *N Engl J Med*. 1996;334:1197.
32. Shaw GM, Velie EM, Schaffer D, et al. Periconceptional intake of vitamin A among women and risk of neural tube defect-affected pregnancies. *Teratology*. 1997;55:132-133.
33. Hendrickx AG, Hummler H, Oneda S. Vitamin A teratogenicity and risk assessment in the cynomolgus monkey (abstract). *Teratology*. 1997;55:68.
34. Bonati M, Nannini S, Addis A. Vitamin A supplementation during pregnancy in developed countries. *Lancet*. 1995;345:736-737.
35. Khoury MJ, Moore CA, Mulinare J. Do vitamin A supplements in early pregnancy increase the risk of birth defects in the offspring? A population-based case-control study (abstract). *Teratology*. 1996;53:91.
36. Lammer EJ, Shaw GM, Wasserman CR, et al. High vitamin A intake and risk for major anomalies involving structures with an embryological cranial neural crest cell component (abstract). *Teratology*. 1996;53:91-92.
37. Mills JL, Simpson JL, Cunningham GC, et al. Vitamin A and birth defects. *Am J Obstet Gynecol*. 1997;177:31-36.
38. Gal I, Sharman IM, Pryse-Davies J. Vitamin A in relation to human congenital malformations. *Adv Teratol*. 1972;5:143-159.
39. Shah RS, Rajalakshmi R. Vitamin A status of the newborn in relation to gestational age, body weight, and maternal nutritional status. *Am J Clin Nutr*. 1984;40:794-800.
40. Baker H, Frank O, Thomson AD, et al. Vitamin profile of 174 mothers and newborns at parturition. *Am J Clin Nutr*. 1975;28:59-65.
41. Baker H, Thind IS, Frank O, et al. Vitamin levels in low-birth-weight newborn infants and their mothers. *Am J Obstet Gynecol*. 1977;129:521-524.
42. Gal I, Parkinson CE. Effects of nutrition and other factors on pregnant women's serum vitamin A levels. *Am J Clin Nutr*. 1974;27:688-695.
43. Wallingford JC, Milunsky A, Underwood BA. Vitamin A and retinol-binding protein in amniotic fluid. *Am J Clin Nutr*. 1983;38:377-381.

44. Brandt RB, Mueller DG, Schroeder JR, et al. Serum vitamin A in premature and term neonates. *J Pediatr*. 1978;92:101-104.
45. Shenai JP, Chytil F, Jhaveri A, et al. Plasma vitamin A and retinol-binding protein in premature and term neonates. *J Pediatr*. 1981:99:302-305.
46. Hustead VA, Gutcher GR, Anderson SA, et al. Relationship of vitamin A (retinol) status to lung disease in the preterm infant. *J Pediatr*. 1984;105:610-615.
47. Kaminetzky HA, Langer A, Baker H, et al. The effect of nutrition in teen-age gravidas on pregnancy and the status of the neonate. I. A nutritional profile. *Am J Obstet Gynecol*. 1973;115:639-646.
48. Gal I, Sharman IM, Pryse-Davies J, et al. Vitamin A as a possible factor in human teratology. *Proc Nutr Soc*. 1969;28:9A-10A.
49. Parkinson CE, Tan JCY. Vitamin A concentrations in amniotic fluid and maternal serum related to neural-tube defects. *Br J Obstet Gynaecol*. 1982; 89:935-939.
50. Hill EP, Longo LD. Dynamics of maternal-fetal nutrient transfer. *Fed Proc*. 1980;39:239-244.
51. Wild J, Schorah CJ, Smithells RW. Vitamin A, pregnancy, and oral contraceptives. *Br Med J*. 1974;1:57-59.
52. Bubb FA. Vitamin A, pregnancy, and oral contraceptives. *Br Med J*. 1974; 1:391-392.
53. Bates C. Vitamin A and infant immunity. *Lancet*. 1993;341:28.
54. Semba RD, Miotti PG, Chiphangwi JD, et al. Maternal vitamin A deficiency and mother-to-child transmission of HIV-1. *Lancet*. 1994;343:1593-1597.
55. Semba RD, Miotti PG, Chiphangwi JD, et al. Infant mortality and maternal vitamin A deficiency during human immunodeficiency virus infection. *Clin Infect Dis*. 1995;21:966-972.
56. Greenberg BL, Semba RD, Vink PE, et al. Vitamin A deficiency and maternal-infant transmission of HIV in two metropolitan areas in the United States. *AIDS*. 1997;11:325-332.
57. Bridbord K, Willoughby A. Vitamin A and mother-to-child HIV-1 transmission. *Lancet*. 1994;343:1585-1586.
58. Semba RD, Miotti P, Chiphangwi JD, et al. Maternal vitamin A deficiency and child growth failure during human immunodeficiency virus infection. *J Acquir Immune Defic Syndr Human Retrovirol*. 1997;14:219-222.
59. World Health Organization. Vitamin A supplementation in HIV-infected women during pregnancy. Accessed October 1, 2023. https://www.who.int/tools/elena/interventions/vitamina-hiv-pregnancy
60. Public Affairs Committee, Teratology Society. Position paper: recommendations for vitamin A use during pregnancy. *Teratology*. 1987;35:269-275.
61. Cohlan SQ. Excessive intake of vitamin A as a cause of congenital anomalies in the rat. *Science*. 1953;117:535-536.
62. Muenter MD. Hypervitaminosis A. *Ann Intern Med*. 1974;80:105-106.
63. Morriss GM. Vitamin A and congenital malformations. *Int J Vitam Nutr Res*. 1976;46:220-222.
64. Fantel AG, Shepard TH, Newell-Morris LL, et al. Teratogenic effects of retinoic acid in pigtail monkeys (*Macaca nemestrina*). *Teratology*. 1977;15:65-72.
65. Vorhees CV, Brunner RL, McDaniel CR, et al. The relationship of gestational age to vitamin A induced postnatal dysfunction. *Teratology*. 1978;17:271-276.
66. Ferm VH, Ferm RR. Teratogenic interaction of hyperthermia and vitamin A. *Biol Neonate*. 1979;36:168-172.
67. Geelen JAG. Hypervitaminosis A induced teratogenesis. *CRC Crit Rev Toxicol*. 1979;6:351-375.
68. Kamm JJ. Toxicology, carcinogenicity, and teratogenicity of some orally administered retinoids. *J Am Acad Dermatol*. 1982;6:652-659.
69. Muenter MD. Hypervitaminosis A. *Ann Intern Med*. 1974;80:105-106.
70. Read AP, Harris R. Spina bifida and vitamins. *Br Med J*. 1983;286:560-561.
71. Bound JP. Spina bifida and vitamins. *Br Med J*. 1983;286:147.
72. Lungarotti MS, Marinelli D, Mariani T, et al. Multiple congenital anomalies associated with apparently normal maternal intake of vitamin A: a phenocopy of the isotretinoin syndrome? *Am J Med Genet*. 1987;27:245-248.
73. Committee on Nutrition, American Academy of Pediatrics. Vitamin and mineral supplement needs in normal children in the United States. *Pediatrics*. 1980;66:1015-1021.

VITAMIN B_1 (THIAMINE)

Vitamin (Water-Soluble Vitamin)

PREGNANCY RECOMMENDATION: Compatible

BREASTFEEDING RECOMMENDATION: Compatible

PREGNANCY SUMMARY

Thiamine (vitamin B_1) is compatible with use during pregnancy, but there is limited data regarding doses above the RDA. The recommended daily allowance for thiamine in pregnancy is 1.4 mg. Thiamine is actively transported across the placenta to the fetus. No animal reproduction studies have been conducted. Vitamin B_1 is water soluble and excess amounts are not stored in the body. Therefore, using this vitamin at the RDA is endorsed by ACOG and AAP.

BREASTFEEDING SUMMARY

Thiamine (vitamin B_1) is excreted into human breast milk. The RDA for thiamine during lactation is 1.4 mg. One group of investigators supplemented well-nourished lactating women with a multivitamin preparation containing 1.7 mg of thiamine. At 6 months postpartum, breast milk concentrations of thiamine did not differ significantly from those of control patients not receiving supplements. Therefore, using this vitamin while breastfeeding at the RDA is only endorsed for those patients with dietary insufficiency.

V

References

1. Product Information. Thiamine Hydrochloride. Dr. Reddy's Laboratories, Inc; 2022.
2. National Institutes of Health Office of Dietary Supplements. Thiamin. Accessed October 8, 2024. https://ods.od.nih.gov/factsheets/Thiamin-HealthProfessional/
3. Frank O, Walbroehl G, Thomson A, et al. Placental transfer: fetal retention of some vitamins. *Am J Clin Nutr*. 1970;23:662-663.
4. Hill EP, Longo LD. Dynamics of maternal-fetal nutrient transfer. *Fed Proc*. 1980;39:239-244.
5. Kaminetzky HA, Baker H, Frank O, Langer A. The effects of intravenously administered water-soluble vitamins during labor in normovitaminemic and hypovitaminemic gravidas on maternal and neonatal blood vitamin levels at delivery. *Am J Obstet Gynecol*. 1974;120:697-703.
6. Baker H, Frank O, Deangelis B, et al. Role of placenta in maternal-fetal vitamin transfer in humans. *Am J Obstet Gynecol*. 1981;141:792-796.
7. Slobody LB, Willner MM, Mestern J. Comparison of vitamin B_1 levels in mothers and their newborn infants. *Am J Dis Child*. 1949;77:736-739.
8. Baker H, Thind IS, Frank O, et al. Vitamin levels in low-birth-weight newborn infants and their mothers. *Am J Obstet Gynecol*. 1977;129:521-524.
9. Heller S, Salkeld RM, Korner WF. Vitamin B_1 status in pregnancy. *Am J Clin Nutr*. 1974;27:1221-1224.
10. Baker H, Frank O, Thomson AD, et al. Vitamin profile of 174 mothers and newborns at parturition. *Am J Clin Nutr*. 1975;28:59-65.
11. Tripathy K. Erythrocyte transketolase activity and thiamine transfer across human placenta. *Am J Clin Nutr*. 1968;21:739-742.

12. Bamji MS. Enzymic evaluation of thiamin, riboflavin and pyridoxine status of parturient women and their newborn infants. *Br J Nutr*. 1976;35:259-265.
13. Dostalova L. Correlation of the vitamin status between mother and newborn during delivery. *Dev Pharmacol Ther*. 1982;4(suppl 1):45-57.
14. Siddall AC. Vitamin B_1 deficiency as an etiologic factor in pregnancy toxemias. *Am J Obstet Gynecol*. 1938;35:662-667.
15. King G, Ride LT. The relation of vitamin B1 deficiency to the pregnancy toxaemias: a study of 371 cases of beri-beri complicating pregnancy. *J Obstet Gynaecol Br Emp*. 1945;52:130-147.
16. Chaudhuri SK, Halder K, Chowdhury SR, Bagchi K. Relationship between toxaemia of pregnancy and thiamine deficiency. *J Obstet Gynaecol Br Commonw*. 1969;76:123-126.
17. Chaudhuri SK. Role of nutrition in the etiology of toxemia of pregnancy. *Am J Obstet Gynecol*. 1971;110:46-48.
18. Thomson AM. Diet in pregnancy. 3. Diet in relation to the course and outcome of pregnancy. *Br J Nutr*. 1959;13:509-525.
19. Roecklein B, Levin SW, Comly M, Mukherjee AB. Intrauterine growth retardation induced by thiamine deficiency and pyrithiamine during pregnancy in the rat. *Am J Obstet Gynecol*. 1985;151:455-460.
20. Fouts PJ, Gustafson GW, Zerfas LG. Successful treatment of a case of polyneuritis of pregnancy. *Am J Obstet Gynecol*. 1934;28:902-907.
21. Willis RS, Winn WW, Morris AT, et al. Clinical observations in treatment of nausea and vomiting in pregnancy with vitamins B_1 and B_6: a preliminary report. *Am J Obstet Gynecol*. 1942;44:265-271.
22. Hunt AD Jr, Stokes J Jr, McCrory WW, Stroud HH. Pyridoxine dependency: report of a case of intractable convulsions in an infant controlled by pyridoxine. *Pediatrics*. 1954;13:140-145.
23. Averback P. Anencephaly associated with megavitamin therapy. *Can Med Assoc J*. 1976;114:995.
24. Reading C. Down's syndrome, leukaemia and maternal thiamine deficiency. *Med J Aust*. 1976;1:505.
25. Thomas MR, Sneed SM, Wei C, et al. The effects of vitamin C, vitamin B6, vitamin B12, folic acid, riboflavin, and thiamin on the breast milk and maternal status of well-nourished women at 6 months postpartum. *Am J Clin Nutr*. 1980;33:2151-2156.
26. Deodhar AD, Rajalakshmi R, Ramakrishnan CV. Studies on human lactation. Part III. Effect of dietary vitamin supplementation on vitamin contents of breast milk. *Acta Paediatr Scand*. 1964;53:42-48.
27. Ford JE, Zechalko A, Murphy J, Brooke OG. Comparison of the B vitamin composition of milk from mothers of preterm and term babies. *Arch Dis Child*. 1983;58:367-372.
28. Nail PA, Thomas MR, Eakin R. The effect of thiamin and riboflavin supplementation on the level of those vitamins in human breast milk and urine. *Am J Clin Nutr*. 1980;33:198-204.
29. Fehily L. Human-milk intoxication due to B1 avitaminosis. *Br Med J*. 1944;2:590-592.
30. Cruickshank JD, Trimble AP, Brown JAH. Interstitial mononuclear pneumonia: a cause of sudden death in Gurkha infants in the Far East. *Arch Dis Child*. 1957;32:279-284.
31. Mayer J. Nutrition and lactation. *Postgrad Med*. 1963;33:380-385.
32. Gunther M. Diet and milk secretion in women. *Proc Nutr Soc*. 1968;27:77-82.
33. Rao RR, Subrahmanyam I. An investigation on the thiamine content of mother's milk in relation to infantile convulsions. *Indian J Med Res*. 1964;52:1198-1201.
34. Debuse PJ. Shoshin beriberi in an infant of a thiamine-deficient mother. *Acta Paediatr*. 1992;81:723-724.

VITAMIN B_2 (RIBOFLAVIN)

Vitamin (Water-Soluble Vitamin)

PREGNANCY RECOMMENDATION: Compatible

BREASTFEEDING RECOMMENDATION: Compatible

PREGNANCY SUMMARY

Several reports describing the use of riboflavin in human pregnancy have been located. The recommended daily allowance (RDA) is 1.4 mg for pregnant patients. Riboflavin crosses the placenta. Deficiency of riboflavin has been associated with preeclampsia and other pregnancy complications. Patients who consume meat or dairy products rarely during pregnancy, which may include some patients who are vegetarian or vegan, may be at risk for low riboflavin levels. No animal reproduction studies have been conducted. Vitamin B_2 is water soluble, and excess amounts are not stored in the body. Therefore, using this vitamin at the RDA is endorsed by ACOG and AAP.

BREASTFEEDING SUMMARY

Riboflavin (vitamin B_2) is excreted into human breast milk. The RDA for riboflavin during lactation is 1.6 mg. Breast milk concentrations were directly proportional to dietary intake. However, using this vitamin while breastfeeding at the RDA is only endorsed for those patients with dietary insufficiency.

References

1. National Institutes of Health. Riboflavin fact sheet for health professionals. Accessed July 29, 2024. https://ods.od.nih.gov/factsheets/Riboflavin-HealthProfessional/
2. AAP Committee on Fetus and Newborn and ACOG Committee on Obstetric Practice. Antepartum care. In: Kilpatrick SJ, Papile LA, Macones GA. eds. *Guidelines for perinatal care*. 8th ed. American Academy of Pediatrics; 2017.
3. National Library of Medicine. Pubchem. Riboflavin. Accessed July 29, 2024. https://pubchem.ncbi.nlm.nih.gov/compound/Riboflavin
4. Hill EP, Longo LD. Dynamics of maternal-fetal nutrient transfer. *Fed Proc*. 1980;39:239-244.
5. Lust JE, Hagerman DD, Villee CA. The transport of riboflavin by human placenta. *J Clin Invest*. 1954;33:38-40.
6. Frank O, Walbroehl G, Thomason A, et al. Placental transfer: fetal retention of some vitamins. *Am J Clin Nutr*. 1970;23:662-663.
7. Kaminetzky HA, Baker H, Frank O, Langer A. The effects of intravenously administered water-soluble vitamins during labor in normovitaminemic and hypovitaminemic gravidas on maternal and neonatal blood vitamin levels at delivery. *Am J Obstet Gynecol*. 1974;120:697-703.
8. Kaminetzky HA, Baker H. Micronutrients in pregnancy. *Clin Obstet Gynecol*. 1977;20:363-380.
9. Baker H, Frank O, Thomason AD, et al. Vitamin profile of 174 mothers and newborns at parturition. *Am J Clin Nutr*. 1975;28:59-65.
10. Baker H, Frank O, Deangelis B, et al. Role of placenta in maternal-fetal vitamin transfer in humans. *Am J Obstet Gynecol*. 1981;141:792-796.
11. Bamji MS. Enzymic evaluation of thiamin, riboflavin and pyridoxine status of parturient women and their newborn infants. *Br J Nutr*. 1976;35:259-265.
12. Baker H, Thind IS, Frank O, et al. Vitamin levels in low-birth-weight newborn infants and their mothers. *Am J Obstet Gynecol*. 1977;129:521-524.
13. Kirshenbaum NW, Dancis J, Levitz M, et al. Riboflavin concentration in maternal and cord blood in human pregnancy. *Am J Obstet Gynecol*. 1987;157:748-752.

14. Dancis J, Lehanka J, Levitz M. Placental transport of riboflavin: differential rates of uptake at the maternal and fetal surfaces of the perfused human placenta. *Am J Obstet Gynecol*. 1988;158:204-210.
15. Dostalova L. Correlation of the vitamin status between mother and newborn during delivery. *Dev Pharmacol Ther*. 1982;4(suppl 1):45-57.
16. Vir SC, Love AHG, Thompson W. Riboflavin status during pregnancy. *Am J Clin Nutr*. 1981;34:2699-2705.
17. Heller S, Salkeld RM, Korner WF. Riboflavin status in pregnancy. *Am J Clin Nutr*. 1974;27:1225-1230.
18. Harpey JP, Charpentier C. Acute fatty liver of pregnancy. *Lancet*. 1983; 1:586-587.
19. Thomas MR, Sneed SM, Wei C, et al. The effects of vitamin C, vitamin B6, vitamin B12, folic acid, riboflavin, and thiamin on the breast milk and maternal status of well-nourished women at 6 months postpartum. *Am J Clin Nutr*. 1980;33:2151-2156.
20. Deodhar AD, Rajalakshmi R, Ramakrishnan CV. Studies on human lactation. Part III. Effect of dietary vitamin supplementation on vitamin contents of breast milk. *Acta Paediatr Scand*. 1964;53:42-48.
21. Ford, JE, Zechalko A, Murphy J, Brooke OG. Comparison of the B vitamin composition of milk from mothers of preterm and term babies. *Arch Dis Child*. 1983;58:367-372.
22. Nail PA, Thomas MR, Eakin R. The effect of thiamin and riboflavin supplementation on the level of those vitamins in human breast milk and urine. *Am J Clin Nutr*. 1980;33:198-204.
23. Gunther M. Diet and milk secretion in women. *Proc Nutr Soc*. 1968;27:77-82.
24. Ronnholm KAR. Need for riboflavin supplementation in small prematures fed human milk. *Am J Clin Nutr*. 1986;43:1-6.

VITAMIN B_6 (PYRIDOXINE)

Vitamin (Water-Soluble Vitamin)

PREGNANCY RECOMMENDATION: Compatible

BREASTFEEDING RECOMMENDATION: Compatible

PREGNANCY SUMMARY

The recommended daily allowance (RDA) of pyridoxine (vitamin B_6) is 1.9 mg. Pyridoxine is actively transported across the placenta to the fetus. Pyridoxine deficiency during pregnancy is a common problem in unsupplemented women. Supplementation with oral pyridoxine reduces but does not eliminate the frequency of deficiency. No definitive evidence has appeared that indicates mild to moderate deficiency of this vitamin is a cause of maternal or fetal complications. Most of the studies with this vitamin have been open and uncontrolled, and were evaluated in treating nausea and vomiting during pregnancy. A significant reduction in nausea and vomiting of pregnancy appears to occur with pyridoxine use. The available data are sufficient to conclude that the combination of pyridoxine and doxylamine is compatible and effective for nausea and vomiting of pregnancy. Vitamin B_6 is water soluble, and excess amounts are not stored in the body. Therefore, using this vitamin at the RDA is endorsed by ACOG and AAP.

BREASTFEEDING SUMMARY

Pyridoxine is excreted into human breast milk, and concentrations in breast milk are directly proportional to intake. In well-nourished women, pyridoxine levels varied depending on intake, from 123 to 314 ng/mL, with peak breast milk levels 3 to 8 hours after ingestion of a vitamin supplement. In lactating women with low nutritional status, supplementation with pyridoxine (0.4-40 mg/d) resulted in mean breast milk concentrations of 80 to 158 ng/mL. However, using this vitamin while breastfeeding at the RDA is only endorsed for those patients with dietary insufficiency.

References

1. National Institutes of Health Office of Dietary Supplements. Vitamin B6. Accessed October 8, 2024. https://ods.od.nih.gov/factsheets/VitaminB6-HealthProfessional/
2. National Library of Medicine. Pubchem. Pyridoxine. Accessed October 8, 2024. https://pubchem.ncbi.nlm.nih.gov/compound/Pyridoxine
3. Frank O, Walbroehl G, Thomson A, et al. Placental transfer: fetal retention of some vitamins. *Am J Clin Nutr*. 1970;23:662-663.
4. Hill EP, Longo LD. Dynamics of maternal-fetal nutrient transfer. *Fed Proc*. 1980;39:239-244.
5. Baker H, Frank O, Deangelis B, et al. Role of placenta in maternal-fetal vitamin transfer in humans. *Am J Obstet Gynecol*. 1981;141:792-796.
6. Wachstein M, Moore C, Graffeo LW. Pyridoxal phosphate (B_6-al-PO_4) levels of circulating leukocytes in maternal and cord blood. *Proc Soc Exp Biol Med*. 1957;96:326-328.
7. Wachstein M, Kellner JD, Ortiz JM. Pyridoxal phosphate in plasma and leukocytes of normal and pregnant subjects following B_6 load tests. *Proc Soc Exp Biol Med*. 1960;103:350-353.
8. Brin M. Thiamine and pyridoxine studies of mother and cord blood. *Fed Proc*. 1966;25:245.
9. Contractor SF, Shane B. Blood and urine levels of vitamin B_6 in the mother and fetus before and after loading of the mother with vitamin B_6. *Am J Obstet Gynecol*. 1970;107:635-640.
10. Brin M. Abnormal tryptophan metabolism in pregnancy and with the oral contraceptive pill. II. Relative levels of vitamin B_6-vitamers in cord and maternal blood. *Am J Clin Nutr*. 1971;24:704-708.
11. Heller S, Salkeld RM, Korner WF. Vitamin B_6 status in pregnancy. *Am J Clin Nutr*. 1973;26:1339-1348.
12. Kaminetzky HA, Baker H, Frank O, Langer A. The effects of intravenously administered water-soluble vitamins during labor in normovitaminemic and hypovitaminemic gravidas on maternal and neonatal blood vitamin levels at delivery. *Am J Obstet Gynecol*. 1974;120:697-703.
13. Brophy MH, Siiteri PK. Pyridoxal phosphate and hypertensive disorders of pregnancy. *Am J Obstet Gynecol*. 1975;121:1075-1079.
14. Bamji MS. Enzymic evaluation of thiamin, riboflavin and pyridoxine status of parturient women and their newborn infants. *Br J Nutr*. 1976;35:259-265.
15. Roepke JLB, Kirksey A. Vitamin B_6 nutriture during pregnancy and lactation. I. Vitamin B_6 intake, levels of the vitamin in biological fluids, and condition of the infant at birth. *Am J Clin Nutr*. 1979;32:2249-2256.
16. Baker H, Thind IS, Frank O, et al. Vitamin levels in low-birth-weight newborn infants and their mothers. *Am J Obstet Gynecol*. 1977;129:521-524.
17. Baker H, Frank O, Thomason AD, et al. Vitamin profile of 174 mothers and newborns at parturition. *Am J Clin Nutr*. 1975;28:59-65.
18. Wachstein M, Gudaitis A. Disturbance of vitamin B_6 metabolism in pregnancy. *J Lab Clin Med*. 1952;40:550-557.
19. Wachstein M, Gudaitis A. Disturbance of vitamin B_6 metabolism in pregnancy. II. The influence of various amounts of pyridoxine hydrochloride

V

upon the abnormal tryptophan load test in pregnant women. *J Lab Clin Med*. 1953;42:98-107.
20. Wachstein M, Gudaitis A. Disturbance of vitamin B_6 metabolism in pregnancy. III. Abnormal vitamin B_6 load test. *Am J Obstet Gynecol*. 1953;66: 1207-1213.
21. Wachstein M, Lobel S. Abnormal tryptophan metabolites in human pregnancy and their relation to deranged vitamin B_6 metabolism. *Proc Soc Exp Biol Med*. 1954;86:624-627.
22. Zartman ER, Barnes AC, Hicks DJ. Observations on pyridoxine metabolism in pregnancy. *Am J Obstet Gynecol*. 1955;70:645-649.
23. Turner ER, Reynolds MS. Intake and elimination of vitamin B_6 and metabolites by women. *J Am Diet Assoc*. 1955;31:1119-1120.
24. Page EW. The vitamin B_6 requirement for normal pregnancy. *West J Surg Obstet Gynecol*. 1956;64:96-103.
25. Coursin DB, Brown VC. Changes in vitamin B_6 during pregnancy. *Am J Obstet Gynecol*. 1961;82:1307-1311.
26. Brown RR, Thornton MJ, Price JM. The effect of vitamin supplementation on the urinary excretion of tryptophan metabolites by pregnant women. *J Clin Invest*. 1961;40:617-623.
27. Hamfelt A, Hahn L. Pyridoxal phosphate concentration in plasma and tryptophan load test during pregnancy. *Clin Chim Acta*. 1969;25:91-96.
28. Rose DP, Braidman IP. Excretion of tryptophan metabolites as affected by pregnancy, contraceptive steroids, and steroid hormones. *Am J Clin Nutr*. 1971;24:673-683.
29. Kaminetzky HA, Langer A, Baker H, et al. The effect of nutrition in teen-age gravidas on pregnancy and the status of the neonate. I. A nutritional profile. *Am J Obstet Gynecol*. 1973;115:639-646.
30. Shane B, Contractor SF. Assessment of vitamin B_6 status. Studies on pregnant women and oral contraceptive users. *Am J Clin Nutr*. 1975;28:739-747.
31. Cleary RE, Lumeng L, Li TK. Maternal and fetal plasma levels of pyridoxal phosphate at term: adequacy of vitamin B_6 supplementation during pregnancy. *Am J Obstet Gynecol*. 1975;121:25-28.
32. Lumeng L, Cleary RE, Wagner R, et al. Adequacy of vitamin B_6 supplementation during pregnancy: a prospective study. *Am J Clin Nutr*. 1976;29:1376-1383. Anonymous. Requirement of vitamin B_6 during pregnancy. *Nutr Rev*. 1976;34:15-16.
33. Dostalova L. Correlation of the vitamin status between mother and newborn during delivery. *Dev Pharmacol Ther*. 1982;4(suppl I):45-57.
34. Hunt IF, Murphy NJ, Martner-Hewes PM, et al. Zinc, vitamin B-6, and other nutrients in pregnant women attending prenatal clinics in Mexico. *Am J Clin Nutr*. 1987;46:563-569.
35. Bapurao S, Raman L, Tulpule PG. Biochemical assessment of vitamin B_6 nutritional status in pregnant women with orolingual manifestations. *Am J Clin Nutr*. 1982;36:581-586.
36. Davis SD. Immunodeficiency and runting syndrome in rats from congenital pyridoxine deficiency. *Nature*. 1974;251:548-50. As cited in Shepard TH. *Catalog of Teratogenic Agents*. 6th ed. The Johns Hopkins University Press; 1989:537-538.
37. Davis SD, Nelson T, Shepard TH. Teratogenicity of vitamin B_6 deficiency: omphalocele, skeletal and neural defects, and splenic hypoplasia. *Science*. 1970;169:1329-1330. As cited in Shepard TH. *Catalog of Teratogenic Agents*. 6th ed. The Johns Hopkins University Press; 1989:537-538.
38. Averback P. Anencephaly associated with megavitamin therapy. *Can Med Assoc J*. 1976;114:995.
39. Sprince H, Lowy RS, Folsome CE, Behrman J. Studies on the urinary excretion of "xanthurenic acid" during normal and abnormal pregnancy: a survey of the excretion of "xanthurenic acid" in normal nonpregnant, normal pregnant, pre-eclamptic, and eclamptic women. *Am J Obstet Gynecol*. 1951;62:84-92.
40. Wachstein M, Graffeo LW. Influence of vitamin B_6 on the incidence of preeclampsia. *Obstet Gynecol*. 1956;8:177-180.
41. Kaminetzky HA, Baker H. Micronutrients in pregnancy. *Clin Obstet Gynecol*. 1977;20:363-380.
42. Diding NA, Melander SEJ. Serum vitamin B_6 level in normal and toxaemic pregnancy. *Acta Obstet Gynecol Scand*. 1961;40:252-261.
43. Hillman RW, Cabaud PG, Nilsson DE, et al. Pyridoxine supplementation during pregnancy. Clinical and laboratory observations. *Am J Clin Nutr*. 1963;12:427-430.
44. Coelingh Bennink HJT, Schreurs WHP. Improvement of oral glucose tolerance in gestational diabetes by pyridoxine. *Br Med J*. 1975;3:13-15.
45. Spellacy WN, Buhi WC, Birk SA. Vitamin B_6 treatment of gestational diabetes mellitus. Studies of blood glucose and plasma insulin. *Am J Obstet Gynecol*. 1977;127:599-602.
46. Perkins RP. Failure of pyridoxine to improve glucose tolerance in gestational diabetes mellitus. *Obstet Gynecol*. 1977;50:370-372.
47. Gillmer MDG, Mazibuko D. Pyridoxine treatment of chemical diabetes in pregnancy. *Am J Obstet Gynecol*. 1979;133:499-502.
48. Snyderman SE, Holt LE, Carretero R, Jacobs K. Pyridoxine deficiency in the human infant. *J Clin Nutr*. 1953;1:200-207.
49. Molony CJ, Parmalee AH. Convulsions in young infants as a result of pyridoxine (vitamin B_6) deficiency. *JAMA*. 1954;154:405-406.
50. Coursin DB. Vitamin B_6 deficiency in infants. *Am J Dis Child*. 1955;90: 344-348.
51. Coursin DB. Effects of vitamin B_6 on the central nervous activity in childhood. *Am J Clin Nutr*. 1956;4:354-363.
52. Scriver CR. Vitamin B_6 deficiency and dependency in man. *Am J Dis Child*. 1967;113:109-114.
53. Hunt AD Jr, Stokes J Jr, McCrory WW, Stroud HH. Pyridoxine dependency: report of a case of intractable convulsions in an infant controlled by pyridoxine. *Pediatrics*. 1954;13:140-145.
54. Bankier A, Turner M, Hopkins IJ. Pyridoxine dependent seizures—a wider clinical spectrum. *Arch Dis Child*. 1983;58:415-418.
55. Bejsovec MIR, Kulenda Z, Ponca E. Familial intrauterine convulsions in pyridoxine dependency. *Arch Dis Child*. 1967;42:201-207.
56. South M. Neonatal seizures after use of pyridoxine in pregnancy. *Lancet*. 1999;353:1940.
57. Willis RS, Winn WW, Morris AT, et al. Clinical observations in treatment of nausea and vomiting in pregnancy with vitamins B1 and B6. A preliminary report. *Am J Obstet Gynecol*. 1942;44:265-271.
58. Weinstein BB, Mitchell GJ, Sustendal GF. Clinical experiences with pyridoxine hydrochloride in treatment of nausea and vomiting of pregnancy. *Am J Obstet Gynecol*. 1943;46:283-285.
59. Hart BF, McConnell WT. Vitamin B factors in toxic psychosis of pregnancy and the puerperium. *Am J Obstet Gynecol*. 1943;46:283.
60. Varas O. Treatment of nausea and vomiting of pregnancy with vitamin B_6. *Bol Soc Chilena Obstet Ginecol*. 1943;8:404. As abstracted in *Am J Obstet Gynecol*. 1945;50:347-348.
61. Weinstein BB, Wohl Z, Mitchell GJ, Sustendal GF. Oral administration of pyridoxine hydrochloride in the treatment of nausea and vomiting of pregnancy. *Am J Obstet Gynecol*. 1944;47:389-394.
62. Dorsey CW. The use of pyridoxine and suprarenal cortex combined in the treatment of the nausea and vomiting of pregnancy. *Am J Obstet Gynecol*. 1949;58:1073-1078.
63. McGanity WJ, McHenry EW, Van Wyck HB, Watt GL. An effect of pyridoxine on blood urea in human subjects. *J Biol Chem*. 1949;178:511-516.
64. Beaton JR, McHenry EW. Observations on plasma glutamic acid. *Fed Proc*. 1951;10:161.
65. Hesseltine HC. Pyridoxine failure in nausea and vomiting of pregnancy. *Am J Obstet Gynecol*. 1946;51:82-86.
66. Sahakian V, Rouse DJ, Rose NB, Niebyl JR. Vitamin B6 for nausea and vomiting of pregnancy (abstract). *Am J Obstet Gynecol*. 1991;164:322.
67. Sahakian V, Rouse D, Sipes S, et al. Vitamin B6 is effective therapy for nausea and vomiting of pregnancy: a randomized double-blind placebo-controlled study. *Obstet Gynecol*. 1991;78:33-36.
68. Vutyavanich T, Wongtra-ngan S, Ruangsri R-A. Pyridoxine for nausea and vomiting of pregnancy: a randomized, double-blind, placebo-controlled trial. *Am J Obstet Gynecol*. 1995;173:881-884.
69. Gardner LI, Welsh-Sloan J, Cady RB. Phocomelia in infant whose mother took large doses of pyridoxine during pregnancy. *Lancet*. 1985;1:636.
70. Jacobsson C, Granstrom G. Effects of vitamin B_6 on beta-aminoproprionitrile-induced palatal cleft formation in the rat. *Cleft Palate Craniofac J*. 1997; 34:95-100.
71. Munger RG, Sauberlich HE, Corcoran C, et al. Maternal vitamin B-6 and folate status and risk of oral cleft birth defects in the Philippines. *Birth Defects Res A Clin Mol Teratol*. 2004;70:464-471.
72. Schuster K, Bailey LB, Mahan CS. Vitamin B_6 status of low-income adolescent and adult pregnant women and the condition of their infants at birth. *Am J Clin Nutr*. 1981;34:1731-1735.
73. Swartwout JR, Unglaub WG, Smith RC. Vitamin B_6, serum lipids and placental arteriolar lesions in human pregnancy. A preliminary report. *Am J Clin Nutr*. 1960;8:434-444.
74. Hillman RW, Cabaud PG, Schenone RA. The effects of pyridoxine supplements on the dental caries experience of pregnant women. *Am J Clin Nutr*. 1962;10:512-515.
75. West KD, Kirksey A. Influence of vitamin B_6 intake on the content of the vitamin in human milk. *Am J Clin Nutr*. 1976;29:961-969.
76. Thomas MR, Kawamoto J, Sneed SM, Eakin R. The effects of vitamin C, vitamin B_6, and vitamin B_{12} supplementation on the breast milk and maternal status of well-nourished women. *Am J Clin Nutr*. 1979;32:1679-1685.

77. Sneed SM, Zane C, Thomas MR. The effects of ascorbic acid, vitamin B_6, vitamin B_{12}, and folic acid supplementation on the breast milk and maternal nutritional status of low socioeconomic lactating women. *Am J Clin Nutr*. 1981;34:1338-1346.
78. Styslinger L, Kirksey A. Effects of different levels of vitamin B-6 supplementation on vitamin B-6 concentrations in human milk and vitamin B-6 intakes of breastfed infants. *Am J Clin Nutr*. 1985;41:21-31.
79. Ford JE, Zechalko A, Murphy J, Brooke OG. Comparison of the B vitamin composition of milk from mothers of preterm and term babies. *Arch Dis Child*. 1983;58:367-372.
80. Deodhar AD, Rajalakshmi R, Ramakrishnan CV. Studies on human lactation. Part III. Effect of dietary vitamin supplementation vitamin contents of breast milk. *Acta Pediatr*. 1964;53:42-48.
81. Thomas MR, Sneed SM, Wei C, et al. The effects of vitamin C, vitamin B_6, vitamin B_{12}, folic acid, riboflavin, and thiamine on the breast milk and maternal status of well-nourished women at 6 months postpartum. *Am J Clin Nutr*. 1980;33:2151-2156.
82. Bessey OA, Adam DJD, Hansen AE. Intake of vitamin B_6 and infantile convulsions: a first approximation of requirements of pyridoxine in infants. *Pediatrics*. 1957;20:33-44.
83. Kirksey A, Roepke JLB. Vitamin B-6 nutriture of mothers of three breast-fed neonates with central nervous system disorders. *Fed Proc*. 1981;40:864.
84. Foukas MD. An antilactogenic effect of pyridoxine. *J Obstet Gynaecol Br Commonw*. 1973;80:718-720.
85. Moretti C, Fabbri A, Gnessi L, et al. Pyridoxine (B6) suppresses the rise in prolactin and increases the rise in growth hormone induced by exercise. *N Engl J Med*. 1982;307:444-445.
86. MacDonald HN, Collins YD, Tobin MJW, Wijayaratne, DN. The failure of pyridoxine in suppression of puerperal lactation. *Br J Obstet Gynaecol*. 1976; 83:54-55.
87. Canales ES, Soria J, Zarate A, Mason M, Molina M. The influence of pyridoxine on prolactin secretion and milk production in women. *Br J Obstet Gynaecol*. 1976;83:387-388.
88. Greentree LB. Dangers of vitamin B_6 in nursing mothers. *N Engl J Med*. 1979;300:141-142.
89. Lande NI. More on dangers of vitamin B_6 in nursing mothers. *N Engl J Med*. 1979;300:926-927.
90. Rivlin RS. More on dangers of vitamin B_6 in nursing mothers. *N Engl J Med*. 1979;300:927.
91. Andon MB, Howard MP, Moser PB, Reynolds RD. Nutritionally relevant supplementation of vitamin B6 in lactating women: effect on plasma prolactin. *Pediatrics*. 1985;76:769-773.

VITAMIN B_{12} (CYANOCOBALAMIN)

Vitamin (Water-Soluble Vitamin)

PREGNANCY RECOMMENDATION: Compatible

BREASTFEEDING RECOMMENDATION: Compatible

PREGNANCY SUMMARY

The RDA and daily recommended intake by the ACOG and AAP for vitamin B_{12} in pregnancy is 2.6 mcg. Vitamin B_{12} crosses the placenta. Severe maternal vitamin B_{12} deficiency may result in megaloblastic anemia with subsequent infertility and poor pregnancy outcome. Less severe maternal deficiency apparently is common and does not pose a significant risk to the mother or fetus. Vitamin B_{12} is water soluble, and excess amounts are not stored in the body. Therefore, using this vitamin at the RDA is endorsed by ACOG and AAP.

BREASTFEEDING SUMMARY

The daily recommended intake by ACOG and AAP for vitamin B_{12} during lactation is 2.8 mcg. If the diet of a lactating woman adequately supplies this amount, maternal supplementation with vitamin B_{12} is not needed. Vitamin B_{12} is excreted into human breast milk. Vitamin B_{12} deficiency in a lactating mother may cause adverse consequences in a nursing infant. Several reports have described megaloblastic anemia in infants exclusively breastfed by vitamin B_{12}-deficient mothers. However, using this vitamin at the RDA is only endorsed for those patients with dietary insufficiency.

References

1. AAP Committee on Fetus and Newborn and ACOG Committee on Obstetric Practice. Antepartum care. In: Kilpatrick SJ, Papile LA, Macones GA, eds. *Guidelines for perinatal care*. 8th ed. American Academy of Pediatrics; 2017.
2. National Institutes of Health. *Vitamin B12 fact sheet for health professionals*. Accessed October 1, 2023. https://ods.od.nih.gov/factsheets/VitaminB12-HealthProfessional/
3. Lexi-Comp, Inc. (Lexi-drugs). Lexi-Comp, Inc; 2023.
4. National Library of Medicine. Pubchem. Vitamin B12. Accessed October 1, 2023.https://pubchem.ncbi.nlm.nih.gov/compound/vitamin-B12
5. Luhby AL, Cooperman JM, Donnenfeld AM, et al. Observations on transfer of vitamin B_{12} from mother to fetus and newborn. *Am J Dis Child*. 1958; 96:532-533.
6. Hill EP, Longo LD. Dynamics of maternal-fetal nutrient transfer. *Fed Proc*. 1980;39:239-244.
7. Kaminetzky HA, Baker H, Frank O, et al. The effects of intravenously administered water-soluble vitamins during labor in normovitaminemic and hypovitaminemic gravidas on maternal and neonatal blood vitamin levels at delivery. *Am J Obstet Gynecol*. 1974;120:697-703.
8. Frank O, Walbroehl G, Thomson A, et al. Placental transfer: fetal retention of some vitamins. *Am J Clin Nutr*. 1970;23:662-663.
9. Luhby AL, Cooperman JM, Stone ML, et al. Physiology of vitamin B_{12} in pregnancy, the placenta, and the newborn. *Am J Dis Child*. 1961;102:753-754.
10. Baker H, Ziffer H, Pasher I, et al. A Comparison of maternal and foetal folic acid and vitamin B_{12} at parturition. *Br Med J*. 1958;1:978-979.
11. Boger WP, Bayne GM, Wright LD, et al. Differential serum vitamin B_{12} concentrations in mothers and infants. *N Engl J Med*. 1957;256:1085-1087.
12. Temperley IJ, Meehan MJM, Gatenby PBB. Serum vitamin B12 levels in pregnant women. *J Obstet Gynaecol Br Commonw*. 1968;75:511-516.
13. Boger WP, Wright LD, Beck GD, et al. Vitamin B_{12}: correlation of serum concentrations and pregnancy. *Proc Soc Exp Biol Med*. 1956;92:140-143.
14. Martin JD, Davis RE, Stenhouse N. Serum folate and vitamin B12 levels in pregnancy with particular reference to uterine bleeding and bacteriuria. *J Obstet Gynaecol Br Commonw*. 1967;74:697-701.
15. Ball EW, Giles C. Folic acid and vitamin B_{12} levels in pregnancy and their relation to megaloblastic anaemia. *J Clin Pathol*. 1964;17:165-174.
16. Izak G, Rachmilewitz M, Stein Y, et al. Vitamin B_{12} and iron deficiencies in anemia of pregnancy and puerperium. *Arch Intern Med*. 1957;99:346-355.
17. Edelstein T, Metz J. Correlation between vitamin B12 concentration in serum and muscle in late pregnancy. *J Obstet Gynaecol Br Commonw*. 1969; 76:545-548.
18. Herbert V. Recommended dietary intakes (RDI) of vitamin B-12 in humans. *Am J Clin Nutr*. 1987;45:671-678.

19. Baker H, Frank O, Thomson AD, et al. Vitamin profile of 174 mothers and newborns at parturition. *Am J Clin Nutr*. 1975;28:59-65.
20. Kaminetzky HA, Baker H. Micronutrients in pregnancy. *Clin Obstet Gynecol*. 1977;20:363-380.
21. Lowenstein L, Lalonde M, Deschenes EB, et al. Vitamin B_{12} in pregnancy and the puerperium. *Am J Clin Nutr*. 1960;8:265-275.
22. Baker SJ, Jacob E, Rajan KT, et al. Vitamin-B_{12} deficiency in pregnancy and the puerperium. *Br Med J*. 1962;1:1658-1661.
23. Killander A, Vahlquist B. The vitamin B_{12} concentration in serum from term and premature infants. *Nord Med*. 1954;51:777-779.
24. Baker H, Thind IS, Frank O, et al. Vitamin levels in low-birth-weight newborn infants and their mothers. *Am J Obstet Gynecol*. 1977;129:521-524.
25. Okuda K, Helliger AE, Chow BF. Vitamin B_{12} serum level and pregnancy. *Am J Clin Nutr*. 1956;4:440-443.
26. Baker H, Frank O, Deangelis B, et al. Role of placenta in maternal-fetal vitamin transfer in humans. *Am J Obstet Gynecol*. 1981;141:792-796.
27. Giugliani ERJ, Jorge SM, Goncalves AL. Serum vitamin B_{12} levels in parturients, in the intervillous space of the placenta and in full-term newborns and their interrelationships with folate levels. *Am J Clin Nutr*. 1985;41:330-335.
28. Giles C. An account of 335 cases of megaloblastic anaemia of pregnancy and the puerperium. *J Clin Pathol*. 1966;19:1-11.
29. Roberts PD, James H, Petrie A, et al. Vitamin B_{12} status in pregnancy among immigrants to Britain. *Br Med J*. 1973;3:67-72.
30. Dostalova L. Correlation of the vitamin status between mother and newborn during delivery. *Dev Pharmacol Ther*. 1982;4(suppl 1):45-57.
31. McGarry JM, Andrews J. Smoking in pregnancy and vitamin B_{12} metabolism. *Br Med J*. 1972;2:74-77.
32. Heaton D. Another case of megaloblastic anemia of infancy due to maternal pernicious anemia. *N Engl J Med*. 1979;300:202-203.
33. Varadi S. Pernicious anaemia and infertility. *Lancet*. 1967;2:1305.
34. Jackson IMD, Doig WB, McDonald G. Pernicious anaemia as a cause of infertility. *Lancet*. 1967;2:1059-1060.
35. Chaudhuri S. Vitamin B_{12} in megaloblastic anaemia of pregnancy and tropical nutritional macrocytic anaemia. *Br Med J*. 1951;2:825-828.
36. Patel JC, Kocher BR. Vitamin B_{12} in macrocytic anaemia of pregnancy and the puerperium. *Br Med J*. 1950;1:924-927.
37. Parr JH, Ramsay I. The presentation of osteomalacia in pregnancy. Case report. *Br J Obstet Gynaecol*. 1984;91:816-818.
38. Streiff RR, Little AB. Folic acid deficiency as a cause of uterine hemorrhage in pregnancy. *J Clin Invest*. 1965;44:1102.
39. Streiff RR, Little AB. Folic acid deficiency in pregnancy. *N Engl J Med*. 1967;276:776-779.
40. Whiteside MG, Ungar B, Cowling DC. Iron, folic acid and vitamin B_{12} levels in normal pregnancy, and their influence on birth-weight and the duration of pregnancy. *Med J Aust*. 1968;1:338-342.
41. Shepard TH. *Catalog of Teratogenic Agents*. 3rd ed. The Johns Hopkins University Press; 1980:348-349.
42. Schorah CJ, Smithells RW, Scott J. Vitamin B_{12} and anencephaly. *Lancet*. 1980;1:880.
43. Ampola MG, Mahoney MJ, Nakamura E, et al. Prenatal therapy of a patient with vitamin-B_{12}-responsive methylmalonic acidemia. *N Engl J Med*. 1975;293:313-317.
44. Morrow G III, Schwarz RH, Hallock JA, et al. Prenatal detection of methylmalonic acidemia. *J Pediatr*. 1970;77:120-123.
45. Samson RR, McClelland DBL. Vitamin B_{12} in human colostrum and milk. *Acta Paediatr Scand*. 1980;69:93-99.
46. Deodhar AD, Rajalakshmi R, Ramakrishnan CV. Studies on human lactation. Part III. Effect of dietary vitamin supplementation on vitamin contents of breast milk. *Acta Paediatr Scand*. 1964;53:42-48.
47. Thomas MR, Kawamoto J, Sneed SM, et al. The effects of vitamin C, vitamin B6, and vitamin B_{12} supplementation on the breast milk and maternal status of well-nourished women. *Am J Clin Nutr*. 1979;32:1679-1685.
48. Sneed SM, Zane C, Thomas MR. The effects of ascorbic acid, vitamin B_6, vitamin B_{12}, and folic acid supplementation on the breast milk and maternal nutritional status of low socioeconomic lactating women. *Am J Clin Nutr*. 1981;34:1338-1346.
49. Sandberg DP, Begley JA, Hall CA. The content, binding, and forms of vitamin B_{12} in milk. *Am J Clin Nutr*. 1981;34:1717-1724.
50. Ford JE, Zechalko A, Murphy J, et al. Comparison of the B vitamin composition of milk from mothers of preterm and term babies. *Arch Dis Child*. 1983;58:367-372.
51. Lampkin BC, Shore NA, Chadwick D. Megaloblastic anemia of infancy secondary to maternal pernicious anemia. *N Engl J Med*. 1966;274:1168-1171.
52. Jadhav M, Webb JKG, Vaishnava S, et al. Vitamin-B_{12} deficiency in Indian infants: a clinical syndrome. *Lancet*. 1962;2:903-907.
53. Lampkin BC, Saunders EF. Nutritional vitamin B_{12} deficiency in an infant. *J Pediatr*. 1969;75:1053-1055.
54. Higginbottom MC, Sweetman L, Nyhan WL. A syndrome of methylmalonic aciduria, homocystinuria, megaloblastic anemia and neurologic abnormalities in a vitamin B_{12}-deficient breast-fed infant of a strict vegetarian. *N Engl J Med*. 1978;299:317-323.
55. Frader J, Reibman B, Turkewitz D. Vitamin B_{12} deficiency in strict vegetarians. *N Engl J Med*. 1978;299:1319.
56. Fleiss PM, Douglass JM, Wolfe L. Vitamin B_{12} deficiency in strict vegetarians. *N Engl J Med*. 1978;299:1319.
57. Hershaft A. Vitamin B_{12} deficiency in strict vegetarians. *N Engl J Med*. 1978; 299:1319-1320.
58. Nyhan WL. Vitamin B_{12} deficiency in strict vegetarians. *N Engl J Med*. 1978; 299:1320.
59. Abdulla M, Aly KO, Andersson I, et al. Nutrient intake and health status of lactovegetarians: chemical analyses of diets using the duplicate portion sampling technique. *Am J Clin Nutr*. 1984;40:325-338.
60. Sklar R. Nutritional vitamin B_{12} deficiency in a breast-fed infant of a vegan-diet mother. *Clin Pediatr*. 1986;25:219-221.

VITAMIN C (ASCORBIC ACID)

Vitamin (Water-Soluble Vitamin)

PREGNANCY RECOMMENDATION: Compatible

BREASTFEEDING RECOMMENDATION: Compatible

PREGNANCY SUMMARY

Several reports describing the use of vitamin C (ascorbic acid) in human pregnancy have been located. The recommended daily allowance (RDA) is 80 mg for pregnant patients 18 years or less and 85 mg for those 19 years or older. Vitamin C crosses the placenta. Vitamin C is water soluble, and excess amounts are not stored in the body. Therefore, using this vitamin at the RDA is endorsed by ACOG and AAP.

BREASTFEEDING SUMMARY

Vitamin C (ascorbic acid) is excreted into breast milk. The recommended daily allowance (RDA) is 115 mg for pregnant patients 18 years or less and 120 mg for those 19 years or older. The upper limit for intake is 2,000 mg/d. Well-nourished lactating women consuming a normal diet will usually excrete sufficient amounts of vitamin C in their breast milk to reach a saturation level. Therefore, using this vitamin at the RDA is only endorsed for those patients with dietary insufficiency.

References

1. National Institutes of Health. Vitamin C fact sheet for health professionals. Accessed October 1, 2023. https://ods.od.nih.gov/factsheets/VitaminC-HealthProfessional/
2. AAP Committee on Fetus and Newborn and ACOG Committee on Obstetric Practice. Antepartum care. In: Kilpatrick SJ, Papile LA, Macones GA, eds. *Guidelines for Perinatal Care*. 8th ed. American Academy of Pediatrics; 2017.
3. American College of Obstetricians and Gynecologists. Nutrition during pregnancy. Accessed October 1, 2023. https://www.acog.org/womens-health/faqs/nutrition-during-pregnancy
4. Lexi-Comp, Inc. (Lexi-drugs). Lexi-Comp, Inc; 2023.
5. National Library of Medicine. Pubchem. Ascorbic acid. Accessed October 1, 2023. https://pubchem.ncbi.nlm.nih.gov/compound/54670067
6. Hill EP, Longo LD. Dynamics of maternal-fetal nutrient transfer. *Fed Proc*. 1980;39:239-44.
7. Streeter ML, Rosso P. Transport mechanisms for ascorbic acid in the human placenta. *Am J Clin Nutr*. 1981;34:1706-1711.
8. Hamil BM, Munks B, Moyer EZ, et al. Vitamin C in the blood and urine of the newborn and in the cord and maternal blood. *Am J Dis Child*. 1947; 74:417-433.
9. Kaminetzky HA, Baker H, Frank O, et al. The effects of intravenously administered water-soluble vitamins during labor in normovitaminemic and hypovitaminemic gravidas on maternal and neonatal blood vitamin levels at delivery. *Am J Obstet Gynecol*. 1974;120:697-703.
10. Snelling CE, Jackson SH. Blood studies of vitamin C during pregnancy, birth, and early infancy. *J Pediatr*. 1939;14:447-451.
11. Adlard BPF, De Souza SW, Moon S. Ascorbic acid in fetal human brain. *Arch Dis Child*. 1974;49:278-282.
12. Braestrup PW. Studies of latent scurvy in infants. II. Content of ascorbic (cevitamic) acid in the blood-serum of women in labour and in children at birth. *Acta Paediatr*. 1937;19:328-334.
13. Braestrup PW. The content of reduced ascorbic acid in blood plasma in infants, especially at birth and in the first days of life. *J Nutr*. 1938;16:363-373.
14. Slobody LB, Benson RA, Mestern J. A comparison of the vitamin C in mothers and their newborn infants. *J Pediatr*. 1946,29:41-44.
15. Teel HM, Burke BS, Draper R. Vitamin C in human pregnancy and lactation. I. Studies during pregnancy. *Am J Dis Child*. 1938;56:1004-1010.
16. Lund CJ, Kimble MS. Some determinants of maternal and plasma vitamin C levels. *Am J Obstet Gynecol*. 1943;46:635-647.
17. Manahan CP, Eastman NJ. The cevitamic acid content of fetal blood. *Bull Johns Hopkins Hosp*. 1938;62:478-481.
18. Raiha N. On the placental transfer of vitamin C. An experimental study on guinea pigs and human subjects. *Acta Physiol Scand*. 1958;45(suppl):155.
19. Khattab AK, Al Nagdy SA, Mourad KAH, et al. Foetal maternal ascorbic acid gradient in normal Egyptian subjects. *J Trop Pediatr*. 1970;16:112-115.
20. McDevitt E, Dove MA, Dove RF, et al. Selective filtration of vitamin C by the placenta. *Proc Soc Exp Biol Med*. 1942;51:289-290.
21. Sharma SC. Levels of total ascorbic acid, histamine and prostaglandins E_2 and $F_{2\alpha}$ in the maternal antecubital and foetal umbilical vein blood immediately following the normal human delivery. *Int J Vitam Nutr Res*. 1982;52: 320-325.
22. Dostalova L. Correlation of the vitamin status between mother and newborn during delivery. *Dev Pharmacol Ther*. 1982;4(suppl 1):45-57.
23. Baker H, Frank O, Thomson AD, et al. Vitamin profile of 174 mothers and newborns at parturition. *Am J Clin Nutr*. 1975;28:59-65.
24. Kaminetzky HA, Langer A, Baker H, et al. The effect of nutrition in teen-age gravidas on pregnancy and the status of the neonate. I. A nutritional profile. *Am J Obstet Gynecol*. 1973;115:639-646.
25. Martin MP, Bridgforth E, McGanity WJ, et al. The Vanderbilt cooperative study of maternal and infant nutrition. X. Ascorbic acid. *J Nutr*. 1957; 62:201-224.
26. Chaudhuri SK. Role of nutrition in the etiology of toxemia of pregnancy. *Am J Obstet Gynecol*. 1971;110:46-48.
27. Wilson CWM, Loh HS. Vitamin C and fertility. *Lancet*. 1973;2:859-860.
28. Vobecky JS, Vobecky J, Shapcott D, et al. Vitamin C and outcome of pregnancy. *Lancet*. 1974;1:630.
29. Nelson MM, Forfar JO. Associations between drugs administered during pregnancy and congenital abnormalities of the fetus. *Br Med J*. 1971;1:523-527.
30. Smithells RW, Sheppard S, Schorah CJ. Vitamin deficiencies and neural tube defects. *Arch Dis Child*. 1976;51:944-950.
31. Cochrane WA. Overnutrition in prenatal and neonatal life: a problem? *Can Med Assoc J*. 1965;93:893-899.
32. Averback P. Anencephaly associated with megavitamin therapy. *Can Med Assoc J*. 1976;114:995.
33. Korner WF, Weber F. Zur toleranz hoher ascorbinsauredosen. *Int J Vitam Nutr Res*. 1972;42:528-544.
34. Ingalls TH, Draper R, Teel HM. Vitamin C in human pregnancy and lactation. II. Studies during lactation. *Am J Dis Child*. 1938;56:1011-1019.
35. Deodhar AD, Rajalakshmi R, Ramakrishnan CV. Studies on human lactation. Part III. Effect of dietary vitamin supplementation on vitamin contents of breast milk. *Acta Paediatr*. 1964;53:42-48.
36. Bates CJ, Prentice AM, Prentice A, et al. The effect of vitamin C supplementation on lactating women in Keneba, a West African rural community. *Int J Vitam Nutr Res*. 1983;53:68-76.
37. Thomas MR, Kawamoto J, Sneed SM, et al. The effects of vitamin C, vitamin B_6, and vitamin B_{12} supplementation on the breast milk and maternal status of well-nourished women. *Am J Clin Nutr*. 1979;32:1679-1685.
38. Thomas MR, Sneed SM, Wei C, et al. The effects of vitamin C, vitamin B_6, vitamin B_{12}, folic acid, riboflavin, and thiamin on the breast milk and maternal status of well-nourished women at 6 months postpartum. *Am J Clin Nutr*. 1980;33:2151-2156.
39. Sneed SM, Zane C, Thomas MR. The effects of ascorbic acid, vitamin B_6, vitamin B_{12}, and folic acid supplementation on the breast milk and maternal nutritional status of low socioeconomic lactating women. *Am J Clin Nutr*. 1981;34:1338-1346.
40. Byerley LO, Kirksey A. Effects of different levels of vitamin C intake on the vitamin C concentration in human milk and the vitamin C intakes of breast-fed infants. *Am J Clin Nutr*. 1985;41:665-671.
41. Salmenpera L. Vitamin C nutrition during prolonged lactation: optimal in infants while marginal in some mothers. *Am J Clin Nutr*. 1984;40:1050-1056.
42. Grewar D. Infantile scurvy. *Clin Pediatr*. 1965;4:82-89.
43. Bank MR, Kirksey A, West K, et al. Effect of storage time and temperature on folacin and vitamin C levels in term and preterm human milk. *Am J Clin Nutr*. 1985;41:235-242.

VITAMIN D (D_2: ERGOCALCIFEROL, D_3: CHOLECALCIFEROL)

Vitamin (Fat-Soluble Vitamin)

PREGNANCY RECOMMENDATION: Compatible

BREASTFEEDING RECOMMENDATION: Compatible

V

PREGNANCY SUMMARY

Several reports describing the use of vitamin D in human pregnancy have been located. The recommended daily allowance (RDA) and daily recommended intake by ACOG and AAP for vitamin D in pregnancy is 15 mcg (600 IU) per day. However, based on evidence that vitamin D deficiency is very common in pregnancy, a much higher dose may be required to prevent and treat a deficiency. Currently, the ACOG practice bulletin states that many experts support that up to 4,000 IU per day is safe. The precursor of active vitamin D, 25-hydroxy vitamin D, crosses the placenta, whereas active vitamin D does not readily cross. Vitamin D is fat soluble and some is stored in the body's fatty tissues and liver.

BREASTFEEDING SUMMARY

Vitamin D is excreted into human breast milk in limited amounts. The recommended daily allowance (RDA) and daily recommended intake by the ACOG and AAP for vitamin D is 15 mcg (600 IU). The CDC Dietary Guidelines for Americans and the AAP both recommend that infants fully or partially breastfed receive 400 IU of vitamin D supplementation each day starting in the first few days of life to prevent vitamin D deficiency.

References

1. National Institutes of Health. Vitamin C fact sheet for health professionals. Accessed October 1, 2023. https://ods.od.nih.gov/factsheets/VitaminC-HealthProfessional/
2. AAP Committee on Fetus and Newborn and ACOG Committee on Obstetric Practice. Antepartum care. In: Kilpatrick SJ, Papile LA, Macones GA. *Guidelines for perinatal care*. 8th ed. American Academy of Pediatrics; 2017.
3. Lexi-Comp, Inc. (Lexi-drugs). Lexi-Comp, Inc;2023.
4. American College of Obstetricians and Gynecologists. Vitamin D: screening and supplementation during pregnancy. Committee Opinion No. 495. *Obstet Gynecol*. 2011;118:197-198.
5. National Library of Medicine. Pubchem. Cholecalciferol. Accessed October 1, 2023. https://pubchem.ncbi.nlm.nih.gov/compound/5280795
6. National Library of Medicine. Pubchem. Ergocalciferol. Accessed October 1, 2023. https://pubchem.ncbi.nlm.nih.gov/compound/5280793
7. Kaludjerovic J, Vieth R. Relationship between vitamin D during perinatal development and health. *J Midwifery Womens Health*. 2010;55:550-560.
8. Goodenday LS, Gordan GS. Fetal safety of vitamin D during pregnancy. *Clin Res*. 1971;19:200.
9. Goodenday LS, Gordan GS. No risk from vitamin D in pregnancy. *Ann Intern Med*. 1971;75:807-808.
10. Sadeghi-Nejad A, Wolfsdorf JI, Senior B. Hypoparathyroidism and pregnancy: treatment with calcitriol. *JAMA*. 1980;243:254-255.
11. Greer FR, Hollis BW, Napoli JL. High concentrations of vitamin D_2 in human milk associated with pharmacologic doses of vitamin D_2. *J Pediatr*. 1984;105:61-64.
12. Pilotti G, Scorta A. Ipervitaminosi A gravidica e malformazioni neonatali dell'apparato urinaria. *Minerva Ginecol*. 1965;17:1103-1108. As cited in Nishimura H, Tanimura T. *Clinical Aspects of the Teratogenicity of Drugs*. American Elsevier; 1976:251-252.
13. Parr JH, Ramsay I. The presentation of osteomalacia in pregnancy. Case report. *Br J Obstet Gynaecol*. 1984;91:816-818.
14. Brooke OG, Brown IRF, Bone CDM, et al. Vitamin D supplements in pregnant Asian women: effects on calcium status and fetal growth. *Br Med J*. 1980;280:751-754.
15. Rosen JF, Roginsky M, Nathenson G, et al. 25-Hydroxyvitamin D: plasma levels in mothers and their premature infants with neonatal hypocalcemia. *Am J Dis Child*. 1974;127:220-223.
16. Watney PJM, Chance GW, Scott P, et al. Maternal factors in neonatal hypocalcaemia: a study in three ethnic groups. *Br Med J*. 1971;2:432-436.
17. Heckmatt JZ, Peacock M, Davies AEJ, et al. Plasma 25-hydroxyvitamin D in pregnant Asian women and their babies. *Lancet*. 1979;2:546-549.
18. Roberts SA, Cohen MD, Forfar JO. Antenatal factors associated with neonatal hypocalcaemic convulsions. *Lancet*. 1973;2:809-811.
19. Purvis RJ, Barrie WJM, MacKay GS, et al. Enamel hypoplasia of the teeth associated with neonatal tetany: a manifestation of maternal vitamin-D deficiency. *Lancet*. 1973;2:811-814.
20. Ford JA, Davidson DC, McIntosh WB, et al. Neonatal rickets in Asian immigrant population. *Br Med J*. 1973;3:211-212.
21. Moncrieff M, Fadahunsi TO. Congenital rickets due to maternal vitamin D deficiency. *Arch Dis Child*. 1974;49:810-811.
22. Watney PJM. Maternal factors in the aetiology of neonatal hypocalcaemia. *Postgrad Med J*. 1975;51(suppl 3):14-17.
23. Cockburn F, Belton NR, Purvis RJ, et al. Maternal vitamin D intake and mineral metabolism in mothers and their newborn infants. *Br Med J*. 1980;2:11-14.
24. Pitkin RM. Calcium metabolism in pregnancy and the perinatal period: a review. *Am J Obstet Gynecol*. 1985;151:99-109.
25. Stimmler L, Snodgrass GJAI, Jaffe E. Dental defects associated with neonatal symptomatic hypocalcaemia. *Arch Dis Child*. 1973;48:217-220.
26. Hillman LS, Haddad JG. Human perinatal vitamin D metabolism. I: 25-hydroxyvitamin D in maternal and cord blood. *J Pediatr*. 1974;84:742-749.
27. Dent CE, Gupta MM. Plasma 25-hydroxyvitamin-D levels during pregnancy in Caucasians and in vegetarian and non-vegetarian Asians. *Lancet*. 1975;2:1057-1060.
28. Weisman Y, Occhipinti M, Knox G, et al. Concentrations of 24,25-dihydroxyvitamin D and 25-hydroxyvitamin D in paired maternal-cord sera. *Am J Obstet Gynecol*. 1978;130:704-707.
29. Steichen JJ, Tsang RC, Gratton TL, et al. Vitamin D homeostasis in the perinatal period: 1,25-dihydroxyvitamin D in maternal, cord, and neonatal blood. *N Engl J Med*. 1980;302:315-319.
30. Birkbeck JA, Scott HF. 25-Hydroxycholecalciferol serum levels in breast-fed infants. *Arch Dis Child*. 1980;55:691-695.
31. Markestad T, Aksnes L, Ulstein M, et al. 25-Hydroxyvitamin D and 1,25-dihydroxyvitamin D of D_2 and D_3 origin in maternal and umbilical cord serum after vitamin D_2 supplementation in human pregnancy. *Am J Clin Nutr*. 1984;40:1057-1063.
32. Kumar R, Cohen WR, Epstein FH. Vitamin D and calcium hormones in pregnancy. *N Engl J Med*. 1980;302:1143-1145.
33. Hillman LS, Haddad JG. Perinatal vitamin D metabolism. II. Serial 25-hydroxyvitamin D concentrations in sera of term and premature infants. *J Pediatr*. 1975;86:928-935.
34. Kumar R, Cohen WR, Silva P, et al. Elevated 1,25-dihydroxyvitamin D plasma levels in normal human pregnancy and lactation. *J Clin Invest*. 1979;63:342-344.
35. Hillman LS, Haddad JG. Perinatal vitamin D metabolism. III. Factors influencing late gestational human serum 25-hydroxyvitamin D. *Am J Obstet Gynecol*. 1976;125:196-200.
36. Turton CWG, Stanley P, Stamp TCB, et al. Altered vitamin-D metabolism in pregnancy. *Lancet*. 1977;1:222-225.
37. Ron M, Levitz M, Chuba J, et al. Transfer of 25-hydroxyvitamin D_3 and 1,25-dihydroxyvitamin D_3 across the perfused human placenta. *Am J Obstet Gynecol*. 1984;148:370-374.
38. Hollis BW, Wagner CL. Assessment of dietary vitamin D requirements during pregnancy and lactation. *Am J Clin Nutr*. 2004;79:717-726.
39. Holick MF. Vitamin D deficiency. *N Engl J Med*. 2007;357:266-281.
40. Ginde AA, Sullivan AF, Mansbach JM, et al Vitamin D insufficiency in pregnant and nonpregnant women of childbearing age in the United States. *Am J Obstet Gynecol*. 2010;202:436.e1-8.
41. Mulligan ML, Felton SK, Riek AE, Bernal-Mizrachi C. Implications of vitamin D deficiency in pregnancy and lactation. *Am J Obstet Gynecol*. 2010;202:429.e1-9.
42. O'Brien J, Rosewasser S, Feingold M, et al. Prenatal exposure to milk with excessive vitamin D supplementation (Abstract). *Teratology*. 1993;47:387.
43. Bimson B, Brustman L, Ibraheemi ZA, et al. Can weekly vitamin d dosing adequately treat vitamin d deficiency in pregnancy? (Abstract). *Am J Obstet Gynecol*. 2017;216(suppl):S380-S381.
44. Friedman WF, Mills LF. The relationship between vitamin D and the craniofacial and dental anomalies of the supravalvular aortic stenosis syndrome. *Pediatrics*. 1969;43:12-18.
45. Rowe, RD, Cooke RE. Vitamin D and craniofacial and dental anomalies of supravalvular stenosis. *Pediatrics*. 1969;43:1-2.
46. Taussig HB. Possible injury to the cardiovascular system from vitamin D. *Ann Intern Med*. 1966;65:1195-1200.
47. Anita AU, Wiltse HE, Rowe RD, et al. Pathogenesis of the supravalvular aortic stenosis syndrome. *J Pediatr*. 1967;71:431-441.
48. Greer FR, Hollis BW, Cripps DJ, et al. Effects of maternal ultraviolet B irradiation on vitamin D content of human milk. *J Pediatr*. 1984;105:431-433.
49. Rothberg AD, Pettifor JM, Cohen DF, et al. Maternal-infant vitamin D relationships during breast-feeding. *J Pediatr*. 1982;101:500-503.
50. Goldberg LD. Transmission of a vitamin-D metabolite in breast milk. *Lancet*. 1972;2:1258-1259.
51. Greer FR, Ho M, Dodson D, et al. Lack of 25-hydroxyvitamin D and 1,25-dihydroxyvitamin D in human milk. *J Pediatr*. 1981;99:233-235.

52. Greer FR, Searcy JE, Levin RS, et al. Bone mineral content and serum 25-hydroxyvitamin D concentration in breast-fed infants with and without supplemental vitamin D. *J Pediatr*. 1981;98:696-701.
53. Greer FR, Searcy JE, Levin RS, et al. Bone mineral content and serum 25-hydroxyvitamin D concentrations in breast-fed infants with and without supplemental vitamin D: one-year follow-up. *J Pediatr*. 1982;100:919-922.
54. Fairney A, Naughten E, Oppe TE. Vitamin D and human lactation. *Lancet*. 1977;2:739-741.
55. Roberts CC, Chan GM, Folland D, et al. Adequate bone mineralization in breast-fed infants. *J Pediatr*. 1981;99:192-196.
56. Chadwick DW. Commentary. Water-soluble vitamin D in human milk: a myth. *Pediatrics*. 1982;70:499.
57. Lakdawala DR, Widdowson EM. Vitamin-D in human milk. *Lancet*. 1977; 1:167-168.
58. Greer FR, Reeve LE, Chesney RW, et al. Water-soluble vitamin D in human milk: a myth. *Pediatrics*. 1982;69:238.
59. Greer FR, Reeve LE, Chesney RW, et al. Commentary. Water-soluble vitamin D in human milk: a myth. *Pediatrics*. 1982;70:499-500.
60. Bunker JWM, Harris RS, Eustis RS. The antirachitic potency of the milk of human mothers fed previously on "vitamin D milk" of the cow. *N Engl J Med*. 1933;208:313-315.
61. O'Connor P. Vitamin D-deficiency rickets in two breast-fed infants who were not receiving vitamin D supplementation. *Clin Pediatr (Phila)*. 1977; 16:361-363.
62. Little JA. Commentary. Water-soluble vitamin D in human milk: a myth. *Pediatrics*. 1982;70:499.
63. Reeve LE, Chesney RW, DeLuca HF. Vitamin D of human milk: identification of biologically active forms. *Am J Clin Nutr*. 1982;36:122-126.
64. Centers for Disease Control and Prevention. Breastfeeding. Vitamin D. Accessed October 1, 2023. https://www.cdc.gov/breastfeeding-special-circumstances/hcp/diet-micronutrients/vitamin-d.html

VITAMIN E (TOCOPHEROL)

Vitamin (Fat-Soluble Vitamin)

PREGNANCY RECOMMENDATION: Compatible

BREASTFEEDING RECOMMENDATION: Compatible

PREGNANCY SUMMARY

Neither deficiency nor excess of vitamin E has been associated with maternal or fetal complications during pregnancy. In a well-nourished woman, adequate vitamin E is consumed in the diet, and supplementation is not required. If dietary intake is poor, supplementation up to the recommended daily allowance (RDA) for pregnancy is recommended. ACOG and the National Institute of Health's RDA for vitamin E during pregnancy is 15 mg, with an upper limit of consumption during pregnancy of 1,000 mg/d. Vitamin E crosses the placenta. Vitamin E is fat soluble and some is stored in the body's fatty tissues and liver.

BREASTFEEDING SUMMARY

Vitamin E is excreted into human breast milk. The ACOG recommended daily allowance (RDA) of vitamin E during lactation is 19 mg, with a tolerable upper limit intake of 1,000 mg/d. Maternal supplementation is recommended only if the diet does not provide sufficient vitamin E to meet the RDA. Human breast milk is more than 5 times richer in vitamin E than cow's milk and is more effective in maintaining adequate serum vitamin E levels in infants up to 1 year of age. One study reported a level of 2.3 mcg/mL of the vitamin in mature breast milk. Breast milk obtained from mothers who delivered preterm was higher. However, using this vitamin at the RDA is only endorsed for those patients with dietary insufficiency.

References

1. National Institutes of Health. Vitamin E fact sheet for health professionals. Accessed October 10, 2023. https://ods.od.nih.gov/factsheets/VitaminE-HealthProfessional/
2. AAP Committee on Fetus and Newborn and ACOG Committee on Obstetric Practice. Antepartum care. In: Kilpatrick SJ, Papile LA, Macones GA, eds. *Guidelines for Perinatal Care*. 8th ed. American Academy of Pediatrics; 2017.
3. National Library of Medicine. Vitamin E. PubChem. Accessed October 10, 2023. https://pubchem.ncbi.nlm.nih.gov/compound/14985
4. Moyer WT. Vitamin E levels in term and premature newborn infants. *Pediatrics*. 1950;6:893-896.
5. Leonard PJ, Doyle E, Harrington W. Levels of vitamin E in the plasma of newborn infants and of the mothers. *Am J Clin Nutr*. 1972;25:480-484.
6. Baker H, Frank O, Thomson AD, et al. Vitamin profile of 174 mothers and newborns at parturition. *Am J Clin Nutr*. 1975;28:59-65.
7. Dostalova L. Correlation of the vitamin status between mother and newborn during delivery. *Dev Pharmacol Ther*. 1982;4(suppl I):45-57.
8. Kaminetzky HA, Baker H. Micronutrients in pregnancy. *Clin Obstet Gynecol*. 1977;20:363-380.
9. Mino M, Nishino H. Fetal and maternal relationship in serum vitamin E level. *J Nutr Sci Vitaminol*. 1973;19:475-482.
10. Haga P, Ek J, Kran S. Plasma tocopherol levels and vitamin E/B-lipoprotein relationships during pregnancy and in cord blood. *Am J Clin Nutr*. 1982;36:1200-1204.
11. Martinez FE, Goncalves AL, Jorge SM, et al. Vitamin E in placental blood and its interrelationship to maternal and newborn levels of vitamin E. *J Pediatr*. 1981;99:298-300.
12. Hill EP, Longo LD. Dynamics of maternal-fetal nutrient transfer. *Fed Proc*. 1980;39:239-244.
13. Martinez FE, Jorge SM, Goncalves AL, et al. Evaluation of plasma tocopherols in relation to hematological indices of Brazilian infants on human milk and cows' milk regime from birth to 1 year of age. *Am J Clin Nutr*. 1984;39:969-974.
14. Mino M, Kitagawa M, Nakagawa S. Red blood cell tocopherol concentrations in a normal population of Japanese children and premature infants in relation to the assessment of vitamin E status. *Am J Clin Nutr*. 1985;41:631-638.
15. Boskovic R, Gargaun L, Oren D, et al. Pregnancy outcome following high doses of vitamin E supplementation. *Reprod Toxicol*. 2005;20:85-88.
16. Kaminetzky HA, Langer A, Baker O, et al. The effect of nutrition in teen-age gravidas on pregnancy and the status of the neonate. I. A nutritional profile. *Am J Obstet Gynecol*. 1973;115:639-646.
17. Hook EB, Healy KM, Niles AM, et al. Vitamin E: teratogen or anti-teratogen? *Lancet*. 1974;1:809.
18. Gyorgy P, Cogan G, Rose CS. Availability of vitamin E in the newborn infant. *Proc Soc Exp Biol Med*. 1952;81:536-538.

19. Kotz J, Parker E, Kaufman MS. Treatment of recurrent and threatened abortion. Report of two hundred and twenty-six cases. *J Clin Endocrinol*. 1941;1:838-849.
20. Shute E. Vitamin E and premature labor. *Am J Obstet Gynecol*. 1942;44:271-279.
21. Oski FA, Barness LA. Vitamin E deficiency: a previously unrecognized cause of hemolytic anemia in the premature infant. *J Pediatr*. 1967;70:211-220.
22. Ritchie JH, Fish MB, McMasters V, et al. Edema and hemolytic anemia in premature infants. A vitamin E deficiency syndrome. *N Engl J Med*. 1968;279:1185-1190.
23. Gross SJ, Gabriel E. Vitamin E status in preterm infants fed human milk or infant formula. *J Pediatr*. 1985;106:635-639.
24. Friedman Z. Essential fatty acids revisited. *Am J Dis Child*. 1980;134:397-408.
25. Mino M, Kijima Y, Nishida Y, et al. Difference in plasma- and red blood cell-tocopherols in breast-fed and bottle-fed infants. *J Nutr Sci Vitaminol*. 1980;26:103-112.
26. Marx CM, Izquierdo A, Driscoll JW, et al. Vitamin E concentrations in serum of newborn infants after topical use of vitamin E by nursing mothers. *Am J Obstet Gynecol*. 1985;152:668-670.

VITAMINS, MULTIPLE

Vitamin

PREGNANCY RECOMMENDATION: Compatible

BREASTFEEDING RECOMMENDATION: Compatible

PREGNANCY SUMMARY

The use of multivitamins up to the recommended daily allowance (RDA) for pregnancy is recommended for the general good health of the mother and the fetus. There is no strong evidence to suggest that vitamin supplementation can prevent cleft lip and palate (CLP). However, a body of evidence has accumulated that supplementation during the first few weeks of gestation, especially with folic acid, may reduce the risk of NTDs (see Folic Acid). The evidence appears particularly strong for the prevention of NTD recurrences. Currently, ACOG recommends 0.4 mg of folic acid supplementation daily for all women planning to become pregnant or capable of becoming pregnant starting at least 1 month prior to pregnancy and continued through 12 weeks' gestation. Additionally, women should receive 4 mg of folic acid daily starting 3 months before conception and continued through 12 weeks' gestation if she has a personal history of, a partner with, or a previous pregnancy affected by NTDs. Women who have had gastric bypass surgery for obesity may be at increased risk for nutritional deficiency, and pregnancy counseling to ensure adequate nutritional intake may be of benefit. See the ACOG bulletin on bariatric surgery and pregnancy for the specific supplementation recommendations for this population.

BREASTFEEDING SUMMARY

Vitamins are naturally present in breast milk (see individual vitamins).

References

1. AAP Committee on Fetus and Newborn and ACOG Committee on Obstetric Practice. Antepartum care. In: Kilpatrick SJ, Papile LA, Macones GA. eds. *Guidelines for Perinatal Care*. 8th ed. American Academy of Pediatrics; 2017.
2. American College of Obstetricians and Gynecologists. Neural tube defects. Practice bulletin No. 187. *Obstet Gynecol*. 2017;130:e279-e290.
3. Douglas B. The role of environmental factors in the etiology of "so-called" congenital malformations. I. Deductions from the presence of cleft lip and palate in one of identical twins, from embryology and from animal experiments. *Plast Reconstr Surg*. 1958;22:94-108.
4. Douglas B. The role of environmental factors in the etiology of "so-called" congenital malformations. II. Approaches in humans; study of various extragenital factors, "theory of compensatory nutrients," development of regime for first trimester. *Plast Reconstr Surg*. 1958;22:214-229.
5. Conway H. Effect of supplemental vitamin therapy on the limitation of incidence of cleft lip and cleft palate in humans. *Plast Reconstr Surg*. 1958;22:450-453.
6. Peer LA, Gordon HW, Bernhard WG. Experimental production of congenital deformities and their possible prevention in man. *J Int Coll Surg*. 1963;39:23-35.
7. Fraser FC, Warburton D. No association of emotional stress or vitamin supplement during pregnancy to cleft lip or palate in man. *Plast Reconstr Surg*. 1964;33:395-399.
8. Peer LA, Gordon HW, Bernhard WG. Effect of vitamins on human teratology. *Plast Reconstr Surg*. 1964;34:358-362.
9. Briggs RM. Vitamin supplementation as a possible factor in the incidence of cleft lip/palate deformities in humans. *Clin Plast Surg*. 1976;3:647-652.
10. Tolarova M. Periconceptional supplementation with vitamins and folic acid to prevent recurrence of cleft lip. *Lancet*. 1982;2:217.
11. Bound JP. Spina bifida and vitamins. *Br Med J*. 1983;286:147.
12. Smithells RW. Spina bifida and vitamins. *Br Med J*. 1983;286:388-389.
13. Main DM, Mennuti MT. Neural tube defects: issues in prenatal diagnosis and counseling. *Obstet Gynecol*. 1986;67:1-16.
14. Rhoads GG, Mills JL. Can vitamin supplements prevent neural tube defects? Current evidence and ongoing investigations. *Clin Obstet Gynecol*. 1986;29:569-579.
15. Lemire RJ. Neural tube defects. *JAMA*. 1988;259:558-562.
16. Smithells RW, Sheppard S, Schorah CJ. Vitamin deficiencies and neural tube defects. *Arch Dis Child*. 1976;51:944-950.
17. Smithells RW, Sheppard S, Schorah CJ, et al. Possible prevention of neural-tube defects by periconceptional vitamin supplementation. *Lancet*. 1980;1:339-340.
18. Smithells RW, Sheppard S, Schorah CJ, et al. Apparent prevention of neural tube defects by periconceptional vitamin supplementation. *Arch Dis Child*. 1981;56:911-918.
19. Smithells RW, Sheppard S, Schorah CJ, et al. Vitamin supplementation and neural tube defects. *Lancet*. 1981;2:1425.
20. Smithells RW, Nevin NC, Seller MJ, et al. Further experience of vitamin supplementation for prevention of neural tube defect recurrences. *Lancet*. 1983;1:1027-1031.
21. Laurence KM, James N, Miller M, et al. Increased risk of recurrence of pregnancies complicated by fetal neural tube defects in mothers receiving poor diets, and possible benefit of dietary counselling. *Br Med J*. 1980;281:1592-1594.
22. Holmes-Siedle M, Lindenbaum RH, Galliard A, et al. Vitamin supplementation and neural tube defects. *Lancet*. 1982;1:276.
23. Holmes-Siedle M. Vitamin supplementation and neural tube defects. *Lancet*. 1983;2:41.
24. Choi NW, Klaponski FA. On neural-tube defects: an epidemiological elicitation of etiological factors. *Neurology*. 1970;20:399-400.
25. Stone DH. Possible prevention of neural-tube defects by periconceptional vitamin supplementation. *Lancet*. 1980;1:647.

26. Smithells RW, Sheppard S. Possible prevention of neural-tube defects by periconceptional vitamin supplementation. *Lancet*. 1980;1:647.
27. Fernhoff PM. Possible prevention of neural-tube defects by periconceptional vitamin supplementation. *Lancet*. 1980;1:648.
28. Elwood JH. Possible prevention of neural-tube defects by periconceptional vitamin supplementation. *Lancet*. 1980;1:648.
29. Anonymous. Vitamins, neural-tube defects, and ethics committees. *Lancet*. 1980;1:1061-1062.
30. Kirke PN. Vitamins, neural tube defects, and ethics committees. *Lancet*. 1980; 1:1300-1301.
31. Freed DLJ. Vitamins, neural tube defects, and ethics committees. *Lancet*. 1980;1:1301.
32. Raab GM, Gore SM. Vitamins, neural tube defects, and ethics committees. *Lancet*. 1980;1:1301.
33. Hume K. Fetal defects and multivitamin therapy. *Med J Aust*. 1980;2: 731-732.
34. Edwards JH. Vitamin supplementation and neural tube defects. *Lancet*. 1982; 1:275-276.
35. Renwick JH. Vitamin supplementation and neural tube defects. *Lancet*. 1982; 1:748.
36. Chalmers TC, Sacks H. Vitamin supplements to prevent neural tube defects. *Lancet*. 1982;1:748.
37. Stirrat GM. Vitamin supplementation and neural tube defects. *Lancet*. 1982; 1:625-626.
38. Kanofsky JD. Vitamin supplements to prevent neural tube defects. *Lancet*. 1982;1:1075.
39. Walsh DE. Vitamin supplements to prevent neural tube defects. *Lancet*. 1982; 1:1075.
40. Meier P. Vitamins to prevent neural tube defects. *Lancet*. 1982;1:859.
41. Smith DE, Haddow JE. Vitamins to prevent neural tube defects. *Lancet*. 1982;1:859-860.
42. Smithells RW, Sheppard S, Schorah CJ, et al Vitamin supplements and neural tube defects. *Lancet*. 1982;1:1186.
43. Anonymous. Vitamins to prevent neural tube defects. *Lancet*. 1982; 2:1255-1256.
44. Lorber J. Vitamins to prevent neural tube defects. *Lancet*. 1982;2:1458-1459.
45. Read AP, Harris R. Spina bifida and vitamins. *Br Med J*. 1983;286:560-561.
46. Rose G, Cooke ID, Polani PE, et al. Vitamin supplementation for prevention of neural tube defect recurrences. *Lancet*. 1983;1:1164-1165.
47. Knox EG. Vitamin supplementation and neural tube defects. *Lancet*. 1983; 2:39.
48. Emanuel I. Vitamin supplementation and neural tube defects. *Lancet*. 1983; 2:39-40.
49. Smithells RW, Seller MJ, Harris R, et al. Vitamin supplementation and neural tube defects. *Lancet*. 1983;2:40.
50. Oakley GP Jr, Adams MJ Jr, James LM. Vitamins and neural tube defects. *Lancet*. 1983;2:798-799.
51. Smithells RW, Seller MJ, Harris R, et al. Vitamins and neural tube defects. *Lancet*. 1983;2:799.
52. Elwood JM. Can vitamins prevent neural tube defects? *Can Med Assoc J*. 1983;129:1088-1092.
53. David TJ. Unusual limb-reduction defect in infant born to mother taking periconceptional multivitamin supplement. *Lancet*. 1984;1:507-508.
54. Blank CE, Kumar D, Johnson M. Multivitamins and prevention of neural tube defects: a need for detailed counselling. *Lancet*. 1984;1:291.
55. Smithells RW. Can vitamins prevent neural tube defects? *Can Med Assoc J*. 1984;131:273-276.
56. Wald NJ, Polani PE. Neural-tube defects and vitamins: the need for a randomized clinical trial. *Br J Obstet Gynecol*. 1984;91:516-523.
57. Seller MJ. Unanswered questions on neural tube defects. *Br Med J*. 1987; 294:1-2.
58. Harris R. Vitamins and neural tube defects. *Br Med J*. 1988;296:80-81.
59. Wild J, Read AP, Sheppard S, et al. Recurrent neural tube defects, risk factors and vitamins. *Arch Dis Child*. 1986;61:440-444.
60. Mulinare J, Cordero JF, Erickson JD, et al. Periconceptional use of multivitamins and the occurrence of neural tube defects. *JAMA*. 1988;260:3141-3145.
61. Holmes LB. Does taking vitamins at the time of conception prevent neural tube defects? *JAMA*. 1988;260:3181.
62. Haddow JE, Hill LE, Kloza EM, et al. Neural tube defects after gastric bypass. *Lancet*. 1986;1:1330.
63. Knudsen LB, Kallen B. Gastric bypass, pregnancy, and neural tube defects. *Lancet*. 1986;2:227.
64. Martin L, Chavez GF, Adams MJ Jr, et al. Gastric bypass surgery as maternal risk factor for neural tube defects. *Lancet*. 1988;1:640-641.
65. Smithells RW, Sheppard S, Wild J, et al. Prevention of neural tube defect recurrences in Yorkshire: final report. *Lancet*. 1989;2:498-499.
66. Mills JL, Rhoads GG, Simpson JL, et al. The absence of a relation between the periconceptional use of vitamins and neural-tube defects. *N Engl J Med*. 1989;321:430-435.
67. Milunsky A, Jick H, Jick SS, et al. Multivitamin/folic acid supplementation in early pregnancy reduces the prevalence of neural tube defects. *JAMA*. 1989;262:2847-2852.
68. Aro T, Haapakoski J, Heinonen OP, et al. Lack of association between vitamin intake during early pregnancy and reduction limb defects. *Am J Obstet Gynecol*. 1984;150:433.

VOCLOSPORIN

Immunologic (Calcineurin Inhibitor)

PREGNANCY RECOMMENDATION: No Human Data—Animal Data Suggest Potential Risk

BREASTFEEDING RECOMMENDATION: Potential Toxicity

PREGNANCY SUMMARY

No reports describing the use of voclosporin in human pregnancy have been located. Based on likely limited placental transfer, fetal exposure is probably small. However, the absence of human pregnancy experience prevents a complete assessment of the embryofetal risk. Embryofetal toxicity was observed in animal studies. Because each capsule contains 21.6 mg of dehydrated ethanol (total daily exposure of 129.6 mg), the manufacturer recommends that the drug not be used during pregnancy. However, there is roughly 14,000 mg of alcohol in one 12-oz beer (5% alcohol), one 5-oz glass of wine (12% alcohol), or one shot (1.5 ounces) of 80-proof liquor (40% alcohol). Therefore, the amount of alcohol that would be consumed daily with voclosporin is less than 1% of these drinks. Nevertheless, a known safety level of daily alcohol exposure during pregnancy has not been defined. Patients with lupus during pregnancy are at increased risk for adverse outcomes, including worsening of underlying disease, spontaneous abortion, preeclampsia, premature delivery, and intrauterine growth restriction. Hypertension was reported in up to 19% of patients treated with this drug in clinical trials. Voclosporin can also prolong the QT interval. Using this drug during pregnancy should be based on the pros and cons of the mother's clinical need for treatment versus any potential fetal risk that might occur from exposure.

BREASTFEEDING SUMMARY

No reports describing the use of voclosporin during human lactation have been located. A limited amount of the drug may appear in breast milk, so some infant exposure will probably occur. Because of the potential for serious adverse reactions that might be seen in a breastfed infant, the manufacturer recommends that women not breastfeed while taking voclosporin and for at least 7 days after the last dose. However, if the clinical decision is to use this drug while breastfeeding, the infant should be monitored for the most common reported adult side effects of headache and abdominal pain (both leading to irritability), hypertension, diarrhea, anemia, cough, urinary tract infection, mouth ulceration, lethargy, tremor, and decreased appetite (monitor growth).

Reference

1. Prescribing Information. Lupkynis. Aurinia Pharma U.S; 2021.

VONOPRAZAN/AMOXICILLIN (DUAL PAK) OR VONOPRAZAN/AMOXICILLIN/CLARITHROMYCIN (TRIPLE PAK)

Gastrointestinal (Potassium-Competitive Acid Blocker/Antibacterial)

PREGNANCY RECOMMENDATION: No Human Data—Animal Data Suggest Potential Risk

BREASTFEEDING RECOMMENDATION: Probably Compatible

PREGNANCY SUMMARY

No reports describing the use of vonoprazan in human pregnancy have been located. In addition, no studies have been located that reported pregnancy outcomes with exposure to the Dual Pak or Triple Pak combinations. Vonoprazan will probably cross the placenta, so some fetal exposure will likely occur. Therefore, the absence of human pregnancy experience prevents a complete assessment of the embryofetal risk. Amoxicillin is considered compatible for use during human pregnancy. Clarithromycin is considered low risk for use in human pregnancy. (See Amoxicillin and Clarithromycin for more details regarding human pregnancy.) Animal studies did show embryofetal toxicity in one species at doses of less than 10 times the RHD for clarithromycin, but not in a second species. Animal studies did not show any embryofetal toxicity for ampicillin or vonoprazan in two species at doses of less than 10 times the RHD. Using this drug during pregnancy should be based on the pros and cons of the mother's clinical need for treatment versus any potential fetal risk that might occur from exposure. Clarithromycin has been associated with the prolongation of the QT interval. Vonoprazan may soon be approved for use as a single-agent drug.

BREASTFEEDING SUMMARY

No reports describing the use of vonoprazan during human lactation have been located. In addition, no studies using the Dual Pak or Triple Pak combinations during human lactation have been located. Amoxicillin and clarithromycin have both been found in human breast milk, though levels for clarithromycin are low. Vonoprazan will probably be found in human breast milk, so some infant exposure will likely occur with this drug as well. Breastfeeding while using these drug combinations should be based on the mother's clinical need for treatment versus any potential infant risks that might occur. If used, the infant should be monitored for the most common reported adult side effects of nausea, headache, and abdominal pain (all leading to irritability), diarrhea, and rash. (See Amoxicillin and Clarithromycin for more details regarding breastfeeding for these two drugs.)

Reference

1. Prescribing Information. Voquezna. Phathom Pharmaceuticals, Inc; 2022.

VORAPAXAR

Hematologic (Antiplatelet)

PREGNANCY RECOMMENDATION: No Human Data—Animal Data Suggest Low Risk

BREASTFEEDING RECOMMENDATION: Potential Toxicity

PREGNANCY SUMMARY

No reports describing the use of vorapaxar in human pregnancy have been located. Some amount of vorapaxar and its active metabolite is likely to cross the placenta, so some fetal exposure will probably occur. Therefore, the absence of

(continued)

human pregnancy experience prevents a complete assessment of embryofetal risk. Animal data in two species did not show embryofetal toxicity at doses of more than 10 times the RHD. The manufacturer recommends discontinuing vorapaxar and starting an appropriate alternative therapy when a pregnancy is detected. Nevertheless, using this drug during pregnancy should be based on the pros and cons of the mother's clinical need for treatment versus any potential fetal risk that might occur from exposure.

BREASTFEEDING SUMMARY

No reports describing the use of vorapaxar during human lactation have been located. The drug and its active metabolite will likely be excreted into breast milk, so some infant exposure will probably occur. The manufacturer recommends not to breastfeed while taking vorapaxar due to a potential for bleeding. Nevertheless, breastfeeding while using this drug should be based on the mother's clinical need for treatment versus any potential infant risks that might occur. If used, the infant should be monitored for the most common reported adult side effects of bruising and bleeding.

Reference

1. Product information. Zontivity. Aralez Pharmaceuticals; 2019.

VORASIDENIB

Antineoplastic (Small-Molecule Inhibitor)

PREGNANCY RECOMMENDATION: No Human Data and No Relevant Animal Data

BREASTFEEDING RECOMMENDATION: Potential Toxicity

PREGNANCY SUMMARY

No reports describing the use of vorasidenib in human pregnancy have been located. The drug will likely cross the placenta, so some fetal exposure will probably occur. Therefore, the absence of human pregnancy experience prevents a complete assessment of the embryofetal risk. Animal studies did show embryofetal toxicity with malformations, but in one species, the doses were more than 10 times the RHD, and in the second species, there was maternal toxicity at doses of 8 times the RHD. However, based on these animal studies and the drug's mechanism of action, the manufacturer recommends that women with reproductive potential use effective contraception during treatment and for 3 months after the last dose. They also recommend that males with female partners of reproductive potential use effective contraception during treatment and for 3 months after the last dose. Nevertheless, using this drug during pregnancy should be based on the pros and cons of the mother's clinical need for treatment versus any potential fetal risk that might occur from exposure. There is a registry for women who are pregnant and have cancer. For more information, women and health care providers are encouraged to contact the Cancer and Pregnancy Registry at 1-877-635-4499.

BREASTFEEDING SUMMARY

No reports describing the use of vorasidenib during human lactation have been located. The drug will likely be found in breast milk, so some infant exposure will likely occur. However, oral bioavailability is only about 35%. Regardless, due to a concern for potential serious adverse effects that might be seen in a breastfed infant, the manufacturer recommends that women not breastfeed while being treated with this drug and for 2 months after the last dose. Nevertheless, breastfeeding while using this drug should be based on the mother's clinical need for treatment versus any potential infant risk that might occur. If used, the infant should be monitored for the most common reported adult side effects of nausea, headache, and musculoskeletal pain (all leading to irritability), diarrhea, fatigue (lethargy), elevated liver function tests, and neutropenia.

Reference

1. Prescribing Information. Voranigo. Sevier Pharmaceuticals; 2024.

VORICONAZOLE

Anti-Infective (Antifungal)

PREGNANCY RECOMMENDATION: No Human Data—Animal Data Suggest Risk

BREASTFEEDING RECOMMENDATION: Potential Toxicity

PREGNANCY SUMMARY

No reports describing the use of voriconazole during human pregnancy have been located. Voriconazole is likely to cross the placenta, so some fetal exposure will probably occur. However, the absence of human pregnancy experience prevents a complete assessment of embryofetal risk. Embryofetal toxicity with malformations was observed in two animal species at doses of less than 10 times the RHD. The animal data also suggested a risk for inhibition of estrogen synthesis. This effect has also been noted in rats treated with another triazole agent, fluconazole. In those studies, the antiestrogen action was thought to be responsible for the observed cleft palate and bone abnormalities (see Fluconazole). Whether this mechanism also applies to voriconazole is unknown. Based on animal studies, the manufacturer recommends that women with reproductive potential use effective contraception during treatment. Nevertheless, using this drug during pregnancy should be based on the pros and cons of the mother's clinical need for treatment versus any potential fetal risk that might occur from exposure.

BREASTFEEDING SUMMARY

No reports describing the use of voriconazole during human lactation have been located. The drug will likely be excreted into breast milk, so some infant exposure will probably occur. Per the manufacturer, breastfeeding while using this drug should be based on the mother's clinical need for treatment versus any potential infant risks that might occur. If used, the infant should be monitored for the most common reported adult side effects of nausea and headache (both leading to irritability), fever, rash, vomiting, tachycardia, and abnormal liver function tests.

References

1. Product information. Voriconazole. Ajanta Pharma Limited; 2022.
2. Moudgal VV, Sobel JD. Antifungal drugs in pregnancy: a review. *Expert Opin Drug Saf*. 2003;2:475-483.
3. Shoai Tehrani M, Sicre de Fontbrune F, Roth P, Allisy C, Bougnoux M-E, Hermine O, Lecuit M, Lortholary O, Charlier C. Case report of exposure to voriconazole in the second and third trimesters of pregnancy. *Antimicrob Agents Chemother*. 2013;57:1094-1095.

VORINOSTAT

Antineoplastic (Histone Deacetylase Inhibitor)

PREGNANCY RECOMMENDATION: No Human Data—Animal Data Suggest Risk

BREASTFEEDING RECOMMENDATION: Potential Toxicity

PREGNANCY SUMMARY

No reports describing the use of vorinostat in human pregnancy have been located. Vorinostat is likely to cross the placenta, so some infant exposure will probably occur. However, the absence of human pregnancy experience prevents a complete assessment of embryofetal risk. Embryofetal toxicity with malformations was observed in two animal species at doses of less than 10 times the human exposure. Based on animal studies and the drug's mechanism of action, the manufacturer recommends that women with reproductive potential use effective contraception during treatment and for 6 months after the last dose. They also recommend that males with female partners of reproductive potential use effective contraception during treatment and for 3 months after the last dose. Nevertheless, using this drug during pregnancy should be based on the pros and cons of the mother's clinical need for treatment versus any potential fetal risk that might occur from exposure. Women who are pregnant and have cancer are encouraged to contact the Cancer and Pregnancy Registry at 877-635-4499. Elevated glucose levels have been reported in patients treated with this drug. Therefore, if used during pregnancy, glucose levels should be monitored.

BREASTFEEDING SUMMARY

No reports describing the use of vorinostat during human lactation have been located. The drug will likely be excreted into breast milk, so some infant exposure will probably occur. Due to a concern for potential serious adverse effects that might be seen in a breastfed infant, the manufacturer recommends that women not breastfeed while being treated with this drug and for at least 1 week after the last dose. Nevertheless, breastfeeding while using this drug should be based on the mother's clinical need for treatment versus any potential infant risks that might occur. If used, the infant should be monitored for the most common reported adult side effects of nausea (leading to irritability), diarrhea, fatigue (lethargy), thrombocytopenia, and decreased appetite (monitor feeding patterns and growth).

Reference

1. Product information. Zolinza. Merck Sharp & Dohme, LLC; 2022.

V

VORTIOXETINE

Mental Health (Antidepressant - Selective Serotonin Reuptake Inhibitor)

PREGNANCY RECOMMENDATION: Limited Human Data—No Relevant Animal Data

BREASTFEEDING RECOMMENDATION: Probably Compatible

PREGNANCY SUMMARY

Limited human data related to the use of vortioxetine in human pregnancy have been reported. A case series of 19 women (1 with twins) exposed to vortioxetine in the first trimester found no malformations in 12 live births. Of the remaining births, two were lost to follow-up, three were spontaneous abortions, two were therapeutic abortions, and one was a fetal demise at 22 weeks of gestation. One termination was for a diagnosis of acrania in a woman who also took carbamazepine and dipyrone. The second termination was for concerns about abnormalities after a cystic hygroma was suspected at 12 weeks' gestation. The drug will probably cross the placenta, so some fetal exposure will likely occur. However, this limited human pregnancy experience prevents a complete assessment of the embryofetal risk. Embryofetal toxicity was observed in animal studies, but dosing was 10 times the MRHD (or greater) and caused maternal toxicity. Vortioxetine is a serotonergic modulator that has similar properties to SSRIs. SSRIs have been extensively studied in pregnant patients. Approximately 30% of neonates exposed to SSRIs late in the third trimester will experience withdrawal symptoms such as tremor, gastrointestinal disturbance, sleep interruption, high-pitched cry, hypertonicity, and tachypnea. Pulmonary hypertension of the newborn has also been suggested as an association with SSRI use in pregnancy. The use of vortioxetine during pregnancy should be based on the mother's need for clinical treatment.

BREASTFEEDING SUMMARY

Vortioxetine is present in breast milk. One case report measured the maximum concentration of vortioxetine in breast milk in three lactating mothers. The RID was found to be 1.1% and 1.7% in mothers taking a dose of 10 mg/d and 20 mg/d, respectively. A second report of a woman taking a vortioxetine dose of 76.1 mcg/kg daily resulted in a RID equal to 1.2% of the mother's weight-adjusted dose. No adverse effects were observed by the mothers in both reports. If vortioxetine is used while breastfeeding, the infant should be monitored for the most common reported adult side effects of nausea (leading to irritability), constipation, and vomiting, along with symptoms of SSRI exposure such as irritability and changes in sleep and feeding patterns.

References

1. Prescribing Information. Trintellix. Takeda Pharmaceuticals America, Inc; 2016.
2. Shweiki S, Diav-Citrin O. Pregnancy outcome after first trimester exposure to vortioxetine: a case series. *Birth Defects Res*. 2021;113:511-515.
3. SSRI withdrawal syndrome in term newborns. *AAP Grand Rounds*. 2006;15: 72-73.
4. Marshall K, Datta P, Rewers-Felkins K, et al. Transfer of the serotonin modulator vortioxetine into human milk: a case series. *Breastfeed Med*. 2021; 16:843-845.
5. Monfort A, Jutras M, Martin B, et al. Simultaneous quantification of 19 analytes in breast milk by liquid chromatography-tandem mass spectrometry (LC-MS/MS). *J Pharm Biomed Anal*. 2021;204:114236.

VOSORITIDE

Miscellaneous (C-Type Natriuretic Peptide)

PREGNANCY RECOMMENDATION: No Human Data—Animal Data Suggest Low Risk

BREASTFEEDING RECOMMENDATION: Probably Compatible

PREGNANCY SUMMARY

No reports describing the use of vosoritide in human pregnancy have been located. The drug is not likely to cross the placenta, so any fetal exposure would probably be clinically insignificant. However, the absence of human pregnancy experience prevents a complete assessment of the embryofetal risk. Animal data did not show any embryofetal toxicity. Using this drug during pregnancy should be based on the pros and cons of the mother's clinical need for treatment versus any potential fetal risk that might occur from exposure.

BREASTFEEDING SUMMARY

No reports describing the use of vosoritide during human lactation have been located. The drug will not likely be excreted into breast milk. However, if the drug were to be found in breast milk, because it is a polypeptide, it would probably be digested in the infant's gastrointestinal tract and not be absorbed. Breastfeeding while using this drug should be based on the mother's clinical need for treatment. If used, the infant should be monitored for the most common reported adult side effects of arthralgia (leading to irritability) and vomiting.

Reference

1. Prescribing Information. Voxzogo. BioMarin Pharmaceutical; 2021.

VOXELOTOR

Hematologic (Hemoglobin S Polymerase Inhibitor)

PREGNANCY RECOMMENDATION: No Human Data—Animal Data Suggest Potential Risk

BREASTFEEDING RECOMMENDATION: Potential Toxicity

PREGNANCY SUMMARY

No reports describing the use of voxelotor in human pregnancy have been located. Voxelotor is likely to cross the placenta, so some fetal exposure will probably occur. Therefore, the absence of human pregnancy experience prevents a complete assessment of embryofetal risk. Embryofetal toxicity with malformations was observed in one animal species at doses of 2.8 times the RHD, but was not observed in a second species at doses of about 0.3 times the RHD. Using this drug during pregnancy should be based on the pros and cons of the mother's clinical need for treatment versus any potential fetal risk that might occur from exposure.

BREASTFEEDING SUMMARY

No reports describing the use of voxelotor during human lactation have been located. The drug will likely be excreted into breast milk, so some infant exposure will probably occur. Due to a concern for potential serious adverse effects that might be seen in a breastfed infant, the manufacturer recommends that women not breastfeed while being treated with this drug and for at least 2 weeks after the last dose. Nevertheless, breastfeeding while using this drug should be based on the mother's clinical need for treatment versus any potential infant risks that might occur. If used, the infant should be monitored for the most common reported adult side effects of headache, abdominal pain, and nausea (all leading to irritability), diarrhea, rash, and pyrexia.

Reference

1. Product information. Oxbryta. Global Blood Therapeutics, Inc; 2023.

VUTRISIRAN

Antineoplastic (Antitransthyretin Small Interfering Ribonucleic Acid Agent)

PREGNANCY RECOMMENDATION: No Human Data—Animal Data Suggest Low Risk

BREASTFEEDING RECOMMENDATION: Probably Compatible

PREGNANCY SUMMARY

No reports describing the use of vutrisiran in human pregnancy have been located. The drug is not likely to cross the placenta in any clinically significant amount. However, the absence of human pregnancy experience prevents a complete assessment of the embryofetal risk. Animal data did not show any embryofetal toxic effects. Using this drug during pregnancy should be based on the pros and cons of the mother's clinical need for treatment versus any potential fetal risk that might occur from exposure. Vutrisiran can decrease serum vitamin A levels, so supplementation is recommended. On the other hand, excessive vitamin A intake during pregnancy can be associated with adverse fetal developmental effects.

BREASTFEEDING SUMMARY

No reports describing the use of vutrisiran during human lactation have been located. Negligible amounts of the drug may be found in breast milk, if any at all. Therefore, infant exposure will probably be clinically insignificant. Breastfeeding while using this drug should be based on the mother's clinical need for treatment. If used, the infant should be monitored for the most common reported adult side effects of arthralgia and extremity pain (both leading to irritability), dyspnea, and decreased vitamin A levels.

Reference

1. Prescribing Information. Amvuttra. Alnylam Pharmaceuticals; 2023.

WARFARIN

Anticoagulant (Vitamin K Antagonist)

PREGNANCY RECOMMENDATION: Human Data Suggest Risk (First Trimester)

BREASTFEEDING RECOMMENDATION: Compatible

PREGNANCY SUMMARY

Since warfarin is the only coumarin derivative currently available in the United States, human data will focus on warfarin. Several reports have described the use of warfarin during pregnancy, and exposure during the first trimester is associated with warfarin embryopathy. Warfarin embryopathy consists of nasal hypoplasia with skeletal abnormalities (including short limbs/digits and epiphyseal stippling), as well as possible eye defects, visual impairment, deafness, mental developmental delay, and other findings. Doses of more than 5 mg/d in the first trimester are primarily associated with these malformations, along with fetal intracranial hemorrhage and fetal loss. During the first trimester, daily doses of 5 mg or less have less than a 3% risk for this teratogenicity, whereas doses over 5 mg daily were associated with more than a 30% risk of embryopathy. The drug crosses the placenta. The manufacturer states that warfarin is contraindicated during pregnancy except in pregnant women with mechanical heart valves, who are at high risk of thromboembolism, and for those for whom the benefits of warfarin may outweigh the risks. Using this drug during pregnancy should be based on the pros and cons of the mother's clinical need for treatment versus any potential fetal risk that might occur from exposure.

The American College of Obstetricians and Gynecologists (ACOG) thromboembolism in pregnancy guidelines note that warfarin embryopathy is associated with exposure at 6 to 12 weeks of gestation, and fetal hemorrhage risk is highest when warfarin is used near term. Due to this, most patients should receive low–molecular-weight heparin instead of warfarin, but warfarin can be considered for patients with mechanical heart valves. The 2020 American College of Cardiology and the American Heart Association (ACC/AHA) guidelines for management of pregnant patients with mechanical heart valves note that three treatment strategies can be considered during pregnancy (continue warfarin throughout pregnancy, use low–molecular-weight heparin throughout pregnancy, or use low–molecular-weight heparin during the first trimester and warfarin during the second and third trimesters). A multidisciplinary approach and detailed discussion with the patient about the risks and benefits of the various treatment options, depending on the patient's gestational age, is recommended. See the guidelines for further detailed information.

BREASTFEEDING SUMMARY

Five publications on warfarin use while breastfeeding have been located, totaling 21 lactating women. From these studies, a total of 14 patients were taking 2 to 12 mg/d warfarin postdelivery, and the drug was not detected in any of the breast milk samples. There were seven cases where infant plasma was assessed, and warfarin was not detected in any of the samples. A total of six infants had blood coagulation analyses performed, and none were abnormal. Lastly, five infants exposed to warfarin from a breastfeeding mother did not show any signs of adverse effects. The manufacturer reports that warfarin has not been detected in human breast milk from their evaluation of published literature. However, due to the potential for adverse effects on the breastfed infant or from the underlying maternal condition, the manufacturer recommends that the developmental and health benefits of breastfeeding should be considered versus the mother's clinical need for warfarin. If used during lactation, the manufacturer reports monitoring the infant for bleeding or bruising. ACOG states that warfarin is compatible with breastfeeding.

References

1. Product information. Warfarin sodium. Taro Pharmaceuticals USA Inc.; 2022.
2. National Library of Medicine. PubChem. Warfarin. Accessed October 26, 2023. https://pubchem.ncbi.nlm.nih.gov/compound/Warfarin
3. American College of Obstetricians and Gynecologists. Thromboembolism in pregnancy. ACOG practice bulletin No. 196. *Obstet Gynecol*. 2018;132:e1-e17.
4. Otto CM, Nishimura RA, Bonow RO, et al. 2020 ACC/AHA guideline for the management of patients with valvular heart disease. *J Am Coll Cardiol*. 2021;77:e25-e197.
5. DiSaia PJ. Pregnancy and delivery of a patient with a Starr-Edwards mitral valve prosthesis. *Obstet Gynecol*. 1966;28:469-471.
6. Hall JG, Pauli RM, Wilson KM. Maternal and fetal sequelae of anticoagulation during pregnancy. *Am J Med*. 1980;68:122-140.
7. Baillie M, Allen ED, Elkington AR. The congenital warfarin syndrome: a case report. *Br J Ophthalmol*. 1980;64:633-635.
8. Harrod MJE, Sherrod PS. Warfarin embryopathy in siblings. *Obstet Gynecol*. 1981;57:673-676.
9. Russo R, Bortolotti U, Schivazappa L, et al. Warfarin treatment during pregnancy: a clinical note. *Haemostasis*. 1979;8:96-98.
10. Biale Y, Cantor A, Lewenthal H, et al. The course of pregnancy in patients with artificial heart valves treated with dipyridamole. *Int J Gynaecol Obstet*. 1980;18:128-132.
11. Moe N. Anticoagulant therapy in the prevention of placental infarction and perinatal death. *Obstet Gynecol*. 1982;59:481-483.

12. Kaplan LC, Anderson GG, Ring BA. Congenital hydrocephalus and Dandy-Walker malformation associated with warfarin use during pregnancy. *Birth Defects*. 1982;18:79-83.
13. Chen WWC, Chan CS, Lee PK, et al. Pregnancy in patients with prosthetic heart valves: an experience with 45 pregnancies. *Q J Med*. 1982;51:358-365.
14. Vellenga E, Van Imhoff GW, Aarnoudse JG. Effective prophylaxis with oral anticoagulants and low-dose heparin during pregnancy in an antithrombin III deficient woman. *Lancet*. 1983;2:224.
15. Michiels JJ, Stibbe J, Vellenga E, et al. Prophylaxis of thrombosis in antithrombin III-deficient women during pregnancy and delivery. *Eur J Obstet Gynecol Reprod Biol*. 1984;18:149-153.
16. Oakley C. Pregnancy in patients with prosthetic heart valves. *Br Med J*. 1983;286:1680-1683.
17. Sheikhzadeh A, Ghabusi P, Hakim S, et al. Congestive heart failure in valvular heart disease in pregnancies with and without valvular prostheses and anticoagulant therapy. *Clin Cardiol*. 1983;6:465-470.
18. Lee C-N, Wu C-C, Lin P-Y, et al. Pregnancy following cardiac prosthetic valve replacement. *Obstet Gynecol*. 1994;83:353-360.
19. Copplestone A, Oscier DG. Heparin-induced thrombocytopenia in pregnancy. *Br J Haematol*. 1987;65:248.
20. Chong MKB, Harvey D, De Swiet M. Follow-up study of children whose mothers were treated with warfarin during pregnancy. *Br J Obstet Gynaecol*. 1984;91:1070-1073.
21. Lee P-K, Wang RYC, Chow JSF, et al. Combined use of warfarin and adjusted subcutaneous heparin during pregnancy in patients with an artificial heart valve. *J Am Coll Cardiol*. 1986;8:221-224.
22. Ayhan A, Yapar EG, Yuce K, et al. Pregnancy and its complications after cardiac valve replacement. *Int J Gynecol Obstet*. 1991;35:117-122.
23. Born D, Martinez EE, Almeida PAM, et al. Pregnancy in patients with prosthetic heart valves: the effects of anticoagulation on mother, fetus, and neonate. *Am Heart J*. 1992;124:413-417.
24. Cola LM, Lavin JP Jr. Pregnancy complicated by Marfan's syndrome with aortic arch dissection, subsequent aortic arch replacement and triple coronary artery bypass grafts. *J Reprod Med*. 1985;30:685-688.
25. Normann EK, Stray-Pedersen B. Warfarin-induced fetal diaphragmatic hernia: case report. *Br J Obstet Gynaecol*. 1989;96:729-730.
26. Campbell JM, Tate G, Scott JS. The use of warfarin in pregnancy complicated by circulating lupus anticoagulant; a technique for monitoring. *Eur J Obstet Gynecol Reprod Biol*. 1988;29:27-32.
27. Ruthnum P, Tolmie JL. Atypical malformations in an infant exposed to warfarin during the first trimester of pregnancy. *Teratology*. 1987;36:299-301.
28. Olthof E, De Vries TW, Touwen BCL, et al. Late neurological, cognitive and behavioural sequelae of prenatal exposure to coumarins: a pilot study. *Ear Hum Develop*. 1994;38:97-109.
29. Orme ML, Lewis PJ, De Swiet M, et al. May mothers given warfarin breast-feed their infants? *Br Med J*. 1977;1:1564-1565.
30. De Swiet M, Lewis PJ. Excretion of anticoagulants in human milk. *N Engl J Med*. 1977;297:1471.
31. McKenna R, Cole ER, Vasan U. Is warfarin sodium contraindicated in the lactating mother? *J Pediatr*. 1983;103:325-327.
32. Ito S, Blajchman A, Stephenson M, et al. Prospective follow-up of adverse reactions in breast-fed infants exposed to maternal medication. *Am J Obstet Gynecol*. 1993;168:1383-1399.
33. Schindler D, Graham TP. Warfarin overdose in a breast-feeding woman. *West J Emerg Med*. 2011;12:216-217.
34. American College of Obstetricians and Gynecologists Committee on Practice Bulletins–Obstetrics. ACOG practice bulletin No. 197: inherited thrombophilias in pregnancy. *Obstet Gynecol*. 2018;132:e18-e34.

X

XENON Xe 129 HYPERPOLARIZED GAS

Radiopharmaceutical Diagnostic Agent

PREGNANCY RECOMMENDATION: No Human Data and No Relevant Animal Data

BREASTFEEDING RECOMMENDATION: Probably Compatible

PREGNANCY SUMMARY

No reports describing the use of xenon Xe 129 hyperpolarized gas in human pregnancy have been located. Based on likely negligible placental transfer, fetal exposure is probably clinically insignificant. However, the absence of human pregnancy experience prevents a complete assessment of the embryofetal risk. No animal data reproduction studies have been conducted with xenon Xe 129 hyperpolarized gas. However, an 80% Xe/20% O_2 gas inhalation did not result in any embryofetal toxicity. Using this drug during pregnancy should be based on the pros and cons of the mother's clinical need for treatment versus any potential fetal risk that might occur from exposure.

BREASTFEEDING SUMMARY

No reports describing the use of xenon Xe 129 hyperpolarized gas during human lactation have been located. The negligible systemic absorption after inhalation and the extremely short elimination half-life should limit any infant exposure. If used while breastfeeding, the infant should be monitored for the most common reported adult side effects of oropharyngeal pain, headache, and dizziness (all leading to irritability).

Reference

1. Product Information. Xenoview. Polarean, Inc; 2022.

Z

ZAFIRLUKAST

Respiratory (Leukotriene Receptor Antagonist)

PREGNANCY RECOMMENDATION: Limited Human Data—Animal Data Suggest Low Risk

BREASTFEEDING RECOMMENDATION: Probably Compatible

PREGNANCY SUMMARY

Two reports describing a total of 33 patients using zafirlukast in human pregnancy have been located. The exposures occurred either in the first or second trimester. Of these patients, there was one (3%) major birth anomaly. This rate falls within the expected rate for birth anomalies in the United States. The drug is likely to cross the placenta, so some fetal exposure will probably occur. Therefore, this limited human pregnancy experience prevents a complete assessment of the embryofetal risk. Animal studies did not show embryofetal toxicity in three species at doses of more than 10 times the recommended human dose (RHD). Using this drug during pregnancy should be based on the pros and cons of the mother's clinical need for treatment versus any potential fetal risk that might occur from exposure. Women who are pregnant and have taken asthma medications during pregnancy are encouraged to contact MotherToBaby Pregnancy Studies at 877–311–8972. The most recent American College of Obstetricians and Gynecologists (ACOG) guideline (published 2008) states that leukotriene inhibitors such as zafirlukast and montelukast are alternative add-on agents if patients are uncontrolled on moderate-dose inhaled steroids; however, long-acting β_2-agonists are preferred because they are more effective as add-on therapy in nonpregnant patients. The 2023 Global Initiative for Asthma (GINA) guidelines state that the advantages of actively treating asthma in pregnancy markedly outweigh the potential risks of asthma medications, and inhaled steroids, β_2-agonists, montelukast, and theophylline have not been associated with harm; however, zafirlukast is not specifically mentioned. Risks of uncontrolled asthma during pregnancy include preterm delivery, low birth weight, increased perinatal mortality, and preeclampsia.

BREASTFEEDING SUMMARY

No reports describing the use of zafirlukast during human lactation have been located. The manufacturer reports that the drug is excreted into breast milk. In healthy women taking twice the normal daily dose, an exclusively breastfed infant would receive about 0.6% of the maternal weight-adjusted dose. The effects on a nursing infant from this exposure are unknown, but likely to be clinically insignificant. The manufacturer recommends that women not use zafirlukast while breastfeeding. Nevertheless, breastfeeding while using this drug should be based on the mother's clinical need for treatment. If used, the infant should be monitored for the most common reported adult side effect of headache (leading to irritability).

References

1. Prescribing Information. Accolate. Par Pharmaceutical; 2018.
2. American College of Obstetricians and Gynecologists. ACOG Practice Bulletin No. 90: asthma in pregnancy. *Obstet Gynecol*. 2008;111:457-464.
3. Global Initiative for Asthma. Global strategy for asthma management and prevention, 2023. Updated July 2023. Accessed July 19, 2023. www.ginasthma.org
4. Bakhireva LN, Jones KL, Schatz M, et al; The Organization of Teratology Information Specialists Collaborative Research Group. Safety of leukotriene receptor antagonists in pregnancy. *J Allergy Clin Immunol*. 2007;119:618-625.
5. Twaites BR, Wilton LV, Shakir SA. Safety of zafirlukast: results of a postmarketing surveillance study on 7976 patients in England. *Drug Saf*. 2007;30:419-429.

ZALEPLON

Central Nervous System (Hypnotic—Nonbenzodiazepine Benzodiazepine Receptor Agonist)

PREGNANCY RECOMMENDATION: Limited Human Data—Animal Data Suggest Potential Risk

BREASTFEEDING RECOMMENDATION: Probably Compatible (With Short-Term Use)

PREGNANCY SUMMARY

Two studies from the Swedish Medical Birth Registry were located that reported the use of zaleplon during pregnancy. The first covered births from 1995–2004, and the second covered births to 2007. The patients in the first study were included in the second. There were 1,318 women who gave birth to 1,341 infants and who reported the use of hypnotic nonbenzodiazepine benzodiazepine receptor agonists during the first trimester. The unexposed group involved 1,106,001 women who gave birth to 1,125,734 infants. The rate of major congenital malformations was similar in the exposed 42/1,341 (3.1%) and the unexposed 36,321/1,125,734 (3.2%) groups. However, only 32 were exposed to zaleplon, and specific data on these were not provided. The drug will probably cross the placenta, so some fetal exposure will likely occur. Therefore, this limited human pregnancy experience prevents a complete assessment of the embryofetal risk. Animal studies did not show any embryofetal toxicity in two species, one at doses of less than 10 times the RHD and the other at more than 10 times the RHD. However, embryofetal toxicity was seen in one species with doses less than 10 times the RHD when it was used throughout the pregnancy and during lactation. The manufacturer states that the drug should not be used during pregnancy due to a lack of data on the drug during human pregnancy. Nevertheless, using this drug during pregnancy should be based on the pros and cons of the mother's clinical need for treatment versus any potential fetal risk that might occur from exposure. Zaleplon has a misuse potential similar to benzodiazepines and benzodiazepine-like hypnotics. The drug is classified as a Schedule IV controlled substance. Women who are pregnant and have taken zaleplon during pregnancy are encouraged to contact the National Pregnancy Registry for Psychiatric Medications at 866–961–2388.

BREASTFEEDING SUMMARY

One study was located that analyzed the use of zaleplon during human lactation in five women. The peak drug level occurred about 1 hour after the dose, and the elimination half-life in breast milk was also about 1 hour (similar to the plasma elimination half-life). Using the mean peak breast milk level for zaleplon, an exclusively breastfed infant would receive about 1.4% of the maternal weight-adjusted dose. It was felt that this small amount would not be clinically significant. However, because the effects on a nursing infant are unknown, the manufacturer recommends that women not breastfeed while using this drug. Nevertheless, breastfeeding while using this drug should be based on the mother's clinical need for treatment. If used, the infant should be monitored for the most common reported adult side effects of headache, back pain, arthralgia, and myalgia (all leading to irritability), constipation, rash, and dry mouth.

References

1. Prescribing Information. Zaleplon. Aurobindo Pharma Limited; 2021.
2. Wikner BN, Stiller CO, Bergman U, et al. Use of benzodiazepines and benzodiazepine receptor agonists during pregnancy: neonatal outcome and congenital malformations. *Pharmacoepidemiol Drug Saf*. 2007;16:1203-1210.
3. Wikner BN, Kallen B. Are hypnotic benzodiazepine receptor agonists teratogenic in humans? *J Clin Psychopharmacol*. 2011;31:356-359.
4. Darwish M, Martin PT, Cevallos WH, et al. Rapid disappearance of zaleplon from breast milk after oral administration to lactating women. *J Clin Pharmacol*. 1999;39:670-674.

ZANAMIVIR

Antiviral (Neuraminidase Inhibitor)

PREGNANCY RECOMMENDATION: Limited Human Data - Animal Data Suggest Low Risk

BREASTFEEDING RECOMMENDATION: Probably Compatible

PREGNANCY SUMMARY

Several reports describing the use of zanamivir in human pregnancy have been located. Over 50 live-born newborns have been reported with first-trimester exposure to zanamivir, with no anomalies reported. More than 150 exposures to the drug have been reported with second/third trimester exposure, and no increased risks for poor pregnancy outcome were identified. A large analysis of neuraminidase inhibitor use during pregnancy, involving data from Scandinavian countries and France, reported on 5,824 exposures compared with 692,232 unexposed pregnancies. Of these, 4,310 were administered oseltamivir and 1,514 were given zanamivir. No increased risks for poor pregnancy outcomes were seen. Of this group, 1,220 had first-trimester exposures, and the rate of congenital anomalies was no different from the control group. However, specific numbers for those exposed to zanamivir versus oseltamivir in the first trimester were not provided. Some amount of the drug may cross the placenta, but with the low systemic absorption following inhalation use, the amount is likely to be small. However, this limited human pregnancy experience still prevents a complete assessment of the embryofetal risk. Animal studies did not show any embryofetal toxicity or malformations in two species at doses of more than 10 times the RHD. ACOG states that pregnant women with suspected or confirmed influenza infection should receive this drug or oseltamivir. The ideal treatment is starting one of these drugs within 48 hours of the onset of symptoms, but treatment should not be withheld if this time is missed. The US Centers for Disease Control and Prevention (CDC) agrees with this treatment schedule; however, it lists oseltamivir as preferred due to more pregnancy studies suggesting it is low risk and beneficial.

BREASTFEEDING SUMMARY

No reports describing the use of zanamivir during human lactation have been located. A limited amount of the drug may be found in breast milk, but the overall infant exposure is likely to be negligible. In addition, the drug is poorly absorbed with oral use. One study estimated that an exclusively breastfed infant of 5 kg would receive about 0.075 mg daily after an inhalation dose of 10 mg by the mother. This would result in a relative infant dose (RID) of less than 1%. Breastfeeding while using this drug should be based on the mother's clinical need for treatment versus any potential infant risks that might occur. If used, the infant should be monitored for the most common reported adult side effects of dizziness and arthralgia (both leading to irritability) and pyrexia.

References

1. Prescribing Information. Relenza. GlaxoSmithKline, LLC; 2021.
2. ACOG Committee Opinion No. 753: assessment and treatment of pregnant women with suspected or confirmed influenza. *Obstet Gynecol*. 2018;132:e169-e173.
3. Centers for Disease Control and Prevention. Guidance: antiviral and obstetric health care. Accessed July 23, 2023. https://www.cdc.gov/flu/professionals/antivirals/avrec_ob.htm
4. Freund B, Gravenstein S, Elliott M, et al. Zanamivir—a review of clinical safety. *Drug Saf*. 1999;21:267-281.
5. Bozzo P, Djokanovic N, Koren G. H1N1 influenza in pregnancy: risks, vaccines, and antivirals. *J Obstet Gynaecol Can*. 2009;31:1172-1175.
6. Tanaka T, Nakajima K, Murashima A, et al. Safety of neuraminidase inhibitors against novel influenza A (H1N1) in pregnant and breastfeeding women. *CMAJ*. 2009;181:55-58.
7. Kiatboonsri S, Kiatboonsri C, Theerawit P. Fatal respiratory events caused by zanamivir nebulization. *Clin Infect Dis*. 2010;50:620.
8. Saito S, Minakami H, Nakai A, et al. Outcomes of infants exposed to oseltamivir or zanamivir in utero during pandemic (H1N1) 2009. *Am J Obstet Gynecol*. 2013;209:130.e1-130.e9.
9. Dunstan HJ, Mill AC, Stephens S, et al. Pregnancy outcome following maternal use of zanamivir or oseltamivir during the 2009 influenza A/H1N1 pandemic: a national prospective surveillance study. *BJOG*. 2014;121:901-906.
10. Ghulmiyyah LM, Alame MM, Mirza FG, et al. Influenza and its treatment during pregnancy: a review. *J Neonatal Perinatal Med*. 2015;8:297-306.
11. Graner S, Svensson T, Beau AB, et al. Neuraminidase inhibitors during pregnancy and risk of adverse neonatal outcomes and congenital malformations: population based European register study. *BMJ*. 2017;356:j629.

ZANUBRUTINIB

Antineoplastic (Bruton Tyrosine Kinase Inhibitor)

PREGNANCY RECOMMENDATION: No Human Data—Animal Data Suggest Potential Risk

BREASTFEEDING RECOMMENDATION: Potential Toxicity

PREGNANCY SUMMARY

No reports describing the use of zanubrutinib in human pregnancy have been located. Based on likely placental transfer, some fetal exposure will probably occur. Therefore, the absence of human pregnancy experience prevents a complete assessment of the embryofetal risk. Embryofetal toxicity with malformations was observed in one of two animal species at doses of less than 10 times the human exposure. Based on animal studies, the manufacturer recommends that women with reproductive potential use effective contraception during treatment and for 1 week after the last dose. They also recommend that males with female partners of reproductive potential use effective contraception during treatment and for 1 week after the last dose. Nevertheless, using this drug during pregnancy should be based on the pros and cons of the mother's clinical need for treatment versus any potential fetal risk that might occur from exposure. Women who are pregnant and have cancer are encouraged to contact the Cancer and Pregnancy Registry at 877–635–4499. Because the drug can produce hypertension, if used during pregnancy, blood pressure should be monitored closely.

BREASTFEEDING SUMMARY

No reports describing the use of zanubrutinib during human lactation have been located. The drug will likely be found in breast milk, so some infant exposure will probably occur. Based on the animal studies, the manufacturer recommends that women withhold breastfeeding while being treated with zanubrutinib and for at least 2 weeks after the last dose. Nevertheless, breastfeeding while using this drug should be based on the mother's clinical need for treatment. If used, the infant should be monitored for the most common reported adult side effects of musculoskeletal pain (leading to irritability), upper respiratory tract infection, hemorrhage, and various laboratory abnormalities (see Prescribing Information [PI]).

Reference

1. Prescribing Information. Brukinsa. Beigene USA; 2023.

ZAVEGEPANT

Pain/Central Nervous System (Antimigraine)

PREGNANCY RECOMMENDATION: No Human Data—Animal Data Suggest Low Risk

BREASTFEEDING RECOMMENDATION: Probably Compatible

PREGNANCY SUMMARY

No reports describing the use of zavegepant in human pregnancy have been located. Based on the likely minimal placental transfer of the drug, fetal exposure will probably be negligible. However, the absence of human pregnancy experience prevents a complete assessment of the embryofetal risk. Animal data did not show any embryofetal toxicity despite being administered subcutaneously in two species at doses of more than 10 times the RHD. Using this drug during pregnancy should be based on the pros and cons of the mother's clinical need for treatment versus any potential fetal risk that might occur from exposure.

BREASTFEEDING SUMMARY

No reports describing the use of zavegepant during human lactation have been located. Very limited amounts of the drug will likely be excreted into breast milk, so some infant exposure might occur. Breastfeeding while using this drug should be based on the mother's clinical need for treatment. If used, the infant should be monitored for the most common reported adult side effects of nausea (leading to irritability) and vomiting.

Reference

1. Prescribing Information. Zavzpret. Pfizer Labs; 2023.

ZICONOTIDE

Pain (Intrathecal Nonopioid Analgesic)

PREGNANCY RECOMMENDATION: Limited Human Data—Animal Data Suggest Low Risk

BREASTFEEDING RECOMMENDATION: Probably Compatible

PREGNANCY SUMMARY

One case report of a single patient with an intrathecal ziconotide pump was located. She had three term deliveries resulting in healthy infants with no complications or congenital anomalies. Based on the likely limited placental transfer, fetal exposure is probably negligible. However, this limited human pregnancy experience prevents a complete assessment of the embryofetal risk. Animal data did not show embryofetal toxicity in two species receiving intravenous (IV) doses much greater than 10 times the maximum recommended human daily intrathecal dose (based on plasma exposure). Using this drug during pregnancy should be based on the pros and cons of the mother's clinical need for treatment versus any potential fetal risk that might occur from exposure.

BREASTFEEDING SUMMARY

No reports describing the use of ziconotide during human lactation have been located. The amount of drug, if any, found in breast milk will likely be clinically insignificant. Additionally, if any of this polypeptide were to be ingested through breastfeeding, it would probably be digested in the infant's gastrointestinal tract and not absorbed. Breastfeeding while using this drug should be based on the mother's clinical need for treatment. If used, the infant should be monitored for the most common reported adult side effects of dizziness and nausea (both leading to irritability) and nystagmus. The manufacturer also recommends monitoring a breastfed exposed infant for sedation, which may result in respiratory depression and/or feeding problems.

References

1. Prescribing Information. Prialt. TerSera Therapeutics; 2023.
2. McDowell GC. Long-term follow-up (>11 years) on successful pregnancies with ziconotide monotherapy for arachnoiditis-related chronic pain. *Neuromodulation*. 2023;26:1263-1265.

ZIDOVUDINE

Antiretroviral (Reverse Transcriptase Inhibitor—Nucleoside Analogue)

PREGNANCY RECOMMENDATION: Human Data Suggest Compatible

BREASTFEEDING RECOMMENDATION: *Contraindicated

PREGNANCY SUMMARY

Numerous publications have been located regarding the use of zidovudine during human pregnancy. From the January 31, 2024, Antiretroviral Pregnancy Registry, 136 (3.2%) fetal anomalies were identified in 4,256 first-trimester exposures. In a recent systematic review and meta-analysis of reported pregnancies with exposure to antiretroviral therapy and the risk for fetal malformations, there were 1,461 (2.7%) infants with birth defects found in 53,186 births. Specific information on zidovudine alone was not provided. However, based on the included studies, a large number of cases were on therapy that included zidovudine. These percentages fall within the expected rate for major congenital birth anomalies, and no specific pattern to the defects has been identified. The drug will cross the placenta, so fetal exposure will occur. Animal studies did not show any teratogenicity in one species at doses of more than 10 times the RHD. Several other animal reproduction studies showed adverse fetal outcomes, but in every case, the amount of drug used was more than 10 times the RHD. Zidovudine is effective in the reduction of maternal-fetal transmission of HIV type 1 (HIV-1) infection with few, if any, adverse effects in the newborns. The 2023 US Department of Health and Human Services AIDS Info guidelines note that zidovudine pharmacokinetics are not significantly changed during pregnancy. They state that, in most cases, patients continue their regimen during pregnancy if it is tolerated, safe, and effective in suppressing viral replication (this includes zidovudine). The guideline recommends that discussion and shared decision-making about the known and potential risks as well as benefits to the mother and fetus, acknowledging that limited data should guide the selection of which antiretrovirals to use during pregnancy. Additionally, treatment initiation should not be delayed due to concerns about teratogenicity with first-trimester exposure. Neonatal anemia, a known toxic effect of zidovudine, may occur and requires monitoring. Providers caring for pregnant patients with HIV and their infants can call the national Perinatal HIV/AIDS hotline (888–448–8765) for free clinical consultation. Additionally, there is a pregnancy exposure registry that monitors pregnancy outcomes in individuals exposed to antiretroviral medicines during pregnancy. Health care professionals are encouraged to register obstetric patients taking zidovudine in the Antiretroviral Pregnancy Registry at 800–258–4263.

BREASTFEEDING SUMMARY

*The 2023 U.S. Department of Health and Human Services AIDS Info guidelines state that using replacement of breast milk through formula or pasteurized donor human breast milk from a milk bank eliminates the risk of postnatal HIV transmission to the infant. Using antiretroviral therapy to achieve and maintain viral suppression during pregnancy and postpartum decreases the risk for infant transmission to less than 1%, but notes that it is not zero. For patients not on therapy or those without viral load suppression during pregnancy (at a minimum of throughout the third trimester) and at delivery, replacement of breast milk is recommended. Patients on antiretroviral therapy who have a sustained undetectable viral load and who choose to breastfeed or use the replacement of breast milk should be supported with this decision. If zidovudine is used during lactation, the drug does cross into breast milk with peak levels occurring about 1 to 2 hours after a dose. Reported breast milk to serum level ratios range from 0.48 to 1.78.

References

1. Prescribing Information. Zidovudine. Aurobindo Pharma Limited; 2021.
2. Liebes L, Mendoza S, Wilson D, et al. Transfer of zidovudine (AZT) by human placenta. *J Infect Dis.* 1990;161:203-207.
3. Bawdon RE, Sobhi S, Dax J. The transfer of anti-human immunodeficiency virus nucleoside compounds by the term human placenta. *Am J Obstet Gynecol.* 1992;167:1570-1574.
4. Schenker S, Johnson RF, King TS, et al. Azidothymidine (zidovudine) transport by the human placenta. *Am J Med Sci.* 1990;299:16-20.
5. Gillet JY, Garraffo R, Abrar D, et al. Fetoplacental passage of zidovudine. *Lancet.* 1989;2:269-270.
6. Lyman WD, Tanaka KE, Kress Y, et al. Zidovudine concentrations in human fetal tissue: implications for perinatal AIDS. *Lancet.* 1990;335:1280-1281.
7. Chavanet P, Diquet B, Waldner A, et al. Perinatal pharmacokinetics of zidovudine. *N Engl J Med.* 1989;321:1548-1549.
8. Pons JC, Taburet AM, Singlas E, et al. Placental passage of azathiothymidine (AZT) during the second trimester of pregnancy: study by direct fetal blood sampling under ultrasound. *Eur J Obstet Gynecol Reprod Biol.* 1991; 40:229-231.
9. O'Sullivan MJ, Boyer PJJ, Scott GB, et al; Zidovudine Collaborative Working Group. The pharmacokinetics and safety of zidovudine in the third trimester of pregnancy for women infected with human immunodeficiency virus and their infants: Phase I Acquired Immunodeficiency Syndrome Clinical Trials group study (protocol 082). *Am J Obstet Gynecol.* 1993;168:1510-1516.
10. Unadkat JD, Pereira CM. Maternal-fetal transfer and fetal toxicity of anti-HIV drugs. A review. *Trophoblast Res.* 1994;8:67-82.
11. Watts DH, Brown ZA, Tartaglione T, et al. Pharmacokinetic disposition of zidovudine during pregnancy. *J Infect Dis.* 1991;163:226-232.
12. Sperling RS, Roboz J, Dische R, et al. Zidovudine pharmacokinetics during pregnancy. *Am J Perinatol.* 1992;9:247-249.
13. Tindall B, Cotton R, Swanson C, et al. Fifth International Conference on the acquired immunodeficiency syndrome. *Med J Aust.* 1990;152: 204-214.
14. Tuntland T, Odinecs A, Pereira CM, et al. In vitro models to predict the in vivo mechanism, rate, and extent of placental transfer of dideoxynucleoside drugs against human immunodeficiency virus. *Am J Obstet Gynecol.* 1999; 180:198-206.
15. Moodley J, Moodley D, Pillay K, et al. Pharmacokinetics and antiretroviral activity of lamivudine alone or when coadministered with zidovudine in human immunodeficiency virus type 1-infected pregnant women and their offspring. *J Infect Dis.* 1998;178:1327-1333.
16. Liebes L, Mendoza S, Lee JD, et al. Further observations on zidovudine transfer and metabolism by human placenta. *AIDS.* 1993;7:590-592.
17. Viscarello RR, DeGennaro NJ, Hobbins JC. Preliminary experience with the use of zidovudine (AZT) during pregnancy. Society of Perinatal Obstetricians Abstracts. *Am J Obstet Gynecol.* 1991;164:248.
18. Cullen MT, Delke I, Greenhaw J, et al. HIV in pregnancy: factors predictive of maternal and fetal outcome. Society of Perinatal Obstetricians Abstracts. *Am J Obstet Gynecol.* 1992;166:386.
19. Taylor U, Bardeguez A. Antiretroviral therapy during pregnancy and postpartum. Society of Perinatal Obstetricians Abstracts. *Am J Obstet Gynecol.* 1992;166:390.

20. Delke I, Greenhaw J, Sanchez-Ramos L, et al. Antiretroviral therapy during pregnancy. Society of Perinatal Obstetricians Abstracts. *Am J Obstet Gynecol.* 1993;168:424.
21. Sperling RS, Stratton P, O'Sullivan MJ, et al. A survey of zidovudine use in pregnant women with human immunodeficiency virus infection. *N Engl J Med.* 1992;326:857-861.
22. Kumar RM, Hughes PF, Khurranna A. Zidovudine use in pregnancy: a report of 104 cases and the occurrence of birth defects. *J Acquir Immune Defic Synd.* 1994;7:1034-1039.
23. Connor EM, Sperling RS, Gelber R, et al; for the Pediatric AIDS Clinical Trials Group Protocol 076 Study Group. Reduction of maternal-infant transmission of human immunodeficiency virus type 1 with zidovudine treatment. *N Engl J Med.* 1994;331:1173-1180.
24. Wade NA, Birkhead GS, Warren BL, et al. Abbreviated regimens of zidovudine prophylaxis and perinatal transmission of the human immunodeficiency virus. *N Engl J Med.* 1998;339:1409-1414.
25. Shaffer N, Chuachoowong R, Mock PA, et al; on behalf of the Bangkok Collaborative Perinatal HIV Transmission Study Group. Short-course zidovudine for perinatal HIV-1 transmission in Bangkok, Thailand: a randomised controlled trial. *Lancet.* 1999;353:773-780.
26. Wiktor SZ, Ekpini E, Karon JM, et al. Short-course oral zidovudine for prevention of mother-to-child transmission of HIV-1 in Abidjan, Côte d'Ivoire: a randomised trial. *Lancet.* 1999;353:781-785.
27. Dabis F, Msellati P, Meda N, et al; for the DITRAME Study Group. 6-month efficacy, tolerance, and acceptability of a short regimen of oral zidovudine to reduce vertical transmission of HIV in breastfed children in Côte d'Ivoire and Burkina Faso: a double- blind placebo-controlled multicentre trial. *Lancet.* 1999;353:786-792.
28. Mofenson LM. Short-course zidovudine for prevention of perinatal infection. *Lancet.* 1999;353:766-767.
29. Lallemant M, Jourdain G, Le Coeur S, et al; for the Perinatal HIV Prevention Trial (Thailand) investigators. A trial of shortened zidovudine regimens to prevent mother-to-child transmission of human immunodeficiency virus type 1. *N Engl J Med.* 2000;343:982-991.
30. Peckham C, Newell ML. Preventing vertical transmission of HIV infection. *N Engl J Med.* 2000;343:1036-1037.
31. McGowan JP, Crane M, Wiznia AA, et al. Combination antiretroviral therapy in human immunodeficiency virus-infected pregnant women. *Obstet Gynecol.* 1999;94:641-646.
32. Guay LA, Musoke P, Fleming T, et al. Intrapartum and neonatal single-dose nevirapine compared with zidovudine for prevention of mother-to-child transmission of HIV-1 in Kampala, Uganda: HIVNET 012 randomised trial. *Lancet.* 1999;354:795-802.
33. Marseille E, Kahn JG, Mmiro F, et al. Cost effectiveness of single-dose nevirapine regimen for mothers and babies to decrease vertical HIV-1 transmission in sub-Saharan Africa. *Lancet.* 1999;354:803-809.
34. Loch M, Carr A, Vasak E, et al. The use of human immunodeficiency virus postexposure prophylaxis after successful artificial insemination. *Am J Obstet Gynecol.* 1999;181:760-761.
35. Watson WJ, Stevens TP, Weinberg GA. Profound anemia in a newborn infant of a mother receiving antiretroviral therapy. *Pediatr Infect Dis J.* 1998; 17:435-436.
36. Shah MM, Li Y, Christensen RD. Effects of perinatal zidovudine on hematopoiesis: a comparison of effects on progenitors from human fetuses versus mothers. *AIDS.* 1996;10:1239-1247.
37. Blanche S, Tardieu M, Rustin P, et al. Persistent mitochondrial dysfunction and perinatal exposure to antiretroviral nucleoside analogues. *Lancet.* 1999;354:1084-1089.
38. Brinkman K, Smeitink JA, Romijn JA, et al. Mitochondrial toxicity induced by nucleoside-analogue reverse-transcriptase inhibitors is a key factor in the pathogenesis of antiretroviral-therapy-related lipodystrophy. *Lancet.* 1999;354:1112-1115.
39. Morris AAM, Carr A. HIV nucleoside analogues: new adverse effects on mitochondria? *Lancet.* 1999;354:1046-1047.
40. Stojanov S, Wintergerst U, Belohradsky BH, et al. Mitochondrial and peroxisomal dysfunction following perinatal exposure to antiretroviral drugs. *AIDS.* 2000;14:1669.
41. Lipshultz SE, Easley KA, Orav EJ, et al; for the Pediatric Pulmonary and Cardiac Complications of Vertically Transmitted HIV Infection Study Group. Absence of cardiac toxicity of zidovudine in infants. *N Engl J Med.* 2000;343:759-766.
42. Richardson MP, Osrin D, Donaghy S, et al. Spinal malformations in the fetuses of HIV infected women receiving combination antiretroviral therapy and co-trimoxazole. *Eur J Obstet Gynecol Reprod Biol.* 2000;93:215-217.
43. Moschovi M, Theodoridou M, Papaevangelou V, et al. Acute lymphoblastic leukaemia in an infant exposed to zidovudine in utero and early infancy. *AIDS.* 2000;14:2410-2411.
44. Hanson IC, Antonelli TA, Sperling RS, et al. Lack of tumors in infants with perinatal HIV-1 exposure and fetal/neonatal exposure to zidovudine. *J Acquir Immune Defic Syndr Hum Retrovirol.* 1999;20:463-467.
45. Culnane M, Fowler MG, Lee SS, et al; for the Pediatric AIDS Clinical Trials Group Protocol 219/076 Teams. Lack of long-term effects of in utero exposure to zidovudine among uninfected children born to HIV-infected women. *JAMA.* 1999;281:151-157.
46. Newschaffer CJ, Cocroft J, Anderson CE, et al. Prenatal zidovudine use and congenital anomalies in a Medicaid population. *J Acquir Immune Defic Syndr.* 2000;24:249-256.
47. Henry K, Chinnock BJ, Quinn RP, et al. Concurrent zidovudine levels in semen and serum determined by radioimmunoassay in patients with AIDS or AIDS-related complex. *JAMA.* 1988;259:3023-3026.
48. Politch JA, Mayer KH, Abbott AF, et al. The effects of disease progression and zidovudine therapy on semen quality in human immunodeficiency virus type 1 seropositive men. *Fertil Steril.* 1994;61;922-928.
49. European Pregnancy and Paediatric HIV Cohort Collaboration (EPPICC) Study Group. Nucleoside reverse transcriptase inhibitor backbones and pregnancy outcomes. *AIDS.* 2019;33:295-304.
50. Tshivuila-Matala COO, Honeyman S, Nesbitt C, et al. Adverse perinatal outcomes associated with antiretroviral therapy regimens: systematic review and network meta-analysis. *AIDS.* 2020;34:1643-1656.
51. Alemu FM, Yalew AW. Does antiretroviral therapy cause congenital malformations? A systematic review and meta-analysis. *Epidemiol Health.* 2021; 43:e2021008.
52. Portwood C, Murray C, Sexton H, et al. Adverse perinatal outcomes associated with HAART and monotherapy. *AIDS.* 2022;36:1409-1427.
53. Kiweewa FM, Tierney C, Butler K, et al. Impact of antiretroviral regimen on pregnancy and infant outcomes in women with HIV/HBV coinfection. *J Acquir Immune Defic Syndr.* 2022;91:79-84.
54. Antiretroviral Pregnancy Registry Steering Committee. Antiretroviral Pregnancy Registry international interim report for 1 January 1989 through 31 January 2023. Registry Coordinating Center. 2023. www.APRegistry.com
55. Panel on Treatment of HIV During Pregnancy and Prevention of Perinatal Transmission. Recommendations for the use of antiretroviral drugs during pregnancy and interventions to reduce perinatal HIV transmission in the United States. Department of Health and Human Services. Accessed July 25, 2023. https://clinicalinfo.hiv.gov/en/guidelines/perinatal
56. Ruff A, Hamzeh F, Lietman P, et al. Excretion of Zidovudine (ZDV) in Human Breast Milk (abstract). Presented at the 34th Interscience Conference on Antimicrobial Agents and Chemotherapy; October, 1994; Orlando, FL.
57. Giuliano M, Guidotti G, Andreotti M, et al. Triple antiretroviral prophylaxis administered during pregnancy and after delivery significantly reduces breast milk viral load. A study within the drug resource enhancement against AIDS and malnutrition program. *J Acquir Immune Defic Syndr.* 2007;44:286-291.
58. Palombi L, Pirillo MF, Andreotti M, et al. Antiretroviral prophylaxis for breastfeeding transmission in Malawi: drug concentration, virological efficacy and safety. *Antiviral Ther.* 2012;17:1511-1519.
59. Davis NL, Corbett A, Kaullen J, et al. Antiretroviral drug concentrations in breastmilk, maternal HIV viral load, and HIV transmission to the infant: results from the BAN study. *J Acquir Immune Defic Syndr.* 2019;80:467-473.

ZILEUTON

Respiratory (Leukotriene Synthesis Inhibitor)

PREGNANCY RECOMMENDATION: No Human Data—Animal Data Suggest Potential Risk

BREASTFEEDING RECOMMENDATION: Probably Compatible

PREGNANCY SUMMARY

No reports describing the use of zileuton in human pregnancy have been located. The drug will likely cross the placenta, so some fetal exposure will probably occur. However, the absence of human pregnancy experience prevents a complete assessment of embryofetal risk. Embryofetal toxicity with malformations was observed in one of two studied animal species with doses of less than 10 times the maximum recommended human dose (MRHD). Using this drug during pregnancy should be based on the pros and cons of the mother's clinical need for treatment versus any potential fetal risk that might occur from exposure. Women who are pregnant and have taken asthma medications during pregnancy are encouraged to contact MotherToBaby Pregnancy Studies at 877–311–8972. Neither the most recent ACOG publication on asthma in pregnancy (published in 2008—reaffirmed in 2020) nor the 2023 GINA guidelines specifically mention zileuton. Both guidelines state that the advantages of actively treating asthma in pregnancy markedly outweigh the potential risks of the medications. Inhaled corticosteroids are usually the first-line treatment for mild to moderate persistent asthma in pregnancy. Listed alternative treatments include cromolyn, theophylline, or leukotriene receptor antagonists. Zileuton is a leukotriene synthesis inhibitor. However, ACOG recommends long-acting β_2-agonists as the preferred add-on drug when pregnant patients are not controlled with inhaled corticosteroids. The reasoning for this is that long-acting inhaled β_2-agonists have been shown to be more effective as an add-on treatment in nonpregnant patients; whereas theophylline has more side effects and requires serum monitoring, and there are minimal data on the leukotriene receptor antagonists in human pregnancy.

BREASTFEEDING SUMMARY

No reports describing the use of zileuton during human lactation have been located. The drug will likely be excreted into breast milk, so some infant exposure will probably occur. Breastfeeding while using this drug should be based on the mother's clinical need for treatment. If used, the infant should be monitored for the most common reported adult side effects of nausea and throat pain (both leading to irritability) and sinusitis.

References

1. Prescribing Information. Zileuton. Lupin Pharmaceuticals, Inc; 2020.
2. American College of Obstetricians and Gynecologists. ACOG Practice Bulletin No. 90: asthma in pregnancy. *Obstet Gynecol*. 2008;111:457-464.
3. Global Initiative for Asthma. Global strategy for asthma management and prevention, 2023. Updated July 2023. Accessed July 19, 2023. www.ginasthma.org

ZILUCOPLAN

Immunologic (Complement Inhibitor)

PREGNANCY RECOMMENDATION: No Human Data—Animal Data Suggest Potential Risk

BREASTFEEDING RECOMMENDATION: Probably Compatible

PREGNANCY SUMMARY

No reports describing the use of zilucoplan in human pregnancy have been located. It appears that the drug will cross the placenta, so fetal exposure will likely occur, especially in the second half of gestation. However, the absence of human pregnancy experience prevents a complete assessment of the embryofetal risk. Animal data did show embryofetal toxicity in one species at doses less than 10 times the RHD. Using this drug during pregnancy should be based on the pros and cons of the mother's clinical need for treatment versus any potential fetal risk that might occur from exposure.

BREASTFEEDING SUMMARY

No reports describing the use of zilucoplan during human lactation have been located. Based on the molecular weight (MW) and high plasma protein binding, the drug will likely not be found in breast milk, despite the long elimination half-life. Furthermore, because it is a peptide of 15 amino acids, if the drug were to be ingested through breastfeeding, it would probably be digested in the infant's gastrointestinal tract and not be absorbed. Breastfeeding while using this drug should be based on the mother's clinical need for treatment versus any potential infant risk. If used, the infant should be monitored for the most common reported adult side effects of diarrhea and upper respiratory tract infection.

Reference

1. Prescribing Information. Zilbrysq. UCB, Inc; 2023.

ZIPRASIDONE

Mental Health (Atypical Antipsychotic)

PREGNANCY RECOMMENDATION: Human Data Suggest Potential Risk (Third Trimester)

BREASTFEEDING RECOMMENDATION: Potential Toxicity

PREGNANCY SUMMARY

Atypical antipsychotics do not appear to increase the risk for congenital malformations as a group. From the National Pregnancy Registry for Atypical Antipsychotics, the rate of birth anomalies was 4.3% (941 in 21,751 first-trimester exposures) compared with a 2.7% rate in the unexposed group (177,165/6,455,324). The rate of anomalies in the unexposed group with mental health conditions was 3.7% (11,647/318,731). Of the 21,751 atypical antipsychotic exposure cases, there were 1,143 with ziprasidone use, but the exact number of anomalies for this specific group was not provided (the anomaly rate was <4%). The manufacturer states that atypical antipsychotics do not have an association with malformations based on data from observational studies, birth registries, and case reports. Additionally, they stated that a large retrospective cohort study using a Medicaid database (n = 9,258) did not result in a higher risk of birth defects in the women exposed to antipsychotics during pregnancy. Specific information on ziprasidone was not provided, and some of these cases are probably included in the National Pregnancy Registry for Atypical Antipsychotics data. However, antipsychotic exposure in the third trimester has been associated with fetal/neonatal adverse reactions of extrapyramidal and/or withdrawal symptoms, including agitation, hypertonia, hypotonia, tremor, somnolence, respiratory distress, and feeding disorder. Duration of onset varies from hours to days, with some infants requiring prolonged hospitalization. Therefore, infants need to be monitored for these symptoms and managed appropriately. Ziprasidone can prolong the QTc interval. The manufacturer recommends avoiding this medication in patients with congenital long QT syndrome and those with a history of cardiac arrhythmias. Additionally, avoid using it in combination with other medications that prolong the QTc interval. In addition, elevated glucose levels have occurred in patients treated with this drug. ACOG guidelines from 2023 state that the risks of uncontrolled schizophrenia and bipolar disorder in pregnancy include preterm delivery, fetal growth restriction, adverse neurodevelopmental outcomes, and postpartum psychosis risk, and therefore, treatment is advised. There is a pregnancy exposure registry that monitors pregnancy outcomes in women using antidepressant drugs. Health care providers are encouraged to call the National Pregnancy Registry for Antidepressants at 1–844–405–6185.

BREASTFEEDING SUMMARY

One study was located that analyzed breast milk for ziprasidone levels. The patient was using the drug postdelivery, and in nearly every sample, ziprasidone was not detected (lower level of detection 10 ng/mL). At the maintenance dose of 160 mg/d, the highest level obtained in breast milk was 11 ng/mL. This is consistent with the MW combined with the very high plasma protein binding. In a case report of a mother using ziprasidone and citalopram while breastfeeding, no adverse infant effects were reported, and the infant was developing normally at 6 months of age. Data from the National Pregnancy Registry for Atypical Antipsychotics have reported on more than 500 breastfeeding patients, and no adverse infant effects have been noted. However, specific information on ziprasidone was not provided. The manufacturer recommends not breastfeeding while using ziprasidone. Nevertheless, breastfeeding while using this drug should be based on the mother's clinical need for treatment versus any potential infant risks that might occur. If used, the infant should be monitored for the most common reported adult side effects of dizziness and asthenia (both leading to irritability), extrapyramidal symptoms (tremors and abnormal muscle movements), somnolence, lethargy, and vomiting. The drug can result in elevated prolactin levels, but this should not produce adverse effects on breastfeeding.

References

1. Prescribing Information. Ziprasidone. Viona Pharmaceuticals, Inc; 2022.
2. Prescribing Information. Ziprasidone mesylate. Dr. Reddy's Laboratories, Inc; 2021.
3. American College of Obstetricians and Gynecologists. Treatment and management of mental health conditions during pregnancy and postpartum: ACOG clinical practice guideline No. 5. *Obstet Gynecol*. 2023;141:1262-1288.
4. Viguera AC, McElheny SA, Caplin PS, et al. Risk of poor neonatal adaptation syndrome among infants exposed to second-generation atypical antipsychotics compared to antidepressants. *J Clin Psychiatry*. 2023;84:22m14492.
5. Viguera A, Freeman MP, Goez-Mogollon L, et al. Reproduction safety of second generation antipsychotics: updated data from the Massachusetts General Hospital National Pregnancy Registry for atypical antipsychotics. *J Clin Psychiatry*. 2021;82:20m13745.
6. Huybrechts KF, Straub L, Karlsson P, et al. Association of in utero antipsychotic medication exposure with risk of congenital malformations in Nordic countries and the US. *JAMA Psychiatry*. 2023;80:156-166.
7. Wang Z, Chan AYL, Coghill D, et al. Association between prenatal exposure to antipsychotics and attention-deficit/hyperactivity disorder, autism spectrum disorder, preterm birth, and small for gestational age. *JAMA Intern Med*. 2021;181:1332-1340.
8. Westin AA, Brekke M, Molden E, et al. Treatment with antipsychotics in pregnancy: changes in drug disposition. *Clin Pharmacol Ther*. 2018;103:477-484.
9. Park Y, Hernandez-Diaz S, Bateman BT, et al. Continuation of atypical antipsychotic medication during early pregnancy and the risk of gestational diabetes. *Am J Psychiatry*. 2018;175:564-574.
10. Kulkarni J, Gurvich C, Gilbert H, et al. The use of first and second generation antipsychotic drugs and the potential to develop gestational diabetes mellitus among perinatal patients with psychosis. *Schizophr Res*. 2023;254:22-26.
11. Heinonen E, Forsberg L, Norby U, et al. Antipsychotic use during pregnancy and risk for gestational diabetes: a national register-based cohort study in Sweden. *CNS Drugs*. 2022;36:529-539.
12. Werremeyer A. Ziprasidone and citalopram use in pregnancy and lactation in a woman with psychotic depression. *Am J Psychiatry*. 2009;166:1298.

13. Peitl MV, Petric D, Peitl V. Ziprasidone as a possible cause of cleft palate in a newborn. *Psychiatr Danub*. 2010;22:117-119.
14. Schlotterbeck P, Saur R, Hiemke C, et al. Low concentration of ziprasidone in human milk: a case report. *Int J Neuropsychopharmacol*. 2009;12:437-438.
15. Viguera AC, Vanderkruik R, Gaccione P, et al. Breastfeeding practices among women taking second-generation antipsychotics: findings from the National Pregnancy Registry for atypical antipsychotics. *Arch Womens Health*. 2022;25:511-516.

ZIV-AFLIBERCEPT

Antineoplastic (VEGF Inhibitor, Fc Portion of IgG1)

PREGNANCY RECOMMENDATION: No Human Data—Animal Data Suggest Potential Risk

BREASTFEEDING RECOMMENDATION: Probably Compatible

PREGNANCY SUMMARY

No reports describing the use of ziv-aflibercept in human pregnancy have been located. Because the drug contains the Fc portion of an immunoglobulin G (IgG) antibody, it likely crosses the placenta in the second half of gestation, so some fetal exposure will probably occur. Therefore, the absence of human pregnancy experience prevents a complete assessment of the embryofetal risk. Embryofetal toxicity with malformations was observed in one animal species receiving doses less than those seen with human exposure. Based on the animal studies and the drug's mechanism of action, the manufacturer recommends that women with reproductive potential use effective contraception during treatment and for 1 month after the last dose. Nevertheless, using this drug during pregnancy should be based on the pros and cons of the mother's clinical need for treatment versus any potential fetal risk that might occur from exposure. Women who are pregnant and have cancer are encouraged to contact the Cancer and Pregnancy Registry at 877–635–4499. Lastly, because the drug can produce hypertension, if used during pregnancy, blood pressure should be monitored closely.

BREASTFEEDING SUMMARY

No reports describing the use of ziv-aflibercept during human lactation have been located. Aflibercept (the intravitreal drug) and ziv-aflibercept are the same molecule with the same MW. The difference is in the osmolality of the solutions, with aflibercept at 300 mOsm/kg versus ziv-aflibercept at 1,000 mOsm/kg. The use of a 2 mg intravitreal aflibercept treatment was evaluated in a postpartum mother, and the drug was detected in the breast milk on day 4 after treatment with a level of about 11 ng/mL. However, because of the IgG antibody and protein nature of the drug, if any were to be ingested through breastfeeding, it would probably be digested in the infant's gastrointestinal tract and not be absorbed. Nevertheless, because of the animal studies and concern for potential adverse reactions that might occur in a breastfed infant, the manufacturer recommends that women not breastfeed while being treated with ziv-aflibercept and for at least 1 month after the last dose. Regardless, breastfeeding while using this drug should be based on the mother's clinical need for treatment. If used, the infant should be monitored for the most common reported adult side effects of abdominal pain and headache (both leading to irritability), lethargy, diarrhea, hypertension, decreased appetite (monitor weight gain), and various laboratory abnormalities (see PI).

References

1. Prescribing Information. Zaltrap. Sanofi-Aventis US; 2020.
2. Juncal VR, Paracha Q, Bamakrid M, et al. Ranibizumab and aflibercept levels in breast milk after intravitreal injection. *Ophthalmology*. 2020;127: 278-280.

ZOLEDRONIC ACID

Bone Health (Bisphosphonate)

PREGNANCY RECOMMENDATION: Limited Human Data—Animal Data Suggest Risk

BREASTFEEDING RECOMMENDATION: Probably Compatible

PREGNANCY SUMMARY

Three case reports of zoledronic acid exposure in pregnancy were located, and no newborn complications or malformations were reported. One patient received treatment at about 13 weeks' gestation for hypercalcemia-induced pancreatitis, the second was treated in the second and third trimesters for metastatic breast cancer, and the third received treatment about 9 months prior to conception. The third case was included because the drug is incorporated into bone matrix with potential release over time, so some fetal exposure may have occurred. A literature review of all bisphosphonates used during

(continued)

pregnancy reported on 65 total cases (this review included one of the cases discussed earlier) and did not identify any serious fetal or neonatal adverse effects. The most commonly used bisphosphonates were alendronate and pamidronate. The drug will likely cross the placenta, so some fetal exposure will probably occur. Therefore, this limited human pregnancy experience prevents a complete assessment of the embryofetal risk. The drug was found to cause embryofetal toxicity with malformations in two animal species at doses less than 10 times the MRHD, but all doses also caused maternal toxicity. Based on the animal studies and the drug's mechanism of action, the manufacturer recommends that women with reproductive potential use effective contraception during and after zoledronic acid treatment for oncology reasons. Nevertheless, using this drug during pregnancy should be based on the pros and cons of the mother's clinical need for treatment versus any potential fetal risk that might occur from exposure. Women who are pregnant and have cancer are encouraged to contact the Cancer and Pregnancy Registry at 877–635–4499. If zoledronic acid is used for osteoporosis or Paget disease, the manufacturer recommends that the drug be discontinued when pregnancy is recognized. Because the drug can produce hypertension, if used during pregnancy, blood pressure should be monitored closely.

BREASTFEEDING SUMMARY

One case report describing the use of zoledronic acid during human lactation has been located. The patient developed severe hip pain at the start of the third trimester and was diagnosed with necrosis of the femoral head about a month after delivery. She was treated with zoledronic acid at about 3 months postpartum, and breastfeeding was held for 1 week. No adverse effects from the treatment were noted in the infant, but no plasma or breast milk drug levels were obtained. The drug will likely be found in breast milk, so some infant exposure will probably occur. However, less than 1% of zoledronic acid is absorbed orally. In addition, the drug has been administered to newborns for the treatment of osteogenesis imperfecta type II and refractory hypercalcemia and has been tolerated well. Nevertheless, due to the concern for potential serious adverse effects that might be seen in a breastfed infant, the manufacturer recommends that women not breastfeed while being treated with this drug for oncology-related conditions. When used for osteoporosis/Paget disease, the manufacturer recommends that the developmental and health benefits of breastfeeding should be considered along with the mother's clinical need for treatment. If the clinical decision is to use this drug while breastfeeding, the infant should be monitored for the most common reported adult side effects of nausea, myalgia, headache, arthralgia, bone pain, and extremity pain (all leading to irritability), anemia, constipation, fever, vomiting, and dyspnea.

References

1. Prescribing Information. Zoledronic acid. Accord Healthcare, Inc; 2020.
2. Prescribing Information. Reclast. Novartis Pharmaceuticals Corporation; 2020.
3. Richi CG, Saad KJ, Chaaban AK, et al. A rare case of hypercalcemia-induced pancreatitis in a first trimester pregnant woman. *Endocrinol Diabetes Metab Case Rep*. 2018;28:17-0175.
4. Andreadis C, Charalampidou M, Diamantopoulos N, et al. Combined chemotherapy and radiotherapy during conception and first two trimesters of gestation in a woman with metastatic breast cancer. *Gynecol Oncol*. 2004;95:252-255.
5. Musacchio E, Sartori L. Zoledronic acid for the treatment of pregnancy-associated femoral head necrosis: a case report. *Case Rep Womens Health*. 2020;26:e00190.
6. Green SB, Pappas AL. Effects of maternal bisphosphonate use on fetal and neonatal outcomes. *Am J Health Syst Pharm*. 2014;71:2029-2036.
7. Djokanovic N, Klieger-Grossmann C, Koren G. Does treatment with bisphosphonates endanger the human pregnancy? *J Obstet Gynaecol Can*. 2008;30:1146-1148.
8. Rakel A, Boucher A, Ste-Marie LG, et al. Role of zoledronic acid in the prevention and treatment of osteoporosis. *Clin Interv Aging*. 2001;6:89-99.
9. Alhousseini A, Mahaseth M, Zeineddine S, et al. A non-lethal osteogenesis imperfecta type II mutation. *Gynecol Obstet Invest*. 2019;84:204-208.
10. Militello MA, Re MP, Vitaliti G, et al. Use of zoledronic acid in a neonate with subcutaneous fat necrosis complicated with severe, refractory hypercalcemia. *Am J Perinatol*. 2019;36:S134-S138.

ZOLMITRIPTAN

Central Nervous System (Antimigraine—Serotonin 5-HT Receptor Agonist)

PREGNANCY RECOMMENDATION: No Human Data—Animal Data Suggest Low Risk

BREASTFEEDING RECOMMENDATION: Probably Compatible

PREGNANCY SUMMARY

No reports describing the use of zolmitriptan in human pregnancy have been located. Based on the likely placental transfer, some fetal exposure will probably occur. However, the absence of human pregnancy experience prevents a complete assessment of the embryofetal risk. No embryofetal toxicity was seen in one animal species at doses of about equal to the MRHD, but embryofetal toxicity was seen at 11 times the MRHD. Using this drug during pregnancy should be based on the pros and cons of the mother's clinical need for treatment versus any potential fetal risk that might occur from exposure. ACOG suggests cautious use of triptans (sumatriptan) for secondary treatment of persistent headache in pregnancy. They report that no studies have evaluated the effects of triptans in pregnancy on potential adverse effects on uterine or fetal blood flow. In addition, because the drug has vasoconstrictive properties, ACOG advises not to use triptans in pregnant patients with hypertension or cardiac disease.

BREASTFEEDING SUMMARY

One report was located that evaluated the use of zolmitriptan during human lactation in four women. The average breast milk concentration was about 2 to 10 ng/mL, with a maximum breast milk concentration of about 3 to 18 ng/mL. The RID based on the maximum concentrations found in breast milk ranged from 1.4% to 9.4% with a mean of 3.6%. It has been shown that using propranolol concomitant with zolmitriptan can elevate the plasma concentrations of zolmitriptan. This could result in higher breast milk levels. One of the four breastfeeding women was also using propranolol, and the levels in her breast milk were the highest obtained at 18 ng/mL. Excluding this woman, the highest breast milk level obtained in the other three women was about 8 ng/mL. Breastfeeding while using this drug should be based on the mother's clinical need for treatment. If used, the infant should be monitored for the most common reported adult side effects of various body pains, headache, paresthesia, and nausea (all leading to irritability), somnolence (leading to lethargy), hypertension, and dry mouth. ACOG states that triptans can be used by lactating patients but recommends a shared decision-making approach regarding the potential need to avoid breastfeeding for a specific timeframe after use.

References

1. Prescribing Information. Zolmitriptan. Ajanta Pharma USA Inc; 2021.
2. Soldin OP, Dahlin J, O'Mara DM. Triptans in pregnancy. *Ther Drug Monit*. 2008;30:1-11.
3. Headaches in pregnancy and postpartum: ACOG Clinical Practice Guideline No. 3. *Obstet Gynecol*. 2021;139:944-972.
4. Amundsen S, Nordeng H, Ole-Martin F, et al. Transfer of triptans into human breast milk and estimation of infant drug exposure through breastfeeding. *Basic Clin Pharmacol Toxicol*. 2021;128:795-804.
5. Peck RW, Seaber EJ, Dixon R, et al. The interaction between propranolol and the novel antimigraine agent zolmitriptan (311C90). *Br J Clin Pharmacol*. 1997;44:595-599.

ZOLPIDEM

Central Nervous System (Hypnotic—Nonbenzodiazepine Benzodiazepine Receptor Agonist)

PREGNANCY RECOMMENDATION: Human Data Suggest Risk (Third Trimester)—Animal Data Suggest Low Risk

BREASTFEEDING RECOMMENDATION: Probably Compatible (With Short-Term Use)

PREGNANCY SUMMARY

Two studies from the Swedish Medical Birth Registry were located that reported the use of zolpidem during pregnancy. The first covered births from 1995–2004, and the second covered births to 2007. The patients in the first study were included in the second. There were 1,318 women who gave birth to 1,341 infants and who reported the use of hypnotic nonbenzodiazepine benzodiazepine receptor agonists during the first trimester. The unexposed group involved 1,106,001 women who gave birth to 1,125,734 infants. The rate of major congenital malformations was similar in the exposed 42/1,341 (3.1%) and the unexposed 36,321/1,125,734 (3.2%) groups. Of the 1,341 infants, 603 were exposed to zolpidem, but specific data for this group were not provided. There was a question of a potential increased risk for intestinal malformations (other than atresia) based on two rare anomalies, but this finding has not been reported in any further analyses to date. In a third large study, 12 (0.5%) anomalies were identified in 2,497 women who took zolpidem during pregnancy. This incidence was no different than the 81 (0.6%) anomalies found in a randomly selected control group of 12,485 pregnancies with no zolpidem exposure. However, these birth anomaly percentages are lower than expected, and specific information on exposure during pregnancy was not provided. Numerous case reports and series were located that describe more than 30 first-trimester exposures to zolpidem with no reported anomalies except for one case of a neural tube defect (NTD) with Chiari malformation. Some publications describe an increased risk for preterm birth, small-for-gestational-age (SGA) infants, and cesarean birth, but this was not consistently found in all reported evaluations. Zolpidem crosses the placenta, so fetal exposure will occur. However, this limited human pregnancy experience still prevents a complete assessment of the embryofetal risk. Animal studies did not show any embryofetal toxicity in two species at doses of less than 10 times the RHD. Third-trimester exposure to zolpidem has been associated with neonates experiencing moderate to severe respiratory depression and sedation with intubation and ventilation in some cases postdelivery. Using this drug during pregnancy should be based on the pros and cons of the mother's clinical need for treatment versus any potential fetal risk that might occur from exposure. The drug is classified as a Schedule IV controlled substance, and it has a misuse potential with dependence similar to benzodiazepines and other benzodiazepine-like hypnotics. Withdrawal symptoms have not been reported in exposed newborns. Women who are pregnant and have taken zolpidem during pregnancy are encouraged to contact the National Pregnancy Registry for Psychiatric Medications at 866–961–2388.

BREASTFEEDING SUMMARY

Three publications have been located evaluating zolpidem use during lactation in nine patients. The drug was found in breast milk in all cases. The RID in one mother/infant pair was calculated to be about 2.7%. In a second evaluation involving five patients administered a single 20-mg dose, the amount of zolpidem in breast milk was calculated to be 0.004% to 0.019% of the maternal dose. In the third study, three postpartum women were using zolpidem (once daily in two women and "as needed" in the third woman). Breast milk levels in the

Z

numerous samples ranged from undetectable to a high of 10 ng/mL. Infant serum was analyzed in these three cases, and the drug was not detected in any case. No adverse events in the infants were reported. The manufacturer recommends holding breastfeeding during treatment and for 23 hours after the last dose. Nevertheless, breastfeeding while using this drug should be based on the mother's clinical need for treatment versus any potential infant risks that might occur. If used, the infant should be monitored for the most common reported adult side effects of dizziness (leading to irritability), diarrhea, sedation, and respiratory depression.

References

1. Prescribing Information. Zolpidem tartrate. Almatica Pharma LLC; 2023.
2. Askew JP. Zolpidem addiction in a pregnant woman with a history of second-trimester bleeding. *Pharmacotherapy*. 2007;27:306-308.
3. Juric S, Newport J, Ritchie JC, et al. Zolpidem (Ambien®) in pregnancy: placental passage and outcome. *Arch Womens Ment Health*. 2009;12: 441-446.
4. Saito J, Tachibana Y, Kawasaki H, et al. Transfer of zolpidem to cord blood and breast milk: a case series evaluating zolpidem serum levels and outcomes in birth and suckling infants. *Breastfeed Med*. 2022;17:1034-1038.
5. Saito J, Tachibana Y, Wada YS, et al. Presence of hypnotics in the cord blood and breast milk with no adverse effects on the infant: a case report. *Breastfeed Med*. 2022;17:349-352.
6. Wilton LV, Pearce GL, Martin RM, et al. The outcomes of pregnancy in women exposed to newly marketed drugs in general practice in England. *Br J Obstet Gynaecol*. 1998;105:882-889.
7. Wang LH, Lin HC, Lin, CC, et al. Increased risk of adverse pregnancy outcomes in women receiving zolpidem during pregnancy. *Clin Pharmacol Ther*. 2010;88:369-374.
8. Wikner BN, Kallen B. Are hypnotic benzodiazepine receptor agonists teratogenic in humans? *J Clin Psychopharmacol*. 2011;31:356-359.
9. Pons G, Francoual C, Guillet P, et al. Zolpidem excretion in breast milk. *Eur J Clin Pharmacol*. 1989;37:245-248.
10. Sharma A, Sayeed N, Khess CRJ, et al. High dose zolpidem induced fetal neural tube defects. *Curr Drug Saf*. 2011;6:128-129.

ZONISAMIDE

Central Nervous System (Antiseizure)

PREGNANCY RECOMMENDATION: Limited Human Data—Animal Data Suggest Risk

BREASTFEEDING RECOMMENDATION: Potential Toxicity

PREGNANCY SUMMARY

There are several reports of zonisamide exposure during pregnancy, with over 100 first-trimester exposures. In this combined group, there were 12 major anomalies but no pattern to the malformations was seen. A few of these publications were from registries where there might be a bias toward the reporting of poor or complicated outcomes. Higher rates of small for gestational age in monotherapy and polytherapy exposure were observed in a few studies, but this was not universally reported. Zonisamide crosses the placenta, so fetal exposure will occur. Animal studies reported embryofetal toxicity with malformations in four species at doses less than 10 times the RHD. Using this drug during pregnancy should be based on the pros and cons of the mother's clinical need for treatment versus any potential fetal risk that might occur from exposure. Because the drug inhibits carbonic anhydrase, it may cause metabolic acidosis. The manufacturer recommends monitoring the mother for metabolic acidosis if zonisamide is used. There is a pregnancy exposure registry that monitors pregnancy outcomes in women using antiseizure drugs. Health care providers are encouraged to call the North American Antiepileptic Drug Pregnancy Registry at 1–888–233–2334.

BREASTFEEDING SUMMARY

Several studies have been located that describe the use of zonisamide during human lactation. The drug was found in human breast milk in all cases. The RIDs in essentially every case were more than 10%, with some calculated values above 50%. In many of these analyses, infant blood was also measured, and zonisamide was detected in several samples. Though the number of cases is small, no adverse infant effects were reported. Because of these reported infant exposure levels, the manufacturer recommends that breastfeeding not occur while using zonisamide, or the drug be discontinued if breastfeeding is elected. Nevertheless, breastfeeding while using this drug should be based on the mother's clinical need for treatment versus any potential infant risks that might occur. If used, the infant should be monitored for the most common reported adult side effects of headache, dizziness, and pruritus (all leading to irritability), somnolence, fatigue (lethargy), and rash. Because the drug inhibits carbonic anhydrase, it may cause metabolic acidosis. The manufacturer recommends monitoring both the mother and infant for metabolic acidosis if zonisamide is used.

References

1. Prescribing Information. Zonisamide. Aurobindo Pharma Limited; 2023.
2. Percucca E, Bialer M. The clinical pharmacokinetics of the newer antiepileptic drugs. *Clin Pharmacokinet*. 1996;31:29-46.
3. Kawada K, Itoh S, Kusaka T, et al. Pharmacokinetics of zonisamide in perinatal period. *Brain Dev*. 2002;24:95-97.
4. Kondo T, Kaneko S, Amano Y, et al. Preliminary report on teratogenic effects of zonisamide in the offspring of treated women with epilepsy. *Epilepsia*. 1996;37:1242-1244.
5. Oles KS, Bell WL. Zonisamide concentration during pregnancy. *Ann Pharmacother*. 2008;42:1139-1141.
6. The Lamotrigine Pregnancy Registry. Final report. Accessed October 29, 2025. https://pregnancyregistry.gsk.com/documents/lam_spring_2010_final_report.pdf 1 September 1992 through 31 March 2010. GlaxoSmithKline, July 2010.
7. Hernandez-Diaz S, Mittendorf R, Smith CR, et al; North American Antiepileptic Drug Pregnancy Registry. Association between topiramate and

zonisamide use during pregnancy and low birth weight. *Obstet Gynecol.* 2014;123:21-28.
8. Reimers A, Helde G, Andersen NB, et al. Zonisamide serum concentration during pregnancy. *Epilepsy Res.* 2018;144:25-29.
9. McCluskey G, Kinney MO, Russell A, et al. Zonisamide safety in pregnancy: data from the UK and Ireland epilepsy and pregnancy register. *Seizure.* 2021;91:311-315.
10. Pennell PB, Karanam A, Meador KJ, et al. Antiseizure medication concentration during pregnancy. Results from the maternal outcomes and neurodevelopmental effects of antiepileptic drugs (MONEAD) study. *JAMA Neurol.* 2022;79:370-379.
11. Shimoyama R, Ohkubo T, Sugawara K. Monitoring of zonisamide in human breast milk and maternal plasma by solid-phase extraction HPLC method. *Biomed Chromatogr.* 1999;13:370-372.
12. Kimura S. [Zonisamide: its placental transport, biological half-life in the newborn, and transport into mother's milk—a study of a case of an infant born of a mother who had been treated with zonisamide alone during pregnancy]. *No To Hattatsu.* 1998;30:350-351.
13. Sugawara K, Shimoyama R, Ohkubo T. Determinations of psychotropic drugs and antiepileptic drugs by high-performance liquid chromatography and its monitoring in human breast milk. *Hirosaki Med J.* 1999;51(suppl):S81-S86.
14. Ohman I, Tomson T. Pharmacokinetics of zonisamide in neonatal period and during lactation. *Basic Clin Pharmacol Toxicol.* 2011;109(suppl 1):73; Abstract P55.
15. Ando H, Matsubara S, Oi A, et al. Two nursing mothers treated with zonisamide: should breast-feeding be avoided? *J Obstet Gynaecol.* 2014; 40:275-278.
16. Birnbaum AK, Meador KJ, Karanam A, et al. Antiepileptic drug exposure in infants of breastfeeding mothers with epilepsy. *JAMA Neurol.* 2020; 77:441-450.

ZURANOLONE

Mental Health (Antidepressant)

PREGNANCY RECOMMENDATION: *Contraindicated

BREASTFEEDING RECOMMENDATION: Probably Compatible

PREGNANCY SUMMARY

No reports describing the use of zuranolone in human pregnancy have been located. The drug will probably cross the placenta, so some fetal exposure will likely occur. Therefore, the absence of human pregnancy experience prevents a complete assessment of the embryofetal risk. Animal studies did show some embryofetal toxicity in one species at doses of less than 10 times the RHD. Based on these animal studies, the manufacturer recommends that women with reproductive potential use effective contraception during treatment and for 1 week after the last dose. *However, based on the drug's US Food and Drug Administration (FDA) approval, it is currently only to be used for treating postpartum depression. Therefore, it is contraindicated for use during an ongoing pregnancy. Zuranolone has an elevated risk of producing physical dependence, which could lead to misuse. It is currently a Schedule IV controlled substance. There is also a pregnancy exposure registry that monitors pregnancy outcomes in women using this drug. Health care providers are encouraged to call the National Pregnancy Registry for Antidepressants at 1–844–405–6185.

BREASTFEEDING SUMMARY

One report describing the use of zuranolone during human lactation has been located. Pharmacokinetic properties were evaluated in 14 healthy lactating women administered a 30-mg daily dose (normal dosing is listed as 50 mg/d). The estimated daily infant dose was 1.25 mcg/kg, resulting in a calculated RID of less than1% (using a daily dose of 50 mg/d). Breastfeeding while using this drug should be based on the mother's clinical need for treatment. If used, the infant should be monitored for the most common reported adult side effects of headache and dizziness (both leading to irritability), somnolence, sedation, and diarrhea.

References

1. Prescribing Information. Zurzuvae. Sage Therapeutics; 2023.
2. Deligiannidis KM, Bullock A, Nandy I, et al. Zuranolone concentrations in the breast milk of healthy, lactating individuals: results from a phase 1 open-labeled study. *J Clin Psychopharmacol.* 2024;44:337-344.

APPENDIX

Classification of Drugs by Pharmacologic Category

1. ANESTHETIC
Benzocaine
Camphor
Desflurane
Etomidate
Isoflurane
Ketamine
Lidocaine
Methohexital Sodium
Nitrous Oxide
Propofol
Ropivacaine
Sevoflurane
Tetracaine

2. ANTIBACTERIAL/ANTIBIOTIC
Amikacin
(Para)-Aminosalicylic Acid
Amoxicillin
Amoxicillin/Clavulanic Acid
Ampicillin
Ampicillin/Sulbactam
Azithromycin
Aztreonam
Bacitracin
Capreomycin
Cefaclor
Cefadroxil
Cefazolin
Cefdinir
Cefditoren
Cefepime
Cefepime/Enmetazobactam
Cefiderocol
Cefixime
Cefotaxime
Cefotetan
Cefoxitin
Cefpodoxime
Cefprozil
Ceftaroline Fosamil
Ceftazidime
Ceftibuten
Ceftobiprole Medocaril
Ceftriaxone
Cefuroxime
Cephalexin
Chloramphenicol
Ciprofloxacin
Clarithromycin
Clindamycin
Clomocycline
Colistimethate
Cycloserine
Dalbavancin
Dapsone
Daptomycin
Delafloxacin
Demeclocycline
Dicloxacillin
Doripenem
Doxycycline
Ertapenem
Erythromycin
Fidaxomicin
Fosfomycin
Gentamicin
Imipenem-Cilastatin
Lefamulin
Levofloxacin
Lincomycin
Linezolid
Mafenide
Meropenem
Methenamine
Metronidazole
Minocycline
Moxifloxacin
Mupirocin
Nafcillin
Neomycin
Nitrofurantoin
Ofloxacin
Omadacycline
Oritavancin
Oxacillin
Ozenoxacin
Penicillin G/Penicillin G Benzathine/
Penicillin V
Piperacillin/Tazobactam
Polymyxin B
Retapamulin
Streptomycin
Sulfadiazine
Sulfamethoxazole/Trimethoprim
Tedizolid
Telavancin
Tetracycline
Tigecycline
Vancomycin

3. ANTIDIABETIC
Acarbose
Albiglutide
Alogliptin
Bexagliflozin
Canagliflozin
Dapagliflozin
Dulaglutide
Empagliflozin
Glimepiride
Glipizide
Glyburide
Insulin, Human
Insulin Aspart
Insulin Degludec
Insulin Detemir
Insulin Glargine
Insulin Glulisine
Insulin Lispro
Linagliptin
Liraglutide
Metformin
Miglitol
Nateglinide
Pioglitazone
Repaglinide
Saxagliptin
Sitagliptin

4. ANTIDOTE
Acamprosate
Acetylcysteine
Amifostine
Atropine
Bezlotoxumab
Black Widow Spider
Antivenin
Centruroides Immune Fab
Dasiglucagon
Dexrazoxane
Diazoxide
Digoxin Immune Fab
Disulfiram
Flumazenil
Fomepizole
Glucagon
Glucarpidase
Idarucizumab
Lanthanum Carbonate
Leucovorin
Levoleucovorin
Lofexidine
Methylene Blue
Naloxone
Naltrexone
Neostigmine
Obiltoxaximab
Physostigmine
Potassium Iodide
Pralidoxime
Protamine

Sevelamer
Succimer

5. ANTIGOUT
Allopurinol
Colchicine
Febuxostat

6. ANTIHISTAMINE
Azelastine
Brompheniramine
Carbinoxamine
Cetirizine
Chlorcyclizine
Chlorpheniramine
Clemastine
Cyproheptadine
Desloratadine
Dexbrompheniramine
Dexchlorpheniramine
Dimenhydrinate
Diphenhydramine
Doxylamine
Fexofenadine
Hydroxyzine
Ketotifen
Levocetirizine
Loratadine
Meclizine
Pyrilamine
Triprolidine

7. ANTIHYPERTENSIVE
Acebutolol
Aliskiren
Aprocitentan
Atenolol
Azilsartan Medoxomil
Benazepril
Betaxolol
Bisoprolol
Candesartan Cilexetil
Captopril
Clevidipine
Clonidine
Enalapril
Eprosartan
Felodipine
Fenoldopam
Fosinopril
Guanfacine
Hydralazine
Indapamide
Irbesartan
Isradipine
Labetalol
Lisinopril
Losartan
Methyldopa
Metoprolol
Metyrosine
Moexipril
Nadolol
Nebivolol
Nicardipine
Nifedipine
Nisoldipine
Nitroprusside
Olmesartan Medoxomil
Perindopril
Phenoxybenzamine
Phentolamine
Propranolol
Quinapril
Ramipril
Telmisartan
Terazosin
Valsartan
Verapamil

8. ANTI-INFECTIVE (ANTIFUNGAL, ETC)
Albendazole
Amphotericin B
Anidulafungin
Artesunate
Atovaquone
Atovaquone/Proguanil
Bedaquiline
Benznidazole
Benzyl Alcohol
Butenafine
Caspofungin
Chlorhexidine
Chloroquine
Ciclopirox
Clavulanate Potassium
Clotrimazole
Econazole
Efinaconazole
Ethambutol
Ethionamide
Fluconazole
Flucytosine
Gentian Violet
Griseofulvin
Hexachlorophene
Hydroxychloroquine
Iodine
Isavuconazonium
Isoniazid
Itraconazole
Ivermectin
Ketoconazole
Mebendazole
Mefloquine
Micafungin
Miconazole
Miltefosine
Naftifine
Nitazoxanide
Nystatin
Palivizumab
Oteseconazole
Oxiconazole
Paromomycin
Penciclovir
Pentamidine
Permethrin
Posaconazole
Povidone Iodine
Praziquantel
Pretomanid
Primaquine
Pyrantel Pamoate
Pyrazinamide
Pyrethrins With Piperonyl Butoxide
Pyrimethamine
Quinidine
Quinine
Rifabutin
Rifampin
Rifamycin
Rifapentine
Rifaximin
Sertaconazole
Sulconazole
Tafenoquine
Tavaborole
Terbinafine
Terconazole
Tinidazole
Tioconazole
Tobramycin
Tolnaftate
Triclabendazole
Trimethoprim
Undecylenic Acid
Voriconazole

9. ANTILIPEMIC
Alirocumab
Atorvastatin
Bempedoic Acid
Benzphetamine HCl
Cholestyramine
Colesevelam
Colestipol
Evolocumab
Ezetimibe
Fenofibrate
Fluvastatin
Gemfibrozil
Lomitapide
Lovastatin
Niacin
Omega-3 Fatty Acids
Pitavastatin
Pravastatin

Rosuvastatin
Simvastatin

10. ANTINEOPLASTIC

Abemaciclib
Abiraterone Acetate
Acalabrutinib
Adagrasib
Ado-Trastuzumab Emtansine
Afatinib
Aldesleukin
Alectinib
Alemtuzumab
Allopurinol
Alpelisib
Amivantamab
Apalutamide
Asciminib
Asparaginase
Asparaginase Erwinia Chrysanthemi
Atezolizumab
Avapritinib
Avelumab
Axitinib
Azacitidine
Belantamab Mafodotin
Belinostat
Belzutifan
Bendamustine
Bevacizumab
Bexarotene
Binimetinib
Bleomycin
Blinatumomab
Bortezomib
Bosutinib
Brentuximab Vedotin
Brigatinib
Busulfan
Cabazitaxel
Cabozantinib
Calaspargase Pegol
Capecitabine
Capivasertib
Capmatinib
Carboplatin
Carfilzomib
Carmustine
Cedazuridine/Decitabine
Cemiplimab
Ceritinib
Cetuximab
Chlorambucil
Cisplatin
Cladribine
Clofarabine
Cobimetinib
Copanlisib
Crizotinib
Cyclophosphamide
Cytarabine
Dabrafenib
Dacarbazine
Dacomitinib
Dactinomycin
Daratumumab
Darolutamide
Dasatinib
Daunorubicin
Decitabine
Deuruxolitinib
Dinutuximab
Docetaxel
Dostarlimab
Doxorubicin
Durvalumab
Duvelisib
Encorafenib
Enfortumab Vedotin
Entrectinib
Enzalutamide
Epirubicin
Erdafitinib
Eribulin
Erlotinib
Etoposide
Everolimus
Exemestane
Fedratinib
Floxuridine
Fludarabine Phosphate
Fluorouracil
Fostamatinib
Fulvestrant
Gefitinib
Gemcitabine
Gilteritinib
Glasdegib
Hydroxyurea
Ibritumomab Tiuxetan
Ibrutinib
Idarubicin
Idelalisib
Ifosfamide
Imatinib
Ipilimumab
Irinotecan
Ivosidenib
Ixabepilone
Lapatinib
Larotrectinib
Lenalidomide
Lenvatinib
Letrozole
Leuprolide
Lorlatinib
Mechlorethamine
Melphalan
Mercaptopurine
Mesna
Methotrexate
Mitomycin
Mitoxantrone
Mogamulizumab
Nelarabine
Nilotinib
Nivolumab
Obinutuzumab
Olaparib
Olutasidenib
Osimertinib
Oxaliplatin
Paclitaxel
Palbociclib
Panitumumab
Pazopanib
Pembrolizumab
Pemetrexed
Pentostatin
Pertuzumab
Pexidartinib
Polatuzumab Vedotin
Ponatinib
Porfimer
Pralatrexate
Procarbazine
Ramucirumab
Ranibizumab
Rasburicase
Regorafenib
Rilonacept
Rituximab
Romidepsin
Ruxolitinib
Selinexor
Siltuximab
Sorafenib
Streptozocin
Sunitinib
Tagraxofusp
Talazoparib
Tamoxifen
Temozolomide
Temsirolimus
Thioguanine
Thiotepa
Topotecan
Trametinib
Trastuzumab
Tretinoin
Valrubicin
Vandetanib
Vemurafenib
Vinblastine
Vincristine
Vinorelbine
Vismodegib
Vorinostat
Zanubrutinib
Ziv-Aflibercept

11. ANTIRETROVIRAL
- Abacavir
- Atazanavir
- Bictegravir/Emtricitabine/Tenofovir
- Cabotegravir and Rilpivirine
- Cobicistat
- Darunavir
- Dolutegravir
- Doravirine
- Efavirenz
- Emtricitabine
- Enfuvirtide
- Entecavir
- Etravirine
- Lamivudine
- Lopinavir
- Nelfinavir
- Nevirapine
- Raltegravir
- Tipranavir
- Zidovudine

12. ANTIVIRAL
- Acyclovir
- Adefovir
- Amantadine
- Ansuvimab
- Atoltivimab/Maftivimab/Odesivimab
- Baloxavir Marboxil
- Cidofovir
- Famciclovir
- Foscarnet
- Ganciclovir
- Ibalizumab
- Maraviroc
- Oseltamivir
- Peramivir
- Ribavirin
- Rilpivirine
- Rimantadine
- Ritonavir
- Sofosbuvir
- Tecovirimat
- Tenofovir Alafenamide
- Tenofovir Disoproxil Fumarate
- Valacyclovir
- Valganciclovir
- Zanamivir

13. AUTONOMIC
- Atenolol
- Atropine
- Benztropine
- Bethanechol
- Carvedilol
- Cevimeline
- Clidinium
- Dicyclomine
- Dihydroergotamine
- Doxazosin
- Droxidopa
- Ephedrine
- Epinephrine
- Glycopyrrolate
- Homatropine
- Hyoscyamine
- Isoproterenol
- Norepinephrine
- Phendimetrazine
- Phentermine
- Pilocarpine
- Vecuronium

14. BONE HEALTH
- Abaloparatide
- Alendronate
- Denosumab
- Ibandronate
- Pamidronate
- Raloxifene
- Risedronate
- Romosozumab
- Zoledronic Acid

15. CARDIOVASCULAR
- Acebutolol
- Acetazolamide
- Adenosine
- Ambrisentan
- Amiloride
- Amiodarone
- Amlodipine
- Amyl Nitrite
- Angiotensin II
- Apomorphine
- Bendroflumethiazide
- Bosentan
- Bumetanide
- Chlorothiazide
- Chlorthalidone
- Digitalis
- Digitoxin
- Digoxin
- Diltiazem
- Disopyramide
- Dobutamine
- Dofetilide
- Dopamine
- Dronedarone
- Esmolol
- Ethacrynic Acid
- Flecainide
- Furosemide
- Hydroflumethiazide
- Ibutilide
- Iloprost
- Isosorbide Dinitrate
- Isosorbide Mononitrate
- Ivabradine
- Lidocaine
- Macitentan
- Mannitol
- Metolazone
- Mexiletine
- Midodrine
- Milrinone
- Minoxidil
- Nitroglycerin
- Pentoxifylline
- Phenylephrine
- Pindolol
- Polidocanol
- Prasugrel
- Prazosin
- Procainamide
- Propafenone
- Protamine
- Ranolazine
- Reteplase
- Sotalol
- Spironolactone
- Tafamidis
- Tenecteplase
- Ticagrelor
- Timolol
- Tirofiban
- Torsemide
- Trandolapril
- Treprostinil
- Triamterene

16. CENTRAL NERVOUS SYSTEM
- Acetazolamide
- Aducanumab
- Almotriptan
- Alprazolam
- Amantadine
- Amphetamine
- Armodafinil
- Atogepant
- Brivaracetam
- Butalbital
- Cannabidiol
- Carbamazepine
- Carbidopa
- Chloral Hydrate
- Chlordiazepoxide
- Clobazam
- Dalfampridine
- Daridorexant
- Daxibotulinumtoxin A
- Deutetrabenazine
- Dexmedetomidine
- Dexmethylphenidate
- Dextroamphetamine
- Diazepam
- Diethylpropion
- Donanemab
- Donepezil
- Eletriptan
- Entacapone
- Erenumab
- Ergotamine

Eslicarbazepine
Estazolam
Eszopiclone
Ethosuximide
Felbamate
Flurazepam
Fremanezumab
Frovatriptan
Gabapentin
Galantamine
Galcanezumab
Istradefylline
Lacosamide
Lamotrigine
Lasmiditan
Levetiracetam
Levodopa
Lorazepam
Magnesium Sulfate
Methocarbamol
Methsuximide
Methylphenidate
Midazolam
Modafinil
Naratriptan
Nimodipine
Ocrelizumab
Ofatumumab
Omaveloxolone
Opicapone
Oxazepam
Oxcarbazepine
Pentobarbital
Perampanel
Phenobarbital
Phenytoin
Pitolisant
Prabotulinum Toxin Type A
Pramipexole
Pregabalin
Primidone
Pyridostigmine
Ramelteon
Rasagiline
Riluzole
Rivastigmine
Rizatriptan
Rocuronium
Ropinirole
Rufinamide
Selegiline
Sodium Oxybate
Sumatriptan
Suvorexant
Tasimelteon
Tetrabenazine
Tiagabine
Tizanidine
Tolcapone
Topiramate
Trihexyphenidyl
Ubrogepant
Valproic Acid
Vigabatrin
Zaleplon
Ziconotide
Zolmitriptan
Zolpidem
Zonisamide

17. CHELATING AGENT

Deferasirox
Deferiprone
Deferoxamine
Dimercaprol
Edetate (Ethylenediamine-tetraacetic acid - EDTA)
Penicillamine
Trientine

18. CORTICOSTEROID

Beclomethasone
Betamethasone
Budesonide
Clobetasol
Cortisone
Deflazacort
Dexamethasone
Flunisolide
Fluocinolone
Fluocinonide
Flurandrenolide
Fluticasone
Halcinonide
Halobetasol
Hydrocortisone
Mometasone
Prednisolone
Prednisone
Triamcinolone

19. DERMATOLOGIC

Abametapir
Abrocitinib
Acitretin
Adapalene
Afamelanotide
Anacaulase
Anthralin
Azficel-T
Berdazimer
Betamethasone
Bimekizumab
Birch Triterpenes
Brodalumab
Calcipotriene
Clascoterone
Clobetasol
Collagenase
Crisaborole
Dapsone
Deucravacitinib
Fluocinolone
Fluocinonide
Flurandrenolide
Hydrocortisone
Hydroquinone
Imiquimod
Iodoquinol
Isotretinoin
Ketoconazole
Luliconazole
Mafenide
Oxymetazoline
Podofilox
Podophyllum
Spinosad
Tazarotene
Tretinoin (Topical)
Trifarotene

20. DIAGNOSTIC

Air Polymer-Type A
Cosyntropin
Deoxycholic Acid
Diatrizoate
Ethiodized Oil
Fluorescein
Gadobenate Dimeglumine
Gadobutrol
Gadopentetate Dimeglumine
Gadoteridol
Indigotindisulfonate
Iodixanol
Iohexol
Iopamidol
Iothalamate Meglumine
Sulfur Hexafluoride
Technetium TC 99M
Thyrotropin Alfa

21. ENDOCRINE/METABOLIC

Ammonium Chloride
Asfotase Alfa
Bromocriptine
Cabergoline
Calcitonin Salmon
Carglumic Acid
Conivaptan
Cosyntropin
Dinoprostone
Lanreotide
Laronidase
Levothyroxine
Liothyronine
Methimazole
Metreleptin
Mifepristone
Miglustat
Octreotide
Osilodrostat
Pasireotide
Pegloticase
Pegvisomant

Pramlintide
Probenecid
Propylthiouracil
Sapropterin
Taliglucerase Alfa
Tesamorelin
Thyrotropin Alfa
Vasopressin
Velaglucerase Alfa

22. GASTROINTESTINAL

Alosetron
Alpha-Galactosidase
Alvimopan
Amisulpride
Aprepitant
Balsalazide
Bisacodyl
Bismuth Subsalicylate
Budesonide
Calcium Carbonate
Casanthranol
Cascara Sagrada
Castor Oil
Chenodiol
Cholic Acid
Cimetidine
Crofelemer
Cromolyn Sodium
Dexlansoprazole
Diphenoxylate
Docusate Calcium
Docusate Potassium
Docusate Sodium
Dolasetron
Dronabinol
Droperidol
Eluxadoline
Esomeprazole
Famotidine
Glycerin
Granisetron
Lactulose
Lansoprazole
Linaclotide
Loperamide
Lubiprostone
Mesalamine
Methscopolamine
Methylnaltrexone
Metoclopramide
Mineral Oil
Misoprostol
Naloxegol
Nizatidine
Obeticholic Acid
Odevixibat
Olsalazine
Omeprazole
Ondansetron
Orlistat
Palonosetron
Pantoprazole
Polyethylene Glycol-3350
Prochlorperazine
Promethazine
Rabeprazole
Rolapitant
Scopolamine
Senna
Simethicone
Sodium Bicarbonate
Sucralfate
Teduglutide
Tenapanor
Trimethobenzamide
Ursodiol

23. GENETIC

Agalsidase Beta
Alglucosidase Alfa
Arimoclomol
Avalglucosidase Alfa
Burosumab
Casimersen
Cerliponase Alfa
Cipaglucosidase Alfa
Cysteamine
Elapegademase
Eliglustat
Elosulfase Alfa
Galsulfase
Golodirsen
Idursulfase
Imiglucerase
Ivacaftor
Lanadelumab
Migalastat
Olipudase Alfa

24. HEMATOLOGIC

Alteplase
Aminocaproic Acid
Anagrelide
Antihemophilic Factor (Human)
Antithrombin (Human/
Recombinant)
Apixaban
Argatroban
Avatrombopag
Axatilimab
Berotralstat
Betrixaban
Bivalirudin
Cangrelor
Caplacizumab
Cilostazol
Clopidogrel
Coumarin Derivatives
Crizanlizumab
Crovalimab
Dabigatran Etexilate
Dalteparin
Danicopan
Daprodustat
Darbepoetin Alfa
Defibrotide
Dipyridamole
Ecallantide
Edoxaban
Eltrombopag
Enoxaparin
Epoetin Alfa
Eptifibatide
Factor XIII Concentrate
Fibrin Sealant
Filgrastim
Fondaparinux
Hemin
Heparin
Luspatercept
Lusutrombopag
Pegfilgrastim
Plerixafor
Rivaroxaban
Romiplostim
Sargramostim
Tranexamic Acid
Vorapaxar
Voxelotor
Warfarin

25. IMMUNOLOGIC

Abatacept
Adalimumab
Anakinra
Anifrolumab
Apremilast
Auranofin
Azathioprine
Baricitinib
Basiliximab
Belatacept
Belimumab
Belumosudil
Canakinumab
Certolizumab Pegol
Corticotropin
Cyclosporine
Daclizumab
Dimethyl Fumarate
Dupilumab
Eculizumab
Elapegademase
Emapalumab
Etanercept
Everolimus
Fingolimod
Glatiramer
Golimumab
Hepatitis B Immune Globulin
Hydroxychloroquine
Immune Globulin
Infliximab
Interferon Beta-1a
Interferon Beta-1b

Interferon Gamma-1b
Leflunomide
Methotrexate
Mycophenolate
Natalizumab
Ozanimod
Peginterferon Beta-1a
Pimecrolimus
Rabies Immune Globulin
Risankizumab
Rituximab
Secukinumab
Siponimod
Sirolimus
Sulfasalazine
Tacrolimus
Teriflunomide
Tetanus Immune Globulin
Thalidomide
Tildrakizumab
Tocilizumab
Tofacitinib
Upadacitinib
Ustekinumab
Varicella-Zoster Immune Globulin
Vedolizumab

26. MEN'S HEALTH

Avanafil
Sildenafil

27. MENTAL HEALTH

Amitriptyline
Amoxapine
Aripiprazole
Asenapine
Atomoxetine
Brexanolone
Brexpiprazole
Bupropion
Buspirone
Cariprazine
Cenobamate
Chlorpromazine
Citalopram
Clomipramine
Clonazepam
Clorazepate
Clozapine
Desipramine
Desvenlafaxine
Doxepin
Droperidol
Duloxetine
Escitalopram
Flibanserin
Fluoxetine
Fluphenazine
Fluvoxamine
Haloperidol
Iloperidone
Imipramine
Isocarboxazid
Lisdexamfetamine
Lithium
Loxapine
Lurasidone
Meprobamate
Milnacipran
Mirtazapine
Nefazodone
Nortriptyline
Olanzapine
Olanzapine/Samidorphan
Paliperidone
Paroxetine
Perphenazine
Phenelzine
Pimozide
Protriptyline
Quazepam
Quetiapine
Risperidone
Sertraline
Solriamfetol
Temazepam
Thioridazine
Thiothixene
Tranylcypromine
Trazodone
Triazolam
Trifluoperazine
Trimipramine
Venlafaxine
Vilazodone
Ziprasidone

28. MISCELLANEOUS

Amifampridine
Avacopan
Bremelanotide
Carboprost
Chondroitin
Cinacalcet
Dehydroepiandrosterone
Desmopressin
Dichlorphenamide
Difelikefalin
Givosiran
Icatibant
Inotersen
Leuprolide
Melatonin
Methoxsalen
Methylergonovine
Ospemifene
Palifermin

29. NUTRITION/NUTRITIONAL SUPPLEMENTS/ELECTROLYTES

Glucosamine
Hyperalimentation
Lipid Emulsion
Lysine
Magnesium Sulfate
Omega-3 Fatty Acids
Potassium Chloride
Potassium Gluconate

30. OPHTHALMIC

Acetazolamide
Aflibercept
Alcaftadine
Apraclonidine
Atropine
Avacincaptad Pegol
Azelastine
Bepotastine Besilate
Besifloxacin
Betamethasone
Betaxolol
Bimatoprost
Brilliant Blue G
Brimonidine
Brinzolamide
Brolucizumab
Bromfenac
Carbachol
Carteolol
Cenegermin
Cetirizine
Ciprofloxacin
Cromolyn Sodium
Cyclopentolate
Cyclosporine
Cysteamine
Dexamethasone
Diclofenac
Difluprednate
Dorzolamide
Echothiophate Iodide
Epinastine Hydrochloride
Fluorometholone
Flurbiprofen
Ganciclovir
Gatifloxacin
Gentamicin
Homatropine
Ketorolac
Ketotifen
Latanoprost
Levobunolol
Levofloxacin
Lidocaine
Loteprednol
Methazolamide
Mitomycin
Moxifloxacin
Naphazoline
Natamycin
Nepafenac
Ofloxacin
Olopatadine
Omidenepag Isopropyl
Oxymetazoline
Pheniramine

Phenylephrine
Pilocarpine
Povidone-Iodine
Prednisolone
Proparacaine
Sulfacetamide
Tafluprost
Tetracaine
Tetrahydrozoline
Timolol
Tobramycin
Travoprost
Triamcinolone
Trifluridine
Tropicamide
Verteporfin

31. PAIN
Acetaminophen
Aspirin
Atracurium
Baclofen
Buprenorphine
Butorphanol
Carisoprodol
Celecoxib
Chlorzoxazone
Codeine
Cyclobenzaprine
Dantrolene
Diclofenac
Diflunisal
Dihydrocodeine
Etodolac
Fenoprofen
Fentanyl
Flurbiprofen
Hydrocodone
Hydromorphone
Ibuprofen
Indomethacin
Ketoprofen
Ketorolac
Levorphanol
Meclofenamate
Mefenamic Acid
Meloxicam
Meperidine
Metaxalone
Methadone
Morphine
Nabumetone
Nalbuphine
Naproxen
Oliceridine
Orphenadrine
Oxaprozin
Oxycodone
Oxymorphone
Pentazocine and Naloxone
Piroxicam
Pramoxine
Remifentanil
Succinylcholine
Sufentanil
Sulindac
Tapentadol
Tolmetin
Tramadol

32. RADIOPHARMACEUTICAL
Choline C 11
Copper CU 64 Dotatate
Florbetaben F18
Fluciclovine F18
Ioflupane Iodine 123
Lutetium Lu 177
Sodium Iodide I 123
Sodium Iodide I 131

33. REPRODUCTIVE
Bazedoxifene and Conjugated Estrogens
Clomiphene
Danazol
Drospirenone and Estetrol
Elagolix
Estradiol
Estrogens, Conjugated
Estrone
Ethinyl Estradiol
Ethynodiol
Magnesium Sulfate
Medroxyprogesterone
Nonoxynol-9
Norethindrone
Oral Contraceptives
Testosterone
Ulipristal

34. RESPIRATORY
Aclidinium Bromide
Albuterol
Aminophylline
Arformoterol
Beclomethasone
Benralizumab
Betamethasone
Budesonide
Ciclesonide
Cromolyn Sodium
Dextromethorphan
Dornase Alfa
Doxapram
Epoprostenol
Fluticasone
Formoterol
Guaifenesin
Ipratropium
Levalbuterol
Mepolizumab
Montelukast
Nintedanib
Olodaterol
Omalizumab
Oxymetazoline
Pirfenidone
Potassium Iodide
Pseudoephedrine
Roflumilast
Salmeterol
Terbutaline
Theophylline
Tiotropium
Varenicline
Zafirlukast
Zileuton

35. TOXINS
Botulinum Toxin Type A and Type B

36. SMOKING CESSATION AIDS
Nicotine Replacement Therapy
Varenicline

37. URINARY
Darifenacin
Fesoterodine
Flavoxate
Hydrochlorothiazide
Mirabegron
Oxybutynin
Pentosan
Phenazopyridine
Potassium citrate
Solifenacin
Tamsulosin
Tolterodine
Tolvaptan
Trospium
Urea

38. VACCINES
Adenovirus Type 4 and Type 7, Live
Anthrax
BCG
Cholera
Haemophilus B Conjugate
Hepatitis A
Hepatitis B Recombinant
Hepatitis B Recombinant Adjuvanted
Human Papillomavirus 9-Valent, Recombinant
Influenza Quadrivalent Inactivated, Influenza Quadrivalent Live
Measles, Mumps, and Rubella
Meningococcal Groups A, C, Y, and W-135
Meningococcal Group B
Pneumococcal 13-, 15-, 20-Valent Conjugate

Pneumococcal 23-Valent Polysaccharide
Poliovirus Inactivated
Rabies for Human Use
Smallpox
Tetanus Toxoid, Reduced Diphtheria Toxoid, Acellular Pertussis
Typhoid, Inactive
Typhoid, Live
Varicella
Yellow Fever

39. VITAMINS

Beta-Carotene
Calcifediol
Calcitriol
Cholecalciferol
Dihydrotachysterol
Ergocalciferol
Folic Acid
Niacin
Niacinamide
Pantothenic Acid (Vitamin B_5)
Paricalcitol
Phytonadione
Vitamin A (Retinol)
Vitamin B_1 (Thiamine)
Vitamin B_2 (Riboflavin)
Vitamin B_6 (Pyridoxine)
Vitamin B_{12} (Cyanocobalamin)
Vitamin C (Ascorbic Acid)
Vitamin D
Vitamin E (Tocopherol)
Vitamins, Multiple

Index

Note: Generic names are shown in **bold** with two sets of page numbers. The first set, also shown in bold, refers to the page number in the text where the monograph is located. The second set, shown in parentheses, refers to the page number in the Appendix where the drug is located by pharmacologic class. The trade names and synonyms are shown with one set of page numbers. These refer to their location in the text.

A

B

C

D

E

F

G

H

I

J

K

L

M

N

O

P

U

V

W

X

Y

Z